D0864092

TIETZ
CLINICAL GUIDE TO
LABORATORY
TESTS

TIETZ
CLINICAL GUIDE TO
LABORATORY
TESTS

FOURTH EDITION

ALAN H.B. WU, PHD, DABCC, FACB

Chief, Clinical Chemistry
San Francisco General Hospital;
Professor, Laboratory Medicine
University of California
San Francisco, California

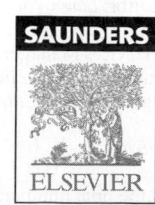

SAUNDERS

ELSEVIER

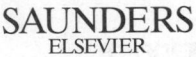

ELSEVIER

11830 Westline Industrial Drive
St. Louis, Missouri 63146

QY
25
C6413
2006

Notice

Clinical chemistry is an ever-changing field. Standard safety precautions must be followed, but as new research and clinical experience broaden our knowledge, changes in treatment and drug therapy may become necessary or appropriate. Readers are advised to check the most current product information provided by the manufacturer of each drug to be administered to verify the recommended dose, the method and duration of administration, and contraindications. It is the responsibility of the treating physician, relying on experience and knowledge of the patient, to determine dosages and the best treatment for each individual patient. Neither the Publisher nor the editor assume any liability for any injury and/or damage to persons or property arising from this publication.

W.B. Saunders

FOURTH EDITION
Previous edition copyrighted 1995, 1990, 1983

Library of Congress Cataloging in Publication Data
Tietz clinical guide to laboratory tests—4th ed. / [edited by] Alan H.B. Wu.
   p. ; cm.
   Rev. ed. of: Clinical guide to laboratory tests / edited by Norbert W. Tietz. 3rd ed. c1995.
   Includes bibliographical references and index.
   ISBN 0-7216-7975-7
   1. Diagnosis, Laboratory—Handbooks, manuals, etc.   I. Title: Clinical guide to laboratory tests.   II. Wu, Alan H. B.   III. Clinical guide to laboratory tests.
   [DNLM: 1. Laboratory Techniques and Procedures—Handbooks. QY 39 T564 2006]
   RB38.2.C55 2006
   616.07′5—dc22   2006042557

Publishing Director: *Andrew Allen*
Executive Editor: *Loren Wilson*
Developmental Editor: *Ellen Wurm*
Publishing Services Manager: *Pat Joiner*
Project Manager: *David Stein*
Senior Designer: *Andrea Lutes*

Printed in USA

Last digit is the print number: 9   8   7   6   5   4   3   2   1

This book is dedicated to my parents, Kina and Hou, my wife, Pamela, and my children Edward, Mark, and Kimberly.

CONTRIBUTORS

Fred S. Apple PhD
Medical Director
Clinical Laboratories Hennepin County
    Medical Center;
Professor of Laboratory Medicine and
    Pathology
University of Minnesota School of Medicine
Minneapolis, Minnesota

Jaber Aslanzadeh, PhD
Associate Professor
University of Connecticut Health Center
Farmington, Connecticut;
Director, Division of Microbiology
Hartford Hospital
Hartford, Connecticut

Enrique Ballesteros, MD
Pathology and Laboratory Medicine/
    Anatomic Pathology
Hartford Hospital
Hartford, Connecticut

Michael J. Bennett, PhD, DABCC, FACB
Professor of Pathology and Laboratory
    Medicine
University of Pennsylvania School of
    Medicine;
Director of Metabolic Disease Laboratory
Children's Hospital of Philadelphia
Philadelphia, Pennsylvania

Roger L. Bertholf, PhD, DABCC, FACB
Associate Professor of Pathology
University of Florida College of Medicine;
Director of Clinical Chemistry and
    Toxicology
Shands Jacksonville Hospital
Jacksonville, Florida

Lawrence W. Bond, PhD, DABCC, FACB
Principle Clinical Scientist and Manager of
    Quality Assurance
Quest Diagnostics, Inc.
St. Louis, Missouri

Larry Broussard, PhD
Professor
Department of Clinical Laboratory Sciences
Louisiana State University Health Sciences
    Center
New Orleans, Louisiana

Dean Carlow, MD, PhD
Assistant Professor
Department of Pathology and Laboratory
    Medicine
University of Pennsylvania School of
    Medicine;
Medical Director, Clinical Chemistry
Children's Hospital of Philadelphia
Philadelphia, Pennsylvania

John H. Contois, PhD, DABCC, FACB
Assistant Professor of Pathology
University of Massachusetts Medical School;
Director of Chemistry; Associate Director,
    Core Laboratory
University of Massachusetts Memorial
    Medical Center
Worcester, Massachusetts

Vanessa Dayton, MD
Clinical Assistant Professor
Laboratory Medicine and Pathology
University of Minnesota School of Medicine;
Faculty Associate
Hennepin County Medical Center;
Staff Pathologist/Hematopathologist
University of Minnesota Medical Center-
    Fairview/Hennepin County Medical Center
Minneapolis, Minnesota

Laurence M. Demers, PhD, DABCC, FACB
Distinguished Professor of Pathology and
    Medicine
Penn State University
College of Medicine, M.S. Hershey Medical
    Center;
Director, Clinical Chemistry and Core
    Endocrine Lab
Hershey, Pennsylvania

D. Robert Dufour, MD
Emeritus Professor of Pathology
George Washington Medical Center
Washington, DC;
Clinical Professor of Pathology
Uniformed Services University of the Health
    Sciences
Bethesda, Maryland;
Consultant, Pathology and Laboratory
    Medicine Service
Veterans Affairs Medical Center
Washington, DC

Karen Earle, MD
Clinical Instructor
Endocrinology and Metabolism
Diabetes Center
University of California San Francisco
San Francisco, California

David B. Endres, PhD
Professor of Clinical Pathology
Keck School of Medicine
University of Southern California
Los Angeles County;
University of Southern California Medical
    Center
Los Angeles, California

Eberhard Fiebig, MD
Acting Director
Chief, Divisions of Hematology / Transfusion
    Medicine
Clinical Laboratory
San Francisco General Hospital;
Associate Professor, Laboratory Medicine
University of California
San Francisco, California

Joyce Liu Flanagan, PhD
Supervisor, Dartmouth Reference Laboratory
Dartmouth Medical School
Lebanon, New Hampshire

Dalia M. Green, PhD
Senior Scientist
Diabetes Care—Blood Glucose Monitoring
BD Diagnostics Preanalytical Systems
Franklin Lakes, New Jersey

Sol F. Green, PhD, FACB
European Director, Clinical Affairs
BD Diagnostics Preanalytical Systems
Franklin Lakes, New Jersey

David G. Grenache, PhD, DABCC, FACTS
Assistant Professor
Department of Pathology and Laboratory
    Medicine
University of North Carolina;
Director, Special Chemistry and Blood Gas
    Laboratories
Associate Director, Core Laboratory
University of North Carolina Hospitals
Chapel Hill, North Carolina

John F. Halsey, PhD
Clinical Associate Professor
Division of Allergy, Immunology and
    Rheumatology
University of Kansas School of Medicine
Kansas City, Kansas;
Laboratory Director
IBT Reference Laboratory
Lenexa, Kansas

Diane C. Halstead, PhD
Clinical Professor
Department of Pediatrics
University of Florida College of Medicine;
Director, Infectious Disease Laboratories
Baptist Health/North Florida Pathology, P.A.
Jacksonville, Florida

Catherine A. Hammett-Stabler, PhD
Associate Professor
Department of Pathology and Laboratory
   Medicine
University of North Carolina;
Director, Toxicology, Clinical Pharmacology,
   Pediatric Metabolism Laboratories
Associate Director, Core Laboratory
University of North Carolina Hospitals
Chapel Hill, North Carolina

Beverly C. Handy, MD, MS
Assistant Professor
The University of Texas M.D. Anderson
   Cancer Center
Houston, Texas

**Ibrahim A. Hashim, MSc, FIBMS, PhD,
   DABCC, FACB**
Associate Professor
Associate Director—Clinical Chemistry
Department of Pathology
University of Texas Southwestern Medical
   Center;
Clinical Consultant and Medical Director
Clinical Chemisty
Parkland Memorial Hospital
Dallas, Texas

Henry A. Homburger, MD
Professor of Laboratory Medicine
Director, Immunology Antibody Laboratory
Mayo Clinic
Rochester, Minnesota

Sidney M. Hopfer, PhD
Professor, Pathology and Laboratory
   Medicine
University of Connecticut School of
   Medicine;
Director, Clinical Core Laboratory
John Dempsey Hospital
Farmington, Connecticut

Dan M. Iancu, MD
Fellow, Chemical Pathology
The University of Texas M.D. Anderson
   Cancer Center
Houston, Texas

Paul J. Jannetto, PhD, MT (ASCP)
Assistant Professor of Pathology
Assistant Director, Clinical
   Chemistry/Toxicology
Director, Rapid Response Lab
Medical College of Wisconsin
Milwaukee, Wisconsin

Karen M. Kloke, BS, MT (ASCP)
Technical Resource Specialist
Mayo Clinic and Foundation
Rochester, Minnesota

Hong Kee Lee, PhD
Postdoctoral Research Associate
Dartmouth Medical School
Lebanon, New Hampshire

Vanda A. Lennon, MD, PhD
Professor of Immunology and Neurology
Departments of Laboratory Medicine and
   Pathology, Immunology and Neurology
Mayo Clinic College of Medicine
Rochester, Minnesota

Chuanyi M. Lu, MD, FCAP
Chief, Hematology and Hematopathology
Laboratory Medicine Service
San Francisco VA Medical Center;
Assistant Professor, Laboratory Medicine
University of California
San Francisco, California

Umesh Masharani MB, BS MRCP (UK)
Associate Clinical Professor
University of California
San Francisco, California

Yvette S. McCarter, PhD, DABMM
Associate Professor of Pathology
Director, Clinical Microbiology Laboratory
University of Florida Health Science Center—
   Jacksonville
Jacksonville, Florida

Joseph P. McConnell, PhD, DABCC
Associate Professor of Laboratory Medicine
Laboratory Director: Cardiovascular
    Laboratory Medicine
Laboratory Director: Immunochemical Care
    Laboratory
Mayo Clinic and Foundation
Rochester, Minnesota

Michael D.D. McNeely, MD, FRCPC,
    FACB, Dip. FA
Senior Clinical Consultant
Provincial Laboratory Coordinating Office
Victoria, British Columbia
Canada

Robert Moore, PhD
Adjunct Faculty
University of Connecticut
Storrs, Connecticut;
Associate Director of Clinical Chemistry,
    Retired
Department of Pathology
Hartford Hospital
Hartford, Connecticut

Ashok Nambiar, MD
Assistant Medical Director
Blood Bank and Donor Center
UCSF Medical Center;
Assistant Professor
Department of Laboratory Medicine
University of California
San Francisco, California

Anthony O. Okorodudu, PhD, DABCC,
    FACB
Professor of Pathology
University of Texas Medical Branch
Director of Clinical Chemistry
UTMB Hospitals
Galveston, Texas

William E. Ottinger, PhD, DABCC, FACB
Technical Director
Quest Diagnostics—Cambridge Business Unit
Cambridge, Massachusetts

Ching-Nan Ou, PhD
Professor of Pathology
Baylor College of Medicine
Director of Clinical Chemistry
Texas Children's Hospital
Houston, Texas

Darryl Erik Palmer-Toy, MD, PhD
Director of Chemistry
Regional Reference Laboratories
Southern California Permanente Medical
    Group
North Hollywood, California

Sherrie L. Perkins, MD, PhD
Professor of Pathology
University of Utah School of Medicine
Director of Hematopathology
University of Utah Health Sciences
Salt Lake City, Utah

Sean J. Pittock, MD
Senior Associate Consultant
Departments of Neurology and Laboratory
    Medicine and Pathology
Mayo Clinic
Rochester, Minnesota

Salvador F. Sena, PhD, DABCC
Clinical Associate
University of Connecticut School of Medicine
Farmington, Connecticut;
Director, Clinical Chemistry
Danbury Hospital
Danbury, Connecticut

Susan E. Sharp, PhD, DABMM
Associate Professor
Department of Pathology
Oregon Health and Sciences University;
Director of Microbiology
Kaiser Permanente
Portland, Oregon

Jennifer A. Snyder, PhD
Clinical Chemistry Fellow
Department of Pathology and Laboratory
  Medicine
University of North Carolina;
Clinical Chemistry Fellow
McLendon Clinical Laboratories
University of North Carolina Hospitals
Chapel Hill, North Carolina

Lori J. Sokoll, PhD
Associate Professor of Pathology
Johns Hopkins University;
Associate Director of Clinical Chemistry
Johns Hopkins Hospital
Baltimore, Maryland

Gregory J. Tsongalis, PhD
Associate Professor
Dartmouth Medical School
Hanover, New Hampshire;
Director, Molecular Pathology
Dartmouth-Hitchcock Medical Center
Lebanon, New Hampshire

**Frank H. Wians, Jr., PhD, MT (ASCP),
  DABCC, FACB**
Professor
Department of Pathology Director
Clinical Chemistry
Division of Clinical Pathology Director
Clinical Chemistry Fellowship Program
  Associate Director
Division of Clinical Pathology Editor-In-
  Chief
Laboratory Medicine
UT Southwestern Medical Center
Dallas, Texas

Jeffrey L. Winters, MD
Assistant Professor of Laboratory Medicine
  and Pathology
Mayo Clinic
Rochester, Minnesota

Steven H.Y. Wong, PhD
Professor of Pathology
Medical College of Wisconsin;
Director, Clinical Chemistry/Toxicology
  Pharmacogenomics and Proteomics
Froedtert Memorial Lutheran Hospital
Milwaukee, Wisconsin

Alan H.B. Wu, PhD, DABCC, FACB
Chief, Clinical Chemistry
San Francisco General Hospital;
Professor, Laboratory Medicine
University of California
San Francisco, California

Jiaxi Wu, PhD, MD
Assistant Professor
Associate Director, Clinical Chemistry
Department of Pathology
Clinical Chemistry Division
University of Texas Southwestern Medical
  Center
Dallas, Texas

Kiang-Teck Yeo, PhD, DABCC, FACB
Professor of Pathology
Dartmouth Medical School;
Director of Clinical Chemistry and
  Endocrinology Laboratories
Dartmouth Hitchcock Medical Center
Lebanon, New Hampshire

REVIEWERS

Valerie Bush, PhD
Director
Clinical Laboratory and Point of Care Testing
Bassett Healthcare
Cooperstown, New York

Carl Garber, PhD, FACB
Director, Technical Statistics Applications
Quest Diagnostics
Lyndhurst, New Jersey

Matthew Meerkin, BSc, MBBS, FRCPA, FAACB, FACB
Consultant Chemical Pathologist
Symbion Health Laverty Pathology;
Adjunct Professor
University of Technology, Sydney
Sydney, Austrailia

Sarstedt AG
Nümbrecht, Germany

Sarstedt Inc.
Newton, North Carolina

Ana K. Stankovic, MD, PhD, MSPH
World Wide Medical Director
BD Diagnostics, Preanalytical Systems
Franklin Lakes, New Jersey

Diane I. Szamosi, MA, MT (ASCP) SH
Technical Marketing Manager
Greiner Bio-One North America, Inc.
PreAnalytics
Monroe, North Carolina

PREFACE

Although Dr. Norbert Tietz has retired from active practice, his name and legacy continues on in his textbooks and in this Fourth Edition of *Clinical Guide to Laboratory Tests*. It has been 11 years since the publication of the last edition. The field of laboratory medicine has exploded with new tests and procedures since the publication of the last edition. The fourth edition highlights four new sections. **Section I,** written by Sol Green, contains preanalytical factors that affect clinical laboratory data including patient status, collection factors, processing and centrifugation, and specimen transportation. This section also generically describes the dozens of blood collection tubes used in modern phlebotomy. **Section VI,** written by C. Mark Lu, consists of an updated catalog of the hundreds of immunophenotyping markers measured by flow cytometry and immunohistochemistry. Part I contains Cluster of Differentiation or "CD" antigens and other immunophenotypic markers, while Part II consists of immunophenotypic markers of hematopoietic and lymphoid neoplasms. **Section VII,** written by Steve Wong and Paul Jannetto, consists of tests useful in the emerging field of pharmacogenetics and pharmacogenomics. Part I consists of Phase I liver drug metabolizing enzymes, Part II consists of Phase II liver drug metabolizing enzymes, Part III consists of drug transporters, and Part IV consists of drug receptor targets. **Section VIII,** written by John Halsey, lists the tests useful for allergy detection. Table VIII-1 lists the various allergens that are commonly tested such as pollens, molds and yeasts, mites, animal proteins, foods, insects, parasites, drugs, and occupational and miscellaneous allergens.

In addition to these new sections, each of the sections from the third edition has been greatly expanded. **Section II** consists of nearly 700 entries of the general clinical laboratory tests, with dozens of new entries and the elimination of many tests that are now obsolete. All entries have been reviewed and updated by contributors largely new to this series. For selected clinical chemistry tests, we have added new data on reference intervals for random urine concentrations, expressed as per gram of creatinine. This is the result of a large database generated by Larry Bond, Bill Ottinger, and Carl Garber for Quest Laboratories. **Section III** on molecular diagnostics tests written by Greg Tsongalis has been greatly expanded to reflect the many changes that this field has undergone in the last decade. In addition to a summary of molecular diagnostic techniques, tests cover the areas of infectious disease, bacteriology, cancer, genetic diseases, and identity testing. **Section IV** consists of therapeutic drugs written by Kiang-Teck Jerry Yeo, Hong Kee Lee, Joyce Liu Flanagan, and Catherine Hammett Stabler, and has been combined with Drugs of Abuse Testing, written by Larry Broussard. As in the previous edition, therapeutic ranges are combined with pharmacokinetic parameters. **Section V,** written by Yvette McCarter, Susan Sharp, Diane Halstead, and Jaber Aslanzadeh, consists of antimicrobial susceptibility tests and combined entries for over 150 microbiology tests for the identification of bacteriological, spirochetal, mycoplasmal, chlamydial, rickettsial, fungal, parasitic, and viral diseases. Tests include cultures, serologies, and special procedures.

Throughout the sections, we have listed the references immediately after each entry to make this guide more user-friendly. Although this book has become a mainstay for clinical laboratories, it was also written for medical practitioners. Thus this book is a *Clinical Guide* to Laboratory Tests. We would like to acknowledge David Stein of Elsevier for his proof-reading assistance.

Alan H.B. Wu
July, 2005

DISCLAIMER

Reference ranges are valuable guides for the clinician, but they should not be regarded as absolute indicators of health and disease. Reference intervals should be used with caution, since values for healthy individuals often overlap significantly with values for persons afflicted with disease. In addition, laboratory values may vary significantly because of differences in methodology and mode of standardization. This is especially true for immunological tests, which use antibodies that may have different characteristics. As a result, laboratory values in individual institutions may differ from those listed in this manual.

Doses for drugs listed as part of the protocol for laboratory tests, as well as their therapeutic and toxic ranges, are those commonly accepted on the basis of present knowledge. The constant acquisition of new knowledge makes it necessary to confirm and compare information supplied in this manual with data furnished by manufacturers. It should also be considered that there are significant differences in drug response among individuals.

INSTRUCTIONS

The following tables provide the content of each of the eight main sections of this book. Below each subsection title is a general description of the contents for each entry. In all sections, specific information related to a particular test method lines up opposite that method. The test index lists test names or diseases from all sections alphabetically. Where appropriate, cross-references are given to other entries. Thin lines serve as guides; double lines separate complete test entries. Cited references are listed below each entry. At the end of the book there is a separate index for disease and keywords.

QUICK REFERENCE TO INFORMATION CONTAINED IN THE *CLINICAL GUIDE TO LABORATORY TESTS*—SECTION I, PHLEBOTOMY TUBES

TUBE TYPE/ MATERIAL	STOPPER COLOR	ADDITIVE/PRESERVATIVE	GENERAL USE
Intended use of tube and material used to make the tube (glass or plastic).	Colors are standardized across the phlebotomy industry.	Chemicals added to perform certain functions (e.g., anticoagulation).	Specific areas within laboratory medicine where the tube is most commonly used.

RECOMMENDED HANDLING CONDITIONS (E.G., MIXING, G FORCE, AND SPIN TIME)	SPECIMEN STABILITY	REMARKS
Handling conditions necessary to ensure optimum stability of test analyte and accuracy of result. Centrifugation speed listed are relative multiples of the gravitational force, g.	General stability information relative to the intended analyte.	Important notes for optimum use of phlebotomy tube.

QUICK REFERENCE TO INFORMATION CONTAINED IN THE *CLINICAL GUIDE TO LABORATORY TESTS*—SECTION I, PREANALYTICAL FACTORS AFFECTING CLINICAL LABORATORY TEST RESULTS

PREANALYTICAL FACTOR	SOURCE OF ERROR OR VARIABILITY	RESULT	REMARKS/OUTCOME/PROCEDURE
Factors listed are patient status, collection procedure, processing and centrifugation, specimen transportation and instrument/method and collection tube compatibility.	These errors are diet, exercise, medication, disease state/patient demographics, body position, endogenous substances, patient identification, tourniquet and draw technique, order of draw, draw volume, mixing, inappropriate use of gel tubes, serum clotting time, centrifugation conditions, common modes of transport, and invalidated preanalytical phase.	The result of the various sources of error or variability listed.	Specific remarks, outcomes, and procedures for the various sources of error or variability are listed.

QUICK REFERENCE TO INFORMATION CONTAINED IN THE *CLINICAL GUIDE TO LABORATORY TESTS*—SECTION II, GENERAL CLINICAL TESTS AND SECTION VIII, ALLERGY TESTING

TEST NAME AND METHOD	SPECIMEN REQUIREMENTS	REFERENCE INTERVAL, CONVENTIONAL [INTERNATIONAL RECOMMENDED UNITS]	CHEMICAL INTERFERENCES AND IN VIVO EFFECTS
Test Name (Synonyms, abbreviations), references related to entire entry. *Method* Important assay conditions; test doses and pretest instructions.	Specimen (anticoagulant). Collection times, storage information, special instructions.	Generally accepted values are listed. Units in brackets usually conform to the SI system (Système International d'Unités). However, units recommended by the International Union of Pure and Applied Chemistry (IUPAC) and the Commission on World Standards of the World Association of Societies of Pathology (COWS of WASP) are used when these units have found wider acceptance in the clinical laboratories and offer advantages over SI units. Factors for converting conventional units to international units are placed between the two ranges and are placed only in the first line of a column of values. Values that line up with a specific procedure were determined using that method. Where appropriate, data are stratified by age and sex, and toxic concentrations are noted where appropriate. Values without designations are ranges for the adult population. Units for the reference range either follow the value or appear at the top of the column of values.	Substances and conditions listed are known to interfere with the test procedure(s). V = *in vivo* effects C = chemical interferences Arrows indicate an increase (↑) or decrease (↓) in value. Abbreviations preceding an arrow indicate the body fluid. For key to abbreviations, see *Abbreviations*.

General comments: Information that pertains to an *entire* entry (test procedure or analyte) begins on the first line of the entry, regardless of the column in which it appears. Related information lines up across the page; thin lines serve as guides. Double lines separate entries. When the name of an entry refers to a group of analytes (e.g., complement components), the individual analytes are also listed in column 1 but are indented.

DIAGNOSTIC INFORMATION	REMARKS
This column lists clinical conditions that manifest a change in the concentration of the analyte or test result. Arrows indicate an increase or a decrease in value. Abbreviations preceding an arrow indicate the specimen; two or more arrows indicate a more pronounced effect.	This column contains general information pertinent to the use of the test procedure. Only information that has specific importance and is not general knowledge is referenced.

QUICK REFERENCE TO INFORMATION CONTAINED IN THE *CLINICAL GUIDE TO LABORATORY TESTS*—SECTION III, MOLECULAR DIAGNOSTICS

TEST METHOD	SPECIMEN AND SPECIAL REQUIREMENTS	CLINICAL COMMENTS AND REMARKS
Disorder, Organism, or Test Name (Synonyms, abbreviations), references related to entire entry.	Specimen. Special instructions for patient preparation and specimen collection and processing.	This column contains general and clinical information pertinent to the use of the test procedure. Only information that has specific importance and is not general knowledge is referenced. The affected target gene is also identified.
Individual disorder name when group is main heading		
Method		

QUICK REFERENCE TO INFORMATION CONTAINED IN THE *CLINICAL GUIDE TO LABORATORY TESTS*—SECTION IV, THERAPEUTIC DRUGS AND DRUGS OF ABUSE

TEST NAME AND METHOD	SPECIMEN	REFERENCE (THERAPEUTIC) INTERVAL, CONVENTIONAL [INTERNATIONAL RECOMMENDED UNITS]	KINETIC VALUES
Test Name (Synonyms, abbreviations), references related to entire entry. *Method* *Molecular weight.*	Specimen (anticoagulant). Collection times, storage information, special instructions.	The most widely used therapeutic and toxic intervals for the drugs are listed.	This column contains specific information about the pharmacokinetic parameters of individual drugs. Parameters such as half-life ($t_{1/2}$) volume of distribution (Vd), clearance (Cl_T), fraction protein bound (PB), free fraction (F), and time to maximum drug concentrations (T_{max}) are listed when well-established values are available. Where available, the enzymes responsible for metabolism are listed. This information is to be used with pharmacogenetic data given in Section VII.

FACTORS INFLUENCING
DRUG DISPOSITION

The column identifies the normal route of drug elimination. Directional arrows indicate changes in the analyte's clearance rate and half-life ($\uparrow$ lengthened, $\downarrow$ shortened, $\rightarrow$ unchanged). Conditions responsible for these changes, such as chronological age, treatment protocols, or disease states are identified. Drugs that are known to cause interactions are also identified. The mechanism of excretion and the effect of dialysis on the removal of the drug are also listed.

REMARKS AND INTERFERENCES

This column contains general information pertinent to the effective use of the drug and factors affecting its laboratory measurement. Only information that has specific importance and is not general knowledge is referenced.

Also listed in this column are substances and conditions known to interfere with the test procedure(s) as well as side effects known to be associated with the use of the drug.

QUICK REFERENCE TO INFORMATION CONTAINED IN THE *CLINICAL GUIDE TO LABORATORY TESTS*—SECTION V, MICROBIOLOGY

TEST NAME OR METHOD	SPECIMEN AND SPECIAL REQUIREMENTS	CLINICAL COMMENTS AND REMARKS
Test Name or Organism (Synonyms, abbreviations), references related to entire entry.	Specimen. Special instructions for patient preparation and specimen collection and processing.	Column contains general and clinical information pertinent to the use of the test procedure. Only information that has specific importance and is not general knowledge is referenced.
Method		
Special tests used to detect the same entity.		

QUICK REFERENCE TO INFORMATION CONTAINED IN THE *CLINICAL GUIDE TO LABORATORY TESTS*—SECTION VI, IMMUNOPHENOTYPING MARKERS

CD MARKERS	OTHER NAMES	MOLECULAR WEIGHT (KDA)
Specific cluster of differentiation (CD) antigen	Common protein name of antigen.	Estimated to the nearest whole kDa.

KNOWN NORMAL DISTRIBUTION	REMARKS
Distribution within normal and cancerous tissues.	General and clinical information pertinent to the CD antigen or immunophenotypic marker.

QUICK REFERENCE TO INFORMATION CONTAINED IN THE *CLINICAL GUIDE TO LABORATORY TESTS*—SECTION VII, PHARMACOGENOMICS

ENZYME NAME	SUBSTRATE	INHIBITORS	INDUCERS	SELECTED MUTATIONS
Name of the enzyme involved in the metabolism.	Drugs that are metabolized by the enzyme.	Other drugs that act as inhibitors of the enzyme, thereby decreasing activity.	Other drugs that act as inducers of the enzyme, thereby increasing activity.	Common mutations and polymorphisms that may have an impact on individual drug concentrations.

PREVALENCE OF VARIANT ALLELE (%, RACE)	NUCLEOTIDE CHANGE	CLINICAL EFFECT (ENZYME ACTIVITY)
The reported prevalence of the variant allele broken down by race. Reference number 22 is used unless otherwise specified.	Specific nucleotide substitution and location of substation on the DNA of the variant allele compared with the wild type allele.	The *in vivo* and *in vitro* effect (if any) that the particular nucleotide change has on the enzyme activity.

CONTENTS

Coagulation
Enrique Ballesteros

Diabetes tests
Ibrahim A. Hashim
Jiaxi Wu
Karen Earle
Umesh Masharani

Endocrinology
Robert Moore

Environmental and chemical toxicology
Roger L. Bertholf

Fertility and pregnancy testing
Frank H. Wians, Jr.
Jiaxi Wu

Fetal lung maturity
David G. Grenache
Jennifer A. Snyder

Fluid analysis
Darryl Erik Palmer-Toy

Gastrointestinal and pancreatic
Michael D. McNeely

Heavy metals
Sidney M. Hopfer

Hematology
Vanessa Dayton

Hemoglobin
Ching-Nan Ou

Hemolytic anemias
Sherrie L. Perkins

In-born errors of metabolism
Michael J. Bennett

Lipids and lipoproteins
John H. Contois

Liver tests
D. Robert Dufour

Proteins
Beverly C. Handy

Renal function and urinalysis
Salvador F. Sena

Thyroid function
Laurence M. Demers

Transfusion medicine
Eberhard Fiebig
Ashok Nambiar

Tumor markers
Lori J. Sokoll

Vitamins and porphyrins
Joseph P. McConnell
Karen M. Kloke

24-hr urine chemistry
Lawrence W. Bond
William E. Ottinger
Carl Garber, Reviewer

SECTION III

MOLECULAR DIAGNOSTICS, *1203*
Gregory J. Tsongalis

SECTION IV

THERAPEUTIC DRUGS AND DRUGS OF ABUSE, *1237*
Larry Broussard
Catherine A. Hammett-Stabler
Kiang-Teck Yeo
Hong Kee Lee
Joyce Liu Flanagan

SECTION V

CLINICAL MICROBIOLOGY, *1519*

Bacteriologic diseases
Diane C. Halstead

Parasitic diseases
Susan E. Sharp

Spirochetal, mycoplasmal, chlamydial, rickettsial, and fungal diseases
Yvette S. McCarter

Virology
Jaber Aslandzadeh

SECTION VI

IMMUNOPHENOTYPING MARKERS, *1633*

Chuanyi M. Lu

SECTION VII

PHARMACOGENOMICS, *1713*

Steven H. Y. Wong
Paul J. Jannetto

SECTION VIII

ALLERGY TESTING, *1743*

John F. Halsey

APPENDIX, *1761*

ABBREVIATIONS

°C	degrees Celcius	AK	adenylate kinase
17-OHCS	17-hydroxycorticosteroids	ALA	aminolevulinic
17-OHP	17-hydroxyprogesterone	ALAD	Aminolevulinate dehydratase
18-OH DOC	18-hydroxydeoxycorticosterone	alb	albumin
1D	1-dimensional	ALCL	anaplastic large cell lymphoma
3-PBA	3-phenoxybenzoic acid	ALG	antilymphocyte globulin
4-NPP	4-nitrophenylphosphate	ALL	acute lymphoid leukemia
5-HIAA	5-hydroxyindolacetic acid	ALP, AP	alkaline phosphatase
5-HTOL	5-hydroxytryptophol	ALT	alanine aminotransferase
6-MP	6-mercaptopurine	AMA	antimitochondrial antibodies
AABB	American Association of Blood Banks	AMI	acute myocardial infarction
AACC	American Association for Clinical Chemistry	AML	acute myeloid leukemia
AAP	alanine aminopeptidase	AMP	amino methyl propanol (2-amino-2-methyl-1-propanol)
AAS	atomic absorption spectrometry	AMV-RT	avian myeloblastosis virus reverse transcriptase
AAT	α_1-antitrypsin	ANA	antinuclear antibody
ab	antibody	ANCA	antineutrophilic cytoplasmic antibodies
ACB	albumin cobalt binding	AND	antideoxyribonuclease
ACCR	amylase creatinine clearance ratio	ANH	atrial natriuretic hormone
ACD	acid-citrate-dextrose	ANLL	acute nonlymphocytic leukemia
ACE	angiotensin converting enzyme	ANNA	antineuronal nuclear antibody
ACIF	anticomplement immunofluorescence	ANP	atrial natriuretic peptide
ACT	activated coagulation time; antichymotrypsin	AO	acridine orange
ACTH	adrenocorticotropic hormone	APA	aspartoacylase
ADA	American Diabetes Association; adenosine deaminase	APC	adenomatous polyposis coli
ADAM	A disintegrin and metalloprotease	APCR	activated protein C resistance
ADCC	antibody-dependent cell-mediated cytotoxicity	APL	acute promyelocytic leukemia
ADH	alcohol dehydrogenase, antidiuretic hormone	APN	aminopeptidase N
ADRB	adrenergic receptor	apo	apoprotein
AED	antiepileptic drugs	APOE	apoprotein E
AF	amniotic fluid	APS	antiphospholipid syndrome
AFB	acid-fast bacteria	aPTT	activated partial thromboplastin time
AFP	α-fetoprotein	ARP	acute phase reacting protein
ag	antigen	ASAL	argininosuccinate lyase
AG	anion gap	ASCA	*Saccharomyces cerevisiae* antibodies
AGP	acid glycoprotein	ascit	ascites
AGT	angiotensin	ASO	antistreptolysin O
AH	antihyaluronidase	AST	aspartate aminotransferase; antimicrobial susceptibility
AHF	antihemolytic factor		test
AI	angiotensin I	ASTRO	American Society for Therapeutic Radiation and
AIDS	acquired immunodeficiency syndrome		Oncology
AIM	activation inducer molecule	AT	antithrombin
AIP	acute intermittent porphyria	ATLL	adult T-cell leukemia/lymphoma
AITL	angioimmunoblastic T-cell lymphoma	AU	arbitrary unit

AUC	area under curve	CDA	congenital dyserythropoietic anemia
AZT	azidothymidine, zidovudine	CDAD	*Clostridium difficile*–associated diarrhea
BAL	British antilewisite; bronchoalveolar lavage	CDC	Centers for Disease Control
BAO	basal acid output	CDK	cyclin-dependent kinase
BAP	bone alkaline phosphatase	CDP	crystalline degradation product
BCYE	buffered charcoal yeast extract agar	CE	capillary electrophoresis
bDNA	branched DNA	CEA	carcinoembryonic antigen
BH4	tetrahydrobiopterin	CEACAM	carcinoembryonic antigen–related cell adhesion
BHI	brain heart infusion		molecules
BLA	Burkitt lymphoma–associated antigen	CEDIA	cloned enzyme donor immunoassay
BL-CAM	B lymphocyte cell adhesion molecule	CEP	congenital erythropoietic porphyria
BLL	blood lead level	CER	cholesterol esterification rate
BMC	Boehringer Mannheim Corporation	CETP	cholesteryl transport protein
BMD	Boehringer Mannheim Diagnostics; Becker muscular	CF	cystic fibrosis; complement fixation
	dystrophy	CFTR	cystic fibrosis transmembrane regulator
BMZ	basement zone	CgA	chromogranin A
BNP	B-type natriuretic peptide	CHD	cold hemagglutinin disease; coronary heart disease
BOHB	β-hydroxybutyrate	CK	creatine kinase
BPG	big plasma glucagon	CKD	chronic kidney disease
BPH	benign prostatic hypertrophy	Cl_2CA	3-(2,2-dichlorovinyl)-2,2-dimethylcyclopropane-
BRCA1 and 2	breast cancer gene 1 and 2		1-carboxylic acid
BT	bleeding time	CLIA	Clinical Laboratory Improvement Act
BTA	bladder tumor antigen	CLL	chronic lymphocytic leukemia
BUN	blood urea nitrogen	CML	chronic myeloid leukemia
BV	bacterial vaginosis	CMML	chronic myelomonocytic leukemia
C	cholesterol	CMP	cytidine monophosphate
C1INH	C1-esterase inhibitor	CMT	Charcot-Marie-Tooth
CA	cold agglutinins; carbonic anhydrase; cancer antigen	CMV	cytomegalovirus
CABG	coronary artery bypass graft	CN	cyanide
CACT	carnitine: acylcarnitine translocase deficiency	CNP	C-type natriuretic peptide
cADPR	cyclic ADP-ribose	CNS	central nervous system
CagA	cytotoxin-associated gene A	COHb	carboxyhemoglobin
CAH	congenital adrenal hyperplasia	COM	catechol-O-methyltransferase
C-ALCL	cutaneous anaplastic large cell lymphoma	COPD	chronic obstructive pulmonary disease
CALLA	common acute lymphoblastic leukemia antigen	CPB	competitive protein binding
cAMP	cyclic adenine monophosphate	CPC	cresolphthalein complexone; ceruloplasmin
CAP	College of American Pathologists	Cp	ceruloplasmin
CAR	cancer-associated retinopathy	CPR	cortisol production rate
CAS	chemical abstract service	cPSA	complexed prostate specific antigen
cAST	cytosolic aspartate aminotransferase	CPT	carnitine palmitoyltransferase
CBG	corticosteroid binding globulin	Cr	creatinine
Cbl	cobalamine binding level	CR	complement receptor
CBS	cystathionine-b-synthase	CRASH	corpus callosum hypoplasia/agenesis, retardation,
CCK-PZ	cholecystokinin-pancreozymin		aphasia, spastic paraplegia/shuffling gait and
CCP	cyclic citrullinated peptide		hydrocephalus
CD	cluster of differentiation	CrCl	creatinine clearance

CRH	cortisol releasing hormone	DNOC	dinitro-o-cresol
CRMP	collapsin response-mediator protein	DOC	deoxycorticosterone
CRP	C-reactive protein	DPD	dihydropyrimidine dehydrogenase; deoxypyridinoline
CS	cell surface; chorionic somatomammotropin	DPG	diphosphoglycerate
CsA	cyclosporine A	DPGM	diphosphoglyceromutase
CSF	cerebrospinal fluid	DPL	diagonal peritoneal lavage
CT	calcitonin; closure time	DRE	digital rectal examination
CTAD	citrate, theophylline, adenosine, and dipyridamole	DRPLA	dentatorubral-pallidoluysian atrophy
CTD	connective tissue disease	dRVVT	dilute Russell viper venom time
cTnI	cardiac troponin I	dsDNA	double stranded DNA
cTnT	cardiac troponin T	DSS	dengue shock syndrome
CTx	C-telopeptide	DVP	differential pulse voltammetry
CV	coefficient of variance	DVT	deep vein thrombosis
CVHD	chronic valve heart disease	E	epinephrine
CZE	capillary zone electrophoresis	E1	estrone
d	days	E2	estradiol
DAF	decay accelerating factor	E3	estriol
DAT	direct antibody test	E4	estetrol
DBS	dried blood spot	EA	ethanolamine; enteric adenovirus; early antigen
DC	dendritic cell	EALT	erythrocyte alanine aminotransferase
DCC	dextran-coated charcoal	EAST	erythrocyte aspartate aminotransferase
DC-SIGN	dendritic cell specific intracellular adhesion molecule-3-grabbing non-integrin	EBA	epidermolysis bullosa acquisita
		EBNA	Epstein-Barr nuclear antigen
DDAVP	desmopressin	EBV	Epstein-Barr virus
DDE	dichlorodiphenyldichloroethylene	EC	enzyme commission
DDR	discoidin domain receptor	ECD	electron capture detector
DDT	dichlorodiphenyltrichloroethane	ECF	extracellular fluid
DEA	diethanolamine; desthylamiodarone; drug enforcement agency	ECG	electrocardiogram
		ECMR	extracellular matrix receptor
DEAE	diethylaminoethyl	ECP	eosinophil cationic protein
DF	dengue fever	EDTA	ethylenediaminetetraacetic acid
DFA	direct fluorescent antigen	EEE	eastern equine encephalitis
DGKC	Deutsche Gesellschaft fur Klinische Chemie	EEG	electroencephalogram
DHEA	dehydroepiandrosterone	EEP	erythropoietic protoporphyria
DHEA-S	dehydroepiandrosterone sulfate	EGF	epidermal growth factor
DHF	dengue hemorrhagic fever	eGFR	estimated glomerular filtration rate
DHPR	dihydropteridine reductase	EGFR	epidermal growth factor receptor
DHT	dihydrotestosterone	EGOT	erythrocyte oxalate transaminase
DIC	disseminated intravascular coagulation	EGPT	erythrocyte glutamate oxalate transaminase
DKA	diabetic ketoacidosis	EGT	euglobulin clot lysis
dL	deciliter	EGTA	ethylenebis(oxyethylenenitrilo)tetraacetic acid
DLBCL	diffuse large B-cell lymphoma	EH	essential hypertension
DM	diabetes mellitus	EHEC	enterohemorrhagic strains of E. coli
DMD	Duchenne muscular dystrophy	EIA	enzyme immunoassay
DMPK	dystrophia myotonica protein kinase	EID	electroimmunodiffusion
DNA	deoxyribonucleic acid	EITB	enzyme-linked immunoelectrotransfer blot

ELAM	endothelial leukocytes adhesion molecule		FPIA	fluorescence polarization immunoassay
ELISA	enzyme-linked immunosorbent assay		FRAX	fragile X
ELVIS	enzyme-linked virus inducible system		FSH	follicle stimulating hormone
EM	electron microscopy		FSI	foam stability index
EMIT	enzyme multipled immunoassay technique		FSP	fibrin split product
EMMPRIN	extracellular matrix metalloproteinase inducer		FT3	free triiodothyronine
enz	enzyme		FT4	free thyroxine
EP	electrophoresis		FT4I	free thyroxine index
EPCR	endothelial cell protein C receptor		FU	fluorouracil
EPO	erythropoietin		FVL	Factor V Leiden
EPP	erythropoietic protoporphyria		G6PD	glucose-6-phosphate
ER	estrogen receptor		G-6-PGM	glucose-6-phosphoglucomutase
Erc	erythrocyte		GA	glutaric acidemia
ERP	estrogen receptor protein		GABA	γ-aminobutyrate
ESBL	extended-spectrum B-lactamase enzyme		GAD	glutamic acid decarboxylase
ESR	erythrocyte sedimentation rate		GADA	glutamic acid decarboxylase autoantibody
ESRD	end-stage renal disease		GAE	granulomatous amebic encephalitis
EtG	ethyl glucuronide		GAPD	glyceraldehyde phosphate dehydrogenase
ETK	erythrocyte transketolase		GAS	group A streptococcus
FA	Fanconi's anemia		GBA	glucocerbrosidase
FAB	French-American-British		GBL	γ- butyrolactone
FAD	flavin adenine dinucleotide		GBM	glomerular basement membrane
FADD	Fas-associated death domain		GBS	group B Streptococcus
FAMA	fluorescent antibody against membrane antigen		GC	gas chromatography
FAP	familial adenomatous polyposis		G-CSF	granulocyte colony stimulating factor
FAST	fast antimicrobial screen test		GDM	gestational diabetes mellitus
FC	follicular carcinoma		GFR	glomerular filtration rate
FCC	small cleaved follicular center-cell lymphoma		GGT	γ-glutamyltransferase
FD	factor D		GH	growth hormone
FDA	Food and Drug Administration		GHB	γ-hydroxybutyrate
FDP	fibrin degradation product		GHRH	growth hormone releasing hormone
FER	fractional esterification rate		GI	gastrointestinal
FES	flame emission spectrometry		GIST	gastrointestinal stromal tumor
FFA	free fatty acids		GLC	gas liquid chromatography
FFP	fresh frozen plasma		GLD	glutamate dehydrogenase
FHIT	fragile histidine triad		GLDH	glutamate dehydrogenase
FID	flame ionization detector		GLI	glucagon-like immunoreactivity
FIGLU	formiminoglutamic acid		Gln	glutamine
FISH	fluoresence-in-situ hybridization		Glu	glutamic acid
fl	fluid		Gly	glycine
FLM	fetal lung maturity		GMS	Giemsa stain; Gomori methenamine silver
Fluor	fluorometry		GnRH	gonadotropin releasing hormone
FMN	flavin mononucleotide		GP	glycoprotein
FN	fibronectin		GPI	glucosephosphate isomerase
F-PBA	4-fluoro-3-phenoxybenzoic acid		GSH	glutathione, reduced
FPG	fasting plasma glucose		GSH-PX	glutathione peroxide

GST	glutathione-S-transferase	HMW	high molecular weight
GTP	guanosine triphosphate	HMWK	high-molecular-weight kininogen
GTT	glucose tolerance test	HNK	human natural killer
GX	glycinexylidide	HNPCC	hereditary nonpolyposis colon cancer
Gβ	globotriaosylceramide	Hp	haptoglobin
h	hours	HPA	human platelet antibody
HAI	hemagglutination inhibition test	hpf	high-power field
HAMA	human antimouse antibodies	HPFH	persistence of fetal hemoglobin
HAS	heat stable antigen	HPLC	high-performance liquid chromatography
HAV	hepatitis A virus	Hpt	haptoglobin
Hb	hemoglobin	HPV	human papillomavirus
HBV	hepatitis B virus	HSA	human serum albumin
HC	hybrid capture	HSP	heat shock protein
hCFH	human complement factor H	HSV	herpes simplex virus
hCFHrp	human complement factor H–related protein	HTGL	hepatic triglyceride lipase
hCG	human chorionic gonadotropin	HTLV	human T-cell lymphotrophic virus
Hci	homocitrulline	HTR	hemolytic transfusion reaction
HCL	hairy cell leukemia	HTT	hydroxytryptamine
HCP	hereditary coproporphyria	HUS	hemolytic uremic syndrome
HCT	hematocrit	HUVS	hypocomplementemic urticarial vasculitis
HCV	hepatitis C virus	HVA	homovanillic acid
HCY	homocysteine	Hx	hemopexin
HD	Huntington's disease	IA	immunoassay; insulin-associated antibody
HDL	high-density lipoprotein	IAA	insulin autoantibody
HDLA	human leukocyte differentiation antigens	IAP	integrin-associated protein
HDN	hemolytic disease of the newborn	IAT	indirect antiglobulin test
HDV	hepatitis D virus	IaTI	inter-α-trypsin inhibitor
HEAA	β-hydroxyethoxyacetic acid	IB	immunoblot
HEP	hepatoerythropoietic porphyria	IBW	ideal body weight
HEV	high endothelial venules	ICAM	intracellular adhesion molecule
H-FABP	human fatty acid binding protein	ICD	isocitrate dehydrogenase
HHH	Hyperornithinemia/hyperammonemia/homocitrullinemia	ICMA	immunochemiluminescence assay
HHV	human herpes virus	ICP	inductively coupled plasma
HI	hemagglutination inhibition	ICSH	International Committee for Standardization in Hematology
His	histidine		
His (p Me)	1-methylhistidine	ID	identification; immunodiffusion
His (τ Me)	3-methylhistidine	IDDM	insulin-dependent diabetes mellitus
HIT	heparin-induced thrombocytopenia	IEF	isoelectric focusing
HIV	human immunodeficiency virus	IEM	immune electron microscopy
HK	hexokinase	IEMA	immunoenzymatic assay
HLA	human leukocyte antigen	IF	intrinsic factor; immunofluorescence
HLR	high-level aminoglycoside resistance	IFCC	International Federation of Clinical Chemistry
HME	human monocytotropic ehrlichiosis	IFG	impaired fasting glucose
hMG	human menopausal gonadotropin	IgA	immunoglobulin A
HMG-CoA	3-hydroxy-3-methylglutaryl	IgD	immunoglobulin D
hML	human mucosal lymphocyte	IgE	immunoglobulin E

IGF	insulin-like growth factor	LDL	low-density lipoprotein
IGF-BP	IGF-specific binding proteins	LE	lupus erythematosus
IgG	immunoglobulin G	Leu	leucine
IgM	immunoglobulin M	LF/FSH-RH	lutropin/follitropin-releasing hormone
IGT	impaired glucose tolerance	LFA	leukocyte function antigen
IHA	indirect hemagglutination	LGL	large granular lymphocyte leukemia
IHC	immunohistochemistry	LGP	lysosomal glycoprotein
IIF	indirect immunofluorescence	LGV	lymphogranuloma venereum
IKAP	IkappaB kinase-associated protein	LH	luteinizing hormone
IL	interleukin	LHRH	leuteinizing hormone-releasing hormone
ILA	induced by lymphocyte activation	LiPA	line probe assays
Ile	isoleucine	Lkcs	leukocytes
IM	intramuscular; infectious mononucleosis	LKM1	liver kidney microsome type 1
IMA	immunometric assay; ischemia-modified albumin	LOAEL	lowest observed adverse effect level
INR	International Normalized Ratio	Lp(a)	lipoprotein (a)
IP	immunoperoxidase	lpf	low-power field
IRG	immunoreactive glucagon	LPI	lysinuric protein intolerance
IRMA	immunoradiometric assay	LPL	lipoprotein lipase
IRP	International Reference Preparation	Lp-PLA2	lipoprotein-associated phospholipase A2
ISA	intrinsic sympathomimetic activity	LPS	lipopolysaccharide
ISE	ion selective electrode	LQTS	long QT syndrome
ISH	in-situ hybridization	LRR	leucine-rich repeat
ISI	International Sensitivity Index	LSD	lysergic acid diethylamide
ITA	immunoturbidimetric assay	LVH	left ventricular hypertrophy
IUD	intrauterine device	LYG	lymphomatoid granulomatosis
IV	intravenous	LyP	lymphomatoid papulosis
IVA	isovaleric acidemia	Lys	lysine
JE	Japanese encephalitis	MAC	membrane attack complex
kat	katal	MALT	mucosa-associated lymphoid tissue
kDa	kilodalton	MAO	monoamine oxidase
KIC	killer inhibitory cell	mAST	mitochondrial aspartate aminotransferase
L	liter	MB	microbiological assay
L/S	lecithin/sphingomyelin ratio	Mb	myoglobin
LA	latex agglutination; lupus anticoagulant	MBC	minimum bactericidal concentration
LAC	California encephalitis	MBP	myelin basic protein
LAD	leukocyte adhesion deficiency	MCAD	medium-chain acyl-COA dehydrogenase deficiency
LAMP	lysosome-associated membrane protein	MCC	methylcrotonyl-CoA carboxylase deficiency
LBC	lamellar body count	MCD	malonyl-CoA decarboxylase deficiency
LC	liquid chromatography	mcg	microgram
LCA	leukocyte common antigen	MCH	mean cell hemoglobin
LCAT	lecithin-cholesterol acyltransferase	MCHC	mean cell hemoglobin concentration
LCHAD	long-chain 3-hydroxyacyl-CoA dehydrogenase deficiency	MCL	mantle cell leukemia
		MCP	membrane cofactor protein
LCM	lymphocytic choriomeningitis; laser capture microdissection	MCTD	mixed connective tissue disease
		MCV	mean cell volume
LD, LDH	lactate dehydrogenase	MD	myotonic dystrophy

MDA	methylenedioxyamphetamine	MSRA	methicillin-resistant *Staphylococcus aureus*
MDEA	methylenedioxyethylamphetamine	MTC	medullary thyroid carcinoma
MDH	malate dehydrogenase	MTf	melanotransferrin
MDMA	methylenedioxymethamphetamine	MTHFR	5,10-methylenetetrahydrofolate reductase
MDR	multiple drug resistance	MUC	mucin-type markers
MDRD	Modification of Diet in Renal Disease	MVE	Murray Valley encephalitis
MEGX	monoethylglycinexylidide	MW	molecular weight
MEIA	microparticle enzyme immunoassay	MZL	marginal zone leukemia
MEKC	micellar electrokinetic chromatography	NAA	neutron activation analysis
MEN	multiple endocrine neoplasia	NACB	National Academy of Clinical Biochemistry
Met	methionine synthase	NAD	nicotinamide adenine dinucleotide
MetHb	methemoglobin	NADH	nicotinamide adenine dinucleotide reduced
MF/SS	mycosis fungoides/Sézary syndrome	NADPH	nicotinamide adenine dinucleotide phosphate
mg	milligram	NAIN	neonatal alloimmune neutropenia
MGC	multiglycosylated core	NAPA	N-acetylprocainamide
MGUS	monoclonal gammapathy of unknown significance	NAPQI	N-acetyl-p-benzoquinone
MHA	Mueller Hinton agar	NASBA	nucleic acid sequence-based amplification
MHC	major histocompatibility complex	NAT	N-acetyltransferase
MHPG	3-methoxy-4-hydroxyphenylglycol	NBT	nitroblue tetrazolium
MI	myocardial infarction	NCAM	neutral cell adhesion molecule; nonspecific cross-
MIC	minimum inhibitory concentration		reacting antigen
MIF	microimmunofluorescence	NCCLS	National Committee for Clinical Laboratory Standards
min	minutes		has changed its name to the Clinical and Laboratory
MIRL	membrane inhibitor of reactive lysis		Standards Institute
mL	milliliter	NCEP	National Cholesterol Education Program
MMA	methylmalonic acid	NCoR	nuclear receptor corepressor
MMF	mycophenolate mofetil	NE	norepinephrine
mo	months	nephelom	nephelometry
MoAB	monoclonal antibody	NF	neurofibromatosis
MODE	3-methoxy-O-demethylencainide	ng	nanogram
mol	mole	NIDA	National Institute on Drug Abuse
MoM	multiples of the median	NIDDM	non–insulin-dependent diabetes mellitus
MOTT	mycobacteria other than tuberculosis	NK	natural killer
MPA	mycophenolic acid	NKDEP	National Kidney Disease Education Program
MPAG	mycophenolic acid glucuronide	NLPHL	nodular lymphocyte predominant Hodgkin lymphoma
MPGM	monophosphoglyceromutase	nm	nanometers
MPL	myeloproliferative leukemia virus	NMR	nuclear magnetic resonance
MPO	myeloperoxidase	NOAEL	no observed adverse effect level
MPP	1-methyl-1,4-phenylpyridinium	non-STEMI	non–ST elevation myocardial infarction
MPS	mucopolysaccharide	NPM	nucleophosmin
MRP	multidrug resistance-associated protein	NSAIDs	nonsteroidal antiinflammatory drugs
MS	mass spectrometry; methionine synthase; multiple	NSCLC	non–small cell lung cancer
	sclerosis	NT	neutralization test
MSAFP	maternal serum α-fetoprotein	NTD	neural tube defect
MSH	melanocyte-stimulating hormone	NTPDase	nucleoside triphosphate diphosphohydrolase
MSP-R	macrophage stimulating protein receptor	NTproBNP	*N*-terminal pro-BNP

NTx	*N*-telopeptide		PEA	phosphoethanolamine
OAT	organic anion transporter		PECAM	platelet endothelial cell adhesion molecule
OC	osteocalcin		PEG	polyethylene glycol
OCT	organic cation transporter		PEL	primary effusion lymphoma
ODE	*O*-demethyl encainide		PETINA	particle-enhanced turbidimetric immunoassay
OGTT	oral glucose tolerance test		PF4	platelet factor 4
OH	hydroxide		PFA	platelet function analyzer
OHP	hydroxyprogesterone		PFGE	pulse field gel electrophoresis
OKT3	anti–T-cell monoclonal antibody		PFIC	progressive familial intrahepatic cholestasis
OLM	ocular larva migrans		PFK	phosphofructokinase
ORNT	ornithine transporter		pg	picogram
ORSA	oxacillin-resistant *Staphylococcus aureus*		PG	phosphatidylglycerol; pepsinogen; pharmacogenetics
OSHA	Occupational Safety and Health Administration		PGH	pituitary glycoprotein hormone
OTC	over-the-counter		PGK	phosphoglycerate kinase
OV	ovarian		PGL	p-selectin glycoprotein ligand
P4	progesterone		PGM	phosphoglucomutase
P5N	pyrimidine 5′-nucleotidase		Pgp	phagocytic glycoprotein
P-5′-P	pyroxidoxal -5′-phosphate		PHA	phytohemagglutinin; passive hemagglutinin
PA	pernicious anemia		Phe	phenylalanine
PABA	para-aminobenzoic acid		PHI	phosphohexose isomerase
PAG	pregnancy-associated glycoprotein		PHPAA	p-hydroxyphenyl acetic acid
PAI	plasminogen activator inhibitor		PHPLA	p-hydroxyphenyl lactic acid
PAM	primary amebic meningoencephalitis		PHPPA	parahydroxyphenylpyruvic acid
PAO	peak acid output		PI	phosphatidylinositol
PAP	prostatic acid phosphatase		Pi	inorganic phosphorus
PAPP-A	pregnancy-associated plasma protein A		PIFT	platelet immunofluorescence test
PAS	periodic acid–Schiff		PK	pharmacokinetics
PB	protein binding		PKU	phenylketonuria
PBB	polybrominated biphenyls; protected bronchial brushing		PL	placental lactogen
PBC	primary biliary cirrhosis		PL	phospholipids
PBDE	polybrominated diphenyl esters		PLAP	placental alkaline phosphatase
PBG	porphobilinogen		pleur	pleural
PBG-D	porphobilinogen deaminase		PLL	prolymphocytic leukemia
PBMC	peripheral blood mononuclear cells		PLP	pyridoxal phosphate
PC	phosphatidylcholine		PMC	pseudomembranous colitis
PCA	Purkinje cell cytoplasmic antibody; parietal cell antibodies		PMN	polymorphonuclear
			PNP	*para*-nitrophenol
PCB	polychlorinated biphenyls		PNS	peripheral nervous system
PCH	paroxysmal cold hemoglobinuria		POMC	pro-opiomelanocortin
PCP	pentachlorophenol; phencyclidine		PP	pancreatic polypeptide
PCR	polymerase chain reaction		PPA	propionic acidemia
PCR-SSP	polymerase chain reaction–sequence specific primers		PPAR	perisome proliferator activated receptor
PCT	porphyria cutanea tarda; prothrombin consumption time		ppm	parts per million
PDH	pyruvate dehydrogenase		PR	progesteron receptor
PE	phosphatidylethanolamine; pulmonary emboli; pleural effusion		PR3	proteinase 3
			PRA	plasma renin activity

PRL	prolactin	RT	room temperature
Pro	proline	RT	reverse transcriptase
PROMM	proximal myotonic myopathy	rT3	reverse triiodothyronine
PRP	progesterone receptor protein	RTA	renal tubular acidosis
PRPP	phosphoribosyl-1-pyrophosphate synthetase	rt-PCR	reverse transcriptase polymerase chain reaction
PSA	prostate specific antigen	RUT	rapid urease test
PSG	pregnancy-specific glycoprotein	RVF	Rift Valley fever
PST	pancreatic Schilling test; peroxisome targeting signal	SA	sialic acid
	type	SAA	serum amyloid A
PT	prothrombin time	SAAG	serum-ascites albumin gradient
PTCA	percutaneous transluminal coronary angioplasty	SAMHSA	Substance Abuse and Mental Health Services
PTH	parathyroid hormone		Administration
PUBS	percutaneous umbilical blood sampling	SAO	sham feeding-stimulated acid output
PUVA	psoralen drug with ultraviolet A	SARS	severe respiratory distress syndrome
PV	plasma volume	SBB	Sudan black B
PYD	pyridinoline	SBMA	spinal and bulbar muscular atrophy
PZP	pregnancy zone protein	SBT	serum bacteriocidal titer
QS	quantitation standard	SCAD	short-chain acyl-CoA dehydrogenase deficiency;
RA	rheumatoid arthritis		spinocerebellar ataxia
RAIU	thyroid uptake of radioactive iodine	SCC	squamous cell carcinoma
RAST	radioallergosorbent test	SCE	Scandinavian Committee on Enzymes
RB	retinoblastoma	SCF	cat scratch fever
RBA	radiobinding assay	SCHAD	short/medium-chain 3-hydroxyacyl-CoA
RBC	red blood cell		dehydrogenase deficiency
RBP	retinal binding protein	sCHE	serum cholinesterase
RCF	relative centrifugal force	SCID	severe combined immunodeficiency
RCM	red cell mass	SCLC	small cell lung cancer
RCV	red cell volume	SCN	thiocyanide
RDA	recommended daily allowance	SD	standard deviation
RDR	relative dose response	SDA	strand displacement amplification
RDS	respiratory distress syndrome	SDH	sorbital dehydrogenase
RDW	red cell distribution of width	SDS	sodium dodecylsulfate
RES	reticuloendothelial system	sec	seconds
RF	rheumatoid factor	SEC, s	squamous epithelial cells
RFLP	restriction fragment length polymorphism	SEM	standard error of the mean
RIA	radioimmunoassay	ser	serine
RIBA	recombinant immunoblot assay	SGOT	serum glutamate oxalate transaminase
RID	radioimmunodiffusion	SGPT	serum glutamate pyruvate transaminase
RLP	remnant lipoprotein	SHBG	sex hormone–binding globulin
RNA	ribonucleic acid	SIADH	syndrome of inappropriate antidiuretic hormone
RNP	ribonuclear protein	SIRP	signal regulatory phosphatase
ROC	receiver-operating characteristic	SIT	serum inhibitory titer
RPFA	rapid platelet function assay	SIV	simian immunodeficiencies virus
RPI	reticulocyte production index	SLAM	signal lymphocyte activation molecule
RPR	rapid plasma reagin	SLE	systemic lupus erythematosus; St. Louis encephalitis
RSV	respiratory syncytial virus	SLL	small lymphocytic lymphoma

SLVL	splenic marginal zone lymphoma with villous lymphocytes	THS	tetrahydrocompound S
		TIBC	total iron-binding capacity
Sm	smooth muscle	TIMI	thrombosis in myocardial infarction
SMA	smooth muscle antibody	titrim	titrimetry
SMRT	silencing mediator of retinoid and thyroid	TLC	thin-layer chromatography
SNP	single nucleotide polymorphism	T-LGL	T-cell large granular lymphocyte leukemia
snRNP	small nuclear ribonucleoproteins	TLV-TWV	threshold limit value–time weighted value
SPS	sodium polyanetholsulfonate	TM	thrombomodulin
SPTCL	subcutaneous panniculitis-like T-cell lymphoma	TMA	transcription-mediated amplification
SRCR	scavenger receptor cysteine-rich	TnC	troponin C
SS	somatostatin	TNF	tissue necrosis factor
SSPE	subacute sclerosing panencephalitis	TNM	tumor node metastasis
SST	serum separator tube	TP	tube precipitin; total protein
STEMI	ST elevation myocardial infarction	t-PA	tissue plasminogen activator
sTfR	serum transferrin receptor, soluble transferrin receptor	TPMT	thiopurine-S-methyltransferase
STn	sialyl-Tn	TPN	total parenteral nutrition
SUR	sulfonylurea receptor	TPO	thrombopoietin; thyroid peroxidase
T3	triiodothyronine	TPO-R	thrombopoietin receptor
T4	thyroxine	TPS	tissue polypeptide-specific antigen
TACTILE	T-cell activation increased late expression	TRALI	transfusion-related acute lung injury
TAPA	target of an antiproliferative antibody	TRAP	tartrate-resistant acid phosphatase
TB	tuberculosis	TRH	thyroid releasing hormone
TBE	tick-borne encephalitis	Trp	tryptophan
TBG	thyroid-binding globulin	TRP	tubular reabsorption of phosphate
TBII	thyroid-binding inhibiting immunoglobulins	TS	Tay-Sachs
TBIM	tyrosine-based inhibitory motifs	TSH	thyroid stimulating hormone
TBPA	thyroxine-binding prealbumin	TSI	thyroid-stimulating immunoglobulins
TBV	total blood volume	TT	thrombin time
TC	total cholesterol	TTA	transtracheal aspirate
TCA	tricyclic antidepressant; tricarboxylic acid cycle	Ttg	tissue transglutaminase
TCE	trichloroethanol	TTI	tissue thromboplastin inhibition
TCR	T-cell receptor	TTP	thrombotic thrombocytopenic purpura
TDE	1,1-dichloro-2,2-bis(p-chlorophenyl) ethane	TU	Todd units
TDM	therapeutic drug monitoring	TURP	transurethral resection of the prostate
TDP	thiamine diphosphate	Tyr	tyrosine
TdT	terminal deoxynucleotidyl transferase	U	unit
TEA	tetraethylammonium	UDG	uridine diphosphate glucuronyl transferase
TeBG	testosterone-estradiol-binding globulin	UDP	uridine diphosphate
Tf	transferrin	uPA	urokinase plasminogen activator
TFP	trifunctional protein deficiency	uPAR	urokinase plasminogen activator receptor
TG	triglyceride; thyroglobulin; thromboglobulin; thyroxine	URL	upper reference limit
TGN	thioguanine	URO-D	uroporphyrinogen decarboxylase
THBR	thyroid hormone–binding ratio	URO-S	uroporphyrinogen III (Co-) synthase
THC	tetrahydrocannabinoid	UTI	urinary tract infection
THF	tetrahydrocortisol	UV	ultraviolet
Thr	threonine	Val	valine

Vd	volume of distribution	VZV	varicella-zoster virus
VDBP	vitamin D-binding protein	WBC	white blood cells
VDHA	watery diarrhea with hypokalemia and achlorhydria	WEE	western equine encephalitis
VEE	Venezuelan equine encephalitis	WG	Wegener's granulomatosis
VIP	vasoactive intestinal polypeptide	WHO	World Health Organization
VLA	very late antigen	WNV	West Nile virus
VLCAD	very-long-chain acyl-CoA dehydrogenase deficiency	WT	wildtype
VLDL	very-low density lipoprotein	y	year
VLM	visceral larva migrans	ZE	Zollinger Ellison
VMA	vanillylmandelic acid	Zn-PP	Zinc-protoporphyrin
VNTR	variable number tandem repeat	ZSR	zero sedimentation ratio
VP	variegate porphyria	α2M	α2-macroglobulin
VRE	vancomycin-resistant enterococci	β2M	β2-microglobulin
vWD	von Willebrand disease		

SECTION I
PREANALYTICAL ASPECTS
OF CLINICAL TESTING

Preanalytical Factors Affecting Clinical Laboratory Test Results

PREANALYTICAL FACTOR	SOURCE OF ERROR OR VARIABILITY	RESULT	REMARKS/OUTCOME/PROCEDURE
Patient Status	Diet	Variation in results based on diet	Metabolic products of food can increase in venous blood. Glucose, lipids, and catecholamines may show variation because of postabsorptive hormonal effects. Caffeine can elevate concentrations of catecholamine and plasma renin.[1] Glucose and lipid profiles require fasting specimens for accurate results. Specimens for chemistry analysis should be collected 12 hours after the last meal.[1]
	Exercise	Variation in results after heavy exercise	Physical activity can have different effects on analyte concentrations, depending on whether it represents isometric or isotonic activity. This is the result of volume shifts between the vascular and interstitial compartments, volume loss by sweating, and changes in hormone concentrations.[2] Differences can be observed in blood chemistry values that occur after heavy exercise (e.g., proteinuria, LD isoenzymes, and elevations in creatine kinase [CK], CK-MB, and testosterone).
	Medication	Variation in results because of timing of blood collection or interference from medication	Therapeutic drug monitoring (TDM) specimen collection should be scheduled according to the time of the last dose. Hepatotoxic drugs can elevate liver function enzymes. Medications affecting plasma volume can affect protein concentrations, complete blood cell count (CBC), blood urea nitrogen (BUN), iron, and calcium concentrations, whereas other medications can interfere with some analytical methods.[3] Drug/drug interactions in vivo can influence the concentration of some drugs by interfering with the volume of distribution and metabolism.
	Disease state/patient demographics	Disease state, patient demographics, and stress can affect laboratory results	Since geriatric, oncology, or other hematological patients can have fragile veins, it is preferable to use a winged blood collection set. The preferable site for venipuncture may be the dorsal part of the hand or wrist area when veins in the antecubital area are not acceptable. Pediatric patients have small veins. Collecting blood from these types of patients can lead to traumatic collection and collapsed veins causing vessel wall injury and hemolysis. Hemolysis caused by turbulent blood flow results in the release of intracellular contents.[4] The use of partial draw vacuum tubes or an aspirated syringe draw may prevent fragile veins from collapsing and may minimize hemolysis.

PREANALYTICAL FACTOR	SOURCE OF ERROR OR VARIABILITY	RESULT	REMARKS/OUTCOME/PROCEDURE
Patient Status—CONT			
			Patient age, body weight, sex, and ethnicity affect analytical results. Physiological variation of veins in obese patients may be difficult to palpate and visualize. Probing with the needle should be avoided because this may lead to erroneous test results and may damage the vein, artery, nerves, and tendons. It is recommended to use a longer needle or select another site. If no other site is available, consider the dorsal part of the hand or wrist.
			Patient anxiety can affect laboratory results. It has been observed to increase secretion of hormones, such as catecholamines and cortisol. Stress is also associated with increased concentrations of albumin, glucose, fibrinogen, insulin, lactate, and cholesterol. Hyperventilation results in respiratory alkalosis with depressed PO_4 and elevated potassium.
	Body position	Increased variability based on body position	Hospital inpatients usually have blood collected while lying down. For outpatients, blood is usually collected with the patient in a blood collection chair or on an examination table. When collecting blood in a home situation, the phlebotomist should ask patients who are not bedridden to sit in a chair that reclines backward as protection from falling if they faint. The position of a patient before and during venipuncture has an effect on laboratory test results. Changing from a supine position to sitting or standing causes constriction of the blood vessels. Changing from sitting to supine causes shifting of water and electrolytes into tissue causing hemoconcentration, affecting serum/plasma levels of total protein, albumin, lipids, and cells to increase. The plasma portion of the patient's blood is filtered into the tissue, resulting in lower plasma volume and elevation of protein concentrations, blood cell counts, BUN, iron, and calcium within the blood.[5]

PREANALYTICAL FACTOR	SOURCE OF ERROR OR VARIABILITY	RESULT	REMARKS/OUTCOME/PROCEDURE

Patient Status—CONT

| | Endogenous substances | Lipemia, icterus, enzyme activity | Lipemic samples: Lipemia is difficult to control by the laboratory. Lipemic specimens occur in nonfasting blood or in patients with hyperlipidemia or receiving total parenteral nutrition (TPN) therapy. Severe hyperlipidemia can result in erroneous results by the displacement of plasma volume and subsequent short sampling. Depending on the extent of lipemia, it can interfere with spectrophotometric, turbidimetric measurements and some immunoassays. It is desirable to collect blood from patients after a period of fasting for many laboratory assays. However, for some patients it may be necessary to pretreat the blood before analysis by ultracentrifugation or enzymatic cleavage to remove lipids.[6] |

Icterus: Visible icterus in the serum occurs when serum bilirubin is >25 mg/L.[7] Bilirubin interferes with several colorimetric assays (e.g., albumin by 2-(4-hydroxyphenylazo) benzoic acid [HABA], cholesterol using ferric chloride reagents, glucose assays based on *o*-toluidine, and biuret total protein methods). In each case, results are elevated but can be corrected by use of appropriate blanking procedures or dual wavelength methods.

Endogenous enzyme activity: Homogeneous immunoassays can be influenced by endogenous enzyme activity that is the same as the enzyme label in the reaction (e.g., alkaline phosphatase). These may be removed by washing as in heterogenous immunoassays.[8]

Heterophile antibodies: Heterophile antibody interferences can occur in both types of immunoassay (homogenous and heterogenous). Heterophile or endogenous antispecies antibodies can bind the assay antibody such that the signal is compromised. Example: Human antimouse antibody (HAMA) will bind to mouse immunoglobulin coating latex microparticles in turbidimetric inhibition assays, with agglutination resulting in falsely elevated signal.[8] HAMA is commonly neutralized by including excess mouse immunoglobulin in the reagent.

PREANALYTICAL FACTOR	SOURCE OF ERROR OR VARIABILITY	RESULT	REMARKS/OUTCOME/PROCEDURE
Patient Status—CONT			
			Metabolites and other proteins: Some proteins and metabolites of drugs can bind nonspecifically with some polyclonal antibodies in immunoassays, causing erroneous results. Example: Rheumatoid factor reacts with the Fc portion of antibody-antigen complexes. In antibody assays with solid-phase adsorbed antigen, this can lead to cross-linking of nonreactive immunoglobulin G (IgG) with subsequent increased signal.[8]
Collection	**Patient Identification** Wrist band, tube label, bar codes	Incorrect, missing, unreadable	Incorrect identification can lead to wrong patient results, delay in patient results, and patient redraw. To avoid these situations, ask for the patient's name, confirm with appropriate identification, match the name with the requisition, correctly label the tubes at the bedside, and ensure that the requisition accompanies the tubes to the laboratory.[9]
Collection	**Tourniquet and Draw Technique** Quality of phlebotomy, placement, and duration	Improper phlebotomy technique	Single-use and latex-free tourniquets are preferred products. Determine if latex sensitivity precautions are necessary. The tourniquet should be placed about 3 to 4 inches above the venipuncture site.[10] Elevations in the concentration of plasma constituents can result when the tourniquet is left on for longer than 1 minute. Hemoconcentration can increase proteins, potassium, and packed cell volume. Traumatic draw as a result of vessel wall injury can cause elevations in CK, myoglobin, and potassium. Blood collections from peripheral catheters may cause hemolysis as a result of circuitous blood flow between the vein and blood collection tube. Use of partial draw tubes will decrease turbulence and specimen hemolysis. Hemolysis rates are higher in acute care settings (e.g., emergency and labor/delivery departments), where peripheral catheter collections are more prevalent. Hemolysis can interfere with results from all laboratory disciplines, especially colorimetric assays.[11-13] Blood collection near the site of infusion may cause elevations of electrolytes and/or other infusion fluids.[14] Decentralization of phlebotomy can double hemolysis rates, specimen rejection rates, and the number of redraws.[1,15,16] Excessive fist clenching can result in elevations in potassium.[17]

PREANALYTICAL FACTOR	SOURCE OF ERROR OR VARIABILITY	RESULT	REMARKS/OUTCOME/PROCEDURE
Collection—CONT			
	Order of Draw	Incorrect order of draw	Improper order of blood collection tube draw can result in incorrect test results. The National Committee for Clinical Laboratory Standards (NCCLS) recommends the following order of draw for glass or plastic tubes[10]: blood culture tubes; coagulation tubes; serum tube with or without clot activator, with or without gel; heparin tube with or without gel plasma separator; EDTA tube and glycolytic inhibitor. Glass serum tubes may be drawn before the coagulation tube. If using a wingset, a discard tube must be drawn before the coagulation tube. The discard tube should be a coagulation or nonadditive tube. In addition, an institution can validate its own order of draw.[18]
			Blood culture specimens should be collected first to prevent contamination from other tubes. Potassium EDTA drawn before a serum tube can cause elevated potassium values. Heparin tubes collected before serum and additive tubes before citrate may effect clotting.
Collection	**Draw Volume**	Incorrect filling of collection tubes will cause an altered blood to additive ratio	**Underfilling:** Inappropriate tube storage conditions prior to blood collection (excessive temperature and/or humidity), as well as tubes used after their expiration date can affect tube vacuum. Blood collection at high altitude can affect draw volume. Premature tube removal from tube holders, vein collapse, and inadequate transfer of blood collected with a syringe to blood collection tubes may also result in suboptimal sample volume, thus altering the correct blood to additive ratio in the tube. Underfilling blood collection tubes can affect red blood cell (RBC) morphology and lipids in EDTA tubes[19-22] and binding of electrolytes and troponin to heparin in some plasma tubes. CK and aminoglycoside values are affected in serum, and erroneous results have been observed in some immunoassays in serum tubes as a result of elevated concentrations of clot activator and/or silicone in blood collection tubes.[23] The anticoagulant to blood ratio for coagulation is usually 9:1. Inadequate filling of the evacuated tube may cause divergence from this ratio, leading to inaccurate results (i.e., the effect of altered sodium citrate concentration on prothrombin time.[24]

PREANALYTICAL FACTOR	SOURCE OF ERROR OR VARIABILITY	RESULT	REMARKS/OUTCOME/PROCEDURE
Collection—CONT			
			Overfilling: An appropriate safety transfer device should be used when transferring blood. Inappropriate transfer of blood from syringe collection to a blood collection tube can result in overfilling blood collection tubes beyond manufacturers' recommended draw volume, causing inadequate anticoagulation, fibrin formation, microclots, platelet clumping, and increased instrument maintenance. It could also lead to a biohazard risk if the tube stopper pops off because of overfilling the tube.
			Liquid additives in blood collection tubes will add a dilution factor compared with dry additives. For example, liquid K_3EDTA causes a dilution of approximately 1% to 2% compared with dry EDTA additive tubes, decreasing white blood cells (WBCs), RBCs, platelets, hematocrit (Hct), and hemoglobin. Therefore institutions should standardize on a single type of EDTA tube, either liquid or dry, to minimize analytical variability.
Mixing	Incorrect number of specimen inversions		Insufficient mixing can cause microclots in blood collection tubes affecting Hct, hemoglobin, and clotting times and causing fibrin formation, leading to instrument probe and/or fluid path obstruction and increased instrument down time. There is greater potential for microclots and platelet clumping with dry additives, which are highly dependent on proper mixing of specimens.
	Excessive inversions or agitation of specimens		Mixing is obtained by gentle inversions of the tube 180 degrees. One inversion is usually defined as gently inverting a specimen upside down and then back right side up. Vigorous inversions may cause foaming or hemolysis. Hemolysis occurs when plasma hemoglobin exceeds 200 mg/L. Hemolysis can cause erroneous test results in nearly all laboratory disciplines (chemistry, hematology, coagulation, and microbiology). Lactate dehydrogenase (LD) and potassium are the most sensitive indicators of hemolysis. Other tests affected by hemolysis are alanine aminotransferase (ALT), aspartate transaminase (AST), hemoglobin, iron, and T_4.[25]

PREANALYTICAL FACTOR	SOURCE OF ERROR OR VARIABILITY	RESULT	REMARKS/OUTCOME/PROCEDURE
Collection—CONT			
	Inappropriate Use of Gel Tubes	Inappropriate blood collection tube for specific analytes	Almost all analytes are stable in gel tubes; however, only some blood collection tube manufacturers validated their use for TDM testing. Analyte stability in gel tubes is dependent on several factors. These include the composition of the gel, gel surface area, volume of sample, time the sample is on the gel, temperature of the specimen, and the chemical structure of the analyte. Hydrophilic analytes are usually stable when specimens are stored in gel tubes for several days at 4° C. Some hydrophobic analytes such as amitriptyline, phenytoin, and progesterone can be underestimated when specimens are stored on the gel over time. Laboratory policies can allow accurate testing of these hydrophobic analytes through monitoring the length of time from specimen collection to analysis and specimen storage temperature, as well as using rejection criteria for short draws and enforcing policies eliminating add-on testing of these tests. Each laboratory should evaluate analyte stability in specimens collected in gel tubes in their laboratory environment before implementing usage.
Processing and Centrifugation	**Serum Clotting Time**	Insufficient clotting time	Serum should be clotted before centrifugation.[26] Clot formation is usually complete within 30 to 60 minutes at room temperature (20 to 25° C). However, some serum tubes may contain a clot activator allowing shorter clotting times. Thrombin presence in collection tubes can usually clot the specimen in as little as 5 minutes. Inadequate clotting time can cause a problem for many instruments because of latent fibrin formation, which may cause instrument probe clogging as well as erroneous results.
		Prolonged contact time with cells before separation	Prolonged contact time of serum/plasma with cells leads to the exchange of compounds in and out of the cell. Serum or plasma should be separated within 2 hours from the time of draw. Particularly critical increases in potassium can be observed.[27,28] Contact time of less than 2 hours is also recommended for adrenocorticotropic hormone (ACTH), cortisol, catecholamines, and lactic acid testing.[29-33] Prolonged cell contact time causing decreases in glucose and increases in CO_2 results from cellular metabolism. Albumin, alkaline phosphatase, ALT, blirubin, calcium, cholesterol, CK, creatinine, magnesium, phosphorus, sodium, total protein, triglycerides, T_3, T_4, urea nitrogen, and uric acid are unaffected at room temperature for as long as 48 hours.[34]

PREANALYTICAL FACTOR	SOURCE OF ERROR OR VARIABILITY	RESULT	REMARKS/OUTCOME/PROCEDURE
Processing and Centrifugation—CONT			
	Centrifugation Conditions	Inappropriate RCF, centrifuge time, and temperature	Recommendations for centrifugation vary according to blood collection tube type, manufacturer, and centrifuge type (swing bucket versus fixed angle). Excessive centrifugation g force (RCF), >3000 g, may cause cell lysis and slight elevations in LD and potassium. Inadequate g force (RCF), <1000 g or less than 10 minutes, may cause incomplete barrier formation in gel tubes or cell contamination of the specimen. Most clinical specimens should be centrifuged at room temperature.[35] Overuse of fixed angle centrifugation can cause rotor heating and affect gel integrity. Platelet poor plasma is required for coagulation testing. Centrifuges should be periodically calibrated. Blood collection tubes should be kept closed at all times.[35]
		Recentrifugation of gel tubes	Recentrifugation of gel tubes may cause serum/plasma under the gel barrier to express up through the gel and mix with the specimen above the gel barrier.[34] Significant elevations in potassium can be observed when gel tubes are recentrifuged after 24 hours.[36]
Specimen Transportation	**Common Modes of Transport** Pneumatic tube, hand carry, ground transport courier, shipment	Excessive time from draw to analysis, excessive vibration, elevated or decreased temperature, and exposure to light	Excessive transport time to analysis can result in hemolysis and elevated LD and potassium values. Most general chemistry tests are stable longer when specimens are centrifuged immediately after blood collection in gel separator tubes or are aliquoted before transport. Transport tubes (double gel) may help during stressed conditions such as specimen centrifugation at low g forces (<1300 g), use of fixed angle centrifuges, minimal spin time, and excessive transport times. These conditions are more prevalent at outpatient drawing stations where specimens should not be transported unspun unless they reach the laboratory with serum/plasma separation within 2 hours of collection.[35] Respinning gel tubes in a core laboratory can cause increased potassium levels (see Centrifugation Conditions).[36] Collection devices containing additives such as sodium fluoride can prevent changes in glucose and concentrations of other analytes over long transport times. Exposure to light can affect bilirubin, vitamin A and B_6, beta-carotene, and porphyrins. These specimens should be protected with aluminum foil, an amber container, or equivalent.[35]

PREANALYTICAL FACTOR	SOURCE OF ERROR OR VARIABILITY	RESULT	REMARKS/OUTCOME/PROCEDURE

Specimen Transportation—CONT

Vibration from some pneumatic tube transport systems can activate platelets affecting prothrombin time (PT) and activated partial thromboplastin time (APTT) testing.[37] Excessive vibration can also cause hemolysis and elevations in LD and potassium.[38] Excessive specimen vibration of arterial blood gas syringes can cause elevations in Po_2 values.[39]

Serum tubes exposed to elevated temperature can affect cryoglobulins, which precipitate at $<37°$ C. Temperatures $>56°$ C will denature proteins, and heated centrifugation can affect gel integrity (see Centrifugation Conditions). Chilling (2 to 8° C) of whole blood specimens is not recommended for whole blood beyond 2 hours.[40-41] It is contraindicated for potassium testing because it causes leakage of potassium from the cells as a result of inhibition of glycolysis. Chilling specimens is required for catecholamines, ammonia, lactic acid, pyruvate, gastrin, and parathyroid hormone (PTH) testing.[42]

Blood collection tubes should be stored and transported in a vertical position to promote complete clot formation and reduce stopper contamination, specimen agitation, and potential hemolysis. Uncontrolled transport conditions can cause inaccurate analytical results. Monitoring patient population results (inpatient versus outpatient), tracking time and temperature from blood collection to analysis, in-servicing proper handling and transport conditions, and establishment of specimen acceptance criteria can help. Cracked or leaking containers allow for contamination of the specimen. Ensure that blood specimens are securely covered and placed in leak-proof plastic bags or lockable rigid containers before transport.

PREANALYTICAL FACTOR	SOURCE OF ERROR OR VARIABILITY	RESULT	REMARKS/OUTCOME/PROCEDURE
Instrument/Method and Collection Tube Compatibility	Invalidated preanalytical phase	Interference between tube additives, environmental conditions, and analytical methodology	Although some blood collection tube manufacturers collaborate with diagnostic manufacturers to ensure compatibility between blood collection tubes and assay reagents, validation of the preanalytical phase and blood collection tubes is crucial. Laboratory environmental variation combined with the growing number of clinical laboratory tests, methodologies, increased assay sensitivity, decreased sample volume, different sample aspiration depths, and different types of blood collection tubes increase the risk of erroneous test results throughout the preanalytical phase. Poor compliance with manufacturers' recommendations, such as short draws, affects the blood to additive ratio in blood collection tubes, increasing the possibility of preanalytical error.

Phlebotomy Tubes

TUBE TYPE/ MATERIAL	STOPPER COLOR	ADDITIVE/PRESERVATIVE	GENERAL USE
Serum/glass	Red or pink	Silicone coating prevents RBCs from adhering to tube walls	General chemistry, blood bank, and serology
Serum/plastic	Red or pink	Silica clot activator/silicone coating	General chemistry, blood bank, and serology
Serum/glass with gel and clot activator	Red/gray or gold	Silica clot activator/silicone coating/gel	General chemistry and serology

*Analyte stability is dependent on time, temperature, transport, processing, and storage conditions. Consult the manufacturer, CLSI, or equivalent standards' body for stability recommendations and/or limitations. If necessary, conduct an evaluation to establish specific claims. Whenever changing any manufacturer's blood collection tube type, size, or storage condition for a particular laboratory assay, the laboratory personnel should review the tube manufacturer's data and their own data to establish/verify the reference range for a specific instrument/reagent system. Based on such information, the laboratory can then decide whether a change is appropropiate.

RECOMMENDED HANDLING CONDITIONS (E.G., MIXING, G FORCE, AND SPIN TIME)	SPECIMEN STABILITY*	REMARKS
No mixing is required for glass serum tubes because glass is a natural clot activator. Allow specimens to clot at room temperature for 30 to 60 minutes before centrifugation. Centrifugation conditions range from 1000 to 3000 g for 10 minutes. Conditions may vary depending on tube manufacturer recommendations.	Most analytes 7 days at 4° C when serum is aliquoted from the clot.	Silicone coatings may interfere with some immunoassays.
For proper additive performance, invert plastic tubes with clot activator 5 to 10 times. Allow specimens to clot at room temperature for 30 to 60 minutes before centrifugation. Centrifugation conditions range from 1000 to 3000 g for 10 minutes. Conditions may vary depending on tube manufacturer recommendations.	Most analytes 7 days at 4° C when serum is aliquoted from the clot.	Silicone coatings may interfere with some immunoassays. Silica is added to plastic tubes to simulate glass clotting because without this addition clotting time would be prolonged. Tubes with clot activator should not to be used as discard tubes for coagulation studies.
For proper additive performance, invert serum tubes 5 to 6 times. Allow specimens to clot at room temperature for 30 to 60 minutes before centrifugation. Centrifugation conditions range from 1000 to 3000 g for 10 minutes. Conditions may vary depending on tube manufacturer recommendations.	Most analytes 7 days at 4° C.	Silicone coatings may interfere with some immunoassays. Silica is added to activate clotting and decrease clotting time. A thixotropic gel is included in these tubes and is present at the tube bottom. The density of this material causes it to move upward during centrifugation to the serum-clot interface, where it forms a barrier separating serum from the clot. Many instruments are configured to sample serum directly from the collection tube, eliminating the need for transfer to another container. Transport tubes contain an additional quantity of gel barrier. This additional material produces a thicker barrier between the serum and cells that may be more stable for shipping from a phlebotomy site to a testing site.

TUBE TYPE/ MATERIAL	STOPPER COLOR	ADDITIVE/PRESERVATIVE	GENERAL USE
Phlebotomy Tubes—CONT			
Serum/plastic with gel and clot activator	Red/gray or gold or red or light brown	Silica clot activator/silicone coating/gel	General chemistry and serology
Plasma/glass Plasma/plastic	Green	Lithium heparin or sodium heparin or ammonium heparin	General chemistry
Plasma/glass with gel Plasma/plastic with gel	Green/gray or light green or green or green/light brown	Lithium heparin/gel	General chemistry

RECOMMENDED HANDLING CONDITIONS (E.G., MIXING, G FORCE, AND SPIN TIME)	SPECIMEN STABILITY*	REMARKS
For proper additive performance, invert serum tubes 5 to 10 times. Allow specimens to clot at room temperature for 30 to 60 minutes before centrifugation. Centrifugation conditions range from 1000 to 3000 g for 10 minutes. Conditions may vary depending on tube manufacturer recommendations.	Most analytes 7 days at 4° C.	Silicone may interfere with some immunoassays. Silica is added to plastic tubes to simulate glass clotting because without this addition clotting time would be prolonged. A thixotropic gel is present at the tube bottom. The density of this material causes it to move upward during centrifugation to the serum-clot interface, where it forms a barrier separating serum from the clot. Serum may be aspirated directly from the collection tube, eliminating the need for transfer to another container. Tubes with clot activator should not be used as discard tubes for coagulation studies.
For proper additive performance, invert heparin additive tubes 5 to 10 times. Centrifugation conditions range from 1000 to 3000 g for 10 to 15 minutes. Conditions may vary depending on tube manufacturer recommendations.	Most analytes 2 hours at room temperature.	Plasma specimens do not require clotting before centrifugation and offer faster turnaround time than serum. Plasma obtained in heparin tubes should be tested or removed from the tube within 2 hours of collection. Do not use tubes containing lithium heparin for lithium measurement. Tubes containing sodium heparin are not recommended for sodium analysis. Lithium heparin may also be used in blood collection syringes for whole blood critical care testing (may contain either reduced or balanced lithium heparin).[43] Do not use ammonium heparin tubes for ammonia measurement.
For proper additive performance, invert all filled additive tubes 5 to 10 times. Centrifugation conditions range from 1000 to 3000 g for 10 to 15 minutes. Conditions may vary depending on tube manufacturer recommendations.	Most analytes 2 hours at room temperature.	Heparin activates antithrombins, thus blocking the coagulation cascade and producing a whole blood/plasma sample. A gel barrier is present at the tube bottom. The density of this material causes it to move upward during centrifugation to the plasma-cell interface, where it forms a barrier separating plasma from cells. Supernatant plasma may be aspirated directly from the collection tube, eliminating the need for manual transfer to another container.

TUBE TYPE/ MATERIAL	STOPPER COLOR	ADDITIVE/PRESERVATIVE	GENERAL USE
Phlebotomy Tubes—CONT			
Plasma/plastic with gel	White or lavender/yellow	K_2EDTA with gel	Plasma testing in molecular diagnostics
Whole blood/glass and plastic	Lavender or pink or lavender/light brown	K_2EDTA or K_3EDTA	Hematology, blood bank, HbA1c, cyclosporin, tacrolimus, and other selected chemistry tests

RECOMMENDED HANDLING CONDITIONS (E.G., MIXING, G FORCE, AND SPIN TIME)	SPECIMEN STABILITY*	REMARKS
For proper additive performance, invert filled additive tubes 8 to 10 times. Centrifugation conditions range from 1000 to 2500 g for 10 minutes. Conditions may vary depending on tube manufacturer recommendations.	Analyte stability varies depending on preanalytical conditions such as sample handling.	For molecular diagnostic testing (e.g., HIV and hepatitis C virus [HCV] viral load testing) and screening nucleic acid test, genotyping blood bank assays, such as but not limited to polymerase chain reaction (PCR) and/or branched DNA (bDNA) amplification techniques, or other procedures, an undiluted plasma specimen is required as determined by the laboratory. Standard centrifugation conditions to generate plasma for testing do not completely sediment all cells. Accordingly, cell-based metabolism, as well as natural degradation *ex vivo*, may affect plasma analyte concentration/activities beyond acellular changes. Blood samples should be centrifuged within 2 hours of collection.
These tubes are used in the collection of blood specimens for whole blood testing that requires no centrifugation. For proper additive performance, invert filled additive tubes 8 to 10 times. Conditions may vary depending on tube manufacturer recommendations.	Routine hematology testing should be conducted within 6 hours of collection, keeping the sample at room temperature.[43]	EDTA is used for a wide range of hematology tests, genetic testing, immunosuppressants, HbA1c, RBC folate, and other selected tests. K_2EDTA, K_3EDTA, Na_2EDTA and serum tubes may be used for routine immunohematology testing such as red cell grouping, Rh typing, and antibody screens.[44] The common types of EDTA used in blood collection tubes are Na_2EDTA, K_3EDTA and K_2EDTA. K_3EDTA is available in both liquid and dry forms. Solubility of EDTA varies. Potassium EDTA is more soluble than the sodium form and liquid EDTA is more soluble than dry. However, liquid K_3EDTA causes a sample dilution of approximately 1-2% of blood. K_3EDTA causes largest amount of RBC shrinkage at increasing EDTA concentrations; therefore K_2EDTA is recommended by NCCLS and International Committee for Standardization in Hematology (ICSH) for blood cell counting and sizing. Other comparative studies using liquid K_3EDTA and the dry form of K_2EDTA have demonstrated either acceptable agreement,[45] no marked differences at optimal conditions,[46] or minimal differences that are not clinically significant.[47] Errors include EDTA-induced platelet-specific antibodies, platelet clamping (pseudothrombocytopenia, EDTA-induced polymorphonuclear leukocyte (PMN), agglutination in vitro, spurious leukopenia, and pseudogranulocytopenia.

TUBE TYPE/ MATERIAL	STOPPER COLOR	ADDITIVE/PRESERVATIVE	GENERAL USE
Phlebotomy Tubes—CONT			
Whole blood/glass	Lavender	Liquid K_3EDTA	Hematology, blood bank, HbA1c, cyclosporin, tacrolimus, and some other chemistry tests
Plasma/glass and plastic	Gray	Glycolytic inhibitor	Glucose and other tests requiring glycolysis inhibition
Serum/glass and plastic	Gray	Glycolytic inhibitor	Glucose and other tests requiring glycolysis inhibition
Serum/glass and plastic	Yellow/gray or orange	Thrombin may contain siliconized coating and/or clot activator	Stat serum testing in chemistry
Plasma/whole blood/glass and plastic	Light blue	May contain siliconized interior with 0.105 to 0.109 mol/L sodium citrate (~3.2% sodium citrate); 9:1 blood to additive ratio	Coagulation testing and platelet function assessment
Plasma/whole blood/glass and plastic	Light blue	0.129 mol/L sodium citrate (equivalent to 3.8% sodium citrate); 9:1 blood to additive ratio	Coagulation testing and platelet function assessment

RECOMMENDED HANDLING CONDITIONS (E.G., MIXING, G FORCE, AND SPIN TIME)	SPECIMEN STABILITY*	REMARKS
These tubes are used in the collection of blood specimens for whole blood testing that requires no centrifugation. For proper additive performance, invert tubes 8 to 10 times. Conditions may vary depending on tube manufacturer recommendations.	Routine hematology testing should be conducted within 6 hours of collection, keeping the sample at room temperature.[43]	Blood collection tubes containing liquid K_3EDTA additive dilute specimens approximately 1% to 2% compared with dry EDTA additives, resulting in a negative bias between the two blood collection tube types. Therefore institutions should standardize on either dry EDTA or liquid and avoid use of both tube types.
For proper additive performance, invert tubes 8 to 10 times. Centrifugation conditions range from 1000 to 3000 g for 10 minutes. Conditions may vary depending on tube manufacturer recommendations.		Various glycolytic inhibitors are available including: potassium oxalate/NaF, EDTA/NaF, sodium heparin/NaF, and iodoacetate. Fluoride and iodoacetate inhibit glycolysis, whereas oxalate, EDTA, and heparin are anticoagulants used to provide plasma specimens. Gray top tubes can also be used for lactate and alcohol determinations.
For proper additive performance, invert tubes 5 to 10 times. Allow specimens to clot at room temperature for 30 to 60 minutes before centrifugation. Centrifugation conditions range from 1000 to 3000 g for 10 minutes. Conditions may vary depending on tube manufacturer recommendations.		Fluoride inhibits glycolysis. Appropriate additive mixing is critical in serum samples due to the absence of an anticoagulant. These tubes can also be used for lactate and alcohol determinations.
For proper additive performance, invert tubes 8 to 10 times. Centrifugation conditions after clot formation range from 1000 to 3000 g for 10 minutes. Conditions may vary depending on tube manufacturer recommendations.	Most analytes 7 days at 4° C, when serum is aliquoted from the clot.	Tube inversions ensure complete clotting usually in 5 minutes.
For proper additive performance, invert tubes three or four times. Vigorous mixing may cause platelet activation. Centrifuge at 1500 to 2500 g for 15 minutes; plasma should contain fewer than 10,000 platelets/mL plasma. Conditions may vary depending on tube manufacturer recommendations.		For clot-based chromogenic and immunological coagulation assays. NCCLS recommends 0.105 to 0.109 mol/L sodium citrate (~3.2% sodium citrate). See NCCLS documents for specimen handling and specific assay recommendations.
For proper additive performance, invert tubes three or four times. Vigorous mixing may cause platelet activation. Centrifuge at 1500 to 2500 g for 15 minutes; plasma should contain fewer than 10,000 platelets/mL plasma. Conditions may vary depending on tube manufacturer recommendations.		For clot-based chromogenic and immunological coagulation assays. NCCLS recommends 0.105 to 0.109 mol/L sodium citrate (~3.2% sodium citrate). See NCCLS documents for specimen handling and specific assay recommendations.

TUBE TYPE/ MATERIAL	STOPPER COLOR	ADDITIVE/PRESERVATIVE	GENERAL USE
Phlebotomy Tubes—CONT			
Plasma/glass and plastic	Light blue	Citrate, theophylline, adenosine, and dipyridamole (CTAD)	Coagulation testing, platelet function studies, and heparin monitoring
Whole blood/glass and plastic	Black	0.105 mol/L sodium citrate solution (equivalent to 3.2% sodium citrate); 4:1 blood to additive ratio	Erythrocyte sedimentation rate (ESR)
Whole blood/glass and plastic	Black	0.129 mol/L sodium citrate solution (equivalent to 3.8% sodium citrate); 4:1 blood to additive ratio	ESR
Activated clotting time (ACT)/glass	Gray	Siliceous earth	ACT
Plasma/glass and plastic	Tan or royal blue or green or lavender	Na_2heparin Na_2EDTA K_2EDTA	Plasma lead testing trace elements/toxicology

RECOMMENDED HANDLING CONDITIONS (E.G., MIXING, G FORCE, AND SPIN TIME)	SPECIMEN STABILITY*	REMARKS
For proper additive performance, invert tubes three or four times. Vigorous mixing may cause platelet activation. Centrifuge at 1500 to 2500 g for 15 minutes; plasma should contain fewer than 10,000 platelets/mL plasma. Conditions may vary depending on tube manufacturer recommendations.		The citrate, theophylline, adenosine, and dipyridamole (CTAD) tube is used for the collection and transport of specimens for hemostasis testing. The CTAD solution is a mixture of sodium citrate, theophylline, adenosine, and dipyridamole. The purpose of the additive is to anticoagulate the specimen and to minimize in vitro platelet activation. CTAD tubes must be protected from artificial and natural light during storage because dipyridamole is light sensitive. Accumulated light exposure in excess of 12 hours can cause additive inactivation. CTAD may result in longer clotting times compared with citrate because of minimization of platelet activation and subsequent neutralization of heparin.
For proper additive performance, invert tube six to eight times. Conditions may vary depending on tube manufacturer recommendations.		ESR determination by Westergren method.
For proper additive performance, invert tube 6 to 8 times. Conditions may vary depending on tube manufacturer recommendations.		ESR determination by Westergren method.
For proper additive performance, invert tube 8 to 10 times. Conditions may vary depending on tube manufacturer recommendations.		The ACT tube is an in vitro diagnostic reagent system used in screening coagulation defects of whole blood, with the exception of platelets (in certain instances) and factor VII (proconvertin). The inert additive siliceous earth provides contact activation resulting in a shortening of the coagulation time and thus creating a uniquely sensitive screening method for detecting coagulation disorders, exclusive of factor VII and platelet deficiencies. As such, the ACT has shown itself to be a simple, sensitive, and reliable test for clotting activity.
For proper additive performance, invert tubes 8 to 10 times. Centrifugation conditions range from 1000 to 3000 g for 10 minutes. Conditions may vary depending on tube manufacturer recommendations.		Some manufacturers' tubes are tested and certified for lead level. Some manufacturers may use special stoppers to eliminate most trace metal contamination.

TUBE TYPE/ MATERIAL	STOPPER COLOR	ADDITIVE/PRESERVATIVE	GENERAL USE
Phlebotomy Tubes—CONT			
Serum/glass and plastic	Royal blue or white	Silicone coated (clot activator in plastic) or no additive	Serum trace elements/ toxicology
Whole blood/glass and plastic	Yellow	Sodium polyanethol sulfonate (SPS)	Whole blood microbiology testing
Whole blood/glass and plastic	Yellow	Acid-citrate-dextrose (ACD) A—trisodium citrate (22 g/L), citric acid (8.0 g/L), dextrose (24.5 g/L)	Blood bank and genetic testing
Whole blood/glass and plastic	Yellow	ACD B—trisodium citrate (13.2 g/L), citric acid (4.8 g/L), dextrose (14.7 g/L)	Blood bank and genetic testing
DNA preparation/plastic	Clear/light blue	DNA additive	DNA extraction
RNA stabilization/plastic	Clear/red or blue	RNA additive	Stabilization of RNA
Urine tube/plastic	Yellow/beige conical and round bottom	No additive	Urine chemistry (urinalysis, dipstick, and sediment) and microbiology

RECOMMENDED HANDLING CONDITIONS (E.G., MIXING, G FORCE, AND SPIN TIME)	SPECIMEN STABILITY*	REMARKS
For proper additive performance, invert tubes 8 to 10 times. Centrifugation conditions after clot formation range from 1000 to 3000 *g* for 10 minutes. Conditions may vary depending on tube manufacturer recommendations.		Some manufacturers may use special stoppers to eliminate most trace metal contamination.
For proper additive performance, invert filled tubes 8 to 10 times. Conditions may vary depending on tube manufacturer recommendations.		For blood culture specimens in microbiology.
For proper additive performance, invert filled tubes 8 to 10 times. Conditions may vary depending on tube manufacturer recommendations.		For blood bank studies, human leukocyte antigen (HLA) phenotyping, DNA, and paternity testing.
For proper additive performance, invert filled tubes 8 to 10 times. Conditions may vary depending on tube manufacturer recommendations.		For blood bank studies, HLA phenotyping, DNA, and paternity testing.
After blood collection, gently invert tube 8 to 10 times. Conditions may vary depending on tube manufacturer recommendations.	DNA profile may remain stable in situ for up to 14 days at 18 to 25° C, 4 weeks at 2 to 8° C, 10 weeks at −20° C, and 10 months at −70/−80° C.	For the collection of whole blood for the isolation of genomic DNA. Molecular test methods that require intact genomic DNA from whole blood. These test methods include, but are not limited to, PCR and Southern blot analysis.
After blood collection, gently invert tube 8 to 10 times. Conditions may vary depending on tube manufacturer recommendations.	RNA profile may remain stable for several days. Stability increases at 4° C and can be further prolonged after freezing. Contact the manufacturer for specific information on stability conditions.	For the collection of whole blood and stabilization of the cellular RNA profile. The RNA tube contains an additive that stabilizes cellular RNA and prepares the sample for RNA purification. Methods include, but are not limited to, reverse transcriptase PCR (RT-PCR) and Northern blot analysis. In stabilized blood, RNA rapidly degrades significantly within hours after blood collection. Furthermore, certain species of RNA, through the process of gene induction, increase once the blood is collected. Both RNA degradation and in vitro gene induction can lead to an underestimation or overestimation of in vivo gene transcript number.
Conditions may vary depending on tube manufacturer recommendations.	Less than 2 hours at room temperature post-collection. Refrigerate specimen if there is a delay of more than 2 hours. Specimen should be at room temperature before testing is performed.[48]	Can be used for automated chemistry on dedicated urinalysis instruments and microscopic analysis of sediments.

TUBE TYPE/ MATERIAL	STOPPER COLOR	ADDITIVE/PRESERVATIVE	GENERAL USE
Phlebotomy Tubes—CONT			
Urine chemistry preservative tube/plastic	Yellow/cherry conical	Urine preservative	Urine chemistry, dipstick, and sediment analysis
Culture and sensitivity urine preservative tube/plastic	Gray/khaki or green/yellow	Urine preservative for microbiology	Microbiology analysis, automated flow cytometry, and sediment analysis
Microcollection/plasma/ plastic	Lavender	May contain silicone, K_2EDTA or K_3EDTA	Hematology

RECOMMENDED HANDLING CONDITIONS (E.G., MIXING, G FORCE, AND SPIN TIME)	SPECIMEN STABILITY*	REMARKS
Shake tubes vigorously to ensure complete dissolution of the preservative. Centrifuge at 600 g for 5 minutes in a swing bucket centrifuge. Conditions may vary depending on tube manufacturer recommendations.	Specimens not tested or preserved within 1 to 2 hours of collection should be refrigerated. Stable up to 72 hours at room temperature.	Urinalysis preservative tube can be used for automated chemistry urinalysis and sediment analysis. Without the presence of a preservative, the bacteria continue to be metabolically active and reproduce, causing changes in the urine chemistry components measured in a routine urinalysis. Because of the instability of bilirubin and urobilinogen in urine when exposed to room temperature and light, testing should be performed as soon as possible. Specimens should be stored in darkness or collected in amber tubes or amber 24-hour containers.
Mix by inverting 8 to 10 times. Conditions may vary depending on tube manufacturer recommendations.	Specimen preserved for 48 hours at room temperature.	Culture and sensitivity for bacteria. Bacteria quantification of clean-voided midstream collected urine is widely used as an aid in evaluating a patient for urinary tract infections. Urine frequently supports the proliferation of bacteria, which may multiply at the same rate as in the nutrient broth. Therefore urine delayed in transit and left at room temperature for an extended period may lead to a false result. As a means of preventing growth of the microorganisms from sources exogenous to the bladder, refrigeration or culturing within 2 hours of micturition is recommended. Timed specimens should be refrigerated between collections. The microbial load in urine from a given patient may be influenced by the time of collection and fluid intake.
For proper additive performance, invert filled additive tubes 8 to 10 times. Tubes must be filled to ensure the proper blood to additive ratio. Conditions may vary depending on tube manufacturer recommendations.	Specimens can be stored up to 4 hours before analysis.	Skin puncture blood specimens for hematologic determinations, WBC, RBC, hemoglobin (Hgb), Hct, reticulocyte, white cell differential count, mean corpuscular hemoglobin (MCH), mean corpuscular hemoglobin concentration (MCHC), mean corpuscular volume (MCV), and platelet count. As with any skin puncture blood system, "milking" the skin puncture site may cause hemolysis and adversely affect the accuracy of the determinations. Some microcollection tubes may contain silcone to facilitate easy removal of the specimen from the container.

TUBE TYPE/ MATERIAL	STOPPER COLOR	ADDITIVE/PRESERVATIVE	GENERAL USE
Phlebotomy Tubes—CONT			
Microcollection/plasma/ plastic	Green	May contain silicone, lithium heparin	General chemistry
Microcollection plasma separator/plastic with gel	Green	May contain silicone, lithium heparin with gel	General chemistry
Microcollection serum separa- tor (amber or clear)/plastic with gel	Gold or red	Silicone with gel	General chemistry
Microcollection/serum/plastic	Red or pink	Silicone	General chemistry

RECOMMENDED HANDLING CONDITIONS (E.G., MIXING, G FORCE, AND SPIN TIME)	SPECIMEN STABILITY*	REMARKS
The sample is inverted 8 to 10 times to ensure dissolution of the anticoagulant. Centrifuge conditions may vary depending on tube manufacturer recommendations.	Most analytes 2 hours at room temperature.	Chemistry values obtained from skin puncture plasma may differ from those obtained from skin puncture serum, venous plasma, or venous serum. Specimens should be centrifuged and processed immediately on arrival in the laboratory. As with any skin puncture blood system, "milking" the skin puncture site may cause hemolysis and adversely affect the accuracy of the determinations. Some microcollection tubes may contain silcone to facilitate easy removal of the specimen from the container.
The sample is inverted 8 to 10 times to ensure dissolution of the anticoagulant. Centrifuge conditions may vary depending on tube manufacturer recommendations.	Most analytes 2 hours at room temperature.	Chemistry values obtained from skin puncture plasma may differ from those obtained from skin puncture serum, venous plasma, or venous serum. Specimens should be centrifuged and processed immediately on arrival in the laboratory. As with any skin puncture blood system, "milking" the skin puncture site may cause hemolysis and adversely affect the accuracy of the determinations. Some microcollection tubes may contain silcone to facilitate easy removal of the specimen from the container.
The sample is allowed to clot for a minimum of 30 minutes. Centrifuge conditions may vary depending on tube manufacturer recommendations.	Most analytes 7 days at 4° C.	Exposure to light can affect bilirubin, vitamin A and B_6, beta-carotene, and porphyrins. These specimens should be protected with an aluminum foil, an amber container, or equivalent.[34]
Allow blood to clot for a minimum of 30 minutes. Centrifuge conditions may vary depending on tube manufacturer recommendations.	Most analytes 7 days at 4° C, when serum is aliquoted from the clot.	Chemistry values obtained from skin puncture serum may differ from those obtained from skin puncture plasma, venous plasma, or venous serum. Specimens should be centrifuged and processed immediately on arrival in the laboratory. As with any skin puncture blood system, "milking" the skin puncture site may cause hemolysis and adversely affect the accuracy of the determinations. Some microcollection tubes may contain silcone to facilitate easy removal of the specimen from the container.

TUBE TYPE/ MATERIAL	STOPPER COLOR	ADDITIVE/PRESERVATIVE	GENERAL USE

Phlebotomy Tubes—CONT

1. Murphy R: Work re-engineering: the benefits and the barriers, an analytical review, *J Soc Health Syst* 5:73-84, 1994.

2. Young DS, Bermes EW: Specimen collection and processing; sources of biologic variation. In Ashwood ER, editor: *Tietz textbook of clinical chemistry,* Philadelphia, 1999, WB Saunders, pp. 42-72.

3. Pippenger CE: Fundamental principles of therapeutic drug monitoring. In Moyer TP, Boeckx RL, editors: *Applied therapeutic drug monitoring, vol 1: Fundamentals,* Washington, DC, 1982, AACC Press, pp. 9-17.

4. Laessig RH, Hassemer DJ, Paskey TA, et al: The effect of 0.1 percent erythrocytes and hemolysis on serum chemistry values, *Am J Clin Pathol* 66:639-644, 1976.

5. Statland BE, Winkel P: Effects of preanalytical factors on the intraindividual variation of analytes in the blood of healthy subjects: consideration of preparation of the subject and time of venipuncture, *CRC Crit Rev Clin Lab Sci* 8:105-144, 1977.

6. Wilde C: Subject preparation, sample collection and handling. In Wild D, editor: *The immunoassay handbook,* New York, 1994, Stockton Press, pp. 243-255.

7. Watson D: A note on the hemoglobin error in some nonprecipitation Diazo-methods for bilirubin determinations, *Clin Chim Acta* 5:613-615, 1960.

8. Davies D: Concepts. In Wild D, editor: *The immunoassay handbook,* New York, 1994, Stockton Press, pp. 84-115.

9. Management of information. In *JCAHO comprehensive accreditation manual for pathology and clinical laboratory services,* Oakbrook Terrace, IL, 2002-2003, Joint Commission Resources, IM.8, IM.10.

10. NCCLS Document H3-A5. *Procedures for the collection of diagnostic blood specimens by venipuncture; approved standard,* ed 5, Wayne, PA, 2003, 23(32) National Committee for Clinical Laboratory Standards, p. 17.

11. Grant MS: The effect of drawing techniques and equipment on the hemolysis of ED laboratory blood samples, *J Emerg Nurs* 29:116-121, 2003.

12. Kennedy C, Angermuller S, King R, et al: A comparison of hemolysis rates using intravenous catheters versus venipuncture tubes for obtaining blood samples, *J Emerg Nurs* 22:566-569, 1996.

13. Sixsmith DM, Weinbaum F, Chan SYA, et al: Reduction of hemolysis of blood specimens drawn from ED patients for routine chemistry tests by use of low vacuum tubes [Abstract], *Acad Emerg Med* 7:524, 2000.

14. Read DC, Viera H, Arkin C: Effect of drawing blood specimens proximal to an in-place but discontinued intravenous solution, *Am J Clin Pathol* 90:702-706, 1988.

15. Lark S: Patient-focused care. Is it working? Is it here to stay? *Lab Med* 28:644-651, 1997.

16. McQueen J: Overcoming the barriers to implementing patient-focused care, *Healthc Inf Manage* 7:17-21, 1993.

17. Don BR, Sebastian A, Cheitlin M, et al: Pseudohyperkalemia caused by fist clenching during phlebotomy, *N Engl J Med* 322:1290-1292, 1990.

18. Calam RR, Cooper MH: Recommended order of draw for collecting blood specimens into additive-containing tubes, *Clin Chem* 28:1399, 1982.

19. Lampasso JA: Error in hematocrit value produced by excessive ethylenediamine tetraacetic acid, *Am J Clin Pathol* 44:109-110, 1965.

20. Lewis SM, Stoddart CTH: Effects of anticoagulants and containers (glass and plastic) on blood count, *Lab Pract* 20:787-792, 1977.

21. Sacker LS: Specimen collection. In Lewis SM, Coster JF, editors: *Quality control in haematology,* New York, 1975, Academic Press, pp. 224-227.

22. Bachorik PS: Collection of blood samples for lipoprotein analysis, *Clin Chem* 28:1375-1378, 1982.

23. Andrejat G, Fitzgibbon L, Gilis R, et al: Heparin interferences in creatine kinase assays, *Clin Chem* 28:1718-1719, 1982.

24. Humphreys RE, McPhedran P: False elevation of partial thromboplastin time and prothrombin time, *JAMA* 214:1702-1704, 1970.

25. Young DS, Pestaner LC, Gibberman V: Effects of drugs on clinical laboratory tests, *Clin Chem* 21:1D-432D, 1975.

26. Zweig MH, Glickman J, Csako G: Analytical interference caused by incompletely clotted serum specimens, *Clin Chem* 40:2325-2326, 1994.

RECOMMENDED HANDLING CONDITIONS (E.G., MIXING, G FORCE, AND SPIN TIME)	SPECIMEN STABILITY*	REMARKS

27. Gourlay NJ, McArthur C: Minimising factitious hyperkalaemia. Centrifuging samples may help prevent false readings, *BMJ* 315:190, 1997.

28. Goodman JR, Vincent J, Rosen I: Serum potassium changes in blood clots, *Am J Clin Pathol* 24:111-113, 1954.

29. Winsten S, Gordesky SE: Transportation of specimens. In Faulkner WR, Maeites S, editors: *Selected methods of clinical chemistry, AACC* 9:11-15, 1982.

30. Adams PC, Woodhouse KW, Adela M, et al: Exaggerated hypokelemia in acute myeloid leukemia, *BMJ* 282:1034-1035, 1981.

31. Boomsma F, Alberts G, VanEijk L, et al: Optimal collection and storage conditions for catecholamine measurement in human plasma and urine, *Clin Chem* 39:2503-2508, 1993.

32. Astles K, Williams CP, Sedor F: Stability of plasma lactate in vitro in the presence of antiglycolytic agents, *Clin Chem* 40:1327-1330, 1994.

33. Laessig RH, Indrikson AA, Hassemer DJ, et al: Changes is serum chemical values as a result of prolonged contact with the clot, *Am J Clin Pathol* 66:598-604, 1976.

34. NCCLS Document H18-A3. *Procedures for the handling and processing of blood specimens.* Approved Guideline, ed 3, Vol 24, No. 28, Wayne, PA, 2004, National Committee for Clinical Laboratory Standards.

35. Hira K, Shimbo T, Fukui T: High serum potassium concentrations after recentrifugation of stored blood specimens, *N Engl J Med* 343:153-154, 2000.

36. Dyszkiewicz-Korpanty A, Quinton R, Yassine J, et al: The effect of a pneumatic tube transport system on PFA-100 trade mark closure time and whole blood platelet aggregation, *J Thromb Haemost* 2:354-356, 2004.

37. Steige H, Jones JD: Evaluation of pneumatic-tube system for delivery of blood specimens, *Clin Chem* 17 (12):1160-1164, 1971.

38. Collinson PO, John CM, Gaze DC, et al: Changes in blood gas samples produced by a pneumatic tube system. *J Clin Pathol* 55 (2):105-107, 2002.

39. Ono T, Kitabuchi K, Takehara M, et al: Serum-constituents analyses: effect of duration and temperature of storage of clotted blood, *Clin Chem* 27:35-38, 1981.

40. Oliver TK, Young GA, Bates GD, et al: Factitial hyperkalemia due to icing before analysis, *Pediatrics* 38:900-902, 1966.

41. Young DS, Bermes EW: Specimen collection and processing; sources of biologic variation. In Tietz NS, editor: *Textbook of clinical chemistry,* Philadelphia, 1986, WB Saunders, pp. 486-494.

42. Toffaletti ME, Hammes R, Gray B, et al: Dry electrolyte-balanced heparinized syringes evaluated for determining ionized calcium and other electrolytes in whole blood, *Clin Chem* 37:1730-1733, 1991.

43. NCCLS Document H35-T. *Additives to blood collection devices: EDTA; tentative standard,* Wayne, PA, 1992, National Committee for Clinical Laboratory Standards, p. 12(17).

44. NCCLS Document H1-A5. *Tubes and additives for venous blood specimen; approved standard,* ed 5, Wayne, PA, 2003, National Committee for Laboratory Standards.

45. Brunson D, Smith BA, Przyk E, et al: Comparing hematology anticoagulants: K_2EDTA vs K_3EDTA, *Lab Hematology* 1:112-119, 1995.

46. Goossens W, Van Duppen V, Verwilghen RL: K_2- or K_3-EDTA: the anticoagulant of choice in routine haematology? *Clin Lab Haematol* 13:291-295, 1992.

47. Van Cott E, Lewandrowski SP, Grzybek DY, et al: A comparison of glass K_3EDTA versus plastic K_2EDTA blood-drawing tubes for complete blood counts, reticulocyte counts, and white blood cell differentials, *Clin Lab Haematol* 9:10-14, 2003.

48. NCCLS Document GP 16-A2: Urinalysis and collection, transportation, and preservation of urine specimens. Approved Guideline-Second Edition, Vol. 21, No. 19, Wayne, PA, 2001.

Section II
General Clinical Tests

TEST NAME AND METHOD	SPECIMEN REQUIREMENTS	REFERENCE INTERVAL, CONVENTIONAL [INTERNATIONAL RECOMMENDED UNITS]			CHEMICAL INTERFERENCES AND IN VIVO EFFECTS
ABO and Rh Typing[1-7] **Testing for minor blood group antigens such as Kell, Duffy, and others is known as red cell phenotyping.** *Agglutination tests using slide, tube, gel card, or microplate formats for ABO, Rh typing.*	Erythrocytes. Clotted blood collected in plain (red stopper) tube without silicon gel[8] or EDTA-anticoagulated blood (pink or lavender top tube). Local laboratory requirements may vary. Store at 4° C. Stable for 5-7 days.	Not applicable.			The presence of fibrin strands, paraproteins, or plasma expanders in serum or Wharton's jelly in cord blood samples may cause pseudoagglutination. Cold-reacting autoantibodies, weakened antigen expression (e.g., variant A genes) or altered antigens (e.g., acquired B phenotype) can give discrepant results. Hematopoietic stem cell transplantation or the presence of transfused red blood cells may give unexpected results.

1. Brecher M, editor: *Technical manual,* ed 15, Bethesda, MD, 2005, AABB.
2. Chapman JF, Elliott C, Knowles SM, et al: Guidelines for compatibility procedures in blood transfusion laboratories, *Transfus Med* 14:59-73, 2004.
3. Issitt P, Anstee D: *Applied blood group serology,* ed 4, Durham, NC, 1998, Montgomery Scientific Publications.
4. Judd W: Red blood cell immunology and compatibility testing. In Simon T, Dzik W, Snyder E, et al, editors: *Rossi's principles of transfusion medicine,* Philadelphia, 2002, Lippincott Williams & Wilkins, pp. 69-88.
5. Shulman IA, Downes KS, Sazama K, et al: Pretransfusion compatibility testing for red blood cell administration, *Curr Opin Hematol* 8:397-404, 2001.
6. Mollison P, Engelfriet C, Contreras M: *Blood transfusion in clinical medicine,* ed 10, Oxford, 1997, Blackwell Scientific Publications.
7. Roitt I, Brostoff J, Male D: *Immunology,* ed 4, London, 1996, Mosby.
8. Geisland JR, Milam JD: Spuriously positive direct antiglobulin tests caused by use of silicone gel, *Transfusion* 20:711-713, 1980.

Test Name and Method	Specimen Requirements		Conventional *mg/L*		International *μmol/L*	Chemical Interferences
Acetaldehyde[1-2] *GLC*	Blood (fluoride/oxalate) 	 Occupational exposure: Toxic range:	<0.2 <0.5 1.0-2.0	× 22.7	[<4.5] [<11.4] [22.7-45.4]	The addition of thiourea to blood inhibits nonenzymatic formation of acetaldehyde.
	Breath	Occupational exposure: After ethanol ingestion: See also *Remarks.*	<0.01 0.007-0.01		[<0.23] [0.16-0.23]	↑ V Disulfiram, some cephalosporins (cefamandole, cefoperazone, moxalactam), chlorpropamide, metronidazole, sulfonylureas.

DIAGNOSTIC INFORMATION	REMARKS

Except for neonates, routine ABO testing requires that the results of red cell typing ("forward type") agree with those of serum testing ("back type"). See *Isoagglutinins.*

Weakened expression of the D antigen, as seen in the "weak D" and some "partial D" variants, may give a false-negative Rh (D) typing result.

ABO discrepancies on the "forward type" may result from weakened antigen expression: leukemia, other malignancies, subgroups of A or B; or from altered antigenic structure: polyagglutination and acquired B phenomena.

ABO discrepancies are resolved by repeat testing or through the use of other immunohematological tests. Until then, group O RBCs are administered. Donor units are issued only after the resolution of any ABO discrepant results.

ABO discrepancies on the "back type" may result from the absence of expected antibodies such as anti-A or anti-B: neonates, elderly patients, congenital or acquired immunodeficiency states; or from the presence of unexpected antibodies: ABO mismatched transplant, cold-reacting autoantibodies or alloantibodies, infusion of IVIG or ABO mismatched platelets; or the presence of interfering substances: fibrin clots, paraproteins, plasma expanders.

Serological determination of minor blood group antigens requires special typing sera. When serological typing is technically not feasible or unreliable (prenatal testing, recent multiple transfusions), blood group genotyping may be helpful. See *Blood Group Genotyping.*

Low to moderate air concentrations (50-200 ppm; 1.14-4.54 mmol/L) cause eye irritation and upper respiratory discomfort. More than 200 ppm may cause dyspnea and CNS depression.

Ethanol is converted by alcohol dehydrogenase (slow) to acetaldehyde, which is then oxidized by acetaldehyde dehydrogenase (fast) to acetic acid. Following administration of an inhibitor of acetaldehyde dehydrogenase such as disulfiram or calcium carbamide, toxic concentrations of acetaldehyde accumulate. Moderate ingestion of ethanol elevates blood acetaldehyde to 0.9-1.3 mg/L [20.4-29.5 μmol/L], whereas in chronic alcoholics concentrations are 1.7-2.5 mg/L [38.6-56.8 μmol/L].

TEST NAME AND METHOD	SPECIMEN REQUIREMENTS	REFERENCE INTERVAL, CONVENTIONAL [INTERNATIONAL RECOMMENDED UNITS]		CHEMICAL INTERFERENCES AND IN VIVO EFFECTS
Acetaldehyde— CONT				
UV/GLC-FID	Urine			

1. Baselt RC: *Biological monitoring methods for industrial chemicals,* Davis, CA, 1980, Biomedical Publications.
2. Baselt RC: *Disposition of toxic drugs and chemicals in man,* ed 7, Foster City, CA, 2004, Biomedical Publications.

TEST NAME AND METHOD	SPECIMEN REQUIREMENTS	REFERENCE INTERVAL, CONVENTIONAL [INTERNATIONAL RECOMMENDED UNITS]		CHEMICAL INTERFERENCES AND IN VIVO EFFECTS
Acetoacetate (ketone body)[1-5] *Reagent strip: Nitroprusside (Bayer Corp. Acetest, Ketostix, Labstix, Multistix; Roche Chemstrip)*[6-8]	Serum or plasma. Cover, deliver to laboratory immediately, and refrigerate until analysis (within 5 days). Avoid hemolysis.	Negative[10]: with overnight fast[1]	<1 mg/dL × 0.098 [<0.1 mmol/L]	S ↑ V Aspirin intoxication, ethanol (IV), levodopa (Ketostix), streptozotocin
	Urine. Analyze immediately or refrigerate to prevent loss due to microbial action. Bring to room temperature before analysis.	Negative		U ↑ C Acetylcysteine, captopril, cysteine, dimercaprol (BAL), 8-hydroxyquinoline (preservative), levodopa, mesna (2-mercaptoethane sulfonate sodium), D-penicillamine, phenazopyridine, phenolphthalein, phenylketones
				U ↑ V Aspirin intoxication, ethanol, ether anesthesia, inositol, isopropanol, metformin, methionine, nicotinic acid, phenformin,[11] valproic acid
Quantitative[9]: *enzymatic*	Plasma (sodium fluoride). Collect on ice; freeze immediately if not assayed on receipt.	0.2-2.0 mg/dL	× 97.95 [20-200 μmol/L]	

DIAGNOSTIC INFORMATION   **REMARKS**

Urinary excretion of acetaldehyde during period of elevated blood level has been suggested but not documented.[2]

↑ Diabetic ketoacidosis, prolonged excessive insulin administration in diabetics, prolonged fasting (so-called ketotic hypoglycemia, most common in children aged 1-6 yr), severe carbohydrate restriction with normal fat intake (weight-reducing diets), anorexia nervosa,[12] persistent vomiting, glycogen storage diseases I, III, and VI, branched-chain ketonuria, methylmalonic acidurla, exercise in untrained subjects,[1] pregnancy,[1] stress,[12] postanesthesia.[13]

↑ States with (1) markedly increased metabolic rate (high fever, severe thyrotoxicosis, active acromegaly); (2) excess of growth hormone, corticotropin, glucocorticoids, hyperinsulinism; or (3) excess of catecholamines causing hyperglycemia, decreased insulin secretion, and increased production of ketone bodies. These conditions (1, 2, and 3) are especially important when diabetes mellitus coexists.

In diabetic ketoacidosis (DKA) β-hydroxybutyrate (BOHB), the predominant ketone, is a better indicator of clinical state than acetoacetate. The BOHB/AcAc ratio is normally 3:1. This ratio will increase to 6:1 or 12:1 during ketoacidosis, particularly if there is associated decreased tissue perfusion, metabolic acidosis, and tissue catabolism. All of these will favor reductive metabolism and hence BOHB production. Acetoacetate may increase during therapy for DKA because BOHB is oxidatively metabolized to acetoacetate.[14]

Hemolysis causes discoloration of test tablets or sticks. Failure to crush Acetest tablets before use with serum may give falsely low results. Moisture reduces sensitivity of Acetest tablets. The lower limit of detection is ~10 mg/dL [1.0 mmol/L] with Acetest tablets.[8]

In some cases of diabetes mellitus with elevated blood ketone levels, no ketone bodies appear in the urine.

False-positive results may be seen with highly pigmented urine specimens and in those preserved with 8-hydroxyquinoline.[8] Detection of urinary ketones may be used to verify compliance with a weight-reducing regimen.[15]

Limits of detection: 5-10 mg/dL [0.5-1.0 mmol/L] acetoacetic acid.[4]

β-Hydroxybutyrate (the predominant ketone) is not measured by reagent strip methods. Acetone is measured only by Chemstrip reagent strip and the Acetest tablet.

Two methods can be used to differentiate false-positive results caused by free sulfhydryl groups from true positive results: (1) add 1 drop of glacial acetic acid to the "positive" test pad (color is removed from false-positive results); (2) monitor the reaction constantly (true positive results develop a purple color with Acetest that intensifies as long as 60 sec; false-positive results develop a purple color that fades, usually completely, within 30 sec).[16]

Quantitative determination of acetoacetate in plasma is only rarely necessary for the workup of metabolic disorders.

TEST NAME AND METHOD	SPECIMEN REQUIREMENTS	REFERENCE INTERVAL, CONVENTIONAL [INTERNATIONAL RECOMMENDED UNITS]			CHEMICAL INTERFERENCES AND IN VIVO EFFECTS

Acetoacetate—CONT

1. Eastham RD: *Biochemical values in clinical medicine,* ed 7, Bristol, UK, 1985, John Wright and Sons, Ltd.
2. Free HM, editor: *Modern urine chemistry,* Elkhart, IN, 1991, Miles Inc., Diagnostics Division.
3. Friedman RB, Anderson RE, Entine SM, et al: Effects of diseases on clinical laboratory tests, *Clin Chem* 26(suppl):1D-476D, 1980.
4. Henry JB, editor: *Clinical diagnosis and management by laboratory methods,* ed 20, Philadelphia, 2001, WB Saunders.
5. Strasinger SK: *Urinalysis and body fluids: a self-instructional text,* ed 2, Philadelphia, 1991, FA Davis.
6. Boehringer Mannheim Corp: *Chemstrip micral urine test strip package insert,* Indianapolis, IN, 1991, Boehringer Mannheim Corp.
7. Bayer Corp., Diagnostics Division: *Multistix package insert,* Elkhart, IN, 1999, Bayer Corp., Diagnostics Division.
8. Bayer Corp., Diagnostics Division: *Acetest reagent tablets package insert,* Elkhart, IN, 1995, Bayer Corp., Diagnostics Division.

TEST NAME AND METHOD	SPECIMEN REQUIREMENTS	REFERENCE INTERVAL, CONVENTIONAL [INTERNATIONAL RECOMMENDED UNITS]			CHEMICAL INTERFERENCES AND IN VIVO EFFECTS
Acetone (ketone body)[1,2] *GLC*	Serum or plasma (fluoride/oxalate). Cover and refrigerate (stable for 7 days) until analysis. Avoid hemolysis.	Ketoacidosis Occupational exposure: Toxic concentration:	*mg/dL* <2.0 10-70 <10 >20	× 0.172	*mmol/L* [<0.34] [1.72-12.04] [<1.72] [>3.44]	
GLC	Urine. Keep refrigerated in a closed container to minimize loss due to evaporation or microbial action.	Occupational exposure:	0.3 >27		[0.05] [>4.65]	
Reagent strip (Roche Diagnostics. Acetest; Chemstrip)[3-7]		Negative				U ↑ C Captopril, levodopa, mesna (2-mercaptoethane sulfonate sodium),[8] other free SH-containing compounds; high levels of phenylketones (Acetest); 8-hydroxyquinoline (preservative)
Semiquantitative	Breath	Occupational exposure:	*mg/L* 0.003 0.006	× 17.2	*μmol/L* [0.052] [0.10]	

1. Henry JB, editor: *Clinical diagnosis and management by laboratory methods,* ed 20, Philadelphia, 2001, WB Saunders.
2. Strasinger SK: *Urinalysis and body fluids: a self-instructional text,* ed 2, Philadelphia, 1991, FA Davis.
3. Roche Diagnostics: *Chemstrip 10 UA package insert,* Indianapolis, IN, 1999, Roche Diagnostics.
4. Free HM, editor: *Modern urine chemistry,* Elkhart, IN, 1991, Miles Inc., Diagnostics Division.

DIAGNOSTIC INFORMATION	REMARKS

9. Li PK, Lee JT, MacGillivray MH, et al: Direct fixed-time kinetic assays for β-hydroxybutyrate and acetoacetate with a centrifugal analyzer or a computer-backed spectrophotometer, *Clin Chem* 26:1713-1717, 1980.

10. Kaplan LA, Kazmierczak SC, Pesce AJ, editors: *Clinical chemistry: theory, analysis and correlation,* ed 4, St. Louis, 2002, CV Mosby.

11. Wallace J, editor: *Interpretation of diagnostic tests,* ed 7, Philadelphia, 2000, JB Lippincott.

12. Newall RG, editor: *Clinical urinalysis,* Buckinghamshire, UK, 1990, Ames Division, Miles Ltd.

13. Newall RG, editor: *Clinical urinalysis,* Buckinghamshire, UK, 1990, Ames Division, Miles Ltd.

14. Krane ES: Diabetic ketoacidosis: biochemistry, physiology treatment and prevention, *Pediatr Clin North Am* 34:935-960, 1987.

15. American Diabetes Association: Position statement: urine glucose and ketone determinations, *Diabetes Care* 19(suppl 1):S35, 1996.

16. Csako G: Causes, consequences, and recognition of false-positive reactions for ketones, *Clin Chem* 36:1388, 1990.

↑ Diabetic or fasting ketoacidosis, 2-propanol poisoning (acetone is a major product of 2-propanol metabolism), starvation, severe carbohydrate restriction

Nitroprusside tests are as much as 10-20 times more sensitive to acetoacetate than to acetone. They do not measure β-hydroxybutyric acid. Strongly positive acetone with normal anion gap, bicarbonate, and plasma glucose suggests rubbing alcohol (isopropanol) intoxication.[9]

Acetest is better suited for serial dilutions in serum because it is formulated with lactose for better color differentiation.[2]

Limits of detection:
Acetest: 20-25 mg acetone/dL [3.4-4.3 mmol/L] of urine

Chemstrip: 40-70 mg acetone/dL [6.9-12.0 mmol/L] of urine

False-negative results may occur with improper specimen handling, which allows acetone to volatilize or be consumed by bacterial action.

The ketone test pad on Multistix reagent strips does not measure acetone.[4,10]

Moisture will adversely affect results obtained from Acetest tablets by reducing sensitivity.

5. Bayer Corp., Diagnostics Division: *Multistix package insert,* Elkhart, IN, 1999, Bayer Corp., Diagnostics Division.

6. Newall RG, editor: *Clinical urinalysis,* Buckinghamshire, UK, 1990, Ames Division, Miles Ltd.

7. Bayer Corp., Diagnostics Division: *Acetest reagent tablets package insert,* Elkhart, IN, 1995, Bayer Corp., Diagnostics Division.

TEST NAME AND METHOD	SPECIMEN REQUIREMENTS	REFERENCE INTERVAL, CONVENTIONAL [INTERNATIONAL RECOMMENDED UNITS]	CHEMICAL INTERFERENCES AND IN VIVO EFFECTS

Acetone—CONT

8. Csako G: False-positive results for ketone with the drug mesna and other free-sulfhydryl compounds, *Clin Chem* 33:289-292, 1987.

9. Jacobs DS, DeMott WR, De Mott WR, editors: *Laboratory test handbook,* ed 5, Stow, OH, 2001, Lexi-Comp, Inc.

Acetonitrile[1,2]
(Methylcyanide;
CAS 140-53-4)

See *Cyanide and Thiocyanate*

Gas chromatography/FID

---

1. Baselt RC: *Biological monitoring methods for industrial chemicals,* Davis, CA, 1980, Biomedical Pub.

2. Caravati EM, Litovitz TL: Pediatric cyanide intoxication and death from acetonitrile-containing cosmetic, *JAMA* 260:3470-3473, 1988.

Test Name and Method	Specimen Requirements	Reference Interval, Conventional [International Recommended Units]		Chemical Interferences
Acetylcholine Esterase (Acetylcholine acetylhydrolase; EC 3.1.1.7; erythrocyte cholinesterase; choline esterase I)	Hemolysate of washed red blood cells (RBCs). Submit whole blood (ACD, EDTA, or heparin). Stable 20 days at 4° C in ACD, 6 days in EDTA or heparin; 5 days at 25° C in ACD, 2 days in EDTA or heparin.	*U/g Hb* 6.9 ± 3.83 (SD) × 0.0645* *U/10^{12} RBCs* 1070 ± 111 × 10^{-3} *U/mL RBCs* 12.5 ± 1.30 × 1.0 Levels lower in newborns[6]	*mU/mol Hb* [2.38 ± 0.23] *nU/RBC* [1.07 ± 0.11] *kU/L RBCs* [12.5 ± 1.30][2]	↓ Organophosphorus insecticides[7]
Ellman et al, acetylthiocholine, 37° C[1]; ICSH, 37° C[2]		Stated reference ranges are derived by calculation from the reference range given in U/g Hb. The conversion factors used in these calculations assume a normal mean corpuscular hemoglobin (MCH) in erythrocytes of 29 × 10^{12} g, e.g., 29 pg/erythrocyte, and a normal mean corpuscular hemoglobin concentration (MCHC) of 34 g/dL. The conversion factors are 0.34 for U/g Hb to U/mL packed RBCs; 29 for U/g Hb to U/10^{12} RBCs.		
		*Conversion factor based on MW of Hb of 64,500.		

			U/g Hb (SD)		*mU/mol Hb*
[1-14C]-Acetylcholine chloride, 37° C[3]	Whole blood (heparin). Avoid hemolysis.	1 wk:	6.7 ± 1.3	× 0.0645	[0.43 ± 0.08]
		1 mo:	7.0 ± 1.2		[0.45 ± 0.08]
		2 mo:	7.3 ± 1.5		[0.47 ± 0.10]
		3 mo:	8.3 ± 1.7		[0.54 ± 0.11]
		>4 mo:	10.2 ± 1.7		[0.66 ± 0.11]

DIAGNOSTIC INFORMATION	REMARKS

10. Miles Inc., Diagnostics Division: *Multistix package insert,* Elkhart, IN, 1992, Miles Inc., Diagnostics Division.

Acetonitrile concentrations in air up to 500 ppm [12.2 mmol/L] cause irritation of mucous membranes. Higher concentrations produce weakness, nausea, convulsions, and death. Urine SCN^- concentration is not significantly elevated after exposure to 160 ppm [3.9 mmol/L] for 4 hr. In biological monitoring, preexposure levels should be established because smokers show elevated concentrations of metabolites. The onset of symptoms is delayed due to metabolic conversion to cyanide. Most poisonings have occurred from fingernail glue remover.

Acetonitrile is not measured in blood and urine, but the metabolites cyanide and thiocyanate are.

↑ Sickle cell anemia[8]

↓ Organophosphate toxicity; paroxysmal nocturnal hemoglobinuria; during relapse of megaloblastic anemia (returns to normal with therapy)[9]; pyridostigmine therapy for myasthenia gravis in parallel with clinical improvement.[10]

Because intraindividual variation in acetylcholinesterase activity is high and the enzyme activity is sensitive to a variety of genetic, physiological, and disease-related factors, use of this assay to diagnose organophosphate poisoning is problematic. Acetylcholinesterase activity may be useful in monitoring exposure to organophosphates, but the clinical diagnosis is usually based on the cholinergic toxidrome.[11]

Erythrocyte cholinesterase recovers more slowly than serum cholinesterase and is thus a more sensitive indicator of chronic organophosphorus poisoning.[12] Recovery is best determined by looking for a plateau in erythrocyte cholinesterase activity and not simply by returning to the reference range.[13]

TEST NAME AND METHOD	SPECIMEN REQUIREMENTS	REFERENCE INTERVAL, CONVENTIONAL [INTERNATIONAL RECOMMENDED UNITS]	CHEMICAL INTERFERENCES AND IN VIVO EFFECTS
Acetylcholine Esterase—CONT			
Polyacrylamide gel EP (qualitative)[4]	Amniotic fluid. Do not freeze; avoid hemolysis.	Negative Positive in open neural tube defects	Cross-reactivity with non-specific cholinesterases
Inhibition[4,5]		Activity differences between uninhibited and BW 284C51 inhibited assay[5]: 5.17 ± 2.63 mU/mL (SD) $\times 1.0$ [5.17 ± 2.63 U/L]	
AE-2 Immunoassay[4,5]		Negative	

1. Ellman GL, Courtney KD, Andres V Jr: A new and rapid colorometric determination of acetylcholinesterase activity, *Biochem Pharmacol* 7:88-95, 1961.

2. Beutler E. Blume KG, Kaplan JC, et al: International Committee for Standardization in Hematology: Recommended methods for red-cell enzyme analysis, *Br J Haematol* 35:331-340, 1977.

3. Lund Karlsen R. Sterri S. Lyngaas S, et al: Reference values for erythrocyte acetylcholinesterase and plasma cholinesterase activities in children: implications for organophosphate intoxication, *Scand J Clin Lab Invest* 41:301-302, 1981.

4. Brock DJH, Barron L: Prenatal diagnosis of neural tube defects with a monoclonal antibody specific for acetyl-cholinesterase, *Lancet* 1:5-7, 1985.

5. Elejalde BR, Peck G, de Elejalde MM: Determination of cholinesterase and acetylcholinesterase in amniotic fluid, *Clin Genet* 29:196-203, 1986.

6. Konrad PN, Valentine WN, Paglia DE: Enzymatic activities and glutathione content of erythrocytes in the newborn: comparison with red cells of older normal subjects and those with comparable reticulocytosis, *Acta Haematol* 48:193-201, 1972.

7. Henry JB, editor: *Clinical diagnosis and management by laboratory methods,* ed 18, Philadelphia, 1991, WB Saunders.

8. Eluwa EO, Obidoa O, Ogan AU, et al: Erythrocyte membrane enzymes in sickle cell anemia. 2. Acetylcholinesterase and ATPase activities, *Biochem Med Metab Biol* 44:234-237, 1990.

9. Miale JB: *Laboratory medicine: hematology,* ed 6, St. Louis, 1982, CV Mosby.

10. Henze T, Neuner M, Michaelis HC: Determination of erythrocyte-bound acetylcholinesterase activity for monitoring pyridostigmine therapy in myasthenia gravis, *J Neurol* 238:225-229, 1991.

11. Kamanyire R, Karalliedde L: Organophosphate toxicity and occupational exposure, *Occup Med* 54:69-75, 2004.

12. Wolf PL: *Practical clinical hematology: interpretations and techniques,* New York, 1973, John Wiley and Sons.

13. Cholinesterases—when to measure and how to interpret, *Lab Report Physicians* 8:25-30, 1986.

DIAGNOSTIC INFORMATION	**REMARKS**

AF ↑ Open neural tube defects

Polyacrylamide gel EP of amniotic fluid for acetyl-cholinesterase is more specific than α-fetoprotein (AFP) determinations and may be used in combination with AFP. Erythrocyte cholinesterase can also be increased in ventral wall defects, omphalocele, other birth defects, and miscarriages. Contamination with fetal serum caused cross-reactivity and false-positive reactions. Inhibition and immunoassay are more specific than EP for determination of true acetylcholinesterase activity.

Because of the variability of the assay, a range of 4.0-8.0 mU/mL [4.0-8.0 U/L] has been proposed. To reliably distinguish normal from affected individuals, separate acetyl-cholinesterase from other cholinesterases by electrophoresis.[5]

TEST NAME AND METHOD	SPECIMEN REQUIREMENTS	REFERENCE INTERVAL, CONVENTIONAL [INTERNATIONAL RECOMMENDED UNITS]				CHEMICAL INTERFERENCES AND IN VIVO EFFECTS
α_1-Acid Glycoprotein (Orosomucoid, AGP)[1] *RID*	Serum. Analyze fresh or store at 4° C for <72 hr. Stable frozen at −20° C for 6 mo, or at −70° C indefinitely. Specimens without lipemia or hemolysis are preferred.	Adult:	*mg/dL* 55-140 (x: 90)	× 0.2439	*μmol/L* [13.4-34.1] [x: 22.0]	S ↑ V Anticonvulsants,[4] glucocorticoids,[3,4] the anabolic steroids danazole,[4,5] and oxymetholone,[4,6] isotretinoin,[4,7] perazine,[4,8] amitriptyline,[4,9] interleukin-6.[4,10] Can be increased in smokers[4,11] and individuals secondarily exposed to tobacco smoke.[4,12]
Nephelometry	Stable at room temperature for up to 6 hr, refrigerated for 1 wk, or at −20° C for 3 mo.	Adult: M, x: Median: F, x: Median:	39-115 83 72 75 64		[9.5-28.0] [20.2] [17.6] [18.3] [15.6]	S ↓V Estrogens,[13] oral contraceptives,[14] penicillamine,[15] tamoxifen,[4,16] mifepristone[4,17]
RID	Urine. Centrifuge and adjust to pH 7.0. Analyze fresh. Stable frozen at −20° C for up to 1 yr.		0.29-0.68 mg/day (x: 0.41)	× 24.39	[7.1-16.6 nmol/day] [x: 10.0]	Diurnal variation (can be absent in elderly individuals)[4,18,19]
	CSF. Centrifuge before analysis. Analyze fresh or store at 4° C for < 72 hr. Stable frozen at −20° C for 6 mo or at −70° C indefinitely. Specimens should not contain blood.		*mg/dL* 0.28-0.54	× 0.2439	*μmol/L* [0.07-0.13]	Excessive turbidity can affect nephelometric methods.

1. Ganrot PO: Variation of the concentrations of some plasma proteins in normal adults, in pregnant women and in newborns, *Scand J Clin Lab Invest* 29(suppl 124):83-88, 1972.

2. Hans P, Brichant JF, Pieron F, et al: Elevated plasma alpha 1-acid glycoprotein levels: lack of connection to resistance to vecurium blockade induced by anticonvulsant therapy, *J Neurosurg Anesthsiol* 9:3-7, 1997.

3. Kulkarni AB, Reinke R, Feigelson P: Acute phase mediators and glucocorticoids elevate alpha 1-acid glycoprotein gene transcription, *J Biol Chem* 260:15386-15389, 1985.

4. Israili ZH, Dayton PG: Human alpha 1-acid glycoprotein and its interactions with drugs, *Drug Metab Rev* 33:161-235, 2001.

5. Laurell C-B, Rannevik GA: Comparison of plasma protein changes induced by danazol, pregnancy, and estrogens, *J Clin Endocrinol Metab* 49:719-725, 1979.

6. Barbosa J, Seal US, Doe RP: Effects of anabolic steroids on haptoglobin, orosomucoid, plasminogen, fibrinogen, transferring, ceruloplasmin, alpha 1-antitrypsin, beta-glucuronidase and total serum proteins, *J Clin Endocrinol Metab* 33:388-398, 1971.

7. Marsden JR, Shuster S, Dennis JD: Antipyrine, clearance and alpha 1-acid glycoprotein levels after isotretinoin, *Hum Toxicol* 4:335-338, 1985.

8. Reuss F, Schleg J, Oerlinghausen B, et al: The relation between serum concentration of alpha 1-acid glycoprotein and clinical characteristics of patients treated with perazine, *Pharmacopsychology* 18:145-146, 1985.

DIAGNOSTIC INFORMATION	REMARKS

S ↑ Acute phase reacting protein, levels increase in response to a variety of events including trauma, surgery, infection, acute illness, burns, chronic inflammatory disorders, some cancers, and variable systemic diseases. Concentrations are frequently increased in the moderately and morbidly obese.[10]

S ↓ Levels can be decreased in pregnancy. Depressed values are also reported in association with pancreatic carcinoma, hepatitis and liver cirrhosis, hyperthyroidism, and conditions affecting protein metabolism such as nephrotic syndrome, cachexia, and states of malnutrition. Values decline in response to successful therapy for conditions associated with increased AGP concentrations, and blunted acute phase reactions can occur in patients with chronic connective tissue disorders.[10]

AGP, also known as orosomucoid, is an acidic, negatively charged member of the lipocalin family of proteins and can be isolated from most body fluids. Retinol-binding protein and α-lactoglobulin are also among the members of the lipocalin family.[4] AGP, like albumin, binds numerous drugs and may have a significant role in the binding of steroids,[4,20] basic, and neutrally charged medications.[4,21] Inflammation can affect glycosylation of AGP,[22,23] and a variety of alleles also exist, which influence drug binding.[4,24] AGP has been shown to display general immunosuppressive abilities including decreasing platelet aggregation,[4,25] phagocytosis,[4,26] neutrophil activation,[4,27] and the proliferation of lymphocytes.[4,28] It has a role in the maintenance of capillary charge selectivity,[4,29] and through its promotion of fibroblast proliferation[1,4] and interaction with collagen[4] supports the healing of wounds.

Quantitation of AGP may be helpful in suspected disease-associated alterations of drug binding that require dosing adjustment.

MW: 41,000
$T_{1/2}$: 5 days

9. Bauman P, Tinguely D, Schopf J, et al: Increase of alpha 1-acid glycoprotein after treatment with amitryptyline, *Br J Clin Pharmacol* 14:102-103, 1982.

10. Banks RE, Forbes MA, Storr M, et al: The acute phase protein response in patients receiving subcutaneous IL-6, *Clin Exp Immunol* 102:217-223, 1995.

11. Benedek IH, Blouin RA, McNamara PJ, et al: Influence of smoking on serum protein composition and the protein binding of drugs, *J Pharm Pharmacol* 36:214-216, 1984.

12. Shima M, Adachi M: Effects of environmental tobacco smoke on serum levels of acute phase proteins in schoolchildren, *Prev Med* 25:617-624, 1996.

13. Tuck CH, Holleran S, Berglund L: Hormonal regulation of lipoprotrin (a) levels: effects of estrogen replacement therapy on lipoprotrin (a) and acute phase reactants in postmenopausal women, *Arterioscler Thromb Vasc Biol* 17:1822-1829, 1997.

14. Wang HP, Chu CY: A solid-phase enzyme-linked immunosorbent assay for the quantitation of human plasma alpha 1-acid glycoprotein, *Clin Chem* 25:546-549, 1979.

15. Borjesson O, Knutsson LP, Svensson B: Penicillamine treatment in rheumatoid arthritis. A retrospective study, *Acta Med Scand* 207:93-96, 1980.

16. Fex G, Adielsson G, Mattson W: Oestrogen-like effects of tamoxifen on the concentration of proteins in plasma, *Acta Endocrinol (Copenh)* 97:109-133, 1981.

TEST NAME AND METHOD	SPECIMEN REQUIREMENTS	REFERENCE INTERVAL, CONVENTIONAL [INTERNATIONAL RECOMMENDED UNITS]	CHEMICAL INTERFERENCES AND IN VIVO EFFECTS

α_1-Acid Glycoprotein—CONT

17. Chen X, Xiao B: Effect of once weekly administration of mifipristone on ovarian function in normal women, *Contraception* 56:175-180, 1997.

18. Yost RL, DeVane CL: Diurnal variation of alpha 1-acid glycoprotein concentration in normal volunteers, *J Pharm Sci* 74:777-779, 1985.

19. Bouvenot G, Bruguerolle B, Arnaud C, et al: Absence of changes in elderly patients of circadian variation of various so-called inflammation proteins, *Ann Biol Clin (Paris)* 47:76-78, 1989.

20. Ganguly M, Carnighan TH, Westphal U: Steroid-protein interactions. XIV. Interaction between human alpha 1-acid glycoprotein and progesterone, *Biochemistry* 6:2803-2814, 1967.

21. Testa B, editor: *Advances in drug research,* London, 1984, Academic Press.

22. Hochepied T, Berger FG, Baumann H, et al: α1-Acid glycoprotein: an acute phase protein with inflammatory and immunomodulating properties, *Cytokine Growth Factor Rev* 14:25-34, 2003.

23. de Graaf TW, Van der Stelt ME, Anbergen MG, et al: Inflammation-induced expression of sialyl Lewis X-containing glycan structures on α1-acid glycoprotein (orosomucoid) in human sera, *J Exp Med* 177:657-666, 1993.

Acrylonitrile (Cyanoethylene; vinyl cyanide; CAS 9003-54-7) See *Cyanide and Thiocyanate.* *Colorimetric (cyanide or thiocyanate metabolites), ion-selective potentiometry (cyanide metabolite)*			
Activated Clotting Time (Activated coagulation time, ACT)[1,2] *ACT analyzers include GEM PCL (Instrumentation Lab., Lexington, MA), Hemochron Jr. Signature (Inter-*	Whole blood (no anticoagulant; draw into tubes containing an activator). Perform test immediately at bedside at 37° C.	*Varies depending on the methodology and the type of surgical/cardiac procedure or therapy.* In general, the accepted goal during cardiopulmonary bypass surgery is ~400-500 sec.	↑ Contamination from a line that contains heparin (especially if drawn from central venous pressure [CVP] line) Hypothermia, hemodilution, and platelet number and function may affect the ACT.

DIAGNOSTIC INFORMATION	REMARKS

24. Eap CB, Cuendet C, Baumann P: Binding of *d*-methedone, *l*-methadone, and *dl*-methadone to proteins in plasma of healthy volunteers: role of the variants of α1-acid glycoprotein, *Clin Pharmacol Ther* 47:338-346, 1990.

25. Costello MJ, Fiedel BA, Gewurz H, et al: Inhibition of platelet aggregation by native and desialised α1-acid glycoprotein, *Nature* 281:677-678, 1979.

26. van Oss CJ, Gillman CF, Bronson PM, et al: Phagocytosis-inhibiting properties of human serum α1-acid glycoprotein, *Immunol Commun* 3:321-328, 1974.

27. Timoshenko AV, Bovin NV, Shiyan SD, et al: Modification of the functional activity of neutrophils treated with acute phase response proteins, *Biochemistry (Mosc)* 63:546-550, 1998.

28. Cheresh DA, Haynes DH, Distasio JA: Interaction of acute phase reactant α1-acid glycoprotein (orosomucoid), with the lymphoid cell surface: a model for non-specific immune suppression, *Immunology* 51:541-548, 1984.

29. Sorensson J, Matejka GL, Ohlson M, et al: Human endothelial cells produce orosomucoid, an important component of the capillary barrier, *Am J Physiol* 276:H530-H534, 1999.

Mild exposure to acrylonitrile results in eye irritation, headache, nausea, and weakness. Severe cases may result in asphyxia and death. The monomer is carcinogenic. In biological monitoring, preexposure levels should be established because smokers show elevated concentrations of metabolites.

Acrylonitrile is not measured in blood or urine; instead, the metabolite cyanide is measured in blood and thiocyanate in urine. Toxicity is due to cyanide formation in vivo.

Kinetic values
$t_{1/2}$: 8 hr

Test is mostly used as "point of care" to monitor high-dose heparin as an anticoagulant during cardiac surgery (extracorporeal circulation), angioplasty, and hemodialysis.

The ACT is also used to determine the dose of protamine sulfate to reverse the heparin effect on completion of the procedure.

Because different methodologies and a number of variables may affect the ACT, this test is not standardized.

TEST NAME AND METHOD	SPECIMEN REQUIREMENTS	REFERENCE INTERVAL, CONVENTIONAL [INTERNATIONAL RECOMMENDED UNITS]	CHEMICAL INTERFERENCES AND IN VIVO EFFECTS
Activated Clotting Time—CONT			
national Techni-dyne Corp., Edison, NJ), the Hepcon HMS (formerly HemTec ACT) (Medtronic Perfusion Systems, Minneapolis, MN), and CoaguChek Pro-DM (Roche Diag., Indianapolis, IN).			Aprotinin can prolong the ACT when *Celite* is used as an activator; the ACT is not prolonged when *kaolin* is used as an activator.

1. Macik BG: Near-site testing in hemostatic disorders. In Kitchens CS, Alving BM, Kessler CM, editors: *Consultative hemostasis and thrombosis,* Philadelphia, 2002, WB Saunders, pp. 535-548.
2. Olson JD, Arkin CF, Brandt JT, et al: College of American Pathologists Conference XXXI on Laboratory Monitoring of Anticoagulant Therapy. Laboratory monitoring of unfractionated heparin therapy, *Arch Pathol Lab Med* 122:782-798, 1998.

TEST NAME AND METHOD	SPECIMEN REQUIREMENTS	REFERENCE INTERVAL, CONVENTIONAL [INTERNATIONAL RECOMMENDED UNITS]	CHEMICAL INTERFERENCES AND IN VIVO EFFECTS
Activated Partial Thromboplastin Time (APTT)[1,2]	Plasma (blue top tube with 3.2% citrate). Centrifuge and remove plasma immediately. Plasma is stable for 1 hr at 4° C, 4 hr on ice, or for 28 days if frozen.	Reference range varies with the reagent-instrument combination used. In general: lower limit of normal 20-25 sec, upper limit <35 sec. Note: The PTT is normally prolonged in newborns/infants. The PTT gradually decreases into the adult range by 6 mo.	↑ Extraneous heparin Traumatic venipuncture may contaminate specimen with tissue thromboplastin and shorten APTT. A difficult draw may also interfere with PTT used for heparin monitoring by neutralizing the heparin effect in sample due to release of PF4 from platelets.

1. Lewis SM, Bain BJ, Bates I, editors: *Dacie and Lewis practical hematology,* ed 9, Edinburgh, 2001, Churchill Livingstone.
2. Jacobs DS, Demott WR, Oxley DK, editors: *Laboratory test handbook,* ed 5, Hudson, OH, 2001, Lexi-Comp, Inc.

DIAGNOSTIC INFORMATION	REMARKS
↑ Intrinsic pathway factor deficiencies VIII, IX, XI, and XII; HMW-kininogen and prekallikrein (rare cause of prolonged APTT); specific inhibitors to above factors; nonspecific inhibitor (lupus anticoagulant); DIC.	The APTT is a clot-based test in which an activator, reagent, and calcium are added to the patient's plasma, and the time for a fibrin clot endpoint to form is measured, typically with optic-based methodology.
↓ Increased factor VIII levels	The APTT is commonly used to monitor heparin therapy. However, the APTT cannot be used with very high doses of heparin (e.g., cardiac bypass surgery) because the test is unclottable.
APTT is also used to adjust heparin, hirudin, and argatroban dosage.	APTT is usually abnormal if the level of any factor is <15-40% of normal, depending on the PTT reagent used.
	Because heparin contamination is a common cause of an unexplained prolonged APTT, heparin neutralization with the enzyme heparinase is recommended to rule out this possibility.
	APTT may be prolonged if anticoagulant volume is not adjusted for increased hematocrit or if the vacuum tube is not filled sufficiently. Freezing of plasma specimen will decrease sensitivity of APTT to lupus anticoagulant and to deficiencies of factors XII, XI, HMW-K, and prekallikrein.

TEST NAME AND METHOD	SPECIMEN REQUIREMENTS	REFERENCE INTERVAL, CONVENTIONAL [INTERNATIONAL RECOMMENDED UNITS]	CHEMICAL INTERFERENCES AND IN VIVO EFFECTS
Activated Protein C Resistance (APCR, factor V Leiden [FVL])[1]	Plasma: stable at room temperature for 4 hr.	Results reported as a ratio of clotting times with and without activated protein C or as a normalized ratio (ratio includes normal pooled plasma).	Lupus anticoagulant, hirudin, and argatroban may interfere with clot-based APCR assay. DNA testing is not affected.

1. Press RD, Bauer KA, Kujovich JL, et al: Clinical utility of factor V Leiden (R506Q) testing for the diagnosis and management of thromboembolic disorders, *Arch Pathol Lab Med* 126:1304-1318, 2002.

Activin A[1]	Serum	Adult,[3] nonpregnant female	*ng/mL*	None found.[2,5]
ELISA[2]		Midcycle:	~0.220	
		Late luteal/early follicular phase:	~0.310	
		Midfollicular phase:	~0.125	
		Midluteal phase:	~0.120	
		Pregnancy Weeks of gestation		
		8:	2.12 ± 0.31	
		8-24:	~2.0	
		38:	25.5 ± 6.0	
	Amniotic fluid	Weeks of gestation[4]	*ng/L*	
		14:	3795	
		15:	4017	
		16:	3860	
		17:	4667	
		18:	5086	

DIAGNOSTIC INFORMATION	REMARKS

Thrombophilia due to the FVL mutation.

FVL is the most common cause of thrombophilia. It is associated with the APCR phenotype.

The original *first generation* APCR functional assay showed poor specificity and was affected by many variables including interference from heparin and lupus anticoagulants. The modified *second generation* APCR assay dilutes the patient plasma with factor V-deficient plasma, thereby eliminating several interfering factors. This latter assay has a very high sensitivity and specificity, can distinguish between heterozygotes and homozygotes, can be interpreted in the presence of heparin or warfarin, in patients with lupus anticoagulant, and in the setting of acute thrombosis and pregnancy.

Initial testing in selected patients may include either the second generation APCR functional assay or a DNA-based testing method. FVL testing is not recommended as a general population screen.

Most patients with a positive APCR assay have the FVL mutation. A small percentage of patients with APCR phenotype using the *first generation* assay do not have a FVL mutation. The significance of this finding is uncertain.

S ↑ Pregnancy, preeclampsia; gestational diabetes; hypothyroidism; hyperthyrodism; cirrhosis; hepatocellular carcinoma; cholangiocarcinoma; metastatic liver cancer

Activins, like inhibins, belong with transforming growth factor β superfamily. Activins are dimers of two β-subunits and hence have three forms: βA-βA (activin A), βB-βB (activin B), and βA-βB (activin AB). Several organs express activin, including gonads, ovary, testis, placenta, brain, pituitary, thyroid, adrenal cortex, bone marrow, liver, and pancreas. However, the contribution of activin A synthesized by these organs to the serum level of activin A is not completely clarified. Activin A may function as a growth factor or a cytokine and have an autocrine or paracrine role to regulate cell growth.

The majority of circulating activin A is bound by α2-macroglobulin and follistatin; the latter is a monomeric glycoprotein structurally unrelated to activins. These binding protein are considered to modulate the biological functions of activin A.

TEST NAME AND METHOD	SPECIMEN REQUIREMENTS	REFERENCE INTERVAL, CONVENTIONAL [INTERNATIONAL RECOMMENDED UNITS]	CHEMICAL INTERFERENCES AND IN VIVO EFFECTS

Activin A[1]—CONT

1. Luisi S, Florio P, Reis FM, et al: Expression and secretion of activin A: possible physiological and clinical implications, *Eur J Endocrinol* 145:225-236, 2001.

2. Evans LW, Muttukrishna S, Knight PG, et al: Development, validation and application of a two-site enzyme-linked immunosorbent assay for activin-AB, *J Endocrinol* 153:221-230, 1997.

3. Muttukrishna S, Fowler PA, George L, et al: Changes in peripheral serum levels of total activin A during the human menstrual cycle and pregnancy, *J Clin Endocrinol Metab* 81:3328-3334, 1996.

4. Wallace EM, D'Antona D, Shearing C, et al: Amniotic fluid levels of dimeric inhibins, pro-alpha C inhibin, activin A and follistatin in Down's syndrome, *Clin Endocrinol (Oxf)* 50:669-673, 1999.

5. Knight PG, Muttukrishna S, Groome NP: Development and application of a two-site enzyme immunoassay for the determination of "total" activin-A concentrations in serum and follicular fluid, *J Endocrinol* 148:267-279, 1996.

TEST NAME AND METHOD	SPECIMEN REQUIREMENTS	REFERENCE INTERVAL, CONVENTIONAL [INTERNATIONAL RECOMMENDED UNITS]			CHEMICAL INTERFERENCES AND IN VIVO EFFECTS
Adenosine Deaminase (EC 3.5.4.4)[1,2]	Serum. Stable at room temperature for 6-12 hr, at 4° C for >1 wk, and at −70° C for 6 mo.	11.5-25.0 U/L	× 0.017	[0.20-0.43 μKat/L]	↓ C p-Chloromercuribenzoate
340 nm, 37° C[3]	Some suggest collection on ice, with serum stored frozen until assay is performed.				
Colorimetric, 37° C[4]		16 ± 3.5 U/L (SD)		[0.27 ± 0.06 μKat/L]	
Colorimetric, 37° C[5]		15.0 ± 4.8 U/L (SD)		[0.25 ± 0.08 μKat/L]	
Kinetic, 37° C[6]			*U/L (2 SD)*	*μKat/L*	
		0-2 yr:	22.4 ± 3.8 × 0.017	[0.38 ± 0.06]	
		3-5 yr:	19.6 ± 4.0	[0.33 ± 0.07]	
		6-8 yr:	18.1 ± 3.1	[0.31 ± 0.05]	
		9-11 yr:	15.8 ± 2.6	[0.27 ± 0.04]	
		12-14 yr:	13.7 ± 2.6	[0.23 ± 0.04]	
		20-30 yr:	12.6 ± 2.0	[0.21 ± 0.03]	
Fluorimetric[7]	Dried blood spots on filter paper. Stable at room temperature ~1 wk, frozen ~1 mo.		*mU/g Hb*	*kU/mol Hb*	
		Neonates:	750-1850 × 0.0645*	[48.4-119.3]	
		Adults:	700-1900	[45.2-122.6]	

DIAGNOSTIC INFORMATION	REMARKS

Serum levels of activin A are similar between men and women aged between 8-15 years and 20-50 years. The activin A level of men increases significantly afterward and peaks at ages 70-90 yr.

The clinical applications remain to be defined.

S ↑ Hepatitis, cirrhosis, hemochromatosis, obstructive jaundice associated with neoplastic disease, cancer of prostate and bladder, hemolytic anemia, rheumatic fever, typhoid fever, gout, thalassemia major, myeloid leukemia, tuberculosis, autoimmune diseases, infectious mononucleosis, heart failure, preeclampsia,[11] hyperemesis gravidarum[12]
S ↓ Type 2 diabetes mellitus[13]
Pleural fluid ↑ tuberculosis[14]

Adenosine deaminase is found in erythrocytes, leukocytes, lung, liver, stomach, genitourinary tract, and serum. The enzyme contains two reactive thiol groups.

The enzyme activities are stated to be much higher in tuberculosis than in any other respiratory disease of children. In tuberculosis, increases may primarily affect isoenzyme 2.[13] Elevations occur during acute exacerbation of chronic sarcoidosis. Adenosine deaminase is one of the few serum enzymes that are consistently low in biliary tract disease and consistently increased in chronic liver disease.[1] There is a negative correlation with age during the first three decades.

Pleural fluid adenosine deaminase is often used in diagnosis of tuberculous pleuritis. Values >100 U/L have high specificity for tuberculosis.

TEST NAME AND METHOD	SPECIMEN REQUIREMENTS	REFERENCE INTERVAL, CONVENTIONAL [INTERNATIONAL RECOMMENDED UNITS]		CHEMICAL INTERFERENCES AND IN VIVO EFFECTS

Adenosine Deaminase—CONT

Spectrophotometry[8-10]	Hemolysate of washed erythrocytes. Submit whole blood (ACD, EDTA, or heparin). Stable for >20 days in ACD or EDTA, >5 days in heparin, at 4° C.	*U/g Hb (SD) (37° C)*	*MU/mol Hb*	
		1.11 ± 0.23	$\times 0.0645*$ $[0.0716 \pm 0.0148]$	
		U/10[12] Ercs	*nU/Ercs*	
		32.3 ± 6.67	$\times 10^{-3}$ $[0.032 \pm 0.0067]$	
		U/mL Ercs	*kU/L Ercs*	
		0.377 ± 0.078	$\times 1.0$ $[0.377 \pm 0.078]$	

U/g Hb $\times$ 29 = U/10[12] Ercs

U/g Hb $\times$ 0.34 = U/mL Ercs†

*Conversion factor based on MW of Hb of 64,500.

†See Note, *Acetylcholinesterase.*

1. Ellis G, Goldberg DM, Spooner RJ, et al: Serum enzyme tests in diseases of the liver and biliary tree, *Am J Clin Pathol* 70:248-258, 1978.

2. Kredich NM, Hershfield MS: Immunodeficiency diseases caused by adenosine deaminase deficiency and purine nucleoside phosphorylase deficiency. In Scriver CR, Beaudet AL, Sly WS, et al, editors: *The metabolic basis of inherited disease,* ed 6, New York, 1989, McGraw-Hill Inc.

3. Ellis G, Goldberg DM: A reduced nicotinamide adenine dinucleotide linked kinetic assay for adenosine deaminase activity, *J Lab Clin Med* 76:507-517, 1970.

4. Storch H, Kruger W, Rotzsch W: Adenosine deaminase activity in plasma and blood cells of patients with haematological and autoimmune diseases, *Acta Haematol* 65:183-188, 1981.

5. Mañá J, Orts J, Fuentas J, et al: Serum adenosine deaminase assay in sarcoidosis has little clinical usefulness, *Clin Chem* 32:1429-1430, 1986.

6. Yasuhara A, Nakamura M, Shuto H, et al: Serum adenosine deaminase activity in the differentiation of respiratory diseases in children, *Clin Chim Acta* 161:341-345, 1986.

7. Orfanos AP, Naylor EW, Guthrie R: Micromethod for estimating adenosine deaminase activity in dried blood spots on filter paper, *Clin Chem* 24:591-594, 1978.

8. Beutler E: *Red cell metabolism: a manual of biochemical methods,* ed 3, New York, 1984, Grune & Stratton.

9. Giusti G, Galanti B: Adenosine deaminase. In Bergmeyer HU, editor: *Methods of enzymatic analysis, vol IV,* ed 3, Weinheim, 1984, Verlag Chemie.

10. Valentine WN, Tanaka KR, Paglia DE: Hemolytic anemias and erythrocyte enzymopathies, *Ann Intern Med* 103:245-257, 1985.

11. Yoneyama Y, Sawa R, Suzuki S, et al: Serum adenosine deaminase activity in women with pre-eclampsia, *Gynecol Obstet Invest* 54:164-167, 2002.

12. Yoneyama Y, Sawa R, Suzuki S, et al: Serum adenosine deaminase activity in women with hyperemesis gravidarum, *Clin Chim Acta* 324:141-145, 2002.

13. Kurtul N, Pence S, Akarsu E, et al: Adenosine deaminase activity in the serum of type 2 diabetic patients, *Acta Medica* 47:33-35, 2004.

14. Sharma S, Suresh V, Mohan A, et al: A prospective study of sensitivity and specificity of adenosine deaminase estimation in the diagnosis of tuberculosis pleural effusion, *Indian J Chest Dis Allied Sci* 43:149-155, 2001.

15. Parkman R, Gelfand EW: Severe combined immunodeficiency disease, adenosine deaminase deficiency and gene therapy, *Curr Opin Immunol* 3:547-551, 1991.

16. Carson DA, Carrera CJ: Immunodeficiency secondary to adenosine deaminase deficiency and purine nucleoside phosphorylation deficiency, *Semin Hematol* 27:260-269, 1990.

DIAGNOSTIC INFORMATION	REMARKS

Values are increased (35-70 times normal) in rare congenital hemolytic anemia (autosomal dominant).[2]

Erc ↓ Severe combined immunodeficiency disease (SCID)

A deficiency of adenosine deaminase is observed in 25% of cases of SCID. SCID accounts for ~85% of observed instances of adenosine deaminase deficiency. SCID is a clinical phenotype in which affected children display absence of antigen-specific T and B lymphocyte immunity, failure to thrive, diarrhea, and recurrent infections.[15,16] Deficiency of adenosine deaminase is the most frequent known cause of SCID; it is observed in 25% of cases. Heterozygotes have normal immune functions and ~50% of normal enzyme activity.

TEST NAME AND METHOD	SPECIMEN REQUIREMENTS	REFERENCE INTERVAL, CONVENTIONAL [INTERNATIONAL RECOMMENDED UNITS]		CHEMICAL INTERFERENCES AND IN VIVO EFFECTS
Adenylate Kinase (AK) in erythrocytes (EC 2.7.4.3)[1-3] *Spectrophotometry*[4]	Hemolysate of washed Ercs. Submit whole blood (ACD, EDTA, or heparin). Stable for >20 days in ACD or EDTA, >5 days in heparin at 4° C.	*U/g Hb (37° C)* 258 ± 29.3 (SD) *U/10^{12} Ercs* 7482 ± 850 *U/mL Ercs* 87.7 ± 9.96	× 0.0645* × 10^{-3} × 1.0	*MU/mol Hb* [16.64 ± 1.89] *nU/Erc* [7.48 ± 0.85] *kU/L Ercs* [87.7 ± 9.96]	None found.

See *Acetylcholinesterase.*

*Conversion factor based on MW of Hb of 64,500.

1. Beutler E: *Red cell metabolism: a manual of biochemical methods,* ed 4, New York, 1986, Grune & Stratton.
2. Brolin SE: Adenylate kinase (myokinase). In Bergmeyer HU, editor: *Methods of enzymatic analysis, vol III,* ed 3, Weinheim, 1983, Verlag Chemie.
3. Colowick SP: Adenylate kinase (myokinase, ADP phosphomutase). In Colowick SP, Kaplan NO, editors: *Methods in enzymology, vol II,* New York, 1955, Academic Press.
4. Corrons JL, Garcia E, Tusell JJ, et al: Red cell adenylate kinase deficiency: molecular study of 3 new mutations (118G>A, 190G>A, and GAC deletion) associated with hereditary nonspherocytic hemolytic anemia, *Blood* 102:353-356, 2003.

Adrenal Autoantibodies[1] *ELISA*[2]	Serum	Negative	Mitochondrial or ribosomal antibodies may interfere using IIF.
CF,[3] *IIF*[4] *(adrenal tissue sections are used for IIF)*		Negative	

1. Ketchum CH, Riley WJ, Maclaren NK: Adrenal dysfunction in asymptomatic patients with adrenocortical autoantibodies, *J Clin Endocrinol Metab* 58:1166-1170, 1984.
2. Stechemesser E, Scherbaum WA, Grossmann T, et al: An ELISA method for the detection of autoantibodies to adrenal cortex, *J Immunol Methods* 80:67-76, 1985.
3. Betterle C, Zanette F, Zanchetta R, et al: Complement-fixing adrenal autoantibodies as a marker for predicting onset of idiopathic Addison's disease, *Lancet* 1:1238-1240, 1983.
4. Bigazzi PE, Burek CL, Rose NR: Antibodies to tissue-specific endocrine, gastrointestinal, and surface-receptor antigens. In Rose NR, deMarcario EC Fakeg JL: editors: *Manual of clinical laboratory immunology,* ed 3, Washington, DC, 1986, American Society for Microbiology.

DIAGNOSTIC INFORMATION	REMARKS
Deficient in rare congenital hemolytic anemia (autosomal recessive)	Although partial deficiencies of AK do not cause hemolytic anemia, recent reports with severe or completely absent AK are associated with mild to severe chronic nonspherocytic hemolytic anemia.[4] $U/g\ Hb \times 29 = U/10^{12}$ Ercs $U/g\ Hb \times 0.34 = U/mL$ Ercs* *See Note, *Acetylcholinesterase*.

↑ Autoimmune adrenal disease	Adrenal autoantibodies are of the IgG class and react with adrenocortical cellular microsomes. This test is used as a marker for predicting the onset of idiopathic Addison's disease; positive titers are seen in ~50% of these patients.[4] Adrenal antibodies are *not* found in adrenal tumors, idiopathic Cushing's syndrome, virilizing adrenal hyperplasia, or tuberculosis of adrenal glands. Patients with autoimmune adrenal disease have higher incidences of other organ-specific autoimmune diseases, e.g., Graves' disease, Hashimoto's thyroiditis, insulin-dependent diabetes mellitus, pernicious anemia, and ovarian failure.
↑ 21 OH antibody in 70% of autoimmune adrenal disease	

TEST NAME AND METHOD	SPECIMEN REQUIREMENTS	REFERENCE INTERVAL, CONVENTIONAL [INTERNATIONAL RECOMMENDED UNITS]		CHEMICAL INTERFERENCES AND IN VIVO EFFECTS
Adrenocortico-tropic Hormone (corticotropin, ACTH)[1-3]	Plasma (EDTA). Place blood immediately in ice water; freeze plasma within 15 min. Store frozen, preferably in plastic tubes at −70° C. Aprotinin (Trasylol), 500 kU/mL, should be added for long-term storage.		*pg/mL*	*pmol/L*	↑ V Aminoglutethimide, amphetamines, hypo-glycemia, insulin, levo-dopa, metoclopramide, metyrapone, pyrogens, RU486, vasopressin (after IV in normals)
		Cord[8]:	50-570 × 0.22	[11-125]	
		Newborn (1 day)[8]:	10-185	[2.2-41]	
RIA[4-6]		Adult[9] 8:00 AM (unrestricted activity):	<120	[<26]	
		4:00-8:00 PM:	<85	[<19]	↓ V Dexamethasone, other corticosteroids, hep-arinized plasma
		Hospitalized volunteers[5] 5:00-7:00 AM (supine):	8-30	[1.8-6.6]	
		12:00 AM (supine):	<10	[<2.2]	
IRMA[7]		Adult[10] 7:00-10:00 AM:	9-52	[2-11]	

		pg/mL (x)[11]		*pmol/L (x)*
RIA	Amniotic fluid	10-18 wk:	209	× 0.22 [46]
		26-30 wk:	430	[95]
		35-36 wk:	162	[36]

1. Findling J, Engeland W, Raff H: The use of immunoradiometric assay for the measurement of ACTH in human plasma, *Trends Endocrinol Metab* 1:283-287, 1990.

2. Goldsmith BM: Adrenocorticotropic hormone (ACTH). In Pesce A, Kaplan LA, editors: *Methods in clinical chemistry,* St. Louis, 1987, CV Mosby.

3. Orth D, Kovacs D, DeBold C: The adrenal cortex. In Wilson JH, Foster DW, editors: *Williams textbook of endocrinology,* ed 8, Philadelphia, 1992, WB Saunders.

4. Marts CJ, Koppeschaar HPF, Veemar W, et al: A direct radioimmunoassay for the determination of adrenocorticotropic hormone (ACTH) and a clinical evaluation, *Ann Clin Biochem* 22:247-256, 1985.

5. Nicholson W, Davis D, Sherrell B, et al: Rapid radioimmunoassay for corticotropin in unextracted human plasma, *Clin Chem* 30:259-265, 1984.

6. Orth D: Adrenocorticotropic hormone (ACTH). In Jaffe BM, Behrman HR, editors: *Methods of hormone radioimmunoas-say,* New York, 1979, Academic Press.

7. Raff H, Findling J: A new immunoradiometric assay for corticotropin evaluated in normal subjects and patients with Cushing's syndrome, *Clin Chem* 35:596-600, 1989.

8. Endocrine Sciences: *Pediatric laboratory services,* Tarzana, CA, 1988, Endocrine Sciences.

9. Vanderbilt Pathology Laboratory Services: *Test catalog,* Nashville, TN, 1989, Vanderbilt Pathology Laboratory Services.

10. Nichols Institute Reference Laboratories: *Test catalog,* San Juan Capistrano, CA, 1993, Nichols Institute Reference Labo-ratories.

DIAGNOSTIC INFORMATION	REMARKS

P ↑ Addison's disease (>1000 pg/mL; >220 pmol/L), congenital adrenal hyperplasia, pituitary-dependent Cushing's disease, ectopic ACTH-producing tumors, Nelson's syndrome

P ↓ Secondary adrenocortical insufficiency, adrenal carcinoma, adenoma, hypopituitarism

Functional tests may be helpful for distinguishing between some causes of increased ACTH secretion. For example, Cushing's disease usually demonstrates suppression of ACTH and cortisol by high-dose dexamethasone, whereas adrenal adenomas, adrenal carcinomas, and ectopic ACTH-producing tumors do not suppress. (See *Dexamethasone Suppression Test, Standard.*)

ACTH is unstable in blood, and proper handling of specimen is important.[12] Most commercial RIAs are insensitive and nonspecific, measuring intact ACTH, precursor molecules, and ACTH fragments. The highly sensitive IRMA recognizes intact ACTH only. RIA is recommended for investigating ectopic ACTH-producing tumors because some of these tumors secrete ACTH precursors and fragments as well as intact ACTH. Immunoradiometric assays are generally more sensitive (and precise) than RIA and are preferred for investigating disorders of the hypothalamic-pituitary-adrenal system.

Pregnancy, menstrual cycle, and stress increase secretion. Nyctohemeral rhythm (sleep-wake cycle): highest levels prevail between 6:00 and 8:00 AM (soon after rising) and lowest levels between 9:00 and 10:00 PM (on retiring to bed), although there may be significant oscillations throughout the day. Periodicity is abolished in all types of hypercortisolism except in occasional cases of adrenal tumors. For meaningful comparisons, blood samples should be drawn at the same time each day, preferably in the early morning. Additional samples taken in the late evening may be helpful in cases of Cushing's syndrome. Sequential assays are useful in monitoring response to therapy.

AF ↓ Anencephalic fetuses

ACTH in amniotic fluid may be of fetal origin. The relatively high concentration of ACTH in the normal fetus may reflect immaturity of hypothalamic regulation.

11.   Tulchinsky D, Ryan KJ, editors: *Maternal-fetal endocrinology,* Philadelphia, 1980, WB Saunders.
12.   Whitley RJ: ACTH assays, *AACC Endo and Metabolism In-Service Training and Continuing Education* 9:7-11, 1990.

TEST NAME AND METHOD	SPECIMEN REQUIREMENTS	REFERENCE INTERVAL, CONVENTIONAL [INTERNATIONAL RECOMMENDED UNITS]			CHEMICAL INTERFERENCES AND IN VIVO EFFECTS
Adrenocortico-tropic Hormone Stimulation Test (after insulin)[1,2]	Serum. Draw at 0, 30, 60, and 90 min after injection.	Cortisol, increase ½ hr after maximum decrease in blood glucose:			See *Cortisol, Total* and *Glucose.*
		>10 mcg/dL	× 27.6	[>276 nmol/L]	
		Peak response:			
		>20 mcg/dL	× 27.6	[>552 nmol/L]	
Dose:					
0.05-0.15 U insulin/kg, IV, after overnight fast		Glucose,			
		≤40 mg/dL	× 0.0555	[<2.2 mmol/L]	
		or signs of hypoglycemia			

1. Alsever RN, Gotlin RW: *Handbook of endocrine tests in adults and children,* ed 2, Chicago, 1978, Year Book Medical Publishers, Inc.
2. Clemmons DR, Van Wyk JJ, Ridgway EG, et al: Evaluation of acromegaly by radioimmunoassay of somatomedin C, *N Engl J Med* 301:1138-1142, 1979.

TEST NAME AND METHOD	SPECIMEN REQUIREMENTS	REFERENCE INTERVAL, CONVENTIONAL [INTERNATIONAL RECOMMENDED UNITS]			CHEMICAL INTERFERENCES AND IN VIVO EFFECTS
Adrenocortico-tropic Hormone Stimulation Test, Prolonged Infusion[1,2]	Serum or plasma (heparin). Store at 4° C for 2 days. Freeze for longer storage.	Cortisol mcg/dL >20	× 27.6	[≥552 nmol/L], peak response:	See *Cortisol, Total.*
Dose, adult[3]: 50 U ACTH or 500 mcg cosyntropin (Cortrosyn), IV, in 500 mL saline for 8 hr on each of 3 days	Urine, 24 hr. Preserve with 1 g boric acid and refrigerate. Stable for at least 2 wk.	17-KGS:* Twofold to fourfold increase 17-KS:† Twofold increase 17-OHCS:‡ Twofold to fivefold increase *17-KGS, 17-ketogenic steroids †17-KS, 17-ketosteroids ‡17-OHCS, 17-hydroxycorticosteroids			S ↑ Estrogens, hydrocortisone See also *Cortisol, Free.*

1. Abboud CF, Laws ER Jr: Clinical endocrinological approach to hypothalamic-pituitary disease, *J Neurosurg* 51:271-291, 1979.
2. Crapo L: Cushing's syndrome: a review of diagnostic tests, *Metabolism* 28:955-977, 1979.
3. Miller RE, Ngai B: *Manual of endocrine diagnostic tests,* ed 4, Lexington, KY, Department of Medicine, 1991, University of Kentucky.

DIAGNOSTIC INFORMATION	REMARKS

Test is used to assess hypothalamic-pituitary-adrenal axis. No response or inadequate response may be due to a hypothalamic lesion or pituitary ACTH deficiency.

Test is also called the insulin-induced hypoglycemia test or insulin tolerance test. In normal individuals, the stress of insulin-induced hypoglycemia induces pituitary ACTH secretion; cortisol is measured as an indicator of ACTH response. Test should be performed only if adrenal responsiveness to ACTH can be assumed or has been demonstrated using the cosyntropin (Cortrosyn) stimulation test. (See *Adrenocorticotropic Hormone Stimulation Test, Rapid.*)

In insulin-resistant patients, give dose of 0.15-0.3 U/kg. For effective ACTH challenge, clinical manifestations of hypoglycemia must be present; if not, repeat dose within 45 min to 1 hr. Risk of the test is serious hypoglycemia. Test is contraindicated in convulsive disorders, ischemic heart disease, or cerebrovascular disease. See *Insulin Tolerance Test.*

Primary adrenal insufficiency (Addison's disease): No or inadequate response

Secondary adrenal insufficiency (hypopituitarism): Delayed but normal response (gradual staircase increase over 2-3 days)

Congenital adrenal hyperplasia due to 21-hydroxylase and 17-hydroxylase deficiency: Increased urinary 17-KGS and 17-KS; little or no change in 17-OHCS or serum cortisol.

In primary adrenal insufficiency, administer 2 mg dexamethasone to prevent adrenal crisis. This stimulation test is not useful in the differential diagnosis of Cushing's syndrome. Adrenal hemorrhages have been reported to occur following ACTH administration to patients with Cushing's syndrome.

TEST NAME* AND METHOD	SPECIMEN REQUIREMENTS	REFERENCE INTERVAL, CONVENTIONAL [INTERNATIONAL RECOMMENDED UNITS]			CHEMICAL INTERFERENCES AND IN VIVO EFFECTS
Adrenocortico-tropic Hormone Stimulation Test, Rapid[1,2]	Serum. Draw at 0, 30, and 60 min after injection.	Cortisol, baseline:	*mcg/dL* >5 × 27.6	*nmol/L* [>138]	↑ V Estrogens, hydrocortisone, cortisone. See also *Cortisol, Total.*
					↑ C Spironolactone (fluorometric procedures)
Dose, adult: 250 mcg cosyntropin (Cortrosyn), IM or IV, after overnight fast		After Cortrosyn, peak response:	>20	[>552]	
Dose, adult: 10 mcg cosyntropin (Cortrosyn), IV bolus, after overnight fast[3]			>19 >20	[>525 at 30 min] [>552 at 60 min]	
		Or increment from baseline cortisol	>7.3	[>200 nmol/L]	

1. Abboud CF, Laws ER Jr: Clinical endocrinological approach to hypothalamic-pituitary disease, *J Neurosurg* 51:271-291, 1979.
2. Alsever RN, Gotlin RW: *Handbook of endocrine tests in adults and children,* ed 2, Chicago, 1978, Year Book Medical Publishers, Inc.
3. González-González JG, De la Garza-Hernández NE, Mancillas-Adame LG, et al: A high-sensitivity test in the assessment of adrenocortical insufficiency 10 vs. 250 μg dose assessment of adrenocortical insufficiency, *J Endocrinol* 159:275-280, 1998.
4. Polderman KH, van Zanten A, Girbes AR: Free cortisol and critically ill patients, *N Engl J Med* 351:395-397, 2004.

Alanine Aminopeptidase (AAP; EC 3.4.11.2)[1]	Serum. Stable at room temperature for 24 hr, at 4° C for 2-3 wk, at −70° C for 6 mo.	≤38 U/L[5] × 0.017		[≤0.65 μKat/L]	S ↑ V: ethanol, tobacco, oral contraceptives[6]
Colorimetric (alanine-4-nitroanilide-hydrochloride), 410 nm[1]					
RIA[2]		M: F:	*mcg/mL (SD)* 1.41 ± 0.30 × 1.0 1.24 ± 0.28	*mg/L* [1.41 ± 0.30] [1.24 ± 0.28]	

*Alanine and β-Alanine are located in the Appendix on p. 1761.

| **DIAGNOSTIC INFORMATION** | **REMARKS** |

This is a screening test only. A normal (positive) response rules out primary and overt secondary adrenal insufficiency, but a partial ACTH deficiency is not excluded. A subnormal response indicates decreased adrenal reserve and a diagnosis of insufficiency, either primary to adrenal failure (e.g., Addison's disease) or secondary to pituitary disease or suppression by steroid medications. To distinguish primary and secondary insufficiency, the prolonged ACTH test and plasma ACTH measurements may be performed. See *Adrenocorticotropic Hormone Stimulation Test, Prolonged Infusion* and *Adrenocorticotropic Hormone*.

A normal response does not rule out partial secondary adrenal insufficiency in patients who cannot maintain sufficient basal ACTH to respond to stress or hypoglycemia. In these cases, the pituitary can be tested with metyrapone or with insulin-induced hypoglycemia. See *Metyrapone Stimulation Test* and *Adrenocorticotropic Hormone Stimulation Test (after Insulin)*.

Total cortisol measurements sensitive to serum protein concentrations.[4]

In adrenal hyperplasia there is a threefold to fivefold increase; in adrenal carcinoma there is little or no response.

S ↑ Hepatobiliary and pancreatic disease, elevation parallels ALP; malignancy[8]; pregnancy, AAP peaks at term.

AAP is also known as microsomal aminopeptidase, in contrast to LAP, which is a cytosolic aminopeptidase.

S ↓ Abortion

Electrophoresis can separate isoenzymes according to tissue origin. Tissues with significant activity are liver, kidney, pancreas, and small intestine. A serum isoform has been noted in subjects on anticonvulsant drugs and abusers of alcohol.[9] Normal serum contains only the liver isoenzyme, whereas normal urine contains only the kidney isoenzyme. The kidney isoenzyme originates from the brush border membranes of the proximal renal tubule.[4] Urinary output of soluble forms of AAP is increased by diuresis.[10] The serum enzyme appears in the urine only in the presence of proteinuria. Urine enzyme activity is most useful when expressed *per g creatinine* rather than as a concentration (per liter) or as output per hour.[11]

TEST NAME AND METHOD	SPECIMEN REQUIREMENTS	REFERENCE INTERVAL, CONVENTIONAL [INTERNATIONAL RECOMMENDED UNITS]		CHEMICAL INTERFERENCES AND IN VIVO EFFECTS

Alanine Aminopeptidase—CONT

Colorimetric (ala-nine-4-nitroanilide-hydrochloride), 410 nm[1]	Urine, 24 hr[1]; use fresh specimen. Collect on ice.	*U/L (SD)* M: 12.6 ± 3.77 × 0.017 F: 7.65 ± 2.46	*μKat/L* [0.21 ± 0.06] [0.13 ± 0.04]	U ↑ V Diatrizoate or man-nitol in patients with ac-tive pyelonephritis.[7]
Colorimetric (alanine-4-nitroanilide), 405 nm, 30° C[3]		*U/mmol creatinine* M: 0.32-0.75 × 1.0 F: 0.24-0.55	*kU/mol creatinine* [0.32-0.75] [0.24-0.55]	U ↓ C Nonspecific in-hibitors in urine. Urine specimen should be fil-tered on Sephadex G50.[1]
Colorimetric (alanine-4-nitroanilide), 405 nm, 37° C[4]		*U/g creatinine (SD)* 8.6 ± 2.4 × 0.113	*kU/mol creatinine* [0.97 ± 0.27]	

1. Jung K, Scholz D: An optimized assay of alanine aminopeptidase activity in urine, *Clin Chem* 26:1251-1254, 1980.

2. Tokioka-Terao M, Hiwada K, Kokubu T: A radioimmunoassay for the measurement of aminopeptidase (microsomal) in human serum, *Enzyme* 33:181-187, 1985.

3. Diener U, Knoll E, Langer B, et al: Urinary excretion of N-acetyl-β-D-glucosaminidase and alanine aminopeptidas in pa-tients receiving amikacin or cis-platinum, *Clin Chim Acta* 112:149-157, 1981.

4. Jung K, Diego J, Strobelt V, et al: Diagnostic significance of some urinary enzymes for detecting acute rejection crises in renal-transplant recipients: alanine aminopeptidase, alkaline phosphatase, γ-glutamyltransferse, N-acetyl-β-D-glucosaminidase, and lysozyme, *Clin Chem* 32:1807-1811, 1986.

5. Neef L, Nilius R, Haschen RJ: Applications of electronic data processing in diagnosis of hepatobiliary diseases. In Schmidt E, Schmidt FW, Trautschold I, et al, editors: *Advances in clinical enzymology,* New York, 1979, S. Karger.

6. Sanderink G, Artur Y, Schiele F, et al: Alanine aminopeptidase in serum: biological variations and reference limits, *Clin Chem* 34:1422-1426, 1988.

7. Dubach UC, Schmidt U, editors: *Diagnostic significance of enzymes and proteins in urine. Current problems in clinical biochemistry, vol 9,* Bern, Switzerland, 1979, Hans Huber Publisher.

8. Severini G, Gentilini L, Tirelli C: Diagnostic evaluation of alanine aminopeptidase as serum marker for detecting cancer, *Cancer Biochem Biophys* 12:199-204, 1991.

9. Taracha E, Habrat B, Lehner M, et al: Alanine aminopeptidase activity in urine: a new marker of chronic alcohol abuse? *Alcohol Clin Exp Res* 28:729-735, 2004.

10. Sanderink GJ, Artur Y, Paille F, et al: Clinical significance of a new isoform of serum alanine aminopeptidase: relationship with liver disease and alcohol consumption, *Clin Chim Acta* 179:23-32, 1989.

11. Jung K, Schulze G: Diuresis-dependent excretion of multiple forms of renal brush-border enzymes in urine, *Clin Chim Acta* 156:77-84, 1986.

12. Jung K, Diego J, Strobelt V: Diagnostic significance of urinary enzymes in detecting acute rejection crises in renal trans-plant recipients depending on expression of results illustrated through the example of alanine aminopeptidase, *Clin Biochem* 18:257-260, 1985.

U ↑ Diseases of the urinary tract, acute and chronic pyelonephritis, glomerulonephritis, immediately following renal transplant (values then decrease and increase again before episodes of rejection)[4]; strongly correlated with dose of prednisolone; after amikacin, gentamicin, and cisplatin; alcohol abuse.[9]

TEST NAME AND METHOD	SPECIMEN REQUIREMENTS	REFERENCE INTERVAL, CONVENTIONAL [INTERNATIONAL RECOMMENDED UNITS]			CHEMICAL INTERFERENCES AND IN VIVO EFFECTS
Alanine Aminotransferase (ALT, L-alanine: 2-oxoglutarate aminotransferase, SGPT; EC 2.6.1.2)[1]	Serum. Enzyme should be assayed on day of collection because activity is lost at room temperature, 4° C, and −40° C.[3]		U/L^4	$\mu Kat/L$	S ↑ V Hepatotoxic drugs or drugs causing cholestasis (see Table II-5). IM injections can cause a slight increase. Many other
		Newborn to 12 mo			drugs can cause increases
		M:	13-45 ×0.017	[0.22-0.77]	that are generally transient
		F:	13-45	[0.22-0.77]	but may, in some cases,
		12 mo to 60 yr			indicate hepatotoxicity.
IFCC, with P-5'-P, 37° C[2]		M:	10-40	[0.17-0.68]	These include acebutolol,
		F:	7-35	[0.12-0.60]	aminoglycosides,
		60-90 yr			azithromycin, bromocrip-
		M:	13-40	[0.22-0.68]	tine, captopril, cephalo-
		F:	10-28	[0.17-0.48]	sporins, clarithromycin,
		>90 yr[5]			clindamycin, clofibrate,
		M:	6-38	[0.10-0.65]	clotrimazole, cy-
		F:	5-24	[0.09-0.41]	closporine, cytarabine,
SCE, 37° C[1]			5-30	[0.09-0.51]	dacarbazine, didanosine, disopyramide, enflurane, ethambutol, fenofibrate, fluoroquinolones (e.g., ciprofloxacin), foscarnet, ganciclovir, heparin, interferon, interleukin 2, labetalol, levamisole, levodopa, lincomycin, mebendazole, mefloquine, metoprolol, nifedipine, omeprazole, ondansetron, penicillins, pentamidine, pindolol, piroxicam, propoxyphene, protriptyline, quinine, ranitidine, retinol, ritodrine, sargramostim, and zimelidine.

S ↓ C *Reflotron:* dopamine, methyldopa

1. Committee on Enzymes of the Scandinavian Society for Clinical Chemistry and Clinical Physiology: Recommended methods for the determination of four enzymes in blood, *Scand J Clin Lab Invest* 33:291-306, 1974.

2. Expert Panel on Enzymes, International Federation of Clinical Chemistry: IFCC methods for the measurement of catalytic concentrations of enzymes, *Clin Chim Acta* 105:147F-154F, 1980.

3. Cuccherini B, Nussbaum SJ, Seff LB, et al: Stability of asparate aminotransferase and alanine aminotransferase activities, *J Lab Clin Med* 102:370-376, 1983.

4. Stranges S, Dorn J, Muti P, et al: Body fat distribution, relative weight, and liver enzyme levels: a population-based study, *Hepatology* 39:754-763, 2004.

DIAGNOSTIC INFORMATION	REMARKS

↑↑ Acute liver cell necrosis of any cause, severe shock, right heart failure, acute anoxia (e.g., status asthmaticus), extensive trauma, left heart failure

↑ Cirrhosis, obstructive jaundice, liver tumors, extensive myocardial infarction, myositis, myocarditis, muscular dystrophy; occasionally in hemolytic disease, preeclampsia, moderate muscle trauma, fatty liver, chronic alcohol abuse, filariasis, severe burns, severe pancreatitis, chronic hepatitis

↓ Pyridoxal phosphate deficiency

ALT is present in very high amounts in liver and kidney and in smaller amounts in skeletal muscle and the heart. Its intracellular location is predominantly cytosolic. There is a mitochondrial isoenzyme, but its half-life in serum is very short. Trace amounts are present in skin, pancreas, spleen, and lung. Activity in erythrocytes is approximately six times the activity in serum.

An ALT level that remains high after an attack of acute hepatitis suggests lack of resolution of the disease and high risk for development of chronic hepatitis.[6,7] Elevated ALT levels are more often due to obesity (particularly in males) or alcohol abuse than to viral hepatitis.[8] Although ALT correlates to body mass index, it correlates better to abdominal fat accumulation.[4] Several studies have suggested basing reference limits for ALT on values found in normal body weight individuals. In such studies, reference limits are typically much lower (30 U/L in men, 19 U/L in women).[9] In blunt abdominal trauma in children, ALT >250 U/L is a good predictor of liver injury.[10] Values are reported to be higher in Hispanics than in other Caucasians.[11,12]

Modern methods incorporate pyridoxal phosphate in the reagent with the result that levels are found ~25% higher than formerly. In some patients on renal dialysis, values may show greater increases.

5. Tietz NW, Shuey DF, Wekstein DR: Laboratory values in fit aging individuals—sexagenarians through centenarians, *Clin Chem* 38:1167-1185, 1992.

6. Jensen DM, Dickerson DD, Linderman MA, et al: Serum alanine aminotransferase levels and prevalence of hepatitis A, B, and delta in outpatients, *Arch Intern Med* 147:1734-1737, 1987.

7. Pastore G, Monno L, Santantonio T, et al: Monophasic and polyphasic pattern of alanine aminotransferase in acute non-A, non-B hepatitis. Clinical and prognostic implications, *Hepatogastroenterology* 32:155-158, 1985.

8. Friedman LS, Dienstag JL, Watkins E, et al: Evaluation of blood donors with elevated serum alanine aminotransferase levels, *Ann Intern Med* 107:137-144, 1987.

TEST NAME AND METHOD	SPECIMEN REQUIREMENTS	REFERENCE INTERVAL, CONVENTIONAL [INTERNATIONAL RECOMMENDED UNITS]	CHEMICAL INTERFERENCES AND IN VIVO EFFECTS

Alanine Aminotransferase—CONT

9. Prati D, Taioli E, Zanella A, et al: Updated definitions of healthy ranges for serum alanine aminotransferase levels, *Ann Intern Med* 137:1-10, 2002.

10. Hennes HM, Smith DS, Schneider K, et al: Elevated liver transaminase levels in children with blunt abdominal trauma: a predictor of liver injury, *Pediatrics* 86:87-90, 1990.

Albumin (Alb)[1-4]	Serum. Analyze fresh		*g/dL*		*g/L*
	or store at 4° C for	0-4 days:	2.8-4.4	× 10	[28-44]
Dye-binding-	<72 hr. Stable frozen	4 days-14 yr:	3.8-5.4		[38-54]
spectrophotometry,	at −20° C for 6 mo or	Adult	3.5-5.2		[35-52]
immunoturbidime-	at −70° C indefinitely.	60-90 yr:	3.2-4.6		[32-46]
try, immunoneph-	Specimens without	>90 yr[4]:	2.9-4.5		[29-45]
elometry	lipemia or hemolysis				
	are preferred.				

S ↓ V L-Asparaginase,[7,8] cisplatin,[9,10] dapsone,[10] dextran perfusion, estrogens, ethanol,[11] ibuprofen, iohexol for intravenous urography,[12] isoniazid, nitrofurantoin, oral contraceptives,[11,13] tamoxifen,[14] valproic acid[15]

In ambulatory patients, values average ∼0.3 g/dL [∼3g/L] higher.

Serum values are typically decreased in pregnancy.

S ↓ C *Bromocresol green method:* Clofibric acid, phenylbutazone

S ↓ C *Bromocresol purple method:* Jaundice, uremia can cause underestimation of albumin concentration[16]

RID	Urine, 24 hr. Use no	3.9-24.4 mg/day	(x: 10.0)	
	preservatives. Store at			
Nephelometric	2-4° C. Freeze for	1-14 mg/dL	× 10	[10-140 mg/L]
	longer storage.			
		At rest:		<80 mg/day
		Ambulatory:		50-80 mg/day

DIAGNOSTIC INFORMATION	REMARKS

11. Robinson D, Whitehead TP: Effect of body mass and other factors on serum liver enzyme levels in men attending for well population screening, *Ann Clin Biochem* 26:393-400, 1989.

12. Saxena S, Shulman IA, Shaw ST Jr, et al: Higher serum alanine aminotransferase levels among Hispanics in a reference population, *Lab Med* 20:264-266, 1989.

S ↑ Any condition causing dehydration

S ↓ *Acute phase reaction and chronic inflammation:* Infection, surgery, trauma, chronic inflammatory diseases, critical illness, malignancy

Decreased hepatic synthesis: Acute and chronic liver disease, amyloidosis, chronic illness, malabsorption, fasting, protein-calorie malnutrition, diabetes mellitus, decreased growth hormone levels, hypothyroidism, hypoadrenalism, carcinoid syndrome, malignancy, disorders associated with a hypergammaglobulinemia,[17] congenital analbuminemia

Increased loss: Nephrotic syndrome/renal dysfunction, thermal burns, exfoliative dermatitis, protein-losing enteropathies, trauma, internal exudate formation, gastrointestinal and lymphatic fistulae, repeated thoracentesis or paracentesis

Increased catabolism: Conditions including therapy with some antimetabolites, radiation treatment, familial hypercatabolic hypoproteinemia, tumors, extensive thermal burns

Plasma volume expansion: Pregnancy, oral contraceptives, congestive heart failure

Albumin is the protein of greatest concentration found in plasma, comprising ~55-60% of the serum protein. Its structure is relatively resistant to denaturation. Other members of the albumin superfamily include vitamin D-binding protein, α-fetoprotein, and afamin. Synthesis is hepatic and is primarily regulated by the colloid osmotic pressure of the interstitial fluid surrounding hepatocytes. Catabolism occurs in nearly all organs, allowing albumin to serve as a source of free amino acids for the body. Approximately 100 variant forms are known. However, with the exception of the syndrome of familial dysalbuminemic hyperthyroxinemia, these are not typically associated with significant alterations in function.[17] The rare condition of analbuminemia, in which serum albumin is almost totally lacking, is usually associated with few symptoms.[21]

Albumin has been demonstrated to serve several functions. It provides the majority of the intravascular oncotic pressure and also contributes to the regulation of fluid concentrations in tissues. It has an important role in the binding and transport of endogenous substances and medications. Hypoalbuminemia can affect free drug concentrations of medications that are highly albumin-bound. There is evidence that albumin has antioxidant activity,[17] may promote wound healing, has a heparin-like anticoagulant effect,[11] and serves as a buffer for acid-base homeostasis.[21]

Antialbumin antibodies are commonly found with hepatic dysfunction and are typically IgA in type.[11]

Ischemia-modified albumin, in which the metal binding capacity of albumin has decreased due to exposure to ischemic events, is a biological marker of myocardial ischemia.[22]

MW: 66,460
$t_{1/2}$: 18-20 days

U ↑ *Functional or benign:* Strenuous exercise/exertion, exposure to cold temperatures, congestive heart failure, substantial fever, postural (orthostatic) proteinuria, pregnancy

Pathological proteinuria: Renal include nephrotic syndrome, nephrosclerosis, amyloidosis and multiple myeloma, glomerulonephritis (acute and chronic), lupus nephritis, infection/pyelonephritis, preeclampsia, diabetic nephropathy,

Urinary protein excretion varies throughout the course of a 24-hr period and can be affected by factors such as administered medications.[23]

Orthostatic (postural) proteinuria can be suspected when a first morning urine sample obtained immediately after rising does not show evidence of proteinuria, whereas a second sample obtained ≥2 hr after upright activity is positive.

TEST NAME AND METHOD	SPECIMEN REQUIREMENTS	REFERENCE INTERVAL, CONVENTIONAL [INTERNATIONAL RECOMMENDED UNITS]				CHEMICAL INTERFERENCES AND IN VIVO EFFECTS

Albumin—CONT

| *Reagent strip*

Latex agglutination inhibition | Urine, random; first morning specimen preferred. Analyze fresh. | **Negative** | | | | U ↑ C *False-positive test strips:* Contamination from quaternary ammonium compounds (detergents), chlorhexidine (cleansers) or amidoamines (fabric softeners)

U ↑ V Nifedipine |

Nephelometric	CSF (lumbar). Centrifuge before analysis. Analyze fresh or store at 4° C for <72 hr. Stable frozen at −20° C for 6 mo or at −70° C indefinitely. Specimens should not contain blood.		*mg/dL*		*mg/L*	
		3 mo-4 yr:	0-45	× 10	[0-450]	
		>4 yr:	10-30		[100-300]	

Spectrophotometric	Peritoneal fluid. Analyze fresh or store at room temperature for up to 1 wk, refrigerated for up to 1 mo, or frozen at −20° C for 6 mo.		*g/dL*		*g/L*	
		Transudates	1.1-2.1	× 10	[11-21]	
		Exudates	0.2-1.0		[2-10]	

DIAGNOSTIC INFORMATION	REMARKS

malignant hypertension, heavy metal exposure, toxic nephropathies, medications, polycystic kidney disease, renal tubular dysfunction, chronic interstitial nephritis, sickle cell nephropathy, rejection of a transplanted kidney

Lower urinary tract: inflammation, infection, tumors

Reagent strips are most sensitive to albumin; consequently globulin, hemoglobin, Bence-Jones protein, or mucoprotein may be present despite a seemingly negative reagent strip result. Tubular proteinuria may also escape detection with reagent strips, in some cases, when only small quantities or no urinary albumin is present. They may also lack sensitivity to detect small concentrations of proteinuria.[24] Urine concentration can also affect sensitivity. Positive (or equivocal) results of screening tests should be confirmed using an alternate methodology.

False-positive results can be seen with very alkaline or highly buffered specimens. Increased salt concentrations can decrease results.

CSF ↑ A breakdown in the blood-brain barrier, decreased CSF flow rate

TEST NAME AND METHOD	SPECIMEN REQUIREMENTS	REFERENCE INTERVAL, CONVENTIONAL [INTERNATIONAL RECOMMENDED UNITS]			CHEMICAL INTERFERENCES AND IN VIVO EFFECTS

Albumin—CONT

Tests for Microal-buminuria[2,3]

Reagent strip

Immunological

Three random urine samples collected over the course of 1 wk (minimizes intraindividual variation). Stable at room temperature for up to 2 days and at 8° C for up to 14 days.

<30 mg/day[5]

Random urine[6]

		mg/dL		mg/L
M:	<40 yr	0.1-14.4	× 10	[10-144]
	≥40 yr	0.1-25.1		[10-251]
F:	<40 yr	0.1-22.6		[10-226]
	≥40 yr	0.1-11.6		[10-116]
M:	<40 yr	1.2-69.8	× 1.0	[12-698]
	≥40 yr	0.8-139.4		[8-1394]
F:	<40 yr	1.3-205.4		[13-2054]
	≥40 yr	1.2-85.6		[12-856]

See *Albumin, urine.*

1. Ritzmann SE, Daniels JC: Serum protein abnormalities in thermal burns. In Lynch JB, Lewis SR, editors: *Symposium on the treatment of burns,* St. Louis, 1973, CV Mosby.

2. Newall RG, editor: *Clinical urinalysis,* Buckinghamshire, UK, 1990, Ames Division, Miles Ltd.

3. Cembrowski GS: Testing for microalbuminuria: promises and pitfalls, *Lab Med* 21:491, 1990.

4. Tietz NW, Shuey DF, Wekstein DR, et al: Laboratory values in fit aging individuals—sexagenarians through centenarians, *Clin Chem* 38:1167-1185, 1992.

5. Sasaki K, Fujita I, Hamasaki Y, et al: Differentiating between bacterial and viral infection by measuring both C-reactive protein and 2'-5'-oligoadenylate synthetase as inflammatory markers, *J Infect Chemother* 8:76-80, 2002.

6. Bond LW, Garber C, Ottinger W, et al: Reference intervals for common analytes in random urine specimens, *Clin Chem* 55:submitted, 2005.

7. Liang DC, Hung IJ, Yang CP, et al: Unexpected mortality from the use of L-asparaginase during remission induction therapy for childhood acute lymphoblastic leukemia: a report from the Taiwan Pediatric Oncology Group, *Leukemia* 13:155-160, 1999.

8. Graham ML, Asselin BL, Herndon JE 2nd, et al: Toxicity, pharmacology and feasibility of administration of PEG-L-asparaginase as consolidation therapy in patients undergoing bone marrow transplantation for acute lymphoblastic leukemia, *Bone Marrow Transplant* 21:879-885, 1998.

9. Nanji AA, Mikhael NZ, Stewart DJ: Hypoalbuminemia in patients receiving cisplatin: correlation between liver platinum and decrease in serum albumin, *Oncology* 43:33-35, 1986.

10. Chang DJ, Lamothe M, Stevens RM, et al: Dapsone in rheumatoid arthritis, *Semin Arthritis Rheum* 25:390-403, 1996.

11. Doweiko JP, Nompleggi DJ: The role of albumin in human physiology and pathophysiology, Part III: albumin and disease states, *JPEN J Parenter Enteral Nutr* 15:476-483, 1991.

12. Brunet WG, Hutton LC, Henderson AR: The effect of nonionic radiographic contrast medium on serum electrolytes and proteins during intravenous urography, *Can Assoc Radiol J* 40:139-141, 1989.

13. Ramcharan S, Sponzilli EE, Wingerd JC: Serum protein fractions. Effects of oral contraceptives and pregnancy, *Obstet Gynecol* 48:211-215, 1976.

14. Grey AB, Evans MC, Kyle C, et al: The anti-oestrogen tamoxifen produces haemodilution in normal postmenopausal women, *J Intern Med* 242:383-388, 1997.

15. Rugino TA, Janvier YM, Baunach JM: Hypoalbuminemia with valproic acid administration, *Pediatr Neurol* 29:440-444, 2003.

16. Calvo R, Carlos R, Erill S: Underestimation of albumin content by bromocresol green, induced by drug displacers and uremia, *Int J Clin Pharmacol Ther Toxicol* 23:76-78, 1985.

DIAGNOSTIC INFORMATION	REMARKS

↑ Is a risk factor for progression to proteinuria and chronic renal failure in both insulin-dependent and non–insulin-dependent diabetic patients.[18] Can also be found in nondiabetic individuals, particularly those who are hypertensive, and is a risk factor for cardiovascular disease and mortality in both nondiabetic hypertensive individuals and diabetic patients.[18-20] Any condition associated with increased urinary albumin concentrations can yield a false-positive result for microalbuminuria.

Microalbuminemia (MA) is most often detected in diabetic individuals who are active smokers, have HbA1c concentrations of >8.0%, and have retinopathy.[18] Evidence suggests that even at urinary albumin concentrations less than those defined as diagnostic of MA, a continuous relationship between the rate of urinary albumin excretion and adverse clinical outcomes exists.[18,25] Regression of MA occurs in some individuals over time.[18]

Medications that act on the renin-angiotensin system may delay onset of renal and cardiovascular disease, making screening for MA important in the care of diabetic patients.[18]

17. Nicholson JP: The role of albumin in critical illness, *Br J Anaesth* 85:599-610, 2000.

18. MacIsaac RJ, Jerums G, Cooper ME: New insights into the significance of microalbuminuria, *Curr Opin Nephrol Hypertens* 13:83-91, 2004.

19. Yudkin JS, Forrest RD, Jackson CA: Microalbuminuria as a predictor of vascular disease in non-diabetic subjects, *Lancet* 2:530-533, 1988.

20. Tsioufis C, Dmitriadis K, Antoniadis D, et al: Inter-relationships of microalbuminuria with other surrogates of the atherosclerotic cardiovascular disease in hypertensive subjects, *Am J Hypertens* 17:470-476, 2004.

21. Doweiko JP, Nompleggi DJ: Role of albumin in human physiology and pathophysiology, *JPEN J Parenter Enteral Nutr* 15:207-211, 1991.

22. Bar-Or D, Lau E, Winkler JV: A novel assay for cobalt-albumin binding and its potential as a marker for myocardial ischemia—a preliminary report, *J Emerg Med* 19:311-315, 2000.

23. Gatalica Z, Vrcic H, Borer WZ: Analbuminemic proteinura: a true but transient finding, *Clin Chem* 37:765-766, 1991.

24. Allen JK, Krauss EA, Deeter RG: Dipstick analysis of urinary protein, *Arch Pathol Lab Med* 115:34-37, 1991.

25. Knight EL, Curhan GC: Editorial review: albuminuria: moving beyond traditional microalbuminuria cut-points, *Curr Opin Nephrol Hypertens* 12:283-284, 2003.

TEST NAME AND METHOD	SPECIMEN REQUIREMENTS	REFERENCE INTERVAL, CONVENTIONAL [INTERNATIONAL RECOMMENDED UNITS]			CHEMICAL INTERFERENCES AND IN VIVO EFFECTS
Alcohol Dehydrogenase (ADH; EC 1.1.1.1)[1-4]	Serum. Stable at room temperature for 1-2 hr, at 4° C for 24 hr, and −70° C for 6 mo.	≤2.8 U/L[2]	× 0.017	[≤0.05 μKat/L]	↑ C Thiourea ↓ C Heavy metals, oxalate, CN⁻; aldehyde as substrate
Bonnichsen and Brink,[1] **Mezey modification, 30° C,** *340 nm*[3]					↑ V Cis-retinoic acid[5]
Shephard et al, 37° C, 340 nm[4]		0-7 U/L[4]		[0.00-0.12 μKat/L]	

1. Bonnichsen RK, Brink NG: Liver alcohol dehydrogenase. In Colowich SP, Kaplan NO, editors: *Methods in enzymology, vol 1,* New York, 1955, Academic Press.
2. Guilbault GG: *Handbook of enzymatic methods of analysis,* New York, 1976, Marcel Dekker, Inc.
3. Mezey E, Cherrick GR, Holt PR: Serum alcohol dehydrogenase: an indicator of intrahepatic cholestasis, *N Engl J Med* 279:241-248, 1968.
4. Shephard MDS, Penberthy L, Berry MN: Adaptation of methods for glutamate dehydrogenase and alcohol dehydrogenase activities to a centrifugal analyzer: assessment of their clinical use in anoxic states of the liver, *J Clin Pathol* 40:1240-1246, 1987.
5. Waladkhani A, Kunz P, Zimmermann W, et al: Changes in human serum alcohol dehydrogenase activity during retinoic acid treatment of cancer patients, *Alcohol Alcohol* 32:739-743, 1997.
6. Chrostek L, Szmitkowski M: Activity of class I and II isoenzymes of alcohol dehydrogenase measured by a fluorometric method in the sera of patients with obstructive jaundice, *Clin Chim Acta* 263:117-122, 1997.
7. Kato S, Ishii H, Kano S, et al: Evidence that "lactate dehydrogenase isoenzyme 6" is in fact alcohol dehydrogenase, *Clin Chem* 30:1585-1586, 1984.
8. Jörnvall H, Hoog JO, von Bahr-Lindstrom H, et al: Mammalian alcohol dehydrogenase of separate classes: intermediates between different enzymes and intraclass isoenzymes, *Proc Natl Acad Sci USA* 84:2580-2584, 1987.
9. Hittle JB, Crabb DW: The molecular biology of alcohol dehydrogenase: implications for the control of alcohol metabolism, *J Lab Clin Med* 112:7-15, 1988.

TEST NAME AND METHOD	SPECIMEN REQUIREMENTS	REFERENCE INTERVAL, CONVENTIONAL			CHEMICAL INTERFERENCES
Aldolase (EC 4,1,2,13) *Enzymatic*	Serum; hemolyzed samples unacceptable; stable at room temperature for 8 hr, refrigerated for 5 days, frozen 6 mo; fasting specimens preferred but not required.	0-30 days: 1 mo-16 yr: ≥17 yr:	6.0-32.0 U/L 3.0-12.0 U/L 1.5-8.1 U/L		

↑ Drug hepatotoxicity, hepatocellular damage, obstructive jaundice,[6] infection, inflammation, and malignancy.

ADH is claimed to be a highly sensitive marker for liver anoxia with centrilobular damage.[4]

ADH is a hepatic cytoplasmic enzyme predominantly located in the centrilobular region. When significantly increased, ADH may sometimes be detected as a sixth band on LDH isoenzyme electrophoresis.[7] ADH isoenzymes specific for liver, gastric mucosa, and kidney have been identified.

ADH is actually a family of closely related enzymes with considerable polymorphism[8] that may influence ethanol elimination rates.[9]

ADH activity is responsible for the metabolic conversion of methanol and ethylene glycol to toxic compounds. Such conversion is inhibited by the administration of ethanol or 4-methylpyrazole.

Highest elevated activities are observed in progressive muscular dystrophy (Duchenne). Lower elevated activities are found in dermatomyositis, polymyositis, and limb-girdle dystrophy. The increase in activities becomes less as muscle mass declines. Aldolase increases have also been observed in myocardial infarction, viral hepatitis, cirrhosis, and obstructive jaundice, prostate tumors, and chronic leukemias.

Creatine kinase (CK) generally provides sufficient diagnostic information; thus aldolase monitoring is not routinely recommended. Increased aldolase activities, in the presence of normal CK activities, have been observed in patients with eosinophilic fasciitis.

TEST NAME AND METHOD	SPECIMEN REQUIREMENTS	REFERENCE INTERVAL, CONVENTIONAL [INTERNATIONAL RECOMMENDED UNITS]			CHEMICAL INTERFERENCES AND IN VIVO EFFECTS
Aldosterone[1-4] RIA	Plasma (heparin or EDTA) or serum. Store frozen. Stable up to 2 yr at $-20°$ C in airtight container.		ng/dL^{5*}	$nmol/L$	P ↑ V Angiotensin, estrogens, laxatives (in chronic abuse with dehydration), loop diuretics (e.g., furosemide), metoclopramide, oral contraceptives, potassium, sodium restriction, spironolactone, thiazide diuretics
		Cord blood:	40-200 × 0.0277	[1.11-5.54]	
		Premature infants			
		31-35 wk, day 4:	19-141	[0.53-3.91]	
		Full-term infants			
		3 days:	7-184	[0.19-5.10]	
		1 wk:	5-175	[0.14-4.85]	
		1-12 mo:	5-90	[0.14-2.49]	
		Children			
		1-2 yr:	7-54	[0.19-1.50]	
		2-10 yr:			P ↓ V Aminoglutethimide,
		Supine:	3-35	[0.08-0.97]	angiotensin-converting inhibitors (e.g., captopril,
		Upright:	5-80	[0.14-2.22]	enalapril, lisinopril), de-
		10-15 yr:			oxycorticosterone, etomi-
		Supine:	2-22	[0.06-0.61]	date, prolonged heparin
		Upright:	4-48	[0.11-1.33]	therapy, indomethacin,
		Adults:			licorice, saline (short-term
		Supine:	3-16	[0.08-0.44]	response if given in hy-
		Upright:	7-30	[0.19-0.83]	pertensives), saralasin (in
		Adrenal vein:	200-800	[5.54-22.16]	sodium-depleted subjects)
		Low-sodium diet[6]: Increases threefold to fivefold over average sodium diet value After fludrocortisone (Florinef) suppression or IV saline infusion[6]: <4 ng/dL × 0.0277 [<0.11 nmol/L]			

	Urine, 24 hr. Refrigerate during collection. Add 50% acetic acid at completion of collection to achieve a pH of between 2 and 4.[5] Store sample frozen. Patient should be without any medication for 3 wk.	*Total urinary Na, mmol/day*	*Urinary aldosterone, mg/day[3]*		*Urinary aldosterone, nmol/day*	U ↑ V Angiotensin, corticotropin, ethacrynic acid, lithium, loop diuretics (e.g., furosemide), oral contraceptives (small number), thiazide diuretics
		<20	35-80	× 2.77	[97-222]	
		50	13-33		[36-91]	
		100	5-24		[14-66]	
		150	3-19		[8-53]	U ↑ C Copper. *Method of*
		200	1-16		[3-44]	*Drewes:* androsterone,
		250	1-13		[3-36]	corticosterone, cortisone, deoxycorticosterone, etio-
		*Early morning samples from subjects on ad libitum sodium intake.				cholanolone, hydrocortisone, progesterone, testosterone, tetrahydro-DOC, tetrahydrocortisol, 17-hydroxy-4-pregnene-3,20-dione, 17,21-dihydroxy-4-pregnene-3,20-dione

DIAGNOSTIC INFORMATION	REMARKS

↑ *Primary aldosteronism* due to aldosterone-secreting adenoma (Conn's syndrome); pseudoprimary aldosteronism (bilateral adrenal hyperplasia); *secondary aldosteronism* in laxative abuse, diuretic abuse, cardiac failure, cirrhosis of the liver with ascites formation, nephrotic syndrome, idiopathic cyclic edema, Bartter's syndrome, hypovolemia due to hemorrhage and transudation, renal juxtaglomerular hyperplasia with potassium wastage and retarded growth, hemangiopericytomas of the kidney that produce renin, renal hypertension during malignant phase, thermal stress, pregnancy, mid and late luteal phases of menstruation, after 10 days of starvation, and in chronic obstructive lung disease

If an upright sample is collected, patient should be upright (standing or seated) for at least 2 hr. Normal secretion depends on multiple factors, including the renin-angiotensin system, potassium, ACTH, magnesium, and sodium. In normal subjects and patients with aldosteronism, there is a significant overlap. The plasma aldosterone level is reduced with age. Also, responses of aldosterone to dietary sodium restriction, upright position, angiotensin II, and potassium are greatly reduced. The decline of aldosterone with age is probably due to the suppression of renin.

A diagnosis of primary aldosteronism may be made (1) by demonstrating suppressed plasma renin activity that cannot be stimulated following sodium restriction (see *Aldosterone Stimulation Test [after Sodium Restriction]*) or administration of a diuretic (see *Furosemide Stimulation Test, Rapid*); and (2) by demonstrating a lack of suppression of aldosterone following saline infusion (see *Aldosterone Suppression Test [after Saline Infusion]*) or treatment with a mineralocorticoid (see *Fludrocortisone Suppression Test* and *Deoxycorticosterone Suppression Test*). Differentiation of hyperplasia from adenoma as the cause of primary aldosteronism can be made by adrenal venous aldosterone sampling. In hyperplasia both adrenals secrete high levels of aldosterone, whereas in adenoma the contralateral adrenal will be suppressed.

Urine specimens should not be acidified with strong mineral acids.

↓ *Without hypertension:* Addison's disease, isolated aldosterone deficiency, syndrome of hypoaldosteronism due to renin deficiency

↓ *With hypertension:* Excess secretion of deoxycorticosterone, corticosterone, or 18-hydroxydeoxycorticosterone; Turner's syndrome (25% of cases); diabetes mellitus; acute alcoholic intoxication (increased during hangover)

TEST NAME AND METHOD	SPECIMEN REQUIREMENTS	REFERENCE INTERVAL, CONVENTIONAL [INTERNATIONAL RECOMMENDED UNITS]	CHEMICAL INTERFERENCES AND IN VIVO EFFECTS
Aldosterone—CONT			U ↓ V Aminoglutethimide, clonidine, deoxycorticosterone, fludrocortisone, glucocorticoids, labetalol, licorice, heparin, metyrapone, propranolol

1. Friedman RB, Young DS: *Effects of disease on clinical laboratory tests,* ed 2, Washington, DC, 1989, American Association for Clinical Chemistry.

2. Biglieri EG, Kater CE: Mineralocorticoids. In Greenspan FS, Forsham PH, editors: *Basic and clinical endocrinology,* East Norwalk, CT, 1992, Appleton & Lange.

3. Kaplan N: Endocrine hypertension. In Wilson JH, Foster DW, editors: *Williams textbook of endocrinology,* ed 8, Philadelphia, 1992, WB Saunders.

4. Saruta T, Suzuki A, Hayashi M, et al: Mechanism of age-related changes in renin and adrenocortical steroids, *J Am Geriatr Soc* 28:210-214, 1983.

5. Endocrine Sciences: *Pediatric laboratory services,* Tarzana, CA, 1992, Endocrine Sciences.

6. Nichols Institute Reference Laboratories: *Test catalog,* San Juan Capistrano, CA, 1987, Nichols Institute Reference Laboratories.

TEST NAME AND METHOD	SPECIMEN REQUIREMENTS	REFERENCE INTERVAL, CONVENTIONAL [INTERNATIONAL RECOMMENDED UNITS]	CHEMICAL INTERFERENCES AND IN VIVO EFFECTS
Aldosterone Stimulation Test (after Sodium Restriction)[1] Patient is hospitalized and receives diet containing 10 mmol Na^+ and 100 mmol K^+ (child: 2 mmol K^+/kg) with ad libitum water intake.	Urine, 12 hr. Collect for creatinine, Na^+, and K^+ measurements until equilibrium with the new Na intake is established, i.e., when Na^+ decreases to <5-6 nmol/12 hr (nmol/12 hr in children). At that point plasma for renin level, after 2 hr of standing by patient is obtained and 24-hr urine for aldosterone, creatinine, and Na^+ is collected.	Plasma renin should be at least: 5-24 ng AI*/ × 1.0 [5-24 mcg AI* × mL/hr $hr^{-1} \times L^{-1}$] Urinary aldosterone increases and may reach: 100 mcg/day × 2.77 [277 nmol/day] *AI, Angiotensin I.	See individual tests.

1. Alsever RN, Gotlin RW: *Handbook of endocrine tests in adults and children,* ed 2, Chicago, 1978, Year Book Medical Publishers, Inc.

DIAGNOSTIC INFORMATION	REMARKS

In primary aldosteronism there is slight or no increase in plasma renin.

In practice, restriction to 20 mmol K^+ in children may be the least amount that can be successfully achieved. A risk of the test is severe volume depletion and orthostatic hypotension. The test should not be used for patients with hypokalemia and heart disease. This test may be combined with the aldosterone suppression test (after saline infusion).

TEST NAME AND METHOD	SPECIMEN REQUIREMENTS	REFERENCE INTERVAL, CONVENTIONAL [INTERNATIONAL RECOMMENDED UNITS]		CHEMICAL INTERFERENCES AND IN VIVO EFFECTS
Aldosterone Suppression Test (after Saline Infusion)[1-5]	Plasma (heparin or EDTA) for aldosterone before and after saline infusion	After saline infusion Plasma aldosterone: <5 ng/dL	× 0.0277 [<140 nmol/L]	See individual test.
Keep patient upright (seated or standing) 2 hr before test; then administer 2 L of normal saline, 0.9 g/dL, over 4 hr to recumbent patient.				
2 g NaCl tablet with each meal for 3 days	24 hr urine			Aldosterone >14 mcg/day and urine Na >200 mmol/24 hr. Diagnostic of 1 degree hyperaldosteronism.

1. Kern DC, Weinherger MH, Mayes DM, et al: Saline suppression of plasma aldosterone in hypertension, *Arch Intern Med* 128:350-386, 1971.
2. McMurray JF, editor: *Manual of endocrine diagnostic tests,* ed 3, Lexington, KY, 1983, Division of Endocrinology, University of Kentucky Medical Center.
3. Gennari FJ: Serum osmolality. Uses and limitations, *N Engl J Med* 310:102-105, 1984.
4. Whitley RJ, Meikle AW, Watts NB: Endocrinology. In Burtis CA, Ashwood ER, editors: *Tietz textbook of clinical chemistry,* ed 2, Philadelphia, 1994, WB Saunders.
5. Holland OB, Brown H, Kuhnert LV, et al: Further evaluation of the saline infusion test for primary aldosteronism, *Hypertension* 6:717-723, 1984.

TEST NAME AND METHOD	SPECIMEN REQUIREMENTS	REFERENCE INTERVAL, CONVENTIONAL [INTERNATIONAL RECOMMENDED UNITS]				CHEMICAL INTERFERENCES AND IN VIVO EFFECTS
Alkaline Phosphatase (ALP, AP; EC 3.1.3.1)[1]	Serum. Analyze within 4 hr. Stable at 0-4° C for 2-3 days, at −25° C for 1 mo.	*King-Armstrong U/dL*[1]			*U/L*	↑ V Hepatotoxic drugs. Many other drugs can cause increases that are generally transient but
King-Armstrong, phenyl phosphate, 37° C	EDTA, oxalate, or citrate anticoagulants cause extensive inhibition. Increases of up to	Birth:	5-15	× 7.1	[36-107]	may, in some cases, indicate hepatotoxicity. These
		Premature:	1.5-2.0	× adult value		include acebutolol,
		1 mo:	10-30		[71-213]	aminoglutethimide,
		3 yr:	10-20		[71-142]	aminoglycosides,
		10 yr:	15-30		[107-213]	
		Adult:	4.5-13		[32-92]	

DIAGNOSTIC INFORMATION	REMARKS

In primary aldosteronism, plasma aldosterone is >10 ng/dL [>277 pmol/L] following saline infusion.

Test is contraindicated in patients with overt or borderline congestive heart failure. Test may be useful for evaluating patients with primary aldosteronism. A diagnosis of autonomous aldosterone overproduction is supported when high aldosterone levels fail to suppress during volume expansion (e.g., saline infusion or treatment with a mineralocorticoid such as fludrocortisone).

Measurement of plasma renin activity is used to confirm the aldosterone response; PRA usually falls to */mL/hr (0.6 mg AI*/L/hr).[5]

See also *Aldosterone Stimulation Test (after Sodium Restriction).*

*AI, Angiotensin I.

↑ *Increased bone formation:* During the healing of a fracture, primary and secondary hyperparathyroidism (if the skeleton is overtly affected), osteomalacia, juvenile rickets (nutritional deficiency of vitamin D)

Bone disease: Metastatic carcinoma in bone, osteogenic sarcoma, myeloma (a slight increase may occur in some cases), Hodgkin's disease if bones are invaded, Gaucher's disease with bone resorption, Paget's disease, Cushing's syndrome; uremic

Origins of the major phosphatases are liver, bone, intestine, endometrium (or placenta), and lung.[1,8] Ingestion of a meal increases the intestinal isoenzyme of ALP in serum, especially in individuals who are blood type O or B and who are Lewis-positive secretors. ALP activity increases in children during periods of rapid growth, in females in the last trimester of pregnancy (decreases to normal within 3-6 wk postpartum), and after menopause.

TEST NAME AND METHOD	SPECIMEN REQUIREMENTS	REFERENCE INTERVAL, CONVENTIONAL [INTERNATIONAL RECOMMENDED UNITS]			CHEMICAL INTERFERENCES AND IN VIVO EFFECTS

Alkaline Phosphatase—CONT

Bowers and McComb (4-NPP, AMP), 29.77° C[1]	30% may occur after thawing frozen samples.	*U/L*		*mKat/L*	bromocriptine, carboplatin, captopril, cephalosporins, clindamycin, clotrimazole, colchicine, cyclosporine, cytarabine, dapsone, desipramine, dicumarol, didanosine, disopyramide, enalapril, ethambutol, etoposide, filgrastim, flucytosine, foscarnet, ganciclovir, gentamicin, interferon, isotretinoin, ketoconazole, labetolol, levamisole, lincomycin, mebendazole, mephenytoin, nifedipine, NSAIDs (e.g., ibuprofen, naproxen), omeprazole, ondansetron, penicillins, phenytoin, propoxyphene, protriptyline, streptozocin, sulfonylureas, thioguanine, ticlopidine, verapamil, and zalcitabine.
		F			
		1-12 yr:	<350 × 0.017	[<5.95]	
		>15 yr:	25-100	[0.43-1.70]	
		M			
		1-12 yr:	<350	[<5.95]	
		12-14 yr:	<500	[<8.50]	
		>20 yr:	25-100	[0.43-1.70]	
		Values may increase up to threefold during puberty.			

		U/L (Central 95th percentile)[5]		
SCE (4-NPP, DEA), 37° C[2]			*M*	*F*
		20-29 yr:	100-320	70-260
		30-39 yr:	90-320	70-260
		40-49 yr:	100-360	80-290
		50-59 yr:	110-390	110-380
		60-69 yr:	120-450	110-380
		>69 yr:	120-460	90-430

		U/L (Central 95th percentile)[6]		
AACC, IFCC reference method (4-NPP, AMP), 30 and 37° C[3]			*30° C*	*37° C*
		20-50 yr		
		M:	38-94	53-128
		F:	28-78	42-98
		≥60 yr		
		M:	43-88	56-119
		F:	40-111	53-141
		60-90 yr[7]		
		M:	—	56-155
		F:	—	43-160

↑ C Ascorbic acid (high doses), magnesium

↓ V Azathioprine, clofibrate, danazol, estrogens, oral contraceptives

		U/L	mKat/L
Kodak (4-NPP, AMP), 37° C		Adult	
		M:	38-126 × 0.017 [0.65-2.14]
		F:	38-126 [0.65-2.14]

↓ C Arsenate, beryllium, citrate, cyanide, EDTA, fluoride, manganese, oxalate, phosphate, sulfhydryl compounds, theophylline, zinc and magnesium salts (in excess)

4-NPP, DEA, 30° C[4]	Amniotic fluid, 15-21 wk gestation	Normal: Phenylalanine-resistant ALP, ≅50% Homoarginine-resistant ALP, ≅80% Cystic fibrosis: Phenylalanine-resistant ALP, >80% Homoarginine-resistant ALP, <65%

DIAGNOSTIC INFORMATION	REMARKS

osteodystrophy, renal tubular disorders associated with phosphate and/or calcium loss resulting in rickets with or without secondary hyperparathyroidism

Renal disease: Renal rickets due to vitamin D-resistant rickets associated with secondary hyperparathyroidism

Liver disease: Infectious mononucleosis, uncomplicated extrahepatic biliary obstruction (more than threefold increase), cytomegalovirus infection in infants, cholangitis and cholangiolitis, hepatocellular necrosis with or without jaundice (less than threefold increase), portal cirrhosis (some cases), liver abscess, primary hepatocellular carcinoma, secondary carcinoma, active regeneration/proliferation of hepatocytes or bile ducts, hepatic nodules (metastatic tumor, cyst, parasitic, amyloid, tubercular, sarcoid, or leukemia); hepatitis due to infection, chemicals, drugs, cardiac failure; chronic use of anticonvulsant drugs

Miscellaneous: Extrahepatic sepsis, ulcerative colitis, regional enteritis, intraabdominal bacterial infections, thyrotoxicosis, benign transient hyperphosphatasemia (children), pulmonary and renal infarction, pancreatitis, presence of Regan or Nagao isoenzymes, phenytoin (dilantin) and alcohol use (enzyme induction)

↓ Hypothyroidism, scurvy, gross anemia, kwashiorkor, achondroplasia, cretinism, deposition of radioactive materials in bone, hypophosphatasemia, hereditary hypophosphatasemia, vitamin B12 deficiency (pernicious anemia), and nutritional deficiency of zinc or magnesium

Total alkaline phosphatase or bone alkaline phosphatase (See *Alkaline Phosphatase, Bone*) is the preferred bone marker in Paget's disease.

Test offers possibility of prenatal detection of cystic fibrosis in the fetus of a mother with a previously affected infant.[4]

TEST NAME AND METHOD	SPECIMEN REQUIREMENTS	REFERENCE INTERVAL, CONVENTIONAL [INTERNATIONAL RECOMMENDED UNITS]	CHEMICAL INTERFERENCES AND IN VIVO EFFECTS

Alkaline Phosphatase—CONT

1. McComb RB, Bowers GN, Posen S: *Alkaline phosphatase,* New York, 1979, Plenum Press.

2. Committee on Enzymes of the Scandinavian Society for Clinical Chemistry and Clinical Physiology: Recommended method for the determination of four enzymes in blood, *Scand J Clin Lab Invest* 33:291-306, 1974.

3. Burtis CA, Ashwood ER, editors: *Tietz textbook of clinical chemistry,* ed 2, Philadelphia, 1994, WB Saunders.

4. Brock DJH: Amniotic fluid alkaline phosphatase isoenzymes in early prenatal diagnosis of cystic fibrosis, *Lancet* 2:941-943, 1983.

5. Gardner MD, Scott R: Frequency distribution and "reference values" of plasma alkaline phosphatase (EC 3.1.3.1) activity in the adult population of a Scottish new town, *J Clin Pathol* 31:1202-1206, 1978.

TEST NAME AND METHOD	SPECIMEN REQUIREMENTS	REFERENCE INTERVAL, CONVENTIONAL [INTERNATIONAL RECOMMENDED UNITS]		CHEMICAL INTERFERENCES AND IN VIVO EFFECTS
Alkaline Phosphatase, Bone (BAP) (EC 3.2.1.2.1)[1-6]	Serum or heparinized plasma. Stable for 2 days at 2-8° C for 2 mo or longer at −70° C.		*ng/mL*	*mcg/L*	↑ V 1,25-dihydroxyvita-min D, thyroid hormones, fluoride, GH
		Adult[13]			
		M:	≤20.1	[≤20.1]	
IRMA (Ostase, Beckman-Coulter)[6-12]		F:			↓ V Glucocorticoids, es-trogens, bisphosphonates, calcitonin
		Premenopausal:	≤14.3	[≤14.3]	
		Postmenopausal:	≤22.4	[≤22.4]	
		Child[14]			
		2-24 mo:	25.4-124.0	[25.4-124.0]	
		2-9 yr:	24.2-89.5	[24.2-89.5]	
		Tanner I-II:	19.5-87.5	[19.5-87.5]	
		Tanner III-IV:	19.5-156.0	[19.5-156.0]	
		Adult			
		M:	8.8-30.0	[8.8-30.0]	
		F:	5.7-22.0	[5.7-22.0]	
Immunoabsorption (BAP, Quidel)[10,11,15]			*U/L*	*U/L*	
		Adult[16]			
		M:	15.0-41.3	[15.0-41.3]	
		F:			
		Premenopausal:	11.6-29.6	[11.6-29.6]	
		Postmenopausal:	14.2-42.7	[14.2-42.7]	

1. Calvo MS, Eyre DR, Gundberg CM: Molecular basis and clinical application of biological markers of bone turnover, *Endocr Rev* 17:333-368, 1996.

2. Naylor KE, Eastell R: Measurement of biochemical markers of bone formation. In Seibel MJ, Robins SP, Bilezikian JP, editors: *Dynamics of bone and cartilage metabolism,* San Diego, 1999, Academic Press, pp. 401-410.

DIAGNOSTIC INFORMATION   **REMARKS**

---

6. Tietz NW, Shuey DF: Reference intervals for alkaline phosphatase activity determined by the IFCC and AACC reference methods, *Clin Chem* 32:1593-1594, 1986.
7. Tietz NW, Shuey DF, Wekstein DR: Laboratory values in fit aging individuals—sexagenarians through centenarians, *Clin Chem* 38:1167-1185, 1992.
8. Simko V: Alkaline phosphatases in biology and medicine, *Dig Dis* 9:189-209, 1991.

↑ Disorders with increased bone formation, Paget's disease (total or bone alkaline phosphatase is best marker), high-turnover osteoporosis, primary and secondary hyperparathyroidism, renal osteodystrophy, hyperthyroidism, osteomalacia, metastatic bone disease, recent bone fractures, acromegaly, children during bone growth, adults >50 yr, menopause

↓ Pregnancy, growth hormone deficiency, hypothyroidism, hypoparathyroidism

BAP, produced by the osteoblast, is a marker of bone formation. Bone, liver, and kidney are isoforms of the same gene product, the tissue-nonspecific gene. BAP is a more sensitive and specific marker of bone formation than total alkaline phosphatase. Consequently, it is more useful in mild metabolic bone diseases such as osteoporosis and early metabolic bone disease. However, because most therapies for osteoporosis and other metabolic bone diseases are antiresorptive, they are usually monitored with collagen telopeptides or cross-links (see *Collagen Cross-Linked Telopeptides and Pyridinium Cross-Links*). Because bone formation and resorption are coupled, formation markers respond to antiresorption therapies, although the response (plateau at 6-12 mo) is delayed compared with resorption markers.

Two methods have been developed using monoclonal antibodies against BAP: an IRMA-measuring mass, and an immunoabsorption assay measuring enzyme activity. These immunoassays exhibit 7-17% cross-reactivity with the liver isoforms. Consequently, current methods overestimate BAP in patients with liver disease with increased concentrations of the liver isoform.

BAP shows the least within-subject variability of bone markers due to its long half-life and the greater reproducibility of serum bone markers. It has several advantages over osteocalcin, the other noteworthy marker of bone formation. Unlike osteocalcin, BAP exhibits little diurnal variation due to its much longer half-life (1-3 days) in vivo. BAP is more useful in patients with impaired renal function. It is more stable in vitro. BAP measurements may not accurately reflect bone formation in patients with liver disease (cross-reactivity of liver isoform), in osteomalacia (mineralizing defect), and with increased concentrations of $1,25(OH)_2D$ (increases synthesis of BAP).

---

3. Seibel MJ, Robins SP, Bilezikian JP: Markers of bone metabolism. In Becker KL, editor: *Principles and practice of endocrinology and metabolism,* ed 3, Philadelphia, 2001, Lippincott Williams & Wilkins, pp. 548-557.
4. Price CP: Multiple forms of human serum alkaline phosphatase: detection and quantitation, *Ann Clin Biochem* 30:355-372, 1993.

TEST NAME AND METHOD	SPECIMEN REQUIREMENTS	REFERENCE INTERVAL, CONVENTIONAL [INTERNATIONAL RECOMMENDED UNITS]	CHEMICAL INTERFERENCES AND IN VIVO EFFECTS

Alkaline Phosphatase, Bone (BAP)—CONT

5. Farley J, Baylink D: Skeletal alkaline phosphatase activity in serum, *Clin Chem* 41:1551-1553, 1995.

6. Kress BC: Bone alkaline phosphatase: methods of quantitation and clinical utility, *J Clin Ligand Assay* 21:139-148, 1998.

7. Garnero P, Delmas PD: Assessment of serum levels of alkaline phosphatase with a new immunoradiometric assay in patients with metabolic bone disease, *J Clin Endocrinol Metab* 77:1046-1053, 1993.

8. Panigrahi K, Delmas PD, Singer F, et al: Characteristics of a two-site immunoassay for alkaline phosphatase in serum, *Clin Chem* 40:822-828, 1994.

9. Withold W, Schulte U, Reinauer H: Method for determination of bone alkaline phosphatase activity: analytical performance and clinical usefulness in patients with metabolic bone disease and malignant bone disease, *Clin Chem* 42:210-217, 1996.

10. Woitge HW, Seibel MJ, Ziegler R: Comparison of total and bone-specific alkaline phosphatase in patients with nonskeletal disorders of metabolic bone disease, *Clin Chem* 42:1796-1804, 1996.

Alkaline Phosphatase Isoenzymes

(ALP isoenzymes; EC 3.1.3.1)[1]

Heat inactivation[2,3]

Serum. Analyze or refrigerate.

Bone and liver I isoenzymes are readily identified in normal serum.

Small amounts of intestinal ALP are occasionally present in individuals with blood types O and B, particularly after meals. Pregnant women have positive placental ALP.

Hepatotoxic drugs may lead to the appearance of liver II and biliary isoenzymes on polyacrylamide gel electrophoresis. See *Alkaline Phosphatase*.

	Percent inactivation,[2] 16 min at 55° C		Fraction inactivation, 16 min at 55° C
Liver:	50-70	× 0.01	[0.50-0.70]
Bone:	90-100		[0.90-1.00]
Intestine:	50-60		[0.50-0.60]
Placenta:	0		[0]
Regan:	0		[0]

	Percent inactivation, 5 min at 65° C		Fraction inactivation, 5 min at 65° C
Liver:	100	× 0.01	[1.00]
Bone:	100		[1.00]
Intestine:	100		[1.00]
Placenta:	0		[0]
Regan:	0		[0]

	Total activity %[3]		Fraction activity
Child and adolescent			
Liver:	5	× 0.01	[0.05]
Bone:	85		[0.85]
Adult (18-30 yr)			
Liver:	40		[0.40]
Bone:	60		[0.60]
Adult (>31 yr)			
Liver:	60		[0.60]
Bone:	40		[0.40]

DIAGNOSTIC INFORMATION	REMARKS

11. Price CP, Milligan TP, Darte C: Direct comparison of performance characteristics of two immunoassays for bone isoforms of alkaline phosphatase in serum, *Clin Chem* 43:2052-2057, 1997.
12. Broyles DL, Nielsen RG, Bussett EM, et al: Analytical and clinical performance and characteristics of tandem-MP Ostase, a new immunoassay for serum bone alkaline phosphatase, *Clin Chem* 44:2139-2147, 1998.
13. *Access Ostase product insert,* Brea, CA, 2001, Beckman Coulter.
14. Alkaline phosphatase, bone specific. In *Quest Diagnostics manual: endocrinology test selection and interpretation,* ed 3, San Juan Capistrano, CA, 2004, Quest-Nichols.
15. Gomez B Jr, Ardakani S, Ju J, et al: Monoclonal antibody assay for measuring bone alkaline phosphatase in serum, *Clin Chem* 41:1560-1566, 1995.
16. *Metra BAP product insert,* San Diego, CA, 2002, Quidel.

↑ *Bone isoenzyme:* Increased bone formation, Paget's disease, bone growth in children, healing of bone fractures, osteomalacia and osteoporosis, postmenopausal osteoporosis, osteomalacia of primary, secondary, and tertiary hyperparathyroidism; nutritional deficiency, e.g., vitamin D rickets, vitamin D-resistant rickets, anticonvulsant-induced iatrogenic rickets, renal tubular acidosis rickets, malabsorption syndrome, osteomalacia; osteosarcoma of bone, metastatic carcinoma of prostate, breast with osteoblastic bone formation, secondary osteoblastic regeneration of healing following successful therapy of osteolytic metastatic bone cancer, lymphoma, leukemia of bone marrow; storage diseases, e.g., Gaucher's disease and Niemann-Pick; bone regeneration following osteoporosis and osteomalacia of Cushing's or chronic adrenal steroids; hyperthyroidism, renal osteodystrophy (uremic bone disease or renal rickets).

↓ Osteopenia due to genetic hypophosphatasemia, cretin hypothyroidism, chronic nutritional deficiency, e.g., magnesium and zinc; vitamin B12 deficiency, pernicious anemia.

↑ *Liver I isoenzyme* (enhanced biosynthesis): Hepatic congestion and decreased clearance of the enzyme, vasculitis, pregnancy

↑ *Liver II isoenzyme* (intracellular enzyme): Parenchymal cell damage

↑ *Biliary ALP:* Cholestasis (high molecule mass lipoprotein-X, ALP

↑ *Intestinal ALP:* Some patients with intestinal disease, some individuals of blood type O or B (particularly after meals); intestinal variant ALP

↑ *Placental ALP:* Appears in maternal serum, especially during the third trimester

See *Alkaline Phosphatase, Bone.*
Various procedures are utilized to assess ALP isoenzymes:
　Heat stability after 56° C for 10 min,
　　Placenta 90% stable
　　Regan 90% stable
　　Liver 50% stable
　　Intestinal 50% stable
　　Bone 10% stable
This technique has important shortcomings because sharp demarcation of heat stability of the ALP isoenzymes does not occur. Presence of very heat-stable isoenzymes (see above) or significant intestinal isoenzyme will alter the heat stability index of the serum. Quantification is difficult when intestinal, placenta, or high concentrations of liver and bone are present. Failure to accurately control the temperature significantly alters findings.

Chemical inhibition: Urea, L-phenylalanine, and other chemicals have been used to differentially inhibit isoenzymes of alkaline phosphatase. Precise quantification of isoenzymes with chemical inhibition has been difficult and is not widely used.

Electrophoresis: Polyacrylamide or agarose gel methods have been used to separate the main ALP isoenzyme groups. An agarose gel technique has been shown to be useful in the detection of bone and liver metastases.[9] The separation of liver and bone is inadequate for precise quantification. Consequently this labor-intensive technique has not been widely used.

Isoelectric focusing[6,7]: IEF has the capability of distinguishing up to 12 ALP isoenzymes/isoforms: biliary, hepatocytic, hepatic reticuloendothelial cell, vascular bed, bone, pulmonary alveolar cells, neutrophil, fetal intestinal (adrenal?), germ cells (testis and ovary), placental or activated T lymphocyte, renal, and intestinal.

TEST NAME AND METHOD	SPECIMEN REQUIREMENTS	REFERENCE INTERVAL, CONVENTIONAL [INTERNATIONAL RECOMMENDED UNITS]	CHEMICAL INTERFERENCES AND IN VIVO EFFECTS

Alkaline Phosphatase Isoenzymes—CONT

Urea and phenyl-alanine inhibition[4]

		% Activity remaining after urea, 2.45 mol/L		Fraction activity remaining after urea, 2.45 mol/L
	Bone:	8	× 0.01	[0.08]
	Liver:	29		[0.29]
	Intestine:	50		[0.50]

		% Activity remaining after phenylalanine, 11.0 nmol/L		Fraction activity remaining after phenylalanine, 11.0 nmol/L
	Bone:	79	× 0.01	[0.79]
	Liver:	80		[0.80]
	Intestine:	22		[0.22]

EP[5]

Bone and liver I isoenzymes are readily identifiable in normal serum. Occasionally intestinal enzyme is present in individuals with B and O blood groups. In pregnancy, the placental enzyme is positive and increases in intensity as pregnancy progresses.

IEF[6,7]

Percentage of total activity[7]

Isoenyme	<1 yr	1-15 yr	Adult	Pregnant women	Pregnant women
Biliary:	3-6	2-5	1-3	1-3	0-12
Liver:	20-34	22-34	17-35	5-17	17-48
Bone:	20-30	21-30	13-19	8-14	7-15
Placental:	8-19	5-17	13-21	53-69	7-15
Renal:	1-3	0-1	0-2	3-6	0-2
Intestinal:	0-2	0-1	0-1	0-1	0-1

Fraction activity

		<1 yr	1-15 yr	Adult	Pregnant women	Pregnant women
Biliary:	× 0.01	[0.03-0.06]	[0.02-0.05]	[0.01-0.03]	[0.01-0.03]	[0.0-0.12]
Liver:		[0.20-0.34]	[0.22-0.34]	[0.17-0.35]	[0.05-0.17]	[0.17-0.48]
Bone:		[0.20-0.30]	[0.21-0.30]	[0.13-0.19]	[0.08-0.14]	[0.08-0.21]
Placental:		[0.08-0.19]	[0.05-0.17]	[0.13-0.21]	[0.53-0.69]	[0.07-0.15]
Renal:		[0.01-0.03]	[0.0-0.01]	[0.0-0.02]	[0.03-0.06]	[0.0-0.02]
Intestinal:		[0.0-0.02]	[0.0-0.01]	[0.0-0.01]	[0.0-0.01]	[0.0-0.01]

↑ *Unidentified isoenzymes:* Frequently of neoplastic origin (e.g., Regan or Nagao isoenzymes). Heat stability and electrophoretic migration of these isoenzymes are similar to those of placental isoenzyme.

Wheat germ lectin precipitation of bone ALP.[8]
This assay was commercialized by Roche outside the U.S. Lectin precipitates ~90% of bone ALP but <5% of nonbone ALP. The robustness of the method has been questioned including lot-to-lot variation in lectin and its stability, the quantitative precipitation of the bone isoenzyme, and coprecipitation of biliary isoenzyme. The method has not been widely used in the U.S.

TEST NAME AND METHOD	SPECIMEN REQUIREMENTS	REFERENCE INTERVAL, CONVENTIONAL [INTERNATIONAL RECOMMENDED UNITS]	CHEMICAL INTERFERENCES AND IN VIVO EFFECTS

Alkaline Phosphatase Isoenzymes—CONT

BMD Iso-ALP
(bone) IFCC
(4-NPP, AMP)
37° C[8]

	U/L
Child, <1 yr:	<800
Prepubertal rise:	800
Adult	
M:	60
F:	50

1. Neef L, Nilius R, Haschen RJ: Applications of electronic data processing in diagnosis of hepatobiliary diseases. In Schmidt E, Schmidt FW, Trautschold I, et al, editors: *Advances in clinical enzymology,* New York, 1979, S. Karger.

2. Stolbach LL: Clinical application of alkaline phosphatase isoenzyme analysis, *Ann NY Acad Sci* 166:760-773, 1969.

3. Whitaker KB, Whitby LG, Moss DW: Activities of bone and liver alkaline phosphatases in serum in health and disease, *Clin Chim Acta* 80:209-220, 1977.

4. O'Carroll D, Statland BE, Steele BW, et al: Chemical inhibition method for alkaline phosphatase isoenzymes in human serum, *Am J Clin Pathol* 63:654-572, 1975.

5. McComb RB, Bowers GN, Posen S: *Alkaline phosphatase,* New York, 1979, Plenum Press.

6. Griffiths J: An alternate origin for the placental isoenzyme of alkaline phosphatase, *Arch Pathol Lab Med* 116:1019-1024, 1992.

7. Griffiths J, Black J: Separation and identification of alkaline phosphatase isoenzymes and isoforms in serum of healthy persons by isoelectric focusing, *Clin Chem* 33:2171-2177, 1987.

8. Rosalki SB, Foo AY, Burlina A, et al: Multicenter evaluation of Iso-ALP test kit for measurement of bone alkaline phosphatase activity in serum and plasma, *Clin Chem* 39:648-652, 1993.

9. Van Hoof VO, Van Oosterom AT, Lepoutre LG, et al: Alkaline phosphatase isoenzyme patterns in malignant disease, *Clin Chem* 38:2546-2551, 1992.

TEST NAME AND METHOD	SPECIMEN REQUIREMENTS	REFERENCE INTERVAL, CONVENTIONAL	CHEMICAL INTERFERENCES AND IN VIVO EFFECTS
Alloantibodies (Atypical, unexpected), Antibody Identification, Red Blood Cell (RBC) [e.g., anti-K (Kell), anti-Jka (Kidd), anti-Fya (Duffy)[1-7]] Indirect antiglobulin test *Agglutination/hemolysis of type O RBCs of known antigen type using tube, gel, or microplate formats.*	Serum or plasma (EDTA). Store at 4° C for 1 wk or up to 6 mo at −30° C. For pretransfusion testing, specimen age must comply with AABB Standards for Blood and Transfusion Services.[1]	Negative	Abnormalities in serum composition such as dysproteinemia and presence of foreign substances (plasma expanders, silicon gel, sodium caprylate, a stabilizer used in albumin preparations) may cause interferences. Some clinically significant antibodies (e.g., those against the Duffy and Kidd blood group antigens) may react only with test erythrocytes homozygous for the corresponding antigen.

Alloantibodies are a result of exposure to foreign erythrocytes by transfusion, pregnancy, or transplantation.

Reactivity in the testing system is dependent on the specificity of the antibody, the titer of the antibody, the antigen profile of the RBCs used for identification, and the test methodology used.

Alloantibodies may be of donor origin, as in the passenger lymphocyte syndrome following hematopoietic stem cell or organ transplantation.[9]

For alloantibody identification, three antigen positive RBCs must demonstrate reactivity to "rule in" the presence of the antibody (probability is 95% that the antibody is present). Three antigen-negative RBCs must demonstrate no reactivity to exclude the presence of an antibody to other antigens (probability is 95% that an antibody to other antigens is not present).

Reaction media may include saline, albumin, low ionic strength solution, or polyethylene glycol, with the addition of antihuman globulin reagent. Procedures including treatment with enzymes or sulfhydryl reagents, adsorption, or neutralization may be done before the application of a detection system such as agglutination.

Alloantibodies due to transfusions or pregnancy may be demonstrable for years after the antigen exposure.[10]

Passively acquired antibodies are usually demonstrable for 4-6 wk, although they may be detectable for up to 6 months.

TEST NAME AND METHOD	SPECIMEN REQUIREMENTS	REFERENCE INTERVAL, CONVENTIONAL [INTERNATIONAL RECOMMENDED UNITS]	CHEMICAL INTERFERENCES AND IN VIVO EFFECTS
Alloantibodies (Atypical, unexpected), Antibody Identification, Red Blood Cell (RBC)—CONT			
			Treatment of red cells with proteolytic enzymes such as ficin or papain may enhance antibody reactivity (e.g., antibodies against Rh, Kidd blood group antigens).
			Duffy, M, N, S, and some other blood group antigens are weakened or destroyed by proteolytic enzymes, whereas sulfhydryl reagents like dithiothreitol have the same effect on Kell and Lutheran blood group antigens, among others. Treatment of test erythrocytes with these agents will result in a decrease in the reactivity of the corresponding antibody.
			Anti-D may be detected in D-negative individuals following RHIG administration.
			Infrequently, other alloantibodies may be passively transferred, e.g., from intravenous immunoglobulin preparations.

1. *Standards for blood banks and transfusion services,* ed 23, Bethesda, MD, 2004, AABB.
2. Brecher M, editor: *Technical manual,* ed 15, Bethesda, MD, 2005, AABB.
3. Chapman JF, Elliott C, Knowles SM, et al: Guidelines for compatibility procedures in blood transfusion laboratories, *Transfus Med* 14:59-73, 2004.
4. Issitt P, Anstee D: *Applied blood group serology,* ed 4, Durham, NC, 1998, Montgomery Scientific Publications.
5. Judd W: Red blood cell immunology and compatibility testing. In Simon T, Dzik W, Snyder E, et al, editors: *Rossi's principles of transfusion medicine,* Philadelphia, 2002, Lippincott Williams & Wilkins, pp. 69-88.
6. Mollison P, Engelfriet C, Contreras M: *Blood transfusion in clinical medicine,* ed 10, Oxford, 1997, Blackwell Scientific Publications.
7. Roitt I, Brostoff J, Male D: *Immunology,* ed 4, London, 1996, Mosby.

DIAGNOSTIC INFORMATION	REMARKS

Autoantibodies may mask the presence of alloantibodies. Autoantibody activity may be removed by adsorbing the serum with pretransfusion autologous erythrocytes to detect underlying alloantibodies. Autoantibodies may be warm or cold reactive and should be tested at appropriate temperatures.

Alloadsorption studies, rather than autoadsorptions, are performed in recently (<3 mo) transfused patients because transfused erythrocytes may carry antigens that may react with and remove important alloantibodies.

See also *Antibody Screen, RBC [Indirect Antiglobulin (Coombs) Test].*

8. Shulman IA, Downes KA, Sazama K, et al: Pretransfusion compatibility testing for red blood cell administration, *Curr Opin Hematol* 8:397-404, 2001.
9. Petz LD: Hemolysis associated with transplantation, *Transfusion* 38:224-228, 1998.
10. Schonewille H, Haak HL, van Zijl AM: RBC antibody persistence, *Transfusion* 40:1127-1131, 2000.

TEST NAME AND METHOD	SPECIMEN REQUIREMENTS	REFERENCE INTERVAL, CONVENTIONAL [INTERNATIONAL RECOMMENDED UNITS]		CHEMICAL INTERFERENCES AND IN VIVO EFFECTS
Alloantibodies, Titer [e.g., anti-D, anti-K (Kell), anti-Jka (Kidd)[1-7]] Indirect antiglobulin test (IAT) *Agglutination of red blood cells of known antigen type using tube, gel, or microplate formats.*	Serum or EDTA plasma. Store at 4° C for 1 wk or at –30° C for up to 6 mo. Retain previous sample for testing with the current sample.	Negative Units: Titer is reported as reciprocal of highest serum dilution showing macroscopic agglutination. Score is a semiquantitative, weighted value reflecting the strength of agglutination in the titration tubes. A difference of >1 dilution step or a score of ≥10 between samples has arbitrarily been deemed significant. A low titer or a titer not increasing during pregnancy usually indicates the fetus is most likely negative for the antigen.		Paraproteins.

1. Brecher M, editors: *Technical manual,* ed 15, Bethesda, MD, 2005, AABB.
2. Chapman JF, Elliott C, Knowles SM, et al: Guidelines for compatibility procedures in blood transfusion laboratories, *Transfus Med* 14:59-73, 2004.
3. Issitt P, Anstee D: *Applied blood group serology,* ed 4, Durham, NC, 1998, Montgomery Scientific Publications.
4. Judd W: Red blood cell immunology and compatibility testing. In Simon T, Dzik W, Snyder E, et al, editors: *Rossi's principles of transfusion medicine,* Philadelphia, 2002, Lippincott Williams & Wilkins, pp. 69-88.
5. Mollison P, Engelfriet C, Contreras M: *Blood transfusion in clinical medicine,* ed 10, Oxford, 1997, Blackwell Scientific Publications.
6. Shulman IA, Downes KA, Sazama K, et al: Pretransfusion compatibility testing for red blood cell administration, *Curr Opin Hematol* 8:397-404, 2001.
7. Roitt I, Brostoff J, Male D: *Immunology,* ed 4, London, 1996, Mosby.
8. Moise KJ Jr: Management of rhesus alloimmunization in pregnancy, *Obstet Gynecol* 100:600-611, 2002.
9. Moise KJ Jr: Non-anti-D antibodies in red-cell alloimmunization, *Eur J Obstet Gynecol Reprod Biol* 92:75-81, 2000.

TEST NAME AND METHOD	SPECIMEN REQUIREMENTS	REFERENCE INTERVAL, CONVENTIONAL		INTERNATIONAL RECOMMENDED UNITS	CHEMICAL INTERFERENCES AND IN VIVO EFFECTS
Aluminum (Al)[1,2] *AAS*	Serum.[3,4] Collect in pretested, metal-free container. Avoid storage in glass. Plasma[5]	*mcg/L* <5.41 Patients on hemodialysis: 20-550 <116[10] 6-7 Patients on Al antacid medication: <30	× 0.037	*μmol/L* [<0.2] [0.74-20.4] [<4.29] [0.22-0.26] [<1.11]	None found.

| DIAGNOSTIC INFORMATION | REMARKS |

Primarily used in prenatal testing to determine alloantibody reactivity in maternal serum, to assess the risk for hemolytic disease of the newborn (HDN).

Precision of the test is poor; technical variables affect results. Previous sample (stored frozen) should be tested in parallel with the current sample.

Titration studies are occasionally of value in antibody identification or in the separation of multiple antibody specificities.

Titration studies are performed without enhancement media.

Titration studies for anti-D antibody are widely used as a guide for noninvasive or invasive interventions in pregnancies at high risk for HDN. Titers between 8 and 32 are frequently considered "significant" or "critical," i.e., may warrant invasive fetal monitoring.[8]

Whereas a very low titer, especially one that does not increase with gestation, correlates in general with a low risk of HDN, close follow up with the obstetric team is recommended. Values for critical titers may vary according to the laboratory that performs the test and have not been well established for non-Rh antibodies.[9]

S ↑ Renal failure, dialysis dementia, Hodgkin's disease, cystic fibrosis; >100 mcg/L [3.7 μmol/L] indicates possible toxicity and >200 mcg/L [7.4 μmol/L] usually shows clinical symptoms of toxicity.

B ↑ Pregnancy, leukemias, liver and bile duct disorders

B ↓ Gastric ulcers, pernicious anemia, diabetes, skin diseases except psoriasis

P, U, Sw ↑ Cystic fibrosis

$Al(OH)_3$ is used in medicine as a gastric antacid and as a phosphate-binding agent in dialysis patients. Al accumulates in patients with renal failure; massive accumulation from long-term intermittent dialysis against high-aluminum dialysate leads to dialysis encephalopathy and vitamin D-resistant osteomalacia. Prolonged IV feeding of preterm infants with Al-containing solutions associated with impaired neurologic function.[11] Role of Al in Alzheimer's disease remains controversial.[12] Al affects bone formation and remodeling and inhibits hemoglobin synthesis.[13] Occupational exposure does not increase serum Al.[14] There are circadian changes of blood Al in normal individuals with highest levels at 9:00 AM and

TEST NAME AND METHOD	SPECIMEN REQUIREMENTS	REFERENCE INTERVAL, CONVENTIONAL [INTERNATIONAL RECOMMENDED UNITS]		CHEMICAL INTERFERENCES AND IN VIVO EFFECTS
Aluminum—CONT				
	Urine, random.[6] *Collect in acid-washed, metal-free plastic container.*	6.5 ± 3.5		[0.24 ± 0.13]
	Dialysis fluid[6]	5.2 ± 1.2		[0.19 ± 0.4]
	Heart[7]	*mcg/g dry wt.* 1.9-19.0	× 0.037	*μmol/g dry wt.* [0.07-0.70]
AAS, NAA	Hair[8]	1-17		[0.04-0.63]
ES	Liver[7]	x: 80		[x: 2.97]
MS	Lung[7]	0.059-410		[0.002-15.21]
	Lymph node[7]	*mg/g dry wt.* 3.2-17.0	× 0.037	*mmol/g dry wt.* [0.12-0.63]
*ICP-MS**	Serum.[9] Collect in pretested, metal-free container.	*mcg/L* 0-15	× 0.037	*μmol/L* [0.00-0.56]
	Dialysis patients:	0-40		[0.00-1.48]
	Toxic	>50		[>1.85]
	Urine.[9] Collect in acid-washed container. Refrigerate during and following collection.	0-7 *mcg/day* 0-10		[0.00-0.26] *μmol/day* [0.00-0.37]

1. Wyngaarden JB, Smith LH Jr, editors: *Cecil textbook of medicine,* ed 18, Philadelphia, 1988, WB Saunders.

2. Piafsky KM, Borga O, Odar-Cederlöf I, et al: Increased plasma protein binding of propranolol and chlorpromazine mediated by disease-induced elevations of α_1-acid glycoprotein, *N Engl J Med* 299:1435-1439, 1978.

3. Ericson SP, McHalsky ML, Rabinow BE, et al: Sampling and analysis techniques for monitoring serum for trace elements, *Clin Chem* 32:1350-1356, 1986.

4. Wang ST, Pizzoloto S, Demshar HP: Aluminum levels in normal human serum and urine as determined by zeeman atomic absorption spectrometry, *J Anal Toxicol* 15:66-70, 1991.

5. Kaehny WD, Hegg AP, Alfrey AC: Gastrointestinal absorption of aluminum from aluminum-containing antacids, *N Engl J Med* 296:1389-1390, 1977.

6. Wilhelm M, Ohnesorge FK: Influence of storage conditions on aluminum concentrations in serum, dialysis fluid, urine, and tap water, *J Anal Toxicol* 14:206-210, 1990.

7. *Chemicals identified in human biological media: a data base. First annual report, vol I, part 2,* ORNL/EIS-1613/V1-P2, Oak Ridge, TN, 1979. Available at National Technical Information Service, U.S. Department of Commerce, Springfield, VA.

8. Jacob RA: Hair as a biopsy material. In Williams DF, editor: *Systemic aspects of biocompatibility,* Boca Raton, FL, 1981, CRC Press, Inc.

DIAGNOSTIC INFORMATION	REMARKS

lowest at 6:00 PM. The aluminum level in serum is claimed to be inversely related to the iron.[10] Serum Al concentrations >100 mcg/L [3.70 μmol/L] are claimed to be a reliable indicator of aluminum-associated osteomalacia.[15]

9.   Associated Regional & University Pathologists, Inc. web site (www.aruplab.com). Specific address Online User's Guide: http://www.aruplab.com/testing/user_guide.jsp. Last accessed 9/2004.

10. Huang I, Huang C, Lim PS, et al: Effect of body iron stores on serum aluminum level in hemodialysis patients, *Nephron* 61:158-162, 1992.

11. Bishop NJ, Morley R, Day JP, et al: Aluminum, neurotoxicity in preterm infants receiving intravenous feeding solutions, *N Engl J Med* 336:1557-1561, 1997.

12. Savory J, Exley C, Forbes WF, et al: Can the controversy of the role of aluminum in Alzheimer's disease be resolved? What are the suggested approaches to this controversy and methodological issues to be considered? *J Toxicol Environ Health* 48:615-635, 1996.

13. Jeffery EH, Abreo K, Burgess E, et al: Systemic aluminum toxicity: effects on bone, hematopoietic tissue, and kidney, *J Toxicol Environ Health* 48:649-665, 1996.

14. de Kom JF, Dissels HM, van der Voet GB, et al: Serum aluminum levels of workers in the bauxite mines, *J Toxicol Clin Toxicol* 35:645-651, 1997.

15. McCarthy JT, Dawn MD, Milliner DS, et al: Interpretation of serum aluminum values in dialysis patients, *Am J Clin Pathol* 86:629-636, 1986.

TEST NAME* AND METHOD	SPECIMEN REQUIREMENTS	REFERENCE INTERVAL, CONVENTIONAL [INTERNATIONAL RECOMMENDED UNITS]		CHEMICAL INTERFERENCES AND IN VIVO EFFECTS
Aminolevulinate Dehydratase (ALAD, porphobilinogen synthase; EC 4.2.1.24)[1-3] **Colorimetric, 38° C**	Erythrocytes.[2] Draw whole blood (heparin; avoid EDTA). Wash freshly drawn Ercs three times in cold saline. Ship Ercs frozen.	108-299 U/mL Ercs[2] × 1.0 ≥4.0 nmol/sec/L Ercs[4]	[108-299 kU/L Ercs]	↓ C EDTA

1. Anderson PM, Desnick RJ: Purification and properties of delta-aminolevulinate dehydratase from human erythrocytes, *J Biochem* 254:6924-6930, 1979.
2. Burch HB, Siegel AL: Improved method for measurement of delta-aminolevulinic acid dehydratase activity of human erythrocytes, *Clin Chem* 17:1038-1041, 1971.
3. Sassa S, Granick S, Bickers DR, et al: Studies on the inheritance of human erythrocyte delta-aminolevulinate dehydratase and uroporphyrinogen synthetase, *Enzyme* 16:326-333, 1973.
4. Mayo Medical Laboratories: *Test catalog,* Rochester, MN, 1993, Mayo Medical Laboratories.
5. Granick JL, Sassa S, Granick S, et al: Studies in lead poisoning II. Correlation between the ratio of activated to inactivated δ-amino levulinic acid dehydratase of whole blood and blood lead level, *Biochem Med* 8:149-159, 1973.

TEST NAME* AND METHOD	SPECIMEN REQUIREMENTS	REFERENCE INTERVAL, CONVENTIONAL [INTERNATIONAL RECOMMENDED UNITS]		CHEMICAL INTERFERENCES AND IN VIVO EFFECTS
δ-Aminolevulinic Acid (d-ALA, DALA, ALA)[1-3] *Spectrophotometric (quantitative)*[2] *Column Chromatography*	Urine, 24 hr. Collect in dark container containing 10 mL HCl, 6 mol/L. Stable refrigerated for 2 wk. Specimen cannot be used for PBG and porphyrins, which need Na_2CO_3 as a preservative. However, some laboratories prefer no HCl or Na_2CO_3 so that all heme precursors can be analyzed on same specimen.	<4.5 mg/L[4] × 7.626 <5.2 mg/day[5] 1.5-7.5 mg/day[1]	[<34 μmol/L] [<34 μmol/day] [11.4-57.2 μmol/day]	↑ C Aminoacetone, ammonia, glucosamine, penicillins ↑ V A number of drugs (see Table I-10) precipitate acute attacks of porphyria in susceptible patients.[6] Lead (Pb) exposure. ↓ V Cisplatin (high dose)

DIAGNOSTIC INFORMATION	REMARKS
↓ Lead poisoning,[5] hereditary tyrosinemia,[6] and ALAD deficiency[7]	Decreased activity of ALAD is a sensitive test for subclinical lead poisoning but has largely been supplanted by direct measurement of blood lead. The enzyme is prone to inactivation during handling of Ercs and the approximate threefold biological variation in normal ALAD values also decreases the test's utility. However, ALAD can be used to follow effectiveness of Pb chelation therapy. Activation of ALAD activity in vitro[5] can help distinguish Pb poisoning from ALAD deficiency and hereditary tyrosinemia. In the latter disorder, it is endogenous succinylacetone that inhibits ALAD and causes increased urine ALA. Hereditary tyrosinemia is associated with neuropathic symptoms similar to those in the acute porphyrias.[6]

6. Sassa S, Kappas A: Hereditary tyrosinemia and the heme biosynthetic pathway—profound inhibition of delta-aminolevulinic acid dehydratase activity by succinylacetone, *J Clin Invest* 71:625-634, 1983.

7. Bird TD, Hamernyik P, Nutter JY, et al: Inherited deficiency of delta-aminolevulinic acid dehydratase, *Am J Hum Genet* 31:662-668, 1979.

↑ Acute porphyrias (acute intermittent, variegate, and hereditary coproporphyria), Pb poisoning, hereditary tyrosinemia, ALAD deficiency (homozygous) Mild increases with diabetic ketoacidosis, pregnancy, porphyria cutanea tarda, use of certain anticonvulsant drugs, and some malignancies.[7] ↓ Alcoholic liver disease	Increased levels of urinary δ-ALA can be used to support a diagnosis of acute porphyria and to follow certain therapies of acute porphyria (e.g., hematin, glucose). An increased δ-ALA with a normal urinary PBG suggests Pb poisoning or hereditary tyrosinemia. However δ-ALA is not a sensitive indicator of Pb poisoning because it does not increase until blood Pb reaches 40 mg/dL [1.93 mmol/L]. For measuring, δ-ALA must be purified and separated from PBG.

TEST NAME AND METHOD	SPECIMEN REQUIREMENTS	REFERENCE INTERVAL, CONVENTIONAL [INTERNATIONAL RECOMMENDED UNITS]	CHEMICAL INTERFERENCES AND IN VIVO EFFECTS

δ-Aminolevulinic Acid—CONT

1. Mayo Medical Laboratories: *Test catalog,* Rochester, MN, 1993, Mayo Medical Laboratories.

2. Mauzerall D, Granick S: The occurrence and determination of delta-aminolevulinic acid and porphobilinogen in urine, *J Biol Chem* 219:435-446, 1956.

3. Poon H, Walker M, Lo YL: Determination of δ-aminolevulinic acid (ALA) and porphobilinogen (PBG) using BIO-RAD columns [Abstract], *Clin Chem* 32:1198, 1986.

4. Valentine WN, Tanaka KR, Paglia DE: Hemolytic anemias and erythrocyte enzymopathies, *Ann Intern Med* 103:245-257, 1985.

Ammonia (NH_3)[1,2]

Enzymatic

Plasma (EDTA or heparin other than ammonium heparinate). Avoid clenching of fist. Place specimen on ice and analyze immediately because concentration increases rapidly on standing. Do not use hemolyzed specimens.

Vitros:

	mcg NH_3/dL		mmol NH_3/L
0-10 days:	170-341	× 0.587	[100-200]
10 days-2 yr:	68-136		[40-80]
>2 yr:	19-60		[11-35]

P,S ↑ V Ammonium salts, asparaginase, barbiturates, diuretics (i.e., acetazolamide, chlorthalidone, ethacrynic acid, furosemide, thiazides), ethanol, narcotic analgesics, parenteral nutrition, tobacco, valproic acid

Resin, enzymatic

	mcg N/dL[2]		μmol N/L
Newborn:	90-150	× 0.714	[64-107]
0-2 wk:	79-129		[56-92]
>1 mo:	29-70		[21-50]
Adult:	15-45		[11-32]

P,S ↑ C Fluorides, oxalate when used as anticoagulants; ammonia in atmosphere

P,S ↓ V Diphenhydramine, kanamycin, lactobacillus acidophilus, lactulose, levodopa, neomycin, cephalothin, smoking

P,S ↓ C *Vitros:* Glucose >600 mg/dL (>33.3 mmol/L)

Urine, 24 hr. Avoid contamination with ammonia and bacteria. Keep at 4-8° C during collection. Analyze without delay.

	mg N/day[3]		mmol N/day
Infant:	560-2900	× 0.0714	[40-207]
Adult:	140-1500		[10-107]

U ↑ V Glycine, methenamine

U ↓ V Acetazolamide, mafenide

1. Brown SS, Mitchell FL, Young DS, editors: *Chemical diagnosis of disease,* Amsterdam, 1979, Elsevier/North Holland Biomedical Press.

2. Burtis CA, Ashwood ER, editors: *Tietz textbook of clinical chemistry,* ed 2, Philadelphia, 1994, WB Saunders.

DIAGNOSTIC INFORMATION	REMARKS

5. Moore MR, McColl KE, Rimington C, et al: Laboratory investigation of the porphyrias. In *Disorders of porphyrin metabolism. Topics in hematology series,* New York, 1987, Plenum Press, 1987.
6. Kappas A, Sassa S, Galbraith RA, et al: The porphyrias. In Scriver CR, Beaudet AL, Sly WS, et al, editors: *The metabolic basis of inherited disease,* ed 6, New York, 1989, McGraw-Hill, Inc.
7. Nuttal KL: Porphyrins and disorders of porphyrin metabolism. In Burtis CA, Ashwood ER, editors: *Tietz textbook of clinical chemistry,* ed 3, Philadelphia, 1999, WB Saunders, pp. 1711-1735.

↑ In fulminant hepatic failure, Reye's syndrome, cirrhosis, gastrointestinal bleeding, portal-systemic shunting of blood, renal disease, GU tract infection with distention and stasis

Several inborn metabolic disorders of the urea cycle and related pathways: With increased fasting NH_3 (hyperammonemia type I, argininemia, ornithinemia), with increase following protein intake (hyperammonemia type II, citrullinuria, argininosuccinic aciduria, lysine intolerance, hyperlysinuria, dibasic aminoaciduria type II)

↑ NH_3 may be an important factor contributing to the pathogenesis of hepatic encephalopathy; however, correlation between plasma NH_3 and the clinical degree of encephalopathy is not always close. Guidelines suggest that ammonia not be used for diagnosis or monitoring of hepatic encephalopathy except in patients in whom the etiology of encephalopathy is not clear.[4]

Blood ammonia measurements are useful in monitoring patients on hyperalimentation therapy.

3. Henry RJ, Cannon DC, Winkelman JW, editors: *Clinical chemistry: principles and techniques,* ed 2, Hagerstown, MD, 1974, Harper and Row.
4. Dufour D, Lott JA, Nolte FS, et al: Diagnosis and monitoring of hepatic injury. I. Performance characteristics of laboratory tests, *Clin Chem* 46:2027-2049, 2000.

TEST NAME AND METHOD	SPECIMEN REQUIREMENTS	REFERENCE INTERVAL, CONVENTIONAL [INTERNATIONAL RECOMMENDED UNITS]	CHEMICAL INTERFERENCES AND IN VIVO EFFECTS
Ammonium Chloride Loading Test (Acid Load Test)[1] Dose: Ammonium chloride, 0.1 g/kg, orally over 1 hr, at 8:00 AM after overnight fast	Urine; collect hourly between 10:00 AM and 4:00 PM. Measure pH immediately.	2-8 hr after the dose: pH should decrease to ≤5.2[1] pH ≤5.3[2] pH ≤5.4[3] At least 30% of hydrogen ion equivalent should be excreted.[3]	None found.

1. Zilva JF, Pannall PR: *Clinical chemistry in diagnosis and treatment,* ed 4, Chicago, 1984, Lloyd-Luke, distributed by Year Book Medical Publishers, Inc.
2. McKinney TD: Renal function tests. In Stein JH, editor: *Internal medicine,* ed 2, Boston, 1987, Little, Brown and Co.
3. Dennis VW: Investigations of renal function. In Wyngaarden JB, Smith LH Jr, Bennett JC, editors: *Cecil textbook of medicine,* ed 19, Philadelphia, 1992, WB Saunders.

TEST NAME AND METHOD	SPECIMEN REQUIREMENTS	REFERENCE INTERVAL, CONVENTIONAL [INTERNATIONAL RECOMMENDED UNITS]	CHEMICAL INTERFERENCES AND IN VIVO EFFECTS
Amylase (Diastase, 1,4-α-D-glucanohydrolase; EC 3.2.1.1)[1-4] *IFCC Method[2] (4,6-ethylidene (G1)-4-nitrophyl (G7)-α-(1→4)-D-maltoheptaoside hydrolyzed to release one molecule of 4-nitrophenol)*	*Serum. Stable at room temperature for 7 days and at 4° C for 1 mo. Store at 4° C.*	Amylase activity is low in infant's blood for the first 2 mo of life; it increases to adult values by the end of the first year of life. 24-65 U/L 0.41-1.10 μKat/L Conversion factor 0.0168 70-300 U/L × 0.017 [1.19-5.10 μKat/L] 33-122 U/L [0.56-2.07 μKat/L] 30-110 U/L [0.51-1.87 μKat/L]	↑ V Drugs causing constriction of sphincter of Oddi (e.g., bethanechol, diphenoxylate, narcotic analgesics), secretin ↓ Calcium binding anticoagulants. ↑ Salivary contamination Some drugs produce increased serum amylase and possibly pancreatitis. These include alcohol, asparaginase, azathioprine, captopril, cimetidine, clofibrate, corticosteroids, cyproheptadine, didanosine, estrogens, ethacrynic acid, furosemide, ibuprofen, indomethacin, mefenamic acid, methyldopa, nitrofurantoin, oral contraceptives, pentamidine, phenylbutazone, sulfonamides, sulindac, tetracycline, thiazide diuretics, valproic acid, and zalcitabine.

Test is indicated in conditions in which there are suspected abnormalities in distal tubular function that are associated with only mild reductions in glomerular filtration rate.[3]

Normal result excludes diagnosis of classic distal renal tubular acidosis (RTA, type I) but does not rule out proximal forms of RTA. In distal RTA type IV, urine may be acidified normally, whereas urinary ammonium ion and net acid excretion are diminished.[2]

Test is not generally done in patients with renal insufficiency. When it is performed, patients usually achieve reduction in urinary pH <5.4, although there is a reduced excretion of ammonium ion and titratable acid.[2]

Sensitivity for acute pancreatitis 72-92%; specificity 20-60%. ↑ 2-12 h after clinical symptoms, peaks at 12-72 h, declines over 3-5 d. Values greater than 3× the upper limit of normal are 60% sensitive and 98% specific.

↑ In any intraabdominal inflammatory event.

S ↑ Parotitis, pancreatitis,[8] intestinal obstruction or infarction, strangulated bowel, ectopic pregnancy, perforated hollow viscus, biliary tract disease of all types, diabetic ketoacidosis, pancreatic cyst and pseudocyst, peritonitis, macroamylasemia, some lung and ovarian tumors, renal failure,[9,10] ERCP,[11] abdominal trauma, head injury, viral infections, postoperative patients, alcohol

S ↓ Pancreatic insufficiency, advanced cystic fibrosis, severe liver disease, pancreatectomy

Tissues with highest amylase activities are parotid glands and the pancreas. Much lower activities are present in ovaries, small and large intestine, and skeletal muscle. Amylase activity is the same in males and females and is not affected by meals or time of day.

PNP-oligosaccharide end-product absorptivity is sensitive to pH, temperature, and protein concentration,[12] and for this reason the 2-chloro-PNP substrates are preferred. The latter are also more sensitive due to reaction products with a higher molarabsorptivity.[12]

See also *Macroamylase.*

TEST NAME AND METHOD	SPECIMEN REQUIREMENTS	REFERENCE INTERVAL, CONVENTIONAL [INTERNATIONAL RECOMMENDED UNITS]		CHEMICAL INTERFERENCES AND IN VIVO EFFECTS
Amylase—CONT				
		≤220 U/L	[≤3.74 μKat/L]	↑ C Contamination of specimen or reaction mixture with saliva
				S ↑ C *Kodak Ektachem:* fluorescein after retinal angiography
		≤225 U/L × 0.017	[≤3.83 μKat/L]	S ↓ V Anabolic steroids
		23-85 U/L	[0.39-1.45 μKat/L]	S ↓ C Lipemia, oxalate, citrate, fluoride, and EDTA. Serum pyruvate at concentrations >1 mmol/L [>8.8 mg/dL] will cause falsely low results with Beckman DS and Sigma methods.
		Adult: 20-104 U/L	[0.34-1.77 μKat/L]	
		>90 yr: 25-147 U/L	[0.43-2.50 μKat/L]	
	Urine, 1 hr or 24 hr. Amylase is very unstable in acid urine. Adjust pH to alkaline range before storage. Store at 4° C.	1-17 U/hr		
		170-2000 U/L × 0.017	[2.89-34.0 μKat/L]	
		5-27 U/hr		
	2- to 4-hr specimen	32-641 U/L × 0.017	[0.54-10.90 μKat/L]	

Random urine[5]:

		U/L		μKat/L
M:				
<40 yr		17-494	× 0.017	[0.29-8.4]
≥40 yr		27-595		[0.46-10.1]
F:				
<40 yr		19-597	× 0.017	[0.32-10.1]
≥40 yr		18-420		[0.31-7.4]

	U/g creatinine	μKat/g creatinine
M:		
<40 yr	21-268	[0.36-4.6]
≥40 yr	26-701	[0.44-11.9]
F:		
<40 yr	43-448	[0.73-7.6]
≥40 yr	37-389	[0.63-6.6]

U ↑ See *Serum.* However, values are normal or low in renal failure and macroamylasemia. Urine amylase may remain elevated for up to 2 wk after an episode of acute pancreatitis and may suggest formation of a pseudocyst.

TEST NAME AND METHOD	SPECIMEN REQUIREMENTS	REFERENCE INTERVAL, CONVENTIONAL [INTERNATIONAL RECOMMENDED UNITS]	CHEMICAL INTERFERENCES AND IN VIVO EFFECTS
Amylase—CONT			
		24 hr: 900 U/day	
		≤1200 U/L [≤20 μKat/L]	
		4-37 U/2 hr × 0.5 [2-19 U/hr]	
	Ascitic or pleural fluids. Stability similar to serum. Store at 4° C.	Ascitic and pleural fluid amylase activity identical to, or slightly less than, serum activity.[6,7]	
CIBA Corning Express (G7-PNP)		Serum: 16-108 U/L [0.27-1.8 μKat/L] Urine: 0-14 U/hr	
Bayer ADVIA (Ethylidene blocked G7-PNP)		Serum/plasma: 20-104 U/L [0.34-1.7 μKat/L] Urine: ≤650 U/L [≤10.9 μKat/L]	
Roche COBAS INTEGRA total (Ethylidene blocked G7-PNP)		Serum/plasma: 28-100 U/L [0.47-1.7 μKat/L] Urine: ≤460 U/L [≤7.7 μKat/L]	
Beckman Coulter SYNCHRON (5ET-G7-PNP)		Serum/plasma: 0-46 U/L [0-0.77 μKat/L] Urine: ≤320 U/L [≤5.4 μKat/L]	
J&J Vitros Slides (dyed amylopectin releasing dyed saccharides)		Serum 30-110 U/L [0.51-1.87 μKat/L]	
Kinetic Infinity (various analyzers) (5E-G7-PNP)		Hitachi Serum: 35-140 U/L @ 37° C [0.59-2.34 μKat/L] 27-108 U/L @ 30° C [0.45-1.81 μKat/L] Urine: 1-17 U/2 hr Olympus Serum: 25-114 U/L @ 37° C [0.42-1.91 μKat/L] Urine: 4-50 U/hr @ 37° C	

DIAGNOSTIC INFORMATION	REMARKS

Ascit fl. ↑ Pancreatitis, intestinal obstruction or infarction, strangulated bowel, perforated hollow viscus, biliary tract disease, carcinoma of ovary, ruptured ectopic pregnancy, disseminated secondary malignant neoplasm, peritonitis, pancreatic cyst, or pseudocyst.[7]

Pleur fl. ↑ Leakage from the abdominal cavity or the presence of an amylase-producing tumor; bronchus, pancreatic, or ovarian tumor; rupture of esophagus, perforation of thoracic duct; pulmonary tuberculosis, embolism, or infarction; congestive heart failure[31]

(Roche) Pancreatic specific method uses salivary amylase antibody inhibition.

(Beckman) Pancreatic specific method uses salivary amylase antibody inhibition.

TEST NAME AND METHOD	SPECIMEN REQUIREMENTS	REFERENCE INTERVAL, CONVENTIONAL [INTERNATIONAL RECOMMENDED UNITS]		CHEMICAL INTERFERENCES AND IN VIVO EFFECTS

Amylase—CONT

1. Tietz NW: Support of the diagnosis of pancreatitis by enzyme tests—old problems, new techniques, *Clin Chim Acta* 257:85-98, 1997.

2. Lorentz K: Approved recommendation on IFCC methods for the measurement of catalytic concentration of enzymes Part 9. IFCC method for α-amylase (1,4-α-D-Glucan 4-glucanhydrolase, EC 3.2.1.1), *Clin Chem Lab Med* 36:185-203, 1998.

3. Yadav D, Agarwal N, Pitchumoni CS: A critical evaluation of laboratory tests in acute pancreatitis, *Am J Gastroenterol* 97:1309-1318, 2002.

4. Burtis CA, Ashwood ER, editors: *Tietz textbook of clinical chemistry,* ed 2, Philadelphia, 1994, WB Saunders.

5. Bond LW, Garber C, Ottinger W, et al: Reference intervals for common analytes in random urine specimens, *Clin Chem* 55: submitted, 2005.

6. Eastham RD: *Biochemical values in clinical medicine,* ed 7, Bristol, UK, 1985, John Wright and Sons, Ltd.

TEST NAME AND METHOD	SPECIMEN REQUIREMENTS	REFERENCE INTERVAL, CONVENTIONAL		[INTERNATIONAL RECOMMENDED UNITS]	CHEMICAL INTERFERENCES AND IN VIVO EFFECTS
Amylase/Creatinine Clearance Ratio (ACCR)[1]	Serum. Store in well-closed container at 4° C or −20° C.	*% Clearance* 1-4[2,3]	× 0.01	*Clearance fraction* [0.01-0.04]	See *Amylase* and *Creatinine.*
	Urine, random. Amylase is very unstable in acid urine. Adjust pH to alkaline range before storage. Store at 4° C.				

1. Swaanenburg JCJM: Is the amylase/creatinine ratio useful as a diagnostic aid for pancreatitis? *Ann Clin Biochem* 24:218-219, 1987.

2. Levitt MD: Clinical use of amylase clearance and isoamylase measurements, *Mayo Clin Proc* 54:428-431, 1979.

3. Lott JA: Inflammatory diseases of the pancreas, *Crit Rev Clin Lab Sci* 17:201-228, 1982.

4. Johnson SG, Ellis CJ, Levitt MD: Mechanism of increased renal clearance of amylase/creatinine in acute pancreatitis, *N Engl J Med* 295:1214-1217, 1976.

5. Recio F, Villamil F, Recio C, et al: Early changes of urinary amylase isoenzymes in diabetes mellitus, *Eur J Clin Chem Clin Biochem* 30:657-662, 1992.

6. Aderka D, Tene M, Graff E, et al: Amylase-creatinine clearance ratio. A simple test to predict gentamicin nephrotoxicity, *Arch Intern Med* 148:1093-1096, 1988.

7. Levitt MD, Ellis CJ: Measurement of serum amylase, urinary amylase and amylase/creatinine clearance using a protein-containing chromogenic substrate, *Am J Gastroenterol* 72:60-64, 1979.

8. Levitt MD, Johnson SG, Ellis CG, et al: Influence of amylase assay technique on renal clearance of amylase-creatinine ratio, *Gastroenterology* 72:1260-1263, 1977.

7.   Friedman RB, Young DS: *Effects of disease on clinical laboratory tests,* ed 2, Washington, DC, 1989, American Association for Clinical Chemistry.

8.   Tietz NW, Huang WY, Rauh DF, et al: Laboratory tests in the differential diagnosis of hyperamylasemia, *Clin Chem* 32:301-307, 1986.

9.   Silva DP, Landt Y, Porter SE, et al: Development and application of monoclonal antibodies to human cardiac myoglobin in a rapid fluorescence immunoassay, *Clin Chem* 37:1356-1364, 1991.

10. Salt WB, Schenker S: Amylase—its clinical significance: a review of the literature, *Medicine* 55:269-289, 1976.

11. Van Deun A, Cobbaert C, Van Orshoven A, et al: Comparison of some recent methods for the differentiation of elevated serum amylase and the detection of macroamylasaemia, *Ann Clin Biochem* 26:422-426, 1989.

12. Foo AY, Rosalki SB: Measurement of plasma amylase activity, *Ann Clin Biochem* 23:624-637, 1986.

↑ Pancreatitis[4] (usually >6%); in some patients with diabetic ketoacidosis, renal insufficiency, duodenal perforation, following extracorporeal circulation, large doses of corticosteroids, hyperemesis of pregnancy, toxemia of pregnancy, after abdominal surgery, pancreatic cancer, myeloma and light-chain disease, and marked hemoglobinuria. Some patients with pancreatitis and macroamylasemia have a normal ratio.[2,3]

Subtile ↑ is an early renal change in diabetes mellitus[5] and gentamycin toxicity.[6]

↓ Macroamylasemia

Ratio is significantly lower for persons <30 yr but otherwise remains constant for both sexes, up to 80 yr.[7]

Ratio is dependent on technique of amylase assay; therefore reference interval must be confirmed for particular methodology.[7,8]

The ratio is calculated as:

$$\frac{\text{Urine amylase}}{\text{Serum amylase}} \times \frac{\text{Serum creatinine}}{\text{Urine creatinine}} \times 100$$

The units used for either test in serum and urine must be the same, e.g., U/L for amylase and mg/dL (or μmol/L) for creatinine. A timed collection of urine is not needed because the rate (mL/min) of urine excretion cancels in the above equation. The change in clearance in some nonpancreatic diseases is probably due to competitive interference of amylase absorption in the tubules by nonspecific proteins with low molecular weights similar to that of amylase.[4]

This test is no longer routinely used in pancreatic disease because clinical experience has not supported earlier publications. It is still useful in the diagnosis of macroamylasemia.

TEST NAME AND METHOD	SPECIMEN REQUIREMENTS	REFERENCE INTERVAL, CONVENTIONAL [INTERNATIONAL RECOMMENDED UNITS]	CHEMICAL INTERFERENCES AND IN VIVO EFFECTS
Amylase Isoenzymes and Isoforms (1,4-α-D-glucanohydrolase; EC 3.2.1.1)[1]	Serum. Analyze promptly or store. See *Amylase.*	Depending on the method, up to three P-type and three S-type isoenzymes have been demonstrated with routine techniques (See *Remarks*). Total S-type accounts for 45-70% (x: 57%) of total activity; the remainder is P-type. Values differ with method. P-type reaches a maximum value in the fourth decade and then declines.	Storage of serum can result in quantitative changes in the isoenzyme patterns observed. Persulfate used to polymerize acrylamide gel can destroy the enzymes.[7]
EP,[2] *IEF,*[2] *selective inhibition,*[3] *RIA,*[4] *immunochemical,*[2,5] *immunoinhibition*[6]	Urine. Amylase is very unstable in acid urine. Adjust pH to alkaline range before storage.	Patterns are essentially the same as for serum except for macroamylase complexes that do not appear in urine. P-type isoamylase is proportionally higher in urine. Reference ranges are much wider than in serum because of the wide variation in diuresis. See also *Macroamylase.*	Improper handling and prolonged storage can produce deamidation products of amylase that exhibit anomalous mobilities on some electrophoretic or isoelectric focusing procedures.[1]
	Ascitic or pleural fluids. Stability similar to serum. Store at 4° C.	Ascitic and pleural fluid isoamylase activity identical to, or slightly less than, serum activity	

1. Zakowski JJ, Bruns DE: Biochemistry of human alpha amylase isoenzymes, *Crit Rev Clin Lab Sci* 21:283-322, 1984.
2. Mifflin TE, Hortin G, Bruns DE: Electrophoretic assays of amylase isoenzymes and isoforms, *Clin Lab Med* 6:583-599, 1986.
3. Huang WY, Tietz NW: Determination of amylase isoenzymes in serum by use of a selective inhibitor, *Clin Chem* 28:1525-1527, 1982.
4. Jalali MT, Laing I, Gowenlock AH, et al: Specific radioimmunoassays for human pancreatic and salivary isoamylases, *Clin Chim Acta* 150:237-246, 1985.
5. Mifflin TE, Benjamin DC, Bruns DE: Rapid quantitative specific measurement of pancreatic amylase in serum with use of a monoclonal antibody, *Clin Chem* 31:1283-1288, 1985.
6. Tietz NW, Burlina A, Gerhardt W, et al: Multicenter evaluation of a specific pancreatic isoamylase assay based on a double monoclonal-antibody technique, *Clin Chem* 34:2096-2102, 1988.
7. Navarro S, Aused R, Casals E, et al: Value of the P_3 amylase fraction as an indicator of the long-term prognosis of acute pancreatitis, *Br J Surg* 74:405-407, 1987.
8. Recio F, Villamil F, Recio C, et al: Early changes of urinary amylase isoenzymes in diabetes mellitus, *Eur J Clin Chem Clin Biochem* 30:657-662, 1992.
9. Fox JG, Guin JD, O'Reilly DS, et al: Assessment of glomerular charge selectivity in man by differential clearance of isoamylases, *Clin Sci* 84:449-454, 1993.

DIAGNOSTIC INFORMATION	REMARKS

Identification of increased S- or P-type isoenzymes is not pathognomonic for a specific disease, although the detection of increased P-type is diagnostically superior to demonstration of elevated total amylase for acute pancreatitis. Abnormal serum salivary amylase is usually present in parotitis but also appears in serum of patients with some types of bronchogenic or serous ovarian tumors and in a variety of abdominal diseases.[1] S-type isoamylase occurs in mumps. If, however, mumps causes pancreatitis, a P-type isoamylase may also be present. Increased P-type isoamylase occurs in diabetic ketoacidosis due either to hyperglycemia or to an associated pancreatitis. S/P ratio is elevated in diabetes possibly because of glomerular changes.[8] S-type isoamylase increases after rupture of the esophagus or of an ectopic pregnancy.

Amylase isoenzyme determinations are helpful in excluding pancreatic causes in postsurgical hyperamylasemia.

Increased P3 amylase has been suggested as an indicator for poor prognosis following acute pancreatitis.[7]

There are two main amylase isoenzymes (P- and S-type), but multiple isoenzymes and isoforms exist because of genetic variants and posttranslational modifications. Up to 17 bands have been observed with high-resolution techniques. Ovarian and bronchogenic tumors produce an amylase that is probably an isoform similar to the S-type isoenzyme.[1]

Observations are highly method dependent.[1] Methods employing the salivary amylase inhibitor from wheat germ or immunoassay with the monoclonal antibody[6] obviate the need for electrophoresis to distinguish S- from P-type amylase (See *Amylase*).

The P-type isoamylase undergoes faster urinary clearance than the S-type isoamylase. The ratio of P-type/S-type urinary clearance is in the range 2.1-6.1 using the monoclonal antibody assay.[9] Note that urinary elevations occur later than serum changes in acute pancreatitis (See *Amylase, serum*). In heavy proteinuria due to primary glomerulopathies, the ratio of P-type/S-type urinary clearance is decreased to the range 0.2-2.2. On remission, the ratio reverts to normal.

TEST NAME AND METHOD	SPECIMEN REQUIREMENTS	REFERENCE INTERVAL, CONVENTIONAL [INTERNATIONAL RECOMMENDED UNITS]			CHEMICAL INTERFERENCES AND IN VIVO EFFECTS
Amyloid A Protein, Serum (SAA) ELISA[1] *RID*	Serum or plasma. Analyze fresh or store at 2-8° C for up to 1 mo, or at −20° C for up to 1 yr. Specimens without lipemia or hemolysis are preferred.	<10 mcg/mL	× 1	[<10 mg/L]	None found.

1. Cunnane G: Amyloid precursors and amyloidosis in inflammatory arthritis, *Curr Opin Rheumatol* 13:67-73, 2001.
2. Sasaki K, Fujita I, Hamasaki Y, et al: Differentiating between bacterial and viral infection by measuring both C-reactive protein and 2'-5'-oligoadenylate synthetase as inflammatory markers, *J Infect Chemother* 8:76-80, 2002.
3. Kisilevsky R, Tam SP: Acute phase amyloid A, cholesterol metabolism, and cardiovascular disease, *Pediatr Pathol Mol Med* 21:291-305, 2002.
4. Ridker P, Hennekens C, Buring J, et al: C-Reactive protein and other markers of inflammation in the prediction of cardiovascular disease in women, *N Engl J Med* 342:836-843, 2000.
5. O'Hanlon D, Lynch J, Cormican M, et al: The acute phase response in breast carcinoma, *Anticancer Res* 22:1289-1293, 2002.
6. Morrow D, Rifai N, Antman E, et al: Serum amyloid A predicts early mortality in acute coronary syndromes: a TIMI 11A substudy, *J Am Coll Cardiol* 35:358-362, 2000.
7. Thurnham DI, McGabe GP, Northrup-Clewes CA, et al: Effects of subclinical infection on plasma retinal concentrations and assessment of prevalence of vitamin A deficiency: meta-analysis. Lancet 62:2052-2058, 2003.
8. Fleck A, Myers MA: Diagnostic and prognostic significance of acute-phase proteins. In Gordon H, Koj A, editors: *The acute-phase response to injury and infection,* Amsterdam, 1985, Elsevier, pp. 249-271.
9. Calvin J, Neale G, Fotherby K, et al: The relative merits of acute-phase proteins in the recognition of inflammatory conditions, *Ann Clin Biochem* 25:60-66, 1988.
10. Riikonen P, Saarinen U, Teppo AM, et al: Cytokine and acute-phase reactant levels in serum of children with cancer admitted for fever and neutropenia, *J Infect Dis* 166:432-436, 1992.
11. Schultz D, Arnold P: Properties of four acute phase proteins: C-reactive protein, serum amyloid A protein, a1-acid glycoprotein, and fibrinogen, *Semin Arthritis Rheum* 20:129-147, 1990.
12. Whicher J, Chambers R, Higgenson J, et al: Acute phase response of serum amyloid A protein and C-reactive protein to the common cold and influenza, *J Clin Pathol* 38:312-316, 1985.
13. Uhlar C, Burgess C, Sharp P, et al: Evolution of the serum amyloid A (SAA) protein superfamily, *Genomics* 19:228-235, 1994.
14. Husebekk A, Skogen B, Husby G, et al: Transformation of amyloid precursor SAA to protein AA and incorporation in amyloid fibrils in vivo, *Scand J Immunol* 21:283-287, 1985.

DIAGNOSTIC INFORMATION	REMARKS

Acute phase-reacting protein. Increased in inflammatory conditions, infection, cardiovascular disease, and malignant tumors.[2-6] Elevated levels associated with adverse outcomes in unstable angina and non-Q wave myocardial infarction.[2,7]

Highly sensitive marker of disease activity, serum concentrations increase within a few hours of an insult.[8-10] Response generally similar to that of C-reactive protein (CRP), although levels may increase when CRP is relatively unaffected.[3,11,12]

SAA is a family of proteins[4,14] that may serve as the precursor molecule for tissue amyloid A protein found in secondary amyloidois.[2,15] Secondary amyloidosis is associated with prolonged increases in SAA, such as those found with rheumatoid arthritis and other chronic inflammatory conditions.[2,16,17] Production of SAA is primarily hepatic, and in circulation it associates with the third fraction of high-density lipoprotein (HDL3).[2] During the acute phase response, it may promote HDL-macrophage binding and decrease HDL-hepatocyte binding.[18] Evidence suggests that SAA can serve immunomodulary functions including up-regulation of adhesion molecules, activation of neutrophils, removal of lipid molecules, acting as a chemotactic agent for inflammatory cells, induction of metalloproteinase production, and affecting platelet function.[18-25]

MW, SAA: 100,000-180,000 (in serum)

MW, AA: 11,685

15. Salazar A, Pinto X, Mana J: Serum amyloid A and high-density lipoprotein cholesterol: serum markers of inflammation in sarcoidosis and other systemic disorders, *Eur J Clin Invest* 31:1070-1077, 2001.

16. De Beer F, Mallya R, Fagan E, et al: Serum amyloid A protein concentration in inflammatory diseases and its relationship to the incidence of reactive systemic amyloidosis, *Lancet* 2:231-234, 1982.

17. Kisilevsky R, Subrahmanyan L: Serum amyloid A changes high density lipoproteins cellular affinity: a clue to serum amyloid A's principle function, *Lab Invest* 66:778-785, 1992.

18. Preciado-Patt L, Hershkoviz R, Fridkin M, et al: Serum amyloid A binds specific extracellular matrix glycoproteins and induces the adhesion of resting CD4+ T cells, *J Immunol* 156:1189-1195, 1996.

19. Badolato R, Wang JM, Stornello SL, et al: Serum amyloid A is an activator of PMN antimicrobial functions: induction of degranulation, phagocytosis and enhancement of anti-Candida activity, *J Leukoc Biol* 67:381-386, 2000.

20. Badolato R, Wang JM, Murphy WJ, et al: Serum amyloid A is a chemoattractant: induction of migration, adhesion and tissue infiltration of monocytes and polymorphonuclear leukocytes, *J Exp Med* 180:203-209, 1994.

21. Badolato R, Wang J, Murphy W, et al: Serum amyloid A is a chemotactic agonist at FPR2, a low affinity N-formylpeptide receptor on mouse neutrophils, *Biochem Biophys Res Commun* 270:331-335, 2000.

22. Olsson N, Siegbahn A, Nilsson G: Serum amyloid A induces chemotaxis of human mast cells by activating a pertussis toxin-sensitive signal transduction pathway, *Biochem Biophys Res Commun* 254:143-146, 1999.

23. Migita K, Kawabe Y, Tominaga M, et al: Serum amyloid A protein induces production of matrix metalloproteinases by human synovial fibroblasts, *Lab Invest* 78:535-539, 1998.

24. Zimlichman S, Danon A, Nathan I, et al: Serum amyloid A, an acute phase protein, inhibits platelet activation, *J Lab Clin Med* 116:180-186, 1990.

25. BioSource International, Inc: *Human serum amyloid A package insert,* Camarillo, CA, 2004, BioSource International, Inc.

TEST NAME AND METHOD	SPECIMEN REQUIREMENTS	REFERENCE INTERVAL, CONVENTIONAL [INTERNATIONAL RECOMMENDED UNITS]			CHEMICAL INTERFERENCES AND IN VIVO EFFECTS
3α-Androstanediol Glucuronide (3-α-diol G)[1] **RIA**	Serum. Freeze.	Prepubertal children: Adult M: F:	*ng/dL*[2] 10-60 × 0.0213 260-1500 60-300	*nmol/L* [0.21-1.28] [5.54-31.95] [1.28-6.39]	None found.

1. Horton R, Hawks D, Lobo R: 3α, 17β-Androstanediol glucuronide in plasma, *J Clin Invest* 69:1203-1206, 1992.
2. Nichols Institute Reference Laboratories: *Test catalog,* San Juan Capistrano, CA, 1993, Nichols Institute Reference Laboratories.

Androstenedione[1,2] *RIA*	Serum. Place specimen on ice and process in 1 hr; store frozen. Specimen should be collected at least 1 wk before or after menstrual period.	Cord: Premature: Newborn (1-7 days): 1-12 mo: Prepubertal (1-10 yr): Puberty (10-17 yr): (varies with Tanner stage and sex)[6] Adult M: F:	*ng/dL*[5] 30-150 × 0.0349 80-446 20-290 6-68 8-50 8-240 75-205 × 0.0349 85-275	*nmol/L* [1.0-5.2] [2.8-15.6] [0.7-10.1] [0.2-2.4] [0.3-1.7] [0.3-8.4] [2.6-7.2] [3.0-9.6]	↑ V Corticotropin, clomiphene, cyproterone acetate, levonorgestrel, metyrapone ↓ V Corticosteroids such as dexamethasone
	Whole blood on filter paper. Stable at room temperature and 4° C for 3 mo. For longer periods, store frozen at 20° C.[3]		114-630[7]	[4.0-22.0]	
	Amniotic fluid	Midpregnancy M fetus: F fetus: Term:	*ng/dL*[8] 1.0 × 34.9 0.7 0.7-3.5	*pmol/L* [34.9] [24.4] [24.4-122.2]	
	Saliva[4]	Prepubertal child: 0.6-7.2 Adult: 4.0-18.1		[21.0-251.4] [139.7-632.1]	

DIAGNOSTIC INFORMATION	REMARKS
↑ *Idiopathic hirsutism, hirsutism associated with polycystic ovary syndrome, acne in females* ↓ Men with disorders of androgen action (e.g., male pseudohermaphroditism)	3-α-diol G (a metabolite of dihydrotestosterone) is an indirect way of testing 5α-reductase activity and is a marker of peripheral androgen conversion. The test is useful in the differential diagnosis of hirsutism, especially when levels of circulating androgens (testosterone, free testosterone, and dihydrotestosterone) are within normal limits. In patients treated for hirsutism, this test is also useful for monitoring clinical response to therapy.
↑ Polycystic ovary syndrome (some cases), hirsutism (some cases), congenital adrenal hyperplasia, Cushing's syndrome, ectopic ACTH-producing tumor, hyperplasia of ovarian stroma or ovarian tumor, osteoporosis in females ↓ Sickle cell anemia, adrenal failure, ovarian failure	Androstenedione is a major precursor in the biosynthesis of androgens and estrogens. It is produced in adrenals and gonads and serves as prohormone for testosterone and estrone, particularly in menopausal females. The test is useful in conjunction with other tests in the evaluation and management of androgen disorders. (See *Testosterone, Free* and *Total; Dihydrotestosterone; Dehydroepiandrosterone Sulfate;* and *17-Ketosteroids.*)
	During the menstrual cycle there are individual differences in plasma androstenedione profiles.[9] During puberty in boys, androstenedione concentrations increase for at least 2 yr before there is a significant increase in serum testosterone.[2] Serum androstenedione testing is gaining popularity for monitoring glucocorticoid treatment of congenital adrenal hyperplasia (CAH) because it reflects control better than 17-hydroxy-progesterone (17-OHP) or any other androgen.
	A great overlap has been observed in values for male and female fetuses.
	A close correlation between salivary and plasma androstenedione levels has been claimed in patients with congenital adrenal hyperplasia.

TEST NAME AND METHOD	SPECIMEN REQUIREMENTS	REFERENCE INTERVAL, CONVENTIONAL [INTERNATIONAL RECOMMENDED UNITS]				CHEMICAL INTERFERENCES AND IN VIVO EFFECTS

Androstenedione—CONT

1. Orth D, Kovacs D, DeBold C: The adrenal cortex. In Wilson JH, Foster DW, editors: *Williams textbook of endocrinology,* ed 8, Philadelphia, 1992, WB Saunders.

2. Pakarinen A, Hammond GL, Vihko R: Serum pregnenolone, progesterone, 17α-hydroxyprogesterone, androstenedione, testosterone, 5α-dihydrotestosterone and androsterone during puberty in boys, *Clin Endocrinol* 11:465-474, 1979.

3. Egan SM, Betts P, Thomson S, et al: A bloodspot androstenedione assay suitable for home-monitoring of steroid replacement therapy in congenital adrenal hyperplasia, *Ann Clin Biochem* 26:262-267, 1989.

4. Otten BJ, Wellen JJ, Rijken JCW, et al: Salivary and plasma androstenedione and 17-hydroxyprogesterone levels in congenital adrenal hyperplasia, *J Clin Endocrinol Metab* 57:1150-1154, 1983.

TEST NAME AND METHOD	SPECIMEN REQUIREMENTS	REFERENCE INTERVAL, CONVENTIONAL		[INTERNATIONAL RECOMMENDED UNITS]	CHEMICAL INTERFERENCES AND IN VIVO EFFECTS
Angiotensin I[1,2] *RIA*	Peripheral venous plasma (Na$_2$EDTA). Patient should be kept in a recumbent position 30 min before collection. Place specimen in ice water and centrifuge at 4° C. Separate plasma and freeze immediately.	<25 pg/mL^3	× 1.0	[<25 ng/L]	See *Renin.*

1. Hermann K, Ganten D, Linger T, et al: Measurement and characterization of angiotensin peptides in plasma, *Clin Chem* 34:1046-1051, 1988.

2. Sealey J: Plasma renin activity and plasma prorenin assays, *Clin Chem* 37:1811-1819, 1991.

3. InterScience Institute: *Current unique and rare endocrine assays. Patient and specimen requirements,* Inglewood, CA, 1988, InterScience Institute.

TEST NAME AND METHOD	SPECIMEN REQUIREMENTS	REFERENCE INTERVAL, CONVENTIONAL		[INTERNATIONAL RECOMMENDED UNITS]	CHEMICAL INTERFERENCES AND IN VIVO EFFECTS
Angiotensin II[1,2] *RIA*	Plasma (Na$_2$ EDTA). Patient should be kept in a recumbent position 30 min before collection. Place specimen in ice water and centrifuge at 4° C. Separate plasma and freeze immediately.	Adult 10-60 pg/mL^3 Pediatric 8.7-21.4 pg/mL	× 1.0	[10-60 ng/L] [8.7-21.4 ng/L]	↓ V Captopril, saralasin, enalapril, lisinopril

1. Simoes E, Silva AC, Diniz JS, et al: The renin angiotensin system in childhood hypertension: selective increase of angiotensin–(1-7) in essential hypertension, *J Pediatrics* 145:93-98, 2004.

2. Oparil S, Haber E: The renin-angiotensin system, *N Engl J Med* 297:389-401, 1974.

3. InterScience Institute: *Current unique and rare endocrine assays,* Inglewood, CA, 1987, InterScience Institute.

DIAGNOSTIC INFORMATION	REMARKS

5. Endocrine Sciences: *Pediatric laboratory services,* Tarzana, CA, 1988, Endocrine Sciences.
6. Tanner J, Whitehouse R: Clinical longitudinal standards for height, weight, height velocity and the stages of puberty, *Arch Dis Child* 51:170, 1976.
7. Thomson S, Wallace A: A ^{125}I-radioimmunoassay for measuring androstenedione in serum and in blood-spot samples from neonates, *Clin Chem* 35:1706-1712, 1989.
8. Tulchinsky D, Ryan KJ, editors: *Maternal-fetal endocrinology,* Philadelphia, 1990, WB Saunders.
9. Wilson JD, Forster DW, editors: *Williams textbook of endocrinology,* ed 7, Philadelphia, 1985, WB Saunders.

See *Renin.*	Patient should be on a normal sodium diet (110 mmol/day).

↑ Hypertension, renin-secreting juxtaglomerular renal tumor, volume depletion, congestive heart failure, cirrhosis	Patient should be on normal sodium diet and be recumbent for 30 min before specimen collection.
↓ Anephric patients, primary aldosteronism, Cushing's syndrome[4]	Angiotensin II is the active hormone of the renin-angiotensin system but is the most difficult component of the renin cascade to measure accurately. Interfering peptides or degradation products must be removed from blood before immunoassay.[5] Great care must be taken in the collection and storage of specimen.

4. Friedman RB, Young DS: *Effects of disease on clinical laboratory tests,* ed 2, Washington, DC, 1989, American Association for Clinical Chemistry.
5. Hermann K, Ganten D, Linger T, et al: Measurement and characterization of angiotensin peptides in plasma, *Clin Chem* 34:1046-1051, 1988.

TEST NAME AND METHOD	SPECIMEN REQUIREMENTS	REFERENCE INTERVAL, CONVENTIONAL [INTERNATIONAL RECOMMENDED UNITS]		CHEMICAL INTERFERENCES AND IN VIVO EFFECTS
Angiotensin-Converting Enzyme (ACE; SACE; EC 3.4.15.1)[1-2]	Serum. Stable at 4° C for 1 wk, at −20° C for 6 mo.	19 ± 6 kU/L (SD)[3] × 17	[323 ± 102 μKat/L]	S ↓ V Captopril, cilazapril, enalapril, lisinopril, perindopril, propranolol, ramipril, trandolapril, and other ACE inhibitors
Hippuryl-L-histidyl-L-leucine, 228 nm, 37° C[3]				S ↓ C Hemolysis, lipemia; EDTA, heavy metals, oxalate
Fluorimetric (hippuryl-L-histidyl-L-leucine substrate with o-phthaldialdehyde), 37° C[4]		*nmol/min/mL* 32.2 ± 9.9 (SD)[4] × 1.0	*U/L* [32.2 ± 9.9]	S ↑ V Triiodothyronine S ↑ C Acetate, bromide, chloride, fluoride, nitrate S ↑ V <20 yr.
Furylacroloyl-phenylalanyl-glycylglycine, 340 nm, 37 ° C[5]		*U/L*[7] 0-2 yr: 5-83 × 0.017 3-7 yr: 8-76 8-14 yr: 6-89 >14 yr: 8-52	*μKat/L* [0.09-1.41] [0.14-1.29] [0.10-1.51] [0.14-0.88]	
Hippuryl-L-histidyl-L-leucine with 4-amino-antipyrine, 505 nm, 37 ° C[6]		*U/L*[8] <1 yr: 10.9-42.1 1-2 yr: 9.4-36.0 3-4 yr: 7.9-29.8 4-9 yr: 9.6-35.4 10-12 yr: 10.3-37.0 13-16 yr: 9.0-33.4 17-19 yr: 7.2-26.6 >>19 yr: 6.1-21.1	*μKat/L* [0.16-0.61] [0.13-0.51] [0.16-0.60] [0.18-0.63] [0.15-0.57] [0.12-0.45] [0.10-0.36]	

1. Allen RK: A review of angiotensin-converting enzyme in health and disease, *Sarcoidosis* 8:95-100, 1991.

2. Rohrbach MS, DeRemee RA: Measurement of angiotensin-converting enzyme activity in serum in the diagnosis and management of sarcoidosis. In Homburger HA, Batsakis JG, editors: *Clinical laboratory annual, vol 1,* New York, 1982, Appleton-Century-Crofts.

3. Ryder KW, Jay SJ, Jackson SA, et al: Characterization of a spectrophotometric assay for angiotensin converting enzyme, *Clin Chem* 27:530-534, 1981.

4. Friedland J, Silverstein E: A sensitive fluorimetric assay for serum angiotensin converting enzyme, *Am J Clin Pathol* 66:416-424, 1976.

5. Holmquist B, Bünning P, Riordan JF: A continuous spectrophotometric assay for angiotensin-converting enzyme, *Anal Biochem* 95:540-548, 1979.

6. Kasahara Y, Ashihara Y: Colorimetry of angiotensin-converting enzyme activity in serum, *Clin Chem* 27:1922-1925, 1981.

7. SmithKline Beecham Clinical Laboratories: Personal communication, 1989.

8. Leavelle DE, editor: *Mayo Medical Laboratories interpretive handbook,* Rochester, MN, 1990, Mayo Medical Laboratories.

DIAGNOSTIC INFORMATION	REMARKS
↑ Sarcoidosis, acute and chronic bronchitis, pulmonary fibrosis (associated with tuberculosis, atypical mycobacterial infection, and some industrially related pneumoconioses), rheumatoid arthritis, cervical adenitis, connective tissue diseases, Gaucher's disease, leprosy, untreated hyperthyroidism, fungal disease, histoplasmosis	Angiotensin-converting enzyme is used almost exclusively when sarcoidosis is suspected.

↓ Far-advanced lung neoplasms

↓ *Anorexia nervosa associated with hypothyroidism*

↑ ED[9]

↑ Laryngeal cancer[10]

9. Hamed EA, Meki AR, Gaafar AA, et al: Role of some vasoactive mediators in patients with erectile dysfunction: their relationship with angiotensin-converting enzyme and growth hormone, *Int J Impot Res* 15:418-425, 2003.

10. Kandpal N, Shukla GK, Bhatia N, et al: Oxidant, vitamin A and angiogenic markers in laryngeal cancer patients, *J Laryngol Otol* 117:871-874, 2003.

TEST NAME AND METHOD	SPECIMEN REQUIREMENTS	REFERENCE INTERVAL, CONVENTIONAL [INTERNATIONAL RECOMMENDED UNITS]	CHEMICAL INTERFERENCES AND IN VIVO EFFECTS
Aniline[1] (Aminobenzene, Arylamine; CAS 62-53-3) See *Methemoglobin.* *Colorimetric*[2]	Urine	*p*-Aminophenol (metabolite) Toxic concentration: >30 mg/L × 9.16 275 μmol/L	

1. Baselt RC: *Biological monitoring methods for industrial chemicals,* Davis, CA, 1980, Biomedical Pub.
2. Van Bocxlaer JF, Clauwaert KM, Lambert WE, et al: Quantitative colorimetric determination of urinary p-aminophenol with an automated analyzer, *Clin Chem* 43:627-634, 1997.
3. Agency for Toxic Substances and Disease Registry: Available at: http://www.atsdr.cdc.gov. Last accessed 2/1/06.

TEST NAME AND METHOD	SPECIMEN REQUIREMENTS	REFERENCE INTERVAL, CONVENTIONAL [INTERNATIONAL RECOMMENDED UNITS]	CHEMICAL INTERFERENCES AND IN VIVO EFFECTS
Anion Gap (AG)[1-5] *Calculation*	Serum, plasma (heparin, NH_4-salt preferred)	$Na^+ - (Cl^- + HCO_3)$: *mEq/L* *mmol/L* 7-16 × 1.0 [7-16] (x̄: 12) [x̄: 12] $(Na^+ + K^+) - (Cl^- + HCO_3)$: 10-20 [10-20] (x̄: 16) [x̄: 16] See *Remarks.*	↑ V Poisoning with ethylene glycol, paraldehyde, methanol, and salicylate; phenformin, fructose administration (causing lactic acidosis); diuretic therapy, combined steroid and diuretic therapy, therapy with sodium salts of strong acids, therapy with certain antibiotics (e.g., penicillin, carbenicillin) ↓ V Bromide toxicity (However, because Br^- is measured as Cl^- in some techniques, this increase in Br^- may not be apparent), polymyxin B, lithium

1. Eastham RD: *Biochemical values in clinical medicine,* ed 7, Bristol, UK, 1985, John Wright and Sons, Ltd.
2. Burtis CA, Ashwood ER, editors: *Tietz fundamentals of clinical chemistry,* ed 5, Philadelphia, 2000, WB Saunders.
3. Bhagavan NV: *Biochemistry,* ed 2, Philadelphia, 1978, JB Lippincott.

Inhaled aniline is rapidly absorbed by the lungs, leading to systemic toxicity. Aniline also is efficiently absorbed through the skin and GI tract. The absorbed compound oxidizes hemoglobin iron to produce methemoglobinemia and is oxidized by the cytochrome P-450 system to p-aminophenol, conjugates of which are excreted in the urine. Exposure to 7-53 ppm aniline vapor for several hours may cause slight symptoms, and concentrations >100-160 ppm produce are toxic. As little as 1 g of ingested aniline can be fatal to humans, but the mean lethal dose is 5-30 g (HSDB 2000).[3]

Aniline measurement in blood is not helpful in monitoring exposure or toxicity. Aniline toxicity is monitored by measuring methemoglobin.

Less than 1% of an absorbed dose of aniline is excreted unchanged in the urine. From 15-60% is oxidized to p-aminophenol, which is excreted in the urine as glucuronide and sulfate conjugates; 89% of the absorbed dose is excreted within 24 hr of exposure.

Acetaminophen may increase urinary p-aminophenol concentrations, but in therapeutic doses the contribution does not exceed the toxic threshold.

↑ *Metabolic acidosis:* Uremia with increase in phosphate, negatively charged amino acids, and sulfate; ketoacidosis (diabetic, alcoholic, and starvation) with increase in β-hydroxybutyrate and acetoacetate; lactic acidosis in shock, muscular exercise, or lactic acid syndrome; salicylate, methanol, ethylene glycol, and paraldehyde poisoning; severe dehydration (increase in plasma protein concentration); greatest increases in anion gap seen in organic acidosis.

The anion gap is normal in hyperchloremic acidosis (e.g., due to gastrointestinal loss of HCO_3) and in some forms of renal tubular acidosis.

↓ Hypokalemia, hypocalcemia; hypomagnesemia; rhabdomyolysis; increase in proteins with less negative charge (hypergammaglobulinemia), decrease in negatively charged proteins (hypoalbuminemia), increase in positively charged proteins (myeloma).

Various dilutional states, disorders associated with hyperviscosity, SIADH

Anion gap is a mathematical approximation of the difference between the unmeasured cations and anions in serum.

The anion gap is also useful for quality control of laboratory results for Na^+, K^+, Cl, and total CO_2.

Changes in methodologies, mainly to ISEs, require a reevaluation of the reference range. For sera from patients with hyperlipemia or severe hyperproteinemia, the solvent exclusion effect will affect the results differently, depending on the specific method used, e.g., direct or indirect potentiometry. Therefore the reference interval may be higher or lower than that given here.

Using the Beckman ASTRA analyzer, Winter et al[5] found an anion gap of 3-11 mmol/L. Dinovo et al[6] conducted a similar study and suggested a reference interval for the anion gap of 5-14 mmol/L.

4. Emmett M, Narins RG: Clinical use of the anion gap, *Medicine* 56:38-54, 1977.
5. Winter SD, Pearson JR, Gabow PA, et al: The fall of the serum anion gap, *Arch Intern Med* 150:311-313, 1990.
6. Dinovo EC, Sansone P, Lee DBN: Changes in the reference range of the serum anion gap, *Clin Chem* 38:935, 1992.

TEST NAME AND METHOD	SPECIMEN REQUIREMENTS	REFERENCE INTERVAL, CONVENTIONAL [INTERNATIONAL RECOMMENDED UNITS]			CHEMICAL INTERFERENCES AND IN VIVO EFFECTS
α_1-Antichy-motrypsin $(\alpha_1 X)$ *RID*[1]	Serum. Analyze fresh or store at 4° C for <72 hr. Stable frozen at −20° C for 6 mo or at −70° C indefinitely. Specimens without lipemia or hemolysis are preferred.	Newborn: Adult:	mg/dL^2 ~1 30-60 x: 45	× 10	mg/L [~10] [300-600] [x: 450]	None found.

1. Ritzmann SE, Tucker ES III: *Protein analysis in disease—current concepts. Workshop manual,* Chicago, 1979, American Society of Clinical Pathologists, Commission for Continuing Education.

2. Tietz NW, editor: *Textbook of clinical chemistry,* Philadelphia, 1999, WB Saunders.

3. Kalsheker N, Morley S, Morgan K: Gene regulation of the serine proteinase inhibitors α_1-antitrypsin and α_1-antichymotrypsin, *Biochem Soc Trans* 30:93-98, 2001.

4. Rubin H: The biology and biochemistry of α_1-antichymotrypsin and its potential role as a therapeutic agent, *Biol Chem Hoppe Seyler* 373:497-502, 1992.

5. Potter H, Wefes I, Nilsson L: The inflammation-induced pathological chaperones ACT and apo-E are necessary catalysts of Alzheimer amyloid formation, *Neurobiol Aging* 22:923-930, 2001.

6. Matsubara E, Hirai S, Amari M, et al: α_1-Antichymotrypsin as a possible biochemical marker for Alzheimer-type dementia, *Ann Neurol* 28:561-567, 1990.

7. Lorier M, Hawes C, Donaldson IM, et al: A case of partial deficiency of α_1-antichymotrypsin, *Clin Chem* 31:1739-1740, 1985.

8. Lindmark B, Arborelius M, Eriksson S: Pulmonary function in middle-aged women with heterozygous deficiency of the serine protease inhibitor alpha 1-antichymotrypsin, *Am Rev Resp Dis* 141:884-888, 1990.

9. Janciauskiene S: Conformational properties of serine proteinase inhibitors (serpins) confer multiple pathophysiological roles, *Biochim Biophys Acta* 1535:221-235, 2001.

10. Kalsheker N: α_1-Antichymotrypsin, *Int J Biochem Cell Biol* 28:961-964, 1996.

11. Lilja H, Cockett A, Abrahamsson P: Prostate specific antigen predominantly forms a complex with α_1-antichymotrypsin in blood, *Cancer* 70(suppl 1):230-234, 1992.

12. Lilja H: Significance of different molecular forms of serum PSA, *Urol Clin North Am* 20:681-686, 1993.

13. Zhang S, Janciauskiene S: Multi-functional capability of proteins: α_1-antichymotrypsin and the correlation with Alzheimer's disease, *J Alzheimers Dis* 4:115-122, 2002.

14. Kilpatrick L, Johnson J, Nickbarg E, et al: Inhibition of human neutrophil superoxide generation by α_1-antichymotrypsin, *J Immunol* 146:2388-2393, 1991.

15. Abraham C: Reactive astrocytes and α_1-antichymotrypsin in Alzheimer's disease, *Neurobiol Aging* 22:931-936, 2001.

↑ Acute phase reacting protein. Increases in inflammatory conditions, infection, malignancy, autoimmunity, burn injuries, acute myocardial infarction, surgery, and liver allograft rejection.[3,4] ↑ Levels found in serum and CSF of patients with Alzheimer's disease.[5,6]

↓ Cases of complete absence of $\alpha_1 X$ have not been reported; however, partial deficiency is known to occur and can be associated with abnormalities of pulmonary function.[4,7,8]

$\alpha_1 X$ is one of the major circulating serine protease inhibitors (serpins). Synthesis is primarily hepatic, although production in other tissues also occurs.[3] It has specific activity against leukocyte cathepsin G, mast cell chymase, and pancreatic chymoytrypsin.[9,10] It also complexes with and inactivates prostate-specific antigen (PSA). PSA complexed with $\alpha_1 X$ is the major form of PSA found in human sera.[11,12] Recent studies indicate that $\alpha_1 X$ may help to mediate oxidative damage by inhibiting oxygen utilization and superoxide production in granulocytes.[4,9,13,14] It is a component of the amyloid plaques found in Alzheimer's disease and shows increased expression in reactive astrocytes.[5,15] It may have a role in the pathogenesis of Alzheimer's disease by binding to amyloid β peptide and catalyzing the formation of amyloid filaments.[5]

MW: 68,000

TEST NAME AND METHOD	SPECIMEN REQUIREMENTS	REFERENCE INTERVAL, CONVENTIONAL [INTERNATIONAL RECOMMENDED UNITS]	CHEMICAL INTERFERENCES AND IN VIVO EFFECTS
Antibody Identification, Red Blood Cell (RBC)[1] *Agglutination/hemolysis of type O test cells of known antigen phenotype, flow cytometry, gel test.*	Serum or plasma (EDTA) 1-6° C for 1 wk and for longer periods at −30° C.	Not applicable.	Plasma expanders, dysproteinemia, silicon gel, sodium caprylate; interferences are removed by adequate washing.

1. Technical manual committee, Brecher ME, editors: *Technical manual,* ed 14, Bethesda, MD, 2002, American Association of Blood Banks.

TEST NAME AND METHOD	SPECIMEN REQUIREMENTS	REFERENCE INTERVAL, CONVENTIONAL [INTERNATIONAL RECOMMENDED UNITS]	CHEMICAL INTERFERENCES AND IN VIVO EFFECTS
Antibody Screen, Red Blood Cell (RBC; erythrocytes) [Indirect Antiglobulin (Coombs) Test][1] *Agglutination/hemolysis of type O test cells, flow cytometry, gel test.*	Serum or plasma (EDTA) 1-6° C for 1 wk and for longer periods at −30° C.	Negative	Plasma expanders, dysproteinemia, silicon gel, sodium caprylate; interferences are removed by adequate washing. See *Antiglobulin Test, Direct,* for drug-induced interferences.

1. Technical manual committee, Brecher ME, editors: *Technical manual,* ed 14, Bethesda, MD, 2002, American Association of Blood Banks.

DIAGNOSTIC INFORMATION	REMARKS

A positive antibody screen should be evaluated by an antibody identification panel.

Reactivity in the testing system is dependent on the specificity of the antibody, the titer of the antibody, the antigen profile of the RBCs used for identification, and the test methodology used.

For alloantibody identification, three antigen-positive RBCs must demonstrate reactivity to "rule in" the presence of the antibody (probability is 95% that the antibody is present). Three antigen-positive RBCs must demonstrate no reactivity to exclude the presence of an antibody to that antigen (probability is 95% that an antibody to this antigen is not present).

Autoantibodies may mask the presence of alloantibodies. Autoantibody activity may be removed by adsorbing the serum with pretransfusion autologous erythrocytes to detect alloantibodies. Autoantibodies may be warm or cold reactive and should be tested at appropriate temperatures. Note that use of a posttransfusion sample is not recommended because transfused erythrocytes may carry antigen that may react with and remove important alloantibody.

See *Antibody Screen, RBC.*

Positive tests may occur after immunization, during pregnancy, or after transfusion with RBCs having antigens foreign to the recipient. Positive test may occur in the presence of RBC autoantibodies.

Drugs may stimulate antibodies, some with Rh-like specificity.

Positive test indicates the presence of one or more atypical antibodies, i.e., alloantibody, to foreign erythrocyte antigens. Allogeneic erythrocyte transfusion and pregnancy are the most frequent sources for these erythrocyte antigens.

Autoantibodies are generally seen in infectious diseases such as infectious mononucleosis or primary atypical pneumonia; collagen vascular disease, especially SLE; and lymphoproliferative diseases such as CLL and lymphocytic lymphomas. Cold autoantibodies may produce cold agglutinin disease, whereas warm autoantibodies may produce a warm autoimmune hemolytic anemia.

Primary response (to first antigen exposure) requires 20-120 days; antibody is largely IgM with a small quantity of IgG. Secondary response requires 1-14 days; antibody is mostly IgG.

Some antibody activity (e.g., anti-Jk^a, anti-E) becomes so weak as to be undetectable but increases rapidly after secondary stimulation with the same antigen.

See also *Alloantibodies (Atypical, Unexpected), Immunoglobulin G (IgG).*

TEST NAME AND METHOD	SPECIMEN REQUIREMENTS	REFERENCE INTERVAL, CONVENTIONAL [INTERNATIONAL RECOMMENDED UNITS]				CHEMICAL INTERFERENCES AND IN VIVO EFFECTS
Anticentromere *Indirect immunofluorescence* *Solid phase EIA*		These antibodies produce a distinctive pattern of speckled nuclear staining on substrates used to detect generic ANA. Results are usually expressed qualitatively as negative or positive.				None known.

1. Tan EM, Rodnan GP, Garcia I, et al: Diversity of antinuclear antibodies in progressive systemic sclerosis. Anti-centromere antibody and its relationship to CREST syndrome, *Arthritis Rheum* 23:617-625, 1980.
2. Kallenberg CG: Anti-centromere antibodies (ACA), *Clin Rheum* 9:136-139, 1990.

TEST NAME AND METHOD	SPECIMEN REQUIREMENTS	*mOsm/kg* *	*pg/mL*		*pmol/L*	CHEMICAL INTERFERENCES
Antidiuretic Hormone (ADH, vasopressin)[1,2] *Immunoassay*[3,4]	Plasma (EDTA).[5] Separate immediately in refrigerated centrifuge and freeze at $-20°$ C.	270-280: 280-285: 285-290: 290-295: 295-300:	<1.5 <2.5 1-5 2-7 4-12	$\times$ 0.926	[<1.4] [<2.3] [0.9-4.6] [1.9-6.5] [3.7-11.1]	↑ V Antipsychotics (e.g., phenothiazines, haloperidol), barbiturates, carbamazepine, chlorpropamide, cisplatin, clofibrate, cyclophosphamide, furosemide (rare), narcotic analgesics, thiazides, tolbutamide, tricyclic antidepressants, vidarabine, vinblastine, vincristine

↓ V Demeclocycline, ethanol, lithium carbonate, phenytoin

*In the SI system, 1 mOsm/kg = 1 mmol osmotically active particles/kg.

1. Young DS: *Effects of drugs on clinical laboratory tests,* ed 3, Washington, DC, 1990, American Association for Clinical Chemistry.
2. Reeves W, Andreoli T: The posterior pituitary and water metabolism. In Wilson JD, Foster DW, editors: *Williams textbook of endocrinology,* ed 8, Philadelphia, 1992, WB Saunders.
3. Crawford G, Gyory A: Measuring arginine vasopressin in children and babies, *Clin Chem* 36:1689, 1990.
4. Jaffe BM, Behrman HR, editors: *Methods of hormone radioimmunoassay,* New York, 1979, Academic Press.
5. Alsever RN, Gotlin RW: Handbook of endocrine tests in adults and children, ed 2, Chicago, 1978, Year Book Medical Publishers. Inc.
6. Zerbe RL, Robertson GL: A comparison of plasma vasopressin measurements with a standard indirect test in the differential diagnosis of polyuria, *N Engl J Med* 305:1539-1546, 1981.

DIAGNOSTIC INFORMATION	REMARKS

Anticentromere antibodies occur in a variant of scleroderma known as CREST syndrome (calcinosis, Raynaud's phenomenon, esophageal dysmotility, sclerodactyly, telangiectasia).[1]

Anticentromere antibodies react with protein antigens associated with the centromere, including CENP-A, -B, and -C that vary in size from 17-80 to 140 kDa, respectively. These autoantibodies occur in up to 96% of patients with CREST syndrome and may antedate the development of symptoms in this disease.[2]

↑ *Inappropriate increase (with respect to plasma osmolality) in syndromes of excessive ADH production (SIADH):* Acute intermittent porphyria, Guillain-Barré syndrome, brain tumor (primary or metastatic), vascular and infectious diseases of the brain, pneumonia, pulmonary tuberculosis, tuberculous meningitis, nephrogenic diabetes insipidus

↑↑↑ Systemic neoplasm (ectopic ADH)

↓ Central diabetes insipidus, psychogenic polydipsia, nephrotic syndrome

To differentiate ADH deficiency (central diabetes insipidus) from renal resistance to ADH (nephrogenic diabetes insipidus) or excess water intake (psychogenic polydipsia), perform dynamic tests.[6] See *Water Deprivation Antidiuretic Hormone Stimulation Test.*

Higher secretion occurs at night; in erect posture; with pain, stress, or exercise; with increased plasma osmolality (e.g., hypertonic saline infusion); and with decrease in effective blood volume or arterial pressure. Lower secretion occurs in recumbency, hypoosmolality, volume expansion, and hypertension. Action of ADH on the kidney is inhibited by lithium, calcium, and demeclocycline. Significant deterioration of ADH occurs with prolonged storage. Plasma samples should not be left at room temperature.

It is important to distinguish SIADH from other conditions that cause dilutional hyponatremia: congestive heart failure, renal insufficiency, glucocorticoid deficiency, hypothyroidism, and drugs that stimulate ADH (e.g., chlorpropamide, thiazide diuretics). Patients with SIADH usually show decreased plasma sodium and plasma osmolality, high urine osmolality relative to plasma osmolality, urine sodium that is neither high nor low, and a reduced ability to excrete a water load. See *Water Loading Antidiuretic Hormone Suppression Test.*

TEST NAME AND METHOD	SPECIMEN REQUIREMENTS	REFERENCE INTERVAL, CONVENTIONAL [INTERNATIONAL RECOMMENDED UNITS]	CHEMICAL INTERFERENCES AND IN VIVO EFFECTS
Anti-dsDNA *Solid phase EIA*		<25 U is negative 25-30 U is equivocal 30-200 U is positive >200 U is strongly positive	None known.
Indirect immunofluorescence on Crithidia luciliae *substrate*		Negative is normal. Sera reactive at dilutions of 1-10 or more are considered positive.	
Immunoprecipitation of radiolabeled (125I) dsDNA		Less than 4.2 U/mL (Wo/80 standard) is normal.	

1. Homburger HA, Larsen SA: Detection of specific antibodies. In Rich RR, Shearer WT, Strober W, et al, editors: *Clinical immunology: principles and practice, vol II,* St. Louis, 1996, Mosby Year Book, Inc., pp. 2096-2109.
2. Kavanaugh A, Tomar R, Reveille J, et al: Guidelines for clinical use of the antinuclear antibody test and tests for specific autoantibodies to nuclear antigens, *Arch Pathol Lab Med* 124:71-81, 2000.

TEST NAME AND METHOD	SPECIMEN REQUIREMENTS	REFERENCE INTERVAL, CONVENTIONAL [INTERNATIONAL RECOMMENDED UNITS]	CHEMICAL INTERFERENCES AND IN VIVO EFFECTS
Antiglobulin Test, Direct (DAT; Direct Coombs Test)[1] *Agglutination, gel test, flow cytometry, ELISA*	Anticoagulated blood (EDTA). Separate red blood cells promptly to prevent adsorption of complement to red cells. Clotted blood should be avoided if possible. If clotted blood is used, keep sample at 37° C until cells have been separated. Store for 1 wk at 4° C.	Negative	Interferences such as hyperviscosity caused by increased immunoglobulins are removed by adequate washing. The following drugs have been reported to cause a positive direct antiglobulin test: Acetaminophen, *p*-aminosalicylic acid, aminopyrine, antihistamines, carbromal, cephalosporins, chlorinated hydrocarbon insecticides, chlorpromazine, chloropropamide, cisplatin, clonisine, dipyrone, ethosuximide, fenfluramine, faudin, hydralazine, hydrochlorothiazide, ibuprofen, insulin, isoniazid, levodopa, mefenamic acid, melphalan, methadone, methyldopa, methysergide, nomifensine,

Anti-dsDNA antibodies of the IgG isotype are characteristic of LE and are rarely found in other CTDs or in drug-induced LE. The levels of anti-dsDNA antibodies fluctuate with disease activity in patients with LE, and elevations of antibody levels may precede clinical exacerbations of disease.[1]

Several different analytic methods are available to detect and measure anti-dsDNA antibodies. Different methods may yield different results depending on the titer and affinity of autoantibodies present. These methods are semiquantitative and should not be relied on to predict exacerbations of disease in patients with LE. Low levels of anti-dsDNA antibodies may occur in diseases other than LE.[2]

The following conditions may cause a positive test:

Autoimmune hemolytic anemia: Warm (37° C) reactive autoantibodies, primary (idiopathic) or secondary, disease-related (e.g., lymphoma and SLE).

Cold reactive autoantibodies:
(1) Cold hemagglutinin disease (CHD), idiopathic or disease-related [e.g., lymphoma, pneumonia (anti-I), and mononucleosis (anti-i)]; and
(2) Paroxysmal cold hemoglobinuria (PCH), idiopathic or disease-related [e.g., viral infections and syphilis (anti-P)].

Drug-induced autoimmune hemolytic anemia:
Drug absorbed onto erythrocytes (e.g., penicillin)
Immune complex formed (e.g., quinidine)
Nonimmunologic adsorptions of proteins (e.g., cephalosporins)
Induction of autoantibodies [e.g., Aldomet (α-methyldopa)]

Alloimmune hemolytic anemia: Hemolytic transfusion reactions (HTRs) and hemolytic disease of the newborn [HDN, maternal antibody (IgG) crossing the placental barrier]; passively acquired antibodies from plasma products (e.g., IV immunoglobulins).

Determination of Ig class, IgG subclass, and complement on affected erythrocytes may aid in establishing etiology and in estimating severity of hemolytic risk.

Autoantibodies often do not show antigenic specificity; when specificity is observed, it is most often in the Rh system and only Rh null cells fail to show agglutination. Alloantibodies are expected to show antigenic specificity or specificities. For this reason antibody elution (removal of antibody bound to RBCs for the purpose of determining antigenic specificity) is generally not informative in the workup of autoimmune hemolytic anemias. Elution studies should be performed, however, in the investigation of HTR and HDN.

TEST NAME AND METHOD	SPECIMEN REQUIREMENTS	REFERENCE INTERVAL, CONVENTIONAL [INTERNATIONAL RECOMMENDED UNITS]	CHEMICAL INTERFERENCES AND IN VIVO EFFECTS
Antiglobulin Test, Direct—CONT			penicillamine, penicillins, phenacetin, phenylbutazone, probenecid, procainamide, quinidine, quinine, rifampin, streptomycin, sulfonamides, sulfonylurea derivatives, tetracycline, triamterene, trimellitic anhydride

1. Technical manual committee, Brecher ME, editors: *Technical manual,* ed 14, Bethesda, MD, 2002, American Association of Blood Banks.

Antihistone *Solid phase EIA*		<1 U is negative 1.0-1.5 U is equivocal	None known.

1. Rubin RL: Antihistone antibodies. In Lahita RG, editor: *Systemic lupus erythematosus,* ed 2, New York, 1987, Churchill Livingstone, pp. 247-271.
2. Totoritis MC, Tan EM, McNally EM, et al: Association of antibody to histone complex H2A-H2B with symptomatic procainamide-induced lupus, *N Engl J Med* 318:1431-1436, 1988.

Anti-Jo 1 (Histidyl tRNA synthetase)			None known.

1. Rubin RL: Antihistone antibodies. In Lahita RG, editor: *Systemic lupus erythematosus,* ed 2, New York, 1987, Churchill Livingstone, pp. 247-271.
2. Totoritis MC, Tan EM, McNally EM, et al: Association of antibody to histone complex H2A-H2B with symptomatic procainamide-induced lupus, *N Engl J Med* 318:1431-1436, 1988.

DIAGNOSTIC INFORMATION	REMARKS

Antihistone antibodies occur in patients with drug-induced LE but are also found in patients with idiopathic LE.[1] Drug-induced LE patients usually do not have antibodies to dsDNA.

Antihistone antibodies in patients with drug-induced LE react with H2A-H2B dimer. Patients with idiopathic LE also have antihistone antibodies that react with these antigens and with other classes of histones.[2] Commercial EIAs do not identify antihistone antibodies with H2A-H2B reactivity exclusively, and the results cannot be relied on to distinguish drug-induced from idiopathic LE.

Anti-Jo 1 antibodies occur in patients with myositis with a frequency that approaches 20%.[1]

Jo-1 protein is a member of the amino-acyl tRNA synthetase family. Anti-Jo1 antibodies are specific for myositis but occur in a minority of patients with this CTD. Myositis is a heterogeneous disease, and anti-Jo-1 antibodies identify a subset of patients who frequently have symmetrical polyarthritis and pulmonary fibrosis.[2]

TEST NAME AND METHOD	SPECIMEN REQUIREMENTS	REFERENCE INTERVAL, CONVENTIONAL [INTERNATIONAL RECOMMENDED UNITS]			CHEMICAL INTERFERENCES AND IN VIVO EFFECTS
Antimony (Sb)[1,2] *Quantitative: NAA*[3]	Plasma. Collect in pretested, metal-free container.	*mcg/dL* 0.052 ± 0.019 (SD)	× 82.1	*nmol/L* [4.3 ± 1.6]	None found.
AAS	Urine, 24 hr. Collect in acid-washed, metal-free container. Stable indefinitely at room temperature.	<10 mcg/L[2] Toxic concentration: >1.0 mg/L	× 8.21 × 8.21	[<82.1 nmol/L] [>8.21 mmol/L]	
AAS, NAA[4]	Liver	*mcg/kg dry wt.* 1.3-76	× 8.21	*nmol/g dry wt.* 11-624	
ICP-MS	Whole blood.[5] Collect in pretested, metal-free container.	*mcg/dL* 0-0.6	× 82.1	*nmol/L* [0.0-49.3]	
	Urine.[5] Collect in acid-washed, metal-free container. Refrigerate during and after collection.	*mcg/L* 0-2 *mcg/day* 0-2.5	× 8.21	*μg/L* [0-16.4] [0-20.5]	

1. Wyngaarden JB, Smith LH Jr, editors: *Cecil textbook of medicine,* ed 18, Philadelphia, 1988, WB Saunders.
2. Klaasen CD, Amdur MO, Doull J, editors: *Casarett and Doull's toxicology. The basic science of poisons,* ed 3, New York, 1986, Macmillan Pub. Co., Inc.
3. Kasperek K, Iyengar GV, Kiem J, et al: Elemental composition of platelets. Part III. Determinations of Ag, Au, Cd, Co, Cr, Cs, Mo, Rb, Sb, and Se in normal human platelets by neutron activation analysis, *Clin Chem* 25:711-715, 1979.
4. Iyengar GV, Woittiez J: Trace elements in human clinical specimens: evaluation of literature data to identify tolerence values, *Clin Chem* 34:474-481, 1988.
5. Associated Regional & University Pathologists, Inc. web site (www.aruplab.com): Available at: http://www.aruplab.com/testing/user_guide.jsp. Last accessed 9/2004.
6. Murray HW: Kala-azar—Progress against a neglected disease (editorial), *N Engl J Med* 347:1793-1794, 2002.
7. Abdulrhaman AA, Ibrahim EA, De Vol EB, et al: Fluconazole for the treatment of cutaneous leishmaniasis caused by leishmania major, *N Engl J Med* 346:891-895, 2002.
8. Environmental Protection Agency Website: Antimony compounds. Available at: http://www.epa.gov/ttnatw01/hlthef/antimony.html. Accessed February 13, 2003.

Antimony compounds are found in a few medications.[6,7] Miners and workers in smelters or ore refineries are exposed to antimony, although industrial poisoning is rare. Vomiting is a prominent symptom of acute poisoning; other symptoms are similar to those of acute arsenic poisoning. Skin lesions called antimony spots (pustular rash around sweat and sebaceous glands).[8] Sb^{3+} is more abundant in erythrocytes; Sb^{5+} is more abundant in plasma. Stibine gas (SbH_3) is highly toxic. (Antimony and nascent H_2 are released by battery plates.) Chronic SbH_3 poisoning results in anemia, weight loss, and dermatitis. Urine is the preferred specimen for assessment of acute exposure.

See Table II-6.

TEST NAME AND METHOD	SPECIMEN REQUIREMENTS	REFERENCE INTERVAL, CONVENTIONAL [INTERNATIONAL RECOMMENDED UNITS]	CHEMICAL INTERFERENCES AND IN VIVO EFFECTS
Antinuclear Antibodies, Specific Autoantibodies *Solid-phase EIA; double immunodiffusion (ID)*	Same as for the generic ANA.	The reference ranges for the EIA method cited below are applicable to all tests for specific ANA autoantibodies except as noted. Different commercial EIA methods may have different reference ranges.	

1. Kavanaugh A, Tomar R, Reveille J, et al: Guidelines for clinical use of the antinuclear antibody test and tests for specific autoantibodies to nuclear antigens, *Arch Pathol Lab Med* 124:71-81, 2000.
2. Homburger HA, Larsen SA: Detection of specific antibodies. In Rich RR, Shearer WT, Strober W, et al, editors: *Clinical immunology: principles and practice, vol II,* St. Louis, 1996, Mosby Year Book, pp. 2096-2109.

Antinuclear Antibody (ANA), Generic *Indirect immunofluorescence (IFA); solid-phase EIA*	Serum. Frozen or refrigerated is preferable.	IFA: Results are expressed as titers (reciprocal of dilution). For example, using HEp2 substrate: Negative at 1-40 dilution is negative. Positive at 1-40 or > dilution is positive. Titers ≥160 are more often associated with detectable specific antibodies to nuclear antigens. EIA: Results are semiquantitative and are expressed in arbitrary units. For example: <1 U: Negative 1-3 U: Weakly positive 3-6 U: Positive >6 U: Strongly positive Results ≥3 U are more often associated with detectable specific antibodies to nuclear antigens.[1]	Positive results may be caused by numerous medications, including adrenergic antagonists. Acute and chronic viral infections (e.g., HIV and HCV) may cause positive results.

1. Homburger HA, Cahen YD, Griffiths J, et al: Detection of antinuclear antibodies: comparative evaluation of enzyme immunoassay and indirect immunofluorescence methods, *Arch Pathol Lab Med* 122:993-999, 1998.
2. Kavanaugh A, Tomar R, Reveille J, et al: Guidelines for clinical use of the antinuclear antibody test and tests for specific autoantibodies to nuclear antigens, *Arch Pathol Lab Med* 124:71-81, 2000.

DIAGNOSTIC INFORMATION	REMARKS
Tests for autoantibodies to specific nuclear antigens are performed to define the specificities of antibodies present in sera that test positive on the generic ANA test.[1]	Several of the specific antinuclear autoantibodies have strong associations with individual CTDs or are prognostic indicators.[1,2] Tests for any of the antibodies listed below are not useful if the test for generic ANA is negative.

The test for generic ANA is the most commonly performed screening test for autoantibodies in patients suspected of having a connective tissue disease (CTD). ANAs occur in both systemic and organic-specific autoimmune diseases. A positive ANA is common in CTD, especially lupus erythematosus for which a positive ANA is a diagnostic criterion. Positive ANAs occur with variable frequency in other CTDs, including rheumatoid arthritis, scleroderma, Sjogren syndrome, mixed connective tissue disease, CREST syndrome, and myositis. A positive ANA result (≥160 titer or ≥3 U) is consistent with the diagnosis of a CTD and indicates an increased likelihood of finding a specific autoantibody on second order testing.[1]

Anti-self-reactivity is an essential feature of the immune system, and low levels of autoantibodies to nuclear antigens are not necessarily an indication of disease. Weakly positive results occur in up to 20% of healthy women aged >40 yr. For purposes of testing in a diagnostic algorithm, it is not indicated to test for specific autoantibodies in sera that give weakly reactive ANA results. IFA and EIA methods are comparable for diagnostic purposes in most clinical situations. Patterns of nuclear fluorescence observed by IFA are not specific for common autoantibodies except centromere (CREST syndrome). As an indicator of disease activity it is not useful to repeat the test for generic ANA in patients with known diagnoses of CTD.[2]

TEST NAME AND METHOD	SPECIMEN REQUIREMENTS	REFERENCE INTERVAL, CONVENTIONAL [INTERNATIONAL RECOMMENDED UNITS]	CHEMICAL INTERFERENCES AND IN VIVO EFFECTS
Antiphospholipid Antibodies (includes antibodies to β-2 glycoprotein 1, anticardiolipin antibodies, and antibodies to phosphatidylserine; includes also IgM, IgG and IgA isotypes) *Solid-phase EIA*	Serum or plasma (citrate anticoagulant). Ambient, refrigerated, or frozen.	Results are reported in arbitrary units, as follows: IgG or IgA antibodies: < or = 15 GPL or APL-negative 15-40 GPL or APL-weakly positive 30-80-GPL or APL-positive >80 GPL or APL-strongly positive IgM antibodies: < or = 10 MPL-negative 10-40 MPL-weakly positive 30 to 80-MPL-positive >80 MPL-strongly positive	Antiphospholipid antibodies have been described in many clinical settings including systemic rheumatic diseases (especially lupus erythematosus), infectious diseases, HIV-positive individuals and may be drug induced. Weakly positive test results have low positive predictive values for APS.[1]

1. Ware Branch D, Khamashta MA: Antiphospholipid syndrome: Obstetric diagnosis, management, and controversies, *Am Coll Obst Gynecol* 101:1333-1344, 2003.
2. Arnout J, Vermylen J: Current status and implications of autoimmune antiphospholipid antibodies in relation to thrombotic disease, *J Thrombos Haemost* 1:931-942, 2003.
3. Bas de Laat H, Derksen Ronald HWN, de Groot PG: β₂-Glycoprotein I, the playmaker of the antiphospholipid syndrome, *Clin Immunol* 112:161-168, 2004.

α₂-Antiplasmin[1,2]	Plasma (blue top-citrate). Stable for 2 hr at 4° C, 4 hr on ice, or store frozen.	*Functional (chromogenic):* 80-120% (0.8-1.2 U/mL) *Antigen (rocket electroimmunoassay):* Antigen: 48-80 mg/dL Antigenic determinations may give proportionally higher or lower values than functional tests.	↓ V Anistreplase, streptokinase, and urokinase

1. Jacobs DS, Demott WR, Oxley DK, editors: *Laboratory test handbook*, ed 5, Hudson, OH, 2001, Lexi-Comp, Inc.
2. Griffin GC, Mammen EF, Sokol RJ, et al: Alpha 2-antiplasmin deficiency. An overlooked cause of hemorrhage, *Am J Pediatr Hematol Oncol* 15:328-330, 1993.

DIAGNOSTIC INFORMATION	REMARKS

Measurement of antiphospholipid antibodies is useful in the evaluation of patients with thrombosis or possible antiphospholipid syndrome (APS), including patients with unexplained thrombosis, recurrent pregnancy loss (usually in the second or third trimester) or thrombocytopenia. APS may account for up to 20% of cases of deep venous thrombosis and up to 33% of strokes in patients <50 y. The diagnosis of APS requires the demonstration of positive or strongly positive tests for IgG or IgM antiphospholipid antibodies on 2 or more occasions at least 6 wk apart in an immunoassay for β_2-glycoprotein 1 dependent antibodies.[1]

Antiphospholipid antibodies react in vitro with a non-covalent complex formed from negatively charged phospholipid and β_2-glycoprotein 1.[1] Several anionic phospholipids, including cardiolipin and phosphatidylserine, have been used as reagents in immunoassays to detect these auto antibodies. Accordingly, the antibodies may be named with reference to the phospholipid antigen, e.g. anticardiolipin antibodies. Antiphospholipid antibodies have specificity for one or more of the 5 antigenic domains of β_2-glycoprotein 1, a 37 kDa protein. These antibodies produce prolongation of phospholipid dependent coagulation tests in vitro, so called lupus anticoagulant activity; and they promote binding of β_2-glycoprotein 1 to platelets and endothelial cells which may promote thrombosis in vivo.[2]

Hereditary α_2-antiplasmin deficiency is associated with a severe bleeding tendency (homozygous) or mild or asymptomatic disorder (heterozygous).

Acquired α_2-antiplasmin deficiency may be seen in liver disease, DIC, thrombolytic therapy, nephrotic syndrome, amyloidosis, or cancer.

Antiplasmin is a component of the fibrinolytic system and serves mainly as a physiologic inhibitor of plasmin. Hereditary deficiency of antiplasmin is rare and is classified as type I (quantitative: decreased antigen and functional levels) and type II (qualitative: normal antigen levels but decreased functional levels).

Homozygotes have severe hemorrhagic manifestations. Heterozygotes, typically with a 30-50% reference range, may have a mild bleeding disorder.

α_2-Antiplasmin levels increase with age. Estrogen from oral contraceptives or pregnancy may also increase plasma concentrations.

TEST NAME AND METHOD	SPECIMEN REQUIREMENTS	REFERENCE INTERVAL, CONVENTIONAL [INTERNATIONAL RECOMMENDED UNITS]	CHEMICAL INTERFERENCES AND IN VIVO EFFECTS
Anti-Scl 70 (Topoisomerase 1)			Weakly positive results for anti-Scl 70 antibodies may occur in sera with high levels of anti-dsDNA antibodies when tests are performed by EIA methods.

1. Homburger HA, Larsen SA: Detection of specific antibodies. In Rich RR, Shearer WT, Strober W, et al, editors: *Clinical immunology: principles and practice, vol II*, St. Louis, 1996, Mosby Year Book, Inc., pp 2096-2109.
2. Kavanaugh A, Tomar R, Reveille J, et al: Guidelines for clinical use of the antinuclear antibody test and tests for specific autoantibodies to nuclear antigens, *Arch Pathol Lab Med* 124:71-81, 2000.

Anti-Sm			None known.

1. Homburger HA, Larsen SA: Detection of specific antibodies. In Rich RR, Shearer WT, Strober W, et al, editors: *Clinical immunology: principles and practice, vol II*, St. Louis, 1996, Mosby Year Book, Inc., pp 2096-2109.

Anti-SSA/Ro		ID: Results are expressed qualitatively. Negative is normal. Presence of a precipitin with identity to a known autoantibody is positive, e.g., anti-SSA/Ro identity. EIA: Results are semiquantitative and are expressed in arbitrary units. For example: <20 U: Negative 20-25 U: Equivocal >25 U: Positive	None known.

1. Homburger HA, Larsen SA: Detection of specific antibodies. In Rich RR, Shearer WT, Strober W, et al, editors: *Clinical immunology: principles and practice, vol II*, St. Louis, 1996, Mosby Year Book, Inc., pp 2096-2109.

DIAGNOSTIC INFORMATION	REMARKS
Anti-Scl 70 antibodies occur in patients with scleroderma (systemic sclerosis) with a frequency that approaches 60% when tests are performed by EIA.[1]	Scl-70 (topoisomerase 1) is a 70 kDa protein antigen. Anti-Scl 70 autoantibodies are specific for scleroderma and are associated with extensive cutaneous disease and an increased risk of interstitial pulmonary fibrosis.[2]
Anti-Sm antibodies occur in patients with LE. The frequency of finding anti-Sm antibodies varies with technique, approaching 30% when tests are performed by EIA.[1]	Sm is a small nuclear ribonucleoprotein comprising several protein antigens that vary in size from 11-26 kDa complexed to snRNAs. The proteins are designated B, B′, D, E, F, and G. Most commercial EIAs do not test specifically for anti-Sm but detect anti-Sm in combination with anti-U1RNP (so-called Sm/RNP reactivity). Specific anti-Sm reactivity is inferred from the finding of a positive result for Sm/RNP with a negative result for U1RNP.
Anti-SSA/Ro antibodies occur in patients with CTDs, including Sjogren syndrome, lupus erythematosus (LE), and rheumatoid arthritis.[1]	SSA/Ro is a saline extractable nuclear antigen comprising protein antigens of 52 and 60 kDa. Presence of anti-SSA/Ro is associated with an increased risk of neonatal LE and congenital complete heart block in infants born to mothers with LE.[2] Anti-SSA/Ro is also associated with features of extraglandular inflammation, including vasculitis, purpura, cytopenias, and adenopathy in patients with LE and other CTDs.

Kavanaugh A, Tomar R, Reveille J, et al: Guidelines for clinical use of the antinuclear antibody test and tests for specific autoantibodies to nuclear antigens, *Arch Pathol Lab Med* 124:71-81, 2000.

TEST NAME AND METHOD	SPECIMEN REQUIREMENTS	REFERENCE INTERVAL, CONVENTIONAL [INTERNATIONAL RECOMMENDED UNITS]	CHEMICAL INTERFERENCES AND IN VIVO EFFECTS
Anti-SSB/La			None known.

1. Homburger HA, Larsen SA: Detection of specific antibodies. In Rich RR, Shearer WT, Strober W, et al, editors: *Clinical immunology: principles and practice, vol II,* St. Louis, 1996, Mosby Year Book, Inc., pp 2096-2109.

TEST NAME AND METHOD	SPECIMEN REQUIREMENTS	REFERENCE INTERVAL, CONVENTIONAL [INTERNATIONAL RECOMMENDED UNITS]	CHEMICAL INTERFERENCES AND IN VIVO EFFECTS
Antithrombin (previously known as Antithrombin III, AT-III)[1]	Plasma (blue top-citrate). Stable up to 4 hr on ice or store frozen.	Variable depending on method. For chromogenic assays, generally 80-120% of standard. Newborns have lower AT levels (~60-80%). For antigenic assays, results may be reported as 21-30 mg/dL × 10 [210-300 mg/L]. Each laboratory should establish its own reference range. Note: Most deficiency cases are heterozygous with levels ~50% of normal (generally levels between 45-75%). In some patients with variant mutations, assay results may be close to normal.	↑ Coumadin, myocardial infarction ↓ Heparin therapy, asparaginase, estrogens, and oral contraceptives

1. Kottke-Marchant K, Duncan A: Antithrombin deficiency. Issues in laboratory diagnosis, *Arch Pathol Lab Med* 126:1326-1336, 2002.

TEST NAME AND METHOD	SPECIMEN REQUIREMENTS	REFERENCE INTERVAL, CONVENTIONAL [INTERNATIONAL RECOMMENDED UNITS]				CHEMICAL INTERFERENCES AND IN VIVO EFFECTS
α_1-Antitrypsin (α_1-Trypsin Inhibitor, α_1-AT, AAT, α_1-Proteinase Inhibitor, α_1-PI)[1-4]	Serum, plasma (EDTA). Stable ≥7 days at 4° C, 3 mo at −70° C. Separate serum immediately and store properly before assay.		*mg/dL*[5]		*g/L*	S ↑ V Estrogens, oral contraceptives, oxymetholone and tamoxifen
		Newborn:	145-270	× 0.01	[1.45-2.70]	
		Adult (M-phenotype):	78-200		[0.78-2.00]	
		>60 yr:	115-200		[1.15-2.00]	

DIAGNOSTIC INFORMATION	REMARKS
Anti-SSB/La antibodies occur in patients with CTDs, including Sjogren syndrome and LE. Anti-SSB/La antibodies are somewhat less common than anti-SSA/Ro in these diseases.[1]	SSB/La is a saline extractable nuclear antigen comprising a 47 kDa protein antigen. This autoantibody is rarely found in the absence of anti-SSA/Ro.

↓ Hereditary deficiency, consumption (thrombosis, DIC, surgery), decreased production (liver disease, L-asparaginase treatment), proteinuria (nephrotic syndrome), and elevated estrogen levels (oral contraceptives, pregnancy).	Antithrombin deficiency, hereditary or acquired, may be associated with an increased risk of thrombosis. Hereditary deficiency is classified as type I quantitative (antigenic) and type II qualitative (functional). Different methods are available to measure antigenic or functional deficiency. The functional assays may be chromogenic or, less commonly, clot based. These assays are based on the reaction with either thrombin or factor Xa (different susceptibility to interferences from thrombin inhibitors such as hirudin). The antigenic assay is immunological (ELISA, immunoelectrophoresis, latex agglutination). A screening functional assay (activity) can be done first; if abnormal, a follow-up antigenic assay can then distinguish between type I and II deficiencies. Because of the many acquired causes of decreased antithrombin levels, an abnormal antithrombin should be repeated, ideally when known conditions of decreased AT (e.g., liver disease) are no longer present. Correlation with family history and testing of relatives may also be informative. Of note, patients with antithrombin deficiency may demonstrate heparin resistance.

↑ Acute phase reacting protein. Increased in inflammation, infection, tissue injury or necrosis, rheumatic diseases, and some malignancies. Also increased with estrogen (oral contraceptives[7]; pregnancy, especially third trimester, when levels can be two times normal[8]) and hepatic inflammation.[9]	α_1-Antitrypsin is normally the major constituent of the α_1-band on routine serum protein electrophoresis. It is an antiprotease that belongs to the serpin family of proteins, which includes α_1-antichymotrypsin, α_2 antiplasmin, plasminogen activator I, thyroxine-binding globulin, cortisol-binding globulin,

TEST NAME AND METHOD	SPECIMEN REQUIREMENTS	REFERENCE INTERVAL, CONVENTIONAL [INTERNATIONAL RECOMMENDED UNITS]	CHEMICAL INTERFERENCES AND IN VIVO EFFECTS
α₁-Antitrypsin—CONT			
Turbidimetric, Nephelometric[5] *RID*[3] *IEP*[3]	Cord blood. Analyze fresh or store at 4° C for <72 hr. Stable frozen at −20° C for 6 mo, or at −70° C indefinitely. Specimens without lipemia or hemolysis are preferred.	Serum AAT levels in inherited deficiency, Pi MS: 80% of Pi MM level Pi MZ, SS, or M null: 50-60% of Pi MM Pi SZ: 35-40% of Pi MM Pi ZZ or Z null: 10-20% of Pi MM Pi null (rare): Undetectable Values are low in fetuses at 25 wk of gestation and reach adult concentrations between 25 wk and term.	False positive: Rheumatoid factor[6]

1. Cox DW, Johnson AM, Fagerhol MK: Report of Nomenclature Meeting for α1-antitrypsin, *Hum Genet* 53:429-433, 1980.

2. Fagerhol MK, Laurell CB: The polymorphism of "prealbumins" and α1-antitrypsin in human sera, *Clin Chim Acta* 16:199-203, 1967.

3. Coakley RJ, Taggart C, O'Neill S, et al: α1-Antitrypsin deficiency, biological answers and clinical questions, *Am J Med Sc* 321:33-41, 2001.

4. Crystal RG: α1-Antitrypsin deficiency, emphysema and liver disease: genetic basis and strategies for therapy, *J Clin Invest* 85:1343-1852, 1990.

5. Tietz NW, Blackburn RH, editors: *Reference ranges and general information,* Lexington, KY, 1986, Clinical Laboratory, AB Chandler Medical Center, University of Kentucky; values partially established at the University of Kentucky Medical Center.

↓ Deficiency states (hereditary). Manifestations include pulmonary emphysema by third or fourth decade of life, COPD, especially in smokers,[3] hepatic disease (hepatitis, cholestasis, eventual cirrhosis or hepatocellular carcinoma) particularly beginning in childhood,[3,10,11] and ulcerative neutrophilic cutaneous panniculitis.[3]

Decreased values can also be caused by excessive catabolism as occurs with idiopathic respiratory distress syndrome of infancy,[12,13] neonatal hepatitis syndrome,[12,14] and severe pancreatic[12,15] or liver disease. Levels are also low with the nephrotic syndrome if inflammation is absent. Consequently, phenotyping studies are recommended to confirm a suspected hereditary deficiency.

angiotensinogen, protease nexin I, kallistatin, and leukocyte inhibitor.[3] The inhibitory activity of α1-AT is against the serine proteases, including neutrophil elastase, cathepsin G, and proteinase 3 released from neutrophil leukocytes during phagocytosis.[3] Most of the serum α_1-AT is hepatic in origin, although it is also produced by other cell types, such as neutrophils, monocytes, and enterocytes.[3,16] Because of its relatively small molecular size, it diffuses readily and is found in nearly all body fluids.[12]

More than 75 allelic variants of α_1-AT are known that are identifiable in serum.[1-3] The gene for α_1-AT is on the q arm of chromosome 14.[3] More than 90% of clinically significant cases of α_1-AT deficiency are caused by the Pi* ZZ mutation.[3] A single amino acid substitution (Gly^{342} to Lys^{342}) appears to be the cause of the Z mutation.[3,17] Genetic deficiency is associated with liver disease, especially in children (neonatal hepatitis syndrome and infantile cirrhosis),[14,18] an increased risk of hepatocellular carcinoma,[3,19] and with chronic lung disease in adults (emphysema, COPD, and chronic bronchitis, especially in smokers).[20]

Therapeutic measures include avoidance of smoking, hepatic transplantation, and exogenous α_1-AT.

Serum or plasma left in contact with leukocytes contaminated with bacteria may show fragmentation of this protein and on assay may give spuriously high or low values.

Indications for quantitation include a visibly diminished α_1-band on serum protein electrophoresis, pulmonary emphysema by the third or fourth decade of life, COPD, hepatic disease in childhood, and ulcerative neutrophilic cutaneous panniculitis.

MW: 54,000
$t_{1/2}$:   4 days

6.   Banks RE, Evans SW, Taylor KF, et al: Measurement of plasma concentrations of polymorphonuclear elastase-α1 proteinase inhibitor (elastase-α1 antitrypsin) in patients with rheumatoid arthritis: interference by rheumatoid factor, *Ann Rheum Dis* 49:18-21, 1990.

7.   Laurell CB, Kullander S, Thorell J: Effect of administration of a combined estrogen-progestin contraceptive on the level of individual plasma proteins, *Scand J Clin Lab Invest* 21:337-343, 1968.

8.   Ganrot PO, Bjerre B: α1-Antitrypsin and α2-macroglobulin concentrations in serum during pregnancy, *Acta Obstet Gynecol Scand* 46:126-137, 1967.

9.   Kindmark CO, Laurell CB: Sequential changes of the plasma protein pattern in inoculation hepatitis, *Scand J Clin Lab Invest* 29(suppl 124):105-115, 1972.

TEST NAME AND METHOD	SPECIMEN REQUIREMENTS	REFERENCE INTERVAL, CONVENTIONAL [INTERNATIONAL RECOMMENDED UNITS]	CHEMICAL INTERFERENCES AND IN VIVO EFFECTS

α₁-Antitrypsin—CONT

10. Eriksson S, Carlson J, Velez R: Risk of cirrhosis and primary liver cancer in α1-antitrypsin deficiency, *N Engl J Med* 314:736-739, 1986.

11. Sveger T: The natural history of liver disease in α1-antitrypsin deficient children, *Acta Pediatr Scand* 77:847-851, 1988.

12. Tietz NW, editor: *Textbook of clinical chemistry,* Philadelphia, 1999, WB Saunders.

13. Evans HE, Levi M, Mandl I: Serum enzyme inhibitor concentrations in the respiratory distress syndrome, *Am Rev Respir Dis* 101:359-363, 1970.

14. Johnson AM, Alper CA: Deficiency of α1-antitrypsin in childhood liver disease, *Pediatrics* 46:921-925, 1970.

15. Dubick MA, Mar G, Mayer AD, et al: Digestive enzymes and protease inhibitors in plasma from patients with acute pancreatitis, *Pancreas* 2:187-194, 1987.

Anti-U1RNP

None known.

1. Homburger HA, Larsen SA: Detection of specific antibodies. In Rich RR, Shearer WT, Strober W, et al, editors: *Clinical immunology: principles and practice, vol II,* St. Louis, 1996, Mosby Year Book, Inc., pp 2096-2109.

2. Kavanaugh A, Tomar R, Reveille J, et al: Guidelines for clinical use of the antinuclear antibody test and tests for specific autoantibodies to nuclear antigens, *Arch Pathol Lab Med* 124:71-81, 2000.

Apolipoprotein A-I (Apo A-I)[1-12]

Immunoassay[1,2,6]

Electrophoresis[1,13,14]

Chromatography[1]

Serum, plasma. Fasting is not required. Stable for 4-7 days at 4° C and for at least 6 mo at −70° C. Avoid repeated freezing and thawing.

	mg/dL[15] 5th-95th Percentile		*g/L* 5th-95th Percentile
4-5 yr			
M:	109-172	× 0.01	[1.09-1.72]
F:	104-163		[1.04-1.63]
6-11 yr			
M:	111-177		[1.11-1.77]
F:	110-166		[1.10-1.66]
12-19 yr			
M:	99-165		[0.99-1.65]
F:	105-180		[1.05-1.80]
20-29 yr			
M:	105-173		[1.05-1.73]
F:	111-209		[1.11-2.09]
30-39 yr			
M:	105-173		[1.05-1.73]
F:	110-189		[1.10-1.89]
40-49 yr			
M:	103-178		[1.03-1.78]
F:	115-195		[1.15-1.95]

↑ V Estrogens, moderate alcohol consumption, HMG CoA reductase inhibitors (statins), niacin, phenobarbital, phenytoin, prednisolone, pregnancy, weight loss in overweight individuals, and exercise.

↓ V Androgens, diuretics (thiazides, chlorothalidone), probucol, stanazolol, cigarette smoking, diets high in carbohydrates or fiber, hospitalization for AMI, stroke, and cardiac catheterization.

DIAGNOSTIC INFORMATION	REMARKS

16. Carlson JA, Rogers BB, Sifers RN, et al: Multiple tissues express α1-antitrypsin in transgenic mice and man, *J Clin Invest* 82:26-36, 1988.
17. Yoshida A, Lieberman J, Gaidulis L, et al: Molecular abnormality of human α1-antitrypsin variant (Pi-ZZ) associated with plasma activity deficiency, *Proc Natl Acad Sci USA* 73:1324-1328, 1976.
18. Sharp HL, Bridges RA, Krivit W, et al: Cirrhosis associated with α1-antitrypsin deficiency, *J Lab Clin Med* 73:934-939, 1969.
19. Erikkson S, Hägerstarnd I: Cirrhosis and malignant hepatoma in α1-antitrypsin deficiency, *Acta Med Scand* 195:451-458, 1974.
20. Eriksson S: Proteases and protease inhibitors in chronic obstructive lung disease, *Acta Med Scand* 203:449-455, 1978.

Anti-U1RNP antibodies occur with varying frequencies in patients with several of the CTDs, especially LE and mixed connective tissue disease (MCTD).[1]

U1RNP is a small nuclear ribonucleoprotein that contains 22, 33, and 70 kDa protein antigens complexed with U1snRNA. When found in isolation (anti-dsDNA and anti-Sm antibodies are undetectable), presence of anti-U1RNP suggests the diagnosis of MCTD. MCTD resembles LE but less frequently has renal involvement.[2]

↑ Familial hyperalphalipoproteinemia, familial cholesteryl ester transfer protein (CETP) deficiency.

↓ Familial hypoalphalipoproteinemia, apo A-I variants (e.g., apo A-I Milano), fish eye disease, familial lecithin-cholesterol acyltransferase (LCAT) deficiency, Tangier disease, familial apo A-I deficiency (with or without apo CIII/apo A-IV deficiency), coronary heart disease, hepatocellular disorders, cholestasis, nephrotic syndrome, chronic renal failure, and malignancy.

Measurement of apo A-I, the major protein component of HDL particles, is useful for characterizing low HDL cholesterol concentrations in individuals and families. Apo A-I measurement may also be useful for assessing CHD risk, although there is debate as to whether apo A-I is better than HDL-cholesterol measurement.

Intraindividual variability in apo A-I measurement averages 7-8%.

Apo A-I methods should be standardized using WHO/IFCC international reference materials.

TEST NAME AND METHOD	SPECIMEN REQUIREMENTS	REFERENCE INTERVAL, CONVENTIONAL [INTERNATIONAL RECOMMENDED UNITS]	CHEMICAL INTERFERENCES AND IN VIVO EFFECTS

Apolipoprotein A-1—CONT

50-59 yr			
M:	107-173	[1.07-1.73]	
F:	117-211	[1.17-2.11]	
60-65 yr			
M:	111-184	[1.11-1.84]	
F:	120-205	[1.20-2.05]	
70+ yr			
M:	119-180	[1.19-1.80]	
F:	118-199	[1.18-1.99]	

Recommended Cutpoint[16]

>120 mg/dL × 0.01 [>1.20 g/L]

1. Bradley WA, Gianturco SH, Segrest JP, editors: *Plasma lipoproteins, part C: quantitation. Methods in enzymology, vol 263,* San Diego, 1996, Academic Press.

2. Laker MF, Evans K: Analysis of apolipoproteins, *Ann Clin Biochem* 33:5-22, 1996.

3. Luc G, Bard JM, Ferrieres J, et al: Value of HDL cholesterol, apolipoprotein A-I, lipoprotein A-I, and lipoprotein A-I/A-II in prediction of coronary heart disease: the PRIME Study, *Arterioscler Thromb Vasc Biol* 22:1155-1161, 2002.

4. Marcovina SM, Albers JJ, Henderson LO, et al: International Federation of Clinical Chemistry standardization project for measurement of apolipoproteins A-I and B. III. Comparability of apolipoprotein A-I values by use of international reference material, *Clin Chem* 39:773-781, 1993.

5. Rader DJ, Hoeg JM, Brewer HB: Quantitation of plasma apolipoproteins in the primary and secondary prevention of coronary artery disease, *Ann Intern Med* 120:1012-1025, 1994.

6. Rifai N, Warnick GR, Dominiczak MH, editors: *Handbook of lipoprotein testing,* ed 2, Washington, DC, 2000, AACC Press.

7. Sniderman AD, Furberg CD, Keech A, et al: Apolipoproteins versus lipids as indices of coronary risk and as targets for statin treatment, *Lancet* 361:777-780, 2003.

8. Walldius G, Jungner I: Apolipoprotein B and apolipoprotein A-I: risk indicators of coronary heart disease and targets for lipid-modifying therapy, *J Intern Med* 255:188-205, 2004.

9. Walldius G, Jungner I, Holme I, et al: High apolipoprotein B, low apolipoprotein A-I, and improvement in the prediction of fatal myocardial infarction (AMORIS study): a prospective study, *Lancet* 358:2026-2033, 2001.

10. Wang M, Briggs MR: HDL: the metabolism, function, and therapeutic importance, *Chem Rev* 104:119-137, 2004.

11. Young DS: *Effects of drugs on clinical laboratory tests,* ed 5, Washington, DC, 2000, AACC Press.

12. Young DS: *Effects of preanalytical variables on clinical laboratory tests,* ed 2, Washington, DC, 1997, AACC Press.

13. Lehmann R, Freiss U, Haring HU, et al: Investigation of a capillary electrophoretic approach for direct quantification of apolipoprotein A-I in serum, *Electrophoresis* 24:1422-1428, 2003.

14. Ordovas JM, editor: *Lipoprotein protocols,* Totowa, NJ, 1998, Humana Press.

15. Bachorik PS, Lovejoy KL, Carroll MD, et al: Apolipoprotein B and AI distributions in the United States, 1988-1991: results of the National Health and Nutrition Examination Survey III (NHANES III), *Clin Chem* 43:2364-2378, 1997.

16. Contois JH, McNamara JR, Lammi-Keefe CJ, et al: Reference intervals for apolipoprotein A-I determined with a commercially available immunoturbidimetric assay: results from the Framingham Offspring Study, *Clin Chem* 42:507-514, 1996.

DIAGNOSTIC INFORMATION	REMARKS

TEST NAME AND METHOD	SPECIMEN REQUIREMENTS	REFERENCE INTERVAL, CONVENTIONAL [INTERNATIONAL RECOMMENDED UNITS]		CHEMICAL INTERFERENCES AND IN VIVO EFFECTS
Apolipoprotein B (Apo B)[1-15] *Immunoassay*[2,4,9] *Electrophoresis*[2,16] *Chromatography*[2]	Serum, plasma. Fasting is not required. Stable for 4-7 days at 4° C and at least 6 mo at −70° C (slight decrease with freezing). Avoid repeated freezing and thawing.	*mg/dL*[17] *5th-95th Percentile*	*g/L* *5th-95th Percentile*	↑ V Androgens (anabolic steroids), β-blockers, cyclosporine, diuretics, retinoids, corticosteroids, high saturated fat and high cholesterol diets, prednisolone, and progestins.
		4-5 yr		
		M: 58-103 × 0.01	[0.58-1.03]	
		F: 58-104	[0.58-1.04]	
		6-11yr		
		M: 56-105	[0.56-1.05]	
		F: 57-113	[0.57-1.13]	↓ V Bile acid sequestrants (resins, e.g., cholestyra-
		12-19 yr		mine, colestipol), estro-
		M: 55-110	[0.55-1.10]	gens, fibric acid deriva-
		F: 53-119	[0.53-1.19]	tives (e.g., clofibrate,
		20-29 yr		gemfibrozil), HMG-CoA
		M: 59-130	[0.59-1.30]	reductase inhibitors
		F: 63-132	[0.63-1.32]	(statins), high poly- and
		30-39 yr		mono-unsaturated fatty
		M: 63-143	[0.63-1.43]	acid and low cholesterol
		F: 59-132	[0.59-1.32]	diets, ketoconazole,
		40-49 yr		neomycin, niacin, probu-
		M: 71-152	[0.71-1.52]	col, thyroxine, hospital-
		F: 70-136	[0.70-1.36]	ization for AMI, stroke, or
		50-59 yr		cardiac catheterization.
		M: 75-160	[0.75-1.60]	
		F: 75-168	[0.75-1.68]	
		60-69 yr		
		M: 81-156	[0.81-1.56]	
		F: 75-173	[0.75-1.73]	
		70+ yr		
		M: 73-152	[0.73-1.52]	
		F: 79-168	[0.79-1.68]	
		Recommended Cutpoints[18]		
		Desirable: <100 mg/dL × 0.01	[<1.00]	
		High risk: >120 mg/dL	[>1.20]	

1. Bairaktari E, Hatzidimou K, Tzallas C, et al: Estimation of LDL cholesterol based on the Friedewald formula and on apo B levels, *Clin Biochem* 33:549-555, 2000.

2. Bradley WA, Gianturco SH, Segrest JP, editors: *Plasma lipoproteins, part C: quantitation. Methods in enzymology, vol 263,* San Diego, 1996, Academic Press.

3. Kronenberg F, Lobentanz E-M, Konig P, et al: Effect of sample storage on the measurement of lipoprotein[a], apolipoproteins B and A-IV, total and high density lipoprotein cholesterol and triglycerides, *J Lipid Res* 35:1318-1328, 1994.

4. Laker MF, Evans K: Analysis of apolipoproteins, *Ann Clin Biochem* 33:5-22, 1996.

5. Marcovina SM, Albers JJ, Kennedy H, et al: International Federation of Clinical Chemistry standardization project for measurement of apolipoproteins A-I and B. IV. Comparability of apolipoprotein B values by use of international reference material, *Clin Chem* 40:586-592, 1994.

6. Packard CJ: Understanding coronary heart disease as a consequence of defective regulation of apolipoprotein B metabolism, *Curr Opin Lipidol* 10:237-244, 1999.

DIAGNOSTIC INFORMATION	REMARKS

↑ Hyperapobetalipoproteinemia (normal LDL-C and elevated apo B), familial combined hyperlipidemia, familial hypercholesterolemia, familial defective apo B-100, polygenic (sporadic) hypercholesterolemia, coronary heart disease, diabetes, hypothyroidism, nephrotic syndrome, chronic renal failure, hepatic obstruction, hepatic disease, and Cushing's syndrome.

↓ Abetalipoproteinemia, hypobetalipoproteinemia, homozygous hypobetalipoproteinemia, hyperthyroidism, malnutrition, intestinal malabsorption, infection, and inflammation.

Apo B exists in two major forms, apo B-48 (synthesized in the intestine) and apo B-100 (synthesized in the liver). The assays commonly in use by clinical laboratories recognize both forms of apo B. Apo B is required for binding of LDL particles to the LDL receptor. Apo B measurement is useful to identify various lipoprotein abnormalities in individuals and families. Many studies indicate that apo B is a better marker for CHD risk than LDL cholesterol. The ratio of apo B/apo A-I also appears superior to the total cholesterol/HDL cholesterol ratio.

One apo B molecule is present on each LDL, IDL, and VLDL particle, and therefore apo B concentration reflects the total number of atherogenic particles in the circulation. Apo B measurement is particularly useful in identifying individuals who have an increased number of small, dense LDL but normal LDL cholesterol concentrations and are at increased risk of CHD.

Intraindividual variability in apo B measurement is ~8-10%. Apo B methods should be standardized using WHO/IFCC international reference materials.

7. Planella T, Cortes M, Martinez-Bru C, et al: Calculation of LDL-cholesterol by using apolipoprotein B for classification of nonchylomicronemic dyslipidemia, *Clin Chem* 43:808-815, 1997.

8. Rader DJ, Hoeg JM, Brewer HB: Quantitation of plasma apolipoproteins in the primary and secondary prevention of coronary artery disease, *Ann Intern Med* 120:1012-1025, 1994.

9. Rifai N, Warnick GR, Dominiczak MH, editors: *Handbook of lipoprotein testing,* ed 2, Washington, DC, 2000, AACC Press.

10. Sniderman AD: How, when, and why to use apolipoprotein B in clinical practice, *Am J Cardiol* 90(suppl):48i-54i, 2002.

11. Sniderman AD, Furberg CD, Keech A, et al: Apolipoproteins versus lipids as indices of coronary risk and as targets for statin treatment, *Lancet* 361:777-780, 2003.

12. Walldius G, Jungner I: Apolipoprotein B and apolipoprotein A-I: risk indicators of coronary heart disease and targets for lipid-modifying therapy, *J Intern Med* 255:188-205, 2004.

TEST NAME* AND METHOD	SPECIMEN REQUIREMENTS	REFERENCE INTERVAL, CONVENTIONAL [INTERNATIONAL RECOMMENDED UNITS]	CHEMICAL INTERFERENCES AND IN VIVO EFFECTS

Apolipoprotein B—CONT

13. Walldius G, Jungner I, Holme I, et al: High apolipoprotein B, low apolipoprotein A-I, and improvement in the prediction of fatal myocardial infarction (AMORIS study): a prospective study, *Lancet* 358:2026-2033, 2001.

14. Young DS: *Effects of drugs on clinical laboratory tests,* ed 5, Washington, DC, 2000, AACC Press.

15. Young DS: *Effects of preanalytical variables on clinical laboratory tests,* ed 2, Washington, DC, 1997, AACC Press.

16. Ordovas JM, editor: *Lipoprotein protocols,* Totowa, NJ, 1998, Humana Press.

Apt (Apt-Downey) Test [Fetal hemoglobin][1,2] *Colorimetric*	Feces, 1 part of stool to 5 or 10 parts of water (tap or distilled). Stool must be grossly bloody (red) and not tarry.	Change of pink hemoglobin solution to brown-yellow in 1-2 min indicates the presence of adult hemoglobin. Persistence of pink color indicates fetal hemoglobin.	None found.

1. Apt L, Downey WS: "Melena" neonatorum: the swallowed blood syndrome, *J Pediatr* 47:6-12, 1955.

Arginase (EC 3.5.3.1)[1-4]	Serum. Avoid hemolysis.	*U/L*		μ*Kat/L*	↑ C Hemolysis, Mn^{2+},
		0.8-7.9	× 0.017	[0.01-0.13]	Co^{2+}, Ni^{2+}, and Mg^{2+}
		M: x̄: 3.0		[0.05]	
Colorimetric, 37° C[2]		F: x̄: 2.9		[0.05]	↓ C Ag^{2+}, Hg^{2+}, Zn^{2+},

L-leucine, and

Fluorimetric, 37° C[3]	Dried blood spots on filter paper; store in freezer.	*U/g Hb (SD)*		*kU/mol Hb*	L-ornithine[2]
		Newborn: 20.9 ± 4.5	× 64.5*	[1348 ± 290]	
		Adult: 18.0 ± 4.2		[1161 ± 271]	

*Conversion factor based on MW of Hb of 64,500.

1. Guilbault GG: *Handbook of enzymatic methods of analysis,* New York, 1976, Marcel Dekker, Inc.

2. Mellerup B: Colorimetric method for rapid determination of serum arginase, *Clin Chem* 13:900-908, 1967.

3. Orfanos AP, Naylor EW, Guthrie R: Fluorometric micromethod for determination of arginase activity in dried blood spots in filter paper, *Clin Chem* 26:1198-1200, 1980.

4. Wilkinson JH: *The principles and practice of diagnostic enzymology,* Chicago, 1976, Year Book Medical Publishers, Inc.

---

*Arginine can be found in the Appendix on p. 1761.

DIAGNOSTIC INFORMATION	REMARKS

17. Bachorik PS, Lovejoy KL, Carroll MD, et al: Apolipoprotein B and AI distributions in the United States, 1988-1991: results of the National Health and Nutrition Examination Survey III (NHANES III), *Clin Chem* 43:2364-2378, 1997.
18. Contois JH, McNamara JR, Lammi-Keefe CJ, et al: Reference intervals for apolipoprotein B determined with a commercially available immunoturbidimetric assay: results from the Framingham Offspring Study, *Clin Chem* 42:515-523, 1996.

Bloody stools containing fetal hemoglobin indicate intrinsic fetal hemorrhage, whereas bloody stools containing Hb A (adult) usually indicate swallowing of maternal blood at parturition.	The test is based on the fact that fetal hemoglobin is more resistant than adult hemoglobin to denaturation with alkali. Bloody stools caused by intrinsic hemorrhage are usually passed 1 day after birth, whereas those caused by ingestion of maternal blood are usually passed within 12 hr after birth. The test can be modified by adding the water and sodium hydroxide directly to a blood-stained diaper. More sensitive spectrophotometric methods may be advantageous.

2. Sherman NJ, Clatworthy HW Jr: Gastrointestinal bleeding in neonates: a study of 94 cases, *Surgery* 62:614-619, 1967.

S ↑ Hepatocellular damage (e.g., cirrhosis, viral or toxic hepatitis, advanced hepatoma, fatty infiltration of the liver, megaloblastic anemias, thalassemia major), malignancy,[5] rheumatoid arthritis,[6] and depression[7]

S ↓ Hyperargininemia

A dried blood specimen represents the activity in erythrocytes and may be used to screen children or infants and potential carriers for arginase deficiency.

Arginase is not a sensitive test of hepatic damage because it increases late in the course of disease.

5. Porembska Z, Skwarek A, Mielczarek M, et al: Serum arginase activity in postsurgical monitoring of patients with colorectal carcinoma, *Cancer* 94:2930-2934, 2002.
6. Huang L, Chang K, Chen C, et al: Arginase levels are increased in patients with rheumatoid arthritis, *Kaohsiung J Med Sci* 17:358-363, 2001.
7. Elgun S, Kumbasar H: Increased serum arginase activity in depressed patients, *Prog Neuropsychopharmacol Biol Psychiatry* 24:227-232, 2000.

TEST NAME AND METHOD	SPECIMEN REQUIREMENTS	REFERENCE INTERVAL, CONVENTIONAL [INTERNATIONAL RECOMMENDED UNITS]			CHEMICAL INTERFERENCES AND IN VIVO EFFECTS
Argininosuccinate Lyase (ASAL; EC 4.3.2.1)[1-2] *Colorimetric*[3]	Serum. Avoid hemolysis. Perform assay within 24 hr of sample collection.	0-4 U/L	× 0.017	[0.00-0.07 μKat/L]	↑ C Hemolysis
Fluorimetric, 37° C[4]		<11 μmol/hr/L	× 0.0167	[<0.18 U/L]	
	Erythrocytes	μmol/hr/L packed Ercs 1120-2420	× 0.0167	U/L [18.7-40.4]	

1. Companini RZ, Tapia RA, Sarnat W, et al: Evaluation of serum argininosuccinate lyase (ASAL) concentrations as an index to parenchymal liver disease, *Clin Chem* 16:44-53, 1970.
2. Levin B: Arginosuccinic aciduria, *Am J Dis Child* 113:162-163, 1967.
3. Sims FH, Rautanen P: Serum argininosuccinate lyase: observations on the sensitivity and specificity of this test in the detection of minimal hepatocellular damage, *Clin Biochem* 8:213-221, 1975.
4. Sherwin JE, Natelson S: Serum and erythrocyte argininosuccinate lyase assay by NADH fluorescence generated from formed fumarate, *Clin Chem* 21:230-234, 1975.
5. Pelli N, Fensom AH, Slade C, et al: Argininosuccinate lyase: a new autoantigen in liver disease, *Clin Exp Immunol* 114:455-461, 1999.
6. Haberle J, Koch H: Genetic approach to prenatal diagnosis in urea cycle defects, *Prenat Diagn* 24:373-383, 2004.
7. Linnebank M, Tschiedel E, Haberle J, et al: Argininosuccinate lyase (ASL) deficiency: mutation analysis in 27 patients and a completed structure of the human ASL gene, *Hum Genet* 111:350-359, 2002.

TEST NAME AND METHOD	SPECIMEN REQUIREMENTS	REFERENCE INTERVAL, CONVENTIONAL [INTERNATIONAL RECOMMENDED UNITS]			CHEMICAL INTERFERENCES AND IN VIVO EFFECTS
Arsenic (As)[1-3] *Quantitative: Colorimetric, AAS, NAA*	Whole blood.[4] Collect in pretested, metal-free container.	*mcg/L* 2-23 Chronic poisoning: 100-500 Acute poisoning: 600-9300	× 0.0133	*μmol/L* [0.03-0.31] [1.33-6.65] [7.98-123.69]	None found.
AAS, NAA	Serum.[5] Collect in metal-free container.	1.7-15.4		[0.02-0.20]	
Colorimetric, AAS	Urine, 24 hr. Collect in acid-washed, metal-free container.	5-50 mcg/day[2,8] (x̄: 15) *mcg/L*[9] Chronic poisoning: 50-5000 Acute poisoning: 1000-20,000	× 0.0133 × 0.0133	[0.067-0.665 μmol/day] [x̄: 0.20] *μmol/L* [0.67-66.50] [13.3-266.0]	May be falsely elevated following ingestion of seafood. Speciation may be required to distinguish toxic from non-toxic forms.[10]

DIAGNOSTIC INFORMATION	REMARKS
↑ Acute viral hepatitis, toxic hepatitis, cirrhosis, diseases with secondary hepatic involvement (e.g., pulmonary disease, diabetes, congestive cardiac failure), post-GI surgical procedures such as cholecystectomy and gastrectomy, neoplastic diseases, and liver metastases	ASAL is more sensitive than ALT or AST in detecting hepatocellular disease.[1,3] Genetic assays now exist for detecting deficiency of this and other urea cycle enzymes.[6,7]
↓ Genetic deficiency of ASAL, mentally deficient patients with argininosuccinic aciduria,[2] and some autoimmune chronic hepatitis associated with antibodies to ASAL.[5]	

Symptoms of acute As poisoning are severe gastric pain, vomiting, and diarrhea, as well as convulsions, cardiovascular collapse, coma, and death. Symptoms of chronic As poisoning are diarrhea, pigmentation and scaling of skin, hyperkeratosis of palms and soles, hepatomegaly, hair loss, peripheral neuropathy, and Mees lines. Hematological changes in chronic arsenic poisoning include anemia, leukopenia, thrombocytopenia, basophilic stippling, disturbed erythropoiesis and myelopoiesis. Epidemiological studies suggest that arsenic is carcinogenic in humans. Experimental corroboration in animals is lacking.	Arsenic is found in house and garden pesticides. As is used as an antiparasitic agent in veterinary medicine and to treat trypanosomiasis and amebiasis in some countries. It occurs naturally in the environment and in food. As^{3+} is more toxic than As^{5+}. Industrial exposure in the manufacture of brass, bronze, ceramics, dye, wood products, and paint may result in As intoxication. As trioxide can induce remission in patients with acute promyelocytic leukemia who have relapsed after other therapies. Urine is the preferred specimen if symptoms are present or in cases of acute exposure. Urine, hair, and nail clippings should be assayed in cases of chronic exposure.

TEST NAME AND METHOD	SPECIMEN REQUIREMENTS	REFERENCE INTERVAL, CONVENTIONAL [INTERNATIONAL RECOMMENDED UNITS]		CHEMICAL INTERFERENCES AND IN VIVO EFFECTS
Arsenic—CONT				
	Hair; at least 1.0 g cut close to the scalp.[6] Wash to remove surface contamination.	*mcg/100 g dry wt.*	*nmol/g dry wt.*	
	Acceptable for industrial exposure:	<65	× 0.133 [<8.65]	
	Chronic poisoning[9]:	100-4700	[13.3-625.1]	
	Acute poisoning[9]:	20,000	[2660]	
	Nail; clippings from all fingers and toes.[6] Wash to remove surface contamination.	20-60	[2.66-7.98]	
	Acceptable for industrial exposure:	<180	[<23.94]	
ICP-MS	Whole blood.[7] Collect in pretested, metal-free container.	*mcg/L* 0-627	*μmol/L* [0.0-0.83]	
	Toxic:	>600	[≥7.98]	
	Urine.[7] Collect in acid-washed, metal-free container. Refrigerate during and after collection.	*mcg/L* 0-35 *mcg/day*[7] 0-50 *mcg/g creatinine* <35	[0.00-0.466] *μmol/day* [0.00-0.665] *μmol/g creatinine* [<0.466]	

1. Henry JB, editor: *Clinical diagnosis and management by laboratory methods,* ed 18, Philadelphia, 1991, WB Saunders.

2. Wyngaarden JB, Smith LH Jr, editors: *Cecil textbook of medicine,* ed 18, Philadelphia, 1988, WB Saunders.

3. Milne DB: Trace elements. In Burtis CA, Ashwood ER, editors: *Tietz textbook of clinical chemistry,* ed 2, Philadelphia, 1994, WB Saunders.

4. Beutler E: *Hemolytic anemia in disorders of red cell metabolism,* New York, 1978, Plenum Pub. Co.

5. Iyengar GV, Woittiez J: Trace elements in human clinical specimens: evaluation of literature data to identify reference values, *Clin Chem* 34:474-481, 1988.

6. Sunshine I, editor: *Methodology for analytical toxicology,* Cleveland, 1975, CRC Press.

7. Associated Regional & University Pathologists, Inc. web site (www.aruplab.com): Available at: http://www.aruplab.com/testing/user_guide.jsp. Last accessed 9/2004.

8. Chappuis P, Thuillier F, Rousselet F: Dosage des oligo-elements dans les humeurs et les tissues, *Gaz Med France* 87:2281-2288, 1980.

9. Baselt RC: *Analytical procedures for therapeutic drug monitoring and emergency toxicology,* ed 2, Littleton, MA, 1987, PSG Publishing Co., Inc.

10. Vahter M: What are the chemical forms of arsenic in urine, and what can they tell us about exposure? (editorial), *Clin Chem* 40:679-680, 1994.

DIAGNOSTIC INFORMATION   **REMARKS**

Surface contamination of hair or nails may not be completely removed by washing. Cutting washed hair into 1-cm segments and analyzing each group of segments separately can give a reliable indication of As concentration in hair versus time of exposure. Concentrations in urine or hair after acute exposure are a function of time.

TEST NAME* AND METHOD	SPECIMEN REQUIREMENTS	REFERENCE INTERVAL, CONVENTIONAL [INTERNATIONAL RECOMMENDED UNITS]	CHEMICAL INTERFERENCES AND IN VIVO EFFECTS
Ascites (Asc) Analysis[1]	Aspirate. Collect 5 mL in each of two EDTA tubes for cell counts and chemistry, aerobic and anaerobic blood culture vials, and up to 100 mL in heparin tubes for cytology. Diagnostic peritoneal lavage (DPL): Either aspirate 15 mL of bloody fluid or infuse 1 L of saline (20 mg/kg for small patients) and withdraw ≥600 mL. Send for cell counts.	(see table below)	Traumatic tap

ANALYSIS TABLE

Cell counts (Asc)	Sterile	Infected		Sterile	Infected
WBC (/μL)	<500	≥500	×0.001	[<0.5 × 10^9/L]	[>0.5 × 10^9/L]
ANC (/μL)	<250	≥250	×0.001	[<0.25 × 10^9/L]	[>0.25 × 10^9/L]
RBC (/μL)	<10^3	>10^5	×0.001	[<1 × 10^9/L]	[>100 × 10^9/L]

Chemistry	Transudate	Exudate		Transudate	Exudate
protein (g/dL)	≤1	≥1	×10	[<11 g/L]	[≥11 g/L]
SAAG (g/dL)	≥1.1	<1.1	×10	[≥11 g/L]	[<11 g/L]
Chol. (mg/dL)	≤55	>55	×0.026	[≤1.4 mmol/L]	[>1.4 mmol/L]

SBP, Spontaneous bacterial peritonitis.
SAAG, Serum–ascites albumin gradient.
ANC, Absolute neutrophil count.

1. Clarke W, Palmer-Toy DE: Clinical chemistry of urine, pleural effusions, and ascites. In Lewandrowski KB, editor: *Clinical chemistry,* Philadelphia, 2002, Lippincott Williams & Wilkins, pp 849-864.

TEST NAME* AND METHOD	SPECIMEN REQUIREMENTS	REFERENCE INTERVAL, CONVENTIONAL [INTERNATIONAL RECOMMENDED UNITS]			CHEMICAL INTERFERENCES AND IN VIVO EFFECTS
Aspartate Aminotransferase (AST, SGOT, L-Aspartate: 2-Oxoglutarate Aminotransferase; EC 2.6.1.1)[1] *Henry, optimized, 340 nm, 30° C*[2] *IFCC, with P-5'-P, 37° C*[3]	Serum. Stable 24 hr at room temperature, 28 days at 4° C, and at least 1 yr at −20° C. Adding pyridoxal phosphate (0.1 mmol/L) improves stability at room temperature to 7 days.[8]		*U/L*[9]		*μKat/L*	S ↑ Hepatotoxic drugs or drugs causing cholestasis (see Table II-5). Many other drugs can cause increases that are generally transient but may, in some cases, indicate hepatotoxicity. These include acebutolol, aminoglutethimide, aminoglycosides, azithromycin, bromocriptine, captopril, carboplatin, carmustine, cephalosporins, cyclosporine, clindamycin, clofibrate, clotrimazole, cytarabine, dacarbazine, dapsone, didanosine, disopyramide, enflurane, ethacrynic acid, ethambutol, etoposide, fenofibrate, fluoroquinolones (e.g., ciprofloxacin), ganci-
		Newborn:	25-75	×0.017	[0.43-1.28]	
		Infant:	15-60		[0.26-1.02]	
		Adult:	8-20		[0.14-0.34]	
		>60 yr				
		M[3]:	11-26		[0.19-0.44]	
		F:	10-20		[0.17-0.34]	
		With P-5'-P:	10-30		[0.17-0.51]	
		0-10 days:	47-150		[0.80-2.55]	
		10 days-24 mo:	9-80		[0.15-1.36]	
		24 mo-60 yr				
		M:	15-40		[0.26-0.68]	
		F:	13-35		[0.22-0.60]	
		60-90 yr				
		M:	19-48		[0.32-0.82]	
		F:	9-36		[0.15-0.61]	
		>90 yr				
		M:	11-38		[0.19-0.65]	
		F:	18-30		[0.31-0.51]	

DIAGNOSTIC INFORMATION	REMARKS

Serum–Asc albumin gradient (SAAG) ≥ 1.1 g/dL implies portal hypertension. Low Chol implies cirrhosis.

Of patients with ascites, 75% have hepatic cirrhosis, 10% have malignancies, and 5% have congestive heart failure.

Low Asc protein increases risk of SBP and portends a worse prognosis once it develops.[2] Elevated ANC is strongly associated with SBP.

Infected Asc almost always has pH < 7.35 or 0.1 units less than arterial pH.

DPL with ↑ RBC or WBC suggests intraabdominal injury.

2. Filik L, Unal S: Clinical and laboratory features of spontaneous bacterial peritonitis, *East Afr Med J* 81:474-479, 2004.

↑↑ Fulminant forms of acute hepatitis, especially viral hepatitis

The enzyme is distributed in all body tissues, but greatest activity occurs in liver, heart, and skeletal muscle and in erythrocytes. Minimal activity occurs in skin, kidney, and pancreas.

↑ Liver cell necrosis or injury of any cause, including cholestatic and obstructive jaundice, chronic hepatitis, drug-induced injury to the liver; alcoholic hepatitis (AST usually > ALT); viral and chronic hepatitis (ALT > AST in most cases; those in whom AST > ALT have poor prognosis)[11]; hepatic metastases and hepatoma; infectious mononucleosis; necrosis or trauma to heart or skeletal muscle; inflammatory disease of heart or skeletal muscle; after acute MI, AST > ALT; severe exercise, heart failure, severe burns, Forbes' disease (children, not adults), heat stroke (mean is 20-fold normal), hypothyroidism (40-90% of cases), intestinal obstruction (may indicate infarction of small intestine), lactate acidosis, legionnaires' disease, malignant hyperthermia, postcommissurotomy syndrome, polymyalgia rheumatica, typhoid fever, thalassemia major, von Gierke's disease, and toxic shock syndrome.[12]

In blunt abdominal trauma in children, AST >450 U/L is a good predictor of liver injury.[13] After severe liver injury in adults, AST peaks within 24 hr and then rapidly decreases during the next 4 days. Elevations prolonged past 4 days should be investigated for a cause.[14]

IgA-AST complexes are frequently found in association with liver malignancies.[15]

Usually normal after IM injections, moderate exercise

Increased or normal in cirrhosis, neurological disease, cerebral infarction or hemorrhage, acute pancreatitis, renal infarction, hemolytic anemia, hemophilia, malnutrition, and obesity

Serum AST activity is increased on the average by ~30% by the addition of pyridoxal-5'-phosphate (P-5'-P) to the reagent or specimen. This increase can be even more striking for patients on chronic hemodialysis. AST values that are abnormal because of heart or liver disease are increased by preincubation of serum with P-5'-P; the effect on the heart enzyme is greater than on the liver enzyme.[16] Note that addition of P-5'-P to reagent systems increases the "blank" reaction.

See also *Aspartate Aminotransferase, Mitochondrial.*

TEST NAME AND METHOD	SPECIMEN REQUIREMENTS	REFERENCE INTERVAL, CONVENTIONAL [INTERNATIONAL RECOMMENDED UNITS]		CHEMICAL INTERFERENCES AND IN VIVO EFFECTS
Aspartate Aminotransferase—CONT				
IFCC, with P-5'-P, 30° C[4]	Adult[7]:	10-30	[0.17-0.51]	clovir, heparin, HMG CoA reductase inhibitors (e.g., lovastatin, simvastatin), idarubicin, interferon, isotretinoin, labetalol, levamisole, levodopa, lincomycin, mebendazole, mefloquine, metoprolol, mexiletine, nifedipine, omeprazole, penicillins, pentamidine, piroxicam, propoxyphene, protriptyline, pyridoxine, ranitidine, ritodrine, sargramostim, streptozocin, sulfonylureas, thiothixene, thiabendazole, thioguanine, ticlopidine, tobramycin, tretinoin, verapamil, and zalcitabine.
				Activity is falsely elevated when AST is complexed with IgG or IgA.[10]
				S ↑ Hemolysis, heparin (Virtos), and iron salts (DuPont *aca*)
SCE, 340 nm, 37° C[5,6] *DGKC, 340 nm, 25° C[7]*	Adult[6]:	7-31 7-18	[0.12-0.53] [0.12-0.31]	S ↓ Ascorbic acid, cyanide, formaldehyde, isoniazid, leucine, mercurochrome, metronidazole, penicillamide, phthalate, succinate, and tartrate

1. Rej R: Measurement of aminotransferases: part I. Aspartate aminotransferase, *Crit Rev Clin Lab Sci* 21:99-186, 1984.

2. Henry RJ, Chiamori N, Golub OJ, et al: Revised spectrophotometric methods for the determination of glutamic-oxalacetic transaminase, glutamic-pyruvic transaminase, and lactic acid dehydrogenase, *Am J Clin Pathol* 34:381-398, 1960.

3. Tietz NW, Shuey DF, Wekstein DR: Laboratory values in fit aging individuals—sexagenarians through centenarians, *Clin Chem* 38:1167-1185, 1992.

4. Committee on Standards, International Federation of Clinical Chemistry: Provisional recommendations on IFCC methods for measurement of catalytic concentrations of enzymes. II. IFCC method for aspartate aminotransferase, *Clin Chim Acta* 70:F19-F42, 1976.

DIAGNOSTIC INFORMATION	REMARKS

5. Committee on Enzymes of the Scandinavian Society for Clinical Chemistry and Clinical Physiology: Recommended methods for the determination of four enzymes in blood, *Scand J Clin Lab Invest* 33:291-306, 1974.

6. Goldberg DM, Remtulla MA, Lustig V: The diagnostic accuracy of three recommended methods for serum aspartate aminotransferase assays in patients suspected by myocardial infarction and hepatobiliary disease, *Clin Biochem* 21:323-328, 1988.

7. Dols JLS, Van Zanten AP: Clinical implications of differences between two recommended procedures for determination of aspartate aminotransferase, *Clin Chem* 29:523-526, 1983.

TEST NAME AND METHOD	SPECIMEN REQUIREMENTS	REFERENCE INTERVAL, CONVENTIONAL [INTERNATIONAL RECOMMENDED UNITS]		CHEMICAL INTERFERENCES AND IN VIVO EFFECTS

Aspartate Aminotransferase—CONT

8. Niblock AE, Leung FY, Henderson AR: Serum aspartate aminotransferase storage and the effect of pyridoxal phosphate, *J Lab Clin Med* 108:461-465, 1986.

9. Burtis CA, Ashwood ER, editors: *Tietz textbook of clinical chemistry,* ed 2, Philadelphia, 1994, WB Saunders.

10. Nagamine M, Okochi K: Complexes of immunoglobulins A and G with aspartate aminotransferase isoenzymes in serum, *Clin Chem* 29:379-381, 1983.

11. Gitlin N: The serum glutamic-oxaloacetic transaminase/serum glutamic pyruvic transaminase ratio as a prognostic index in severe acute viral hepatitis, *Am J Gastroenterol* 77:2-4, 1982.

12. Wallach J, editor: *Interpretation of diagnostic tests,* ed 4, Boston, 1986, Little, Brown and Co.

TEST NAME AND METHOD	SPECIMEN REQUIREMENTS	REFERENCE INTERVAL, CONVENTIONAL	[INTERNATIONAL RECOMMENDED UNITS]	CHEMICAL INTERFERENCES AND IN VIVO EFFECTS
Aspartate Aminotransferase, Mitochondrial (mAST; EC 2.6.1.1)[1] *Precipitation of cAST (Rej) and assay at 37° C (no P-5'-P)*[2]	Serum. Stable 2 hr at room temperature; 2 days at −60° C.[7] Because activity increases at 4° C and −20° C over 20 days, store for no more than 7 days at 4° C and 30 days at −20° C.[8]	0.11-2.98 U/L × 0.017 (1-97.5 percentile)	[<0.01-0.05 μKat/L]	↑ Nonspecific binding in RIA, minimized by absorbing antisera with albumin ↓ Chromatographic analysis may introduce inhibitory salts or buffers; cycloserine.
Precipitation of cAST (Leung) and assay at 37° C (no P-5'-P)[3]		6.9 ± 2.1 U/L (SD)	[0.12 ± 0.04 μKat/L]	
RIA by precipitation of cAST (Leung) and assay[3]		53.9 ± 22.6 mcg/L (SD)		
Precipitation of cAST and assay at 37° C (no P-5'-P)[4]		0.93-2.64 U/L × 0.017 (2.5-97.5 percentile)	[0.02-0.04 μKat/L]	
Precipitation of cAST and assay at 30° C with P-5'-P[5]		0.43 ± 0.37 U/L (SD)	[± 0.006 μKat/L]	
RIA[6]		18-70 mcg/L		
Immunoprecipitation[6]		<7 U/L × 0.017	[<0.12 μKat/L]	

1. Rej R: Measurement of aminotransferases: part I. Aspartate aminotransferase, *Crit Rev Clin Lab Sci* 21:99-186, 1984.

2. Jung K, Pergande M, Rej R, et al: Mitochondrial enzymes in human serum: comparative determinations of glutamate dehydrogenase and mitochondrial aspartate aminotransferase in healthy persons and patients with chronic liver diseases, *Clin Chem* 31:239-243, 1985.

| DIAGNOSTIC INFORMATION | REMARKS |

13. Hennes HM, Smith DS, Schneider K, et al: Elevated liver transaminase levels in children with blunt abdominal trauma: a predictor of liver injury, *Pediatrics* 86:87-890, 1990.

14. Cogbill TH, Moore EE, Feliciano DV, et al: Hepatic enzyme response and hyperpyrexia after severe liver injury, *Am Surg* 58:395-399, 1992.

15. Moriyama T, Nobuoka M, Makino M: Incidence and properties of aspartate aminotransferase-immunoglobulin complexes in patients with a high serum aspartate to alanine aminotransferase ratio, *Clin Chim Acta* 790:47-56, 1990.

16. Rosalki SB, Bayoumi RA: Activation by pyridoxal 5-phosphate of aspartate transaminase in serum of patients with heart and liver disease, *Clin Chim Acta* 59:357-360, 1975.

↑↑ Acute liver disease, myocardial infarction; increase reflects severity of disease, organ damage, and prognosis.

The release and clearance of mAST are slower than for cAST; after infarction, mAST values reach a peak in serum later than do cAST values, and abnormal values persist longer.

↑ Chronic alcohol abuse, alcoholic hepatitis, fulminant viral hepatitis, myocardial infarction, severe heart failure, and liver injury.

Isoenzymes of AST are cAST (cytosolic form) and mAST (mitochondrial). In human liver and most other organs, mAST represents 80% of the total, but in serum it is usually <10%.[1] Most immunological methods measure residual catalytic activity of serum mAST after precipitation of cAST with specific antibody. An alternative approach involves digestion of cAST by proteinase K, which does not inactivate mAST.[9] The kinetic assay for total AST is optimized for cAST, although substrate requirements for mAST are much higher. Furthermore, mAST is activated to a greater degree by P-5′P than is cAST, so that omission of P-5′P from reagent will underestimate the contribution of mAST to total AST activity. Alcohol can lead to expression of mAST on the surface of hepatocytes,[10] a mechanism that may be responsible for the greater percentage increase in mAST in alcoholic liver disease.[11]

3. Leung FY, Niblock AE, Henderson AR: Radioimmunoassay of aspartate aminotransferase isoenzymes in human serum, *Clin Chem* 30:1361-1365, 1984.

4. Parkman R, Gelfand EW: Severe combined immunodeficiency disease, adenosine deaminase deficiency and gene therapy, *Curr Opin Immunol* 3:547-551, 1991.

TEST NAME* AND METHOD	SPECIMEN REQUIREMENTS	REFERENCE INTERVAL, CONVENTIONAL [INTERNATIONAL RECOMMENDED UNITS]	CHEMICAL INTERFERENCES AND IN VIVO EFFECTS

Aspartate Aminotransferase, Mitochondrial—CONT

5. Nalpas B, Vassault A, Le Guillou A, et al: Serum activity of mitochondrial aspartate aminotransferase: a sensitive marker of alcoholism with or without alcoholic hepatitis, *Hepatology* 4:893-896, 1984.

6. Niblock AE, Jablonsky G, Leung FY, et al: Changes in mass and catalytic activity concentrations of aspartate aminotransferase isoenzymes in serum after a myocardial infarct, *Clin Chem* 32:496-500, 1986.

7. Panteghini M, Malchiodi A, Calarco M, et al: Clinical and diagnostic significance of aspartate aminotransferase isoenzymes in sera of patients with liver disease, *J Clin Chem Clin Biochem* 22:153-158, 1984.

8. Boyde TRC, Kwong EML: Aspartate aminotransferase isoenzymes—differential kinetic assay in serum, *Clin Chim Acta* 128:95-102, 1983.

Atrial Natriuretic Hormone (ANH)[1] *RIA*[2]	Plasma (K₂EDTA). Collect blood into prechilled tubes and deliver to lab on ice. Centrifuge in a refrigerated centrifuge, and freeze plasma promptly. Stable for 4 wk at −25° C.	20-77 pg/mL[3] × 1.0 [20-77 ng/L]	↓ V Prazosin, urapidil, xipamide

1. Leavelle DE, editor: *Mayo Medical Laboratories interpretive handbook,* Rochester, MN, 1990, Mayo Medical Laboratories.

2. Ogawa K, Ito T, Hashimoto M, et al: Plasma atrial natriuretic factor in CHF [letter]. *Lancet* 7:106, 1986.

3. de Zeeuw D, Janssen WM, de Jong PE: Atrial natriuretic factor: its (patho) physiological significance in humans, *Kidney Int* 4I:1115-1133, 1992.

B-type Natriuretic Peptide (BNP) *Immunoassay*[1,2] *Point-of-care immunoassays also available.*[3] *Biosite (POCT), Beckman, Bayer, Abbott, Shionogi, Tosoh*[3]	EDTA plasma collected in plastic tubes. Samples stable for 4 hr at room temperature, 24 hr at 2-8° C and >3 days at −20° C.[4]	*mcg/L x* *pmol/L* Cutoff concentration for heart failure (HF): 0-100 × 3.472 [0-347][5] There are several practical issues regarding the use of plasma/whole blood monitoring of BNP intervals that vary depending on (1) which assay is used, and (2) the relative impact of these factors in relation to the degree of left ventricle dysfunction remains to be debated. When BNP concentrations are monitored in the age decades of >60 yr, reference concentrations >100 ng/L, the cutoff that has demonstrated a high negative predictive value (NPV) in ruling out HF. There is an inverse relationship between values and body mass index.[6]	Assays may differ in their susceptibility to analytical interferences. Interferences from rheumatoid factors or heterophilic antibodies may lead to false test results. Formulation of immunoassay kits remains very important in minimizing interference from heterophilic antibodies, and in some situations only addition of the non-

*Aspartic Acid can be found in the Appendix on p. 1761.

DIAGNOSTIC INFORMATION	REMARKS

9. Panteghini M, Bonora R, Pagani F: Automated measurement of mitochondrial aspartate aminotransferase by selective proteolysis with proteinase K, *Clin Chem* 39:2199-2200, 1993.

10. Zhou S, Gordon RE, Bradbury M, et al: Ethanol up-regulates fatty acid uptake and plasma membrane expression and export of mitochondrial aspartate aminotransferase in HepG2 cells, *Hepatology* 27:1064-1074, 1998.

11. Macchia T, Mancinelli R, Gentili S, et al: Mitochondrial aspartate aminotransferase isoenzyme: a biochemical marker for the clinical management of alcoholics? *Clin Chim Acta* 263:79-96, 1997.

↑ Congestive heart failure, cardiovascular disease with elevated cardiac filling pressure, asymptomatic cardiac volume overload, atrial pacing, paroxysmal atrial tachycardia.[4]

ANH is an endogenous antihypertensive agent secreted from the cardiac atria. This hormone enhances salt and water excretion, blocks aldosterone and renin secretion, inhibits the action of angiotensin II and vasopressin, and inhibits smooth muscle contraction. Its net effect is to decrease blood volume and reduce blood pressure.

Side-by-side studies have shown that ANP and NT-proANH are not as useful for congestive heart failure as are B-type natriuretic peptide or NT-proBNP.[4]

See *B-type natriuretic peptide and NT-proBNP.*

---

4. Doust JA, Glasziou PP, Pietrzak E, et al: A systematic review of the diagnostic accuracy of natriuretic peptides for heart failure, *Arch Intern Med* 164:1978-1984, 2004.

Increased concentrations of BNP and NT-proBNP occur in patients with HF.[6] They are also increased in asymptomatic left ventricular dysfunction (LVD), arterial and pulmonary hypertension, cardiac hypertrophy, valvular heart disease, arrhythmia, and acute coronary syndrome.[7] NPs are useful for prognosis for guiding and monitoring HF therapy.[8] However, BNP and NT-proBNP are increased in a variety of cardiac diseases; thus the clinician has to be conscious in interpreting results. In the management of cardiology patients, clinicians need to know (1) the form of the biomarker, (2) the immunoassays used are lacking standardization, (3) the discrimination limits are dependent on age, gender, and biological variation, (4) the diagnostic time window (admission or serial sampling to obtain peak value), (5) the clinical setting (used by the general practitioner, ED, CCU, etc.), (6) the diagnostic use (early

BNP has biologic effects similar to those of atrial natriuretic peptide (ANP) and is stored mainly in the myocardium of the cardiac ventricles. Blood levels of BNP are elevated in hypervolemic states such as CHF and hypertension.[6]

Natriuretic peptides (NPs) are secreted to regulate fluid volume, blood pressure, and electrolyte balance. They have activity in both the central and peripheral nervous systems. ANP was the first described in 1981.[3] BNP was discovered 7 yr later in the porcine brain.[12] However, in humans, the main source of circulatory BNP is the heart ventricles. Other members of the NP family include C-type natriuretic peptide (CNP) and urodilatin. Although these hormones are not produced by myocardium, they are released with ANP and BNP in patients with volume overload, hypertension, and hyponatremia.

TEST NAME AND METHOD	SPECIMEN REQUIREMENTS	REFERENCE INTERVAL, CONVENTIONAL [INTERNATIONAL RECOMMENDED UNITS]			CHEMICAL INTERFERENCES AND IN VIVO EFFECTS

B-type Natriuretic Peptide (BNP)—CONT

Antibody recognition: Assay	Antigen	Capture Ab	Detection Ab	
Abbott AxSym	a.a. 1-32 3-32	Scios (ring)	Shionig (C-term)	
Bayer Centaur	a.a. 1-32 3-32	Shionigi (ring)	Shinogi (C-term)	
Biosite Triage (Beckman Access)	a.a. 1-32	Scios (ring)	Biosite (N-term)	
Shionogi	a.a. 1-32 a.a. 3-32	Shionigi (ring)	Shionigi (C-term)	

immune serum from the animal species that was used to raise the antibodies is effective.

↑ Icteric and hemolyzed samples might also be a problem in certain immunoassays with fluorimetric detection of the signal. Some analyzers may be particularly susceptible to the presence of particles (e.g., fibrin strands) or bubbles in the sample thereby causing erroneous test results.

1. Wu AH, Packer M, Smith A, et al: Analytical and clinical evaluation of the Bayer ADVIA Centaur automated B-type natriuretic peptide assay in patients with heart failure: a multisite study, *Clin Chem* 50:867-873, 2004.

2. Wieczorek SJ, Wu AH, Christenson R, et al: A rapid B-type natriuretic peptide assay accurately diagnoses left ventricular dysfunction and heart failure: a multicenter evaluation, *Am Heart J* 144:834-839, 2002.

3. Clerico A, Del Ry S, Giannessi D: Measurement of cardiac natriuretic hormones (atrial natriuretic peptide, brain natriuretic peptide, and related peptides) in clinical practice: the need for a new generation of immunoassay methods, *Clin Chem* 46:1529-1534, 2000.

4. Kelly P, Foreman P, Taylor V, et al: Stability of BNP in whole blood and plasma, *Clin Chem* 50:A3, 2004. [Abstract]

5. Maisel AS, Krishnaswamy P, Nowak RM, et al: Rapid measurement of B-type natriuretic peptide in the emergency diagnosis of heart failure, *N Engl J Med* 347:161-167, 2002.

6. Wang TJ, Larson MG, Levy D, et al: Impact of obesity on plasma natriuretic peptide levels [see comment], *Circulation* 109:594-600, 2004.

7. Munagala VK, Burnett JC Jr, Redfield MM: The natriuretic peptides in cardiovascular medicine, *Curr Probl Cardiol* 29:707-769, 2004.

8. Cowie MR, Jourdain P, Maisel A, et al: Clinical applications of B-type natriuretic peptide (BNP) testing, *Eur Heart J* 24:1710-1718, 2003.

| DIAGNOSTIC INFORMATION | REMARKS |

and/or late, rule-in, rule-out, definitive for ACS, CHF, LVD [diastolic or systolic dysfunction], asymptomatic LVD, etc.), prognostic use (importance of increased level at admission, peak-value, risk stratification), or for therapeutic guidance (titration of therapies of the biomarkers used), (7) possible confounding diseases, and (8) biological variability. The BV indicate a change of 130% for BNP and 90% for NT-proBNP is necessary before results of serially collected data can be considered statistically significant.[9,10]

There are no primary reference materials to standardize BNP assays, and different antibodies are used that detect different forms of NPs.

Clinical laboratory testing in the setting of CHF focuses on several goals: (1) to determine the cause of diagnostic symptoms, (2) to estimate the degree of severity of heart failure, (3) to estimate the risk of disease progression and risk, and (4) to screen for less symptomatic disease.[11]

The NPs should be tested to (1) to confirm HF in patients presenting with ambiguous clinical features or confounding pathology etiologies, such as chronic obstructive pulmonary disease, (2) to assist/improve the diagnostic accuracy for HF, and (3) assist in ruling out HF with a normal NP. However, plasma NPs testing in patients with obvious HF (e.g., NYHA class IV) is not necessary. The NPs are "not a stand-alone diagnostic test"; it must be used and interpreted with regard to the clinical presentation, specifically pertaining to the age and gender of the patient.

ANP and BNP are released in response to atrial/ventricular stretch from volume overload, wall tension, and myocardial stretching. Blood NPs increase in all diseases with volume overload, including renal and liver diseases, as well as some endocrine disorders (e.g., Cushing's, primary hyperaldosteronism).[13] NPs increase cardiac output by decreasing systemic and pulmonary vascular resistance. Additionally, NPs reduce production of renin and aldosterone by increasing renal blood flow, GFR, and urine output. Overall, NPs regulate blood pressure and volume status. They also have direct effects on the myocardium interstitium.

BNP synthesis mostly relies primarily on gene expression and initial up-regulation of mRNA.

9. Doust JA, Pietrzak E, Dobson A, et al: How well does B-type natriuretic peptide predict death and cardiac events in patients with heart failure: systematic review, *BMJ* 330:625, 2005.

10. Wu AHB, Smith A, Wieczorek S, et al: Biological variation for N-terminal pro- and B-type natriuretic peptides and implications for therapeutic monitoring of patients with congestive heart failure, *Am J Cardiol* 92:628-631, 2003.

11. Apple FS, Panteghini M, Ravkilde J, et al: Quality specifications for B-type natriuretic peptide assays, *Clin Chem* 51:486-493, 2005.

12. Sonnenberg H, Chong CK, Veress AT: Cardiac atrial factor—an endogenous diuretic? *Can J Physiol Pharmacol* 59:1278-1279, 1981.

13. Sudoh T, Kangawa K, Minamino N, et al: A new natriuretic peptide in porcine brain, *Nature* 332:78-81, 1988.

TEST NAME AND METHOD	SPECIMEN REQUIREMENTS	REFERENCE INTERVAL, CONVENTIONAL [INTERNATIONAL RECOMMENDED UNITS]			CHEMICAL INTERFERENCES AND IN VIVO EFFECTS
Base Excess (BE)[1-3] *Nomogram*	Whole blood, arterial. Collect anaerobically in heparinized syringe.	Newborn: Infant: Child: Adult:	*mEq/L* −10 to −2 −7 to −1 −4 to +2 −2 to +3	× 1.0	*mmol/L* [−10 to −2] [−7 to −1] [−4 to +2] [−2 to +3]	↑ V Carbenicillin, diuretics (chlorthalidone, ethacrynic acid, thiazides) ↓ V Methoxyflurane

1. Eastham RD: *Biochemical values in clinical medicine,* ed 7, Bristol, UK, 1985, John Wright and Sons, Ltd.
2. Siggaard-Andersen O: *The acid-base status of the blood,* ed 4, Copenhagen, 1974, Munksgaard.
3. Heusel JW, Siggaard-Andersen O, Scott MG: Physiology and disorders of water, electrolyte, and acid-base metabolism. In Burtis CA, Ashwood ER, editors: *Tietz textbook of clinical chemistry,* ed 3, Philadelphia, 1999, WB Saunders.

Benzene[1] *GLC, colorimetric (for phenol metabolite), GC-FID[2] (measures benzene directly); UV (measures phenol metabolite) HPLC,LC/ ESI-NI/MS (measures S-phenylmercapturic acid metabolite)[3]*	Serum (refrigerate) Urine[1] Breath[1]	Toxic concentration: As phenol: Toxic concentration, as phenol: As S-PMA Not considered useful for low (<1 ppm) exposures. Occupational exposure:	*mg/L* >1.0 <20.0 >30.0 <25 mcg/g creatinine 0.05 ppm	× 12.8 × 10.6 × 10.6 × 12.8	*μmol/L* [>13] [<213] [>319] [1 μmol/L]	Substances producing phenol as a metabolite can interfere with colorimetric assay (e.g., Pepto-Bismol, Chloraseptic). S-PMA is increased in smokers.

1. Baselt RC: *Biological monitoring methods for industrial chemicals,* Davis, CA, 1980, Biomedical Pub.
2. Collom WD, Winek CL: Detection of glue constituents in fatalities due to "glue sniffing," *Clin Toxicol* 3:125-130, 1970.
3. Pieri M, Miraglia N, Acampora A, et al: Determination of urinary S-phenylmercapturic acid by liquid chromatography-tandem mass spectrometry, *J Chromatogr* 795:347-354, 2003.

↑ Metabolic alkalosis, acute respiratory alkalosis

↓ Metabolic acidosis, acute respiratory acidosis

Values of BE may have some clinical utility in determining the extent of fluid treatment in acid-base disorders.

This parameter represents the base concentration of whole blood on titration with strong acid to pH 7.4 at a P_{CO_2} of 40 mm Hg [5.32 kPa] at 37° C. BE and buffer base can be derived from a nomogram (see Fig. II-1) or can be read directly from those blood gas instruments with computing capabilities.

Benzene exposure has been associated with acute nonlymphocytic leukemia, aplastic anemia, and degenerative changes in the bone marrow. In addition to industrial uses, benzene is a component of gasoline and tobacco smoke.

The threshold limit–time-weighted value (TLV-TWA) is 0.5 ppm in air. Benzene is classified as a group A1 carcinogen by the American Conference of Governmental Industrial Hygenists.

See Table II-6.

TEST NAME AND METHOD	SPECIMEN REQUIREMENTS	REFERENCE INTERVAL, CONVENTIONAL [INTERNATIONAL RECOMMENDED UNITS]		CHEMICAL INTERFERENCES AND IN VIVO EFFECTS
Beryllium (Be)[1,2] *Fluorimetric,[2] AAS[3]*	Urine, 24 hr. Collect in acid-washed, metal-free container.	Toxic concentration:	$<1\ mcg/day$[4] $\times 0.11$ [<0.11 μmol/day] >20 mcg/L [>2.22 μmol/L]	None found.
	Lung		*mcg/kg dry wt.* *μmol/kg dry wt.* 3-10 $\times 0.11$ [0.33-1.11]	
		Beryllium disease:	4-45,700 [0.33-5073]	

1. Aller AJ: The clinical significance of beryllium, *J Trace Elem Electrol Health Dis* 4:1-6, 1990.
2. Venugopal B, Luckey TD: *Metal toxicity in mammals, vol 2,* New York, 1978, Plenum Press.
3. Baselt RC: *Biological monitoring methods for industrial chemicals,* ed 2, Littleton, MA, 1988, PSG Publishing.
4. Jacobs DS, Kasten BL, DeMott WR, et al, editors: *Laboratory test handbook,* ed 2, Stow, OH, 1990, LexiComp, Inc.
5. Beckett WS: Occupational respiratory disease (review article), *N Engl J Med* 342:406-413, 2004.

TEST NAME AND METHOD	SPECIMEN REQUIREMENTS	REFERENCE INTERVAL, CONVENTIONAL [INTERNATIONAL RECOMMENDED UNITS]			CHEMICAL INTERFERENCES AND IN VIVO EFFECTS
Bicarbonate (HCO_3^-)[1,2] *Calculation*	Plasma, arterial, or venous. Collect sample anaerobically. Heparin is the preferred anticoagulant.	Arterial: Venous:	*mEq/L*[2] 21-28 22-29	$\times 1.0$	*mmol/L* [21-28] [22-29]	↑ V Morphine, barbiturates (if respiratory depression occurs); corticosteroids (long term); diuretics (e.g., thiazides, chlorthalidone, ethacrynic acid, furosemide, metolazone), overuse of laxatives
	Whole blood, arterial	Cord blood[4,5] Arterial: Venous: Newborn: Infant: 2 mo-2 yr: Adult:	 21-28 22-29 17-24 19-24 16-24 22-26		 [21-28] [22-29] [17-24] [19-24] [16-24] [22-26]	↓ V Ammonium chloride, acetazolamide, cholestyramine, cyclosporine; poisoning with ethylene glycol, methanol, paraldehyde, phenformin, salicylate (late toxicity)
	Peritoneal fluid[3]		24-29		[24-29]	
	Pancreatic fluid[3]		66-127		[66-127]	
	Duodenal fluid[3]		4-21		[4-21]	

1. Burtis CA, Ashwood ER, editors: *Tietz fundamentals of clinical chemistry,* ed 5, Philadelphia, 2000, WB Saunders.
2. Scott MG, Heusel JW, LeGrys VA, et al: Electrolyte and blood gases. In Burtis CA, Ashwood ER, editors: *Tietz textbook of clinical chemistry,* ed 3, Philadelphia, 1999, WB Saunders.
3. Altman PL, Dittmer DS, editors: *Blood and other body fluids,* Bethesda, MD, 1971, Federation of American Societies for Experimental Biology.

Toxicity from beryllium exposure is latent; symptoms develop from inhalation of or contact with Be salts or metal dust. Potentially reversible symptoms of acute toxicity include eye ulcers and inflammation of the lungs, airways, and skin. Other acute responses are hyperemia, edema, hemorrhage with mild edema of the brain, liver inflammation, and focal hemorrhage of the spleen. Chronic inhalation will lead to berylliosis. Beryllium can enter the bloodstream through the lungs and will cause cellular death in tissues in which it accumulates. Beryllium toxicity has been associated with an increased incidence of pulmonary cancers.

Beryllium exposure is an industrial hazard for workers in metal extraction and refining plants; exposure to Be may occur near rocket bases or nuclear plants, or where coal is burned extensively. Urinary excretion is variable in exposed workers and does not correlate well with beryllium disease. Be disease diagnosed on history of exposure, finding of noncaseating granulomas in lung, and T lymphocytes sensitized to Be obtained from blood or lavage fluid.[5]

↑ Compensated respiratory acidosis, metabolic alkalosis

↓ Metabolic acidosis, compensated respiratory alkalosis

See also *Carbon Dioxide, Total.*

Bicarbonate can be determined directly by titration, but this is rarely done. Bicarbonate is generally calculated using the Henderson-Hasselbalch equation or a nomogram based on this equation.

$$HCO_3^- = Total\ CO_2 - H_2CO_3$$

Small amounts of CO_3^- and carbamino compounds present in plasma are customarily included in this fraction.

The HCO_3^- is the largest fraction contributing to the total carbon dioxide. Therefore both parameters change usually in the same direction.

The standard bicarbonate is the concentration of bicarbonate in whole blood at 38° C equilibrated at a P_{CO_2} of 40 mm Hg [5-32 kPa] with the blood Hb fully oxygenated.

4. Burtis CA, Ashwood ER, editors: *Tietz textbook of clinical chemistry,* ed 3, Philadelphia, 1999, WB Saunders.
5. Yeomans ER, Hauth JC, Gilstrap LC III, et al: Umbilical cord pH, PCO_2, and bicarbonate following uncomplicated term vaginal deliveries, *Am J Obstet Gynecol* 151:798-800, 1985.

TEST NAME AND METHOD	SPECIMEN REQUIREMENTS	REFERENCE INTERVAL, CONVENTIONAL [INTERNATIONAL RECOMMENDED UNITS]		CHEMICAL INTERFERENCES AND IN VIVO EFFECTS
Bile Acid Breath Test (^{14}C-Cholyl-glycine Breath Test; CO_2 Breath Test)[1-3] Dose: 10 μCi cholyl[1-^{14}C]-glycine in 30 mL 20% ethanol, administered with 5 oz of a liquid nutrient	Breath. Determine radioactivity of $^{14}CO_2$ in breath samples at 2 and 4 hr by liquid scintillation spectroscopy and correct for body wt.[1]	*Cumulative excretion of $^{14}CO_2$ in breath* *% of* *dose (SD)* 2 hr after dose: 0.11 ± 0.15 4 hr after dose: 0.52 ± 0.09	*Fraction* *of dose* × 0.01 [0.0011 ± 0.0015] [0.0052 ± 0.0009]	V ↑ Cimetidine[4]

1. Fromm H, Hoffman AF: Breath test for altered bile-acid metabolism, *Lancet* 2:621-625, 1971.

2. King CE, Toskes PP, Guilarte TR, et al: Comparison of the one-gram α-[^{14}C] xylose breath test to the [^{14}C] bile acid breath test in patients with small-intestine bacterial growth, *Dig Dis Sci* 25:53-58, 1980.

3. Yamada T, editor: *Textbook of gastroenterology,* Philadelphia, 1991, JB Lippincott.

4. Shindo K, Yamazaki R, Koide K, et al: Alteration of bile acid metabolism by cimetidine in healthy humans, J Investig Med 44:462-469, 1996.

5. Toskes PO, Donaldson RM Jr: The blind loop syndrome. In Sleisenger MH, Fordtran JS, editors: *Gastrointestinal disease: pathophysiology, diagnosis, management,* ed 4, Philadelphia, 1989, WB Saunders.

6. Kiss Z, Wolfling J, Csati S, et al: The ursodeoxycholic acid-p-aminobenzoic acid deconjugation test, a new tool for the diagnosis of bacterial overgrowth syndrome, *Eur J Gastroenterol Hepatol* 9:679-682, 1997.

| **Bile Acids, Individual**[1,2]

GLC | Serum, fasting | *mcg/mL*[3]
Deoxycholic: 0.22 ± 0.13
Chenode-oxycholic: 0.31 ± 0.32
Cholic: 0.20 ± 0.17 | *μmol/L*
× 2.547 [0.56 ± 0.33]
× 2.547 [0.79 ± 0.82]
× 2.448 [0.49 ± 0.42] | V ↓ (Deoxycholic) Rifampin[6] |

Conjugated Acid *RIA*			*mcg/mL*	*μmol/L**
		Choric:	0.12-0.61	× 2.448 [0.3-1.5][4]
		Chenodeoxycholic:	0.16-0.98	× 2.547 [0.4-2.5][4]
		Cholylglycine:	0.13 ± 0.01 (SD)	× 2.151 [0.28 ± 0.02][5]
		Chenodeoxycholylglycine:	0.09 ± 0.01 (SD)	× 2.222 [0.2 ± 0.02][5]
		Deoxycholylglycine:	0.03 ± 0.005 (SD)	× 2.222 [0.07 ± 0.01][5]
		Sulfolithocholylglycine:	0.01 ± 0.005 (SD)	× 1.949 [0.06 ± 0.01][5]

*mmol glycine-conjugated bile acids/L

DIAGNOSTIC INFORMATION	REMARKS

↑ GI bacterial overgrowth associated with stasis, ileal dysfunction (disease, bypass, or surgical resection)

The bile acid breath test does not differentiate bacterial overgrowth from ileal damage or resection. This creates clinical difficulties because bacterial overgrowth may be superimposed on ileal damage in conditions such as Crohn's disease, lymphoma, and radiation enteritis. False-negative results have been described in 30-40% of patients with culture-proven overgrowth.[5] An alternative version of the test uses ursodeoxycholic acid conjugated to p-aminobenzoic acid and measures urinary excretion of hippurate. Results of the two versions are often discordant in bacterial overgrowth, suggesting that use of both methods may be helpful.[6]

This is a rapid, simple outpatient procedure in which values are elevated 10-fold with increased bacterial bile acid deconjugation. Fecal radioactivity measurement permits separation of bile acid malabsorption from bacterial overgrowth and will also identify patients with a negative breath test despite bile acid malabsorption.[1]

The ^{14}C-D-xylose breath test is the test of choice to detect bacterial overgrowth.[5] See *[14]C-D-Xylose Breath Test.*

Determination of the ratio of cholylglycine to chenodeoxycholylglycine may be of diagnostic value because ~80% of patients with hepatocellular disease have a ratio <1, whereas ~80% of patients with cholestatic disease have a ratio >1.

S ↑ (Ursodeoxycholic acid) Cystic fibrosis[7]

TEST NAME AND METHOD	SPECIMEN REQUIREMENTS	REFERENCE INTERVAL, CONVENTIONAL [INTERNATIONAL RECOMMENDED UNITS]	CHEMICAL INTERFERENCES AND IN VIVO EFFECTS

Bile Acids, Individual—CONT

1. Brown SS, Mitchell FL, Young DS, editors: *Chemical diagnosis of disease,* Amsterdam, 1979, Elsevier/North Holland Biomedical Press.
2. Demers L: Diagnostic use of serum bile acid measurements, *Lab Management* May:43-50, 1979.
3. Sandberg D, Sjövall J, Sjövall K, et al: Measurement of human serum bile acids by gas-liquid chromatography, *J Lipid Res* 6:182-192, 1965.
4. Roda A, Roda E, Aldini R, et al: Results with six "kit" radioimmunoassays for primary bile acids in human serum intercompared, *Clin Chem* 26:1677-1682, 1980.

TEST NAME AND METHOD	SPECIMEN REQUIREMENTS	REFERENCE INTERVAL, CONVENTIONAL	[INTERNATIONAL RECOMMENDED UNITS]	CHEMICAL INTERFERENCES AND IN VIVO EFFECTS
Bile Acids, Total[1,2] *Enzymatic (3α-hydroxysteroid dehydrogenase)*	Serum, fasting. Stable for 6 mo at 4° C in the absence of bacterial growth.	*mcg/mL* Na tauro-cholate: 1.25-3.41 Na cheno-deoxycholate: 2.4 ± 0.83	*μmol/L* × 2.0 [2.5-6.8][5] × 2.547 [6.1 ± 2.1][6]	S ↑ V Cyclosporine, isoniazid, methotrexate, rifampin S ↑ C *Enzymatic:* Fusidic acid
GLC	Serum, 2-hr postprandial	3.6 ± 2.0 (SD)	[9.2 ± 5.1][6]	S ↓ V Cholestyramine
	Serum, fasting	0.3-2.3 mcg/mL[3] × 2.448*	[0.73-5.63 μmol/L]	
	Serum, 1-hr postprandial	1.8-3.2 mcg/mL[3]	[4.41-7.83 μmol/L]	
	Feces	120-225 mg/day[4] × 2.448*	[294-551 μmol/day]	F ↑ V Cholestyramine, neomycin F ↓ V Clofibrate, rifampin,[7] high-carbohydrate diet (IV)
		*Conversion factor based on MW of cholic acid of 408.6.		

1. Brown SS, Mitchell FL, Young DS, editors: *Chemical diagnosis of disease,* Amsterdam, 1979, Elsevier/North Holland Biomedical Press.
2. Demers L: Diagnostic use of serum bile acid measurements, *Lab Management* May:43-50, 1979.
3. Sandberg D, Sjövall J, Sjövall K, et al: Management of human serum bile acids by gas-chromotography, *J Lipid Res* 6:182-192, 1978.
4. Grandy S, Ahrens E, Miettinen T: Quantitative isolation and gas chromatographic analysis of total fecal bile acids, *J Lipid Res* 6:397-410, 1990
5. Skrede S, Solberg H, Bloomhoff J, et al: Bile acids measured in serum during fasting as a test for liver disease, *Clin Chem* 24:1095-1099, 1978.
6. Kobayashi K, Allen R, Bloomer J, et al: Enzymatic fluorometry for estimating serum total bile acid concentrations, *JAMA* 241:2043-2045, 1979.
7. Lutjohann D, Hahn C, Prange W, et al: Influence of rifampin on serum markers of cholesterol and bile acid synthesis in men, *Int J Clin Pharmacol Ther Toxicol* 42:307-313, 2004.
8. Jimenez F, Monte MJ, El-Mir MY, et al: Chronic renal failure-induced changes in serum and urine bile acid profiles, *Dig Dis Sci* 47:2398-2406, 2002.

5. Demers L, Hepner G: Radioimmunoassay of bile acids in serum, *Clin Chem* 22:602-606, 1976.
6. Lutjohann D, Hahn C, Prange W, et al: Influence of rifampin on serum markers of cholesterol and bile acid synthesis in men, *Int J Clin Pharmacol Ther Toxicol* 42:307-313, 2004.
7. Smith J, Lewindon P, Hoskins A, et al: Endogenous ursodeoxycholic acid and cholic acid in liver disease due to cystic fibrosis, *Hepatology* 39:1673-1682, 2004.

S ↑ Viral hepatitis, alcoholic liver disease, cirrhosis, cholestasis, hepatocellular carcinoma, drug-induced liver injury, cystic fibrosis, neonatal hepatitis syndrome, biliary atresia, chronic renal failure.[8]

Also increased in cholestasis of pregnancy, and levels may predict adverse fetal outcomes.[9]

In all forms of hepatobiliary dysfunction, postprandial values exceed the upper limit of reference ranges. Thus postprandial measurement of serum bile acids may prove to be a very sensitive test of hepatobiliary function. The enzymatic method measures unconjugated and conjugated bile acids with the exception of bile acids sulfated at the C3-position.

The total concentration of bile acids in serum is extremely variable. Although elevated in a variety of liver disorders, knowledge of their concentration may provide little additional diagnostic value in liver disease.

Examining patterns of individual bile acids and their state of conjugation may provide more useful information; however, these assays are more difficult to perform.[10]

9. Glants A, Marshall HV, Mattson LA: Intrahepatic cholestasis of pregnancy: relationship between bile acid levels and total complication rates, *Hepatology* 40:467-474, 2004.
10. Matsui A, Setchell KDR: Serum bile acid analysis, *Clin Chim Acta* 127:1-17, 1983.

TEST NAME AND METHOD	SPECIMEN REQUIREMENTS	REFERENCE INTERVAL, CONVENTIONAL [INTERNATIONAL RECOMMENDED UNITS]		CHEMICAL INTERFERENCES AND IN VIVO EFFECTS
Bilirubin[1,2] *Total* *Diazotization, spectrophotometric*	Serum. Protect from light.	*Premature full-term*[8] *mg/dL* Cord: <2.0 <2.0 × 17.1 0-1 day: <8.0 1.4-8.7 1-2 days: <12.0 3.4-11.5 3-5 days: <16.0 1.5-12.0 >5 days- 60 yr[9]: 0.3-1.2 60-90 yr: 0.2-1.1 >90 yr: 0.2-0.9	*Premature full-term* μ*mol/L* [<34] [<34] [<137] [24-149] [<205] [58-197] [<274] [26-205] [5-21] [3-19] [3-15]	↑ C Aminosalicylic acid (Vitros); hemoglobin; levodopa (Vitros), lipemia (levels depend on specific method) S ↑ V Transfusion (transient).[1] See Table II-5, for cholestatic hepatotoxic drugs and Table II-4, for drugs causing hemolysis. S ↓ C Aminophenazone S ↓ V Oral contraceptives,[10] smoking[11]
Reagent Strip (Bayer Ictotest, Bili-Labstix, Multistix; BMC Chemstrips)[3-6]	Urine, fresh random. Protect from light. Refrigerated specimen stable for 1 day.	Negative		U ↑ C Large amounts of phenothiazines; metabolites of phenazopyridine (Pyridium), ethoxazene (Serenium), and etodolac (Lodine) and high levels of urobilin, indican, metabolites of antiinflammatory drugs nefenamic and flufenamic acid, or salicylates may cause an orange-to-red color. U ↓ C Large amounts of ascorbic acid, nitrite (in urinary tract infections)
Oxidation method (Harrison spot test, Fouchet's test)	Urine, fresh or acidified.	Negative		U ↓ (color masking) High levels of indican, salicylates, urobilin, or urobilinogen may cause purple, brown-purple, or gray-purple color.

DIAGNOSTIC INFORMATION	REMARKS

S ↑ Hepatocellular damage (inflammatory, toxic, neoplastic), intrahepatic and extrahepatic biliary tree obstruction, hemolytic diseases, neonatal physiological jaundice, Crigler-Najjar syndrome, Gilbert's disease, Dubin-Johnson syndrome, fructose intolerance; breast-milk jaundice syndrome, hypothyroidism, and transient familial hyperbilirubinemia in infants

The direct spectrophotometric method can be applied only to specimens from infants <6 wk because cartenoids cause positive interference.

Transcutaneous measurement of bilirubin using direct spectrophotometry is available for measurement of bilirubin in neonates and correlates reasonably well with serum bilirubin measurement using the diazo reaction.[12,13]

U ↑ Conditions that have an elevated serum conjugated bilirubin (see above)

Qualitative tests are clinically satisfactory. Extrahepatic biliary tract obstruction is the classic cause of bilirubinuria. Urine bilirubin and urobilirubin are useful in the differential diagnosis of jaundice; bilirubinuria is present in liver disease, both obstructive and hepatocellular, but absent in hemolytic jaundice. In infants, early urine testing to aid in the diagnosis of biliary atresia may avoid early death, allow timely successful surgery, and obviate the need for transplants.[15] In viral hepatitis bilirubin may appear in the urine before the appearance of jaundice and typically clears before its disappearance. Excretion of bilirubin is enhanced by alkalosis.

Levels of sensitivity:
BMC Chemstrip: 0.5 mg/dL [9 μmol/L]
Bayer Bili-Labstix: 0.4-0.8 mg/dL [7-14 μmol/L]
Ictotest: 0.05-0.1 mg/dL [0.8-1.7 μmol/L]

Rifampin and large amounts of chlorpromazine metabolites may cause false-positive results. Wash-through method may differentiate bilirubin from drugs causing false-positive results.[16]

TEST NAME AND METHOD	SPECIMEN REQUIREMENTS	REFERENCE INTERVAL, CONVENTIONAL [INTERNATIONAL RECOMMENDED UNITS]			CHEMICAL INTERFERENCES AND IN VIVO EFFECTS
Bilirubin—CONT					
Diazotization, spectrophotometric	Amniotic fluid. Protect from light.	*mg/dL* 28 wk: <0.075 40 wk: <0.025 or	× 17.1	*μmol/L* [<1.3] [<0.4]	AF ↑ C Bilirubin or hemoglobin from maternal or fetal blood as a result of trauma during amniocentesis
		ΔA_{450} 28 wk: <0.048 40 wk: <0.02			
Conjugated *Diazotization, spectrophotometric*	Serum. Protect from light.	<0.2 mg/dL[8]	× 17.1	[<3.4 μmol/L]	
Vitros[7]	Serum or heparinized plasma. Protect from light.	<0.3 mg/dL	× 17.1	[<5 μmol/L]	Amphotericin B, biliverdin, hemoglobin, levodopa, methotrexate, nitrofurantoin, phenazopyridine, piroxicam, sulfasalazine (spectral interferents) Exposure to light will form photobilirubin, which will be measured as conjugated bilirubin and will increase conjugated bilirubin by as much as 1 mg/dL [17 μmol/L]. S ↑ V Carbamazepine, isotretinoin, phenobarbital, phenytoin
Unconjugated *Ektachem[7]*	Serum or heparinized plasma. Protect from light.	<1.1 mg/dL	× 17.1	[<19 μmol/L]	See *Bilirubin, Conjugated.*

DIAGNOSTIC INFORMATION	REMARKS

AF ↑ Erythroblastosis, maternal infectious hepatitis, maternal sickle cell crisis

Positive interference by moderate amounts of hemoglobin can be mathematically corrected.[2]

S ↑ Intrahepatic and extrahepatic biliary tree obstruction, hepatocellular damage (especially late in the disease process), cholestasis (for drugs causing cholestasis, see Table II-5), Dubin-Johnson syndrome, Rotor's syndrome

The portion of bilirubin detected with traditional methods consists of conjugated and δ-bilirubin, and a small fraction of unconjugated bilirubin. Typically, 70-90% of conjugated and δ-bilirubin react directly. The proportion of unconjugated bilirubin that reacts directly is increased by exposure to light,[17] alkaline pH, presence of detergent or other surfactants,[18] and varies widely from one method to another in proficiency surveys,[19] probably related to matrix effects.[20]

Normal adults have very low conjugated bilirubin levels, usually <0.1 mg/dL [<1.7 μmol/L] (lower limit of detection).

Vitros: Because conjugated bilirubin measured by this method does not include the δ-fraction as does the direct bilirubin, conjugated bilirubin is a better indicator than direct bilirubin during the resolving phase of hepatic and cholestatic disorders.[20]

S ↑ Hemolytic disorders or those associated with breakdown of hemoglobin such as large resolving hematomas; convalescent phase of acute hepatitis and sepsis; transient neonatal hyperbilirubinemia, Gilbert's syndrome, Criglar-Najjar syndrome, and ineffective erythropoiesis as seen in B_{12} and folate deficiencies and cirrhosis.[12,13]

Unconjugated bilirubin is measured by the same slide (by differential light absorption) as conjugated bilirubin but is not reported by many laboratories and is used only in the calculation of δ-bilirubin.

TEST NAME* AND METHOD	SPECIMEN REQUIREMENTS	REFERENCE INTERVAL, CONVENTIONAL [INTERNATIONAL RECOMMENDED UNITS]			CHEMICAL INTERFERENCES AND IN VIVO EFFECTS
Bilirubin—CONT					
δ-Bilirubin *(Delta Bilirubin)*	Serum. Protect from light.	<0.2 mg/dL	× 17.1	[<3 μmol/L]	See *Bilirubin, Total* and *Bilirubin, Conjugated.*

1. Henry JB, editor: *Clinical diagnosis and management by laboratory methods,* ed 18, Philadelphia, 1991, WB Saunders.
2. Tietz NW, editor: *Fundamentals of clinical chemistry,* ed 3, Philadelphia, 1987, WB Saunders.
3. Boehringer Mannheim Corp: *Chemstrip 10 UA package insert,* Indianapolis, IN, 1992, Boehringer Mannheim Corp.
4. Free HM, editor: *Modern urine chemistry,* Elkhart, IN, 1991, Miles Inc., Diagnostics Division.
5. Miles Inc., Diagnostics Division: *Multistix package insert,* Elkhart, IN, 1992, Miles Inc., Diagnostics Division.
6. Strasinger SK: *Urinalysis and body fluids: a self-instructional text,* ed 2, Philadelphia, 1991, FA Davis.
7. Rosner W, Polimeni S, Khan MS: Radioimmunoassay for human corticosteroid-binding globulin, *Clin Chem* 29:1389-1391, 1983.
8. Wiesen A, Byrd J, Hospenthal D, et al: Transient abnormalities in serum bilirubin and lactate dehydrogenase levels following red blood cell transfusions in adults, *Am J Med* 104:144-147, 1998.
9. Tietz NW, Shuey DF, Wekstein DR: Laboratory values in fit aging individuals—sexagenarians through centenarians, *Clin Chem* 38:1167-1185, 1992.
10. Schiele F, Vincent-Viry M, Fournier B, et al: Biological effects of eleven combined oral contraceptives on serum triglycerides, gamma-glutamyltransferase, alkaline phosphatase, bilirubin and other biochemical variables, *Clin Chem Lab Med* 36:871-878, 1998.
11. Schwertner H: Association of smoking and low serum bilirubin antioxidant concentrations, *Atherosclerosis* 136:383-387, 1998.
12. Robertson A, Kazmierczak S, Vos P: Improved transcutaneous bilirubinometry: comparison of SpectR(X) BiliCheck and Minolta Jaundice Meter JM-102 for estimating total serum bilirubin in a normal newborn population, *J Perinatol* 22:12-14, 2002.
13. Bhutani V, Gourley GR, Adler S, et al: Noninvasive measurement of total serum bilirubin in a multiracial predischarge newborn population to assess the risk of severe hyperbilirubinemia, *Pediatrics* 106:E17, 2000.
14. Weiss JS, Gautam A, Lauff JJ, et al: The clinical importance of a protein-bound fraction of serum bilirubin in patients with hyperbilirubinemia, *N Engl J Med* 309:147-150, 1983.
15. Newall RG, editor: *Clinical urinalysis,* Buckinghamshire, UK, 1990, Ames Division, Miles Ltd.
16. Henry JB, editor: *Clinical diagnosis and management by laboratory methods,* ed 18, Philadelphia, 1991, WB Saunders.
17. Ihara H, Nakamura H, Aoki Y, et al: In vitro effects of light on serum bilirubin subfractions measured by high-performance liquid chromatography: comparison with four routine methods, *Clin Chem* 38:2124-2129, 1992.
18. Doumas B, Wu T: The measurement of bilirubin fractions in serum, *Crit Rev Clin Lab Sci* 28:415-445, 1991.
19. Lott J, Doumas B: "Direct" and total bilirubin tests: contemporary problems, *Clin Chem* 39:641-647, 1993.
20. Lo S, Doumas B, Ashwood E: Performance of bilirubin determinations in US laboratories—revisited, *Clin Chem* 50:190-194, 2004.

*Biotin and Biotinidase can be found in the Appendix on p. 1761.

DIAGNOSTIC INFORMATION	**REMARKS**

S ↑ Hepatobiliary disorders; may remain elevated after conjugated and unconjugated bilirubin have returned to normal. Thus conjugated bilirubin is a better indicator during resolution of disease than direct or total bilirubin.[14]

This derived test (total bilirubin minus conjugated plus unconjugated bilirubin) should not be calculated on neonatal patients (<14 days).

δ-Bilirubin is a form of bilirubin that is covalently bound to albumin. It has a longer half-life than other forms of bilirubin; thus it remains elevated during the convalescent phases of hepatic disorders when the conjugated and unconjugated bilirubin have already begun to decline or have returned to normal.[21]

TEST NAME AND METHOD	SPECIMEN REQUIREMENTS	REFERENCE INTERVAL, CONVENTIONAL [INTERNATIONAL RECOMMENDED UNITS]			CHEMICAL INTERFERENCES AND IN VIVO EFFECTS
Bismuth (Bi) *Quantitative: AAS*	Whole blood.[1] Collect in pretested, metal-free container.	*mcg/L* 1-12	× 4.785	*nmol/L* [4.8-57.4]	None found.
	Plasma (heparin). Collect in metal-free container.	0.1-3.5[3]		[0.5-16.7]	
	Urine, 24 hr. Collect in acid-washed, metal-free container. Stable indefinitely at room temperature.	0.3-4.6		[1.4-22.0]	
ICP-MS	Whole blood[2]	*mcg/L* 0-5	× 4.785	*nmol/L* [0.00-23.93]	
		0-2		[0.00-9.57]	
	Urine[2]	*mcg/day* 0-3		*nmol/day* [0.00-14.36]	

1. Serfontein WJ, Mekel R, Bank S, et al: Bismuth toxicity in man. I. Bismuth blood and urine levels in patients after administration of a bismuth protein complexes, *Res Commun Chem Pathol Pharmacol* 26:383-389, 1979.
2. Associated Regional & University Pathologists, Inc. web site (www.aruplab.com): Online User's Guide available at: http://www.aruplab.com/testing/user_guide.jsp. Last accessed 9/2004.
3. Froomes PRA, Wan AT, Harrison PM, et al: Improved assay for bismuth in biological samples by atomic absorption spectrophotometry with hydride generation, *Clin Chem* 34:382-384, 1988.

TEST NAME AND METHOD	SPECIMEN REQUIREMENTS	REFERENCE INTERVAL, CONVENTIONAL [INTERNATIONAL RECOMMENDED UNITS]			CHEMICAL INTERFERENCES AND IN VIVO EFFECTS
Bisphospho-glyceromutase (Diphospho-glyceromutase, DPGM) in Erythrocytes (EC 2.7.5.4)[1-3] *ICSH, 37° C*[3]	Hemolysate of washed Ercs. Submit whole blood (ACD, EDTA, or heparin). Stable 5 days at 25° C in ACD or heparin, 2 days in EDTA; stable for 20 days at 4° C in ACD, 6 days in EDTA or heparin.	*U/g Hb* 4.78 ± 0.65 (SD) *U/10[12] Ercs* 139 ± 18.8 *U/mL Ercs* 1.63 ± 0.22	× 0.0645* × 10⁻³ × 1.0	*MU/mol Hb* [0.31 ± 0.04] *nU/Ercs* [0.14 ± 0.02] *kU/L Ercs* [1.63 ± 0.22]	None found.

See *Acetylcholinesterase.*

*Conversion factor based on MW of Hb of 64,500.

1. Beutler E: *Hemolytic anemia in disorders of red cell metabolism,* New York, 1978, Plenum.
2. Beutler E: *Red cell metabolism: a manual of biochemical methods,* ed 4, New York, 1986, Grune & Stratton.
3. Beutler E, Blume KG, Kaplan JC, et al: International committee for standardization in haematology: recommended methods for red-cell enzyme analysis, *Br J Haematol* 35:331-340, 1977.
4. Kralovics R, Prchal JT: Congenital and inherited polycythemia, *Curr Opin Pediatr* 12:29-34, 2000.

DIAGNOSTIC INFORMATION	REMARKS
Symptoms from chronic exposure include weakness, decreased appetite, fever, rheumatic-like pain, foul breath, renal damage, black gum line, anuria, diarrhea, and bone changes.	Workers in cosmetic, disinfectant, pigment, and solder industries may be exposed to bismuth. Bi poisoning may occur as a consequence of therapy for syphilis. Bismuth is included in some drug products and over-the-counter medications (i.e., bismuth subsalicylate). See Table II-6.

Homozygous deficiency may be a rare cause of polycythemia.[4]	The same enzyme has 2,3-DPG phosphatase activity. U/g Hb $\times$ 29 = U/10^{12} Ercs U/g Hb $\times$ 0.34 = U/mL Ercs* *See Note, *Acetylcholinesterase.*

TEST NAME AND METHOD	SPECIMEN REQUIREMENTS	REFERENCE INTERVAL, CONVENTIONAL [INTERNATIONAL RECOMMENDED UNITS]	CHEMICAL INTERFERENCES AND IN VIVO EFFECTS
Bladder Tumor–Associated Antigen (BTA)[1,2] *Immunoassay*	Urine. Voided or catheterized specimen. Stable at room temperature for 48 hr, 2-8° C for 7 days, 24 wk at −20° C; avoid repeated freezing and thawing.	*Quantitative (BTA TRAK)* ≤14 U/mL × 1.0 [≤14 kU/L] *Qualitative (BTA stat)* None detected.	↑ Hematuria, potential false-positive results with gross hematuria caused by circulating blood antigens.[3]

1. Konety BR, Getzenberg RH: Urine based markers of urological malignancy, *J Urol* 165:600-611, 2001.
2. Fritsche HA: Bladder cancer and urine tumor marker tests. In Diamandis EP, Fritsche HA, Lilja H, et al, editors: *Tumor markers. Physiology, pathobiology, technology, and clinical applications,* Washington, DC, 2002, AACC Press.
3. Oge O, Kozaci D, Gemalmaz H: The BTA stat test is nonspecific for hematuria: an experimental hematuria model, *J Urol* 167:1318-1319, 2002.

TEST NAME AND METHOD	SPECIMEN REQUIREMENTS	REFERENCE INTERVAL, CONVENTIONAL [INTERNATIONAL RECOMMENDED UNITS]	CHEMICAL INTERFERENCES AND IN VIVO EFFECTS
Bleeding Time (BT)[1-4]	None—performed at the bedside or in office.	Generally 2-9 min, depending on the method used.	↑ V Aspirin, alcohol, allopurinol, some antibiotics, anticoagulants, asparaginase, dextran, diltiazem hydrochloride, halothane, nifedipine, nonsteroidal antiinflammatory drugs, propranolol, streptokinase and urokinase, and valproic acid ↓ V Desmopressin, epoetin (erythropoetin)

1. Lewis SM, Bain BJ, Bates I, editors: *Dacie and Lewis practical hematology,* ed 9,Edinburgh, 2001, Churchill Livingstone.
2. Jacobs DS, Demott WR, Oxley DK, editors: *Laboratory test handbook,* ed 5, Hudson, OH, 2001, Lexi-Comp, Inc.
3. Rodgers RP, Levin J: A critical reappraisal of the bleeding time, *Semin Thromb Hemost* 16:1-20, 1990.

DIAGNOSTIC INFORMATION	REMARKS

Clinical use in detecting bladder cancer recurrence. Monitoring sensitivity of 57-83% and specificity of 68-72% for BTA *stat* and sensitivity of 66-78% and specificity of 50-75% for BTA TRAK.[1]

Positive result or elevated values observed with renal stones, nephritis, urinary tract infections, cystitis, renal cancer, and recent bladder or urinary tract trauma, including cystoscopy.

The antigen in bladder tumor–associated antigen detected in the BTA *stat* and TRAK assays is human complement factor H–related protein (hCFHrp), which has similarity to human complement factor H (hCFH), also detected in the assays. hCFH functions in the alternative complement pathway by interacting with complement factor C3b to prevent cell lysis. Bladder tumor–associated antigen may allow tumor cells to evade the host immune system.

The qualitative point-of-care BTA *stat* assay (Bion Diagnostic Sciences, Inc., Cortlandt Manor, NY) is an immunochromatographic assay utilizing two monoclonal antibodies to hCFRrp. The quantitative BTA TRAK assay has an EIA format. Both tests have FDA-approved indications for use as an aid in the management of bladder cancer patients in conjunction with cystoscopy.

↑ Platelet function disorder, both hereditary (Glanzmann's thrombasthenia, Bernard-Soulier syndrome, storage pool disorder) and acquired (uremia, paraprotein, drugs), von Willebrand's disease, thrombocytopenia, and vascular abnormalities such as Ehlers-Danlos syndrome.

The bleeding time measures overall platelet function. It is neither a sensitive nor a specific test, and its use has overall declined with time.

The BT is subject to many variables (constant blood pressure, length of incision, blotting technique). Only experienced individuals should perform the test; ideally the same individual/team should do the test for consistency.

Although the BT time may be informative in evaluating a patient with a bleeding history, it should not be used as a perioperative screening test in an individual without a history of bleeding.

The original BT was known as the Duke BT, in which the earlobe was pierced. Subsequent modifications include the Ivy BT and the template methods (Surgicutt and Simplate). In both methods a blood pressure cuff is used on the upper arm and inflated to 40 mm Hg to increase capillary pressure in the forearm, and either a puncture wound (Ivy) or a linear incision (template) is made in the forearm.[5]

4. Peterson P, Hayes TE, Arkin CF, et al: The preoperative bleeding time test lacks clinical benefit, *Arch Surg* 133:134-139, 1998.
5. Lind SE: The bleeding time does not predict surgical bleeding, *Blood* 77:2547-2552, 1991.

TEST NAME AND METHOD	SPECIMEN REQUIREMENTS	REFERENCE INTERVAL, CONVENTIONAL [INTERNATIONAL RECOMMENDED UNITS]		CHEMICAL INTERFERENCES AND IN VIVO EFFECTS
Blood Volume, Total (TBV)[1,2] *(1) Sum of* [125]*I-albumin plasma volume (PV) plus* [51]*Cr red cell volume (RCV)*	See *Red Cell (Erythro-cyte) Mass* and *Plasma Volume.*	60-80 mL/kg[1]		See *Plasma Volume.*
(2) Calculation from RCV and Hct				

1. Dacie J, Lewis S, editors: *Practical haematology,* ed 8, Edinburgh, 1995, Churchill Livingstone.
2. International Committee for Standardization in Haematology: Recommended methods for measurement of red-cell and plasma volume, *J Nucl Med* 21:793-800, 1980.
3. Winters J, Pineda A: Hemapheresis. In Henry J, editor: *Clinical diagnosis and management by laboratory methods,* Philadelphia, 2001, WB Saunders, pp. 776-805.

TEST NAME AND METHOD	SPECIMEN REQUIREMENTS	REFERENCE INTERVAL, CONVENTIONAL				[INTERNATIONAL RECOMMENDED UNITS]	CHEMICAL INTERFERENCES AND IN VIVO EFFECTS
Borate[1] *Boric acid; Sodium borate (Borax)* *Colorimetric*	Serum. Do not use borosilicate glassware.	Child: Adult, M: Toxic concentration:	*mg/L* <7 <2 >20	× 16.4		*μmol/L* [<115] [<33] [<329]	High concentrations of Sb, Fe, Cu, and oxidizing acids may interfere.

1. Baselt RC: *Biological monitoring methods for industrial chemicals,* Davis, CA, 1980, Biomedical Pub.
2. Wester RC, Hui X, Maibach HI, et al: In vivo percutaneous absorption of boron as boric acid, borax, and disodium octaborate tetrahydrate in humans: a summary, *Biol Trace Elem Res* 66:101-109, 1998.
3. Linden CH, Hall AH, Kulig KW, et al: Acute ingestions of boric acid, *J Toxicol Clin Toxicol* 24:264-279, 1986.

| DIAGNOSTIC INFORMATION | REMARKS |

↑ TBV

Polycythemia vera, pulmonary disease, severe starvation, acidosis, thyrotoxicosis, vasodilatation, cardiac failure, overhydration, renal insufficiency, congenital cardiac disorders, pregnancy, recumbent posture, athletes

↓ TBV

Hemorrhage, burns, severe anemia, pheochromocytoma, chronic infection, chronic azotemia, vomiting, diarrhea, dehydration, salt deficiency, diabetes, starvation, old age, bed rest, exercise, cold, standing, apprehension, obesity (fat is relatively avascular)

Determination of TBV by laboratory methods is rarely indicated in clinical medicine, including hemapheresis.[3] Usually estimation from nomograms or mathematical formulas suffices.

If accurate determination of the TBV is critical, calculation from the sum of measured red cell and plasma volumes is the recommended method. In this approach a disproportionate high white cell count may underestimate the true TBV.

The alternative method of calculating TBV from RCV and Hct uses a correction factor (0.9) to account for the mean Hct difference between whole-body and venous Hct.

$$TBV = \frac{RCV}{0.9 \times Hct}$$

The Hct difference in individuals varies widely around this mean, both in healthy persons and in disease states, most notably in splenomegaly (↑) and, to some extent, in severe anemia (↓). At Hct >55% [>0.55], this method underestimates TBV. When TBV is based on total body water or lean body mass (instead of body weight), there is no difference between the values for obese and lean persons.

Orally administered borate is rapidly distributed throughout body water, is not metabolized, and has an elimination half-life of 21 hr.

Dermal absorption of borate is minimal and significantly less than dietary exposure.[2]

Boric acid and sodium borate are used in cleaning agents, preservatives, and fungicides. Serum boric acid levels correlate poorly with development of symptoms in acute, single ingestions.[3]

The NOAEL and LOAEL for borate are 55 and 7 mg/kg/day, respectively.

See Table II-6.

TEST NAME AND METHOD	SPECIMEN REQUIREMENTS	REFERENCE INTERVAL, CONVENTIONAL [INTERNATIONAL RECOMMENDED UNITS]	CHEMICAL INTERFERENCES AND IN VIVO EFFECTS
BRCA1, BRCA2 *Molecular testing* *Breast cancer antigen*	Whole blood (EDTA) at room temperature	*Interpretation of test results is individual and method specific.*	

1. Welcsh PL, King M-C: *BRCA1* and *BRCA2* and the genetics of breast and ovarian cancer, *Hum Mol Genet* 10:705-713, 2001.

2. Genetic/familial high-risk assessment: breast and ovarian. Clinical practice guidelines in oncology, *National Comprehensive Cancer Network.* Available at: www.nccn.org. v1.2005. Last accessed 2/22/05.

3. Ozcelik H, Glendon G: BRCA1 and BRCA2: genes that predispose to breast and ovarian cancer. In Diamandis EP, Fritsche HA, Lilja H, et al, editors: *Tumor markers. Physiology, pathobiology, technology, and clinical applications,* Washington DC, 2002, AACC Press.

BRCA1 and *BRCA2* are tumor suppressor genes that function in DNA damage repair and transcriptional regulation. *BRCA1* and *BRCA2* are located on chromosomes 17q21 and 13q12.3, respectively, and are inherited in an autosomal-dominant fashion.[1] Germline mutations in these genes result in a predisposition to breast and ovarian cancers, and these mutations account for the majority of families with hereditary susceptibility to breast and ovarian cancer. *BRCA2* is associated with male breast cancer and may be associated with prostate and pancreas cancers.[2,3]

Hereditary breast cancer accounts for 5-10% of all breast cancer cases, and approximately 10% of epithelial ovarian cancers are related to genetic mutations. *BRCA1* and *BRCA2* mutation carriers have an estimated lifetime risk of breast cancer ranging from 55-85% compared with a lifetime risk of 13% in the general population. Founder mutations, exhibiting specific patterns, have been identified in the Ashkenazi Jewish population and in other populations including those in Iceland and the Netherlands.[1,2,4]

Candidates for *BRCA1* and *BRCA2* testing include probands at high risk for *BRCA1* or *BRCA2* cancer-predisposing mutations or at-risk relatives of an individual with an identified mutation. Genetic counseling for risk assessment and test interpretation, taking into account family history, is part of the pretesting and posttesting process.[4,5] Typically, testing is performed on genomic DNA isolated from peripheral blood lymphocytes. Testing for mutations in *BRCA1* and *BRCA2* includes sequence analysis and mutation analysis. Comprehensive analysis (Myriad Genetics, Inc., Salt Lake City, UT) includes full *BRCA1* and *BRCA2* gene sequencing and detection of five genomic rearrangements of the *BRCA1* gene. Mutation-specific analysis (single and multisite) can include testing for specific familial mutations if a deleterious familial mutation is known or for population-specific mutations such as the three common mutations associated with Ashkenazi Jewish ancestry. Sites performing testing can be found at www.genetests.org.[2,5,6]

4. Meyskens FL: Cancer prevention, screening, and early detection. In Abeloff MD, Armitage JO, Niederhuber JE, et al, editors: *Clinical oncology,* Philadelphia, 2004, Elsevier Churchill Livingstone.

5. Petrucelli N, Daly MB, Burke W, et al: BRCA1 and BRCA2 hereditary breast/ovarian cancer, *GeneReviews.* Available at: www.genetests.org. 2004. Last accessed 2/22/05.

6. Myriad Genetics, Inc. Available at: www.myriad.com. Last accessed 2/22/05.

TEST NAME AND METHOD	SPECIMEN REQUIREMENTS	REFERENCE INTERVAL, CONVENTIONAL [INTERNATIONAL RECOMMENDED UNITS]	CHEMICAL INTERFERENCES AND IN VIVO EFFECTS
Breath Hydrogen Test (for bacterial intestinal overgrowth)[1,2] *GC* Dose: 10 g lactulose in 200 mL water	Take test meal in evening (see *Remarks*). After 10-hr fast, administer lactulose and collect end-expiratory breath samples at 15 min, 30 min, 60 min, 90 min, and 120 min. On a separate day give glucose load and measure 2-hr H_2 excretion.	H_2 excretion *ppm (SD)* *Volume fraction* Fasting: 4.6 ± 5.1 $\times 1.0$ $4.6 \times 10^{-6} \pm 5.1 \times 10^{-6}$ After lactulose Early increase <12 $<12 \times 10^{-6}$ Lactulose causes a colonic response in most subjects >30 min after ingestion.	None found.

1. Kerlin P, Wong L: Breath hydrogen testing in bacterial overgrowth of the small intestine, *Gastroenterology* 95:982-988, 1988.
2. Yamada T, editor: *Textbook of gastroenterology,* Philadelphia, 1991, JB Lippincott.
3. Riordan SM, McIver CJ, Duncombe VM, et al: Evaluation of the rice breath hydrogen test for small intestinal bacterial overgrowth, *Am J Gastroenterol* 95:2858-2864, 2000.
4. Bauer TM, Schwacha H, Steinbruckner B, et al: Diagnosis of small intestinal bacterial overgrowth in patients with cirrhosis of the liver: poor performance of the glucose breath hydrogen test, *J Hepatol* 33:382-386, 2000.
5. Stotzer PO, Kilander AF: Comparison of the 1-gram (14)C-D-xylose breath test and the 50-gram hydrogen glucose breath test for diagnosis of small intestinal bacterial overgrowth, *Digestion* 61:165-171, 2000.
6. Riordan SM, McIver CJ, Walker BM, et al: The lactulose breath hydrogen test and small intestinal bacterial overgrowth, *Am J Gastroenterol* 91:1795-1803, 1996.

C-Peptide[1-5] *RIA*	Serum, fasting. Store at $-70°$ C. Stable for 30 days when frozen.	0.78-1.89 ng/mL$^2 \times 0.333$* [0.26-0.63 nmol/L] *Conversion factor based on MW of C-peptide of 3000.	↑ V Chloroquine, danazol, ethinyl estradiol, oral contraceptives
Immunometeric assays "Chemiluminescent"		0.9-4.3 ng/mL 0.28-1.42 nmol/L	↓ Proinsulin (some assays) ↓ EDTA (15-20%) ↓ Hemolysis

DIAGNOSTIC INFORMATION	REMARKS
A high fasting breath H_2 level and an increase of at least 12 ppm [12×106] within 30 min after lactulose challenge are indicative of bacterial overgrowth in the small intestine. The increase must precede the colonic response.	Bacterial overgrowth is defined as a jejunal culture yielding at least 105 organisms/mL.
	No antibiotics, laxatives, or enemas for 1 wk before the test.
False-positive tests can be expected in patients without overgrowth if there is accelerated gastric emptying and rapid transit of substrate to the cecum. Therefore avoid laxatives. False-negative breath tests are observed in patients receiving antibiotics and in nonhydrogen producers.	The test meal consists of meat and rice taken the evening before the test. Avoid foods high in fiber.
	The test originally used a glucose challenge and was reported to have a sensitivity of 93% and specificity of 78%.[1] More recent studies show sensitivities of 20-58%, specificities of 36-91%, and PPV from 63-75%.[3-6] The test is questionable for routine diagnosis. The lactulose is diagnostically similar but is much easier to perform.

↑ Insulinoma, pancreas or β-cell transplants, ingestion of oral hypoglycemic drugs, renal failure, non–insulin-dependent (type II) diabetes mellitus	A strong correlation exists between serum levels of insulin and C-peptide. However, C-peptide is biologically inactive. Insulin does not cross-react in C-peptide assays; proinsulin may cross-react but typically contributes <1% to the C-peptide values.
↓ Factitious hypoglycemia due to insulin administration, radical pancreatectomy, insulin-dependent (type I) diabetes mellitus	A molar ration of C-peptide/insulin >5 in the peripheral circulation is probably due to the longer half-life of C-peptide over that of insulin in circulation (20 min vs. 5-10 min) and to the fact that C-peptide is not significantly metabolized by the liver. Unlike insulin, the majority of C-peptide is degraded in the kidney and partially excreted in the urine.
Other applications are (1) to assess β-cell function and endogenous insulin secretion in the presence of exogenous insulin or when circulating insulin antibodies preclude measurement of insulin, and (2) to facilitate the interpretation of peripheral insulin levels when hepatic insulin extraction may be variable.	Both C-peptide and insulin should be in same units (i.e., pmol/L) for ratio calculation.
Measurements of C-peptide before and after glucagon stimulation may be of value in assessing insulin treatment in diabetes mellitus. (See also *C-Peptide Stimulation Test.*)	

TEST NAME AND METHOD	SPECIMEN REQUIREMENTS	REFERENCE INTERVAL, CONVENTIONAL [INTERNATIONAL RECOMMENDED UNITS]			CHEMICAL INTERFERENCES AND IN VIVO EFFECTS

C-Peptide—CONT

| | Urine, 24 hr. Neutralize to pH 7.0-7.5, and store at $-15°$ C. Stable at $-70°$ C for ≥ 1 yr. | *mcg/day* 64.6 ± 20.5 (SD)[3] | × 0.333* | *nmol/day* [21.5 ± 6.8] | |

		mcg/g creatinine[6]		*nmol/mmol creatinine*
	2-7 yr:	14-129	× 0.0377	[0.53-4.86]
	Adult:	11-53		[0.41-2.00]

*Conversion factor based on MW of C-peptide of 3000.

1. Bonser AM, Garcia-Webb P: C-peptide measurement: methods and clinical utility, *Crit Rev Clin Lab Sci* 19:297-352, 1983.

2. Hoogwerf BJ, Goetz FC: Urinary C-peptide—a simple measure of integrated insulin production with emphasis on the effects of body size, diet and corticosteroids, *J Clin Endocrinol Metab* 56:60-67, 1982.

3. Horwitz DL, Starr JE, Mako ME, et al: Proinsulin, insulin and C-peptide concentrations in human portal and peripheral blood, *J Clin Invest* 55:1278-1283, 1975.

4. Morrisey JL, Shihabi ZK: Assay of 4-hydroxy-3-methoxyphenylacetic (homovanillic) acid by liquid chromatography with electrochemical detection, *Clin Chem* 25:2045-2047, 1979.

5. Polonsky K, Frank B, Pugh W, et al: The limitations to and valid use of C-peptide as a marker of the secretion of insulin, *Diabetes* 35:379-386, 1986.

6. Nichols Institute Reference Laboratories: *Test catalog,* San Juan Capistrano, CA, 1993, Nichols Institute Reference Laboratories.

7. Tillil H, Shaprio ET, Given BD, et al: Reevaluation of urine C-peptide as measure of insulin secretion, *Diabetes* 37:1195-1200, 1988.

C-Peptide Stimulation Test[1-5] Dose: 1 mg glucagon, IV	Serum, fasting. Draw basal and 6 min after glucagon stimulation (glucose, insulin, and C-peptide).	C-peptide			None found.

		ng/mL[1]		*nmol/L*
	Baseline:	0.78-1.89	× 0.333*	[0.26-0.63]
	After glucagon:	2.73-5.64		[0.91-1.88]

*Conversion factor based on MW of C-peptide of 3000.

1. Hoekstra JBL, van Rijn HJM, Erkelens DW, et al: C-peptide [review], *Diabetes Care* 5:438-446, 1982.

2. Koskinen PJ, Viikari JS, Irjala KMA, et al: Plasma and urinary C-peptide in the classification of adult diabetics, *Scand J Clin Lab Invest* 46:655-663, 1986.

3. Koskinen PJ, Viikari JS, Irjala KMA: Glucagon-stimulated and postprandial plasma C-peptide values as measures of insulin secretory capacity, *Diabetes Care* II:318-322, 1988.

4. Madsbad S, Krarup T, McNair P, et al: Practical clinical value of the C-peptide response to glucagon stimulation in the choice of treatment of diabetes mellitus, *Acta Med Scand* 210:153-156, 1981.

5. Singer D, Coley C, Samet J, et al: Tests of glycemia in diabetes mellitus. Their use in establishing a diagnosis and in treatment, *Ann Intern Med* 110:25, 1989.

DIAGNOSTIC INFORMATION

REMARKS

This test is useful when continuous assessment of β-cell function is desirable or frequent blood sampling is not practical.

Urine C-peptide values correlate well with fasting serum levels but not with insulin secretory rate.[7]

In subjects with diabetes mellitus, those with values >1.8 ng/mL [>0.60 nmol/L] after glucagon stimulation can often be managed without insulin treatment.

Determines insulin secretory reserve, can help distinguish patients with T1DM from T2DM because T1DM patients will usually have low or undetectable C-peptide levels after stimulation.

TEST NAME AND METHOD	SPECIMEN REQUIREMENTS	REFERENCE INTERVAL, CONVENTIONAL [INTERNATIONAL RECOMMENDED UNITS]	CHEMICAL INTERFERENCES AND IN VIVO EFFECTS
C-Reactive Protein (CRP)[1-3] *RID, EIA, RIA* *Turbidimetric, Nephelometric*	Serum. Analyze fresh or store at 4° C for <72 hr. Stable frozen at −20° C for 6 mo or at −70° C indefinitely. Specimens without lipemia or hemolysis are preferred.	<1 mg/dL × 10 [<10 mg/L] Lower 95th percentile[1]: 20-610 mg/dL [× 0.01 = 0.20-6.10 mg/L]	Excessive turbidity can affect nephelometric methods.

	mcg/dL		*mcg/L*
Cord:	1-35	× 10	[10-350]
Median:	7.2		[72]
$\bar{x}$:	10.9		[109]
Adult:	6.8-820		[68-8200]
Median:	58		[580]
$\bar{x}$:	134		[1340]
Newborn[4]:	1.3-44.4		[13-444]

High sensitivity-CRP (hs-CRP)[5,6]

CHD risk level

	mg/L
Low	<1
Average	1-3
High	>3 (up to 10)

Noncardiovascular cause should be considered if values are >10 mg/L with repeat measurements.

1. Kindmark C-O: The concentration of C-reactive protein in sera from healthy individuals, *Scand J Clin Lab Invest* 29:407-411, 1972.

2. Du Clos TW: Function of C-reactive protein, *Ann Med* 32:274-278, 2000.

3. Maksimowicz-McKinnon K, Bhatt DL, Calabrese LH: Recent advances in vascular inflammation: C-reactive protein and other inflammatory biomarkers, *Curr Opin Rheumatol* 16:18-24, 2004.

4. Soldin SJ, Brugnara C, Wong EC, editors: *Pediatric reference ranges,* ed 4, Washington, DC, 2003, AACC Press.

5. Quest Diagnostics Directory of Services: Available at: http://www.questdiagnostics.com/. Last accessed 9/28/04.

6. Pearson TA, Mensah GA, Alexander RW, et al: Marker of inflammation and cardiovascular disease. Application to clinical and public health practice: a statement for healthcare professionals from the Centers of Disease Control and Prevention and the American Heart Association, *Circulation* 107:499-511, 2003.

7. Walls DH, Krohn MA, Wener MH, et al: C-reactive protein in normal pregnancy, *Obstet Gynecol* 77:176-180, 1991.

8. Sabel K-G, Hanson LA: The clinical usefulness of C-reactive protein (CRP) determinations in bacterial meningitis and septicemia in infancy, *Acta Pediatr Scand* 63:381-388, 1974.

DIAGNOSTIC INFORMATION

↑ Acute phase reacting protein. Rapid, marked increases occur with inflammation, infection, trauma and tissue necrosis, malignancies, and autoimmune diseases.[2,3] Unlike other acute phase (AP) proteins, such as α1-antitrypsin and haptoglobin, CRP is essentially unaffected by hormones (whether endogenous, as in pregnancy, or exogenous).[7] CRP values increase very quickly and dramatically in response to stimuli, and then decrease substantially with resolution of the disorder.[2] Because concentrations typically increase more markedly than do those of other AP proteins, CRP is exceptionally useful in assessing the acute phase response.

Levels of CRP do not increase consistently in viral or spirochetal infections. Consequently, in the absence of other causes, very high levels may be indicative of a bacterial infection.[8-10] The CRP response has been found to be particularly helpful in the neonatal period in the diagnosis of bacterial sepsis.[8] In patients with bacterial meningitis, very high initial levels may also be predictive of neurological sequelae.[11] Sequential levels are valuable to monitor response to antimicrobial therapy.[11] Similarly, because levels are increased initially after surgery but decrease rapidly in the absence of bacterial infection, sequential levels are useful to monitor for postoperative infection.[12]

CRP levels are valuable in the clinical assessment of chronic inflammatory disorders such as rheumatoid arthritis,[13] systemic lupus erythematosus,[14] vasculitis syndromes, and inflammatory bowel disease.[15] Therapeutic nonsteroidal antiinflammatory medications decrease the CRP response.[16]

↓ No deficiency states have been identified.[15]

REMARKS

C-reactive protein (CRP) is a member of the pentraxin protein family.[2] Hepatic secretion is stimulated in response to inflammatory cytokines such as interleukin 6 (IL-6).[2] CRP is believed to have a role in the innate immune response. CRP activates the complement system, binds to Fc receptors, and serves as an opsonin for some microorganisms.[2] In a calcium-dependent mechanism, it has been shown to bind pathogens such as *Haemophilus influenzae, Leishmania donovani,* and the C-polysaccharide of the pneumococcal cell wall.[2] Evidence suggests that CRP may also have a role in the clearance of nuclear antigens and damaged cell membranes.[2,18]

It binds phosphatidylcholine on damaged cell membranes,[2,17] exposed chromatin,[2,18] and small nuclear ribonucloproteins (snRNPs), which may be involved in autoimmunity.[2,19] CRP is actively transported into cell nuclei.[2] Studies in mice have demonstrated a protective effect against the development of autoimmunity[2,20] and the lethal effects of infection.[2,21]

High sensitivity measurements of CRP are useful in assessing vascular inflammation and cardiovascular risk stratification.[3] Studies indicate that CRP may be involved in the atherogenesis,[393] and elevated levels can decrease endothelial cell expression and activity of nitric oxide synthase.[3,21] CRP level has been shown to be an independent risk factor for atherosclerotic disease, and increases predicted are associated with increased cardiovascular morbidity and mortality in patients with coronary artery disease.[3]

There is a good correlation with the erythrocyte sedimentation rate (ESR), but CRP appears and disappears earlier than changes in ESR.

MW: 105,000-114,700

9. McCarthy PL, Frank AL, Ablow RC, et al: Value of the C-reactive protein test in the differential of bacterial and viral pneumonia, *J Pediatr* 92:454-456, 1978.

10. Peltola HO: C-reactive protein for rapid monitoring of infectious of the central nervous system, *Lancet* 1:980-982, 1982.

11. Valmari P, Peltola H, Ruuskanen O: C-reactive protein as a predictor of sequelae of meningitis, *Lancet* 1:741-742, 1984.

12. Fischer CL, Gill C, Forrester MG, et al: Quantitation of acute phase proteins postoperatively: value in detection of complications, *Am J Pathol* 66:840-846, 1976.

13. Rowe IF, Sheldon J, Riches PG, et al: Comparative studies of serum and synovial fluid C-reactive protein concentrations, *Ann Rheum Dis* 46:721-726, 1987.

14. Spronk PE, ter Borg EJ, Kallenberg CG: Patients with systemic lupus erythematosus and Jaccoud's arthropathy: a clinical subset with increased C-reactive protein response, *Ann Rheum Dis* 51:358-361, 1992.

15. Pepys MB: C-reactive protein fifty years on, *Lancet* 1:653-657, 1981.

16. Cush JJ, Lipsky PE, Postlethwaite AE, et al: Correlation of serological indicators of inflammation with effectiveness of nonsteroidal anti-inflammatory drug therapy in rheumatoid arthritis, *Arthritis Rheum* 33:19-28, 1990.

TEST NAME AND METHOD	SPECIMEN REQUIREMENTS	REFERENCE INTERVAL, CONVENTIONAL [INTERNATIONAL RECOMMENDED UNITS]	CHEMICAL INTERFERENCES AND IN VIVO EFFECTS

C-Reactive Protein—CONT

17. Volanakis JE, Wirtz KWA: Interaction of C-reactive protein with artificial phosphatidylcholine bilayers, *Nature* 281:155-157, 1979.

18. Robey FA, Jones KD, Tanaka T, et al: Binding of C-reactive protein to chromatin and nucleosome core particles. A possible physiological role of C-reactive protein, *J Biol Chem* 259:7311-7316, 1984.

19. Du Clos TW: C-reactive protein reacts with the U1 small nuclear ribonucleoprotein, *J Immunol* 143:2553-2559, 1989.

20. Du Clos TW, Zlock L, Hicks PS, et al: Decreased autoantibody levels and enhanced survival of (NZB X NZW) F1 mice treated with C-reactive protein, *Clin Immunol Immunopathol* 70:22-27, 1994.

TEST NAME AND METHOD	SPECIMEN REQUIREMENTS	REFERENCE INTERVAL, CONVENTIONAL			[INTERNATIONAL RECOMMENDED UNITS]	CHEMICAL INTERFERENCES AND IN VIVO EFFECTS
Cadmium (Cd)[1] *AAS*	Whole blood (heparin, EDTA).[2] Collect in pretested, metal-free container.	Nonsmokers: Smokers:	*mcg/L*[3] 0.3-1.2 0.6-3.9	× 8.897	*nmol/L* [2.7-10.7] [5.3-34.7]	↑ C Sodium salts
		Toxic range:	100-3000	× 0.0089	*μmol/L* [0.9-26.7]	
	Urine.[3] Collect in metal-free container. Use no preservatives. Stable for 7 days at room temperature.	0.5-4.7 mcg/L Exposed to Cd: 10-580 mcg/L See also Table II-12.	× 8.897 × 0.0089	[4.4-41.8 nmol/L] [0.09-5.16 μmol/L]		U ↑ V EDTA U ↓ V Antacids, antibiotics, antituberculosis therapy
ICP-MS	Whole blood.[4] Collected in pretested, metal-free container. Urine.[4] Collect in acidwashed, metal-free container. Refrigerate during and following collection.	*mcg/L* 0-5 0.0-2.6 mcg/L 0.0-3.3 mcg/day 0.0-3.0 mcg/g creatinine	× 8.897	*nmol/L* [0.0-44.5] [0.0-23.13 nmol/L] [0.0-29.36 nmol/day] [0.0-26.69 nmol/g creatinine]		

1. Wyngaarden JB, Smith LH Jr, editors: *Cecil textbook of medicine,* ed 18, Philadelphia, 1988, WB Saunders.

2. Baselt RC: *Analytical procedures for therapeutic drug monitoring and emergency toxicology,* ed 2, Littleton, MA, 1987, PSG Publishing Co., Inc.

3. Iyengar GV, Woittiez J: Trace elements in human clinical specimens: evaluation of literature data to identify tolerence values, *Clin Chem* 34:474-481, 1988.

4. Associated Regional & University Pathologists, Inc. web site (www.aruplab.com): Online User's Guide available at: http://www.aruplab.com/testing/user_guide.jsp. Last accessed 9/2004.

21. Mold C, Nakayama S, Holzer TJ, et al: C-reactive protein is protective against *Streptococcus pneumoniae* infection in mice, *J Exp Med* 154:1703-1708, 1981.
22. Venugopal S, Devaraj S, Yuhanna I, et al: Demonstration that C-reactive protein decreases eNOS expression and bioactivity in human aortic endothelial cells, *Circulation* 106:1439-1441, 2002.

Acute exposure from inhalation (industrial settings) results in acute respiratory symptoms including pulmonary edema, proliferative interstitial pneumonia, and cardiovascular collapse; permanent lung damage may occur. Cd can be ingested from food stored or prepared in cadmium-plated containers. Acute poisoning from ingestion results in a sudden onset of violent GI symptoms within 30 min after eating. Chronic ingestion results in severe osteomalacia and Fanconi-like renal dysfunction. OSHA recommends three laboratory tests to monitor exposure to cadmium: whole blood cadmium, urine cadmium, and urine β_2-microglobulin (β_2-M). (See Table II-12, for 1999 revised standard.)

Cd accumulates in tissue, concentrating primarily in the kidney and liver. More than 95% of blood Cd is in erythrocytes. Smokers have higher blood cadmium levels than nonsmokers. See Table II-12 for OSHA-recommended action levels for workers exposed to cadmium.

See Table II-6.

TEST NAME AND METHOD	SPECIMEN REQUIREMENTS	REFERENCE INTERVAL, CONVENTIONAL [INTERNATIONAL RECOMMENDED UNITS]			CHEMICAL INTERFERENCES AND IN VIVO EFFECTS
Calcitonin (CT)[1-5] *RIA*[6] *EIA*[6] *IRMA*[6]	Serum or plasma (heparin), fasting; freeze immediately at 20° C or lower.	Serum[7*] Cord blood: x̄: 83 Newborn (1-7 days) x̄: 223 Child: x̄: 38 Adult: x̄: 44	*pg/mL* 25-150 70-348 <70 <150	× 1.0	*ng/L* [25-150] [x̄: 83] [70-348] [x̄: 223] [<70] [x̄: 38] [<150] [x̄: 44]	↑ V Calcium infusion, epinephrine, estrogens, glucagon, pentagastrin, sincalide (cholecystokinin), oral contraceptives Gross lipemia and hemolysis may interfere.
		Plasma (heparin)[8] Adult M: F:	≤19 ≤14		[≤19] [≤14]	

*Method standardized with WHO calcitonin preparation 70/234.

1. Austin LA, Heath H III: Calcitonin: physiology and pathophysiology, *N Engl J Med* 304:269-278, 1981.
2. Mathé G, editor: *A symposium on physiological levels of calcitonin in man,* New York, 1984, Masson Publishing USA.
3. Mendelsohn G, Baylin SB: Medullary thyroid carcinoma: diagnostic and clinical features, *Lab Management* 21:21-35, 1983.
4. Sizemore GW, Go VL: Stimulation tests for diagnosis of medullary thyroid carcinoma, *Mayo Clin Proc* 50:53-56, 1975.
5. Talmage RV, Cooper CW, Toverud SU: The physiological significance of calcitonin, *Bone Miner Res* 1:74-143, 1983.
6. Endres DB, Rude RK: Physiology and disorders of water, electrolyte, and acid-base metabolism. In Burtis CA, Ashwood ER, editors: *Tietz textbook of clinical chemistry,* ed 3, Philadelphia, 1999, WB Saunders.
7. Endocrine Sciences: *Pediatric laboratory services,* Tarzana, CA, 1992.
8. Mayo Medical Laboratories: *Interpretive handbook,* Rochester, MN, 2001, Mayo Medical Laboratories.
9. Behrman RE, Kliegman RM, Nelson WE, editors: *Nelson textbook of pediatrics,* ed 14, Philadelphia, 1992, WB Saunders.
10. Ashwond ER: Clinical chemistry of pregnancy. In Burtis CA, Ashwood ER, editors: *Tietz textbook of clinical chemistry,* ed 2, Philadelphia, 1994, WB Saunders.
11. Grauer A, Raue F, Gagel R: Changing concepts in the management of hereditary and sporadic medullary thyroid carcinoma, *Endocrinol Metab Clin North Am* 19:613-635, 1990.

| Calcitonin Stimulation Test (after Pentagastrin)[1-5] Dose: 0.5 mcg pentagastrin/kg IV push | Plasma (heparin), fasting. Draw baseline, 1.5, 2, and 5 min after pentagastrin injection. | Calcitonin[6] Maximum response after pentagastrin M: F: | *pg/mL* ≤110 ≤30 | × 1.0 | *ng/mL* [≤110] [≤30] | See *Calcitonin.* |

DIAGNOSTIC INFORMATION	REMARKS

↑ Medullary thyroid carcinoma (MTC); C-cell hyperplasia; in some patients with carcinoma of lung, breast, or pancreas; Z-E syndrome; pernicious anemia; chronic renal failure; pseudohypoparathyroidism; tumors of APUD cells; carcinoid syndrome; alcoholic cirrhosis; patients with pancreatitis and thyroiditis.

Elevations may be observed in pregnancy and benign diseases of the lung. Calcitonin may also be ectopically produced by numerous cancers, particularly those of a neuroendocrine nature.[9]

Test is useful in monitoring response to therapy and predicting recurrences of disease in individuals with medullary thyroid carcinoma; it is also useful as a screening test for family members of patients with medullary carcinoma (20% of these cancers have a familial pattern).[10,11]

Calcitonin is a peptide hormone produced by the perifollicular C cells of the thyroid gland. Its physiologic function is as an antagonist of parathyroid hormone to inhibit osteoclastic bone activity and to decrease serum calcium. It is a 32-amino acid chain with an MW of 3400.

Values for healthy subjects vary depending on the particular immunoassay used. CT levels decrease gradually with age but increase during pregnancy and lactation. Values in serum are higher than in plasma. Clinically the test is useful as a tumor marker for MTC, especially in following patients with the disease or screening asymptomatic relatives of MTC patients. About 10% of cases appear as a component of multiple endocrine neoplasia (MEN) type IIA or IIB. Some patients may have normal or borderline elevated basal calcitonin values; in these cases provocative agents such as pentagastrin or calcium may be used to stimulate calcitonin secretion and demonstrate the abnormalities [see *Calcitonin Stimulation Test (after Calcium Infusion)* and *Calcitonin Stimulation Test (after Penta-gastrin)*].

↑ Medullary thyroid carcinoma (MTC)

Test is not needed for patients with diagnostically high basal calcitonin (CT). It is most useful in screening family members of patients with familial medullary carcinoma. In patients with MTC, maximum responses usually occur within 2 min after pentagastrin injection; a 5- to 36-fold increase in calcitonin over basal values is typically produced. In patients with elevated calcitonin levels and nonthyroidal malignancies, responses after pentagastrin are not as vigorous.

TEST NAME AND METHOD	SPECIMEN REQUIREMENTS	REFERENCE INTERVAL, CONVENTIONAL [INTERNATIONAL RECOMMENDED UNITS]	CHEMICAL INTERFERENCES AND IN VIVO EFFECTS

Calcitonin Stimulation Test (after Pentagastrin)—CONT

1. Endres DB, Rude RK: Mineral and bone metabolism. In Burtis CA, Ashwood ER, editors: *Tietz textbook of clinical chemistry,* ed 3, Philadelphia, 1999, WB Saunders.

2. Gharib H, Kao PC, Heath H III: Determinations of silica purified plasma calcitonin for the detection and management of medullary thyroid carcinoma: comparison of two provocative tests, *Mayo Clin Proc* 62:373-378, 1987.

3. Hay ID, Klee GG: Thyroid dysfunction, *Endocrinol Metab Clin North Am* 17:473-509, 1988.

4. Lavin N: *Manual of endocrinology and metabolism,* Boston, 1986, Little, Brown and Co.

5. Sizemore GW, Go VL: Stimulation tests for diagnosis of medullary thyroid carcinoma, *Mayo Clin Proc* 50:53-56, 1975.

6. Mayo Medical Laboratories: *Test catalog,* Rochester, MN, 2001, Mayo Medical Laboratories.

TEST NAME AND METHOD	SPECIMEN REQUIREMENTS	REFERENCE INTERVAL, CONVENTIONAL [INTERNATIONAL RECOMMENDED UNITS]			CHEMICAL INTERFERENCES AND IN VIVO EFFECTS
Calcitonin Stimulation Test (after Calcium and Pentagastrin Infusion)[1-5]	Serum, fasting. Draw baseline, 1, 2, and 5 min after calcium and pentagastrin infusion.	Calcitonin After calcium and pentagastrin M:	pg/mL^6	ng/L	See *Calcitonin Stimulation Test (after Calcium Infusion)* and *Calcitonin Stimulation Test (after Pentagastrin).*
		1 min:	<324 × 1.0	[<324]	
Dose: Ca (2 mg/kg)		2 min:	10-491	[10-491]	
IV infusion for		5 min:	8-343	[8-343]	
1 min, followed by		10 min:	<112	[<112]	
pentagastrin					
(0.5 mcg/kg) IV		F:			
infusion for		1 min:	<41	[<41]	
5-10 sec.		2 min:	<70	[<70]	
		5 min:	<39	[<39]	

1. Cibull M, Whitley R: Boy with thick lips. In Tietz NW, editor: *Applied laboratory medicine,* Philadelphia, 1992, WB Saunders.

2. Emmertsen K: Medullary thyroid carcinoma and calcitonin, *Dan Med Bull* 32:1-28, 1985.

3. Rude RK, Singer FR: Comparison of serum calcitonin levels after a 1-minute calcium injection and after pentagastrin injection in the diagnosis of medullary thyroid carcinoma, *J Clin Endocrinol Metab* 44:980-983, 1977.

4. Saad M, Ordonez N, Rashid R, et al: Medullary carcinoma of the thyroid, *Medicine* 63:319-342, 1984.

DIAGNOSTIC INFORMATION	REMARKS
	For the detection and management of MTC, pentagastrin is considered by some to be the provocative agent of choice. Side effects of pentagastrin (e.g., nausea, headache, epigastric and chest discomfort) are common but usually very brief. A few patients with MTC, however, do not respond to pentagastrin, and a calcium infusion test—alone or in combination with pentagastrin—may also be needed. [See *Calcitonin Stimulation Test (after Calcium Infusion).*] In some cases it may be necessary to carry out these stimulation tests over a period of months or years to confirm or rule out a diagnosis.
See *Calcitonin Stimulation Test (after Calcium Infusion)* and *Calcitonin Stimulation Test (after Pentagastrin).*	See *Calcitonin Stimulation Test (after Calcium Infusion)* and *Calcitonin Stimulation Test (after Pentagastrin).*

5. Sizemore GW, Go VL: Stimulation tests for diagnosis of medullary thyroid carcinoma, *Mayo Clin Proc* 50:53-56, 1975.
5. Quest Diagnostics Nichols Institute Reference Manual: *Services and information, tests and methods, specimen requirements, guidelines for interpretation of results,* San Juan Capistrano, CA, 1998/1999, Quest Diagnostics Nichols Institute.

TEST NAME AND METHOD	SPECIMEN REQUIREMENTS	REFERENCE INTERVAL, CONVENTIONAL [INTERNATIONAL RECOMMENDED UNITS]			CHEMICAL INTERFERENCES AND IN VIVO EFFECTS
Calcitonin Stimulation Test (after calcium infusion)[1-3] Dose: Ca (as gluconate), 2 mg/kg IV infusion for 1 min or 2.4 mg Ca/kg IV push	Plasma (heparin), fasting. Draw baseline, 5, and 10 min after calcium injection.	Calcitonin[4] Maximum response after calcium M: F:	*pg/mL* ≤190 ≤130	× 1.0	*ng/L* [≤190] [≤130]	See *Calcitonin.*

1. Mendelsohn G, Baylin SB: Medullary thyroid carcinoma: diagnostic and clinical features, *Lab Management* 21:21-35, 1983.
2. Rude RK, Singer FR: Comparison of serum calcitonin levels after a 1-minute calcium injection and after pentagastrin injection in the diagnosis of medullary thyroid carcinoma, *J Clin Endocrinol Metab* 44:980-983, 1977.
3. Wells SA, Baylin SB, Linehan WM, et al: Provocative agents and the diagnosis of medullary carcinoma of the thyroid gland, *Ann Surg* 188:139, 1978.
4. Mayo Medical Laboratories: *Interpretive handbook,* Rochester, MN, 2001, Mayo Medical Laboratories.

TEST NAME AND METHOD	SPECIMEN REQUIREMENTS	REFERENCE INTERVAL, CONVENTIONAL [INTERNATIONAL RECOMMENDED UNITS]			CHEMICAL INTERFERENCES AND IN VIVO EFFECTS
Calcium, Ionized (CaI)[1-8] *ISE*	Collect blood anaerobically; draw without stasis or after circulation has been restored for >1 min. Place on ice and deliver to the lab immediately. Plasma or serum can be stored in a tightly sealed container at 4° C for several days or at −20° C for 6 mo.				↑ V Decreased plasma pH, hydrochlorothiazide (chronic use), lithium ↓ V Anticonvulsants, danazol, foscarnet, furosemide (initial effect); increased ionic strength and increased plasma pH ↓ C Ca-binding agents (e.g., citrate, oxalate, EDTA, heparin)
	Whole blood (heparin) 18-60 yr:[11] 60-90 yr: >90 yr:	*mg/dL* 4.60-5.08 4.64-5.16 4.48-5.28	× 0.25	*mmol/L* [1.15-1.27] [1.16-1.29] [1.12-1.32]	
	Plasma (heparin) >18 yr[12]:	4.12-4.92		[1.03-1.23]	

DIAGNOSTIC INFORMATION	REMARKS

↑ Medullary thyroid carcinoma, pseudohypoparathyroidism

Regardless of age, increase in calcitonin (CT) in response to Ca infusion is greater in men than in women, but basal levels of CT and the response to Ca wane with age in both sexes. The 4-hr calcium infusion test (15 mg Ca/kg) can be unpleasant for patients (e.g., causing fatigue, nausea, vomiting) and is no longer routinely used. A 10-min calcium infusion test (3 mg/kg) is also available, but the 1-min infusion is commonly employed. This short test is relatively free of side effects. A combined calcium-pentagastrin infusion test is considered by some to be more effective and reliable than either pentagastrin or calcium infusion alone.

↑ Primary hyperparathyroidism, PTH-producing tumors, excess intake of vitamin D, various malignancies (elevations may be seen even when total Ca is normal)

↓ Primary hypoparathyroidism (both Ca fractions), pseudohypoparathyroidism, vitamin D deficiency, magnesium deficiency; after transfusions with blood containing anions that complex free Ca (e.g., citrate); after major surgery, trauma, sepsis, burns, pancreatitis, multiple organ failure; after hemodialysis with low-calcium dialysate; alkalemia or increases in ionic strength (e.g., increased Na)

See also *Calcium, Total.*

Test is useful in determining the "physiologically active" or free Ca level in patients with altered proteins (chronic renal failure, nephrotic syndrome, malabsorption, multiple myeloma) and in disturbances of acid-base metabolism. Ionized Ca values reflect Ca metabolism better than total Ca values, and many clinicians prefer CaI over total Ca for evaluating Ca abnormalities. A significant decrease in CaI regardless of total Ca level may lead to an increase in neuromuscular irritability and thus to tetany.

Differences in specimen preparation and electrode selectivity are probably responsible for differences in reported reference ranges. Heparin itself causes a 0.04 mg/dL [0.01 mmol/L] decrease in CaI for each unit added per milliliter of blood. Adjusting the pH of the specimen to pH 7.4 at the time of measurement is not necessary if the specimen is collected anaerobically.

Various formulas are available for calculating CaI using total calcium, total protein, and albumin values. However, these formulas may not apply in some situations; their use is discouraged.[14]

TEST NAME AND METHOD	SPECIMEN REQUIREMENTS	REFERENCE INTERVAL, CONVENTIONAL [INTERNATIONAL RECOMMENDED UNITS]		CHEMICAL INTERFERENCES AND IN VIVO EFFECTS

Calcium, Ionized—CONT

	Serum[9,10]		*mg/dL*		*mmol/L*	
		Neonates				
		Cord blood:	5.20-6.40	× 0.25	[1.30-1.60]	
		2 hr:	4.84-5.84		[1.21-1.46]	
		24 hr:	4.40-5.44		[1.10-1.36]	
		3 days:	4.60-5.68		[1.15-1.42]	
		5 days:	4.88-5.92		[1.22-1.48]	
		Youth:	4.80-5.52		[1.20-1.38]	
		Adults:	4.64-5.28		[1.16-1.32]	
	Capillary blood	Newborn, full-term[13]:				
		Day 1 (6-36 hr):	4.20-5.48		[1.05-1.37]	
		Day 2 (60-84 hr):	4.40-5.68		[1.10-1.42]	
		Day 5 (108-132 hr):	4.80-5.92		[1.20-1.48]	

1. Boink AB, Buckley BM, Christiansen TF, et al: IFCC recommendation—recommendation on sampling, transport and storage for the determination of the concentration of ionized calcium in whole blood, plasma and serum, *Clin Chim Acta* 202:S13-S22, 1991.

2. Bowers GN Jr, Brassard C, Sena SF: Measurement of ionized calcium in serum with ion-selective electrodes: a mature technology that can meet the daily service needs, *Clin Chem* 32:1437-1447, 1986.

3. Buckley BM, Russell LJ: The measurement of ionized calcium in blood plasma, *Ann Clin Biochem* 25:447-465, 1988.

4. Burritt MF, Pierides AM, Offord KP: Comparative studies of total and ionized serum calcium values in normal subjects and patients with renal disorders, *Mayo Clin Proc* 55:606-613, 1980.

5. Engel K, Pedersen KO, Nielson SP, et al, editors: Ionized calcium workshop no. 1, *Scand J Clin Lab Invest* 43(suppl):165, 1983.

6. Gray TA, Paterson CR: The clinical value of ionized calcium assays, *Ann Clin Biochem* 25:210-219, 1988.

7. Wandrup J: Critical analytical and clinical aspects of ionized calcium in neonates, *Clin Chem* 35:2027-2033, 1989.

8. Wandrup J, Kroner J, Pryds O, et al: Age-related reference values for ionized calcium in the first week of life in premature and full-term neonates, *Scand J Clin Lab Invest* 48:255-260, 1988.

9. Longhead JL, Mimouni F, Tsang RC: Serum ionized calcium concentrations in normal neonates, *Am J Dis Child* 142:516-518, 1988.

10. Toffaletti JG: Duke University Medical Center. Personal communication.

11. Tietz NW, Shuey DF, Wekstein DR: Laboratory values in fit aging individuals—sexagenarians through centenarians, *Clin Chem* 38:1167-1185, 1992.

12. Burtis CA, Ashwood ER, editors: *Tietz textbook of clinical chemistry,* ed 2, Philadelphia, 1994, WB Saunders.

13. Nelson N, Finnström O, Larsson L: Neonatal reference values for ionized calcium, phosphate and magnesium. Selection of reference population by optimality criteria, *Scand J Clin Lab Invest* 47:111-117, 1987.

14. Halvorsen PR, Gross TL: Laboratory and clinical evaluation of a rapid slide agglutination test for phosphatidylglycerol, *Am J Obstet Gynecol* 151:1061-1066, 1985.

DIAGNOSTIC INFORMATION   **REMARKS**

Values may differ slightly with the use of different electrodes for measurement.

TEST NAME AND METHOD	SPECIMEN REQUIREMENTS	REFERENCE INTERVAL, CONVENTIONAL [INTERNATIONAL RECOMMENDED UNITS]			CHEMICAL INTERFERENCES AND IN VIVO EFFECTS
Calcium, Total (CaT)[1-8] *Spectrophotometric (CPC), AAS*	Serum, fasting; obtain blood with minimal venous occlusion and without exercise or after restoring circulation for >1 min.	Cord: Premature: 0-10 days: 10 days-24 mo: 24 mo-12 yr: 12 yr-18 yr: Adults[9] 18-60 yr: 60-90 yr: >90 yr:	*mg/dL* 8.2-11.2 6.2-11.0 7.6-10.4 9.0-11.0 8.8-10.8 8.4-10.2 8.6-10.0 8.8-10.2 8.2-9.6	× 0.25	*mmol/L* [2.05-2.80] [1.55-2.75] [1.90-2.60] [2.25-2.75] [2.20-2.70] [2.10-2.55] [2.15-2.50] [2.20-2.55] [2.05-2.40]	S ↑ V Alkaline antacids, androgens, Ca salts, calusterone, danazol, diethylstilbestrol (rapid increase in 24 hr in patients with breast cancer), dihydrotachysterol, diuretics chronically administered (including chlorthalidone, ethacrynic acid, furosemide, thiazides), ergocalciferol, isotretinoin, lithium, progesterone, PTH, tamoxifen, testolactone, vitamin D, vitamin A.

S ↑ Ca salts (possible contamination of distilled water), chlorpropamide (*o*-cresolphthalein complex-one method), fat emulsions

S ↓ V Albuterol, alprostadil, aminoglycocides (e.g., gentamicin), asparaginase, barbiturates in elderly, calcitonin, carbamazepine, carbenoxolone, carboplatin, corticosteroids; diuretics (initial effect) including acetazolamide, ethacrynic acid, furosemide, ergocalciferol, gastrin, glucagon, glucose, indapamide, insulin, isoniazid, laxatives (excessive use), magnesium salts, methicillin, phenytoin, phosphates, plicamycin, saline (effect of isotonic solution in hypercalcemia), tetracycline (in pregnancy)

S ↓ C Fluorides, oxalate, protein (with AAS unless added to standards), sulfates

DIAGNOSTIC INFORMATION	REMARKS

S ↑ Primary and tertiary hyperparathyroidism, malignant disease with bone involvement (in particular metastatic carcinoma of the breast, lung, kidney, multiple myeloma, lymphomas, and leukemia), malignant diseases without bone involvement (particularly in squamous cell carcinoma of lung, carcinoma of kidney), malignant neoplasms of esophagus, pancreas, bladder; malignant neoplasm of liver, polycythemia vera, pheochromocytoma (associated parathyroid hyperplasia), sarcoidosis, vitamin D intoxication, milk-alkali syndrome, Paget's disease with immobilization, thyrotoxicosis, acromegaly, diuretic phase of acute tubular necrosis, "idiopathic" hypercalcemia of infancy, dehydration (e.g., from vomiting, diarrhea, alcohol), familial hypocalciuric hypercalcemia, iatrogenic hypercalcemia

S ↓ Idiopathic, surgical, or congenital hypoparathyroidism; pseudohypoparathyroidism; vitamin D deficiency (in particular nutritional malabsorption); chronic renal failure; magnesium deficiency; prolonged anticonvulsant therapy; acute pancreatitis; hyperphosphatemia; massive blood transfusion; leprosy; anterior pituitary hypofunction; cystinosis; osteomalacia (advanced disease); proximal and distal renal tubular disease; alcoholism; hepatic cirrhosis; hypoalbuminemia; neonatal prematurity; inadequate nutrition

The lowest values are observed at 2:00-4:00 AM and the highest at 8:00 PM. Concentrations of Ca vary with age and are highest in the neonatal period. There is a gradual decrease of Ca levels in males >50 yr. Upright position for 15 min causes an increase of 4-7% in Ca level (minimal change in ionized calcium, CaI). Total serum Ca level is altered by changes in protein concentration. A change of 1 g/dL [10 g/L] of protein (albumin) corresponds to a parallel change in total Ca concentration of ≤0.8 mg/dL [≤0.2 mmol/L]. False elevations of serum Ca are caused by venous stasis during collection and by prolonged storage of blood. Use carefully prepared syringes, containers, and glassware for blood collection because Ca soaps adhere to glass. Repeated determinations of serum Ca should be made for diagnosis of hyperparathyroidism; at times the total Ca is normal and the CaI is elevated. Tetany may occur if total serum Ca is <6.0-7.0 mg/dL [1.50-1.75 mmol/L]; in both metabolic and respiratory alkalemia, tetany may occur with normal serum total Ca level (but low CaI).

See also *Parathyroid Hormone* and Figure II-3.

TEST NAME AND METHOD	SPECIMEN REQUIREMENTS	REFERENCE INTERVAL, CONVENTIONAL [INTERNATIONAL RECOMMENDED UNITS]	CHEMICAL INTERFERENCES AND IN VIVO EFFECTS

Calcium, Total—CONT

| | Urine, 24 hr. Collect in a bottle containing 10 mL of HCl, 6 mol/L, or acidify after collection to pH <2.0 to dissolve Ca salts. | Infant and child[10]:
Up to 6.0 mg/kg/day × 0.025 [0.15 mmol/kg/day] | U ↑ V Acetazolamide, amiloride, ammonium chloride, asparaginase, cadmium, calcitonin, Ca salts, cholestyramine, corticosteroids, corticotropin, dehydrotachysterol; initial effect of diuretics including ethacrynic acid, furosemide, mannitol, metolazone, thiazides, triamterene; ergocalciferol, glucose, growth hormone, mithramycin, nandrolone, PTH (bone mobilization), sodium chloride, spironolactone (pharmacological doses contain 40 mg Ca), vitamin D |

			mg/day[11]		*mmol/day*	
		Ca-free diet:	5-40	× 0.025	[0.13-1.00]	
		Low to average*				
		Ca diet:	50-150		[1.25-3.75]	
		Average*				
		Ca diet:	100-300		[2.50-7.50]	

Random urine[12]:

		mg/dL		*mmol/L*
	M:	0.9-37.9	× 0.25	[0.225-9.47]
	F:	0.5-35.7		[0.125-8.92]

		mg/g creatinine		*mmol/g creatinine*
	M:	12-244	× 0.025	[0.30-6.10]
	F:	9-328		[0.225-8.20]

*Average Ca diet, 800 mg/day [20 mmol/day].

U ↑ C Ca salts (possible contamination of distilled water)

U ↓ V Bicarbonates; chronic effect of diuretics including chlorthalidone, thiazides; estrogens, lithium, neomycin, oral contraceptives, PTH (can increase tubular reabsorption)

U ↓ C Alkaline urine (due to precipitated Ca salts), oxalate (may be incomplete precipitation). Urine acidification prevents such losses.

	CSF	4.2-5.4 mg/dL × 0.25 [1.05-1.35 mmol/L]	See *Interferences* for serum.

AAS	Feces	420-560 mg/day × 0.025 [10.5-14.0 mmol/day]	

DIAGNOSTIC INFORMATION	REMARKS

U ↑ Increased exposure to sunlight, hyperparathyroidism, osteolytic bone metastases (carcinoma, sarcoma), myeloma; osteoporosis (especially after immobilization, in Cushing's syndrome, in acromegaly), vitamin D intoxication (hypercalciuria occurs in many cases before serum Ca increases), distal renal tubular acidosis, idiopathic hypercalciuria, thyrotoxicosis, Paget's disease, Fanconi's syndrome, hepatolenticular degeneration, schistosomiasis, sarcoidosis, malignant neoplasm of breast or bladder, osteitis deformans, immobilization

U ↓ Hypoparathyroidism, pseudohypoparathyroidism, rickets, osteomalacia, all cases in which serum Ca is low (other than renal disease), many cases of nephrosis, acute nephritis, malignant neoplasm in bone, osteoblastic metastases, hypothyroidism, celiac sprue disease, steatorrhea, hypocalciuric hypercalcemia

Values in both healthy and sick individuals span a wide range. Calcium and protein intake and phosphate excretion alter urinary Ca excretion. Urine Ca decreases in late normal pregnancy. About one third of hyperparathyroid patients have normal urine output. Test has little practical value in differential diagnosis.

The rate of Ca excretion can also be expressed as a calcium/creatinine ratio. In healthy individuals with constant muscle mass, urinary Ca (mg/dL)/Cr (mg/dL) is usually 0.14 [Ca(mmol/L)/Cr (mmol/L) = < 0.40]. Values >0.57 (mmol/L units) or >0.20 (mg/dL units) suggest hypercalciuria.

In cases of hypercalciuria, e.g., Ca >350 mg/day [>8.75 mmol/day], some investigators collect a 2-hr urine sample after a 12-hr fast to determine whether a decrease in dietary Ca changes the hypercalciuria. In absorptive hypercalciuria (i.e., too much Ca from GI absorption), values < 20 mg Ca/2 hr [<0.50 mmol/2 hr] are found. In nonabsorptive hypercalciuria, > 30 mg Ca/2 hr [>0.75 mmol/2 hr] suggests some other problem such as hyperparathyroidism.[13]

See *Calcium, Ionized.*

Values correlate very closely with serum ionized Ca concentrations. CSF does not reflect serum Ca changes in hypoparathyroidism. Increases in total and ionized CSF calcium appear in conditions in which the CSF protein is also increased.

Values for fecal excretion assume an average Ca intake of 700 mg/day [17.5 mmol/day] and net absorption of 20-40%.

TEST NAME AND METHOD	SPECIMEN REQUIREMENTS	REFERENCE INTERVAL, CONVENTIONAL [INTERNATIONAL RECOMMENDED UNITS]	CHEMICAL INTERFERENCES AND IN VIVO EFFECTS

Calcium, Total—CONT

1.   Burtis CA, Ashwood ER , editors: *Tietz textbook of clinical chemistry,* ed 3, Philadelphia, 1999, WB Saunders.
2.   Eastham RD: *Biochemical values in clinical medicine,* ed 7, Bristol, UK, 1985, John Wright and Sons, Ltd.
3.   Bringhurst FR: Calcium and phosphate distribution, turnover, and metabolic actions. In DeGroot LJ, editor: *Endocrinology, vol 2,* ed 2, Philadelphia, 1989, WB Saunders.
4.   Burritt MF, Pierides AM, Offord KP: Comparative studies of total and ionized serum calcium values in normal subjects and patients with renal disorders, *Mayo Clin Proc* 55:606-613, 1980.
5.   Gosling P: Analytical reviews in clinical biochemistry: calcium measurement, *Ann Clin Biochem* 23:146-156, 1986.
6.   Iqbal SJ, Giles M, Ledger S, et al: Need for albumin adjustments of urgent total serum calcium, *Lancet* 2:1477-1478, 1988.
7.   Johnson KR, Mascall GC, Howarth AT: Differential laboratory diagnosis of hypercalcemia, *Crit Rev Clin Lab Sci* 21:51-97, 1984.

| **Calcium Suppression Test (after Corticosteroid)**[1,2]

Dose: 200 mg hydrocortisone (40 mg prednisone) daily for 6-10 days. | Serum, 1 day before and daily during hydrocortisone administration. | Decrease in serum Ca (total) during cortisone administration of >2.0 mg/dL [× 0.25 = >0.50 mmol/L] or into the normal range is strong evidence for a diagnosis other than primary hyperparathyroidism. | None found. |

1.   Aurbach GD, Marx SJ, Spiegel AM: Parathyroid hormone, calcitonin, and the calciferols. In Wilson JD, Foster DW, editors: *Williams textbook of endocrinology,* ed 8, Philadelphia, 1992, WB Saunders.
2.   Watson L, Moxham J, Frase P: Hydrocortisone suppression test and discriminant analysis in differential diagnosis of hypercalcemia, *Lancet* 1:1320-1325, 1980.

| **Cancer Antigen 15-3 (CA15-3)**[1,2]

Immunoassay | Serum or plasma (EDTA, heparin). Stable up to 5 days at 2-8° C. For longer periods, freeze at −20° C or colder. Avoid repeated freeze-thaw cycles. | <30 U/mL   × 1.0   [<30 kU/L] | None found. |

8. Wong ET, Freier EF: The differential diagnosis of hypercalcemia. An algorithm for more effective use of laboratory tests, *JAMA* 247:75-80, 1982.

9. Tietz NW, Shuey DF, Wekstein DR: Laboratory values in fit aging individuals—sexagenarians through centenarians, *Clin Chem* 38:1167-1185, 1992.

10. Burtis CA, Ashwood ER, editors: *Tietz textbook of clinical chemistry,* ed 2, Philadelphia, 1994, WB Saunders.

11. Mayo Medical Laboratories: *Test catalog,* Rochester, MN, 2001, Mayo Medical Laboratories.

12. Bond LW, Garber C, Ottinger W, et al: Reference intervals for common analytes in random urine specimens, *Clin Chem* 55:submitted, 2005.

13. Leavelle DE, editor: *Mayo Medical Laboratories interpretive handbook,* Rochester, MN, 1990, Mayo Medical Laboratories.

In hyperparathyroidism, no response.

A marked decrease will be observed in hypercalcemia secondary to sarcoidosis, vitamin D intoxication, breast cancer and myeloproliferative disorders, hypercalcemia due to immobilization, and Addison's disease. Patients with metastatic tumors or nonmetastatic malignant disease show a variable response.

Correction of hypercalcemia generally rules out primary hyperparathyroidism. Because fluid retention may produce some decrease in serum Ca, correction for protein concentration should be made. Because of the general availability of other diagnostic tests such as PTH and vitamin D metabolites, this test is rarely used.

S ↑ In ~80% of women with metastatic breast cancer. Test may be useful to predict recurrence of disease and to evaluate response to therapy. The clinical sensitivity is 0.60, the specificity 0.87, and the positive predictive value 0.91. In addition to breast cancer, elevated concentrations also found in pancreas, lung, ovarian, colorectal, and liver cancers and in benign liver and breast diseases.[1,3-5]

CA 15-3 is a mucin-type high-molecular-weight glycoprotein, localized to the apical side of alveoli and ducts of mammary glands, and is present as a circulating antigen. The test utilizes two antibodies (Fujirebio Diagnostics, Inc., Malvern, PA), 115D8 raised against antigens of human milk fat-globule membranes and DF3 prepared against a membrane-enriched fraction from a human breast cancer cell line. CA 15-3 FDA indications are for serial testing in conjunction with other clinical and diagnostic procedures as an aid in the early detection of recurrence in previously treated stage II and III breast cancer patients and for monitoring response to therapy in metastatic breast cancer patients. Considered equivalent to the CA 27.29 mucin marker.

TEST NAME AND METHOD	SPECIMEN REQUIREMENTS	REFERENCE INTERVAL, CONVENTIONAL [INTERNATIONAL RECOMMENDED UNITS]			CHEMICAL INTERFERENCES AND IN VIVO EFFECTS

Cancer Antigen 15-3—CONT

1. Hayes DF, Zurawski VR, Kufe DW: Comparison of circulating CA 15-3 and carcinoembryonic antigen in patients with breast cancer, *J Clin Oncol* 4:1541-1550, 1986.

2. Duffy MJ: CA 15-3 and related mucins as circulating markers in breast cancer, *Ann Clin Biochem* 36:579-586, 1999.

3. Dnistrian AM, Schwartz MK, Greenberg EJ, et al: CA 15-3 and carcinoembryonic antigen in the clinical evaluation of breast cancer, *Clin Chim Acta* 200:81-94, 1991.

TEST NAME AND METHOD	SPECIMEN REQUIREMENTS	REFERENCE INTERVAL, CONVENTIONAL		[INTERNATIONAL RECOMMENDED UNITS]	CHEMICAL INTERFERENCES AND IN VIVO EFFECTS
Cancer Antigen 27.29 (CA 27.29)[1,2] *Immunoassay*	Serum. Stable up to 2 days at 2-8° C. For longer periods, freeze at −20° C or colder. Avoid repeated freeze-thaw cycles.	<38 U/mL	× 1.0	[<38 kU/L]	None found.

1. Berveridge RA: Review of clinical studies of CA 27.29 in breast cancer management, *Int J Biol Markers* 14:36-39, 1999.

2. Chan DW, Sell S: Tumor markers. In Burtis CA, Ashwood ER, editors: *Tietz textbook of clinical chemistry,* ed 3, Philadelphia, 1999, WB Saunders.

3. Bon GG, von Mensdorff-Pouilly S, Kenemans P, et al: Clinical and technical evaluation of ACS BR serum assay of MUC1 gene-derived glycoprotein in breast cancer, and comparison with CA 15-3 assays, *Clin Chem* 43:585-593, 1997.

4. Chan DW, Berveridge RA, Nuss H, et al: Use of Truquant BR radioimmunoassay for early detection of breast cancer recurrence in patients with stage II and stage III disease, *J Clin Oncol* 15:2322-2328, 1997.

TEST NAME AND METHOD	SPECIMEN REQUIREMENTS	REFERENCE INTERVAL, CONVENTIONAL		[INTERNATIONAL RECOMMENDED UNITS]	CHEMICAL INTERFERENCES AND IN VIVO EFFECTS
Cancer Antigen 72-4 (CA 72-4, TAG-72, tumor-associated glyco-protein 72)[1] *Immunoassay*	Serum. Stable up to 24 hr at 2-8° C. For longer periods, freeze at −20° C or colder. Avoid repeated freeze-thaw cycles.	<4.0 ng/mL	× 1.0	[<4.0 mcg/L]	None found.

DIAGNOSTIC INFORMATION	REMARKS

4. Dnistrian AM, Schwartz MK, Greenberg EJ, et al: Evaluation of CA M26, CA M29, CA 15-3 and CEA as circulating tumor markers in breast cancer patients, *Tumor Biol* 12:82-90, 1991.

5. Chan DW, Sell S: Tumor markers. In Burtis CA, Ashwood ER, editors: *Tietz textbook of clinical chemistry,* ed 3, Philadelphia, 1999, WB Saunders.

S ↑ In approximately 75% of women with metastatic breast cancer. Test may be useful to predict recurrence of disease and to evaluate response to therapy.[1,3] The clinical sensitivity is 57.7%, the specificity 97.9%, the positive predictive value 83.3%, and the negative predictive value 92.6% for detecting recurrence in patients with stage II and III disease. In addition to breast cancer, elevated concentrations also found in pancreas, lung, ovarian, colorectal, and liver cancers and in benign liver and breast diseases.[4]

CA 27.29 (BR 27.29) is a mucin-type high-molecular-weight glycoprotein, localized to the apical side of alveoli and ducts of mammary glands, and is present as a circulating antigen. The competitive CA 27.29 assay utilizes the B27.29 monoclonal antibody generated against the 20 amino acid tandem repeat backbone of the MUC-1 mucin core. The B27.29 reactive sequence overlaps with one of the two antibodies (DF3) in the CA 15-3 tumor marker assay.[2]

CA 27.29 FDA indications are for serial testing in conjunction with other clinical and diagnostic procedures as an aid in the early detection of recurrence in previously treated stage II and III breast cancer patients and for monitoring response to therapy in metastatic breast cancer patients. CA 27.29 is considered equivalent to the CA 15-3 mucin marker.

A greater percentage of patients with metastatic gastric carcinoma demonstrate elevated levels of TAG 72 compared with CEA or CA 19-9. Increased levels are not observed in benign gastric disease but are seen in >50% of patients with gastric cancers.[1] Although useful for monitoring gastric carcinoma after treatment, sensitivity is improved combining CA 72-4, CEA, and CA 19.9.[2]

TAG-72 is a high-molecular-weight (MW 220-1000 kDa), mucin-like, tumor-associated antigen. It is assayed with two monoclonal antibodies, CC49 prepared against highly purified TAG-72 and B72-3, which is directed against a membrane fraction from a human breast cancer cell line. The antigen is found primarily in adenocarcinomas of the gastrointestinal tract and in ovary and breast tissues. Assays do not have FDA approval for clinical use.

TEST NAME AND METHOD	SPECIMEN REQUIREMENTS	REFERENCE INTERVAL, CONVENTIONAL [INTERNATIONAL RECOMMENDED UNITS]		CHEMICAL INTERFERENCES AND IN VIVO EFFECTS

Cancer Antigen 72-4—CONT

1. Byrne DJ, Browning MCK, Cuschieri A: CA 72-4: a new tumor marker for gastric cancer, *Br J Surg* 77:1010-1013, 1992.

| **Cancer Antigen 125** (CA 125)[1-3] *Immunoassay* | Serum. Stable up to 5 days at 2-8° C. For longer periods, freeze at −20° C or lower. | <35 U/mL | × 1.0   [<35 kU/L] | Assay interferences may result from heterophilic antibodies particularly as a result of therapeutic or diagnostic use of monoclonal antibodies. |

1. Jacobs I, Bast RC Jr: The CA 125 tumour-associated antigen: a review of the literature, *Hum Reprod* 4:1-12, 1989.
2. Bast RC Jr, Xu FJ, Yu YH, et al: CA 125: the past and the future, *Int J Biol Markers* 13:179-187, 1998.
3. Shih IM, Sokoll LJ, Chan DW: Ovarian cancer. In Diamandis EP, Fritsche HA, Lilja H, et al, editors: *Tumor markers. Physiology, pathobiology, technology, and clinical applications*, Washington, DC, 2002, AACC Press.

2. Hammarström S, Stigbrand T: Gastric cancer. In Diamandis EP, Fritsche HA, Lilja H, et al, editors: *Tumor markers. Physiology, pathobiology, technology, and clinical applications,* Washington, DC, 2002, AACC Press.

↑ Serous, endometrial, clear-cell, and undifferentiated ovarian carcinoma, adenocarcinoma of the endometrium or fallopian tube, some nongynecological malignancies, certain nonmalignant conditions (pregnancy, menstruation, peritoneal or pleural inflammation, ovarian cysts, endometriosis), and other cancers including those of the uterus, colorectal, liver, and lung. This test is approved by the FDA as an aid in monitoring response to therapy for patients with epithelial ovarian cancer. CA 125 was initially approved as an aid in the detection of residual ovarian cancer in women who have undergone first-line therapy and are considered for diagnostic second-look procedures. However, second-look laparotomy is now considered to be controversial. Because of lack of sensitivity and specificity, CA 125 is not approved by the FDA or recommended for screening.[1-3]

CA 125 is a high-molecular-weight glycoprotein (MW 200,000 to >1,000,000). It was first detected with a monoclonal antibody derived from a papillary serous-cyst adenocarcinoma of the ovary. The CA 125 antigen was found to be produced by epithelial ovarian carcinoma cell lines but not by normal cells. The CA 125 II sandwich assay utilized the CA 125 and M11 monoclonal antibodies.

CA 125 is present in normal endometrial tissue and in serous and mucinous uterine fluids. It does not enter the circulation except in instances of destruction of natural barriers. Serum levels may double during menses, especially with endometriosis. Higher serum levels can be found in the first trimester of pregnancy. Increased levels may also be observed in 1% of healthy controls, 6% of patients with certain nonmalignant conditions, and in some patients with nongynecological malignancies.

In both ovarian and endometrial malignancies, a persistently increasing CA 125 value may be associated with progressive malignant disease and poor therapeutic response, whereas a declining CA 125 value indicates a favorable prognosis and good therapeutic response. Elevated CA 125 is also a predictor of the presence of an intraperitoneal tumor or a recurrence. Normal levels do not rule out recurrence or the presence of extensive tumor.[1,2]

TEST NAME AND METHOD	SPECIMEN REQUIREMENTS	REFERENCE INTERVAL, CONVENTIONAL [INTERNATIONAL RECOMMENDED UNITS]			CHEMICAL INTERFERENCES AND IN VIVO EFFECTS
Captopril Stimulation Test[1] Dose: 25 mg captopril orally after overnight fast; patient should be seated during the test.	Plasma (Na$_2$EDTA) before and 2 hr after captopril. Place in ice water. Separate plasma and freeze promptly at $-20°$ C. Stable for up to 1 yr.	After captopril[2] Aldosterone <15 ng/dL Renin >2 ng AI*/ mL/hr *AI, Angiotensin I.	$\times 0.0277$ $\times 1.0$	[<0.42 nmol/L] [$>>2$ mcg AI* $\times$ hr^{-1} $\times$ L^{-1}]	See *Aldosterone* and *Renin*.

1. Lyons DF, Kem DC, Brown RD, et al: Single dose captopril as a diagnostic test for primary aldosteronism, *J Clin Endocrinol Metab* 57:892-896, 1983.
2. Miller RE, Ngai B: *Manual of endocrine diagnostic tests,* ed 4, Lexington, KY, 1991, Department of Medicine, University of Kentucky.

TEST NAME AND METHOD	SPECIMEN REQUIREMENTS	REFERENCE INTERVAL, CONVENTIONAL [INTERNATIONAL RECOMMENDED UNITS]			CHEMICAL INTERFERENCES AND IN VIVO EFFECTS
Carbaryl[1] *(Carbamic acid, methyl-, 1-napthyl ester; CAS 63-25-2)* *Colorimetric*	Blood Urine	See *Cholinesterase.* 1-Naphthol (metabolite): Occupational exposure: Toxic concentration:	*mg/L* <0.3 >4.0 >65	*μmol/L* [<1.4] [>18.4] [>299]	None found.

$\times 4.60$ applies to the 1-Naphthol (metabolite) row.

1. Baselt RC: *Biological monitoring methods for industrial chemicals,* Davis, CA, 1980, Biomedical Pub.
2. Cranmer MF: Carbaryl: a toxicological review and risk analysis, *Neurotoxicology* 7:247-272, 1986.

TEST NAME AND METHOD	SPECIMEN REQUIREMENTS	REFERENCE INTERVAL, CONVENTIONAL [INTERNATIONAL RECOMMENDED UNITS]			CHEMICAL INTERFERENCES AND IN VIVO EFFECTS
Carbohydrate Antigen 19-9 (CA 19-9)[1-3] *Immunoassay*	Serum or plasma (assay dependent). Serum stable up to 24 hr at 2-8° C. For longer periods, freeze serum at $-20°$ C or colder.	<37.0 U/mL	$\times 1.0$	[<37.0 kU/L]	None found.

1. Ritts RE, Pitt HA: CA 19-9 in pancreatic cancer, *Surg Oncol Clin N Am* 7:93-101, 1998.
2. Eskelinen M, Haglund U: Serological tumor markers in pancreatic cancer. In Diamandis EP, Fritsche HA, Lilja H, et al, editors: *Tumor markers. Physiology, pathobiology, technology, and clinical applications,* Washington, DC, 2002, AACC Press.

DIAGNOSTIC INFORMATION	REMARKS
In primary aldosteronism, plasma aldosterone remains high and plasma renin activity remains low after captopril.	Occasional patients with essential hypertension (EH) have high aldosterone levels, and many with EH have low renin. The ratio of aldosterone to PRA after captopril (>50 in primary aldosteronism, <50 in EH) provides the best discrimination.
Symptoms of exposure are typical of cholinergic toxins and include blurred vision, salivation, sweating, nausea, vomiting, and convulsions.	This insecticide (Sevin) is a carbamate derivative that inhibits cholinesterase enzymes. Because the insecticide is rapidly metabolized to 1-naphthol, measurement of the parent compound is not helpful. 1-naphthol is excreted primarily in conjugated forms in the urine. Occasionally, phenolic metabolites may be detected in urine as long as 2-3 days after significant pesticide absorption.[2]
↑ All forms of gastrointestinal cancer and other adenocarcinomas. Most frequently elevated marker in pancreatic cancer (sensitivity 70-95%). Amount of elevation has no relation to tumor mass, but test can be used to monitor the course of disease. Elevations are also seen in acute and chronic pancreatitis, cholangitis, and cirrhosis.[1-3]	CA 19-9 is a derivative of the Lewis blood group. Individuals with blood group Le[a-b-] do not synthesize CA 19-9 (5-10% of the population). CA 19-9 is a high-molecular-weight glycoprotein (MW 1,000,000). CA 19-9 alone is the preferred test for patients with pancreatic cancer; CEA is the preferred test for patients with colorectal cancer. Also useful for monitoring in gastric cancer. CA 19-9 is approved for use by the FDA for serial testing as an aid in monitoring patients with pancreatic cancer who have measurable CA 19-9 results over the course of their disease.[1-3]

3. Chan DW, Sell S: Tumor markers. In Burtis CA, Ashwood ER, editors: *Tietz textbook of clinical chemistry,* ed 3, Philadelphia, 1999, WB Saunders.

TEST NAME AND METHOD	SPECIMEN REQUIREMENTS	REFERENCE INTERVAL, CONVENTIONAL [INTERNATIONAL RECOMMENDED UNITS]			CHEMICAL INTERFERENCES AND IN VIVO EFFECTS
Carbon Dioxide, Total (tCO$_2$, CO$_2$T, CO$_2$ Content)[1-3] *Potentiometric, colorimetric,*[3] *enzymatic,*[4] *pH differential*[5]	Plasma or serum, venous. Collect the sample anaerobically. Heparin is the preferred anticoagulant. To avoid dilutional errors and pH changes, do not use excess liquid heparin. For Vitros analyzers, do not use specimens from patients receiving sodium diatrizoate.	*mEq/L* Adult: 23-29 >60 yr: 23-31 >90 yr: 20-29[7]	× 1.0	*mmol/L* [23-29] [23-31] [20-29]	↑V Aldosterone, bicarbonates, carbenicillin, carbenoxolone, corticosteroids, diuretics (e.g., thiazides, chlorthalidone, ethacrynic acid, furosemide, metolazone). *Vitros:* Bromide, iodide, lactate (above normal levels), organic acids (hippurate, *p*-hydroxyphenyllactate, *p*-hydroxyphenylbutyrate, acetoacetate), nitrate (burn patients receiving silver nitrate), x-ray contrast agents (diatrizoates).[8] *CX3:* Acetoacetate (Li), ≥200 mmol/L; sodium azide, ≥50 ppm.
	Plasma (heparin), capillary[2]	Premature 1 wk: 14-27 Newborn: 13-22 Infant: 20-28 Child: 20-28 Adult: 22-28		[14-27] [13-22] [20-28] [20-28] [22-28]	
	Whole blood	Arterial: 19-24 Venous: 22-26		[19-24] [22-26]	↓V Acetazolamide, ammonium chloride, methicillin, nitrofurantoin, tetracycline, triamterene; lactic acidosis with phenformin, fructose; acidosis with methanol, paraldehyde, dimercaprol. *CX3:* Glutathione, ≥20 mmol/L; *N*-acetylcysteine, ≥20 mmol/L; α-ketoglutarate, ≥10 mg/dL; histidine, ≥10 mg/dL.[5]
	Cord blood[6]	14-22		[14-22]	

1. Eastham RD: *Biochemical values in clinical medicine,* ed 7, Bristol, UK, 1985, John Wright and Sons, Ltd.

2. Burtis CA, Ashwood ER, editors: *Tietz fundamentals of clinical chemistry,* ed 5, Philadelphia, 2000, WB Saunders.

3. Scott MG, Heusel JW, LeGrys VA, et al: Electrolyte and blood gases. In Burtis CA, Ashwood ER, editors: *Tietz textbook of clinical chemistry,* ed 3, Philadelphia, 1999, WB Saunders.

4. Ortho-Clinical Diagnostics: *Vitros product ECO$_2$ slides, Pub. no. MP2-89,* Raritan, NJ, 2003, Ortho-Clinical Diagnostics.

5. Beckman Instruments, Inc.: *Synchron CX3 clinical system manual,* Brea, CA, 1991, Beckman Instruments, Inc.

6. Burtis CA, Ashwood ER, editors: *Tietz textbook of clinical chemistry,* ed 2, Philadelphia, 1994, WB Saunders.

7. Tietz NW, Shvey DF, Wekstein DR: Laboratory values in fit aging individuals—sexagenarians through centarians, *Clin Chem* 38:1167-1185, 1982.

8. Ortho-Clinical Diagnostics: *Vitros product CO$_2$ DT slides, Pub. no. C-308,* Raritan, NJ, 2003, Ortho-Clinical Diagnostics.

↑ Respiratory acidosis, especially compensated, caused by poor gas exchange (emphysema, pneumonia, cardiac failure with pulmonary congestion, cystic fibrosis) or depression of respiratory center; generalized respiratory disease; metabolic alkalosis, e.g., after severe vomiting in pyloric stenosis, hypokalemic states, excessive alkali intake.

↓ Compensated respiratory alkalosis, metabolic acidosis in diabetes mellitus, renal glomerular or tubular failure, renal tubular acidosis, and intestinal loss of alkali with coexisting increase in Cl and normal anion gap (in acidosis due to most other obscure causes, the chloride is normal or low and anion gap is increased), ureteric transplantation into ileum or colon, hypotension, dehydration or other states with poor tissue perfusion.

Arteriovenous difference varies with the metabolic activity of the organ or tissue from which the venous blood is obtained. Therefore arterial blood is preferred for many studies.

TEST NAME AND METHOD	SPECIMEN REQUIREMENTS	REFERENCE INTERVAL, CONVENTIONAL [INTERNATIONAL RECOMMENDED UNITS]			CHEMICAL INTERFERENCES AND IN VIVO EFFECTS
Carbon Dioxide, Partial Pressure $[P_{CO_2}, P(a)_{CO_2}]$[1-3] *Potentiometric*[3]	Whole arterial blood (heparinized syringe). Place in ice water and deliver to the lab immediately. To avoid dilutional errors and pH changes, do not use excess liquid heparin.		*mm Hg*[1,3]	*kPa*	See *Bicarbonate*.
		Newborn:	27-40 × 0.133	[3.59-5.32]	
		Infant:	27-41	[3.59-5.45]	↑ V Diazepam, midazolam, narcotic analgesics
		Adult			
		M:	35-48	[4.66-6.38]	
		F:	32-45	[4.26-5.99]	↓ V Tromethamine
		All values apply to sea level; values are lower at high altitudes. Decrease is:			
	Freely flowing capillary blood, collected in a heparinized capillary tube, can be used as an adequate substitute for arterial blood.	3 mm Hg/km × 0.133		[0.40 Pa/m]	
		5 mm Hg/mile × 0.08		[0.40 Pa/m]	
	Venous blood (right atrium)[3]	6-7 mm Hg [0.80-0.93 kPa] higher than the arterial P_{CO_2}			
	Cord blood[4]		*mm Hg*	*kPa*	
		Arterial:	49.2 ± 8.4 (SD) × 0.133	[6.54 ± 1.12]	
		Venous:	38.2 ± 5.6	[5.08 ± 0.74]	

1. Henry JB, editor: *Clinical diagnosis and management by laboratory methods,* ed 20, Philadelphia, 2001, WB Saunders.
2. Bhagavan NV: *Biochemistry,* ed 2, Philadelphia, 1978, JB Lippincott.
3. Scott MG, Heusel JW, LeGrys VA, et al: Electrolyte, and blood gases. In Burtis CA, Ashwood ER, editors: *Tietz textbook of clinical chemistry,* ed 3, Philadelphia, 1999, WB Saunders.
4. Yeomans ER, Hauth JC, Gilstrap LC III, et al: Umbilical cord pH, PCO₂, and bicarbonate following uncomplicated term vaginal deliveries, *Am J Obstet Gynecol* 151:798-800, 1985.

Carbon Disulfide	Blood (fluoride/oxalate). Refrigerate.	Negative			None found.
(Carbon bisulfide; CAS 75-15-0)		Occupational	*mg/L*	*mmol/L*	
		exposure:	<0.3 × 13.1	[<3.9]	
GLC,[1] *colorimetric (metabolites)*[2]	Urine	Toxic:	>0.5	[>6.6]	

1. Sunshine I, editor: *Methodology for analytical toxicology,* Cleveland, 1975, CRC Press.
2. Baselt RC: *Biological monitoring methods for industrial chemicals,* Davis, CA, 1980, Biomedical Pub.

DIAGNOSTIC INFORMATION   REMARKS

↑ *Respiratory acidosis (hypercapnia):* Increased P_{CO_2} in inspired air (e.g., rebreathing air); decreased alveolar ventilation due to diseases of the lungs and bronchial tree, foreign body in the airways, allergic laryngeal edema, asthmatic shock, chronic bronchitis, pulmonary tuberculosis or emphysema, chronic obstructive lung disease; disturbances in respiratory control center (e.g., brain tumor, depression of the respiratory center by drugs like opiates and barbiturates); disturbances in neuromuscular apparatus of breathing (e.g., poliomyelitis, curare intoxication, severe electrolyte disturbances, acute intermittent porphyria, severe hypothyroidism); myopathy; cardiac disease; metabolic alkalosis (with compensatory hypoventilation). P_{CO_2} values >80 mm Hg [>10.64 kPa] may cause narcosis.

↓ *Respiratory alkalosis (hypocapnia):* Increased alveolar ventilation caused by mechanical artificial ventilation or by stimulation of the respiratory center due to one or more of the following factors: hypoxia, salicylates, anxiety, hyperthermia, head injury with damage to respiratory center.

Respiratory conditions will primarily affect the P_{CO_2}, whereas metabolic disturbances are first reflected in the HCO_3.

With the patient in a sitting or standing position, the values are slightly lower (2-4 mm Hg; 0.27-0.53 kPa) than in the supine position. The difference between arterial blood and peripheral venous blood varies considerably, depending on the skin temperature, length of stasis, and muscular activity.

Sources of error are exposure of the blood to air and acid formation by metabolic processes in the erythrocytes and leukocytes during storage. Glycolysis and oxidative metabolism increase P_{CO_2} by 5 mm Hg/hr [0.67 kPa/hr] at 37° C and 0.5 mm Hg/hr [0.07 kPa/hr] at 2-4° C. P_{CO_2} values measured at 37° C must be corrected to the actual body temperature because P_{CO_2} increases with increase of temperature. See nomogram, Figure II-2. The bicarbonate concentration can be computed by the P_{CO_2} and the pH (see Figure II-1).

Acute exposure causes irritation to eyes, skin, and mucous membranes. Chronic exposure may result in headache, polyneuritis, emotional disturbances, psychosis, atherosclerosis, coronary heart disease, hypertension, central scotoma, red-green color blindness, anorexia, weight loss, Parkinson-like syndrome, fatigue, anemia, blood and protein in the urine, and liver damage.

Exposure is usually by inhalation of vapor or absorption of liquid CS_2 through the skin.

Carbon disulfide is a metabolite of disulfiram and other thiocarbamates.[2]

TEST NAME AND METHOD	SPECIMEN REQUIREMENTS	REFERENCE INTERVAL, CONVENTIONAL [INTERNATIONAL RECOMMENDED UNITS]		CHEMICAL INTERFERENCES AND IN VIVO EFFECTS
Carbonic Anhydrase (CA, carbonate dehydratase, carbonate hydrolyase) (EC 4.2.1.1)	Plasma (heparin). Store at −20° C.	*mg/mL (SEM)* CA-B: 0.63 ± 0.12 CA-C: 0.20 ± 0.02	*mg/L* × 1.0 [0.63 ± 0.12] [0.20 ± 0.02]	↑ V Oral contraceptives ↓ V Acetazolamide, sulfonamides and sulthiame; ethanol
	Hemolyzed erythrocytes. Store at −20° C.	*mg/g Hb (SEM)* CA-B: 12.1 ± 0.53 CA-C: 1.5 ± 0.6	*g/mol Hb* × 64.5* [780 ± 34.2] [97 ± 38.7]	↓ C 5-Methyl-1,10-phenanthroline
Radioassay				

IE[1,2]		*g/L Ercs*
		Infant (cord blood)[2]
		CA-B: 0.009-0.67
		        (x̄: 0.29)
		CA-C: 0.030-0.095
		        (x̄: 0.067)
		
		Adult[2]
		CA-B: (x̄: 4.89)
		CA-C: (x̄: 0.60)		

		mg/g Hb
		Adult[1]
		CA-B: 11.5-20.7
		        (x̄: 16.4)
		CA-C: 2.6-5.4
		        (x̄: 3.9)
			g/mol Hb
			× 64.5* [742-1335]
			        [x̄: 1058]
			[168-348]
			[x̄: 252]	

Colorimetric[3]		*mmol/ min/g Hb* CA-B (x̄; n = 3): 6.3 CA-C (x̄; n = 3): 4.3	*kU/mol Hb* × 64.5* [406] [277]	
Titrimetric[3]		CA-B (x̄; n = 3): 4.5 CA-C (x̄; n = 3): 2.7	[290] [174]	

*Conversion factor based on MW of Hb of 64,500.

1. Magid E: Determination of erythrocyte carbonic anhydrase B and C: an aid in the diagnosis of thyroid disorders? *Scand J Clin Invest* 26:257-262, 1970.

2. Mondrup M, Anker N, Christensen F: Carbonic anhydrase isoenzyme determination: an aid to the diagnosis of "small-for-date" infants, *Clin Chim Acta* 100:107-112, 1980.

3. Shapira E, Ben-Yoseph Y, Eyal FG, et al: Enzymatically inactive red cell carbonic anhydrase B in a family with renal tubular acidosis, *J Clin Invest* 55:59-63, 1974.

4. Yoshida K, Kiso Y, Watanabe T, et al: Clinical utility of red blood cell carbonic anhydrase 1 and zinc concentration: in patients with thyroid disease, *Metabolism* 40:1048-1051, 1991.

DIAGNOSTIC INFORMATION	REMARKS

↑ Pregnancy (CA-B isoenzyme)

↓ Renal tubular acidosis; hyperthyroidism (↓CA-B with normal CA-C) in proportion to the length of time thyroid hormones are elevated.[4]

Activity is low in umbilical cord blood. CA exists primarily as isoenzymes B and C (CA-B, CA-C). Activity is very low in neonatal erythrocytes.

TEST NAME AND METHOD	SPECIMEN REQUIREMENTS	REFERENCE INTERVAL, CONVENTIONAL [INTERNATIONAL RECOMMENDED UNITS]		CHEMICAL INTERFERENCES AND IN VIVO EFFECTS
Carboxyhemoglo-bin (COHb)[1] *Colorimetric, GLC*[2]	Whole blood (heparin). Stable >4 mo in filled, well-capped tube.[3] Note: Do not use oxalate. Collect specimen before treatment with oxygen is started.	*%* *Saturation* *of Hb* Nonsmokers: Smokers 1-2 packs/day: Heavy smokers >2 packs/day: Toxic[4]: Lethal:	0.5-1.5 × 0.01 4-5 8-9 >20 >50	*Fraction* *of Hb* *saturation* [0.005-0.015] [0.04-0.05] [0.08-0.09] [>0.20] [>0.50]	None found.

1. Burtis CA, Ashwood ER, editors: *Tietz textbook of clinical chemistry,* ed 2, Philadelphia, 1994, WB Saunders.
2. Baselt RC: *Analytical procedures for therapeutic drug monitoring and emergency toxicology,* ed 2, Littleton, MA, 1987, PSG Publishing Co., Inc.
3. Ocak A, Valentour JC, Blanke RV: The effects of storage conditions on the stability of carbon monoxide in postmortem blood, *J Anal Toxicol* 9:202-206, 1985.
4. Burtis CA, Ashwood ER, editors: *Tietz fundamentals of clinical chemistry,* ed 5, Philadelphia, 2000, WB Saunders.
5. Baselt RC: *Biological monitoring methods for industrial chemicals,* Davis, CA, 1980, Biomedical Pub.
6. Steinke JM, Shepherd AP: Effect of temperature on optical absorbance spectra of oxy-, carboxy-, and deoxy-hemoglobin, *Clin Chem* 37:1633-1638, 1991.

| **Carcinoembryonic Antigen** (CEA)[1-3] *Immunoassay* | Serum. Stable up to 24 hr at 2-8° C. For longer periods, freeze at −20° C or colder. Plasma may be used in some methods. | *ng/mL*[2] Nonsmokers: Smokers: Reference ranges may be method dependent. | <3.0 × 1.0 <5.0 | *mcg/L* [<3.0] [<5.0] |

DIAGNOSTIC INFORMATION	REMARKS

↑ CO poisoning, hemolytic disease, blood in intestine, reactions of intestinal bacteria, calorie reduction, following exercise.

In CO poisoning, COHb <10% [<0.10] may increase disturbances of cognitive function or aggravate preexisting heart disease; 15-25% [0.15-0.25] may cause dizziness and nausea.[5]

COHb is increased by exposure to gases from defective furnaces, automobile exhaust, coal gas, water gas, and most combustibles. CO is lower in rural areas. Procedure may also be performed on a cooximeter, which also determines total Hb, % oxyhemoglobin, and % methemoglobin and calculates O_2 content.

Temperature affects optical absorbance.[6]

CO is a metabolite of methylene chloride.[5]

Screening tests are insensitive. They are useful only for severe acute poisoning.

$t_{1/2}$

With O_2 administration:	80 min
With O_2 at 3 atm:	24 min[5]

Levels are slightly higher in smokers than in nonsmokers. In malignant disease, elevated values are related to the stage and extent of the disease. Increased values have been observed in cancer of the colon, rectum, lung, breast, liver, pancreas, stomach, and ovary. Lesser elevations have been reported in benign liver disease (hepatitis, cirrhosis), benign gastric and intestinal disease (polyposis, ulcerative colitis), benign breast disease, pulmonary infection, emphysema, and renal failure. CEA is useful in monitoring patients with colon, breast, and gastric cancers. Preoperative concentrations of CEA correlate with prognosis and development of metastasis in colorectal cancer and serial measurements have a sensitivity of ~80% and a specificity of ~70% for detecting recurrence. CEA should not be used for screening/early detection of malignant disease.[1-3]

CEA is a tumor-associated, oncofetal antigen observed in embryonic and fetal tissues. The CEA family is a heterogeneous group of cell-surface glycoproteins, and up to 36 different glycoproteins have been identified. Because of structural similarities CEA is classified as a member of the immunoglobulin gene super g family. CEA has a molecular mass of ~200 kDa and a high carbohydrate content (50-60%). Because of the heterogeneity of CEA and differences in antibodies, numerical values will differ with different assay techniques. It is essential that the same method be used for longitudinal monitoring. Concordance between methods may be very poor in specimens with elevated values. Factors cannot be applied to convert values from one method to those of another.

TEST NAME* AND METHOD	SPECIMEN REQUIREMENTS	REFERENCE INTERVAL, CONVENTIONAL [INTERNATIONAL RECOMMENDED UNITS]		CHEMICAL INTERFERENCES AND IN VIVO EFFECTS

Carcinoembryonic Antigen—CONT

1. Schwartz MK: Tumor markers for colorectal cancer. In Diamandis EP, Fritsche HA, Lilja H, et al, editors: *Tumor markers. Physiology, pathobiology, technology, and clinical applications,* Washington, DC, 2002, AACC Press.

2. Chan DW, Sell S: Tumor markers. In Burtis CA, Ashwood ER, editors: *Tietz textbook of clinical chemistry,* ed 3, Philadelphia, 1999, WB Saunders.

Carnosine (Car)[1-5] *Ion-exchange chromatography*	Urine, 24 hr. Add 20 mL of toluene at the start of collection. (Alternatively, refrigerate specimen during collection.) Store frozen at −70° C.	*mg/day* 3-16 yr: 7.7-49.8 Adult: 3.6-28.3	× 4.42	$\mu mol/day$[6] [34-220] [16-125]	None found.

1. Friedman RB, Young DS: *Effects of disease on clinical laboratory tests,* ed 2, Washington, DC, 1989, American Association for Clinical Chemistry.

2. Scriver CR, Beaudet AL, Sly WS, et al, editors: *The metabolic basis of inherited disease,* ed 6, New York, 1989, McGraw-Hill Publishing Co.

3. Young DS: *Effects of drugs on clinical laboratory tests,* ed 3, Washington, DC, 1990, American Association for Clinical Chemistry.

4. Bremer HJ, Duran M, Kamerling JP, et al: *Disturbances of amino acid metabolism: clinical chemistry and diagnosis,* Baltimore, 1981, Urban and Schwarzenburg.

5. Nyhan W, Sakait N: *Diagnostic recognition of genetic disease,* Philadelphia, 1987, Lea & Febiger.

6. Mayo Medical Laboratories: *Test catalog,* Rochester, MN, 1993, Mayo Medical Laboratories.

β-Carotene *HPLC*[1-3] *LC-tandem mass spectrometry*[4,5]	Serum. Avoid hemolysis; protect from light. Freeze. Fasting specimen. Stable for years at −70° C.[6]	10-85 mcg/dL 3-115 mcg/dL	× 0.0186 × 0.0186	[0.19-1.58 μmol/L] [0.05-2.14 μmol/L][7]	↓ V Kanamycin, metformin, mineral oil, canola oil, neomycin, oral contraceptives ↓ C Citrate, hemolysis ↑ C Canthaxanthine

DIAGNOSTIC INFORMATION	REMARKS

3. Duffy MJ: Carcinoembryonic antigen as a marker for colorectal cancer: is it clinically useful? *Clin Chem* 47:624-630, 2001.

U ↑ Carnosinemia, high-meat diet (especially poultry)	Carnosine is present in the skeletal muscles of almost all animals.

↑ Liver disease, diabetes mellitus, hypothyroidism, high dietary intake, essential hyperlipemia, pregnancy, subacute thyroiditis, hyperlipoproteinemia (types I, IIA, and IIB), myxedema, chronic nephritis, nephrotic syndrome ↓ High fever, rheumatoid arthritis, liver disease, acquired immune deficiency syndrome (AIDS), Tangier disease, small bowel disease, Zollinger-Ellison syndrome, Whipple's disease, enteritis, pancreatitis, pancreatic cancer, cystic fibrosis, malabsorption with excess loss of fat or vitamin A; levels <30 mcg/dL [<0.56 μmol/L] in severe malabsorption.	β-Carotene is a precursor of vitamin A and has received attention as a preventive agent for certain cancers, although most recent trials have not demonstrated benefit and some report harmful primary endpoints.[8] Its level does not always reflect vitamin A status and varies with dietary intake. High values can be used to rule out steatorrhea, but low-normal levels lack specificity. Total serum carotenoids, normally 60-200 mcg/dL [0.60-2.00 mg/L], vary with dietary intake and can be measured photometrically after extraction into hexane-ethanol. Excessive dietary intakes are not toxic but can cause hypercarotenemia and carotenodermia in the nasolabial folds, hands, and feet; color of the sclera is unaffected. Carotenemia can be confused with jaundice. β-Carotene may be administered to reduce the severity of photosensitivity reactions in patients with erythropoietic protoporphyria (EPP).[9]

TEST NAME AND METHOD	SPECIMEN REQUIREMENTS	REFERENCE INTERVAL, CONVENTIONAL [INTERNATIONAL RECOMMENDED UNITS]	CHEMICAL INTERFERENCES AND IN VIVO EFFECTS

β-Carotene—CONT

1. Lee BL, New AL, Ong CN: Simultaneous determination of tocotrienols, tocopherols, retinol, and major carotenoids in human plasma, *Clin Chem* 49:2056-2066, 2003.
2. Epler KS, Ziegler RG, Craft NE: Liquid chromatographic method for the determination of carotenoids, retinoids and tocopherols in human serum and in food, *J Chromatogr* 619:37-48, 1993.
3. Nierenberg DW, Nann SL: A method for determining concentrations of retinol, tocopherol, and five carotenoids in human plasma and tissue samples, *Am J Clin Nutr* 56:417-426, 1992.
4. Van Breemen: Electrospray liquid chromatography-mass spectrometry of carotenoids, *Anal Chem* 67:2004-2009, 1995.
5. Andreoli R, Manini P, Poli D, et al: Development of a simplified method for the simultaneous determination of retinol, alpha-tocopherol, and beta-carotene in serum by liquid chromatography-tandem mass spectrometry with atmospheric pressure chemical ionization, *Anal Bioanal Chem* 378:987-994, 2004.

TEST NAME AND METHOD	SPECIMEN REQUIREMENTS	REFERENCE INTERVAL, CONVENTIONAL [INTERNATIONAL RECOMMENDED UNITS]	CHEMICAL INTERFERENCES AND IN VIVO EFFECTS
Catalase (EC 1.11.1.6)[1,2] *Titrimetry*[1]	Washed erythrocytes prepared from whole blood (EDTA, heparin)	34.5-48.3 mEq H_2O_2 decomposed in 10 sec/mL Ercs (x̄: 41.9) [× 6.0 = 207-290 MU/L Ercs; x: 251] 3061-4173 mEq H_2O_2 decomposed in 10 sec/1012 Ercs (x̄: 3644) [× 0.006 = 18.4-25.0 mU/Erc; x: 21.9] 1.04-1.40 mEq H_2O_2 decomposed in 10 sec/0.01 g Hb (x̄: 1.22) [× 38.7* = 40.2-54.2 GU/mol Hb; x: 47.2] See *Acetylcholinesterase*.	
Disc flotation time[3]	Urine collected under aseptic conditions using pHisoHex (hexachlorophene) and benzalkonium chloride (1:2000).	Not established. Zero flotation time corresponds to no detectable catalase activity.	U ↑ Sustained after renal artery injection of acetrizoate.

1. Chakraborty D, Bhattacharyya M: Antioxidant defense status of red blood cells of patients with beta-thalassemia and Ebeta-thalassemia, *Clin Chim Acta* 305:123-129, 2001.
2. Gerli GC, Beretta L, Bianchi M, et al: Erythrocyte superoxide dismutase, catalase and glutathione peroxidase activities in β-thalassemia (major and minor), *Scand J Haematol* 25:87-92, 1980.
3. Braude AI, Berkowitz H: Detection of urinary catalase by disk flotation, *J Lab Clin Med* 57:490-494, 1961.
4. Yasmineh WG, Chung MY, Caspers JI: Determination of serum catalase activity on a centrifugal analyzer by an NADP/NADPH coupled enzyme reaction system, *Clin Biochem* 25:21-27, 1992.

6. Craft NE, Brown ED, Smith JC Jr: Effects of storage and handling conditions on concentrations of individual carotenoids, retinol, and tocopherol in plasma, *Clin Chem* 34:44-48, 1998. Erratum: *Clin Chem* 34:1505, 1998.
7. Armstrong NC, Paganga G, Brunner E, et al: Reference values for alpha-tocopherol and beta-carotene in the Whitehall II study, *Free Radic Res* 27:207-219, 1997.
8. Cohen V, Khuri FR: Chemoprevention of lung cancer, *Curr Opin Pulm Med* 10:279-283, 2004.
9. Alemzadeh R, Feehan T: Variable effects of beta-carotene therapy in a child with erythropoietic protoporphyria, *Eur J Pediatr* 163:547-549, 2004.

Ercs ↑↑ β-Thalassemia minor

α-Thalassemia and HB Lepore α-Thalassemia major and glucose-6-phosphate dehydrogenase deficiency

Ercs near normal in β-thalassemia major (2 of 7 cases)

Ercs ↓ Iron deficiency anemia; acatalasemia (acatalasia), an autosomal recessive disorder characterized in homozygotes by ulcerations of gums or tonsils and by oral mucosal necrosis on exposure to H_2O_2 (Takahara's disease).

U ↑ Proteinuria (damaged renal tubular cells), pernicious anemia, pyuria, and hematuria.

TEST NAME AND METHOD	SPECIMEN REQUIREMENTS	REFERENCE INTERVAL, CONVENTIONAL [INTERNATIONAL RECOMMENDED UNITS]			CHEMICAL INTERFERENCES AND IN VIVO EFFECTS
Catecholamines, Fractionated[1-6] *HPLC (free amines)*[7-9] *LC-MS/MS (free amines)*[10]	Urine, 24 hr. Preserve with 20 mL of HCl, 6 mol/L; refrigerate. See also *Remarks*.	*Epinephrine (E)*[11]			U ↑ V Caffeine, epineph-rine, ethanol, isopro-terenol, levodopa, nico-tine, nitroglycerin, reserpine (initial effect), theophylline
		mcg/day		*nmol/day*	
		<1 yr:	0-2.5	× 5.46	[0-14]	
		1 yr:	0-3.5		[0-19]	
		2-3 yr:	0-6.0		[0-33]	
		4-9 yr:	0.2-10		[1-55]	
		10-15 yr:	0.5-20		[3-109]	
		≥16 yr:	0-20		[0-109]	U ↓ V Clonidine, guanethidine, ouabain, prazosin, radiographic agents, reserpine (chronic), bretylium
		mcg/g creatinine[12]		*μmol/mol*	
		0-11 mo:	0-375	× 0.617	[0-231]	
		1-4 yr:	0-82		[0-51]	
		4-10 yr:	5-93		[3-57]	
		10-18 yr:	3-58		[2-36]	
		>18 yr:	1-44		[0.6-27]	
		Norepinephrine (NE)[11]			
		mcg/day		*nmol/day*	
		<1 yr:	0-10	× 5.91	[0-59]	
		1 yr:	1-17		[6-100]	
		2-3 yr:	4-29		[24-171]	
		4-6 yr:	8-45		[47-266]	
		7-9 yr:	13-65		[77-384]	
		≥10 yr:	15-80		[89-473]	
		mcg/g creatinine[12]		*μmol/mol*	
		0-11 mo:	25-310	× 0.669	[17-207]	
		1-4 yr:	25-290		[17-194]	
		4-10 yr:	27-108		[18-72]	
		10-18 yr:	4-105		[3-70]	
		>18 yr:	9-112		[6-75]	
		Dopamine (DA)[11]			
		mcg/day		*nmol/day*	
		<1 yr:	0-85	× 6.53	[0-555]	
		1 yr:	10-140		[65-914]	
		2-3 yr:	40-260		[261-1697]	
		≥4 yr:	65-400		[424-2612]	
		mcg/g creatinine[12]		*μmol/mol*	
		0-11 mo:	240-1290	× 0.738	[177-952]	
		1-4 yr:	80-1220		[59-900]	
		4-10 yr:	220-720		[162-531]	
		10-18 yr:	120-450		[89-332]	
		>18 yr:	30-350		[22-258]	

↑ In catecholamine-secreting neurochromaffin tumors such as pheochromocytoma, paraganglioma, and neuroblastoma (neuroblastoma is not associated with increased epinephrine); anxiety, intense physical activity.

↓ Autonomic neuropathy including diabetes, parkinsonism; orthostatic hypotension.

HPLC with electrochemical detection methods are prone to interference by several drugs. If possible, the patient should discontinue all drugs at least 1 wk before testing. The preferred specimen is a 24-hr urine collection. Shorter, timed collections (e.g., 12 hr) or random spot urines collected during an acute hypertensive episode have also been suggested, provided the catecholamine excretion is normalized to creatinine excretion. HPLC methods with tandem mass spectrometry are free of interferences from drugs and drug metabolites.

Exercise, stress, smoking, and pain induce physiologic increase of catecholamines. Excretion levels are significantly lower during the night. E and NE excretion increase during the luteal phase of the menstrual cycle, then decrease to a minimum during the ovulatory period. Similar changes occur in vanillylmandelic acid (VMA).

Simultaneous determination of homovanillic acid (HVA) and VMA may be helpful for the diagnosis of neural crest tumors. Measurements of VMA and catecholamines in urine are more specific (fewer false-positive results) but less sensitive (more false-negative results) than urine metanephrines for pheochromocytoma. Increased dopamine is particularly characteristic of neuroblastoma.

The measurement of plasma free metanephrines is recommended as the initial screening test for pheochromocytoma (high diagnostic sensitivity and specificity). See *Metanephrines, Fractionated.*

TEST NAME AND METHOD	SPECIMEN REQUIREMENTS	REFERENCE INTERVAL, CONVENTIONAL [INTERNATIONAL RECOMMENDED UNITS]		CHEMICAL INTERFERENCES AND IN VIVO EFFECTS

Catecholamines, Fractionated—CONT

HPLC	Plasma (heparin or EDTA), fasting. Chill specimens immediately in ice water. Plasma should be separated in a refrigerated centrifuge within 30 min of collection and then frozen immediately at $-20°$ C in plastic vials. Stable for 8 mo at $-70°$ C. See also *Remarks.*	pg/mL[11]
		Epinephrine
		  Supine: <110
		  Standing: <140
		Norepinephrine
		  Supine: 70-750
		  Standing: 200-1700
		
		Dopamine (no postural change):
		
		<30 pg/mL
			$pmol/L$
			
			$\times 5.46$ [<601]
			         [<764]
			
			$\times 5.91$ [414-4433]
			         [1182-10,047]
			
			$\times 6.53$ [<196 pmol/L]
				P ↑ V Ajmaline, diazoxide, ethanol, ether, isoproterenol (inhaled, effect slight), MAO inhibitors, nitroglycerin, phentolamine, propranolol, theophylline, upright posture, exercise, stress
				
				P ↑ C Levodopa, methyldopa.
				
				P ↓ V Clonidine

1. Benowitz NL: Pheochromocytoma, *Adv Intern Med* 35:195-220, 1990.

2. Krakoff LR, Garbouit D: Adreno-medullary hypertension: a review of syndrome, pathophysiology, diagnosis, and treatment, *Clin Chem* 37:1849-1853, 1991.

3. Hernandez FC, Sanchez M, Alvarez A, et al: A five-year report on experience in the detection of pheochromocytoma, *Clin Biochem* 33:649-655, 2000.

4. Pacak K, Linehan WM, Eisenhofer G, et al: Recent advances in genetics, diagnosis, localization, and treatment of pheochromocytoma, *Ann Intern Med* 134:315-329, 2001.

| DIAGNOSTIC INFORMATION | REMARKS |

In pheochromocytoma there is a higher level of NE than E in plasma.[13]

Most assays measure only free catecholamines, but a few measure both free and conjugated types. Free amines are more closely associated with tumor load than are conjugated amines. Conditions of sampling are important and should be standardized. The collection of samples with metabisulfite or glutathione is sometimes recommended to prevent oxidation of catecholamines. Blood catecholamines are raised by many variables, including the stress of venipuncture and upright posture. Ideally blood should be collected through an indwelling venous catheter after 30 min of rest in a supine position.

The use of epinephrine, norepinephrine, or dopamine must be discontinued for ≥ 12 hr before specimen collection. Discontinue drugs that are known to stimulate the release of catecholamines for 3-7 days. Patients should not eat, use tobacco, or drink caffeinated beverages for at least 4 hr before collection

Plasma catecholamines (total) are often >1000 pg/mL in patients with pheochromocytoma but may be less (or even normal) in normotensive patients between acute attacks. This test is frequently used in subjects with high suspicion for the disease but who have urine results that are borderline or normal. Pharmacologic tests to suppress or stimulate catecholamine release may be considered if measurements of catecholamines and metabolites fail to provide a diagnosis. (See *Clonidine Suppression Test.*) Plasma catecholamines have also been utilized for tumor localization by selective venous sampling. Measurements of plasma norepinephrine are useful in diagnosing patients with orthostatic hypotension. Failure to increase the supine norepinephrine concentration on standing suggests a sympathetic nervous system disorder.

This is not the preferred test for detection of pheochromocytoma as plasma catecholamines may not be consistently increased. This test may be useful in patients whose plasma or urine metanephrine concentrations do not exclude the diagnosis.

5. Alexander F: Neuroblastoma, *Urol Clin North Am* 27:383-392, vii, 2000.

6. Lenders JW, Pacak K, Walther MM, et al: Biochemical diagnosis of pheochromocytoma: which test is best? *JAMA* 287:1427-1434, 2000.

7. Bouloux P, Perrett D, Besser GM: Methodological considerations in the determination of plasma catecholamines by high-performance liquid chromatography with electrochemical detection, *Ann Clin Biochem* 22:194-203, 1985.

8. Moyer TP, Jiang NS, Tyce GM, et al: Analysis for urinary catecholamines by liquid chromatography with amperometric detection methodology and clinical interpretation of results, *Clin Chem* 25:256-263, 1979.

TEST NAME AND METHOD	SPECIMEN REQUIREMENTS	REFERENCE INTERVAL, CONVENTIONAL [INTERNATIONAL RECOMMENDED UNITS]		CHEMICAL INTERFERENCES AND IN VIVO EFFECTS

Catecholamines, Fractionated—CONT

9. Rosano TG, Swift TA, Hayes LW: Advances in catecholamine and metabolite measurements for diagnosis of pheochromocytomas, *Clin Chem* 37:1854-1867, 1991.

10. Kushnir MM, Urry FM, Frank EL, et al: Analysis of catecholamines in urine by positive-ion electrospray tandem mass spectrometry, *Clin Chem* 48:323-331, 2002.

11. Mayo Medical Laboratories: *Test catalog,* Rochester, MN, 2004, Mayo Medical Laboratories.

CD40 ligand[1-5] *Immunoassay*	Serum. CD40 ligand is readily released from activated platelets. Samples should be collected on ice and centrifuged immediately to produce platelet-poor plasma.	Healthy population: Cutoff for risk stratification for acute coronary syndromes:	*mcg/L* 0.03 and 3.98 5.0

1. Prasad KS, Andre P, Yan Y, et al: The platelet CD40L/GP IIb-IIIa axis in atherothrombotic disease, *Curr Opin Hematol* 10:356-361, 2003.

2. André P, Nannizzi-Alaimo L, Prasad SK, et al: The switch hitting player of cardiovascular disease, *Circulation* 106:896-899, 2002.

3. Varo N, de Lemos JA, Libby P, et al: Soluble CD40L: risk prediction after acute coronary syndromes, *Circulation* 108:1049-1052, 2003.

4. Heeschen C, Dimmeler S, Hamm CW, et al: Soluble CD40 ligand in acute coronary syndromes, *N Engl J Med* 348:1104-1111, 2003.

5. Heeschen C, Dimmeler S, Fichtlscherer S, et al: Prognostic value of placental growth factor in patients with acute chest pain, *JAMA* 291:435-441, 2004.

Test Name and Method	Specimen	Reference (mg/dL[1])			mg/L	Chemical Interferences
Ceruloplasmin (Cp, copper oxidase; EC 1.16.3.1)[1-4] *Nephelometry*[5] *Turbidimetry* *RID*	Serum. Analyze fresh or store for 3 days at 4° C, 4 wk at –20° C. Specimens without lipemia or hemolysis are preferred.	1 day-3 mo: 6-12 mo: 12 mo-7 yr: >7 yr:	5-18 33-43 24-56 18-45	× 10	[50-180] [330-430] [240-560] [180-450]	S ↑ V Anticonvulsant therapy (carbamazepine, phenobarbital, phenytoin, valproic acid),[8] estrogens,[9] methadone,[10] oral contraceptives,[9] smoking,[5] tamoxifen.

During pregnancy, levels gradually increase and can peak at values 2-3× normal.[6,7]

S ↓ V L-Asparaginase

Excessive turbidity can affect nephelometric methods.

12. Rosano TG: Liquid-chromatographic evaluation of age-related changes in the urinary excretion of free catecholamines in pediatric patients, *Clin Chem* 30:301-303, 1984.
13. Shapiro B, Fig LM: Management of pheochromocytoma, *Endocrine Metab Clin North Am* 18:443-481, 1989.

CD40 ligand has been shown to be useful for risk stratification of patients with acute coronary syndrome. In the Opus-TIMI16 Trial, increased CD40 ligand was associated with a higher incidence of death or nonfatal myocardial infarction.[3] In the CAP-TURE trial, patients with high CD40 ligand who were treated with abciximab (glycoprotein IIb/IIIa inhibitor) had a lower incidence of death or myocardial infarction than patients with high CD40l who were not treated.[4] The highest odds ratio was obtained when CD40 ligand was combined with other markers such as placental growth factor.[5]

CD40 is a receptor found on leukocytes, endothelial and smooth muscle cells, and platelets. CD40 ligand is a soluble protein ligand that is shed from activated leukocytes and platelets. Given the role of platelets and monocytes in the pathophysiology of acute coronary syndromes, CD40 ligand has been suggested as a marker for risk stratification.

S ↑ Acute phase reacting protein. Increased in inflammation, infection, tissue injury, cardiovascular disease, and some malignancies. Elevations of ceruloplasmin occur very gradually, typically peaking in 4-20 days.[11]

Pregnancy: levels may increase to approximately double the baseline values during the third trimester.[6]

S ↓ Hepatolenticular degeneration (Wilson's disease). Autosomal-recessive disease involving copper metabolism. A lack of, or a defective copper transporting P-type ATPase (ATP7B) results in impaired incorporation of copper into apoceruloplasmin and subsequent impairment of biliary excretion.[12] Affected individuals experience hepatic copper accumulation, hepatic and neurological disease.[13]

Ceruloplasmin (CP), an α_2-globulin, is a member of the multi-copper oxidase family of proteins. This serum ferroxidase contains ~95% or more of the plasma copper.[16] It has a role in both iron and copper metabolism.

Immunonephelometric methods may measure both the inactive apo-CP and serum CP; consequently, assessment of oxidase activity may be useful for clinical diagnosis.[17]

Epidemiological evidence suggests that CP may be an independent risk factor for cardiovascular disease, possibly due to oxidative alteration of low density lipoprotein.[4]

Indications for quantitation include evaluation of the acute phase response and assessment for possible Wilson's disease,

TEST NAME AND METHOD	SPECIMEN REQUIREMENTS	REFERENCE INTERVAL, CONVENTIONAL [INTERNATIONAL RECOMMENDED UNITS]	CHEMICAL INTERFERENCES AND IN VIVO EFFECTS
Ceruloplasmin—CONT			
RID	Urine, 24 hr. Centrifuge and adjust to pH 7.0. Analyze fresh. Stable frozen at −20° C for up to 1 yr.	0.006-0.040 mg/day ($\bar{x}$: 0.056)	

1. Tietz NW, editor: *Textbook of clinical chemistry,* Philadelphia, 1999, WB Saunders.

2. Denko CW, Gabriel P: Age and sex-related levels of albumin, ceruloplasmin, alpha-1-antitrypsin, alpha-1-acid glycoprotein and transferring, *Ann Clin Lab Sci* 2:63-68, 1981.

3. Hellman NE, Gitlin JD: Ceruloplasmin metabolism and function, *Annu Rev Nutr* 22:439-458, 2002.

4. Fox PL, Mukhopadhyay C, Ehrenwald E: Structure, oxidant activity, and cardiovascular mechanism of human ceruloplasmin, *Life Sci* 56:1749-1758, 1995.

5. Davidoff GN, Votaw ML, Coon WW, et al: Elevations in serum copper, erythrocytic copper, and ceruloplasmin concentrations in smokers, *Am J Clin Pathol* 70:790-792, 1978.

6. Laurell CB, Rannevik G: A comparison of plasma protein changes induced by danazol, pregnancy, and estrogens, *J Clin Endocrinol Metab* 49:719-725, 1979.

7. Putnam FW, editors: *The plasma proteins: structure, functions and genetic control,* ed 2, vol 1-3, New York, 1977, Academic Press.

8. Tutor-Crespo MJ, Hermida J, Tutor JC: Assessment of copper status in epileptic patients treated with anticonvulsant drugs by measuring specific oxidase activity of ceruloplasmin, *Epilepsy Res* 56:147-153, 2003.

9. Kluft C, Leuven JA, Helmerhorst FM, et al: Pro-inflammatory effects of oestrogens during oral contraceptives and hormone replacement treatment, *Vascul Pharmacol* 39:149-154, 2002.

10. Bastomsky CH, Dent RR, Tolis G, et al: Elevated serum concentrations of thyroxine-binding globulin and caeruloplasmin in methadone-maintained patients, *Clin Biochem* 10:124-126, 1977.

11. Aronsen K-F, Ekelund G, Kindmark CO, et al: Sequential changes of plasma proteins after surgical trauma, *Scand J Clin Invest* 29(suppl 124):127-136, 1972.

12. Loudianos G, Gitlin JD: Wilson's disease, *Semin Liver Dis* 20:353-364, 2000.

13. Ferenci P: Review article: diagnosis and current therapy of Wilson's disease, *Alim Pharmacol Ther* 19:157-165, 2004.

14. Menkes JH: Kinky hair disease: twenty-five years later, *Brain Dev* 10:77-79, 1988.

15. Xu X, Pin S, Gathinji M, et al: Aceruloplasminemia: an inherited neurodegenerative disease with impairment of iron homeostasis, *Ann NY Acad Sci* 1012:299-305, 2004.

16. Hellman NE, Gitlin JD: Ceruloplasmin metabolism and function, *Annu Rev Nutr* 22:439-458, 2002.

DIAGNOSTIC INFORMATION	REMARKS

Menkes' kinky hair syndrome: A sex-linked disorder caused by defective gastrointestinal copper absorption. Clinical features include cognitive decline, seizures, and bone deformities.[14]

Aceruloplasminemia. An autosomal-recessive disease involving excess tissue iron deposition. Patients experience neurological degeneration, blepharospasm, pancreatic and retinal symptoms.[15]

Early diagnosis of these disorders is important for therapeutic intervention.

Concentrations of urinary copper are typically increased in Wilson's disease.

Menkes' kinky hair syndrome, aceruloplasminemia, or other conditions associated with decreased CP levels (i.e., dietary).

MW: 132,000
$t_{1/2}$: 4.5 days

17.   Walshe JM: Wilson's disease: the importance of measuring serum caeruloplasmin non-immunologically, *Ann Clin Biochem* 40(Pt 2):115-121, 2003.

TEST NAME AND METHOD	SPECIMEN REQUIREMENTS	REFERENCE INTERVAL, CONVENTIONAL [INTERNATIONAL RECOMMENDED UNITS]			CHEMICAL INTERFERENCES AND IN VIVO EFFECTS
Cesium (Cs)	Serum. Collect in metal-free container.	*mcg/L (SD)* 1.0 ± 0.4	× 7.52	*nmol/L* [7.52 ± 3 .0]	None found.
NAA[1,2]					
	Plasma (citrate). Collect in metal-free container.	0.85 ± 0.22		[6.39 ± 1.65]	
	Platelets (pure).[2] Collect in metal-free container.	*ng/g wet wt.* 54.8 ± 19.2	× 7.52	*pmol/g wet wt.* [412 ± 144]	
	Erythrocytes[1]	5-10 mcg/kg	× 7.52	[38-75 nmol/kg]	
	Urine, 24 hr.[1] Collect in metal-free container.	8-20 mcg/day	× 7.52	[60-150 nmol/day]	
	Liver[1]	*mcg/kg dry wt.* 10-20	× 7.52	*nmol/kg dry wt.* 75-150	
	Hair[1]	*mg/kg dry wt.* 0.1-1.0	× 7.52	*µmol/kg dry wt.* 0.75-7.52	

1. Iyengar GV, Woittiez J: Trace elements in human clinical specimens: evaluation of literature data to identify reference values, *Clin Chem* 34:474-481, 1988.
2. Kasperek K, Iyengar GV, Kiem J, et al: Elemental composition of platelets. Part III. Determinations of Ag, Au, Cd, Co, Cr, Cs, Mo, Rb, Sb, and Se in normal human platelets by neutron activation analysis, *Clin Chem* 25:711-715, 1979.
3. Neulieb R: Effect of oral intake of cesium chloride: a single case report, *Pharmacol Biochem Behav* 21(suppl 1):15-16, 1984.
4. Pinter A, Dorian P, Newman D: Cesium-induced torsades de pointes, *N Engl J Med* 346:383, 2002.
5. Brachmann J, Scherlag BJ, Rosenshtraukh LV, et al: Bradycardia-dependant triggered activity: relevance to drug-induced multiform ventricular tachycardia, *Circulation* 68:845-856, 1983.

TEST NAME AND METHOD	SPECIMEN REQUIREMENTS	REFERENCE INTERVAL, CONVENTIONAL [INTERNATIONAL RECOMMENDED UNITS]			CHEMICAL INTERFERENCES AND IN VIVO EFFECTS
Chloride (Cl)[1-5]	Serum or plasma. Avoid hemolysis.		*mEq/L*[5]	*mmol/L*	S ↑ V Acetazolamide, androgens, cholestyramine, diazoxide, estrogens, guanethidine, methyldopa, oxyphenbutazone, phenylbutazone, thiazides (prolonged therapy), triamterene (nephrotoxic effect)
Coulometric, colorimetric, ISE		Cord:	96-104	× 1.0 [96-104]	
		Premature:	95-110	[96-110]	
		0-30 days:	98-113	[98-113]	
		Thereafter:	98-107(108)	[98-107]	
		>90 yr:	98-111[7]	[98-111]	

S ↑ C Bromides, iodides, *Kone Microlyte:* aspirin; *Hitachi:* sodium bicarbonate

DIAGNOSTIC INFORMATION	REMARKS

No adverse effects from industrial exposure have been reported. Nausea, diarrhea, and torsades de pointes have been reported in patients receiving naturopathic therapy for cancer.[3,4]

The serum level of cesium may be influenced by platelet destruction during the clotting process. Increased K levels facilitate Cs excretion. Hemolysis will increase serum or plasma Cs because erythrocytes have 6.5 times higher levels of Cs than does plasma. Cesium chloride blocks the inward-rectifying potassium channel.[5]

S ↑ Dehydration, renal tubular acidosis, acute renal failure, diabetes insipidus, metabolic acidosis associated with prolonged diarrhea with loss of $NaHCO_3$, salicylate intoxication, respiratory alkalosis, some cases of primary hyperparathyroidism, following head injury associated with hypothalamic stimulation or damage, adrenocortical hyperfunction

Except in emergencies, the specimen should be collected when the patient is in a fasting state. There is a slight decrease in chloride ions after meals. Factors similar to those provoking hypernatremia also cause hyperchloremia. In bromide intoxication, Br^- replaces Cl^-. The resulting hypochloremia may not be detected because some laboratory methods are nonspecific.

S ↓ Excessive sweating, prolonged vomiting from any cause or gastric suction, persistent gastric secretion, salt-losing nephritis, Addisonian crisis, metabolic acidosis associated with increase in organic anions, aldosteronism, potassium depletion associated with alkalosis, respiratory acidosis, cerebral salt wasting after head injury, water intoxication and other conditions with expansion of the extracellular fluid volume, acute intermittent porphyria, SIADH

Direct ISE measurements do not give the volume displacement error in specimens with high lipid or protein content, as indirect ISE and flame measurements do.

TEST NAME AND METHOD	SPECIMEN REQUIREMENTS	REFERENCE INTERVAL, CONVENTIONAL [INTERNATIONAL RECOMMENDED UNITS]		CHEMICAL INTERFERENCES AND IN VIVO EFFECTS

Chloride—CONT

CX3: N-acetylcysteine, ≥20 mmol/L; ammonium carbonate, ≥50 mmol/L; ascorbic acid, ≥20 mg/dL; cysteine, ≥20 mmol/L; gluathione, ≥5 mmol/L; guanidine, ≥1 mg/dL[10]; procainamide-HCL, ≥10 mcg/mL; sodium azide, ≥500 ppm

S ↓ V Bicarbonates, carbenoxolone, corticotropin, diuretics (e.g., bumetanide, ethacrynic acid, furosemide, mannitol, metolazone, thiazides, triamterene), laxatives (chronic abusers), theophylline

Urine, 24 hr.

		mEq/day		*mmol/day*
Infant:		$2\text{-}10^5$	× 1.0	[2-10]
Child <6 yr:		$15\text{-}40^8$		[15-40]
6-10 yr				
M:		36-110		[36-110]
F:		18-74		[18-74]
10-14 yr				
M:		64-176		[64-176]
F:		36-173		[36-173]
Adult:		$110\text{-}250^5$		[110-250]
>60 yr:		95-195		[95-195]

Values vary greatly with Cl intake.

Random urine[9]:

	mEq/L		*mmol/L*
M: <40 yr	27-371	× 1.0	[27-371]
≥40 yr	30-260		[30-260]
F: <40 yr	20-295		[20-295]
≥40 yr	24-255		[24-255]

	mEq/g creatinine		*mmol/g creatinine*
M:	25-253	× 1.0	[25-253]
F:	39-348		[39-348]

U ↑ V Diuretics (e.g., amiloride, ammonium chloride, bumetanide, chlorthalidone, ethacrynic acid, furosemide, metolazone, spironolactone, thiazides, triamterene), digitalis, isosorbide, viomycin

U ↑ C Bromides, iodides

U ↓ V Acetazolamide, clopamide, corticosteroids, diazoxide, epinephrine, levaterenol, mafenide

DIAGNOSTIC INFORMATION	REMARKS

U ↑ Increased salt intake; postmenstrual diuresis (physiological); massive diuresis from any cause, e.g., salt-losing nephritis (Cl is excreted along with cations); potassium depletion; adrenocortical insufficiency, tubulointerstitial disease, Bartter's syndrome

U ↓ Reduced salt intake, premenstrual salt and water retention (physiological), excessive extrarenal chloride loss (e.g., vomiting, intestinal fistula, severe diarrhea, excessive sweating with poor NaCl intake), adrenocortical hyperfunction, postoperative chloride retention, any kind of salt retention (e.g., formation of edema, brain damage)

Normally the urine chloride excretion approximates the dietary intake.

TEST NAME AND METHOD	SPECIMEN REQUIREMENTS	REFERENCE INTERVAL, CONVENTIONAL [INTERNATIONAL RECOMMENDED UNITS]			CHEMICAL INTERFERENCES AND IN VIVO EFFECTS
Chloride—CONT					
	CSF		*mEq/L*		*mmol/L*
		Infant:	110-130	× 1.0	[110-130][1]
		Adult:	118-132		[118-132][5]
	Erythrocyte fluid[2]		49-54		[49-54]
	Whole blood[2]		77-87		[77-87]
	Tissue cells[2]		~1		[~1]
	Feces, 24 hr.	*mEq/day*			*mmol/day*
		~2[1]		× 1.0	[~2]
		3.2 ± 0.7[3]			[3.2 ± 0.7]
Coulometric, colorimetric[6]	Sweat (iontophoresis) An applied electric field drives pilocarpine into the skin, inducing local sweating. Sweat is collected and chloride concentration measured.		*mEq/L*		*mmol/L*
		Normal:	5-35	× 1.0	[5-35]
		Marginal:	30-70		[30-70]
		Cystic fibrosis:	60-200		[60-200]
	Saliva[6]	Without stimulation:	5-20		[5-20]
		After stimulation:	x̄: 44		[x̄: 44]

1. Eastham RD: *Biochemical values in clinical medicine,* ed 7, Bristol, UK, 1985, John Wright and Sons, Ltd.

2. Burtis CA, Ashwood ER, editors: *Tietz fundamentals of clinical chemistry,* ed 5, Philadelphia, 2000, WB Saunders.

3. Wallace J, editor: *Interpretation of diagnostic tests,* ed 7, Philadelphia, 2000, Lippincott Williams & Wilkins.

4. Chan MK, Varghese L, Moorhead JF: Urinary chloride excretion in suspected Bartter's syndrome, *N Engl J Med* 301:1450, 1979.

5. Scott MG, Heusel JW, LeGrys VA, et al: Electrolyte, and blood gases. In Burtis CA, Ashwood ER, editors: *Tietz textbook of clinical chemistry,* ed 3, Philadelphia, 1999, WB Saunders.

6. Soergel KH: Acute pancreatitis. In Sleisenger MH, Fordtran JS, editors: *Gastrointestinal disease: pathophysiology, diagnosis, management,* ed 4, Philadelphia, 1989, WB Saunders.

7. Awdeh ZL, Alper CA: Inherited structural polymorphism of the fourth component of human complement, *Proc Natl Acad Sci USA* 77:3576-3580, 1980.

8. Liappis N, Reimnitz P: Referenzwerte der natrium-, kalium-, kalzium-, chlorid-, und anorganischen phosphat-ausscheidung im 24 h-urin gesunder kinder, *Klin Padiatr* 196:367-369, 1984.

DIAGNOSTIC INFORMATION	REMARKS

CSF ↑ Any condition with elevated serum chloride

CSF ↓ Any condition with decreased serum Cl level, tuberculous meningitis, other bacterial meningitides (nonspecific, test reflects systemic hypochloremia)

F ↑ Severe diarrhea (up to 500 mmol of chloride can be lost in 24 hr), congenital chloridorrhea (very rare condition), idiopathic proctocolitis, ileostomy

---

Sw ↑ Cystic fibrosis (in 98% of patients), untreated adrenal insufficiency, familial hypoparathyroidism, familial ectodermal dysplasia with sensorineural deafness, nephrogenic diabetes insipidus, hypothyroidism, fucosidosis, G6PD deficiency, mucopolysaccharidosis, hereditary nephrogenic diabetes, familial cholestasis, alcoholic pancreatitis, some cases of renal disease.[11] Most of these conditions are rare and are clinically distinct from cystic fibrosis.

The sweat test with iontophoretic stimulation is considered the most reliable single test in the diagnosis of cystic fibrosis. Test becomes positive between 3 and 5 wk in most affected infants. Test may be normal in patients with salt depletion, e.g., during periods of hot weather. Additional electrolyte studies prevent misinterpretations. Sweat conductivity performs comparable to sweat chloride concentration in diagnosing CF.[12,13]

Sweat chloride increases by 10 mmol/L during a lifetime.

Skin lesions or rash can cause increase in values.

At least 75 mg of sweat should be collected.[14]

Sal ↑ Cystic fibrosis

Sal ↓ Congestive heart failure, adrenocortical hyperfunction

Results obtained with the saliva test are inconsistent and not as reliable as those obtained with the sweat test.

---

9.   Bond LW, Garber C, Ottinger W, et al: Reference intervals for common analytes in random urine specimens, *Clin Chem* 55: submitted, 2005.

10. Beckman Instruments, Inc: *Synchron CX3 clinical system manual,* Brea, CA, 1991, Beckman Instruments, Inc.

11. Tietz NW, Pruden EL, Siggaard-Andersen O: Electrolytes. In Burtis CA, Ashwood ER, editors: *Tietz textbook of clinical chemistry,* ed 2, Philadelphia, 1994, WB Saunders.

12. Lezana JL, Vargas MH, Karam-Bechara J, et al: Sweat conductivity and chloride titration for cystic fibrosis diagnosis in 3834 subjects, *J Cyst Fibros* 2:1-7, 2003.

13. Heeley ME, Woolf DA, Heeley AF: Indirect measurements of sweat electrolyte concentration in the laboratory diagnosis of cystic fibrosis, *Arch Dis Child* 82:420-424, 2000.

14. Sweat Testing: Sample collection and quantitative analysis; approved guidelines, NCCLS C34-A, Wayne, PA, 1994, National Committee for Clinical Laboratory Standards.

TEST NAME AND METHOD	SPECIMEN REQUIREMENTS	REFERENCE INTERVAL, CONVENTIONAL [INTERNATIONAL RECOMMENDED UNITS]			CHEMICAL INTERFERENCES AND IN VIVO EFFECTS
Chlorinated Hydrocarbon Solvents *GC-FID, GC-ECD*[1]	Blood (fluoride/oxalate). Refrigerate.	*Carbon tetrachloride* Occupational exposure: Toxic concentration:	*mg/L* <1 >20	× 6.49	µ*mol/L* [<7] [>130]	None found.
		Chloroform Occupational exposure: Toxic concentration:	<5 >10	× 8.38	[<42] [>84]	
		Methylene chloride Occupational exposure: Toxic concentration:	<12 >200	× 11.8	[<142] [>2360]	
		Trichloroethane Occupational exposure:	<1.5	× 7.51	[<11]	
		Trichloroethylene Occupational exposure:	<7	× 7.61	[<53]	
		Tetrachloroethylene Occupational exposure:	<3	× 6.03	[<18]	
	Breath	Occupational exposure Carbon tetrachloride: Methylene chloride: Trichloroethane: Trichloroethylene: Tetrachloroethylene:	*ppm* <3 <33 <50 <1 <15	× 6.5 × 11.8 × 7.51 × 7.61 × 6.03	µ*mol/L* [<20] [<389] [<375.5] [<8] [<90]	

1. Reddrop CJ, Riess W, Slater TF: Two rapid methods for the simultaneous gas-liquid chromatographic determination of carbon tetrachloride and chloroform in biological material and expired air, *J Chromatogr* 193:71-82, 1980.

2. Baselt RC: *Biological monitoring methods for industrial chemicals,* Davis, CA, 1980, Biomedical Pub.

Chlorinated hydrocarbons show varying degrees of toxicity, but all are CNS depressants and with prolonged exposure produce liver and kidney damage. Some of the chlorinated hydrocarbons are suspected carcinogens.

The chlorinated hydrocarbons are widely used solvents and are absorbed by inhalation or cutaneously. Dichloromethane is metabolized in part to CO with resulting elevation of carboxyhemoglobin concentration. Trichloroethane, trichloroethylene, and tetrachloroethylene are partially metabolized to trichloroethanol and trichloracetic acid, both of which can be monitored by GLC.[2]

TEST NAME AND METHOD	SPECIMEN REQUIREMENTS	REFERENCE INTERVAL, CONVENTIONAL [INTERNATIONAL RECOMMENDED UNITS]				CHEMICAL INTERFERENCES AND IN VIVO EFFECTS
Chlorophenoxy-acetic Acids[1]	Serum		*mg/L*		*μmol/L*	None found.
		Occupational exposure[3]:	5-40	× 4.52	[23-181]	
2,4-Dichlorophen-oxyacetic acid		Toxic concentration:	>400		[>1808]	
(2,4-D)	Urine	Occupational exposure[3]:	50-100		[226-452]	
GC-FID, GC-ECD[2]		Toxic concentration:	>200		[>904]	
2,4,5-Trichlorophe-	Serum	Asymptomatic[1]:	<88	× 3.91	[<344]	
noxyacetic acid						
(2,4,5-T)	Urine	Asymptomatic[1]:	<3.6		[<14]	
GC-FID, GC-ECD[2]						

1. Baselt RC: *Biological monitoring methods for industrial chemicals,* Davis, CA, 1980, Biomedical Pub.
2. Smith AE, Hayden BJ: Method for the determination of 2,4-dichlorophenoxyacetic acid residues in urine, *J Chromatogr* 171:482-485, 1979.
3. Baselt RC: *Analytical procedures for therapeutic drug monitoring and emergency toxicology,* ed 2, Littleton, MA, 1987, PSG.

TEST NAME AND METHOD	SPECIMEN REQUIREMENTS	REFERENCE INTERVAL, CONVENTIONAL [INTERNATIONAL RECOMMENDED UNITS]			CHEMICAL INTERFERENCES AND IN VIVO EFFECTS
Cholecystokinin-pancreozymin (CCK-PZ, CCK)[1-3] *RIA*[4]	Plasma, fasting. Collect blood in special tube containing heparin and Trasylol. Separate plasma in a refrigerated centrifuge within 30 min of collection and then freeze immedi-ately.	<80 pg/mL[5]	× 1.0	[<80 ng/L]	Secretion of CCK-PZ is completely inhibited by somatostatin infusion.

1. Henderson AR, Tietz NW, Rinker AD: Gastric, pancreatic, and intestinal function. In Burtis CA, Ashwood ER, editors: *Tietz textbook of clinical chemistry,* ed 2, Philadelphia, 1994, WB Saunders.
2. Morgan LM, Marks VL: The gastrointestinal hormones. In Pennington GW, Naik S, editors: *Hormone analysis: methodology and clinical interpretation, vol 2,* Boca Raton, FL, 1981, CRC Press.
3. Walsh JH: Gastrointestinal hormones. In Johnson LR, editor: *Physiology of the gastrointestinal tract,* ed 2, New York, 1987, Raven Press.

DIAGNOSTIC INFORMATION	REMARKS

Lethal exposures cause convulsions, vomiting, multiorgan failure, and neurodegenerative changes. Nonlethal toxic exposures cause irritation in the mouth, throat, and GI tract, vomiting, chest and abdominal pain, diarrhea, and muscle fasciculation, tenderness, and stiffness.

Kinetic values

2,4-D
$t_{1/2}$[3]:   4-140 hr
V_d: 0.1 L/kg
Lethal dose in man is estimated to be 28 g.

2,4,5-T
$t_{1/2}$[3]:   23 hr
V_d: 0.08 L/kg
99% protein bound
Low toxicity.

↑ Patients with pancreatic exocrine and celiac disease (up to 8500 pg/mL [8500 ng/L]). CCK values are also of possible interest in fatty food intolerance, gastric ulcer, postgastrectomy states, and irritable bowel syndromes. There is no defined clinical diagnostic purpose for this test.

There are various stimulating agents and protocols.[6] Variation in reference ranges among laboratories is large.

CCK, like gastrin, exists in several different molecular forms; unlike gastrin, a sulfated form occurs naturally and is required for biological activity. Cholecystokinin and pancreozymin are not different substances but are the same hormone with a dual action.

The CCK half-life in vivo has been reported as 2.5 min or 5-7 min. Because CCK is responsible for a number of important actions on the GI tract, notably gall bladder contraction and pancreatic enzyme secretion, disturbances in its secretion or actions may be important in various clinical disorders of these organs (e.g., pancreatic insufficiency, celiac disease, Z-E syndrome). Levels of CCK increase following ingestion of a test meal; responses are more rapid in patients with duodenal ulcers and diabetes than in healthy subjects.

---

4. Chang T-M, Chey WY: Radioimmunoassay of cholecystokinin, *Dig Dis Sci* 28:456-468, 1983.

5. InterScience Institute: *Current unique and rare endocrine assays. Patient and specimen requirements,* Inglewood, CA, 1988, InterScience Institute.

6. Chowdhury RS, Forsmark CR: Pancreatic function testing, *Aliment Pharmacol Ther* 17:733-750, 2003.

TEST NAME AND METHOD	SPECIMEN REQUIREMENTS	REFERENCE INTERVAL, CONVENTIONAL [INTERNATIONAL RECOMMENDED UNITS]	CHEMICAL INTERFERENCES AND IN VIVO EFFECTS

Cholesterol, Total (TC)[1-12]
 	
Enzymatic[10,13-15]
	Serum, plasma (EDTA or heparin but not oxalate, fluoride, or citrate); fasting ≥12 hr is recommended; nonfasting specimen is acceptable if TC is not part of a fasting lipid profile. Patient should be sitting for 5 min before blood draw; avoid prolonged tourniquet use. Stable 4-7 days at 4° C. Avoid repeated freezing and thawing.	*Recommended cutpoints, adults*[3]
		Desirable:
		  <200 mg/dL × 0.0259 [<5.18 mmol/L]
		Borderline high:
		  200-239 mg/dL [5.18-6.19 mmol/L]
		High:
		  ≥240 mg/dL [≥6.22 mmol/L]
		
		Recommended cutpoints, children[7]
		Acceptable:
		  <170 mg/dL [<4.40 mmol/L]
		Borderline:
		  170-199 mg/dL [4.40-5.15 mmol/L]
		High:
		  ≥200 mg/dL [≥5.18 mmol/L]
			↑ C β-hydroxysterols, hemolysis (method-specific)
			
			↑ V ACTH, bile salts, amiodarone, androgens, carbamazepine, retinoids, corticosteroids, cigarette smoking, cyclosporine, levodopa, HIV protease inhibitors, thiazide diuretics, phenothiazines, pregnancy, high saturated fat and high cholesterol diets.
			
			↓ C Ascorbic acid (method-specific), bilirubin (method-specific), EDTA plasma concentrations are 3-6% lower than serum.

	mg/dL[16,17] 5th-95th percentile		mmol/L 5th-95th percentile	
Non-Hispanic white				↓ V Asparaginase, bile acid sequestrants (resins, e.g., cholestyramine, colestipol), cyproterone acetate, doxazosin, fibric acid derivatives (e.g., clofibrate, gemfibrozil), estrogens, heparin, HMG-CoA reductase inhibitors (statins), ketoconazole, neomycin, prazosin, probucol, sitosterols, tacrolimus, thyroid hormone replacement therapy, low cholesterol and high polyunsaturated fat diets, long-term alcohol consumption, weight loss in overweight individuals, acute myocardial infarction.
4-5 yr				
M:	130-197	× 0.0259	[3.37-5.10]	
F:	128-208		[3.32-5.39]	
6-11 yr				
M:	128-216		[3.32-5.59]	
F:	128-212		[3.32-5.49]	
12-19 yr				
M:	116-205		[3.00-5.31]	
F:	118-227		[3.06-5.88]	
20-29 yr				
M:	125-239		[3.24-6.19]	
F:	133-243		[3.44-6.29]	
30-39 yr				
M:	142-267		[3.68-6.92]	
F:	139-249		[3.60-6.45]	
40-49 yr				
M:	152-275		[3.94-7.12]	
F:	150-274		[3.89-7.10]	
50-59 yr				
M:	155-286		[4.01-7.41]	
F:	171-304		[4.43-7.87]	
60-69 yr				
M:	157-283		[4.07-7.33]	
F:	173-309		[4.48-8.00]	
70+ yr				
M:	146-273		[3.78-7.07]	
F:	166-308		[4.30-7.98]	

DIAGNOSTIC INFORMATION	REMARKS

↑ Familial hypercholesterolemia, familial dysbetalipoproteinemia (type III), familial combined hyperlipidemia, familial defective apo-B-100, polygenic (sporadic) hypercholesterolemia, coronary heart disease, hypercholesterolemia secondary to obstructive liver disease, primary biliary cirrhosis, nephrotic syndrome, chronic renal failure, Cushing's syndrome, type 2 diabetes, hypothyroidism, obesity, pregnancy, certain glycogen storage diseases.

↓ Hypo-α-lipoproteinemias (e.g., Tangier disease), abetalipoproteinemia, hypobetalipoproteinemias, hepatocellular necrosis, malignancy, hyperthyroidism, malabsorption, malnutrition, severe acute illness, inflammation, infection.

The National Cholesterol Education Program (NCEP) recommends that all adults >20 yr be screened for CHD risk with measurement of TC, HDL-cholesterol, LDL-cholesterol, and triglyceride concentrations.

The pediatric NCEP report also confirmed a strong correlation between juvenile and adult cholesterol concentrations and recommended selective screening of children who have a family history of premature heart disease or at least one parent with high blood cholesterol. An initial TC measurement ≥200 mg/dL should lead to a complete lipoprotein profile as a follow-up evaluation.

Intraindividual variability in total cholesterol is ~6% over ≥1 month. Seasonal variation in cholesterol levels has also been observed; levels are ~2.2 (men) and 6.0 (women) mg/dL higher in winter than in summer (greater difference in hypercholesterolemics). Because of biological and analytical variation at least two serial samples may be necessary for clinical decision-making.

The goal for cholesterol measurement, as defined by the NCEP Laboratory Standardization Panel, is a total error <9%, consistent with a precision <3% CV, and a bias ±3% relative to the CDC reference method.

TEST NAME AND METHOD	SPECIMEN REQUIREMENTS	REFERENCE INTERVAL, CONVENTIONAL [INTERNATIONAL RECOMMENDED UNITS]		CHEMICAL INTERFERENCES AND IN VIVO EFFECTS
Cholesterol, Total (TC)—CONT				
		Non-Hispanic black		
		4-5 yr		
		M:	122-211	[3.16-5.46]
		F:	121-220	[3.13-5.70]
		6-11 yr		
		M:	128-224	[3.32-5.80]
		F:	131-227	[3.39-5.88]
		12-19 yr		
		M:	119-220	[3.08-5.70]
		F:	120-229	[3.11-5.93]
		20-29 yr		
		M:	133-249	[3.44-6.45]
		F:	129-253	[3.34-6.55]
		30-39 yr		
		M:	134-262	[3.47-6.79]
		F:	132-248	[3.42-6.42]
		40-49 yr		
		M:	143-285	[3.70-7.38]
		F:	141-269	[3.65-6.97]
		50-59 yr		
		M:	136-309	[3.52-8.00]
		F:	152-302	[3.94-7.82]
		60-69 yr		
		M:	148-294	[3.83-7.61]
		F:	170-322	[4.40-8.34]
		70+ yr		
		M:	141-289	[3.65-7.49]
		F:	156-304	[4.04-7.87]
		Mexican Americans		
		4-5 yr		
		M:	119-204	[3.08-5.28]
		F:	121-206	[3.13-5.34]
		6-11 yr		
		M:	128-215	[3.32-5.57]
		F:	126-209	[3.26-5.41]
		12-19 yr		
		M:	119-213	[3.08-5.52]
		F:	120-224	[3.11-5.80]
		20-29 yr		
		M:	130-250	[3.37-6.48]
		F:	132-245	[3.42-6.35]
		30-39 yr		
		M:	141-274	[3.65-7.10]
		F:	136-266	[3.52-6.89]
		40-49 yr		
		M:	150-290	[3.89-7.51]
		F:	149-282	[3.86-7.30]

DIAGNOSTIC INFORMATION   REMARKS

TEST NAME AND METHOD	SPECIMEN REQUIREMENTS	REFERENCE INTERVAL, CONVENTIONAL [INTERNATIONAL RECOMMENDED UNITS]	CHEMICAL INTERFERENCES AND IN VIVO EFFECTS
Cholesterol, Total (TC)—CONT			
	50-59 yr		
	M:	146-279	[3.78-7.23]
	F:	158-294	[4.09-7.61]
	60-69 yr		
	M:	160-285	[4.14-7.38]
	F:	165-297	[4.27-7.69]
	70+ yr		
	M:	144-273	[3.73-7.07]
	F:	153-295	[3.96-7.64]

1. Cohn JS, McNamara JR, Cohn SD, et al: Postprandial plasma lipoprotein changes in human subjects of different ages, *J Lipid Res* 29:469-479, 1988.

2. Cooper GR, Myers GL, Smith J, et al: Blood lipid measurements: variations and practical utility, *JAMA* 267:1652-1660, 1992.

3. Expert Panel on Detection, Evaluation, and Treatment of High Blood Cholesterol in Adults: Executive summary of the Third Report of the National Cholesterol Education Program (NCEP) Expert Panel on detection, evaluation, and treatment of high blood cholesterol in adults (Adult Treatment Panel III), *JAMA* 285:2486-2497, 2001.

4. Henkin Y, Como JA, Oberman A: Secondary dyslipidemia: inadvertent effects of drugs in clinical practice, *JAMA* 267:961-968, 1992.

5. Henry JB, editor: *Clinical diagnosis and management by laboratory methods,* ed 19, Philadelphia, 1996, WB Saunders.

6. National Cholesterol Education Program: *Recommendations for improving cholesterol measurement: a report from the Laboratory Standardization Panel of the National Cholesterol Education Program,* NIH Publication No. 90-2964, Bethesda, MD, 1990, National Cholesterol Education Program.

7. National Cholesterol Education Program (NCEP): Highlights of the report of the expert panel on blood cholesterol levels in children and adolescents, *Pediatrics* 89:495-501, 1992.

8. Ockene IS, Chiriboga DE, Stanek EJ, et al: Seasonal variation in serum cholesterol levels, *Arch Intern Med* 164:863-870, 2004.

9. Rader DJ: Lipid disorders. In Topol EJ, editor: *Textbook of cardiovascular medicine,* ed 2, Philadelphia, PA, 2002, Lippincott Williams & Wilkins.

10. Rifai N, Warnick GR, Dominiczak MH, editors: *Handbook of lipoprotein testing,* ed 2, Washington, DC, 2000, AACC Press.

11. Young DS: *Effects of drugs on clinical laboratory tests,* ed 5, Washington, DC, 2000, AACC Press.

12. Young DS: *Effects of preanalytical variables on clinical laboratory tests,* ed 2, Washington, DC, 1997, AACC Press.

13. Allain CC, Poon LS, Chan CSG, et al: Enzymatic determination of total serum cholesterol, *Clin Chem* 20:470-475, 1974.

14. Witte DL, Brown LF, Feld RD: Enzymatic analysis of serum cholesterol and triglycerides: a brief review, *Lab Med* 9:39-44, 1978.

15. Zak B, Artiss JD: Some observations on cholesterol measurement in the clinical laboratory, *Microchem J* 41:251-270, 1990.

16. NHANES III, 1988-94: Available at: www.cdc.gov/nchs/data/nhanes/cholfem.pdf. Accessed June 3, 2004.

17. NHANES III, 1988-94: Available at: www.cdc.gov/nchs/data/nhanes/cholmal.pdf. Accessed June 3, 2004.

DIAGNOSTIC INFORMATION   **REMARKS**

TEST NAME AND METHOD	SPECIMEN REQUIREMENTS	REFERENCE INTERVAL, CONVENTIONAL [INTERNATIONAL RECOMMENDED UNITS]			CHEMICAL INTERFERENCES AND IN VIVO EFFECTS
Cholinesterase (S-Pseudocholine esterase, choline esterase II, SChE, acylcholine acylhydrolase; EC 3.1.1.8)[1-3]	Serum. Avoid hemolysis. Stable at room temperature for 6 hr, 1 wk at 4° C, 6 mo at −70° C. Avoid repeated freezing and thawing.	4.9-11.9 U/mL $\times 1.0$ [4.9-11.9 kU/L] Values are low at birth and for the first 6 mo of life, increasing to 30-50% above adult values until 5 yr and then gradually decreasing to adult values by puberty.[8]			↓ V Anabolic steroids, carbamates, cimetidine, cyclophosphamide, echothiopate iodide, estrogens, glucocorticoids, lithium, neostigmine, neuromuscular relaxants (e.g., pancuronium, succinylcholine), oral contraceptives, organophosphorus insecticides, phenelzine, phenothiazines, physostigmine, radiographic agents (e.g., iopanoic acid), ranitidine, streptokinase, testosterone
Colorimetric (propionylthiocholine), 37° C[4]					
Du Pont aca (butylthiocholine), 37° C[5]		7-19 U/mL $\times 1.0$ [7-19 kU/L]			
Inhibition: Ellman reaction with and without inhibitors[4,6,7]			*% Inhibition[6]*	*Fraction inhibited*	↓ C Borate, citrate anticoagulant, detergents, fluoride, heavy metals, pyrophosphate, serum separators, tertiary and quaternary amines
		Dibucaine:	79-84 $\times 0.01$	[0.79-0.84]	
		Fluoride:	58-64	[0.58-0.64]	
		RO 02-0683:	94-98	[0.94-0.98]	
Kodak Ektachem (butylthiocholine), 37° C		M:	5.9-12.2 kU/L		
		F:	4.7-10.4 kU/L		

1. Burtis CA, Ashwood ER, editors: *Tietz textbook of clinical chemistry,* ed 2, Philadelphia, 1994, WB Saunders.
2. Ellman GL, Courtney KD, Andres V Jr, et al: A new and rapid colorimetric determination of acetylcholinesterase activity, *Biochem Pharmacol* 7:88-95, 1961.
3. Evans RT, Wroe J: Is serum cholinesterase activity a predictor of succinylcholine sensitivity? An assessment of four methods, *Clin Chem* 24:1762-1766, 1978.
4. Dietz AA, Rubenstein HM, Lubrano T: Colorimetric determination of serum cholinesterase and its genetic variants by the propionylthiocholine-dithiobis (nitrobenzoic acid) procedure, *Clin Chem* 19:1309-1313, 1973.
5. Westgard JO, Hunt MR, Lahmeyer BI: *Estimates of normal ranges for 15 determinations on the Du Pont Automatic Clinical Analyzer,* Wilmington, DE, 1972, Du Pont Co., Instrument Products Automatic Clinical Analysis Division.
6. Evans RT: Cholinesterase phenotyping: clinical aspects and laboratory application, *Crit Rev Clin Lab Sci* 23:35-64, 1986.
7. Silk E, King J, Whittaker M: Assay of cholinesterase in clinical chemistry, *Ann Clin Biochem* 16:57-75, 1979.
8. Meites S, editor: *Pediatric clinical chemistry,* ed 3, Washington, DC, 1989, American Association for Clinical Chemistry.
9. Kamolz LP, Andel H, Greher M, et al: Serum cholinesterase activity in patients with burns, *Clin Chem Lab Med* 40:60-64, 2002.

↑ Type IV hyperlipoproteinemia, nephrosis, obesity (including diabetics), psychosis, breast cancer

↓ Genetic CHE variants (see *Remarks*); organophosphorus insecticide poisoning (the most important application). Enzyme is also decreased in hepatitis, cirrhosis, hepatic metastases, hepatic congestion of heart failure, hepatic amebiasis, malnutrition, anemias, acute infections, burns,[9] myocardial infarction, pulmonary embolism, plasmapheresis, dermatomyositis, muscular dystrophy, after surgery, chronic renal disease, late pregnancy, conditions with low serum albumin (e.g., malabsorption), exfoliative dermatitis.

The SChE assay can be used in conjunction with in vitro enzyme inhibition (by dibucaine, fluoride, and RO 02-0683 to give the respective "inhibitor numbers") to detect several atypical SChE variants (at least 15 different phenotypes are known). Phenotypes at risk include UA (usually only during pregnancy); AF, FS, and FF (moderate risk); and AA, AS, and SS (severe risk). Succinylcholine anesthesia in these individuals may result in prolonged anesthesia and/or apnea, and its use in such cases should be avoided.[1]

The assay of serum SChE is of most interest clinically in the detection of possible insecticide poisoning, evaluation of liver function, and atypical enzyme variants (succinylcholine sensitivity). The decrease of SChE in liver disease generally parallels that of serum albumin levels. SChE should not be confused with the erythrocyte enzyme acetylcholinesterase (EC 3.1.1.7).

See *Acetylcholinesterase.*

Serum $t_{1/2}$: 12-14 days

TEST NAME AND METHOD	SPECIMEN REQUIREMENTS	REFERENCE INTERVAL, CONVENTIONAL [INTERNATIONAL RECOMMENDED UNITS]	CHEMICAL INTERFERENCES AND IN VIVO EFFECTS
Chorionic Gonadotropin **(hCG)**[1-4] *Qualitative* *Agglutination inhibition (slide or tube tests)*	Urine; freshly voided first-morning specimen preferred. Centrifuge at 900*g* for 10 min. Store at 2-8° C for up to 48 hr.	Negative; pregnancy is detected 8-14 days after first missed menstrual period.	False-positive results: Menotropins (pergonal, LH with FSH), chorionic gonadotropin (Follutein) U ↑ Proteinuria, hematuria, gross bacterial contamination, detergents Variable effects of phenothiazines have been reported.
Immunometric assay	Urine (see above) or serum. Store serum at 2-8° C for up to 24 hr. Otherwise, freeze at −20° C.	Negative; pregnancy is detected in urine 1 wk after implantation or 4-5 days before first missed menstrual period.	

DIAGNOSTIC INFORMATION	REMARKS

Human chorionic gonadotopin (hCG) is composed of two non-covalently bound glycoprotein subunits, α and β. Sera from normal pregnant women contain hCG in many forms, including intact (92-98%), α-subunit (0-7%), β-subunit (0-3%), and partially degraded (e.g., nicked hCG and β-core fragments). Urine from early pregnancy contains mostly β-core fragments ($\sim$50%) and to a lesser degree intact hCG ($\sim$35%) and nicked hCG ($\sim$10%).[6,7] hCG assays measure only the intact molecule. Assays specific for the β-subunit may be used for those situations in which subunit production should be monitored. (See *Chorionic Gonadotropin, β-Subunit.*)

Sensitivity of the agglutination inhibition tube assay[8]: >150 mU/mL [>150 U/L]

Slide tests are more rapid but less sensitive than tube tests for the detection of pregnancy. Neither test is sensitive enough to detect ectopic or abnormal intrauterine pregnancies. Cross-reactions with LH (as in menopause, mid-cycle LH peak) may give false-positive values. These tests are infrequently used and have been replaced by more sensitive immunometric assays.

Home pregnancy test kits are commonly used. Most kits use an immunometric technique; detection limits in urine are $\sim$50 mU/mL [50 U/L], making these tests suitable for detecting hCG just after the first missed menstrual period.[8] Home tests require 2-30 min to perform.

Sensitivity of the qualitative *laboratory immunometric assay:* 25-50 mU/mL [25-50 U/L]

Assay is rapid (3-15 min) and specific for the intact hCG. The assay has good correlation with positive, negative, equivocal results of quantitative serum hCG.[9] The rapidity and simplicity of the test make it most useful on an emergency basis for determining pregnancy in patients with pelvic pain. However, this test may miss the diagnosis of very early or abnormal pregnancy.

TEST NAME AND METHOD	SPECIMEN REQUIREMENTS	REFERENCE INTERVAL, CONVENTIONAL [INTERNATIONAL RECOMMENDED UNITS]		CHEMICAL INTERFERENCES AND IN VIVO EFFECTS

Chorionic Gonadotropin—CONT

Quantitative

Immunometric assay

Serum. Store at 2-8° C for up to 24 hr. Otherwise, freeze at −20° C.

Males and nonpregnant females:

mU/mL*   *U/L*

<5.0   × 1   [<5]

See *Chorionic Gonadotropin, β-Subunit.*

Female[5] After Fertilization	After LMP	mU/mL*	U/L
2 wk	4 wk	5-100	5-100
3 wk	5 wk	200-3000	200-3000
4 wk	6 wk	10,000-80,000	10,000-80,000
5-12 wk	7-14 wk	90,000-500,000	90,000-500,000
13-24 wk	15-26 wk	5000-80,000	5000-80,000
26-28 wk	27-40 wk	3000-15,000	3000-15,000
Trophoblastic disease	>100,000	>100,000	

*Values based on the Second International Standard for CG.

LMP, Last menstrual period.

1. Ashwood ER: Clinical chemistry of pregnancy. In Burtis CA, Ashwood ER, editors: *Tietz textbook of clinical chemistry,* ed 3, Philadelphia, 1999, WB Saunders.

2. Braunstein GD, Rasor J, Adler D, et al: Serum human chorionic gonadotropin levels throughout normal pregnancy, *Am J Obstet Gynecol* 126:678-681, 1976.

3. Hussa RO: Human chorionic gonadotropin, a clinical marker. Review of its biosynthesis, *Ligand Rev* 2(suppl 2):1, 1981.

4. Keller PJ: Biochemical methods for monitoring risk pregnancies. In Keller PJ, editor: *Contributions to gynecology and obstetrics, vol 2,* Zurich, 1976, S. Karger.

5. Painter PC, Cope JY, Smith JL: Reference information for the clinical laboratory. In Burtis CA, Ashwood ER, editors: *Tietz textbook of clinical chemistry,* ed 3, Philadelphia, 1999, WB Saunders.

6. Cole L, Kardana A, Birken S: The isomers, subunits and fragments of hCG. In Bellet D, Bidart J-M, editors: *Structure-function relationship of gonadotropins (Serono symposia publications from Raven Press, vol 65),* New York, 1989, Raven Press.

7. Ozturk M, Bellet D, Manil L, et al: Physiological studies of human chorionic gonadotropin (hCG), α-hCG, and β-hCG as measured by specific monoclonal immunoradiometric assays, *Endocrinology* 120:549-558, 1987.

8. Ashwond ER: Clinical chemistry of pregnancy. In Burtis CA, Ashwood ER, editors: *Tietz textbook of clinical chemistry,* ed 2, Philadelphia, 1994, WB Saunders.

9. Norman RJ, Buck RH, Rom L, et al: Blood or urine measurement of human chorionic gonadotropin for detection of ectopic pregnancy? A comparative study of quantitative and qualitative methods in both fluids, *Obstet Gynecol* 71:315-318, 1988.

10. Braunstein GD, Karow W, Gentry W, et al: First-trimester chorionic gonadotropin measurements as an aid in the diagnosis of early pregnancy disorders, *Am J Obstet Gynecol* 131:25-32, 1978.

11. Pittaway D, Reish R, Wnetz A: Doubling times of human chorionic gonadotropin increase in early viable intrauterine pregnancies, *Am J Obstet Gynecol* 152:299-302, 1985.

Sensitivity of the quantitative immunometric assay:
1-2 mU/mL [1-2 U/L]; assay time: 0.2-1 hr

Test is specific for intact hCG and has little or no cross-reactivity with LH. It is used to diagnose very early pregnancy (6-8 days after conception) and estimate gestational age. This sensitive test may also be used to detect ectopic hCG-producing tissue.

Because there is considerable variability in hCG concentration among gravid women, a single value cannot be used to date the gestational stage accurately. Nor can a single determination be used to determine fetal viability. Serial determinations may be helpful when abnormal pregnancy is suspected.[10] In normal intrauterine pregnancy, hCG rapidly increases, with a doubling time of 1.5 days during weeks 2-5. In ectopic pregnancy or spontaneous abortion, hCG concentrations increase more slowly or decrease.[11]

TEST NAME AND METHOD	SPECIMEN REQUIREMENTS	REFERENCE INTERVAL, CONVENTIONAL [INTERNATIONAL RECOMMENDED UNITS]			CHEMICAL INTERFERENCES AND IN VIVO EFFECTS
Chorionic Gonadotropin (hCG) Stimulation Test[1,2] Dose, adult and child, Male: 1500 U* hCG, IM, on days 1, 3, and 5	Two consecutive morning serum specimens for testosterone before hCG administration; on the sixth day, serum for testosterone.	*ng/dL*^{2} *Testosterone* Before hCG stimulation 1 wk-6 mo: 1-8 yr: Puberty Stage 1: 2: 3: 4: 5: After hCG stimulation 1 wk-6 mo: 1-8 yr: Puberty Stage 1: 2: 3: 4: 5:	 4-530 <12 5-60 19-195 82-400 130-550 120-805 180-735 85-370 75-600 140-1030 460-1505 570-1950 980-2200	*nmol/L* × 0.0347 [0.1-18.4] [<0.4] [0.2-2.1] [0.7-6.8] [2.8-13.8] [4.5-19.1] [4.2-27.9] [6.2-25.5] [2.9-12.8] [2.6-20.8] [4.9-35.7] [16.0-52.2] [19.8-67.7] [34.0-76.3]	↑ V Barbiturates ↑ C Cholesterol (CPB method), dihydrotestosterone ↓ V Pyproterone, dexamethasone (women), digoxin (males, chronic administration), ethanol (in male alcoholics), metyrapone (males), spironolactone (males).
Female: 2000-3000 U* hCG, IM, q 24 hr × 2 *Referenced to the World Health Organization's Second International Standard.	Serum before first and 4 hr after last hCG injection for testosterone.	Female: 0- to 5-fold increase^2			

1. Alsever RN, Gotlin RW: *Handbook of endocrine tests in adults and children,* ed 2, Chicago, 1978, Year Book Medical Publishers, Inc.
2. Endocrine Sciences: *Pediatric laboratory services,* Tarzana, CA, 1992, Endocrine Sciences.

DIAGNOSTIC INFORMATION	REMARKS
No response or inadequate response in primary hypogonadism (e.g., anorchia, Leydig cell agenesis, Leydig cell hypoplasia).	The hCG stimulation test is also helpful in the diagnosis of steroid 5α-reductase deficiency.[2]
A positive response is seen in cryptorchidism (undescended testes).	The test is of little value in the diagnosis of women with androgen excess. Suppression tests are more useful.

TEST NAME AND METHOD	SPECIMEN REQUIREMENTS	REFERENCE INTERVAL, CONVENTIONAL [INTERNATIONAL RECOMMENDED UNITS]			CHEMICAL INTERFERENCES AND IN VIVO EFFECTS
Chorionic Gonadotropin, β-Subunit (β-hCG)[1,2] *Immunoassay*	Serum. Stable up to 7 days at 2-8° C. For longer periods, freeze at −20° C or colder. Avoid specimens that are hemolyzed, turbid, or that contain particulate matter.	<2 ng/mL or: <5 ng/mL	× 1.0	[<2 mcg/L] [<5 U/L]	None found.
		Units expressed in mU/mL [U/L] depend on a conversion factor related to an appropriate international reference standard. These conversion factors are method dependent.[5]			
	Amniotic fluid[3]	See *Remarks*.			
ICMA	CSF[4]	<1.5 mU/L	× 1.0	[<1.5 U/L]	

1. Ashwond ER: Clinical chemistry of pregnancy. In Burtis CA, Ashwood ER, editors: *Tietz textbook of clinical chemistry,* ed 2, Philadelphia, 1994, WB Saunders.

2. Cole L, Kardana A, Birken S: The isomers, subunits and fragments of hCG. In Bellet D, Bidart J-M, editors: *Structure-function relationship of gonadotropins (Serono symposia publications from Raven Press, vol 65),* New York, 1989, Raven Press.

3. Tulchinsky D, Ryan KJ, editors: *Maternal-fetal endocrinology,* Philadelphia, 1980, WB Saunders.

4. Mayo Medical Laboratories: *Test catalog,* Rochester, MN, 1994, Mayo Medical Laboratories.

5. Nisselbaum JS, Bosl G, Schwartz MK: Argument in favor of using mass units to calibrate and report concentrations of human choriogonadotropin, *Clin Chem* 32:1998-2000, 1986.

6. Bosl GJ, Geller NL, Cirrincione C, et al: Multivariate analysis of prognostic variables in patients with metastatic testicular cancer, *Cancer Res* 43:3403-3417, 1983.

7. Jones WF, Lewis JL, Lehr M: Monitoring of chemotherapy in gestational trophoblastic neoplasm by radioimmunoassay of the beta-subunit of human chorionic gonadotropin, *Am J Obstet Gynecol* 12:669-673, 1975.

DIAGNOSTIC INFORMATION	REMARKS

↑ Choriocarcinoma, hydatidiform mole, and nontrophoblastic cancers, particularly germ cell tumors of the ovary and testes. In germ cell tumors, both β-hCG and AFP are elevated; the increase and decrease reflect the course of the disease. Detection of increased levels facilitates initial diagnosis, but during recurrence, only one of the two markers may be elevated. Using multivariate analysis, the combination of LDH and β-hCG levels and the total number of metastatic sites predicts whether there will be a response to the therapy. During therapy, a decrease in level is a good prognostic indicator. Increases are also observed in 100% of trophoblastic tumors, 70% of men with nonseminomatous testicular tumors, and 10% with seminomas.[6-10]

The β-subunit of hCG is a sialoglycoprotein that contains 180 amino acids and has an MW of 25,000-30,000. The first 150 amino acids have an 80% homology with luteinizing hormone. hCG is synthesized by trophoblastic cells of the developing blastocysts and later by syncytiotrophoblastic cells. The biological half-life ($t_{1/2}$) is 12-36 hr.

Serial determinations in neoplasms that produce hCG indicate both a response to treatment by surgery or chemotherapy and recurrences. In some tumors variable amounts of free α- or β-subunits of the hormone have been identified.[11] Increased concentration of hCG is also found in patients without tumors but with a variety of benign diseases with enhanced cellular proliferation. The detection limit for serum is 1-3 mU/mL [1-3 U/L].

Values up to 50 mU/mL [50 U/L] may occur in pregnant women during the first week following conception. Maximum values (up to 290,000 mU/mL [290,000 U/L]) are reached by the second or third month, and then there is a gradual decrease to values as low as 4000 mU/mL [4000 U/L].

Most assays for β-hCG are designed to measure the intact hCG molecule and the free β-hCG molecule. When hCG is assayed as a tumor marker, a method measuring total β-subunits (free and intact) must be used.

S ↓ Threatened abortion, ectopic pregnancy

AF ↑ Severe erythroblastosis fetalis (some reports)

CSF ↑ Spinal fluid dysgerminomas and meningeal carcinomatosis

The pattern of change in hCG levels in amniotic fluid mimics that observed in maternal serum. The mean concentration of hCG in the maternal peripheral circulation at term is 40-100 times higher than in the amniotic fluid, which in turn is at least 10-fold greater than that measured in umbilical blood.

8. Mann K, Lamerz R, Hellmann T, et al: Use of human chorionic gonadotropin and alpha fetoprotein radioimmunoassays: Specificity and apparent half-life after delivery in patients with germ cell tumors, *Oncodev Biol Med* 1:301-311, 1980.

9. Seckl MJ, Rustin GJS, Bagshawe KD: Frequency of serum tumor marker monitoring in patients with non-seminomatous germ cell tumors, *Br J Cancer* 61:916-918, 1990.

10. Toner GC, Geller NL, Tan C, et al: Serum tumor marker half-life during chemotherapy allows early prediction of complete response and survival in nonseminomatous germ cell tumors, *Cancer Res* 50:5904-5910, 1990.

11. Schwarz S, Berger P, Wick G: Epitope-selective, monoclonal-antibody-based immunoradiometric assay of predictable specificity for differential measurement of choriogonadotropin and its subunits, *Clin Chem* 31:1322-1328, 1985.

TEST NAME AND METHOD	SPECIMEN REQUIREMENTS	REFERENCE INTERVAL, CONVENTIONAL [INTERNATIONAL RECOMMENDED UNITS]			CHEMICAL INTERFERENCES AND IN VIVO EFFECTS
Chromium (Cr)[1,2] *AAS, NAA*	Whole blood.[3] Collect in pretested, metal-free container.	*mcg/L* 0.7-28.0	× 19.2	*nmol/L* [13.4-538]	U ↑ V EDTA
	Serum.[4,5] Collect in pretested, metal-free container.	<0.05-0.5		[1-10]	
	Erythrocytes[6]	20-36		[384-692]	
	Urine, 24 hr.[3,7] Collect in acid-washed, metal-free container; use no preservatives.	0.1-2.0		[1.9-38.4]	
	Hair.[3] Cut specimens close to scalp in 2- to 5-cm lengths; wash in acetone solution and digest in 70% ultrapure nitric acid.	*mcg/g dry wt.* 0.10-4.10	× 19.2	*nmol/g dry wt.* [1.9-78.7]	
ICP-MS	Serum.[8] Collect in pretested, metal-free container.	*mcg/L* 0.5-2.1	× 19.2	*nmol/L* [9.6-40.3]	
	Urine.[8] Collect in acid-washed, metal-free container. Refrigerate during and following collection.	0.0-5.0 mcg/L 0.0-6.0 mcg/day		[0.0-96 nmol/L] [0.0-115.2 nmol/day]	

1. Henry JB, editor: *Clinical diagnosis and management by laboratory methods,* ed 18, Philadelphia, 1991, WB Saunders.

2. Milne DB: Trace elements. In Burtis CA, Ashwood ER, editors: *Tietz textbook of clinical chemistry,* ed 2, Philadelphia, 1994, WB Saunders.

3. Iyengar GV, Woittiez J: Trace elements in human clinical specimens: evaluation of literature data to identify telerence values, *Clin Chem* 34:474-481, 1988.

4. Bro S, Jorgensen PJ, Christensen JM, et al: Concentration of nickel and chromium in serum: influence of blood sampling technique, *J Trace Elem Electrolytes Health Dis* 2:31-35, 1988.

5. Veillon C, Patterson KY, Bryden NA: Determination of chromium in human serum by electrothermal atomic absorption spectrometry, *Anal Chim Acta* 164:67-76, 1984.

6. Johnson HL, Sauberlich HE: Trace element analysis in biological samples. In Prasad AS, editor: *Clinical, biochemical, and nutritional aspects of trace elements,* New York, 1982, Alan R. Liss, Inc.

7. Veillon C, Patterson KY, Bryden NA: Chromium in urine as measured by atomic absorption spectrometry, *Clin Chem* 28:2309-2311, 1982.

8. Associated Regional & University Pathologists, Inc. web site (www.aruplab.com). Available at: Online User's Guide: http://www.aruplab.com/testing/user_guide.jsp. Last accessed 9/2004.

DIAGNOSTIC INFORMATION	**REMARKS**

↓ Pregnancy, diabetic children

Toxicity is mostly from occupational exposure in electroplating, welding, steelmaking, leather tanning, photography, dyeing, and chemical manufacture operations. Exposure of the skin results in dermatitis and ulceration. Ingestion results in vertigo, abdominal pain, vomiting, anuria, convulsions, shock, or coma.

Chromium as Cr^{3+} is a required cofactor in the initiation of the action of insulin in peripheral tissues (GTF; glucose tolerance factor). Reduced Cr intake can be an aggravating factor in the disturbed glucose tolerance of marasmic infants, maturity-onset diabetic patients, and some elderly persons. Metallic chromium is not allergenic or toxic, but Cr^{3+} and Cr^{6+} are toxic in excess, although carcinogenic effects are thought to be due to Cr^{6+}. Cr^{6+} is more toxic than Cr^{3+}.

Glucose intolerance and neuropathy due to chromium deficiency have been documented in patients receiving Cr-deficient IV solutions for long periods.

Hair ↓ Diabetes (0.07 ± 0.05 mcg/g; 1.3 ± 1.0 nmol/g)

TEST NAME AND METHOD	SPECIMEN REQUIREMENTS	REFERENCE INTERVAL, CONVENTIONAL [INTERNATIONAL RECOMMENDED UNITS]			CHEMICAL INTERFERENCES AND IN VIVO EFFECTS
Chromogranin A (CgA)[1-3] *Immunoassay (ELISA, RIA)*	Serum. Stable up to 1 wk at 2-8° C. For longer periods, store frozen at −20° C or colder.[4] *Specimen requirements are assay specific.*	*ng/mL*[4] M: 0-76 F: 0-51 *ELISA, reference ranges are assay specific.*	× 1.0	*mcg/L* 0-76 0-51	S ↑ V proton pump inhibitors Icteric and lipemic samples are unacceptable.

1. Nobels FRE, Kwekkeboom DJ, Bouillon R, et al: Chromogranin A: its clinical value as a marker of neuroendocrine tumours, *Eur J Clin Invest* 28:431-440, 1998.

2. Eriksson B, Öberg K, Stridsberg M: Tumor markers in neuroendocrine tumors, *Digestion* 62(suppl 1):33-38, 2000.

3. Öberg K, Stridsberg M: Neuroendocrine tumors. In Diamandis EP, Fritsche HA, Lilja H, editors: *Tumor markers. Physiology, pathobiology, technology, and clinical applications,* Washington, DC, 2002, AACC Press.

4. Chromogranin A. ARUP user's guide. Available at: www.aruplab.com. Last accessed 1/31/05.

5. Stridsberg M, Eriksson B, Öberg K, et al: A comparison between three commercial kits for chromogranin A measurements, *J Endocrinol* 177:337-341, 2003.

Chymotrypsin (EC 3.4.21.1)[1] *RIA*[2,3]	Serum, plasma (EDTA and polybrene). Store at 4° C or −20° C.	~10 mcg/L[3] 14.7-77.5 mcg/L (x̄: 37.5)	↑ Oral enzyme preparations ↓ C Aromatic hydrocarbons, diethyl ether organophosphorus compounds, heavy metal ions

DIAGNOSTIC INFORMATION	REMARKS

↑ Carcinoid tumors, pheochromocytomas, neuroblastomas, small cell lung cancers, hyperparathyroid adenomas, pituitary tumors, prostate cancers, pancreatic islet tumors including multiple endocrine neoplasia (MEN) I and II syndromes, pancreatic islet cell syndromes including insulinomas, glucagonomas, somatostatinomas, Zollinger-Ellison syndrome, Verner-Morrison syndrome, pancreatic polypeptide-producing tumors, and nonfunctioning neuroendocrine tumors. Concentrations correlate with tumor burden.

Nontumor-associated increases include renal insufficiency, liver disease, atrophic gastritis, inflammatory bowel disease, and stress.[2,3]

Chromogranin A (CgA) is a 48-kDa acidic glycoprotein that is part of a family of proteins found in neuroendocrine cells and in neuronal cells in the central and peripheral nervous system, thus explaining their role in neuroendocrine tumors. On stimulation, CgA, in addition to peptide hormones and neuropeptides, is released from the secretory granules of neuroendocrine cells. CgA can be processed by neuroendocrine cells into a number of bioactive peptides that may differ by cell type. N-terminal peptides have vasodilatory functions, whereas mid- and C-terminal peptides have autocrine or paracrine inhibitory functions.

CgA is used as an aid in the diagnosis and monitoring of carcinoid tumors, pheochromocytoma, neuroblastoma, endocrine pancreatic tumors, and small cell lung cancers. May be useful in nonfunctioning neuroendocrine tumors that do not secrete other hormones.[1-3]

Several non–FDA-approved commercial assays for CgA are available that are primarily in use outside the United States. These assays have different formats (ELISA, RIA), types of antibodies, standards, and units. Assays measure different forms of the molecule and therefore give different results and differ in clinical performance.[3,5]

S ↑ Acute pancreatitis, chronic renal failure can also be found with gastric or pancreatic cancer[10] and junctional epidermlysis bullosa.[11]

S ↓ Chronic pancreatitis, late cystic fibrosis

Fecal chymotrypsin tests provide a noninvasive method to evaluate for suspected pancreatic exocrine insufficiency. They can also be used to monitor adequacy of treatment. Evidence suggests that assays of fecal elastase-1 concentrations may be more sensitive for the diagnosis of moderate and severe disease.[9] Direct, invasive functional assays like the pancreozymin-secretin test are frequently considered the "gold standard" and can be used to provide definitive diagnosis.[9]

TEST NAME AND METHOD	SPECIMEN REQUIREMENTS	REFERENCE INTERVAL, CONVENTIONAL [INTERNATIONAL RECOMMENDED UNITS]		CHEMICAL INTERFERENCES AND IN VIVO EFFECTS

Chymotrypsin—CONT

Titrimetric (N-acetyl- L-tyrosine ethyl ester), pH 7.8, 25° C[4]	Stool, diluted ×10 with NaCl, 0.15 mol/L, homogenized and filtered; stable 1 wk at room temperature.	*mcg/kg stool* 120-1265 (x̄: 290) 74-1200[8] (x̄: 340)	× 1.0	*mcg/g stool* [120-1265] [x̄: 290] [74-1200] [x̄: 340]	↓ Diarrhea, lactose malabsorption, irritable bowel syndrome[9]

Photometric, 405 nm, p-nitro- anilide, 25° C[5]	100 mg stool homogenized in buffered lauryl trimethyl ammonium chloride and centrifuged. Perform assay on supernatant.	*U/g stool* Premature: 16.5 ± 10 (SD) Infant: 19 ± 12	
25° C[6]		*U/g stool* 0-3 mo: 32 ± 6 (SD) 3-6 mo: 35 ± 9 6-12 mo: 36 ± 16 1-5 yr: 34 ± 8 5-10 yr: 32 ± 5	
37° C[7]		1-60 yr: >>11.5	

1. Tietz NW, editor: *Textbook of clinical chemistry,* Philadelphia, 1999, WB Saunders.

2. Iwaki K, Ogawa M, Tanaka S, et al: Radioimmunoassay for human pancreatic chymotrypsin and measurement of serum immunoreactive chymotrypsin contents in various diseases, *Res Commun Chem Pathol Pharmacol* 40:489-496, 1983.

3. Geokas MC, Largman C, Brodrick JW, et al: Immunoreactive forms of human pancreatic chymotrypsin in normal plasma, *J Biol Chem* 254:2775-2781, 1979.

4. Ammann RW, Tagwecher E, Kashiwagi H, et al: Diagnostic value of fecal chymotrypsin and trypsin assessment for the detection of pancreatic disease, *Am J Diag Dis* 13:123-146, 1968.

5. Dockter G, Hoppe-Seyler F, Appel W, et al: Determination of chymotrypsin in stool by a new photometric method, *Clin Biochem* 19:329-332, 1986.

6. de Pedro C, Codoceo R, Vazquez P, et al: Fecal chymotrypsin levels in children with pancreatic insufficiency, *Clin Biochem* 19:338-340, 1986.

7. Melzi d'Eril GV, Pavesi F, Lotzniker M, et al: Fecal chymotrypsin: a new colorimetric test, *J Lab Med* 13:17-20, 1986.

8. Haverback BJ, Dyce BJ, Gutentag PJ, et al: Measurement of trysin and chymotrypsin in stool, *Gastroenterology* 44:588-597, 1963.

9. Luth S, Teyssen S, Forssmann K, et al: Fecal elastase-1 determination: "gold standard" of indirect pancreatic test? *Scand J Gastroenterol* 36:1092-1099, 2001.

10. Heng MC, Barrascout CE, Rasmus W, et al: Elevated serum chymotrypsin levels in a patient with junctional epidermolysis bullosa. Normalization after UVB therapy with good clinical response, *Int J Dermatol* 26:385-388, 1987.

11. Jodl J, Korufalt R, Svenningsen NW, et al: Chymotryptic activity in stool of low-birth weight infants in the first week of life, *Acta Paediatr Scand* 64:619-623, 1975.

DIAGNOSTIC INFORMATION	REMARKS

F ↓ Chronic pancreatitis, cystic fibrosis, end-stage renal disease, Schwachman's syndrome, small-for-gestational age neonates.[11]

TEST NAME AND METHOD	SPECIMEN REQUIREMENTS	REFERENCE INTERVAL, CONVENTIONAL [INTERNATIONAL RECOMMENDED UNITS]			CHEMICAL INTERFERENCES AND IN VIVO EFFECTS
Circulating Immune Complexes *C1q-binding assays* *Liquid-phase RIA*[1]	Serum. Stable for 1 mo at −20° C.	<75 U/mL	× 1.0	[<75 kAU*/L]	↓ Anti-C1q antibodies, IV administration of g-emitting radioisotope
Solid-phase EIA[2,3]		<20 mcg equivalent/mL			↓ Anti-C1q antibodies
Raji cell assay[4]		<38 mcg aggregated human γ-globulin equivalent/mL			↓ Antilymphocyte antibodies
		AU, Arbitrary unit.			

1. Zubler RH, Lange G, Lambert PH, et al: Detection of immune complexes in unheated sera by a modified ^{125}I-C1q binding test. Effect of heating on the binding of C1q by immune complexes and application of the test to systemic lupus erythematosus, *J Immunol* 116:232-235, 1976.
2. Agnello V, Mitamura T: Detection of immune complexes in systemic lupus erythematosus with the C11 solid phase assay: Correlation with nDNA antibodies and hypocomplementemia, *Clin Immunol Immunopathol* 42:338-343, 1987.

TEST NAME AND METHOD	SPECIMEN REQUIREMENTS	REFERENCE INTERVAL, CONVENTIONAL [INTERNATIONAL RECOMMENDED UNITS]			CHEMICAL INTERFERENCES AND IN VIVO EFFECTS
Citrate, Citric Acid *Enzymatic*[1-2]	Serum, plasma. Stable in whole blood for 90 min at room temperature.	*mg/dL* 1.5-3.2	× 0.0526	*mmol/L* [0.08-0.17][2]	↓ V High protein diet, chronic metabolic acidosis induced by chronic diarrhea, renal tubular acidosis, carbonic andydrase inhibitors, ureteral diversion
Enzymatic,[2] *capillary electrophoresis*[3]	Urine, 24 hr. Add 10 g of boric acid or 10 mL of 6N HCl at start of collection or adjust pH to ≤2.	Adult M: 0.6-4.8 mmol/24 hr[4] Adult F: 1.3-6.0 mmol/24 hr[4]			

Random urine[5]:

	mg/dL		*mmol/L*
M:			
<40 yr	0.94-86.4	× 0.0526	[0.049-4.54]
≥40 yr	0.7-113		[0.037-5.94]
F:			
<40 yr	4.0-193		[0.021-10.2]
≥40 yr	1.0-156		[0.053-8.20]

	mg/g *creatinine*		*mmol/g* *creatinine*
M:	3.0-72.2	× 0.00526	[0.016-0.38]
F:	5.4-95.5		[0.028-0.50]

DIAGNOSTIC INFORMATION	REMARKS
Each of the C1q-binding assays detects antigen-antibody complexes that activate complement by the classical pathway.	Anti-C1q antibodies occur in some patients with SLE. The test has clinical utility in studying immune complex diseases.
Solid-phase EIA detects activating complexes only in the classical pathway.	
Raji cell assay also detects activating complexes in the alternative pathway.	Antilymphocyte antibodies occur in many patients with SLE.

3. Hay FC, Nineham LJ, Roitt IM: Routine assay for the detection of immune complexes of known immunoglobulin class using solid phase C1q, *Clin Exp Immunol* 24:396-400, 1976.
4. Cook L, Agnello V: Detection of immune complexes. In Rose NR, Friedman H, Fahey JL, editors: *Manual of clinical immunology,* Washington, DC, 1992, American Society for Microbiology.

↓ In kidney stone formers	Citrate in urine is a principal inhibitor of kidney stone formation. Citrate combines with calcium in the tubular lumen to form a soluble complex (thereby reducing the concentration of free calcium available to combine with oxalate) and also appears to inhibit the process of crystal agglomeration, in which individual calcium oxalate crystals combine to form a stone. Hypocitraturia is considered a risk factor for kidney stone formation and occurs in isolation in stone formers or in association with hypercalciuria, hyperoxaluria, or hyperuricosuria.[6]

TEST NAME* AND METHOD	SPECIMEN REQUIREMENTS	REFERENCE INTERVAL, CONVENTIONAL [INTERNATIONAL RECOMMENDED UNITS]		CHEMICAL INTERFERENCES AND IN VIVO EFFECTS

Citrate, Citric Acid—CONT

1. McWhinney BC, Cowley DM, Chalmers AH: An automated method for measuring plasma citrate without protein precipitation, *Clin Chem* 31:1578-1579, 1985.

2. Tompkins D, Toffaletti J: Enzymic determination of citrate in serum and urine, with use of the Worthington "ultrafree" device, *Clin Chem* 28:192-195, 1982.

3. Holmes RP: Measurement of urinary oxalate and citrate by capillary electrophoresis and indirect ultraviolet absorbance, *Clin Chem* 41:1297-1301, 1995.

Classical Pathway Components *C1* *Functional hemolytic assay*[1]	Serum. Collect and store at $-70°$ C as for CH_{50}.	U/mL 70,000-200,000 $C1H_{50}$ $\times$ 0.001	MU/L [70-200]	$\downarrow$ C EDTA, EGTA, or other calcium chelators

C1q *RID*[1,2]		mg/dL Newborn[2]: 9-20 (x = 12.4) $\times$ 10 Maternal: 9-24.8 (x = 16.4) Adult: 14.9-22.1 (x = 18.5) Adult[1]: 83-125 mcg/mL $\times$ 1000 [83-125]	mg/L [90-200] [90-248] [149-221]	None found.

C1q				

---

4. Samuell CT, Kasidas GP: Biochemical investigation in renal stone formers, *Ann Clin Biochem* 32:112-122, 1995.

5. Bond LW, Garber C, Ottinger W, et al: Reference intervals for common analytes in random urine specimens, *Clin Chem* 55: submitted, 2005.

6. Rose BD, Curhan G: *Risk factors for idiopathic calcium stones, UpToDate, v. 13.3,* Available at: www.utdol.com. Accessed Feb 13, 2006.

S ↓ *Congenital:* Inherited deficiency of C1q, C1r, or C1s

Acquired: Reflects complement consumption resulting from activation by immune complexes, cryoglobulinemia, or other autoimmune process, severe malnutrition, and lymphopenia. C1 function is decreased in serum from patients with acquired but not hereditary angioedema. Hypocomplementemic urticarial vasculitis (HUVS) and SLE may be associated with autoantibodies to the collagen-like region of C1q.[10]

S ↑ *Acquired:* Acute phase response

The complement system, as a component of the innate immune response, comprises >30 individual proteins located in plasma or on cellular surfaces.[19]

The C1 molecular complex consists of one C1q subunit, two C1r subunits, and two C1s subunits held together by Ca^{2+} ions. Most of the circulating C1 is produced by intestinal epithelial cells, although mononuclear phagocytes and fibroblasts also make active C1.[4] The functional assay measures the hemolytic activity of intact C1. The $C1H_{50}$ is defined as the reciprocal of the dilution that lyses 50% of the cells.

S ↓ *Congenital:* Inherited deficiency of C1q, hypogammaglobulinemia

Acquired: Complement consumption resulting from immune complexes, autoimmune processes, cryoglobulinemia, HUVS, and lymphopenia

S ↑ *Acquired:* Increased C1q levels have been associated with kala-azar (*Leishmania donovani* infection).[11]

C1q, the recognition unit for the classical pathway, binds to immunoglobulin in immune complexes ($IgM>IgG_3>$- $IgG_1>IgG_2$, but not IgA, IgE, or IgG_4). C1q is therefore used in tests for the presence of immune complexes. Nonimmunological activators of C1q include DNA, IgG bound to staphylococcal protein A, complexes of C-reactive protein with polysaccharide, membranes of subcellular organelles (mitochondria), some enveloped viruses, monosodium urate crystals (in gout), and lipid A of bacterial lipopolysaccharide.[20-24]

S ↓ *Congenital:* Inherited deficiency of C1q, linked to immune complex disease with and without recurrent infections

Acquired: C1q is often low in patients with hypogammaglobulinemia; the decrease is thought to be caused by hypercatabolism of C1q rather than by primary deficiency. Other causes for low C1q are complement consumption resulting from formation of immune complexes, cryoglobulinemia or other autoimmune processes, hypocomplementemic urticarial vasculitis syndrome (HUVS), and lymphopenia.

The C1q molecule is made up of 18 polypeptide chains: six A chains (MW 26,500 each), six B chains (MW 26,500 each), and six C chains (MW 24,000 each), arranged into six subunits of three chains each (1A:1B:1C).[25] The N-terminal ends have collagen-like amino acid sequences that form a single "stalk," whereas the C-terminal ends are globular and spread out from each other in a configuration that resembles a bouquet of flowers. The binding sites for immunoglobulin Fc are in these globular heads, whereas the collagen-like tail portion reacts with C1q receptors.

C1q is produced by epithelial cells, primarily in the intestine but also in the lung and other tissues.[26] The $t_{1/2}$ of C1q in the circulation is ~40 hr, with a fractional catabolic rate of 2.7-2.8% of the plasma pool per hour and a synthesis rate of 140-190 mg/kg body wt./hr. Approximately 50-75% of the C1q is in the intravascular space.[27]

TEST NAME AND METHOD	SPECIMEN REQUIREMENTS	REFERENCE INTERVAL, CONVENTIONAL [INTERNATIONAL RECOMMENDED UNITS]		CHEMICAL INTERFERENCES AND IN VIVO EFFECTS

Classical Pathway Components—CONT

Functional *hemolytic assay*[1]		*U/mL* 2500-9500 $C1qH_{50}$[1] $\times 0.001$	*MU/L* [2.5-9.5]	
Turbidimetric[3]		34-63[3]	[0.034-0.63]	
C1r *RID*[1]	Serum; plasma (EDTA, EGTA, citrate [ACD]). Collect and store at $-70°$ C as for CH_{50}.	0.025-0.10 mg/mL[4] $\times 1.0$ Mean serum concentration Adults: 34 mcg/mL[5] $\times 1.0$ 48 mcg/mL[6]	[0.025-0.10 g/L] [34 mg/L] [48 mg/L]	None found.
C1s *(C1-esterase)* *RID*[1]	Serum; plasma (EDTA, heparin, EGTA, cit-rate). Collect and store at $-70°$ C as for CH_{50}.	0.05-0.10 mg/mL[7] $\times 1.0$ Mean serum concentration Adults: 31 mcg/mL[4] $\times 1.0$ 34 mcg/mL[5]	[0.05-0.10 g/L] [31 mg/L] [34 mg/L]	None found.
C2 *RID*[1]		1.6-3.6 mg/dL[7] $\times 10$ Mean serum concentration Adults: 25 mcg/mL[5] $\times 1.0$ 20 mcg/mL[8]	[16-36 mg/L] [25 mg/L] [20 mg/L]	

DIAGNOSTIC INFORMATION	REMARKS
	This test measures the function of C1q in a hemolytic assay using sensitized sheep erythrocytes (EA), serial dilutions of the test serum or plasma, and serum depleted by affinity chromatography of C1q (but not other complement components). C1q function is lost rapidly when serum is heated $>37°$ C and is irreversibly destroyed by heating at $56°$ C for 30 min. Serum samples that have not been collected or stored properly may have low C1q function.
S ↓ *Congenital:* C1r deficiency is associated with SLE-like disease, renal disease, recurrent infections, and rheumatoid arthritis. C1r-deficient patients may also have low C1s. *Acquired:* Immune complex diseases, autoimmune processes, bacterial and viral infections, and severe trauma and burns. Activation of the classical pathway leads to rapid binding of C1INH to the C1r and C1s enzymes and clearance of C1r-C1INH and C1s-C1INH complexes.	Under physiological conditions, C1r forms dimers (C1r$_2$) that associate with C1q and dimers of C1s to form C1qr$_2$s$_2$. C1r is a serine protease that remains inactive in the C1qr2s2 complex but is converted to an active enzyme C1r when C1q binds to an immune complex or other activator. The substrates of C1r are other C1r molecules and C1s. When cleaved by C1r, C1s also becomes an active serine esterase. C1r and C1s share a high degree of homology and presumably evolve from gene duplication. C1r and C1s are inactivated in serum by C1-esterase inhibitor (C1-INH), to which they covalently bind, and the C1r-C1INH and C1s-C1INH complexes are subsequently removed from the circulation. Serum C1s is synthesized by epithelial cells of the intestine and bladder and to some extent by fibroblasts, monocytes, and macrophages in other tissues.[28] The binding of C1INH to C1r masks the antigenic site of C1r recognized by many antisera used for the detection and quantitation of C1r, thus making the C1r "invisible" to detection by immunochemical means.[29]
S ↓ *Congenital:* C1s deficiency (rare), associated with SLE-like disease, renal disease, recurrent infections, and rheumatoid arthritis. C1s deficiency is usually linked to C1r deficiency. *Acquired:* Immune complex diseases, autoimmune processes, bacterial and viral infections, and severe trauma and burns. Activation of the classical pathway leads to rapid binding of C1INH to the C1r and C1s enzymes and clearance of C1r-C1INH and C1s-C1INH complexes.	In serum, C1s forms calcium-dependent dimers that associate with C1r dimers and C1q to form macromolecular C1qr2s2. C1s is a serine esterase that remains inactive in the C1qrs complex but is converted to its active form when cleaved by C1r. The substrates of C1s are C4 and C2, which combine to form the classical pathway C3 convertase (C4b2a). C1s is inactivated by C1-esterase inhibitor (C1INH), leading to C1s-C1INH complexes that are cleared from the circulation. Serum C1s is synthesized by epithelial cells of the intestine and bladder and to some extent by fibroblasts, monocytes, and macrophages in other tissues.[28]
S ↓ *Congenital:* C2 deficiency is the most common complement deficiency in Caucasian populations (the frequency of the C2 null gene is 0.01, incidence of deficiency is 1 in 10,000). Type I C2 deficiency is a defect in synthesis of C2 protein, and little or no C2 is detectable in the circulation. Type II C2 defi-	C2 is a proenzyme that becomes active after cleavage by C1s. The larger fragment (C2a) combines with C4b to form the enzyme site of C3 and C5 convertases, and the smaller fragment (C2b) may be further cleaved to produce the kinin-like activity in angioedema patients.[30]

TEST NAME AND METHOD	SPECIMEN REQUIREMENTS	REFERENCE INTERVAL, CONVENTIONAL [INTERNATIONAL RECOMMENDED UNITS]			CHEMICAL INTERFERENCES AND IN VIVO EFFECTS

Classical Pathway Components—CONT

		U/mL		MU/L	
Functional hemolytic assay[1]		15,350-46,240 C2H$_{50}$[1]	× 0.001	[15.4-46.2]	

		mg/dL		mg/L	
C4					↑ V Cimetidine (in ARC
	Cord serum:	13.7-44.9[2]	× 10	[137-449]	patients), cyclophos-
Turbidimetric,		24.0-37.2[8]		[240-372]	phamide (in SLE pa-
Nephelometric,		6.6-23[9]		[66-230]	tients), and danazol
RID[1]	1 mo:	27.5-47.3[8]		[275-473]	
	6 mo:	30.5-58.7[8]		[305-587]	
	Adults:	28.7-67.5[2]		[287-675]	
		37.4-64.4[8]		[374-644]	
		15-45[9]		[150-450]	

DIAGNOSTIC INFORMATION   **REMARKS**

ciency is a defect in C2 protein secretion and is associated with low levels of protein in the circulation.[11] Heterozygous individuals have half-normal levels. C2-deficient patients may be asymptomatic or may present with SLE-like disease, renal disease, rheumatoid arthritis, and recurrent infections (usually with *Streptococcus pneumoniae, Staphylococcus pneumoniae,* and *Haemophilus influenzae*).[12]

Acquired: Hereditary and acquired angioedema patients have low C2 and low C4 because of uncontrolled expression of C1 activity. C2 is also decreased in patients with immune complex diseases, bacteremia, viremia, autoimmune disorders, severe trauma, burns, and severe malnutrition.

S ↑ *Congenital:* Patients with deficiencies of C1q, C1r, or C1s often have elevated C2, C4, and C1INH levels and functions.[13]

Acquired: Acute phase response

C2 is synthesized by hepatocytes and by monocytes and macrophages in blood and other tissues.[28] The genes for C2 are linked to those of factor B and C4 in the HLA domain on chromosome 6, and there are multiple alleles giving rise to different C2 isotypes in the population. The most common of these, C2 C, is found in ~96% of the population.[31]

The hemolytic activity of C2 is extremely heat sensitive and can be destroyed by heating serum at 50° C for 30 min. Loss of C2 activity can occur on improper handling or storage of the specimen. The hemolytic assay for C2 function uses sensitized sheep erythrocytes precoated with C1 and C4. The $C2H_{50}$ is the reciprocal of the dilution of test material that lyses 50% of the cells in 1 mL of the assay mixture.

S ↑ *Congenital:* Presence of more than four C4 alleles. Deficiency of C1q, C1r, or C1s is associated with increases in C2, C4, and C1 INH.

Acquired: Acute phase reaction, certain malignancies

S ↓ *Congenital:* Total C4 deficiency is rare, but partial C4 deficiency is common (see *Remarks*). Partial and complete C4 deficiency and certain C4 haplotypes have been associated with immune complex diseases, SLE, autoimmune thyroiditis, and juvenile dermatomyositis.[14-16] Onset of SLE in C-deficient patients is often early (preteens) and tends to be somewhat less severe than that in patients with normal complement; ANA titers are negative in these patients. Infections associated with C4 deficiency include bacterial or viral meningitis, *Streptococcus* and *Staphylococcus* sepsis, and pneumonia.

C4 is a glycoprotein, MW 205,000, that participates in the classical pathway of activation. Precursor C4 is synthesized as a single polypeptide chain that is posttranslationally cleaved into three disulfide-linked chains (a, b, and g). C4 is produced primarily by hepatocytes but can also be made by other cell types (monocytes, fibroblasts, macrophages). Complement activation produces several C4 split products that have different biological activities: C4a is a weak anaphylatoxin, C4b is part of the enzyme that cleaves C3, C4b, iC4b, and C4d are opsonins that bind to CR1, CR3, and CR2 receptors, respectively. C4c is an inactive product found in the fluid phase.

The fragments of C4, C4a, and C4d can be measured by RIA, rocket electrophoresis, or ELISA techniques. These fragments provide very sensitive measures of in vivo complement activation. Activation of as little as 1% of the classical pathway can be detected by comparing the ratio of C4a or C4d with C4 in the plasma. By measuring fragments of factor B, C3, and C5, one can determine which pathway has been activated and to what extent. Previous objections to using complement mea-

TEST NAME AND METHOD	SPECIMEN REQUIREMENTS	REFERENCE INTERVAL, CONVENTIONAL [INTERNATIONAL RECOMMENDED UNITS]			CHEMICAL INTERFERENCES AND IN VIVO EFFECTS
Classical Pathway Components—CONT					
C4					
Functional hemolytic assay		*kU/mL* 400-43,000 C4H$_{50}$	× 1.0	*MU/L* [400-43,000]	None found.
Alternative Pathway Components **Factor D** *RIA,*[1] *ELISA*[2]	Serum; plasma (EDTA, EGTA, citrate). Collect and store at −70° C as for CH$_{50}$.	1-5 mcg/mL[6]	× 1.0	[1-5 mg/L]	None found.

DIAGNOSTIC INFORMATION	REMARKS

surements to follow a patient's disease progress were related only to C4 and C3 levels, which are relatively insensitive because most patients with inflammation also mount an acute-phase response that can mask complement consumption. Use of complement split-product measurements should make it much easier and more accurate to monitor trends and predict flares in a patient's disease.

Acquired: Hereditary and acquired angioedema, complement activation resulting from immune complex diseases, decreased synthesis (liver disease), increased consumption in glomerulonephritis, SLE, rheumatoid arthritis, respiratory distress syndrome, autoimmune hemolytic anemia, cryoglobulinemia, and sepsis.

There are two separate genes for C4: C4A and C4B. They are class III MHC genes located near the genes for C2, factor B, and 21-hydroxylase on the short arm of chromosome 6. There are many different alleles of C4A and C4B, which were identified previously as C4F (fast) and C4S (slow) by their electrophoretic mobility and as the Chido (C4B) and Rodgers (C4A) blood group antigens.[32] Null alleles that produce no protein are common. Sixty-nine to 76% of Caucasians express all four alleles, 13-24,5% express three alleles, and ~10% express only two alleles. Expression of only one or no alleles is rare.

C4 has an internal thiolester group that becomes exposed when the molecule undergoes cleavage during complement activation. This cleavage allows formation of bonds with nearby nucleophile groups where C4A preferentially binds to amino groups and C4B preferentially binds to carboxyl groups. The wide range of titers reflects the variation of C4A and C4b haplotypes in the population. The distribution of titers among the population tends to be triphasic, with C4B having higher titers than C4A. C4A is a more efficient opsonin for immune complexes, which may be why deficiency of C4A is linked with SLE and other diseases in which immune complexes play a role. C4 function is sensitive to treatment by chaotropic agents, hydrazine, hydroxylamine, ionic detergents (SDS), and denaturants such as urea and guanidine HCl.

S ↓ *Congenital:* Factor D deficiency is very rare. AH_{50} is abnormal, but CH_{50} is normal. Patients often have infections resulting from *N. meningitidis, H. influenzae, Proteus* sp., and *Pseudomonas* sp.

S ↑ *Acquired:* End-stage kidney disease with loss of filtration leads to increased factor D levels in plasma, in correlation with serum creatinine levels.[17] SLE patients with renal disease, polycystic kidney disease, and rheumatoid arthritis with secondary amyloidosis.[18]

Factor D (FD) is an MW 25,000 serine esterase with specificity for factor B when the latter is bound to C3b or C3b-like C3. It is the only complement enzyme that circulates in its active state. It is essential for triggering the alternative pathway of activation and is the rate-limiting factor in this pathway. FD is identical to the enzyme adipsin, produced in adipocytes, and involved in lipid metabolism.[33] Its primary site of synthesis in vivo is not known, but it is produced in culture by monocytes and macrophages and by HepG2 cells.[34]

TEST NAME AND METHOD	SPECIMEN REQUIREMENTS	REFERENCE INTERVAL, CONVENTIONAL [INTERNATIONAL RECOMMENDED UNITS]	CHEMICAL INTERFERENCES AND IN VIVO EFFECTS

Classical Pathway Components—CONT

1. Fudenberg HH, Sites DP, Caldwell JJ, et al: *Basic and clinical immunology,* ed 3, Los Altos, CA, 1980, Lange Medical Publications.

2. Kohler PF: Human complement system. In Samter M, editors: *Immunological diseases,* ed 3, Boston, 1978, Little, Brown and Co.

3. Mayo Medical Laboratories: *Test catalog,* Minneapolis, MN, 2004, Mayo Medical Laboratories.

4. Behring Diagnostics, Inc.: *Table of blood plasma proteins,* Somerville, NJ, 1992, Behring Diagnostics, Inc.

5. Ziccardi RJ, Cooper NR: The subunit composition and sedimentation properties of human C1, *J Immunol* 118:2047-2052, 1977.

6. Lachmann PJ, Peters DK: Complement. In Lachmann PJ, Peters DK, editors: *Clinical aspects of immunology,* vol 1, ed 4, Oxford, UK, 1982, Blackwell Scientific Publications.

7. SmthKline Beecham: *Clinical laboratories: directory of services,* Van Nuys, CA, 1992, SmithKline Beecham.

8. Davis CA, Vallota EH, Forristal J: Serum complement levels in infancy: age related changes, *Pediatr Res* 13:1042-1046, 1979.

9. Meites S, editor: *Pediatric clinical chemistry: reference (normal) values,* Washington, DC, 1979, American Association for Clinical Chemistry.

10. Wisnieski JJ, Jones SM: Comparison of the autoantibodies to the collagen-like region of C1q in hypocomplementemic urticarial vasculitis syndrome and systemic lupus erythmatosus, *J Immunol* 148:1396-1403, 1992.

11. Johnson CA, Densen P, Wetsel RA, et al: Molecular heterogeneity of C2 deficiency, *N Engl J Med* 326:871-874, 1992.

12. Ruddy S: Complement deficiencies. 3. The second component, *Prog Allergy* 39:250-266, 1986.

13. Loos M, Heinz HP: Complement deficiencies. 1. The first component: C1q, C1r, C1s, *Prog Allergy* 39:212-231, 1986.

14. Fielder AH, Walport MJ, Batchelor JR, et al: Family study of major histocompatibility complex in patients with systemic lupus erythematosus: importance of null alleles of C4A and C4B in determining disease susceptibility, *Br Med J (Clin Res Ed)* 286:425-428, 1983.

15. Ratanachaiyavong LL, McGregor AM: C4A gene deletion. Association with Graves' disease, *J Mol Endocrinol* 3:145-153, 1989.

16. Robb SA, Fielder AH, Saunders CE, et al: C4 complement allotypes in juvenile dermatomyositis, *Hum Immunol* 22:31-38, 1988.

17. Volanakis JE, Barnum SR, Giddens M, et al: Renal filtration and catabolism of complement protein D, *N Engl J Med* 312:395-398, 1985.

| Clomiphene (Clomid) Stimulation Test[1-4] Dose: Clomid, 50 mg orally b.i.d. × 7 | Collect serum for baseline measurement and after clomiphene administration (day 8). See *Remarks.* | After clomiphene: *LH:* Mean increase >120% above baseline [× 0.01 = >1.20, fraction increase] Range: 30-300% [0.30-3.00, concentration fraction] *FSH:* Mean increase >40% above baseline [>0.40, fraction increase] Range: 20-60% [0.20-0.60, concentration fraction] | See individual tests. |

DIAGNOSTIC INFORMATION   **REMARKS**

18. Laurell AB: Complement determinations in clinical diagnosis. In Rother K, Till GO, editors: *The complement system,* Berlin, 1988, Springer-Verlag.

19. Walport MJ: Advances in immunology: complement (first of two parts), *N Engl J Med* 344:1058-1066, 2001.

20. Cooper NR, Morrison DC: Binding and activation of the first component of complement by the lipid A region of lipopolysaccharide, *J Immunol* 120:1862-1868, 1978.

21. Cooper NR, Nemerow GR: Complement, viruses and virus-infected cells, *Springer Semin Immunopathol* 6:327-347, 1983.

22. Giclas PC, Ginsberg MH, Cooper NR: IgG-independent activation of the classical complement pathway by monosodium urate crystals, *J Clin Invest* 63:759-764, 1979.

23. Pinckard RN, Olson MS, Giclas PC, et al: Consumption of classical pathway components by heart subcellular membranes in vitro and in patients after acute myocardial infarction, *J Clin Invest* 56:740-750, 1975.

24. Volanakis JE: Complement activation by C-reactive protein complexes, *Ann NY Acad Sci* 389:235-250, 1982.

25. Law SKA, Reid KBM: *Complement,* Oxford, UK, 1988, IRL Press.

26. Rabson A: Enumeration of T-cell subsets in patients with HIV infection, *AIDS Clin Care* 7:1-3, 1995.

27. Gitlin D, Kumate J, Urrusti J, et al: The selectivity of the human placenta in the transfer of proteins from mother to fetus, *J Clin Invest* 43:1938-1951, 1964.

28. Cole FS, Colten HR: Complement biosynthesis. In Rother K, Till GO, editors: *The complement system,* Berlin, 1988, Springer-Verlag.

29. Ziccardi RJ, Cooper NR: Development of an immunochemical test to assess C1 inactivator function in human serum and its use for diagnosis of hereditary angioedema, *Clin Immunol Immunopathol* 15:465-471, 1979.

30. Donaldson VH, Rosen FS, Bing DH: Role of the second component of complement (C2) and plasmin in kinin release in hereditary angioneurotic edema (HANE) plasma, *Trans Assoc Am Physicians* 90:174-183, 1977.

31. Jahn I, Uring-Lambert B, Arnold D, et al: C2 reference typing report, *Complement Inflamm* 7:175-182, 1990.

32. Awdeh ZL, Alper CA: Inherited structural polymorphism of the fourth component of human complement, *Proc Natl Acad Sci USA* 77:3576-3580, 1980.

33. White RJ, Foristal J, Davis CA, et al: Isolation and characterization of DNA clones for human complement factor D [abstract], *Complement* 6:415, 1989.

34. Burger R: Factors of the alternative pathway. In Rother K, Till GO, editors: *The complement system,* Berlin, 1988, Springer-Verlag.

In hypothalamic-pituitary dysfunction there is no response; in prepubertal state, anorexia nervosa, and postmenopausal females, there is no or inadequate response.

A normal response essentially rules out organic impairment of gonadotropin secretion (e.g., pituitary tumor) and may be of value in assuring patients with delayed puberty that sexual maturity will ensue. An abnormal response suggests an organic lesion.

In healthy individuals clomiphene blocks estrogen feedback mechanisms in the hypothalamus, thus leading to an increase in gonadotropin-releasing hormone and, consequently, circulating LH and FSH.[5]

Because of the pulsatile nature of pituitary gonadotropin secretion, obtain three separate blood samples 20 min apart for baseline and poststimulation specimens. Aliquots of the sera on each day may be pooled.

In prepubertal children and in early puberty, clomiphene suppresses rather than stimulates gonadotropin release; therefore this test has little usefulness in these situations. In females, risks include hyperstimulation of the ovaries, cystic ovarian changes, and multiple pregnancies. There are no significant risks in men.

TEST NAME AND METHOD	SPECIMEN REQUIREMENTS	REFERENCE INTERVAL, CONVENTIONAL [INTERNATIONAL RECOMMENDED UNITS]	CHEMICAL INTERFERENCES AND IN VIVO EFFECTS
Clomiphene (Clomid) Stimulation Test—CONT			

1. Alsever RN, Gotlin RW: *Handbook of endocrine tests in adults and children,* ed 2, Chicago, 1978, Year Book Medical Publishers, Inc.
2. Ismail AA: *Biochemical investigations in endocrinology,* London, 1981, Academic Press.
3. Miller RE, Ngai B: *Manual of endocrine diagnostic tests,* ed 4, Lexington, KY, 1991, Department of Medicine, University of Kentucky.

TEST NAME AND METHOD	SPECIMEN REQUIREMENTS	REFERENCE INTERVAL, CONVENTIONAL [INTERNATIONAL RECOMMENDED UNITS]	CHEMICAL INTERFERENCES AND IN VIVO EFFECTS

Clonidine Suppression Test[1]
 	
Dose: 4.3 mcg clonidine/kg orally after overnight fast
	Plasma (heparin or EDTA), fasting, before and 3 hr after clonidine. Draw samples from indwelling catheter after 30 min of rest in a supine position. See *Catecholamines, Fractionated.*	Norepinephrine at 3 hr:
		  Within established reference range[1,2]
		  Decrease to <50% of baseline concentration[2,3]
			See *Catecholamines, Fractionated.*

1. Bravo E, Tarazi R, Found F, et al: Clonidine suppression test: a useful aid in the diagnosis of pheochromocytoma, *N Engl J Med* 305:623-626, 1981.
2. Grossman E, Goldstein DS, Hoffman A, et al: Glucagon and clonidine testing in the diagnosis of pheochromocytoma, *Hypertension* 17:733-741, 1991.
3. Elliott WJ, Murphy MB: Reduced specificity of the clonidine suppression test in patients with normal plasma catecholamine levels, *Am J Med* 84:419-424, 1988.
4. Eisenhofer G, Goldstein DS, Walther MM, et al: Biochemical diagnosis of pheochromocytoma: how to distinguish true- from false-positive test results, *J Clin Endocrinol Metab* 88:2656-2666, 2003.

4. Santen RJ, Leonard JM, Sherins RS, et al: Short- and long-term effects of clomiphene citrate on the pituitary-testicular axis, *J Clin Endocrinol Metab* 33:970-979, 1971.
5. Carr BR: Disorders of the ovary and female reproductive tract. In Wilson JD, Foster DW, editors: *Williams textbook of endocrinology,* ed 8, Philadelphia, 1992, WB Saunders.

Lack of a decrease in norepinephrine is suggestive of pheochromocytoma.

Clonidine inhibits neurogenic catecholamine release and will cause a decrease of plasma norepinephrine into the reference interval in hypertensive subjects without pheochromocytoma.

Intermittent catecholamine secretion by a pheochromocytoma may also give a false-negative response.

In patients without pheochromocytoma, the majority of plasma metanephrine is derived from norepinephrine released by sympathetic nerves and is therefore decreased in response to clonidine. The inclusion of plasma normetanephrine measurements has been shown to increase the sensitivity of the clonidine stimulation test, particularly when used in patients with only slight elevations of plasma metanephrines.[4]

TEST NAME AND METHOD	SPECIMEN REQUIREMENTS	REFERENCE INTERVAL, CONVENTIONAL [INTERNATIONAL RECOMMENDED UNITS]	CHEMICAL INTERFERENCES AND IN VIVO EFFECTS
Coagulation Factors Assays (II, V, VII, VIII, IX, X, XI, and XII)[1-5]	Plasma (blue top-citrate). Place on ice immediately. Stable for 2 hr at room temperature or for 4 hr at 2-8° C. Freeze if assay is delayed >2 hr.	Results are expressed in percent of normal plasma activity or international units. One unit is the average factor activity present in 1 mL of normal human plasma. The reference interval is typically 60-150%. Neonates/Infants: All coagulation factors, except for factor VIII, are decreased compared with adult levels. The factor levels progressively increase to adult levels by ~6 mo.	For all factors: ↓ C Heparin (interferes mainly with PTT based assays) ↓ C Lupus anticoagulant (interferes mainly with PTT based assays) ↓ V Anabolic steroids, androgens, antibiotics ↑ V Estrogens, oral contraceptives

1. Lewis SM, Bain BJ, Bates I, editors: *Dacie and Lewis practical hematology,* ed 9, Edinburgh 2001, Churchill Livingstone.
2. Jacobs DS, Demott WR, Oxley DK, editors: *Laboratory test handbook,* ed 5, Hudson, OH, 2001, Lexi-Comp, Inc.
3. Lusher JM, Hillman-Wiseman C, Hurst D: In vivo recovery with products of very high purity—assay discrepancies, *Haemophilia* 4:641-645, 1998.
4. Alving BM: The antiphospholipid syndrome: clinical presentation, diagnosis, and patient management. In Kitchens CS, Alving BM, Kessler CM, editors: *Consultative hemostasis and thrombosis,* Philadelphia, 2002, WB Saunders, pp. 269-278.
5. Choufani EB, Sanchorawala V, Ernst T, et al: Acquired factor X deficiency in patients with amyloid light-chain amyloidosis: incidence, bleeding manifestations, and response to high-dose chemotherapy, *Blood* 97:1885-1887, 2001.

Cobalt (Co)[1,2] *NAA, AAS*	Serum. Collect in pretested, metal-free container.		*mcg/L* 0.11-0.45[3] × 16.97	*nmol/L* [1.9-7.6]	None found.
		Therapeutic range[2]:	4.0-10.0	[67.9-169.7]	
		Toxicity has been reported for doses >5 mg/day [× 16.97 = 85 μmol/day][1]			
	Urine. Collect in acid-washed, metal-free container.	1-2 mcg/L	× 16.97	[17-34 nmol/L]	

DIAGNOSTIC INFORMATION	REMARKS

↓ Hereditary deficiency (rare hereditary combined deficiencies may be seen)

Factor VIII deficiency: in addition to decreased levels in hemophilia, patients with von Willebrand disease may also have low FVIII.

Acquired deficiency:
Specific inhibitors may arise to virtually any coagulation factor. Most common specific inhibitors are antibodies to FVIII and IX.

Multiple factor deficiencies: liver disease (except factor VIII), DIC.

Factors II, VII, IX, and X: vitamin K deficiency or warfarin.

Of note, heparin, hirudin, and argatroban can act as "inhibitors" and interfere with specific factor assays.

Factor II: rare patients with lupus anticoagulant

Factor X: acquired factor X deficiency may occur in patients with amyloidosis.

The PTT and the PT are the basis for these factor assays. Factors VIII, IX, XI, and XII are PTT based. Factors II, V, VII, and X are PT based. The test is based on the ability of patient plasma to correct the PTT or PT of specific factor-deficient plasma. Quantitative results are obtained from comparing with a standard curve made from dilutions of normal reference plasma and specific factor-deficient plasma.

Nonspecific and specific inhibitors can interfere with a factor assay; therefore multiple dilutions should be performed to dilute out the effect of the inhibitor. A common example is an acquired inhibitor to FVIII that interferes with the FIX assay, resulting in a falsely decreased FIX value. With additional dilutions the specific factor VIII inhibitor will be diluted out, and the factor IX assay will normalize.

Although the factor assays are typically clot-based (PTT or PT), chromogenic and immunologic assays do exist for some of the factors, including FVIII. Differences between the standard PTT-based FVIII assay compared with the chromogenic FVIII have been noticed in the monitoring of the B-domain–deleted recombinant factor VIII concentrate, with PTT assay levels ~50% of chromogenic activities.

Toxic effects due to excess cobalt intake have been noted in renal patients receiving erythropoietic agents and in very heavy drinkers of beer with added cobalt. Toxic effects include thyroid gland hyperplasia, myxedema, cardiomyopathy (particularly in alcoholism), polycythemia, and nerve damage. Co deficiency has not been reported in humans. Cobalt exposure or inhalation of Co dust in industrial settings may produce allergic dermatitis, asthma, and pulmonary symptoms.

Co is an integral component of vitamin B_{12}. It is found in most foods and is readily absorbed from the gastrointestinal tract. Co concentrations may be increased in individuals with deteriorating orthopedic implants.[5,6] Cobalt chloride is used in the treatment of some refractory anemias, including sickle cell anemia,[7] but use has decreased since the introduction of erythropoietin as a therapeutic agent. Co is used in treating cancer of the oral cavity, pharynx, and larynx, rhabdomyosarcoma, carcinoma of the penis, and radiosensitive but widespread tumors. Samples collected to assess occupational exposure should be collected at the end of shift on the last day of the work week.

TEST NAME AND METHOD	SPECIMEN REQUIREMENTS	REFERENCE INTERVAL, CONVENTIONAL [INTERNATIONAL RECOMMENDED UNITS]		CHEMICAL INTERFERENCES AND IN VIVO EFFECTS
Cobalt—CONT				
	Erythrocytes[3]	*mcg/kg* 16-46	× 16.97	*nmol/kg* [272-781]
	Hair[3]	*mcg/kg dry wt.* 0.4-500		*nmol/kg dry wt.* [7-8485]
ICP-MS	Serum.[4] Collect in pretested, metal-free container.	*mcg/L* 0.1-0.4 mcg/L	× 16.97	*nmol/L* [1.7-6.8 nmol/L]
	Whole blood.[4] Collect in pretested, metal-free container.	0.5-3.9 mcg/L		[8.5-66.2 nmol/L]
	Urine.[4] Collect in acid-washed, metal-free container. Refrigerate during and following collection.	0.1-2.0 mcg/L	× 16.97	[1.7-33.9 nmol/L]

1. Williams WJ, Beutler E, Erslev AJ, et al, editors: *Hematology,* ed 4, New York, 1990, McGraw-Hill Publishing Co.
2. Wyngaarden JB, Smith LH Jr, editors: *Cecil textbook of medicine,* ed 18, Philadelphia, 1988, WB Saunders.
3. Iyengar GV, Woittiez J: Trace elements in human clinical specimens: evaluation of literature data to identify telerence values, *Clin Chem* 34:474-481, 1988.
4. Associated Regional & University Pathologists, Inc. web site (www.aruplab.com): Specific address Online User's Guide: http://www.aruplab.com/testing/user_guide.jsp. Last accessed 9/2004.

Collagen Telopeptides and Pyridinium Crosslinks[1-18]				↑ V Thyroid hormones, glucocorticoids, growth hormone, 1,25-dihydroxyvitamin D
N-telopeptide (NTx)				↓ V Bisphosphonates, estrogens, calcitonin
ELISA[5,19,20,22]	Serum. Refrigerate for up to 24 hr. Store frozen.	*nmol BCE*/L* Adult M: F, premenopausal:	10.7-22.9 8.7-19.8	
ELISA[5,21,22]	Urine, second morning void. Refrigerate. Store frozen.	*nmol BCE*/mmol creatinine* Adult M: F, premenopausal:	11-103 10-110	

DIAGNOSTIC INFORMATION	REMARKS

5. Taylor A: Detection and monitoring of disorders of essential trace elements [review], *Ann Clin Biochem* 33:486-510, 1996.
6. Sunderman FW Jr, Hopfer SM, Swift T, et al: Cobalt, chromium, and nickel concentrations in body fluids of patients with porous-coated knee or hip prosthesis, *J Orthop Res* 7:307-315, 1989.
7. Nichols Institute Reference Laboratories: *Test catalog,* San Juan Capistrano, CA, 1987, Nichols Institute Reference Laboratories.

↑ High-turnover osteoporosis, Paget's disease, primary hyperparathyroidism, osteomalacia, renal osteodystrophy, hyperthyroidism, acromegaly, bone metastases, liver disease, bone growth (children and adolescents), menopause, age (>45-50 yr)

↓ Hypoparathyroidism

Collagen pyridinium cross-links and cross-linked telopeptides are formed during maturation of type I collagen, the protein accounting for 90% of organic matrix of bone. Type I collagen is a triple helix of two identical and one closely related amino acid chains. During collagen maturation, intermolecular N- and C-telopeptide cross-links are formed between 2 hydroxylysyl and 1 lysyl or 3 hydroxylysl sidechains of neighboring fibrils forming deoxypyridinoline (DPD) or pyridinoline (PYD), respectively. During bone resorption, these collagen telopeptides and pyridinium cross-links are released into the circulation and excreted in urine. DPD (found in bone and dentine) is a more sensitive and specific marker of bone resorption than PYD (also found in cartilage, tendons, and vascular tissue).

Telopeptides in serum or urine are measured by immunoassays, whereas DPD is measured by immunoassay or HPLC. DPD immunoassays recognize primarily free DPD, not DPD colla-

TEST NAME AND METHOD	SPECIMEN REQUIREMENTS	REFERENCE INTERVAL, CONVENTIONAL [INTERNATIONAL RECOMMENDED UNITS]		CHEMICAL INTERFERENCES AND IN VIVO EFFECTS

Collagen Telopeptides and Pyridinium Crosslinks—CONT

	Urine, 24 hr. Refrigerate. Store frozen.	*nmol BCE*/mmol creatinine*		
		Adult		
		M:	5-87	
		F, premenopausal:	5-79	

*BCE, Bone collagen equivalent. Calibrated using a standard of bacterial collagenase-digested human bone collagen.

C-telopeptide (CTx) (β-Cross-Laps)[6,23-25]

ECLIA[26]	Serum, fasting morning specimen. Refrigerate up to 24 hr. Store frozen.	*pg/mL*	*ng/L*
		Adult	
		M	
		30-50 yr: ≤584	[≤584]
		>50-70 yr: ≤704	[≤584]
		>70 yr: ≤854	[≤584]
		F	
		Premenopausal: ≤573	[≤573]
		Postmenopausal: ≤1008	[≤1008]

Collagen Pyridinium Crosslinks

Deoxypyridino-line, Free[27,28]

ICMA[29]	Urine, second morning void. Refrigerate. Store frozen.	*nmol/mmol creatinine*	
		Adult	
		M:	2.3-5.4
		F:	3.0-7.4

Deoxypyridinoline, Total[3,30,31]

HPLC[32]	Urine, 24 hr. Preserve with 25 mL of HCl, 6 mol/L; refrigerate. Store frozen.	*nmol/mmol creatinine*	
		Child	
		2-10 yr:	31-112
		11-14 yr:	17-101
		15-17 yr:	≤59
		Adult	
		M:	3.7-19
		F, premenopausal:	4.4-21

gen peptides. Total DPD and PYD can be measured by HPLC following acid hydrolysis of urine. N-telopeptide (NTx) and C-telopeptide (CTx) immunoassays recognize the N-telopeptide cross-links and β-isomerized C-telopeptide cross-links, respectively.

NTx, CTx, and DPD are specific and sensitive markers of bone resorption and can be used to measure bone resorption in osteoporosis and other metabolic bone diseases. In osteoporosis, although they are potentially useful for predicting bone loss and fracture risk and for selecting patients for therapy, they have been most useful in monitoring the effectiveness of antiresorptive therapy. Even for monitoring the efficacy of treatment, their usefulness has been compromised by preanalytical and analytical variation.

Most bone markers exhibit a significant diurnal variation with peak in the early morning and a nadir in the afternoon, a result of the nocturnal peak in bone turnover. Consequently, specimens should be collected at a specific time of day to minimize the impact of diurnal variation when comparing specimens with previous results (monitoring) or with reference intervals. A second morning void is usually recommended for urinary markers. Because urinary markers are normalized by dividing by urinary creatinine, the variability between creatinine measurements, within-subject variability in creatinine, and its dependence on muscle mass all contribute to overall variability. Less within-subject variation is observed with the serum telopeptides.

Reference intervals depend on the reason for ordering the test. For osteoporosis, reference intervals should be based on healthy premenopausal women and healthy men <50 yr because of the aged-related increase in bone resorption, osteopenia, and osteoporosis. Depending on the bone marker, a reduction of 30-60% should be observed after 3-6 mo of antiresorptive therapy. NTx and CTx decrease faster and to a greater extent than DPD.

Pyridinium cross-links have largely replaced hydroxyproline as a marker of bone resorption.[33] (See *Hydroxyproline, Total.*)

TEST NAME AND METHOD	SPECIMEN REQUIREMENTS	REFERENCE INTERVAL, CONVENTIONAL [INTERNATIONAL RECOMMENDED UNITS]		CHEMICAL INTERFERENCES AND IN VIVO EFFECTS

Collagen Telopeptides and Pyridinium Crosslinks—CONT

Pyridinoline, Total[3,30,31]

HPLC[32]

	Urine, 24 hr. Preserve with 25 mL of HCl, 6 mol/L; refrigerate. Store frozen.	*nmol/mmol creatinine*	
		Child	
		2-10 yr:	158-442
		11-14 yr:	107-398
		15-17 yr:	42-200
		Adult	
		M:	20-61
		F, premenopausal:	22-89

1. Rossert J, de Crombrugghe B: Type I collagen: structure, synthesis, and regulation. In Belezikian JP, Raisz LG, Rodan GA, editors: *Principles of bone biology,* ed 2, vol 1, San Diego, 2002, Academic Press, pp. 189-210.

2. Robins SP, Brady JD: Collagen cross-linking and metabolism. In Bilezikian JP, Raisz LG, Rodan GA, editors: *Principles of bone biology,* ed 2, vol 1, San Diego, 2002, Academic Press, pp. 211-223.

3. James IT, Walne AJ, Perrett D, et al: The measurement of pyridinium crosslinks: a methodological overview, *Ann Clin Biochem* 33:397-420, 1996.

4. Fraser WD: The collagen crosslinks pyridinoline and deoxypyridinoline: a review of their biochemistry, physiology, measurement, and clinical applications, *J Clin Ligand Assay* 21:102-110, 1998.

5. Mallinak NJS, Clemens D: Crosslinked N-telopeptides of bone collagen: a marker of bone resorption, *J Clin Ligand Assay* 21:111-117, 1998.

6. Pedersen BJ, Ravn P, Bonde M: Type I collagen C-telopeptide degradation products as bone resorption markers, *J Clin Ligand Assay* 21:118-127, 1998.

7. Seibel MJ: Biochemical markers of bone remodeling, *Endocrinol Metab Clin N Am* 32:83-113, 2003.

8. Garnero P, Gineyts E, Arbault P, et al: Different effects of bisphosphonates and estrogen therapy on free and peptide-bound bone cross-links excretion, *J Bone Miner Res* 10:641-649, 1995.

9. Kamel S, Brazier M, Neri V, et al: Multiple molecular forms of pyridinoline cross-links excreted in human urine evaluated by chromatographic and immunoassay methods, *J Bone Miner Res* 10:1385-1392, 1995.

10. Vesper H, Cosman F, Endres DB, et al: Application of biochemical markers of bone turnover in the assessment and monitoring of bone diseases, Approved Guideline, C48-A, Wayne, PA, 2004, NCCLS.

11. Calvo MS, Eyre DR, Gundberg CM: Molecular basis and clinical application of biological markers of bone turnover, *Endocr Rev* 17:333-368, 1996.

12. Garnero P, Delmas PD: Biochemical markers of bone turnover in osteoporosis. In Marcus R, Feldman D, Kelsey J, editors: *Osteoporosis,* ed 2, San Diego, 2001, Academic Press, pp. 459-477.

13. Woitge HW, Seibel MJ: Risk assessment for osteoporosis II: biochemical markers of bone turnover: bone resorption indices, *Clin Lab Med* 20:503-525, 2000.

14. Woitge HW, Pecherstorfer M, Li Y, et al: Novel serum markers of bone resorption: clinical assessment and comparison with established urinary indices, *J Bone Miner Res* 14:782-801, 1999.

15. Fall PM, Kennedy D, Smith JA, et al: Comparison of serum and urine assays for biochemical markers of bone resorption in postmenopausal women with and without hormone replacement therapy and in men, *Osteoporos Int* 11:481-485, 2000.

16. Ebeling PR, Atley LM, Guthrie JR, et al: Bone turnover markers and bone density across the menopausal transition, *J Clin Endocrinol Metab* 81:3366-3371, 1996.

17. Seibel MJ: Biochemical markers of bone metabolism in the assessment of osteoporosis: useful or not? *J Endocrinol Invest* 26:464-471, 2003.

DIAGNOSTIC INFORMATION	REMARKS

18. Klee G, Brown D, Kophor R, et al: Biochemical markers for bone turnover in osteoporosis. Institute for Clinical Systems Improvement Technology Assessment Report #53. Available at: www.icsi.org,

19. Clemens JD, Herrick MV, Singer FR, et al: Evidence that serum NTx (collagen type I N-telopeptides) can act as an immunochemical marker of bone resorption, *Clin Chem* 43:2058-2063, 1997.

20. Gertz B, Clemens D, Holland SD, et al: Application of a new serum assay for type I collagen crosslinked N-telopeptides: assessment of clinical changes in bone turnover with and without alendronate treatment, *Calcif Tissue Int* 63:102-106, 1996.

21. Hansen DA, Weiss MAE, Bollen A-M, et al: A specific immunoassay for monitoring human bone resorption: quantitation of type I collagen cross-linked N-telopeptides in urine, *J Bone Miner Res* 7:1251-1258, 1992.

22. Collagen cross-linked N-telopeptides (NTx), serum or urine. In *Quest Diagnostics manual: endocrinology test selection and interpretation,* ed 3, San Juan Capistrano, CA, 2004, Quest-Nichols, p. 40.

23. Bonde M, Garnero P, Fledeluis C, et al: Measurement of bone degradation products in serum using antibodies reactive with an isomerized form of an 8 amino acid sequence of the C-telopeptide of type I collagen, *J Bone Miner Res* 12:1028-1034, 1997.

24. Rosenquist C, Fledeluis C, Christgau S, et al: Serum crosslaps one step ELISA. First application of monoclonal antibodies for measurement in serum of bone-related degradation products of C-terminal telopeptides of type I collagen, *Clin Chem* 44:2281-2289, 1998.

25. Garnero P, Borel O, Delmas PD: Evaluation of a fully automated serum assay for C-terminal cross-linking telopeptide of type I collagen in osteoporosis, *Clin Chem* 47:694-702, 2001.

26. β-*CrossLaps/serum product insert,* Indianapolis, IN, 2003, Roche Diagnostics.

27. Robins SP, Woitge H, Hesley R, et al: Direct, enzyme-linked immunoassay for urinary deoxypyridinoline as a specific marker for measuring bone resorption, *J Bone Miner Res* 9:1643-1649, 1994.

28. Gomez B Jr, Ardakani S, Evans BJ, et al: Monoclonal antibody assay for free urinary pyridinium cross-links, *Clin Chem* 42:1168-1175, 1996.

29. *Pyrilinks-D Immulite 2000 product insert,* Los Angeles, 2004, Diagnostic Products.

30. Black D, Duncan A, Robins SP, et al: Quantitative analysis of pyridinium crosslinks of collagen in urine using ion-paired reversed-phase high-performance liquid chromatography, *Anal Biochem* 169:197-203, 1988.

31. Fraser WD: The collagen crosslinks pyridinoline and deoxypyridinoline: a review of their biochemistry, physiology, measurement and clinical applications, *J Clin Ligand Assay* 21:102-110, 1998.

32. Pyridinium collagen cross-links, urine (PYD and DPYD). In *Quest Diagnostics manual: endocrinology test selection and interpretation,* ed 3, San Juan Capistrano, CA, 2004, Quest-Nichols, p. 141.

33. Endres DB: Biochemical markers of bone metabolism, *AACC Endo and Metabolism In-Service Training and Continuing Education* 11:27-29, 1993.

TEST NAME AND METHOD	SPECIMEN REQUIREMENTS	REFERENCE INTERVAL, CONVENTIONAL [INTERNATIONAL RECOMMENDED UNITS]			CHEMICAL INTERFERENCES AND IN VIVO EFFECTS

Complement, Total Hemolytic

CH_{50}[1,2]

Quantitative functional assay

Serum; CNS, pleural, or synovial fluid (pair with serum sample collected at the same time for comparison). Collect blood in plain redtop tube and allow to clot for 30 min. Do not let blood or body fluid stand at room temperature or 37° C for >1 hr. Centrifuge sample and transfer cell-free and clot-free serum or fluid to clean tube. Store at −70° C (−20° C acceptable for overnight only). Ship on dry ice. Avoid repeated freeze/thaw cycles.

$$
\begin{array}{cccc}
 & CH_{50}\ U/mL & & CH_{50}\ kU/L \\
\text{Serum:} & 26\text{-}58^{3} & \times 1000 & [26\text{-}58] \\
 & 33\text{-}61^{4} & & [33\text{-}61]
\end{array}
$$

Normal synovial, pleural, or CNS fluid complement[4] = 70% of serum complement after correction for protein:

$$\frac{\text{Fluid C}}{\text{Serum C}} \div \frac{\text{Fluid protein}}{\text{Serum protein}} \times 100$$

Synovial fluid: ≥33% of matching serum CH_{50}.[5]

↓ C EDTA, EGTA, ACD (Calcium chelators may decrease the CH_{50} due to dissociation of the C1qrs complex.)

↑ V Cyclophosphamide (in SLE patients), danazol

S ↓ *Congenital:* Inherited deficiency of complement component or control protein

Acquired: Mixed cryoglobulinemia, C1q-precipitin syndrome, acquired C1-INH deficiency, and type II membranoproliferative glomerulonephritis can cause very low or absent CH_{50}. Complement consumption due to immune complex disease, infectious processes, autoimmune processes, malignancy, trauma, burns, hypocomplementemic urticarial vasculitis, partial lipodystrophy, and liver disease can also cause low CH_{50}.

Fluid ↓ Decreases <70% of serum value, after correction for protein, are indicative of local consumption and are seen in synovial fluid from patients with seropositive rheumatoid arthritis or acute rheumatic fever and in pleural effusions from SLE patients.[4]

S ↑ *Acquired:* Acute phase response

Fluid ↑ CH_{50} and complement components may exceed 70% of serum values, after correction for protein concentration, in synovial and pleural fluids from patients with osteoarthritis and congestive heart failure with effusions.[4]

The CH_{50} measures total hemolytic activity of the classical pathway of complement (C1, C2, C4, C3, C5, C6, C7, C8, and C9). There is interlaboratory variability, similar to other bioassays, in the ranges reported. The quantitative functional hemolytic assay uses sheep erythrocytes (E) that have been coated with rabbit antisheep erythrocyte antibodies (A) to form sensitized erythrocytes (EA). After incubation, the unlysed EA are removed by centrifugation, and the percentage of cells lysed is determined from the amount of hemoglobin in the supernatants.

The CH_{50} unit is defined as the reciprocal of the dilution of serum that will lyse 50% of the cells in 1 mL of the suspension.

The CH_{50} is useful for detecting complement deficiencies and for monitoring complement consumption in patients with immune complex diseases such as vasculitis or systemic lupus erythematosus. The CH_{50} is less sensitive to changes due to complement activation than is measurement of complement split products that are produced only during activation. Complement function can be evaluated by assessing deposition of activation products on serum activation with immobilized complement-activating molecules (IgM for classical pathway, LPS for alternative pathway, or mannose for the lectin pathway).[5] The CH_{50} depends on the classical pathway (C1, C4, C2) for activity and shares the terminal components (C3, C5-C9) with the alternative pathway. If there is a complete deficiency of one of the components (C1q, C1r, C1s, C4, C2, C3, C5, C6, C7, or C8), then the CH_{50} will be 0 U/mL. C9 deficiency causes the CH_{50} to be low but usually not absent. If tested together with the AH_{50} (Total Alternative Pathway Activity), the CH_{50} can be used to narrow the search for the missing component:

If both the CH_{50} and the AH_{50} = 0 U/mL (kU/L), then the defect is in one of the late components (test C3, C5, C6, C7, and C8).

If the CH_{50} is 0 U/mL (kU/L) and the AH50 is normal, then the defect is in one of the classical pathway components (test C1q, C1r, C1s [or C1 function], C2, and C4).

If the CH_{50} is normal and the AH_{50} = 0 U/mL (kU/L), then one of the alternative pathway components is deficient (test factors D and B and properdin).

TEST NAME AND METHOD	SPECIMEN REQUIREMENTS	REFERENCE INTERVAL, CONVENTIONAL [INTERNATIONAL RECOMMENDED UNITS]			CHEMICAL INTERFERENCES AND IN VIVO EFFECTS
Complement, Total Hemolytic—CONT					
CH_{100} *Radial diffusion*	Serum; plasma (EDTA)	>70 U/mL CH_{100}	× 1000	[>70 kU/L]	↓C EDTA, EGTA, ACD (Calcium chelators may decrease the CH_{50} due to dissociation of the C1qrs complex.)
Alternative Pathway, Total Hemolytic AH_{50} *Functional hemolytic assay*	Serum; plasma (EDTA). Collect cell-free serum or plasma. Store at −70° C (−20° C acceptable for overnight only). Ship on dry ice.	28-144 AH_{50} U/mL[6]	× 1000	[28-144 kU/L]	None found.

DIAGNOSTIC INFORMATION	REMARKS
	If the CH_{50} and/or AH_{50} are low but not absent or if more than one component is low, then the most likely reason is depletion of complement due to *in vivo* activation; however, the patient may be heterozygous for a complement deficiency. Test for complement split products for evidence of activation, for factor H or factor I in the case of suspected congenital deficiency, or follow the above suggestions to identify the pathway involved in heterozygous deficiency.
	The rate-limiting components in the CH_{50} reaction are C2, C5, C3, and C4, and the main heat-labile components are C1q and C2.
	Note: Absence of C9 causes the CH_{50} and AH_{50} to be low but not usually as low as 0 U/mL. Deficiencies of factors H or I result in uncontrolled complement activation, with significant decreases in C3 and the late components.
	This test is semiquantitative and is used as a screen for hemolytic complement activity (See *CH_{50}*). A variation on this method measures alternative pathway activity by incorporating rabbit erythrocytes into the agarose gel. The CH_{100} test can be used as a rapid screen for complement deficiency or to monitor complement activity in patients with SLE or other immune complex disorders.
The AH_{50} requires all of the components of the alternative pathway and the terminal pathway (Factor D, Factor B, properdin, C3b, C3, C5, C6, C7, C8, and C9). The assay is most useful in helping to decide which complement component is missing in a complement-deficient patient, as described under CH_{50}, or in evaluating the performance of the alternative pathway as a whole.	The AH_{50} hemolytic assay uses rabbit or guinea pig erythrocytes (Erab, Egp) that have not been sensitized with antibodies and a buffer containing EGTA (to block the Ca^+-dependent classical pathway activity) plus Mg^{2+} (required by the alternative pathway). The percentage of cells lysed is determined from the amount of hemoglobin in the supernatants.
S $\downarrow$ *Congenital:* Inherited deficiency of complement component or control protein	The AH_{50} unit is defined as the reciprocal of the dilution of serum that will lyse 50% of the cells in 1 mL of the suspension.
S $\downarrow$ *Acquired:* Complement consumption due to immune complex disease, infectious process, autoimmune process, malignancy, cryoglobulinemia, trauma, burns	
S $\uparrow$ *Acquired:* Acute phase response.	

TEST NAME AND METHOD	SPECIMEN REQUIREMENTS	REFERENCE INTERVAL, CONVENTIONAL [INTERNATIONAL RECOMMENDED UNITS]		CHEMICAL INTERFERENCES AND IN VIVO EFFECTS

Complement, Total Hemolytic—CONT

1. Kabat EA, Mayer MM: *Experimental immunochemistry,* Springfield, IL, 1961, Charles C Thomas.
2. Kirschfink M, Mollnes TE: Modern complement analysis, *Clin Diagn Lab Immunol* 10:982-989, 2003.
3. Fudenberg HH, Sites DP, Caldwell JJ, et al: *Basic and clinical immunology,* ed 3, Los Altos, CA, 1980, Lange Medical Publications.
4. Kohler PF: Human complement system. In Samter M, editor: *Immunological diseases,* ed 3, Boston, 1978, Little, Brown and Co.

Copper (Cu)[1-3]

AAS; colorimetric, cuprizone

Serum.[5] Collect in pretested, metal-free container or draw into plastic syringe using a stainless steel needle. Keep sample in plastic vial or metal-free tube. There is diurnal variation with highest levels in the morning.

	mcg/dL		*μmol/L*
Birth-6 mo:	20-70	× 0.157	[3.1-11.0]
6 yr:	90-190		[14.1-29.8]
12 yr:	80-160		[12.6-25.1]
Adult			
M:	70-140		[11.0-22.0]
F:	80-155		[12.6-24.3]
>60 yr			
M:	85-170		[13.3-26.7]
F:	85-190		[13.3-29.8]
Pregnancy at term:	118-302		[18.5-47.4]

Values for African-Americans are 8-12% higher.

P,S ↑ V Carbamazepine, estrogens, oral contraceptives, phenobarbital, phenytoin

---

Plasma (EDTA),[6] separate red cells immediately. Keep sample in plastic vial.

Adult		
M:	56-111	[8.8-17.5]
F:	69-169	[10.7-26.6]
F, oral contraceptives:	100-200	[15.7-31.5]

Erythrocytes[5]; whole blood (heparin). Separate red cells immediately; wash in saline.

90-150 mcg/dL   × 0.157   [14.1-23.6 μmol/L]

Urine, 24 hr. Collect in acid-washed metal-free container. Acidify to pH 2.0 with HCl or nitric acid.

2-80 mcg/L 2056 × 0.0157 [0.03-1.26 μmol/L]
3-35 mcg/day [0.047-0.55 μmol/day]

↑ V Cisplatin

5. Hedberg H: Studies on the depressed hemolytic complement activity of synovial fluid in adult rheumatoid arthritis, *Acta Rheum Scand* 9:165-193, 1963.
6. Delk AS: A rapid sensitive immunologic agglutination test for phosphatidylglycerol (PG), *Am Clin Prod Rev* 10:8-13, 1984.

S ↑ Age, infections and inflammation, pregnancy, leukemia, biliary cirrhosis, typhoid fever, Hodgkin's disease, pellagra, pulmonary tuberculosis, most anemias, thalassemia major and minor, rheumatic fever, acute myocardial infarction, brain infarction, ankylosing spondylitis, rheumatoid arthritis, hypothyroidism and hyperthyroidism, collagen diseases, SLE, complications of renal dialysis and neonatal transfusions; trauma and malignant neoplasms of the GI tract, lung, bone, breast, cervix, and hematopoietic system

S ↓ Wilson's disease (40-60 mcg/dL; 6.3 9.4 μmol/L), GI disease (sprue, small bowel, celiac), cystic fibrosis, nephrotic syndrome, Menkes' syndrome, ACTH or prednisone-induced remission of leukemia, some iron-deficiency anemias, burns, disproteinemia, protein malnutrition, chronic ischemic heart disease.

During estrogen therapy (and pregnancy), the synthesis of ceruloplasmin in the liver is greatly increased. As a result, plasma Cu is about twice the normal level. Plasma ceruloplasmin is also increased during administration of oral contraceptives or antiepileptics (carbamazepine, phenobarbital, and phenytoin).

Ercs ↑ Pulmonary tuberculosis (characteristic), lead toxicity

Ercs ↓ Protein malnutrition

U ↑ Wilson's disease (>100 mg/day, >1.57 mmol/day; may be lower in young presymptomatic siblings),[12] chronic active hepatitis, biliary cirrhosis, rheumatoid arthritis, proteinuria

U ↓ Protein malnutrition

90-95% of plasma Cu is in the copper oxidase enzyme ceruloplasmin. Plasma Cu and/or ceruloplasmin oxidase activity can be used as a measure of body copper status. Copper absorption may be impaired in patients with diffuse small bowel disease and in those with high intakes of the competing ions zinc and cadmium. Cu deficiency has been observed in infants (especially premature) on Cu-deficient milk diets, in patients receiving long-term TPN with solutions deficient in trace metals, and in patients receiving zinc therapy or copper chelators such as penicillamine. Symptoms of copper deficiency include neutropenia, anemia (iron-unresponsive), osteoporosis, various bone/joint abnormalities, decreased skin pigmentation, and possibly neurological and cardiac abnormalities. Genetically determined diseases of copper metabolism include Wilson's disease (hepatolenticular degeneration), a Cu accumulation disease, and the rare Menkes' steely-hair syndrome, an infant copper deficiency disease. Indian childhood cirrhosis may also reflect an inherited metabolic disease requiring high concentrations of environmental Cu.[14]

Cu is increased in CSF of persons with brain infarction and in synovial fluid of persons with rheumatoid arthritis. Symptoms of Cu salt poisoning include nausea, vomiting, headache, diarrhea, and abdominal pain. Liver injury, jaundice, and hemolytic shock may follow. Copper toxicity may occur, owing to ingestion of Cu-contaminated solutions, use of Cu IUDs, or exposure to Cu fungicides. Serum total Cu and ceruloplasmin are reduced in Wilson's disease, owing to decreased hepatic synthesis of ceruloplasmin, whereas serum ionized calcium, urinary Cu excretion, and liver Cu levels are increased.

Assay of urine is useful only in diagnosing or assessing treatment for Wilson's disease.

TEST NAME AND METHOD	SPECIMEN REQUIREMENTS	REFERENCE INTERVAL, CONVENTIONAL [INTERNATIONAL RECOMMENDED UNITS]		CHEMICAL INTERFERENCES AND IN VIVO EFFECTS
Copper—CONT				
AAS	Liver (needle biopsy)	*mcg/g dry wt.*[10] 10-35 (Higher in infants aged <6 mo)	× 0.0157	*mmol/g dry wt.* [0.16-0.55]
		mcg/g wet wt.[11] 3.2-9.9	× 0.0157	*mmol/g wet wt.* [0.05-0.16]
	Hair.[7,8] Cut specimens close to the scalp in 2- to 5-cm lengths. Wash in acetone solution and digest in 70% ultrapure nitric acid.	Proximal segments: Whole hair or distal ends:	*mcg/g dry wt.* 4-16 20-60	× 0.0157	*μmol/g dry wt.* [0.06-0.25] [0.31-0.94]
X-ray fluorescence[4]	Bronchoalveolar lavage fluid	*ng/10³ macrophages* <0.55	× 15.7	*fmol/macrophage* [<8.6]
ICP-MS	Serum.[9] Collect in pretested, metal-free container.	Birth-6 mo: 6 mo-18 yr: Adult M: F:	*mcg/dL* 20-70 90-190 70-140 80-155	× 0.157	*μmol/L* [3.1-11.0] [14.1-29.0] [11.0-22.0] [12.6-24.3]
	Urine.[9] Collect in acid-washed, metal-free container. Refrigerate during and following collection.	0.2-8.0 mcg/dL 3-50 mg/day	× 0.157	[0.03-1.26 mmol/L] [0.47-7.85 mmol/day]
	Liver[9]	15-55 mcg/g liver		

1. Henry JB, editor: *Clinical diagnosis and management by laboratory methods,* ed 18, Philadelphia, 1991, WB Saunders.

2. Milne DB: Trace elements. In Burtis CA, Ashwood ER, editors: *Tietz textbook of clinical chemistry,* ed 2, Philadelphia, 1994, WB Saunders.

3. O'Dell BL: Copper. In Brown ML, editor: *Present knowledge in nutrition,* ed 6, Washington, DC, 1990, International Life Sciences Institute, Nutrition Foundation.

4. Maier EA, Rastegar F, Heimburger R, et al: Simultaneous determination of trace elements in lavage fluids from human bronchial alveoli by energy dispersive X-ray fluorescence. 1: Technique and determination of the normal reference interval *Clin Chem* 31:551-555, 1985.

5. Tietz NW, editor: *Fundamentals of clinical chemistry,* ed 3, Philadelphia, 1987, WB Saunders.

6. Milne DB, Johnson PE: Assessment of copper status: effect of age and gender on reference ranges in healthy adults, *Clin Chem* 39:883-887, 1993.

7. Jacob RA: Hair as a biopsy material. In Williams DF, editor: *Systemic aspects of biocompatibility,* Boca Raton, FL, 1981, CRC Press, Inc.

DIAGNOSTIC INFORMATION	REMARKS
Liver ↑ Wilson's disease (>250 mcg/g dry wt.; >3.9 μmol/g dry wt.),[13] sarcoidosis, biliary cirrhosis	See Table II-6.
Hair ↓ Diabetes	Hair Cu concentrations increase from proximal (scalp) to distal ends of the hair shaft. Reported higher levels in females may be due to analysis of more distal segments. Because of exogenous contamination and other factors, hair Cu is not a reliable measure of Cu status.

8. Associated Regional & University Pathologists, Inc. web site (www.aruplab.com). Specific address Online User's Guide: http://www.aruplab.com/testing/user_guide.jsp. Last accessed 9/2004.

9. Mayo Medical Laboratories: *Test catalog,* Rochester, MN, 1993, Mayo Medical Laboratories.

10. Hair analysis for mercury, *Lab Rep Phys* 2:85-87, 1980.

11. Conn RB, editor: *Current diagnosis,* ed 7, Philadelphia, 1985, WB Saunders.

12. Wyngaarden JB, Smith LH Jr, editors: *Cecil textbook of medicine,* ed 18, Philadelphia, 1988, WB Saunders.

13. Barceloux DG: Copper, *Clin Toxicol* 37:217-230, 1999.

TEST NAME AND METHOD	SPECIMEN REQUIREMENTS	REFERENCE INTERVAL, CONVENTIONAL [INTERNATIONAL RECOMMENDED UNITS]	CHEMICAL INTERFERENCES AND IN VIVO EFFECTS
Coproporphyrin-Isomers[1] *HPLC, Fluorimetric*[1-4]	Urine, 24 hr.[1] Collect in dark container with 5 g sodium carbonate. Store at 4° C during collection. Stable up to 7 days at −20° C.	*Coprophrphyrin I* Males: 10-40 mcg/24 hr × 1.53 [15.3-61.2 nmol/24 hr][1] Females: 2-30 mcg/24 hr × 1.53 [3.1-45.9 nmol/24 hr][1] *Coproporphyrin III* Males: 15-110 mcg/24 hr × 1.53 [23.0-168.3 nmol/24 hr][1] Females: 6-80 mcg/24 hr × 1.53 [9.2-122.4 nmol/24 hr][1] *%Coproporphyrin I* Males: 20-45% of total urinary coproporphyrins[1] Females: 20-45% of total urinary coproporphyrins[1]	↓ C Loss of analyte due to exposure to light, or to pH <6.0.

1. Mayo Medical Laboratories: *Test catalog,* Rochester, MN, 2004, Mayo Medical Laboratories.
2. Lim CK, Peters TJ: High performance liquid chromatography of uroporphyrin and coproporphyrin isomers, *Methods Enzymol* 123:383-389, 1986.
3. Kuhnel A, Gross U, Jacob K, et al: Studies on coproporphyrin isomers in urine and feces in the porphyries, *Clin Chim Acta* 282:45-58, 1999.
4. Jacob K, Egeler E, Hennel B, et al: The isomer ratios of urinary coproporphyrins I–IV are pH-dependent, *Eur J Clin Chem Clin Biochem* 29:115-119, 1991.
5. Mayo Medical Laboratories: *Interpretative handbook,* Rochester, MN, 2001, Mayo Medical Laboratories.
6. Wolkoff A, Wolpert E, Pascasio F, et al: Rotor's syndrome. A distinct inheritable pathophysiologic entity, *Am J Med* 60:173-179, 1976.

TEST NAME AND METHOD	SPECIMEN REQUIREMENTS	*mg/L*		*nmol/L*	CHEMICAL INTERFERENCES
Corticosteroid-Binding Globulin (CBG, Transcortin)[1-3] *Radioassay*[3]	Serum. Store frozen at −20° C.	Child M: F: Adult M: F: Pregnancy: Oral contraceptives:	 18.3-28.3 14.3-26.7 18.8-25.2 14.9-22.9 31.5-60.0 20.2-52.3	× 17.18*	↑ V Estrogens, lynestrenol, oral contraceptives ↓ Testosterone

Reference intervals (nmol/L column): Child M: [314-486]; F: [246-458]; Adult M: [323-433]; F: [256-393]; Pregnancy: [541-1031]; Oral contraceptives: [347-899]

*Conversion factor based on an MW of 58,200.

DIAGNOSTIC INFORMATION	REMARKS

↑ %Coproporphyrin I[5-7] Dubin-Johnson syndrome >80%
Rotor syndrome 60-80%

Porphyrins are intermediate metabolites of the heme synthetic pathway, which occurs in the liver and bone marrow. The three clinically important types of porphyrins are uroporphyrins, protoporphyrins, and coproporphyrins. In biologic fluids, porphyrins can exist as different configurations of the same compound (isomers).

Dubin-Johnson and Rotor syndromes are rare hereditary disorders with impaired intrahepatic bile excretion and hyperbilirubinemia (conjugated). Other than jaundice, affected individuals are typically asymptomatic.

One characteristic of both Dubin-Johnson and Rotor syndrome is chronic hepatic retention of coproporphyrin III. This retention diminishes the urinary excretion of coproporphyrin III.[4,8]

7. Frank M, Doss M, de Carvalho D: Diagnostic and pathogenetic implications of urinary coproporphyrin excretion in the Dubin-Johnson syndrome, *Hepatogastroenterology* 37.147-151, 1980.
8. Koskelo P, Mustajoki P: Altered coproporphyrin-isomer excretion in patients with the Dubin-Johnson syndrome, Int J Biochem 12:975-978, 1980.

↑ Ovarian hyperfunction, estrogen therapy, pregnancy, chronic active hepatitis, during treatment with anticonvulsant drugs.[4]

↓ Ovarian hypofunction, complicated pregnancies after the first trimester, fetal death, septic shock, CBG familial deficiency, inflammation, chronic liver diseases, hyperthyroidism, nephrosis, other protein-losing conditions.[5]

CBG, a glycoprotein primarily synthesized in the liver, binds and transports cortisol, corticosterone, progesterone, 17α-hydroxyprogesterone, and, to a much lesser degree, testosterone. However, dexamethasone does not bind to CBG. The protein is polymorphic with inheritance expressed as autosomal codominant.

Concentration in blood is sensitive to exogenous estrogens in a dose-responsive manner. CBG concentrations in patients with endometrial cancer are claimed to be higher than in normal premenopausal women. There is no diurnal variation and no changes during the menstrual cycle.

MW: 55,700
$t_{1/2}$:   5 days

TEST NAME AND METHOD	SPECIMEN REQUIREMENTS	REFERENCE INTERVAL, CONVENTIONAL [INTERNATIONAL RECOMMENDED UNITS]	CHEMICAL INTERFERENCES AND IN VIVO EFFECTS

Corticosteroid-Binding Globulin—CONT

1. Robinson PA, Langley MS, Hammond GL: A solid-phase radioimmunoassay for human CBG, *J Endocrinol* 104:259-267, 1985.
2. Rosner W, Polimeni S, Khan MS: Radioimmunoassay for human corticosteroid-binding globulin, *Clin Chem* 29:1389-1391, 1983.
3. Wilson EA: Corticosteroid-binding globulin and estrogens in maternal and cord blood, *Am J Obstet Gynecol* 135:215-218, 1979.

TEST NAME AND METHOD	SPECIMEN REQUIREMENTS	REFERENCE INTERVAL			CHEMICAL INTERFERENCES
Corticosterone (Compound B)[1,2] *RIA*	Serum. Separate within 1 hr; store frozen.		Ng/dL^3	$nmol/L$	None found.
		Cord blood:	235-1080 $\times$ 0.0289	[7-31]	
		Newborn (1-7 days):	70-850	[2-25]	
		Child (1-16 yr)			
		8:00 AM:	135-1860	[4-54]	
		4:00 PM:	70-620	[2-18]	
		Adult			
		8:00 AM:	130-820	[4-24]	
		4:00 PM:	60-220	[2-6]	
EIA		Adult[4]			
		M:	320-760	[9.2-22]	
		F:	90-390	[2.6-11]	

1. Holsboer F, Haack D, Gerken A, et al: Plasma dexamethasone concentrations and differential suppression response of cortisol and corticosterone in depressives and controls, *Biol Psychiatry* 19:281-291, 1984.
2. Saruta T, Suzuki A, Hayashi M, et al: Mechanism of age-related changes in renin and adrenocortical steroids, *J Am Geriatr Soc* 28:210-214, 1983.
3. Endocrine Sciences: *Pediatric laboratory services,* Tarzana, CA, 1992, Endocrine Sciences.
4. Cayman Chemical Co.: *Assay insert,* Ann Arbor, MI, 2004, Cayman Chemical Co.
5. Brown SS, Mitchell FL, Young DS, editors: *Chemical diagnosis of disease,* Amsterdam, 1979, Elsevier/North Holland Biomedical Press.

TEST NAME AND METHOD	SPECIMEN REQUIREMENTS	REFERENCE INTERVAL	CHEMICAL INTERFERENCES
Corticotropin-Releasing Hormone (CRH) Stimulation Test[1-3] Dose: 1 mcg/kg ovine CRH, IV at 9:00 AM to 8:00 PM After dexamethasone suppression	Dose: 0.5 mg dexamethasone every 6 hr for 2 days; 2 hr after last dose 1 mcg/kg CRH given IV. Samples drawn after 15 min.	Twofold to fourfold increase in mean baseline concentrations of ACTH or cortisol. Cortisol > 1.4 mcg/L virtually 100% specific and 100% diagnostic.	See *Adrenocorticotropic Hormone* and *Cortisol, Total.*

DIAGNOSTIC INFORMATION	REMARKS

4. Orth D, Kovacs D, DeBold C: The adrenal cortex. In Wilson JH, Foster DW, editors: *Williams textbook of endocrinology,* ed 8, Philadelphia, 1992, WB Saunders.
5. Sava L, Zouaghi H, Carli A, et al: Serum depletion of corticosteroid-binding activities: an early marker for human septic shock, *Biochem Biophys Res Commun* 102:411-419, 1981.

↑ Adrenogenital syndrome with 17-hydroxylase deficiency, congenital 18-hydroxylation defect with salt-losing syndrome, adrenal adenomas.

The ratio of cortisol/corticosterone (range, 5.9-59.1; x̄: 21.0) decreases when ACTH is given.[5] There is no significant change in corticosterone level with age.

Concurrent determinations of corticosterone and cortisol increase the sensitivity of the dexamethasone suppression test in patients with endogenous depression. See *Dexamethasone Suppression Test, Overnight.*

Normal or exaggerated response: Pituitary Cushing's disease

No response: Ectopic ACTH-secreting tumor

A positive response to CRH or a suppressed response to high-dose dexamethasone has a 97% positive predictive value for Cushing's disease. However, a lack of response to either test excludes Cushing's disease in only 64-78% of patients. When the tests are considered together, negative responses from both have a 100% predictive value for ectopic ACTH secretion.

ACTH concentrations reach a peak 10 or 15 min after CRH injection; peak values are higher in the morning than in the evening.[4] Serum cortisol reaches a peak 30-60 min after CRH injection; peak values are the same at both times of day.

This test works as well as the standard dexamethasone suppression test (high-dose) in distinguishing pituitary Cushing's disease from ectopic ACTH secretion. The CRH test is less time consuming and may be performed on an outpatient basis.

Sensitivity decreases from 94% to 88% and specificity increases from 86% to 100% when cortisol response only is considered.

TEST NAME AND METHOD	SPECIMEN REQUIREMENTS	REFERENCE INTERVAL, CONVENTIONAL [INTERNATIONAL RECOMMENDED UNITS]	CHEMICAL INTERFERENCES AND IN VIVO EFFECTS

Corticotropin-Releasing Hormone (CRH) Stimulation Test—CONT

| | Blood (heparin) for plasma ACTH from both inferior petrosal sinus (IPS) veins and from a peripheral vein, before and 2, 5, 10, and 15 min after CRH injection. | Ratio of IPS to peripheral venous ACTH concentration: <3 to 1[3] | |

1. Nieman LK, Chrousos GP, Oldfield EH, et al: The ovine corticotropin releasing hormone stimulation test and the dexamethasone suppression test in the differential diagnosis of Cushing's syndrome, *Ann Intern Med* 105:862-867, 1986.

2. Nusynowitz ML: Screening tests and the free thyroxine index, *Arch Intern Med* 140:1017, 1980.

3. Whitley RJ, Meikle AW, Watts NB: Endocrinology. In Burtis CA, Ashwood ER, editors: *Tietz textbook of clinical chemistry,* ed 2, Philadelphia, 1994, WB Saunders.

TEST NAME AND METHOD	SPECIMEN REQUIREMENTS	REFERENCE INTERVAL, CONVENTIONAL			[INTERNATIONAL RECOMMENDED UNITS]	CHEMICAL INTERFERENCES AND IN VIVO EFFECTS
Cortisol, Free[1-2] *RIA (extracted)*	Urine, 24 hr. Preserve with 1 g boric acid. Freeze for long-term storage.	Child[5] 1-10 yr: 11-20 yr: Adult[6]:	*mcg/day* 2-27 5-55 20-90	× 2.76	*nmol/day* [6-74] [14-152] [55-248]	↑ V Cortisone acetate, danazol, hydrocortisone, oral contraceptives
HPLC[3,4]		Child[3] 2-11 yr: 12-16 yr: Adult[3]:	1-21 2-38 ≤50		[3-58] [6-105] [≤138]	↓ V Dexamethasone, ethacrynic acid, ketoconazole, thiazides
RIA	Amniotic fluid	Term:	26 ng/mL[7]	× 2.76	[72 nmol/L]	
	Saliva. Stable for 1 wk at 4° C and for 4 mo when frozen. Freezing is recommended.[1]	Child and adult 7:00 AM: 10:00 PM:	*ng/mL*[8] 1.4-10.1 0.7-2.2	× 2.76	*nmol/L* [4-28] [2-6]	
Equilibrium dialysis/ICMA	Serum	Adult[3] 8:00 AM: 4:00 PM:	*mcg/dL* 0.6-1.6 0.2-0.9	× 2.76	*nmol/L* [1.7-4.4] [0.6-2.5]	

1. Moore A, Aitken R, Gaskell S, et al: Cortisol assays: guidelines for the provision of a clinical biochemistry service, *Ann Clin Biochem* 22:435-454, 1985.

2. Schöneshöfer M, Fenner A, Dulce HJ: Interferences in the radioimmunological determination of urinary free cortisol, *Clin Chim Acta* 101:125-134, 1980.

<3 to 1: Pituitary Cushing's disease
>3 to 1: Ectopic ACTH-secreting tumor or adrenal tumors

This test is usually reserved for differentiating difficult cases of Cushing's disease and ectopic ACTH-secreting tumors.

4. Orth D, Kovacs D, DeBold C: The adrenal cortex. In Wilson JH, Foster DW, editors: *Williams textbook of endocrinology,* ed 8, Philadelphia, 1992, WB Saunders.

↑ Cushing's syndrome, late pregnancy, stress
ACTH-secreting tumor, pseudo-Cushing's syndrome.

↓ Addison's disease, congenital adrenal hyperplasia
(adrenogenital syndromes), hypopituitarism.

Test is extremely useful for discriminating Cushing's syndrome from simple obesity. Urinary free cortisol is proportional to the free (nonprotein-bound) cortisol in blood and is the most sensitive and specific test for initial screening of Cushing's syndrome. Nyctohemeral variations are not seen in 24-hr urine collections. Test is not recommended for diagnosis of Addison's disease.

See *Cortisol, Total.*

Salivary cortisol reflects the unbound cortisol in serum; it shows nyctohemeral variations similar to those in serum. Morning salivary cortisol values are decreased in adrenal insufficiency; evening values are increased in Cushing's syndrome.[9]

3. Nichols Institute Reference Laboratories: *Test catalog,* San Juan Capistrano, CA, 1993, Nichols Institute Reference Laboratories.

4. Canalis E, Reardon G, Caldarella A: A more specific, liquid-chromatographic method for free cortisol in urine, *Clin Chem* 28:2418-2420, 1982.

TEST NAME AND METHOD	SPECIMEN REQUIREMENTS	REFERENCE INTERVAL, CONVENTIONAL [INTERNATIONAL RECOMMENDED UNITS]	CHEMICAL INTERFERENCES AND IN VIVO EFFECTS

Cortisol, Free—CONT

5. Meites S, editor: *Pediatric clinical chemistry,* ed 2, Washington, DC, 1981, American Association for Clinical Chemistry.

6. Healthcare Corporation: *Package insert for clinical assays Gamma Coat [^{125}I] Cortisol radioimmunoassay kit,* Cambridge MA, 1990.

7. Tulchinsky D, Ryan KJ, editors: *Maternal-fetal endocrinology,* Philadelphia, 1980, WB Saunders.

TEST NAME AND METHOD	SPECIMEN REQUIREMENTS	REFERENCE INTERVAL, CONVENTIONAL			[INTERNATIONAL RECOMMENDED UNITS]	CHEMICAL INTERFERENCES AND IN VIVO EFFECTS
Cortisol, Total (free and bound)[1-4]	Serum or plasma (heparin). Store at 4° C for 2 days. Freeze for longer storage.		*mcg/dL*[6]		*nmol/L*	↑ V Amphetamines, corticotropin, cortisone acetate, estrogens, ethanol (IV, oral), hydrocortisone, interferon (gamma), methoxamine, metoclopramide, naloxone, nicotine (heavy smoking), oral contraceptives, vasopressin
		Cord blood:	5-17	× 27.6	[138-469]	
RIA		0-2 yr[7]:	1-35		[27.6-966]	
		2-6 yr:	1-26		[27.6-718]	
		6-11 yr:	1-38		[27.6-1049]	
		11-15 yr:	2-25		[55.2-690]	
		15-19 yr:	1-31		[27.6-856]	
		Adult				
		8:00 AM:	5-23		[138-635]	↑ C *Fluorimetric:*
		4:00 PM:	3-16		[83-441]	Mepacrine, quinacrine,
		8:00 PM[1]:	<50%		[<0.50]	spironolactone; *RIA:* Estrogen, prednisolone, prednisone
					of 8:00 AM	
		Maternal				
		(at birth)[8]:	54.3 ± 3.1		[1500 ± 86]	
						↓ V Aminoglutethimide, beclomethasone, betamethasone valerate, danazol, desoximetasone, dexamethasone, etomidate, ketoconazole, levodopa, lithium carbonate, methylprednisolone (depot), metyrapone, morphine, phenytoin (women), trilostane

	Amniotic fluid[5]	Term:	100-210 ng/mL × 2.76 [276-579 nmol/L]	

8. Riad-Fohmy D, Read G, Walker R, et al: Steroids in saliva for assessing endocrine function, *Endocr Rev* 3:367, 1982.
9. Orth D, Kovacs D, DeBold C: The adrenal cortex. In Wilson JH, Foster DW, editors: *Williams textbook of endocrinology,* ed 8, Philadelphia, 1992, WB Saunders.

↑ Cushing's (pituitary) disease, adrenal adenoma, carcinoma

↑↑ Ectopic ACTH syndrome

↓ Addison's disease, congenital adrenal hyperplasia (adrenogenital syndromes), hypopituitarism (need for functional tests)

Most assays displace cortisol from binding proteins to measure total hormone (free and bound). Increased secretion is seen in hypoglycemia, stress, ether narcosis, pregnancy, obesity, depression, and hyperthyroidism. Decreased secretion can be seen in hypothyroidism, cirrhosis, and hepatitis. Blood cortisol levels, however, may be normal in these conditions due to altered clearance rates. Cortisol secretion does not change with age. In pregnancy there is a progressive rise (due to increased cortisol-binding globulin); in late pregnancy there is a 2.5-fold increase.

There is a diurnal variation in secretion of cortisol; the level at 8:00 PM is normally 50% of the level at 8:00 AM. Random cortisol determinations are not very helpful. Loss of diurnal variation is often seen in Cushing's syndrome. The etiology of Cushing's syndrome may be established using various tests and protocols.

(See *Dexamethasone Suppression Test, Standard;* and *Andrenocorticotropic Hormone.*)

For cases of hypocortisolism, adrenal reserve of cortisol may be demonstrated using ACTH stimulation tests.

In primary adrenal insufficiency (Addison's disease), inadequate responses are seen following administration of cosyntropin (Cortrosyn). (See *Andrenocorticotropic Hormone Stimulation Test, Rapid* and *Prolonged*). Hypopituitarism with ATH deficiency gives a delayed but normal response to prolonged exogenous ACHT stimulation but does not respond to a variety of other stimulation tests. (See *Andrenocorticotropic Hormone Stimulation Test [after Insulin]* and *Metyrapone Stimulation Test.*)

AF ↑ Cortisol/cortisone ratio in lung maturation (reliability of L/S ratio exceeds that of the cortisol/cortisone ratio)

Decreases in AF have been reported in pregnancies with anencephalic fetuses.[5]

It has been reported that the competitive protein binding assay following chromatography yields concentrations of AF unconjugated cortisol that correlate poorly with maternal cortisol levels and highly with the duration of labor and the weight of the fetus.[5] There is disagreement regarding the increase of corticoids during the last 10 wk of pregnancy. Those who found increasing levels of cortisol toward the end of pregnancy also found a good correlation between total cortisol and the L/S

TEST NAME AND METHOD	SPECIMEN REQUIREMENTS	REFERENCE INTERVAL, CONVENTIONAL [INTERNATIONAL RECOMMENDED UNITS]	CHEMICAL INTERFERENCES AND IN VIVO EFFECTS

Cortisol, Total—CONT

1. Alsever RN, Gotlin RW: *Handbook of endocrine tests in adults and children,* ed 2, Chicago, 1978, Year Book Medical Publishers.
2. Loraine JA, Bell ET: *Hormone assays and their clinical application,* New York, 1976, Churchill Livingstone.
3. Moore A, Aitken R, Gaskell S, et al: Cortisol assays: guidelines for the provision of a clinical biochemistry service, *Ann Clin Biochem* 22:435-454, 1985.
4. Whitley RJ, Meikle AW, Watts NB: Endocrinology. In Burtis CA, Ashwood ER, editors: *Tietz textbook of clinical chemistry,* ed 2, Philadelphia, 1994, WB Saunders.
5. Tulchinsky D, Ryan KJ, editors: *Maternal-fetal endocrinology,* Philadelphia, 1980, WB Saunders.
6. Endocrine Sciences: *Pediatric laboratory services,* Tarzana, CA, 1988, Endocrine Sciences.
7. Soldin OP, Hoffman EG, Waring MA, et al: Pediatric reference intervals for FSH, LH, estradiol, T3, free T3, cortisol and growth hormone on the DPC Immulite 1000, *Clin Chim Acta* in press, 2005.
8. Predine J, Merceron L, Barrier G, et al: Unbound cortisol in umbilical cord plasma and maternal plasma: a reinvestigation, *Am J Obstet Gynecol* 135:1104-1108, 1979.

TEST NAME AND METHOD	SPECIMEN REQUIREMENTS	REFERENCE INTERVAL, CONVENTIONAL	[INTERNATIONAL RECOMMENDED UNITS]	CHEMICAL INTERFERENCES AND IN VIVO EFFECTS
Cortisol Production Rate (CPR)[1,2] *Isotope dilution* Dose: 0.2 µCi ^{14}C-cortisol, IV, at 8:00 AM	Urine, 24 hr, after injection. Refrigerate during collection.	*mg/day* 10-25 × 2.76 Lean subjects: 13-35 Obese subjects: 13-52 Lean and obese subjects: 4-19 mg/g creatinine × 0.312	*µmol/day* [28-69] [36-97] [36-144] [1.2-5.9 mmol/mol]	See *Cortisol, Total.*

1. Esteban NV, Loughlin T, Yergey AL, et al: Daily cortisol production rate in man determined by stable isotope dilution/mass spectrometry, *J Clin Endocrinol Metab* 72:39-45, 1991.
2. Boehringer Mannheim Corp.: *Chemstrip Micral Urine Test Strip package insert,* Indianapolis, IN, 1991, Boehringer Mannheim Corp.

| DIAGNOSTIC INFORMATION | REMARKS |

ratio. This suggests that amniotic fluid total cortisol may reflect initiation of fetal lung maturation. The ratio of amniotic fluid cortisol to cortisone bears a stronger relation to gestational age and lung maturity than do cortisol concentrations alone. The origin of amniotic fluid steroids is not well understood.[5]

↑ Cushing's syndrome, 33-182 mg/day [91-502 μmol/day]; 28-228 mg/g creatinine [8.7-71.2 mmol/mol creatinine].

Testing for CPR is not generally available and remains primarily a research tool. CPR is calculated by dividing the total dose of ^{14}C-cortisol injected by the specific activity of ^{14}C-labeled urinary cortisol metabolites. Obese subjects tend to have an elevated CPR compared with lean subjects. The effect can be eliminated by expressing the CPR as mg/g urine creatinine [mmol/mol creatinine].

TEST NAME AND METHOD	SPECIMEN REQUIREMENTS	REFERENCE INTERVAL, CONVENTIONAL [INTERNATIONAL RECOMMENDED UNITS]	CHEMICAL INTERFERENCES AND IN VIVO EFFECTS
Creatine kinase (CK), Total (EC 2.7.3.2)[1-4] *Enzymatic*	Serum or heparinized plasma; stable at room temperature for 4 hr, refrigerated for 5 days, frozen for 1-2 mo (maybe longer if frozen at −80° C).	*Reference range, U/L* Newborn and pediatric: 145-1578 (median, 382 U/L) Alter cesarean births[4]: 2-3× adult values 4 days: 3× adult values 6 wk-12 yr[5]: Adult values Adult males >19 yr: 20-200 U/L Adult females >19 yr: 20-180 U/L (Normal range can be assay and instrument dependent.) Heterogeneity of serum CK activities have been described among racial groups. African-American men > Caucasian men > African-American women > Caucasian women; 97.5th percentiles were as follows: 520 U/L, 370 U/L, 290 U/L, and 145 U/L, respectively.[6]	S ↑ V Muscular exercise (significant elevations), aminocaproic acid, amphotericin B, bucindolol, captopril, carbenoxolone, carbromal, carteolol, chlorpromazine, clofibrate, clonidine, colchicine, cyclopropane, diethyl ether, ethanol (alcoholics), gemfibrozil, halofenate, haloperidol, halothane, HMG CoA reductase inhibitors (e.g., lovastatin), isotretinoin, labetalol, lidocaine, lithium, D-penicillamine, perphenazine, pindolol, prochlorperazine, propranolol, quinidine; halothane and succinylcholine administered together during anesthesia; poisoning with barbiturates, carbon monoxide, drugs of abuse (e.g., cocaine, lysergide, phencyclidine), ethchlorvynol, tricyclics; drugs given by IM injection. S ↑ C Hemolysis, serum Hb >39 mg/dL [>4.65 µmol/L] due to adenylate kinase. Some methods (e.g., SMAC) are very sensitive to adenylate kinase interference. Bilirubin, lipemia, and heparin do not interfere. S ↓ Exposure of specimen to direct sunlight or to fluorescent light; loss of CO_2.

S,B ↑ Trauma, surgery, myocardial infarction, and loss of blood supply to any muscle, myopathic disorders of any cause (e.g., rhabdomyolysis, polymyositis, dermatomyositis, myocarditis, alcoholism), muscular dystrophies of all types (especially Duchenne dystrophy in early stages), Reye's syndrome, poisoning with coma, malignant hyperpyrexia and prolonged hypothermia, hypothyroidism, infectious diseases (e.g., typhoid fever), arrhythmias (infrequently), direct-current countershock, congestive heart failure, tachycardia, pulmonary emboli, tetanus, generalized convulsions, extensive brain infarction (may mask concomitant MI), pregnancy, hypoxic shock, neoplasms of prostate, bladder, and GI tract, pulmonary edema, delirium tremens, acute psychotic reaction, head injury, infarction of GI tract.

Most increases relate to diseases of skeletal or heart muscle, rarely to diseases of smooth muscle. Oral contraceptives cause lower activities.

Lower than normal values probably have no meaning but reflect either small muscle mass, sedentary lifestyle, or both. MI may occur in frail, elderly persons with CK remaining below the upper reference limit (URL).[8-16] Bed rest, even overnight, can lower CK activity by ≥20%.

Following MI, CK activity increases 4-8 hr after acute onset, activities peak at 12-36 hr, and usually return to normal activities in 3-4 days. Although total CK has been used as a diagnostic tool for MI detection, along with CK MB, it has predominantly been replaced with cardiac troponin I or T, due to the lack of myocardial tissue specificity. In developing countries, where cost is of primary concern, total CK still is a cost effective screening and diagnostic tool; however, clinical specificity is sacrificed (range, 70-80%).

The use of an optimized CK assay is encouraged because it possesses optimal reagent stability and maximally reactivates CK activity.

In the context of a cardiac (or coronary) care unit population, increased total CK has a sensitivity of ~97% and a specificity of 67% for the diagnosis of MI. Test performance varies with the selected decision threshold.[17-20]

TEST NAME AND METHOD	SPECIMEN REQUIREMENTS	REFERENCE INTERVAL, CONVENTIONAL [INTERNATIONAL RECOMMENDED UNITS]	CHEMICAL INTERFERENCES AND IN VIVO EFFECTS
Creatine kinase (CK), Total—CONT			S ↓ C Very high or low Mg level; contamination with oxidizing agents (e.g., hypochlorite), heparin. CK activity is found to the greatest extent in striated muscle (skeletal) and heart muscle. Therefore any type of injury to the muscle—skeletal or heart—will cause an elevation in serum CK, whether traumatic or pathologic.

1. Hørder M, Elser RC, Gerhardt W, et al: Approved IFCC recommendation on methods for the measurement of catalytic concentration of enzymes: Part 7. IFCC method for creatine kinase (ATP: creatine N-phosphotransferase, EC 2.7.3.2), *Eur J Clin Chem Clin Biochem* 29:435-456, 1991.

2. Committee on Enzymes of the Scandinavian Society for Clinical Chemistry and Clinical Physiology: Recommended method for the determination of creatine kinase in blood modified by the inclusion of EDTA, *Scand J Clin Lab Invest* 39:1-5, 1979.

3. Gerhardt W: Creatine kinase. In Bergmeyer HU, editor: *Methods of enzymatic analysis, vol III*, ed 3, Weinheim, 1983, Verlag Chemie.

4. Gruber W: Inhibition of creatine kinase activity by Ca^{2+} and reversing effect of ethylenediaminetetraacetate, *Clin Chem* 24:177-178, 1978.

5. Joupilla R, Joupilla P, Koivisto M, et al: Maternal, foetal, and neonatal blood-creatine-phosphokinase activities and creatine-phosphokinase isoenzymes after labour with and without epidural analgesia and after Caesarean section, *Acta Anaesthesiol Scand* 22:491-496, 1978.

6. Cherian AG, Hill JG: Age dependence of serum enzymatic activities (alkaline phosphatase, aspartate aminotransferase, and creatine kinase) in healthy children and adolescents, *Am J Clin Pathol* 70:783-789, 1978.

7. Black HR, Quallich H, Gareleck CB: Racial differences in serum creatine kinase levels, Am J Med 81:479-487, 1986.

8. Bilodeau L, Preese LM, Apple FS: Does low total creatine kinase rule out myocardial infarction? *Ann Intern Med* 116:523-524, 1992.

9. Clyne CA, Medeiros LJ, Marton KI: The prognostic significance of immunoradiometric CK-MB assay (IRMA) diagnosis of myocardial infarction in patients with low total CK and elevated MB isoenzymes, *Am Heart J* 118:901-906, 1989.

10. Cook JC, Wong E, Haywood JLJ: Creatine kinase: race-gender differences in patients hospitalized for suspected myocardial infarction, *J Natl Med Assoc* 82:249-254, 1990.

11. Dillon MC, Calbreath DF, Dixon AM, et al: Diagnostic problem in acute myocardial infarction. CK-MB in the absence of abnormally elevated total creatine kinase levels, *Ann Intern Med* 142:33-38, 1982.

12. Heller GV, Blaustein AS, Wei JY: Implications of increased myocardial isoenzyme level in the presence of normal serum creatine kinase activity, *Am J Cardiol* 57:24-27, 1983.

13. McQueen MJ, Strickland RD, Mori L: Detection of ischemic myocardial injury in patients with normal, or moderately elevated, serum CK and AST activities, *Clin Biochem* 15:138-140, 1982.

14. Vladutiu AO, Schachner A: Increased creatine kinase (CK) MB isoenzyme in patients with "normal" total CK activity suspected of acute myocardial infarction, *J Med* 20:73-81, 1989.

15. White RD, Grande P, Califf L, et al: Diagnostic and prognostic significance of minimally elevated creatine kinase-MB in suspected acute myocardial infarction, *Am J Cardiol* 55:1478-1484, 1985.

16. Yusuf S, Collins R, Lin L, et al: Significance of elevated MB isoenzyme with normal creatine kinase in acute myocardial infarction, *Am J Cardiol* 59:245-250, 1987.

17. Lee TH, Goldman L: Serum enzyme assays in the diagnosis of acute myocardial infarction: recommendations based on a quantitative analysis, *Ann Intern Med* 105:221-233, 1986.

18. Leung FY, Galbraith LV, Jablonsky G, et al: Re-evaluation of the diagnostic utility of serum total creatine kinase and creatine kinase-2 in myocardial infarction, *Clin Chem* 35:1435-1440, 1989.

19. Lott JA: Serum enzyme determinations in the diagnosis of acute myocardial infarction: an update, *Hum Pathol* 15:706-710, 1984.

20. Lott JA, Stang JM: Serum enzymes and isoenzymes in the diagnosis and differential diagnosis of myocardial ischemia and necrosis, *Clin Chem* 26:1241-1250, 1980.

TEST NAME AND METHOD	SPECIMEN REQUIREMENTS	REFERENCE INTERVAL, CONVENTIONAL [INTERNATIONAL RECOMMENDED UNITS]			CHEMICAL INTERFERENCES AND IN VIVO EFFECTS
Creatine Kinase Isoforms (CK Isoforms)[1-3] *EP*[4,5]	Serum. Store between −4 and −70° C. Add EDTA or EGTA to give a concentration of 5 mmol/L to prevent in vitro isoform generation.	*% of total activity* CK-MM$_1$[5]: 42-75 CK-MM$_2$: 18-51 CK-MM$_3$: 2-14	× 0.01	*Fraction of total activity* [0.42-0.75] [0.18-0.51] [0.02-0.14]	None found.

1. Apple FS: Acute myocardial infarction and coronary reperfusion—serum cardiac markers for the 1990s, *Am J Clin Pathol* 97:217-226, 1992.

2. Armbruster DA: The genesis and clinical significance of creatine kinase isoforms, *Lab Med* 22:325-334, 1991.

3. Wu AHB: Creatine kinase MM and MB isoforms, *Lab Med* 23:303-305, 1992.

4. Panteghini M, Cuccia C, Malchiodi A, et al: Isoforms of creatine kinase MM and MB in acute myocardial infarction: a clinical evaluation, *Clin Chim Acta* 155:1-10, 1986.

5. Wu AHB, Gornet TG, Wu VH, et al: Early diagnosis of acute myocardial infarction by rapid analysis of creatine kinase isoenzyme-3 (CK-MM) subtypes, *Clin Chem* 33:358-362, 1987.

6. Jaffe AS, Serota H, Grace A, et al: Diagnostic changes in plasma creatine kinase isoforms early after the onset of acute myocardial infarction, *Circulation* 74:105-109, 1986.

7. Bhayana V, Cohoe S, Leung FY, et al: Diagnostic evaluation of the assays for creatine kinase-2 mass and creatine kinase-3 and -2 isoform ratios in the early diagnosis of acute myocardial infarction, *Clin Chem* 39:488-495, 1993.

8. Wu AH, Wang XM, Gornet TG, et al: Creatine kinase MB isoforms in patients with skeletal muscle injury: ramifications for early detection of acute myocardial infarction, *Clin Chem* 38:2396-2400, 1992.

9. Annesley AM, Strongwater SL, Schnitzer TJ: MM subisoenzymes of creatine kinase as an index of disease activity in polymyositis, *Clin Chem* 31:402-406, 1985.

Following AMI, the CK-MM$_3$ and the CK-MM$_3$/MM$_1$ ratio peak 18 and 10-12 hr, respectively, after chest pain. After reperfusion (spontaneously, or after treatments such as angioplasty or infusions with streptokinase or tissue plasminogen activator), peaks occur at 5-12 and 4-10 hr. Isoform profiles change before changes in total CK and CK-MB activities occur.[6]

ROC-curve analysis shows that the CK-MM isoform ratio (CK-MM$_3$/CK-MM$_1$) has greater diagnostic efficiency than CK-MB activity between 3 and 9 hr after the onset of chest pain, whereas the reverse is true for the period between 10 and 18 hr.[5] ROC-curve analysis also shows that the CK-MB and CK-MM isoform ratios have diagnostic efficiencies equivalent to the CK-2 mass assay in the 4-18 hr after onset of chest pain.[7]

Acute skeletal muscle injury produces an abnormal CK-2 isoform ratio during the first 12 hr following injury.[8]

In polymyositis, the isoform profile can reliably distinguish between a clinically stable (or improving) condition and clinical deterioration.[9]

Muscular exercise may cause significant elevations of CK-MM$_3$. Levels increase within 2 hr, peak at 6 hr, and then return to baseline values. Total CK does not increase significantly until 6 hr after exercise.

The gene products are CK-MMc (or CK-MM$_3$) and CK-MB$_2$. In blood, the C-terminal lysine residues of the M-subunits are removed one at a time by the action of the plasma enzymes carboxypeptidase N (arginine carboxypeptidase, EC 3.4.17.3) or B (EC 3.4.17.2) to produce the more anodic CK-MM$_2$ and then the most anodic form, CK-MM$_1$.

In the case of CK-MB, there are two isoforms, CK-MB$_2$ and CK-MB$_1$, the latter being the more anodic form.

CK isoforms are not widely used in clinical practice today due to the use of myoglobin, CK-MB mass, and cardiac troponins.

TEST NAME AND METHOD	SPECIMEN REQUIREMENTS	REFERENCE INTERVAL, CONVENTIONAL [INTERNATIONAL RECOMMENDED UNITS]		CHEMICAL INTERFERENCES AND IN VIVO EFFECTS

Creatine Kinase (CK) MB (CK-MB)

Immunoassay[1,2]

Point-of-care immunoassays assays also available[3]

Electrophoresis, immunoinhibition[4]

Serum, plasma (anticoagulant specifics can be found in manufacturers' package inserts), and whole blood for several POC assays have been shown to be acceptable.[5]

Assay	*LLD*	*95th or 99th*
Abbott AxSYM (n)	0.7	3.8
Bayer Centaur (s)	0.18	4.8
Beckman Access (p)	0.3	4.0
Dade-Behring Dimension (s)	0.5	3.1
DPC Immulite (s)	0.2	3.5
Ortho Vitros ECi (p)	0.6	3.4
Tosoh AIA 600II (b)	0.5	5.8
Roche Elecsys 2010 (s)	0.1	2.9
Biosite Triage (p)	1.0	4.3

All results in mcg/L. Specimen types as indicated in the manufacturer's package inserts used for determination of 99th percentile reference ranges; s = serum, p = heparin plasma, b = both, n = not specified. Most commercial assays use the "Conan" anti-CK-MB antibody licensed from Washington University.[6]

All concentrations >99th limit are designated as irreversible myocardial injury. In the presence of the clinical setting of ischemia, an increased cTn >99th percentile indicative of acute myocardial infarction (MI).

CK-MB, as has been recognized for years for total CK, demonstrates a significant 1.5- to 3-fold higher 99th percentile reference limits for males versus females.

Reference range at the 99th percentile						
Assay	*All*	*M*	*F*	*White*	*Black*	*Hispanic*	*Asian*
AxSYM	7.6	8.7	4.8	5.9	9.6	3.7	7.0
Centaur	3.28	4.38	1.68	1.78	4.75	0.89	1.15
Access	7.9	8.2	5.6	6.6	9.3	3.4	5.4
Dimension	3.9	4.2	3.1	3.5	4.2	2.5	3.3
Vitros ECi	4.1	4.2	2.9	4.1	4.0	1.9	3.7
AIA 600II	5.7	5.6	3.6	5.3	6.1	3.2	3.3
Elecsys 2010	7.0	7.6	4.7	4.1	4.0	1.9	3.7

A standard reference material for CK-MB is available.[7]

No interferences from other proteins have been documented.

Although the measurement of CK-MB in serum or plasma has been replaced in many medical centers with cTnT or cTnI,[8] it is still a useful laboratory test for the diagnosis of AMI, assessment of reinfarction, and detection of injury following PCI and recommended as an acceptable alternative to cardiac troponin. The classic time versus CK-MB level (activity or mass concentration) pattern observed following the onset of chest pain in AMI shows an initial increase takes 4-6 hr to increase above the upper reference limit. Peak levels occur at ~24 hr.[9] Return to normal (baseline) takes 48-72 hr ($t_{1/2}$ of CK-MB is 10-12 hr). Factors that may affect the classic pattern include size of infarction, CK-MB composition in the myocardium, concomitant skeletal muscle injury, and reperfusion (spontaneous, following thrombolytics, or following angioplasty). The lack of tissue specificity and differentiation of increased CK-MB due to the heart or skeletal muscle becomes important because a normal percentage of CK-MB of total CK activity may be misleading if concomitant injury occurs in skeletal muscle coincident with an AMI. The fractional amount of CK-MB release from the heart would be obscured by the large release of total CK from skeletal muscle injury.

Clinical studies comparing CK-MB mass to activity assays have shown that CK-MB mass measurements provide earlier detection of abnormal CK-MB levels following AMI. Thus clinical sensitivity is improved without sacrificing specificity. Because >50% of patients with AMI present to emergency departments with a nondiagnostic ECG (NSTEMI), rapid and sensitive assays for the measurement of CK-MB will help clarify the diagnosis in those patients. As described by the ESC/ACC consensus document on the redefinition of AMI, sampling at a minimal 6-9 hr after presentation is suggested before ruling out AMI. The improved immunoassays are able to quantitate significant changes during the early hours after the onset of chest pain within the normal range for CK-2 to facilitate earlier AMI detection.

Clinical use of the percent relative index (%RI; %RI = [CK-MB mass/total CK activity × 100]) or %CK-MB (CK-MB activity/total CK × 100) aids in the interpretation of CK-MB concentrations for the detection of AMI. Although not absolute, an increased %CK-MB or %RI points toward the heart as the source of CK-MB in serum. However, the %RI and %CK-MB should not be used for interpretation when the total CK activity remains within the reference interval because of the potential of falsely elevated values. It is also confounded if there is any concomitant skeletal muscle injury because the sensitivity for the detection of cardiac events is lost.[10]

Three cytosolic isoenzymes (CK-MM, CK-MB, CK-BB) and one mitochondrial isoenzyme (CK-Mt) of CK (~MW 80 kDa for all) have been identified and can be separated by electrophoresis. Three different genes have been identified that encode for and are specific for CK-M, CK-B, and mitochondrial CK subunits.[11] Although CK-MM is predominant in both heart and skeletal muscle, CK-MB has been shown to be more specific for the myocardium, which contains 10-20% of its total CK activity as CK-MB, compared with amounts varying from 2-5% in skeletal muscle.

Early studies involving animal hearts or specimens obtained at autopsy from human hearts suggested a uniform distribution of CK-MB ranging from 5-50% of the total CK activity. However, it has been shown that the proportion of CK-MB was 6-15% lower in the surrounding normal areas of tissue than in infarcted myocardium in humans. Further, in response to acute and chronic coronary artery occlusion in a dog model, myocardium showed twofold to threefold increases in CK-MB in both ischemic and nonischemic myocardium. When studied more completely in humans, CK-MB concentrations ranged from 15-24% of total CK in myocardial tissue obtained from patients with left ventricular hypertrophy (LVH) due to aortic stenosis, from patients with CAD without LVH, and from patients with CAD and LVH due to aortic stenosis. In contrast, patients with normal left ventricular tissue had a low percentage of CK-MB (<2%). These data suggest that changes in the CK isoenzyme distribution are dynamic and occur in hypertrophied and diseased human myocardium. Diseased cells also have less total CK per cell.

Normal skeletal muscle, depending on its location, contains very little CK-MB. Percentages as high as 5-7% have been reported, but <2% is much more common.[12] There are some differences related to slow versus fast twitch muscle and thus to race. Severe skeletal muscle injury following trauma or surgery can lead to absolute elevations of CK-MB above the upper reference limit of CK-MB in serum. However, the percent CK-MB in serum would be low (percentages advocated vary but when comparing activity to activity a percentage or <5% is often used and when one compares CK activity to CK-MB mass, a percentage of <2.5% is usually advocated). Increases in serum total CK and CK-MB in several patient groups often present a diagnostic challenge to the clinician. Persistent elevations of serum CK-MB resulting from chronic muscle disease occur in patients with muscular dystrophy, end stage renal disease, polymyositis, and in healthy subjects who undergo extreme exercise or physical activities.[13] The increase in serum CK-MB in runners, for example, may be related to the adaptation by the skeletal muscle during regular training and after

TEST NAME AND METHOD	SPECIMEN REQUIREMENTS	REFERENCE INTERVAL, CONVENTIONAL [INTERNATIONAL RECOMMENDED UNITS]	CHEMICAL INTERFERENCES AND IN VIVO EFFECTS
Creatine Kinase (CK) MB (CK-MB)—CONT			
Immunochemical, CK-2 + CK-1 (Ortho Vitros), 37° C	Serum. Store at 4 or −20° C.	16 U/L; 4-25% [0.04-0.25, fraction] of total CK activity	The assay is specific for B-subunit activity, i.e., it will detect CK-2, CK-1, and macro CK (type 1) activities.

1. Uettwiller-Geiger D, Wu AHB, Apple FS, et al: Multicenter evaluation of an automated assay for troponin I, *Clin Chem* 48:869-876, 2002.

2. Apple FS, Maturen AJ, Mullins RE, et al: Multicenter clinical and analytical evaluation of the AxSYM troponin-I immunoassay to assist in the diagnosis of myocardial infarction, *Clin Chem* 45:206-212, 1999.

3. Apple FS, Christenson RH, Valdes R Jr, et al: Simultaneous rapid measurement of whole blood myoglobin, creatine kinase MB, and cardiac troponin I by the triage cardiac panel for detection of myocardial infarction, *Clin Chem* 45:199-205, 1999.

4. Wu AH, Bowers GN Jr: Evaluation and comparison of immunoinhibition and immunoprecipitation methods for differentiating MB and BB from macro forms of creatine kinase isoenzymes in patients and healthy individuals, *Clin Chem* 28:2017-2021, 1982.

5. Buttery JE, Stuart S, Pannall PR: Stability of the CK-MB isoenzyme on routine storage, *Clin Biochem* 25:11-13, 1992.

6. Vaidya HC, Maynard Y, Dietzler DN, et al: Direct measurement of creatine kinase-MB activity in serum after extraction with a monoclonal antibody specific to the MB isoenzyme, *Clin Chem* 32:657-663, 1986.

7. Christenson RH, Vaidya H, Landt Y, et al: Standardization of creatine kinase-MB (CK-MB) mass assays: the use of recombinant CK-MB as a reference material, *Clin Chem* 45:1414-1423, 1999.

8. Falahati A, Sharkey SW, Christensen D, et al: Implementation of serum cardiac troponin I as marker for detection of acute myocardial infarction [see comment], *Am Heart J* 137:332-337, 1999.

9. Wu AHB, Apple FS, Gibler WB, et al: National Academy of Clinical Biochemistry Standards of Laboratory Practice: recommendations for use of cardiac markers in coronary artery diseases, *Clin Chem* 45:1104-1121, 1999.

10. el Allaf M, Chapelle JP, el Allaf D, et al: Differentiating muscle damage from myocardial injury by means of the serum creatine kinase (CK) isoenzyme MB mass measurement/total CK activity ratio, *Clin Chem* 32:291-295, 1986.

11. Perryman MB, Strauss AW, Buettner TL, et al: Molecular heterogeneity of creatine kinase isoenzymes, *Biochim Biophys Acta* 747:284-290, 1983.

12. Orth HD: The cytoplasmic isoenzyes from human tissues. In Lang H, editor: *Creatine kinase isoenzymes. Pathophysiology and clinical application,* Berlin, 1982, Springer-Verlang.

13. Ionasescu V, Ionasescu R, Feld R, et al: Alterations in creatine kinase in fresh muscle and cell cultures in Duchenne dystrophy, *Ann Neurol* 9:394-399, 1981.

14. Apple FS, Rogers MA, Sherman WM, et al: Profile of creatine kinase isoenzymes in skeletal muscles of marathon runners, *Clin Chem* 30:413-416, 1984.

15. Hood D, Van Lente F, Estes M: Serum enzyme alterations in chronic muscle disease. A biopsy-based diagnostic assessment, *Am J Clin Pathol* 95:402-407, 1991.

acute exercise, resulting in increased CK-MB tissue concentrations.[14] The mechanism responsible for increased CK-MB in skeletal muscle following chronic muscle disease or injury is thought to be due to the regeneration process of muscle, with reexpression of CK-B genes similar to those found in the heart; thus giving rise to increased CK-MB levels in skeletal muscle. Thus skeletal muscle can become like heart muscle in its CK isoenzyme composition, with up to 50% CK-MB in some patients with severe polymyositis.[15]

Ion-exchange chromatography and electrophoresis have largely been replaced with immunoassays, although immunoinhibition techniques are still being used.

TEST NAME AND METHOD	SPECIMEN REQUIREMENTS	REFERENCE INTERVAL, CONVENTIONAL [INTERNATIONAL RECOMMENDED UNITS]			CHEMICAL INTERFERENCES AND IN VIVO EFFECTS
Creatinine[1-5] *Colorimetric, Jaffé* *(after adsorption);* *enzymatic*[6,7] *Jaffé, kinetic*[8]	Serum or plasma (fluoride or heparin). Stable refrigerated for 24 hr. Freeze for longer storage. (Fluoride and ammonium heparinate are not suitable for enzymatic method.)		*mg/dL*	μ*mol/L*	S ↑ V Drugs causing nephrotoxicity (Table II-6).
		Cord:	0.6-1.2 × 88.4	[53-106]	
		Newborn			S ↑ C Acetoacetate, acetohexamide (*ASTRA,* Beckman CX series, *aca*), acetone, ascorbic acid, cefaclor, cefamandole, cefazolin, ceforanide, cefoxitin, cephalothin, creatine (Vitros), flucytosine, lidocaine *(Vitros),* fructose, glucose, ibuprofen (deproteinization), levodopa, methyldopa, nitrofurantoin and piperacillin (Beckman *Seralyzer),* proline *(Vitros),* pyruvate, uric acid
		1-4 days:	0.3-1.0	[27-88]	
		Infant:	0.2-0.4	[18-35]	
		Child:	0.3-0.7	[27-62]	
		Adolescent:	0.5-1.0	[44-88]	
		18-60 yr[8]			
		M:	0.9-1.3	[80-115]	
		F:	0.6-1.1	[53-97]	
		60-90 yr			
		M:	0.8-1.3	[71-115]	
		F:	0.6-1.2	[53-106]	
		>90 yr			
		M:	1.0-1.7	[88-150]	
		F:	0.6-1.3	[53-115]	
					S ↓ C N-Acetylcysteine, bilirubin, cephalothin *(aca),* dipyrone, hemoglobin, lipemia
Enzymatic (creatinine amidohydrolase, sarcosine oxidase)[9]			*mg/dL*	μ*mol/L*	S ↑ C Bilirubin, benzyl alcohol
		0-1 yr:	0.04-0.33 × 88.4	[4-29]	
		2-5 yr:	0.04-0.45	[4-40]	
		6-9 yr:	0.20-0.52	[18-46]	S ↓ C Pyruvate with high LDH
		10 yr:	0.22-0.59	[19-52]	
		Adult			
		M:	0.62-1.10	[55-96]	
		F:	0.45-0.75	[40-66]	
Jaffé, manual	Urine, 24 hr. Stable if refrigerated up to 4 days. Freeze for longer storage.		*mg/kg/day*	μ*mol/kg/day*	U ↑ V Captopril, corticosteroids
		Infant:	8-20 × 8.84	[71-177]	
		Child:	8-22	[71-194]	
		Adolescent:	8-30	[71-265]	U ↑ C Ascorbic acid, cefamandole, cefazolin, cefoxitin, cephalothin, fructose, levodopa, methyldopa, nitrofurans
		Adult			
		M:	14-26	[124-230]	
		F:	11-20	[97-177]	
		Declines with age to 10 mg/kg/day [88.4 μmol/kg/day] at age 90 yr. Decline starts in fifth decade.			U ↓ V Androgens and anabolic steroids, thiazides
		Or			
			mg/day	*mmol/day*	
		M:	800-2000 × 0.00884	[7.1-17.7]	
		F:	600-1800	[5.3-15.9]	

DIAGNOSTIC INFORMATION	REMARKS

S ↑ Renal function impairment, both acute and chronic, from any cause (perfusion deficits, intrinsic renal diseases, and postrenal obstruction to urine flow); active acromegaly and gigantism, hyperthyroidism, meat meals

Creatinine is not a sensitive indicator of early renal disease. Plasma creatinine is less affected than urea by dietary intake. Lipemia and hemolysis cause false elevations on the *aca*. Ketosis causes false elevations with Beckman CX series.

S ↓ Debilitation (due to increased age or decreased muscle mass), pregnancy (especially first and second trimester)

For each 50% reduction in GFR, serum creatinine doubles. In chronic renal disease, the plasma level may be more sensitive to changes in glomerular function than creatinine clearance, which may be factitiously higher than the true value.[1]

Reaction temperatures >30° C cause overestimation of creatinine because of effects of interfering substances. With enzymatic methods, prompt separation of cells and serum is required to avoid ammonia production in sample.

U ↑ Exercise, acromegaly, gigantism, diabetes mellitus, infections, hypothyroidism, meat meals

U ↓ Hyperthyroidism, anemia, paralysis, muscular dystrophy, diseases with decreased muscle mass (e.g., neurogenic atrophy, polymyositis, etc.), inflammatory disease affecting muscle, metabolic disease affecting muscle, advanced renal disease, leukemia, vegetarian diets

Creatinine is decreased unilaterally in urine from a kidney affected by renal stenosis.

Determination of urine creatinine concentrations is of little or no help in evaluation of renal function unless it is done as part of a creatinine clearance test. Because the excretion of creatinine in one given person is relatively constant (assuming a constant diet), 24-hr urine creatinine levels are used as an approximate check on the completeness of a 24-hr urine collection, especially in serial collections.

TEST NAME AND METHOD	SPECIMEN REQUIREMENTS	REFERENCE INTERVAL, CONVENTIONAL [INTERNATIONAL RECOMMENDED UNITS]		CHEMICAL INTERFERENCES AND IN VIVO EFFECTS

Creatinine—CONT

Random urine[10]:

		mg/dL		mmol/L
M				
	<40 yr:	24-392	× 0.0884	[2.12-3.46]
	≥40 yr:	22-328		[1.94-2.90]
F				
	<40 yr:	16-327		[1.41-2.89]
	≥40 yr:	15-278		[1.32-2.46]

Amniotic fluid. Refrigerate. Freeze if analysis is delayed >24 hr.

>37 wk: >2.0 mg/dL × 88.4 [>177 μmol/L]

1. Eastham RD: *Biochemical values in clinical medicine,* ed 7, Bristol, UK, 1985, John Wright and Sons, Ltd.
2. Friedman RB, Anderson RE, Entine SM, et al: Effects of diseases on clinical laboratory tests, *Clin Chem* 26(suppl), 1980.
3. Henry JB, editor: *Clinical diagnosis and management by laboratory methods,* ed 18, Philadelphia, 1991, WB Saunders.
4. Jacobs DS, Kasten BL, DeMott WR, et al, editors: *Laboratory test handbook,* ed 2, Stow, OH, 1990, LexiComp, Inc.
5. Wallach J, editor: *Interpretation of diagnostic tests,* ed 5, Boston, 1992, Little, Brown and Co.
6. Henry RJ, Cannon DC, Winkelman JW, editors: *Clinical chemistry: principles and techniques,* ed 2, Hagerstown, MD, 1974, Harper and Row.
7. Tietz NW, editor: *Fundamentals of clinical chemistry,* ed 3, Philadelphia, 1987, WB Saunders.
8. Tietz NW, Shuey DF, Wekstein DR: Laboratory values in fit aging individuals—sexagenarians through centenarians, *Clin Chem* 38:1167-1185, 1992.
9. Sugita O, Uchiyama K, Yamada T, et al: Reference values of serum and urine creatinine, and of creatimne clearance by a new enzymatic method, *Ann Clin Biochem* 29:523-528, 1992.
10. Bond LW, Garber C, Ottinger W, et al: Reference intervals for common analytes in random urine specimens, *Clin Chem* 55: submitted, 2005.

TEST NAME AND METHOD	SPECIMEN REQUIREMENTS	REFERENCE INTERVAL, CONVENTIONAL [INTERNATIONAL RECOMMENDED UNITS]			CHEMICAL INTERFERENCES AND IN VIVO EFFECTS
Creatinine Clearance (Endogenous)[1-5]	Serum or plasma. Collect at midpoint of the test period. See *Creatinine.*	*Mean creatinine clearance mL/min/1.73 m²*		*Mean creatinine clearance mL/sec/m²*	↑ V Amino acids, furosemide, methylprednisone, carbenoxolone
	Urine.[5] Complete collection during precisely timed intervals (4, 12, or 24 hr). Keep sample refrigerated or on ice during collection and refrigerate until analysis.	0-1 yr[5]:	72 × 0.00963	[0.69]	↑ C Levodopa (Jaffé method)
		1 yr:	45	[0.43]	
		2 yr:	55	[0.53]	↓ V Diazoxide, thiazides, triamterene, transient effect of cannabis and heroin; nephrotoxic drugs (Table II-6). See also *Glomerular Filtration Rate.*
		3 yr:	60	[0.58]	
		4 yr:	71	[0.68]	
		5 yr:	73	[0.70]	
		6 yr:	64	[0.62]	
		7 yr:	67	[0.65]	
		8 yr:	72	[0.69]	
		9 yr:	83	[0.80]	
		10 yr:	89	[0.86]	

DIAGNOSTIC INFORMATION	REMARKS
AF ↑ Diabetic mothers and preeclampsia (implies greater maturity than actually attained by fetus)	Amniotic fluid creatinine >2.0 mg/dL [>177 μmol/L] is an index of fetal maturity if the maternal serum creatinine is normal.
See *Glomerular Filtration Rate.*	The patient must be adequately hydrated before and throughout the test to provide urine flow >2 mL/min [0.03 mL/sec]. Correct for body surface area of the patient. Avoid tea, coffee, and drugs during the test. Stop treatment with ACTH, cortisone, or thyroxine before the test. Avoid vigorous exercise during the test. In severe renal impairment, the serum creatinine level is more indicative of GFR than is the creatinine clearance value, which is factitiously higher than the true clearance value.

TEST NAME AND METHOD	SPECIMEN REQUIREMENTS	REFERENCE INTERVAL, CONVENTIONAL [INTERNATIONAL RECOMMENDED UNITS]	CHEMICAL INTERFERENCES AND IN VIVO EFFECTS

Creatinine Clearance (Endogenous)—CONT

11 yr:	92	[0.89]
12 yr:	109	[1.05]
13-14 yr:	86	[0.83]
20-29 yr
M:	94-140	[0.91-1.35]
F:	72-110	[0.69-1.06]
30-39 yr
M:	59-137	[0.57-1.32]
F:	71-121	[0.68-1.17]

For each decade thereafter, values decrease
~6.5 mL/min based on 1.73 m^2 body surface
[~0.06 mL/sec/m^2].[6]

Impairment	*mL/min/ 1.73 m^2*		*mL/sec/m^2*
Borderline:	62.5-80	×0.00963	[0.60-0.77]
Slight:	52-63		[0.50-0.60]
Mild:	42-52		[0.41-0.50]
Moderate:	28-42		[0.27-0.40]
Marked:	<28		[<0.27]

1. Eastham RD: *Biochemical values in clinical medicine,* ed 7, Bristol, UK, 1985, John Wright and Sons, Ltd.
2. Henry JB, editor: *Clinical diagnosis and management by laboratory methods,* ed 18, Philadelphia, 1991, WB Saunders.
3. Jacobs DS, Kasten BL, DeMott WR, et al, editors: *Laboratory test handbook,* ed 2, Stow, OH, 1990, LexiComp, Inc.
4. Tietz NW, editor: *Fundamentals of clinical chemistry,* ed 3, Philadelphia, 1987, WB Saunders.
5. Wallach J, editor: *Interpretation of diagnostic tests,* ed 5, Boston, 1992, Little, Brown and Co.
6. Rowe JW: The influence of age on renal function, *Res Staff Phys* 24:49-55, 1978.

CSF Pressure[1,2]	CSF. Before collecting three 2- to 4-mL samples in sterile tubes, always measure the opening pressure. If pressure is >180 mm of water, do not remove more than 1-2 mL of fluid.[1]	50-180 mm water, for adult patient in the lateral recumbent position *10-100 mm water, for children aged <8 yr*	Inhalational anaesthetics will increase CSF pressure by cerebral vasodilation.[3]

DIAGNOSTIC INFORMATION	REMARKS

↑ Mass lesions (e.g., tumor abscess or intracerebral hemorrhage), cerebral edema, meningitis (tuberculous, acute pyogenic, or cryptococcal), coccidioidomycosis, intracranial venous sinus thrombosis, impaired CSF resorption secondary to elevated CSF protein or subarachnoid hemorrhage, acute blood hyposmolality, congestive heart failure, acute superior vena cava obstruction, choroid plexus tumor, toxoplasmosis, lead encephalopathy, amebic meningoencephalitis with elevations in CSF proteins.

Cerebellar herniation or spinal cord compression above the puncture site is suggested if CSF pressure decreases by 25-50% on removal of 1-2 mL fluid.

CSF pressure is directly related to jugular and vertebral venous pressures, and therefore minor variations (5-10 mm) occur with respiration. Any increase in abdominal pressure (coughing, sneezing, straining, or breath-holding) may cause an artifactual elevation of CSF pressure. If the initial pressure is normal and there is clinical suspicion of subarachnoid block, spinal cord tumor, obstruction at the foramen magnum, or sinus thrombosis, a jugular compression (Queckenstedt test) may be performed. (Compression of both jugular veins normally increases CSF pressure rapidly to >300 mm, with rapid return to normal values on cessation of compression. In a "positive" Queckenstedt test, the increase in CSF pressure is decreased or delayed. About 80% of patients with cord compression have a positive Queckenstedt test.)[1]

TEST NAME AND METHOD	SPECIMEN REQUIREMENTS	REFERENCE INTERVAL, CONVENTIONAL [INTERNATIONAL RECOMMENDED UNITS]				CHEMICAL INTERFERENCES AND IN VIVO EFFECTS

CSF Pressure—CONT

1. Henry JB, editor: *Clinical diagnosis and management by laboratory methods,* ed 18, Philadelphia, 1991, WB Saunders.
2. Wallach J, editor: *Interpretation of diagnostic tests,* ed 5, Boston, 1992, Little, Brown and Co.
3. Gallagher A, Pike M, Berg S: Beware CSF pressure measured under general anaesthesia, *Arch Dis Child* 89:691, 2004.
4. Mokri B: Spontaneous low cerebrospinal pressure/volume headaches, *Curr Neurol Neurosci Rep* 4:117-124, 2004.

Cyanide[1]	Serum. Store at 4-8° C.		*mg/L*		*μmol/L*	Sulfide interferes with
		Nonsmokers[3]:	0.004	× 38.4	[0.15]	some methods using ion-
Colorimetric,		Smokers:	0.006		[0.23]	selective electrodes.
ion-selective		Nitroprusside				
potentiometry,[2]		therapy:	0.01-0.06		[0.38-2.30]	↑ V Nitroprusside
microdiffusion,		Toxic				(excessive rate of
GC (electron		concentration:	>0.1		[>3.84]	administration)
capture or						
nitrogen-	Blood (fluoride/ox-	Nonsmokers:	0.016		[0.61]	
phosphorus	alate). Store at 4-8° C.	Smokers:	0.041		[1.57]	
detector),		Nitroprusside				
GC-MS, HPLC[3]		therapy:	0.05-0.50		[1.92-19.20]	
		Toxic				
		concentration:	>1.00		[>38.40]	

1. Baselt RC: *Biological monitoring methods for industrial chemicals,* Davis, CA, 1980, Biomedical Pub.
2. Baselt RC: *Analytical procedures for therapeutic drug monitoring and emergency toxicology,* ed 2, Littleton, MA, 1987, PSG Publishing Co., Inc.
3. Toida T, Togawa T, Tanabe S, et al: Determination of cyanide and thiocyanate in blood plasma and red cells by high-performance liquid chromatography with fluorometric detection, *J Chromatogr* 308:133-142, 1984.

3',5'-Cyclic	Plasma (EDTA). Do		*ng/mL*[2]		*nmol/L*	↑ V A number of drugs
Adenosine	not use heparin or cit-	M:	4.6-8.6	× 3.04	[14-26]	and hormones exert their
Monophosphate	rate. Separate within	F:	4.3-7.6		[13-23]	pharmacological action by
(cAMP)[1]	1 hr of collection and					increasing the concentra-
	freeze.					tion of cAMP at the tissue
RIA						

DIAGNOSTIC INFORMATION	REMARKS

↓ CSF leakage (e.g., dural tear, CSF rhinorrhea, previous lumbar puncture), complete spinal subarachnoid block (e.g., neoplasms, abscess, herniated intervertebral disc, vertebral fracture, adhesions), circulatory collapse, severe dehydration, acute blood hyperosmolality, diabetic coma,[2] spontaneous intracranial hypotension syndrome[4]

Adverse effects include dizziness, weakness, mental and motor impairment, and sudden death.

Exposure to cyanide may occur by inhalation of hydrocyanic acid or ingestion of salts. Fumes from burning nitrogen-containing products contain cyanide and are a hazard to firefighters. Ingestion of cyanogenetic foods (some fruit seeds) or Laetrile (*l*-mandelonitrile-β-glucuronic acid) may produce cyanide poisoning. Eighty percent of a cyanide dose is converted to thiocyanate via rhodanase in the liver.

Kinetic values
$t_{1/2}$: 44-66 hr

See *Thiocyanate*.

Limited clinical utility except in calculating the nephrogenous portion of the total urinary cAMP.

A small circadian rhythm has been demonstrated in plasma with a peak at 12:00 PM and lowest level at late evening. In urine, this diurnal variation is unimportant. In normal individuals, about half of the total urinary cAMP is derived from glomerular filtration of plasma cAMP. The remaining urinary

TEST NAME AND METHOD	SPECIMEN REQUIREMENTS	REFERENCE INTERVAL, CONVENTIONAL [INTERNATIONAL RECOMMENDED UNITS]		CHEMICAL INTERFERENCES AND IN VIVO EFFECTS

3′,5′-Cyclic Adenosine Monophosphate—CONT

	Urine, random, 2 hr, or 24 hr. Collect timed specimens with boric acid or thymol as preservative. Store frozen at −20° C.	*mg/g creatinine*[3]	*μmol/mol creatinine*	level. These include ADH, corticotropin, glucagon, parathyroid hormone, phenothiazines, prostaglandins, thyrotropin, and xanthines (theophylline). At present, data are lacking to substantiate an effect on plasma levels. Parathyroid hormone can increase urinary levels.
		Total: 0.29-2.10 × 344	[100-723] [or 0.89-6.38 μmol/g creatinine]	
		mg/day[4] 0.33-3.58 × 3.04	*μmol/day* [1.0-10.9]	
		mcg/dL glomerular filtrate[1] 0.60-1.50 × 30.4	*nmol/L glomerular filtrate* [18.3-45.5]	
		mmol/g creatinine[5]	*nmol/mol creatinine*	
		Nephrogenous: <3.1 × 113.1	[<351]	
		mcg/dL glomerular filtrate[1] 0.09-0.92 × 30.4	*nmol/L glomerular filtrate* [2.9-28.1]	
	CSF	4.9-9.9 ng/mL × 3.04	[15-30 nmol/L][6]	

1. Aurbach GD, Marx SJ, Spiegel AM: Parathyroid hormone, calcitonin, and the calciferols. In Wilson JD, Foster DW, editors: *Williams textbook of endocrinology,* ed 8, Philadelphia, 1992, WB Saunders.
2. Chiang CS, Kowalski AJ: cAMP radioimmunoassay without interference from calcium or EDTA, *Clin Chem* 28:150-152, 1982.
3. Turner GA, Ellis RD, Guthrie D, et al: Levels of adenosine 3′,5′ cyclic monophosphate and guanosine 3′,5′ cyclic monophosphate in single urine specimens collected from a large population of healthy subjects, *Ann Clin Biochem* 19:77-82, 1982.
4. Sato T, Saito K, Takezawa J, et al: Urinary excretion of cyclic nucleotides and principal electrolytes in healthy humans of different ages, *Clin Chim Acta* 110:215-225, 1981.
5. SmithKline Beecham Clinical Laboratories: *Southwest service manual,* Tucker, GA, 1986, SmithKline Beecham Clinical Laboratories.
6. Eastham RD: *Biochemical values in clinical medicine,* ed 7, Bristol, UK, 1985, John Wright and Sons, Ltd.

DIAGNOSTIC INFORMATION	REMARKS

U ↑ Primary hyperparathyroidism (about 85% of patients), humoral hypercalcemia of malignancy (~50% of patients), osteomalacia due to vitamin D deficiency, calcium malabsorption, calcium urolithiasis associated with hypercalciuria, type II pseudohypoparathyroidism, mania, familial Mediterranean fever

U ↓ Hypoparathyroidism, type I pseudohypoparathyroidism, depression

portion is synthesized by the kidney and excreted by renal tubular cells. This latter portion of the total urinary cAMP is known as nephrogenous cAMP and is under direct influence of PTH. Plasma cAMP assays have limited clinical utility except in calculating the nephrogenous portion of the total urinary cAMP. Total urinary cAMP can be expressed as a rate per unit time or per gram creatinine. Because rates can vary with illness or sex, it is preferable to express total cAMP as a function of GFR using urine and serum creatinine levels:

$$cAMP_u \times \left(\frac{Cr_s}{Cr_u}\right) = cAMP_u \text{ (total)}$$

$cAMP_u$ (total) = nmol/dL glomerular filtrate
Cr_s = serum creatinine in mg/dL
Cr_u = urine creatinine in g/L
$cAMP_u$ = urine cAMP in mmol/L

Nephrogenous cAMP can be calculated by subtracting the amount of cyclic AMP filtered (plasma cAMP × creatinine clearance) from the total urinary cAMP.

In routine clinical testing, urinary cAMP corrected for GFR is almost as good as nephrogenous cAMP for discriminating parathyroid secretory states. Because increased urinary cAMP excretion is associated with many cancers, this test should be used cautiously in a clinical diagnosis of hyperparathyroidism (see *Parathyroid Hormone*). The test, however, is very useful in evaluating states of PTH resistance and degrees of hypoparathyroidism.

CSF ↓ After intracranial hemorrhage or trauma

TEST NAME* AND METHOD	SPECIMEN REQUIREMENTS	REFERENCE INTERVAL, CONVENTIONAL [INTERNATIONAL RECOMMENDED UNITS]	CHEMICAL INTERFERENCES AND IN VIVO EFFECTS
Cyclic citrullinated peptide antibodies (CCP) *Solid phase EIA*	Serum, frozen or refrigerated is preferable.	<5 U: Negative >5 U: Positive Results are expressed in arbitrary units. Reference ranges may vary with reagent manufacturer.	None known.

1. Visser H, le Cessie S, Vos K, et al: How to diagnose rheumatoid arthritis early: a prediction model for persistent (erosive) arthritis, *Arthritis Rheum* 46:357-365, 2002.
2. Schellekens GA, Visser H, De Jong BA, et al: The diagnostic properties of rheumatoid arthritis antibodies recognizing a cyclic citrullinated peptide, *Arthritis Rheum* 43:155-163, 2000.

TEST NAME* AND METHOD	SPECIMEN REQUIREMENTS	REFERENCE INTERVAL, CONVENTIONAL [INTERNATIONAL RECOMMENDED UNITS]	CHEMICAL INTERFERENCES AND IN VIVO EFFECTS
CYFRA 21-1[1,2] *Immunoassay*	Serum, EDTA and heparinized plasma in some assays. Stable up to 4 wk at 2-8° C. For longer periods, freeze at −20° C or colder. Avoid repeated freeze-thaw cycles.	<3.3 ng/mL[3] × 1.0 [<3.3 mcg/L] *Reference ranges are assay specific.*	None found.

1. Barak V, Goike H, Panaretakis KW, et al: Clinical utility of cytokeratins as tumor markers, *Clin Biochem* 37:529-540, 2004.
2. Schneider PM, Metzger R, Brabender J, et al: Lung cancer. In Diamandis EP, Fritsche HA, Lilja H, et al, editors: *Tumor markers. Physiology, pathobiology, technology, and clinical applications,* Washington, DC, 2002, AACC Press.
3. Rastel D, Ramaioli A, Cornillie F, et al: CYFRA 21.1, a sensitive and specific new tumour marker for squamous cell lung cancer. Report of the first European multicentre evaluation, *Eur J Cancer* 30:601-606, 1994.
4. Nisman B, Barak V, Shapiro A, et al: Evaluation of urine CYFRA 21-1 for the detection of primary and recurrent bladder cancer, *Cancer* 94:2914-2922, 2002.

*Cystathionine can be found in the Appendix on p. 1761.

DIAGNOSTIC INFORMATION	REMARKS

Testing for CCP antibodies is useful for evaluating patients suspected of having rheumatoid arthritis (RA). Positive results occur in 60-80% of RA patients depending on disease severity.[1] False-positive results are uncommon, and the positive predictive value of CCP antibodies for RA is greater than rheumatoid factor. CCP antibodies occur in up to 30% of patients with seronegative RA (rheumatoid factor negative disease).

CCP autoantibodies react with epitopes that contain citrulline, including synthetic cyclic peptide fragments.[2] CCP autoantibodies may occur in patients with other connective tissue diseases, especially LE.

In non–small cell lung cancer (NSCLC), comprising squamous cell carcinoma, adenocarcinoma, and large cell carcinoma, the marker has utility for monitoring the course of disease and has prognostic value.[1,2] Applications of CYFRA 21-1 in urine may also exist for bladder cancer.[4] Serum concentrations may also be increased in patients with renal failure, liver cirrhosis, benign pulmonary disease such as fibrosis, tuberculosis, and chronic obstructive pulmonary disease. Levels are not affected by smoking status.[1,2]

Intermediate filament proteins of the cell cytoskeleton, types I (acidic proteins) and II (basic proteins), constitute the cytokeratins of which >20 proteins have been identified. Intact cytokeratins have low solubility; however, degraded fragments are soluble, and cytokeratins can be detected in blood, urine, cyst, fluids, ascites, pleural effusions, and CSF after release from tumor cells.[1,2]

CYFRA 21-1 measures fragments of cytokeratin 19 defined by the monoclonal antibodies KS19.1 and BM19.21 (Fujirebio Diagnostics, Inc., Malvern, PA). This test does not have FDA approval for clinical use.

TEST NAME AND METHOD	SPECIMEN REQUIREMENTS	REFERENCE INTERVAL, CONVENTIONAL [INTERNATIONAL RECOMMENDED UNITS]		CHEMICAL INTERFERENCES AND IN VIVO EFFECTS
Cystatin C[1] *Particle-enhanced nephelometric immunoassay (PENIA)*[2-5]	Serum or plasma (heparin or EDTA) Stable 7 days at −20 to 20° C, 6 mo at −80° C.[8] 3% difference in EDTA or Li heparin plasma values compared with serum.[9]	24-36 wk (premature): <1 yr: 1-17 yr: Adult: >65 yr:	*mg/L* 0.4-2.8 0.6-2.0 0.5-1.3 0.5-1.0 0.9-3.4	None found (PENIA).
Particle-enhanced turbidimetric immunoassay (PETIA)[6,7]	Significant (15%) reduction observed after multiple freeze/thaw cycles.[9]	0.2-18 yr: Adult:	0.7-1.4 0.5-1.2	↑ C hemolysis (PETIA)[11] ↑ C lipemia (PETIA)[11]
Particle-enhanced nephelometric immunoassay (PENIA)	Urine	<0.28 mg/L		None found.

1. Laterza OF, Price CP, Scott MG: Cystatin C: An improved estimator of glomerular filtration rate? *Clin Chem* 48:699-707, 2002.
2. Finney H, Newman DJ, Thakkar H, et al: Reference ranges for plasma cystatin C and creatinine measurements in premature infants, neonates, and older children, *Arch Dis Child* 82:71-75, 2000.
3. Finney H, Newman DJ, Price CP: Adult reference ranges for serum cystatin C, creatinine and predicted creatinine clearance, *Ann Clin Biochem* 37:49-59, 2000.
4. Uhlmann EJ, Hock KG, Issitt C, et al: Reference intervals for plasma cystatin C in healthy volunteers and renal patients, as measured by the Dade Behring BN II system, and correlation with creatinine, *Clin Chem* 47:2031-2033, 2001.
5. Finney H, Bates CJ, Price CP: Plasma cystatin C determinations in a healthy elderly population, *Arch Gerontol Geriatr* 29:75-94, 1999.
6. Bókenkamp A, Domanetzki M, Zinck R, et al: Cystatin C—a new marker of glomerular filtration rate in children independent of age and height, *Pediatrics* 101:875-881, 1998.
7. Erlandsen EJ, Randers E, Kristensen JH: Reference intervals for serum cystatin C and serum creatinine in healthy adults, *Clin Chem Lab Med* 36:393-397, 1998.
8. Erlandsen EJ, Randers E, Kristensen JH: Evaluation of the Dade Behring N Latex Cystatin C assay on the Dade Behring Nephelometer II system, *Scand J Clin Lab Invest* 59:1-8, 1999.
9. Finney H, Newman DJ, Gruber W, et al: Initial evaluation of cystatin C measurement by particle-enhanced immunonephelometry on the Behring nephelometer systems (BNA, BN II), *Clin Chem* 43:1016-1022, 1997.
10. Herget-Rosenthal S, Feldkamp T, Volbracht L, et al: Measurement of urinary cystatin C by particle-enhanced nephelometric immunoassay: precision, interferences, stability and reference range, *Ann Clin Biochem* 41:111-118, 2004.
11. Lewis AV, James TJ, McGuire JB, et al: Improved immunoturbidimetric assay for cystatin C, *Ann Clin Biochem* 38:111-114, 2001.

Cystatin C can be used to diagnose impaired renal function; its concentration in serum or plasma is increased in patients with reduced glomerular filtration rate (GFR). The reciprocal of serum cystatin C concentration has been shown to be more strongly correlated with GFR (as determined by "gold standard" methods measuring the clearance of exogenous substances like inulin or ^{51}Cr-EDTA) than the reciprocal of serum creatinine. Cystatin C increases more rapidly than creatinine in the early stages of GFR impairment.

Cystatin C is a low molecular weight (13 kD) cysteine protease inhibitor that is produced at a constant rate by all nucleated cells. It is freely filtered by the glomerulus and reabsorbed (but not secreted) by the renal tubules with no extrarenal excretion. Its concentration is not affected by diet, muscle mass, or acute inflammation, giving it an apparent advantage over serum creatinine and other proteins as a marker of renal function, particularly in pediatric patients, where near-adult levels are reached early in childhood. Cystatin C has been found to have improved clinical utility compared with serum creatinine in monitoring for early renal damage in patients receiving chemotherapy, patients with cirrhosis, rheumatoid arthritis, IgA nephropathy, and renal transplant patients.

Increased excretion in renal disorders. Good predictor of the severity of acute tubular necrosis.

TEST NAME AND METHOD	SPECIMEN REQUIREMENTS	REFERENCE INTERVAL, CONVENTIONAL [INTERNATIONAL RECOMMENDED UNITS]			CHEMICAL INTERFERENCES AND IN VIVO EFFECTS
Cystine [(Cys)2][1-5] *Ion-exchange chromatographic*	Plasma (heparin) or serum, fasting. Place blood in ice water immediately; separate and freeze within 1 hr of collection. Stable for 1 wk at $-20°$ C; for longer periods deproteinize and store at $-70°$ C.[6,7]		*mg/dL*	*μmol/L*	
		Premature 1 day:	0.78 ± 0.12 (SD) $\times 83.3$	$[65 \pm 10]$[10]	
		Newborn 1 day:	0.43-1.01	$[36-84]$[10]	
		1-3 mo:	0.65 ± 0.25 (SD)	$[54 \pm 21]$[10]	
		2-6 mo:	0.64-0.97	$[53-81]$[10]	
		3-10 yr:	0.54-0.92	$[45-77]$[10]	
		6-18 yr:	0.43-0.70	$[36-58]$[10]	
		Adult:	0.40-1.40	$[33-117]$[10]	
	Urine, 24 hr. Add 20 mL of toluene at start of collection. (Alternatively, refrigerate specimen during collection.) Store frozen at $-20°$ C.[8]		*mg/day*	*μmol/day*[10]	U ↑ V Cycloleucine, histidine, progesterone
		10 days-7 wk:	2.16-3.37 $\times 8.32$	$[18-28]$	
		3-12 yr:	4.9-30.9	$[41-257]$	
		Adult:	*mg/g* creatinine	*mmol/mol* creatinine	U ↓ V Ascorbic acid (after large intake),[11] penicillamine
		Or	8 ± 3(SD) $\times 0.94$	$[7.5 \pm 2.8]$	
			μmol/g creatinine[9]	*mmol/mol creatinine*	
		0-1 mo:	64-451 $\times 0.113$	$[7-51]$	
		1-6 mo:	66-375	$[7-42]$	
		6 mo-1 yr:	70-316	$[8-36]$	
		1-2 yr:	53-244	$[6-28]$	
		2-3 yr:	62-246	$[7-28]$	

1. Friedman RB, Young DS: *Effects of disease on clinical laboratory tests,* ed 2, Washington, DC, 1989, American Association for Clinical Chemistry.
2. Scriver CR, Beaudet AL, Sly WS, et al, editors: *The metabolic basis of inherited disease,* ed 6, New York, 1989, McGraw-Hill Publishing Co.
3. Young DS: *Effects of drugs on clinical laboratory tests,* ed 3, Washington, DC, 1990, American Association for Clinical Chemistry.
4. Bremer HJ, Duran M, Kamerling JP, et al: *Disturbances of amino acid metabolism: clinical chemistry and diagnosis,* Baltimore, 1981, Urban and Schwarzenburg.
5. Nyhan W, Sakait N. *Diagnostic recognition of genetic disease,* Philadelphia, 1987, Lea & Febiger.
6. Cummings JG: Routine amino acids analysis in the clinical laboratory, *Am Clin Prod Rev* Feb:20-25, 1988.
7. Schaefer A, Piquard F, Haberey P: Plasma amino acids analysis: effects of delayed samples preparation and of storage, *Clin Chim Acta* 164:163-169, 1987.
8. Pesce A, Kaplan L, editors: *Methods in clinical chemistry,* St. Louis, 1987, CV Mosby.
9. Mayo Medical Laboratories: *Test catalog,* Rochester, MN, 1993.
10. Shih V: *Laboratory techniques for the detection of hereditary metabolic disorders,* Boca Raton, FL, 1973, CRC Press.
11. Tsao C, Muyashita K: Effect of large intake of ascorbic acid on the urinary excretion of amino acids and related compounds, *IRCS Med Sci* 13:855-856, 1985.

DIAGNOSTIC INFORMATION	REMARKS
P ↑ Septic patients,[12] chronic renal failure P ↓ 1-2 days following abdominal surgery,[13] protein malnutrition	Results are expressed in terms of the half-cystine residues responsible for the disulfide linkage in proteins. Cysteine [(Cys)] is very unstable and undergoes spontaneous oxidation to the disulfide cystine [(Cys)2] in solution. Therefore the total (Cys)2 measured by most chromatographic methods always includes Cys. To measure Cys, the sulfhydryl group may be stabilized with iodoacetate or *N*-ethylmaleimide; this derivative can then be separated and measured. In cystinosis, plasma cystine is usually normal, but increased cystine may be found in tissues and cells.
U ↑ Cystinosis, cystinurias, cystinlysinuria, in first trimester of pregnancy (levels decrease thereafter) U ↓ Severely burned patients[14]	Urinary excretion is age-dependent. It is high in the first months of life but decreases thereafter. High levels of arginine, ornithine, and lysine are also seen in the cystinurias, cystine excretion is normal in dibasic aminoaciduria.

12. Freund H, Atamian S, Holyroyde J, et al: Plasma amino acids as predictors of the severity and outcome of sepsis, *Ann Surg* Nov:571-576, 1979.

13. Jain KM, Rush BF Jr, Seelig RF, et al: Changes in plasma amino acid profiles following abdominal operations, *Surg Gynecol Obstet* 152:302-306, 1981.

14. Mårtensson J, Larsson J, Norström H: Amino acid metabolism during the anabolic phase of severely burned patients: with special reference to sulfur amino acids, *Eur J Clin Invest* 17:130-135, 1987.

TEST NAME AND METHOD	SPECIMEN REQUIREMENTS	REFERENCE INTERVAL, CONVENTIONAL [INTERNATIONAL RECOMMENDED UNITS]	CHEMICAL INTERFERENCES AND IN VIVO EFFECTS
D-Dimer[1-5]	Plasma (citrate). Whole blood for SimpliRed D-dimer	Negative <0.5 mcg/mL FEU × 500 <0.25 ng/mL D-DU	None found.

1. Lewis SM, Bain BJ, Bates I, editors: *Dacie and Lewis practical hematology,* ed 9, Edinburgh, 2001, Churchill Livingstone.
2. Jacobs DS, Demott WR, Oxley DK, editors: *Laboratory test handbook,* ed 5, Hudson, OH, 2001, Lexi-Comp, Inc.
3. Keeling DM, Wright M, Baker P, et al: D-dimer for the exclusion of venous thromboembolism:comparison of a new automated latex particle immunoassay (MDA D-dimer) with an established enzyme-linked fluorescent assay (VIDAS D-dimer), *Clin Lab Haemost* 21:359-362, 1999.
4. Cunningham MT, Olson JD: Proficiency testing finds too-high cutoffs and more, *CAP Today* 19:54, 2005.
5. Freyburger G, Trillaud H, Labrouche S: D-dimer strategy in thrombosis exclusion: a gold standard approach in 100 patients suspected of deep venous thrombosis or pulmonary embolism: 8 DD methods compared, *Thromb Haemost* 79:32-37, 1998.

Deferoxamine Test[1-3] *Colorimetric, AAS* Dose: 15 mg deferoxamine mesylate/kg, IM[2]	Urine, 24 hr. Collect in iron-free container.	0.4-2.0 mg Fe/day × 17.91 [7.2-36.0 μmol Fe/day]	See *Iron.*

1. Henry JB, editor: *Clinical diagnosis and management by laboratory methods,* ed 18, Philadelphia, 1991, WB Saunders.
2. Edwards CQ, Carroll M, Bray P, et al: Hereditary hemochromatosis: diagnosis in siblings and children, *N Engl J Med* 297:7-13, 1977.
3. Edwards CQ, Du done MM, Skolnick MH, et al: Hereditary haemochromatosis, *Baillieres Clin Haematol* 11:411-435, 1982

DIAGNOSTIC INFORMATION	REMARKS

↑ Primary and secondary fibrinolysis; during thrombolytic therapy with tissue plasminogen activator; thrombosis, including deep vein thrombosis, pulmonary embolism, arterial thromboembolism, and DIC; vasoocclusive crises of sickle cell anemia; pregnancy (especially postpartum period); malignancy; surgery

Increased levels of D-dimer indicate a fibrin clot was formed and subsequently degraded by plasmin. Essentially, a D-dimer is present whenever the coagulation system has been activated, followed by fibrinolysis; therefore although a very sensitive test, it is not very specific.

The D-dimer can be measured by a variety of methods, semi-quantitative and quantitative, manual and automated, latex agglutination versus ELISA. The use of automated quantitative methods such as an automated latex particle immunoassay or a enzyme-linked fluorescent assay on modern coagulation analyzers have increased significantly over the past few years.[3]

These highly sensitive automated D-dimer tests reportedly may be used to exclude PE and DVT: a negative test essentially rules out thrombosis, but a positive test does not confirm the diagnosis, and further testing is recommended.[5]

↑ Genetic hemochromatosis (>10 mg Fe/day; >179 μmol Fe/day), other iron overload disorders

Test is an adjunctive test in detecting iron overload. Deferoxamine is a chelating agent with a high affinity for iron; it is used therapeutically in treating iron poisoning.

TEST NAME AND METHOD	SPECIMEN REQUIREMENTS	REFERENCE INTERVAL, CONVENTIONAL [INTERNATIONAL RECOMMENDED UNITS]			CHEMICAL INTERFERENCES AND IN VIVO EFFECTS
Dehydroepian-drosterone Sulfate (DHEA-S, DHEA-SO4)[1-3]	Serum or plasma (EDTA). Stable for 2 days at 4° C or for 2 mo at −20° C.	*mcg/dL*[4]		*μmol/L*	↑ V Clomiphene, danazol
		1-5 days			↓ V Dexamethasone,
		M: 108-406	× 0.027	[2.9-10.9]	prednisone, other gluco-
		F: 10-248		[0.3-6.7]	corticoids
		1 mo-5 yr			
RIA		M: 1-41		[0.03-1.1]	
		F: 5-55		[0.1-1.5]	See also *Dehydroepian-drosterone, Unconjugated.*
		6-9 yr			
		M: 2.5-145		[0.07-3.9]	
		F: 2.5-140		[0.07-3.8]	
		10-11 yr			
		M: 15-115		[0.4-3.1]	
		F: 15-260		[0.4-7.0]	
		12-17 yr			
		M: 20-555		[0.5-15.0]	
		F: 20-535		[0.5-14.4]	
		Puberty Tanner stage			
		1			
		M: 5-265		[0.1-7.2]	
		F: 5-125		[0.1-3.4]	
		2			
		M: 15-380		[0.4-10.3]	
		F: 15-150		[0.4-4.0]	
		3			
		M: 60-505		[1.6-13.6]	
		F: 20-535		[0.5-14.4]	
		4			
		M: 65-560		[1.8-15.1]	
		F: 35-485		[0.9-13.1]	
		5			
		M: 165-500		[4.4-13.5]	
		F: 75-530		[2.0-14.3]	
		Adults			
		M			
		19-30 yr: 125-619		[3.4-16.7]	
		31-50 yr: 59-452		[1.6-12.2]	
		51-60 yr: 20-413		[0.5-11.1]	
		61-83 yr: 10-285		[0.3-7.7]	
		F			
		19-30 yr: 29-781		[0.8-21.1]	
		31-50 yr: 12-379		[0.8-10.2]	
		Postmeno-pausal: 30-260		[0.8-7.0]	
	Amniotic fluid	10-50 ng/mL	× 2.71	[27-136 nmol/L]	

DIAGNOSTIC INFORMATION	REMARKS

↑ Females with hirsutism, acne; congenital adrenal hyperplasia, adrenal cortex tumors (values higher in adrenal carcinomas than in adrenal adenomas), Cushing's disease, ectopic ACTH-producing tumors; polycystic ovary syndrome

↑ Precocious puberty

↓ Adrenal insufficiency (primary or secondary)

DHEA-S originates almost exclusively in the adrenals, although some may be derived from the testes; none is produced by the ovaries. DHEA-S is weakly androgenic but is metabolized in peripheral tissues to testosterone and dihydrotestosterone. Plasma levels of DHEA-S are >1000 times those of DHEA and 10 times those of cortisol. Unlike DHEA, DHEA-S does not exhibit a marked diurnal variation and has a low clearance rate. Unlike testosterone, DHEA-S does not circulate bound to sex hormone.

Testing for DHEA-S instead of 17-KS in urine has been suggested for estimating adrenal androgen production. DHEA-S levels in men and women decline progressively with age.

Levels are increased in cord blood during pregnancy and decrease precipitously on delivery. Levels in premature infants are generally much higher than in full-term infants. Pregnancy and oral contraceptives induce a moderate decrease. Virilizing ovarian tumors rarely produce DHEA-S.

In addition to DHEA-S, other plasma markers of androgen excess are available. See *Testosterone, Total; Testosterone, Free; Dihydrotestosterone; Androstenedione;* and *3α-Androstanediol Glucuronide.*

AF ↓ Anencephaly

TEST NAME AND METHOD	SPECIMEN REQUIREMENTS	REFERENCE INTERVAL, CONVENTIONAL [INTERNATIONAL RECOMMENDED UNITS]		CHEMICAL INTERFERENCES AND IN VIVO EFFECTS

Dehydroepiandrosterone Sulfate—CONT

1. Haning RV: Using DHEAS to monitor androgen disorders, *Contemp Obstet Gynecol* 18:117-132, 1981.
2. Korth-Schultz S, Levine LS, New ME: DHEA-S levels. A rapid test for abnormal adrenal androgen secretion, *J Clin Endocrinol Metab* 42:1005-1013, 1976.
3. Lobo RA, Paul WL, Goebelsmann U: Dehydroepiandrosterone sulfate as an indicator of adrenal androgen function, *Obstet Gynecol* 57:69-73, 1981.

TEST NAME AND METHOD	SPECIMEN REQUIREMENTS	REFERENCE INTERVAL, CONVENTIONAL	[INTERNATIONAL RECOMMENDED UNITS]	CHEMICAL INTERFERENCES AND IN VIVO EFFECTS
Dehydroepian-drosterone (DHEA), Unconjugated[1] *RIA*[2]	Serum. Samples may be stored refrigerated for 2 days or for 2 mo if frozen at −20° C.	*ng/dL*[5] Cord: 200-1590 × 0.0347 (x̄: 600) Premature: 80-3150 (x̄: 811) Newborn, 3 days: 65-1250 (x̄: 570) 1-30 days: 50-760 (x̄: 285) 1-6 mo: 26-385 (x̄:113) *ng/dL*[5] 6-12 mo: 18-95 × 0.0347 (x̄: 36) 1-6 yr: (x̄: 29) 6-8 yr: (x̄: 93) 8-10 yr: 31-345 (x̄: 156) Puberty Tanner stage 1 M: 31-345 (x̄: 156) F: 31-345 (x̄: 156) 2 M: 110-495 (x̄: 300) F: 150-570 (x̄: 330) 3 M: 170-585 (x̄: 390) F: 200-600 (x̄: 385)	*nmol/L* [6.9-55.1] [x̄: 20.8] [2.8-109.3] [x̄: 28.1] [2.3-43.4] [x̄: 19.8] [1.7-26.3] [x̄: 9.9] [0.9-13.4] [x̄: 3.9] *nmol/L* [0.6-3.3] [x̄: 1.3] [x̄: 1.0] [x̄: 3.2] [1.1-12.0] [x̄: 5.4] [1.1-12.0] [x̄: 5.4] [1.1-12.0] [x̄: 5.4] [3.8-17.2] [x̄: 10.4] [5.2-19.8] [x̄: 11.4] [5.9-20.3] [x̄: 13.5] [6.9-20.8] [x̄: 13.3]	S ↑ V Clomiphene, corticotropin S ↓ V Carbamazepine, testosterone, other glucocorticoids

4. Nichols Institute Reference Laboratories: *Test catalog,* San Juan Capistrano, CA, 1993, Nichols Institute Reference
    Laboratories.

↑ Adrenogenital syndrome due to deficiency of
3β-dehydrogenase, 21-hydroxylase, and 11β-hydroxylase; hirsutism, polycystic ovary syndrome, virilizing adrenal tumors, Cushing's disease, ectopic ACTH-producing tumors

↓ With increased age in men and women, hyperlipidemia, psychosis,[7] psoriasis. See *Dehydroepiandrosterone Sulfate.*

DHEA may be of value in assessing adrenarche and delayed puberty. During childhood and adolescence DHEA excretion is gradually increased. DHEA excretion increases rapidly after puberty, peaks at age 20 yr, and then decreases. It decreases in the elderly to a greater extent than do the other steroids. There is a moderate decrease during pregnancy.

DHEA is peripherally interconvertible with its sulfated conjugate (DHEA-S). DHEA has a diurnal variation (highest in morning), does not circulate bound to sex hormone binding globulin (SHBG), and is only weakly androgenic.

TEST NAME AND METHOD	SPECIMEN REQUIREMENTS	REFERENCE INTERVAL, CONVENTIONAL [INTERNATIONAL RECOMMENDED UNITS]		CHEMICAL INTERFERENCES AND IN VIVO EFFECTS

Dehydroepiandrosterone (DHEA), Unconjugated—CONT

	4		
	M:	160-640	[5.5-22.2]
		($\bar{x}$: 395)	[$\bar{x}$: 13.7]
	F:	200-780	[6.9-27.0]
		($\bar{x}$: 430)	[$\bar{x}$: 14.9]
	5		
	M:	250-900	[8.7-31.2]
		($\bar{x}$: 505)	[$\bar{x}$: 17.5]
	F:	215-850	[7.5-29.5]
		($\bar{x}$: 540)	[$\bar{x}$: 18.7]
	Adult		
	M[6]:	180-1250	[6.2-43.3]
	F:	130-980	[4.5-34.0]

Amniotic fluid[4]   Term: 1.5-15 ng/mL   × 3.47   [5.2-52.0 nmol/L]

GLC[3]

Urine, 24 hr. Preserve with boric acid. Store refrigerated.

	mg/day		*mmol/day*
Child			
0-1 yr:	<0.2	× 3.47	[<0.3]
1-2 yr:	<0.1		[<0.3]
3-5 yr:	<0.1		[<0.3]
6-9 yr:	<0.2		[<0.7]
10-15 yr:	<0.4		[<1.4]
Adult			
M:	<3.1		[<10.8]
F:	<1.5		[<5.2]

DHEA production rate:
8 mg/day   × 3.47   [28 μmol/day]

U ↑ V Corticotropin

U ↓ V Ampicillin (by 75%, after 6-day administration to pregnant females), dexamethasone, other glucocorticoids, oral contraceptives

1. Orth D, Kovacs D, DeBold C: The adrenal cortex. In Wilson JH, Foster DW, editors: *Williams textbook of endocrinology,* ed 8, Philadelphia, 1992, WB Saunders.
2. de Peretti E, Forest MG: Unconjugated dehydroepiandrosterone plasma levels in normal subjects from birth in adolescence in humans: the use of a sensitive radioimmunoassay, *J Clin Endocrinol Metab* 43:982-987. 1976.
3. Mayo Medical Laboratories: *Test catalog,* Rochester, MN, 1993, Mayo Medical Laboratories.
4. Tulchinsky D, Ryan KJ, editors: *Maternal-fetal endocrinology,* Philadelphia, 1980, WB Saunders.
5. Endocrine Sciences: *Pediatric laboratory services,* Tarzana, CA, 1992, Endocrine Sciences.
6. Nichols Institute Reference Laboratories: *Test catalog,* San Juan Capistrano, CA, 1993, Nichols Institute Reference Laboratories.
7. Erb JL, Kadane JB, Tourney G: Discrimination between schizophrenic and control subjects by means of plasma dehydroepiandrosterone measurements, *J Clin Endocrinol Metab* 52:181-186, 1981.

DIAGNOSTIC INFORMATION	REMARKS
AF ↑ Sulfatase deficiency in placenta (↑ DHEA-S, normal DHEA)	There is a normal increase of serum estradiol after IV infusion of DHEA-S. The increase distinguishes congenital adrenal hypoplasia from placental sulfatase deficiency where there is no increase in estradiol excretion.
AF ↓ Congenital adrenal hypoplasia	

TEST NAME AND METHOD	SPECIMEN REQUIREMENTS	REFERENCE INTERVAL, CONVENTIONAL [INTERNATIONAL RECOMMENDED UNITS]			CHEMICAL INTERFERENCES AND IN VIVO EFFECTS
11-Deoxycortico-sterone (DOC; 11-desoxycortico-sterone)[1] *RIA*	Plasma (heparin) or serum. Separate within 1 hr; store frozen.	Ad libitum diet, 8:00 AM	*ng/dL*	*nmol/L*	↑ V Spironolactone
		Cord[2]:	111-372 × 0.0303	[3.4-11.3]	
		2 hr postpartum[3]:	152-1870	[4.6-56.6]	
			ng/dL[2]	*pmol/L*	
		7 days:	<3-45 × 30.3	[<91-1360]	
		2 wk-7 yr:	<3-37	[<91-1120]	
		7-11 yr:	<3-23	[<91-696]	
		11-15 yr:	<3-19	[<91-575]	
		Adult (8:00 AM)[3]:	2-19	[61-576]	
	Urine, 24 hr. Store refrigerated.	<10 mcg/D × 3.03		[<30 nmol/day]	

1. Loraine JA, Bell ET: *Hormone assays and their clinical application,* New York, 1976, Churchill Livingstone.
2. Endocrine Sciences: *Pediatric laboratory services,* Tarzana, CA, 1992, Endocrine Sciences.
3. Sippell WG, Dorr HG, Bidlingmaier F, et al: Plasma levels of aldosterone, corticosterone, 11-deoxycorticosterone, progesterone, 17-hydroxyprogesterone, cortisol, and cortisone during infancy and childhood, *Pediatr Res* 74:39-46, 1980.
4. Friedman RB, Young DS: *Effects of disease on clinical laboratory tests,* ed 2, Washington, DC, 1989, American Association for Clinical Chemistry.

TEST NAME AND METHOD	SPECIMEN REQUIREMENTS	REFERENCE INTERVAL			CHEMICAL INTERFERENCES
11-Deoxycortisol (Compound S)[1-3] *RIA*	Serum. Separate within 1 hr and store frozen.		*mcg/dL[1]*	*µmol/L*	↑ V Metyrapone
		Cord blood:	295-554 × 0.0289	[9-16]	↓ V All glucocorticoids
		Premature infant, 31-35 wk, day 4:	48-579	[1-17]	(e.g., hydrocortisone,
		Newborn (3 day):	13-147	[0.4-4]	dexamethasone, pred-
		1-12 mo:	<10-156	[<0.3-4.5]	nisone)
		1-10 yr, 8:00 AM:	20-155	[0.6-4.5]	
		Adult, 8:00 AM:	12-158	[0.3-4.6]	

1. Endocrine Sciences: *Pediatric laboratory services,* Tarzana, CA, 1993, Endocrine Sciences.
2. Jubiz W, Matsukura S, Meikle AW, et al: Plasma metyrapone, adrenocorticotropic hormone, cortisol, and deoxycortisol levels. Sequential changes during oral and intravenous metyrapone administration, *Arch Intern Med* 125:468-471, 1970.
3. Jubiz W, Meikle AW, West CD, et al: Single-dose metyrapone test, *Arch Intern Med* 125:472-474, 1970.

DIAGNOSTIC INFORMATION	REMARKS

↑ Adrenogenital syndromes due to 17- and 11-hydroxylase deficiencies. DOC increases in pregnancy from 23 wk to a maximum value at term.

↓ Preeclampsia[4]

Normal secretion is dependent on ACTH and is suppressible by dexamethasone. There is a circadian rhythm with mean evening levels <50% of morning levels. There is a massive increase after administration of 11β-hydroxylase inhibitor (metyrapone). Sodium depletion or angiotensin infusions do not increase plasma DOC.

↑ Adrenocortical hyperplasia due to 11-hydroxylase defect, adrenal carcinoma

See also *Tetrahydrodeoxycortisol.*

Measurement of compound S has been associated with the metyrapone test for evaluating pituitary-adrenal reserve. See *Metyrapone Stimulation Test.*

Whereas most immunoassays for 11-deoxycortisol are adequate for monitoring the metyrapone test, more sensitive assays are needed for evaluating adrenocortical hyperplasia. Significant cross-reactivity with 17-hydroxyprogesterone may be encountered in direct (no extraction) immunoassays.

TEST NAME AND METHOD	SPECIMEN REQUIREMENTS	REFERENCE INTERVAL, CONVENTIONAL [INTERNATIONAL RECOMMENDED UNITS]			CHEMICAL INTERFERENCES AND IN VIVO EFFECTS
Dexamethasone Suppression Test, Overnight[1,2]	Serum for cortisol, drawn at 8:00 AM on following morning	Cortisol, suppression to:			↑ V Estrogens
		<3 mcg/dL	× 0.0276	[<0.08 µmol/L]	↓ V Phenytoin
Dose: 1 mg dexamethasone orally at 11:00 PM or 12:00 AM					
Dose: 4 mg dexamethasone orally at 11:00 PM or 12:00 AM		Cortisol, Suppression to:			
		<50% of baseline	× 0.01	[<0.50]	

1. Crapo L: Cushing's syndrome: a review of diagnostic tests, *Metabolism* 28:955-977, 1979.
2. Whitley RJ, Meikle AW, Watts NB: Endocrinology. In Burtis CA, Ashwood ER, editors: *Tietz textbook of clinical chemistry,* ed 2, Philadelphia, 1994, WB Saunders.
3. Butler PW, Besser GM: Pituitary-adrenal function in severe depressive illness, *Lancet* 1:1234-1236, 1968.
4. Dexamethasone suppression test lacks sensitivity and specificity when used to screen for endogenous depression, *Lab Rep Phys* 6:7-8, 1984.
5. Crapo L: Cushing's syndrome: a review of diagnostic tests, *Metabolism* 28:955-977, 1979.
6. Meikle AW: Dexamethasone suppression test: usefulness of simultaneous measurement of plasma cortisol and dexamethasone, *Clin Endocrinol (Oxf)* 16:401-408, 1982.

TEST NAME AND METHOD	SPECIMEN REQUIREMENTS	REFERENCE INTERVAL, CONVENTIONAL [INTERNATIONAL RECOMMENDED UNITS]			CHEMICAL INTERFERENCES AND IN VIVO EFFECTS
Dexamethasone Suppression Test, Standard[1,2]	For 6 days collect serum (8:00 AM and 8:00 PM) and 24-hr urine for baseline measurements (days 1 and 2) and during dexamethasone administration (days 3-6).	Serum cortisol, Suppression on day 4 to			↓ V Nonsuppression may occur with alcohol (chronic), barbiturates, carbamazepine, indomethacin, meprobamate, phenytoin, and rifampin.
		<50% of baseline	× 0.01	[<0.50]	
Dose, adult, low dose: 0.5 mg dexamethasone orally q 6 hr × 8 on days 3 and 4		or to <5 mcg/dL	× 27.6	[138 nmol/L]	
		Urine 17-KGS, Suppression on day 4 to			
		<7 mg/day	× 3.47	[<24 µmol/day]	Enhanced suppression may occur with amphetamine, benzodiazepines, and corticosteroids.
		Urine 17-OHCS, Suppression on day 4 to			
		<4.5 mg/day	× 2.76	[<12.4 µmol/day]	See also individual tests.
		Urine-free cortisol, Suppression on day 4 to			
		<50%	× 0.01	[0.50]	

DIAGNOSTIC INFORMATION	REMARKS
Cushing's syndrome: >10 mcg/dL [>276 nmol/L] Half of patients with endogenous depression have suppression test values >5 mcg/dL [>138 nmol/L].[3]	1.1% of normals, 13% of obese, and 23% of hospitalized or chronically ill controls give false-positive results. Test is easy to perform on ambulatory patients and serves as a screening test for subjects suspected of having Cushing's syndrome. Test may be abnormal if patient is stressed or pregnant. Because many conditions can invalidate the test, its use as a routine marker for endogenous depression may not be valid.[4] Some patients with Cushing's disease have false-negative results with this low dose of dexamethasone. A 24-hr urine free cortisol determination also serves as a useful screening test for Cushing's syndrome. (See *Cortisol, Free.*)
Most patients with pituitary Cushing's disease demonstrate suppression, whereas patients with adrenal adenoma, carcinoma, and ectopic ACTH-producing tumors do not.	False-negative test results with the low-dose overnight test can be assessed with a high (4 mg) or high-high (8-24 mg) dose of dexamethasone. With high-high dose testing, <10% of patients with pituitary Cushing's disease fail to suppress.[5] Simultaneous measurement of cortisol and dexamethasone in the 8:00 AM blood sample improves reliability of this test for Cushing's syndrome.[6]
The low dose distinguishes normals from patients with Cushing's syndrome, in whom incomplete or no suppression occurs.	A dose of 20 mg/kg/day should be used for children and obese subjects.

TEST NAME AND METHOD	SPECIMEN REQUIREMENTS	REFERENCE INTERVAL, CONVENTIONAL [INTERNATIONAL RECOMMENDED UNITS]		CHEMICAL INTERFERENCES AND IN VIVO EFFECTS

Dexamethasone Suppression Test, Standard—CONT

High dose: 2.0 mg dexamethasone orally q 6 hr × 8 on days 5 and 6		Serum cortisol, Suppression on day 6 to <10 mcg/dL	× 27.6	[<276 nmol/L]	
		Urine cortisol, 17-KGS, and 17-OHS, Suppression on day 6 to <50% of baseline	× 0.01	[<0.50]	

1. Alsever RN, Gotlin RW: *Handbook of endocrine tests in adults and children,* ed 2, Chicago, 1978, Year Book Medical Publishers Inc.
2. Abboud CF, Laws ER Jr: Clinical endocrinological approach to hypothalamic-pituitary disease, *J Neurosurg* 51:271-291, 1979.

p-**Dichloro-benzene**[1] *(1,4-Dichloroben-zene; CAS 106-46-7)*	Urine	Negative Occupational exposure, as *p*-dichlorophenol: <233 mg/L	× 0.0614	[<14.3 mmol/L]	Colorimetric procedure is nonspecific and may show interference by other phenolic substances.[3]
Colorimetric					
GC-FID, GC-ECD[2]	Whole blood (oxalate)	10 mg/L	× 0.0614	[0.614 mmol/L]	

1. Baselt RC: *Biological monitoring methods for industrial chemicals,* Davis, CA, 1980, Biomedical Pub.
2. Morita M, Ohi G: Para-dichlorobenzene in human tissue and atmosphere in Tokyo metropolitan area, *Environ Pollut* 8:269-274, 1975.
3. Pagnotto LD, Walkley JE: Urinary dichlorophenol as an index of para-dichlorobenzene exposure, *Am Ind Hyg Assoc J* 26:137-142, 1965.

Dihydropteridine Reductase (DHPR; EC 1.6.99.7)[1-3]	Whole blood (heparin)	*nmol/min/mg Hb (SD)*		*kU/mol Hb*	None found.
		1 mo-40 yr: 3.20 ± 0.70	× 64.5	[206 ± 45]	
Spectrophotometric, 550 nm, 25° C[4]	Whole blood on filter paper. Stable for 10 days at 30° C, for 2 mo at 4° C.	*nmol/min/5-mm filter paper disc*[4] *(SD)*		*mU/5-mm filter paper disc (SD)*	
		Newborn: 5.77 ± 1.16	× 1.0	[5.77 ± 1.16]	
		1 mo-40 yr: 3.77 ± 0.72		[3.77 ± 0.72]	

DIAGNOSTIC INFORMATION

REMARKS

High dose: 90% of patients with Cushing's disease demonstrate suppression, whereas patients with adrenal adenoma, carcinoma, and ectopic ACTH-producing tumors do not.

Exposure is most commonly by inhalation, although accidental and intentional ingestions have been reported. Chronic oral exposure may cause a microcytic anemia. Respiratory exposure may be associated with eye, nose, and skin irritation; headache; nausea; anemia; and hepatotoxicity.

p-Dichlorobenzene is used as a disinfectant, insecticide, and deodorant in restroom and animal facilities.

Occupational exposure

TLV = 75 ppm [450 mg/m^3]

↓ Tetrahydrobiopterin-deficient hyperphenylalaninemia (cofactor variant of classic PKU)

Hyperphenylalaninemia can result from a deficiency of phenylalanine hydroxylase (classic PKU) or from defects associated with the enzyme cofactor tetrahydrobiopterin (BH$_4$). BH$_4$ defects can be caused by a deficiency of DHPR or by a defect in biopterin biosynthesis. BH$_4$ defects account for 1-3% of patients with hyperphenylalaninemia. In addition to DHPR assays, cofactor variant screening also involves measurement of urine pteridines.

TEST NAME AND METHOD	SPECIMEN REQUIREMENTS	REFERENCE INTERVAL, CONVENTIONAL [INTERNATIONAL RECOMMENDED UNITS]			CHEMICAL INTERFERENCES AND IN VIVO EFFECTS

Dihydropteridine Reductase—CONT

1. Narisawa K, Arai N, Kayakawa H, et al: Diagnosis of variant forms of hyperphenylalaninemia using filter paper spots of blood and urine. In Naruse H, Iria M, editors: *Neonatal screening,* Amsterdam, 1983, Excerpta Medica.

2. Naylor E: Screening for PKU cofactor variants. In Carter T, Willey A, editors: *Genetic disease. Screening and management,* New York, 1986, Alan R. Liss, Inc.

Test	Specimen		*ng/dL*[4]		*nmol/L*	Interferences
Dihydrotestosterone (DHT; 5-α-dihydrotestosterone; 5AD)[1-3]	Serum. Separate within 1 hr. Store frozen.	Cord blood:	2-8	× 0.0344	[0.07-0.28]	See *Testosterone, Total.*
		Premature				
		M:	10-53		[0.34-1.82]	
		F:	2-13		[0.07-0.45]	
		Newborn				
RIA		M:	5-60		[0.17-2.06]	
		F:	<2-15		[<0.07-0.52]	
		Prepubertal				
		Child (1-10 yr):	<3		[<0.10]	
		Puberty Tanner stage				
		1				
		M:	<3		[<0.10]	
		F:	<3		[<0.10]	
		2				
		M:	3-17		[0.10-0.58]	
		F:	5-12		[0.17-0.41]	

	ng/day[4]		*nmol/L*
Puberty Tanner stage			
3			
M:	8-33	× 0.0344	[0.27-1.14]
F:	7-19		[0.24-0.65]
4			
M:	22-52		[0.76-1.79]
F:	4-13		[0.14-0.45]
5			
M:	24-65		[0.83-2.24]
F:	3-18		[0.10-0.62]
Adult			
M:	30-85		[1.03-2.92]
F:	4-22		[0.14-0.76]

		mcg/day		*nmol/day*
Urine, 24 hr	Adult[5]			
	M:	20-50	× 3.44	[68-172]
	F:	<8		[<27]

DIAGNOSTIC INFORMATION	REMARKS

3. Niederwieser A, Curtius H-Ch: Tetrahydrobiopterin deficiencies in hyperphenylalaninemia. In Bickel H, Wachtel U, editors: *Inherited diseases of amino acid metabolism,* Stuttgart, 1985, Thieme, Inc.

4. Arai N, Narisau K, Hayakawa H, et al: Hyperphenylalaninemia due to dihydropteridine reductase deficiency: diagnosis by enzyme assays on dried blood spots, *Pediatrics* 70:426-430, 1982.

See *Testosterone, Total.*

↓ 5α-Reductase deficiency, hypogonadism

↑ Hirsutism

DHT is largely derived from peripheral tissue conversion of testosterone catalyzed by a steroid 5α-reductase enzyme.

Serum levels of dihydrotestosterone decrease rapidly in males during the first week after birth; they then increase between 30 and 60 days to 12-85 ng/dL [0.41-2.92 nmol/L] and gradually decrease to 3 ng/dL [0.10 nmol/L] by 7 mo. In females, DHT decreases to prepubertal levels during the first month.

Serum concentrations of dihydrotestosterone are closely related to those of testosterone but are lower. There is a decrease in the ratio of dihydrotestosterone to testosterone throughout pregnancy.

DHT is the primary active metabolite of testosterone that is responsible for hair growth. Measurements of circulating DHT may not be useful in evaluating hirsutism because serum concentrations reflect intracellular concentrations poorly. However, DHT is metabolized to a 3α-androstanediol glucuronide (3α-diol). See *Testosterone, Free;* and *3α-Androstanediol Glucuronide.*

TEST NAME AND METHOD	SPECIMEN REQUIREMENTS	REFERENCE INTERVAL, CONVENTIONAL [INTERNATIONAL RECOMMENDED UNITS]		CHEMICAL INTERFERENCES AND IN VIVO EFFECTS

Dihydrotestosterone—CONT

1. Griffin JE, Wilson JD: Disorders of the testes and male reproductive tract. In Wilson JD, Foster DW, editors: *Williams textbook of endocrinology,* ed 8, Philadelphia, 1992, WB Saunders.
2. Pakarinen A, Hammond GL, Vihko R: Serum pregnenolone, progesterone, 17α-hydroxyprogesterone, androstenedione, testosterone, 5α-dihydrotestosterone and androsterone during puberty in boys, *Clin Endocrinol* 11:465-474, 1979.

Dimethylfor-mamide (*N,N-Dimethylforma-mide; DMF; CAS 68-12-2*) *GLC*	Blood (fluoride/ox-alate)		*mg/L*		*μmol/L*	None found.
		Occupational exposure:	3	× 13.7	[41]	
		Methylformamide (metabolite):	2	× 16.9	[34]	
	Urine, 24 hr		*mg/day*		*mmol/d*	
		Formamide (metabolite):	6.9	× 22.2	[153]	
		Methylformamide (metabolite):	24	× 16.9	[406]	
			mg/g creatinine		*mmol/mol creatinine*	
		DMF-creatinine ratio[1]:	>40	× 1.54	[>62]	

1. Lauwerys RR: *Industrial chemical exposure. Guidelines for biological monitoring,* Davis, CA, 1983, Biomedical Pub.

Dinitro-*o*-cresol[1] (*4,6-Dinitro-o-cresol; DNOC; CAS CAS 534-52-1*) *Colorimetric*[2]	Plasma (EDTA)		*mg/L*		*μmol/L*	None found.
		Occupational exposure:	4.3	× 5.05	[22]	
		Toxic concentration:	>15		[>76]	
	Blood (EDTA)[3]	Occupational exposure:	1.4-4.3		[7-22]	
		Toxic concentration:	20		[>101]	

1. Baselt RC: *Biological monitoring methods for industrial chemicals,* Davis, CA, 1980, Biomedical Pub.
2. Lauwerys RR: *Industrial chemical exposure. Guidelines for biological monitoring,* Davis, CA, 1983, Biomedical Pub.
3. Ocak A, Valentour JC, Blanke RV: The effects of storage conditions on the stability of carbon monoxide in postmortem blood, *J Anal Toxicol* 9:202-206, 1985.
4. Available at: http://www.epa.gov/ttn/atw/hlthef/di-creso.html. Last accessed 2/1/06.

DIAGNOSTIC INFORMATION	REMARKS

3. Whitley RJ: Free testosterone: the bearded woman, *AACC Endo Metabolism In-Service Training Continuing Education* 11:63-65, 1993.
4. Endocrine Sciences: *Pediatric laboratory services,* Tarzana, CA, 1992, Endocrine Sciences.
5. Hicks JM, Young DS: *DORA '87: directory of rare analyses,* Washington, DC, 1987, AACC Press.

Adverse effects can occur after inhalation, skin absorption, or ingestion. These include nausea, abdominal pain, hepatomegaly, and hepatic necrosis.

Methylformamide persists longer than the parent compound and is more conveniently measured for biological monitoring. Metabolism involves sequential N-demethylation to methylformamide and formamide, which are excreted by the kidney. It is likely that a portion is excreted in expired breath.

Kinetic values
$t_{1/2}$: 2-6 hr

Symptoms of acute (short-term) and chronic (long-term) toxicity include profuse sweating, increased pulse and respiratory rates, thirst, fatigue, headache, appetite loss, and greenish-yellow pigmentation of the conjunctivae in humans. Effects to the respiratory, cardiovascular, gastrointestinal, and central nervous system (CNS) of chronically exposed workers have been reported.[4]

DNOC was used as a pesticide until its registration was removed by the EPA in 1991.

Kinetic values
$t_{1/2}$: 5-6 days

TEST NAME AND METHOD	SPECIMEN REQUIREMENTS	REFERENCE INTERVAL, CONVENTIONAL [INTERNATIONAL RECOMMENDED UNITS]			CHEMICAL INTERFERENCES AND IN VIVO EFFECTS
Dioxane *(1,4-Dioxane; CAS 123-9-1)*	Plasma	Occupational exposure: HEAA* (metabolite):	*mg/L* <12 <10	× 11.4 × 8.33	μ*mol/L* [<137] [<83]	None found.
GC-FID[1]	Urine	HEAA:*	*mg/L* <8 <113	× 11.4 × 8.33	μ*mol/L* [<91] [<6772]	

*HEAA, β-Hydroxyethoxyacetic acid.

1.　Braun WH: Rapid method for the simultaneous determination of 1,4-dioxan and its major metabolite, beta-hydroxyethoxyacetic acid, concentrations in plasma and urine, *J Chromatogr* 115:263-266, 1977.

Disaccharide Absorption Tests[1-3] Dose: Individual disaccharide, orally, 50 g/m² body surface, or 1 g/kg body wt. to a total of 25 g.	Serum. Draw samples at 0, 30, 60, 90, and 120 min.	Change in glucose from fasting value: Inconclusive: Abnormal:	*mg/dL* >30 20-30 <20	× 0.055	*mmol/L* [>1.7] [1.1-1.7] [<1.1]	See *Glucose.* False-positive (low increase) result in 20-30% because of tight insulin control.
	Breath: End-expiratory air at 0, 30, 60, 90, and 120 min.	H₂ > 20 ppm above the baseline level but before a colonic response.				False-positive results can occur with excessive oral dose. Positive tests should be repeated with 50% dosage.

1.　Bondy PK, Rosenberg LE, editors: *Metabolic control and disease,* ed 8, Philadelphia. 1980, WB Saunders.

2.　Burtis CA, Ashwood ER, editors: *Tietz textbook of clinical chemistry,* ed 2, Philadelphia, 1994, WB Saunders.

3.　Mishkin D, Sablauskas L, Yalovsky M, et al: Fructose and sorbitol malabsorption in ambulatory patients with functional dyspepsia: comparison with lactose maldigestion/malabsorption, *Dig Dis Sci* 42:2591-2598, 1997.

Dioxane is a skin and mucous membrane irritant with relatively low acute toxicity. Deaths associated with dioxane exposure have resulted from liver and kidney failure, and sublethal acute exposures resulted in nausea, vomiting, and irritation of the eyes and respiratory tract.

A widely used solvent, dioxane is absorbed by inhalation and by the skin. The bulk of absorbed dioxane is metabolized to β-hydroxyethoxyacetic acid and excreted by the kidneys. A substantial portion of dioxane may be expired in breath.

Kinetic values
TLV: 25 ppm (90 mg/m^3)
$t_{1/2}$,
Dioxane: 1 hr
HEAA: 3 hr

Impairment of carbohydrate absorption may occur as a result of mucosal damage or dysfunction as in sprue, celiac disease, or acute gastroenteritis, or as a result of a deficiency of a single or all brush border oligosaccharidases.

These tests are used to diagnose malabsorption due to specific or generalized disaccharidase deficiencies (lactose, fructose, sorbitol). The most common form is lactase deficiency. (See *Lactose Tolerance Test.*) To eliminate misinterpretations of serum test results, a glucose tolerance test and absorption tests of the component monosaccharides may be needed to rule out monosaccharide malabsorption. Diagnosis of disaccharidase deficiencies is confirmed by assay of the disaccharidase in a small-intestinal biopsy specimen.

Breath testing is highly sensitive and specific.

TEST NAME AND METHOD	SPECIMEN REQUIREMENTS	REFERENCE INTERVAL, CONVENTIONAL [INTERNATIONAL RECOMMENDED UNITS]			CHEMICAL INTERFERENCES AND IN VIVO EFFECTS
2,3-Diphospho-glycerate (2,3-DPG) in Erythrocytes[1-5] *Krimsky and Beutler (UV), 25° C*[13]	Hemolysate of washed Ercs. Submit whole blood (ACD, EDTA, or heparin). Perform extraction immediately.	*μmol/g Hb* 12.3 ± 1.87 (SD) *μmol/10[12] Ercs* 356 ± 54 *μmol/mL Ercs* 4.2 ± 0.64	× 0.0645* × 1.0 × 1.0	*mol/mol Hb* [0.79 ± 0.12] *mmol/L Erc* [356 ± 54] *mmol/L Ercs* [4.2 ± 0.64]	None found.

Levels are lower in newborns and even more decreased in premature infants.[7]

Grisolin et al, modified (Auto-Analyzer, colorimetric)[6]	Hemolysate of washed Ercs. Submit whole blood (heparin).	*Years* *μmol/g Hb (SD)* 18-24: 14.9 ± 1.6 25-34: 14.4 ± 1.3 35-44: 14.3 ± 1.5 45-54: 14.2 ± 1.5 55-64: 14.9 ± 1.8 65-74: 13.8 ± 1.9 75-84: 13.9 ± 2.4 >85: 12.8 ± 2.0	× 0.0645*	*mol/mol Hb* [0.96 ± 0.10] [0.93 ± 0.08] [0.92 ± 0.10] [0.92 ± 0.10] [0.96 ± 0.12] [0.89 ± 0.12] [0.90 ± 0.15] [0.82 ± 0.13]	

See *Acetylcholinesterase.*

*Conversion factor based on MW of Hb of 64,500.

1. Beutler E: *Hemolytic anemia in disorders of red cell metabolism,* New York, 1978, Plenum Pub. Co.
2. Beutler E: *Red cell metabolism: a manual of biochemical methods,* ed 4, New York, 1986, Grune & Stratton.
3. Friedman RB, Anderson RE, Entine SM, et al: Effects of diseases on clinical laboratory tests, *Clin Chem* 26:1-46D, 1980.
4. Miale JB: *Laboratory medicine: hematology,* ed 6, St. Louis, 1982, CV Mosby Co.
5. Williams JJ, Beutler E, Ersley JJ, et al, editors: *Manual of hematology,* ed 6, New York, 2003, McGraw-Hill Publishing Co.
6. Purcell Y, Brozovic B: Red cell 2,3-diphosphoglycerate concentration in man decreases with age, *Nature* 251:511-512, 1974.
7. Oski FA: Red cell metabolism in the newborn infant. V. Glycolytic intermediates and glycolytic enzymes, *Pediatrics* 44:84-91, 1969.

Donath-Landsteiner (D-L) Test for Paroxysmal Cold Hemoglobinuria (PCH)[1-3]	*Screening test:* Whole blood, part allowed to clot at 37° C, part chilled in melting ice and then warmed to 37° C.	Normal: No hemolysis	↓ Complement may mask positive result (extrinsic C may be added).

DIAGNOSTIC INFORMATION	REMARKS

↑ Anemia, pyruvate kinase deficiency, uremia, cirrhosis, and in conditions of hypoxia, e.g., obstructive lung disease, congenital cyanotic heart disease, and after vigorous exercise; hyperthyroidism, cystic fibrosis (pulmonary involvement),[3] chronic renal failure (secondary to anemia)

In general, 2,3-DPG increases in response to hypoxia or anemia and decreases in acidosis.

$$\text{mmol/g Hb} \times 29 = \text{mmol/10}^{12} \text{ Ercs}$$

$$\text{mmol/g Hb} \times 0.34 = \text{mmol/mL Ercs*}$$

↓ Polycythemia, hexokinase deficiency, phosphofructokinase deficiency, respiratory distress syndrome,[3] 2,3-diphosphoglyceromutase deficiency

*See Note, *Acetylcholinesterase.*

Hemolysis in blood that has been chilled and then warmed indicates the presence of bithermic cold hemolysins or Donath-Landsteiner antibodies (D-L Ab). D-L Ab are IgG immunoglobulins, typically with anti-P specificity, although other specificities such as anti-I or anti-HI may occur very rarely. PCH itself is rare. Originally described in congenital or late syphilis, PCH is usually acute, transient, and associated with viral infections but may be idiopathic.

Hemolysis is complement dependent, and a fresh source of complement may be needed to demonstrate the D-L Ab. The D-L Ab is a nonagglutinating IgG that binds complement in the cold and lyses erythrocytes at 37° C.

TEST NAME AND METHOD	SPECIMEN REQUIREMENTS	REFERENCE INTERVAL, CONVENTIONAL [INTERNATIONAL RECOMMENDED UNITS]	CHEMICAL INTERFERENCES AND IN VIVO EFFECTS

Donath-Landsteiner (D-L) Test for Paroxysmal Cold Hemoglobinuria (PCH)—CONT

1. Hall R, Malia RG: *Medical laboratory haematology,* ed 2, London, 1991, Butterworths.
2. Williams JJ, Beutler E, Ersley JJ, et al, editors: *Manual of hematology,* ed 6, New York, 2003, McGraw-Hill Publishing Co.

Elastase[1] ELISA	Spot stool	Normal pancreatic exocrine function >200 mcg/g stool	

1. Phillips IJ, Rowe DJ, Dewar P, et al: Faecal elastase 1: a marker of exocrine pancreatic insufficiency in cystic fibrosis, *Ann Clin Biochem* 36:739-742, 1999.

Endomysial antibodies (IgA)[1,2] *Indirect immuno-fluorescence*	Serum. Stable 1 week RT, 2 wk at 4° C, 1 year frozen.	Negative is normal. Sera reactive at a dilution of 1 to 5 or > are positive. Sera that contain SMA may produce indeterminate results.	None known. Testing in children is not as useful because celiac disease antibodies may not have developed. May be negative in patients taking gluten-free diets. Reappears with gluten challenge. 2.6% of patients will be negative because of selective IgA deficiency. A serum IgA should be carried out and, if abnormal, IgG-based testing carried out.

1. Wong RC, Steele RH, Reeves GE, et al: Antibody and genetic testing in coeliac disease, *Pathology* 35: 285-304, 2003.
2. Devlin SM, Andrews CN, Beck PL: Celiac disease: CME update for family physicians, *Can Fam Physician* 50: 719-725, 2004.
3. Kapuscinska A, Zalewski T, Chorzelski TP, et al: Disease specificity and dynamics of changes in IgA class anti-endomysial antibodies in celiac disease, *J Pediatr Gastroenterol Nutr* 6:529-534, 1987.

DIAGNOSTIC INFORMATION	REMARKS

3. Petz LD, Garratty G: *Acquired immune hemolytic anemias,* ed 2, New York, 2004, Churchill Livingstone.

<200 mcg/g stool exocrine pancreatic insufficiency. For pancreatic insufficiency sensitivity is 63% for mild and 100% moderate/severe, and 93% specific. Considered the best marker of exocrine pancreatic deficiency in cystic fibrosis.	Serum test has no advantage over standard markers of pancreatitis.
Endomysial antibodies (IgA) are specific for celiac disease (85-98% sensitive; 97-100% specific). 70% in dermatitis herpetiformis, Testing for endomysial antibodies is indicated in patients suspected of having celiac disease or dermatitis herpetiformis 70% sensitivity).[3]	The test for endomysial antibodies detects antibodies to tissue transglutaminase, the principal auto antigen reactive with endomysial antibodies in tissue substrate sections, e.g. monkey esophagus (cf. Tissue transglutaminase antibodies, IgA and IgG isotypes for further information). Celiac disease is an immune disorder found in 1% of the NA population that is stimulated by gluten. It is characterized by typical GI symptoms and a variety of less common symptoms. This antibody is against the endomyosium, an area of connective tissue surrounding smooth muscle cells. Many labs do not use this test as it employs monkey esophagus as a substrate. Small bowel biopsy is needed for definitive diagnosis. More than 97% of people with celiac disease have DQ2 and/or DQ8 HLA haplotypes compared with 40% of the population *See: Reticulin Antibody, Tissue Transglutaminase Antibody, and Gliadin Antibody.*

TEST NAME AND METHOD	SPECIMEN REQUIREMENTS	REFERENCE INTERVAL, CONVENTIONAL [INTERNATIONAL RECOMMENDED UNITS]			CHEMICAL INTERFERENCES AND IN VIVO EFFECTS
β-Endorphin[1-3] *RIA*	Plasma (EDTA). Collect on ice; refrigerate during centrifugation. Freeze immediately.	6:00-10:00 AM: 16-48 pg/mL[4]	× 1.0	[16-48 ng/L]	None found.

1. Endocrine Sciences: Pediatric Laboratory Services. Tarzana, CA, 1988.
2. Adams ML, Brasr DA, Welch SP, et al: The role of endogenous peptides in the action of opioid analgesics, *Ann Emerg Med* 15:65-68, 1986.
3. Kiritsy-Roy JA, Van Loon GR: Endogenous opioid peptides in neuroendocrine regulation. In Collu R, Brown GM, Van Loon GR, editors: *Clinical neuroendocrinology,* Boston, 1988, Blackwell Scientific Publications.
4. Nichols Institute Reference Laboratories: *Test catalog,* San Juan Capistrano, CA, 1993, Nichols Institute Reference Laboratories.
5. Young E: Endogenous opioid peptides in neuroendocrine regulation, *AACC Endo and Metabolism In-service Training and Continuing Education* 8:7-13, 1990.

Enolase (EC 4.2.1.11) *340 nm, 37° C[1]*	Serum. Stable at room temperature for 6-12 hr, at 4° C for 48 hr, and at −20° C for 6 mo.	13 ± 4 U/L (SD)			S ↑ C Hemolysis
ICSH, 37° C[2]	Hemolysate of washed erythrocytes. Submit whole blood (ACD, EDTA, or heparin). Stable for >20 days at 4° C, >5 days at 25° C.	*U/g Hb (SD)* 5.39 ± 0.83 *U/10[12] Ercs* 156 ± 24 *U/mL Ercs* 1.83 ± 0.28 Activity higher in newborns[11,12]	× 64.5* × 10[−3] × 1.0	*kU/mol Hb* [348 ± 54] *nU/Erc* [0.16 ± 0.02] *kU/L Ercs* [1.83 ± 0.28]	

*Conversion factor based on MW of Hb of 64,500.

DIAGNOSTIC INFORMATION	REMARKS
↑ Physical and emotional stress, exercise, surgery, pregnancy and labor, electroconvulsive therapy; newborns during first 24 hr of life.[3]	β-Endorphin is a 31-amino acid opioid peptide derived from proopiomelanocortin (POMC). Adrenocorticotropin (ACTH), α-melanocytestimulating hormone (α-MSH), β-lipotropin, and several other peptides are also derived from POMC. High concentrations of β-endorphin are found in the pituitary gland and the hypothalamus. Plasma levels show a circadian pattern that is synchronous with that of ACTH. In addition to being an analgesic, β-endorphin is known to modulate a number of hormones. No diseases are clearly associated with disordered β-endorphin levels, but increased plasma levels may accompany pituitary Cushing's disease and depression.[5]
↑ Myocardial infarct, muscle disease, hepatitis	Enolase is a dimer of three peptides: α, β, and γ. αα is widely distributed; ββ and αβ exist mainly in heart and skeletal muscle. γγ and αα are located in nerve tissue. Activity is slightly higher in infants than in adults. The γγ dimer is widely referred to as NSE. This isoenzyme consists of two identical polypeptide chains each with an MW of 39,000.
There are no reliable reports of deficiency.[11,13]	Activity is normal or slightly increased in young erythrocytes.[16] U/g Hb × 29 = U/10^{12} Ercs U/g Hb × 0.34 = U/mL Ercs* *See Note, *Acetylcholinesterase.*

TEST NAME AND METHOD	SPECIMEN REQUIREMENTS	REFERENCE INTERVAL, CONVENTIONAL [INTERNATIONAL RECOMMENDED UNITS]		CHEMICAL INTERFERENCES AND IN VIVO EFFECTS

Enolase—CONT

TEST NAME AND METHOD	SPECIMEN REQUIREMENTS	REFERENCE INTERVAL, CONVENTIONAL	[INTERNATIONAL RECOMMENDED UNITS]	CHEMICAL INTERFERENCES AND IN VIVO EFFECTS
Neuron-specific Enolase (NSE, Neuron-specific Isoenzyme of Enolase, gg-Enolase)[3-6] IEMA (Roche), RIA (Pharmacia), bioluminescence[4]	Serum. Stable up to 48 hr at 2-8° C. For longer periods, freeze at ≤20° C. Avoid repeated freeze-thaw cycles. Avoid hemolysis; separate serum from erythrocytes in <60 min.	0-9 ng/mL (Pharmacia)[6] × 1.0 0-22 ng/mL (Roche)[6]	[0-9 mcg/L] [0-22 mcg/L]	NSE is also found in erythrocytes, plasma cells, and platelets. Specimens containing particulate matter must be clarified.

EIA[7]			*ng/mL*		*mcg/L*	
		Child:	2.6-10.8	× 1.0	[2.6-10.8]	
		Adult:	1.4-5.7		[1.4-5.7]	

RIA[8]				
	Adult:	6 ± 5 (SE)	[6 ± 5]	

RIA[9]				
	<1 yr:	7.5 ± 2.1 (SE)	[7.5 ± 2.1]	
	Adult:	5.2 ± 1.1	[5.2 ± 1.1]	

EIA[10]				
	<1 mo:	2.7 ± 1.2 (SD)	[2.7 ± 1.2]	
	1 mo-1 yr:	4.0 ± 1.4	[4.0 ± 1.4]	
	1-2 yr:	4.1 ± 1.6	[4.1 ± 1.6]	
	2-3 yr:	4.5 ± 2.1	[4.5 ± 2.1]	
	3-5 yr:	5.4 ± 1.3	[5.4 ± 1.3]	
	5-10 yr:	5.1 ± 1.6	[5.1 ± 1.6]	

1. Herraez-Dominguez M, Goldberg DM, Anderson AJ, et al: Serum enolase and pyruvate kinase activities in the diagnosis of myocardial infarction, *Enzyme* 21:211-224, 1976.

2. Beutler E: *Red cell metabolism: a manual of biochemical methods,* ed 3, New York, 1984, Grune & Stratton.

3. Jorgensen LGM, Husch FR, Skov EG, et al: Occurrence of neuron-specific enolase in tumor tissue and serum in small cell lung cancer, *Br J Cancer* 63:151-153, 1991.

4. Notami T, Morikawa J, Kata K, et al: Radioimmunoassay development for human neuron-specific enolase: with some clinical results in lung cancer and neuroblastoma, *Tumor Biol* 6:57-63, 1985.

5. Platt MS, Potter JL, Boeckman CR, et al: Elevated GGTP/SGOT ratio. An early indicator of infantile obstructive cholangiopathy, *Am J Dis Child* 735:834-836, 1981.

6. Savoia M, Schwartz D, Smith C et al: NSE as a tumor marker [abstract], *Clin Chem* 33:928, 1987.

7. Ishiguro Y, Kato K, Shimizu A, et al: High levels of immunoreactive nervous system-specific enolase in sera of patients with neuroblastoma, *Clin Chim Acta* 121:173-180, 1982.

8. Akoun GM, Scarna HM, Milleron BJ, et al: Serum neuron-specific enolase. A marker for disease extent and response to therapy for small-cell lung cancer, *Chest* 87:39-43, 1985.

9. Zeltzer PM, Marangos PJ, Evans AE, et al: Serum neuron-specific enolase in children with neuroblastoma. Relationship to stage and disease course, *Cancer* 57:1230-1234, 1986.

10. Ishiguro Y, Kato K, Ito T, et al: Nervous system-specific enolase in serum as a marker for neuroblastoma, *Pediatrics* 72:696-700, 1983.

DIAGNOSTIC INFORMATION	REMARKS

S ↑ 90-100% of patients with neuroblastoma and 70-90% of individuals with small cell cancer of the lung (SCCL). In SCCL, elevations are related to extent of disease and are observed in only 50-60% of patients with limited disease. Enzyme activity shows excellent correlation to clinical status when used in monitoring. There is significantly lower survival in SCCL patients with markedly elevated values. Elevations may also be observed in septic shock, pneumonia, or neural trauma.

NSE is also increased in patients with stroke.[14,15] NSE concentrations are a predictor of the extent of neural damage and neurological deficits.

NSE is a specific serum marker for the family of neuroendocrine tumors of the APUD series (amine precursor uptake and decarboxylation). These include neuroblastoma and retinoblastoma, medullary carcinoma of the thyroid, pancreatic islet cell carcinoma, carcinoid, pheochromocytoma, and SCCL. The test is intended for research (investigational) use only and does not have FDA approval for general clinical application.

11. Williams WJ, Beutler E, Erslev AJ, et al, editors: *Hematology,* ed 4, New York, 1990, McGraw-Hill Publishing Co.

12. Konrad PN, Valentine WN, Paglia DE: Enzymatic activities and glutathione content of erythrocytes in the newborn: comparison with red cells of older normal subjects and those with comparable reticulocytosis, *Acta Haematol* 48:193-201, 1972.

13. Beutler E: Red cell enzyme defects as nondiseases and as disease, *Blood* 54:1-7, 1979.

14. Cunningham RT, Watt M, Winder J, et al: Serum neurone-specific enolase as an indicator of stroke volume, *Eur J Clin Invest* 26;298-303, 1996.

15. Oh SH, Lee JG, Na SJ, et al: Prediction of early clinical severity and extent of neuronal damage in anterior-circulation infarction using the initial serum neuron-specific enolase level, *Arch Neurol* 60:37-41, 2003.

16. Beutler E: *Hemolytic anemia in disorders of red cell metabolism,* New York, 1978, Plenum Pub. Co.

TEST NAME AND METHOD	SPECIMEN REQUIREMENTS	REFERENCE INTERVAL, CONVENTIONAL [INTERNATIONAL RECOMMENDED UNITS]		CHEMICAL INTERFERENCES AND IN VIVO EFFECTS
Erythrocyte Count (Erc Count, Red Blood Cell Count, RBC)[1-4] Automated Methods: **Electronic impedance:** *Coulter STKS, MAXM, GEN-S Abbott Cell-Dyn 3500R, 3700, 4000* *Hydrodynamic focusing, laser light scatter: Bayer Advia 1200* *Hydrodynamic focusing and direct current detection: Sysmex SF-3000, SF-9000, XE-2100*	Whole blood (EDTA). Stable 24 hr at 23° C, 48 hr at 4° C. Fetal blood. Collect by percutaneous umbilical blood sampling.		$\times\,10^6$ *cells/μL*	$\times\,10^{12}$ *cells/L*	$\downarrow$ C The presence of cold agglutinins may cause falsely decreased erythrocyte (RBC) counts. A hemolyzed specimen will falsely lower the automated count. $\uparrow$ C Marked leukocytosis (WBC > 100,000/μL) can falsely increase RBC count on automated counters.
		Fetal[6]		
		18-20 wk:	2.66 ± 0.29 (SD)	[2.66 ± 0.29]
		21-22 wk:	2.96 ± 0.26	[2.96 ± 0.26]
		23-25 wk:	3.06 ± 0.26	[3.06 ± 0.26]
		26-30 wk:	3.52 ± 0.32	[3.52 ± 0.32]
		Cord blood[7]:	3.9-5.5 (2 SD)	[3.9-5.5]
			$\times\,10^6$ *cells/μL*	$\times\,10^{12}$ *cells/L*
		0.5 mo[8]:	3.9-5.9	[3.9-5.9]
		1 mo:	3.3-5.3	[3.3-5.3]
		4 mo:	3.5-5.1	[3.5-5.1]
		6 mo:	3.9-5.5	[3.9-5.5]
		9 mo:	4.0-5.3	[4.0-5.3]
		12 mo:	4.1-5.3	[4.1-5.3]
		1-2 yr[9]:	3.8-4.8 (95% range)	[3.8-4.8]
		3-5 yr:	3.7-4.9	[3.7-4.9]
		6-8 yr:	3.8-4.9	[3.8-4.9]
		9-11 yr:	3.9-5.1	[3.9-5.1]
		12-14 yr		
		M:	4.1-5.2	[4.1-5.2]
		F:	3.8-5.0	[3.8-5.0]
		15-17 yr		
		M:	4.2-5.6	[4.2-5.6]
		F:	3.9-5.1	[3.9-5.1]
		18-44 yr		
		M:	4.3-5.7	[4.3-5.7]
		F:	3.8-5.1	[3.8-5.1]
		45-64 yr		
		M:	4.2-5.6	[4.2-5.6]
		F:	3.8-5.3	[3.8-5.3]
		65-74 yr		
		M:	3.8-5.8	[3.8-5.8]
		F:	3.8-5.2	[3.8-5.2]
	Capillary[5]	1 day:	5.1 ± 0.7 (SD)	[5.1 ± 0.7]
		4 day:	5.0 ± 0.6	[5.0 ± 0.6]
		7 day:	4.9 ± 0.6	[4.9 ± 0.6]
		1-2 wk:	4.8 ± 0.8	[4.8 ± 0.8]
		3-4 wk:	4.0 ± 0.6	[4.0 ± 0.6]
		5-6 wk:	3.6 ± 0.2	[3.6 ± 0.2]
		7-8 wk:	3.4 ± 0.4	[3.4 ± 0.4]
		9-10 wk:	3.6 ± 0.3	[3.6 ± 0.3]
		11-12 wk:	3.7 ± 0.3	[3.7 ± 0.3]

1. Henry JB, editor: *Clinical diagnosis and management by laboratory methods,* ed 20, Philadelphia, 2001, WB Saunders.
2. Lee BR, Luekens JN, et al: *Wintrobe's clinical hematology,* ed 11, Philadelphia, 2003, Lippincott Williams & Wilkins.

DIAGNOSTIC INFORMATION

REMARKS

↑ Polycythemia: Relative polycythemia: hemoconcentration, excitement, Gaisbock syndrome. Absolute polycythemia: Primary polycythemia (congenital or neoplastic [Polycythemia vera]) Secondary polycythemia (decreased tissue oxygenation, increased erythropoietin, iron deficiency, thalassemia traits, microcytic hemoglobinopathies, androgen abuse)

↓ Anemia, recumbency, drugs that cause aplastic anemia or that cause hemolysis, either in G6PD deficiency or by an immune mechanism (specific agents listed in Table II-4)

Erythrocyte (RBC) counts are slightly lower between 5:00 PM and 7:00 AM and after meals (up to 10% lower); they are up to 5.7% lower if drawn from a recumbent patient. Falsely high results may occur due to prolonged venous stasis during venipuncture. A slight but significant decrease occurs in the lower reference limit of erythrocytes in men aged 65-74 yr. There is no significant change in men or women aged >85 yr compared with those aged 65-74 yr.[10]

Erythrocyte count is not affected by excess EDTA. Electronic counts are considerably more precise than hemocytometer counts, which are obsolete.

. Beutler E, Lichtman MA, Coller B, editors: *Williams hematology,* ed 6, New York, 2000, McGraw-Hill.

. Rodak BF, editor: *Hematology; clinical principles and applications,* ed 2, Philadelphia, 2002, WB Saunders.

TEST NAME AND METHOD	SPECIMEN REQUIREMENTS	REFERENCE INTERVAL, CONVENTIONAL [INTERNATIONAL RECOMMENDED UNITS]	CHEMICAL INTERFERENCES AND IN VIVO EFFECTS

Erythrocyte Count—CONT

5. Matoth Y, Zaizon R, Varsano I: Postnatal changes in some red cell parameters, *Acta Paediatr Scand* 60:317-323, 1971.
6. Nathan DG, Orkin SH, Ginsburg D, et al: *Hematology of infancy and childhood,* ed 6, Philadelphia, 2003, WB Saunders.
7. Saarinen UM, Siimes MA: Development changes in red blood cell counts and indices of infants after exclusion of iron deficiency by laboratory criteria and continuous iron supplementation, *J Pediatr* 92:412-416, 1978.

TEST NAME AND METHOD	SPECIMEN REQUIREMENTS	REFERENCE INTERVAL, CONVENTIONAL [INTERNATIONAL RECOMMENDED UNITS]		CHEMICAL INTERFERENCES AND IN VIVO EFFECTS
Erythrocyte Sedimentation Rate (ESR, Sed Rate)[1-4] *Westergren*[3,4] ─────── *Westergren, modified (ICSH recommended method)*[3,4]	Whole blood (Na citrate). Stable 2 hr at 25° C, 12 hr at 4° C.	*mm/hr* Child: 0-10 Adult <50 yr M: 0-15 F: 0-20 >50 yr, M: 0-20 F: 0-30		↑ V Dextran, fat emulsions, anemia, macrocytosis, hemolysis ↓ V Corticotropin, cortisone, cyclophosphamide, hypogammaglobulinemia, spherocytic red cells, microcytic red cells ↑ C Fluorides, glucose, oxalate, quinine; false increase with oxalate or heparin anticoagulated blood
MicroESR[4,5]	Capillary blood (EDTA), whole blood (EDTA).			
Wintrobe[2]	Do not use heparin.	*mm/hr* Child: 0-13 Adult M: 0-9 F: 0-20		
ZSR (Zeta sedimentation ratio)[6]	Whole blood (EDTA). Stable 2 hr at 25° C, 12 hr at 4° C.	41-54% *AU*, Arbitrary unit.	× 1.0	[41-54 AU*]

1. Henry JB, editor: *Clinical diagnosis and management by laboratory methods,* ed 20, Philadelphia, 2001, WB Saunders.
2. Green JP, Foerster J, Lukens W, et al: *Wintrobe's clinical hematology,* ed 11, Philadelphia, 2003, Lippincott Williams & Wilkins.
3. International Committee for Standardization in Haematology (ICSH): Recommendation for measurement of erythrocyte sedimentation rate of human blood, *Am J Clin Pathol* 68:505-507, 1977.
4. Rodak BF, editor: *Hematology: clinical principles and applications,* ed 2, Philadelphia, 2002, WB Saunders.
5. Barrett BA, Hill PI: A micromethod for erythrocyte sedimentation suitable for use on venous or capillary blood, *Am J Clin Pathol* 33:1118-1122, 1980.
6. Bull BS, Brailsford JD: The zeta sedimentation ratio, *Blood* 40:550-558, 1972.
7. Bull BS, Brecher G: An evaluation of the relative merits of the Wintrobe and Westergren sedimentation methods including hematocrit correction, *Am J Clin Pathol* 65:502-510, 1974.
8. Sox HC Jr, Liang MH: The erythrocyte sedimentation rate. Guidelines for rational use, *Ann Intern Med* 104:515-523, 1986.

DIAGNOSTIC INFORMATION	REMARKS

8. Yip R, Johnson C, Dallman PR: Age-related changes in laboratory values used in the diagnosis of anemia and iron deficiency, *Am J Clin Nutr* 39:427-436, 1984.
9. Zauber NP, Zauber AG: Hematologic data of healthy very old people, *JAMA* 257:2181-2184, 1987.

↑ Infections, inflammatory disease, tissue destruction, and other conditions leading to increased plasma fibrinogen or globulins (asymmetrical molecules) such as malignant neoplasms, paraproteinemia (e.g., macroglobulinemia, multiple myeloma); anemia, increasing with severity

↓ *Conditions in which the ESR does not increase with conditions listed above:* Polycythemia, sickle cell anemia, spherocytosis, hypofibrinogenemia

The ESR correlates well with the plasma fibrinogen level and depends on rouleaux formation of erythrocytes. Poikilocytosis therefore tends to inhibit sedimentation; conversely, increased flattening of erythrocytes, as in obstructive liver disease, tends to accelerate sedimentation. The sensitivity of the ESR in detecting plasma protein abnormalities is best in the absence of anemia; in anemia, the ZSR has an advantage. The Wintrobe method is more sensitive in the normal to slightly elevated range, whereas the Westergren is more sensitive in the elevated range.[7] The micromethod may be useful in pediatric patients.

The ESR should not be used to screen asymptomatic patients for disease. When the ESR is increased, a careful history and physical examination will usually disclose the cause. The test is useful and is indicated for the diagnosis and monitoring of temporal arteritis and polymyalgia rheumatica. The ESR is included in the Jones Criteria for diagnosis of rheumatic fever. The ESR has little diagnostic value in rheumatoid arthritis but may be useful in monitoring disease activity when clinical findings are equivocal. Because the test is often normal in patients with neoplasms, infection, and connective tissue disease, the ESR cannot be used to exclude these diseases in patients with vague complaints.[8]

The ZSR is not affected by anemia, in contrast to the Westergren and Wintrobe methods.

The ZSR requires a special instrument.

TEST NAME AND METHOD	SPECIMEN REQUIREMENTS	REFERENCE INTERVAL, CONVENTIONAL [INTERNATIONAL RECOMMENDED UNITS]			CHEMICAL INTERFERENCES AND IN VIVO EFFECTS
Erythropoietin[1,2] *Chemiluminescent Assay*[3] *Automated Immunochemilu-minometric Assay (ICMA)*[3]	Serum or non-EDTA plasma. Stable at room temperature for 8 hr; refrigerated 1 wk; frozen 2 mo.	5-30 mU/mL	× 1.0	[5-30 U/L]	↑ V Anabolic steroids; exogenous erythropoietin (such as Epogen). ↓ V Amphotericin B inhibits usual erythropoietin response in anemic patients. HIV patients on AZT have lower erythropoietin levels.[4]

1. Lee BR, Luekens JN, et al: *Wintrobe's clinical hematology,* ed 11, Philadelphia, 2003, Lippincott Williams & Wilkins, 2003.
2. Erslev AJ, Caro J, Miller O, et al: Plasma erythropoietin in health and disease, *Ann Clin Lab Sci* 10:250-257, 1980.
3. Benson EW, Hardy R, Chaffin C, et al: New automated chemiluminescent assay for erythropoietin, *J Clin Lab Anal* 14:271-273, 2000.
4. Rischl M, Galpin JE, Levine JED, et al: Recombinant human erythropoietin for patients with AIDS treated with zidovudine, *N Engl J Med* 322:1488-1493, 1990.
5. Erslev AJ, Wilson J, Caro J: Erythropoietin titers in anemia, nonuremic patients, *J Lab Clin Med* 709:429-433, 1987.
6. Wilber RL: Detection of DNA-recombinant human epoeitin-alfa as a pharmacological ergonogenic aid, *Sports Med* 32:125-142, 2002.

TEST NAME AND METHOD	SPECIMEN REQUIREMENTS	REFERENCE INTERVAL, CONVENTIONAL [INTERNATIONAL RECOMMENDED UNITS]			CHEMICAL INTERFERENCES AND IN VIVO EFFECTS
Estetrol (E₄), Unconjugated[1,2] *RIA*	Plasma	*Weeks of gestation* *pg/mL* 20-26: 175 ± 30 (SE) 30: x̄: 350 36: x̄: 900 40: 1200 ± 110	× 0.00329	*nmol/L* [0.58 ± 0.10] [x̄: 1.15] [x̄: 2.96] [3.95 ± 0.36]	None found.
	Amniotic fluid[3]	*Weeks of gestation* *ng/mL* 32: 0.8 40-42: 13	× 3.29	*nmol/L* [2.6] [42.7]	

E₄ makes up 0.5-2.0% of total unconjugated estrogens at term [× 0.01 = 0.005-0.020, mass fraction].

1. Alsever RN, Gotlin RW: *Handbook of endocrine tests in adults and children,* ed 2, Chicago, 1978, Year Book Medical Publishers, Inc.
2. Tulchinsky D, Frigoletto F, Ryan KJ, et al: Plasma estetrol as an index of fetal well-being, *J Clin Endocrinol Metab* 40:560-567, 1975.

DIAGNOSTIC INFORMATION	**REMARKS**

↑ Anemias (including aplastic anemia), secondary polycythemia (e.g., high-altitude hypoxia, chronic obstructive pulmonary disease, pulmonary fibrosis), erythropoietin-producing tumors (e.g., cerebellar hemangioblastomas, pheochromocytomas, renal tumors), pregnancy (striking change), polycystic kidney disease, kidney transplant rejection (early manifestation?), following moderate bleeding of a normal individual

↓ Renal failure, primary polycythemia (Polycythemia vera)

Erythropoietin is a glycoprotein hormone that regulates erythropoiesis. Erythropoietin levels in anemia are primarily determined by the degree of anemia and not by any specific effect of the underlying illness on the production of erythropoietin.[5] This test is useful in differentiating primary from secondary polycythemia and in detecting recurrence of erythropoietin-producing tumors. It has been suggested that morning values are higher than afternoon values because of the diurnal rhythm of secretion.

Electrophoretic mobility methods have been recommended for detection of DNA-recombinant human erythropoietin when use is suspected by competitive athletes.[6]

See *Estriol, Free;* and *Estriol, Total.*

Estetrol (15α-hydroxyestriol), contrary to earlier expectations, does not appear to be a better indicator than estriol (E_3) for detecting fetal distress during the third trimester.[4] In contrast to E_3, negligible E_4 is contributed by the placenta. E_4 (as well as E_3) increases throughout gestation, with threefold to sevenfold increase between the 24th and 40th weeks.

3. Davis PJ: Aging and endocrine function, *Clin Endocrinol Metab* 8:603-619, 1979.
4. Casey ML, MacDonald PC, Simpson ER: Endocrinological changes of pregnancy. In Wilson JD, Foster DW, editors: *Williams textbook of endocrinology,* ed 8, Philadelphia, 1992, WB Saunders.

TEST NAME AND METHOD	SPECIMEN REQUIREMENTS	REFERENCE INTERVAL, CONVENTIONAL [INTERNATIONAL RECOMMENDED UNITS]		CHEMICAL INTERFERENCES AND IN VIVO EFFECTS
Estradiol (E$_2$), Unconjugated[1,2] *RIA*	Serum. Specimen may be stored at 2-8° C for 2 days in glass tubes. Otherwise, freeze and store at −20° C. Give the time of sampling with reference to the menstrual cycle.	Cord blood: 3000-29,000 pg/mL [× 3.67 = 11,010-106,430 pmol/L]		S ↑ V Clomiphene, diazepam
				S ↓ V Oral contraceptives (inhibit physiological increase), megestrol
		pg/mL	*pmol/L*	
		Prepubertal child[4]		
		30-60 days		
		M: 10-32 × 3.67	[37-117]	
		F: 5-50	[18-184]	
		6 mo-10 yr: <15	[<55]	
		Puberty[5]		
		Tanner stage		
		1		
		M: 3-15	[11-55]	
		F: 5-10	[18-37]	
		2		
		M: 3-10	[11-37]	
		F: 5-115	[18-422]	
		3		
		M: 5-15	[18-55]	
		F: 5-180	[18-661]	
		4		
		M: 3-40	[11-147]	
		F: 25-345	[92-1266]	
		5		
		M: 15-45	[55-165]	
		F: 25-410	[92-1505]	
		Adult[5]		
		M: 10-50	[37-184]	
		F, early follicular phase: 20-150	[73-551]	
		F, late follicular phase: 40-350	[147-1285]	
		F, midcycle peak: 150-750	[551-2753]	
		F, luteal phase: 30-450	[110-1652]	
		F, postmenopausal: ≤20	[≤73]	
	Urine, 24 hr. Preserve with boric acid.	*mcg/day*[6]	*nmol/day*	U ↑ V Spironolactone (in males)
		Children		
		M and		
		prepubertal		U ↓ V Oral contraceptives, probenecid
		F: <5 × 3.67	[<18.4]	
		Adult		
		M: 1-4	[3.7-14.7]	
		F, follicular: 1-13	[3.7-47.7]	
		F, midcycle: 4-20	[14.7-73.4]	
		F, luteal: 1-17	[3.7-26.1]	
		F, Postmenopausal: 0-4	[0-14.7]	
GLC-MS[3]	Amniotic fluid	Term: 0.8-1.9 ng/mL × 3.67	[2.9-7.0 nmol/L]	

DIAGNOSTIC INFORMATION	REMARKS

S ↑ Feminization in children, estrogen-producing tumors, gynecomastia, hepatic cirrhosis, hyperthyroidism

S ↓ Primary and secondary hypogonadism

Estradiol is the most active of endogenous estrogens. The test is of value, together with gonadotropins, in evaluating menstrual and fertility problems in adult females. Measurement is also useful in the evaluation of gynecomastia or feminization states due to estrogen-producing tumors, menstrual cycle irregularities, and sexual maturity in females and in monitoring of hMG (Pergonal) therapy.

Direct (no extraction) assays for E_2 in serum or plasma may give inaccurate results, particularly in prepubertal children or subjects receiving oral estrogen replacement therapy.[7] E_2 levels are markedly elevated at birth and decrease rapidly during the first week. In females, serum estradiol levels increase progressively throughout puberty. During the normal ovulatory cycle, estradiol is secreted in a biphasic pattern, with midcycle and luteal phase peaks. In males, estradiol levels increase during puberty as a result of peripheral testosterone conversion.[8]

TEST NAME AND METHOD	SPECIMEN REQUIREMENTS	REFERENCE INTERVAL, CONVENTIONAL [INTERNATIONAL RECOMMENDED UNITS]	CHEMICAL INTERFERENCES AND IN VIVO EFFECTS

Estradiol (E_2), Unconjugated—CONT

1. Landgren B, Aedo A, Diczfalusy E: Hormonal changes associated with ovulation and luteal function. In Flamigni C, Givens J, editors: *The gonadotropins: basic science and clinical aspects in females,* London, 1982, Academic Press.

2. Ratcliffe W, Carter G, Dowsett M, et al: Oestradiol assays: applications and guidelines for the provision of a clinical biochemistry service, *Ann Clin Biochem* 25:466-483, 1988.

3. Siegel AL, Adlercreutz H, Luukkainen T: Gas chromatographic and mass spectrometric identification of neutral and phenolic steroids in amniotic fluid, *Ann Med Exp Biol Fenn* 47:22-32, 1969.

4. Endocrine Sciences: *Pediatric laboratory services,* Tarzana, CA, 1992, Endocrine Sciences.

5. Nichols Institute Reference Laboratories: *Test catalog,* San Juan Capistrano, CA, 1993, Nichols Institute Reference Laboratories.

Estriol (E_3), Free (Unconjugated)[1-5]

RIA

Serum. Stable 4 days at 4° C. Specify weeks of gestation.

	ng/mL		*nmol/L*
M and nonpregnant F[7]:	<2.0	× 3.47	[<6.9]

Pregnancy Weeks of gestation[4]	ng/mL		nmol/L
22:	2.6-8.0	× 3.47	[9.0-27.8]
26:	2.5-13.5		[8.7-46.8]
30:	3.5-19.0		[12.1-65.9]
34:	5.3-18.3		[18.4-63.5]
35:	5.2-26.4		[18.0-91.6]
36:	8.2-28.1		[28.4-97.5]
37:	8.0-30.1		[27.8-104.4]
38:	8.6-38.0		[29.8-131.9]
39:	7.2-34.3		[25.0-119.0]
40:	9.6-28.9		[33.3-100.3]

Amniotic fluid[6]

Weeks of gestation	ng/mL (95% range)		nmol/L (95% range)
16-20:	1.0-3.2	× 3.47	[3.5-11]
20-24:	2.1-7.8		[7.3-27]
24-28:	2.1-7.8		[7.3-27]
28-32:	4.0-13.6		[14-47]
32-36:	3.6-15.5		[12-54]
36-38:	4.6-18.0		[16-62]
38-40:	5.4-19.8		[19-69]

S ↓ V Ampicillin, dinoprost tromethamine ($PGF_{2\alpha}$), penicillin

See also *Estriol, Total.*

---

1. Cuckle H: Measuring unconjugated estriol in maternal serum to screen for fetal Down syndrome [editorial], *Clin Chem* 38:1687-1789, 1992.

2. Johnson TR, Moore WM, Jefferies JE: *Children are different: developmental physiology,* ed 2, Columbus, OH, 1978, Ross Laboratories.

3. O'Shea G: Plasma estriols, *Can J Med Technol* 41:E132-E134, 1979.

DIAGNOSTIC INFORMATION	REMARKS

6. Joupilla R, Joupilla P, Koivisto M, et al: Maternal, foetal, and neonatal blood-creatine-phosphokinase activities and creatine-phosphokinase isoenzymes after labour with and without epidural analgesia and after Caesarean section, *Acta Anaesthesiol Scand* 22:491-496, 1978.
7. Diver MJ: Plasma estradiol concentrations in neonates, *Clin Chem* 33:1934, 1987.
8. Howanitz JH, Howanitz PJ: Hormones. In Howanitz JH, Howanitz PJ, editors: *Laboratory medicine: test selection and interpretation,* New York, 1991, Churchill Livingstone.

↑ Sharp increase if delivery is imminent

↓ In about half of pregnancies in which the fetus has major malformations of CNS not involving anterior pituitary; congenital heart disease, Down syndrome

Free E_3 measurements are more specific than total E_3 for monitoring the output of the fetoplacental unit at the time of phlebotomy.

Values vary widely from patient to patient; serial determinations are recommended. AM concentrations are higher than PM; therefore specimens should be drawn at the same time of day to allow comparison of values. E_3 increases progressively during pregnancy. (See *Estriol, Total.*) The surge in unconjugated serum E_3 levels during the 35th-36th weeks has proved useful in estimating fetal age.

Subnormal levels or a decrease in serum concentration in two or more successive measurements suggests fetal distress. Unfortunately, the sensitivity and specificity of this test for predicting fetal distress are very poor; thus its use for this purpose has been largely abandoned. However, serum determinations of E_3 in combination with β-hCG and AFP (triple test) or with β-hCG, AFP, and inhibin A (quadruple test)[8] are used for maternal screening for Down syndrome at 16-18 wk gestation. A great number of drugs interfere with the chemical determination of estriol; thus the RIA test is preferred for this and other analytical reasons.

Saliva is used as an alternative testing sample for free E_3 analysis.[9-11]

See *Estriol, Total;* and *Placental Lactogen.*

4. Ashwood ER: Clinical chemistry of pregnancy. In Burtis CA, Ashwood ER, editors: *Tietz textbook of clinical chemistry,* ed 3, Philadelphia, 1999, WB Saunders.
5. Tulchinsky D, Little AB, editors: *Maternal-fetal endocrinology,* Philadelphia, 1994, WB Saunders.
6. Younglai EV, Effer SB, Pelletier C: Amniotic fluid progestins and estrogens in relation to length of gestation, *Am J Obstet Gynecol* 111:833-839, 1971.

TEST NAME AND METHOD	SPECIMEN REQUIREMENTS	REFERENCE INTERVAL, CONVENTIONAL [INTERNATIONAL RECOMMENDED UNITS]		CHEMICAL INTERFERENCES AND IN VIVO EFFECTS

Estriol (E_3), Free (Unconjugated)—CONT

7. SmithKline Beecham Clinical Laboratories: *Directory of services,* Atlanta, GA, 1991, SmithKline Beecham Clinical Laboratories.

8. Jung K, Schulze G: Diuresis-dependent excretion of multiple forms of renal brush-border enzymes in urine, *Clin Chim Acta* 156:77-84, 1986.

9. Evans JJ, Wilkinson AR, Aickin DR: Salivary estriol concentrations during normal pregnancies, and a comparison with plasma estriol, *Clin Chem* 30:120-121, 1984.

TEST NAME AND METHOD	SPECIMEN REQUIREMENTS	REFERENCE INTERVAL, CONVENTIONAL		[INTERNATIONAL RECOMMENDED UNITS]	CHEMICAL INTERFERENCES AND IN VIVO EFFECTS
Estriol (E_3), Total[1,2] *RIA*	Serum or plasma (EDTA). Separate immediately and store frozen. Specify gestational age.	*Weeks of gestation* *ng/mL*[5] 28-30: 38-140 30: 31-140 32: 35-330 34: 45-260 36: 48-350 38: 59-570 40: 95-460	× 3.47	*nmol/L* [132-486] [108-486] [121-1145] [156-902] [167-1215] [205-1978] [330-1596]	S ↓ V Ampicillin, dinoprost tromethamine ($PGF_{2\alpha}$), penicillin
	Urine, 24 hr.[3] Collect with 1 g boric acid or preserve with thimerosal (25 mg/L); refrigerate during and after collection. Specify gestational age.	*mcg/day*[6] M: 1.0-11.0 F, follicular phase: 0-15.0 F, ovulatory phase: 13.0-54.0 F, luteal phase: 8.0-60.0 F, postmenopausal: 0-11.0 Pregnancy 1st trimester: 0-800 2nd trimester: 800-12,000 3rd trimester: 5000-50,000	× 3.47	*nmol/day* [3.5-38.2] [0-52.0] [45.1-187.4] [27.8-208.2] [0-38.2] [0-2776] [2776-41,640] [17,350-173,500]	U ↑ V Corticotropin (in pregnancy), spironolactone (males) U ↓ V Ampicillin, neomycin, oral contraceptives, probenecid, thyroxine
GLC	Amniotic fluid[4]	*Weeks of gestation* *ng/mL* 21-32: 5-50 33-35: 90-240 36-41: 150-213	× 3.47	*nmol/L* [17-174] [312-833] [521-739]	

DIAGNOSTIC INFORMATION	REMARKS

10. Jung K, Diego J, Strobelt V: Diagnostic significance of urinary enzymes in detecting acute rejection crises in renal transplant recipients depending on expression of results illustrated through the example of alanine aminopeptidase, *Clin Biochem* 18:257-260, 1985.
11. Jung K, Diego J, Strobelt V, et al: Diagnostic significance of some urinary enzymes for detecting acute rejection crises in renal-transplant recipients: alanine aminopeptidase, alkaline phosphatase, γ-glutamyltransferse, N-acetyl-β-D-glucosaminidase, and lysozyme, *Clin Chem* 32:1807-1811, 1986.

$\downarrow$ High-risk pregnancies involving diabetes, postmaturity, preeclampsia, fetal growth retardation, Rh immunization, intrauterine fetal death, anemia, malnutrition, pyelonephritis, intestinal disease and hemoglobinopathies, hypoplasia of fetal adrenals, anencephalic fetus; decreased in pregnancy with fetus affected by virilizing form of congenital adrenal hyperplasia; decreased in placental sulfatase deficiency or 16α-hydroxylase deficiency.

The predominant urinary estrogen during pregnancy is E_3. Serial measurement reflects the integrity of the fetoplacental complex. E_3 measurements are sometimes useful in following the high-risk pregnant patient. Declining values indicate fetal jeopardy, particularly if present over several days. A single determination cannot be interpreted in a meaningful fashion. Unfortunately, in some high-risk pregnancies, estriol values may not be reduced. In recent years E_3 measurements have been used less frequently in clinical practice in favor of ultrasound determinations and evaluations of maternal blood pressure, renal function, or carbohydrate metabolism. When serial measurements are performed, serum samples should be collected at the same time of day. Highest serum levels are seen at midday. See *Estrogens, Total;* and *Placental Lactogen.*

AF $\downarrow$ Anencephaly, erythroblastosis fetalis

At term E_3 represents >90% of the total amniotic fluid estrogens because it increases 5- to 10-fold in its mean values. Unconjugated E_3 is ~10% of total E_3 in amniotic fluid. The demonstration of a good correlation between E_3 levels in the amniotic fluid and in maternal urine would suggest no specific advantage of amniotic fluid over urinary E_3 determination. Decreases of amniotic E_3 closely parallel the severity of the hemolytic process in the fetus. It is claimed that amniotic fluid concentrations of E_3 of <100 ng/mL [<350 nmol/L] indicate that the fetus is in jeopardy. A highly significant correlation exists between amniotic fluid E_3 levels and the weight of the infant and placenta. Meconium in the amniotic fluid may give erroneously high E_3 levels. E_3 in a single amniotic fluid specimen is of limited value.

TEST NAME AND METHOD	SPECIMEN REQUIREMENTS	REFERENCE INTERVAL, CONVENTIONAL [INTERNATIONAL RECOMMENDED UNITS]	CHEMICAL INTERFERENCES AND IN VIVO EFFECTS

Estriol (E$_3$), Total—CONT

1. Miller RE, Ngai B: *Manual of endocrine diagnostic tests,* ed 4, Lexington, KY, 1991, Department of Medicine, University of Kentucky.
2. O'Shea G: Plasma estriols, *Can J Med Technol* 41:E132-E134, 1979.
3. Pesce A, Kaplan L, editors: *Methods in clinical chemistry,* St. Louis, 1987, CV Mosby.

TEST NAME AND METHOD	SPECIMEN REQUIREMENTS	REFERENCE INTERVAL, CONVENTIONAL [INTERNATIONAL RECOMMENDED UNITS]	CHEMICAL INTERFERENCES AND IN VIVO EFFECTS
Estrogen (Estradiol) Receptor Protein (ERP)[1-3] *Immunohisto-chemistry*	Tissue, frozen or formalin-fixed paraffin embedded. Tumor and biopsy, including core and fine-needle aspirates, specimens acceptable.	Subjective interpretation dependent on intensity of staining and number of positive cells. Only the staining of the cell nuclei is considered positive. Reported as positive or negative or as percent of positive cells. Favorable response >20% of cells stain; borderline, 11-20%; unfavorable, <10%.	In fine-needle aspirates, false-negative results due to air-drying artifacts or inadequate nuclei.

		fmol/mg cytosol protein		nmol/kg cytosol protein	
Ligand binding: dextran-coated charcoal method (DCC)[4]	Tissue, 0.1-1 g. Tissue must be dissected to be free of fat and normal tissue, cut into small pieces, placed in a plastic tube, and snap frozen in liquid nitrogen within 30 min of surgical removal. Store at −70° C. Frozen tissue is stable for several months.	Negative: Borderline: (or inhibition <60% by unlabeled hormone) Positive: (with K$_d$ >5 × 10^{-9} mol/L)	<6 6-10 >10	× 1.0	[<6] [>10]	↓ V Endogenous estrogens saturating receptor sites. Potentially falsely low results in fibrotic tumors, samples with low protein concentrations, from degradation of thermolabile receptor proteins.

		fmol/mg cytosol protein		nmol/kg cytosol protein
EIA		Negative: <15 Positive: >15	× 1.0	[<15] [>15]

---

1. Chan DW, Sell S: Tumor markers. In Burtis CA, Ashwood ER, editors: *Tietz textbook of clinical chemistry,* ed 3, Philadelphia, 1999, WB Saunders.
2. Spyratos F: Prognostic and predictive markers for breast cancer. In Diamandis EP, Fritsche HA, Lilja H, et al, editors: *Tumor markers. Physiology, pathobiology, technology, and clinical applications,* Washington, DC, 2002, AACC Press.
3. Elledge RM, Allred DC: Clinical aspects of estrogen and progesterone receptors. In Harris JR, Lippman ME, Morrow M, et al, editors: *Diseases of the breast,* ed 3, Philadelphia, 2004, Lippincott Williams & Wilkins.
4. Menendez-Botet CJ, Schwartz MK: A review of methodology for estrogen and progesterone receptor protein analysis, *J Int Fed Clin Chem* 4:94-99, 1992.
5. Fleisher M, Dnistrian AM, Sturgein CM, et al: Practice guidelines and recommendations for use of tumor markers in the clinic. In Diamandis EP, Fritsche HA, Lilja H, et al, editors: *Tumor markers. Physiology, pathobiology, technology, and clinical applications,* Washington, DC, 2002, AACC Press.

DIAGNOSTIC INFORMATION	REMARKS

4. Tulchinsky D, Ryan KJ, editors: *Maternal-fetal endocrinology,* Philadelphia, 1980, WB Saunders.
5. Goebelsmann U, Katagiri H, Stanczyk F, et al: Estriol assays in obstetrics, *J Steroid Biochem* 6:703-709, 1975.
6. ARUP-Cleveland Clinic Laboratory: *Reference manual,* Cleveland, OH, 1991, ARUP-Cleveland Clinic Laboratory.

Test is used primarily for identifying patients with breast cancers likely to respond to either additive or ablative hormone therapies.

Patients positive for both ERP and progesterone receptor protein (PRP, see also *Progesterone Receptor Protein*) have a higher percentage (75-80%) response to hormonal therapy than do women positive for either ERP or PRP alone. Only 40-50% of ERP-positive, PRP-negative patients respond; 25-30% of ERP-negative, PRP-positive show a response. Response is observed in only 10% or fewer of patients who are negative for both ERP and PRP. The percentage of positive specimens is greater in postmenopausal women than in those who are premenopausal. Receptor status is also influenced by age.

Patients who are hormone-receptor positive have a better prognosis for both disease-free survival and overall survival than those who are receptor negative.

The definition of positive or negative may vary from one laboratory to the next. Results can vary due to tissue and antibody treatment and antibody specificity.[3,5]

Estrogen receptors are a part of the nuclear steroid hormone receptor family and play a role in hormone directed transcriptional activation. There are two estrogen receptor isoforms: ERα (classic ER) and ERβ, which have 96% homology and 58% homology for DNA and ligand-binding domains, respectively. Ligand-binding properties and biological activities are different for the two isoforms with ERα playing a more predominant role in breast cancer.[1-3,5]

Estrogen receptors can be measured by quantitative ligand-binding assays (DCC) and immunoassays and semiquantitative/qualitative immunocytochemical assays. IHC measures receptors in the invasive carcinoma cells and not intraductal carcinoma or normal breast tissue in contrast to ligand-binding methods and are not influenced by the presence of estrogens, antiestrogens, or steroid-binding proteins.

Although clinical data and guidelines for the use of estrogen receptors were primarily developed using older techniques such as DCC, immunohistochemistry is considered equivalent or superior and is the preferred method in clinical practice.[3,6,7]

The American Society for Clinical Oncology, among other groups, recommends measurement of estrogen and progesterone receptors in primary breast cancers.[5,6]

6. Bast RC, Ravdin P, Hayes DF, et al: 2000 update of recommendations for the use of tumor markers in breast and colorectal cancer: clinical practice guidelines of the American Society of Clinical Oncology, *J Clin Oncol* 19:1865-1878, 2001.
7. Harvey JM, Clark GM, Osborne CK, et al: Estrogen receptor status by immunohistochemistry is superior to the ligand-binding assay for predicting response to adjuvant endocrine therapy in breast cancer, *J Clin Oncol* 17:1474-1481, 1999.

TEST NAME AND METHOD	SPECIMEN REQUIREMENTS	REFERENCE INTERVAL, CONVENTIONAL [INTERNATIONAL RECOMMENDED UNITS]			CHEMICAL INTERFERENCES AND IN VIVO EFFECTS
Estrogens, Total[1,2] *RIA*	Serum. Freeze immediately.	*Estrone plus estradiol*			↑ V Digoxin, estrogens, oral contraceptives
			pg/mL[3]	*ng/L*	
		Cord blood:	7500-65,000 × 1.0	[7500-65,000]	
		Prepuberty (1-10 yr):	<25	[<25]	
		Puberty Tanner stage 1			
		M:	10-38	[10-38]	
		F:	10-46	[10-46]	
		2			
		M:	17-45	[17-45]	
		F:	22-63	[22-63]	
		3			
		M:	22-55	[22-55]	
		F:	24-110	[24-110]	
		4			
		M:	27-80	[27-80]	
		F:	40-180	[40-180]	
		5			
		M:	25-80	[25-80]	
		F:	60-280	[60-280]	
		Adult			
		M:	20-80	[20-80]	
		F, follicular phase:	60-200	[60-200]	
		F, luteal phase:	160-400	[160-400]	
		F, postmeno-pausal[4]:	<130	[<130]	
	Urine, 24 hr. Preserve with boric acid. Keep refrigerated during collection.	*Estrone plus estradiol plus estriol*			U ↑ V Acetazolamide (in pregnancy), clomiphene, corticotropin, gonadotropin, hydrochlorothiazide (in pregnancy), testosterone
			mcg/day[5]	*Same*	
		Child:	<10		
		Adult			
		M:	15-40		
		F, premenopausal:	15-80		
		F, postmenopausal:	<20		U ↑ C *Fluorimetric, colorimetric:* Anthraquinone, levodopa, licorice, phenolphthalein; *Brown's and Kober's procedures:* Cortisone, meprobamate, methenamine, phenolphthalein, senna

↑ Ovarian tumors producing estrogens, granulosa cell and theca cell tumors, testicular tumors; some tumors or hyperplasia of adrenal cortex, chorioepithelioma

↓ Ovarian agenesis, primary ovarian malfunction, hypopituitarism, hypofunction of adrenal cortex, menopause, anorexia nervosa, psychogenic stress, GnRH deficiency

The serum assay does not measure estriol and should not be used in pregnancy or to assess fetal well-being. In addition to assessing gonadal hypofunction and hormonally active tumors, this test is used to evaluate sexual precocity, induction of ovulation, and oocyte recovery in in vitro fertilization.[6,7]

Plasma estrogen levels gradually increase during the follicular phase. A sharp midcycle peak is followed by a short ovulatory lowering (nadir) and then a second, rather broad, luteal increase corresponding more or less to the increase exhibited by 17-hydroxy-progesterone or progesterone. With the advent of immunoassay techniques, total estrogen measurements have been largely replaced by more specific methods.

TEST NAME AND METHOD	SPECIMEN REQUIREMENTS	REFERENCE INTERVAL, CONVENTIONAL [INTERNATIONAL RECOMMENDED UNITS]	CHEMICAL INTERFERENCES AND IN VIVO EFFECTS
Estrogens, Total—CONT			U ↓ V Ampicillin, dexamethasone, neomycin, oral contraceptives, penicillin, phenothiazines
			U ↓ C Axcetazolamide, fructose, falactose, glucose, inulin, methanamine, sucrose, and phenolphthalein affect hydrolysis of estrogen conjugates
			Colorimetric, fluorimetric: Corticotropin, danthron, hydrocholothiazide, vitamin B complex
			The following drugs cause interference with colorimetic/fluorometric procedures, but the effect has been reported both as an increase and a decrease: cascara, diethylstilbestrol, ethinyl estradiol.

1. Diczfalusy E: Circulating steroids and menstrual cycle. In Vokaer R, DeMaubeuge M, editors: *Sexual endocrinology,* New York, 1978, Masson Publishing USA.

2. Whitley RJ, Meikle AW, Watts NB: Endocrinology. In Burtis CA, Ashwood ER, editors: *Tietz textbook of clinical chemistry,* ed 2, Philadelphia, 1994, WB Saunders.

3. Endocrine Sciences: *Pediatric laboratory services,* Tarzana, CA, 1992, Endocrine Sciences.

4. Nichols Institute Reference Laboratories: *Test catalog,* San Juan Capistrano, CA, 1993, Nichols Institute Reference Laboratories.

5. Painter PC, Cope JY, Smith JL: Reference information for the clinical laboratory. In Burtis CA, Ashwood ER, editors: *Tietz textbook of clinical chemistry,* ed 3, Philadelphia, 1999, WB Saunders.

6. Taymor ML, Yussman MA, Gminski D: Estrogen monitoring in ovulation induction, *Fertil Steril* 21:759-762, 1970.

7. Thomas C, van den Berg R, Segers M: Time-resolved fluoroimmunoassay for unconjugated estrogen in urine: comparison with a fluorometric assay for total estrogen and application in an in vitro fertilization program, *Clin Chem* 36:1774-1778, 1990.

DIAGNOSTIC INFORMATION	REMARKS

TEST NAME AND METHOD	SPECIMEN REQUIREMENTS	REFERENCE INTERVAL, CONVENTIONAL [INTERNATIONAL RECOMMENDED UNITS]		CHEMICAL INTERFERENCES AND IN VIVO EFFECTS
Estrone (E_1)[1,2]	Serum. Freeze and store at $-20°$ C.		ng/dL^4 $pmol/L$	S ↑ V Digoxin, estrogens
RIA		Cord blood:	380-3100 $\times$ 37 [14,000-115,000]	
		Prepubertal child		
		1-10 yr:	<1.5 [<56]	
		Puberty Tanner stage		
		1		
		M:	0.5-1.7 [18-63]	
		F:	0.4-2.9 [15-107]	
		2		
		M:	1.0-2.5 [37-92]	
		F:	1.0-3.3 [37-122]	
		3		
		M:	1.5-2.5 [55-92]	
		F:	1.5-4.3 [55-159]	
		4		
		M:	1.5-4.5 [56-166]	
		F:	1.6-7.7 [59-285]	
		5		
		M:	2.0-4.5 [74-166]	
		F:	2.9-10.5 [107-388]	
		Adult[5]		
		M:	1.5-6.5 [55-240]	
		F, Early follicular phase:	1.5-15 [55-555]	
		F, Late follicular phase:	10-25 [370-925]	
		F, Luteal phase:	1.5-20 [55-740]	
		F, Postmeno-pausal:	1.5-5.5 [55-204]	
	Urine, 24 hr. Use 1 g boric acid as preservative. Stable 7 days at $4°$ C.		mcg/day $nmol/day$	U ↓ V Probenecid
		Adult[6]		
		M:	3-8 $\times$ 3.70 [11-30]	
		F, ovulatory peak:	11-31 [41-115]	
		F, luteal phase:	10-23 [37-85]	
		F, postmenopausal:	1-7 [4-26]	
GLC-MS[3]	Amniotic fluid	38-40 wk:	2.3-4.0 ng/mL $\times$ 3.7 [9-15 nmol/L]	

1. Loraine JA, Bell ET: *Hormone assays and their clinical application,* New York, 1976, Churchill Livingstone.
2. Radfan N, Ansusingha K, Kenny F: Estradiol and estrone during normal and precocious growth, *J Pediatr* 89:719, 1976.
3. Tulchinsky D, Ryan KJ, editors: *Maternal-fetal endocrinology,* Philadelphia, 1980, WB Saunders.
4. Endocrine Sciences: *Pediatric laboratory services,* Tarzana, CA, 1992, Endocrine Sciences.

DIAGNOSTIC INFORMATION	REMARKS

Estrone increases 10-fold in pregnancy from the 24th to the 41st wk. E_1 (but not estradiol, E_2) in nonpregnant women and in men shows significant diurnal rhythm. See *Estrogens, Total; and Estradiol, Unconjugated.*

Values are very high at birth but decrease after 7 days to prepubertal levels.

E_1 is a more potent estrogen than estriol (E_3) but is less potent than estradiol (E_2). E_1 is the major circulating estrogen after menopause. E_2/E_1 ratios change appreciably during the menstrual cycle. Most E_1 is in the form of the sulfate conjugate.[7]

There is no increase in concentration of E_1 and E_2 between 12 and 40 wk of gestation. Amniotic fluid concentrations of these steroids may reflect their concentration in fetal blood.

5. Nichols Institute Reference Laboratories: *Test catalog,* San Juan Capistrano, CA, 1993, Nichols Institute Reference Laboratories.

6. Painter PC, Cope JY, Smith JL: Reference information for the clinical laboratory. In Burtis CA, Ashwood ER, editors: *Tietz textbook of clinical chemistry,* ed 3, Philadelphia, 1999, WB Saunders.

7. Rémy-Martin A, Prost O, Nicollier M, et al: Estrone sulfate concentrations in plasma of normal individuals, postmenopausal women with breast cancer, and men with cirrhosis, *Clin Chem* 29:86-89, 1983.

TEST NAME AND METHOD	SPECIMEN REQUIREMENTS	REFERENCE INTERVAL, CONVENTIONAL [INTERNATIONAL RECOMMENDED UNITS]		CHEMICAL INTERFERENCES AND IN VIVO EFFECTS
Ethanolamine (EA)[1,2] *Ion-exchange chromatographic*	Urine, 24 hr. Add 10 mL of 6 mol/L HCl at start of collection. (Alternatively, refrigerate specimen during collection.) Store frozen at $-20°$ C.[3]	*mg/g creatinine* Newborn[5]: 110	*mmol/mol creatinine* $\times$ 1.85 [203.5]	None found.
		mg/dL	$\mu mol/L^6$	
		Child: 0.73-2.54 $\times$ 163.7	[120-416]	
		Adult: 1.81-4.90	[297-802]	
		1 day-1 mo 5.1-20.7	[840-3400][7]	
		1 mo-2 yr 0-13.6	[0-2230][7]	
		2 yr-18 yr 0-3.2	[0-530][7]	
		Adult 0-3.1	[0-520][7]	
	CSF. Collect in sterile tubes; store frozen. Stable at $-20°$ C for 1 wk or at $-70°$ C for 2 mo.[4]	*mg/dL* Neonate: 0.118 ± 0.04 (SEM) $\times$ 163.7 3 mo-2 yr: 0.038 ± 0.011 2 yr-10 yr: 0.048 ± 0.014 Adult: 0.074 ± 0.009	$\mu mol/L$ $[19.3 \pm 6.6]^8$ $[6.2 \pm 1.8]^9$ $[7.8 \pm 2.3]^9$ $[12.1 \pm 1.5]^{10}$	

1. Scriver CR, Beaudet AL, Valle D, et al, editors: *The metabolic and molecular bases of inherited disease,* ed 8, New York, 2001, McGraw-Hill.

2. Bremer HJ, Duran M, Kamerling JP, et al: *Disturbances of amino acid metabolism: clinical chemistry and diagnosis,* Baltimore, 1981, Urban and Schwarzenburg.

3. Pesce A, Kaplan LA, editors: *Methods in clinical chemistry,* St. Louis, 1987, Mosby.

4. Heiblim DI, Evans HE, Glass L, et al: Amino acid concentrations in cerebrospinal fluid, *Arch Neurol* 35:765-768, 1978.

5. Saifer A: Rapid screening methods for the detection of inherited and acquired aminoacidopathies, *Adv Clin Chem* 14:145-218, 1971.

6. Meites S, editor: *Pediatric clinical chemistry,* ed 3, Washington, DC, 1989, American Association for Clinical Chemistry.

7. Slocum RH, Cummings JG: Amino acid analysis of physiological samples. In Hommes FA, editor: *Techniques in human biochemical genetics,* New York, 1991, Wiley-Liss, pp. 87-126.

8. Heiblim DI, Evans HE, Glass L, et al: Amino acid concentrations in cerebrospinal fluid, *Arch Neurol* 35:765-768, 1978.

9. Goldsmith RF, Earl JW, Cunningham AM: Determination of δ-aminobutyric acid and other amino acids in cerebrospinal fluid of pediatric patients by reversed-phase liquid chromatography, *Clin Chem* 33:1736-1740, 1987.

10. Shih V: *Laboratory techniques for the detection of hereditary metabolic disorders,* Boca Raton, FL, 1973, CRC Press.

Ethyl glucuronide (EtG)[1] *Chromatographic methods, ELISA*	Serum	Undetectable ($<$0.1 mg/L)[3,4]	Unknown.
	Urine, stable for 4 days at room temperature.[2]	Undetectable ($<$0.1 mg/L)[5]	

DIAGNOSTIC INFORMATION	REMARKS

U ↑ Hyperlysinemia, primary hepatoma, ethanolaminosis

Relatively high concentrations of free EA are present in human tissues, especially in the brain, lung, and liver. In urine a very high excretion occurs on the first day of life.

Values in children (3 mo-10 yr) were measured using reversed-phase liquid chromatography.

↑ Alcohol intake.

Ethyl glucuronide (EtG) is a highly specific but minor metabolite of ethanol. It is generated by conjugation of ethanol with glucuronide in the liver. Shortly after intake of even small amounts of ethanol, EtG is detectable, peaks at 2-3.5 hr in blood and subsequently decreases exponentially. The half-life ranges from 2-3 hr. EtG is eliminated through urine excretion.

EtG is nonvolatile, water-soluble, and stable. It can be detected up to 80 hr after the complete elimination of ethanol from the body. It is used as a sensitive and specific marker for detecting recent alcohol use and a marker for detecting lapse/relapse.

TEST NAME AND METHOD	SPECIMEN REQUIREMENTS	REFERENCE INTERVAL, CONVENTIONAL [INTERNATIONAL RECOMMENDED UNITS]	CHEMICAL INTERFERENCES AND IN VIVO EFFECTS

Ethyl glucuronide—CONT

1. Wurst FM, Skipper GE, Weinmann W: Ethyl glucuronide—the direct ethanol metabolite on the threshold from science to routine use, *Addiction* 98(suppl 2):51-61, 2003.
2. Stephanson N, Dahl H, Helander A, et al: Direct quantification of ethyl glucuronide in clinical urine samples by liquid chromatography-mass spectrometry, *Ther Drug Monit* 24:645-651, 2002.
3. Schmitt G, Droenner P, Skopp G, et al: Ethyl glucuronide concentration in serum of human volunteers, teetotalers, and suspected drinking drivers, *J Forensic Sci* 42:1099-1102, 1997.

Euglobulin Clot Lysis (EGT, Euglobulin Lysis Time)[1]	Test performed on freshly drawn platelet-poor plasma (citrate). Laboratory must be notified in advance, and the sample must be centrifuged within 30 min at 4° C.	Tubes should be inspected every 15 min for clot lysis. In most individuals clot lysis will be complete between 90 min and 4 hr. A normal control should always be run in parallel. <90 min: increased (abnormal) fibrinolytic activity	↓ V Alteplase (t-PA), anistreplase, asparaginase, clofibrate, dextran, streptokinase, urokinase Note: Arrow indicates decreased lysis *time* (=increased fibrinolysis).

1. Lewis SM, Bain BJ, Bates I, editors: *Dacie and Lewis practical hematology,* ed 9, Edinburgh, 2001, Churchill Livingstone.

Factor Inhibitors (specific)[1,2] *Bethesda method for quantitation of factor inhibitors*	Plasma (citrate). Stable on ice for up to 4 hr. Stable indefinitely frozen.	Specific inhibitors to factors VIII and IX are typically measured in Bethesda units. One Bethesda unit is defined as the amount of inhibitor that inactivates 50% of the factor VIII or IX in an equal mixture of normal and patient plasma in 2 hr at 37° C.	↑ Other anticoagulants such as heparin or lupus anticoagulant

1. Lewis SM, Bain BJ, Bates I, editors: *Dacie and Lewis practical hematology,* ed 9, Edinburgh, 2001, Churchill Livingstone.
2. Jacobs DS, Demott WR, Oxley DK, editors: *Laboratory test handbook,* ed 5, Hudson, OH, 2001, Lexi-Comp, Inc.

DIAGNOSTIC INFORMATION	REMARKS

4. Schmitt G, Aderjan R, Keller T, et al: Ethyl glucuronide: an unusual ethanol metabolite in humans. Synthesis, analytical data, and determination in serum and urine, *J Anal Toxicol* 19:91-94, 1995.
5. Dahl H, Stephanson N, Beck O, et al: Comparison of urinary excretion characteristics of ethanol and ethyl glucuronide, *J Anal Toxicol* 26:201-204, 2002.

Lysis is marked and rapid in primary fibrinolysis but is only minimal or is not present in conditions associated with secondary fibrinolysis (e.g., liver disease, DIC).

Increased fibrinolysis (shortened lysis time) may be associated with severe stress (exercise, surgery, cancer), α_2-antiplasmin deficiency,[2] or plasminogen activator inhibitor-1 deficiency.

A falsely low lysis time may be seen in DIC due to low fibrinogen.

The Euglobin clot lysis time (EGT) is a global test of the fibrinolytic system. When plasma is diluted and acidified, the precipitate formed contains plasminogen and its activators but is devoid of most of the plasmin inhibitors. When this precipitate is redissolved, the ability to lyse a fibrin clot is then assessed.

EGT is a screening test for determining fibrinolysis in the absence of inhibitors. This test may also be used to monitor therapy with urokinase, streptokinase, and tissue plasminogen activator. If fibrinogen is low, no clot may form unless fibrinogen is added to the sample. If plasminogen has been depleted, test may be normal. Heparin therapy does not affect the results. Lysis time may be shortened in healthy persons after exercise. Prolonged venous occlusion by tourniquet may increase fibrinolytic activity. Traumatic venipuncture may cause an increase in fibrinolytic activity.

2. Aoki N, Saito H, Kamiya T, et al: Congenital deficiency of α_2 plasmin inhibitor associated with severe hemorrhagic tendency, *J Clin Invest* 63:877-884, 1979.

Specific factor inhibitors may arise against any coagulation factor.

Specific inhibitors to factors VIII and IX are by far the most common. A specific inhibitor may arise in patients with known hereditary factor deficiency or rarely in nonhemophiliac patients. These antibodies may arise spontaneously or in association with drugs or autoimmune disorders. Specific inhibitors to other factors are very rare. Specific factor inhibitors may be associated with severe clinical bleeding.

The presence of an inhibitor to factor VIII or factor IX is usually suspected with a prolonged APTT in the presence of a normal PT and a mixing study with a "no correction" pattern (immediate and/or at 2 hr incubation).

The classic Bethesda quantitative inhibitor assay is typically described for factor VIII inhibitors. The Bethesda assay may be modified as follows: *porcine* factor VIII may be used to determine whether the factor VIII inhibitor cross-reacts with porcine factor VIII; the incubation time of 2 hr is not necessary to quantify a factor IX inhibitor; the normal plasma may be substituted by factor VIII concentrate (Oxford method).

TEST NAME AND METHOD	SPECIMEN REQUIREMENTS	REFERENCE INTERVAL, CONVENTIONAL [INTERNATIONAL RECOMMENDED UNITS]	CHEMICAL INTERFERENCES AND IN VIVO EFFECTS
Factor XIII Screen (Fibrin-stabilizing Factor, FSF, Clot solubility test)[1] *Screen of clot solubility, 37° C (urea, 5 mol/L)*	Plasma (blue top-citrate). Stable for 2 hr at 4° C, on ice for 4 hr, or store frozen.	In a patient with hemostatic levels of factor XIII, the clot will remain stable for 24 hr. In the absence of factor XIII, the clot will dissolve, often within ≤2-3 hr.	None found.

1. Anwar R, Miloszewski KJ: Factor XIII deficiency, *Br J Hematol* 107:468-484, 1999.

Fat, Fecal[1-4] *Gravimetric*[3,4]	Feces, 72 hr. Refrigerate during collection. Avoid urinary contamination. Do not use wax-coated containers.	*g/day* Infant Breast-fed: <1 0-6 yr: <2 Adult: <7 Adult (fat-free diet): <4 Stool fats are heterogeneous results that should be reported in g/day rather than in mmol/day.	↑ V Aminosalicylic acid (high dose), azathioprine, bisacodyl (prolonged use), cholestyramine (dose >15 g/day), kanamycin, neomycin, tetracycline
Titrimetric[1,3,4]		Adult: <6	↓ C Medium-chain triglyceride supplements

Colorimetric[5]

		% of dry wt.	Mass fraction (dry wt.)
Infant			
Breast-fed:		9-38	× 0.01 [0.09-0.38]
Formula-fed:		27-52	[0.27-0.52]
Adult:		15-25	[0.15-0.25]

	Coefficient of fat absorption (%)[3]	Absorbed fraction
Infant		
Breast-fed:	>93	× 0.01 [>0.93]
Formula-fed:	>83	[>0.83]
>1 yr:	≥95	[≥0.95]

DIAGNOSTIC INFORMATION	REMARKS

Positive: Hereditary factor XIII deficiency

Rare acquired factor XIII inhibitors (some associated with isoniazid, penicillin, or phenytoin).

Hereditary factor XIII deficiency is rare. Symptomatic patients usually have <1% activity. Factor XIII deficiency typically causes delayed bleeding and poor wound healing. In the neonate it can present as umbilical stump bleeding.

The factor XIII screen evaluates clot stability in 5 mol/L urea. This test will detect most symptomatic patients. Kits for confirmatory quantitative assays for factor XIII antigen are now available.

↑ Fat malabsorption results from three disorder categories: pancreatic insufficiency (loss of lipase and inability to split triglycerides), hepatobiliary (bile deficiency and inadequate emulsification), and intestinal (rapid transit, inadequate absorptive surface, etc.); thus small-bowel diseases with fat malabsorption, viral hepatitis, diabetes mellitus, peptic ulcer disease, carcinoid syndrome, α-β-lipoproteinemia, cystic fibrosis, multiple sclerosis, gastroduodenal fistula, regional enteritis, extrahepatic biliary obstruction, psoriasis, progressive systemic sclerosis, dumping syndrome, pancreatic insufficiency or obstruction, Whipple's disease, malnutrition, celiac disease, tropical sprue, thyrotoxicosis, pernicious anemia, Addison's disease, liver cirrhosis, increased intestinal motility

A dietary fat intake of 50-150 g/day of long-chain triglyceride should be maintained for at least 2 days before and during the collection period for the fecal fat determination. Patients should consume 30 mL corn or olive oil with each meal. Butter is composed of short chain FA and does not count.

Procedures without hydrolysis measure only total fatty acids, which represent 60-80% of total fecal lipids. Variation among methods depends on which fatty acid is used as the standard.

Various lipid tolerance tests (ingestion of lipid followed by serum measurements) are not useful.

$$\text{Coefficient of fat absorption } (\%) = \frac{\text{Fat ingested} - \text{fat excreted}}{\times 100 \text{ Fat ingested}}$$

TEST NAME AND METHOD	SPECIMEN REQUIREMENTS	REFERENCE INTERVAL, CONVENTIONAL [INTERNATIONAL RECOMMENDED UNITS]	CHEMICAL INTERFERENCES AND IN VIVO EFFECTS
Fat, Fecal—CONT			
Microscopic screen[4,6]	Random stool sample	An average of 2.5 fat droplets per high power field in normal individuals.	

1. Behrman RE, Kliegman RM, Nelson WE, et al, editors: *Nelson textbook of pediatrics,* ed 14, Philadelphia, 1992, WB Saunders.
2. Brown SS, Mitchell FL, Young DS, editors: *Chemical diagnosis of disease,* Amsterdam, 1979, Elsevier/North Holland Biomedical Press.
3. Henry RJ, Cannon DC, Winkelman JW, editors: *Clinical chemistry: principles and technics,* ed 2, Hagerstown, MD, 1974, Harper and Row.
4. Tietz NW, editor: *Fundamentals of clinical chemistry,* ed 5, Philadelphia, 2001, WB Saunders.
5. Massion CG, McNeely MD: Accurate method for estimation of both medium- and long-chain fatty acids and triglycerides in fecal fat, *Clin Chem* 19:499-505, 1973.
6. Fine KD, Ogunji F: A new method of quantitative fecal fat microscopy and its correlation with chemically measured fecal fat output, *Am J Clin Pathol* 113:528-534, 2000.

TEST NAME AND METHOD	SPECIMEN REQUIREMENTS	REFERENCE INTERVAL, CONVENTIONAL [INTERNATIONAL RECOMMENDED UNITS]	CHEMICAL INTERFERENCES AND IN VIVO EFFECTS
Fatty Acid Binding Protein, Heart Type (H-FABP)[1-4]	Serum or plasma	*mcg/L*	
		Reference interval (HyCult) 0-1.6	
Immunoassay		Myoglobin/H-FAPB ratio[1]	
		Heart 4-5	
		Skeletal muscle 20-70 (depending on source)	
		Serum cutoff <10	

1. Glatz JF, van de Vusse GJ, Simoons ML, et al: Fatty acid-binding protein and the early detection of acute myocardial infarction, *Clin Chim Acta* 272:87-92, 1998.
2. Ghani F, Wu AHB, Petry C, et al: Role of heart type fatty acid-binding protein in early detection of acute myocardial infarction, *Clin Chem* 46:718-719, 2000.
3. Van Nieuwenhoven FA, Kleine AH, Wodzig WH, et al: Discrimination between myocardial and skeletal muscle injury by assessment of the plasma ratio of myoglobin over fatty acid-binding protein, *Circulation* 92:2848-2854, 1995.
4. Glatz JFC, Vander Putten RFM, Hermans WT, et al: Fatty acid binding protein as an early plasma marker of myocardial ischemia and risk stratification. In Wu AHB, editor: *Cardiac markers,* ed 2, Totowa, NJ, 2003, Humana Press.

Patients with steatorrhea have, on average, 10 times as many fat droplets per standard volume of stool as healthy controls.

Screening methods are 98% sensitive when performed with great care. Routine performance of this test generally does not provide results equivalent to those reported in the medical literature.

The ability of assays to distinguish total, split, and neutral fats is overemphasized because bowel flora can hydrolyze triglyceride. Total fat, regardless of form, is the clinically important value.

Heart-type fatty acid binding protein is released into blood after irreversible myocardial damage and is an early marker of myocardial infarction. H-FABP is released with the same kinetics as myoglobin, i.e., first increased within 3-6 hr and returns to normal within 24 hr.[2] However, H-FABP is more specific to cardiac damage, as the ratio of heart to skeletal muscle for H-FABP is higher (~7) than for myoglobin (~0.6).[3] Some have advocated the use of a myoglobin to H-FABP ratio.[4]

Fatty acid binding protein is a low molecular weight protein (14-15 kDa) found in the cytoplasm of most cells. There are at least nine isoenzymes, including heart (H), liver (L), and intestinal (I).[4] Whereas the heart type is found in the highest concentration in the myocardium, H-FABP is also found in skeletal muscles, distal renal tubules, and the brain.

TEST NAME AND METHOD	SPECIMEN REQUIREMENTS	REFERENCE INTERVAL, CONVENTIONAL [INTERNATIONAL RECOMMENDED UNITS]		CHEMICAL INTERFERENCES AND IN VIVO EFFECTS
Fatty Acid Profile[1-3] *GLC*[1,2]	Serum, plasma (EDTA, heparin), fasting ≥12 hr. Collect on ice and send to laboratory without delay.	*Nonesterified fatty acids, % of total*	*Fraction of total nonesterified fatty acids*	
		Oleic: 26-45 × 0.01	[0.26-0.45]	
		Palmitic: 23-25	[0.23-0.25]	
		Stearic: 10-14	[0.10-0.14]	
		Linoleic: 8-16	[0.08-0.16]	
		Linoleate[4]: ≥25	[≥0.25]	
		Arachidonate: ≥6	[≥0.06]	
		Ratio, % linoleic to % palmitic	*Ratio, fraction of linoleic to palmitic*	
		Normal: ≥0.70 × 0.01	[≥0.007]	
		Chronic malabsorption of linoleic: <0.70	[<0.007]	
		Ratio, % eicosatrienoic to % arachidonic[5]: <0.40 × 0.01	[<0.004, fraction]	
		This ratio is the hallmark of essential fatty acid deficiency.		

1. Tietz NW, editor: *Fundamentals of clinical chemistry,* ed 5, Philadelphia, 2001, WB Saunders.
2. Nelson GJ, editor: *Blood lipids and lipoproteins: quantitation, composition, and metabolism,* New York, 1972, Wiley-Interscience.
3. Cunnane SC: Problems with essential fatty acids: time for a new paradigm? *Prog Lipid Res* 42:544-568, 2003.
4. Leavelle DE, editor: *Mayo Medical Laboratories interpretive handbook,* Rochester, MN, 1988, Mayo Medical Laboratories.
5. Cleveland Clinic Foundation. Division of Laboratory Medicine: *Guide to laboratory services,* Cleveland, 1979-1980, Cleveland Clinic Foundation.

TEST NAME AND METHOD	SPECIMEN REQUIREMENTS	REFERENCE INTERVAL, CONVENTIONAL	[INTERNATIONAL RECOMMENDED UNITS]	CHEMICAL INTERFERENCES AND IN VIVO EFFECTS
Fatty Acids, Free (FFA, NEFA)[1,2] *Colorimetric*[1,2] *HPLC*[3]	Plasma (heparin or EDTA), fasting ≥12 hr. Separate from cells under refrigerated conditions and analyze without delay. Blood from heparinized patients is	*mg/dL*[2] Adult: 8-25 × 0.0354* Child and obese adult: <31	*mmol/L* [0.28-0.89] [<1.10]	↑ V Amphetamines, benzquinamide, caffeine, carbutamide, chlorpromazine, desipramine, diazoxide, endotoxin, epinephrine, ethanol, glucose, hGH, heparin,

DIAGNOSTIC INFORMATION	REMARKS
	See also *Phytanic Acid, Fatty Acids, Free and Omega-3 and Omega-6 Fatty Acids.*
	The test has limited clinical application. Used in nutritional and lipid research.
	Using the FA profile to adjust dietary intake in otherwise normal persons is not widely accepted.
↓ Acrodermatitis enteropathica	This condition is seen with impaired absorption and metabolism of essential fatty acids.
	Potential decrease in severe fat malabsorption, alcoholism, infants not breast-fed, and TPN.
	Omega-3 and -6 fatty acids may be considered part of an FA profile.
↑ Anything that causes a release of lipolytic substances (e.g., ACTH, epinephrine, glucagons, growth hormone, norepinephrine, thyrotropin, thyroxin); thus starvation, fasting, stress, exercise, diabetes (out of control), late pregnancy (placental hormones), pheochromocytoma, thyrotoxicosis, von Gierke's disease, most metabolic disturbances.	Most fatty acids have an even number of C atoms and are present in anionic form. They are carried largely by albumin and to some extent by lipoproteins.
	Even when plasma is refrigerated, FFA increases 12-25% in 24 hr. However, fatty acids in heptane extracts are stable for several days if refrigerated.

TEST NAME AND METHOD	SPECIMEN REQUIREMENTS	REFERENCE INTERVAL, CONVENTIONAL [INTERNATIONAL RECOMMENDED UNITS]	CHEMICAL INTERFERENCES AND IN VIVO EFFECTS
Fatty Acids, Free—CONT	unsuitable for analysis. Specimen unstable; see *Remarks*.		isoproterenol, levodopa, lysergide, mescaline, molindone, nicotine, oral contraceptives, phenformin, prazosin, reserpine, theophyline, tolbutamide, thyroxine
			↑ C *Colorimetric:* acetic acid, acetoacetic acid, β-hydroxybutyric acid, lactic acid, phospholipids
		*Conversion factor based on MW for oleic acid of 282.47.	↓ V Asparaginase, aspirin, β-blockers, clofibrate, enflurane, glibormuride, glisoxepid, glucose, glyburide, insulin, neomycin, niacin, nicotinyl alcohol, phenformin, streptozotocin, sucrose

1. Henry RJ, Cannon DC, Winkelman JW, editors: *Clinical chemistry: principles and technics,* ed 2, Hagerstown, MD, 1974, Harper and Row.
2. Tietz NW, editor: *Fundamentals of clinical chemistry,* ed 5, Philadelphia, 2001, WB Saunders.
3. Mehta A, Oeser AM, Carlson MG: Rapid quantification of free fatty acids in human plasma by high-performance liquid chromatography, *J Chromatogr B Biomed Sci Appl* 719:9-23, 1998.
4. Kitchell BB, Lazar JD, Whorton AR, et al: Some pitfalls in the quantitation and comparison of plasma free fatty acids, *Clin Chem* 27:356-357, 1981.
5. Jeevanandam M, Hsu Y-C, Ramias L, et al: A rapid, automated micromethod for measuring free fatty acids in plasma/serum, *Clin Chem* 35:2228-2231, 1989.

TEST NAME AND METHOD	SPECIMEN REQUIREMENTS	REFERENCE INTERVAL, CONVENTIONAL [INTERNATIONAL RECOMMENDED UNITS]	CHEMICAL INTERFERENCES AND IN VIVO EFFECTS
Ferric Chloride Test ($FeCl_3$)[1-4]	Urine, fresh random	Negative	↑ C Aminosalicylic acid, clioquinol, levodopa, phenazone, phenothiazines, salicylates

1. Hicks JM, Boeckx RL, editors: *Pediatric clinical chemistry,* Philadelphia, 1984, WB Saunders.
2. Kaplan LA, Pesce AJ, editors: *Clinical chemistry: theory, analysis and correlation,* ed 2, St. Louis, 1989, CV Mosby.

DIAGNOSTIC INFORMATION	REMARKS

↓ Cystic fibrosis

FFA determinations offer no clinically useful diagnostic information but are used in metabolic research.

Because some plasma components interfere with colorimetric procedures, previous extraction of the specimen will improve accuracy.[4]

Enzymatic methods have the advantage that no extraction step is needed and that the reactions are specific for FFA.[5]

Positive: Ketonuria, phenylketonuria, tyrosinemia (green); homogentisuria (blue-green); maple syrup urine disease (gray-green); melanoma (gray turning black)[1]

The colors obtained in this test are highly variable, primarily as a result of color masking by the urinary pigments. This is not a specific test and is very insensitive. Positive results for metabolic disorders or for drugs must be confirmed by methods with higher specificity, particularly methods based on GC-MS or LC-MS-MS. Negative tests do not exclude the possibility of abnormal urinary constituents.

3.   Pesce A, Kaplan L, editors: *Methods in clinical chemistry,* St. Louis, 1987, CV Mosby.

4.   Hommes FA, editor: *Techniques in diagnostic human biochemical genetics,* New York, 1991, Wiley-Liss.

TEST NAME AND METHOD	SPECIMEN REQUIREMENTS	REFERENCE INTERVAL, CONVENTIONAL [INTERNATIONAL RECOMMENDED UNITS]				CHEMICAL INTERFERENCES AND IN VIVO EFFECTS
Ferritin[1,2] *RIA, EIA, IRMA*	Serum. Stable 7 days at 2-8° C, 6 mo at −20° C. Avoid repeated freezing and thawing. Do not thaw frozen specimens in a 37° C bath. Violent mixing may denature ferritin.		*ng/mL*[2,3]		*mcg/L*	S ↑ V Ethanol (alcoholics), iron salts, oral contraceptives
		Newborn:	25-200	× 1.0	[25-200]	
		1 mo:	200-600		[200-600]	
		2-5 mo:	50-200		[50-200]	
		6 mo-15 yr:	7-140		[7-140]	S ↓ V Erythropoietin
		Adult				
		M:	20-250		[20-250]	
		F:	10-120		[10-120]	
		Iron overload				
		Adult M:	>400		[>400]	
		Adult F:	>200		[>200]	
		See also *Remarks*.				

1. Nuttall KL, Klee GG: Analytes of hemoglobin metabolism—porphyrin, iron, and bilirubin. In Burtis CA, Ashwood ER, editors: *Fundamentals of clinical chemistry,* ed 5, Philadelphia, 2001, WB Saunders.
2. Williams WJ, Beutler E, Erslev AJ, et al, editors: *Hematology,* ed 3, New York, 1983, McGraw-Hill Book Co.
3. Seamonds B, Anderson K, Whitaker B: Reference intervals for ferritin: age dependence, *Clin Chem* 26:1515-1516, 1980.

Fetal Hemoglobin (Hb F)[1-4]	Hemolysate prepared from whole blood (EDTA, citrate, heparin)		*% Hb F*		*Mass fraction Hb F*	None found.
Alkali denaturation (White)		1 day:	77.0 ± 7.3	× 0.01	[0.770 ± 0.073]	
		5 days:	76.8 ± 5.8		[0.768 ± 0.058]	
		3 wk:	70.0 ± 7.3		[0.700 ± 0.073]	
		6-9 wk:	52.9 ± 11.0		[0.529 ± 0.110]	
		3-4 mo:	23.2 ± 16.0		[0.232 ± 0.160]	
EP, pH 8.4-8.6		6 mo:	4.7 ± 2.2		[0.047 ± 0.022]	
		8-11 mo:	1.6 ± 1.0		[0.160 ± 0.010]	
		Adult:	<2.0		[<0.020]	
Cation exchange Chromatography[5-7]						

DIAGNOSTIC INFORMATION	REMARKS

↑↑ Iron overload (e.g., hemochromatosis, certain liver diseases)

↑ Fasting or inanition, acute leukemia, inflammatory diseases (e.g., pulmonary infections, osteomyelitis, chronic urinary tract infections, rheumatoid arthritis, SLE, burns), certain acute and chronic hepatocellular diseases (e.g., alcoholic and inflammatory liver disease), acute myeloblastic and lymphoblastic leukemia, Hodgkin's disease, breast carcinoma. Increase in serum or plasma ferritin due to inflammatory conditions (acute phase response) can mask a diagnostically low result.

↓ Iron deficiency. Ferritin levels <10 ng/mL [<10 mcg/L] usually indicate iron deficiency anemia.

Ferritin originates in the reticuloendothelial system (RES). It consists of a protein shell, apoferritin (MW 445,000), containing varying amounts of iron in its core as ferric hydroxide-phosphate complexes.

Serum ferritin contains 20-25% iron; its concentration is a good measure of iron stores in normal persons and in individuals with iron deficiency; 1 ng/mL [1 mcg/L] of serum ferritin is equivalent to 8 mg [143 μmol] of stored iron.

Fe uptake by ferritin requires previous oxidation of Fe^{2+} to Fe^{3+}. The measurement of serum ferritin is a good indicator of available iron stores in uncomplicated iron-deficiency states, idiopathic hemochromatosis, and transfusion siderosis. In conditions of iron overload and in some chronic diseases, serum ferritin is an unreliable estimate of the storage iron. Median values and the variability of serum ferritin levels increase with age in adults.[3]

Serum ferritin concentration is a very sensitive and early indicator of iron deficiency that is uncomplicated by other concurrent disease. However, in the case of iron overload, serum ferritin is less sensitive than serum iron concentration, TIBC, or percent transferrin saturation.

↑ *Hereditary disorders:* Homozygous β-thalassemia (20-100% Hb F [0.200-1.000, mass fraction of Hb F]), heterozygous β-thalassemia (up to 5% [0.050] Hb F in some cases), hereditary persistence of Hb F (homozygotes 100% [1.000], heterozygotes 15-35% [0.150-0.350]), sickle cell anemia (1-30% [0.010-0.300]), trisomy D

Acquired disorders (up to 10% Hb F): Pernicious anemia, PNH, refractory normoblastic anemia, sideroblastic anemia, pure red cell aplasia, aplastic anemia, pregnancy, molar pregnancy, hyperthyroidism, juvenile chronic myeloid leukemia (Philadelphia chromosome negative, marked elevation of Hb F), acute leukemias, erythroleukemia, benign monoclonal gammopathies, cancer with marrow metastases, chronic renal disease.[11]

↓ Hemolytic anemia in the newborn

30% of Hb F inhibits the sickling reaction of Hb S. Hb F is resistant to alkali denaturation (as are Hb Bart's, J, Rainier, and Bethesda). This technique is most useful for screening and for cases in which the percentage of Hb F is low (<15% [<0.150, mass fraction]). It is unreliable, usually falsely low, at higher levels of Hb F.

Electrophoresis is useful for confirmation of the alkali denaturation test and is more reliable at higher levels of Hb F.

Cation-exchange chromatography is the best method for quantitation of high levels of Hb F. However, depending on the $^G\gamma\!:^A\gamma$ ratio, the retention time of Hb F may shift slightly. The $^G\gamma$ is eluted faster than the $^A\gamma$ and is enriched in newborn hemoglobin.

TEST NAME AND METHOD	SPECIMEN REQUIREMENTS	REFERENCE INTERVAL, CONVENTIONAL [INTERNATIONAL RECOMMENDED UNITS]	CHEMICAL INTERFERENCES AND IN VIVO EFFECTS
Fetal Hemoglobin—CONT			
Kleihauer-Betke (acid elution)[8-10]	Whole blood (EDTA or heparin), fresh or stored at 4° C for <10 days, or fresh peripheral smears.	Only few erythrocytes (<1% [<0.01, mass fraction]) in adult whole blood contain Hb F with this method.	
F cells, IF[9]	Whole blood (ETDA or heparin), fresh or stored, at 4° C for <10 days.	Adult: 0.5-0.7% [0.005-0.070, mass fraction], or erythrocytes are F cells (contain Hb F).	

1. Miale JB: *Laboratory medicine: hematology,* ed 6, St. Louis, 1982, CV Mosby.
2. Burtis CA, Ashwood ER, editors: *Tietz textbook of clinical chemistry,* ed 3, Philadelphia, 1999, WB Saunders.
3. Williams WJ, Beutler E, Erslev AJ, et al, editors: *Hematology,* ed 4, New York, 1990, McGraw-Hill Publishing Co.
4. Weatherall DJ, Clegg JB: *The thalassaemic syndromes,* ed 3, Oxford, 1981, Blackwell Scientific Publications.
5. Papadea C, Cate JC IV: Identification and quantification of hemoglobins A, F, S, and C by automated chromatography, *Clin Chem* 42:57-63, 1996.
6. Riou J, Godart C, Hurtreal D, et al: Cation-exchange HPLC evaluated for presumptive identification of hemoglobin variants, *Clin Chem* 43:34-39, 1997.
7. Ou CN, Rognerud CL: Rapid analysis of hemoglobin variants by cation-exchange HPLC, *Clin Chem* 39:820-824, 1993.
8. Henry JB, editor: *Clinical diagnosis and management by laboratory methods,* ed 20, Philadelphia, 2001, WB Saunders.
9. Huisman THJ, Jonxis JHP: *The hemoglobinopathies: techniques of identification,* New York, 1977, Marcel Dekker, Inc.
10. Blight LE, Judd SJ, White GH: Relative diagnostic value of serum non-SHBG-bound testosterone, free androgen index and free testosterone in the assessment of mild to moderate hirsutism, *Ann Clin Biochem* 26: 311-316, 1989.
11. Brosius EM, Schmidt RM: Quantitation of hemoglobin F, *Am J Clin Pathol* 72:421-425, 1979.

TEST NAME AND METHOD	SPECIMEN REQUIREMENTS	REFERENCE INTERVAL, CONVENTIONAL [INTERNATIONAL RECOMMENDED UNITS]		CHEMICAL INTERFERENCES AND IN VIVO EFFECTS
Fetal Lung Maturity Test by Fluorescence Polarization	Amniotic fluid, 1 mL. Samples should be uncentrifuged. Storage at room temperature for up to 16 hr or at 4° C for 24 hr does not affect test results.[6]	<260 mP:* 260-290 mP: >290 mP:	Mature[7] Transitional Immature	Blood >0.5% increases low values for mP and decreases high values.[9]
Fluorescence polarization (NBD-phosphatidylcholine)[1-3]		*P (an arbitrary unit) is the degree of fluorescence polarization.		

DIAGNOSTIC INFORMATION

REMARKS

↑ Fetomaternal hemorrhage; infants who are small for gestational age or with chronic anoxia. In blacks, hereditary persistence of fetal hemoglobin (HPFH) has a uniform distribution of Hb F among erythrocytes. In other forms of HPFH and in thalassemia and acquired conditions, Hb F is unevenly distributed among erythrocytes.

The Kleihauer-Betke acid elution technique can be modified to optimize detection and quantitation of fetal cells on a maternal blood smear or to distinguish between various types of congenital and acquired increases in fetal hemoglobin. The laboratory must always be notified of the suspected diagnosis so that the appropriate screening can be performed. Accurate quantitation of fetal/maternal hemorrhage is necessary for dosing of Rh immune globulin. Visual observation of distribution of fetal hemoglobin in red cells is a simple and inexpensive method for subtyping HPFH.

The immunofluorescent determination is a more sensitive and more reproducible test for F cells than is the acid elution method.

Using 260 mP as the cutoff, this test has a sensitivity of 94% and a specificity of 84%. Supplemental use of the L/S ratio is not beneficial.[13]

NBD-phosphatidylcholine binds to albumin and to surfactant phospholipids. The resulting fluorescence polarization is a function of the surfactant/albumin ratio.[18]

TEST NAME AND METHOD	SPECIMEN REQUIREMENTS	REFERENCE INTERVAL, CONVENTIONAL [INTERNATIONAL RECOMMENDED UNITS]		CHEMICAL INTERFERENCES AND IN VIVO EFFECTS

Fetal Lung Maturity Test by Fluorescence Polarization—CONT

Fluorescence polarization (PC-16)[4,5] (TDX-FLMII)	Same as above.	≤39 mg surfactant/g albumin: 40-54 mg surfactant/g albumin: ≥55 mg surfactant/g albumin:	Immature[8] Indeterminate Mature	Blood increases immature result by 5.8 mg surfactant/g albumin for every 0.1×10^{12} erythrocytes, has a minimal effect on intermediate results, and will decrease the result from a mature specimen.[6,10] Vaginally collected specimens result in values that are on average 35% lower than those collected via amniocentesis.[11] Specimens with visible meconium contamination and those contaminated with maternal urine can generate either false-positive or false-negative results and should not be used.[6,12]

1. Ashwood E, Tait J, Foerder C, et al: Improved fluorescence polarization assay for use in evaluating fetal lung maturity. III. Retrospective clinical evaluation and comparison with the lecithin/sphingomyelin ratio, *Clin Chem* 32:260-264, 1986.

2. Foerder C, Tait J, Franklin R, et al: Improved fluorescence polarization assay for use in evaluating fetal lung maturity. II. Analytical evaluation and comparison with the lecithin/sphingomyelin ratio, *Clin Chem* 32:255-259, 1986.

3. Tail J, Franklin R, Simpson J, et al: Improved fluorescence polarization assay for use in evaluating fetal lung maturity. I. Development of the assay procedure, *Clin Chem* 32:248-254, 1986.

4. Ashwood E, Palmer S, Lenke K: Rapid fetal lung maturity testing: commercial versus NBD-phosphatidylcholine assay, *Obstet Gynecol* 81:1048-1053, 1992.

5. Russell JC: A calibrated fluorescence polarization assay for assessment of fetal lung maturity, *Clin Chem* 33:1177-1184, 1987.

6. Grenache DG, Parvin CA, Gronowskim AM: Preanalytical factors that influence the Abbott TDx Fetal Lung Maturity II assay, *Clin Chem* 49:935-939, 2003.

7. Chen C, Roby P, Weiss N, et al: Clinical evaluation of the NBD-PC fluorescence polarization assay for prediction of fetal lung maturity, *Obstet Gynecol* 80:688-692, 1992.

8. Abbott Laboratories: *TDx/TDxFLx Fetal Lung Maturity II,* Abbott Park, IL, 1996, Abbott Laboratories.

9. Tail J, Franklin R, Simpson J, et al: Improved fluorescence polarization assay for use in evaluating fetal lung maturity. I. Development of the assay procedure, *Clin Chem* 32:248-254, 1986.

10. Carlan SJ, Gearity D, O'Brien WF: The effect of maternal blood contamination on the TDx-FLM II assay, *Am J Perinatol* 14:491-494, 1997.

11. Cleary-Goldman J, Connelly T, Chelmow D, et al: Accuracy of the TDx-FLM assay of amniotic fluid: a comparison of vaginal pool samples with amniocentesis, *J Matern Fetal Neonatal Med* 11:374-377, 2002.

12. Russell JC, Cooper CM, Ketchum CM, et al: Multicenter evaluation of TDx test for assessing fetal lung maturity, *Clin Chem* 35:1005-1010, 1989.

DIAGNOSTIC INFORMATION	REMARKS

A cutoff of ≥45 mg surfactant/g albumin for maturity has been shown to increase specificity from 72% to 84% with no change in sensitivity (100%).[14] There is evidence to support a risk-based approach to clinical interpretation that accounts for gestational age.[15,16]

After 31 wk, results from twin pregnancies are on average 22 mg surfactant/g albumin higher than those from singleton pregnancies.[17]

This version of the assay uses the dye PC-16.[19]

Gently remix specimen if centrifuging has occurred.[6]

13. Ashwood ER: Clinical chemistry of pregnancy. In Burtis CA, Ashwood ER, editors: *Tietz textbook of clinical chemistry*, ed 2, Philadelphia, 1994, WB Saunders.

14. Fantz CR, Powell C, Karon B, et al: Assessment of the diagnostic accuracy of the TDx-FLM II to predict fetal lung maturity, *Clin Chem* 48:761-765, 2002.

15. Kaplan LA, Chapman JF, Bock JL, et al: Prediction of respiratory distress syndrome using the Abbott FLM-II amniotic fluid assay, *Clin Chim Acta* 326:61-68, 2002.

16. Parvin CA, et al: Predicting respiratory distress syndrome using gestational age and fetal lung maturity by fluorescent polarization, *Am J Obstet Gynecol* 192:199-207, 2005.

17. McElrath TF, Norwitz ER, Robinson JN, et al: Differences in TDx fetal lung maturity assay values between twin and singleton gestations, *Am J Obstet Gynecol* 182:1110-1112, 2000.

18. Ashwood E, Chamberlain B: Binding of fluorescent phosphatidylcholine in amniotic fluid, *Obstet Gynecol* 71:370-374, 1988.

19. Russell J: A calibrated fluorescence polarization assay for assessment of fetal lung maturity, *Clin Chem* 33:1177-1184, 1987.

TEST NAME AND METHOD	SPECIMEN REQUIREMENTS	REFERENCE INTERVAL, CONVENTIONAL [INTERNATIONAL RECOMMENDED UNITS]		CHEMICAL INTERFERENCES AND IN VIVO EFFECTS
Fetal Lung Maturity Test by Foam Stability *Foam Stability Index (FSI)*[1-10]	Amniotic fluid, 5 mL. *(See L/S ratio for additional information)*	*Probability of RDS*[2,3,5] *FSI value* 44 45 46 47 48 50	*(in %)* 70 40 15 <1 <1 <1	↑ C Blood ($\geq$1%) or meconium ($\geq$4%) increases the FSI value.[2] Amniotic fluid collected vaginally increases the incidence of false mature results.[6]
Shake Test[8]		Negative: Intermediate: Positive:	Fetal lung immaturity Transitional maturity Fetal lung maturity	↑ C Blood or meconium produces false mature or intermediate results.[8,9]

1. Brown LM, Duck-Chong CG: Methods of evaluating fetal lung maturity, *Crit Rev Clin Lab Sci* 16:85-159, 1982.
2. Sher G, Statland BE: Assessment of fetal pulmonary maturity by the Lumadex foam stability index test, *Obstet Gynecol* 61:444-449, 1983.
3. Sher G, Statland BE, Freer DE: Clinical evaluation of the quantitative foam stability index test, *Obstet Gynecol* 55:617-620, 1980.
4. Sher G, Statland BE, Freer DE, et al: Assessing fetal lung maturity by the foam stability index test, *Obstet Gynecol* 52:673-679, 1978.
5. Ashwood ER: Clinical chemistry of pregnancy. In Burtis CA, Ashwood ER, editors: *Tietz textbook of clinical chemistry*, Philadelphia, 1999, WB Saunders, pp. 1736-1775.
6. Brown LM, Duck-Chong CG: Methods of evaluating fetal lung maturity, *Crit Rev Clin Lab Sci* 16:85-159, 1982.
7. The American College of Obstetricians and Gynecologists: *Assessment of fetal lung maturity*, ACOG Educational Bulletin, Washington, DC, 1996, The American College of Obstetricians and Gynecologists.
8. Clements JA, Platzker AC, Tierney DF, et al: Assessment of the risk of the respiratory-distress syndrome by a rapid test for surfactant in amniotic fluid, *N Engl J Med* 286:1077-1081, 1972.
9. Keniston RC, Noland GL, Pernoll ML: The effect of blood, meconium, and temperature on the rapid surfactant test, *Obstet Gynecol* 48:442-446, 1976.
10. Bhagwanani SG, Fahmy D, Turnbull AC: Bubble stability test compared with lecithin assay in prediction of respiratory distress syndrome, *BMJ* 1:697-700, 1973.

DIAGNOSTIC INFORMATION	REMARKS
The incidence of false-immature results is high but the predictive value of a mature (FSI = 48) result is close to 100%.[6]	Provides a functional measure of fetal lung maturity based on the surface tension properties of surfactant phospholipids. The FSI test uses the same methodology as the older shake test, except the concentration of ethanol used is varied over several tubes. The FSI value is the highest concentration of ethanol that supports a stable ring of foam. The advantage of the FSI over the shake test is improved quantitation of results.[6] To avoid false-positive results, care must be taken to ensure tubes and stoppers used are kept clean and free of detergents.[5] Siliconized collection tubes will produce stable foam and should not be used.[7] The 95% ethanol used as a reagent is hygroscopic. Water absorption must be avoided to preserve the proper ethanol concentration.[5]
Many results are intermediate and have little value in predicting RDS.[6,10] *(See above).*	At 1:1 and 1:2 dilutions of amniotic fluid with 95% ethanol, a positive result is the presence of a complete ring of bubbles with both dilutions; an intermediate result is the presence of a complete ring of bubbles at the 1:1 dilution but not the 1:2 dilution; and a negative result is the absence of a complete ring of bubbles at either dilution.[6,8]

TEST NAME AND METHOD	SPECIMEN REQUIREMENTS	REFERENCE INTERVAL, CONVENTIONAL [INTERNATIONAL RECOMMENDED UNITS]					CHEMICAL INTERFERENCES AND IN VIVO EFFECTS

α-Fetoprotein (AFP)

Immunoassay

Serum. Store at 2-8° C if assay is to be performed within 24 hr; otherwise freeze at −20° C or colder.

	ng/mL^1		mcg/L
Wk gestation	(Median)		(Median)
14	25.6	× 1.0	[25.6]
15	29.9		[29.9]
16	34.8		[34.8]
17	40.6		[40.6]
18	47.3		[47.3]
19	55.1		[55.1]
20	64.3		[64.3]
21	74.9		[74.9]

None found. Turbid samples or those containing particulate material should be clarified.

Amniotic fluid

	mg/mL^1		mg/L
Wk gestation	(Median)		(Median)
15	16.3	× 1.0	[16.3]
16	14.5		[14.5]
17	13.4		[13.4]
18	12.0		[12.0]
19	10.7		[10.7]
20	8.1		[8.1]

DIAGNOSTIC INFORMATION	REMARKS

$\uparrow$ Maternal serum levels >2× the median should be investigated by ultrasound examination to rule out incorrectly estimated gestational age, multiple gestation, fetal death, or obvious malformation (e.g., anencephaly). Increased AFP concentrations in maternal serum and amniotic fluid are associated with open neural tube defects (NTD, e.g., anencephaly, spina bifida), omphalocele, esophageal or duodenal atresia, Meckel's syndrome, fetal hepatic necrosis secondary to viral infection, and other conditions.[8]

$\downarrow$ Down syndrome (trisomy 21),[9,10] fetal demise, molar pregnancy, spontaneous abortion, trisomy 18, overestimated gestational age

AF $\downarrow$ Toxemia

AFP is synthesized in the liver. Some fetal AFP enters the maternal circulation. The serum AFP in maternal blood reaches its maximum at the 30th wk of pregnancy, then decreases rapidly to <2% of the maximum at 34-36 wk of pregnancy.

Owing to the very steep concentration gradient between fetal serum, amniotic fluid, and maternal serum, very slight contamination of either amniotic fluid or maternal serum with fetal serum will cause very high apparent values. Only 44 μL of fetal blood in 10 mL or amniotic fluid can double the AFP concentration at 16 wk gestation.[11]

Maternal serum AFP (MSAFP) values are expressed as multiples of the median (MoM) by dividing the patient's AFP value by the median AFP for a normal pregnancy of the same gestational age. These MoMs are then corrected for maternal weight according to the following formula[10]: Weight-adjusted MoM $= 10^{[0.2658\,(0.00188\,\times\,\text{maternal weight, pounds})]}$

Values for maternal insulin-requiring diabetic patients should be adjusted by dividing by 0.8; values for black patients should be adjusted by dividing by 1.1. If the patient is known to be carrying twins, divide the MoM by 2.13.

Maternal serum AFP (MSAFP) values are expressed as multiples of the median (MoM) by dividing the patient's AFP value by the median AFP for a normal pregnancy of the same gestational age. These MoMs are then corrected for maternal weight according to the following formula[10]:

Weight-adjusted MoM $= 10^{[0.2658\,(0.00188\,\times\,\text{maternal weight, pounds})]}$

Values for maternal insulin-requiring diabetic patients should be adjusted by dividing by 0.8; values for black patients should be adjusted by dividing by 1.1. If the patient is known to be carrying twins, divide the MoM by 2.13.

Maternal serum AFP values should be reported to the clinician as absolute concentrations and as adjusted multiples of the median for the stated gestational age. For various conditions, estimates of *a priori* and *a posteriori* risks should be calculated and reported.[1] To improve the detection rate of Down syndrome, some screening programs use multiple serum markers (e.g., AFP, hCG, and estriol).[12]

TEST NAME AND METHOD	SPECIMEN REQUIREMENTS	REFERENCE INTERVAL, CONVENTIONAL [INTERNATIONAL RECOMMENDED UNITS]			CHEMICAL INTERFERENCES AND IN VIVO EFFECTS

α-Fetoprotein—CONT

1. Ashwood ER: Clinical chemistry of pregnancy. In Burtis CA, Ashwood ER, editors: *Tietz textbook of clinical chemistry,* ed 3, Philadelphia, 1999, WB Saunders.

2. Chan DW, Sell S: Tumor markers. In Burtis CA, Ashwood ER, editors: *Tietz textbook of clinical chemistry,* ed 3, Philadelphia, 1999, WB Saunders.

3. Johnson PJ: Tumor markers in primary malignancies of the liver. In Diamandis EP, Fritsche HA, Lilja H, et al, editors: *Tumor markers. Physiology, pathobiology, technology, and clinical applications,* Washington, DC, 2002, AACC Press.

4. Bosl GJ, Geller NL, Cirrincione C, et al: Multivariate analysis of prognostic variables in patients with metastatic testicular cancer, *Cancer Res* 43:3403-3417, 1983.

5. Mann K, Lamerz R, Hellmann T, et al: Use of human chorionic gonadotropin and alpha fetoprotein radioimmunoassays: specificity and apparent half-life after delivery in patients with germ cell tumors, *Oncodev Biol Med* 1:301-311, 1980.

6. Seckl MJ, Rustin GJS, Bagshawe KD: Frequency of serum tumor marker monitoring in patients with non-seminomatous germ cell tumors, *Br J Cancer* 61:916-918, 1990.

7. Toner GC, Geller NL, Tan C, et al: Serum tumor half-life during chemotherapy allows early prediction of complete response and survival in nonseminomatous germ cell tumors, *Cancer Res* 50:5904-5910, 1990.

TEST NAME AND METHOD	SPECIMEN REQUIREMENTS	REFERENCE INTERVAL, CONVENTIONAL		[INTERNATIONAL RECOMMENDED UNITS]	CHEMICAL INTERFERENCES AND IN VIVO EFFECTS
Fibrin(ogen) Degradation Products [FDP, Fibrin(ogen) Split Products, FSP][1]	Serum. Collect 2 mL whole blood in a special tube that contains thrombin and soybean trypsin inhibitor (see *Remarks*). Allow to clot at 37° C for 30 min.	Normal: DIC:	<10 mcg/mL generally	× 1.0	[<10 mg/L] >40 mcg/mL	↑ V Plasminogen activators Increased levels of rheumatoid factor may cause false-positive results in some assays. Heparin and dysfibrinogenemia will give a false-positive result.

1. Garvey MB, Black JM: The detection of a fibrinogen-fibrin degradation products by means of a new antibody coated latex particle, *J Clin Pathol* 25:680-682, 1972.

DIAGNOSTIC INFORMATION	REMARKS

The presence in amniotic fluid of the isoenzyme of acetyl-cholinesterase from neutral tissue should be sought whenever there is a question of an open NTD.[13] Elevated serum levels of AFP with normal amniotic fluid levels are associated with poor perinatal outcome, particularly with low birth weight and/or with premature delivery.[14]

8. Adams MJ, Windham GC, James LM, et al: Clinical interpretation of maternal serum α-fetoprotein concentrations, *Am J Obstet Gynecol* 148:241-254, 1984.

9. Cuckle HS, Nanchahal K, Wald NJ, et al: Estimating a woman's risk of having a pregnancy associated with Down's syndrome using her age and serum alpha-fetoprotein level, *Br J Obstet Gynecol* 94:387-402, 1987.

10. Knight GJ, Palomaki GE, Haddow JE: Use of maternal serum alpha-fetoprotein measurements to screen for Down's syndrome, *Clin Obstet Gynecol* 31:306-327, 1988.

11. Doran TA, Allen LC, Pirani BB, et al: False-positive amniotic fluid alpha fetoprotein level resulting from contamination with fetal blood: results of an experiment, *Am J Obstet Gynecol* 127:759-762, 1977.

12. Haddow J, Palnmali G, Knight G, et al: Prenatal screening for Down's syndrome with use of maternal serum markers, *N Engl J Med* 327:588-593, 1992.

13. Brock DJH, Barron L, van Hegningen V: Prenatal diagnosis of neural-tube defects with monoclonal antibody specific for acetylcholinesterase, *Lancet,* 1:5-7, 1985.

14. Brock DJH, Barron L, Jelen P, et al: Maternal serum alpha-fetoprotein measurements as an early indicator of low birth weight, *Lancet* 2:267-268, 1977.

↑ Fibrinolysis associated with DIC, thrombolytic therapy, myocardial infarction, venous thrombosis, pulmonary embolism.

Elevations are less marked (usually between 10 and 40 μg/mL) in malignancy, infection, and liver disease.

The fibrinolytic enzyme, plasmin, degrades fibrinogen into fibrinogen degradation products and the fibrin clot into fibrin degradation products, including the D-dimer. The FDP assay will detect end-products (X, Y, D, and E) from fibrinogen and fibrin.

The measurement of fibrinogen/fibrin degradation products is based on a semiquantitative latex agglutination test by which different dilutions are tested until macroscopic agglutination is no longer seen *(Thrombo-Wellcotest).*

The D-dimer is more sensitive for evidence of clot formation and degradation, whereas the FDP will also detect degradation of fibrinogen (primary fibrinogenolysis). FDPs are most commonly used as part of a laboratory workup for DIC.

TEST NAME AND METHOD	SPECIMEN REQUIREMENTS	REFERENCE INTERVAL, CONVENTIONAL [INTERNATIONAL RECOMMENDED UNITS]	CHEMICAL INTERFERENCES AND IN VIVO EFFECTS
Fibrinogen[1-5]	Plasma (blue top-citrate). Samples can be stored at room temperature up to 4 hr; frozen ($-70°$ C) for 18 mo.	*Clauss* method: Generally 1.5-4.0 g/L (150-400 mg/dL). Reference range may depend on the reagent-instrument combination. Reference intervals should be established by each laboratory.	↑ V Estrogens, oral contraceptives ↓ V Anabolic steroids, androgens, asparaginase, fish oil, plasminogen activators, valproic acid ↓ C Inhibitors of fibrin polymerization; heparin at high concentration (recommend removing heparin from patient sample)

1. Lewis SM, Bain BJ, Bates I, editors: *Dacie and Lewis practical hematology,* ed 9, Edinburgh, 2001, Churchill Livingstone.

2. Jacobs DS, Demott WR, Oxley DK, editors: *Laboratory test handbook,* ed 5, Hudson, OH, 2001, Lexi-Comp, Inc.

3. Mackie IJ, Kitchen S, Machin SJ, et al: Guidelines on fibrinogen assays, *Br J Haematol* 121:396-404, 2003.

4. Lowe GDO, Rumley A: Use of fibrinogen and D-dimer in prediction of arterial thrombotic events, *Thromb Haemost* 82:667-672, 1999.

5. Clauss A: Gerinnungsphysiologische Schnellmethode zur Bestimmung des Fibrinogens, *Acta Haematol* 17:237-240, 1957.

Fibronectin (FN, Cold-Insoluble Globulin, Cell Surface Protein, Opsonic α_2-Surface Binding Protein)[1,2] *EID*	Plasma. Analyze fresh or store at 4° C for <72 hr. Stable frozen at $-20°$ C for 6 mo, or at $-70°$ C indefinitely. Specimens without lipemia or hemolysis are preferred.	300 ± 100 mcg/mL × 1.0 [300 ± 100 mg/L] Neonates, especially preterm and sick full-term[4]: × 210 mg/L	None found.

DIAGNOSTIC INFORMATION	REMARKS

↑ Fibrinogen is a sensitive acute phase reactant. Increased levels are also seen in pregnancy, oral contraception, postmenopausal women, smoking, and exercise.

↓ Inherited deficiency, resulting in an abnormal (dysfibrinogenemia), reduced (hypofibrinogenemia) or absent fibrinogen (afibrinogenemia).

Acquired deficiency: liver disease, consumptive coagulopathies such as DIC, and hemodilution.

Fibrinogen is typically performed in the investigation for unexplained bleeding, prolonged PT/PTT, or as part of a DIC panel.

An elevated fibrinogen has also been used as a predictor of arterial thrombotic events.

Fibrinogen is generally measured by a clot based functional (activity) assay. The clot based assays performed on modern automated coagulation analyzers typically use photooptical technology. The older manual instruments (fibrometer) were based on electromechanical methods. The *Clauss* assay,[5] based on a high concentration of thrombin added to dilute patient plasma, is the most commonly used method.

The less frequently used immunological (antigenic) assays (ELISAs, RID) measure protein concentration but not functional activity.

↑ FN in synovial fluid is present in higher concentration than in the paired serum. Doubt remains as to whether FN is or is not a positive acute phase reactant. In severe infection FN levels may decrease markedly.

↓ In circumstances where protein loss is manifest (e.g., in coagulopathies, trauma, and vascular collapse), splenomegaly. Decreases may indicate sequestration of FN in association with other serum proteins, immune complexes, and platelets.[5]

Fibronectins are large adhesive glycoproteins that are integral parts of cell surfaces, extracellular matrices, and also occur in intravascular and extravascular fluids. FN molecules in plasma and in other fluids differ by virtue of their carbohydrate composition.[6] The proteins are synthesized by a variety of cells, including endothelium, macrophages, synoviocytes, and hepatocytes.

FN is a dimer whose chains are interconnected by disulfide bridges. It binds to collagen, gelatin, heparin, and a variety of lectins through specific binding sequences. It also binds variably to glass and plastics, a factor that complicates its analysis. In addition, FN binds to immune complexes, C1q, IgM rheumatoid factors, cryoprecipitates, and fibrin. It can also be found bound to precipitates of denatured proteins and to proteins precipitated with polyethylene glycol.[5] Its intensely adhesive nature may be one of the specific roles of FN in ridding the body of such materials.

TEST NAME AND METHOD	SPECIMEN REQUIREMENTS	REFERENCE INTERVAL, CONVENTIONAL [INTERNATIONAL RECOMMENDED UNITS]	CHEMICAL INTERFERENCES AND IN VIVO EFFECTS
Fibronectin—CONT			
Fibronectin, fetal[3] *ELISA*	Cervicovaginal fluid. Collect specimen with a swab. Saturate the swab ($\sim$150 μL) and place it into 750 μL of buffer.	$\leq$50 ng/mL	

1. Luban NLC: Fibronectin, *Clin Chem* 27:965-966, 1981.
2. Mosesson MW, Amrani DL: The structure and biologic activities of plasma fibroneclin, *Blood* 56:145-158, 1980.
3. Ashwood ER: Clinical chemistry of pregnancy. In Burtis CA, Ashwood ER, editors: *Tietz textbook of clinical chemistry,* ed 3, Philadelphia, 1999, WB Saunders.
4. Delpuech P, Desch G, Hassanaly F, et al: Fibronectin concentrations in plasma of healthy preterm, full-term, and sick full-term neonates, *Clin Chem* 34:592, 1988.
5. Herbert KE, Coppock JS, Griffiths AM, et al: Fibronectin and immune complexes in rheumatic diseases, *Ann Rheum Dis* 46:734-740, 1987.
6. Carrieri P, Orifice G, Indaco A: No effect of acetylsalicylic acid on β-thromboglobulin and platelet factor 4 plasma levels in patients with transient ischemic attacks, *Stroke* 17:1153-1155, 1986.

TEST NAME AND METHOD	SPECIMEN REQUIREMENTS	REFERENCE INTERVAL, CONVENTIONAL [INTERNATIONAL RECOMMENDED UNITS]	CHEMICAL INTERFERENCES AND IN VIVO EFFECTS
Fludrocortisone (9α-Fluorohydro-cortisone) Suppression[1] Dose, adult: Patient on normal diet receives 0.1 mg fludrocortisone orally q 6 hr $\times$ 12 Child: 0.05-0.1 mg q 12 hr $\times$ 6	Collect 24-hr urine for Na$^+$, K$^+$, creatinine, and aldosterone 1 day before fludrocortisone and on day 3. Collect plasma for renin and aldosterone after 2-hr standing position for baseline measurements and at end of fludrocortisone administration.	After fludrocortisone, Plasma aldosterone: $<$4 ng/dL $\times$ 27.7 [$<$111 pmol/L] Plasma renin: $<$6 ng AI*/mL/hr $\times$ 1.0 [$<$6 mcg AI $\times$ h^{-1} $\times$ L^{-1}] Urinary aldosterone: $<$20 mcg/day $\times$ 2.77 [$<$55 nmol/day] *AI*, Angiotensin I.	See individual tests.

1. Alsever RN, Gotlin RW: *Handbook of endocrine tests in adults and children,* ed 2, Chicago, 1978, Year Book Medical Publishers, Inc.

DIAGNOSTIC INFORMATION	REMARKS
	FN is degraded by proteolytic enzymes to its monomer; the biological activity of the monomer is different from activity of the dimer in enhancing opsonization. The presence of fibronectin on cell surfaces promotes cell-cell interactions and also plays a role in clot retraction.
	MW: 440,000-500,000
↑ During second and third trimesters twofold to fourfold higher risk for preterm delivery	Testing should be done sometime between 24 and 30 wk gestations. A negative test result following a positive test decreases the risk. Two negative test results reduce the risk to baseline.
	The majority of patients with positive results will repair placental disruptions and successfully continue the pregnancy.
In primary aldosteronism, there is no aldosterone suppression. See also *Aldosterone Suppression Test (after Saline Infusion).*	Fludrocortisone, a potent mineralocorticoid, will suppress plasma renin activity and plasma aldosterone in normal subjects but not in subjects with primary aldosteronism. Fludrocortisone should be administered with caution to patients with hypokalemia and heart or renal failure.[2]

2.   Watts NB, Keffer JH: *Practical endocrinology,* ed 4, Philadelphia, 1989, Lea & Febiger.

TEST NAME AND METHOD	SPECIMEN REQUIREMENTS	REFERENCE INTERVAL, CONVENTIONAL [INTERNATIONAL RECOMMENDED UNITS]			CHEMICAL INTERFERENCES AND IN VIVO EFFECTS
Fluoride[1]	Plasma (heparin).[2] Avoid glass.	*mg/L* 0.01-0.20	× 52.6	*mmol/L* [0.5-10.5]	↑ C Fluoride contamination in chemicals, water, and glassware
Ion-selective potentiometry, GLC[2]	Urine. Avoid glass; collect in polyethylene.	Adult[3]: 0.2-3.2 Occupational exposure[4]: <8.0		[10.5-168] [<421]	

1. Baselt RC: *Biological monitoring methods for industrial chemicals,* Davis, CA, 1980, Biomedical Pub.
2. Baselt RC: *Analytical procedures for therapeutic drug monitoring and emergency toxicology,* ed 2, Littleton, MA, 1987, PSG Publishing Co.
3. Baselt RC, Cravey RH: *Disposition of toxic drugs and chemicals in man,* ed 3, Chicago, 1989, Year Book Medical Pub.
4. Lauwerys RR: *Industrial chemical exposure. Guidelines for biological monitoring,* Davis, CA, 1983, Biomedical Pub.
5. Czerwinski E, Nowak J, Dabroska P, et al: Bone and joint pathology in fluoride-exposed workers, *Arch Environ Health* 43:340-343, 1988.
6. Menkes CJ: Clinical manifestations and etiology of osteomalacia. http://www.uptodate.com.searchterm.fluoride. Accessed September 14, 2004.
7. Arnow PM, Bland LA, Garcia-Houchins S, et al: An outbreak of fatal fluoride intoxication in a long-term hemodialysis unit, *Ann Intern Med* 121:339, 1994.
8. Ekstrand J, Alvang J, Boreus LO, et al: Pharmacokinetics of fluoride in man after single and multiple oral doses, *Eur J Clin Pharmacol* 12: 311-317, 1977.

Fluorocarbons	Plasma (fluoride/oxalate). Draw quickly and freeze immediately.	Concentrations found in blood after use of inhalers utilizing fluorocarbons:	None found.
GLC-FID[1]			

	mg/L	*mmol/L*
Fluorocarbon[2] (trichlorofluoromethane):	0.5-4.5 × 7.28	[3.6-32.8]
Toxic concentration:	>2.0	[>14.6]
Fluorocarbon[3] (dichlorodifluoromethane):	0.2-4.7 × 8.27	[1.7-38.9]
Toxic concentration:	>1.0	[>8.3]

1. Garriott J, Petty CS: Death from inhalant abuse: toxicologic and pathologic evaluation of 34 cases, *Clin Toxicol* 76:305-315, 1980.
2. Behrman RE, Kliegman RM, Nelson WE, et al, editors: *Nelson textbook of pediatrics,* ed 14, Philadelphia, 1992, WB Saunders.

DIAGNOSTIC INFORMATION	REMARKS

Adverse effects include irritation, respiratory distress, neurological abnormalities, gastrointestinal pain, muscular fibrillation, and tetany.[1] Death is usually due to respiratory paralysis. X-rays for diagnosis of chronic fluorosis show increased bone density and mineral deposits in ligaments and tendons.[5]

High doses of fluorides can inhibit mineralization and produce osteomalacia.[6]

Individuals undergoing hemodialysis may be at risk for toxicity.[7]

Fluoride is encountered as hydrogen fluoride and its inorganic salts. These salts are used in industry and as insecticides. An organic form, monofluoroacetic acid, is extremely toxic.

Average daily dietary intake is 0.5-5 mg [26-263 μmol] as F^-. Drinking water is fortified with F^- to 1 mg/L [52.6 μmol/L] in some areas. Plasma contains 72% of whole blood fluoride in ionic form. Fifty percent is excreted in urine, 10% in feces, and 20% in sweat. The rest is retained primarily in bone.[1]

Minimum toxic or lethal dose is not well established. There are wide variations in response to a given dose among individuals.[8]

Kinetic values
$t_{1/2}$:   2-9 hr
Vd: 0.5-0.7 L/kg

The abuse of fluorocarbons has led to fatalities associated with freezing of the larynx or sensitization of the myocardium with subsequent ventricular fibrillation and sudden death.

Plasma levels of fluorinated hydrocarbon are not clinically useful.[4]

These compounds in a variety of formulations are used as refrigerants and aerosol propellants. They are highly volatile; 90% of an ingestion is excreted in expired breath in 1 hr.

Kinetic values
Fluorocarbon[2]
$t^{1/2}$:   1.5 hr

3.   Beutler E: *Hemolytic anemia in disorders of red cell metabolism,* New York, 1978, Plenum Pub.

4.   POISINDEX Toxicologic Management: *Fluorinated hydrocarbons,* vol 75, Denver, CO, 1993, Micromedex, Inc.

TEST NAME AND METHOD	SPECIMEN REQUIREMENTS	REFERENCE INTERVAL, CONVENTIONAL [INTERNATIONAL RECOMMENDED UNITS]			CHEMICAL INTERFERENCES AND IN VIVO EFFECTS
Folate MB (L. casei)[1-3]	Serum or plasma (sodium citrate, heparin, or oxalate); freeze if assay is delayed. Avoid exposure to sunlight. Specimens stable 24 hr at 4° C or 6-8 wk at −20° C. Dried blood spot or dried serum spot.[7,8] Stable 1 yr at −20° C stored in a plastic bag with desiccant sachet.	Folate-responsive megaloblastic anemia:	ng/mL 5-16 × 2.265 <3	nmol/L [11-36] [<7]	S ↓ V Drugs causing megaloblastic anemia (including folic acid antagonists), methotrexate, pentamidine, pyrimethamine, triamterene, trimethoprim; drugs that impair absorption (aminosalicylic acid, anticonvulsants [e.g., carbamazepine, phenobarbital, phenytoin, primidone, valproic acid], colchicine, cycloserine, estrogens, glutethimide, isoniazid, mefenamic acid, met-
Immunometric (automated)[4,5]	Serum or plasma (heparin); freeze if assay delayed >8 hr. Reject if moderately hemolyzed.		>3.5	[>7.8]	formin, neomycin, nitrofurans, oral contraceptives, phenacetin, phenformin); alcohol, antacids, bicarbonate, cholestyramine, sulfasalazine S ↓ C Antibiotics (MB assay) Heterophile antibodies (IM)
CPB radioassay[6]	Erythrocyte hemolysate; collect whole blood (EDTA). Determine hematocrit value, then hemolyze (2 mL 0.2% ascorbic acid/100 mL blood at room temperature for 90 min; protect from light). Stable 4 hr at 8° C or 8 wk at −20° C. Avoid repeated freezing and thawing.	2-16 yr: >16 yr:	>160 140-628	[>362] [317-1422]	Ercs ↓ V Anticonvulsants (phenytoin, phenobarbital, primidone), oral contraceptives Ercs ↓ Heparin may interfere with the IM assays Drugs affecting serum folate levels may affect erythrocyte level also. See listing under serum.

DIAGNOSTIC INFORMATION	REMARKS

S ↑ Blind loop syndrome, vegetarian diet, distal small bowel disease, PA, B_{12} deficiency

S ↓ Untreated folate deficiency (usually resulting in megaloblastic anemia), infantile hyperthyroidism, alcoholism, malnutrition, scurvy, deficiency of certain enzymes, liver disease, B_{12} deficiency, dietary amino acid excess, Lesch-Nyhan syndrome, achlorhydria, chronic hemodialysis, adult celiac disease, tropical sprue, Crohn's disease, sometimes in ulcerative colitis, malabsorption, hemolytic anemias, carcinomas, myelofibrosis (decreased in >50% of patients), vitamin B6 deficiency anemia, disorders of glutathione metabolism, sideroblastic anemia, pregnancy, regional enteritis, Whipple's disease, amyloidosis, extensive intestinal resection, severe exfoliative dermatitis

Ercs ↓ Untreated folate deficiency, usually associated with megaloblastic anemia (<140 ng/mL; <317 nmol/L); decrease in Ercs is also seen in 60% of uncomplicated vitamin B_{12} deficiency. See also above.

Folate deficiency is the most common vitamin deficiency and is prevalent in alcoholic liver disease, pregnancy, and the elderly. Folate deficiency may result from poor intestinal absorption (absence of intestinal microorganisms, in celiac disease or sprue, or after surgical intestinal resection), nutritional deficiency, excessive demands (pregnancy, liver disease, or malignancy), and in response to certain drugs (methotrexate, anticonvulsant therapy, especially during pregnancy).[4]

The sequence of abnormalities that occur in the development of folate deficiency is as follows: low serum levels (3 wk), hypersegmentation of neutrophils (11 wk), increased urinary excretion of FIGLU (13 wk), low erythrocyte folate levels (17 wk), macroovalocytosis of erythrocytes (18 wk), megaloblastic bone marrow (19 wk), and megaloblastic anemia (19-20 wk). There is also a decrease in granulocytes and thrombocytes and an increase in plasma homocysteine.

Erythrocyte levels are better indicators of tissue stores of folate than are serum levels, which are responsive to recent dietary intakes. Except during pregnancy, the presence of neutrophil hypersegmentation (≥1 six-lobed PMN/100 cells) is a useful indicator of folate deficiency and a reliable predictor of megaloblastic bone marrow. However, megaloblastosis can occur despite normal folate levels in serum and erythrocytes. Only 50% of pregnant women with megaloblastosis have low levels of folate in erythrocytes.

Folate-responsive disorders include homocystinuria type II and formiminotransferase deficiency. Hyperhomocysteinemia, as a result of folate or vitamin B_{12} deficiency, is an independent risk factor for occlusive vascular disease. The therapeutic dose for treating megaloblastic anemia is 100 mcg/day; toxicity does not occur even at doses of 15 mg/day. Patients with low erythrocyte folate levels or with megaloblastic anemia should be evaluated for vitamin B_{12} deficiency.

Folate deficiency during pregnancy has been associated with the increased occurrence of neural tube defects. In a retrospective study of pregnant women without folate supplementation, neural tube defects were 4× more likely to occur than in women with supplementation.[10]

TEST NAME AND METHOD	SPECIMEN REQUIREMENTS	REFERENCE INTERVAL, CONVENTIONAL [INTERNATIONAL RECOMMENDED UNITS]		CHEMICAL INTERFERENCES AND IN VIVO EFFECTS
Folate—CONT				
Immunometric (automated)[4,5]	Prepare hemolysate from whole blood (heparin or EDTA); determine hematocrit.	0-11 mo: 1-11yr: >12 yr:	$74\text{-}995^9$ $96\text{-}362^9$ >280	[168-2254] [218-820] [>634]

1. Wilson SD, Horne DW: Use of glycerol-cryoprotected Lactobacillus casei for microbiological assay of folic acid, *Clin Chem* 28:1198-1200, 1982.

2. Molloy AM, Scott JM: Microbiological assay for serum, plasma, and red cell folate using cryopreserved, microtiter plate method, *Methods Enzymol* 281:43-53, 1997.

3. O'Broin S, Kelleher B: Microbiological assay on microtiter plates of folate in serum and red cells, *J Clin Pathol* 45:344-347, 1992.

4. Fairbanks VF, Klee GG: Biochemical aspects of hematology. In Burtis CA, Ashwood ER, editors: *Tietz textbook of clinical chemistry,* Philadelphia, 1999, WB Saunders, pp. 1690-1698

5. Bayer Diagnostics: *Bayer Advia: Centaur Folate, package insert,* East Walpole, MA, 2002, Bayer Diagnostics.

6. Thorpe SJ, Sands D, Heath AB, et al: An International Standard for whole blood folate: evaluation of a lyophilised haemolysate in an international collaborative study, *Clin Chem Lab Med* 42:533-539, 2004.

7. O'Broin S, Gunter E: Dried-serum spot assay for folate, *Clin Chem* 48:1128-1130, 2002.

8. O'Broin S, Gunter E: Screening of folate status with use of dried blood spots on filter paper, *Am J Clin Nutr* 70:359-67, 1999.

9. Mayo Medical Laboratories: *Test catalog,* Rochester, MN 2004, Mayo Medical Laboratories.

10. Milunsky A, Jick H, Jick SS, et al: Multivitamin/folic acid supplementation in early pregnancy reduces the prevalence of neural tube defects, *JAMA* 262:2847-2852, 1989.

11. Klee GG: Cobalamin and folate evaluation: measurement of methylmalonic acid and homocysteine vs vitamin B(12) and folate, *Clin Chem* 46:1277-1283, 2000.

Test Name and Method	Specimen Requirements	Reference Interval	*mU/mL**	*U/L*	Chemical Interferences
Follitropin (Follicle-Stimulating Hormone, FSH)[1-4] *Immunoassay*	Serum. Store refrigerated or frozen. Stable for 8 days at room temperature or for 14 days at 4° C.[5,6]	Prepubertal child 2-11 mo M: F: 1-10 yr M: F: Puberty Tanner stage 1-2 M: F:	0.19-11.3 0.10-11.3 0.3-4.6 0.68-6.7 0.30-4.6 0.68-6.7	× 1.0 [0.19-11.3] [0.10-11.3] [0.3-4.6] [0.68-6.7] [0.30-4.6] [0.68-6.7]	S ↑ V Cimetidine, clomiphene, digitalis, levodopa S ↓ V Corticosteroids, estrogens (effects depend on dose and duration; large doses decrease and small doses may increase), gonadotropin-releasing hormone analogs (continuous administration), megestrol, oral contraceptives, phenothiazines, stanozolol

Testing for homocysteine and methylmalonic acid determinations may help distinguish between B_{12} and folate deficiency states. In folate deficiency, homocysteine levels are elevated and methylmalonic acid levels are normal. In vitamin B_{12} deficiency, both homocysteine levels and methylmalonic acid (MMA) levels are elevated.[9] It has been suggested that early assessment of vitamin B_{12} and folate status by measuring homocysteine and MMA may have advantages over measuring folate and B_{12}.[11]

S,U ↑ Primary gonadal failure, ovarian or testicular agenesis, Klinefelter's syndrome, Reifenstein's syndrome, castration, alcoholism, menopause, orchitis, gonadotropin-secreting pituitary tumors

S,U ↓ Anterior pituitary hypofunction, hypothalamic disorders, pregnancy, anorexia nervosa, polycystic ovary disease, hemochromatosis, sickle cell anemia, severe illness, hyperprolactinemia

In hypogonadism, FSH and LH levels lower than normal for the patient's age indicate hypothalamic or pituitary problems; higher levels indicate a primary gonadal defect.

Peak levels at midcycle are lower and shorter than for LH. Because of the episodic, circadian, and cyclic nature of pituitary gonadotropin secretion, clinical evaluation may require determinations of FSH in pooled blood specimens, multiple serial blood specimens, or timed urine specimens. For example, obtain three separate blood samples at 15- to 30-min intervals and pool equal volumes of serum.

In males there is less variation, and no values similar to the midcycle surge in females are normally seen. In males, correlations between sperm count and FSH are relatively poor. In the first year of life, gonadotropin levels are relatively high, then decrease to very low levels after 1-2 yr, and finally increase throughout puberty until adult levels are attained.

TEST NAME AND METHOD	SPECIMEN REQUIREMENTS	REFERENCE INTERVAL, CONVENTIONAL [INTERNATIONAL RECOMMENDED UNITS]		CHEMICAL INTERFERENCES AND IN VIVO EFFECTS
Follitropin—CONT				
		3-4		
		M: 1.24-15.4	[1.24-15.4]	
		F: 1.0-7.4	[1.0-7.4]	
		5		
		M: 1.53-6.8	[1.53-6.8]	
		F: 1.0-9.2	[1.0-9.2]	
		Adult		
		M: 1.42-15.4	[1.42-15.4]	
		F, follicular phase: 1.37-9.9	[1.37-9.9]	
		F, ovulatory peak: 6.17-17.2	[6.17-17.2]	
		F, luteal phase: 1.09-9.2	[1.09-9.2]	
		F, postmenopausal: 19.3-100.6	[19.3-100.6]	
	Urine, 24 hr. Use no preservatives. Store frozen.	U/day^+		U ↑ V Clomiphene
		Prepubertal child		U ↓ V Digitalis, estrogens
		M, F: <1.0-3.4		(comments above apply),
		1, M, F: <1.3		oral contraceptives
		2, M: 1-7		
		F: 2-6		
		3, M: 2-9		
		F: 3-8		
		4, M: 2-10		
		F: 3-9		
		5, M: 3-12		
		F: 2-11		
		Adult,		
		M: 3-11		
		F, Non-midcycle: 2-15		
	Amniotic fluid	mU/mL $(IRP\text{-}2\text{-}hMG)^7$	U/L	
		Fetus-3 mo		
		M: 1.0	× 1.0 [1.0]	
		F: 1.0	[1.0]	
		3-6 mo		
		M: 1-1.2	[1-1.2]	
		F: 4.3 ± 3.8 (1 SD)	[4.3 ± 3.8]	
		6-9 mo		
		M: 2.2 ± 1.2	[2.2 ± 1.2]	
		F: 1.4 ± 0.4	[1.4 ± 0.4]	

*World Health Organization, second International
Reference Preparation of FSH/LH 78/549.[8]
+World Health Organization, first International
Reference Preparation of FSH/LH 69/104.[9]

DIAGNOSTIC INFORMATION   **REMARKS**

Owing to variation in purity of standards, many assays express concentrations in terms of international units of either the World Health Organization's International Reference Preparations of FSH/LH or the 2nd International Reference Preparation of human menopausal gonadotropin. Recently, highly purified pituitary reference material has been used for assay standardization (WHO 1st International Standard 83/575).[3]

AF ↑ Alcoholism

AF ↓ Anterior pituitary hypofunction

TEST NAME AND METHOD	SPECIMEN REQUIREMENTS	REFERENCE INTERVAL, CONVENTIONAL [INTERNATIONAL RECOMMENDED UNITS]	CHEMICAL INTERFERENCES AND IN VIVO EFFECTS

Follitropin—CONT

1. Beastall G, Ferguson K, O'Reilly D, et al: Assays for follicle-stimulating hormone and luteinizing hormone: guidelines for the provision of a clinical biochemistry service, *Ann Clin Biochem* 24:246-262, 1987.

2. Vermes I, Bonte H, Veer G, et al: Interpretations of five monoclonal immunoassays of lutropin and follitropin: effects of normalization with WHO standards, *Clin Chem* 37:415-421, 1991.

3. Whitley RJ, Meikle AW, Watts NB: Endocrinology. In Burtis CA, Ashwood ER, editors: *Tietz textbook of clinical chemistry,* ed 2, Philadelphia, 1994, WB Saunders.

4. Wiedemann G, Jonetz-Mentzel L: Establishment of reference ranges for prolactin in neonates, infants, children, and adolescents, *Eur J Chem Clin Biochem* 31:447-451, 1993.

5. Kubasik NP, Ricotta M, Hunter T, et al: Effect of duration and temperature of storage on serum analyte stability: examination of 14 selected radioimmunoassay procedures, *Clin Chem* 28:164-165, 1982.

TEST NAME AND METHOD	SPECIMEN REQUIREMENTS	REFERENCE INTERVAL, CONVENTIONAL [INTERNATIONAL RECOMMENDED UNITS]		CHEMICAL INTERFERENCES AND IN VIVO EFFECTS
Free Thyroxine Index (FT_4I)[1-6]		$FT_4\ index$[7]	*(x)*	↑ V Amiodarone, in the presence of anti-T_4 antibodies or increased T_4 binding by thyroxine-binding prealbumin (TBPA)
	Cord blood: Newborn	6.0-13.2	(9.8)	
Calculation	1-3 day:	9.9-17.5	(13.9)	
$FTI = TT_4 \times$	1 wk:	7.5-15.1	(11.2)	
THBR	1-12 mo:	5.0-13.0	(8.4)	
	1-3 yr:	5.4-12.5	(8.1)	
	3-10 yr:	5.7-12.8	(8.2)	↓ V Anticonvulsants (carbamazepine, phenytoin); in some nonthyroidal illnesses in which a serum inhibitor interferes with binding of T_4 more than T_3.
	Pubertal child and adult:	4.2-13.0	(8.0)	

1. Alsever RN, Gotlin RW: *Handbook of endocrine tests in adults and children,* ed 2, Chicago, 1978, Year Book Medical Publishers, Inc.

2. Committee on Nomenclature of the American Thyroid Association: Revised nomenclature for tests of thyroid hormones and thyroid-related proteins in serum, *J Clin Endocrinol Metab* 64:1089-1094, 1987.

3. Felicetta JV, Green WL: Value of free thyroxine index, *N Engl J Med* 302:1480-1481, 1980.

4. Demers LM, Spencer C: Laboratory medicine practice guidelines for the laboratory support of the thyroid, *Thyroid* 13:4-104, 2003.

5. Larsen PR, Davies TF, Schlumberger MJ, et al: The thyroid gland. In Larsen PR, Kronenberg HM, Malmed S, et al, editors: *Williams textbook of endocrinology,* ed 10, Philadelphia, 1992, WB Saunders.

6. Nusynowitz ML: Screening tests and the free thyroxine index, *Arch Intern Med* 140:1017, 1980.

7. Endocrine Sciences: *Pediatric laboratory services,* Tarzana, CA, 1988, Endocrine Sciences.

6. Livesey JH, Hodgkinson SC, Roud AR, et al: Effect of time, temperature and freezing on the stability of immunoreactive LH, FSH, TSH, growth hormone, prolactin and insulin in plasma, *Clin Biochem* 13:151-155, 1980.
7. Johnson TR, Moore WM, Jefferies JE: *Children are different: developmental physiology,* ed 2, Columbus, OH, 1978, Ross Laboratories.
8. Nichols Institute Reference Laboratories: *Test catalog,* San Juan Capistrano, CA, 1993, Nichols Institute Reference Laboratories.
9. Endocrine Sciences: *Pediatric laboratory services,* Tarzana, CA, 1992, Endocrine Sciences.

↑ Hyperthyroidism, dysalbuminemic hyperthyroxinemia, congenital TBG excess, T_4 autoantibody

↓ Hypothyroidism, severe nonthyroidal illness, congenital TBG deficiency

The FT_4I correlates well with free thyroxine except in severe illness and dysalbuminemic hyperthyroxinemia and provides an estimate of the biologically active (free) T_4. It is calculated by multiplying total T_4 by THBR. (See *Thyroid Hormone Binding Ratio.*) The resulting value has a reference range close to the normal range for total T_4. Calculations of FT_4I using the percentage T_3 resin uptake are now considered obsolete.

In most instances, FT_4I is more convenient and less expensive than FT_4 estimate tests but has a lower sensitivity and specificity for the diagnosis of hyperthyroidism and hypothyroidism than a FT_4 E test.

FT_4I provides results that are comparable with reference methods for FT_4 (e.g., direct equilibrium dialysis; see *Thyroxine, Free*) in healthy subjects, hyperthyroid and hypothyroid patients, and patients with only mild abnormalities in TBG. However, the diagnostic accuracy of FT_4I can be variable in euthyroid patients with extreme abnormalities in TBG or TBPA concentrations (e.g., congenital TBG excess or deficiency).

TEST NAME AND METHOD	SPECIMEN REQUIREMENTS	REFERENCE INTERVAL, CONVENTIONAL [INTERNATIONAL RECOMMENDED UNITS]		CHEMICAL INTERFERENCES AND IN VIVO EFFECTS
Fructosamine[1-6] *Colorimetric NBT; affinity chromatography*	Serum. Store at −70° C.[8] Hemolyzed (moderate-gross) and icteric samples not suitable	*% of Total protein* 1-2	× 0.01	*Fraction of total protein* [0.01-0.02]
NBT; Colorimetric (Roche Diagnostics)[7]		Child: 5% below adult levels 18-60 yr: 202-282 μmol/L [Fructosamine]$_{corrected for albumin}$ = 191-265 μmol/L		↑ C Bilirubin, triglycerides, ↑↓ C Hemoglobin ↓ C Ascorbic acid ↓ V Pyridoxine

1. Armbruster DA: Fructosamine: structure, analysis, and clinical usefulness (review), *Clin Chem* 33:2153-2163, 1987.

2. Austin GE, Mullins RH, Morin LG: Non-enzymic glycation of individual plasma proteins in normoglycemic and hyperglycemic patients, *Clin Chem* 33:2220-2224. 1987.

3. Cefalu WT, Parker TB, Johnson CR: Validity of scrum fructosamine as index of short-term glycemic control in diabetic outpatients, *Diabetes Care* 11:662-664, 1988.

4. Guillausseau PJ, Charles MA, Godard V, et al: Comparison of fructosamine glycated hemoglobin as an index of glycemic control in diabetic patients, *Diabetes Res* 13:127-131, 1990.

5. Mendelovic DB, Whitehouse FW, Foreback CC: The why and wherefore of fructosamine, *Henry Ford Hosp Med J* 40:149-151, 1992.

6. Lin M-J, Hoke C, Ettinger B, et al: Technical performance evaluation of BM/Hitachi 747-200 serum fructosamine assay, *Clin Chem* 42:2, 244-248, 1996.

7. DeSchepper J, Derde M-P, Goubert P, et al: Reference values for fructosamine concentrations in children's sera: influence of protein concentration, age, and sex, *Clin Chem* 34:2444-2447, 1988.

8. Koskinen P, Irjala K: Stability of serum fructosamine during storage, *Clin Chem* 34:2545-2546, 1988.

9. Howanitz JH, Howanitz PJ, editors: *Laboratory medicine: test selection and interpretation,* New York, 1991, Churchill Livingstone.

10. Cefalu WT, Bell-Farrow AD, Petty M, et al: Clinical validation of a second generation fructosamine assay, *Clin Chem* 37:1252-1256, 1991.

Fructosamine reflects the mean glucose concentration in blood over recent period of 2-3 wk, whereas glycohemoglobin (HbA$_{1c}$) is indicative of the concentration of blood glucose over intermediate to long term 4-8 wk. See *Glycated Hemoglobin(s) (glycohemoglobin)*.

The fructosamine assay shows some promise for the assessment of short-term glycemic control in diabetic patients, especially in newborns and in nonpregnant women.[1]

It may also be of value in patients with hematological disorders affecting red blood cell half-life.

"Fructosamine" describes serum proteins that have been glycated, i.e., are derivatives of the nonenzymatic reaction product of a sugar (glucose) and one of the serum proteins (albumin).

Severe hypoproteinemic states (albumin[9] may falsely lower fructosamine concentrations. Interpret results with caution in patients with abnormal rates of serum protein turnover.

Correcting for changes in protein concentration improves correlation with fasting glucose and HbA$_{1c}$.[6,10] Correction can be either for albumin and/or total protein using the following formulas [Fructosamine]$_{corrected for total protein}$ = (fructosamine/total protein) $\times$ 70 g/L

[Fructosamine]$_{corrected for albumin}$ = (fructosamine/albumin) $\times$ 41g/L (70 and 41 g/L represent mean values for diabetic population).

Hemoglobin, ascorbic acid, and ceruloplasmin inhibit fructosamine generation.[9]

Method is unaffected by hemoglobin variants.

TEST NAME AND METHOD	SPECIMEN REQUIREMENTS	REFERENCE INTERVAL, CONVENTIONAL [INTERNATIONAL RECOMMENDED UNITS]		CHEMICAL INTERFERENCES AND IN VIVO EFFECTS
Fructose (Levulose)[1,2] *Colorimetric*[2]	Serum. Store at $-20°$ C. Stable for >6 mo.	1-6 mg/dL	$\times$ 55.5 [55.5-333 μmol/L]	
	Urine. Store at $-20°$ C. Stable for >6 mo.	30-65 mg/day	$\times$ 5.55 [170-360 μmol/day][1]	U ↑ C Ingestion of fruits, honey, syrups, sucrose
Seminal Fructose Qualitative: Resorcinol[3]	Semen. Store at $-20°$ C. Stable for >6 mo.	Normal: Positive		
Quantitative *Spectrophotometric, Resorcinol*		>150 mg/dL	$\times$ 55.5 [>325 μmol/L][4]	
Corrected Seminal Fructose		2.5-8.0 mg fructose per 10^6 spermatozoa/mL		

1. Henry JB, editor: *Clinical diagnosis and management by laboratory methods,* ed 18, Philadelphia, 1991, WB Saunders.
2. Henry RJ, Cannon DC, Winkelman JW, editors: *Clinical chemistry: principles and technics,* ed 2, Hagerstown, MD, 1974, Harper and Row.
3. Keel BA, Webster BW: *CRC Handbook of the Laboratory Diagnosis and treatment of infertility,* Boca Raton, FL, 1990, CRC Press, pp. 49.
4. *ARUP-Cleveland Clinic Laboratory: Reference manual,* Cleveland, OH, 1991, Endocrine Sciences.
5. Gonzales GF, Villena A: True corrected seminal fructose level: a better marker of the function of seminal vesicles in infertile men, *Int J Androl* 24:255-260, 2001.

TEST NAME AND METHOD	SPECIMEN REQUIREMENTS	REFERENCE INTERVAL, CONVENTIONAL [INTERNATIONAL RECOMMENDED UNITS]	CHEMICAL INTERFERENCES AND IN VIVO EFFECTS
Fructose Tolerance Test[1,2] Dose: 200 mg/kg, IV	Serum or whole blood. Draw before dose and every half hour thereafter to 2 hr. Determine glucose, CO_2, phosphate, and lactate in each sample.	See *Diagnostic Information* and *Remarks*.	See individual methods.

1. Hicks JM, Boeckx RL, editors: *Pediatric clinical chemistry,* Philadelphia, 1984, WB Saunders.
2. Scriver CR, Beaudet AL, Sly WS, et al, editors: *The metabolic basis of inherited disease,* ed 6, New York, 1989, McGraw-Hill Publishing Co.

DIAGNOSTIC INFORMATION	REMARKS

S ↑ Essential fructosuria, hereditary fructose intolerance

U ↑ Essential fructosuria, hereditary fructose intolerance, hepatic failure

Fructose is a reducing sugar. It reacts in Seliwanoff's resorcinol test and can be identified by TLC.

Fresh specimens are required because fructose can undergo conversion to glucose in an alkaline medium.

See also *Fructose Tolerance Test.*

Fructose may be absent in some congenital abnormalities of the male genital tract. It is produced in the male reproductive tract by the seminal vesicles. Fructose is the energy source for sperm motility. Its measurement is useful in investigation of azospermia, and it is used as a marker of the seminal vesicles. The use of corrected fructose levels is said to improve its diagnostic value.[5] Corrected fructose is calculated by multiplying the log of motile sperm concentration by seminal fructose concentration.

Patients with fructose-1,6,-diphosphatase deficiency and hereditary fructose intolerance (fructose-1-phosphate aldolase deficiency) show a decrease in glucose, CO_2, and phosphate levels, whereas lactate levels increase.

Because of the ill effects of oral fructose loads on patients with one or another of the deficiencies, the oral loading test is not recommended.[2] Most clinicians use either enzymatic assays or DNA testing to make these diagnoses.

TEST NAME AND METHOD	SPECIMEN REQUIREMENTS	REFERENCE INTERVAL, CONVENTIONAL [INTERNATIONAL RECOMMENDED UNITS]	CHEMICAL INTERFERENCES AND IN VIVO EFFECTS
Furosemide Stimulation Test, Rapid[1-4] Dose: 60 mg furosemide orally after overnight fast. Patient should be on normal diet without medications the week before the test.	Plasma (Na$_2$EDTA) for renin values before and 5 hr after furosemide administration. Patient should be kept in an up-right position (sitting, standing, walking).	Renin: 1-6 ng AI */mL/hr × 1.0 [1-6 mg AI × hr^{-1} × L^{-1}] *AI, Angiotensin I.	See *Renin.*

1. Miller RE, Ngai B: *Manual of endocrine diagnostic tests,* ed 4, Lexington, KY, 1991, Department of Medicine, University of Kentucky.
2. Samloff IM: Pepsinogens I and II: purification from gastric mucosa and radioimmunoassay in serum, *Gastroenterology* 82:26-33, 1982.
3. Wallach L, Ildiko N, Dawson KG: Stimulated renin: a screening test for hypotension, *Ann Intern Med* 82:27-34, 1975.
4. Watts NB, Keffer JH: *Practical endocrinology,* ed 4, Philadelphia, 1989, Lea & Febiger.

Galactose[1] *Enzymatic*[2]	Whole blood or plasma. Collect blood into heparin. Heparinized samples can be shipped overnight. Do not freeze whole blood. Separate and store plasma at −20° C.[3]	*mg/dL*[5] Newborn: 0-20 × 0.0555 Thereafter: <5 Whole blood 0-8.1 Plasma 0-5.4	*mmol/L* ↑ Ascorbic acid [0-1.11] [<0.28] [0-0.45][3] [0-0.3]
	Urine. Store at −20° C. Newborn: Newborn: 1-2 wk: Adults:	≥60 0-27 0-19.8 0-5.4	[≥3.33] U ↑ V Lactose [0-1.5][3] [0-0.1.1] [0-0.3]
		Adult: <14 mg/day × 0.00555 [<0.08 mmol/day]	
	Urine. Collect 2 hr after patient drinks a glass of milk.[4]	Nondetectable[4]	

1. Henry RJ, Cannon DC, Winkelman JW, editors: *Clinical chemistry: principles and technics,* ed 2, Hagerstown, MD, 1974, Harper and Row.
2. Dahlqvist A, Svenningsen NW: Galactose in the urine of newborn infants, *J Pediatr* 75:454-462, 1969.
3. Slocum RH, Shin GS: Galactose metabolites and disorders of galactose metabolism. In *Techniques in human biochemical genetics,* New York, 1991, Wiley-Liss, pp. 87-126.

DIAGNOSTIC INFORMATION	REMARKS
Stimulated response: Renin-dependent forms of hypertension (such as renovascular hypertension), high-renin essential hypertension, Bartter's syndrome, pheochromocytoma	This test is a screening procedure only and may be done on an outpatient basis. Furosemide (Lasix) diuresis is a potent stimulus to renin secretion.
No response: Hypertension from mineralocorticoid excess (such as primary aldosteronism), hyporeninemic hypoaldosteronism, low-renin essential hypertension	
S ↑ Galactokinase-deficient and galactose-1-phosphate uridyltransferase–deficient galactosemias	Galactose is a reducing sugar and can be identified by TLC and quantitated by a specific enzymatic assay.

Because of the transient galactosemia and galactosuria that can occur in galactokinase deficiency, blood and urine specimens may need to be collected shortly after a galactose-containing meal or glass of milk to demonstrate abnormally elevated galactose levels. |
| U ↑ Neonates ≥6 days old, premature infants, late pregnancy, lactation, children with high milk consumption, galactokinase-deficient and gal-1-P uridyltransferase–deficient galactosemias, hepatitis, biliary atresia of the newborn | See also *Galactosemia Screening.* |

4. Mayo Medical Laboratories: *Test catalog,* Rochester, MN, 2005, Mayo Medical Laboratories.

5. Behrman RE, Kliegman RM, Nelson WE, et al, editors: *Nelson textbook of pediatrics,* ed 18, Philadelphia, 1992, Elsevier.

TEST NAME AND METHOD	SPECIMEN REQUIREMENTS	REFERENCE INTERVAL, CONVENTIONAL [INTERNATIONAL RECOMMENDED UNITS]	CHEMICAL INTERFERENCES AND IN VIVO EFFECTS
Galactose-1-Phosphate *Microplate, colorimetric*[1,2]	Dried blood spots on filter paper. Stable 30 days at 4° C.	*mmol/L* <0.74	
Microplate, fluorimetric[3]	Dried blood spots on filter paper.	<80 mg/L total galactose + gal-1-P	
Enzymatic[1]	Washed red blood cells.	*mg/dL* < 0.3	

1. Shin Y: Galactose metabolites and disorders of galactose metabolism. In Hommes FA, editor: *Techniques in human biochemical genetics,* New York, 1991, Wiley-Liss, pp. 267-283.
2. Diepenbrock F, Heckler R, Schickling H, et al: Colorimetric determination of galactose and galactose-1-phosphate from dried blood, *Clin Biochem* 25:37-39, 1992.
3. Yamaguchi A, Fukushi M, Shimuzi Y, et al: Microassay for newborn screening for galactosemia with use of a fluorometric microplate reader, *Clin Chem* 35:1962-1964, 1989.

α-D-Galactose-1-Phosphate Uridylyltransferase in Erythrocytes (UDP-G-1-P; EC 2.7.7.12)[1-3] *Radiometric after DEAE separation*[3]	Hemolysate of washed Ercs. Submit whole blood (EDTA, heparin). Stable 14 days at room temperature, 4 wk at 4° C. Do not freeze.		*mmol/hr/mL*[3] 5.9-9.5 (x̄: 7.3)		*U/L* [98-158] [x̄: 122]	None found.
		Galactosemia heterozygotes:	2.0-4.8 (x̄: 3.7)		[33-80] [x̄: 62]	
		Galactosemia homozygotes:	0.0		[0.0]	

UDPG consumption assay, 37° C[4]

U/g Hb		*MU/mol Hb*
18.5-28.5	× 0.0645*	[1.19-1.84]
U/10^{12} Ercs		*nU/Erc*
537-827	× 10^{-3}	[0.54-0.83]
U/mL Ercs		*kU/L Ercs*
6.29-9.69	× 1.0	[6.29-9.69]

*Conversion factor based on MW of Hb of 64,500.

	U/g Hb[4]		*MU/mol Hb*
Heterozygotes (Duarte variant):	13.5-18.5	× 0.0645*	[0.87-1.19]
Galactosemia heterozygotes and homozygotes for the Duarte variant:	8.5-13.5		[0.55-0.87]

DIAGNOSTIC INFORMATION	REMARKS
↑ Galactosemia because of deficiency of α-D-galactose-1-phosphate-uridylyl-transferase (EC 2.7.7.12) or UDP-glucose-4-epimerase (EC 5.1.3.2).	These screening tests should be performed immediately to enable institution of diet treatment if results are positive. Assay based on washed red cells is preferable for confirming diagnosis of galactosemia and for subsequent monitoring of response to therapy.
Galactosemia associated with decreased UDP-G-1-P activity may be responsible for the development of hepatic and renal disease, cataracts, and other abnormalities.	The enzyme catalyzes the conversion of galactose-1-phosphate and UDP-glucose to glucose-1-phosphate and UDP-galactose. Galactosemia is an inborn error of metabolism characterized by the inability to convert galactose to glucose and clinically by cirrhosis and cataracts. Activity is expressed as the total amount (micromole) of galactose-1-phosphate converted by 1 mL of packed erythrocytes/hr. Can be used to diagnose galactosemia in patients transfused with normal erythrocytes. U/g Hb × 29 = U/10^{12} Ercs U/g Hb × 0.34 = U/mL Ercs* *See Note, *Acetylcholinesterase.*

TEST NAME AND METHOD	SPECIMEN REQUIREMENTS	REFERENCE INTERVAL, CONVENTIONAL [INTERNATIONAL RECOMMENDED UNITS]	CHEMICAL INTERFERENCES AND IN VIVO EFFECTS
α-D-Galactose-1-Phosphate Uridylyltransferase in Erythrocytes—CONT			
		Double hetero-zygotes for galactosemia and the Duarte variant: 3.5-8.5 [0.23-0.55] See *Acetylcholinesterase*.	

1. Kalckar HM, Anderson EP, Isselbacher KJ: Galactosemia, a congenital defect in a nucleotide transferase, *Biochim Biophys Acta* 20:262-268, 1956.
2. Weatherall DJ: ABC of clinical haematology. The hereditary anaemias, *BMJ* 314:492-496, 1197.
3. Ng WG, Bergren WR, Donnell GN: An improved procedure for the assay of hemolysate galactose-1-phosphate uridyl transferase activity by the use of ^{14}C-labeled galactose-1-phosphate, *Clin Chim Acta* 15:489-492, 1967.
4. Beutler E: *Red cell metabolism: a manual of biochemical methods,* ed 4, New York, 1986, Grune & Stratton.

TEST NAME AND METHOD	SPECIMEN REQUIREMENTS	REFERENCE INTERVAL, CONVENTIONAL [INTERNATIONAL RECOMMENDED UNITS]	CHEMICAL INTERFERENCES AND IN VIVO EFFECTS
Galactosemia Newborn Screening[1-6] *Metabolite Assays (galactose)* *Inhibition assay*[7]	Whole blood on filter paper	Bacterial growth. Inhibition of growth indicates the presence of galactose.	False-positive result: antibiotics, increased valine
Paigen assay	Whole blood on filter paper; cord or capillary blood (heparin) from newborn	No bacterial growth. Inhibition of bacterial growth is directly proportional to galactose concentration.	False-negative result: antibiotics
Gal-1-P Uridylltransferase Assay (Beutler) *Qualitative, fluorimetric*[8]	Whole blood on filter paper	Bright fluorescence at 1 and 2 hr (assuming no other enzyme is deficient).	False-positive result at 2 hr: inactivation of transferase because of shipping conditions, transferase variants (e.g., Duarte). However, heterozygotes for galactosemia and homozygotes for the Duarte variant may exhibit less fluorescence at 1 hr.

DIAGNOSTIC INFORMATION	REMARKS

Deficiency of any one of three erythrocyte enzymes leads to galactosemia and galactosuria: galactose-1-P uridyltransferase (classic galactosemia), galactokinase, or UDP galactose-4-epimerase.

Metabolite assays are sensitive to increased galactose (inhibition assay) or increased galactose or gal-1-P (Paigen) and thus detect any of the three types of galactosemia. Difficulties with the inhibition assay are encountered because of characteristics of the bacteria used in the assay.

↓ Transferase-deficient galactosemia

Transferase assays are specific for transferase-deficient galactosemia. Because these assays use intrinsic erythrocyte enzymes, low G6PD or G-6-PGM activities may delay the appearance of fluorescence or dye decolorization. Only severe G6PD or G-6-PGM deficiencies will give false-positive results. The qualitative assay detects only the presence or absence of transferase deficiency and is subject to a high incidence of false-positive results.

TEST NAME AND METHOD	SPECIMEN REQUIREMENTS	REFERENCE INTERVAL, CONVENTIONAL [INTERNATIONAL RECOMMENDED UNITS]		CHEMICAL INTERFERENCES AND IN VIVO EFFECTS

Galactosemia Newborn Screening—CONT

Quantitative, fluorimetric[8] — Whole blood; cord or capillary blood (heparin) from newborn

	$\mu mol/hr/g$ Hb	kU/mol Hb	
	$18\text{-}30^4$ $\times 1.075$	[19-32]	False-negative result: blood transfusion
Homozygote:	<3	[<3.2]	
Heterozygote:	Intermediate values		

1. Henry JB, editor: *Clinical diagnosis and management by laboratory methods,* ed 20, Philadelphia, 2001, WB Saunders.
2. Pesce A, Kaplan L, editors: *Methods in clinical chemistry,* St. Louis, 1987, CV Mosby.
3. Beutler E: Galactosemia: screening and diagnosis, *Clin Biochem* 24:293-300, 1991.
4. Burman D, Holton JB, Pennock CA, editors: *Inherited disorders of carbohydrate metabolism,* Baltimore. 1978, University Park Press.
5. Donnell SN, editor: *Galactosemia,* Washington, DC, 1993, National Institutes of Health 93-3438.
6. Levy HL, Hammersen G: Newborn screening for galactosemia and other galactose metabolic defects, *J Pediatr* 92:871-877, 1978.
7. Mayes JS, Guthrie R: Detection of heterozygotes for galactokinase deficiency in a human population, *Biochem Genet* 2:219-230, 1968.
8. O'Brien D, Ibbott FA, Rodgerson DO: *Laboratory manual of pediatric microbiochemical techniques,* New York, 1968, Harper and Row.

Gastric Analysis (Gastric Content)[1]

Volume — Gastric residue (total content after 12-hr fast). Patient should not smoke, chew gum, or exercise.

20-100 mL (usually <50 mL)	× 0.001	[0.020-0.100 L] [<0.05 L]	↓ V Atropine, ganglionic blocking agents, insulin, diazepam, 5-hydroxytryptamine

Consistency, color, odor, bile

Consistency:	Fluid, may be slightly viscous from mucus
Color:	Colorless
Odor:	Sour
Bile:	Present in 25% of normals

DIAGNOSTIC INFORMATION	REMARKS

Quantitative assays, in addition to diagnosing transferase deficiency, can identify heterozygous transferase-deficient carriers and homozygous transferase variants. In addition to these screening assays, presumptive diagnosis of galactosemia may be made by the presence of serum and urine non–glucose-reducing substance with identification by TLC. Blood for galactosemia screening should be obtained as early in life as possible, and no later than 3-4 days. Positive screening tests should be rapidly confirmed by the assay of the specific enzyme as soon as possible and begin appropriate dietary therapy if necessary.

↑ Delayed emptying of stomach (e.g., pyloric obstruction, carcinoma of stomach), increased gastric secretion (e.g., duodenal ulcer, Z-E syndrome), regurgitation of duodenal content

The analysis of gastric content (basal and after stimulation) was once an important diagnostic procedure. However, the widespread use of fiberoptic endoscopy has rendered the test obsolete except for research investigations. Knowledge of normal stomach content is useful for identifying abnormal stomach aspirates.[2]

Antacids and H_2-receptor antagonists should be avoided 24-48 hr before testing. Tricyclic antidepressants, anticholinergics, and reserpine should be avoided 12-72 hr before testing.[3]

Bile is frequently present after partial gastrectomy or gastroenterostomy, after regurgitation, and with obstructing lesions of the small intestine distal to the ampulla of Vater.

Excess mucus is found in cases of gastritis and pyloric obstruction.

TEST NAME AND METHOD	SPECIMEN REQUIREMENTS	REFERENCE INTERVAL, CONVENTIONAL [INTERNATIONAL RECOMMENDED UNITS]	CHEMICAL INTERFERENCES AND IN VIVO EFFECTS
Gastric Analysis—CONT			
Blood		Negative	
HCl, free		No stimulation: Up to 40 mmol/L; 4% of normals and 25% of individuals >60 yr have no free HCl in unstimulated state.	↑ V Caffeine, calcium salts, corticotropin, ethanol, rauwolfia, reserpine, tolazoline
			↓ V Acetazolamide (large doses), atropine, diazepam, ganglionic blocking agents, glucagon, H$_2$-receptor antagonists (e.g., cimetidine, ranitidine), insulin, oxyphencyclimine, omeprazole, propranolol, secretin, 5-hydroxytryptamine
Total acidity		10-50 mmol/L	
pH		1.5-3.5	
Chloride		45-155 mmol/L	
Organic acids		Negative	

1. Henderson AR, Tietz NW, Rinker AD: Gastric, pancreatic, and intestinal function. In Burtis CA, Ashwood ER, editors: *Tietz textbook of clinical chemistry,* ed 2, Philadelphia, 1994, WB Saunders.
2. Rosenfeld L: Gastric tubes, meals, acid, and analysis: rise and decline, *Clin Chem* 43:837-842, 1997.
3. Jacobs DS, Kasten BL, DeMott WR, et al, editors: *Laboratory test handbook,* ed 2, Stow, OH, 1990, LexiComp, Inc.

DIAGNOSTIC INFORMATION	REMARKS
Blood may be positive in gastric carcinoma, gastric ulcer, or gastritis. Bleeding gums can also cause a positive test.	In the presence of free HCl, hematin is formed, with brown, coffee grounds-like appearance.
	Fresh blood is red and may be caused by trauma or fresh bleeding from lesions (e.g., ulcer, carcinoma).
↑ Duodenal ulcer, some cases of gastric ulcer, Z-E syndrome. The test is negative in those with pernicious anemia.	Diagnosis of achlorhydria is confirmed only if no free HCl is found after maximum stimulation; false achlorhydria may occur if free HCl is secreted but subsequently neutralized (e.g., by food, regurgitated material).
In those with pernicious anemia, pH is >7.0.	Red color after addition of Toepfer's reagent indicates the presence of HCl and a pH <3.0.
	Chloride measurements are helpful to detect false achlorhydria.
Lactate and butyrate are positive if pH is neutral or alkaline for >6 hr (e.g., carcinoma, pyloric stenosis).	

TEST NAME AND METHOD	SPECIMEN REQUIREMENTS	REFERENCE INTERVAL, CONVENTIONAL [INTERNATIONAL RECOMMENDED UNITS]			CHEMICAL INTERFERENCES AND IN VIVO EFFECTS
Gastrin[1-6]	Serum, fasting; freeze immediately. For long-term storage freeze at −70° C.		*pg/mL*	*pmol/L*	↑ V Amino acids (oral), calcium carbonate (oral), calcium chloride (IV), catecholamines, cimetidine (meal stimulated), coffee, insulin, omeprazole
RIA		Cord[7]:	20-290 0.475	[9.5-138]	
		0-4 days:	120-183	[57-87]	
		Child[7]:	<10-125	[<5-59]	
		Adult			
		16-60 yr:	25-90	[12-43]	
		>60 yr:	<100	[<48]	
					↓ V Atropine (IM), secretin (normals)

1. Feldman M: Clinical significance of serum gastrin: fasting and stimulated, *Clin Chem* 31:890-891, 1985.

2. Henderson AR, Tietz NW, Rinker AD: Gastric, pancreatic, and intestinal function. In Burtis CA, Ashwood ER, editors: *Tietz textbook of clinical chemistry,* ed 2, Philadelphia, 1994, WB Saunders.

3. Malagelada J-R, Davis CS, O'Fallon WM, et al: Laboratory diagnosis of gastrinoma. I. A prospective evaluation of gastric analysis and fasting serum gastrin levels, *Mayo Clin Proc* 57:211-218, 1982.

4. Malagelada J-R, Glanzman SL, Go VLW: Laboratory diagnosis of gastrinoma. II. A prospective study of gastrin challenge tests, *Mayo Clin Proc* 57:219-226, 1982.

5. McGuigan JE: The Zollinger-Ellison syndrome. In Sleisenger MH, Fordtran JS, editors: *Gastrointestinal disease: pathophysiology, diagnosis, management,* ed 4, Philadelphia, 1989, WB Saunders.

6. Wolfe MM, Jensen RT: Zollinger-Ellison syndrome: current concepts in diagnosis and management, *N Engl J Med* 317:1200-1209, 1987.

7. Endocrine Sciences: *Pediatric laboratory services,* Tarzana, CA, 1992, Endocrine Sciences.

DIAGNOSTIC INFORMATION	**REMARKS**

↑ Zollinger-Ellison (Z-E) syndrome (frequently caused by pancreatic gastrinoma), antral G-cell hyperplasia, pyloric obstruction, vagotomy without gastric resection, retained antrum, chronic atrophic gastritis, pernicious anemia, chronic renal failure, gastric carcinoma, gastric ulcer

↓ Antrectomy with vagotomy, hypothyroidism

The principal forms of gastrin in blood are G-34 (big gastrin; $t_{1/2}$, 42 min), G-17 (little gastrin; $t_{1/2}$, 5 min), and G-14 (minigastrin; $t_{1/2}$, 5 min). Each of these polypeptides circulates in nonsulfated (I) or sulfated (II) forms.

Gastrin values follow a circadian rhythm (lowest 3:00 to 7:00 AM, highest during the day) or fluctuate physiologically in relation to meals. Increasing gastrin levels in older subjects may indicate a decline in the production of acid rather than atrophic gastritis. Basal gastric acid output is inversely related to gastrin levels. Interpretation of elevated levels requires knowledge of gastric acid secretion.

Most Z-E patients have fasting gastrin levels >500 pg/mL [> 225 pmol/L] and high basal gastric acid secretion, but up to 40% of Z-E patients may have gastrin values between 100-500 pg/mL [45-225 pmol/L]. About 20% of Z-E patients also have parathyroid and pituitary adenomas (MEN type I or Werner's syndrome). About 90% of Z-E patients with borderline fasting gastrin levels (i.e., 100-500 pg/mL) [45-225 pmol/L] will show an increase of >200 pg/mL [95 pmol/L] above the baseline in response to secretin stimulation; a calcium infusion test gives similar responses in patients with gastrinomas.

See also *Gastrin Stimulation Test (after Secretin)* and *Gastrin Stimulation Test (after Calcium Infusion)*.

TEST NAME AND METHOD	SPECIMEN REQUIREMENTS	REFERENCE INTERVAL, CONVENTIONAL [INTERNATIONAL RECOMMENDED UNITS]		CHEMICAL INTERFERENCES AND IN VIVO EFFECTS
Gastrin Stimulation Test (after Calcium Infusion)[1-3] Dose: 15 mg Ca/kg in 500 mL normal saline over 4 hr	Serum. Draw in fasting state before infusion and at 1, 2, 3, and 4 hr (through indwelling needle in the contralateral arm).	Gastrin: Calcium:	Little or no increase over baseline Linear increase over baseline. Average after 4 hr, 13.3 ± 0.2 mg/dL (SEM)[1] $[\times 0.25 = 3.33 \pm 0.05$ mmol/L]	See *Gastrin.*

1. Malagelada J-R, Glanzman SL, Go VLW: Laboratory diagnosis of gastrinoma. II. A prospective study of gastrin challenge tests, *Mayo Clin Proc* 57:219-226, 1982.
2. McGuigan JE: Peptic ulcer and gastritis. In Isselbacher KJ, Braunwald E, Wilson JD, et al, editors: *Harrison's principles of internal medicine,* ed 13, New York, 1994, McGraw-Hill Publishing Co.
3. Romanus ME, Neal JA, Dilley WG, et al: Comparison of four provocative tests for the diagnosis of gastrinoma, *Ann Surg* 197:608-616, 1983.
4. Frucht H, Howard JM, Slaff JI, et al: Secretin and calcium provocative tests in the Zollinger-Ellison syndrome. A prospective study, *Ann Intern Med* 111:713-722, 1989.

TEST NAME AND METHOD	SPECIMEN REQUIREMENTS	REFERENCE INTERVAL, CONVENTIONAL [INTERNATIONAL RECOMMENDED UNITS]	CHEMICAL INTERFERENCES AND IN VIVO EFFECTS
Gastrin Stimulation Test (after Secretin)[1-4] Dose: 2-3 U/kg secretin injected over 30 sec	Serum. Draw in fasting state before injection and at 5-min intervals for 30 min after injection.	Gastrin: No response or slight suppression[5]	See *Gastrin.* Discontinue proton pump inhibitors 5 days before or H2 receptor antagonists 24 hr before the test.

1. Brady CE: Secretin provocation test in the diagnosis of Zollinger-Ellison syndrome, *Am J Gastroenterol* 86:129-134, 1991.
2. McGuigan JE: Peptic ulcer and gastritis. In Isselbacher KJ, Braunwald E, Wilson JD, et al, editors: *Harrison's principles of internal medicine,* ed 13, New York, 1994, McGraw-Hill Publishing Co.
3. McGuigan JE, Wolfe MM: Secretin injection test in the diagnosis of gastrinoma, *Gastroenterology* 79:1324-1331, 1980.
4. Romanus ME, Neal JA, Dilley WG, et al: Comparison of four provocative tests for the diagnosis of gastrinoma, *Ann Surg* 197:608-616, 1983.
5. Henderson AR, Tietz NW, Rinker AD: Gastric, pancreatic, and intestinal function. In Burtis CA, Ashwood ER, editors: *Tietz textbook of clinical chemistry,* ed 2, Philadelphia, 1994, WB Saunders.
6. Malagelada J-R, Glanzman SL, Go VLW: Laboratory diagnosis of gastrinoma. II. A prospective study of gastrin challenge tests, *Mayo Clin Proc* 57:219-226, 1982.

DIAGNOSTIC INFORMATION	**REMARKS**

↑ Gastrinoma (Z-E syndrome, gastrin >400 pg/mL; >400 ng/L)

Slight ↑ Duodenal ulcer (gastrin <400 pg/mL; <400 ng/L)

↓ Pernicious anemia, atrophic gastritis

Serum calcium is measured to ensure that adequate calcium has been given. In patients with Z-E syndrome, gastrin levels increase more than twofold above baseline during Ca infusion. In one study the highest gastrin concentrations reached during Ca infusion were as follows: 620-66,000 pg/mL [620-66,000 ng/L] for gastrinoma; 44-328 pg/mL [44-328 ng/L] for duodenal ulcer.

Test is useful in patients without marked elevation in basal gastrin levels. Test is more time consuming than the secretin stimulation test and may cause unpleasant side effects. The test should be reserved for patients with a negative secretin test, gastric acid hypersecretion, and a strong clinical suspicion of the Zollinger-Ellison syndrome.[4]

↑ Gastrinoma (Zollinger-Ellison syndrome)

↓ Duodenal ulcer, antral G-cell hyperplasia, achlorhydria

In 95% of patients with gastrinomas, gastrin levels increase paradoxically by 100-200 pg/mL [48-95 pmol/L] 5 min after secretin injection. In one study, the highest gastrin concentrations reached after secretin injections were 759-103,335 pg/mL [759-103,335 ng/L] for gastrinoma and 43-317 pg/mL [43-317 ng/L] for duodenal ulcer.[6] (See *Gastrin and Gastrin Stimulation Test [after Calcium Infusion].*) The gastrin stimulation test (after secretin) is the preferred provocative test for patients suspected of having Zollinger-Ellison syndrome. (See *Gastric Stimulation Test.*)

TEST NAME AND METHOD	SPECIMEN REQUIREMENTS	REFERENCE INTERVAL, CONVENTIONAL [INTERNATIONAL RECOMMENDED UNITS]	CHEMICAL INTERFERENCES AND IN VIVO EFFECTS
Gliadin Antibodies, IgA and IgG *Solid-phase EIA*	Serum, frozen or refrigerated is preferable.	Results are age dependent and are expressed in arbitrary units. Reference ranges may vary with reagent manufacturer. IgA or IgG: <3 yr of age: >3 yr of age: <20 U: negative <25 U: negative 20-25 U: equivocal 25-50 U: equivocal >25 U: positive >50 U: positive	None known.

1. NIH Consensus Development Conference on Celiac Disease. http://consensus.nih.gov/2004/2004celiacdisease118html.htm. Last accessed 1/31/06.

Glomerular Basement Membrane (GBM) Antibody *EIA, ELISA*[1-5]	Serum	IgG: ≤5 EU/mL: Negative 5.1-20.0 EU/mL: Borderline >20.0 EU/mL: Positive	None found.
IFA[4]		IgA: Negative IgG: Negative	

1. Peter JB, Shen GQ, Lin H-C: A sensitive enzyme immunoassay (EIA) for detection of antibodies to glomerular basement membranes (GBM) [abstract], *Am J Clin Pathol* 91:367, 1989.
2. Saxena R, Isaksson B, Bygren P, et al: A rapid assay for circulating anti-glomerular basement membrane antibodies in Goodpasture syndrome, *J Immunol Methods* 18:73-78, 1989.
3. Westman KW, Bygren PG, Eilert I, et al: Rapid screening assay for anti-GBM antibody and ANCAs; an important tool for the differential diagnosis of pulmonary renal syndromes, *Nephrol Dial Transplant* 12:1863-1868, 1997.
4. Mayo Medical Laboratories: *Interpretive handbook,* Rochester, MN, 2001, Mayo Medical Laboratories.
5. Jaskowski TD, Martins TB, Litwin CM, et al: Comparison of four enzyme immunoassays for the detection of immunoglobulin G antibody against glomerular basement membrane, *J Clin Lab Anal* 16:143-145. 2002.
6. Pusey CD: Anti-glomerular basement membrane disease, *Kidney Int* 64:1535-1550, 2003.

DIAGNOSTIC INFORMATION	REMARKS

Testing for gliadin antibodies is useful to monitor compliance with a gluten-free diet in patients with celiac disease. Gliadin antibodies occur in patients with celiac disease but are not as specific for this disease as Ttg antibodies.[1]

A decrease in the level of gliadin antibodies (IgA and IgG) after institution of a gluten-free diet is indicative of a favorable response in patients with celiac disease.

GBM antibodies are found in the serum of most individuals with active Goodpasture's syndrome when measured with sensitive and specific ELISAs and are not present in healthy subjects. Compared with clinical diagnosis, ELISA has been shown to have a sensitivity of 87% and a specificity of 98%. A small percentage of patients with other renal diseases (systemic lupus erythematosus, mixed connective tissue disease, systemic vasculitis) may have borderline titers.

IFA is less sensitive and specific than ELISA, with ~75% sensitivity in patients with confirmed Goodpasture's syndrome. False-positive results can occur because of background fluorescence caused by nonspecific IgG in the human kidney used to prepare the fluorescent antibody.

In anti-GBM antibody disease, circulating autoantibodies are directed against an antigen (primarily the globular domain of the type IV collagen chains) in the glomerular basement membrane, resulting in acute and rapidly progressive glomerulonephritis that is typically associated with crescent formation.[6] The antibody type is usually IgG or IgA, but IgM has also occasionally been found. Goodpasture's syndrome is a rapidly progressive autoimmune disorder that consists of the clinical constellation of acute glomerulonephritis, pulmonary hemorrhage, and anti-GBM antibodies. The pulmonary damage is caused by cross-reactivity of the GBM antibodies with the alveolar basement membranes.

TEST NAME AND METHOD	SPECIMEN REQUIREMENTS	REFERENCE INTERVAL, CONVENTIONAL [INTERNATIONAL RECOMMENDED UNITS]		CHEMICAL INTERFERENCES AND IN VIVO EFFECTS
Glomerular Filtration Rate (GFR), Estimated *MDRD equation*[1-3] *(Modification of Diet in Renal Disease)*	See *Creatinine, Serum or Plasma.*	*Age (yr)* 20-29 30-39 40-49 50-59 60-69 ≥70	*Average GFR (mL/min/1.73 m^2)*[3] 116 107 99 93 85 75	See *Creatinine, Serum or Plasma.*

Chronic kidney disease: <60 mL/min/1.73 m^2
Kidney failure: <15 mL/min/1.73 m^2

1. Manjunath G, Sarnak MJ, Levey AS: Prediction equations to estimate glomerular filtration rate: an update, *Curr Opin Nephrol Hyperten* 10:785-792, 2001.
2. Levey AS, Bosch JP, Lewis JB, et al: A more accurate method to estimate glomerular filtration rate from serum creatinine: a new prediction equation, *Ann Intern Med* 130:461-470, 1999.

DIAGNOSTIC INFORMATION	REMARKS

See *Glomerular Filtration Rate (measured).*

MDRD equation[2,3]:

$$\text{GFR (mL/min/1.73 m}^2) = 186* \times (P_{cr})^{-1.154} \times (\text{Age})^{-0.203} \times (0.742 \text{ if female}) \times (1.210 \text{ if African American})$$

where:

GFR = glomerular filtration rate

P_{cr} *= serum or plasma creatinine in mg/dL*

Age = age in years

The National Kidney Disease Education Program (NKDEP)[3,4] recommends the use of the MDRD equation to estimate or predict GFR from serum creatinine in adults with chronic kidney disease (CKD) and those at risk for CKD (diabetes, hypertension, and family history of kidney failure) and advocate routine reporting by laboratories of GFR estimates with serum creatinine.

The primary reasons for these recommendations are:
- GFR and creatinine clearance are poorly inferred from the serum creatinine alone because they are related inversely (nonlinearly) to serum creatinine and the effects of age, sex, and race on creatinine production complicate interpretation;
- Creatinine is more often measured than urinary albumin in practice;
- Measurement of kidney function (GFR or creatinine clearance) is essential once albuminuria is discovered;
- The MDRD equation is the most thoroughly validated equation and is superior to other methods of approximating GFR such as the Cockroft-Gault equation and even 24-hr urine collections;
- Nephrologists routinely use an equation to estimate GFR because the laboratory reference limits for serum creatinine are crude; and
- The MDRD equation does not require weight as a variable and yields an estimated GFR normalized to 1.73 m^2 body surface area.

The MDRD equation is most accurate for GFRs ≤ 60 mL/min/1.73 m^2. It is recommended that values >60 mL/min/1.73 m^2 be reported as "greater than 60."

*For laboratories who have creatinine concentrations calibrated to the NIST standard or traceable to isotope dilation mass spectrometry, use a coeffcient of 175 instead of 186.

3. National Kidney Disease Education Program.: *Steps to routine laboratory of estimates GFR,* Available at: http://www.nkdep.nih.gov. Calculators for estimating GFR in adults using the WORD equation are available at: http://www.nkdep.gov/professionals/gfr_calculators/index.htm. A calculator for estimating GFR in children using the Schwartz equation is available at: http://www.nkdep.gov/professionals/gfr_calculators/gfr_children.htm. Last accessed 3/1/06.

4. Levey AS, Coresh J, Balk E, et al: National Kidney Foundation practice guidelines for chronic kidney disease: evaluation, classification and stratification, *Ann Intern Med* 139:137-147, 2003.

TEST NAME AND METHOD	SPECIMEN REQUIREMENTS	REFERENCE INTERVAL, CONVENTIONAL [INTERNATIONAL RECOMMENDED UNITS]	CHEMICAL INTERFERENCES AND IN VIVO EFFECTS
Glomerular Filtration Rate, Measured (GFR)[1-6]		Average normal (after 2 yr): 130 mL/min/1.73 m² [× 0.00963 = 1.25 mL/sec/m²] Newborn: 70-80% less than above value	↑ V Amino acids, carbon monoxide, clonidine, diltiazem (IV), glucocorticoids
Inulin clearance	See *Inulin Clearance (Exogenous).*	For age-related changes, see *Inulin Clearance* and *Creatinine Clearance.*	↓ V Cortisone, diazoxide, diuretics (e.g., furosemide, thiazides, tri-
Creatinine clearance	See *Creatinine Clearance (Endogenous).*		amterene), enalapril; epinephrine and levarterenol both have a slight effect;
51Chromium edetic acid (radioisotope test)[7] Dose: IV injection 0.5-1.0 MCi51Cr-EDTA/kg in 10 mL of 5% dextrose	Plasma. Draw at 2 and 4 hr.		ganglionic blocking agents, histamine, isoproterenol, lisinopril, nephrotoxic drugs (Table II-6), oxprenolol, propranolol, somatostatin

1. Eastham RD: *Biochemical values in clinical medicine,* ed 7, Bristol, UK, 1985, John Wright and Sons, Ltd.
2. Friedman RB, Anderson RE, Entine SM, et al: Effects of diseases on clinical laboratory tests, *Clin Chem* 26:(suppl), 1980.
3. Henry JB, editor: *Clinical diagnosis and management by laboratory methods,* ed 18, Philadelphia, 1991, WB Saunders.
4. Tietz NW, editor: *Fundamentals of clinical chemistry,* ed 3, Philadelphia, 1987, WB Saunders.
5. Wallach J, editor: *Interpretation of diagnostic tests,* ed 5, Boston, 1992, Little, Brown and Co.
6. Hagstam K, Nordenfelt I, Svensson L, et al: Comparison of different methods for determination of glomerular filtration rate in renal disease, *Scand J Clin Lab Invest* 34:31-36, 1974.
7. Chantler C, Barratt TML: Estimation of glomerular filtration rate from plasma clearance of 51 chromium editic acid, *Arch Dis Child* 47:613-617, 1972.
8. Brown SS, Mitchell FL, Young DS, editors: *Chemical diagnosis of disease,* Amsterdam, 1979, Elsevier/North Holland Biomedical Press.

Glucagon[1-5] *RIA*	Plasma (EDTA); freeze. Stable for up to 74 days at −20° C.	Cord: 1-3 days: 4-14 yr: Adult:	*pg/mL*[7] 0-215 (x̄: 83) 0-1750 (x̄: 270) 0-148 (x̄: 70) 20-100	× 1.0	*ng/L* [0-215] [x̄: 83] [0-1750] [x̄: 270] [0-148] [x̄: 70] [20-100]	↑ V Amino acids (e.g., arginine), cholecystokinin-pancreozymin, danazol, gastrin, glucocorticoids, insulin, nifedipine, sympathomimetic amines ↓ V Atenolol, pindolol, propranolol, secretin

↑ High cardiac output, pregnancy, burns, carbon monoxide toxicity, high-protein diet, hypercatabolic states, anemia

↓ *Decreased renal blood flow:* shock, hemorrhage, dehydration, congestive heart failure; intrinsic renal disease, glomerulonephritis, nephrotic syndrome, pyelonephritis, amyloidosis, acute tubular dysfunction, interstitial nephritis, papillary necrosis, postrenal obstruction to urinary flow; also decreased in malaria, multiple myeloma, adrenocortical hypofunction, cystinosis, hepatolenticular degeneration, vitamin D–resistant rickets, chronic obstructive lung disease, hepatic failure, eclampsia, and preeclampsia.

Inulin clearance is the best test for GFR, but no routine methods are available. Proteinuria and advanced renal failure make creatinine clearance an unreliable method for measuring GFR. When serum creatinine concentrations are elevated, tubular secretion results in overestimation of GFR by the creatinine clearance test. Urea clearance is a measure of total renal function and not a sensitive measure of GFR. It is greatly affected by urinary flow rate.[51]Cr-EDTA shows excellent agreement with inulin clearance and requires no urine collection. Tests on edematous patients may require extra blood samples when GFR is measured by isotope tests.[8] The[51]Cr-EDTA method is suitable for measuring GFR of infants with obstructive uropathy.[7]

GFR can also be reliably estimated from the serum creatinine, age, sex, and race using the MDRD equation. The National Kidney Disease Education Program recommends this approach for adults with kidney disease or at risk for kidney disease. (See *Glomerular Filtration Rate, Estimated.*)

↑ *Glucagonoma:* 900-7800 pg/mL [900-7800 ng/L]

Diabetes mellitus: Mean levels 1525 ± 578 pg/mL [1525 ± 578 ng/L]; true pancreatic glucagon levels predominantly increased.

Chronic renal failure: Mean basal levels 540 ± 40 pg/mL [540 ± 40 ng/L]; predominant elevation in proglucagon

Hyperlipoproteinemia, types III and IV

The amount of pancreatic glucagon found in plasma will depend on specificity of the antiserum used.

Some investigators prefer to collect blood samples in prechilled tubes containing EDTA and a proteinase inhibitor such as Trasylol to prevent possible loss of immunoreactivity.

Glucagon is a polypeptide hormone secreted by the islet α-cells in the pancreas; it stimulates the production of glucose in the liver and the oxidation of fatty acids. Glucagon secretion is stimulated by low levels of plasma glucose.

TEST NAME AND METHOD	SPECIMEN REQUIREMENTS	REFERENCE INTERVAL, CONVENTIONAL [INTERNATIONAL RECOMMENDED UNITS]	CHEMICAL INTERFERENCES AND IN VIVO EFFECTS
Glucagon—CONT			*Familial hyperglucagonemia* (predominant elevation in proglucagon) *Others:* acromegaly, cirrhosis, Cushing's syndrome, severe pancreatitis ↓ Cystic fibrosis, chronic pancreatitis, postpancreatectomy Glucagon deficiency may reflect a general loss of pancreatic tissue caused by inflammatory disease, neoplastic replacement of the pancreas, or its surgical removal.

DIAGNOSTIC INFORMATION	REMARKS

Severe stress, including infections, trauma, burns, surgery, acute hypoglycemia

Glucagon-like polypeptides of varying molecular weights are also found in stomach and intestinal tissues. Glucagon-like peptide-1 (7-36) is secreted into the circulation after a glucose load and is highly insulinotropic. Insulin-like effects of this peptide have also been reported.[4,5]

Plasma pancreatic glucagon is heterogeneous and consists of four fractions: true pancreatic glucagon (MW 3500), proglucagon (MW 9000), small glucagon (MW 2000), and big plasma glucagon (MW 160,000). The latter may represent binding of the 3500-MW glucagon to plasma protein. This 3500-MW fraction is considered to be the biologically active hormone.

Measuring glucagon after ethanol extraction eliminates interference from big plasma glucagon (BPG).

Empirically, glucagon and glucagon-like polypeptides are classified based on their reactivity toward antibodies of known regional specificity. True pancreatic glucagons and other polypeptides that react with C-terminal antibodies are termed *immunoreactive glucagons,* or IRG; glucagon-like polypeptides that react only with N-terminal-specific antibodies are termed *glucagon-like immunoreactivity,* or GLI.[8] Although it is probably an oversimplification, IRG is often associated with the pancreas and GLI with the gut. In healthy individuals, ~40-50% of circulating IRG is biologically active (3500-MW fraction). Most of the remainder consists of big glucagons.

In glucagons deficiency there is a failure of plasma glucagons to increase during arginine infusion. In contrast to normals, glucagon secretion in diabetic patients does not decrease after ingestion of a carbohydrate meal, whereas arginine infusion causes significantly greater increase of glucagon secretion. (See *Glucagon Stimulation Test [after Arginine]* and *Glucagon Suppression Test [after Glucose Load].)* Abnormally elevated fasting levels of glucagons in patients with chronic renal failure return to normal after successful renal transplantation. Renal rejection has resulted in a dramatic increase in plasma glucagons several days before changed in blood creatinine levels. Fasting and moderate or severe exercise cause a glucagon release, and this may play an important part in neonatal hypoglycemia in these babies.

Hypoglycemic stimulation of glucagon release is lost in insulin-dependent diabetes.

In gastrectomized subjects, oral loads of glucose, galactose, and fructose all produce significant increases in plasma glucagons; glucose has the greatest effect, and fructose has the least. See *Glucagon Suppression Test (after Glucose Load).*

TEST NAME AND METHOD	SPECIMEN REQUIREMENTS	REFERENCE INTERVAL, CONVENTIONAL [INTERNATIONAL RECOMMENDED UNITS]	CHEMICAL INTERFERENCES AND IN VIVO EFFECTS

Glucagon—CONT

Amniotic fluid[6]

	pg/mL (SEM)		ng/L
Midgestation:	43 ± 10	× 1.0	[43 ± 10]
Term:	117 ± 38		[117 ± 38]

1. Eastham RD: *Biochemical values in clinical medicine,* ed 7, Bristol, UK, 1985, John Wright and Sons Ltd.
2. Buchanan KD: The gastrointestinal hormones: general concepts, *Clin Endocrinol Metab* 8:249-263, 1979.
3. Hendriks T, Benraad TJ: On the stability of immunoreactive glucagon in plasma samples, *Diabelologia* 20:553-557, 1981.
4. Kreymann B, Ghatei M, Williams G, et al: Glucagon-like peptide-1 7-36: a physiological incretion in man, *Lancet* 2:1300-1304, 1987.
5. Orskov C: Glucagon-like peptide-1, a new hormone of the entero-insular axis, *Diabetologia* 35:701-711, 1992.
6. Tulchinsky D, Ryan KJ, editors: *Maternal-fetal endocrinology,* Philadelphia, 1980, WB Saunders.
7. Nichols Institute Reference Laboratories: *Test catalog,* San Juan Capistrano, CA, 1993, Nichols Institute Reference Laboratories.
8. Orskov C, Holst J: Radioimmunoassays for glucagon-like peptides 1 and 2 (GLP-1 and GLP-2), *Scand J Clin Lab Invest* 47:165-174, 1987.

TEST NAME AND METHOD	SPECIMEN REQUIREMENTS	REFERENCE INTERVAL, CONVENTIONAL [INTERNATIONAL RECOMMENDED UNITS]	CHEMICAL INTERFERENCES AND IN VIVO EFFECTS
Glucagon Stimulation Test (after Arginine)[1] Dose: After overnight fast, IV infusion of 0.5 g arginine/kg (but not >30 g) over 30 min	Plasma (EDTA), fasting. Draw at 15, 30, 45, and 60 min from a venous line maintained with a slow saline drip.	Peak glucagons concentration, at 30 min: 100-1500 pg/mL × 1.0 [100-1500 ng/L]	↑ V Clofibrate See *Glucagon.*

1. Alsever RN, Gotlin RW: *Handbook of endocrine tests in adults and children,* ed 2, Chicago, 1978, Year Book Medical Publishers Inc.

TEST NAME AND METHOD	SPECIMEN REQUIREMENTS	REFERENCE INTERVAL, CONVENTIONAL [INTERNATIONAL RECOMMENDED UNITS]				CHEMICAL INTERFERENCES AND IN VIVO EFFECTS
Glucose[1-13] *Hexokinase* ―――――― *Glucose oxidase/oxygen consumption* ―――――― *Glucose oxidase/hydrogen peroxide (Trinder)*	Serum. Separate from cells rapidly to avoid loss. Stable for 8 hr at 25° C, 72 hr at 4° C. Plasma. Preserve with sodium fluoride or iodoacetate. Stable for 24 hr at room temperature.		*mg/dL*		*mmol/L*	S ↑ V ACTH, asparaginase, β-adrenergic agonists (e.g., albuterol, isoproterenol, terbutaline), caffeine, calcitonin (salmon), corticosteroids, diazoxide, diuretics (acetazolamide, chlorthalidone, ethacrynic acid, furosemide, thiazides, triamterine), dopamine, epinephrine,
		Cord:	45-96	× 0.0555	[2.5-5.3]	
		Premature:	20-60		[1.1-3.3]	
		Neonate:	30-60		[1.7-3.3]	
		Newborn				
		1 day:	40-60		[2.2-3.3]	
		>1 day:	50-80		[2.8-4.4]	
		Child:	60-100		[3.3-5.6]	
		Adult[19]:	74-106		[4.1-5.9]	
		60-90 yr:	82-115		[4.6-6.4]	
		>90 yr:	75-121		[4.2-6.7]	

DIAGNOSTIC INFORMATION	REMARKS
	The source of amniotic fluid glucagon (predominantly big glucagon) is unknown.
Exaggerated response in diabetes, chronic renal failure, and liver failure.	Arginine also stimulates insulin secretion. The failure of glucagons to increase after arginine stimulation is seen in glucagon deficiencies such as cystic fibrosis and chronic pancreatitis. This test is of rare clinical utility.

S ↑ *Primary:* Diabetes mellitus (adult and juvenile)

Physiological: Strenuous exercise, strong emotion, increased epinenphrine from injection, shock, burns; infection (?)

Endocrine disorders: Pheochromocytoma, thyrotoxicosis, acromegaly, gigantism, Cushing's syndrome, glucagonoma, somatostatinoma

Pancreatic disease: Acute and chronic pancreatitis; pancreatitis resulting from mumps, cystic fibrosis, hemochromatosis; neoplasms of pancreas

Glucose can be measured in whole blood, serum, or plasma, but plasma is recommended for diagnosis of diabetes mellitus. Furthermore, it is the WHO/ADA criteria and not reference ranges that are used for diagnosis of diabetes mellitus.

Concentration of glucose is higher in arterial than in venous samples. For fasting samples, a 6- to 8-hr fast is required.

The enzymatic hexokinase method is the basis for the reference method for the determination of glucose in serum or plasma.

TEST NAME AND METHOD	SPECIMEN REQUIREMENTS	REFERENCE INTERVAL, CONVENTIONAL [INTERNATIONAL RECOMMENDED UNITS]	CHEMICAL INTERFERENCES AND IN VIVO EFFECTS
Glucose—CONT			
	If sodium fluoride is used as a preservative, a decrease of 9 mg/dL [0.5 mmol/L] is seen during the first 2 hr. Stable after 2 hr.	Glucose oxidase/oxygen consumption values are slightly lower. *WHO/ADA criteria for diagnosis of diabetes mellitus* Fasting: ≥126 mg/dL (7.0 mmol/L) 2-hr post–glucose load ≥200 mg/dL (11.1 mmol/L)	estrogens, fructose, glucagon, indomethacin, lithium carbonate, morphine, nicotinic acid (large doses), octreotide (somatostatin), oral contraceptives, phenothiazines, phenytoin, rifampin, streptozotocin, theophylline, thiabendazole, D-thyroxine
Glucose oxidase, potentiometric or amperometric[14]	Whole blood. Preserve with sodium fluoride if not analyzed immediately; otherwise, anticoagulate with heparin.	Whole blood glucose levels are 90% of plasma glucose.[14]	
Spectrophotometric	Whole blood.	65-95 mg/dL ×0.0555 [3.5-5.3 mmol/L]	S ↑ C *Beckman (glucose oxidase):* 2-Deoxyglucose, hydroxyethyl starch

S ↓ V Acetaminophen (toxic dose), β-adrenergic blockers (see *Remarks*), anabolic steroids (effect in diabetics), antihistamines, aspirin (toxic doses), bezafibrate, captopril, cyproterone, disopyramide, ethanol, fenfluramine (diabetics), guanethidine analogs, indomethacin (variable effects), marijuana, MAO inhibitors, nifedipine (inconclusive), pentamidine (after several days), pivampicillin, protionamide, spironolactone, tromethamine

S ↓ C *Glucose oxidase peroxidase:* Acetaminophen, levodopa

Trinder's glucose oxidase: Substances oxidized by hydrogen peroxide (e.g., ascorbate, bilirubin, and uric acid)

Hexokinase: Glucose-1-phosphate, fructose-6-phosphate, glutathione (NADP$^+$ yeast G6PD direct method) |

Related to other disorders: Cerebrovascular accident, acute myocardial infarction or severe angina, chronic liver disease, chronic renal disease

Related to insulin receptor antibodies: Acanthosis nigricans

Vitamin B₁ deficiency: Wernicke's encephalopathy

S ↓ *Pancreatic disorders:* Islet cell tumor, glucagon deficiency

Tumors: Carcinoma of adrenal gland, carcinoma of stomach, fibrosarcoma

Severe hepatic disorders: Poisoning (e.g., arsenic, carbon tetrachloride, chloroform, cinchophen, phosphorus, alcohol, salicylates, phenformin, antihistamines)

Endocrine disorders: Hypopituitarism, Addison's disease, hypothyroidism

Functional disorders: Postgastrectomy, gastroenterostomy, autonomic nervous system disorders

Pediatric anomalies: Prematurity, infant of diabetic mother, ketotic hypoglycemia, Zetterstrom's syndrome, idiopathic leucine sensitivity

Enzyme deficiency diseases: von Gierke's syndrome, galactosemia, maple syrup urine disease, fructose intolerance.

The glucose oxidase/oxygen consumption method correlates best with reference methodology. It has high precision and accuracy.

There are many variations of the glucose oxidase/hydrogen peroxide procedure, some of which employ an indicator dye to measure the production of hydrogen peroxide. These dyes may be subject to oxidation and cause a positive bias. Thus it is important to recognize that different methods within this method classification may produce significantly different results.

Nonselective β-blockers (e.g., propranolol) impair glycogenolysis and the hyperglycemic response to endogenous epinephrine. Hypoglycemia may persist or recovery be delayed particularly in diabetic patients. The release of insulin in response to hyperglycemia is decreased, particularly with nonselective agents.

TEST NAME AND METHOD	SPECIMEN REQUIREMENTS	REFERENCE INTERVAL, CONVENTIONAL [INTERNATIONAL RECOMMENDED UNITS]				CHEMICAL INTERFERENCES AND IN VIVO EFFECTS

Glucose—CONT

						↑ C Other hexoses, especially mannose and galactose; high levels of urea
Reagent strips (Miles Inc. Dextrostix, Glucostix, Wisidex II; Roche Chemstrip BG)[15,16]	Whole blood. Avoid fluoride preservative.		*mg/dL*		*mmol/L*	B ↓ C Acetaminophen, ascorbic acid, salicylic acid, sodium fluoride, bilirubin, uric acid
		Fasting:	<100	× 0.0555	[<5.6]	
		2-hr OGTT:				
		Venous:	<120		[<6.7]	
		Capillary:	<140		[<7.8]	
One Touch, Accuchek (glucose oxidase-peroxidase–based dry reagent reflectometry)		Fasting	60-130		[3.3-7.2]	
Electrochemistry (sensor electrodes) (e.g., Abbott, Roche, Bayer)						
Noninvasive or minimally invasive glucose analyses,[17] Glucose Watch Biographer (Cygnus); Continuous Glucose Monitoring System (MiniMed)		Glucose levels variable.				

Quantitative (Hexokinase, O_2 consumption)	Urine. Collect in dark bottle; keep on ice. Preserve 24-hr sample with 5 mL of glacial acetic acid or 5 g of sodium benzoate or sodium fluoride. Analyze at room temperature.	<0.5 g/day		× 5.55	[<2.78 mmol/day]	U ↑ V Carbamazepine, corticosteroids, D-thyroxine, diuretics (e.g., acetazolamide, chlorthalidone, ethacrynic acid, furosemide, thiazides), EDTA, lithium carbonate, nicotinic acid
		1-15 mg/dL		× 0.0555	[0.1-0.8 mmol/L]	
		Random urine[20]:				
			mg/dL		*mmol/L*	
		M:	1-42	× 0.0555	[0.055-2.33]	
		F:	0-33		[0-18.3]	
			mg/g creatinine		*mmol/g creatinine*	
		<40 yr				
		M:	3-181	× 0.00555	[0.017-1.00]	
		F:	5-203		[0.028-1.13]	
		≥40 yr				
		M:	19-339		[0.10-1.89]	
		F:	8-331		[0.044-1.84]	

DIAGNOSTIC INFORMATION	REMARKS

Hematocrit >55% causes decreased result. Hematocrit <35% causes increased result. Dextrostix and Glucostix may be read visually.

Accuracy of some of the reagent strip tests is greatly increased if strips are read in specially designed meters.

The performances of semiquantitative glucose systems have been compared by Jacobs et al.[21] These authors recommend that a conventional test be used to validate blood glucose levels when handheld units provide glucose values >500 mg/dL or when hematocrit values are >55%.

Useful in detecting unsuspected hypoglycemia. Continuous monitoring up to 72 hr or frequent measurement up to 12 hr. Calibration with reference plasma glucose value is required.

U ↑ Any cause of increased blood glucose, especially rapid intestinal absorption (postgastrectomy dumping, normal pregnancy) and endocrine disorders (diabetes mellitus, thyrotoxicosis, gigantism, acromegaly, Cushing's syndrome, adrenocortical hyperplasia); major trauma, stroke, MI or circulatory collapse, oral steroid therapy, burns, infection, pheochromocytoma.[9]

Decreased renal threshold: Tubulointerstitial diseases, phenothiazines, lead poisoning in infants and children.

U ↑ C Hydrogen peroxide, hypochlorite (bleach) or detergents used to wash containers.

Reagent strip tests may show false-negative results with decreased urine pH and increased ketones and salt concentrations. Diabetic patients may have increased renal threshold (glucose >250 mg/dL; >13.9 mmol/L).[6]

Reactivity of Clinistix, Diastix, and Multistix: High specific gravity depresses color development, whereas low specific gravity intensifies it.[18,19,23]

Chemstrip allows quantitation of glucose in a range of 60 mg/dL to 5 g/dL [3.3-278 mmol/L]; Chemstrip multistrip detects glucose levels of 40 mg/dL [2.2 mmol/L]; the Diastix, Multistix lower limit of detection is 75-125 mg/dL [4.2-6.9 mmol/L] glucose.

TEST NAME AND METHOD	SPECIMEN REQUIREMENTS	REFERENCE INTERVAL, CONVENTIONAL [INTERNATIONAL RECOMMENDED UNITS]			CHEMICAL INTERFERENCES AND IN VIVO EFFECTS

Glucose—CONT

Qualitative: *Reagent strips* *(Miles Inc. Clini-* *stix; Lilly Tes-* *Tape)*[18]	Random sample. Ana- lyze immediately or store at 2-4° C. Analyze at room temperature.	Negative			

Semiquantitative: *Reagent strips* *(Miles Inc. Multi-* *stix, Diastix, Lab-* *stix, Combistix,* *Uristix,* *Ketodiastix*[19]*;* *Roche Chem-* *Strip*[18]*)*		Negative			

			mg/dL		*mmol/L*
Enzymatic	CSF. Process immedi- ately to avoid falsely low results. Store at −20° C.	Infant, child: Adult:	60-80 40-70	× 0.0555	[3.3-4.4] [2.2-3.9]

1. Boehringer Mannheim Corp: *Chemstrip 10 UA package insert,* Indianapolis, IN, 1992, Boehringer Mannheim Corp.
2. Boehringer Mannheim Corp: *Urinalysis today,* Indianapolis, IN, 1991, Boehringer Mannheim Corp.
3. Burtis CA, Ashwood ER, editors: *Tietz textbook of clinical chemistry,* ed 2, Philadelphia, 1994, WB Saunders.
4. Eastham RD: *Biochemical values in clinical medicine,* ed 7, Bristol, UK, 1985, John Wright and Sons Ltd.
5. Free HM, editor: *Modern urine chemistry,* Elkhart, IN, 1991, Miles Inc., Diagnostics Division.
6. Henry JB, editor: *Clinical diagnosis and management by laboratory methods,* ed 18, Philadelphia, 1991, WB Saunders.
7. Kaplan LA, Pesce AJ, editors: *Clinical chemistry: theory, analysis and correlation,* ed 2, St. Louis, 1989, CV Mosby.
8. Miles Inc., Diagnostics Division: *Multistix package insert,* Elkhart, IN, 1992, Miles Inc., Diagnostics Division.
9. Newall RG, editor: *Clinical urinalysis,* Buckinghamshire, UK, 1990, Ames Division, Miles Ltd..
10. Pesce A, Kaplan L, editors: *Methods in clinical chemistry,* St. Louis, 1987, CV Mosby.
11. Strasinger SK: *Urinalysis and body fluids: a self-instructional text,* ed 2, Philadelphia, 1991, FA Davis.
12. Tietz NW, editor: *Fundamentals of clinical chemistry,* ed 3, Philadelphia, 1987, WB Saunders.
13. Sacks DB, Bruns DE, Goldstein DE, et al: Guidelines and recommendations for laboratory analysis in the diagnosis and management of diabetes mellitus, *Clin Chem* 48:436-472, 2002.
14. Kost GJ, Wiese DA, Bowen TP: New whole blood methods and instruments: glucose measurements and test menus for critical care, *J Int Fed Clin Chem* 3:160-172, 1991.
15. Ames Division, Miles Laboratories: *Dextrostix package insert,* Elkhart, IN, 1988, Ames Division, Miles Laboratories.

DIAGNOSTIC INFORMATION	REMARKS

U ↓ C Ascorbic acid (at glucose levels[11]), levodopa, mercurial diuretics, tetracycline prepared with ascorbic acid, 5-HIAA, dipyrone.

Prolonged exposure of a urine sample to room temperature may lower glucose results because of glycolysis resulting from microbial contamination.

Specific gravity >1.020 plus increased pH causes reduced sensitivity and falsely low glucose values.

Acidification of urine causes Chemstrip to turn black.[2] Ketones do not interfere with Chemstrip measurement.

In unstable diabetic patients, urine testing may be misleading, and home blood glucose monitoring should be advocated.

False-negative results are associated with use of sodium fluoride as preservative.

CSF ↑ Diabetic hyperglycemia, epidemic encephalitis, CNS syphilis, increased serum glucose.

In pyogenic meningitis, CSF glucose may return to normal rapidly after antibiotic therapy.

CSF ↓ Slight: Subarachnoid hemorrhage, nonbacterial meningoencephalitis

Prolonged exposure of CSF sample to room temperature may lower glucose results because of glycolysis resulting from microbial contamination.

CSF ↓↓ Acute pyogenic meningitis, TB meningitis, cryptococcal meningitis, primary amebic meningoencephalitis, mumps, encephalitis, primary or metastatic tumor of meninges, sarcoidosis.

16. Ames Division, Miles Laboratories: *Glucostix package insert,* Elkhart, IN, 1987, Ames Division, Miles Laboratories.

17. Khalil OS: Spectroscopic and clinical aspects of noninvasive glucose measurements, *Clin Chem* 45:165-177, 1999.

18. Boehringer Mannheim Corp: *Urinalysis today,* Indianapolis, IN, 1986, Boehringer Mannheim Corp.

19. Tietz NW, Shuey DF, Wekstcin DR: Laboratory values in fit aging individuals—sexagenarians through centenarians, *Clin Chem* 38:1167-1185, 1992.

20. Bond LW, Garber C, Ottinger W, et al: Reference intervals for common analytes in random urine specimens, *Clin Chem* 55:submitted, 2005.

21. Jacobs E, Vadasdi E, Roman S, et al: The influence of hematocrit, uremia, and hemodialysis on whole blood glucose analysis, *Lab Med* 24:295-300, 1993.

22. Ames Division, Miles Laboratories: *Factors Affecting Urine Chemistry Tests.* Elkhart, IN, 1986.

TEST NAME AND METHOD	SPECIMEN REQUIREMENTS	REFERENCE INTERVAL, CONVENTIONAL [INTERNATIONAL RECOMMENDED UNITS]	CHEMICAL INTERFERENCES AND IN VIVO EFFECTS
Glucose, 2-hr Postprandial[1-3] *Enzymatic* Patient consumes a breakfast, lunch, or glucose solution (75 g) and remains at rest during the following 2 hr.	Serum, 2 hr after meal. For preparation of patient, see *Glucose Tolerance Test, Oral.*	<140 mg/dL[3]　　$\times$ 0.0555　　[<7.8 mmol/L]	See *Glucose* and *Glucose Tolerance Test, Oral.*

1. Sacks DB, Bruns DE, Goldstein DE, et al: Guidelines and recommendations for laboratory analysis in the diagnosis and management of diabetes mellitus, *Clin Chem* 48:436-472, 2002.
2. Alsever RN, Gotlin RW: *Handbook of endocrine tests in adults and children,* ed 2, Chicago, 1978, Year Book Medical Publishers Inc.
3. Burtis CA, Ashwood ER, editors: *Tietz textbook of clinical chemistry,* ed 2, Philadelphia, 1994, WB Saunders.

TEST NAME AND METHOD	SPECIMEN REQUIREMENTS	REFERENCE INTERVAL, CONVENTIONAL [INTERNATIONAL RECOMMENDED UNITS]	CHEMICAL INTERFERENCES AND IN VIVO EFFECTS
Glucose Tolerance Test, Intravenous (IV GTT)[1-6] For 3 days before test, patient should maintain a diet containing at least 150 g of carbohydrate/day, followed by an overnight fast (> 10 hr). Dose: 0.5 g glucose/kg given as 25 g/100 mL solution, IV, within 1-2 min	Serum or plasma. Fasting, 3, 5, 10, 20, 30, 45, and 60 min after the end of infusion for glucose. For plasma insulin (if desired), collect blood at 2, 3, and 5 min.	Newborn: Normal glucose disappearance rate is less than that in older infants and adults. Plasma insulin response on first day is characterized by a small spike and large wave. Adult: K_t^* $>1.5\%$/min [>0.015, fraction/min]; K_t declines by $\sim0.09\%$/min/decade [0.0009/min/decade] over 50 yr. Shortly after infusion, glucose concentration of 250 mg/dL [13.9 mmol/L] may be seen. Fasting level is regained by 90 min, subfasting level by 2 hr, returning to fasting level by 3 hr. Some glycosuria is expected because of blood glucose concentrations above the renal threshold. Insulin reaches a peak during the first 5 min.[7]	See *Glucose Tolerance Test, Oral;* and *Insulin, Immunoreactive.*

	K_t %/min (SEM)	K_t fraction/min (SEM)
Term infants[7]		
First 6 hr:	$0.80 \pm 0.23 \times 0.01$	[0.008 ± 0.002]
2-5 days:	1.41 ± 0.5	[0.014 ± 0.005]
6 mo-10 yr:	2.8 ± 0.55	[0.028 ± 0.006]
14-16 yr:	1.7 ± 0.3	[0.017 ± 0.003]

*K_t, Mean rate of glucose disappearance.

DIAGNOSTIC INFORMATION	REMARKS

↑ Diabetes mellitus (>200 mg/dL; >11.10 mmol/L)

See also *Glucose Tolerance Test, Oral.*

Individuals with values between 140 mg/dL [7.8 mmol/L] and 200 mg/dL [11.1mmol/L] need to be studied further.

General use of this test is not recommended because of many factors that influence the results. For differences in capillary and venous blood, see *Glucose Tolerance Test, Oral.*

K_t <1%/min is considered suggestive of diabetes. Results of the IVGTT often fail to correlate with results of the oral glucose tolerance test. In liver disease the decrease from the peak values is delayed, and fasting levels are regained by 3-5 hr. In Addison's disease and hypopituitarism, the peak levels are normal, but severe hypoglycemia follows. In cases of G6PD deficiency, the oral test is normal, but IV test results are significantly higher. Hyperinsulinemia is characteristic of erythroblastosis and β-cell neoplasia or hyperplasia; the condition is also seen in infants of gestational diabetic patients and those who are small-for-date.

This test is not currently used to diagnose diabetes but is often used in clinical research studies to evaluate first phase insulin release. As the number of β cells decreases, there is a loss of insulin secretion. The Diabetes Prevention Trial type 1[6] found that subjects often had an abnormal IVGTT before onset of diabetes. The most consistent abnormality of diabetic patients appears to be a blunting of the early insulin peak in the first few minutes after IV glucose injection.

Test may be performed to eliminate factors related to rate of glucose absorption from the GI tract. For example, some patients cannot tolerate an oral carbohydrate load; others may have had previous gastric surgery.

No difference is observed in mean rate of glucose disappearance (K_t) whether 0.5 or 1.0 g/kg glucose is given.[7]

Blood glucose levels decrease exponentially. The rate of glucose disappearance *(K)* can be calculated as follows:

$$\frac{70}{K} = t_{1/2}$$

where $t_{1/2}$ is the number of minutes required for the blood glucose to decrease to one half of the 10-min level, and *K* is the rate of disappearance of blood glucose, expressed as %/min.[4]

The presence of insulin antibodies in the plasma may invalidate measurements of plasma insulin by conventional RIA. The preparation of the patient is similar to that described for the OGTT. (See *Glucose Tolerance Test, Oral.*)

TEST NAME AND METHOD	SPECIMEN REQUIREMENTS	REFERENCE INTERVAL, CONVENTIONAL [INTERNATIONAL RECOMMENDED UNITS]	CHEMICAL INTERFERENCES AND IN VIVO EFFECTS

Glucose Tolerance Test, Intravenous—CONT

1. Alsever RN, Gotlin RW: *Handbook of endocrine tests in adults and children,* ed 2, Chicago, 1978, Year Book Medical Publishers Inc.
2. Eastham RD: *Biochemical values in clinical medicine,* ed 7, Bristol, UK, 1985, John Wright and Sons Ltd.
3. Elahi D, Andersen DK, Tobin JD, et al: Discrepant performance on oral and intravenous glucose tolerance tests: the role of gastric inhibitory polypeptide, *J Clin Endocrinol Metab* 52:1199-1203, 1981.
4. Miller RE, Ngai B: *Manual of endocrine diagnostic tests,* ed 4, Lexington, KY, 1991, Department of Medicine, University of Kentucky.

TEST NAME AND METHOD	SPECIMEN REQUIREMENTS	REFERENCE INTERVAL, CONVENTIONAL [INTERNATIONAL RECOMMENDED UNITS]	CHEMICAL INTERFERENCES AND IN VIVO EFFECTS
Glucose Tolerance Test, Oral (OGTT)[1-5] *Hexokinase and glucose oxidase* 3 days before test patient receives diet containing at least 150 g of carbohydrate/day and overnight fast of 8-14 hr Dose, nonpregnant adult: 75 g orally Pregnant female: 100 g orally Child: 1.75 g/kg IBW up to maximum of 75 g	Serum. Nonpregnant adult: draw at fasting and 120 min after glucose administration. Pregnant female: draw at fasting, 60, 120, and 180 min after glucose.	Adult (nonpregnant) or children *mg/dL* / *mmol/L* Fasting: <100 [< 5.6] 120 min: <140 [< 7.8] Adult (pregnant)* *mg/dL* / *mmol/L* Fasting: 95 [5.3] 60 min: 180 [10.0] 120 min: 155 [8.6] 180 min: 140 [7.8] Two or more of the venous plasma concentrations must be met or exceeded for a positive diagnosis of gestational diabetes mellitus (GDM).	A number of drugs affect insulin secretion and action and in the susceptible individual induce glucose intolerance or frank diabetes. Glucocorticoids, β-agonists, growth hormone, and nicotinic acid principally interfere with insulin action. Tacrolimus, β-blockers, diazoxide, and diphenylhydantoin principally affect insulin secretion. Thiazide diuretics, cyclosporine, and atypical antipsychotics (olanzapine, clozapine, quetiapine, and resperidone) affect both insulin secretion and action. Intravenous pentamidine is a β-cell toxin and can induce permanent diabetes.

1. Eastham RD: *Biochemical values in clinical medicine,* ed 7, Bristol, UK, 1985, John Wright and Sons Ltd.
2. American Diabetes Association, Inc.: *The physician's guide to type ii diabetes (NIDDM): diagnosis and treatment,* New York, 1984, American Diabetes Association, Inc.
3. Miller RE, Ngai B: *Manual of endocrine diagnostic tests,* ed 4, Lexington, KY, 1991, Department of Medicine, University of Kentucky.
4. Sacks DB: Carbohydrates. In Burtis CA, Ashwood ER, editors: *Tietz textbook of clinical chemistry,* ed 2, Philadelphia, 1994, WB Saunders.
5. Genuth S, Alberti KG, Bennett P, et al: Follow-up report on the diagnosis of diabetes mellitus, *Diabetes Care* 26:3160-3167, 2003.
6. National Diabetes Data Group: Classification and diagnosis of diabetes mellitus and other categories of glucose intolerance, *Diabetes* 28:1039-1057, 1979.

5. Sacks DB: Carbohydrates. In Burtis CA, Ashwood ER, editors: *Tietz textbook of clinical chemistry,* ed 2, Philadelphia, 1994, WB Saunders.

6. Diabetes Prevention Trial–Type 1 Diabetes Study Group: Effects of insulin in relatives of patients with type 1 diabetes mellitus, *N Engl J Med* 346:1685-1691, 2002.

7. Johnson TR, Moore WM, Jefferies JE: *Children are different: developmental physiology,* ed 2, Columbus, OH, 1978, Ross Laboratories.

Diabetes mellitus (DM) in nonpregnant adult[6]: The 120-min sample must be ≥200 mg/dL [≥11.1 mmol/L]; 120-min values of 140-199 mg/dL (7.8-11.1 mmol/L) are defined as impaired glucose tolerance (IGT). The test should be confirmed on another day.

Fasting plasma glucose of >126 mg/dL (7.0 mmol/L) after a fast of at least 8 hr on two occasions is diagnostic of diabetes mellitus. Fasting plasma glucose of 100-125 mg/dL (5.6-6.9 mmol/L) is defined as impaired fasting glucose (IFG)

A random plasma glucose of >200 mg/dL (11.1 mmol/L) with symptoms of diabetes is diagnostic. A confirmatory FPG test or OGTT should be completed on a different day if the clinical condition of the patient permits.

Two-step approach to screening for gestational diabetes mellitus. A glucose challenge test: 50 g oral glucose load is administered between 24th and 28th wk gestation without regard to time of day or time of meal. A 1-hr venous plasma glucose of ≥130 mg/dL (7.2 mmol/L) indicates need for a 100-g oral glucose tolerance test.

Patients with IFG and/or IGT are referred to as having "prediabetes" because of their high risk of developing the disease in the future. These patients are also at high risk for cardiovascular disease.

Risk assessment for gestational diabetes mellitus should be undertaken at the first prenatal visit. Women at high risk (obesity, personal history of GDM, glycosuria, strong FH of diabetes) should undergo testing as soon as possible. If negative, then retest at 24-28 wk. Women at average risk should be tested at 24-28 wk of gestation.

For proper interpretation of test results, careful selection and preparation of patient are required. In addition to receiving adequate food intake, the patient must not be stressed (e.g., must have had no recent surgery, infection, or illness), endocrine function should be evaluated (e.g., adrenal, thyroid, and growth hormone), and nonessential medications should be discontinued. An 8- to 14-hr fast is recommended; no coffee or smoking is allowed.

Test should be performed on ambulatory patients. Patient should not be exercising during test. Test should be initiated before 10:00 AM. When capillary blood is used for OGTT, levels may be 20-70 mg/dL [1.1-3.9 mmol/L] higher than those in venous blood.

TEST NAME AND METHOD	SPECIMEN REQUIREMENTS	REFERENCE INTERVAL, CONVENTIONAL [INTERNATIONAL RECOMMENDED UNITS]		CHEMICAL INTERFERENCES AND IN VIVO EFFECTS
Glucose-6-Phosphate Dehydrogenase (G6PD) in Erythrocytes (EC 1.1.1.49)[1-9]	Hemolysate of washed Ercs. Submit whole blood (ACD, EDTA, or heparin). Do not use oxalate or fluoride. Stable >20 days at 4° C, 5 days at 25° C.	*U/g Hb* 12.1 ± 2.09 (SD) *U/10^{12} Ercs* 351 ± 60.6 *U/mL k* 4.11 ± 0.71	× 0.0645* × 10^{-3} × 1.0	*MU/mol Hb* [0.78 ± 0.13] *nU/Erc* [0.35 ± 0.06] *U/L Ercs* [4.11 ± 0.71]

None found.

Bishop, modified (UV), 30° C[10]

3.4-8.0 U/g Hb	× 0.0645*	[0.22-0.52 MU/mol Hb]
98.6-232 U/10^{12} Ercs	× 10^{-3}	[0.10-0.23 nU/Erc]
1.16-2.72 U/mL Ercs	× 1.0	[1.16-2.72 kU/L Ercs]

Newborn: 50% higher

*Conversion factor based on MW of Hb of 64,500.

Zinkham (UV), 30° C[11]

Newborn
7.8-14.4 U/g Hb	× 0.0645*	[0.50-0.93 MU/mol Hb]
226-418 U/10^{12} Ercs	× 10^{-3}	[0.23-0.42 nU/Erc]
2.65-4.90 U/mL Ercs	× 1.0	[2.65-4.90 kU/L Ercs]

Adult
5.5-9.3 U/g Hb	× 0.0645*	[0.35-0.60 MU/mol Hb]
160-270 U/10^{12} Ercs	× 10^{-3}	[0.16-0.27 nU/L Ercs]
1.87-3.16 U/mL Ercs	× 1.0	[1.87-3.16 kU/L Ercs]

See *Acetylcholinesterase.*

*Conversion factor based on MW of Hb of 64,500.

1. Beutler E: *Hemolytic anemia in disorders of red cell metabolism,* New York, 1978, Plenum Pub Co.

2. Miale JB: *Laboratory medicine: hematology,* ed 6, St. Louis, 1982, CV Mosby.

3. Mehta A, Mason PJ, Vulliamy TJ: Glucose-6-phosphate dehydrogenase deficiency, *Baillieres Best Pract Res Clin Haematol* 13:21-38, 2000.

4. Konrad PN, Valentine WN, Paglia DE: Enzymatic activities and glutathione content of erythrocytes in the newborn: comparison with red cells of older normal subjects and those with comparable reticulocytosis, *Acta Haematol* 48:193-201, 1972.

5. Weatherall DJ: ABC of clinical haematology. The hereditary anaemias, *BMJ* 314:492-496, 1197.

6. Simmons A: *Technical hematology,* ed 3, Philadelphia, 1980, JB Lippincott.

7. Miwa S, Fujii H: Molecular basis of erythroenzymopathies associated with hereditary hemolytic anemia: tabulation of mutant enzymes, *Am J Hematol* 51:122-132, 1996.

DIAGNOSTIC INFORMATION   REMARKS

Deficiency causes hemolytic anemia after ingestion of 8-aminoquinoline antimalarials, nalidixic acid, nitrofurantoin, phenacetin, large doses of vitamin C, and some sulfonamides and sulfones.[12] (See Table I-4.) Hemolytic episodes may also occur after exposure to fava beans in diabetic acidosis and in infections. Deficiency may be the cause of hemolytic disease of newborns in Asians and Mediterraneans.

Three G6PD variants are of high frequency and have clinical consequences in different ethnic groups. They are defined by electrophoretic and kinetic criteria as:

G6PD A−: Common in blacks (10% of males). Associated with moderately severe self-limited hemolysis after ingestion of 8-aminoquinolines, such as primaquine, and other drugs.

G6PD Mediterranean: Common particularly in Iraqis, Kurds, Sephardic Jews, and Lebanese; less common in Greeks, Italians, Turks, North Africans, Spaniards, Portuguese, and Ashkenazic Jews; associated with severe and sometimes fatal hemolysis after exposure to fava beans; may also cause hemolytic disease of the newborn (HDN).

G6PD Mahidol: Common in Southeast Asians (22% of males). Associated with hemolysis after ingestion of 8-aminoquinolines, such as chloroquine; also associated with HDN.

Some G6PD variants, such as G6PD A+, have no clinical importance. There are many other common clinically important variants caused by several different mutations.[12]

Activity is higher in young Ercs.[1] Testing of reticulocyte-depleted blood may be necessary after recent hemolysis to detect deficiency. Deficiency is usually difficult to detect in female heterozygotes and immediately after hemolytic episodes in persons with G6PD A−.[13] Heterozygotes for any G6PD-deficiency variants are often impossible to identify except by pedigree analysis.

Mutation analysis is available to diagnose variation in G6PD.

U/g Hb × 29 = U/10^{12} Ercs
U/g Hb × 0.34 = U/mL Ercs*

*See Note, *Acetylcholinesterase.*

8. Wilkinson JH: *The principles and practice of diagnostic enzymology,* Chicago, 1976, Year Book Medical Publishers, Inc.
9. Wolf PL: *Practical clinical hematology: interpretations and techniques,* New York, 1973, John Wiley and Sons.
10. Tietz NW, editor: *Fundamentals of clinical chemistry,* ed 5, Philadelphia, 2001, WB Saunders.
11. Zinkham WH: An in-vitro abnormality of glutathione metabolism in erythrocytes from normal newborns: mechanism and clinical significance, *Pediatrics* 23:18-32, 1959.
12. Beutler E: G6PD: population genetics and clinical manifestations, *Blood Rev* 10:45-52, 1996.

TEST NAME AND METHOD	SPECIMEN REQUIREMENTS	REFERENCE INTERVAL, CONVENTIONAL [INTERNATIONAL RECOMMENDED UNITS]		CHEMICAL INTERFERENCES AND IN VIVO EFFECTS
Glucosephosphate Isomerase (GPI, Phosphohexose Isomerase, PHI) in Erythrocytes (EC 5.3.1.9)[1] *ICSH, 37° C*[1]	Hemolysate of washed Ercs. Submit whole blood (ACD, EDTA, or heparin). Stable >20 days at 4° C, >5 days at 25° C.	*U/g Hb* 60.8 ± 11.0 (SD) *U/10^{12} Ercs* 1763 ± 322 *U/mL Ercs* 20.7 ± 3.77	× 0.0645* × 10^{-3} × 1.0	*MU/mol Hb* [3.92 ± 0.72] *nU/Erc* [1.76 ± 0.32] *kU/L Ercs* [20.7 ± 3.77]	None found.

Activity higher in newborns.[2,3]

See *Acetylcholinesterase*.

*Conversion factor based on MW of Hb of 64,500.

1. Beutler E: *Red cell metabolism: a manual of biochemical methods,* ed 4, New York, 1986, Grune & Stratton.
2. Williams JJ, Beutler E, Ersley JJ, et al, editors: *Manual of hematology,* ed 6, New York, 2003, McGraw-Hill Publishing Co.
3. Konrad PN, Valentine WN, Paglia DE: Enzymatic activities and glutathione content of erythrocytes in the newborn: comparison with red cells of older normal subjects and those with comparable reticulocytosis, *Acta Haematol* 48:193-201, 1972.

TEST NAME AND METHOD	SPECIMEN REQUIREMENTS	REFERENCE INTERVAL, CONVENTIONAL [INTERNATIONAL RECOMMENDED UNITS]			CHEMICAL INTERFERENCES AND IN VIVO EFFECTS
α-Glucosidase (α-D-glucoside glucohydrolase; also known as acid maltase. EC 3.2.1.20)[1] *Fluorimetric (4-methyl-umbelliferyl-α-D-glucopyra-noside), 37° C*[2,3]	Amniotic fluid cells (cultured)[2]	*nmol/hr/mg* *Before heating* pH 4: 43-263 pH 4/pH 6: 0.3-2.6 *After heating* pH 4: 38-258 pH 4/pH 6: 2.5-3.7	× 16.67	*mU/g* *Before heating* [717-4384] [5-43] *After heating* [633-4301] [42-62]	None found.
	Fibroblasts from skin (cultured)	*nmol/hr/mg* *Before heating* pH 4: 214-580 pH 4/pH 6: 1.0-3.5 *After heating* pH 4: 120-580 pH 4/pH 6: 2.2-3.5	× 16.67	*mU/g* *Before heating* [3567-9669] [17-58] *After heating* [2000-9669] [37-58]	

Fluorimetric (pyridyl-aminomaltotrisacch-aride with HPLC separation), 37° C[4]

pH 4.5: 152 ± 36 (mean ± SD) nmol/mg protein/hr
[× 16.67 = 253 ± 600 mU/g protein]

DIAGNOSTIC INFORMATION	**REMARKS**

↓ Congenital nonspherocytic hemolytic anemia (autosomal recessive)

Activity is higher in young erythrocytes or reticulocytes.[1] May need to test reticulocyte-depleted blood if there is active hemolysis with increase reticulocytes.

U/g Hb × 29 = U/10^{12} Ercs
U/g Hb × 0.34 = m/L Ercs*

*See Note, *Acetylcholinesterase.*

↓↓ In Pompe's disease (glycogen storage disorder type II), acid form is low or absent. The neutral form (pH 6.0) is increased in a variety of unrelated disorders, but greatest increases occur in acutely ill patients with cystic fibrosis and necrotizing pancreatitis.[3]

α-Glucosidase activity measured at pH 4 increases with age of amniotic cell culture. If time of incubation is short and if the pH 4/pH 6 ratio is used without the thermal treatment, there is a potential for misdiagnosis of an affected fetus as normal.[2,10]

Pompe's disease (type II glycogenosis)[1] is characterized by the accumulation of glycogen in all body tissues as a result of the deficiency of lysosomal acid α-glucosidase. This enzyme has a pH optimum of ~4. An additional form of α-glucosidase not deficient in Pompe's disease shows an optimum of ~pH 6 with overlap at pH 4. Specificity of the pH 4 form is achieved by heat denaturing the pH 6 form, which is more heat labile. Prenatal diagnosis of Pompe's disease is facilitated by the analysis of α-glucosidase in cells cultured from amniotic fluid. Absence of this enzyme has also been demonstrated in heart, skeletal muscle, liver, skin, fibroblasts, urine, and leukocytes of patients with Pompe's disease.

No activity detected in Pompe's disease.

TEST NAME AND METHOD	SPECIMEN REQUIREMENTS	REFERENCE INTERVAL, CONVENTIONAL [INTERNATIONAL RECOMMENDED UNITS]		CHEMICAL INTERFERENCES AND IN VIVO EFFECTS

α-Glucosidase—CONT

Colorimetric (p-nitro-phenyl-α-glucoside with use of immobilized antibodies to liver acid α-glucosidase), 37° C[5]	Urine, fresh. Store at −20° C.	Total α-glucosidase (pH 4): Acid α-glucosidase (pH 4):	*mU/mL* 0.11-3.00 × 1.0 (x̄: 1.49) 0.79-2.73 (x̄: 1.45)	*U/L* [0.11-3.00] [x̄: 1.49] [0.79-2.73] [x̄: 1.45]
Fluorimetric (4-methyl-umbelliferyl-α-D-glucopyrano-side before and after inhibition with antibody to placental acid α-glucosidase), pH 4.0, 37° C[6]		85.9 ± 4.8 (mean ± SD) nmol/hr/mg creatinine		
Colorimetric (p-nitro-phenyl-α-glucopyrano-side), 37° C[7]	Seminal plasma. Use immediately or store at −80° C.	*mAU*/g protein* 467 ± 135 (SD) × 1.0	*µU/g protein* [467 ± 135]	
Fluorimetric (4-methyl-umbelliferyl-α-D-glucopyr-anoside), 37° C[8,9]	Serum. Centrifuge blood at 4° C, then store at −20° C.	Reference range not well established. *AU, pmol/min/mL incubation medium.		

1. Hirschorn R, Reuser AJJ: Glycogen storage disease type II. In Scriver CR, Beaudet AL, Valle D, et al, editors: *The metabolic and molecular bases of inherited disease,* ed 8, New York, 2001, McGraw-Hill Inc.

2. Fujimoto A, Fluharty AL, Stevens RL, et al: Two alpha-glucosidases in cultured amniotic fluid cells and their differentiation in the prenatal diagnosis of Pompe's disease, *Clin Chim Acta* 68:177-186, 1976.

3. Porter WH, Jennings CD, Wilson HD: Measurement of α-glucosidase activity in serum from patients with cystic fibrosis or pancreatitis, *Clin Chem* 32:652-565, 1986.

4. Midorikawa M, Okada S, Kato T, et al: Diagnosis of Pompe's disease using pyridylaminomaltooligosaccharides as substrates of α-14,4-glucosidase, *Clin Chim Acta* 147:97-102, 1985.

5. Schram AW, Brouwer-Kelder B, Donker-Koopman WE, et al: Use of immobilized antibodies in investigating acid a-glucosidase in urine in relation to Pompe's disease, *Biochim Biophys Acta* 567:370-383, 1979.

6. Tsuji A, Yang R-C, Omura K, et al: A simple differential immunoprecipitation of urinary acid and neutral a-glucosidases for glycogenosis II, *Clin Chim Acta* 167:313-320, 1987.

7. Chapdelaine P, Tremblay RR, Dube JY: p-Nitrophenol-α-D-glucopyranoside as substrate for measurement of maltase activity in human semen, *Clin Chem* 24:208-211, 1978.

DIAGNOSTIC INFORMATION	REMARKS

Little or no activity detected in Pompe's disease.

↓ Male infertility disorders (i.e., varicocele, azoospermia) and often vasectomy

↑ Cystic fibrosis, pancreatitis

8. Casola L, DiMatteo G, Romano M, et al: Glycosidases in serum of cystic fibrosis patients, *Clin Chim Acta* 94:83-88, 1979.

9. Hultberg B, Ceder O, Kollberg H: Acid hydrolases in sera and plasma from patients with cystic fibrosis, *Clin Chim Acta* 112:167-175, 1981.

10. Fujimoto A, Fluharty AL: The change in the pH 4 and pH 6 forms of α-glucosidase in cultured amniotic fluid cells and its implication in prenatal diagnosis of Pompe's disease, *Clin Chim Acta* 90:157-161, 1978.

TEST NAME AND METHOD	SPECIMEN REQUIREMENTS	REFERENCE INTERVAL, CONVENTIONAL [INTERNATIONAL RECOMMENDED UNITS]			CHEMICAL INTERFERENCES AND IN VIVO EFFECTS
β-Glucuronidase (EC 3.2.1.31)[1-3] *Colorimetric (4-nitrophenyl-β-D-glucuronide), 405 nm, 37° C*[4]	Serum. Stable at room temperature for 24 hr, at 4° C for 1 wk, and at −70° C for 6 mo.	2.44 ± 0.89 U/L (SD)			S ↑ V Anabolic steroids, androgens, chlorpromazine, estrogens, ethanol (acute alcoholism), oral contraceptives, rifampin S ↓ C Hg^{2+}, Cu^{2+}, Ag^+, Ni^{2+}, Zn^{2+}, Sn^{2+9}
Fluorimetric (4-methyl-umbelliferyl-β-D-glucuronide), 37° C[5]		nmol/hr/mL (SEM) 0-12 yr: 87.6 ± 14.9 12-18 yr: 67.9 ± 4.7 >19 yr: 62.9 ± 6.2	× 0.0167	U/L [1.46 ± 0.25] [1.13 ± 0.08] [1.05 ± 0.10]	
Fluorimetric (4-methyl-umbelliferyl-β-D-glucuronide), 37° C[6]		nmol/hr/mL (SD) Cord M: 195 ± 64 F: 188 ± 67 1-4 yr M: 150 ± 62 F: 130 ± 63 5-9 yr M: 85 ± 36 F: 72 ± 16 10-14 yr M: 57 ± 17 F: 62 ± 19 15-19 yr M: 86 ± 24 F: 96 ± 23 20-24 yr M: 116 ± 33 F: 111 ± 34 25-49 yr M: 116 ± 48 F: 75 ± 25 50-74 yr M: 131 ± 50 F: 110 ± 45	× 0.0167	U/L [3.25 ± 1.07] [3.13 ± 1.12] [2.50 ± 1.03] [2.17 ± 1.05] [1.42 ± 0.60] [1.20 ± 0.27] [0.95 ± 0.28] [1.03 ± 0.32] [1.43 ± 0.40] [1.60 ± 0.38] [1.93 ± 0.55] [1.85 ± 0.57] [1.93 ± 0.80] [1.25 ± 0.42] [2.18 ± 0.83] [1.83 ± 0.75]	
Fluorimetric[7]	Fibroblasts, skin biopsy (4-mm punch)	363 +/− 85 nmol/n/mg protein			
Colorimetric[8]	Spinal fluid. Freeze until analyzed.	Normal: >70 mU/L Interminate: 49-70 Suspicious: <70 mU/L			

DIAGNOSTIC INFORMATION	REMARKS

S ↑ I-Cell disease. Viral or toxic hepatitis with extensive cell necrosis, cirrhosis; malignancies of pancreas, breast, colon, cervix, or liver; pregnancy (3rd trimester); diabetic patients >12 yr (activity of β-glucuronidase in serum correlates with HbA1c)[5]; hypertension

S ↓ Mucopolysaccharidosis VII, severe liver failure, Marfan's syndrome

β-Glucuronidase is a lysosomal hydrolase. Its absence is responsible for mucopolysaccharidosis VII (Sly syndrome)[3] and can be confirmed by measuring the enzyme in leukocytes or cultured fibroblasts. Serum activity tends to increase in deficiencies of other lysosomal hydrolases. It is present in urine and increases nonspecifically in many renal tract disorders. Tissue levels increase in many cancers, giving increased activity in body fluids, e.g., pleural fluid (lung cancer), gastric juice (stomach cancer), and vaginal fluid (cervical cancer).[8]

Detects mucopolysaccharidosis VII. Patients have no or little detectable activity.

Marker of metastatic leptomeningeal carcinoma.

TEST NAME AND METHOD	SPECIMEN REQUIREMENTS	REFERENCE INTERVAL, CONVENTIONAL [INTERNATIONAL RECOMMENDED UNITS]		CHEMICAL INTERFERENCES AND IN VIVO EFFECTS

β-Glucuronidase—CONT

1. Fishman WH, Kato K, Antiss CL, et al: Human serum β-glucuronidase: Its measurement and some of its properties, *Clin Chim Acta* 15:435-447, 1967.

2. Goldbarg JA, Pineda EP, Blanks BM, et al: A method for the colorimetric determination of β-glucuronidase in urine, serum and tissue: assay of enzymatic activity in health and disease, *Gastroenterology* 36:193-201, 1959.

3. Neufeld EF, Muenzer J: The mucopolysaccharidoses. In Scriver CR, Beaudet AL, Valle D, et al, editors: *The metabolic and molecular bases of inherited disease,* ed 8, New York, 2001, McGraw-Hill Inc.

4. Koskinen H, Jarvisalo J, Huuskonen MS, et al: Serum lysosomal enzyme activities in silicosis and asbestosis, *Eur J Resp Dis* 64:182-188, 1983.

5. Merimee TJ, Kennedy AL, Mehl TD, et al: Serum glycosidase activity in diabetes mellitus, *Diabetes* 30:115-118, 1981.

6. Lombardo A, Gor GC, Marchesini S, et al: Influence of age and sex on five human plasma lysosomal enzymes assayed by automated procedures, *Clin Chim Acta* 113:141-152, 1981.

Test Name and Method	Specimen Requirements	Reference Interval	Conventional	[Intl]	Chemical Interferences
Glutamate Dehydrogenase (GLD, GLDH; EC 1.4.1.3)[1]	Serum or plasma (EDTA ~2 mmol/L, citrate ~10 mmol/L, and heparin ~7.5 μmol/L). Stable at 4° C for 48 hr or at −20° C for 2 wk.	*U/L*		*μKat/L*	↑ V Ethanol, oral contraceptives, streptokinase
		<30 days: ≤6.6	× 0.017	[≤0.11]	
		1-6 mo: ≤4.3		[≤0.07]	
		7-12 mo: ≤3.5		[≤0.06]	↑ C ADP
Spectrophotometric, 340 nm, 25° C[1]		1-2 yr: ≤2.8		[≤0.05]	
		2-3 yr: ≤2.6		[≤0.04]	↓ V Elevated thyroxine
		3-15 yr: ≤3.2		[≤0.05]	
		Adult			↓ C Chelating agents and metal ions, lipidemia, increased pyruvate levels
		M: ≤4.0		[≤0.07]	
		F: ≤3.0		[≤0.05]	
Spectrophotometric, 340 nm, 37° C[2,3]		≤7.9[3]		[≤0.13]	
		≤4.0[4]		[≤0.07]	

1. Schmidt ES, Schmidt FW: Glutamate dehydrogenase: biochemical and clinical aspects of an interesting enzyme, *Clin Chim Acta* 43:43-56, 1988.

2. Ellis G, Goldberg DM: Optimal conditions for the kinetic assay of serum glutamate dehydrogenase activity at 37 °C, *Clin Chem* 18:523-527, 1972.

3. Schmidt ES, Schmidt FW: Glutamatedehydrogenase. In Bergmeyer HU, editor: *Methods of enzymatic analysis, vol III,* ed 3, Weinheim, 1983, Verlag Chemie.

4. Ellis G, Goldberg DM, Spooner RJ, et al: Serum enzyme tests in diseases of the liver and biliary tree, *Am J Clin Pathol* 70:248-258, 1978.

5. Salaspuro M: Use of enzymes for the diagnosis of alcohol-related organ damage, *Enzyme* 37:87-107, 1987.

6. Jenkins WJ, Rosalki SB, Foo Y, et al: Serum glutamate dehydrogenase is not a reliable marker of liver cell necrosis in alcoholics, *J Clin Pathol* 35:207-210, 1982.

7. Mills PR, Spooner RJ, Russell RI, et al: Serum glutamate dehydrogenase as a marker of hepatocyte necrosis in alcoholic liver disease, *BMJ* 283:754-755, 1981.

8. Holt JT, Arvan DA, Mayer TK: Masking by enzyme inhibitor of raised serum glutamate dehydrogenase activity in Reye's syndrome, *Lancet* 2:4-7, 1983.

9. Holt JT, Arvan DA, Mayer TK, et al: Glutamate dehydrogenase in Reye's syndrome. Evidence for the presence of an altered enzyme in serum with increased susceptibility to inhibition by GTP, *Biochim Biophys Acta* 749:42-46, 1983.

DIAGNOSTIC INFORMATION	REMARKS

7. Wenger DA, Williams C: Screening for lysosomal disorders. In Hommes FA, editor: *Techniques in diagnostic biochemical genetics,* New York, 1991, Wiley-Liss.

8. Goldberg, D.M., Watts, C., and Hart, D.M.: Evaluation of several enzyme tests in vaginal fluid as aids to the diagnosis of invasive and preinvasive cervical cancer, *Am J Obstet Gynecol* 107: 465-471, 1970.

9. Guilbault GG: *Handbook of enzymatic methods of analysis,* New York, 1976, Marcel Dekker, Inc.

GLD is abnormal in all categories of hepatic and biliary tract diseases.[4,5] Others have shown that GLD activities do not differentiate between patients with and those without alcoholic hepatitis or hepatocyte necrosis.[6,7]

GLD is a mitochondrial enzyme present in highest concentration in liver, where it is found particularly in the central areas of the liver lobule. It is also present in erythrocytes.

Serum GLD is markedly inhibited by guanosine triphosphate in Reye's syndrome so that serum activities are low. Dialysis removes the inhibitor; therefore the ratio of dialyzed to undialyzed activity markedly increases (up to 700-fold). Increase in this ratio is diagnostic for Reye's syndrome.[8,9]

TEST NAME AND METHOD	SPECIMEN REQUIREMENTS	REFERENCE INTERVAL, CONVENTIONAL [INTERNATIONAL RECOMMENDED UNITS]		CHEMICAL INTERFERENCES AND IN VIVO EFFECTS
Glutamic Acid (Glu)[1-5] *Ion-exchange chromatography*	Plasma (heparin) or serum, fasting. Place blood in ice water immediately; separate and freeze within 1 hr of collection. Stable for 1 wk at −20° C; for longer periods deproteinize and store at −70° C.[6,7]	*mg/dL* Premature First 6 wk 1.57-4.05 1 day-1 mo 0.91-9.11 6 mo-3 yr: 0.28-1.47 3-10 yr: 0.34-3.68 6-18 yr: 0.10-0.96 Adult: 0.21-2.82	μ*mol/L* [107-276][10] [62-620][10] [19-100][11] [23-250][12] [7-65][11] [14-192][12]	P ↑ V Testosterone P ↓ V Oral contraceptives
	Urine, 24 hr. Add 10 mL of 6 mol/L HCl at start of collection. (Alternatively, refrigerate specimen during collection.) Store frozen at −20° C.[8]	*mg/day* 10 days-7 wk: 0.3-1.5 × 6.80 Adult: <33.8 *mg/g creatinine* or 4 ± 1 (SD) × 0.77	μ*mol/day*[12] [2-10] [<230] *mmol/mol creatinine* [3.1 ± 0.8]	
	CSF. Collect in sterile tubes; store frozen. Stable at −20° C for 1 wk or at −70° C for 2 mo.[9]	*mg/dL* Neonate: 0.26 ± 0.27 (SEM) 3 mo-2 yr: 0.0068 ± 0.0025 (SD) 2-10 yr: 0.0090 ± 0.0025 Adult: 0.025 ± 0.004	μ*mol/L* ×68.0 [17.7 ± 18.4][9] [0.46 ± 0.17][13] [0.61 ± 0.17][13] [1.7 ± 0.3][12]	

1. Burtis CA, Ashwood ER, Bruce DE, editors: *Tietz textbook of clinical chemistry and molecular diagnostics,* ed 2, Philadelphia, 2005, WB Saunders.

2. Friedman RB, Young DS: *Youngs effects on line,* 2006, American Association for Clinical Chemistry.

3. Scriver CR, Beaudet AL,Valle D, et al, editors: *The metabolic and molecular bases of inherited disease,* ed 8, New York, 2001, McGraw-Hill.

4. Bremer HJ, Duran M, Kamerling JP, et al: *Disturbances of amino acid metabolism: clinical chemistry and diagnosis,* Baltimore, 1981, Urban and Schwarzenburg.

5. Nyhan W, Sakait N: *Diagnostic recognition of genetic disease,* Philadelphia, 1987, Lea & Febiger.

6. Cummings JG: Routine amino acids analysis in the clinical laboratory, *Am Clin Prod Rev* Feb:20-25, 1988.

7. Schaefer A, Piquard F, Haberey P: Plasma amino acids analysis: effects of delayed samples preparation and of storage, *Clin Chim Acta* 164:163-169, 1987.

8. Pesce A, Kaplan L, editors: *Methods in clinical chemistry,* St. Louis, 1987, CV Mosby.

9. Heiblim DI, Evans HE, Glass L, et al: Amino acid concentrations in cerebrospinal fluid, *Arch Neurol* 35:765-768, 1978.

10. Slocum RH, Cummings JG: Amino acid analysis of physiological samples. In *Techniques in human biochemical genetics,* New York, 1991, Wiley-Liss, pp. 83-126.

11. Meites S, editor: *Pediatric clinical chemistry,* ed 3, Washington, DC, 1989, American Association for Clinical Chemistry.

12. Shih V: *Laboratory techniques for the detection of hereditary metabolic disorders,* Boca Raton, FL, 1973, CRC Press.

13. Goldsmith RF, Earl JW, Cunningham AM: Determination of δ-aminobutyric acid and other amino acids in cerebrospinal fluid of pediatric patients by reversed-phase liquid chromatography, *Clin Chem* 33:1736-1740, 1987.

14. Jain KM, Rush BF Jr, Seelig RF, et al: Changes in plasma amino acid profiles following abdominal operations, *Surg Gynecol Obstet* 152:302-306, 1981.

DIAGNOSTIC INFORMATION	REMARKS
P ↑ Malignant neoplasm of pancreas, gout, glutamic acidemia, rheumatoid arthritis	Glutamic acid content of erythrocytes is much higher than that of plasma.
P ↓ Histidinemia, 4 days after abdominal surgery,[14] chronic renal failure	Improper storage of specimens may lead to decomposition of glutamine and formation of high concentrations of glutamic acid. See also Table II-2.
U ↑ Dicarboxylic aminoaciduria	Excretion in newborns is usually low. Aspartic acid is also significantly increased in dicarboxylic aminoaciduria.
CSF ↑ Bacterial meningitis, meningoradiculitis Garin-Bujadoux-Bannwarth, carcinomatous meningitis[15]	Values in children (3 mo-10 yr) were measured using reversed-phase liquid chromatography.

15. Schott KJ, Meier D: Free amino acid pattern of cerebrospinal fluid in meningeal pathology, *Acta Neurol Scand* 75:304-309, 1987.

TEST NAME AND METHOD	SPECIMEN REQUIREMENTS	REFERENCE INTERVAL, CONVENTIONAL [INTERNATIONAL RECOMMENDED UNITS]			CHEMICAL INTERFERENCES AND IN VIVO EFFECTS
Glutamine (Gln)[1-8] *Ion-exchange chromatography*	Plasma (heparin) or serum, fasting. Place blood in ice water immediately; separate and freeze within 1 hr of collection. Stable for 1 wk at $-20°$ C; for longer periods deproteinize and store at $-70°$ C.[9,10]		*mg/dL* Premature 3.62-12.41 1 day-1 mo 5.49-10.35 3 mo-6 yr: 6.93-10.89 $\times$ 68.5 6-18 yr: 5.26-10.80 Adult: 5.78-10.38	$\mu mol/L$[8,13] [248-850] [376-709] [475-746] [360-740] [396-711]	P $\downarrow$ V Asparaginase P $\uparrow$ V Phenobarbital and phenytoin (in children)
	Urine, 24 hr. Add 10 mL of 6 mol/L HCl at start of collection. (Alternatively, refrigerate specimen during collection.) Store frozen at $-20°$ C.[11]		*mg/day* 10 days-7 wk: 12.4-25.8 $\times$ 6.85 3-12 yr: 20.4-113.7 Adult: 43.8-151.8 *mg/g creatinine* or 40 $\pm$ 19 (SD)[13] $\times$ 0.77	$\mu mol/day$ [85-177][14] [140-779][14] [300-1040][15] *mmol/mol creatinine* [30.8 $\pm$ 14.6]	
	CSF. Collect in sterile tubes; store frozen. Stable at $-20°$ C for 1 wk or at $-70°$ C for 2 mo.[12]		*mg/dL* Neonate: 10.34 $\pm$ 3.60 (SEM) $\times$ 68.5 3 mo-2 yr: 7.27 $\pm$ 1.30 (SD) 2-10 yr: 6.76 $\pm$ 1.20 Adult: 8.61 $\pm$ 0.50	$\mu mol/L$ [708 $\pm$ 246][16] [498 $\pm$ 89][12] [463 $\pm$ 82][12] [590 $\pm$ 34][14]	

1. Burtis CA, Ashwood ER, Bruns DE, editors: *Tietz textbook of clinical chemistry and molecular diagnostics,* ed 4, Philadelphia, 2005, WB Saunders.

2. Friedman RB, Young DS: *Youngs effects on line,* 2006, American Association for Clinical Chemistry.

3. Jacobs DS, Kasten BL Jr, DeMott WR, et al, editors: *Laboratory test handbook,* Stow, OH/St. Louis, 1988, LexiComp/Mosby.

4. Scriver CR, Beaudet AL, Valle D, et al, editors: *The metabolic and molecular bases of inherited disease,* ed 8, New York, 2001, McGraw-Hill.

5. Young DS: *Effects of drugs on clinical laboratory tests,* ed 3, Washington, DC, 1990, American Association for Clinical Chemistry.

6. Bremer HJ, Duran M, Kamerling JP, et al: *Disturbances of amino acid metabolism: clinical chemistry and diagnosis,* Baltimore, 1981, Urban and Schwarzenburg.

7. Nyhan W, Sakait N: *Diagnostic recognition of genetic disease,* Philadelphia, 1987, Lea & Febiger.

8. Slocum RH, Cummings JG: Amino acid analysis of physiological samples. In Hommes FA, editor: *Techniques in diagnostic human biochemical genetics,* New York, 1991, Wiley Liss, pp. 87-126.

9. Cummings JG: Routine amino acids analysis in the clinical laboratory, *Am Clin Prod Rev* Feb:20-25, 1988.

10. Schaefer A, Piquard F, Haberey P: Plasma amino acids analysis: effects of delayed samples preparation and of storage, *Clin Chim Acta* 164:163-169, 1987.

11. Pesce A, Kaplan L, editors: *Methods in clinical chemistry,* St. Louis, 1987, CV Mosby.

12. Heiblim DI, Evans HE, Glass L, et al: Amino acid concentrations in cerebrospinal fluid, *Arch Neurol* 35:765-768, 1978.

13. Meites S, editor: *Pediatric clinical chemistry,* ed 3, Washington, DC, 1989, American Association for Clinical Chemistry.

DIAGNOSTIC INFORMATION	REMARKS

P ↑ Hyperammonemia caused by any of the following: hepatic coma, Reye's syndrome, meningitis, cerebral hemorrhage, total parenteral nutrition, urea cycle defects ornithine transcarbamylase deficiency, carbamoylphosphate synthetase deficiency, citrullinemia, argininosuccinic aciduria, and HHH syndrome. Some cases of hyperlysinemia type I, lysinuric protein intolerance.

In hepatic encephalopathy, values correlate better with the clinical course than do values for blood ammonia. Glutamine is the storage form of ammonia in tissues.

See also Table II-2.

P ↓ Rheumatoid arthritis

U ↑ Hartnup disease, generalized aminoaciduria, rheumatoid arthritis

---

CSF ↑ Bacterial meningitis, meningoradiculitis Garin-Bujadoux-Bannwarth, carcinomatous meningitis,[17] histidinemia

Glutamine is the most prominent amino acid in CSF. CSF glutamine and blood ammonia levels are used in the diagnosis of hepatic encephalopathy.

Values in children (3 mo-10 yr) were measured using reversed-phase liquid chromatography.

---

14. Shih V: *Laboratory techniques for the detection of hereditary metabolic disorders,* Boca Raton, FL, 1973, CRC Press.

15. Mayo Medical Laboratories: *Test catalog,* Rochester, MN, 1993, Mayo Medical Laboratories.

16. Goldsmith RF, Farl JW, Cunningham AM: Determination of δ-aminobutyric acid and other amino acids in cerebrospinal fluid of pediatric patients by reverse-phase liquid chromatography, *Clin Chem* 33:1736-1740, 1987.

17. Schott KJ, Meier D: Free amino acid pattern of cerebrospinal fluid in meningeal pathology, *Acta Neurol Scand* 75:304-309, 1987.

TEST NAME AND METHOD	SPECIMEN REQUIREMENTS	REFERENCE INTERVAL, CONVENTIONAL [INTERNATIONAL RECOMMENDED UNITS]		CHEMICAL INTERFERENCES AND IN VIVO EFFECTS
γ-Glutamylcysteine Synthetase in Erythrocytes (EC 6.3.2.2)[1,2]	Hemolysate of washed Ercs. Submit whole blood (heparin). Stability is not known.	6.9-12.7 μmol Pi/hr/10^{10} Ercs (37° C) (n = 5) [× 0.00167 = 0.0115-0.0212 nU/Erc]		None found.

1. Ristoff E, Mayatepek E, Larsson A: Long-term clinical outcome in patients with glutathione synthetase deficiency, *J Pediatr* 139:79-84, 2001.
2. Weatherall DJ: ABC of clinical haematology. The hereditary anaemias, *BMJ* 314:492-496, 1197.

TEST NAME AND METHOD	SPECIMEN REQUIREMENTS	REFERENCE INTERVAL, CONVENTIONAL [INTERNATIONAL RECOMMENDED UNITS]				CHEMICAL INTERFERENCES AND IN VIVO EFFECTS
γ-Glutamyltransferase (GGT, Glutamyl Transpeptidase; EC 2.3.2.2)[1]	Serum. Stable 1 mo at 4° C or 1 yr at −20° C.	*U/L* M: 22.1 ± 11.7 (SD) F: 15.4 ± 6.58 (SD)	× 0.017	*μKat/L* [0.38 ± 0.20] [0.26 ± 0.11]		↑ V Acetaminophen (poisoning), barbiturates, captopril (rare), cephalosporins, cimetidine, estrogens, ethanol (observed in moderate or
Rosalki, 37° C[1]						heavy drinkers), isotretinoin, methotrexate,
RIA[2]		2.03-5.52 mcg/mL	× 1.0	[2.03-5.52 mg/L]		oral contraceptives (and pregnancy), phenytoin,
SCE, 37° C[3]		*U/L* *(2.5-97.5 percentile)*		*μKat/L*		primidone, propoxyphene, streptokinase, smoking; See also Table II-5.
		20-24 yr M: 7-45 F: 4-27	× 0.017	[0.12-0.77] [0.07-0.46]		Heparin causes an increase with the SCE and a decrease with the IFCC
		25-29 yr M: 5-43 F: 4-26		[0.09-0.73] [0.07-0.44]		method.[5]
		30-34 yr M: 5-60 F: 3-37		[0.09-1.02] [0.05-0.63]		↓ V Ascorbic acid (1 g/day for long term), bezafibrate, clofibrate,
		35-39 yr M: 5-96 F: 3-25		[0.99-1.63] [0.05-0.43]		fenofibrate
		40-44 yr M: 5-82 F: 3-30		[0.09-1.39] [0.05-0.51]		↓ C *Reflotron:* acetaminophen (high doses)
		45-49 yr M: 5-53 F: 4-44		[0.09-0.90] [0.07-0.75]		
		50-54 yr M: 7-64		[0.12-1.09]		

DIAGNOSTIC INFORMATION   **REMARKS**

Deficient in very rare congenital hemolytic anemia (autosomal recessive)

↑↑ Obstructive liver disease and posthepatic obstruction[6]

↑ Liver disease (inflammation, cirrhosis, space-occupying lesions), obesity, infectious mononucleosis, renal transplant, hyperthyroidism, myotonic dystrophy, diabetes mellitus, pancreatitis, alchohol-induced liver disease

↓ Hypothyroidism

γ-Glutamyltransferase is useful as a marker for pancreatic cancer, prostatic cancer, and hepatoma because levels reflect remission and recurrence.[7] The enzyme is also used in ratio with HDL cholesterol (alcohol abuse), alkaline phosphatase (alcoholic liver disease), and aspartate aminotransferase (distinguishes neonatal hepatitis from biliary atresia).[8,9]

The test has been useful in detection of male (but not in female) early-risk drinkers[10] and is probably most applicable as part of an alcoholic-screening panel[11] or as follow-up on patients with chronic alcoholism undergoing treatment.[12] It is said to be a more sensitive indicator of liver disease in children than is alkaline phosphatase.[1]

GGT may form complexes with apolipoproteins and immunoglobulin A.[13]

Enzyme activity is an index of exposure to enzyme-inducing drugs such as phenytoin and phenobarbital, as well as ethanol. GGT is related to body weight and body mass index but is most highly correlated to abdominal fat.[14] Activity decreases after meals but increases with prolonged fasting.

The serum enzyme shows heterogeneity on electrophoresis, electrofocusing, and lectin-affinity chromatography. Isoforms are attributed to variation in carbohydrate content.[15]

Claims have been made for the existence of cancer-specific forms, especially in hepatoma and colorectal carcinoma, but sensitivity is too low for the test to be useful.[16,17]

TEST NAME AND METHOD	SPECIMEN REQUIREMENTS	REFERENCE INTERVAL, CONVENTIONAL [INTERNATIONAL RECOMMENDED UNITS]		CHEMICAL INTERFERENCES AND IN VIVO EFFECTS

γ-Glutamyltransferase—CONT

		U/L	μKat/L	
Szasz, 37° C,[4]				
L-g-glutamyl-	Cord blood:	11-194	[0.19-3.30]	
p-nitroanilide	0-1 mo:	0-151	[0.00-2.57]	
	1-2 mo:	0-114	[0.00-1.94]	
	2-4 mo:	0-81	[0.00-1.38]	
	4-7 mo:	0-34	[0.00-0.58]	
	7-12 mo:	0-23	[0.00-0.39]	
	1-2 yr:	0-24	[0.00-0.41]	
	2-5 yr:	1-20	[0.02-0.34]	
	5-10 yr:	3-22	[0.05-0.37]	
	10-15 yr			
	M:	3-25	[0.05-0.43]	
	F:	3-20	[0.05-0.34]	
	Adult			
	M:	2-30	[0.03-0.51]	
	F:	1-24	[0.02-0.41]	
Beckman, 37° C, *L-g-glutamyl-* *p-nitroanilide*		7-64	[0.12-1.09]	
BMC, 37° C, *L-g-glutamyl-* *p-nitroanilide*[4]	M:	11-49	[0.19-0.83]	
	F:	7-32	[0.12-0.54]	
OCD Vitros, 37° C, *L-g-glutamyl-* *p-nitroanilide*		8-78	[0.14-1.33]	

1. Rosalki SB: Gamma-glutamyl transpeptidase, *Adv Clin Chem* 17:53-107, 1975.

2. Masuike M, Ogawa M, Kitahara T, et al: Development of radioimmunoassay for gamma-glutamyltransferase using pancreatic enzyme, *Ann Clin Biochem* 20:247-250, 1983.

3. Arnesen E, Huseby HE, Brenn T, et al: The Tromsø Heart Study: distribution of, and determinants for, gamma-glutamyltransferase in a free-living population, *Scand J Clin Lab Invest* 46:63-70, 1986.

4. Knight JA, Raymond RE: γ-Glutamyltransferase and alkaline phosphatase activities compared in serum of normal children and children with liver disease, *Clin Chem* 27:48-51, 1981.

5. Strømme JH, Theodorsen L: Heparin interferences in the measurement of γ-glutamyltransferase activity with the Scandinavian and the IFCC recommended method, *Scand J Clin Lab Invest* 45:437-442, 1985.

6. Reichling JJ, Kaplan MM: Clinical use of serum enzymes in liver disease, *Dig Dis Sci* 33:1601-1614, 1988.

7. Sahm DF, Murray JL, Munson PL, et al: Gamma-glutamyltranspeptidase levels as an aid in the management of human cancer, *Cancer* 52:1673-1678, 1983.

8. Fung KP, Lau SP: γ-Glutamyl transpeptidase activity and its serial measurement in differentiation between extrahepatic biliary atresia and neonatal hepatitis, *J Pediatr Gastroenterol Nutr* 4:208-213, 1985.

9. Platt MS, Potter JL, Boeckman CR, et al: Elevated GGTP/SGOT ratio. An early indicator of infantile obstructive cholangiopathy, *Am J Dis Child* 735:834-836, 1981.

10. Nilssen O, Førde OH: The Tromsø Heart Study: the positive predictive value of gamma-glutamyltransferase and an alcohol questionnaire in the detection of early-stage risk drinkers, *J Intern Med* 229:497-500, 1991.

11. Salaspuro M: Use of enzymes for the diagnosis of alcohol-related organ damage, *Enzyme* 37:87-107, 1987.

12. Artur Y, Wellman-Bednawska M, Jacquier A, et al: Associations between serum gamma-glutamyltransferase and apolipoproteins: relationships with hepatobiliary diseases, *Clin Chem* 30:1318-1321, 1984.

13. Stranges S, Dorn J, Muti P, et al: Body fat distribution, relative weight, and liver enzyme levels: a population-based study, *Hepatology* 39:754-762, 2004.

14. Schuckit MA, Irwin M: Diagnosis of alcoholism, *Med Clin North Am* 72:1133-1153, 1988.

15. Delanghe JR, De Buyzere ML, De Sheerder IK, et al: Lectin-affinity chromatography of serum gamma glutamyltransferase in liver disease, *Clin Chim Acta* 162:311-318, 1987.

16. Huseby N-E, Eide TJ: Variant γ-glutamyltransferases in colorectal carcinomas, *Clin Chim Acta* 135:301-307, 1983.

17. Xu K-C, Meng X-Y, Shi Y-C, et al: The diagnostic value of a hepatoma-specific band of serum gamma-glutamyltransferase, *Int J Cancer* 36:667-669, 1985.

TEST NAME AND METHOD	SPECIMEN REQUIREMENTS	REFERENCE INTERVAL, CONVENTIONAL [INTERNATIONAL RECOMMENDED UNITS]		CHEMICAL INTERFERENCES AND IN VIVO EFFECTS
Glutathione, Reduced (GSH), in Erythrocytes[1-4] *Beutler, 25° C, colorimetric*[2]	Hemolysate of washed Ercs. Submit whole blood (ACD, EDTA, or heparin). Stability at 4° C: ACD, >20 days; EDTA and heparin, 1 day. Stability at 25° C: ACD, 5 days; EDTA, 1 day; heparin, 2 days.	$\mu mol/g\ Hb$ 6.57 ± 1.04 (SD) $\mu mol/10^{12}\ Ercs$ 190 ± 30.2 $\mu mol/mL\ Ercs$ 2.23 ± 0.35 See *Acetylcholinesterase.* *Conversion factor based on MW of Hb of 64,500.	× 0.0645* × 1.0 × 1.0	*mol/mol Hb* [0.42 ± 0.07] *mmol/L Ercs* [190 ± 30.2] *mmol/L Ercs* [2.23 ± 0.35] None found.

1. Beutler E: *Hemolytic anemia in disorders of red cell metabolism,* New York, 1978, Plenum Pub. Co.

2. Beutler E: *Red cell metabolism: a manual of biochemical methods,* ed 4, New York, 1986, Grune & Stratton.

3. Konrad PN, Valentine WN, Paglia DE: Enzymatic activities and glutathione content of erythrocytes in the newborn: comparison with red cells of older normal subjects and those with comparable reticulocytosis, *Acta Haematol* 48:193-201, 1972.

4. Wilkinson JH: *The principles and practice of diagnostic enzymology,* Chicago, 1976, Year Book Medical Publishers, Inc.

5. Hunaiti AA, Soud M: Effect of lead concentration on the level of glutathione, glutathione S-transferase, reductase and peroxidase in human blood, *Sci Total Environ* 248:45-50, 2000.

6. Dincer Y, Akcay T, Alademir Z, et al: Effect of oxidative stress on glutathione pathway in red blood cells from patients with insulin-dependent diabetes mellitus, *Metabolism* 51:1360-1362, 2002.

7. Fang YZ, Yang S, Wu G: Free radicals, antioxidants, and nutrition, *Nutrition* 18:872-879, 2002.

8. Vesovic D, Borjanovic S, Markovic S, et al: Strenuous exercise and action of antioxidant enzymes, *Med Lav* 93:540-550, 2002.

Glutathione Peroxidase (GSH-Px) in Erythrocytes (EC 1.11.1.9)[1-4] *UV, 37° C*[2]	Hemolysate of washed Ercs. Submit whole blood (EDTA). Stable 20 days at 4° C, 5 days at 25° C.	U.S.-Northern European and U.S.-African adults: $U/g\ Hb$ 30.8 ± 4.73 (2 SD) $U/10^{12}\ Ercs$ 893 ± 137 *U/mL Ercs* 10.5 ± 1.61	× 0.0645* × 10^{-3} × 1.0	*MU/mol Hb* [1.99 ± 0.31] *nU/Erc* [0.89 ± 0.14] *kU/L Ercs* [10.5 ± 1.61]	Activity may decrease in iron deficiency anemia and selenium deprivation.
	Hemolysate of washed Ercs. Submit whole blood (ACD).	$U/g\ Hb$ 32.1 ± 3.84 (2 SD) $U/10^{12}\ Ercs$ 930 ± 111 *U/mL Ercs* 10.9 ± 1.31 *Conversion factor based on MW of Hb of 64,500.	× 0.0645* × 10^{-3} × 1.0	*MU/mol Hb* [2.07 ± 0.25] *nU/Erc* [0.93 ± 0.11] *kU/L Ercs* [10.9 ± 1.31]	

DIAGNOSTIC INFORMATION	REMARKS

$\uparrow$ Myelofibrosis and deficiency of pyrimidine-5′-nucleotidase

$\downarrow$ In deficiencies of G6PD, GSH synthetase, and g-glutamyl synthetase; lead exposure,[5] diabetes mellitus,[6,7] and acute exercise[8]

mmol/g Hb $\times$ 29 = mmol/10^{12} Ercs
mmol/g Hb $\times$ 0.34 = mmol/mL Ercs*

*See Note, *Acetylcholinesterase.*

$\uparrow$ G6PD deficiency, α-thalassemia, polyunsaturated fatty acids supplementation,[5] acute lymphocytic leukemia[6]

$\downarrow$ Iron deficiency anemia, lead exposure,[7] sickle cell anemia,[8] selenium deficiency[9,10] (including treatment diet for phenylketonuria)[11]

The relationship between enzyme deficiency and nonspherocytic hemolytic anemia and hemolytic disease of the newborn (HDN) has not been established.[4]

There are considerable ethnic differences in activity.[12]

GSH-Px is a selenium-requiring enzyme.

U/g Hb $\times$ 29 = U/10^{12} Ercs
U/g Hb $\times$ 0.34 = U/mL Ercs*

*See Note, *Acetylcholinesterase.*

TEST NAME AND METHOD	SPECIMEN REQUIREMENTS	REFERENCE INTERVAL, CONVENTIONAL [INTERNATIONAL RECOMMENDED UNITS]		CHEMICAL INTERFERENCES AND IN VIVO EFFECTS

Glutathione Peroxidase (GSH-Px) in Erythrocytes—CONT

| | Hemolysate of washed Ercs. Submit whole blood (heparin). | *U/g Hb*
34.2 ± 4.77 (2 SD)
U/10[12] Ercs
992 ± 138
U/mL Ercs
11.6 ± 1.62 | × 0.0645*

× 10⁻³

× 1.0 | *MU/mol Hb*
[2.21 ± 0.31]
nU/Erc
[0.99 ± 0.14]
kU/L Ercs
[11.6 ± 1.62] |

1. Beutler E: *Hemolytic anemia in disorders of red cell metabolism,* New York, 1978, Plenum Pub. Co.
2. Beutler E: *Red cell metabolism: a manual of biochemical methods,* ed 4, New York, 1986, Grune & Stratton.
3. Beutler E, Matsumoto F: Ethnic variations in red cell glutathione peroxidase activity, *Blood* 46:103-110, 1975.
4. Weatherall DJ: ABC of clinical haematology. The hereditary anaemias, *BMJ* 314:492-496, 1997.
5. Bellisola G, Galassini S, Moschini G, et al: Selenium and glutathione peroxidase variations induced by polyunsaturated fatty acids oral supplementation in humans, *Clin Chim Acta* 205:75-85, 1992.
6. Devi GS, Prasad MH, Saraswathi I, et al: Free radicals antioxidant enzymes and lipid peroxidation in different types of leukemias, *Clin Chim Acta* 293:53-62, 2000.
7. Hunaiti AA, Soud M: Effect of lead concentration on the level of glutathione, glutathione S-transferase, reductase and peroxidase in human blood, *Sci Total Environ* 248:45-50, 2000.
8. Chan AC, Chow CK, Chiu D: Interaction of antioxidants and their implication in genetic anemia, *Proc Soc Exp Biol Med* 222:274-282, 1999.
9. Thomson CD: Assessment of requirements for selenium and adequacy of selenium status: a review, *Eur J Clin Nutr* 58:391-402, 2004.
10. Maehira F, Luvo GA, Miyagi I, et al: Alterations of serum selenium concentrations in the acute phase of pathological conditions, *Clin Chim Acta* 31:137-146, 2002.
11. Jochum F, Terwolbeck K, Meinhold H, et al: Effects of a low selenium state in patients with phenylketonuria, *Acta Paediatr* 86:775-777, 1997.
12. Beutler E, Matsumoto F: Ethnic variations in red cell glutathione peroxidase activity, *Blood* 46:103-110, 1975.

| **Glutathione Reductase in Erythrocytes** (EC 1.6.4.2)[1]

ICSH, 37° C[1] | Hemolysate of washed erythrocytes. Submit whole blood (ACD, EDTA, or heparin). Stable >20 days at 4° C, 5 days at 25° C; prepare erythrocyte hemolysate. | Reaction without added flavin adenine dinucleotide, FAD:

U/g Hb
7.18 ± 1.09 (SD)
U/10[12] Ercs
208 ± 31.6
U/mL Ercs
2.44 ± 0.37

Reaction using FAD:
U/g Hb
10.4 ± 1.5 (SD)
U/10[12] Ercs
302 ± 43.5
U/mL Ercs
3.54 ± 0.51 |

× 0.0645*

× 10⁻³

× 1.0

× 0.0645*

× 10⁻³

× 1.0 | Hemoglobin C,[4] valproic acid[5]

MU/mol Hb
[0.46 ± 0.07]
nU/Erc
[0.21 ± 0.03]
kU/L Ercs
[2.44 ± 0.37]

MU/mol Hb
[0.67 ± 0.10]
nU/Erc
[0.30 ± 0.04]
kU/L Ercs
[3.54 ± 0.51] |

DIAGNOSTIC INFORMATION	REMARKS

↑ In diabetes, in G6PD deficiency, and after administration of nicotinic acid,[6] exercise training[7]

Rare case of severe hereditary deficiency caused hemolysis after ingestion of fava beans.[6]

See also *Riboflavin.*

↓ Thalassemia[8]

Glutathione reductase activity is chiefly a reflection of the state of riboflavin nutrition.[9,10]

T_3 and T_4 stimulate FAD production.

This assay is not valid in subjects with impaired activity of G6PD.

U/g Hb × 29 = U/10^{12} Ercs
U/g Hb × 0.34 = U/mL Ercs*

*See Note, *Acetylcholinesterase.*

TEST NAME AND METHOD	SPECIMEN REQUIREMENTS	REFERENCE INTERVAL, CONVENTIONAL [INTERNATIONAL RECOMMENDED UNITS]	CHEMICAL INTERFERENCES AND IN VIVO EFFECTS

Glutathione Reductase in Erythrocytes—CONT

See *Acetylcholinesterase.*

*Conversion factor based on MW of Hb of 64,500.

Enzymatic, spec-trophotometric,[2] automated[3]

Activation coefficient as an index of riboflavin sufficiency
Normal: 1.0-1.4
Riboflavin deficiency: >1.45

$$\text{Activation coefficient} = \frac{\text{Activity with added FAD}}{\text{Activity without added FAD}}$$

1. Beutler E: *Red cell metabolism: a manual of biochemical methods,* ed 4, New York, 1986, Grune & Stratton.
2. Tietz NW, editor: *Textbook of clinical chemistry,* Philadelphia, 1986, WB Saunders.
3. Vuilleumier JP, Keller HE, Keck E: Clinical chemical methods for the routine assessment of the vitamin status in human populations. 3. The apoenzyme stimulation tests for vitamin-B$_1$, vitamin-B$_2$, and vitamin-B$_6$ adapted to the Cobas-Bio analyzer, *Int J Vit Nutr Res* 60:126-135, 1990.
4. Bessis M: *Blood smears reinterpreted,* Brecher G, translator. New York, 1976, Springer-Verlag.
5. Bennett JM, Catovsky D, Daniel MT, et al: Proposals for the classification of chronic (mature) B and T lymphoid leukaemias, *J Clin Pathol* 42:567-584, 1989.
6. Arun P, Padmakumaran Nair KG, Manojkumar V, et al: Decreased hemolysis and lipid peroxidation in blood during storage in the presence of nicotinic acid, *Vox Sang* 76:220-225, 1999.
7. Evelo CTA, Palmen NGM, Artur Y, et al: Changes in blood glutathione concentrations and in erythrocyte glutathione reductase and glutathione s-transferase activity after running training and after participation in contests, *Eur J Appl Physiol* 64:354-358, 1992.
8. Chakraborty D, Bhattacharyya M: Antioxidant defense status of red blood cells of patients with beta-thalassemia and Ebeta-thalassemia, *Clin Chim Acta* 305:123-129, 2001.
9. Beutler E: Red cell enzyme defects as nondiseases and as disease, *Blood* 54:1-7, 1979.
10. Wilkinson JH: *The principles and practice of diagnostic enzymology,* Chicago, 1976, Year Book Medical Publishers, Inc.

| **Glutathione Synthetase in Erythrocytes** (EC 6.3.2.3)[1] | Hemolysate of washed Ercs. Submit whole blood (ACD, EDTA, or heparin). Stable for >20 days in ACD or EDTA, >5 days in heparin, at 4° C. | 3.3-7.1 mmol Pi/hr/10^{10} Ercs (37° C) (n = 5) [× 1.67 = 5.5-11.8 pU/Erc] | Not known. |

1. Ristoff E, Mayatepek E, Larsson A: Long-term clinical outcome in patients with glutathione synthetase deficiency, *J Pediatr* 139:79-84, 2001.
2. Miwa S, Fujii H: Molecular basis of erythroenzymopathies associated with hereditary hemolytic anemia: tabulation of mutant enzymes, *Am J Hematol* 51:122-132, 1996.

DIAGNOSTIC INFORMATION	REMARKS

Deficient in rare congenital hemolytic anemia (autosomal recessive)

Some chemicals and drugs that cause hemolytic anemia in G6PD deficiency may also cause anemia in glutathione synthetase deficiency.[2] See *Glucose-6-Phosphate Dehydrogenase in Erythrocytes.*

Pancellular deficiency of glutathione synthetase characterizes 5-oxoprolinuria, a severe neurological disorder that is accompanied by mild hemolytic anemia.[3]

3.   Konrad PN, Richards F II, Valentine WN, et al: γ-Glutamyl-cysteine synthetase deficiency. A cause of hereditary hemolytic anemia, *N Engl J Med* 286:557-561, 1972.

TEST NAME AND METHOD	SPECIMEN REQUIREMENTS	REFERENCE INTERVAL, CONVENTIONAL [INTERNATIONAL RECOMMENDED UNITS]			CHEMICAL INTERFERENCES AND IN VIVO EFFECTS
Glycated Hemoglobin(s)[1-8] *Hemoglobin A*$_{1c}$ *IEF*[1,3,5]	Washed erythrocytes or hemolysate. Collect whole blood (EDTA, heparin, or oxalate). Stable 4-7 days at 4° C, 30 days at 70° C.	*%* *Total Hb* 4.0-5.2	× 0.01	*Hb fraction* [0.040-0.052]	↑ V Carbamylated hemoglobin (formed in uremic patients), hydrochlorothiazide, indapamide, morphine, propranolol
Hemoglobin A$_1$ *Agar gel EP*[1,7]		5.0-7.5		[0.050-0.075]	↑ V Hb F and labile intermediates may cause false elevations. Hemolytic processes may cause falsely low results because of increased erythrocyte turnover.
Column chromatography, cation exchange[1,3,5]		4.5-8.5		[0.045-0.085]	↑ V Hb F, lactescence ↓ V Hemoglobinopathies, hemolytic processes ↓ C Salicylate, carbamate, galactose
HPLC[1,3,5] e.g., BioRad Variant II Affinity Chromatography (Boronate), e.g., Abbott IMx		4.5-5.7		[0.045-0.057]	↑ V Hb F ↓ V Hemoglobinopathies, hemolytic processes
Colorimetric, thiobarbituric acid[1,3,5]		*nmol/10 g Hb* 20-22	× 6.45	*μmol/mol Hb* [129-142]	None found.
Column or affinity chromatographic[1,3]		*% Total Hb* 5.3-7.5		*Hb fraction* [0.053-0.075]	↑ V Aldimine intermediates may interfere.

Glycated hemoglobins are increased as a reflection of hyper-glycemia during the lifespan of erythrocytes (120 days).

Note: Different analytical methods may measure different glycated hemoglobins. Caution must be exercised in the inter-pretation of results.

This test, although not useful for the diagnosis of diabetes mellitus, has been shown to be useful in monitoring its long-term control. Glycated hemoglobin concentration appears to reflect the mean blood glucose concentration over the previous 4-8 wk. Note that improvement in glucose control occurring in the 4 wk before the drawing of the sample is not well reflected in the result because formation of glycated hemoglobin is irreversible. Agar gel EP and HPLC measure HbA$_1$; isoelectric focusing, Hb A$_{1c}$.

Labile forms may be removed by overnight incubation in saline at room temperature, by incubation for 5 hr at 37° C, or by incubation in a pH 5 buffer for 15 min at 37° C.[1]

See also *Fructosamine*.

This method measures Hb A$_1$ and Hb A$_{1c}$. Like HPLC, it is particularly sensitive to variations in temperature and pH.

This method is usually a cationic exchange procedure and measures Hb A$_{1c}$ and Hb A$_{1a+b}$. The procedure is highly sensitive to variations in temperature and pH.

This method measures A$_1$ and non-A$_1$-glycohemoglobins. Note also that units differ from those of other glycated hemoglobin procedures.

Column or affinity chromatography measures total glycated hemoglobins. Results tend to be slightly higher than with other methods.

TEST NAME AND METHOD	SPECIMEN REQUIREMENTS	REFERENCE INTERVAL, CONVENTIONAL [INTERNATIONAL RECOMMENDED UNITS]	CHEMICAL INTERFERENCES AND IN VIVO EFFECTS

Glycated Hemoglobin(s)—CONT

Immunoassay
Turbidimetric/
immunoinhibition
(Antibody-
mediated inhibition
of latex agglutina-
tion), e.g., Roche,
Bayer DA-2000

4.0-6.0%

1. Burtis CA, Ashwood ER, editors: *Tietz textbook of clinical chemistry,* ed 2, Philadelphia, 1994, WB Saunders.

2. Kaplan LA, Pesce AJ, editors: *Clinical chemistry: theory, analysis and correlation,* ed 2, St. Louis, 1989, CV Mosby.

3. Pesce A, Kaplan L, editors: *Methods in clinical chemistry,* St. Louis, 1987, CV Mosby.

4. Tietz NW, editor: *Fundamentals of clinical chemistry,* ed 3, Philadelphia, 1987, WB Saunders.

5. Goldstein DE, Little RR, Wiedmeyer HM, et al: Glycated hemoglobin: methodologies and clinical applications, *Clin Chem* 32:B64-B70, 1986.

6. Guillausseau PJ, Charles MA, Godard V, et al: Comparison of fructosamine glycated hemoglobin as an index of glycemic control in diabetic patients, *Diabetes Res* 13:127-131, 1990.

7. Menard I, Dempsey ME, Blankstein LA, et al: Quantitative determination of glycosylated hemoglobin A_1 by agar gel electrophoresis, *Clin Chem* 26:1598-1602, 1980.

8. Nathan DM: Labile glycosylated hemoglobin contributes to hemoglobin A_1 as measured by liquid chromatography and electrophoresis, *Clin Chem* 27:1261-1263, 1981.

TEST NAME AND METHOD	SPECIMEN REQUIREMENTS	REFERENCE INTERVAL, CONVENTIONAL	[INTERNATIONAL RECOMMENDED UNITS]	CHEMICAL INTERFERENCES AND IN VIVO EFFECTS
Glyceraldehyde Phosphate Dehydrogenase (GAPD) in Erythrocytes (EC 1.2.1.12)[1] *ICSH, 37° C*[1]	Hemolysate of washed Ercs. Submit whole blood (ACD, EDTA, or heparin). Stable 6 days at 4° C, >5 days at 25° C.	*U/g Hb* 226 ± 41.9 (SD) × 0.0645* *U/10[12] Ercs* 6554 ± 1215 × 10[−3] *U/mL Ercs* 76.8 ± 14.2 × 1.0 Higher in newborns[2] See *Acetylcholinesterase.*	*MU/mol Hb* [14.6 ± 2.70] *nU/Erc* [6.6 ± 1.22] *kU/L Ercs* [76.8 ± 14.2]	None found.

*Conversion factor based on MW of Hb of 64,500.

1. Beutler E: *Red cell metabolism: a manual of biochemical methods,* ed 4, New York, 1986, Grune & Stratton.

2. Williams JJ, Beutler E, Ersley JJ, et al, editors: *Manual of hematology,* ed 6, New York, 2003, McGraw-Hill Publishing Co.

3. Beutler E: Red cell enzyme defects as nondiseases and as disease, *Blood* 54:1-7, 1979.

4. Beutler E: *Hemolytic anemia in disorders of red cell metabolism,* New York, 1978, Plenum Pub. Co.

DIAGNOSTIC INFORMATION **REMARKS**

GAPD has no role in hemolytic anemia.[3]

Activity is slightly higher in young erythrocytes.[4]

U/g Hb $\times$ 29 = U/10^{12} Ercs

U/g Hb $\times$ 0.34 = U/mL Ercs*

*See Note, *Acetylcholinesterase.*

TEST NAME AND METHOD	SPECIMEN REQUIREMENTS	REFERENCE INTERVAL, CONVENTIONAL [INTERNATIONAL RECOMMENDED UNITS]				CHEMICAL INTERFERENCES AND IN VIVO EFFECTS
Glyceric Acid *Gas chromatography mass spectrometry*	Urine, random. Store at $-20°$ C. Analyze as per urine organic acid protocol.	 Normal Patients with L-glyceric aciduria			*μmol/mmol creatinine* <10 >100	None found.
Glycerol, Free[1-5] *Enzymatic*[2,4]	Plasma (EDTA), fasting ≥12 hr, resting. Separate plasma immediately. Freeze at $-20°$ C. Avoid vacuum tubes with glycerol-coated stoppers and repeated freezing and thawing.	3-10 yr: 11-80 yr:	*mg/dL* 0.56-2.14 (x̄: 1.33) 0.29-1.72 (x̄: 0.81)	× 0.1086	*mmol/L* [0.06-0.23] [x̄: 0.14] [0.03-0.19] [x̄: 0.09]	↑ C Glycerol-coated stoppers used in vacuum tubes, use of heparin anticoagulated samples. ↑ V Ethanol, epinephrine, mannitol infusion, nitroglycerin, glucagon, thyroxine, growth hormone, total parenteral nutrition, heparin (IV), stress. ↓ V Amino acids, sulfonylureas, e.g., glyburide, tolbutamide.

1. Brown SS, Mitchell FL, Young DS, editors: *Chemical diagnosis of disease,* Amsterdam, 1979, Elsevier/North Holland Biomedical Press.

2. Tietz NW, editor: *Fundamentals of clinical chemistry,* ed 3, Philadelphia, 1987, WB Saunders.

3. Pecora P, Suraci C: Blood glycerol: are there normal values? *IRCS Med Sci Libr Compend* 8:62-63, 1980.

4. Rifai N, Warnick GR, editors: *Methods for clinical laboratory measurements of lipid and lipoprotein risk factors,* Washington, DC, 1991, AACC Press.

5. Roy AV: Free glycerol interferences on the enzymic determination of serum triglycerides [abstract], *Clin Chem* 25:1073, 1979.

6. Hellerud C, Burlina A, Gabelli C, et al: Glycerol metabolism and the determination of triglycerides—clinical, biochemical and molecular findings in six subjects, *Clin Chem Lab Med* 41:46-55, 2003.

7. Elin RJ: The variability of the glycerol concentration in human serum [abstract], *Clin Chem* 29:1174, 1983.

DIAGNOSTIC INFORMATION	REMARKS
↑ Primary hyperoxaluria, type II (L-glyceric aciduria)	See also *Oxalate*.

↑ Hyperthyroidism, chronic renal failure, diabetes mellitus, liver cirrhosis, liver disorders, obesity, stress, glycerol kinase deficiency.[6] The glycerol concentration varies greatly in healthy controls (0-16 mg/dL; 0-1.74 mmol/L), unselected patients (0-47.3 mg/dL; 0-5.14 mmol/L), and selected patients with liver diseases (7-449 mg/dL; 0.76-48.76 mmol/L).[7]	Poor blood-drawing techniques (causing epinephrine effect or stress), acute exercise, and other metabolically stressful disease states will cause elevation in glycerol.

TEST NAME AND METHOD	SPECIMEN REQUIREMENTS	REFERENCE INTERVAL, CONVENTIONAL [INTERNATIONAL RECOMMENDED UNITS]		CHEMICAL INTERFERENCES AND IN VIVO EFFECTS
Glycine (Gly)[1-7] *Ion-exchange chromatographic*	Plasma (heparin) or serum, fasting. Place blood in ice water immediately; separate and freeze within 1 hr of collection. Stable for 1 wk at −20° C; for longer periods deproteinize and store at −70° C.[8,9]	*mg/dL* Premature 1 day: 3.45 ± 2.06 (SD) Newborn 1 day: 1.68-3.86 1 day-1 mo 1.74-5.55 1-3 mo: 1.23 ± 0.22 (SD) 2-6 mo: 1.31-2.22 9 mo-2 yr: 0.42-2.31 3-10 yr: 0.88-1.67 6-18 yr: 1.18-2.27 Adult: 0.90-4.16	*µmol/L*[12] × 133.3 [460 ± 275] [224-514] [232-740][13] [164 ± 29] [175-296] [56-308] [117-223] [158-302][14] [120-554]	P ↑ V Histidine (after oral load), valproate P ↓ V Oral contraceptives
	Urine, 24 hr. Add 10 mL of 6 mol/L HCl at start of collection. (Alternatively, refrigerate specimen during collection.) Store frozen at −20° C.[10]	*mg/day* 10 days-7 wk: 14.6-59.2 3-12 yr: 12.4-106.8 Adult: 59.0-294.6 *mg/g creatinine* or 60 ± 24 (SD) *µmol/g creatinine*[15] 0-1 mo: 1017-10,417 1-6 mo: 1315-8804 6 mo-1 yr: 1422-5754 1-2 yr: 1025-4596 2-3 yr: 1026-4310	*µmol/day*[12] × 13.3 [194-787] [165-1420] [785-3918] *mmol/mol creatinine* × 1.51 [90.6 ± 36.2] *mmol/mol creatinine* × 0.113 [114.9-1177.1] [148.6-994.9] [160.7-650.2] [115.8-519.3] [115.9-487.0]	U ↑ V Niacinamide, valproate U ↓ V Ascorbic acid (after large intake),[17] niacin
	CSF. Collect in sterile tubes; store frozen. Stable at −20° C for 1 wk or at −70° C for 2 mo.[11]	*mg/dL* Neonate: 0.083 ± 0.032 (SEM) 3 mo-2 yr: 0.036 ± 0.015 (SD) 2-10 yr: 0.034 ± 0.011 Adult: 0.044 ± 0.002	*µmol/L* ×113.3 [11.0 ± 4.2][11] [4.8 ± 2.0][16] [4.6 ± 1.5][16] [5.8 ± 0.3][12]	

1. Burtis CA, Ashwood ER, Bruns DE, editors: *Tietz textbook of clinical chemistry and molecular diagnostics,* ed 4, Philadelphia, 2005, WB Saunders.

2. Friedman RB, Young DS: *Youngs effect on line,* 2006, American Association for Clinical Chemistry.

3. Scriver CR, Beaudet AL, Valle D, et al, editors: *The metabolic and molecular bases of inherited disease,* ed 8, New York, 2001, McGraw-Hill.

4. Young DS: *Effects of drugs on clinical laboratory tests,* ed 3, Washington, DC, 1990, American Association for Clinical Chemistry.

5. Bremer HJ, Duran M, Kamerling JP, et al: *Disturbances of amino acid metabolism: clinical chemistry and diagnosis,* Baltimore, 1981, Urban and Schwarzenburg.

6. Cynober L, Dinh FN, Blonde F, et al: Plasma and urinary amino acid pattern in severe burn patients: evolution throughout the healing period, *Am J Clin Nutr* 36:416-425, 1982.

DIAGNOSTIC INFORMATION	REMARKS
P ↑ Septicemia, hypoglycemia, nonketotic hyperglycinemia, hyperammonemia type I, severe burns,[18,19] iminoglycinuria type II, starvation, propionic acidemia, methylmalonic acidemia, carbamoylphosphate synthetase deficiency, kwashiorkor, chronic renal failure, lysinuric protein intolerance	Glycine is one of the main amino acids in all body fluids. Glycine concentrations in plasma depend on nutritional state and duration of fasting.
	See also Table II-2.
P ↓ Gout, diabetes mellitus, following abdominal surgery[20]	
U ↑ Hypoglycemia, cystinuria, Hartnup disease, pregnancy, cystathioninuria, hyperprolinemia, glycinuria, Joseph's syndrome (severe prolinuria and hydroxyprolinuria), burn patients,[6] nonketotic hyperglycinemia, familial iminoglycinuria type I, generalized aminoaciduria, propionic acidemia, methylmalonic acidemia, carbamoylphosphate synthetase deficiency, vitamin D–resistant rickets, rheumatoid arthritis	High levels of proline and hydroxyproline are also seen in the aminoglycinurias.
CSF ↑↑ nonketotic hyperglycinemia	Values in children (3 mo-10 yr) were measured using reversed-phase liquid chromatography.
CSF ↑ Bacterial meningitis,[21] aseptic meningitis, meningoradiculitis Garin-Bujadoux-Bannwarth, carcinomatous meningitis	Measurement of the CSF: plasma glycine ratio is the optimal way to diagnose nonketotic hyperglycinemia.

7. Nyhan W, Sakait N: *Diagnostic recognition of genetic disease,* Philadelphia, 1987, Lea & Febiger.
8. Cummings JG: Routine amino acids analysis in the clinical laboratory, *Am Clin Prod Rev* Feb:20-25, 1988.
9. Schaefer A, Piquard F, Haberey P: Plasma amino acids analysis: effects of delayed samples preparation and of storage, *Clin Chim Acta* 164:163-169, 1987.
10. Pesce A, Kaplan L, editors: *Methods in clinical chemistry,* St. Louis, 1987, CV Mosby.
11. Heiblim DI, Evans HE, Glass L, et al: Amino acid concentrations in cerebrospinal fluid, *Arch Neurol* 35:765-768, 1978.
12. Shih V: *Laboratory techniques for the detection of hereditary metabolic disorders,* Boca Raton, FL, 1973, CRC Press.
13. Slocum RH, Cummings JG: Amino acid analysis of physiological samples. In Hommes FA, editor: *Techniques in diagnostic human biochemical genetics,* New York, 1991, Wiley Liss, pp. 87-126.
14. Meites S, editor: *Pediatric clinical chemistry,* ed 3, Washington, DC, 1989, American Association for Clinical Chemistry.

TEST NAME AND METHOD	SPECIMEN REQUIREMENTS	REFERENCE INTERVAL, CONVENTIONAL [INTERNATIONAL RECOMMENDED UNITS]			CHEMICAL INTERFERENCES AND IN VIVO EFFECTS

Glycine—CONT

15. Mayo Medical Laboratories: *Test catalog*, Rochester, MN, 2005, Mayo Medical Laboratories.
16. Goldsmith RF, Earl JW, Cunningham AM: Determination of δ-aminobutyric acid and other amino acids in cerebrospinal fluid of pediatric patients by reversed-phase liquid chromatography, *Clin Chem* 33:1736-1740, 1987.
17. Tsao C, Muyashita K: Effects of large intake of ascorbic acid on the urinary excretion of amino acids and related compounds, *IRCS Med Sci* 13:855-856, 1985.
18. Cynober L, Dinh FN, Blonde F, et al: Plasma and urinary amino acid pattern in severe burn patients: evolution throughout the healing period, *Am J Clin Nutr* 36:416-425, 1982.

Glycolic Acid[1-6]	Serum, plasma.	$\mu mol/L$ ~8			None found.
Colorimetric, enzymatic, GLC, GC-MS	Urine, 24 hr. Refrigerate.	*mg/day* 15-60	$\times$ 0.0131	*mmol/day* 0.20-0.79	
MW 76					

1. Porter WH, Rutter PW, Bush BA, et al: Ethylene glycol toxicity: the role of serum glycolic acid in hemodialysis, *J Toxicol Clin Toxicol* 39:607-615, 2001.
2. Maeda-Nakai E, Ichiyama A: A spectrophotometric method for the determination of glycolate in urine and plasma with glycolate oxidase, *J Biochem* 127:279-287, 2000.
3. Fraser AD: Importance of glycolic acid analysis in ethylene glycol poisoning, *Clin Chem* 44:1769-1770, 1998.
4. Yao HH, Porter WH: Simultaneous determination of ethylene glycol and its major toxic metabolite, glycolic acid, in serum by gas chromatography, *Clin Chem* 42:292-297, 1998.
5. Fraser AD, MacNeil W: Colorimetric and gas chromatographic procedures for glycolic acid in serum: the major toxic metabolite of ethylene glycol, *Clin Toxicol* 31:397-405, 1993.
6. Porter WH, Rutter PW, Yao HH: Simultaneous determination of ethylene glycol and glycolic acid in serum by gas chromatography-mass spectrometry, *J Anal Toxicol* 23:591-597, 1999.

α₂-HS-Glycoprotein (α₂-HS, Ba-α₂-Glycoprotein)[1-5] *RID*[1] *ELISA*[5]	Serum or plasma. Analyze fresh or store at 4° C for < 72 hr. Stable frozen at −20° C for 6 mo or at −70° C indefinitely. Specimens without lipemia or hemolysis are preferred.	*mg/dL* 40-85 ($\bar{x}$: 60) M: $\bar{x}$: 62[6]	$\times$ 10	*mg/L* [400-850] [$\bar{x}$: 600] [$\bar{x}$: 617]	None found.
EID[4]	Urine, 24 hr. Centrifuge and adjust to pH 7.0. Analyze fresh. Stable frozen at −20° C for up to 1 yr.	5-95 percentile: Median:	0.07-1.12 mg/day 0.23		

DIAGNOSTIC INFORMATION	**REMARKS**

19. Cynober L, Dinh FN, Saizy R, et al: Plasma amino acid levels in the first few days after burn injury and their predictive value, *Intensive Care Med* 9:325-331, 1983.

20. Jain KM, Rush BF Jr, Seelig RF, et al: Changes in plasma amino acid profiles following abdominal operations, *Surg Gynecol Obstet* 152:302-306, 1981.

21. Schott KJ, Meier D: Free amino acid pattern of cerebrospinal fluid in meningeal pathology, *Acta Neurol Scand* 75:304-309, 1987.

Glycolic acid is increased in all nonuremic patients with primary hyperoxaluria type I (usually >100 mg/day; >1.31 mmol/day). In patients with hyperoxaluria type II (L-glyceric aciduria) the excretion of glycolic acid is within the reference range.

Glycolic acid is the principal toxic metabolite of ethylene glycol and should be monitored in addition to ethylene glycol concentrations after ethylene glycol poisoning. It accounts for >90% of the anion gap in ethylene glycol–poisoned patients. Initial glycolic acid concentrations $\geq$10 mmol/L predict acute renal failure.

See also *Ethylene Glycol and Oxalate.*

Negative acute phase reacting protein.[7-9]

$\downarrow$ Inflammatory conditions, infection, and malnutrition.[9-12] Levels also decreased with some hematological malignancies.[13]

$\uparrow$ In serum and peritoneal fluid of women with endometriosis.[14,15] Antibodies to α_2-HS are also increased in the serum of patients with endometriosis.[16]

α_2-HS accumulates in bone and dentin[17-19] and appears to be involved with regulating calcium metabolism.[18-21] This protein has been shown to promote opsonization and to decrease insulin receptor tyrosine kinase activity.[8,22,23]

MW: 49,000

TEST NAME AND METHOD	SPECIMEN REQUIREMENTS	REFERENCE INTERVAL, CONVENTIONAL [INTERNATIONAL RECOMMENDED UNITS]		CHEMICAL INTERFERENCES AND IN VIVO EFFECTS

α_2-HS-Glycoprotein—CONT

	CSF. Centrifuge before analysis. Analyze fresh or store at 4° C for <72 hr. Stable frozen at −20° C for 6 mo or at −70° C indefinitely. Specimens should not contain blood.	0.17 mg/dL	× 10	[1.7 mg/L]

1. Ritzmann SE, Tucker ES III: *Protein analysis in disease—current concepts. Workshop manual,* Chicago, 1979, American Society of Clinical Pathologists, Commission for Continuing Education.

2. Schwick H-G, Haupt H: Chemistry and function of human plasma proteins, *Angew Chem* 191:87-99, 1980.

3. Haralambie G: Biochemical changes in blood (at rest) induced by exercise and training. In Siest G, editor: *Reference values in human chemistry,* Basel, Switzerland, 1973, S. Karger.

4. Weeke EOB: Urinary serum proteins. *Protides Biol Fluids,* 21:363-369, 1974.

5. Mathur SP, Lee JH, Arnaud P, et al: Levels of transferrin and alpha 2-HS glycoprotein in women with and without endometriosis, *Autoimmunity* 29:121-127, 1999.

6. Burgl W, Simonen S, Bardner S, et al: Unusually high concentrations of $Zn\alpha$2HS-glcyprotein in human ejaculates, *Clin Chem* 35:1649-1650, 1989.

7. Daveau M, Christian-Davrinche, Julen N, et al: The synthesis of human alpha-2-HS glycoprotein is down-regulated by cytokines in hepatoma HepG2 cells, *FEBS Lett* 241:191-194, 1988.

8. Lebreton JP, Joisel F, Raoult JP, et al: Serum concentration of human alpha 2 HS glycoprotein during the inflammatory process: evidence that alpha 2 HS glycoprotein is a negative acute-phase reactant, *J Clin Invest* 64:1118-1129, 1979.

9. Abiodun PO, Olomu IN: Serum alpha 2-HS-glycoprotein levels in neonatal infections, *Biol Neonate* 60:114-117, 1991.

10. Jersmann HP, Dransfiel I, Hart SP: Fetuin/alpha 2-HS glycoprotein enhances phagocytosis of apoptotic cells and macropinocytosis by human macrophages, *Clin Sci* 105:273-278, 2003.

11. Abiodun PO, Olomu IN: Alpha 2 HS-glycoprotein levels in children with protein-energy malnutrition and infections, *J Pediatr Gastroenterol Nutr* 6:271-275, 1987.

12. Abiodun PO, Ihongbe JC, Dati F: Decreased levels of apha 2 HS-glycoprotein in children with protein-energy malnutrition, *Eur J Pediatr* 144:368-369, 1985.

13. Kalabay L, Cseh K, Benedek S, et al: Serum alpha 2-HS glycoprotein concentration in patients with hematological malignancies, *Ann Hematol* 63:264-269, 1991.

14. Mathur SP: Autoimmunity in endometriosis: relevance to infertility, *Am J Reprod Immunol* 44:89-95, 2000.

15. Mathur SP, Lee JH, Arnaud P, et al: Levels of transferrin and alpha 2-HS glycoprotein in women with and without endometriosis, *Autoimmunity* 29:121-127, 1999.

16. Mathur SP, Holt VL, Lee JH, et al: Levels of antibodies to transferrin and alpha 2-HS glycoprotein in women with and without endometriosis, *Am J Reprod Immunol* 40:69-73, 1998.

17. Jahnen-Dechent W, Trindl A, Godovac-Zimmermann J, et al: Posttranslational processing of human alpha 2-HS glycoprotein (human fetuin). Evidence for the production of a phosphorylated single-chain form by hepatoma cells, *Eur J Biochem* 226:59-69, 1994.

18. Nishio S, Hatanaka M, Takeda H, et al: Calcium phosphate crystal-associated proteins: α-2-HS-glycoprotein, prothrombin fragment 1 and osteopontin, *Int J Urol* 8:S58-S62, 2001.

19. Heiss A, DuChesne A, Denecke B, et al: Structural basis of calcification inhibition by α-2-HS-glycoprotein/fetuin-A, *J Biol Chem* 278:13333-13341, 2003.

20. Lin KH, Lee HY, Shih CH, et al: Plasma protein regulation by thyroid hormone, *J Endocrinol* 179:367-377, 2003.

21. Jahnen-Dechent W, Schafer C, Heiss A, et al: Systemic inhibition of spontaneous calcification by the serum protein alpha 2-HS glycoprotein/fetuin, *Z Kardiol* 90:47-56, 2001.

22. Srinivas PR, Wagner AS, Reddy LV, et al: Alpha 2-HS-glycoprotein is an inhibitor of the human insulin receptor at the tyrosine kinase level, *Mol Endocrinol* 7:1445-1455, 1993.

23. Kalabay L, Cseh K, Pajor A, et al: Correlation of maternal serum fetuin/alpha 2-HS glycoprotein concentration with maternal insulin resistance and anthropometric parameters of neonates in normal pregnancy and gestational diabetes, *Eur J Endocrinol* 147:243-248, 2002.

TEST NAME AND METHOD	SPECIMEN REQUIREMENTS	REFERENCE INTERVAL, CONVENTIONAL [INTERNATIONAL RECOMMENDED UNITS]			CHEMICAL INTERFERENCES AND IN VIVO EFFECTS
3.8S α_2-Glycopro-tein (Histidine-rich α_2-Glycoprotein)[1-5] *RID*[2]	Serum. Analyze fresh or store at 4° C for <72 hr. Stable frozen at −20° C for 6 mo or at −70° C indefinitely. Specimens without lipemia or hemolysis are preferred.	5-15 mg/dL x̄: 9.0	× 10	[50-150 mg/L] [x̄: 90]	None found.

1. Ritzmann SE, Daniels JC, editors: *Serum protein abnormalities, diagnostic and clinical aspects,* Boston, 1975, Little, Brown and Co.

2. Ritzmann SE, Tucker ES III: *Protein analysis in disease—current concepts. Workshop manual,* Chicago, 1979, American Society of Clinical Pathologists, Commission for Continuing Education.

3. Schwick H-G, Haupt H: Chemistry and function of human plasma proteins, *Angew Chem* 191:87-99, 1980.

4. Saigo K, Yoshida A, Ryo R, et al: Histidine-rich glycoprotein as a negative acute phase reactant, *Am J Hematol* 34:149-150, 1990.

5. Lijnen H, Jacobs G, Collen D: Histidine-rich glycoprotein in a normal and clinical population, *Thromb Res* 22:519-523, 1981.

6. Leebeek F, Kluft C, Knot E, et al: Histidine-rich glycoprotein is elevated in mild liver cirrhosis and decreased in moderate and severe liver cirrhosis, *J Lab Clin Med* 113:493-497, 1989.

7. Omri A, Kruithof E, Bachmann F: Histidine-rich glycoprotein during pregnancy, *Thromb Haemost* 59:341, 1988.

8. Halbmayer WM, Hopmeier P, Feichtinger C, et al: Histidine-rich glycoprotein (HRG) in uncomplicated pregnancy and mild and moderate preeclampsia, *Thromb Haemost* 67:585-586, 1992.

9. Shigekiyo T, Yoshida H, Matsumoto K, et al: HRG Tokushima: molecular and cellular characterization if histidine-rich glycoprotein (HRG) deficiency, *Blood* 91:128-133, 1998.

10. Souto J, Gari M, Falkon L, et al: A new case of hereditary histidine-rich glycoprotein deficiency with familial thrombophilia, *Thromb Haemost* 75:374-375, 1996.

11. Hennis BC, Van Boheemen PA, Koeleman BP, et al: A specific allele of the histidine-rich glycoprotein (HRG) locus is linked with elevated plasma levels of HRG in a Dutch family with thrombosis, *Br J Haematol* 89:845-852, 1995.

12. Ehrenforth S, Aygoren-Pursun E, Hach-Wunderle V, et al: Prevalence of elevated histidine-rich glycoprotein in patients with thrombophilia—a study of 695 patients, *Thromb Haemost* 71:160-161, 1994.

13. Hoffmann JJML, Hennis BC, Kluft C, et al: Hereditary increase of plasma histidine-rich glycoprotein associated with abnormal heparin binding (HRG Eindhoven), *Thromb Haemost* 70:894-899, 1993.

14. Gorgani NN, Smith BA, Kono H, et al: Histidine-rich glycoprotein binds to DNA and FcγRI and potentiates the ingestion of apoptotic cells by macrophages, *J Immunol* 169:4745-4751, 2002.

15. Kluszynski BA, Kim C, Faulk WP: Zinc as a cofactor for heparin neutralization by histidine-rich glycoprotein, *J Biol Chem* 272:13541-13547, 1997.

16. Lijnen HR, Hoylaerts M, Collen D: Isolation and characterization of a human plasma protein with affinity for the lysine binding sites in plasminogen. Role in the regulation of fibrinolysis and identification as histidine-rich glycoprotein, *J Biol Chem* 255:10214-10222, 1980.

17. Leung LL: Interaction of histidine-rich glycoprotein with fibrinogen and fibrin, *J Clin Invest* 77:1305-1311, 1986.

18. Gorgani NN, Parish CR, Altin JG: Differential binding of histidine-rich glycoprotein (HRG) to human IgG subclasses and IgG molecules containing κ and λ light chains, *J Biol Chem* 274:29633-29640, 1999.

May be a negative acute-phase protein.[4] Serum concentrations decrease in liver disease, septicemia, and during pregnancy.[4-8] Hereditary states of deficiency[9,10] and excess[11-13] have been associated with increased risk of thrombosis.

3.8S α_2-Glycoprotein is primarily synthesized by the liver[14] and is found in both plasma and platelets.[9,15] This protein interacts with a variety of molecules, including heparin, plasminogen, fibrinogen, IgG, and immunoglobulin free light chains, in addition to the surfaces of several cell types, including T lymphocytes and macrophages.[14-21] It can decrease heparin activity,[15] suppress activation of T lymphocytes,[20] and promote macrophage phagocytosis of apoptotic cells.[14] Data suggest it may have a role in modulating insoluble immune complex formation by rheumatoid factor.[22]

MW: 75,000

19. Jones A, Hulett MD, Parish CR: Histidine-rich glycoprotein binds to cell-surface heparan sulfate via its N-terminal domain following zinc chelatin, *J Biol Chem* 279:30114-30122, 2004.

20. Shatsky M, Saigo K, Burdach S, et al: Histidine-rich glycoprotein blocks T cell rosette formation and modulates both T cell activation and immunoregulation, *J Biol Chem* 264:8254-8259, 1989.

21. Saigo K, Shatsky M, Leung LK: Interaction of histidine-rich glycoprotein with human T lymphocytes, *J Biol Chem* 264:8249-8253, 1989.

22. Gorgani NN, Altin JG, Parish CR: Histidine-rich glycoprotein prevents formation of insoluable immune complexes by rheumatoid factor, *Immunology* 98:456-463, 1999.

TEST NAME AND METHOD	SPECIMEN REQUIREMENTS	REFERENCE INTERVAL, CONVENTIONAL [INTERNATIONAL RECOMMENDED UNITS]			CHEMICAL INTERFERENCES AND IN VIVO EFFECTS
β₂-Glycoprotein I (β₂GpI, apolipoprotein H)[1,2] *RID* ELISA[3]	Serum. Analyze fresh or store at 4° C for <72 hr. Stable frozen at −20° C for 6 mo or at −70° C indefinitely. Specimens without lipemia or hemolysis are preferred.	15-30 mg/dL[1] (x̄: 24)	× 10	[150-300 mg/L] [x̄: 240]	None found.
	Urine, 24 hr. Centrifuge and adjust to pH 7.0. Analyze fresh. Stable frozen at −20° C for up to 1 yr.	0.21-0.44 mg/day		(x̄: 0.33)[4]	

1. Ritzmann SE, Tucker ES III: *Protein analysis in disease—current concepts, workshop manual,* Chicago, 1979, American Society of Clinical Pathologists, Commission for Continuing Education.

2. Merten M, Motamedy S, Ramamurthy S, et al: Sulfatides: targets for antiphospholipid antibodies, *Circulation* 108:2082-2087, 2003.

3. Yasuda S, Atsumi T, Ieko M, et al: Nicked beta2-glocoprotein I: a marker of cerebral infarct and a novel role in the negative feedback pathway of extrinsic fibrinolysis, *Blood* 103:3766-3772, 2004.

4. Pesce AJ, First MR: *Proteinuria—an integrated review,* New York, 1979, Marcel Dekker.

5. Lapsley M, Flynn FV, Sansom PA: Beta 2-glycoprotein-1 (apolipoprotein H) excretion in chronic renal tubular disorders: comparison with other protein markers of tubular malfunction, *J Clin Pathol* 44:812-816, 1991.

6. Norden AG, Fulcher LM, Lapsley M, et al: Excretion of beta-2-glycoprotein 1 (apolipoprotein H) in renal tubular disease, *Clin Chem* 37:74-77, 1991.

7. Flynn, FV, Lapsley M, Sansom PA, et al: Urinary excretion of beta 2-glycoprotein 1 (apolipoprotein H) and other markers of tubular malfunction in "non-tubular" renal disease, *J Clin Pathol* 45:561-567, 1992.

8. Crook M, Chng SI, Lumb P, et al: Serum apolipoprotein H and its relationship to blood pressure, serum lipids, fasting plasma glucose and insulin in normal individuals, *Ann Clin Biochem* 38:494-498, 2001.

9. Cavallo PP, Gruden G, Giunti S, et al: Apolipoprotein H is increased in type 2 diabetic patients with microalbuminuria, *Nutr Metab Cardiovasc Dis* 10:311-314, 2000.

10. Pettingale KW, Tee DE: Serum protein changes in breast cancer: a prospective study, *J Clin Pathol* 30:1048-1052, 1977.

11. Hoeg JM, Segal P, Gregg RE, et al: Characterization of plasma lipids and lipoproteins in patients with beta-2-glycoprotein 1 (apolipoprotein H) deficiency, *Atherosclerosis* 55:25-34, 1985.

12. Sepehrnia B, Kamboh MI, Adams-Campbell LL, et al: Genetic studies of human apolipoproteins. VIII. Role of the apolipoprotein H polymorphism in relation to serum lipoprotein concentrations, *Hum Genet* 82:118-122, 1989.

13. George J, Harats D, Gilburd B, et al: Immunolocalization of beta2-glycoprotein 1 (apolipoprotein H) to human atherosclerotic plaques: potential implications for lesion progression, *Circulation* 99:2227-2230, 1999.

14. Mehdi H, Naqvi A, Kamboh MI: A hydrophobic sequence at position 313-316 (Lue-Ala-Phe-Trp) in the fifth domain of apolipoprotein H (beta2-glycoprotein 1) is crucial for cardiolipid binding, *Eur J Biochem* 267:1770-1776, 2000.

15. Hunt J, Krilis S: The fifth domain of beta-2-glycoprotein 1 contains a phospholipid binding site (Cys281-Cys288) and a region recognized by anticardiolipin antibodies, *J Immunol* 152:653-659, 1994.

16. Merten M, Motamedy S, Ramamurthy S, et al: Sulfatides: targets for antiphospholipid antibodies, *Circulation* 108:2082-2087, 2003.

↑ Significantly increased renal excretion is found in renal tubular disease and in some causes of renal dysfunction that are nontubular in origin.[5-7] Elevated serum levels can be found with diabetes mellitus,[8] with dyslipidemias,[9] and with malignant breast tumors.[10]

↓ S Hereditary deficiency.[11]

β_2-Glycoprotein I may have a role in lipid metabolism as it associates with very low-density lipoprotein, low-density lipoprotein, high-density lipoprotein, and chylomicrons.[12] It is found in atherosclerotic plaques.[13]

This protein also binds negatively charged phospholipids[14,15] and surface-bound sulfatides.[16] Evidence indicates it is involved in autoimmune activity as it has been identified as an antigen for antiphospholipid antibodies[17] and serves as a cofactor for some antiphospholipid antibody-anionic phospholipid-interactions.[18] Antibodies to β_2Gp$_I$ have been shown to be associated with increased risk of thrombotic events[19] and interference with protein C action.[20] β_2Gp$_I$ inhibits Hageman factor and FXI activation.[21,22]

MW: 50,000

17. McNeil HP, Simpson RJ, Chesterman CN, et al: Antiphospholipid antibodies are directed against a complex antigen that includes a lipid-binding inhibitor of coagulation: beta-2-glycoprotein 1 (apolipoprotein H), *Proc Natl Acad Sci USA* 87:4120-4124, 1990.

18. Jones JV, James H, Tan MH, et al: Antiphospholipid antibodies require beta-2-glycoprotein 1 (apolipoprotein H) as a cofactor, *J Rheumatol* 19:1397-1402, 1992.

19. Ebeling F, Petaja J, Alanko S, et al: Infant stroke and of beta-2-glycoprotein 1 antibodies: six cases, *Eur J Pediatr* 162:678-681, 2003.

20. Chen WH, Kao YF, Lan MY, et al: A perturbation of antithrombin-III and protein C coupling associates with an increase of anti-beta2-glycoprotein 1 antibody in non-antiphospholipid antibody syndrome cerebral ischemia, *Blood Coagul Fibrinolysis* 13:703-709, 2002.

21. Henry ML, Everson B, Ratnoff OD: Inhibition of Hageman factor (factor XII) by beta-2-glycoprotein 1, *J Lab Clin Med* 111:519-523, 1988.

22. Shi T, Iverson GM, Qi JC, et al: Beta-2-glycoprotein 1 binds factor XI and inhibits its activation by thrombin and factor XIIa: loss of inhibition by clipped beta-2-glycoprotein 1, *Proc Natl Acad Sci USA* 101:3939-3944, 2004.

TEST NAME AND METHOD	SPECIMEN REQUIREMENTS	REFERENCE INTERVAL, CONVENTIONAL [INTERNATIONAL RECOMMENDED UNITS]		CHEMICAL INTERFERENCES AND IN VIVO EFFECTS
Gold (Au)[1]	Serum. Collect in metal-free container.		mg/dL^4 $\mu mol/L$ <10 × 0.00508 [<0.5]	None found.
AAS		Therapeutic range:	100-200 [5.1-10.2]	
Dose (therapeutic),[2] 50% gold sodium thiomalate: *mg, IM* Wk 1: 10 Wk 2: 25 Wk 3-20: 50		Initially the serum gold concentration will peak 2-6 hr after each injection and then gradually decrease through the week. It will plateau in 6-8 wk. Thereafter a 50-mcg [254 μmol] injection will produce a peak concentration of 400-800 mcg/dL [20.3-40.6 μmol/L], which will decrease by ~60% over the next 6 days. There is considerable individual variation. When gold is administered every 3-4 wk, the serum concentration will remain 75-125 mcg/dL [3.8-6.3 μmol/L].		
Therapy is continued at a maintenance level with 50-mg injections (IM) given at increasingly longer intervals.	Whole blood.[3] Collect in metal-free container.	<0.5 mcg/L × 0.00508 [<0.0026 μmol/L]		
	Urine, 24 hr.[4] Collect in metal-free container. Use no preservatives.	<1 mcg/day × 5.08 [<5.1 nmol/day]		↑ V Dimercaprol

1. Wyngaarden JB, Smith LH Jr, editors: *Cecil textbook of medicine,* ed 18, Philadelphia, 1988, WB Saunders.
2. McGarty DJ: *Arthritis and allied conditions,* ed 10, Philadelphia, 1985, Lea & Febiger.
3. Perrelli G, Piolatto G: Tentative reference values for gold, silver and platinum: literature data analysis, *Sci Total Environ* 120:93-96, 1992.
4. Mayo Medical Laboratories: *Test catalog,* Rochester, MN, 1993, Mayo Medical Laboratories.
5. Jones G, Brooks PM: Injectable gold compounds: an overview, *Br J Rheumatol* 35:1154-1158, 1996.
6. Lacaille D, Stein HB, Rabound J, et al: Longterm therapy of psoriatic arthritis: intramuscular gold or methotrexate? *J Rheumatol* 27:1922-1927, 2000.

Gonadotropin- Releasing Hormone (GnRH) Test [Lutropin/Follitropin-Releasing Hormone (LH/FSH-RH) Test, Luteinizing Hormone-Releasing Hormone (LRH, LHRH) Test][1-3]	Serum drawn at 0, +30, +60, +90, and +120 min with respect to the administration of GnRH for LH and FSH measurements.	Peak LH response[4] Prepubertal child: Puberty and adult: Peak FSH response[4] Prepubertal child: Puberty and adult:	Absent or minimal response 3- to 10-fold increase above baseline Absent or minimal response 1.5- to 3-fold increase above baseline	See individual tests.

DIAGNOSTIC INFORMATION	REMARKS

At least 35% of patients undergoing chrysotherapy develop some degree of Au toxicity. The most common manifestation of toxicity is dermatitis with eosinophilia. Other common side effects are pruritus and albuminuria. More adverse reactions ascribed to gold therapy are enterocolitis, intrahepatic cholestasis, skin hyperpigmentation, peripheral neuropathy, chrysiasis, and diffuse pulmonary infiltrates.

Other effects are leukopenia, hematuria, and thrombocytopenia. Aplastic anemia may be life threatening.[5]

Gold salts are used in the treatment of rheumatoid arthritis. Au appears to accumulate in different tissue compartments at varying rates, and there is evidence that long-term maintenance therapy is superior to larger doses for a shorter period. Au is detectable in serum 10 mo after cessation of treatment. Correlations between therapeutic doses, serum or urine concentration, and clinical effects are not well established. It has been suggested that only serum levels >300 mcg/dL [15.2 μmol/L] are effective in the treatment of rheumatoid arthritis.

Methotrexate may be superior to Au therapy for treatment of psoriatic arthritis.[6]

See Tables II-5 and II-6.

In a majority of patients with pituitary disease there is an absent or blunted response. In hypothalamic disease there is a normal or prepubertal response, but repeated stimulation may be necessary. In anorexia nervosa the peak response is reduced. In delayed puberty there is no response, or response is greater for FSH than for LH. In primary gonadal failure the response is exaggerated and prolonged. In children with true sexual precocity, GnRH-induced LH release is in the pubertal range. In children with precocious thelarche or adrenarche, LH responses are prepubertal.[5]

Because of considerable overlap of response in patients with hypothalamic or pituitary diseases, the test is more useful in assessing pituitary gonadotropin reserve than in localizing the site of dysfunction. In patients with pituitary tumors, response to GnRH may be normal, and absent responses can be seen in patients with hypothalamic disease. Release of LH (after GnRH) is dose dependent; in normal men 10 mg of GnRH gives significant increase, and further increase is observed with increase in dose to 150 mcg. The lowest dose evoking FSH release is 100 mcg of GnRH. Peak responses for both LH and FSH occur between 15 and 30 min. Because of the pulsatile secretion of gonadotropins, two baseline values for LH and FSH

TEST NAME AND METHOD	SPECIMEN REQUIREMENTS	REFERENCE INTERVAL, CONVENTIONAL [INTERNATIONAL RECOMMENDED UNITS]	CHEMICAL INTERFERENCES AND IN VIVO EFFECTS
Gonadotropin-Releasing Hormone (GnRH) Test—CONT			
Dose: GnRH, 2.5 mg/kg (100 mg maximum), by rapid IV bolus			

1. Alsever RN, Gotlin RW: *Handbook of endocrine tests in adults and children,* ed 2, Chicago, 1978, Year Book Medical Publishers Inc.
2. Ismail AA: *Biochemical investigations in endocrinology,* London, 1981, Academic Press.
3. Johnson TR, Moore WM, Jefferies JE: *Children are different: developmental physiology,* ed 2, Columbus, OH, 1978, Ross Laboratories.
4. Watts NB, Keffer JH: *Practical endocrinology,* ed 4, Philadelphia, 1989, Lea & Febiger.
5. Endocrine Sciences: *Pediatric laboratory services,* Tarzana, CA, 1992, Endocrine Sciences.
6. Nichols Institute Reference Laboratories: *Test catalog,* San Juan Capistrano, CA, 1993, Nichols Institute Reference Laboratories.

TEST NAME AND METHOD	SPECIMEN REQUIREMENTS	REFERENCE INTERVAL, CONVENTIONAL [INTERNATIONAL RECOMMENDED UNITS]	CHEMICAL INTERFERENCES AND IN VIVO EFFECTS
Granulocyte Antibodies[1,2]	Serum. Store at −20° C.	Negative.	Antibodies with nongranulocyte specificity, e.g., anti-HLA antibodies.
1) Agglutination, using tube, capillary, or microplate formats			
2) Immunofluorescence, using fluorescence microscopy or flow cytometry			
3) Chemiluminescence			

| **DIAGNOSTIC INFORMATION** | **REMARKS** |

are obtained before GnRH administration. Third-generation LH and FSH assays, with sensitivities of 0.01 mU/mL, are recommended for prepubertal GnRH testing.[6]

LH increases 15-30 min after GnRH. Peak LH excretion is slight in prebuteral children (both sexes), increases during puberty, and increases still further in adulthood. However, there is no clear correlation between the stage of puberty and the magnitude of the response to the GnRH. Females usually show a significant variability during the menstrual cycle, with greater stimulation of LH during the luteal phase. Pituitary release of LH is biphasic in prepubertal subjects, suggesting either a second intragonadotrope LH pool that is more slowly mobilized or new LH synthesis during the prolonged infusion. FSH release is greatest in prepubertal females.

Responses to GnRH may be used to monitor treatment of sexual precocity.

| | |

Useful in identifying and monitoring patients previously immunized by transfusions, pregnancies, or allografts.

Can be helpful in confirming the diagnosis in immune-mediated neutropenia, including neonatal alloimmune neutropenia (NAIN),[4] and in transfusion-related acute lung injury (TRALI).[5]

In most granulocyte antibody assays fresh purified granulocytes from normal subjects are used as substrate, which make these tests challenging to perform and therefore limited to special laboratories.

TEST NAME AND METHOD	SPECIMEN REQUIREMENTS	REFERENCE INTERVAL, CONVENTIONAL [INTERNATIONAL RECOMMENDED UNITS]	CHEMICAL INTERFERENCES AND IN VIVO EFFECTS
Granulocyte Antibodies—CONT			
4) Monoclonal antibody-specific immobilization of granulocyte antigen (MAIGA) assay			
Granulocyte Antigens			
Polymerase Chain Reaction-Sequence Specific Primers (PCR-SSP)[3]	Whole blood (EDTA). Transport at 2-6° C. Maternal and paternal samples should preferably be tested concurrently in cases of neonatal alloimmune neutropenia (NAIN).	Not applicable.	PCR inhibition by sample contaminants (heparin, EDTA).

1. Stroncek D: Granulocyte antigens and antibody detection, *Vox Sang* 87(suppl 1):91-94, 2004.

2. Dacie J, Lewis S, editors: *Practical haematology,* ed 8, Edinburgh, 1995, Churchill Livingstone.

3. Hessner MJ, Curtis BR, Endean DJ, et al: Determination of neutrophil antigen NA gene frequencies in five different ethnic groups by polymerase chain reaction with sequence-specific primers, *Transfusion* 36:895-899, 1996.

4. Davoren A, Saving K, McFarland JG, et al: Neonatal neutropenia and bacterial sepsis associated with placental transfer of maternal neutrophil-specific autoantibodies, *Transfusion* 44:1041-1046, 2004.

5. Kleinman S, Caulfield T, Chan P, et al: Toward an understanding of transfusion-related acute lung injury: statement of a consensus panel, *Transfusion* 44:1774-1789, 2004.

6. Davoren A, Curtis BR, et al: TRALI due to granulocyte-agglutinating human neutrophil antigen-3a (5b) alloantibodies in donor plasma: a report of 2 fatalities, *Transfusion* 43:641-645, 2003.

DIAGNOSTIC INFORMATION	REMARKS

Determination of the neutrophil antigen type in babies with NAIN and other patients with immune neutropenia confirms the specificity of the granulocyte antibody.

Parental genotyping is required to assess the risk of NAIN in subsequent pregnancies.

When donor-derived granulocyte antibody is implicated in TRALI, neutrophil antigen typing of the recipient confirms antibody specificity.[6]

Serologic typing of granulocyte antigens has been largely replaced by DNA-based genotyping methods. All neutrophil antigen variants may not be detected by currently available PCR-SSP assays.

Genotyping methods allow the determination of neutrophil antigen type even in severely neutropenic patients.

TEST NAME AND METHOD	SPECIMEN REQUIREMENTS	REFERENCE INTERVAL, CONVENTIONAL [INTERNATIONAL RECOMMENDED UNITS]				CHEMICAL INTERFERENCES AND IN VIVO EFFECTS
Growth Hormone (GH, Soma-tropin)[1-5]	Serum; refrigerate immediately. Patient must be fasting and at complete rest 30 min before test. Avoid stress during collection. EDTA plasma gives lower values with some methods.[6] Stable for 8 hr at 2-8° C or longer at −20° C.		*ng/mL**		*mcg/L*	↑ V β-Adrenergic blockers (e.g., atenolol, metoprolol, propranolol), amphetamines, arginine, baclofen, bromocriptine (transient effect, normals), clonidine (transient), corticotropin, estrogens, glucagon, guanfacine (transient), insulin, levodopa, methylphenidate, metoclopramide, metyrapone (large doses, e.g., 6 g), nalorphine, nicotinic acid (IV), oral contraceptives, oxprenolol, vasopressin
		Cord blood:	8-41	× 1.0	[8-41]	
		0-7 yr[8]	1-13.6		[1-13.6]	
		7-11 yr	1-16.4		[1-16.4]	
RIA		11-15 yr	1-14.4		[1-14.4]	
		15-19 yr	1-13.4		[1-13.4]	
		Adult				
		M[3]:	0-4		[0-4]	
		F:	0-18		[0-18]	
		>60 yr				
		M:	1-9		[1-9]	
		F:	1-16		[1-16]	

*Calibrated against the World Health Organization First International Reference Preparation for GH, 66/217.

↓ V Bromocriptine (acromegaly), corticosteroids, glucose, phenothiazines, pirenzepine, probucol

Amniotic fluid[7]	20 wk, x̄:	10 ng/mL	× 1.0	[10 mcg/L]
	Term, x̄:	30 ng/mL		[30 mcg/L]

1. Baumann G: Growth hormone binding proteins and various forms of growth hormone: implications for measurements, *Acta Paediatr Scand* 370(suppl):72-80, 1990.

2. Rudd B: Growth, growth hormone and the somatomedins: an historical perspective and current concepts, *Ann Clin Biochem* 28:542-555, 1991.

3. Smith C, Norman M: Prolactin and growth hormone: molecular heterogeneity and measurement in serum, *Ann Clin Biochem* 27:542-550, 1990.

4. Underwood LE, editor: *Human growth hormone: progress and challenges,* New York, 1988, Marcel Dekker, Inc.

5. Whitley RJ, Meikle AW, Watts NB: Endocrinology. In Burtis CA, Ashwood ER, editors: *Tietz textbook of clinical chemistry,* ed 2, Philadelphia, 1994, WB Saunders.

6. Bauman JE: Comparison of radioimmunoassay results in serum and plasma, *Clin Chem* 26:676-677, 1980.

7. Tulchinsky D, Ryan KJ, editors: *Maternal-fetal endocrinology,* Philadelphia, 1980, WB Saunders.

DIAGNOSTIC INFORMATION	REMARKS

S ↑ Pituitary gigantism, acromegaly (to 400 ng/mL [400 mcg/L]), Laron dwarfism (defective GH receptor), ectopic GH secretion (neoplasms of stomach, lung), malnutrition, renal failure, cirrhosis, stress, exercise, prolonged fasting, uncontrolled diabetes mellitus, anorexia nervosa

S ↓ Pituitary dwarfism, hypopituitarism, adrenocortical hyperfunction

Secretion of GH is episodic and pulsatile; transient levels up to 40 ng/mL [40 mcg/L] have been observed in healthy subjects. Highest values occur during periods of deepest sleep. In acromegaly and gigantism, rhythmicity is lost. Test is also useful for evaluating the efficacy of acromegaly treatment. In obesity, release of GH is reduced, and response of GH to insulin, arginine, sleep, or exercise may be impaired. Ability to secrete GH in response to a conventional challenge declines with age.[9]

Random levels of GH provide little diagnostic information; GH secretion is best assessed during tests that stimulate or suppress release. Patients with acromegaly, for example, have subnormal GH responses to glucose load. (See *Growth Hormone Suppression Test [after Glucose]*.) Patients with GH-producing pituitary tumors often release GH in response to TRH or GnRH, and patients with suspected GH deficiencies have subnormal responses to stimulation tests. (See *Growth Hormone Suppression Test [after Arginine], Growth Hormone Suppression Test [after Insulin], Growth Hormone Suppression Test [after L-Dopa], Growth Hormone Suppression Test [after Glucagon and Propranolol],* and *Insulin Tolerance Test.*) Continuous or intermittent GH sampling over a 24-hr period, however, has been used to identify partial GH deficiency overlooked with stimulation tests; such procedures are laborious and expensive.

The presence of GH variants in serum often leads to discrepancies among the results given by different immunoassay systems. To prevent misdiagnosis, reference values for GH and cutoff values for GH stimulation tests should be established separately for each method proposed for routine use.[10,11]

AF ↓ Anencephalic fetus

The progressive increase of GH levels in amniotic fluid correlates well with both increased pituitary content and fetal serum concentration of GH and contrasts with the lack of change in maternal serum GH throughout gestation.

8. Soldin OP, Hoffman EG, Waring MA, et al: Pediatric reference ntervals for FSH, LH, estradiol, T3, free T3, cortisol and growth hormone on the DPC Immulite 1000, *Clin Chim Acta* 355:205-210, 2005.

9. Davis PJ: Aging and endocrine function, *Clin Endocrinol Metab* 8:603-619, 1979.

10. Banfi G, Marinelli M, Casari E, et al: Isotopic and nonisotopic assays for measuring somatotropin compared: re-evaluation of cut off values in provocative tests, *Clin Chem* 37:273-276, 1991.

11. Reiter E, Morris A, MacGilivray M, et al: Variable estimates of serum growth hormone concentrations by different radioassay systems, *J Clin Endocrinol Metab* 66:68-71, 1988.

TEST NAME AND METHOD	SPECIMEN REQUIREMENTS	REFERENCE INTERVAL, CONVENTIONAL [INTERNATIONAL RECOMMENDED UNITS]			CHEMICAL INTERFERENCES AND IN VIVO EFFECTS
Growth Hormone Releasing Hormone (GHRH, Somatocrinin)[1-4] *RIA*	Plasma (heparin). Separate immediately, and freeze at −20° C.	<50 pg/mL[4]	× 1.0	[<50 ng/L]	None found.

1. Frohman LA, Jansson JO: Growth hormone-releasing hormone, *Endocr Rev* 7:223-253, 1986.
2. Thorner MO, Frohman LA, Leong DA, et al: Extrahypothalamic growth hormone-releasing factor (GRF) is a rare cause of acromegaly: plasma GRF levels in 177 acromegalic patients, *J Clin Endocrinol Metab* 59:846-849, 1984.
3. Vance ML, Thorner MO: Some clinical considerations of growth hormone and growth hormone-releasing hormone. In Martini L, Ganong WF, editors: *Frontiers in neuroendocrinology, vol 10,* New York, 1988, Raven Press.
4. Nichols Institute Reference Laboratories: *Test catalog,* San Juan Capistrano, CA, 1993, Nichols Institute Reference Laboratories.

TEST NAME AND METHOD	SPECIMEN REQUIREMENTS	REFERENCE INTERVAL, CONVENTIONAL [INTERNATIONAL RECOMMENDED UNITS]			CHEMICAL INTERFERENCES AND IN VIVO EFFECTS
Growth Hormone Stimulation Test (after Arginine)[1-3] Dose: Arginine HCl, IV, 0.5 g/kg over 30 min	Serum, fasting. Draw baseline and 30, 60, and 90 min after infusion has been started.	Growth hormone Baseline: After arginine Increase above baseline: Peak response:	*ng/mL* <5 >5 >10	*mcg/L* × 1.0 [<5] [>5] [>10]	See *Growth Hormone.*

1. Miller RE, Ngai B: *Manual of endocrine diagnostic tests,* ed 4, Lexington, KY, 1991, Department of Medicine, University of Kentucky.
2. Watts NB, Keffer JH: *Practical endocrinology,* ed 4, Philadelphia, 1989, Lea & Febiger.
3. Whitley RJ, Meikle AW, Watts NB: Endocrinology. In Burtis CA, Ashwood ER, editors: *Tietz textbook of clinical chemistry,* ed 2, Philadelphia, 1994, WB Saunders.

DIAGNOSTIC INFORMATION	REMARKS

↑ Acromegaly caused by GHRH secretion by neoplasms (e.g., pancreatic islet tumors, bronchial or thymic carcinoid tumors, neuroendocrine tumors) | GHRH is produced by the hypothalamus and stimulates the release of GH from the pituitary. Hypersecretion of GHRH is a rare cause of acromegaly. Excessive production of GHRH may be caused by a hypothalamic tumor, or more commonly, by peripheral tumors. Chronic stimulation of the pituitary by GHRH causes pituitary hyperplasia, which cannot be distinguished from a GH-secreting pituitary tumor by imaging techniques. Circulating levels of GHRH are useful in differentiating between a pituitary tumor and ectopic GHRH hypersecretion. |

Hypopituitarism, no response (all levels <5 ng/mL [<5 mcg/L]) | Arginine HCl should be given with caution to patients with severe liver or renal disease and acidosis. If the fasting GH level is >5 ng/mL [>5 mcg/L], no increase may be seen. Release of GH is augmented in normal male subjects by pretreatment with diethylstilbestrol, 2.5 mg, twice a day for 2 days. The main advantage of this test is the absence of significant side effects. A subnormal response should be confirmed by performing another provocative test (e.g., stimulation with insulin, glucagon, clonidine, or L-dopa) because ~20% of healthy individuals may not respond to arginine.

For initial testing of GH deficiency, a vigorous exercise test is considered by many investigators to be a simple, relatively risk-free stimulus for assessing GH reserve, particularly in children. However, much controversy surrounds the use of all GH stimulation tests, and a diagnosis of GH deficiency must be considered in the context of the clinical picture. |

TEST NAME AND METHOD	SPECIMEN REQUIREMENTS	REFERENCE INTERVAL, CONVENTIONAL [INTERNATIONAL RECOMMENDED UNITS]				CHEMICAL INTERFERENCES AND IN VIVO EFFECTS
Growth Hormone Stimulation Test (after Glucagon and Propranolol)[1-3]	Serum for GH baseline at 9:00 AM (before glucagon), 11:00 AM, and 12:00 PM.	After glucagon, Growth hormone,	*ng/mL*		*mcg/L*	See *Growth Hormone.*
		Increase above baseline:	>5	× 1.0	[>5]	
		Peak response:	>10		[>10]	
Dose, adult: 0.75 mg/kg propranolol, orally, at 7:00 AM (fast from midnight); 0.03 mg/kg glucagon, IM, at 9:00 AM.						

1. Abboud CF, Laws ER Jr: Clinical endocrinological approach to hypothalamic-pituitary disease, *J Neurosurg* 51:271-291, 1979.
2. Miller RE, Ngai B: *Manual of endocrine diagnostic tests,* ed 4, Lexington, KY, 1991, Department of Medicine, University of Kentucky.
3. Whitley RJ, Meikle AW, Watts NB: Endocrinology. In Burtis CA, Ashwood ER, editors: *Tietz textbook of clinical chemistry,* ed 2, Philadelphia, 1994, WB Saunders.

TEST NAME AND METHOD	SPECIMEN REQUIREMENTS	REFERENCE INTERVAL, CONVENTIONAL [INTERNATIONAL RECOMMENDED UNITS]				CHEMICAL INTERFERENCES AND IN VIVO EFFECTS
Growth Hormone Stimulation Test (after Insulin)[1-4]	Serum, fasting. Draw at 30, 60, and 90 min through an indwelling needle.	After insulin: Glucose				Values are reduced by cyproheptadine, methysergide, and phentolamine; they are augmented by propranolol. See also *Growth Hormone.*
		Decrease: <50% of baseline [<0.5 fraction] and <40 mg/dL × 0.0555 [<2.2 mmol/L]				
Dose, adult: Regular insulin, 0.1-0.15 U/kg, IV. When hypopituitarism is strongly suspected, a dose of 0.05 U/kg should be used.			*ng/mL*		*mcg/L*	
		Growth hormone				
		Increase above baseline:	>5	× 1.0	[>5]	
		Peak response:	>10		[>10]	
			mcg/dL		*µmol/L*	
		Cortisol				
Child: 0.05 U/kg		Increase above baseline:	>7	× 0.0276	[>0.19]	
		Peak response:	>20		[>0.55]	

DIAGNOSTIC INFORMATION	REMARKS

Hypopituitarism: No response or inadequate response (all levels <5 ng/mL [<5 mcg/L])

Test is contraindicated in heart disease, bronchial asthma, and diabetes mellitus. Glucagon is not a potent stimulus for GH release, and although propranolol augments the response, other stimulation tests are often preferred (e.g., with arginine, L-dopa, insulin, or clonidine).

No response or inadequate response is seen in hypothalamic or anterior pituitary dysfunction (e.g., growth hormone and ACTH deficiencies).

Blood glucose level must fall below 40 mg/dL [2.2 mmol/L] and/or adrenergic signs must be observed. If such criteria are not met within 45 min to 1 hr after insulin, a repeat dose should be given. Risks are severe hypoglycemia with seizures, cardiac arrhythmias, and coma. A solution of 50% dextrose for IV administration should be available. Patients with resistance to insulin (e.g., those who have Cushing's syndrome, diabetes, obesity, or acromegaly) may require a higher dose of insulin (0.15-0.3 U/kg) for this test.

For initial testing of growth hormone deficiency, a vigorous exercise test is considered by many investigators to be a simple, relatively risk-free stimulus for assessing GH reserve, particularly in children. For subsequent testing, a subnormal GH response to insulin-induced hypoglycemia should be confirmed by performing another provocative test (e.g., stimulation with glucagons, L-dopa, arginine, or clonidine) because ~20% of healthy individuals may not respond to insulin. Much controversy surrounds the use of all GH stimulation tests, and a diagnosis of GH deficiency must be considered in the context of the clinical picture.

TEST NAME AND METHOD	SPECIMEN REQUIREMENTS	REFERENCE INTERVAL, CONVENTIONAL [INTERNATIONAL RECOMMENDED UNITS]				CHEMICAL INTERFERENCES AND IN VIVO EFFECTS

Growth Hormone Stimulation Test (after Insulin)—CONT

1. Abboud CF, Laws ER Jr: Clinical endocrinological approach to hypothalamic-pituitary disease, *J Neurosurg* 51:271-291, 1979.
2. Miller RE, Ngai B: *Manual of endocrine diagnostic tests,* ed 4, Lexington, KY, 1991, Department of Medicine, University of Kentucky.
3. Watts NB, Keffer JH: *Practical endocrinology,* ed 4, Philadelphia, 1989, Lea & Febiger.
4. Whitley RJ, Meikle AW, Watts NB: Endocrinology. In Burtis CA, Ashwood ER, editors: *Tietz textbook of clinical chemistry,* ed 2, Philadelphia, 1994, WB Saunders.

TEST NAME AND METHOD	SPECIMEN REQUIREMENTS	REFERENCE INTERVAL, CONVENTIONAL [INTERNATIONAL RECOMMENDED UNITS]				CHEMICAL INTERFERENCES AND IN VIVO EFFECTS
Growth Hormone Stimulation Test (after L-Dopa)[1-4] Dose, adult: 500 mg L-dopa, orally. Child: 10 mg/kg	Serum, fasting from midnight. Draw baseline and 30, 60, 90, and 120 min after L-dopa. Keep patient at rest.	Growth hormone after L-dopa Increase above baseline: Peak response (at 90 min):	*ng/mL* >5 >10	× 1.0	*mcg/L* [>5] [>10]	Release is inhibited by phenothiazines and TRH. See also *Growth Hormone.*

1. Abboud CF, Laws ER Jr: Clinical endocrinological approach to hypothalamic-pituitary disease, *J Neurosurg* 51:271-291, 1979.
2. Miller RE, Ngai B: *Manual of endocrine diagnostic tests,* ed 4, Lexington, KY, 1991, Department of Medicine, University of Kentucky.
3. Watts NB, Keffer JH: *Practical endocrinology,* ed 4, Philadelphia, 1989, Lea & Febiger.
4. Whitley RJ, Meikle AW, Watts NB: Endocrinology. In Burtis CA, Ashwood ER, editors: *Tietz textbook of clinical chemistry,* ed 2, Philadelphia, 1994, WB Saunders.

DIAGNOSTIC INFORMATION	REMARKS

This test should not be performed if primary adrenal insufficiency is likely because an adrenal crisis may be precipitated.

See *Insulin Tolerance Test.*

Hypopituitarism: No response (all levels <5 ng/mL [<5 mcg/L])

Patients should be tested while fasting; a negative response is obtained if blood glucose levels are >120 mg/dL [× 0.0555 = 6.7 mmol/L].

Risks are vertigo and nausea during the first 30 min of the test. If results are abnormal, other provocative tests with insulin, arginine, glucagon, or clonidine are indicated because ~20% of normal subjects may not respond to L-dopa. A paradoxical decrease in GH may be observed in acromegaly. Tolerance to the test dose of L-dopa may be improved by giving 250 mg L-dopa orally with meals 3 times a day for 2 days before the test and by giving the 500-mg test dose with food.

TEST NAME AND METHOD	SPECIMEN REQUIREMENTS	REFERENCE INTERVAL, CONVENTIONAL [INTERNATIONAL RECOMMENDED UNITS]	CHEMICAL INTERFERENCES AND IN VIVO EFFECTS
Growth Hormone Suppression Test (after Glucose)[1-3] Dose: 100 g or 1.75 g glucose/kg orally after overnight fast.	Serum, fasting. Draw baseline and 60 and 120 min after glucose load.	Growth hormone after glucose Suppression to <2 ng/mL or undetectable levels $\times 1.0$ [<2 mcg/L]	See *Growth Hormone*.

1. Miller RE, Ngai B: *Manual of endocrine diagnostic tests,* ed 4, Lexington, KY, 1991, Department of Medicine, University of Kentucky.
2. Watts NB, Keffer JH: *Practical endocrinology,* ed 4, Philadelphia, 1989, Lea & Febiger.
3. Whitley RJ, Meikle AW, Watts NB: Endocrinology. In Burtis CA, Ashwood ER, editors: *Tietz textbook of clinical chemistry,* ed 2, Philadelphia, 1994, WB Saunders.

Guanine Deaminase (Guanase; EC 3.5.4.3)[1,2] *Colorimetric (guanine), 37° C*[1]	Serum. Stable at room temperature for 6 hr, at 4° C for 1 wk, and at −15° C for 6 mo.	Generally, very low to undetectable activity <3 U/L $\times 0.017$ [<0.05 µKat/L]	S ↑ V Drugs causing acute hepatocellular damage. See Table II-5.

Colorimetric (8-azaguanine), 37° C[3]		U/L	µKat/L
		M: 1.2 ± 0.8 $\times 0.017$	[0.02 ± 0.01]
		F: 1.2 ± 0.7	[0.02 ± 0.01]

Kinetic (guanine), 30° C	0-1.02 U/L[5]	[0.00-0.02 µKat/L]
	0.4-1.8 U/L (mean $\pm$ 2 SD)[6]	[0.01-0.03 µKat/L]

Radiometric (14° C), 37° C[4]	Adult: <0.74 U

1. Henry RJ, Cannon DC, Winkelman JW, editors: *Clinical chemistry: principles and technics,* ed 2, Hagerstown, MD, 1974, Harper and Row.
2. Ellis G, Goldberg DM: Assay of human serum and liver guanase activity with 8-aza-guanine as substrate, *Clin Chim Acta* 37:47-52, 1972.
3. Ito S, Takaota T, Mori H, et al: A sensitive new method for measurement of guanase with 8-azaguanine in bicine bis-hydroxy ethyl glycine buffer as substrate, *Clin Chim Acta* 115:135-144, 1981.
4. Kuzmits R, Seyfried H, Wolf A, et al: Evaluation of serum guanase in hepatic diseases, *Enzyme* 25:148-152, 1980.
5. Nishikawa Y, Fukumoto K: Kinetic measurement of guanine deaminase in serum with a centrifugal analyzer, *Clin Chem* 27:560-561, 1981.
6. Yasminch WG: Simple ultraviolet spectrophotometric method for the determination of serum guanase activists, *Clin Biochem* 21:239-243, 1988.

There is no or incomplete suppression from the high basal level in gigantism or acromegaly. Subjects with acromegaly typically have baseline values >10 ng/mL [>10 mcg/L].

Paradoxical increases of GH are possible in patients with acromegaly. Subjects with liver disease, uremia, or heroin addiction may fail to suppress. Partial suppression is sometimes seen in patients with anorexia nervosa.

↑ Viral hepatitis, extrahepatic obstructive jaundice, metastatic hepatic disease, heavy metal toxicity with hepatic or cerebral damage

Increased half-life in shock is inversely correlated with survival.[5] Guanine deaminase is relatively specific for liver disease.[7]

This enzyme is used in Japan to screen donor blood units with levels >3.6 U/L rejected for transfusion.[8] With introduction of such use, incidence of posttransfusion hepatitis decreased from 17% to 7%.[9,10]

7. Tanaka K, Ichihara A: Clinical value of the determination of serum guanase activity. Studies on patients and experimental data from mongrel dogs and cultured rat hepatocytes, *Gasteroenterology* 83:1102-1108, 1981.

8. Ito S, Yasuhiro T, Iwasake A, et al: Relationship between guanase activity in donor blood and the incidence of posttransfusional non-A, non-B hepatitis, and a possible method for preventing posttransfusional hepatitis, *Hepatology* 6:990-993, 1986.

9. Ito S, Kitagawa N, Akihiko I, et al: Clinical value of the guanase screening test in donor blood for prevention of posttransfusional non-A, non-B hepatitis, *Hepatology* 8:383-384, 1988.

10. Ito S, Takaota T, Mori H, et al: A sensitive new method for measurement of guanase with 8-azaguanine in bicine bishydroxy ethyl glycine buffer as substrate, *Clin Chim Acta* 115:135-144, 1981.

TEST NAME AND METHOD	SPECIMEN REQUIREMENTS	REFERENCE INTERVAL, CONVENTIONAL [INTERNATIONAL RECOMMENDED UNITS]			CHEMICAL INTERFERENCES AND IN VIVO EFFECTS
Haptoglobin (Hp, HPT, Hemoglobin-binding Protein)[1-3]	Serum. Avoid hemolysis. Stable 2 wk at $-20°$ C.		mg/dL^1	mg/L	S $\uparrow$ V Androgens (anabolic steroids)
		Newborn:	5-48 $\times 10$	[50-480]	
		Adult:	26-185	[260-1850]	
		>60 yr:			S $\downarrow$ V Agents causing
Nephelometric		M:	35-164	[350-1640]	hemolytic anemia (e.g.,
		F:	40-175	[400-1750]	dapsone, methyldopa, sulfasalazine) estrogens, oral contraceptives, tamoxifen

The average HP concentrations obtained from the serum of healthy individuals shows considerable interlaboratory variation.[3]

Excessive turbidity can affect nephelometric methods.

1. Tietz NW, editor: *Textbook of clinical chemistry,* Philadelphia, 1999, WB Saunders.
2. Putnam FW, editor: *The plasma proteins: structure, functions and genetic control, vol 1-3,* ed 2, New York, 1977, Academic Press.
3. Dobryszcka W: Biological functions of haptoglobin—new pieces to an old puzzle, *Eur J Clin Chem Biochem* 35:647-654, 1997.

DIAGNOSTIC INFORMATION	REMARKS

↑ Inflammation, infection, tissue injury, trauma, major depressive episodes, malignancies.[3]

↓ Hepatic dysfunction, any cause of hemolysis, including autoimmune, mechanical (artificial heart valves, hypersplenism), transfusion reactions, hemoglobinopathies (sickle cell, hemoglobin C, thalassemias).[3] Can also be decreased with ineffective erythropoiesis, disaggregation of internal hematomas,[3] red cell membrane or metabolic defects (G6PD deficiency, hereditary spherocytosis, paroxysmal nocturnal hemoglobinuria).

Haptoglobin (Hp) is a positive acute phase reacting protein (APR), which covalently binds free hemoglobin. The subsequent haptoglobin-hemoglobin complexes are quickly cleared from circulation by the reticuloendothelial system, allowing recycling of iron. Consequently, rapid decreases in HP concentrations are a sensitive marker of hemolysis. In patients experiencing both hemolysis and an acute phase response, which can complicate interpretation of HP values, HP levels frequently decrease faster than the simultaneous acute phase increase. Assessment of other APRs within the specimen that are not affected by hemolysis should be helpful in these cases. HP is found in nearly all body fluids. Synthesis is not confined to the liver but also takes place in the adipose tissue and lung, where it serves in an antimicrobial and antioxidant capacity. By complexing with hemoglobin, the generation of lipid peroxide and hydroxyl radical promoted by hemoglobin in sites of inflammation are avoided.[3] Evidence suggests that HP promotes angiogenesis and cholesterol crystallization.[3]

Three main phenotypes of haptoglobin are known, Hp 1-1, 2-1, and 2-2. Hp 1-1 circulates as a monomer, and 2-1 and 2-2 are polymers. Ahaptoglobimemia is not typically associated with any clinical manifestations and is frequently noted in neonates and infants (up to the age of 3 mo).[3]

Indications for quantitation include evaluation for suspected hemolysis, pregnancy-associated hypertension,[2] transfusion reactions (comparison of pretransfusion and posttransfusion results), assessing disease status. Interpretation of Hp values should be performed with regard to the overall clinical findings, given that many factors affect results. Subtyping has been useful for forensic and paternity testing purposes.[3]

MW, Type 1-1:	85,000-100,000
Type 2-1:	86,018 plus polymers
Type 2-2:	>200,000 (multiple polymers)

$t_{1/2}$: 2 days

TEST NAME AND METHOD	SPECIMEN REQUIREMENTS	REFERENCE INTERVAL, CONVENTIONAL [INTERNATIONAL RECOMMENDED UNITS]	CHEMICAL INTERFERENCES AND IN VIVO EFFECTS
Heinz Body Preparation[1,2] *Phase contrast microscopy or supravital stain (methyl violet or crystal violet)*	Whole blood (heparin, EDTA, or citrate)	Negative Heinz bodies are not present in normal blood except in a few cells in some newborn infants or in splenectomized individuals.	↑ V Oxidant drugs in sufficient dosage may cause Heinz bodies and hemolysis in healthy individuals. These include aminosalicylic acid, aniline, chlorates, dapsone, hydroxylamine, naphthalene, nitrobenzene, nitrofurantoin, phenacetin, phenol derivatives, phenylhydrazine, phenylsemicarbazide, resorcin, salicylazosulfidine, sodium sulfoxone, sulfamethoxypyridine, sulfonamides, and sulfones.

1. Dacie JV, Lewis SM: *Practical haematology,* ed 8, Edinburgh, 1995, Churchill Livingstone.
2. Williams WJ, Beutler E, Erslev AJ, et al, editors: *Hematology,* ed 4, New York, 1990, McGraw-Hill Publishing Co.

TEST NAME AND METHOD	SPECIMEN REQUIREMENTS	REFERENCE INTERVAL, CONVENTIONAL [INTERNATIONAL RECOMMENDED UNITS]			CHEMICAL INTERFERENCES AND IN VIVO EFFECTS
Hematocrit (HCT, Hct)[1-4] *Calculation from MCV and Ercs (electronic counters)*	Whole blood (EDTA). Stable 48 hr at 4° C, 6 hr at 23° C. Fetal blood. Collect by percutaneous umbilical blood sampling (PUBS).		*%Packed Ercs volume (V Ercs/V whole blood × 100)*	*Volume fraction (V Ercs/V whole blood)*	↓ C Drugs that cause aplastic anemia or that cause hemolysis in G6PD deficiency or by an immune mechanism (specific agents listed in Table II-4).
		Fetal[5]			
		18-20 wk:	35.86 ± 3.29 (SD) × 0.01	[0.36 ± 0.03]	
		21-22 wk:	38.53 ± 3.21	[0.39 ± 0.03]	
		23-25 wk:	38.59 ± 2.41	[0.39 ± 0.02]	
		26-30 wk:	41.54 ± 3.31	[0.42 ± 0.03]	↓ V Cold agglutinins can falsely decrease calculated HCT. Low plasma proteins will falsely decrease HCT measured by conductivity.
Conductivity of whole blood (Point of Care analyzers)			*%Packed Ercs volume (V Ercs/V whole blood × 100)*	*Volume fraction (V Ercs/V whole blood)*	
		Cord blood[6]:	42-60 × 0.01	[0.42-0.60]	↑ V Increased WBC will falsely increase HCT measured by conductivity.
		0.5 mo[7]:	41-65	[0.41-0.65]	
		1 mo:	33-55	[0.33-0.55]	
		2 mo:	28-42	[0.28-0.42]	
		4 mo:	32-44	[0.32-0.44]	
		6 mo:	31-41	[0.31-0.41]	
		9 mo:	32-40	[0.32-0.40]	
		12 mo:	33-41	[0.33-0.41]	
		1-2 yr[8]:	32-40	[0.32-0.40]	
			(95% range)		
		3-5 yr:	32-42	[0.32-0.42]	

↑ In G6PD deficiency and other enzyme deficiencies of hexose monophosphate shunt, Heinz bodies and hemolysis may be caused by lower doses of the oxidant drugs listed under *Interferences* and by designated drugs in Table II-4.

↑ Unstable hemoglobin disorders (congenital Heinz body anemia), after splenectomy, or when challenged with oxidant drugs.

↑ Homozygous β-thalassemia

Heinz bodies are precipitated hemoglobin, either oxidatively denatured or inherently unstable. They are usually invisible on Wright's stained, air-dried films.

Visualization requires phase microscopy or supravital staining. With methyl violet or crystal violet, Heinz bodies stain purple and the precipitated RNA in the reticulocytes does not stain. In reticulocyte preparations utilizing brilliant cresyl blue or new methylene blue, Heinz bodies stain pale blue, and the precipitated RNA in the reticulocytes stains purple. Heinz bodies tend to adhere to the erythrocyte membrane.

↑ Polycythemia, extreme physical exercise or excitement, hemoconcentration, high altitude

↓ Anemia, recumbency

A calculated HCT is ~2% lower than a microhematocrit resulting from trapped plasma in a centrifuged column of erythrocytes. Healthy pregnant women usually have slightly lower hematocrit than do nonpregnant women. HCT is ~2% lower in deoxygenated than in fully oxygenated blood. Immediately after blood loss or transfusion, the HCT is not a reliable estimate of anemia.

Hb, HCT, and erythrocytes (RBCs) are slightly lower between 5:00 PM and 7:00 AM and after meals (up to 10% lower); they are up to 5.7% lower if drawn from a recumbent patient. Falsely high results may occur because of prolonged venous stasis during venipuncture. A slight but significant decrease occurs in the lower reference limit of Hb, HCT, and erythrocytes (RBCs) in men aged 65-74 yr. There is no significant change in men or women over age 85 yr compared with ages 65-74 yr.[10]

TEST NAME AND METHOD	SPECIMEN REQUIREMENTS	REFERENCE INTERVAL, CONVENTIONAL [INTERNATIONAL RECOMMENDED UNITS]		CHEMICAL INTERFERENCES AND IN VIVO EFFECTS
Hematocrit—CONT				
		6-8 yr:	33-41	[0.33-0.41]
		9-11 yr:	34-43	[0.34-0.43]
		12 -14 yr		
		M:	35-45	[0.35-0.45]
		F:	34-44	[0.34-0.44]
		15-17 yr		
		M:	37-48	[0.37-0.48]
		F:	34-44	[0.34-0.44]
		18-44 yr		
		M:	39-49	[0.39-0.49]
		F:	35-45	[0.35-0.45]
		45-64 yr		
		M:	39-50	[0.39-0.50]
		F:	35-47	[0.35-0.47]
		65-74 yr		
		M:	37-51	[0.37-0.51]
		F:	35-47	[0.35-0.47]
Centrifugation (microhematocrit)	Capillary whole blood (heparin)	*%Packed Ercs volume (V Ercs/V whole blood × 100)*[9]	*Volume fraction (V Ercs/V whole blood)*	↑ V Sickle cell anemia and other disorders with decreased red cell deformability
		1 day: 61 ± 7.41 (SD)	[0.61 ± 0.07]	
		4 days: 57 ± 8.1	[0.57 ± 0.08]	↓ C Excess anticoagulant
		7 days: 56 ± 9.4	[0.56 ± 0.09]	(cell shrinkage)
		1-2 wk: 54 ± 8.3	[0.54 ± 0.08]	
		3-4 wk: 43 ± 5.7	[0.43 ± 0.06]	
		5-6 wk: 36 ± 6.2	[0.36 ± 0.06]	
		7-8 wk: 33 ± 3.7	[0.33 ± 0.04]	
		9-10 wk: 32 ± 2.7	[0.32 ± 0.03]	
		11-12 wk: 33 ± 3.3	[0.33 ± 0.03]	

1. Henry JB, editor: *Clinical diagnosis and management by laboratory methods,* ed 20, Philadelphia, 2001, WB Saunders.

2. Green JP, Foerster J, Lukens JN: *Wintrobe's clinical hematology,* ed 11, Philadelphia, 2003, Lippincott, Williams & Wilkins.

3. Beutler E, Lichtman MA, Coller B, editors: *Williams hematology,* ed 6, New York, 2000, McGraw-Hill.

4. Rodak BF, editor: *Hematology; clinical principles and applications,* ed 2, Philadelphia, 2002, WB Saunders.

5. Forestier F, Daffos F, Galacteros F, et al: Hematologic values of 163 normal fetuses between 18 and 30 weeks of gestation, *Pediatr Res* 20:342-346, 1986.

6. Nathan DG, Orkin SH, Ginsburg D, et al: *Hematology of infancy and childhood,* ed 6, Philadelphia, 2003, WB Saunders.

7. Saarinen UM, Siimes MA: Development changes in red blood cell counts and indices of infants after exclusion of iron deficiency by laboratory criteria and continuous iron supplementation, *J Pediatr* 92:412-416, 1978.

8. Yip R, Johnson C, Dallman PR: Age-related changes in laboratory values used in the diagnosis of anemia and iron deficiency, *Am J Clin Nutr* 39:427-436, 1984.

9. Matoth Y, Zaizon R, Varsano I: Postnatal changes in some red cell parameters, *Acta Paediatr Scand* 60:317-323, 1971.

10. Zauber NP, Zauber AG: Hematologic data of healthy very old people, *JAMA* 257:2181-2184, 1987.

DIAGNOSTIC INFORMATION

REMARKS

TEST NAME AND METHOD	SPECIMEN REQUIREMENTS	REFERENCE INTERVAL, CONVENTIONAL [INTERNATIONAL RECOMMENDED UNITS]			CHEMICAL INTERFERENCES AND IN VIVO EFFECTS
Hemoglobin, Bart's (Hb Bart's, $\gamma 4$)[1,2]	Hemolysate prepared from whole blood (EDTA, citrate, or heparin). Use fresh or keep at 4° C.	*% of total Hb* Newborn: <0.5 (disappears during the first few months of life)	× 0.01	*Mass fraction of total Hb* [<0.005]	None found.
Cellulose acetate or agarose gel EP, pH 8.6		Child and adult: None present			
Cellulose acetate or agarose gel EP, pH 6.5-7.0					
HPLC (cation exchange, CM-52)[3-5]					

1. Fairbanks VP: *Hemoglobinopathies and thalassemias: laboratory methods and case studies,* New York, 1980, Thieme-Stratton, Inc.
2. Weatherall DJ, Clegg JB: *The thalassaemic syndromes,* ed 3, Oxford, 1981, Blackwell Scientific Publications.
3. Abraham E, Abraham A, Stallings M: High-pressure liquid chromatographic separation of glycosylated and acetylated minor hemoglobins in newborn infants and in patients with sickle cell disease, *J Lab Clin Med* 104:1027-1034, 1984.
4. Van der Dijs FPL, van den Berg GA, Schermer JG, et al: Screening cord blood for hemoglobinopathies and thalassemia by HPLC, *Clin Chem* 38:1864-1869, 1992.
5. Fucharoen S, Winichagoon P, Wisedpanichkij R, et al: Prenatal and postnatal diagnoses of thalassemias and hemoglobinopathies by HPLC, *Clin Chem* 44:740-748, 1998.

TEST NAME AND METHOD	SPECIMEN REQUIREMENTS	REFERENCE INTERVAL, CONVENTIONAL [INTERNATIONAL RECOMMENDED UNITS]			CHEMICAL INTERFERENCES AND IN VIVO EFFECTS
Hemoglobin (Hb) Electrophoresis[1-4]	Hemolysate prepared from whole blood (EDTA, citrate, or heparin). Use fresh or refrigerated at 4° C.	*% Hemoglobin* Hb A: >95 Hb A_2: 1.5-3.7 Hb F: <2	× 0.01	*Hb fraction* [>0.95] [0.015-0.037] [<0.02]	Blood transfusions may obscure or dilute abnormal Hb for 3-4 mo.
		For newborns and infants, see *Fetal Hemoglobin.*			
Cellulose acetate or agarose gel EP, pH 8.4-8.6					
Citrate agar gel EP, pH 6.0-6.5					

DIAGNOSTIC INFORMATION	REMARKS

↑ α-*Thalassemia (α-thal) syndromes, Hb Bart's measured in cord blood:* 100% [1.00] in Hb Bart's hydrops fetalis syndrome (homozygous α°-thal, deletion of 4 α-genes); 19-27% [0.19-0.27] in Hb H disease (double heterozygosity for α°-thal and α⁺-thal, deletion of 3 α-genes); 3-6% [0.03-0.06] in α-thalassemia minor (homozygous α⁺-thal or heterozygous α°-thal, deletion of 2 α-genes); 1-3% [0.01-0.02] in the silent carrier state (heterozygous α⁺-thal, deletion of 1 α-gene).

The levels of Hb Bart's in cord blood as given correspond only approximately to proposed genotypes of α-thalassemia. It is not possible to predict the genotype from the level of Hb Bart's in cord blood.

There is considerable overlap in the levels of Hb Bart's in cord blood in the various α-thalassemia syndromes, especially in different populations.

Cellulose acetate at pH 8.6 is a screening procedure; at alkaline pH, Hb Bart's migrates anodally to Hb A, between Hb A and Hb H.

This is the best method for demonstrating small amounts. At acid pH, Hb Bart's migrates cathodally (with Hb F) and Hb H migrates cathodally (with Hb A).

This technique allows rapid quantitation of Hb Bart's on small sample size.

↑ Hb S,
  A>S: Sickle trait (Hb AS), sickle-α-thalassemia
  S, F, no A: Sickle cell anemia, sickle-β°-thalassemia, sickle- δβ°-thalassemia, sickle-HPFH
  S>A, F: Sickle-β⁺-thalassemia

Several hemoglobin variants migrate like S on cellulose acetate at pH 8.6 (D and G, most common), but of these only Hb S gives a positive sickling or solubility test. Iron deficiency or α-thalassemia may decrease the relative proportions of hemoglobins S, C, and A₂.

↑ Hb C,
  A>C: Hb C trait (Hb AC)
  C, F, no A: Hb C disease, Hb C-β°-thalassemia, Hb C- δβ°-thalassemia, Hb C-HPFH
  C>A: Hb C-β⁺-thalassemia

It is possible with paper electrophoresis to separate hemoglobins A, S, C, A₂, and others, but resolution is not sharp.

This is the traditional method of choice for screening for common variants, but small amounts of Hb A or Hb F are difficult to detect.

↑ Hb F (see *Fetal Hemoglobin*)

↑ Hb A₂ (see *Hemoglobin A₂*)

Citrate agar at acid pH separates Hb S from Hb D and G and separates Hb C from O-Arab and E; these groups have similar migrations at pH 8.4-8.6.

↑ Hb H (see *Hemoglobin H*)

TEST NAME AND METHOD	SPECIMEN REQUIREMENTS	REFERENCE INTERVAL, CONVENTIONAL [INTERNATIONAL RECOMMENDED UNITS]	CHEMICAL INTERFERENCES AND IN VIVO EFFECTS
Hemoglobin (Hb) Electrophoresis—CONT			
Starch gel EP, pH 8.8-9.0			
Starch gel EP, pH 6.8-7.0			
Globin-chain EP, pH 6.3 and 8.9			
IEF, pH 6-8[3,5]			
Cation-exchange HPLC[4,6-9]			

1. Williams WJ, Beutler E, Erslev AJ, et al, editors: *Hematology,* ed 4, New York, 1990, McGraw-Hill Publishing Co.
2. Fairbanks VP: *Hemoglobinopathies and thalassemias: laboratory methods and case studies,* New York, 1980, Thieme-Stratton, Inc.
3. Huisman THJ: *The hemoglobinopathies. Methods in hematology, vol 15,* Edinburgh, 1986, Churchill Livingstone.
4. Hoyer JD, Kroft SH, editors: *Color atlas of hemoglobin disorders—a compendium based on proficiency testing,* Northfield, IL, 2003, College of American Pathologists.
5. Burtis CA, Ashwood ER, editors: *Tietz textbook of clinical chemistry,* ed 3, Philadelphia, 1999, WB Saunders.
6. Papadea C, Cate JC IV: Identification and quantification of hemoglobins A, F, S, and C by automated chromatography, *Clin Chem* 42:57-63, 1996.
7. Riou J, Godart C, Hurtreal D, et al: Cation-exchange HPLC evaluated for presumptive identification of hemoglobin variants, *Clin Chem* 43:34-39, 1997.
8. Ou CN, Rognerud CL: Rapid analysis of hemoglobin variants by cation-exchange HPLC, *Clin Chem* 39:820-824, 1993.
9. Ou CN, Rognerud CL: Diagnosis of hemoglobinopathies:electrophoresis vs. HPLC, *Clin Chim Acta* 313:187-194, 2001.

TEST NAME AND METHOD	SPECIMEN REQUIREMENTS	REFERENCE INTERVAL, CONVENTIONAL [INTERNATIONAL RECOMMENDED UNITS]	CHEMICAL INTERFERENCES AND IN VIVO EFFECTS
Hemoglobin H (Hb H, β4)[1] *Isopropanol precipitation[2,3]*	Whole blood (ACD, EDTA, or heparin). Use fresh.	No precipitation at 40 min.	↑ Hb F (>5%; >0.05, mass fraction) may cause false-positive results.

DIAGNOSTIC INFORMATION	REMARKS

Starch gel at pH 8.8-9 may be a better general method for resolution and reproducibility; it is especially useful for resolving minor fractions.

This starch gel method separates Hb H and Hb Bart's from other hemoglobins.

Globin-chain electrophoresis identifies variants not distinguishable by other electrophoretic techniques. It is particularly useful for identifying Hb D-Punjab, Hb G-Philadelphia, and Hb Hasharon.

IEF is increasingly used in identifying mutant hemoglobins; it enables detection of variants that migrate with Hb A.

HPLC possesses both the high resolution and sensitivity for detection of hemoglobin variants and has been increasingly used in the routine clinical laboratories.

↑ *Hb H disease:* Slight opacity appears at 10 min; precipitation   Blood older than 3 days may give false-positive result.
occurs before 40 min.

TEST NAME AND METHOD	SPECIMEN REQUIREMENTS	REFERENCE INTERVAL, CONVENTIONAL [INTERNATIONAL RECOMMENDED UNITS]	CHEMICAL INTERFERENCES AND IN VIVO EFFECTS
Hemoglobin H—CONT			
Inclusion bodies, brilliant cresyl blue[4]	Whole blood (ACD, EDTA, or heparin).	Negative. No Hb H inclusions are detected at 1-4 hr after incubation.	↑ Heinz bodies resulting from other causes (e.g., drugs, chemicals, homozygous-β-thalassemia) may be present but are usually preformed.
			↓ C Some lots of brilliant cresyl blue fail to induce Hb H precipitates.
Starch gel or starch block EP, pH 6.8-7.0[5,6]	Whole blood (ACD, EDTA, or heparin).	No Hb H detected.	

1. Altman P, Dittmer D: *Blood and other body fluids,* Washington, DC, 1961, Federation of American Societies for Experimental Biology.

2. Fairbanks VP: *Hemoglobinopathies and thalassemias: laboratory methods and case studies,* New York, 1980, Thieme-Stratton, Inc.

3. Huisman THJ: *The hemoglobinopathies. Methods in hematology, vol 15,* Edinburgh, 1986, Churchill Livingstone.

4. Jones JA, Broszeit HK, LeCrone CN, et al: An improved method for detection of red cell hemoglobin H inclusions, *Am J Med Technol* 47:94-96, 1981.

5. Henry JB, editor: *Clinical diagnosis and management by laboratory methods,* ed 20, Philadelphia, 2001, WB Saunders.

6. Williams WJ, Beutler E, Erslev AJ, et al, editors: *Hematology,* ed 4, New York, 1990, McGraw-Hill Publishing Co.

7. Jandl JH: *Blood: textbook of hematology,* Boston, 1987, Little, Brown and Co.

TEST NAME AND METHOD	SPECIMEN REQUIREMENTS	REFERENCE INTERVAL, CONVENTIONAL [INTERNATIONAL RECOMMENDED UNITS]	CHEMICAL INTERFERENCES AND IN VIVO EFFECTS
Hemoglobin (Hb), Plasma[1-3] *Colorimetric*[3]	Whole blood (heparin, ACD, EDTA). Use butterfly set with 18-gauge needle. Discard first 4 mL, and then collect blood for test. Store plasma at 4° C.	<3 mg/dL ×0.155* [<0.47 μmol/L] With meticulous technique, the value should be <1 mg/dL ×0.155* [<0.16 μmol/L] *Conversion factor based on MW of Hb of 64,500.	↑ Hemolysis during or after venipuncture; alglucerase ↑ V Drugs causing hemolysis in G6PD-deficient individuals or through an immune mechanism, e.g., analgesics, antimalarials, cinchona alkaloids, nitrofurans, sulfonamides, sulfones; specific agents are listed in Table I-4. ↓ V Anistreplase, α-interferon

DIAGNOSTIC INFORMATION	REMARKS
↑ *Hb H disease:* 10-100% of erythrocytes develop pale blue inclusions by 1 hr (single, large inclusions are present after splenectomy). ↑ *a-Thalassemia trait* (some cases): A very few erythrocytes may contain inclusions. ↑ *Unstable hemoglobin disorders:* If spleen is intact, inclusions develop later than Hb H; after splenectomy, Heinz bodies (inclusions) are preformed.	This method utilizes the reticulocyte-rich fraction of erythrocytes, concentrating the Hb H-positive cells, which are found more easily in α-thalassemia minor. Reticulocyte precipitates of RNA are dark purple; Hb H precipitates are pale blue.
Hb H disease: In adults, 2-40% of total hemoglobin is Hb H. The occurrence of Hb H may be an acquired disorder in some cases of erythroleukemia and other myeloproliferative diseases.[7]	Starch gel or starch block EP, pH 6.8-7.0, gives better separation of Hb H from Hb A than an alkaline pH.
↑↑ Intravascular hemolysis (e.g., PNH, PCH), major transfusion reaction, traumatic hemolytic anemia, falciparum malaria, cold hemagglutinins, violent exercise, burns, March hemoglobinuria. ↑ Extravascular hemolysis, transfusion reaction; slight elevations in sickle cell anemia, β-thalassemia major, warm-type autoimmune hemolytic anemia.	Measurement of free Hb in plasma is of no practical value in the diagnosis of chronic hemolytic anemias. Hemolysis in the process of blood collection is an important variable that limits the value of an isolated estimation of plasma hemoglobin. Serial estimations may be of greatest use.[4]

TEST NAME AND METHOD	SPECIMEN REQUIREMENTS	REFERENCE INTERVAL, CONVENTIONAL [INTERNATIONAL RECOMMENDED UNITS]		CHEMICAL INTERFERENCES AND IN VIVO EFFECTS

Hemoglobin (Hb), Plasma—CONT

1. Dacie JV, Lewis SM: *Practical haematology,* ed 8, Edinburgh, 1995, Churchill Livingstone.
2. Lee GR, Bithell TC, Foerster J, et al: *Wintrobe's clinical hematology,* ed 11, Philadelphia, 2003, Lea & Febiger.

Hemoglobin (Hb), Total[1-3]	Whole blood (EDTA). Stable 48 hr at 4° C, 24 hr at 23° C.		*g/dL*	*g/L*	↑ C Hypertriglyceridemia; marked leukocytosis
		Fetal[6]			(WBC >100,000/μL).
Cyanmethemoglo-		18-20 wk:	11.47 ± 0.78 (SD)	[115 ± 7.8]	False elevations may be
bin (HiCN), light		21-22 wk:	12.28 ± 0.89	[123 ± 8.9]	found in the presence of
absorbance	Fetal blood. Collect by	23-25 wk:	12.40 ± 0.77	[124 ± 7.7]	Hb C or Hb S, advanced
(Coulter, Abbott,	percutaneous umbilical	26-30 wk:	13.35 ± 1.17	[134 ± 11.7]	liver disease, and easily
Bayer automated	blood sampling	Cord blood[7]:	12.5-20.5 (SD)	[135-205]	precipitated globulins,
methods)[3]	(PUBS).	0.5 mo[8]:	13.4-19.8	[134-198]	e.g., in multiple myeloma
		1 mo:	10.7-17.1	[107-171]	or Waldenstrom's
		2 mo:	9.4-13.0	[94-130]	macroglobulinemia (trans-
Sodium Laurel		4 mo:	10.3-14.1	[103-141]	cutaneous method not
Sulfate-hemoglobin		6 mo:	11.1-14.1	[111-141]	affected).[4]
(SLS-hemoglobin),		9 mo:	11.4-14.0	[114-140]	
light absorbance		12 mo:	11.3-14.1	[113-141]	
(Sysmex automated		0.5-2 yr[9]:	11.0-14.0	[110-140]	↑ V Heavy smoking be-
analyzer)[3]		2-5 yr:	11.0-14.0	[110-140]	cause of the presence of
		5-9 yr:	11.5-14.5	[115-145]	COHb, which is
Transcutaneous		9-12 yr:	12.0-15.0	[120-150]	nonfunctional.
method using near					
infrared spec-			*g/dL*	*g/L*	
troscopy[4]			*(95% range)*		
		12-14 yr			
		M[9]:	12.0-16.0	[120-160]	
		F:	11.5-15.0	[115-150]	
		15-17 yr			
		M:	11.7-16.6	[123-166]	
		F:	11.7-15.3	[117-153]	
		18-44 yr			
		M:	13.2-17.3	[132-173]	
		F:	11.7-15.5	[117-155]	
		45-64 yr			
		M:	13.1-17.2	[131-172]	
		F:	11.7-16.0	[117-160]	
		65-74 yr			
		M:	12.6-17.4	[126-174]	
		F:	11.7-16.1	[117-161]	

DIAGNOSTIC INFORMATION   REMARKS

3. Tietz NW, editor: *Textbook of clinical chemistry,* Philadelphia, 1986, WB Saunders.
4. Hall R, Malia RG: *Medical laboratory haematology,* ed 2, London, 1991, Butterworths.

↑ Polycythemia, after vigorous exercise or excitement, hemoconcentration (as in dehydration, burns, severe vomiting, intestinal obstruction)

↓ Anemia, recumbency; drugs that cause aplastic anemia or that cause hemolysis, either in G6PD deficiency or by an immune mechanism (specific agents listed in Table II-4)

The cyanmethemoglobin technique is the method of choice selected by the International Committee for Standardization in Hematology (ICSH). The method measures all hemoglobin derivatives except sulfhemoglobin by hemolyzing the specimen and adding a reducing agent. As such, this method does not distinguish between intracellular versus extracellular hemoglobin (hemolysis).

Hb at birth is usually lower in premature infants than in term infants. The mean Hb in black persons is 0.4-1.0 g/dL [4-10 g/L] lower than in whites after the first decade of life.[9]

Hb, Hct, and erythrocyte count are slightly lower between 5:00 PM and 7:00 AM and after meals (up to 10% lower); values are up to 5.7% lower in recumbency. Falsely high results may occur because of prolonged venous stasis during venipuncture. A slight but significant decrease occurs in the lower reference limit of Hb in men aged 65-74 yr. There is no significant change in men or women >age 85 yr as compared with ages 65-74 yr.[10]

TEST NAME AND METHOD	SPECIMEN REQUIREMENTS	REFERENCE INTERVAL, CONVENTIONAL [INTERNATIONAL RECOMMENDED UNITS]		CHEMICAL INTERFERENCES AND IN VIVO EFFECTS

Hemoglobin (Hb), Total—CONT

			g/dL	*g/L*	
Oxyhemoglobin	Capillary blood (heparin)[5]	1 day:	19.0 ± 2.2 (SD)	[190 ± 22]	
		4 days:	18.6 ± 2.1	[186 ± 21]	
		7 days:	17.9 ± 2.5	[179 ± 25]	
		1-2 wk:	17.3 ± 2.3	[173 ± 23]	
		3-4 wk:	14.2 ± 2.1	[142 ± 21]	
		5-6 wk:	11.9 ± 1.5	[119 ± 15]	
		7-8 wk:	11.1 ± 1.1	[111 ± 11]	
		9-10 wk:	11.2 ± 0.9	[112 ± 9]	
		11-12 wk:	11.3 ± 0.9	[113 ± 9]	
		M:	14-18	[140-180]	
		F:	12-16	[120-160]	
Gasometric	Whole blood (EDTA, oxalate, or heparin)	M:	14-18	[140-180]	
		F:	12-16	[120-160]	

1. Green JP, Foerster J, Lukens JN: *Wintrobe's clinical hematology,* ed 11, Philadelphia, 2003, Lippincott, Williams & Wilkins.
2. Beutler E, Lichtman MA, Coller B, editors: *Williams hematology,* ed 6, New York, 2000, McGraw-Hill.
3. Rodak BF, editor: *Hematology; clinical principles and applications,* ed 2, Philadelphia, 2002, WB Saunders.
4. Saigo T, Imoto S, Hashimoto M, et al: Noninvasive monitoring of hemoglobin, *Am J Clin Pathol* 121:51-55, 2004.
5. Matoth Y, Zaizon R, Varsano I: Postnatal changes in some red cell parameters, *Acta Paediatr Scand* 60:317-323, 1971.
6. Forestier F, Daffos F, Galacteros F, et al: Hematologic values of 163 normal fetuses between 18 and 30 weeks of gestation, *Pediatr Res* 20:342-346, 1986.
7. Nathan DG, Orkin SH, Ginsburg D, et al: *Hematology of infancy and childhood,* ed 6, Philadelphia, 2003, WB Saunders.
8. Saarinen UM, Siimes MA: Development changes in red blood cell counts and indices of infants after exclusion of iron deficiency by laboratory criteria and continuous iron supplementation, *J Pediatr* 92:412-416, 1978.
9. Yip R, Johnson C, Dallman PR: Age-related changes in laboratory values used in the diagnosis of anemia and iron deficiency, *Am J Clin Nutr* 39:427-436, 1984.
10. Zauber NP, Zauber AG: Hematologic data of healthy very old people, *JAMA* 257:2181-2184, 1987.

Hemoglobin (Hb), Urine[1-6]	Urine, fresh random. First morning specimen is preferred. Examine immediately. Refrigerate to prevent microbial growth if analysis is delayed >1 hr. Mix well before testing to suspend intact erythrocytes.	Negative (<0.03 mg free Hb/dL or <10 Ercs/μL) [<0.3 mg free Hb/L or <10 × 10⁶ Ercs/L]		↑ C Oxidizing contaminants (e.g., hypochlorites used for cleaning bedpans, urinals), microbial peroxidase associated with urinary tract infections, iodine
Reagent strips (Miles Inc. Multistix, Labstix, Hemacombistix, Hemastix[7]; BMC Chemstrips)[8]				↑ V A large number of drugs have been reported

DIAGNOSTIC INFORMATION	REMARKS

↓ V Lower values may be found in smokers because of the presence of carboxyhemoglobin (not measured by either oxy-hemoglobin method or gasometric method).

This method measures only physiologically active Hb capable of carrying oxygen; it does not measure methemoglobin, sulfhemoglobin, or carboxyhemoglobin. It is rarely used except for standardization in hemoglobinometry.

All causes of hematuria (see *Sediment, Urinary* for complete list), renal calculi, tumors, exposure to toxic agents[6]

Intravascular hemolysis: Pregnancy and the puerperium, extensive burns, transfusion reactions, kidney infarction, PCH, PNH, transurethral prostatectomy, drugs and poisons (e.g., sulfonamides, quinine, phenylhydrazine), oxidant drugs and fava beans in G6PD-deficient patients, bites of poisonous snakes and spiders, infections (malaria, blackwater fever, gas gangrene, typhus fever, anthrax, yellow fever), direct or in-

Reagent strip testing for urine hemoglobin has been shown to reliably replace microscopy in detection of hematuria.[5] These tests detect both intracellular and extracellular hemoglobin and myoglobin (Mb) but are more sensitive to the free Hb and Mb than to intact erythrocytes. A positive result merits further investigation. Sensitivity is reduced in urines with high specific gravity. Erythrocyte lysis occurs at a specific gravity.[9] Also, Mb is soluble in 80% (w/v) saturated ammonium chloride, whereas Hb is not.[10]

TEST NAME AND METHOD	SPECIMEN REQUIREMENTS	REFERENCE INTERVAL, CONVENTIONAL [INTERNATIONAL RECOMMENDED UNITS]	CHEMICAL INTERFERENCES AND IN VIVO EFFECTS

Hemoglobin (Hb), Urine—CONT

to cause hematuria, including ciprofloxacin, cyclophosphamide, fenoprofen, gold salts, mebendazole, polymyxin B, and suprofen. Drugs causing hemolysis may also cause hematuria (see Table II-4). False-positive results occasionally are seen in menstruating women.

↓ C Ascorbic acid (not with Chemstrips), gentisic acid, use formalin as preservative for urine, proteinuria, excessive amounts of urinary nitrite, urine pH <5

1. Boehringer Mannheim Corp: *Urinalysis today,* Indianapolis, IN, 1991, Boehringer Mannheim Corp.
2. DeGowin EL, DeGowin RL: *Bedside diagnostic examination,* ed 5, New York, 1987, Macmillan Pub. Co.
3. Free HM, editor: *Modern urine chemistry,* Elkhart, IN, 1991, Miles Inc., Diagnostics Division.
4. Henry JB, editor: *Clinical diagnosis and management by laboratory methods,* ed 20, Philadelphia, 2001, WB Saunders.
5. Newall RG, editor: *Clinical urinalysis,* Buckinghamshire, UK, 1990, Ames Division, Miles Ltd.
6. Strasinger SK: *Urinalysis and body fluids: a self-instructional text,* ed 2, Philadelphia, 1991, FA Davis.
7. Miles Inc., Diagnostics Division: *Multistix package insert,* Elkhart, IN, 1992, Miles Inc., Diagnostics Division.
8. Boehringer Mannheim Corp.: *Chemstrip 10 UA package insert,* Indianapolis, IN, 1992, Boehringer Mannheim Corp.
9. Wilson JD, Braunwald E, Isselbacher KJ, et al, editors: *Harrison's principles of internal medicine,* ed 12, New York, 1991, McGraw-Hill Publishing Co.
10. Williams WJ, Beutler E, Erslev AJ, et al, editors: *Hematology,* ed 4, New York, 1990, McGraw-Hill Publishing Co.

TEST NAME AND METHOD	SPECIMEN REQUIREMENTS	REFERENCE INTERVAL, CONVENTIONAL	[INTERNATIONAL RECOMMENDED UNITS]	CHEMICAL INTERFERENCES AND IN VIVO EFFECTS
Hemoglobins, Unstable[1,2] *Heat denaturation (screen), 50° C for 2 hr, Tris buffer*	Whole blood (ACD, EDTA, or heparin). Use fresh.	*Percent precipitation* <5 at 2 hr × 0.01	*Precipitated fraction* <0.05 at 2 hr	↑ V Heinz bodies resulting from another cause, e.g., oxidant drugs, G6PD deficiency; iron deficiency may cause false-positive results.

travascular trauma to erythrocytes (exercise, cardiac valve prostheses, severe aortic regurgitation, necrotizing arteriolitis); microangiopathic hemolytic anemia (hemolytic uremic syndrome, thrombotic thrombocytopenic purpura, DIC, renal cortical necrosis); hemolysis from donor's blood because of improper storage, heating, freezing, or additives.

Myoglobinuria may give positive results (see *Myoglobin*). Presence of nitrate in large quantities will delay the reaction.

Sensitivity:
Chemstrips, 5-10 Ercs/μL urine [5-10 $\times$ 10^6 Ercs/L][1]; Hb 0-3 Ercs

Hemastix, 5-20 Ercs/μL urine [5-20 $\times$ 10^6 Ercs/L][7]; 0.015-0.06 mg/dL free Hb [15-60 mg/L free Hb]

$\uparrow$ Congenital Heinz body anemia (10-40% of the hemoglobin is a structurally abnormal, unstable Hb.)

False-negative and false-positive results are a problem. Comparing absorbance of supernatant before and after denaturation permits estimation of the amount of unstable Hb.

Unstable hemoglobins will precipitate faster than normal hemoglobin.

TEST NAME AND METHOD	SPECIMEN REQUIREMENTS	REFERENCE INTERVAL, CONVENTIONAL [INTERNATIONAL RECOMMENDED UNITS]	CHEMICAL INTERFERENCES AND IN VIVO EFFECTS
Hemoglobins, Unstable—CONT			
Heat denaturation (screen), 60-65° C for 30 min, phosphate buffer[3]		Minimal precipitation of Hb at 30 min Percent denatured Hb is estimated at 0, 2, 4, 6, 8, 10, 15, 20, 25, and 30 min in patient and control samples.	↑ C Old sample
Isopropanol precipitation		No precipitation at 40 min Hb H: Slight opacity at 10 min	↑ V Hb F (>5%; >0.05, mass fraction) or slightly unstable hemoglobin (e.g., Hb E, Hb H) may cause positive test.

1. Williams WJ, Beutler E, Erslev AJ, et al, editors: *Hematology,* ed 4, New York, 1990, McGraw-Hill Publishing Co.
2. Huisman THJ: *The hemoglobinopathies. Methods in hematology, vol 15,* Edinburgh, 1986, Churchill Livingstone.
3. Huisman THJ, Jonxis JHP: *The hemoglobinopathies: techniques of identification,* New York, 1977, Marcel Dekker.

TEST NAME AND METHOD	SPECIMEN REQUIREMENTS	REFERENCE INTERVAL, CONVENTIONAL [INTERNATIONAL RECOMMENDED UNITS]	CHEMICAL INTERFERENCES AND IN VIVO EFFECTS

Hemopexin (Hx, Hpx)[1-6]
 	
RID
	Serum. Analyze fresh or store at 4° C for <72 hr. Stable frozen at −20° C for 6 mo or at −70° C indefinitely. Specimens without lipemia or hemolysis are preferred.	Fetus, term[3]: >30% [× 0.01 = >0.30, fraction]
		      of mean adult concentration or
		      >18% [>0.18] of maternal
		      concentration
		
		Adult: 50-115 mg/dL × 0.01 [0.50-1.15 g/L]
		         (x̄: 75) [x̄: 0.75]
		Maternal: >1.5 × that of nonpregnant female
			None found.

	Urine, 24 hr. Centrifuge and adjust to pH 7.0. Analyze fresh. Stable frozen at −20° C for up to 1 yr.	x̄: 0.2 mg/day[4]	

1. Brown SS, Mitchell FL, Young DS, editors: *Chemical diagnosis of disease,* Amsterdam, 1979, Elsevier/North Holland Biomedical Press.
2. Henry JB, editor: *Clinical diagnosis and management by laboratory methods,* ed 20, Philadelphia, 2001, WB Saunders.
3. Putnam FW, editor: *The plasma proteins: structure, function and genetic control, vol 1-3,* ed 2, New York, 1977, Academic Press.
4. Müller-Eberhard U, Liem HH: Hemopcxin, the heme-binding serum β-glycoprotein, *Ric Clin Lab* 5:275-291, 1975.

DIAGNOSTIC INFORMATION	REMARKS
	The difference in percent denatured Hb between patient and control at 10 min is a semiquantitative estimate of the amount of unstable Hb.
	Isopropanol precipitation is a more sensitive test than heat denaturation (50° C, Tris buffer). Unstable hemoglobins begin precipitation at 5 min and become flocculent after 20 min. To exclude a false-negative test, incubation should be continued until precipitation of the control occurs.
	See also *Heinz Body Preparation* and *Hemoglobin H.*
↓ During intense hemolytic processes Hemopexin is a weak acute phase reactant with levels rarely increasing more than twofold over resting levels.	This polymorphic protein is synthesized by hepatocytes. Hemopexin binds heme/metheme with high affinity at a 1:1.11 (mg/g) ratio. The complex is cleared from the circulation by the liver, in contrast to the hemoglobin-haptoglobin complex that is cleared by the reticuloendothelial system. Hemopexin also binds porphyrins other than heme. The heme-hemopexin complex, once processed in the liver, releases hemopexin for return to the circulation, unlike haptoglobin, which is destroyed once complexed with hemoglobin. Serial analysis of hemopexin may be a better index of hemolysis than is haptoglobin analysis during processes where haptoglobin is consumed (e.g., after surgery in which extracorporeal blood oxygenation is employed, and decreasing hemopexin levels indicate continued erythrocyte destruction). MW: 60,000

5. Ritzmann SE, Tucker ES III: *Protein analysis in disease—current concepts, Workshop manual,* Chicago, 1979, American Society of Clinical Pathologists, Commission for Continuing Education.
6. Schwick H-G, Haupt H: Chemistry and function of human plasma proteins, *Angew Chem* 191:87-99, 1980.

TEST NAME AND METHOD	SPECIMEN REQUIREMENTS	REFERENCE INTERVAL, CONVENTIONAL [INTERNATIONAL RECOMMENDED UNITS]	CHEMICAL INTERFERENCES AND IN VIVO EFFECTS
Hemosiderin[1,2] *Prussian blue sediment staining*	Urine, fresh random.	Negative	None found.

1. Henry JB, editor: *Clinical diagnosis and management by laboratory methods,* ed 20, Philadelphia, 2001, WB Saunders.
2. Lee GR, Bithell TC, Foerster J, et al: *Wintrobe's clinical hematology,* ed 11, Philadelphia, 2003, Lea & Febiger.

TEST NAME AND METHOD	SPECIMEN REQUIREMENTS	REFERENCE INTERVAL, CONVENTIONAL [INTERNATIONAL RECOMMENDED UNITS]	CHEMICAL INTERFERENCES AND IN VIVO EFFECTS
Heparin Anti-Xa Assay[1,2]	Plasma (blue top citrate). Separate plasma as soon as possible to minimize effect of released platelet factor 4 from platelets, which may cause falsely low values. Stable for 2 hr at room temperature or for 8 hr at 2-8° C. Do not centrifuge at refrigerated temperatures because this disrupts platelets and releases PF4. May also store frozen.	*Unfractionated heparin* No heparin: <0.05 U/mL Therapeutic heparin: 0.3-0.7 U/mL	Platelet factor 4 released from platelets neutralizes heparin, LMWH, or danaparoid.

1. Jacobs DS, Demott WR, Oxley DK, editors: *Laboratory test handbook,* ed 5, Hudson, OH, 2001, Lexi-Comp, Inc.
2. Olson JD, Arkin CF, Brandt JT, et al: College of American Pathologists Conference XXXI on Laboratory Monitoring of Anticoagulant Therapy. Laboratory monitoring of unfractionated heparin therapy, *Arch Path Lab Med* 122:782-798, 1998.

DIAGNOSTIC INFORMATION	REMARKS

↑ *Hemolytic anemias associated with intravascular hemolysis:* Hemolytic transfusion reactions, cold hemagglutinin disease, paroxysmal cold hemoglobinuria, paroxysmal nocturnal hemoglobinuria, microangiopathic hemolytic anemia, mechanical trauma to erythrocyte (heart valve hemolysis), hemolysis caused by body burns, hemolysis associated with oxidant drugs (with or without G6PD deficiency), thalassemia major, sickle cell anemia, severe megaloblastic anemia, and clostridial exotoxemia.

The presence of hemosiderin in the urine indicates the recent or chronic release of free hemoglobin into the circulating plasma and the depletion of hemopexin and haptoglobin. Hemosiderin is usually attributable to intravascular hemolysis but may originate from conditions such as hemorrhagic pancreatitis in which breakdown of blood cells occurs in the peritoneal cavity.

Hemosiderin is not detected in alkaline urine.[1]

↑ Hemochromatosis

This test can be used to monitor heparin therapy. It is also useful for determining heparin overdose. It can establish precisely the level of heparin in plasma.

Although the aPTT is the most commonly used test for monitoring heparin therapy, the heparin anti-Xa assay is increasingly being used and in some laboratories has replaced the aPTT. Proposed advantages of the anti-X assay include obtaining therapeutic levels more rapidly, differentiating patients at risk of bleeding, and less influence from biologic variables that affect the aPTT.

LMWH and danaparoid generally do not prolong the aPTT; therefore the anti-Xa assay is also used for monitoring these anticoagulants when indicated.

The anti-X assay is a chromogenic assay that measures heparin concentration indirectly. Antithrombin and factor Xa are used as the assay reagents. Heparin in the patient's plasma binds with the added excess antithrombin and inhibits excess factor Xa. The quantity of residual factor Xa is measured using a chromogenic substrate, and the released colored compound is measured spectrophotometrically. The quantity of residual enzyme is inversely proportional to the amount of heparin present in plasma.

TEST NAME AND METHOD	SPECIMEN REQUIREMENTS	REFERENCE INTERVAL, CONVENTIONAL [INTERNATIONAL RECOMMENDED UNITS]	CHEMICAL INTERFERENCES AND IN VIVO EFFECTS
Heparin-Induced Thrombocytopenia (Platelet factor 4)[1,2]	Plasma (blue top citrate). Stable for 24 hr at room temperature.	The magnitude of a positive result for HIT antibodies may be diagnostically important when taken together with the pretest probability of HIT. *Serotonin release assay* Negative: <20% Weak: 20-50% Strong platelet activation: >50% *Antigen assay* (Optical density [OD] reading): Negative: <0.45 Weak: 0.45-1.0 Strong: >1.0	High fibrinogen may cause a false-positive reaction in the platelet aggregation test.

1. Warkentin TE: Platelet count monitoring and laboratory testing for heparin-induced thrombocytopenia. Recommendations of the College of American Pathologists, *Arch Pathol Lab Med* 126:1415-1423, 2002.

2. Brandt JT: Diagnosing heparin-induced thrombocytopenia, *CAP Today* 15(5):40-52, 2000.

TEST NAME AND METHOD	SPECIMEN REQUIREMENTS	REFERENCE INTERVAL, CONVENTIONAL [INTERNATIONAL RECOMMENDED UNITS]	CHEMICAL INTERFERENCES AND IN VIVO EFFECTS
Hepatitis A Antibody (Anti-HA, Anti-HAV, Total Anti-HA, IgG-anti-HA, IgM-anti-HA) *Total (IgG + IgM) Anti-HA*[1] *IRMA, IEMA*	Serum. Stable for 7 days at room temperature and indefinitely at 4° C or 20° C.	Negative.	None found.

Heparin-induced thrombocytopenia.

Note: The diagnosis should be made if there are clinical abnormalities present and HIT antibodies are detected. Negative testing for HIT antibodies using two assays (ideally one activation and one antigen assay) essentially rules out HIT.

HIT is a serious clinicopathologic syndrome (thrombocytopenia, thrombosis) associated with heparin therapy or even small amounts of heparin (e.g., heparin-coated lines). The HIT antibodies are directed at neoepitopes on platelet factor 4 (PF4), which appear on exposure to heparin. However, only a minority of patients who form HIT antibodies actually develop thrombocytopenia or thrombosis. Testing for HIT should be performed when clinically suspected.

Two types of assays are used for a diagnosis of HIT. The functional (platelet activation) assays are based on the patient antibodies activating test platelets in the presence of heparin. These assays include the platelet aggregation method, the washed platelet activation assays (serotonin release assay and heparin-induced platelet agglutination), and flow cytometry. The washed platelet activation assays have greater diagnostic specificity but are technically demanding and usually done in reference laboratories.

The antigenic assay (ELISA) is based on detection of antibody binding to PF4/heparin (usually IgG). However, they may detect nonpathogenic IgA and IgM antibodies. A particle gel immunoassay (ID-H/PF4 test) is also available.

The antigen assays are more widely available. The ELISA assay is generally considered the most sensitive test. However, the activation assays have a greater diagnostic specificity than antigen assays.

Hepatitis A, formerly called *infectious hepatitis,* is a picornavirus usually transmitted through either oral or fecal contact (but rarely transmitted parenterally[3]) that can cause either asymptomatic infection or symptomatic clinical hepatitis. Both IgG and IgM antibodies occur early in the acute infection (see Fig. II-4) with IgG persisting for years. Diagnosis of acute HAV infection requires positivity for IgM-anti-HA (see Table II-7). After an acute infection, IgM-anti-HA usually disappears in 3-4 mo but may persist up to 10 mo. With increasing use of vaccination, most positive IgM anti-HA results are false positive; CPC recommends the test only be used in the setting of acute hepatitis.[4] Patients with IgG-anti-HA are

A high percentage of the population has protective antibody to the hepatitis A virus (total anti-HA) acquired from clinically unapparent infections. This is why *standard immune globulin* has been effective as prophylaxis for hepatitis A exposures.

See Table II-7.

TEST NAME AND METHOD	SPECIMEN REQUIREMENTS	REFERENCE INTERVAL, CONVENTIONAL [INTERNATIONAL RECOMMENDED UNITS]	CHEMICAL INTERFERENCES AND IN VIVO EFFECTS
Hepatitis A Antibody—CONT *IgM-anti-HA*[1] *Anti-m capture*[2]			

1. Gerlich WH, Thomssen R: Terminology, structure, and laboratory diagnosis of hepatitis viruses. In McIntyre N, Benhamou J-P, Bircher J, et al, editors: *Oxford textbook of clinical hepatology,* New York, 1991, Oxford University Press.
2. Duermeyer W, Wielaard F, van der Veen J: A new principle for the detection of specific IgM antibodies applied in an ELISA for hepatitis A, *J Med Virol* 4:25-32, 1979.
3. Richardson L, Evatt B: Risk of hepatitis A virus infection in persons with hemophilia receiving plasma-derived products, *Transf Med Rev* 14:64-73, 2000.
4. Dominguez A, Bruguera M, Plans P, et al: Prevalence of hepatitis antibodies in school children in Catalonia after the introduction of universal hepatitis A vaccination, *J Med Viral* 73:172-176, 2004.
5. Centers for Disease Conrol and Prevention: Positive results for active hepatitis A virus infection among persons with no recent history of acute hepatitis—United States, 2002-2004, *Morb Mortal Wkly Rep* 54:453-465, 2005.

TEST NAME AND METHOD	SPECIMEN REQUIREMENTS	REFERENCE INTERVAL, CONVENTIONAL [INTERNATIONAL RECOMMENDED UNITS]	CHEMICAL INTERFERENCES AND IN VIVO EFFECTS
Hepatitis B Core Antibody (Anti-HBc, Total anti-HBc, IgM-anti-HBc) *Total (IgG + IgM) Anti-HBc*[1] *IRMA, IEMA, MEA, CA* *IgM-anti-HBc*[1] *Anti-m Capture*[2]	Serum. Stable for 7 days at room temperature and indefinitely at 4° C or 20° C.	Negative.	C ↑ Influenza vaccine

1. Gerlich WH, Thomssen R: Terminology, structure, and laboratory diagnosis of hepatitis viruses. In McIntyre N, Benhamou J-P, Bircher J, et al, editors: *Oxford textbook of clinical hepatology,* New York, 1991, Oxford University Press.
2. Duermeyer W, Wielaard F, van der Veen J: A new principle for the detection of specific IgM antibodies applied in an ELISA for hepatitis A, *J Med Virol* 4:25-32, 1979.
3. Seeff L, Beebe G, Hoofnagle J, et al: A serologic follow-up of the 1942 epidemic of post-vaccination hepatitis in the United States Army, *N Engl J Med* 316:965-970, 1987.
4. Dufour D, Talastas M, Fernandez MD, et al: Low positive anti-hepatitis C virus enzyme immunoassay results: an important predictor of low likelihood of hepatitis C infection, *Clin Chem* 49:479-486, 2003.
5. Czaja A, Shiels MT, Taswell HF, et al: Frequency and significance of immunoglobulin M antibody to hepatitis B core antigen in corticosteroid-treated severe chronic active hepatitis B, *Mayo Clin Proc* 63:119-125, 1988.

protected from the virus. Hepatitis A never causes a chronic infection, but acute relapses occasionally occur. Antibody is detectable in almost all immunized individuals.[5]

Hepatitis B (HBV) core protein forms the capsid of the virus
and is a potent immunogen.[1] Anti-HBc assay is the first antibody test to become positive with exposure to HBV and persists the longest after resolution of acute infection.[3] In acute
HBV infection, both total and IgM anti-HBc are positive,
whereas only total anti-HBc is typically present in chronic and
resolved infection (see Table II-7 and Fig. II-5). Many years
after exposure, anti-HBc[1] may be the only marker present,
particularly in those who also are positive for HCV RNA.[4]

Low levels of IgM-anti-HBc can sometimes be present in
chronic hepatitis B, particularly during flares of activity and at
times of conversion from positive antigen to positive antibody.[5]
In these cases it is necessary to retest patients after several
months (or years) to differentiate *acute* from *chronic*
infections.

TEST NAME AND METHOD	SPECIMEN REQUIREMENTS	REFERENCE INTERVAL, CONVENTIONAL [INTERNATIONAL RECOMMENDED UNITS]	CHEMICAL INTERFERENCES AND IN VIVO EFFECTS
Hepatitis B DNA (HBV-DNA)[1] *Polymerase chain reaction*[2]	Serum. Freeze if test cannot be run immediately. Stable for at least 7 days at 20° C.	Negative (Limits of detection: 100 U/mL)	None found.

1. Gerlich WH, Thomssen R: Terminology, structure, and laboratory diagnosis of hepatitis viruses. In McIntyre N, Benhamou J-P, Bircher J, et al, editors: *Oxford textbook of clinical hepatology,* New York, 1991, Oxford University Press.

2. Lok A, McMahon B: Chronic hepatitis B, *Hepatology* 34:1225-1241, 2001.

3. Mommeja-Marin H, Mondou E, Blum MR, et al: Serum HBV DNA as a marker of efficacy during therapy for chronic HBV infection: analysis and review of the literature, *Hepatology* 37:1309-1319, 2003.

4. Motsuyanagi H, Yasuda K, Iino S, et al: Persistent viremia after recovery from self-limited acute hepatitis B, *Hepatology* 27:1377-1382, 1998.

5. Plentz A, Koller G, Weinberger KM, et al: Precision and stability of hepatitis B virus DNA levels in chronic surface antigen carriers, *J Med Virol* 73:522-528, 2004.

6. Saldanha J, Gerlich W, Lelie N, et al: An international collaborative study to establish a World Health Organization international standard for hepatitis B virus DNA nucleic acid amplification techniques, *Vox Sang* 80:63-71, 2001.

TEST NAME AND METHOD	SPECIMEN REQUIREMENTS	REFERENCE INTERVAL, CONVENTIONAL [INTERNATIONAL RECOMMENDED UNITS]	CHEMICAL INTERFERENCES AND IN VIVO EFFECTS
Hepatitis B Surface Antibody (Anti-HBs, HBsAb)[1] *IRMA, IEMA, MEIA, CA*	Serum. Stable for 7 days at room temperature and indefinitely at 4° C or 20° C.	Negative (Limits of detection: 2-10 U/L)	None found.

| DIAGNOSTIC INFORMATION | REMARKS |

The presence of HBV-DNA in serum confirms active hepatitis B infection and implies infectivity of serum. Current use of the assay is primarily for assessing responses of hepatitis B to therapy, such as interferon-α, lamivudine, or adefovir.[3] HBV-DNA measurement is also important in persons infected by mutant strains of HBV that do not make antigen or normal surface antigen. HBV-DNA is also used before and after liver transplantation to detect low-level viral replication. HBV-DNA typically can be detected using very sensitive techniques even in those thought to have recovered from HBV infection and positive for anti-HBs and anti-HBc.[4] Viral load fluctuates over time in most patients and may vary by as much as 10^2-10^4 in serial measurements.[5]

Hepatitis B (HBV)-DNA and -RNA can also be detected in tissues using molecular biological techniques, but these tests are not generally available. A variety of methods are used, separated into amplified and nonamplified methods. The detection limit for nonamplified methods is typically on the order of 10^4 U/mL, but most have detection limits $>10^5$ U/mL. Polymerase chain reaction (PCR) assays are generally the most sensitive amplified methods, but current branched DNA assays have detection limits of $\sim 10^3$ U/mL. Differences between assays may exceed one log.[5]

The World Health Organization has recognized an international standard for HBV-DNA quantification,[6] and assays are commonly reported in International Units based on comparison with the standard. Correlation between copies/mL (or genome equivalents) and International Units are not the same for all assays, and the conversion factor can differ with viral load even with the same assay. On a theoretical basis, 1 pg of genomic HBV-DNA is equivalent to 2.85×10^5 copies of virus.

See also *Section II, Hepatitis B Virus.*

See Table II-7.

With naturally occurring hepatitis B infections, anti-HBs usually appear in the serum several weeks after disappearance of HBsAg (see Fig. II-5). The presence of anti-HBs generally means there is protection against hepatitis B infection. However, convalescent anti-HBs may fall below limits of detection. A qualitative anti-HBs test is usually adequate to assess natural immunity, but a quantitative finding of >10 U/L for postvaccine testing is the accepted concentration that confers protection.

Anti-HBs is now mainly used to assess efficacy of hepatitis B vaccine but remains an adjunct test along with anti-HBc for determining whether subjects have immunity because of a naturally acquired infection or whether chronic hepatitis B may exist in an HBsAg-negative patient.

See Table II-7.

TEST NAME AND METHOD	SPECIMEN REQUIREMENTS	REFERENCE INTERVAL, CONVENTIONAL [INTERNATIONAL RECOMMENDED UNITS]	CHEMICAL INTERFERENCES AND IN VIVO EFFECTS
Hepatitis B Surface Antibody—CONT			

1. Gerlich WH, Thomssen R: Terminology, structure, and laboratory diagnosis of hepatitis viruses. In McIntyre N, Benhamou J-P, Bircher J, et al, editors: *Oxford textbook of clinical hepatology,* New York, 1991, Oxford University Press.

TEST NAME AND METHOD	SPECIMEN REQUIREMENTS	REFERENCE INTERVAL, CONVENTIONAL [INTERNATIONAL RECOMMENDED UNITS]	CHEMICAL INTERFERENCES AND IN VIVO EFFECTS
Hepatitis B Surface Antigen (HBsAg)[1] *IRMA, IEMA, MEIA, CA*	Serum. Stable for 7 days at room temperature and indefinitely at 4° C or 20° C.	Negative (Limits of detection: 0.02-1.0 ng/mL; typical positive quantitation: 10^4-10^5 ng/mL)	None found.

1. Gerlich WH, Thomssen R: Terminology, structure, and laboratory diagnosis of hepatitis viruses. In McIntyre N, Benhamou J-P, Bircher J, et al, editors: *Oxford textbook of clinical hepatology,* New York, 1991, Oxford University Press.

2. Bloomberg BS, Gerstley BJ, Hungertad DA, et al: A serum antigen (Australia antigen) in Down's syndrome, leukemia, and hepatitis, *Ann Intern Med* 66:924-933, 1967.

3. Coleman P, Chen Y, Mushahwar I: Immunoassay detection of hepatitis B surface antigen mutants, *J Med Virol* 59:19-24, 1999.

4. Locarnini S, Gish R: Studying the treatment of chronic hepatitis B viral infection in special populations. In Hamatake R, Lau J, editors: *Hepatitis B and D protocols. Volume II: immunology, model systems, and clinical studies,* Totowa, NJ, 2004, Humana Press, pp. 457-498.

5. Francois G, Kew M, Van DP, et al: Mutant hepatitis B viruses: a matter of academic interest only or a problem with far-reaching implications? *Vaccine* 19:3799-3815, 2001.

HBsAg is the surface lipoprotein coat of the hepatitis B virus. It was originally discovered by Blumberg[2] and was called *Australian antigen.* Antigenic differences in HBsAg characterize the eight genotypes (A-H) of the hepatitis B virus. These are composed of a common a determinant, an a, d, or y determinant, and either an r or w determinant.

Hepatitis B is a DNA virus of the *Hepadnaviridae* family that replicates via an RNA intermediate using reverse transcriptase. It can cause persistent infection leading to cirrhosis and hepatocellular carcinoma. It has a unique partially double-stranded, circular DNA that utilizes the same nucleotide sequences to code for different proteins by frame-shifting. The virus infects hepatocytes, which then produce complete viral particles and excess HBsAg. The hepatitis B virus is not cytopathic. Instead, the host immune reaction to foreign viral proteins lyses infected hepatocytes and causes hepatitis. Because of immature host immunity, infected neonates and young children are much more likely to become chronic carriers of hepatitis B than adults. (See Fig. II-5 for the serological responses and the various outcomes of hepatitis B infections.)

HBsAg comprises three proteins (SHBs, encoded by the S domain of the hepatitis B genome; MHBs, encoded by S + preS1; and LHBs, encoded by S + preS1 + preS2). Detection of HBsAg is usually the first detectable marker of hepatitis B infection and remains positive in persistent infections (see Fig. II-5). Therefore HBsAg should be tested in the clinical settings of both acute and chronic hepatitis.

HBsAg produced by recombinant DNA techniques in yeast is used as a highly effective vaccine. Original vaccines used purified HBsAg harvested from chronic hepatitis B carriers.

Quantitation of HBsAg is possible but not usually performed. With acute hepatitis B a 50% decrease in HBsAg serum concentrations after 1 mo indicates resolving infection, whereas an increase implies persistence.[1]

Assays for HBsAg typically detect the common a determinant, as do antibodies induced by the hepatitis B vaccine. There are rare mutations in the a determinant that affect recognition by the antigen-binding region of anti-HBs. These variants may result in falsely negative HBsAg assays.[1] Such variants may also escape detection by antibody induced by the vaccine, producing infection in anti-HBs-positive individuals. Such mutations do not typically occur in genotype A, owing to differences in folding of the surface antigen that do not favor production of such mutants.[3,4]

A number of reports have documented chronic hepatitis B infections without HBsAg detectable in serum, largely because of such variants.[5] Although this is rare, the presence of the virus can be deduced by testing for anti-HBc, anti-HBs, and HBV-DNA (see Table II-7).

TEST NAME AND METHOD	SPECIMEN REQUIREMENTS	REFERENCE INTERVAL, CONVENTIONAL [INTERNATIONAL RECOMMENDED UNITS]	CHEMICAL INTERFERENCES AND IN VIVO EFFECTS
Hepatitis B$_e$ Antigen and Antibody (HB$_e$Ag; Anti-HB$_e$, HB$_e$Ab) *EIA*[1]	Serum. Stable for 7 days at room temperature and indefinitely at 4° C or 20° C.	Negative.	None found.

1. Gerlich WH, Thomssen R: Terminology, structure, and laboratory diagnosis of hepatitis viruses. In McIntyre N, Benhamou J-P, Bircher J, et al, editors: *Oxford textbook of clinical hepatology,* New York, 1991, Oxford University Press.

2. Chu C, Yeh CT, Chiu CT, et al: Precore mutant of hepatitis B virus prevails in acute and chronic infections in an area in which hepatitis B is endemic, *J Clin Microbiol* 34:1815-1818, 1996.

3. Hunt C, McGill J, Allen M, et al: Clinical relevance of hepatitis B virus mutations, *Hepatology* 31:1037-1044, 2000.

4. Locarnini S, Gish R: Studying the treatment of chronic hepatitis B viral infection in special populations. In Hamatake R, Lau J, editors: *Hepatitis B and D protocols. Volume II: immunology, model systems, and clinical studies,* Totowa, NJ, 2004, Humana Press, pp. 457-498.

5. Chen R, Edwards R, Shaw T, et al: Effect of the G1896A precore mutation on drug sensitivity and replication yield of lamivudine-resistant HBV in vitro, *Hepatology* 37:27-35, 2003.

HB$_e$Ag and anti-HB$_e$ are ordered together and should only be studied in patients who are chronically HB$_s$Ag positive. There is no rationale for ordering these studies in patients with acute hepatitis. The HB$_e$ gene includes part of the HB$_c$ gene along with a "core promotor" region and an upstream "precore" region that generates a signal peptide causing carboxy-terminal truncation of the core protein. The resulting HB$_e$Ag is produced along with infectious viral particles but is not incorporated into virus. Its exact function is unknown, but some believe it may function to induce host immune tolerance, especially in congenital or neonatal infection. In general, active hepatitis B viral replication is associated with infective serum that is HB$_e$Ag positive and anti-HB$_e$ negative. On conversion to a nonreplicative state, anti-HB$_e$ appears in the serum and HB$_e$Ag disappears. Mutants in the precore region (particularly insertion of a stop codon by a G to A mutation at nucleotide 1896)[2] prevent expression of HB$_e$Ag, but anti-HB$_e$ and infectious viral particles are still produced. These precore mutants are responsible for the majority of infections in Asia, Africa, and Southern Europe but are less common in Northern Europe and North America[2,3] because they do not occur in the endemic genotype A hepatitis B strain.[4]

The main utility of testing for HB$_e$Ag and anti-HB$_e$ is to assess response of the hepatitis B infection to therapy.

See Table II-7.

Presence of HB$_e$Ag implies that infective hepatitis B virus is present in serum. However, its absence on conversion to anti-HB$_e$ does not rule out infectivity, especially in persons infected with genotypes other than A. HB$_e$Ag-negative strains respond similarly to antiviral treatment.[5] Measurement of HBV-DNA is now recommended, especially in persons with increased ALT but negative HB$_e$Ag.

TEST NAME AND METHOD	SPECIMEN REQUIREMENTS	REFERENCE INTERVAL, CONVENTIONAL [INTERNATIONAL RECOMMENDED UNITS]	CHEMICAL INTERFERENCES AND IN VIVO EFFECTS
Hepatitis C Antibody (Anti-HCV)[1,2] *EIA, CA, MEIA recombinant immunoblot assay (RIBA)*	Serum. Stable for 7 days at room temperature and indefinitely at 4° C or 20° C.	Negative.	C ↑ influenza vaccination

1. Alter HJ: Descartes before the horse: I clone, therefore I am: the hepatitis C virus in current perspective, *Ann Intern Med* 115:644-649, 1991.

2. Gerlich WH, Thomssen R: Terminology, structure, and laboratory diagnosis of hepatitis viruses. In McIntyre N, Benhamou J-P, Bircher J, et al, editors: *Oxford textbook of clinical hepatology,* New York, 1991, Oxford University Press.

3. Alter MJ, Margolis HM, Krzysztof K, et al: The natural history of community-acquired hepatitis C in the United States, *N Engl J Med* 327:1899-1905, 1992.

4. Kim W, Brown R, Terrault N, et al: Burden of liver disease in the United States: summary of a workshop, *Hepatology* 36:227-242, 2002.

5. Seeff LB, Buskell-Bales Z, Wright BC, et al: Long-term mortality after transfusion-associated non-A, non-B hepatitis, *N Engl J Med* 327:1906-1911, 1992.

6. Choo QL, Kuo G, Weiner AJ, et al: Isolation of a cDNA clone derived from a blood-borne non-A, non-B viral hepatitis genome, *Science* 244:359-362, 1989.

7. Gretch D: Diagnostic tests for hepatitis C, *Hepatology* 26:43S-47S, 1997.

The hepatitis C virus (HCV) is a single-stranded RNA virus of the *Flaviviridae* family that is now known to be responsible for >95% of the cases of "non-A, non-B" hepatitis (see Fig. II-6). The most common mode of acquisition of HCV is through injection drug use, but transfusion before effective blood donor testing was available (1992) and noninjection drug use are also common risk factors. Transmission by needlestick or transmission to a fetus by an infected mother occurs in ~3-5% of exposures. Sexual transmission is rare. Hepatitis C is the most common cause of chronic hepatitis, cirrhosis,[3] and hepatocellular carcinoma and is the major cause of cryoglobulinemia.[4] However, long-term follow-up evaluation (~18 yr) of patients with transfusion-acquired non-A, non-B hepatitis (most of whom presumably had hepatitis C infections) did not show an increase in overall mortality, although there was a slight increase in liver-related mortality.[5]

The hepatitis C genome was discovered using molecular techniques, although the virus had not been isolated.[6] The second-generation EIA and RIBA tests use the c100-3, c200, c22, and c33c antigens, whereas third-generation EIA and CA tests utilize c22, c33, c100, and NS-5 antigens. Antibody becomes detectable an average of 9 weeks after exposure with third-generation assays and 12 weeks after exposure using second-generation assays; ~40-50% of those with acute HCV infection have negative anti-HCV at the time of diagnosis.[7] Approximately half of those with acute HCV clear virus and some of these never develop anti-HCV. In the remainder, ~15-30% subsequently lose anti-HCV over 15-20 yr of follow-up evaluation.[8,9] Most (90%) of those truly positive for anti-HCV are chronically infected.[10] Presence of anti-HCV does not imply protective immunity.

Usually anti-HCV is obtained first to diagnose HCV (see Table II-7). RIBA is equivalent to Western blot in confirming true positive anti-HCV. Samples that are weakly positive (signal to cutoff value ratio <3.9 for ELISA, <8.0 for CA, or <10.0 for MEIA) are usually negative on RIBA,[10,11] and CDC guidelines recommend confirmation with RIBA before reporting these as positive.[12] Samples that are strongly positive are almost never RIBA negative. HCV-RNA can also be obtained if there is high clinical suspicion of HCV despite a negative anti-HCV, especially in immunosuppressed individuals or in the setting of acute hepatitis. Anti-HCV and the RIBA often do not become positive during an acute infection; thus repeat testing several months later is required if HCV-RNA is negative.

8. Rodger A, Thomson JA, Thompson SC, et al: Assessment of long-term outcomes of hepatitis C virus infection in a cohort of patients with acute hepatitis in 1971-1975: results of a pilot study, *J Gastroenterol Hepatol* 14:269-273, 1999.

9. Seeff L, Hollinger FB, Alter HJ, et al: Long-term mortality and morbidity of transfusion-associated non-A, non-B, and type C hepatitis: a National Heart, Lung, and Blood Institute collaborative study, *Hepatology* 33:455-463, 2001.

10. Dufour D, Talastas M, Fernandez MD, et al: Low positive anti-hepatitis C virus enzyme immunoassay results: an important predictor of low likelihood of hepatitis C infection, *Clin Chem* 49:479-486, 2003.

11. Dufour D, Talastas M, Fernandez MD, et al: Chemiluminescence assay improves specificity of hepatitis C antibody detection, *Clin Chem* 49:940-944, 2003.

12. Alter M, Kuhnert W, Finelli L: Guidelines for laboratory testing and results reporting of antibody to hepatitis C virus, *MMWR Morb Mortal Wkly Rep* 52 (RR-3):1-15, 2003.

TEST NAME AND METHOD	SPECIMEN REQUIREMENTS	REFERENCE INTERVAL, CONVENTIONAL [INTERNATIONAL RECOMMENDED UNITS]	CHEMICAL INTERFERENCES AND IN VIVO EFFECTS
Hepatitis C Core Antigen (HCV-Ag)[1-4] *ELISA*	Serum or plasma. Stable at 4° C for 7 days; minimal loss at 25° C for 7 days. Stable at −20° C indefinitely.	<2 pg/mL	None reported.

1. Alter HJ: Descartes before the horse: I clone, therefore I am: the hepatitis C virus in current perspective, *Ann Intern Med* 115:644-649, 1991.
2. Gerlich WH, Thomssen R: Terminology, structure, and laboratory diagnosis of hepatitis viruses. In McIntyre N, Benhamou J-P, Bircher J, et al, editors: *Oxford textbook of clinical hepatology,* New York, 1991, Oxford University Press.
3. Alter MJ, Margolis HM, Krzysztof K, et al: The natural history of community-acquired hepatitis C in the United States, *N Engl J Med* 327:1899-1905, 1992.
4. Strader D, Wright T, Thomas DL, et al: Diagnosis, management, and treatment of hepatitis C, *Hepatology* 39:1147-1171, 2004.

TEST NAME AND METHOD	SPECIMEN REQUIREMENTS	REFERENCE INTERVAL, CONVENTIONAL [INTERNATIONAL RECOMMENDED UNITS]	CHEMICAL INTERFERENCES AND IN VIVO EFFECTS
Hepatitis C RNA (HCV-RNA)[1,2] *Reverse-Transcriptase PCR (rt-PCR), branched DNA (b-DNA), transcription-mediated amplification (TMA)*	Plasma (ACD or EDTA; avoid heparin). Separate plasma and freeze at −20° C within 4 hr of collection. Analysis should be within 2 wk. At least for b-DNA methods, separation of serum from cells within 1-2 hr of collection allows storage at room temperature up to 24 hr, at 4° C for up to 1 wk, and at −70° C indefinitely and through several freeze-thaw cycles.[3]	Negative.	Cross-contamination with RNA from other specimens causing false-positive results is possible, particularly with target amplification techniques.

1. Hu KQ, Yu CH, Vierling JM: Direct detection of circulating hepatitis C virus RNA using probes from the 5′-untranslated region, *J Clin Invest* 89:2040-2045, 1992.
2. Kato N, Yokosura O, Hosoda K, et al: Quantification of hepatitis C virus by competitive reverse transcription-polymerase chain reaction: increase of the virus in advanced liver disease, *Hepatology* 18:16-20, 1993.
3. Davis G, Lau J, Urdea M, et al: Quantitative detection of hepatitis C virus RNA with a solid-phase signal amplification method: definition of optimal conditions for specimen collection and clinical application in interferon-treated patients, *Hepatology* 19:1337-1341, 1994.
4. Strader D, Wright T, Thomas DL, et al: Diagnosis, management, and treatment of hepatitis C, *Hepatology* 39:1147-1171, 2004.

DIAGNOSTIC INFORMATION	REMARKS

See *Hepatitis C Antibody* for information regarding the virus and its clinical course. HCV antigen appears at about the same time as HCV-RNA with acute infection and increases in parallel to it. There is a strong correlation between core antigen and HCV-RNA, with 1 pg/mL of core antigen approximately equivalent to 8000 U/mL of HCV-RNA. HCV antigen becomes undetectable with successful treatment but is not as sensitive at detecting residual virus as are HCV-RNA assays with detection limits <50 U/mL.

HCV core antigen has similar sensitivity in infection with all genotypes of HCV. Assays detect total HCV antigen and require dissociation of antigen from antibody before measurement.

See Table II-7.

See *Hepatitis C Antibody* for information regarding the virus and its clinical course. Detection of HCV-RNA is used to confirm current infection and to monitor treatment with interferon-α (with or without ribavirin). The most widely used genomic area for detection by PCR seems to be a well conserved 5'-noncoding region, although newer assays also use the NS5b region.

Assays for HCV-RNA are typically divided into qualitative and quantitative forms. Qualitative assays have generally had lower detection limits, but real-time PCR and TMA quantitative assays are generally replacing qualitative assays. Quantitative assays (viral load) are needed pretreatment to assess response (<2 log decrease after 12-wk treatment indicates lack of response).[4]

RNA is very susceptible to degradation; thus improper specimen handling can cause false-negative results. Monitoring of treatment at time points beyond 12 wk requires use of assays with lower detection limits ≤50 U/mL.[5] Assays are now generally reported in U/mL, with standardization using the WHO reference material.[6] Although this improves reproducibility between methods, it does not eliminate differences.[7]

There are six genotypes of HCV, with <70% homology in nucleic acid sequence. Determination of genotype, either by line probe analysis or direct sequencing of either the 5'-noncoding or NS5b region, is critical pretreatment, as genotypes 2/3 respond to lower doses and shorter duration of treatment than do other genotypes.[4]

See Table II-7.

5. Seeff L, Hoofnagle J: National Institutes of Health Consensus Development Conference: management of hepatitis C: 2002, *Hepatology* 36:S1-2, 2002.
6. Saldanha J, Heath A, Lelie N, et al: Calibration of HCV working reagents for NAT assays against the HCV international standard. The Collaborative Study Group, *Vox Sang* 78:217-224, 2000.
7. Saldanha J, Gerlich W, Lelie N, et al: An international collaborative study to establish a World Health Organization international standard for hepatitis B virus DNA nucleic acid amplification techniques, *Vox Sang* 80:63-71, 2001.

TEST NAME AND METHOD	SPECIMEN REQUIREMENTS	REFERENCE INTERVAL, CONVENTIONAL [INTERNATIONAL RECOMMENDED UNITS]	CHEMICAL INTERFERENCES AND IN VIVO EFFECTS
Hepatitis Delta Antigen and Antibody (HDAg; anti-HD)[1]	Serum. Stable for 7 days at room temperature and indefinitely at 4° C or 20° C.	Negative.	None found.
Solid-phase EIA[2,3]			

1. Gerlich WH, Thomssen R: Terminology, structure, and laboratory diagnosis of hepatitis viruses. In McIntyre N, Benhamou J-P, Bircher J, et al, editors: *Oxford textbook of clinical hepatology,* New York, 1991, Oxford University Press.
2. Dubois F, Goudeau A: Kinetics of delta antigen and delta antibody in acute delta hepatitis: evaluation with different enzyme immunoassays, *J Clin Microbiol* 26:1339-1342, 1988.
3. Rizzetto M, Shih JW-K, Gerin JL: The hepatitis B virus-associated δ antigen: isolation from liver, development of solid-phase radioimmunoassays for δ antigen and anti-δ and partial characterization of δ antigen, *J Immunol* 725:318-324, 1980.

TEST NAME AND METHOD	SPECIMEN REQUIREMENTS	REFERENCE INTERVAL, CONVENTIONAL [INTERNATIONAL RECOMMENDED UNITS]	CHEMICAL INTERFERENCES AND IN VIVO EFFECTS
Her-2/*neu* **(c-*erb*B-2)** *Immunohisto-chemistry (IHC)* *Fluorescence in situ hybridization (FISH)*	Formalin-fixed, paraffin-embedded tissue.	*Score* *Interpretation* 0 None 1+ Partial in at least 10% of tumor cells 2+ Weak, complete pattern in at least 10% of tumor cells 3+ Strong, complete pattern in at least 10% of tumor cells Negative for gene amplification (method specific)	*Membranous Staining Pattern* Negative Negative Weakly positive Strongly positive
Immunoassay[1]	Serum. Stable up to 8 hr at room temperature and up to 24 hr at 2-8° C. For longer periods, store frozen at −20° C or colder.	*ng/mL* <15 × 1.0	*mcg/L* <15

DIAGNOSTIC INFORMATION	REMARKS

Hepatitis Delta is a replication-defective RNA virus or virusoid that requires the surface coat of hepatitis B (HBsAg) to become an infectious virus. After transcription of the RNA into mRNA, the virus produces a protein, HDAg, which may interfere with translation of other mRNAs and produce cell damage. When hepatitis D infection occurs simultaneously with hepatitis B, the course of both infections tends to be more severe, but self-limited. However, in the case of acute hepatitis D superinfection of an established hepatitis B infection, there is much more hepatitis D replication, and a more severe clinical hepatitis occurs. In this situation, the hepatitis D infection usually becomes chronic, and HBV replication is suppressed. Anti-HD does not necessarily indicate active infection, but the presence of HDAg does.

The role of testing for either HDAg or anti-HD is currently controversial because the incidence of infection with HDV has declined markedly in the U.S. with use of HBV vaccine. Generally one tests for hepatitis D only in patients positive for HBsAg. It has been suggested, for prognostic reasons, that all patients with chronic hepatitis B be tested for anti-HD, especially if there is exacerbation of a stable hepatitis.

See also *Section II, Hepatitis Delta Virus.*

See Table II-7.

Her-2/*neu* gene amplification and overexpression of the Her-2/*neu* protein is found in 25-30% of primary breast cancers. The protein is expressed on normal epithelial cells and is overexpressed in other epithelial tumors, including lung, hepatocellular, pancreatic, colon, stomach, ovarian, cervical, and bladder cancers.[1-4]

The Her-2 (human epidermal growth factor receptor-2)/*neu* oncogene, located on the long arm of chromosome 17, encodes a 185 kDa transmembrane protein (p185) that is part of the epidermal growth factor receptor family (EGFR) and has tyrosine kinase activity. Binding of ligand, including EGR, EGF-like ligands, and neuregulins, to the receptor causes dimerizations, which initiates an intracellular signaling cascade leading to cell proliferation. The extracellular domain of the protein (p105) is a glycoprotein that is shed into the circulation.[1-4]

Trastuzumab (Herceptin) is a humanized monoclonal antibody against the extracellular domain of Her-2/*neu* that acts by inhibiting the activated proliferation signal. High levels of Her-2/*neu* expression or amplification in tissue are recommended to identify patients with metastatic, recurrent, and/or treatment-refractory unresectable locally advanced breast cancer for trastuzumab treatment.[5] Her-2/*neu* expression may also have negative prognostic value. Tumors scored as weakly positive (2+) using IHC (scale 0-3+) are typically sent for additional testing using FISH.[1-4]

TEST NAME AND METHOD	SPECIMEN REQUIREMENTS	REFERENCE INTERVAL, CONVENTIONAL [INTERNATIONAL RECOMMENDED UNITS]		CHEMICAL INTERFERENCES AND IN VIVO EFFECTS
Her-2/neu (c-erbB-2)—CONT				

1. Payne RC, Allard JW, Anderson-Mauser L, et al: Automated assay for Her-2/neu in serum, *Clin Chem* 46:175-182, 2000.
2. Spyratos F: Prognostic and predictive markers for breast cancer. In Diamandis EP, Fritsche HA, Lilja H, et al, editors: *Tumor markers. Physiology, pathobiology, technology, and clinical applications,* Washington, DC, 2002, AACC Press.
3. Kunz GM, Sokoll LJ: Her-2/neu testing, *Clin Lab News* 30:12-14, 2004.
4. Carney WP, Neumann R, Lipton A, et al: Potential clinical utility of serum Her-2/neu oncoprotein concentrations in patients with breast cancer, *Clin Chem* 49:1579-1598, 2003.
5. *Her-2/neu package insert,* ADVIA Centaur, Tarrytown, NY, Bayer HealthCare.

TEST NAME AND METHOD	SPECIMEN REQUIREMENTS	REFERENCE INTERVAL, CONVENTIONAL		[INTERNATIONAL RECOMMENDED UNITS]	CHEMICAL INTERFERENCES AND IN VIVO EFFECTS
Hexachlorophene	Whole blood (heparin, oxalate, or EDTA)		*mg/L*	*mmol/L*	None found.
(2,2'-Dihydroxy- 3,3', 5,5', 6,6'- hexachlorodi- phenylmethane; CAS 70-30-4)		Infant: Adult: After topical use:	<0.182 × 2.46 <0.089 0.1-0.655	[<0.048] [<0.219] [0.246-1.611]	
	Milk		<0.009 mg/L × 2.46	[<0.022 μmol/L]	
GLC	Fat		<0.05 mg/kg × 2.46	[<0.123 μmol/kg]	

1. Goutieres F, Aicardi J: Accidental percutaneous hexachlorophene intoxication in children, *BMJ* 2:663-665, 1977.
2. POISINDEX Toxocologic Management: *Hexachlorophene, vol 78,* Denver, CO, 1993, Micromedex, Inc.

DIAGNOSTIC INFORMATION	REMARKS

FDA-cleared assays for measurement of the Her-2/*neu* protein in serum are available for use in the follow-up evaluation and monitoring of patients with metastatic breast cancer in patients with a Her-2/*neu* concentration >15 ng/mL (Oncogene Science microtiter ELISA and ADVIA Centaur and Immuno 1, Bayer HealthCare). The test may also have clinical utility in assessing prognosis, predicting response to therapy, and detecting early disease progression. Trastuzumab does not cross-react in the Her-2/*neu* assay.[4]

Repeated exposure of newborn infants to high concentrations of hexachlorophene is associated with vascular encephalopathy of the brainstem reticular formation. Other adverse effects include diplopia, irritability, muscular fasciculations,[1] vomiting, and seizures.

This is an antibacterial agent that was once widely used in soaps, cosmetics, and antiseptic solutions. Excretion by the kidney is minimal, but disposition in man has not been studied.

Plasma hexachlorophene levels have not been demonstrated to correlate well with clinical effects.[2]

Kinetic values
$t_{1/2}$:   24 hr

TEST NAME AND METHOD	SPECIMEN REQUIREMENTS	REFERENCE INTERVAL, CONVENTIONAL [INTERNATIONAL RECOMMENDED UNITS]		CHEMICAL INTERFERENCES AND IN VIVO EFFECTS
Hexokinase (HK) in Erythrocytes (EC 2.7.1.1)[1] *ICSH, 37° C*[1-3]	Hemolysate of washed Ercs. Submit whole blood (ACD, EDTA, or heparin). Stable >20 days at 4° C, 5 days at 25° C.	*U/g Hb* 1.27 ± 0.18 (SD) × 0.0645* *U/10^{12} Ercs* 36.8 ± 5.2 × 1.0 *U/mL Ercs* 0.43 ± 0.06 × 1.0 Activity higher in infants.[4] See *Acetylcholinesterase.* *Conversion factor based on MW of Hb of 64,500.	*MU/mol Hb* [0.08 ± 0.01] *pU/Erc* [36.8 ± 5.2] *kU/L Ercs* [0.43 ± 0.06]	↓ In the presence of copper unless EDTA (400 μmol/L) is also present.

1. Beutler E: *Red cell metabolism: a manual of biochemical methods,* ed 4, New York, 1986, Grune & Stratton.
2. Beutler E, Blume KG, Kaplan JC, et al: International committee for standardization in haematology: recommended methods for red-cell enzyme analysis, *Br J Haematol* 35:331-340, 1977.
3. Miwa S, Fujii H: Molecular basis of erythroenzymopathies associated with hereditary hemolytic anemia: tabulation of mutant enzymes, *Am J Hematol* 51:122-132, 1996.
4. Oski FA: Red cell metabolism in the newborn infant. V. Glycolytic intermediates and glycolytic enzymes, *Pediatrics* 44:84-91, 1969.
5. Valentine WN, Tanaka KR, Paglia DE: Hemolytic anemias and erythrocyte enzymopathies, *Ann Intern Med* 103:245-257, 1985.
6. Beutler E: *Hemolytic anemia in disorders of red cell metabolism,* New York, 1978, Plenum Pub. Co.
7. Staal GEJ, Rijksen G: The role of red cell aging in the diagnosis of glycolytic enzyme defects. In Magnani M, De Flora A, editors: Red blood cell aging, *Adv Exp Med Biol* 507:239-249, 1991.

TEST NAME AND METHOD	SPECIMEN REQUIREMENTS	REFERENCE INTERVAL, CONVENTIONAL [INTERNATIONAL RECOMMENDED UNITS]			CHEMICAL INTERFERENCES AND IN VIVO EFFECTS
Hexosaminidase A (EC 3.2.1.52)[1] *DEAE chromatography, fluorimetric, 37° C*[2]	Serum; allow blood to clot at 3° C and centrifuge at 3° C. Store at −20° C.		*nmol/hr/ mL (SD)*	*U/L*	S ↑ V Oral contraceptives[6,7]
		Noncarriers:	524 ± 68 × 0.0167	[8.75 ± 1.13]	
		Obligate heterozygotes:	260 ± 63	[4.34 ± 1.05]	
		Tay-Sachs (TS) homozygotes:	0	[0]	

	Percent activity as hexosaminidase A		*Fraction activity*
Noncarriers:	80 ± 5.8	× 0.01	[0.80 ± 0.06]
Obligate heterozygotes:	58 ± 5.6		[0.58 ± 0.06]
TS homozygotes:	0		[0]

		nmol/hr/mL (SD)		*U/L*
Thermal inactivation (indirect), fluorimetric, 37° C[2] *Fluorimetric (MU-β-Glc Nac-6-S), 37° C*[3]	Noncarriers:	448 ± 87	× 0.0167	[7.48 ± 1.45]
	Obligate heterozygotes:	239 ± 35		[3.99 ± 0.58]
	TS homozygotes:	41		[0.68]

DIAGNOSTIC INFORMATION	REMARKS
Deficiency is a rare cause of congenital nonspherocytic hemolytic anemia (autosomal recessive).[5]	Activity in young erythrocytes is much higher; therefore one should question normal enzyme activity in the presence of reticulocytosis and may require testing of reticulocyte-depleted samples.[6,7] $U/g\ Hb \times 29 = U/10^{12}\ Ercs$ $U/g\ Hb \times 0.34 = U/mL\ Ercs*$ *See Note, *Acetylcholinesterase.*
S ↑ Pregnancy, diabetes[6,7] S ↓↓ (or absent) Tay-Sachs homozygotes (both absolute hexosaminidase A and percent of total hexosaminidase) S ↓ Tay-Sachs heterozygotes (both absolute hexosaminidase A and percent hexosaminidase A) See also Table II-8.	Three predominant isoenzymes of hexosaminidase have been identified in serum hexosaminidases A, B, and S. Hexosaminidase A activity is used to distinguish normal subjects from Tay-Sachs heterozygote carriers and from homozygotes. Heterozygotes show a decrease in hexosaminidase A with an increase in hexosaminidases S and B. Homozygotes show virtually no hexosaminidase A but a substantial increase in hexosaminidases S and B.

TEST NAME AND METHOD	SPECIMEN REQUIREMENTS	REFERENCE INTERVAL, CONVENTIONAL [INTERNATIONAL RECOMMENDED UNITS]	CHEMICAL INTERFERENCES AND IN VIVO EFFECTS

Hexosaminidase A—CONT

		Percent activity as hexosaminidase A		*Fraction activity*
Noncarriers:		60 ± 8.2	$\times 0.01$	$[0.60 \pm 0.08]$
Obligate heterozygotes:		42 ± 5.4		$[0.42 \pm 0.05]$
TS homozygotes:		4		$[0.04]$

	nmol/hr/mL (SD)		*U/L*
Controls:	130 ± 25	$\times 0.0167$	$[2.17 \pm 0.41]$
(range)	(93-180)		$[1.55-3.00]$
TS carriers:	71.4 ± 7.0		$[1.19 \pm 0.11]$
(range)	(58.8-83.5)		$[0.98-1.39]$
TS patients:	1.26 ± 0.74		$[0.021 \pm 0.012]$
(range)	(0.38-2.33)		$[0.063-0.039]$

Fluorimetric (MU-β-Gal Nac-6-S), 37° C[3]	Leukocytes isolated from 5-10 mL of heparinized blood and stored frozen at −20° C. Blood should be kept on ice and separated within 24 hr.	*U/L*	
		20-30 yr	
		F:	6.2 ± 2.0
		M:	7.0 ± 1.3
		31-40 yr	
		F:	7.7 ± 1.9
		M:	6.5 ± 1.9
		41-50 yr	
		F:	7.9 ± 2.5
		M:	8.1 ± 1.7
		51-60 yr	
		F:	7.8 ± 1.7
		M:	8.5 ± 2.2
		61-70 yr	
		F:	8.2 ± 3.1
		M:	8.7 ± 1.9
		71-80 yr	
		F:	9.0 ± 1.9
		M:	8.7 ± 2.3

Fluorimetric (MU-β-GalNAcS) Total and percentage hex A heat denaturation method		*nmol/hr/mg protein*	*%A[5]*
	Control	801 ± 190	55-72
	Tay-Sachs	367-930	0-8
	B1 variant	189-1621	10-52
	Sandhoff	21-91	85-100

EIA (4-nitrophenyl-2-acetomido-2-deoxy-β-D-glucopyranoside), 37° C[4]			
	Controls:	21.7 ± 4.7	$[0.36 \pm 0.08]$
	(interval)	(16.8-28.0)	$[0.28-0.47]$
	TS carriers:	12.8 ± 1.8	$[0.21 \pm 0.03]$
	(interval)	(9.8-16.4)	$[0.16-0.27]$
	TS patients:	0.22 ± 0.12	$[0.004 \pm 0.002]$
	(interval)	(0.05-0.30)	$[0.0008-0.005]$

DIAGNOSTIC INFORMATION	REMARKS

The sulfated substrate used in this method is specifically cleaved by hexosaminidase A and allows direct assay of enzyme activity ($<2.5\%$ of activity in unfractionated serum is caused by hexosaminidase B). They are likely to replace thermal inactivation over the next few years.

The leukocyte assay is preferable to the serum assay. Testing can also be performed on tissues and amniotic fluid cells.

Hexosaminidase A accounts for 50-60% of total serum hexosaminidase activity.

In pregnancy, total serum hexosaminidase increases by fivefold, mainly because of hexosaminidase B, which is ~75% of total activity. After birth, total activity and the proportion of the B form decrease to reference intervals within 1 wk.

TEST NAME AND METHOD	SPECIMEN REQUIREMENTS	REFERENCE INTERVAL, CONVENTIONAL [INTERNATIONAL RECOMMENDED UNITS]	CHEMICAL INTERFERENCES AND IN VIVO EFFECTS

Hexosaminidase A—CONT

1. Gravel RA, Kabeck MM, Proia RL, et al: The G_{M2} gangliosidoses. In Scriver CR, Beaudet AL, Valle D, et al, editors: *The metabolic and molecular bases of inherited disease,* ed 8, New York, 2001, McGraw-Hill Inc.

2. Nakagawa S, Kumin S, Nitowsky HM: Human hexosaminidase isoenzymes: chromatographic separation as an aide to heterozygote identification, *Clin Chim Acta* 75:181-191, 1977.

3. Ben-Yoseph Y, Reid JE, Shapiro B, et al: Diagnosis and carrier detection of Tay-Sachs disease: direct determination of hexosaminidase A using 4-methylumbelliferyl derivatives of β-N-acetylglucosamine-6-sulfate, *Am J Hum Genet* 37:733-740, 1985.

4. Isaksson A, Hultberg B: Immunoassay of β-hexosaminidase isoenzymes in serum in patients with raised total activities, *Clin Chim Acta* 183:155-162, 1989.

5. Wenger DA, Williams C: Screening for lysosomal disorders. In Hommes FA, editor: *Techniques in diagnostic human biochemical genetics,* New York, 1991, Wiley-Liss, pp. 587-617.

6. Lowden JA: Serum β-hexosaminidases in pregnancy, *Clin Chim Acta* 93:409-417, 1979.

7. Nitowsky HM, Davis J, Nakagawa S, et al: Human hexosaminidase isoenzymes. IV. Effects of oral contraceptive steroids on serum hexosaminidase activity, *Am J Obstet Gynecol* 134:642-647, 1979.

Hexosaminidase B (EC 3.2.1.52)[1] *DEAE chromatographic, fluorimetric, 37° C*[2]	Serum, clotted and centrifuged at 3° C. Store at −20° C.			↑ Oral contraceptives[4]
			nmol/hr/ mL (SD)	*U/L*
		Noncarriers:	22 ± 10.2 × 0.0167	0.37 ± 0.17
		Obligate heterozygotes:	51 ± 30.0	0.85 ± 0.50
		Tay-Sachs homozygotes (n = 2):	305	5.09
			Activity, % of total	*Fraction of total activity*
		Noncarriers:	3 × 0.01	0.03
		Obligate heterozygotes:	11	0.11
		Tay-Sachs homozygotes (n = 2):	36	0.36

In biliary obstruction, total hexosaminidase increases about fourfold because of an increase in the proportion of the B form to ~60% of total activity; after relief of the obstruction, the proportion of the B form decreases.

↑↑ Tay-Sachs disease (homozygotes)

↑ Tay-Sachs disease (heterozygote carriers), diabetes, pregnancy.[5]

↓↓ (or absent) Sandhoff disease (homozygotes)

↓ Sandhoff disease (heterozygote carriers)

See also Table II-8.

Three predominant isoenzymes of hexosaminidase have been identified in serum hexosaminidases A, B, and S. Hexosaminidases B and S are heat stable and therefore must be separated chromatographically. Hexosaminidase B is the major heat-stable isoenzyme in platelets.

Hexosaminidase B accounts for 40-50% of total serum hexosaminidase activity.

In pregnancy, total serum hexosaminidase increases by fivefold, mainly because of hexosaminidase B, which is ~75% of total activity. After birth, total activity and the proportion of the B form decrease to reference ranges within 1 wk.

In biliary obstruction, total hexosaminidase increases about fourfold because of an increase in the proportion of the B form to ~60% of total activity; after relief of the obstruction, the proportion of the B form decreases.

TEST NAME AND METHOD	SPECIMEN REQUIREMENTS	REFERENCE INTERVAL, CONVENTIONAL [INTERNATIONAL RECOMMENDED UNITS]	CHEMICAL INTERFERENCES AND IN VIVO EFFECTS
Hexosaminidase B—CONT			
EIA (4-nitrophenyl-2-acetomido-2-deoxy-β-D-glucopyranoside)[3]		*U/L*	
		20-30 yr	
		F: 4.2 ± 1.6	
		M: 4.2 ± 1.7	
		31-40 yr	
		F: 5.6 ± 1.7	
		M: 5.1 ± 1.4	
		41-50 yr	
		F: 5.5 ± 1.7	
		M: 5.5 ± 1.9	
		51-60 yr	
		F: 6.2 ± 2.0	
		M: 6.3 ± 2.0	
		61-70 yr	
		F: 7.0 ± 2.8	
		M: 6.6 ± 1.6	
		71-80 yr	
		F: 7.4 ± 2.3	
		M: 8.0 ± 2.4	
Fluorimetric (MU-β-GalNAcS) total and percentage hex A heat denaturation method	Leukocytes isolated from 5-10 mL of heparinized blood. Separation must be within 24 hr.	*nmol/hr/mg protein* *%A* Control 801 ± 190 55-72 Tay-Sachs 367-930 0-8 B1 variant 189-1621 10-52 Sandhoff 21-91 85-100	

1. Gravel RA, Kabeck MM, Proia RL, et al: The G_{M2} gangliosidoses. In Scriver CR, Beaudet AL, Valle D, et al, editors: *The metabolic and molecular bases of inherited disease,* ed 8, New York, 2001, McGraw-Hill Inc.

2. Nakagawa S, Kumin S, Nitowsky HM: Human hexosaminidase isoenzymes: chromatographic separation as an aide to heterozygote identification, *Clin Chim Acta* 75:181-191, 1977.

3. Isaksson A, Haltberg B: Immunoassay of hexosaminidase isoenzymes in serum in patients with raised total activities, *Clin Chim Acta* 183:155-162, 1989.

4. Nitowsky HM, Davis J, Nakagawa S, et al: Human hexosaminidase isoenzymes. IV. Effects of oral contraceptive steroids on serum hexosaminidase activity, *Am J Obstet Gynecol* 134:642-647, 1979.

5. Lowden JA: Serum β-hexosaminidases in pregnancy, *Clin Chim Acta* 93:409-417, 1979.

Hexosaminidase, Total (β-*o*-Acetyl-glucosaminidase; β-*N*-Acetyl-glucosaminidase, NAG; β-*N*-Acetyl-hexosaminidase; EC 3.2.1.52)	Serum; allow blood to clot at 3° C and centrifuge at 3° C. Store at −20° C.	*nmol/hr/* *mL (SD)* *U/L* Noncarriers: 772 ± 183 × 0.0167 [12.89 ± 3.06] Obligate heterozygotes: 570 ± 105 [9.52 ± 1.75] Tay-Sachs homozygotes (n = 2): 1027 [17.15]	S ↑ V Ethanol, isoniazid, oral contraceptives,[12] rifampicin S ↓ C Acetate

DIAGNOSTIC INFORMATION

REMARKS

See *Hexosamonidase A.*

The leukocyte assay is preferred to serum assay.

S ↑ Hepatic disease with hepatocellular necrosis and cirrhosis, gastric cancer, neoplasia, myeloma, myocardial infarct, pregnancy, symptomatic porphyria, vascular complications of diabetes mellitus.[13]

S ↓ Sandhoff disease

Sensitive marker for heavy drinking

Hexosaminidase, β-*N*-acetylglucosaminidase, and *N*-acetyl-β-D-glucosaminidase (NAG) are alternative names used for the same lysosomal enzyme.[6] The name *hexosaminidase* has traditionally been used in conjunction with the diagnosis of Tay-Sachs and Sandhoff diseases, for which isoenzyme separation is necessary, although the use of specific substrates may render such separation unnecessary. In the context of other pathological conditions, the enzyme is more commonly referred to as *N*-acetyl-β-D-glucosaminidase.

TEST NAME AND METHOD	SPECIMEN REQUIREMENTS	REFERENCE INTERVAL, CONVENTIONAL [INTERNATIONAL RECOMMENDED UNITS]		CHEMICAL INTERFERENCES AND IN VIVO EFFECTS

Hexosaminidase, Total—CONT

Fluorimetric (4-methylumbellif- eryl-2-acetamido- 2-deoxy- β-D-glucopyrano- side), 37° C[1]

		U/L		*μKat/L*
Fluorimetric (4-methylumbellif- eryl-2-acetamido- 2-deoxy- β-D-glucopyrano- side), 37° C[2]		0.67 ± 0.23 (SD) × 0.017		[0.01 ± 0.004]

Fluorimetric (4-methylumbellif- eryl-glucopyrano- side), 37° C[3]	Plasma (heparinized, platelet-free). Stable for 15 days at 4° C.	0.55-0.91		[0.01-0.02]

Photometric (4-nitrophenyl- 2-acetamido- 2-deoxy- β-D-glucopyrano- side), 405 nm, 37° C[4]		24.8 ± 6.3 (SD)		[0.42 ± 0.11]

Fluorimetric (4-methylumbellif- eryl- β-D-N-acetylglu- cosaminide), 37° C[5]		*nmol/hr/ mL (SD)*		*U/L*
		Cord blood		
		M:	1381 ± 363 × 0.0167	[23.0 ± 6.1]
		F:	1267 ± 310	[21.2 ± 5.2]
		1-4 yr		
		M:	910 ± 315	[15.2 ± 5.3]
		F:	690 ± 261	[11.5 ± 4.4]
		5-9 yr		
		M:	698 ± 185	[11.7 ± 3.1]
		F:	675 ± 207	[11.3 ± 3.5]
		10-14 yr		
		M:	486 ± 88	[8.1 ± 1.5]
		F:	481 ± 83	[8.0 ± 1.4]
		15-19 yr		
		M:	740 ± 137	[12.4 ± 2.3]
		F:	663 ± 292	[11.1 ± 4.9]
		20-24 yr		
		M:	968 ± 191	[16.1 ± 3.2]
		F:	1045 ± 222	[17.4 ± 3.7]

DIAGNOSTIC INFORMATION	REMARKS
	Three predominant isoenzymes of lysosomal hexosaminidase have been identified in serum: hexosaminidase A (or acid form), hexosaminidase B (or basic form), and hexosaminidase S. Separation is readily accomplished by DEAE cellulose chromatography or isoelectric focusing. Alternatively, the isoenzymes may be distinguished as the thermolabile hexosaminidase A and thermostable components, hexosaminidases B and S. Distinction by thermostability consistently yields a lower absolute and lower relative hexosaminidase A than does column separation. The enzyme exists as the following dimers: S ($\alpha\alpha$), A ($\alpha\beta$), and B ($\beta\beta$). Newly developed specific substrates may distinguish the separate isoenzymes characteristic of Tay-Sachs and Sandhoff diseases.
	For the diagnosis of Tay-Sachs disease, total hexosaminidase determinations are of no value. Tay-Sachs victims lack the A isoenzyme but may have increased D and/or S. Hexosaminidase is usually determined in serum. It has also been reported in platelets, peripheral blood leukocytes, urine, saliva, tears, and fibroblast cultures from skin.[17] Amniotic fluid and fetal blood obtained at fetoscopy have been used for the antenatal diagnosis of Tay-Sachs disease (by demonstrating the absence of the heat-labile hexosaminidase A isoenzyme) and for Sandhoff disease, in which hexosaminidases A and B are absent.
	See also *Hexosaminidase A* and *Hexosaminidase B*.

TEST NAME AND METHOD	SPECIMEN REQUIREMENTS	REFERENCE INTERVAL, CONVENTIONAL [INTERNATIONAL RECOMMENDED UNITS]			CHEMICAL INTERFERENCES AND IN VIVO EFFECTS
Hexosaminidase, Total—CONT					
		25-49 yr			
		M:	870 ± 196	[14.5 ± 3.3]	
		F:	743 ± 144	[12.4 ± 2.4]	
		50-74 yr			
		M:	951 ± 218	[15.9 ± 3.6]	
		F:	866 ± 182	[14.4 ± 3.0]	
Fluorimetric (4-methylumbelliferyl-glucopyranoside), 37° C[6]	Urine, random. Collect without preservatives at 4° C and assay immediately or store at −20° C. Stable 1 mo at −20° C. Gel filtration is recommended to remove inhibitors. Fibroblast-like cells isolated from amniotic fluid.	*nmol/hr/mg creatinine* 40-120 × 1.89 (See *Remarks.*)		*U/mol creatinine* [76-227]	U ↑ V Drugs causing proximal tubular damage. Some examples are aminoglycosides (e.g., gentamicin, tobramycin, amikacin), amphotericin, and cisplatin.
Colorimetric (4-nitrophenyl-N-acetyl-β-D-glucosaminide), 405 nm, 37° C		3.8 ± 2.3 U/L (SD)[10] × 0.017 [0.06 ± 0.04 μKat/L] *U/mmol creatinine*[11] 0-20 × 1.0		*kU/mol creatinine* [0-20]	
Fluorimetric (4-methylumbelliferyl-β-D glucosaminide), 37° C[7]		*U/g creatinine* 0-2.5 × 113		*U/mol creatinine* [0-283]	
Fluorimetric (4-methylumbelliferyl-N-acetyl-β-D-glucosaminide), 37° C[8]		*nmol/hr/mg creatinine* 29 ± 16 (SD) × 1.89		*U/mol creatinine* [54.8 ± 30.2]	
Colorimetric (2-methoxy-4-[2'-nitro-vinyl]-phenyl-2-acetamide-2-deoxy-β-D-glucopyranoside)[9]		14.6 ± 8.2 μmol/30 min/mmol creatinine			

DIAGNOSTIC INFORMATION	REMARKS

U ↑ Glomerulopathies, nephrotic syndrome, Goodpasture's disease, direct injury to renal cells, acute renal transplant rejection, immunosuppressive nephrotoxicity, thrombosis of donor renal artery or vein as a result of ischemia or nephrotoxicity, urinary tract infection; active phase of acute tubular necrosis, heavy metal poisoning, active glomerulonephritis, analgesic nephropathy, aminoglycoside toxicity, chronic pyelonephritis, renal injury resulting from hypotension or anoxia.

Diseases with secondary renal involvement: renal artery stenosis in hypertensives, rheumatoid arthritis, degenerative joint disease, diabetes mellitus, stroke, myocardial infarction, carotid thrombosis, chronic liver disease, after surgery, burns, cardiac bypass operation, hypertension, multiple myeloma, and chemotherapy.[14,15]

NAG is the most widely assayed urinary enzyme used for the detection and diagnosis of renal disease.[18] This is because of its stability in urine, its high molecular weight (130,000), which prevents glomerular filtration, and its very high activity in tubular lysosomes. An increase in urinary activity therefore indicates renal damage. Increased urinary NAG activity resulting from renal damage by antibiotics or chemotherapy appears earlier than elevations in serum creatinine or decreased creatinine clearance. However, analytically sensitive assays are necessary because of its low activity in health.

Urinary excretion of NAG provides an early warning of rejection episodes for renal transplants. The urine reference interval shows an almost linear increase in NAG activity from ages 10 yr to >70 yr, from 40-90 nmol/hr/mg creatinine [75.6-170 U/mol creatinine]. Children >40 nmol/hr/mg creatinine [>75.6 U/mol creatinine].[6]

Changes have also been observed in the urinary pattern of NAG isoenzymes in renal disease. When using ion-exchange chromatography several isoenzyme forms, B_1, I_1, I_2, and A^S, are detected between the main A and B hexosaminidases. For example, after renal transplantation, no change in the urinary isoenzyme profile is observed in the stable transplant, whereas reversible rejection shows a marked increase in the I_2 form with a decrease in the relative proportion of the A form; the profile normalizes when rejection is treated. When patients do not respond to treatment, both the B and I forms increase, whereas the A form decreases.[18]

This chromophore has a higher molar absorbance than 4-nitrophenol; therefore 15-fold urine dilution can be used, and the effect of endogenous inhibitors thus is eliminated.

TEST NAME AND METHOD	SPECIMEN REQUIREMENTS	REFERENCE INTERVAL, CONVENTIONAL [INTERNATIONAL RECOMMENDED UNITS]	CHEMICAL INTERFERENCES AND IN VIVO EFFECTS

Hexosaminidase, Total—CONT

1. Nakagawa S, Kumin S, Nitowsky HM: Human hexosaminidase isoenzymes: chromatographic separation as an aide to heterozygote identification, *Clin Chim Acta* 75:181-191, 1977.

2. Whiting PH, Ross IS, Borthwick L: Serum and urine N-acetyl-β-D-glucosaminidase in diabetics on diagnosis and subsequent treatment, and stable insulin dependent diabetics, *Clin Chim Acta* 92:459-463, 1979.

3. Woollen JW, Walker PG: The fluorometric estimation of N-acetyl-β-glucosaminidase and β-galactosidase in blood plasma, *Clin Chim Acta* 12:647-658, 1965.

4. Koskinen H, Jarvisalo J, Huuskonen MS, et al: Serum lysosomal enzyme activities in silicosis and asbestosis, *Eur J Resp Dis* 64:182-188, 1983.

5. Lombardo A, Gor GC, Marchesini S, et al: Influence of age and sex on five human plasma lysosomal enzymes assayed by automated procedures, *Clin Chim Acta* 113:141-152, 1981.

6. Tucker SM, Boyd PIR, Thompson AE, et al: Automated assay of W-acetyl-p-glucosaminidase in normal and pathological human urine, *Clin Chim Acta* 62:333-339, 1975.

7. Powell SC, Scaro J, Wilson E, et al: Assay of urinary N-acetyl-beta-glucosaminidase in a centrifugal analyzer, *Clin Chem* 29:1717-1719, 1983.

8. Alderman MH, Melcher L, Drayer DE, et al: Increased excretion of urinary N-acetyl-β-glucosaminidase in essential hypertension and its decline with antihypertensive therapy, *N Engl J Med* 309:1213-1217, 1983.

9. Yuen C-T, Price RG, Chattagoon L, et al: Colorimetric assays for N-acetyl-β-D-glucosaminidase and β-D-galactosidase in human urine using newly-developed ω-nitrostyryl substrates, *Clin Chim Acta* 124:195-204, 1982.

High-Density Lipoprotein Cholesterol (HDL-C)[1-12]

Homogeneous/ direct[8,13-19,20,21]

Lipoprotein precipitation[8,22,23]

Electrophoresis[8,24-26]

Ultracentrifugation[8,27]

Chromatography[8,27]

Serum, plasma (EDTA or heparin but not oxalate, fluoride, or citrate). Fasting ≥12 hr is recommended; nonfasting specimen is acceptable if HDL-C is not part of a fasting lipid profile. Patient should be sitting for 5 min before blood draw, and prolonged tourniquet use should be avoided. Stable 1-7 days at 4° C. Avoid repeated freezing and thawing.

	Recommended Cutpoints[3]		
Low:	<40 mg/dL	× 0.0259	[<1.04 mmol/L]
High:	≥60 mg/dL		[≥1.55 mmol/L]

	5th-95th percentile mg/dL[6,28]		*5th-95th percentile mmol/L*
Non-Hispanic White			
4-5 yr			
M:	30-66	× 0.0259	[0.78-1.71]
F:	30-68		[0.78-1.76]
6-11 yr			
M:	34-73		[0.88-1.89]
F:	32-68		[0.83-1.76]
12-19 yr			
M:	31-63		[0.80-1.63]
F:	32-70		[0.83-1.81]
20-29 yr			
M:	28-69		[0.73-1.79]
F:	36-86		[0.93-2.23]
30-39 yr			
M:	26-68		[0.67-1.76]
F:	33-82		[0.85-2.12]
40-49 yr			
M:	26-72		[0.67-1.86]
F:	37-79		[0.96-2.05]

↓ C EDTA plasma concentrations are 3-6% lower than serum.

↑ V Carbamazepine, estrogens, moderate alcohol intake, fibric acid derivatives (e.g., clofibrate, gemfibrozil, fenofibrate), HMG CoA reductase inhibitors (statins), bile acid sequestrants (resins, e.g., cholestyramine, colestipol), niacin (or nicotinic acid), phenobarbital, phenytoin, weight loss in overweight individuals, and exercise.

10. Horak E, Hopfer SM, Sunderman FW Jr: Spectrophotometric assay for urinary N-acetyl-β-D-glucosaminidase activity, *Clin Chem* 27:1180-1185, 1981.

11. Sri Krishna K, Kirubakaran MG, Pandey AP, et al: Urinary N-acetyl-β-D-glucosaminidase and aminopeptidase N in the diagnosis of graft rejection after live donor renal transplantation, *Clin Chim Acta* 150:69-85, 1985.

12. Nitowsky HM, Davis J, Nakagawa S, et al: Human hexosaminidase isoenzymes. IV. Effects of oral contraceptive steroids on serum hexosaminidase activity, *Am J Obstet Gynecol* 134:642-647, 1979.

13. Lowden JA: Serum β-hexosaminidases in pregnancy, *Clin Chim Acta* 93:409-417, 1979.

14. Coward RA, DeLamore IW, Mallick NP, et al: Urinary N-acetyl-β-D-glucosaminidase as an indicator of tubular damage in multiple myeloma, *Clin Chim Acta* 138:293-298, 1984.

15. Johnston IDA, Jones NF, Scobie JE, et al: The diagnostic value of urinary enzyme measurements in hypertension, *Clin Chim Acta* 133:317-325, 1983.

16. Gravel RA, Kabeck MM, Proia RL, et al: The G_{M2} gangliosidoses. In Scriver CR, Beaudet AL, Valle D, et al, editors: *The metabolic and molecular bases of inherited disease,* ed 8, New York, 2001, McGraw-Hill Inc.

17. Vladutiu AO, Schachner A: Increased creatine kinase (CK) MB isoenzyme in patients with "normal" total CK activity suspected of acute myocardial infarction, *J Med* 20:73-81, 1989.

18. Price RG: Measurement of N-acetyl-β-glucosaminidase and its isoenzymes in urine: methods and clinical applications, *Eur J Clin Chem Clin Biochem* 30:693-705, 1992.

↑ Familial hyperalphalipoproteinemia. Secondary increase because of primary biliary cirrhosis, chronic hepatitis, and alcoholism.

↓ Familial hypoalphalipoproteinemia, Tangier disease, or other apo A-I variants, fish-eye disease, familial lecithin-cholesterol acyltransferase (LCAT) deficiency, familial cholesteryl ester transfer protein (CETP) deficiency, familial apo A-I deficiency (with or without apo CIII/apo A-IV deficiency), and coronary heart disease.

The following can lead to secondary decrease in HDL-C: hypertriglyceridemia, Cushing's syndrome, type 2 diabetes, hepatocellular disorders, cholestasis, nephrotic syndrome, chronic renal failure, obesity, and malignancy.

HDL particles are antiatherogenic; they promote cellular cholesterol efflux and reverse cholesterol transport, and they also appear to have antiinflammatory, antioxidant, and anticoagulant properties.

Epidemiological studies demonstrate an inverse association between HDL-C concentration and coronary heart disease (CHD). The measurement of HDL-C is useful in identifying lipoprotein disorders and assessing CHD risk. The National Cholesterol Education Program (NCEP) recommends that all adults >20 yr be screened for CHD risk with measurement of fasting total cholesterol, HDL-C, LDL-C, and triglyceride concentrations. According to NCEP guidelines, HDL-C<40 mg/dL is a risk factor for CHD. HDL-C ≥60 mg/dL is a "negative" risk factor; its presence subtracts one risk factor from the total count.

It is suggested that for every 5-mg/dL [0.13 mmol/L] decrease in HDL-C below the mean, the risk of CHD increases 25%.

Intraindividual variation in HDL-C is ~7% over 1-12 months. Because of biological and analytical variation, at least two serial samples may be necessary for clinical decision making.

TEST NAME AND METHOD	SPECIMEN REQUIREMENTS	REFERENCE INTERVAL, CONVENTIONAL [INTERNATIONAL RECOMMENDED UNITS]	CHEMICAL INTERFERENCES AND IN VIVO EFFECTS

High-Density Lipoprotein Cholesterol—CONT

50-59 yr			↓ V Anabolic steroids
M:	26-74	[0.67-1.92]	(e.g., danazol), androgens,
F:	34-87	[0.88-2.25]	β-blockers, cyclosporine,
60-69 yr			diuretics (thiazides,
M:	28-71	[0.73-1.84]	chlorothalidone), gluco-
F:	31-86	[0.80-2.23]	corticoids, retinoids, inter-
70+ yr			feron, interleukin, probu-
M:	28-72	[0.73-1.86]	col, progestins, HIV
F:	32-83	[0.83-2.15]	protease inhibitors, diet
Non-Hispanic Black			high in carbohydrates or
4-5 yr			polyunsaturated fatty
M:	36-75	[0.93-1.94]	acids, diet low in total fat,
F:	35-76	[0.91-1.97]	lack of exercise, infection,
6-11 yr			inflammation, cigarette
M:	40-86	[1.04-2.23]	smoking, hospitalization
F:	36-78	[0.93-2.02]	for AMI, stroke, or car-
12-19 yr			diac catheterization.
M:	36-73	[0.93-1.89]	
F:	36-80	[0.93-2.07]	
20-29 yr			
M:	35-82	[0.91-2.12]	
F:	37-84	[0.96-2.18]	
30-39 yr			
M:	32-83	[0.83-2.15]	
F:	36-85	[0.93-2.20]	
40-49 yr			
M:	30-91	[0.78-2.36]	
F:	34-86	[0.88-2.23]	
50-59 yr			
M:	29-86	[0.75-2.23]	
F:	35-85	[0.91-2.20]	
60-69 yr			
M:	30-80	[0.78-2.07]	
F:	34-89	[0.88-2.31]	
70+ yr			
M:	33-95	[0.85-2.46]	
F:	35-92	[0.91-2.38]	
Mexican Americans			
4-5 yr			
M:	29-72	[0.75-1.86]	
F:	32-65	[0.83-1.68]	
6-11 yr			
M:	35-75	[0.91-1.94]	
F:	34-73	[0.88-1.89]	
12-19 yr			
M:	31-67	[0.80-1.74]	
F:	35-76	[0.91-1.97]	

DIAGNOSTIC INFORMATION   **REMARKS**

The goal for HDL cholesterol measurement, as defined by the Working Group on Lipoprotein Measurement of NCEP, is a total error ≤13%, consistent with a precision ≤4% CV and a bias ±5%.

TEST NAME AND METHOD	SPECIMEN REQUIREMENTS	REFERENCE INTERVAL, CONVENTIONAL [INTERNATIONAL RECOMMENDED UNITS]		CHEMICAL INTERFERENCES AND IN VIVO EFFECTS

High-Density Lipoprotein Cholesterol—CONT

20-29 yr			
M:	30-66	[0.78-1.71]	
F:	34-77	[0.88-1.99]	
30-39 yr			
M:	27-74	[0.70-1.92]	
F:	31-77	[0.80-1.99]	
40-49 yr			
M:	28-66	[0.73-1.71]	
F:	32-70	[0.83-1.81]	
50-59 yr			
M:	28-80	[0.73-2.07]	
F:	34-87	[0.88-2.25]	
60-69 yr			
M:	30-66	[0.78-1.71]	
F:	32-81	[0.83-2.10]	
70+ yr			
M:	28-67	[0.73-1.74]	
F:	34-80	[0.88-2.07]	

1. Cohn JS, McNamara JR, Cohn SD, et al: Postprandial plasma lipoprotein changes in human subjects of different ages, *J Lipid Res* 29:469-479, 1988.

2. Cooper GR, Myers GL, Smith J, et al: Blood lipid measurements: variations and practical utility, *JAMA* 267:1652-1660, 1992.

3. Expert Panel on Detection, Evaluation, and Treatment of High Blood Cholesterol in Adults: Executive Summary of the Third Report of the National Cholesterol Education Program (NCEP) Expert Panel on Selection, Evaluation, and Treatment of High Blood Cholesterol in Adults (Adult Treatment Panel III), *JAMA* 285:2486-2497, 2001.

4. Henkin Y, Como JA, Oberman A: Secondary dyslipidemia: inadvertent effects of drugs in clinical practice, *JAMA* 267:961-968, 1992.

5. Kimberly M, Leary E, Cole T, et al: Selection, validation, standardization, and performance of a designated comparison method for HDL cholesterol for use in the cholesterol reference method laboratory network, *Clin Chem* 45:1803-1812, 1999.

6. Ockene IS, Chiriboga DE, Stanek EJ, et al: Seasonal variation in serum cholesterol levels, *Arch Intern Med* 164:863-870, 2004.

7. Rader DJ: Lipid disorders. In Topol EJ, editor: *Textbook of cardiovascular medicine,* ed 2, Philadelphia, PA, 2002, Lippincott Williams & Wilkins.

8. Rifai N, Warnick GR, Dominiczak MH, editors: *Handbook of lipoprotein testing,* ed 2, Washington, DC, 2000, AACC Press.

9. Wang M, Briggs MR: HDL: the metabolism, function, and therapeutic importance, *Chem Rev* 104:119-137, 2004.

10. Warnick GR, Wood PD: National Cholesterol Education Program recommendations for measurement of high-density lipoprotein cholesterol: executive summary. The National Cholesterol Education Program Working Group on Lipoprotein Measurement, *Clin Chem* 41:1427-1433, 1995.

11. Young DS: *Effects of drugs on clinical laboratory tests,* ed 5, Washington, DC, 2000, AACC Press.

12. Young DS: *Effects of preanalytical variables on clinical laboratory tests,* ed 2, Washington, DC, 1997, AACC Press.

13. Halloran P, Roetering H, Pisani T, et al: Reference standardization and analytical performance of a liquid homogeneous high-density lipoprotein cholesterol method compared with chemical precipitation method, *Arch Pathol Lab Med* 123:317-326, 1999.

14. Harris N, Galpachian V, Rifai N: Three routine methods for measuring high-density-lipoprotein cholesterol compared with the reference method, *Clin Chem* 42:738-743, 1996.

15. Harris N, Galpachian V, Thomas J, et al: Three generations of high-density lipoprotein cholesterol assays compared with ultracentrifugation/dextran sulfate-Mg2+ method, *Clin Chem* 43:816-823, 1997.

16. Nauck M, Graziani M, Jarausch J, et al: A new liquid homogeneous assay for HDL cholesterol determination evaluated in seven laboratories in Europe and the United States, *Clin Chem Lab Med* 37:1067-1076, 1999.

17. Nauck M, Marz W, Jarausch J, et al: Multi-center evaluation of a homogeneous assay for HDL-cholesterol without sample pre-treatment, *Clin Chem* 43:1622-1629, 1997.

18. Nauck M, Marz W, Wieland H: New immunoseparation based homogeneous assay for HDL-cholesterol compared with three homogeneous and two heterogeneous methods for HDL-cholesterol, *Clin Chem* 44:1443-1451, 1998.

19. Okamoto Y, Tanaka S, Nakano H: Direct measurement of HDL cholesterol preferable to precipitation method, *Clin Chem* 41:1784, 1995.

20. Simo JM, Castellano I, Ferre N, et al: Evaluation of a homogeneous assay for high-density lipoprotein cholesterol: limitations in patients with cardiovascular, renal, and hepatic disorders, *Clin Chem* 44:1233-1241, 1998.

21. Sugiuchi H, Uji Y, Okabe H, et al: Direct measurement of high-density-lipoprotein cholesterol in serum with polyethylene-glycol-modified enzymes and sulfated alpha-cyclodextrin, *Clin Chem* 41:717-723, 1995.

22. Albers JJ, Segrest JP, editors: *Plasma lipoproteins, part B: characterization, cell biology, and metabolism. Method in enzymology, vol 129,* Orlando, FL, 1986, Academic Press.

23. Warnick G, Benderson J, Albers JJ: Dextran sulfate-Mg2+ precipitation procedure for quantitation of high density lipoprotein cholesterol, *Clin Chem* 28:1379-1388, 1982.

24. Contois JH, Gillmor R, Moore R, et al: Quantitative determination of cholesterol in lipoprotein fractions by electrophoresis, *Clin Chim Acta* 282:1-14, 1999.

25. Lynch GJ, Arbuckle GB, Cowley DM, et al: Routine lipid screening by cholesterol staining electrophoresis-including lipoprotein(a) cholesterol (Lp(a)-c), *Aust J Med Sci* 19:123-126, 1998.

26. Nauck M, Winkler K, Marz W, et al: Quantitative determination of high-, low-, and very-low density lipoproteins and lipoprotein(a) by agarose gel electrophoresis and enzymatic cholesterol staining, *Clin Chem* 41:1761-1767, 1995.

27. Ordovas JM, editor: *Lipoprotein protocols,* Totowa, NJ, 1998, Humana Press.

28. NHANES III, 1988-94: Available at: www.cdc.gov/nchs/data/nhanes/hdlmale.pdf. Accessed June 3, 2004.

TEST NAME AND METHOD	SPECIMEN REQUIREMENTS	REFERENCE INTERVAL, CONVENTIONAL [INTERNATIONAL RECOMMENDED UNITS]	CHEMICAL INTERFERENCES AND IN VIVO EFFECTS
High-Molecular-Weight Kininogen (HMWK, Fitzgerald Factor, Williams Factor, Flaujeac Factor)[1]	Plasma (blue-top-citrate). Stable for 2 hr at 4° C or 28 days if frozen.	HMWK factor assay: reference range generally 50-150% of normal. This test is similar to other aPTT-based factor assays; for HMWK, the patient plasma is incubated with HMWK-deficient plasma. HMWK deficiency plasma corrects after addition of normal plasma (mixing study).	See *Activated Partial Thromboplastin Time.*

1. Jacobs DS, Demott WR, Oxley DK, editors: *Laboratory test handbook,* ed 5, Hudson, OH, 2001, Lexi-Comp, Inc.
2. La Follette L, Gordon EM, Mazur CA, et al: Hyperprolactinemia and reduction in plasma tilers of Hageman factor, prekallikrein, and high molecular weight kininogen in patients with acute myocardial infarction, *J Lab Clin Med* 110:318-321, 1987.

Histidine (His)[1-6] *Ion-exchange chromatographic*	Plasma (heparin) or serum, fasting. Place blood in ice water immediately; separate and freeze within 1 hr of collection. Stable for 1 wk at −20° C; for longer periods deproteinize and store at −70° C.[7,8]		*mg/dL*	*µmol/L*[11]
		Premature		
		1 day:	0.78 ± 0.31 (SD) × 64.5	[50 ± 20]
		Newborn		
		1 day:	0.76-1.77	[49-114]
		1 day-1 mo	0.46-2.13	[30-138][12]
		1-3 mo:	0.98 ± 0.16 (SD)	[63 ± 10]
		2-6 mo:	1.49-2.12	[96-137]
		9 mo-2 yr:	0.37-1.74	[24-112]
		3-10 yr:	0.37-1.32	[24-85]
		6-18 yr:	0.99-1.64	[64-106][13]
		Adult:	0.50-1.66	[32-107]

	Urine, 24 hr. Add 10 mL of 6 mol/L HCl at start of collection. (Alternatively, refrigerate specimen during collection.) Store frozen at −20° C.[9]		*mg/day*	*µmol/day*[11]	U ↑ V Protein, tetracycline
		10 days-7 wk:	16.0-38.6 × 6.45	[103-249]	
		3-12 yr:	47.4-199.2	[306-1285]	
		Adult:	72.9-440.8	[470-2843]	U ↓ V Estrogens (male)
			mg/g creatinine	*mmol/mol creatinine*	
		or	71 ± 35 (SD) × 0.73	[51.8 ± 25.6]	

DIAGNOSTIC INFORMATION	REMARKS
↓ Hereditary HMWK deficiency. Functional levels of HMW-kininogen are also significantly decreased in acute myocardial infarction and in association with elevation of serum levels of prolactin.[2]	HMW-kininogen is a contact factor of the intrinsic pathway of the coagulation system. HMW-kininogen, together with kallikrein, enhances the activation of factor XII. Similar to deficiencies of factor XII and prekallikrein, HMW-kininogen deficiency may cause a prolonged PTT but no bleeding. A deficiency of HMW-kininogen can be initially suspected with a mixing study: a correction of aPTT would support a factor deficiency. If there is no history of bleeding, a factor XII assay will be commonly performed in most laboratories. If factor XII is normal, both prekallikrein and HMW kininogen assays should be ordered (these are usually send-out tests done in a few reference laboratories).
P ↑ Histidinemia, pregnancy, transient histidinemia of newborns, hemolysis P ↓ 1-16 days after abdominal surgery,[17] rheumatoid arthritis	In pregnancy, plasma histidine increases ~50%. Histidinemia results from an inherited absence of histidase. This is regarded as a benign inborn error of amino acid metabolism. See also Table II-2.
U ↑ Histidinemia, Hartnup disease, pregnancy, generalized aminoaciduria	Increases in urinary levels may follow heavy meat ingestion.

TEST NAME AND METHOD	SPECIMEN REQUIREMENTS	REFERENCE INTERVAL, CONVENTIONAL [INTERNATIONAL RECOMMENDED UNITS]		CHEMICAL INTERFERENCES AND IN VIVO EFFECTS

Histidine—CONT

		$\mu mol/g$ creatinine[14]		$mmol/mol$ creatinine	
	0-1 mo:	365-2857	× 0.113	[41.2-322.8]	
	1-6 mo:	727-3167		[82.2-357.9]	
	6 mo-1 yr:	877-3346		[99.1-378.1]	
	1-2 yr:	850-3005		[96.0-339.6]	
	2-3 yr:	1009-2524		[114.0-285.2]	

		mg/dL		$\mu mol/L$	
CSF. Collect in sterile tubes; store frozen. Stable at −20° C for 1 wk or at −70° C for 2 mo.[10]	Neonate:	0.398 ± 0.226 (SEM)	× 64.5	[25.7 ± 14.6][15]	
	3 mo-2 yr:	0.205 ± 0.040 (SD)		[13.2 ± 2.6][16]	
	2-10 yr:	0.153 ± 0.037		[9.9 ± 2.4][16]	
	Adult:	0.186 ± 0.008		[12.0 ± 0.5][11]	

1. Burtis CA, Ashwood ER, Bruns DE, editors: *Tietz textbook of clinical chemistry and molecular diagnostics,* ed 4, Philadelphia, 2005, WB Saunders.
2. Friedman RB, Young DS: *Youngs effect on line,* 2006, American Association for Clinical Chemistry.
3. Scriver CR, Beaudet AL, Valle D, et al, editors: *The metabolic and molecular bases of inherited disease,* ed 8, New York, 2001, McGraw-Hill.
4. Young DS: *Effects of drugs on clinical laboratory tests,* ed 3, Washington, DC, 1990, American Association for Clinical Chemistry.
5. Bremer HJ, Duran M, Kamerling JP, et al: *Disturbances of amino acid metabolism: clinical chemistry and diagnosis,* Baltimore, 1981, Urban and Schwarzenburg.
6. Nyhan W, Sakait N: *Diagnostic recognition of genetic disease,* Philadelphia, 1987, Lea & Febiger.
7. Cummings JG: Routine amino acids analysis in the clinical laboratory, *Am Clin Prod Rev* Feb:20-25, 1988.
8. Schaefer A, Piquard F, Haberey P: Plasma amino acids analysis: effects of delayed samples preparation and of storage, *Clin Chim Acta* 164:163-169, 1987.
9. Pesce A, Kaplan L, editors: *Methods in clinical chemistry,* St. Louis, 1987, CV Mosby.
10. Heiblim DI, Evans HE, Glass L, et al: Amino acid concentrations in cerebrospinal fluid, *Arch Neurol* 35:765-768, 1978.
11. Shih V: *Laboratory techniques for the detection of hereditary metabolic disorders,* Boca Raton, FL, 1973, CRC Press.
12. Slocum RH, Cummings JG: Amino acid analysis of physiological samples. In Hommes FA, editor: *Techniques in human biochemical genetics,* New York, 1991, Wiley-Liss, pp. 87-126.
13. Meites S, editor: *Pediatric clinical chemistry,* ed 3, Washington, DC, 1989, American Association for Clinical Chemistry.
14. Mayo Medical Laboratories: *Test catalog,* Rochester, MN, 1993, Mayo Medical Laboratories.
15. Heiblim DI, Evans HE, Glass L, et al: Amino acid concentrations in cerebrospinal fluid, *Arch Neurol* 35:765-768, 1978.
16. Goldsmith RF, Earl JW, Cunningham AM: Determination of δ-aminobutyric acid and other amino acids in cerebrospinal fluid of pediatric patients by reversed-phase liquid chromatography, *Clin Chem* 33:1736-1740, 1987.
17. Jain KM, Rush BF Jr, Seelig RF, et al: Changes in plasma amino acid profiles following abdominal operations, *Surg Gynecol Obstet* 152:302-306, 1981.

DIAGNOSTIC INFORMATION	REMARKS

CSF ↑ Histidinemia

Values in children (3 mo-10 yr) were measured using reversed-phase liquid chromatography.

TEST NAME AND METHOD	SPECIMEN REQUIREMENTS	REFERENCE INTERVAL, CONVENTIONAL [INTERNATIONAL RECOMMENDED UNITS]			CHEMICAL INTERFERENCES AND IN VIVO EFFECTS
Homocitrulline (Hci)[1-4]	Urine, 24 hr. Add 10 mL of 6 mol/L HCl at start of collection.	Adult:	*mg/day*[6] <11	× 5.29	*μmol/day* [<58]	None found.
Ion-exchange chromatography	(Alternatively, refrigerate specimen during collection.) Store frozen at −20° C.[5]		*mg/g creatine* <17		*μmol/g* [<90]	

1. Valle D, Simell O: The hyperornithinemias. In Scriver CR, Beaudet AL, Sly WS, et al, editors: *The metabolic and molecular bases of inherited disease,* New York, 2001, McGraw-Hill, pp. 1882-1888.

2. Burtis CA, Ashwood ER, Bruns DE, editors: *Tietz textbook of clinical chemistry and molecular diagnostics,* ed 4, Philadelphia, 2005, WB Saunders.

3. Scriver CR, Beaudet AL, Valle D, et al, editors: *The metabolic and molecular bases of inherited disease,* ed 8, New York, 2001, McGraw-Hill.

4. Bremer HJ, Duran M, Kamerling JP, et al: *Disturbances of amino acid metabolism: clinical chemistry and diagnosis,* Baltimore, 1981, Urban and Schwarzenburg.

5. Pesce A, Kaplan L, editors: *Methods in clinical chemistry,* St. Louis, 1987, CV Mosby.

6. Shih V: *Laboratory techniques for the detection of hereditary metabolic disorders,* Boca Raton, FL, 1973, CRC Press.

TEST NAME AND METHOD	SPECIMEN REQUIREMENTS	REFERENCE INTERVAL, CONVENTIONAL [INTERNATIONAL RECOMMENDED UNITS]		CHEMICAL INTERFERENCES AND IN VIVO EFFECTS
Homocysteine (Hcys)[1-20]	Urine, random.	Negative.		↑ C Cystine (with the cyanide-nitroprusside test)
Nitroprusside[4]				↑ V Folate antagonists (e.g., methotrexate), nitrous oxide, metformin, niacin, theophylline,
TLC[4]				
HPLC[19,21,22]	Plasma (EDTA, heparin, or citrate) or serum. Gel	*μmol/L*[28] *5th-95th percentile*		L-dopa, androgens, aminoglutethimide, cy-
GC/MS[19,23]	barrier tubes are acceptable. Serum results are	12-19 yr M:	4.3-9.9	closporine, fibric acid derivatives, and diuretics.
FPIA/EIA[24-26]	5-10% higher than EDTA or heparin	F: 20-39 yr	3.3-7.2	↓ V Penicillamine,
Enzymatic[27]	plasma, whereas citrated plasma results are 5-15% lower. Tubes containing adenosine analogs (e.g., DS30 tubes, Drew Scientific) are effective stabilizers but are not compatible with assays using SAH hydrolase (e.g., FPIA). Fasting is not required, but Hcy can in-	M: F: 40-59 yr M: F: 60+ yr M: F: Recommended cutpoints: M: F:	5.2-11.4 3.7-10.4 5.7-12.9 4.1-10.2 5.9-15.3 4.9-11.6 ≤11.4 μmol/L ≤10.4 μmol/L	*N*-acetylcysteine, mesna, estrogens, tamoxifen, betaine, and simvastatin.

DIAGNOSTIC INFORMATION	REMARKS

U ↑ Hyperornithinemia-hyperammonemia-homocitrullinuria (HHH) syndrome, hyperlysinemia, saccharopinuria[3]

Excretion decreases gradually with age; only traces are found in older children and adults.

See also Table II-2C.

↑ Homocystinuria (defects in cystathionine-β-synthase [CBS], methionine synthase [MS], MS reductase, or intracellular cobalamin metabolism).

↑ Homocystinuria, heterozygous CBS defect, MTHFR 677C→T homozygosity, vitamin B_{12} deficiency, folate deficiency, vitamin B_6 deficiency, cigarette smoking, coffee consumption, renal failure, hypothyroidism, hyperproliferative disorders, diabetes, psychiatric disorders, impaired cognitive function in elderly persons, pregnancy complications (e.g., preeclampsia, low birth weight, premature delivery, recurrent pregnancy loss, placental abruption), and birth defects (e.g., neural tube defects).

↓ Down syndrome, pregnancy, hyperthyroidism, and early diabetes.

Homocystinuria refers to an inborn error of metabolism associated with the excretion of large amounts of Hcy and greatly elevated plasma Hcy levels (typically >100 μmol/L). Although the most common defect is CBS deficiency, other enzymes and factors involved in the metabolism of homocysteine may be involved.

Serum or plasma homocysteine is used as a functional test for vitamin B_{12}, folate, and/or vitamin B_6 deficiency. Elevated Hcy is also an independent risk factor for cardiovascular disease.

Hcy measurement in conjunction with methionine load testing is generally considered a research tool and of limited clinical utility.

Intraindividual variability is ~8% over a 1-yr period, although it can be as much as 25% in patients with hyperhomocysteinemia. Generally, a single measurement is considered adequate to determine Hcy status.

TEST NAME AND METHOD	SPECIMEN REQUIREMENTS	REFERENCE INTERVAL, CONVENTIONAL [INTERNATIONAL RECOMMENDED UNITS]	CHEMICAL INTERFERENCES AND IN VIVO EFFECTS
Homocysteine—CONT	crease 10-15% 6-8 hr after a high protein meal. Separate plasma or serum from red cells within 1 hr of collection. After separation of serum or plasma from red cells, specimens are stable for at least 4 days at room temperature, several weeks at 4° C, and years if frozen. Urine (random or aliquot from a well-mixed 24-hr urine collection).	Individuals in the reference sample were vitamin replete with normal kidney function (vitamin B12 and folate ≥ median; serum creatinine <110 and <90 μmol/L for males and females, respectively).	

1. Andersson A, Isaksson A, Hultberg B: Homocysteine export from erythrocytes and its implication for plasma sampling, *Clin Chem* 38:1311-1315, 1992.

2. Berwanger CS, Jeremy JY, Stansby G: Homocysteine and vascular disease, *Br J Surg* 82:726-731, 1995.

3. Bostom AG, Shemin D, Lapane KL, et al: Hyperhomocysteinemia, hyperfibrinogenemia, and lipoprotein(a) excess in maintenance dialysis patients: a matched case-control study, *Atherosclerosis* 125:91-101, 1996.

4. Burtis CA, Ashwood ER, editors: *Tietz textbook of clinical chemistry,* ed 3, Philadelphia, 1999, WB Saunders.

5. Fiskerstrand T, Refsum H, Kvalheim G, et al: Homocysteine and other thiols in plasma and urine: automated determination and sample stability, *Clin Chem* 39:263-271, 1993.

6. Genest JJ, McNamara JR, Upson B, et al: Prevalence of familial hyperhomocyst(e)inemia in men with premature coronary artery disease, *Arterioscl Thromb* 11:1129-1136, 1991.

7. Hill DM, Johnson LJ, Burns PJ, et al: Effects of temperature on stability of blood homocysteine in collection tubes containing 3-deazoadenosine, *Clin Chem* 48:2017-2022, 2002.

8. Landgren F, Israelsson B, Lindgren A, et al: Plasma homocysteine in acute myocardial infarction: homocysteine-lowering effect of folic acid, *J Intern Med* 237:381-388, 1995.

9. Langman LJ, Cole DEC: Homocysteine: cholesterol of the 90s? *Clin Chim Acta* 286:63-80, 1999.

10. Malinow MR, Ducimetiere P, Luc G, et al: Plasma homocyst(e)ine levels and graded risk for myocardial infarction: findings in two populations at contrasting risk for coronary heart disease, *Atherosclerosis* 126:27-34, 1996.

11. Mills JL, McPartlin JM, Kirke PN, et al: Homocysteine metabolism in pregnancies complicated by neural tube defects, *Lancet* 345:149-151, 1995.

12. Motulsky AG: Nutritional ecogenetics: homocysteine-related arteriosclerotic vascular disease, neural tube defects, and folic acid, *Am J Hum Genet* 58:17-20, 1996.

13. Rasmussen K, Moller J: Total homocysteine determination in clinical practice, *Ann Clin Biochem* 37:627-648, 2000.

14. Refsum H, Smith AD, Ueland PM, et al: Facts and recommendations about total homocysteine determinations: an expert opinion, *Clin Chem* 50:3-32, 2004.

15. Rifai N, Warnick GR, Dominiczak MH, editors: *Handbook of lipoprotein testing,* ed 2, Washington, DC, 2000, AACC Press.

16. Schnyder G, Roffi M, Pin R, et al: Decreased rate of coronary restenosis after lowering of plasma homocysteine levels, *N Engl J Med* 345:1593-1600, 2001.

17. Scriver CR, Beaudet AR, Sly W, et al, editors: *The metabolic and molecular bases of inherited disease,* ed 8, New York, 2001, McGraw-Hill.

18. Seshadri S, Beiser A, Selhub J, et al: Plasma homocysteine as a risk factor for dementia and Alzheimer's disease, *N Engl J Med* 346:476-483, 2002.

19. Ueland PM, Refsum H, Stabler SP, et al: Total homocysteine in plasma or serum: methods and clinical applications, *Clin Chem* 39:1764-1779, 1993.

20. Verhoef P, Stampfer MJ, Buring JE, et al: Homocysteine metabolism and risk of myocardial infarction: relation with vitamins B6, B12, and folate, *Am J Epidemiol* 143:845-859, 1996.

21. Burtis CA, Ashwood ER, editors: *Tietz textbook of clinical chemistry,* ed 3, Philadelphia, 1999, WB Saunders.

22. Jacobsen DW, Gatautis VJ, Green R: Determination of plasma homocysteine by high-performance liquid chromatography with fluorescence detection, *Anal Biochem* 178:208-214, 1989.

23. Stabler SP, Marcell PD, Podell ER, et al: Quantitation of total homocysteine, total cysteine, and methionine in normal serum and urine using capillary gas chromatography-mass spectrometry, *Anal Biochem* 162:185-196, 1987.

24. Axis Biochemicals: *Homocysteine EIA package insert,* Oslo, Norway, 2004, Axis Biochemicals.

25. Shipchandler MT, Moore EG: Rapid, fully automated measurement of plasma homocyst(e)ine with the Abbott Imx analyzer, *Clin Chem* 41:991-994, 1995.

26. Wu AHB, Holtman V, Apple FS, et al: Multicenter analytical evaluation of an automated immunoassay for total plasma homocysteine, *Ann Clin Lab Sci* 30:185-190, 2000.

27. Tan Y, Tang L, Sun X, et al: Total homocysteine enzymatic assay, *Clin Chem* 46:1686-1688, 2000.

28. Sehlub J, Jacques PF, Rosenberg IH, et al: Serum total homocysteine concentrations in the Third National Health and Nutrition Survey (1991-1994): Population reference ranges and contribution of vitamin status to high serum concentrations, *Ann Intern Med* 131:331-339, 1999.

TEST NAME AND METHOD	SPECIMEN REQUIREMENTS	REFERENCE INTERVAL, CONVENTIONAL [INTERNATIONAL RECOMMENDED UNITS]			CHEMICAL INTERFERENCES AND IN VIVO EFFECTS
Homogentisic Acid[1] *Gas chromatography-mass spectrometry*[2]	Urine, fresh random. For storage, acidify to pH 3 and store frozen.[3] Measured as part of urine organic acid profile.	Normal; none detected Alkaptonuria: ≥2.0 g/day			No interference by gentisic acid, 3,4-dihydroxyphenylacetic acid, ascorbic acid, and L-dopa.

1. Hicks JM, Boeckx RL, editors: *Pediatric clinical chemistry,* Philadelphia, 1984, WB Saunders.
2. Chalmers RA, Lawson AM: *Organic acids in man,* London, 1982, Chapman and Hall.
3. Feldman JM, Bowman J: Urinary homogentisic acid: determination by thin-layer chromatography, *Clin Chem* 19:459-462, 1973.

TEST NAME AND METHOD	SPECIMEN REQUIREMENTS	REFERENCE INTERVAL, CONVENTIONAL [INTERNATIONAL RECOMMENDED UNITS]			CHEMICAL INTERFERENCES AND IN VIVO EFFECTS
Homovanillic Acid (3-Methoxy-4-hydroxyphenylacetic acid; HVA)[1,2]	Urine, 24 hr. Collect with 20 mL of HCl, 6 mol/L.	3-6 yr: 6-10 yr: 10-16 yr: 16-83 yr:[13]	*mg/day*[12] 1.4-4.3 2.1-4.7 2.4-8.7 1.4-8.8	× 5.49	*μmol/day* [8-24] [12-26] [13-48] [8-48]	↑ V Disulfiram, L-dopa, pyridoxine, and reserpine (maximum during second day of treatment)
HPLC[3-7] *GC*[8,9] *GC-MS*[10] *LC-MS/MS*[11]		0-3 mo: 3-12 mo: 1-2 yr: 2-5 yr: 5-10 yr: 10-15 yr: >15 yr:	*mcg/mg creatinine*[14] 11.3-35.0 8.4-44.9 12.2-31.8 3.4-32.0 6.8-23.7 3.2-13.6 3.2-9.6	× 0.621	*mmol/mol creatinine* [7.0-21.7] [5.2-27.9] [7.6-19.7] [2.1-19.9] [4.2-14.7] [2.0-8.4] [2.0-6.0]	↓ V Moclobemide

1. Rosano TG, Whitley RJ: Catecholamines and serotonin. In Burtis CA, Ashwood ER, editors: *Tietz textbook of clinical chemistry,* Philadelphia, 1999, WB Saunders.
2. Monsaingeon M, Perel Y, Simonnet T, et al: Comparative values of catecholamines and metabolites for the diagnosis of neuroblastoma, *Eur J Pediatr* 162:397-402, 2003.
3. Morrisey JL, Shihabi ZK: Assay of 4-hydroxy-3-methoxyphenylacetic (homovanillic) acid by liquid chromatography with electrochemical detection, *Clin Chem* 25:2045-2047, 1979.
4. Soldin SJ, Hill JG: Simultaneous liquid chromatographic analysis of 4-hydroxy-3-methoxymandelic acid and 4-hydroxy-3-methoxyphenylacetic acid in urine, *Clin Chem* 26:291-294, 1980.
5. Bonfigli AR, Coppa G, Testa R, et al: Determination of vanillylmandelic, 5-hydroxyindoleacetic and homovanillic acid in urine by isocratic liquid chromatography, *Eur J Clin Chem Clin Biochem* 35:57-61, 1997.

DIAGNOSTIC INFORMATION	REMARKS

↑ Alkaptonuria

Darkening of urine on exposure to air and sunlight, although characteristic of alkaptonuria, takes many hours and must be distinguished from darkening caused by other substances.

↑ Neuroblastoma, pheochromocytoma, and paraganglioma.

HVA is the major terminal metabolite of dopamine and is frequently used to diagnose and monitor patients with neuroblastoma. For the diagnosis of neuroblastoma it is important to carry out simultaneous determinations of HVA and VMA because either or both may be elevated. In patients with neuroblastoma, a HVA/VMA ratio <1 or >2 had an unfavorable prognosis.[15]

The preferred specimen is a 24-hr urine collection. Shorter timed collections (e.g., 12-hr) or random urines have also been used, provided the HVA excretion is normalized to the creatinine excretion.

Because chromatographic methods are not prone to interferences seen with older photometric methods, dietary restrictions during urine collection are not required.

Other tests may be helpful in screening, diagnosis, or monitoring therapy (see *Catecholamines, Fractionated;* and *Vanillylmandelic Acid*).

6. Fujita K, Maruta K, Ito S, et al: Urinary 4-hydroxy-3-methoxymandelic (vanillylmandelic) acid, 4-hydroxy-3-methoxyphenylacetic (homovanillic) acid, and 5-hydroxy-3-indoleacetic acid determined by liquid chromatography with electrochemical detection, *Clin Chem* 29:876-878, 1983.

7. Gironi A, Seghieri G, Niccolai M, et al: Simultaneous liquid-chromatographic determination of urinary vanillylmandelic acid, homovanillic acid, and 5-hydroxyindoleacetic acid, *Clin Chem* 34:2504-2506, 1988.

8. Brewster MA, Berry DH, Moriarty M: Urinary 3-methoxy-4-hydroxyphenylacetic (homovanillic) and 3-methoxy-4-hydroxymandelic (vanillylmandelic) acids: gas-liquid chromatographic methods and experience with 13 cases of neuroblastoma, *Clin Chem* 23:2247-2249, 1977.

9. Tuchman M, Crippin PJ, Krivit W: Capillary gas-chromatographic determination of urinary homovanillic acid and vanillylmandelic acid, *Clin Chem* 29:828-831, 1983.

TEST NAME AND METHOD	SPECIMEN REQUIREMENTS	REFERENCE INTERVAL, CONVENTIONAL [INTERNATIONAL RECOMMENDED UNITS]			CHEMICAL INTERFERENCES AND IN VIVO EFFECTS

Homovanillic Acid—CONT

10. Fauler G, Leis HJ, Huber E, et al: Determination of homovanillic acid and vanillylmandelic acid in neuroblastoma screening by stable isotope dilution GC-MS, *J Mass Spectrom* 32:507-514, 1997.

11. Magera MJ, Thompson AL, Matern D, et al: Liquid chromatography-tandem mass spectrometry method for the determination of vanillylmandelic acid in urine, *Clin Chem* 49:825-826, 2003.

12. Prémel-Cabic A, Turcant A, Allain P: Normal reference intervals for free catecholamines and then acid metabolites in 24-h urines from children, as determined by liquid chromatography with amperometric detection, *Clin Chem* 32:1585-1587, 1986.

TEST NAME AND METHOD	SPECIMEN REQUIREMENTS	REFERENCE INTERVAL, CONVENTIONAL			[INTERNATIONAL RECOMMENDED UNITS]	CHEMICAL INTERFERENCES AND IN VIVO EFFECTS
Hydrogen Sulfide *Colorimetric,*[1] *ion-selective potentiometry,*[2] *ion chromatography*[3]	Blood (fluoride/oxalate). Freeze. Specimens must be analyzed promptly.	As sulfide: Lethal concentration:	*mg/L* <0.05 >0.90	× 29.3	*μmol/L* [<1.5] [>26.4]	Cyanide may interfere with the ion-selective potentiometric method.[2]

1. Baselt RC, Cravey RH: *Disposition of toxic drugs and chemicals in man,* ed 3, Chicago, 1989, Year Book Medical Pub.

2. Baselt RC: *Biological monitoring methods for industrial chemicals,* Davis, CA, 1980, Biomedical Pub.

3. Richardson CJ, Magee EAM, Cummings JH: A new method for the determination of sulphide in gastrointestinal contents and whole blood by microdistillation and ion chromatography, *Clin Chim Acta* 293:115-125, 2000.

TEST NAME AND METHOD	SPECIMEN REQUIREMENTS	REFERENCE INTERVAL, CONVENTIONAL			[INTERNATIONAL RECOMMENDED UNITS]
β-Hydroxybutyric Acid (Ketone Body)[1,2] *Ketosite (Stanbio Lab); enzymatic*[3]	Whole blood, serum, or plasma (EDTA, heparin, oxalate, citrate); store in refrigerator for up to 12 hr. Freeze serum or plasma for longer storage.	0.21-2.81 mg/dL	× 96.05		[20-270 μmol/L]
Enzymatic-kinetic[4]	Serum, refrigerated or on ice water (not frozen).	<3.02 mg/dL			[290 μmol/L]

DIAGNOSTIC INFORMATION	REMARKS

13. Gerlo A, Malfait R: High-performance liquid chromatographic assay of free norepinephrine, epinephrine, dopamine, vanillylmandelic acid and homovanillic acid, *J Chromatogr* 343:9-20, 1985.

14. Tuchman M, Morris C, Ramnaraine M, et al: Value of random urinary homovanillic acid and vanillylmandelic acid in the diagnosis and management of patients with neuroblastoma: comparison with 24-h urine collections, *Pediatrics* 75:324-328, 1985.

15. Nishi M, Miyake H, Takeda T, et al: The relationship between homovanillic/vanillylmandelic acid ratios and prognosis in neuroblastoma, *Oncol Rep* 5:631-633, 1998.

Like cyanide, sulfide inhibits cytochrome oxidase and produces cellular anoxia. Death occurs rapidly at concentrations of 1000 ppm [29.3 mmol/L].	Sulfide is widely used in industry; hydrogen sulfide gas is produced by decomposing protein, e.g., sewer gas or marsh gas. Its odor is easily detected at a concentration of 0.03 ppm [0.9 µmol/L], but at 150 ppm [4.4 mmol/L], the olfactory nerves are paralyzed.
	Sulfide is partially oxidized in erythrocytes and liver to thiosulfate; a portion is excreted by lungs as hydrogen sulfide.

β-Hydroxybutyrate (BOHB) (the predominant ketone) is a better indicator of clinical state than acetoacetate in diabetic ketoacidosis (DKA). The BOHB/AcAc ratio is normally 3:1. This ratio will increase to 6:1 or 12:1 during ketoacidosis, particularly if there is associated decreased tissue perfusion, metabolic acidosis, and tissue catabolism. All of these will favor reductive metabolism and hence BOHB production. Acetoacetate may increase during therapy for DKA because BOHB is oxidatively metabolized to acetoacetate.[5]	β-Hydroxybutyric acid is not detectable by common tests for ketone bodies (Acetest, Chemstrip, and Ketostix). β-Hydroxybutyrate is an extremely reliable guide for monitoring the progress of insulin therapy in the treatment of diabetic ketoacidosis. During successful therapy, total ketones and β-hydroxybutyrate decrease, but acetoacetate increases. β-Hydroxybutyrate measurements quantitate this decrease; Acetest, Ketostix, Chemstrip, and Multistix results show an initial increase reflecting the acetoacetate activity.
↑ Alcoholic ketoacidosis, lactic acidosis (shock, renal failure), liver disease, infections, phenformin, and salicylate poisoning.	The hallmark of alcoholic ketoacidosis is ketoacidosis without marked hyperglycemia; β-hydroxybutyrate component is markedly increased, not acetoacetate. Therefore the reagent strip tests for ketoacidosis will appear normal in alcoholic ketoacidosis.[6]
	No interferences from mesna, acetylcysteine, cysteine, dimercaprol, captopril, or D-penicillamine, which cause false-positive results with urinary reagent strips.

TEST NAME AND METHOD	SPECIMEN REQUIREMENTS	REFERENCE INTERVAL, CONVENTIONAL [INTERNATIONAL RECOMMENDED UNITS]	CHEMICAL INTERFERENCES AND IN VIVO EFFECTS

β-Hydroxybutyric Acid—CONT

1. Strasinger SK: *Urinalysis and body fluids: a self-instructional text,* ed 2, Philadelphia, 1991, FA Davis.
2. Burtis CA, Ashwood ER, editors: *Tietz fundamentals of clinical chemistry,* ed 5, Philadelphia, 2000, WB Saunders.
3. Stanbio Laboratory: *Ketosite package insert,* Boerne, TX, 2002, Stanbio Laboratory.
4. Koch DD, Feldbruegge DH: Optimized kinetic method for automated determination of β-hydroxybutyrate, *Clin Chem* 33:1761-1766, 1987.

**17-Hydroxycorti-
costeroids**
(17-OHCS)[1,2]

*Colorimetric
(Porter-Silber)*

1. Crapo L: Cushing's syndrome: a review of diagnostic tests, *Metabolism* 28:955-977, 1979.
2. Whitley RJ, Meikle AW, Watts NB: Endocrinology. In Burtis CA, Ashwood ER, editors: *Tietz textbook of clinical chemistry,* ed 2, Philadelphia, 1994, WB Saunders.

**18-Hydroxycorti-
costerone**[1-2]

RIA

1. Biglieri EG, Schambelan M: The significance of elevated levels of plasma 18-hydroxycorticosterone in patients with primary aldosteronism, *J Clin Endocrinol Metab* 49:377-380, 1979.
2. Kaplan N: Endocrine hypertension. In Wilson JH, Foster DW, editors: *Williams textbook of endocrinology,* ed 8, Philadelphia, 1992, WB Saunders.

18-Hydroxydeoxy-corticosterone (18-OH DOC)[1] *RIA*[2]	Serum. Separate within 1 hr. Store frozen.	*ng/dL* Ad libitum diet 8:00 AM: 3-16 × 0.0289 4:00 PM: 2-5 Premature infants (31-35 wk) <380 ng/dL Term infants, 3 days <942 ng/dL	*nmol/L* [0.09-0.46] [0.06-0.14]	See *H-Deoxycorticosterone.*

| DIAGNOSTIC INFORMATION | REMARKS |

5. Krane EJ: Diabetic ketoacidosis: biochemistry, physiology, treatment, and prevention, *Pediatr Clin North Am* 34:935-960, 1987.

6. Palmer JP: Alcoholic ketoacidosis: clinical and laboratory presentations, pathophysiology and treatment, *Clin Endocrinol Metab* 12:1983, 1987.

Although valuable in specific circumstances, this test has largely been replaced by plasma and urine cortisol assays.

See *Cortisol, Total* and *Cortisol, Free.*

Although plasma 18-hydroxycorticosterone is increased in a majority of patients with aldosterone-producing adenomas, this test is of limited value for an individual patient.

Radiographic studies and adrenal vein aldosterone sampling are preferred for the differential diagnosis of primary aldosteronism.

Excessive secretion of 18-OH DOC has been demonstrated in four forms of hypertension with suppressed PRA: in 17α-hydroxylase deficiency, Cushing's syndrome, primary aldosteronism, and essential hypertension (a small number of patients).[5]

↓ Ratio aldosterone/DOC + 18-DOC with malignant adrenocortical tumors.[6]

Secretion of 18-OH DOC appears to be primarily ACTH-dependent, but small increments in 18-OH DOC secretion may possibly be associated with activation of the zona glomerulosa by sodium depletion.

TEST NAME AND METHOD	SPECIMEN REQUIREMENTS	REFERENCE INTERVAL, CONVENTIONAL [INTERNATIONAL RECOMMENDED UNITS]		CHEMICAL INTERFERENCES AND IN VIVO EFFECTS
18-Hydroxydeoxycorticosterone—CONT				
GLC[3]		20-160	[0.58-4.62]	
	Urine, 24 hr.[4] Store frozen.	<3.0 mcg/day × 2.89	[<8.67 µmol/day]	

1. Melby JC, Dale SL, Grekin RJ, et al: 18-Hydroxy-11-deoxycorticosterone (18 OH DOC) secretion in experimental and human hypertension, *Recent Prog Horm Res* 28:287-337, 1972.
2. Dale SL, Komanicky P, Pratt JH, et al: Radioimmunoassay of 18-hydroxy-11-deoxycorticosterone in plasma, *J Clin Endocrinol Metab* 43:803-809, 1976.
3. Loraine JA, Bell ET: *Hormone assays and their clinical application,* New York, 1976, Churchill Livingstone.
4. Hicks JM, Young DS: *DORA '87: directory of rare analyses,* Washington, DC, 1987, AACC Press.
5. Agrin RJ, Dale SL, Holbrook M, et al: Urinary free 18-hydroxy-11-desoxycorticosterone excretion in normal and hypertensive patients, *J Clin Endocrinol Metab* 47:877-884, 1978.
6. Aupetit-Faisant B, Blanchouin-Emeric N, Battaglia C: Dysfunction of aldosterone pathway in adrenal carcinoma: a biochemical mean to distinguish non-malignant (NMT) and malignant (MT) adrenocortical tumors, *Cancer Detect Preven* 20, 1996.

TEST NAME AND METHOD	SPECIMEN REQUIREMENTS	REFERENCE INTERVAL, CONVENTIONAL [INTERNATIONAL RECOMMENDED UNITS]		CHEMICAL INTERFERENCES AND IN VIVO EFFECTS
5-Hydroxy-indoleacetic Acid (5-HIAA)[1-3] *Qualitative* *Colorimetric*[4]	Urine, fresh random. Patient should abstain from medication and over-the-counter drugs for 72 hr before test.	Negative: <25 mg/day × 5.23 [<131 µmol/day]		↑ V Atenolol, fluorouracil, melphalan, pindolol, rauwolfia alkaloids (e.g., reserpine, slight effect) ↑ C Acetaminophen, foods high in hydroxyindole content (avocados,
Quantitative *Colorimetric,*[5,6] *HPLC*[3]	Urine, 24 hr. Patient should abstain from medication and over-the-counter drugs for 72 hr before test. Collect without preservatives, but refrigerate during collection. Adjust pH between 2 and 3 by adding HCl, 6 mol/L. Acidified urine can be stored at 4° C for 2 wk and at −20° C for longer periods.	2-7 mg/day[7] × 5.23	[10.5-36.6 µmol/day]	bananas, tomatoes, plums, walnuts, pineapples, and eggplant), guaiacol (glyceryl guaiacolate, a common ingredient in cough syrups), mephenesin, methocarbomol, phanacetin; naproxen, oxprenolol, and pindolol interfere with nitronaphthol method. ↓ V Corticotropin, ethanol, imipramine, isoniazid, levodopa, MAO inhibitors, and methyldopa

DIAGNOSTIC INFORMATION	REMARKS

↑ Midgut carcinoid tumors (e.g., ileal carcinoids), foregut carcinoid tumors (e.g., pancreatic, duodenal, or biliary carcinoids), ovarian carcinoid tumors, celiac sprue, tropical sprue, Whipple's disease, oat cell carcinoma of the bronchus, and bronchial adenoma of carcinoid type

↓ Depressive illness, small intestinal resection, mastocytosis, PKU, and Hartnup disease

Estimations of urinary 5-HIAA are generally more useful than measurements of the parent hormone (serotonin) for diagnosing carcinoid tumors. When dietary sources of 5-hydroxyindoles (e.g., walnuts, bananas, avocados, eggplants, pineapples, plums, and tomatoes) are excluded, urinary 5-HIAA excretion >25 mg/day [>130 μmol/day] is diagnostic of the carcinoid syndrome. Functioning metastatic carcinoid tumors may show striking 5-HIAA elevations, often exceeding 350 mg/day [1820 μmol/day]. In such cases, a qualitative screening test gives a positive result.

When tumors are small and have not metastasized, a sensitive and specific quantitative test is needed. If normal or borderline results are seen in patients with clinical evidence of carcinoid syndrome, blood levels of serotonin or 5-hydroxytryptophan should be assessed. In some cases, 5-HIAA secretion may be intermittent, and repeat urine collections may be needed to document a clinical diagnosis. (See also *Substance P.*)

Hindgut tumors (rectal carcinoids) rarely secrete 5-HIAA and are often not associated with the carcinoid syndrome. Foregut carcinoids frequently produce other hormones such as catecholamines, ACTH, insulin, and growth hormone. They are also associated with multiple endocrine neoplasia (MEN type I).

TEST NAME AND METHOD	SPECIMEN REQUIREMENTS	REFERENCE INTERVAL, CONVENTIONAL [INTERNATIONAL RECOMMENDED UNITS]	CHEMICAL INTERFERENCES AND IN VIVO EFFECTS
5-Hydroxyindoleacetic Acid—CONT			↓ C Acetic acid, dihydriozyphenylacetic acid, formaldehyde (from methenamine compounds), gentisic acid, homogentisic acid, L-dopa, methenamine, phenothiazines, and salicylates (fluorimetric method)

1. Feldman JM, O'Dorisio TM: Role of neuropeptides and serotonin in the diagnosis of carcinoid tumors, *Am J Med* 81(suppl 6B):41-48, 1986.

2. Roberts LJ, Dates JA: Disorders of vasodilator hormones: the carcinoid syndrome and mastocytosis. In Wilson JD, Foster DW, editors: *Williams textbook of endocrinology,* ed 8, Philadelphia, 1992, WB Saunders.

3. Rosano TG, Whitley RJ: Catecholamines and serotonin. In Burtis CA, Ashwood ER, editors: *Tietz textbook of clinical chemistry,* ed 3, Philadelphia, 1999, WB Saunders.

4. Sjoerdsma A, Weissbach H, Udenfriend S: Simple test for diagnosis of metastatic carcinoid (argentaffinoma), *JAMA* 159:397, 1955.

5. Goldenberg H: Specific photometric determination of 5-hydroxyindolcacetic acid in urine, *Clin Chem* 19:38-44, 1973.

6. Udenfriend S, Titus E, Weissbach H: The identification of 5-hydroxy-3-indoleacetic acid in normal urine and a method for its assay, *J Biol Chem* 276:499-505, 1955.

7. Burtis CA, Ashwood ER, editors: *Tietz textbook of clinical chemistry,* ed 3, Philadelphia, 1999, WB Saunders.

TEST NAME AND METHOD	SPECIMEN REQUIREMENTS	REFERENCE INTERVAL, CONVENTIONAL [INTERNATIONAL RECOMMENDED UNITS]	CHEMICAL INTERFERENCES AND IN VIVO EFFECTS
21-Hydroxylase antibodies; adrenal antibodies	Serum, frozen or refrigerated, is preferable.	<1 U: negative >1 U: positive Results are expressed in arbitrary units and may vary with reagent manufacturer.	None known.
Solid phase EIA (21-hydroxylase antibodies)		Negative is normal. Sera reactive at ≥1-4 dilution are positive.	
Indirect immunofluorescence (adrenal antibodies)			

1. Tanaka H, Perez M, Powell M, et al: Steroid 21-hydroxylase autoantibodies: measurements with a new immunoprecipitation assay, *J Clin Endocrinol Metab* 82:1440-1446, 1997.

DIAGNOSTIC INFORMATION

REMARKS

Antibodies to 21-hydroxylase (adrenal antibodies) occur in patients with primary adrenal insufficiency (Addison's disease). Results may be positive in patients with autoimmune polyendocrine syndromes I or II and less frequently in patients with autoimmune thyroid diseases.[1]

21-Hydroxylase is a microsomal enzyme with a molecular size of 55 kDa.

TEST NAME AND METHOD	SPECIMEN REQUIREMENTS	REFERENCE INTERVAL, CONVENTIONAL [INTERNATIONAL RECOMMENDED UNITS]			CHEMICAL INTERFERENCES AND IN VIVO EFFECTS
17-Hydroxypreg-nenolone[1]	Serum. Store frozen at −20° C.	*ng/dL*		*nmol/L*	None found.
		Premature[3] (26-28 wk)			
RIA		Day 4:	375-3559 × 0.0301	[11.3-107.1]	
		(31-35 wk)			
		Day 4:	64-2380	[1.9-71.6]	
		Full term[3]			
		3 days:	10-829	[0.3-24.9]	
		1-6 mo:	36-763	[1.1-23]	
		1-12 mo:	42-540	[1.3-16.3]	
		Prepubertal child (2-8 yr)[4]:	≤100 × 0.0301	[≤3.0]	
		Adult[5]			
		M:	41-183	[1.2-5.5]	
		F,			
		Follicular:	45-1185	[1.3-35.7]	
		Luteal:	42-450	[1.3-13.5]	
		Postmenopausal:	18-48	[0.5-1.4]	
	Urine, 24 hr.[2] Preserve with 1 g of boric acid.	*mg/day*		*nmol/day*	
		M:	<2.8 × 3.01	[<8.4]	
		F:	<5.2	[<15.7]	

1. McKenna TJ, Miller RB, Liddle GW: Plasma pregnenolone and 17-OH pregnenolone in patients with adrenal tumors, ACTH excess, or idiopathic hirsutism, *J Clin Endocrinol Metab* 44:231-236, 1977.
2. InterScience Institute: *Current unique and rare endocrine assays,* Inglewood, CA, 1987, InterScience Institute.
3. Esoterix Laboratory: *Test information,* Austin, TX, Esoterix, Inc.
4. Nichols Institute Reference Laboratories: *Test catalog,* San Juan Capistrano, CA, 1993, Nichols Institute Reference Laboratories.
5. Radioassay Systems Laboratories: ICN Biomedicals, Inc., Costa Mesa, CA. Personal communication.

TEST NAME AND METHOD	SPECIMEN REQUIREMENTS	REFERENCE INTERVAL, CONVENTIONAL [INTERNATIONAL RECOMMENDED UNITS]			CHEMICAL INTERFERENCES AND IN VIVO EFFECTS
17-Hydroxypro-gesterone (17-OHP)[1,2]	Serum. Freeze immediately; early morning specimen preferred.	*ng/dL*[4]		*nmol/L*	None found.
		Cord blood:	900-5000 × 0.03	[27.3-151.5]	
	Store at 4° C for up to	Premature:	26-568	[0.8-17.0]	
	4 days or at 20° C for	Newborn (3 days):	7-77	[0.2-2.3]	
RIA	up to 1 mo.	Prepubertal child:	3-90	[0.1-2.7]	
		Puberty			
		Tanner stage			
		1			
		M:	3-90	[0.1-2.7]	
		F:	3-82	[0.1-2.5]	
		2			
		M:	5-115	[0.2-3.5]	
		F:	11-98	[0.3-3.0]	

DIAGNOSTIC INFORMATION	REMARKS
↑ Congenital adrenal hyperplasia caused by 21-hydroxylase deficiency and 3β-hydroxysteroid dehydrogenase-isomerase deficiency, idiopathic hirsutism, and adrenal carcinomas ↓ Adrenal insufficiency	
↑ Congenital adrenal hyperplasia caused by 21-hydroxylase (P-450$_{C21}$) deficiency (values 4000-22,000 ng/dL [121-666 nmol/L]); 11β-hydroxylase (P-450$_{C11}$) deficiency associated with modest elevations; and some cases of adrenal or ovarian neoplasms ↓ Male pseudohermaphrodites [17β-hydroxylase (P-450$_{C17}$) deficiency]; Addison's disease	17-OHP has a marked circadian variation in secretion (highest value in morning). The luteal phase elevation indicates corpus luteum activity. There is a significant increase 1 day before the LH peak, followed by a peak that coincides with that of the LH midcycle peak. This is followed by a short decrease and increase, which correlate with those of estradiol and progesterone. Highest values are found in patients with 21-hydroxylase deficiency. Increased basal and ACTH-stimulated serum 17-OHP concentrations are used to diagnose classic and nonclassic forms of 21-hydroxylase deficiency and their carrier states.[5,6] Test may be useful in monitoring patients with CAH who are receiving glucocorticoid treatment. Cross-reacting substances present in neonatal and infant serum specimens may interfere in direct (nonextraction) assays.[7]

TEST NAME AND METHOD	SPECIMEN REQUIREMENTS	REFERENCE INTERVAL, CONVENTIONAL [INTERNATIONAL RECOMMENDED UNITS]			CHEMICAL INTERFERENCES AND IN VIVO EFFECTS
17-Hydroxyprogesterone—CONT					
		3			
		M:	10-138	[0.3-4.2]	
		F:	11-155	[0.3-4.7]	
		4			
		M:	29-180	× 0.03 [0.9-5.4]	
		F:	18-230	[0.5-7.0]	
		5			
		M:	24-175	[0.7-5.3]	
		F:	20-265	[0.6-8.0]	
		Adult			
		M:	27-199	[0.8-6.0]	
		F,			
		Follicular phase:	15-70	[0.4-2.1]	
		Luteal phase:	35-290	[1.0-8.7]	
		Pregnancy: 800	200-1200	[6.0-36.0]	
		Post-ACTH:	<320	[<9.6]	
		Postmenopausal:	<70	[<2.1]	
	Amniotic fluid[3]		*ng/mL*	*nmol/L*	
		12-19 wk:	0.4-2/5	× 3.03 [1.2-7.6]	
		Term:	0.3-0.6	[0.9-1.8]	

1. Hughes IA, Riad-Fahmy D, Griffiths K: Plasma 17-OH progesterone concentrations in newborn infants, *Arch Dis Child* 54:347-349, 1979.
2. Orth D, Kovacs D, DeBold C: The adrenal cortex. In Wilson JH, Foster DW, editors: *Williams textbook of endocrinology,* ed 8, Philadelphia, 1992, WB Saunders.
3. Tulchinsky D, Ryan KJ, editors: *Maternal-fetal endocrinology,* Philadelphia, 1980, WB Saunders.
4. Endocrine Sciences: *Pediatric laboratory services,* Tarzana, CA, 1992, Endocrine Sciences.
5. White PC, New MI, Dupont B: Congenital adrenal hyperplasia. Part 1, *N Engl J Med* 316:1519-1524, 1987.
6. White PC, New MI, Dupont B: Congenital adrenal hyperplasia. Part 2, *N Engl J Med* 316:1580-1586, 1987.
7. Wong T, Shackleton C, Covey T, et al: Identification of the steroids in neonatal plasma that interfere with 17α-hydroxyprogesterone in radioimmunoassays, *Clin Chem* 38:1830-1837, 1992.

TEST NAME AND METHOD	SPECIMEN REQUIREMENTS	REFERENCE INTERVAL, CONVENTIONAL [INTERNATIONAL RECOMMENDED UNITS]			CHEMICAL INTERFERENCES AND IN VIVO EFFECTS
Hydroxyproline, Free[1-4]	Plasma (heparin) or serum, fasting. Place blood in ice water immediately; separate and freeze within 1 hr of collection. Stable for 1 wk at −20° C; for longer periods deproteinize and store at −70° C.[5,6]	*mg/dL*		*μmol/L*	None found.
		Premature			
Ion-exchange chromatography		1 day:	0.52 ± 0.52 (SD)	× 76.3 [40 ± 40][9]	
		6-18 yr			
		M:	<0.66	[<50][10]	
		F:	<0.58	[<44][10]	
		Adult			
		M:	<0.55	[<42][10]	
		F:	<0.48	[<34][10]	

DIAGNOSTIC INFORMATION	REMARKS

This test has replaced urinary pregnanetriol as the best screening test for CAH. Patients with CAH may also have increased 17-ketosteroids. 11-Deoxycortisol measurements may help distinguish 11β- and 21-hydroxylase deficiencies.

See *17-Ketosteroids, Pregnanetriol* and *11-Deoxycortisol.*

AF ↑ Congenital adrenal hyperplasia (CAH) caused by 21-hydroxylase deficiency

P ↑ Hydroxyprolinemia, uremia, and cirrhosis

Less than 5% of total hydroxyproline is free. Total hydroxyproline is a measure of total collagen turnover. (See *Hydroxyproline, Total.*)

TEST NAME AND METHOD	SPECIMEN REQUIREMENTS	REFERENCE INTERVAL, CONVENTIONAL [INTERNATIONAL RECOMMENDED UNITS]	CHEMICAL INTERFERENCES AND IN VIVO EFFECTS
Hydroxyproline, Free—CONT			
	CSF. Collect in sterile tubes; store frozen. Stable at $-20°$ C for 1 wk or at $-70°$ C for 2 mo.[7]	0.090 ± 0.008 (SD)	$[6.9 \pm 0.6]$[11]
Colorimetric	Urine, 24 hr. Add 20 mL of toluene at start of collection. (Alternatively, refrigerate specimen during collection.) Store frozen at $-20°$ C.[8]	Adult: ≤1.3 mg/day[12] $\times 7.63$ [≤10 μmol/day]	U ↑ V Aminopropionitrile, growth hormone, parathyroid hormone, phenobarbital, phenytoin, tolbutamide, and vitamin D

U ↓ V Ascorbic acid, calcitonin, corticosteroids, diphosphonates, estrogens, mithramycin, oral contraceptives, progesterone, and propranolol |

1. Friedman RB, Young DS: *Effects of disease on clinical laboratory tests,* ed 2, Washington, DC, 1989, American Association for Clinical Chemistry.

2. Scriver CR, Beaudet AL, Sly WS, et al, editors: *The metabolic basis of inherited disease,* ed 6, New York, 1989, McGraw-Hill Publishing Co.

3. Young DS: *Effects of drugs on clinical laboratory tests,* ed 3, Washington, DC, 1990, American Association for Clinical Chemistry.

4. Nyhan W, Sakait N: *Diagnostic recognition of genetic disease,* Philadelphia, 1987, Lea & Febiger.

5. Cummings JG: Routine amino acids analysis in the clinical laboratory, *Am Clin Prod Rev* Feb:20-25, 1988.

6. Schaefer A, Piquard F, Haberey P: Plasma amino acids analysis: effects of delayed samples preparation and of storage, *Clin Chim Acta* 164:163-169, 1987.

7. Heiblim DI, Evans HE, Glass L, et al: Amino acid concentrations in cerebrospinal fluid, *Arch Neurol* 35:765-768, 1978.

8. Pesce A, Kaplan L, editors: *Methods in clinical chemistry,* St. Louis, 1987, CV Mosby.

9. Shih V: *Laboratory techniques for the detection of hereditary metabolic disorders,* Boca Raton, FL, 1973, CRC Press.

10. Meites S, editor: *Pediatric clinical chemistry,* ed 3, Washington, DC, 1989, American Association for Clinical Chemistry.

11. Kruse T, Reiber H, Neuhoff V: Amino acid transport across the human blood-CSF barrier, *J Neurol Sci* 70:129-138, 1985.

12. Mayo Medical Laboratories: *Test catalog,* Rochester, MN, 1993, Mayo Medical Laboratories.

13. Behrman RE, Kliegman RM, Nelson WE, et al, editors: *Nelson textbook of pediatrics,* ed 14, Philadelphia, 1992, WB Saunders.

DIAGNOSTIC INFORMATION	REMARKS

CSF ↑ Bacterial meningitis[13]

U ↑ Hydroxyprolinemia, iminoglycinuria types I and II

Urinary excretion of free hydroxyproline increases during the first 10-14 days after birth. Only very low levels are seen after age 1 yr. In addition to hydroxyproline, proline and glycine are also excreted in the iminoglycinurias. Free hydroxyproline increases in urine during periods of rapid growth and increased collagen turnover (See *Hydroxyproline, Total*).

TEST NAME AND METHOD	SPECIMEN REQUIREMENTS	REFERENCE INTERVAL, CONVENTIONAL [INTERNATIONAL RECOMMENDED UNITS]			CHEMICAL INTERFERENCES AND IN VIVO EFFECTS
Hydroxyproline, Total[1-3] *Colorimetric*	Urine, 24 hr; refrigerate during collection. Add 25 mL of HCl, 6 mol/L, to ensure pH <2. Keep patient on gelatin-free and low-collagen diet for 24-48 hr.	*mg/day*[4] Child 3 days: 8-20 1 mo: 32-63 1-10 yr: 15-150 11-14 yr: 68-169 Adult M: 9-73 F: 7-49	× 0.0076	*mmol/day* [0.06-0.15] [0.24-0.48] [0.11-1.14] [0.52-1.28] [0.07-0.55] [0.05-0.37]	↑ V Bed rest, growth hormone, parathyroid hormone, phenobarbital, pregnancy (last trimester), sulfonylureas, thyroid hormone, and vitamin D ↓ V Antineoplastic agents, ascorbic acid, aspirin (100 mg/kg in children has significant effect), calcitonin, calcium gluconate, corticosteroids, diphosphonate, estradiol, estriol, glucocorticoids (in rheumatoid patients under treatment), mithramycin, and propranolol
		mcg/mg[5] *creatinine* Child <5 yr: 100-400 5-12 yr: 100-150 13-18 yr: 25-150 Adults 19-36 [values decrease with increasing age]	× 0.863	*mmol/mol creatinine* [86-345] [86-129] [22-129] [16-31]	
HPLC[6,7]		*mg/day* Adults: 16-49	× 0.0076	*mmol/day*[8] [0.12-0.37]	

1. Epstein S: Serum and urinary markers of bone remodeling: assessment of bone turnover, *Endocr Rev* 9:437-449, 1988.
2. Gasser A, Celada A, Courvoisier B, et al: The clinical measurement of urinary total hydroxyproline excretion, *Clin Chim Acta* 95:487-497, 1979.
3. Calvo MS, Eyre DR, Gundberg CM: Molecular basis and clinical application of biological markers of bone turnover, *Endocr Rev* 17;333-368, 1996.
4. Hydroxyproline, free and total, urine. In *Quest Diagnostics manual: endocrinology test selection and interpretation,* ed 3, San Juan Capistrano, CA, 2004, Quest-Nichols, p. 96.
5. Allison DJ, Walker A, Smith QC: Urinary hydroxyproline: creatinine ratio of normal humans at various ages, *Clin Chim Acta* 14:729-734, 1966.
6. Paroni R, DeVecchi E, Fremo I, et al: Total urinary hydroxyproline determined with rapid and simple high-performance liquid chromatography, *Clin Chem* 38:407-411, 1992.
7. Reed P, Holbrook IB, Gardner ML, et al: Simple, optimized liquid chromatographic for measuring totat hydroxyproline in urine evaluated, *Clin Chem* 37:285-290, 1991.
8. Hughes H, Hagen L, Sutton RA: Liquid-chromatographic determination of 4-hydroxyproline in urine, *Clin Chem* 32:1002-1004, 1986.

TEST NAME AND METHOD	SPECIMEN REQUIREMENTS	REFERENCE INTERVAL, CONVENTIONAL [INTERNATIONAL RECOMMENDED UNITS]	CHEMICAL INTERFERENCES AND IN VIVO EFFECTS
5-Hydroxytryptophol **(5-HTOL)**[1,2] *Chromatographic methods, ELISA*	Urine.[3] Store at 4°, 25°, and 30° C for 1 wk, and at −80° C for several months.[4]	0.03-0.25 μmol 3-10 nmol/mmol creatinine[4] 4-17 (<20) pmoles 5-HTOL/nmoles 5-HIAA ratio[5]* *To compensate for urine dilution and dietary intake of serotonin.	Unknown.

DIAGNOSTIC INFORMATION	REMARKS

↑ Acromegaly, hyperthyroidism, hyperparathyroidism, Paget's disease, rickets and osteomalacia, extensive fractures, bony metastases, osteoporosis, sarcoidosis, severe burns, acute osteomyelitis, congenital hypophosphatasia, fibrous dysplasia, growth spurts, and in elderly persons

↓ Hypopituitarism, hypothyroidism, hypoparathyroidism, malnutrition, and muscular dystrophy (chronic)

Hydroxyproline, produced by the posttranslational hydroxylation of proline, constitutes ~13% of the collagen molecule. Urinary total hydroxyproline excretion reflects total collagen turnover. Approximately half of total body collagen is in bone with the remainder in skin, muscle, and other tissues. Hydroxyproline is also found in serum proteins, notably C1q, a component of complement. During collagen degradation, ~10% of hydroxyproline is excreted in urine, mainly as small peptides. Urinary hydroxyproline is increased by ingestion of meat, fish, and other foods or products containing gelatin or collagen. There is a diurnal rhythm of excretion of hydroxyproline with highest excretion at night.

Total hydroxyproline is measured after acid hydrolysis. Although total hydroxyproline was used as a marker of bone resorption, hydroxyproline is also produced during collagen synthesis (collagen propeptides). Collagen telopeptides and cross-links (see *Collagen Telopeptides and Pyridinium Cross-links*) are more sensitive and specific markers of bone resorption. Consequently, hydroxyproline is no longer routinely used to measure bone resorption.

U ↑ Alcohol intake or serotonin-rich food (such as bananas). 5-HTOL/5-HIAA ratio increases after alcohol intake but not bananas.[6]

Serotonin is metabolized to 5-hydroxytryptophol-3-acetic acid (5-HIAA) and 5-hydroxytryptophol (5-HTOL), both of which are normal constituents of urine. Under normal physiological condiditons, 5-HIAA is the major metabolite. Alcohol dose-dependently shifts serotonin metabolism toward 5-HTOL and leads to the increase of urinary 5-HTOL and 5-HTOL/5-HIAA ratio. The 5-HTOL/5-HIAA ratio is usually monitored to compensate for urine dilution and dietary intake of serotonin.

TEST NAME AND METHOD	SPECIMEN REQUIREMENTS	REFERENCE INTERVAL, CONVENTIONAL [INTERNATIONAL RECOMMENDED UNITS]	CHEMICAL INTERFERENCES AND IN VIVO EFFECTS

5-Hydroxytryptophol *(5-HTOL)*—CONT

1. Helander A, Beck O, Borg S: The use of 5-hydroxytryptophol as an alcohol intake marker, *Alcohol Alcohol Suppl* 2:497-502, 1994.
2. Beck O, Helander A: 5-hydroxytryptophol as a marker for recent alcohol intake, *Addiction* 98(suppl 2):63-72, 2003.
3. Stephanson N, Dahl H, Helander A, et al: Direct quantification of ethyl glucuronide in clinical urine samples by liquid chromatography-mass spectrometry, *Ther Drug Monit* 24:645-651, 2002.
4. Helander A, Beck O, Borg S: Determination of urinary 5-hydroxytryptophol by high-performance liquid chromatography with electrochemical detection, *J Chromatogr* 579:340-345, 1992.
5. Voltaire A, Beck O, Borg S: Urinary 5-hydroxytryptophol: a possible marker of recent alcohol consumption, *Alcohol Clin Exp Res* 16:281-285, 1992.
6. Helander A, Wikstrom T, Lowenmo C, et al: Urinary excretion of 5-hydroxyindole-3-acetic acid and 5-hydroxytryptophol after oral loading with serotonin, *Life Sci* 50:1207-1213, 1992.

IgG Index[1,2]	CSF, serum	Index: 0.3-0.6	None found.
Calculation			

1. Tietz NW, editor: *Textbook of clinical chemistry,* Philadelphia, 1986, WB Saunders.
2. Killingsworth LM, Cooney SK, Tyllia MM, et al: Deciphering cerebrospinal fluid patterns, *Diagn Med* March/April:23-29, 1982.
3. Sharief MK, Hentges R, Chiardi M: Intrathecal immune response in patients with the post-polio syndrome, *N Engl J Med* 325:749-755, 1991.
4. Lunding J, Midgard R, Vedeler CA: Oligoclonal bands in cerebrospinal fluid: a comparative study of isoelectric focusing, agarose gel electrophoresis and IgG index, *Acta Neurol Scand* 102:322-325, 2000.

The increased 5-HTOL/5-HIAA ratio reflects alcohol intake in the past 24 hr and to remain elevated for 6-15 hr after blood returned to normal. The ratio is highly sensitive and specific and has been proposed as a marker for detecting recent alcohol intake, monitoring lapses into drinking during outpatient treatment, evaluating treatment effects, and so on.

↑ Multiple sclerosis (MS) and other CNS demyelinating processes, infectious processes of the CNS such as neurosyphilis, Lyme borreliosis, acute bacterial meningitis, schistosomiasis, and neurocysticercosis.

$$\text{IgG index} = \frac{\text{IgG, CSF/IgG, serum}}{\text{albumin, CSF/albumin, serum}}$$

A recent clinical study has shown that IgM is a more specific indicator of disease in the post-polio syndrome than the IgG index.[3]

The IgG index is age dependent and less sensitive for detecting juvenile MS. It provides an evaluation of local IgG synthesis, a finding that is equivalent to detecting the presence of oligoclonal bands, especially in MS. The index also helps to distinguish between exudation of serum IgG into CSF and synthesis of IgG within the CNS, although isoelectric focusing may serve better in this regard.[4]

TEST NAME AND METHOD	SPECIMEN REQUIREMENTS	REFERENCE INTERVAL, CONVENTIONAL [INTERNATIONAL RECOMMENDED UNITS]	CHEMICAL INTERFERENCES AND IN VIVO EFFECTS
IgG Synthesis Rate[1]	CSF, serum	-9.9 to $+3.3$ mg/day ($\bar{x}$: -3.3)	None found.
Calculation[2]			

1. Tietz NW, editor: *Textbook of clinical chemistry,* Philadelphia, 1986, WB Saunders.
2. Tourtellotte WW, Ma BI: Multiple sclerosis: the blood-brain barrier and the measurement of de novo central nervous system IgG synthesis, *Neurology* 28(suppl):76-83, 1978.
3. Reiber H, Thompson EJ, Grimsley G, et al: Quality assurance for cerebrospinal fluid protein analysis: international consensus by an Internet-based group discussion, *Clin Chem Lab Med* 41:331-337, 2003.

Test Name	Specimen		*mg/dL*			*mg/L*	Chemical Interferences
Immunoglobulin A (IgA)	Serum. Analyze fresh or store at 4° C for <72 hr. Stable frozen at −20° C for 6 mo or at −70° C indefinitely. Specimens without lipemia or hemolysis are preferred.	Cord serum:	1-4	× 10		[10-40]	S ↓ V Anticonvulsants (Carbamazepine,[10] phenytoin,[11] and valproic acid[12]), some oral contraceptive formulations,[13] methylprednisolone,[14] gold compounds,[15] penicillamine,[16] and L-asparaginase
Nephelometric, RID[1]		1 mo:	2-50			[20-500]	
		2-5 mo:	4-80			[40-800]	
		6-9 mo:	8-80			[80-800]	
		10-12 mo:	15-90			[150-900]	
		1 yr:	15-110			[150-1100]	
		2-3 yr:	18-150			[180-1500]	
		4-5 yr:	25-160			[250-1600]	
		6-8 yr:	35-200			[350-2000]	
		9-12 yr:	45-250			[450-2500]	Excessive turbidity can affect nephelometric methods.
		>12 yr:	40-350			[400-3500]	

Values compiled from multiple sources.[6-9]

DIAGNOSTIC INFORMATION	REMARKS

The CNS synthesis rate of IgG by B cells infiltrating areas of active demyelination is a useful parameter for monitoring disease activity in multiple sclerosis.[2]

See also *IgG Index.*

Synthesis rate (mg/day) =

$$\left[\left(IgG_{CSF} - \frac{IgGs}{369}\right) - \left(Alb_{CSF} - \frac{Albs}{230}\right)\left(\frac{IgGs}{Albs}\right) \times (0.43)\right] \times 5$$

where:

IgG_{CSF} = concentration of IgG in cerebrospinal fluid in mg/dL

IgG_S = concentration of IgG in serum in mg/dL

Alb_{CSF} = concentration of albumin in cerebrospinal fluid in mg/dL

Alb_S = concentration of albumin in serum in mg/dL

369 = ratio of serum/CSF IgG concentrations in normal subjects

230 = ratio of serum/CSF albumin concentrations in normal subjects

0.43 = MW albumin/MW IgG

5 = average volume (in dL) of CSF normally formed in 24 hr

Alternative formulas may perform better.[3]

S ↑ *Polyclonal:* Increased serum IgA concentrations are found in chronic inflammatory disorders, infectious processes, and in association with tumors. These include rheumatoid arthritis, inflammatory bowel disease, ankylosing spondylitis,[17] mixed connective tissue disease,[18] and chronic liver conditions of both infectious and noninfectious etiology. Elevated levels have been reported in patients with malignancies of diverse organ sites and in patients with Wiskott-Aldrich syndrome.

Monoclonal: Multiple myeloma, solitary plasmacytoma, alpha-heavy chain disease, monoclonal gammopathy of undetermined significance (MGUS), lymphoma, and chronic lymphocytic leukemia.

S ↓ Selective IgA deficiency is one of the most frequently encountered primary immunodeficiencies. Although clinical manifestations are absent in many cases, it can be associated with infectious, autoimmune, and allergic complications,[17] gastric carcinoma, and lymphoma.[20]

IgA is present in both monomeric and dimeric forms and is the predominant immunoglobulin type found in secretions. It activates complement by the alternative pathway. Two subclasses have been identified (IgA₁, IgA₂). Secretory IgA, which provides mucosal protection, consists of a dimer, a joining J-chain, and a secretory component obtained from epithelial cells. The secretory component may provide some resistance to enzymatic cleavage.

IgA cannot cross the placenta. Although it can be produced by infants, their serum values are typically low.[24,25] Demonstration of increased concentrations in cord blood has been used as evidence of maternal blood contamination when performing serological assessment for possible intrauterine infection. Secretory IgA of maternal origin in colostrum and milk provides breast-fed infants with protection against infection within the intestinal tract.

TEST NAME AND METHOD	SPECIMEN REQUIREMENTS	REFERENCE INTERVAL, CONVENTIONAL [INTERNATIONAL RECOMMENDED UNITS]			CHEMICAL INTERFERENCES AND IN VIVO EFFECTS

Immunoglobulin A—CONT

EID ELISA[2]	Urine, 24 hr. Centrifuge and adjust to pH 7.0. Analyze fresh. Stable frozen at −20° C for up to 1 yr.	0.08-0.42 mg/day			

		mg/dL (SD)		*mg/L*	
RIA[3]	CSF. Centrifuge before analysis. Analyze fresh or store at 4° C for <72 hr. Stable frozen at −20° C for 6 mo or at −70° C indefinitely. Specimens should not contain blood.	15-20 yr: 0.07 ± 0.04 21-40 yr: 0.07 ± 0.03 41-60 yr: 0.10 ± 0.03 61-87 yr: 0.11 ± 0.06	× 10	[0.7 ± 0.4] [0.7 ± 0.3] [1.0 ± 0.3] [1.1 ± 0.6]	

		mg/dL		*mg/L*	
RID[4] ――――――― *Nephelometric*[4]	Saliva. Centrifuge before analysis. Analyze fresh or store at 4° C for <72 hr. Stable frozen at −20° C for 6 mo or at −70° C indefinitely.	Secretory IgA: 1.7-29.2 (x̄: 7.7) 3.5-36.8 (x̄: 11.4)	× 10	[17-292] [x̄: 77] [35-368] [x̄: 114]	

RID	Colostrum. Centrifuge before analysis. Analyze fresh or store at 4° C for <72 hr. Stable frozen at −20° C for 6 mo or at −70° C indefinitely.	~450 mg/dL	× 0.01	[~4.5 g/L]	

1. Rizmann SE, Aquanno JJ, Finney MA, et al: Quantitation of normal and abnormal serum immunoglobulins G, A, and M by radial immunodiffusion, nephelometry, and turbidimetry. In Ritzmann SE, editor: *Protein abnormalities, vol 1. Physiology of immunoglobulins: diagnostic and clinical aspects,* New York, 1982, Alan R. Liss, Inc.

2. Floege J, Boeddeker M, Dreikhausen U, et al: Quantification of human urinary free secretory component, secretory and nonsecretory IgA by ELISA, *Clin Physiol Biochem* 7:165-175, 1989.

DIAGNOSTIC INFORMATION   **REMARKS**

Decreased or undetectable levels of IgA may be a component of other immunodeficiency states such as hyper-IgM, common variable immunodeficiency,[21] and ataxia telangiectasia,[22] or secondary to conditions such as thermal burns or suppression of uninvolved polyclonal immunoglobulins when a non-IgA M-protein is present.

U↑ IgA nephropathy (Berger's disease), severe nephrotic syndrome, surgical neobladder[23]

Sal .↑ Can be increased rheumatoid arthritis, Sjögren's syndrome, or other autoimmune conditions.

IgA is the second most frequent type of monoclonal immunoglobulin (M-protein) identified in multiple myeloma (10-15%).[26] In standard serum protein electrophoretic studies, IgA M-proteins commonly migrate within the beta region or near the beta-gamma junction; consequently, their presence can be obscured by the beta bands. Quantitated IgA concentrations can also be normal or low despite the presence of an IgA M-protein. Serum immunofixation studies should be performed if an IgA monoclonal immunoglobulin is suspected. Polymerization commonly occurs with these M-proteins, resulting in multiple bands in electrophoretic studies. Complex formation with other serum proteins and enzymes are not infrequent and may complicate isoenzyme identification because of changes in migration characteristics.[27]

Isolated IgA deficiency is reportedly the most frequently identified primary immunodeficiency (estimated at 1:400 to 1:3000 blood donors).[28] Some of these individuals will have anti-IgA antibodies and can experience an anaphylactic reaction if transfused with IgA-containing blood products. Anaphylactic transfusion reactions related to IgA deficiency, however, are relatively uncommon. Antibodies can be directed against the alpha chain or a specific subclass. Quantitated total IgA values can be within the normal interval despite a subclass deficiency with antisubclass antibodies.

Immunochemical methods do not differentiate monoclonal from polyclonal immunoglobulin concentrations. Serum electrophoresis and immunofixation should be performed for quantitation of M-proteins. For optimum avoidance of antigen excess, serum dilutions resulting in IgA concentrations of 50-100 mg/dL (500-1000 mg/L) have been recommended.

Indications for quantitation include assessment for possible immunodeficiency, investigation of an anaphylactic transfusion reaction, diagnosis and serial monitoring of patients with monoclonal gammopathies, and evaluation for ataxia telangiectasia.

MW: 160,000 (monomer)
$t_{1/2}$:   6 days.

3.   Nerenberg ST, Prasad R: Radioimmunoassays for Ig classes G, A, M, D, and E in spinal fluids: normal values of different age groups, *J Lab Clin Med* 86:887-898, 1975.

4.   Goodwin CL, Ritzmann SE: Quantitiation of secretory IgA by laser nephelometry. American Society of Clinical Pathologist, Dallas, TX, March 22, 1978, *Am J Clin Pathol* 70:327-328, 1978.

TEST NAME AND METHOD	SPECIMEN REQUIREMENTS	REFERENCE INTERVAL, CONVENTIONAL [INTERNATIONAL RECOMMENDED UNITS]		CHEMICAL INTERFERENCES AND IN VIVO EFFECTS

Immunoglobulin A—CONT

5. Allansmith M, McClellan BH, Butterworth M, et al: The development of immunoglobulin levels in man, *J Pediatr* 72:276-290, 1968.

6. Buckley CE III, Dorsey FC: Serum immunoglobulin levels throughout the life span of healthy man, *Ann Intern Med* 75:673-682, 1971.

7. Jolliff CR, Cost KM, Stivrins PC, et al: Reference intervals for serum IgG, IgA, IgM, C3, and C4 as determined by rate nephelometry, *Clin Chem* 28:126-128, 1982.

8. Maddison SE, Stewart CC, Farshy CE, et al: The relationship of race, sex, and age to concentration of serum immunoglobulins expressed in international units in healthy adults in the U.S.A, *Bull World Health Organ* 52:179-185, 1975.

9. Putnam FW: Immunoglobulins I, II, III. In Putnam FW, editor: *The plasma proteins, vol II*, ed 2, New York, 1977, Academic Press.

10. Basaran N, Hincal F, Kansu E, et al: Humoral and cellular immune parameters in untreated and phenytoin- or carbamazepine-treated epileptic patients, *Int J Immunopharmacol* 16:1071-1077, 1994.

11. Pereira LF, Sanchez JF: Reversible panhypogammaglobulinemia associated with phenytoin treatment, *Scand J Infect Dis* 34:785-787, 2002.

12. Joubert PH, Aucamp AK, Potgieter GM, et al: Epilepsy and IgA deficiency—the effect of sodium valproate, *S Afr Med J* 52:642-644, 1977.

13. Klinger G, Graser T, Mellinger U, et al: A comparative study of the effects of two oral contraceptives containing dienogest or desogestrel on the human immune system, *Gynecol Endocrinol* 14:15-24, 2000.

14. Forster PJ, Grindulis KA, Neumann V, et al: High-dose intravenous methylprednisolone in rheumatoid arthritis, *Ann Rheum Dis* 41:444-446, 1982.

15. Lorber A, Simon TM, Leeb J, et al: Effect of chrysotherapy on parameters of immune response, *J Rheumatol Suppl* 5:82-90, 1979.

16. Williams A, Scott DL, Greenwood A, et al: The clinical value of measuring immunoglobulins when assessing penicillamine therapy in rheumatoid arthritis, *Clin Rheumatol* 7:347-353, 1988.

TEST NAME AND METHOD	SPECIMEN REQUIREMENTS	REFERENCE INTERVAL, CONVENTIONAL [INTERNATIONAL RECOMMENDED UNITS]			CHEMICAL INTERFERENCES AND IN VIVO EFFECTS
Immunoglobulin D (IgD)[1-3] *Nephelometric, RID*[1]	Serum. Analyze fresh or store at 4° C for <72 hr. Stable frozen at −20° C for 6 mo or at −70° C indefinitely. Specimens without lipemia or hemolysis are preferred.	*mg/dL* Cord:	>2	× 10	*mg/L* [>20]	None found.
		mg/dL[5] Newborn: Adult:	0-1.0 0-8.0	× 10	*mg/L* [0-10] [0-80]	Excessive turbidity can affect nephelometric methods.
RIA[4]	CSF. Centrifuge before analysis. Analyze fresh or store at 4° C for <72 hr. Stable frozen at −20° C for 6 mo or at −70° C indefinitely. Specimens should not contain blood.	*U/mL (2 SD)* 15-20 yr: 21-40 yr: 41-60 yr: 61-87 yr:	3.56 ± 2.0 3.02 ± 1.3 2.96 ± 0.88 3.20 ± 0.9	× 1.0	*kU/L (2 SD)* [3.56 ± 2.0] [3.02 ± 1.3] [2.96 ± 0.88] [3.20 ± 0.9]	

1. Ritzmann SE, Tucker ES III: *Protein analysis in disease—current concepts. Workshop manual,* Chicago, 1979, American Society of Clinical Pathologists, Commission for Continuing Education.

DIAGNOSTIC INFORMATION	REMARKS

17. Wendling D, Didier JM, Seilles E: Serum secretory immunoglobulins in ankylosing spondylitis, *Clin Rheumatol* 15:590-593, 1996.

18. Bakri Hassan A, Ronnelid J, Gunnarsson I, et al: Increased serum levels of immunoglobulins, C-reactive protein, type 1 and type 2 cytokines in patients with mixed connective tissue disease, *J Autoimmun* 11:503-508, 1998.

19. French MA, Dawkins RL: Central MHC genes, IgA deficiency and autoimmune disease, *Immunol Today* 11:271-274, 1990.

20. Cunningham-Rundles C: Physiology of IgA and IgA deficiency, *J Clin Immunol* 21:303-309, 2001.

21. Sutor G, Fabel H: Sarcoidosis and common variable immunodeficiency. A case of sarcoidosis in conjunction with severe impairment of the cellular and humoral immune system, *Respiration* 67:204-208, 2000.

22. Schwartzman JS, Sole D, Naspitz CK: Ataxia-telangiectasia: a clinical and laboratory review study of 14 cases, *Allergol Immunopathol (Madr)* 18:105-111, 1990.

23. d'Addessi A, Racioppi M, Fanasca A, et al: Long-term behavior of secretory immunity in ileocecal and ileal orthotopic neobladders, *Urol Int* 67:41-45, 2001.

24. Gitlin D, Kumate J, Urrusti J, et al: The marked selectivity of the human placenta in the transfer of proteins from mother to fetus, *J Pediatr* 63:870-871, 1963.

25. Gitlin D, Kumate J, Urrusti J, et al: The selectivity of the human placenta in the transfer of proteins from mother to fetus, *J Clin Invest* 43:1938-1951, 1964.

26. Schur PH, Kyle RA, Bloch KJ, et al: IgG subclasses: relationship to clinical aspects of multiple myeloma and frequency distribution among M-components, *Scand J Haematol* 12:60-68, 1974.

27. Murthy VV: Identification of false-positive CK-MB activity in an elderly patient, *Am J Clin Pathol* 99:97-100, 1993.

28. Cunningham-Rundles C: Physiology of IgA and IgA deficiency, *J Clin Immunol* 21:303-309, 2001.

S ↑ *Polyclonal:* Smoking,[6] infections, including AIDS,[3] acute viral hepatitis,[7] chronic obstructive pulmonary disease,[8] hyperIgD and periodic fever syndrome,[8] after allogeneic bone marrow transplant (children).[9,10]

Monoclonal: IgD multiple myeloma, monoclonal gammopathy of undetermined significance

S ↓ Hereditary or acquired deficiency syndromes.

IgD exists in both a secreted and a membrane-bound form. It is sensitive to proteolytic cleavage and has a relatively short half-life of 2.8 days in the serum.[2] Membrane-bound IgD is found on the surface of mature B-cells and appears to have an immunoregulatory function. Antibody activity against a variety of antigens has been identified.[3] Autoantibodies of the IgD type can be found in some patients with autoimmune diseases.[11]

IgD multiple myeloma (mm) is estimated to represent ~2% of all myelomas.[12] The majority is of the λ light chain type, and a Bence Jones proteinuria, typically heavy, is present in >90% of cases.[12,13] An increased incidence of amyloidosis, renal insufficiency, and shorter overall survival has been reported with the IgD type as compared with other types of mm.[12]

MW: 175,000.

2. Putnam FW, editor: *The plasma proteins: structure, functions and genetic control,vol 1-3,* ed 2, New York, 1977, Academic Press.

TEST NAME AND METHOD	SPECIMEN REQUIREMENTS	REFERENCE INTERVAL, CONVENTIONAL [INTERNATIONAL RECOMMENDED UNITS]	CHEMICAL INTERFERENCES AND IN VIVO EFFECTS

Immunoglobulin D—CONT

3. Preud'homme J-L, Petit I, Barra A, et al: Structural and functional properties of membrane and secreted IgD, *Mol Immunol* 37:871-887, 2000.

4. Nerenberg ST, Prasad R: Radioimmunoassays for Ig classes G, A, M, D, and E in spinal fluids: normal values of different age groups, *J Lab Clin Med* 86:887-898, 1975.

5. Tietz NW, editor: *Textbook of clinical chemistry,* Philadelphia, 1999, WB Saunders.

6. Bahna SL, Heiner DC, Myhre BA: Changes in serum IgD in cigarette smokers, *Clin Exp Immunol* 51:624-630, 1983.

7. Rostenberg I, Penaloza R: Serum IgG and IgD levels in some infectious and non-infectious diseases, *Clin Chim Acta* 85:319-321, 1978.

8. Offord KP, Gleich GJ, Barbee RA, et al: Serum IgD in subjects with and without chronic obstructive pulmonary disease: a previous finding restudies, *Am Rev Respir Dis* 126:118-120, 1982.

Immunoglobulin G (IgG)[1-3]

Nephelometric, turbidimetric

Serum. Analyze fresh or store at 4° C for <72 hr. Stable frozen at −20° C for 6 mo or at −70° C indefinitely. Specimens without lipemia or hemolysis are preferred.

565-1765 mg/dL   1820 × 0.01   [5.65-17.65 g/L]

x̄: 1047   [x̄: 10.47]

	mg/dL		*g/L*
Cord:	650-1600	× 0.01	[6.5-16.0]
1 mo:	250-900		[2.5-9.0]
2-5 mo:	200-700		[2.0-7.0]
6-9 mo:	220-900		[2.2-9.0]
10-12 mo:	290-1070		[2.9-10.7]
1 yr:	340-1200		[3.4-12.0]
2-3 yr:	420-1200		[4.2-12.0]
4-6 yr:	460-1240		[4.6-12.4]
>6 yr:	650-1600		[6.5-16.0]

Values compiled from various sources.[5-7]

S ↑ V L-Asparaginase, nitrofurantoin, and propylthiouracil

S ↓ V Dextran,[10] gold compounds,[11] methylprednisolone,[12] and phenytoin[13]

Excessive turbidity can affect nephelometric methods.

RID, ELISA

Reference values are available by age:

Subclass	mg/dL		g/L
IgG1	500-1200	× 0.01	[5-12]
IgG2	200-600		[2-6]
IgG3	50-100		[0.5-1.0]
IgG4	50-100		[0.5-1.0]

The subclasses can also be reported as a percent of the total IgG.[8]

9. d'Addessi A, Racioppi M, Fanasca A, et al: Long-term behavior of secretory immunity in ileocecal and ileal orthotopic neobladders, *Urol Int* 67:41-45, 2001.

10. Korver K, Radl J, Schellekaus PT, et al: Transient increase of serum IgD levels after allogeneic bone-marrow transplantation, *Clin Exp Immunol* 72:337-343, 1988.

11. Luster MI, Leslie GA, Bardana EJ Jr: Structure and biological functions of human IgD. VII. IgD antinuclear antibodies in sera of patients with autoimmune disorders, *Int Arch Allergy Appl Immunol* 52:212-218, 1976.

12. Blade J, Kyle RA: Nonsecretory myeloma, immunoglobulin D myeloma, and plasma cell leukemia, *Hematol Oncol Clin North Am* 13:1259-1272, 1999.

13. Blade J, Kyle RA: Immunoglobulin D multiple myeloma: presenting features, response to therapy, and survival in a series of 53 cases, *J Clin Oncol* 12:2398-2404, 1994.

S ↑ *Polyclonal:* Chronic or recurrent infections. Autoimmune disorders including rheumatoid arthritis, sarcoidosis, Sjögren's syndrome, systemic lupus erythematosus, autoimmune pancreatitis, autoimmune hepatitis, and idiopathic portal hypertension. Some intrauterine contraceptive devices.[14]

Monoclonal: Multiple myeloma, solitary plasmacytoma, gamma-heavy chain disease, monoclonal gammopathy of undetermined significance (MGUS), lymphoma, and chronic lymphocytic leukemia.

S ↓ Primary immunodeficiency states including severe combined immunodeficiency, X-linked agammaglobulinemia, common variable immunodeficiency, hyper-IgM syndrome, and Nijmegen breakage syndrome.[15] Conditions secondarily affecting serum immunoglobulin levels, such as protein-losing enteropathies, the nephrotic syndrome, thermal burns, myotonic dystrophy, treatment with immunosuppressant drug regimens, or suppression of uninvolved polyclonal immunoglobulins when a non-IgG M-protein is present. Quantitated total IgG values can be increased or within the normal range, or a generalized hypergammaglobulinemia can be present despite an IgG subclass deficiency.[16] The clinical presentation of a subclass deficiency is variable, ranging from asymptomatic to recurrent infections and other signs of immunodeficiency.

Concentrations are variable with HIV infection. They are often elevated, however, a hypogammaglobulinemia can be present, or there may be deficiencies of one or more IgG subclasses.

Representing 70-80% of the total serum immunoglobulins in the normal adult, immunoglobulin G (IgG) is the major circulating immunoglobulin. It exists in four subclasses (IgG_1, IgG_2, IgG_3, IgG_4), with IgG_1 predominating at ~65% of total IgG. During the secondary immune response, IgG is the major antibody type produced.[1] Deficient individuals typically experience recurrent pyogenic infections.

IgG is the most frequent type of heavy chain identified in multiple myeloma, representing 50% of whole immunoglobulin M-proteins.[19] Similar to the normal distribution of immunoglobulins, the majority of these (~70%) are IgG_1.[20] Monoclonal IgG proteins, usually at levels of ≥4000 mg/dL [40 g/L], can be associated with the hyperviscosity syndrome consisting of variable cardiovascular, neurologic, and bleeding complications.[21]

IgG of maternal origin provides passive immunity to the neonate. It is the only class of immunoglobulin transported across the placenta, and this appears to be Fc receptor mediated. Although initially very low, maternally derived IgG increases during the second and third trimesters in the fetus, eventually surpassing maternal levels by term in most cases.[2] IgG_1 is transported preferentially, with IgG_2 shown to have the lowest capacity for placental transfer.[3] After birth, IgG of maternal origin progressively decreases as the infant's immune system matures, with total IgG levels lowest at ~3 months of age.[17] Small-for-gestational age and premature infants are at increased risk of immunodeficiency because of lower initial IgG levels.[2,17] IgG_2 and IgG_4 levels have been reported to mature relatively slower; consequently, evaluation of decreased values may be difficult in patients <2 yr of age.[16,22]

TEST NAME AND METHOD	SPECIMEN REQUIREMENTS	REFERENCE INTERVAL, CONVENTIONAL [INTERNATIONAL RECOMMENDED UNITS]				CHEMICAL INTERFERENCES AND IN VIVO EFFECTS

Immunoglobulin G—CONT

RIA^4	CSF. Centrifuge before analyze fresh or store at 4° C for <72 hr. Stable frozen at −20° C for 6 mo or at −70° C indefinitely. Specimens should not contain blood.		mg/dL $(2\ SD)^9$			mg/L
		15-20 yr:	3.5 ± 2.0	$\times\ 10$		$[35 \pm 20]$
		21-40 yr:	4.2 ± 1.4			$[42 \pm 14]$
		41-60 yr:	4.7 ± 1.0			$[47 \pm 10]$
		61-87 yr:	5.8 ± 1.6			$[58 \pm 16]$

1. Rose NR, et al, editors: *Manual of clinical laboratory immunology,* ed 6, Washington, DC, 2002, ASM Press.

2. Simister NE: Placental transport of immunoglobulin G, *Vaccine* 21:3365-3369, 2003.

3. Malek A: Ex vivo placenta models: transport of immunoglobulin G and its subclasses, *Vaccine* 21:3362-3364, 2003.

4. Nerenberg ST, Prasad R: Radioimmunoassays for Ig classes G, A, M, D, and E in spinal fluids: normal values of different age groups, *J Lab Clin Med* 86:887-898, 1975.

5. Allansmith M, McClellan BH, Butterworth M, et al: The development of immunoglobulin levels in man, *J Pediatr* 72:276-290, 1968.

6. Buckley CE III, Dorsey FC: Serum immunoglobulin levels throughout the life span of healthy man, *Ann Intern Med* 75:673-682, 1971.

7. Maddison SE, Stewart CC, Farshy CE, et al: The relationship of race, sex, and age to concentration of serum immunoglobulins expressed in international units in healthy adults in the U.S.A, *Bull World Health Organ* 52:179-185, 1975.

8. Schur PH, Alpert E, Alper C: Gamma G subgroups in human fetal, cord, and maternal sera, *Clin Immunol Immunopathol* 2:62-66, 1973.

9. Daha M, Van ES LA: *Enhanced decay of classical pathway C3 convertase activity and of stabilized C42 (F-42) by C4-binding protein (C4bp) [Abstract],* Paris, 1990, Proc. 4th Int. Congr. Immunol.

10. Bergman A, Andreen M, Blomback M: Plasma substitution with 3% dextran-60 in orthopedic surgery: influence on plasma colloid osmotic pressure, coagulation parameters, immunoglobulins and other plasma constituents, *Acta Anaesthesiol Scand* 34:21-29, 1990.

11. Lorber A, Simon TM, Leeb J, et al: Effect of chrysotherapy on parameters of immune response, *J Rheumatol Suppl* 5:82-90, 1979.

Immunochemical methods do not differentiate monoclonal from polyclonal immunoglobulin concentrations. Serum electrophoresis and immunofixation should be performed for quantitation of M-proteins. For optimum avoidance of antigen excess, serum dilutions resulting in IgG concentrations of 100-200 mg/dL [1000-2000 mg/L] have been recommended.

Indications for quantitation include assessment for possible immunodeficiency and the diagnosis and serial monitoring of patients with monoclonal gammopathies. IgG subclasses evaluation may be helpful if other causes of immunodeficiency cannot be identified.

MW: 150,000 (monomer)

$t_{1/2}$:   24 days.

CSF↑ Increased intrathecal synthesis is found in most cases of multiple sclerosis. It can also be found in other inflammatory conditions involving the CNS such as Guillain-Barre syndrome, infections, and subacute sclerosing panencephalitis, and less frequently in various disorders such as CNS neoplasms and cerebrovascular diseases.[17,18]

Increased CSF IgG values can be caused by intrathecal synthesis or alternately may reflect the presence of blood-derived immunoglobulins resulting from elevated plasma levels or an increased permeability of the blood-brain barrier (BBB). Evaluation of the BBB and investigation of suspected intrathecal IgG synthesis involve assessment of the CSF/serum albumin ratio, CSF/serum IgG ratio, and IgG index or IgG synthesis rate. CSF protein electrophoretic studies showing bands of restricted heterogeneity (oligoclonal) in the gamma region that are not present in serum electrophoretic studies are evidence of immunoglobulin production within the CNS.[18]

12. Forster PJ, Grindulis KA, Neumann V, et al: High-dose intravenous methylprednisolone in rheumatoid arthritis, *Ann Rheum Dis* 41·444-446, 1982.

13. Pereira LF, Sanchez JF: Reversible panhypogammaglobulinemia associated with phenytoin treatment, *Scand J Infect Dis* 34:785-787, 2002.

14. Eissa MK, Sparks RA, Newton JR: Immunoglobulin levels in the serum and cervical mucus of tailed copper IUD users, *Contraception* 32:87-95, 1985.

15. van Engelen BG, Hiel JA, Gabreels FJ, et al: Decreased immunoglobulin class switching in Nijmegen breakage syndrome due to DNA repair defect, *Hum Immunol* 62:1324-1327, 2001.

16. Shield JP, Strobel S, Levinsky RJ, et al: Immunodeficiency presenting as hypergammaglobulinemia with IgG2 subclass deficiency, *Lancet* 340:448-450, 1992.

17. Tietz NW, editor: *Textbook of clinical chemistry,* Philadelphia, 1999, WB Saunders.

18. Correale J, de los Milagros Bassani Molinas M: Oligoclonal bands and antibody responses in multiple sclerosis, *J Urol* 249:375-389, 2002.

19. Knowles DM, editor: *Neoplastic hematopathology,* ed 2, Philadelphia, 2001, Lippincott Williams & Wilkins.

20. Kyle RA, Gleich GJ: IgG subclasses in monoclonal gammopathy of undetermined significance, *J Lab Clin Med* 100:806-814, 1982.

21. Mehta J, Singhal S: Hyperviscosity syndrome in plasma cell dyscrasias, *Semin Thromb Hemost* 29:467-471, 2003.

22. Morgan G, Levinsky RJ: Clinical significance of IgG subclass deficiency, *Arch Dis Child* 63:771-773, 1985.

TEST NAME AND METHOD	SPECIMEN REQUIREMENTS	REFERENCE INTERVAL, CONVENTIONAL [INTERNATIONAL RECOMMENDED UNITS]				CHEMICAL INTERFERENCES AND IN VIVO EFFECTS
Immunoglobulin M (IgM)[1-4] *Nephelometric*[5]	Serum. Analyze fresh or store at 4° C for <72 hr. Stable frozen at −20° C for 6 mo or at −70° C indefinitely. Specimens without lipemia or hemolysis are preferred.	Cord:* 1 mo: 2-5 mo: 6-9 mo: 10-12 mo: 1-8 yr: 9-12 yr: >12 yr:	*mg/dL* <25 20-80 25-100 35-125 40-150 45-200 50-250 50-300	× 0.01	*g/L* [<250] [200-800] [250-1000] [350-1250] [400-1500] [450-2000] [500-2500] [500-3000]	S ↑V Chronic chlorpromazine administration S ↓ V Dextran,[11] phenytoin,[12] or carbamazepine[13] therapy, treatment with gold compounds,[14] and L-asparaginase

Results vary with standard preparation. Values compiled from various sources.[7-10]

Excessive turbidity can affect nephelometric methods.

*Cord blood IgM must be evaluated in the light of cord blood IgA levels. If cord IgA is >5 mg/dL [>50 mg/L], contamination of newborn serum by maternal blood renders IgM falsely elevated and uninterpretable.

RIA[6]	CSF. Centrifuge before analysis. Analyze fresh or store at 4° C for <72 hr. Stable frozen at −20° C for 6 mo or at −70° C indefinitely. Specimens should not contain blood.	15-20 yr: 21-40 yr: 41-60 yr: 61-87 yr:	*mg/dL (SD)* 0.02 ± 0.009 0.016 ± 0.003 0.017 ± 0.004 0.017 ± 0.005	× 10	*mg/L (SD)* [0.2 ± 0.09] [0.16 ± 0.03] [0.17 ± 0.04] [0.17 ± 0.05]	

1. Ritzmann SE, Tucker ES III: *Protein analysis in disease—current concepts, Workshop manual,* Chicago, 1979, American Society of Clinical Pathologists, Commission for Continuing Education.

S ↑ *Polyclonal:* A selective increase in IgM concentration can represent a response to infection. Increases in antigen-specific IgM commonly occur on exposure to a diverse variety of viral (including HAV, HBV, CMV, EBV, and other viruses) bacterial or parasitic agents. Chronic inflammatory conditions such as rheumatoid arthritis and primary biliary cirrhosis can also be associated with increased serum IgM values. "Classical" rheumatoid factors (RF) are IgM autoantibodies against IgG[15]; however, RF can be other immunoglobulin types. Serum IgM concentrations can be elevated secondary to the nephrotic syndrome or with the inherited hyper-IgM syndrome.

S ↑ *Monoclonal:* Waldenström's macroglobulinemia, lymphoma, chronic lymphocytic leukemia, μ-heavy chain disease (rare), multiple myeloma (also very rare), Schnitzler's syndrome,[16] cold IgM antibody agglutinin, monoclonal gammopathy of undetermined significance (MGUS).

S ↓ Selective IgM deficiency is uncommon and can be associated with autoimmune disorders.[17] Recurrent infection is a typical manifestation. Decreased levels are more frequently seen in conjunction with general immunodeficiency states such as occurs with monoclonal gammopathies, splenectomy,[18] enteric protein loss or some other causes of protein deficiency, thermal burns, or treatment with immunosuppressive drug regimens.

CSF ↑ Levels >3.0 mg/dL [>30 mg/L] suggest bacterial rather than viral meningitis.[19]

During B-cell development, IgM is the first immunoglobulin type produced and becomes a component of the B-cell surface receptor. It is also the initial antibody type secreted during the primary humoral response to antigen. The majority of "natural antibodies" that bind antigens not previously exposed to the individual are IgM in nature. On antigenic exposure, the typical antibody response sequence consists of an increase in antigen-specific IgM, isotype switching, and then subsequent increases in antigen-specific immunoglobulins of other classes.[3] IgM levels peak, then frequently decline, but can remain elevated.

Because of its pentameric structure (five subunits with a joining J-chain, 10 sites available for antigen binding), IgM is an effective activator of complement.[3] Most cold-reactive autoantibodies are IgM. Low molecular weight monomeric and oligomeric forms can be found in patients with lymphoproliferative, infectious, and autoimmune disorders.[4] Small amounts of these forms may be detected in normal sera using sensitive methods.[20]

IgM can be produced by the fetus and cannot cross the placenta. Consequently, serological assessment of antigen-specific IgM in fetal cord blood or in serum during the immediate postnatal period is used in the diagnosis of congenital infection. A substantial fraction of total IgM in neonates can be in the low molecular weight form.[21]

Monoclonal IgM proteins, usually at levels of ≥3000 mg/dL [30 g/L], can be associated with the hyperviscosity syndrome, consisting of variable cardiovascular, neurologic, and bleeding complications.[22] Immunochemical methods do not differentiate monoclonal from polyclonal immunoglobulin concentrations. Serum electrophoresis and immunofixation should be performed for quantitation of M-proteins. For optimum avoidance of antigen excess, serum dilutions resulting in IgM concentrations of 50-100 mg/dL [500-1000 mg/L] have been recommended.

Indications for quantitation include the diagnosis of infection, assessment for possible immunodeficiency, and the diagnosis and serial monitoring patients with monoclonal gammopathies.

MW: 900,000
$t_{1/2}$:   5 days.

2. Putnam FW, editor: *The plasma proteins: structure, functions and genetic control, vols 1-3,* ed 2, New York, 1977, Academic Press.

TEST NAME AND METHOD	SPECIMEN REQUIREMENTS	REFERENCE INTERVAL, CONVENTIONAL [INTERNATIONAL RECOMMENDED UNITS]	CHEMICAL INTERFERENCES AND IN VIVO EFFECTS

Immunoglobulin M—CONT

3. Boes M: Role of natural and immune IgM antibodies in immune responses, *Mol Immunol* 37:1141-1149, 2000.

4. Schwarz JA, Kaboth U, Reikowski H, et al: Monomeric IgM in acute and chronic liver diseases, *Klin Wochenschr* 53:535-538, 1975.

5. Rizmann SE, Aguanno JJ, Finney MA, et al: Quantitation of normal and abnormal serum immunoglobulins G, A, and M by radial immunodiffusion, nephelometry, and turbidimetry. In Ritzmann SE, editor: *Protein abnormalities, vol 1. Physiology of immunoglobulins: diagnostic and clinical aspects,* New York, 1982, Alan R. Liss, Inc.

6. Nerenberg ST, Prasad R: Radioimmunoassays for Ig classes G, A, M, D, and E in spinal fluids: normal values of different age groups, *J Lab Clin Med* 86:887-898, 1975.

7. Allansmith M, McClellan BH, Butterworth M, et al: The development of immunoglobulin levels in man, *J Pediatr* 72:276-290, 1968.

8. Buckley CE III, Dorsey FC: Serum immunoglobulin levels throughout the life span of healthy man, *Ann Intern Med* 75:673-682, 1971.

9. Maddison SE, Stewart CC, Farshy CE, et al: The relationship of race, sex, and age to concentration of serum immunoglobulins expressed in international units in healthy adults in the U.S.A., *Bull World Health Organ* 52:179-185, 1975.

10. Alford CA Jr: Immunoglobulin determination in the diagnosis of fetal infection, *Pediatr Clin N Am* 18:99-113, 1971.

11. Bergman A, Andreen M, Blomback M: Plasma substitution with 3% dextran-60 in orthopedic surgery: influence on plasma colloid osmotic pressure, coagulation parameters, immunoglobulins and other plasma constituents, *Acta Anaesthesiol Scand* 34:21-29, 1990.

12. Pereira LF, Sanchez JF: Reversible panhypogammaglobulinemia associated with phenytoin treatment, *Scand J Infect Dis* 34:785-787, 2002.

Immunological Monitoring (T-Cell Subsets)[1-3]

Flow cytometry

Whole blood (Na heparin or EDTA). Specimen must be <8 hr old. Do not refrigerate. Leukocyte and differential count should be reported in absolute numbers.

↓ V Corticosteroids and immunosuppressive drugs (such as cyclosporin, azathioprin, and mycophenolate) decrease numbers of circulating T-lymphocytes.

Age	CD_3^+	CD_4^+	CD_8^+	CD_{19}^+	CD_{56}^+	
0-6 mo[4]	3.5-5.0	2.8-3.9	0.35-2.5	0.43-3.3	0.2-0.6	$\times 10^9 cells/L$
6-12 mo	3.4-4.6	2.6-3.5	0.35-2.5	0.43-3.3	0.2-0.6	
12-18 mo	3.2-3.9	2.3-2.9	0.35-2.5	0.43-3.3	0.2-0.6	
18-24 mo	2.8-3.5	1.9-2.5	0.35-2.5	0.43-3.3	0.2-0.6	
24-30 mo	2.3-3.3	2.6-3.5	0.35-2.5	0.43-3.3	0.2-0.6	
30-36 mo	1.9-3.1	1.2-2.0	0.35-2.5	0.43-3.3	0.2-0.6	
36 mo to Adult[3,5]	0.79-2.19	0.49-1.44	0.27-0.66	0.17-0.41	0.098-0.325	

0-36 mo values based on measurements from 66 infant whole blood samples using Coulter STKS for total leukocyte count measurement and Becton-Dickinson FACScan for flow cytometric immunophenotyping.

---

1. Nathan DG, Orkin SH, Ginsburg D, et al: *Hematology of infancy and childhood,* ed 6, Philadelphia, 2003, WB Saunders.

2. Greer JP, Foerster J, Lukens JN, et al: *Wintrobe's clinical hematology,* ed 11, Philadelphia, 2003, Lippincott Williams & Wilkins.

3. Crosson J, Montgomery R: Normal ranges for blood B-lymphocytes, T-lymphocytes and subsets in adults. Unpublished data, Minneapolis, MN, 2004, Hennepin County Medical Center.

13. Basaran N, Hincal F, Kansu E, et al: Humoral and cellular immune parameters in untreated and phenytoin- or carbamazepine-treated epileptic patients, *Int J Immunopharmacol* 16:1071-1077, 1994.

14. Lorber A, Simon TM, Leeb J, et al: Effect of chrysotherapy on parameters of immune response, *J Rheumatol Suppl* 5:82-90, 1979.

15. Terness P, Opelz G: Natural anti-immunoglobulin autoantibodies: irrelevant by-products or immunoregulatory molecules? *Int Arch Immunol* 115:270-277, 1998.

16. Lim W, Shumak KH, Reis M, et al: Malignant evolution of Schnitzler's syndrome—chronic uticaria and IgM monoclonal gammopathy: report of a new case and review of the literature, *Leuk Lymphoma* 43:181-186, 2002.

17. Takeuchi T, Nakagawa T, Maeda Y, et al: Functional defect of B lymphocytes in a patient with selective IgM deficiency associated with systemic lupus erythematosus, *Autoimmunity* 34:115-122, 2001.

18. Eibl M: Immunological consequences of splenectomy, *Prog Pediatr Surg* 18:139-145, 1985.

19. Gitlin D, Kumate J, Urrusti J, et al: The marked selectivity of the human placenta in the transfer of proteins from mother to fetus, *J Pediatr* 63:870-871, 1963.

20. Xu HJ, Umapathysivam K, McNeilage J, et al: An enhanced chemiluminescent detection system combined with a modified immunoblot technique for the detection of low molecular weight IgM in sera of healthy adults and neonates, *J Immunol Methods* 146:241-247, 1992.

21. Roberts-Thomson PJ, Kennedy A, Koh LY, et al: Frequency of low molecular weight IgM in human cord blood, *J Reprod Immunol* 11:321-325, 1987.

22. Mehta J, Singhal S: Hyperviscosity syndrome in plasma cell dyscrasias, *Semin Thromb Hemost* 29:467-471, 2003.

There is a decrease in total T-lymphocytes (CD_3^+), normal or increased B-lymphocytes (CD_{19}^+), and normal or increased natural killer cells (CD_3-CD_{56}^+) in congenital severe combined immunodeficiency.

T-helper cells (CD_4^+) are depleted in HIV/AIDS, and CD_4^+ lymphocyte levels are used as a marker of prognosis and response to therapy.

An increase in total T-lymphocytes (CD_3^+) or cytotoxic lymphocytes (CD_8^+) is associated with acute renal allograft rejection, with severe viral infection (especially cytomegalovirus and Epstein-Barr virus), and with large granular lymphocytic leukemia. A decrease in total T-cells (CD_3^+) is associated with the effectiveness of therapy with antilymphocyte globulin (ALG) or anti–T-cell monoclonal antibody (OKT_3).

Current published reference intervals should be used with caution. Interlaboratory variations can result from differences in antibodies and equipment utilized, as well as whether the absolute numbers are calculated using a dual-platform method (total leukocyte count measured by separate automated counter multiplied by cell fraction measured by flow cytometry) versus a single-platform method (absolute count measured and calculated by single-flow cytometry method).

4. Setterlung LK, Berglund C, Kruchten S, et al: Analysis of lymphocyte subsets in young infants and children. Unpublished data, Minneapolis and St. Paul, MN, 2004, Children's Hospitals and Clinics.

5. Rodak BF, editor: *Hematology; clinical principles and applications,* ed 2, Philadelphia, 2002, WB Saunders.

TEST NAME AND METHOD	SPECIMEN REQUIREMENTS	REFERENCE INTERVAL, CONVENTIONAL [INTERNATIONAL RECOMMENDED UNITS]		CHEMICAL INTERFERENCES AND IN VIVO EFFECTS
Inhibin[1,2]	Serum		*pg/mL*	None found.
		Adult[5]		
ELISA[3,4]		M:	1.0-3.6	
		F:		
		Nonpregnant,		
		early follicular phase:	5.5-28.2	
		mid follicular phase:	7.9-34.5	
		late follicular phase:	19.5-102.3	
		mid cycle:	49.9-155.5	
		Early L		
		luteal:	35.9-132.7	
		mid luteal:	13.2-159.6	
		late luteal:	7.3-89.9	
		IVF-peak levels:	354.2-1690.0	
		PCOS-ovulatory:	5.7-16.0	
		postmenopausal:	1.0-3.9	

1. Tong S, Wallace EM, Burger HG: Inhibins and activins: clinical advances in reproductive medicine, *Clin Endocrinol (Oxf)* 58:115-127, 2003.
2. Groome NP, Evans LW: Does measurement of inhibin have a clinical role? *Ann Clin Biochem* 37:419-431, 2000.
3. Groome NP, Illingworth PJ, O'Brien M, et al: Detection of dimeric inhibin throughout the human menstrual cycle by two-site enzyme immunoassay, *Clin Endocrinol (Oxf)* 40:717-723, 1994.
4. Groome NP, Illingworth PJ, O'Brien M, et al: Measurement of dimeric inhibin B throughout the human menstrual cycle, *J Clin Endocrinol Metab* 81:1401-1405, 1996.
5. Available at: http://www.aruplab.com/guides/clt/tests/clt_a19b.jsp. Last accessed 2/1/06.

TEST NAME AND METHOD	SPECIMEN REQUIREMENTS	REFERENCE INTERVAL, CONVENTIONAL		[INTERNATIONAL RECOMMENDED UNITS]	CHEMICAL INTERFERENCES AND IN VIVO EFFECTS
Inositol, Free (Myoinositol)[1-3]	Serum	7.0 mcg/mL	× 5.551	[39 μmol/L]	
GLC[4]	Urine, 24 hr[5]	30 mg/day	× 5.551	[166 μmol/day]	U ↑ Glucose (IV)[6]

1. Shils ME, Olson JA, Shike M, editors: *Modern nutrition in health and disease,* ed 8, Philadelphia, 1994, Lea & Febiger.
2. Jyonouchi H, Sun S, Iijima K, et al: Effects of anti-7,8-dihydroxy-9,10-epoxy-7,8,9,10-tetrahydrobenzo[α]pyrene on human small airway epithelial cells and the protective effects of myo-inisitol, *Carcinogenesis* 20:139-145, 1999.
3. Hallman M, Bry K, Hoppu K, et al: Inositol supplementation in premature infants with respiratory distress syndrome, *N Engl J Med* 326:1233-1239, 1992.
4. Lewin LM, Melmed S, Passwell JH, et al: Myoinositol in human neonates: serum concentrations and renal handling, *Pediatr Res* 12:3-6, 1978.

DIAGNOSTIC INFORMATION	REMARKS

S ↑ Normal pregnancy, ovarian (granulosa cell) cancers, preeclamptic toxemia, Down syndrome pregnancy.

S ↓ Ovarian aging.

Inhibins, like activins, belong with the transforming growth factor-β family, sharing structural homology through the β subunit. Inhibins are heterodimers and hence have two forms: α-βA (inhibin A) and α-βB (inhibin B).

The synthesis and secretion of dimeric inhibins seem confined to the ovary (granulosa cells), testis (Sertoli cells), and placenta. Physiologically, inhibins inhibit the release of FSH from the anterior pituitary, serving as a negative feedback regulator for FSH.

Circulating inhibins bind to α2-macroglobulin with a low affinity, which does not seem to interfere with the current ELISA assay.

The current clinical applications are mainly limited to the second trimester screening for Down syndrome by inhibin A and the detection and monitoring of ovary granulosa cell tumors.

↑ Impaired renal function, diabetes.[6,7]

Myoinositol is found in many foods.[8] It has been shown to have a chemopreventative effect against tumorigenesis.[2,9]

Studies indicate that it may also be important for fetal development, and serum values are higher in the fetus and the neonate compared with adult concentrations.[10] Inositol supplementation can improve outcomes in premature infants with respiratory distress syndrome.[3]

5. Melmed S, Lewin LM, Bank H: Myoinositol clearance in renal failure and patient with normal kidney function, *Am J Med Sci* 274:55-59, 1977.

6. Daughaday WH, Larner J: The renal excretion of inositol in normal and diabetic human beings, *J Clin Invest* 33:326-332, 1954.

7. Clements RS, Reynertson R: Myoinositol metabolism in diabetes mellitus. Effect of insulin treatment, *Diabetes* 26:215-221, 1977.

TEST NAME AND METHOD	SPECIMEN REQUIREMENTS	REFERENCE INTERVAL, CONVENTIONAL [INTERNATIONAL RECOMMENDED UNITS]			CHEMICAL INTERFERENCES AND IN VIVO EFFECTS

Inositol, Free—CONT

8. Clements RS Jr, Darnell B: Myo-inositol content of common foods: development of high myo-inositol diet, *Clin Nutr* 33:1954-1967, 1980.

9. Wattenberg IW, Estensen RD: Chemoprevention effects of myo-inisitol and dexamethasone on beno[α]pyrene and 4-(methyInitrosoamino)-1-(3)pyridyl)-1-butanone-induced pulmonary carcinogenesis in female A/J. mice, *Cancer Res* 56:5132-5135, 1996.

TEST NAME AND METHOD	SPECIMEN REQUIREMENTS	REFERENCE INTERVAL, CONVENTIONAL [INTERNATIONAL RECOMMENDED UNITS]			CHEMICAL INTERFERENCES AND IN VIVO EFFECTS
Insecticides	Serum. Avoid plastic containers.		mg/L^8	$\mu mol/L$	Most interferences can be removed by Florisil column chromatography.
		Dieldrin:	<0.025 × 2.63	[<0.066]	
Organochlorine		Chlordecone:	<0.010 × 2.04	[<0.20]	
		DDE:*	<0.5 × 3.14	[<1.57]	
GLC-ECD[1]		DDT:†	<0.2 × 2.82	[<0.56]	
		Heptachlor-Expoxide:	<0.4 × 2.57	[<0.10]	
		Lindane:	<0.0 × 3.44	[<0.07]	
		Methoxychlor:	<0.04 × 2.89	[<0.12]	
		TDE:††	<0.07 × 3.12	[<0.22]	
		Toxic concentration:	Variable		
	Fat		mg/kg	$\mu mol/kg$	
		Dieldrin:	<0.21 × 2.63	[<0.55]	
		DDT:	<28 × 2.82	[<79]	
		DDE:	<5 × 3.14	[<16]	
Organophosphate	Whole blood (EDTA)	See *Acetylcholinesterase*.			None found.
Colorimetric,[2]					
GC-FID, ECD[1]	Urine. Analyze promptly or freeze.	*Organophosphate metabolites (as diethylphosphoric acid)*			
		Normal concentration:	<0.1 × 6.49	[<0.65]	
		Toxic concentration			
		Diazinon:	>0.1	[>0.65]	
		Dichlorvos:	>0.1	[>0.65]	
		Malathion:	>0.2	[>1.3]	
		Methylparathion:	>0.2	[>1.3]	
		Parathion:	>0.2	[>1.3]	
		p-Nitrophenol:	>1 × 7.19	[>7.2]	
		(metabolite of methylparathion and parathion)			

*DDE, Dichlorodiphenyldichloroethylene.
†DDT, Dichlorodiphenyltrichloroethane.
††TDE, 1,1-Dichloro-2,2-bis(*p*-chlorophenyl) ethane.

DIAGNOSTIC INFORMATION	REMARKS

10.   Quirk JG, Bleasdale JE: Myo-inositol in the human fetus, *Obstet Gynecol* 62:41-44, 1983.

Toxicity is low for some members of this group (e.g., DDT) and high for others (e.g., lindane). Exposure may cause non-specific symptoms such as nausea, vomiting, and apprehension. High doses produce CNS symptoms, including behavioral changes, sensory disturbances, convulsions, and coma. Myocardial sensitization to catecholamines may lead to ventricular arrhythmias.[10]

Organochlorine compounds are lipophilic[8] and may be stored in adipose tissue for long periods. Occupational exposure may result in relatively high serum or fat concentrations without symptoms of toxicity. Many organochlorine compounds induce their own metabolism, leading to altered $t_{1/2}$. Hepatic disease generally increases toxicity, $t_{1/2}$, and plasma concentration.

Kinetic values
$t_{1/2}$[11]

Dieldrin:	90 days
Chlordecone:	150 days

Symptoms of toxicity are typical of the anticholinergic toxidrome, including miosis, blurred vision, salivation, sweating, nausea, and diarrhea.

Organophosphates interfere with acetylcholinesterase activity. Toxicity resulting from organophosphate exposure is ordinarily monitored by measuring cholinesterase activity in plasma (pseudocholinesterase) or erythrocytes (acetylcholinesterase). Measurement of individual organophosphate compounds is not usually helpful because blood and urine concentrations do not correlate well with symptoms of toxicity.

p-Nitrophenol is a metabolite of the parathion derivatives only.[2] Rapid metabolism of these substances necessitates prompt analysis.[12]

See also *Acetylcholinesterase.*

TEST NAME AND METHOD	SPECIMEN REQUIREMENTS	REFERENCE INTERVAL, CONVENTIONAL [INTERNATIONAL RECOMMENDED UNITS]			CHEMICAL INTERFERENCES AND IN VIVO EFFECTS

Insecticides—CONT

Pyrethrins and pyrethroids *HPLC*[3]*; GC-ECD*[4]*; GC-FID*[5]*; GC-MS*[6,7]	Urine (metabolites stable for up to 1 yr frozen)[5]	*Occupational exposure*[9]:			Specimens are pretreated by acid hydrolysis and extraction on a reversed-phase column.
		Pyrethroid metabolite	*mcg/g creatinine*	*nmol/g creatinine*	
		cis-Cl_2CA*	1.0-13.9 × 4.78	[4.78-66.4]	
		trans-Cl_2CA†	3.7-70.3 × 4.78	[17.7-336]	
		3-PBA††	2.5-42.5 × 4.67	[11.7-198]	

95th percentile in population without occupational exposure[9]:

Br_2CA†††	0.35 × 3.36	[1.18]
cis-Cl_2CA*	0.58 × 4.78	[2.77]
trans-Cl_2CA†	1.40 × 4.78	[6.69]
F-PBA‡	0.40 × 4.31	[1.72]

*cis-3-(2,2-dichlorovinyl)-2,2-dimethylcyclopropane-1-carboxylic acid

†trans-3-(2,2-dichlorovinyl)-2,2-dimethylcyclopropane-1-carboxylic acid

††3-phenoxybenzoic acid

†††cis-3-(2,2-dibromovinyl)-2,2-dimethylcyclopropane-1-carboxylic acid

‡4-fluoro-3-phenoxybenzoic acid

1. Steentoft A: A case of fatal dieldrin poisoning, *Med Sci Law* 19:268-269, 1979.

2. Baselt RC: *Analytical procedures for therapeutic drug monitoring and emergency toxicology,* ed 2, Littleton, MA, 1987, PSG Publishing Co., Inc.

3. Wintersteiger R, Ofner B, Juan H, et al: Determination of traces of pyrethrins and piperonyl butoxide in biological material by high-performance liquid chromatography, *J Chromatogr* 660:205-210, 1994.

4. Leng G, Kühn K-H, Wieseler B, et al: Metabolism of (S)-bioallethrin and related compounds in humans, *Toxicol Lett* 107:109-121, 1999.

5. Junting L, Chuichang F: Solid phase extraction method for rapid isolation and clean-up of some synthetic pyrethroid insecticides from human urine and plasma, *Forensic Sci Int* 51:89-93, 1991.

6. Leng G, Lewalter J, Röhrig B, et al: The influence of individual susceptibility in pyrethroid exposure, *Toxicol Lett* 107:123-130, 1999.

7. Angerer J, Ritter A: Determination of metabolites of pyrethroids in human urine using solid phase extraction and gas chromatography-mass spectrometry, *J Chromatogr B Biomed Appl* 695:217-226, 1997.

8. Taylor JR, Calabrese VP, Blanke RV: Organochlorine and other insecticides. In Vinken PJ, Bruyn GW, editors: *Handbook of clinical neurology, vol 36: intoxications of the nervous system, part 1,* New York, 1979, North-Holland Publishing Co.

9. Heudorf U, Angerer J: Metabolites of pyrethroid insecticides in urine specimens: current exposure in an urban population in Germany, *Environ Health Perspect* 109:213-217, 2001.

10. Fenton JJ: *Toxicology: a case-oriented approach,* Boca Raton, FL, 2002, CRC Press, pp. 285-286.

11. Baselt RC: *Biological monitoring methods for industrial chemicals,* Davis, CA, 1980, Biomedical Pub.

12. Thompson JF, editor: *Analysis of pesticide residues in human and environmental samples,* Research Triangle Park, NC, 1977, U.S.E.P.A., Health Effects Research Lab, Environmental Toxicology Division.

DIAGNOSTIC INFORMATION

REMARKS

Skin and lungs are most likely routes of exposure. Toxicity in mammals is low. Topical exposure may cause local irritation. Headache, nausea, and paresthesia have been reported after human exposure to pyrethroids. Massive exposure may cause convulsions and death from respiratory and circulatory failure.

Pyrethrins and pyrethroids are rapidly metabolized, so blood concentrations of these compounds are not helpful. Urinary metabolites have been measured in occupationally exposed individuals, but monitoring is not common because of the low toxicity of these compounds in humans compared with other insecticidal agents.

TEST NAME AND METHOD	SPECIMEN REQUIREMENTS	REFERENCE INTERVAL, CONVENTIONAL [INTERNATIONAL RECOMMENDED UNITS]	CHEMICAL INTERFERENCES AND IN VIVO EFFECTS
Insulin and Glucose Response to 72-hr Fasting[1-3] Patient is allowed no food but should have water or calorie-free and caffeine-free beverages during fast. Patient should stay active throughout fast.	Obtain capillary glucose measurements with a reflectance meter every 4 hr until values <60 mg/dL. Then increase frequency to each hour. When capillary glucose value is <49 mg/dL and/or symptoms of neuroglycopenia send off venous sample for glucose, insulin, proinsulin, C-peptide measurements, and sulfonylurea levels.	>40 mg glucose/dL during a 72-hr period of fasting [× 0.0555 = >2.2 mmol glucose/L] Values are slightly lower in females. Insulin (RIA): <5 µU/mL × 6.945 [34.7 pmol/L] or undetectable C-peptide (ICMA): <0.2 nmol/L Proinsulin (ICMA): < 5 pmol/L	See individual tests.

1. Alsever RN, Gotlin RW, editors: *Handbook of endocrine tests in adults and children,* ed 2, Chicago, 1978, Year Book Medical Publishers. Inc.
2. Miller RE, Ngai B: *Manual of endocrine diagnostic tests,* ed 4, Lexington, KY, 1991, Department of Medicine, University of Kentucky.
3. Service FJ, Dale AJD, Elveback LR, et al: Insulinoma: clinical and diagnostic features of 60 consecutive cases, *Mayo Clin Proc* 51:417-429, 1976.

TEST NAME AND METHOD	SPECIMEN REQUIREMENTS	REFERENCE INTERVAL, CONVENTIONAL [INTERNATIONAL RECOMMENDED UNITS]	CHEMICAL INTERFERENCES AND IN VIVO EFFECTS
Insulin Antibodies (Anti-Insulin Ab)[1-5] *Radiobinding assay*	Serum, separated from cells and frozen. Do not use plasma.	<3% binding of labeled human, beef, or pork insulin by patient's serum.[1]	None found.

Concentrations of <45 mg glucose/dL [<2.5 mmol glucose/L] with a simultaneous serum insulin value (RIA) >6 μU/mL [>41.7 pmol/L] (>3 μU/mL on ICMA insulin assay) is diagnostic of insulinoma. C-peptide levels of ≥200 pmol/L and proinsulin levels of ≥5 pmol/L are consistent with hyperinsulinemia molar ratio of C-peptide and insulin is 0.2. An elevated insulin level with very low or undetectable C-peptide suggests factitious insulin use.

This is a very sensitive test for insulinoma; >90% of insulinoma patients will show hypoglycemia ≤48 hr of fasting. Test is indicated if patient has significant symptoms of fasting hypoglycemia and has fasting serum glucose <60 mg/dL [<3.3 mmol/L]. The fast is terminated when the patient develops significant symptoms of hypoglycemia and/or has plasma glucose value <45 mg/dL [<2.5 mmol/L]. There is no advantage to prolonging the fast beyond 72 hr. Patients with insulinoma have suppressed levels of plasma beta hydroxybutyrate (<2.7 nmol), whereas levels are higher in normals. At the end of the 72-hr fast, if plasma glucose is ≤60 mg/dL, 1 mg of glucagons IV is administered, and plasma glucose is measured after 10, 20, and 30 min. Patients with insulinoma have an increment of ≥25 mg/dL increase in glucose over the terminal fasting plasma glucose. Normal individuals have lower increments.

↑ Immune insulin resistance, pre–type I diabetes (before insulin treatment), polyendocrine autoimmune syndromes

Insulin antibodies are produced in nearly all diabetic patients treated with exogenous (bovine or porcine) insulin and in surreptitiously administered insulin.

Binding of >10% indicates significant insulin antibody levels and affinity.

The most common type of anti-insulin Ab is IgG, but IgA, IgM, IgD, and IgE have been reported. Most of these insulin antibodies have low affinity and do not cause clinical problems. However, their presence will interfere with and complicate most insulin immunoassays. In this case, measurements of C-peptide may be indicated because C-peptide is not found in commercial insulin preparations. Occasionally high-affinity insulin antibodies may bind to exogenous insulin and interfere with its action. The widespread use of human insulin, plus improvements in the purity of animal insulins, has led to significant reductions in the production of interfering antibodies.

A sensitized radiobinding assay and a direct ELISA solid-phase assay have been designed to detect insulin autoantibodies in prediabetic (type I) patients and others with autoimmune disorders.[6]

Insulin resistance can also be caused by antibodies to the insulin receptor.[7] These antibodies have varying effects on circulating blood glucose, ranging from hypoglycemia to hyperglycemia. Antibodies to insulin receptors have been found in

TEST NAME AND METHOD	SPECIMEN REQUIREMENTS	REFERENCE INTERVAL, CONVENTIONAL [INTERNATIONAL RECOMMENDED UNITS]	CHEMICAL INTERFERENCES AND IN VIVO EFFECTS
Insulin Antibodies—CONT			

1. Armitage M, Wilkin T, Wood P, et al: Insulin autoantibodies and insulin assay, *Diabetes* 37:1932-1936, 1988.
2. Asplin CM, Hollander P, Pecorarco RE, et al: Insulin, pancreatic polypeptide, and glucagon antibodies in insulin-dependent diabetes mellitus, *Diabetes Care* 4:337-342, 1981.
3. Atkinson MA, Maclaren NK, Riley JW, et al: Are insulin autoantibodies markers for insulin-dependent diabetes mellitus? *Diabetes* 35:894-898, 1986.
4. Reeves WG: Insulin antibody determination: theoretical and practical considerations, *Diabetologia* 24:399-403, 1983.
5. Wilkin T: The measurement of insulin antibodies and its interpretation. In Pal S, editor: *Immunoassay technology, vol 2,* Berlin, 1986, Walter de Gruyter.

TEST NAME AND METHOD	SPECIMEN REQUIREMENTS	REFERENCE INTERVAL, CONVENTIONAL [INTERNATIONAL RECOMMENDED UNITS]	CHEMICAL INTERFERENCES AND IN VIVO EFFECTS
Insulin Autoantibodies (IAA) *Radioimmunoassay* *Radioimmunoprecipitation assay (or radiobinding assay [RBA])* *ELISA*	Serum	Negative	Exogenous insulin from insulin therapy

1. Palmer JP, Asplin CM, Clemons P, et al: Insulin antibodies in insulin-dependent diabetics before insulin treatment, *Science* 222:1337-1339, 1983.
2. Schatz D, Krischer J, Horne G, et al: Islet cell antibodies predict insulin-dependent diabetes in United States school age children as powerfully as in unaffected relatives, *J Clin Invest* 93:2403-2407, 1994.
3. Ziegler AG, Ziegler R, Vardi P, et al: Life-table analysis of progression to diabetes of anti-insulin autoantibody-positive relatives of individuals with type I diabetes, *Diabetes* 38:1320-1325, 1989.
4. Feeney SJ, Myers MA, Mackay IR, et al: Evaluation of ICA512As in combination with other islet cell autoantibodies at the onset of IDDM, *Diabetes Care* 20:1403-1407, 1997.
5. Bingley PJ, Bonifacio E, Williams AJ, et al: Prediction of IDDM in the general population: strategies based on combinations of autoantibody markers, *Diabetes* 46:1701-1710, 1997.

patients with non–insulin-dependent diabetes (type II), renal diseases, systemic lupus erythematosus, insulin resistance with acanthosis nigricans, and other immunologic disorders.[8]

6. Mayo Medical Laboratories: Test catalog, Rochester, MN, 1994.
7. Wilkin T: Insulin antibodies as markers for type I diabetes, *Endocr Rev* 11:92-104, 1990.
8. Flier JS, Kahn CR, Roth J, et al: Antibodies that impair insulin receptor binding in an unusual diabetic syndrome with severe insulin resistance, *Science* 190:63-68, 1976.
9. Nichols Institute Reference Laboratories: *Test catalog,* San Juan Capistrano, CA, 1993, Nichols Institute Reference Laboratories.

The presence of islet cell antibodies indicates ongoing β-cell destruction. The test is helpful in the early diagnosis of type 1a diabetes mellitus and in the identification of patients at high risk for type 1a diabetes.

To date, insulin is the only β-cell-specific autoantigen.[1] However, IAA by itself is a weak predictor of type 1 diabetes.[2] The combination of IAA and ICA improves risk prediction for type 1 diabetes.[3]

Children at onset of type 1 diabetes are more commonly IAA positive than adults.[4,5] Up to 80% of new-onset type 1 diabetic patients before the age of 5 yr have IAA compared with only ~30% for adults.[6] IAAs appear to be inversely correlated with age for both new-onset type 1 diabetic patients and their high-risk nondiabetic relatives.[7]

IAA measured by ELISA should be avoided because IAA detected by ELISA does not correlate with autoimmune diabetes.[8,9]

IAA should be determined before insulin therapy because insulin antibodies (IA) will develop 5-7 days after insulin introduction; the concentrations induced by exogenous insulin are often ≥10-fold than those by IAA.

6. Kersalainer J, Knip M, Mustonen A, et al: Relation between insulin antibody and complement fixing islet cell antibody at clinical diagnosis of IDDM, *Diabetes* 35:620-622, 1986.
7. Vardi P, Ziegler AG, Mathews JH, et al: Concentration of insulin autoantibodies at onset of type I diabetes: inverse log-linear correlation with age, *Diabetes Care* 11:736-739, 1988.
8. Kuglin B, Kolb IT, Palmer J: Insulin antoantibodies—which method? *Lancet* 334:622-623, 1989.
9. Levy-Marchal C, Bridel MP, Socloyez-Goffaux F, et al: Superiority of radiobinding assay over ELISA for detection of IAAs in newly diagnosed type I diabetic children, *Diabetes Care* 14:61-63, 1991.
10. Wilkins T, Mirza I, Armitage M, et al: Insulin autoantibody polymorphisms with greater discrimination of diabetes in humans, *Diabetologia* 31:670-674, 1988.

TEST NAME AND METHOD	SPECIMEN REQUIREMENTS	REFERENCE INTERVAL, CONVENTIONAL [INTERNATIONAL RECOMMENDED UNITS]			CHEMICAL INTERFERENCES AND IN VIVO EFFECTS
Insulin, Free[1-3]	Serum, fasting; separate from cells as soon	$\mu U/mL$[4]		$pmol/L$	See *Insulin, Immunoreactive.*
RIA	as possible. Freeze immediately; store frozen.	Infant and prepubertal child:	<13 × 6.945*	[<90]	Anti-insulin antibodies
		Pubertal child and adult:	<17	[<118]	
		*Conversion factor based on MW of insulin of 6000 and on 1 U of insulin being equal to			
Immunometric assay chemiluminescence		0.04167 mg of the WHO Fourth International Standard.			
		1.4-14.0 μU/mL			

1. Arnqvist H, Olsson P, von Schenck H: Free and total insulin as determined after precipitation with polyethylene glycol: analytical characteristics and effects of sample handling and storage, *Clin Chem* 33:93-96, 1987.
2. Kuzuya H, Blix PM, Hornitz DL, et al: Determination of free and total insulin and C-peptide in insulin-treated diabetes, *Diabetes* 26:22-29, 1977.
3. Rudkowski R, Antony G: The effect of immediate polyethylene glycol precipitation on free insulin measurements in diabetic patients with insulin antibodies, *Diabetes* 35:253-257, 1986.
4. Endocrine Sciences: *Pediatric laboratory services,* Tarzana, CA, 1992, Endocrine Sciences.

TEST NAME AND METHOD	SPECIMEN REQUIREMENTS	REFERENCE INTERVAL, CONVENTIONAL [INTERNATIONAL RECOMMENDED UNITS]			CHEMICAL INTERFERENCES AND IN VIVO EFFECTS
Insulin, Immunoreactive[1-7]	Serum, fasting. Freeze. Stable for 3 mo at −20° C.	mU/mL		$pmol/L$	↑ V Acetohexamide, albuterol, amino acids, calcium gluconate (newborn), chlorpropamide, cyproheptadine (nondiabetic patients), danazol, fructose, glucagon, glucose, growth hormone, levodopa (during therapy of Parkinsonism), medroxyprogesterone, niacin (high doses), oral contraceptives, pancreozymin (IV infusion), phentolamine (infusion), prednisolone, quinidine, secretin (IV), spironolactone, sucrose, terbutaline, tolazamide, and tolbutamide
RIA		Child, 2-12 yr:	<10 × 6.945*	[<69]	
		Adult:	<35	[<243]	
		Insulin ($\mu U/mL$): glucose (mg/dL) ratio[9]: <0.3 [× 125 = <38 × 10^{-9} (mole ratio)]			
Immunometric assay		$\mu U/mL$		$pmol/L$[10]	
		Adult:	0.7-9.0 × 6.945	[5-63]	
		Type II diabetic:	0.7-25.0	[5-174]	

DIAGNOSTIC INFORMATION	REMARKS

↑ Insulin overdose, insulin resistance syndromes, and endogenous hyperinsulinemia

↓ Inadequately treated type I diabetes mellitus

Free (bioactive) insulin is measured after PEG precipitation of insulin antibodies and their bound insulin. Total insulin (free insulin plus antibody-bound inactive insulin) can be measured using the same immunoassay if the sample is acidified to dissociate insulin from endogenous insulin antibodies before treatment with PEG. If insulin antibodies are not present, the free and total insulin assays are equivalent.

Circulating insulin antibodies develop after diabetic patients are treated with exogenous insulin preparations. Insulin antibodies not only interfere with insulin assays but also they reduce the amount of active insulin present in circulation by binding exogenous insulin. Free insulin assays therefore have proved valuable in monitoring insulin therapy. In insulin-dependent diabetic patients, free insulin levels are usually ≤10% of total insulin, and values up to 100 μU/mL [694 pmol/L] can be found.

↑ Insulinoma (pancreatic islet cell tumor), non–insulin-dependent (type II) diabetes mellitus, liver disease, acromegaly, Cushing's syndrome, dystrophia myotonica, familial fructose and galactose intolerance, obesity (may be twice normal), surreptitious use of insulin or oral hypoglycemic agents

↓ Insulin-dependent (type I) diabetes mellitus (<20 μU/mL [<139 pmol/L]), hypopituitarism. An insulin-glucose ratio >0.3 [>38 × 10⁻⁹] is presumptive evidence of insulinoma.

From a clinical standpoint, measurement of insulin has little value except in the diagnosis of fasting hypoglycemia. Accordingly, fasting hypoglycemia associated with inappropriately high serum insulin concentrations strongly suggests an islet cell tumor (insulinoma). (See *Insulin and Glucose Response to 72-hr Fasting.*) To distinguish insulinoma from factitious hypoglycemia resulting from insulin administration, serum C-peptide values are recommended. (See *C-Peptide.*)

Insulin assays are not included in diagnostic criteria for DM, and insulin values may range from low (IDDM) to high (NIDDM); however, insulin measurements during an OGTT may help in the diagnosis of early prehyperglycemic DM.[11] It is claimed that insulin levels obtained after a 75-g oral glucose load may be useful in predicting degenerative complications of DM (e.g., retinopathy) or in predicting the benefits of insulin therapy.[12] (For an alternative strategy, see *C-Peptide Stimulation Test.*)

TEST NAME AND METHOD	SPECIMEN REQUIREMENTS	REFERENCE INTERVAL, CONVENTIONAL [INTERNATIONAL RECOMMENDED UNITS]	CHEMICAL INTERFERENCES AND IN VIVO EFFECTS
Insulin, Immunoreactive—CONT			↓ V β-Adrenergic blockers (e.g., propranolol), asparaginase, bezafibrate, calcitonin, chloropropamide (when initial level high), cimetidine, clofibrate, diazoxide, doxazosin, ethacrynic acid, ethanol, ether, furosemide, metformin, nifedipine, phenformin, phenobarbital, phenytoin, thiazide diuretics, and tolbutamide (in some patients)
			↓ C Hemolysis (in RIA). Heparin in sample may alter results depending on amount of heparin, use of single or double antibody, and the presence of EDTA.
	Amniotic fluid[8]	<16 wk: undetectable Term, x̄: 11.3 μU/mL × 6.945 [78 pmol/L] *Conversion factor based on MW of insulin of 6000 and on 1 U of insulin being equal to 0.04167 mg of the WHO Fourth International Standard.	

1. Eastham RD: *Biochemical values in clinical medicine,* ed 7, Bristol, UK, 1985, John Wright and Sons Ltd.

2. Gerbitz VK-D: Pancreatische B-zellen Peptide: Kinetic and Konzentration von Proinsulin Insulin and C-Peptid in Plasma and Urin Probleme der Mezmethoden Klinische Aussage und Literaturubersicht, *J Clin Chem Clin Biochem* 18:313-326, 1980.

3. Reaven GM, Chen YD, Hollenbeck CB, et al: Plasma insulin, C-peptide, and proinsulin concentrations in obese and nonobese individuals with varying degrees of glucose tolerance, *J Clin Endocrinol Metab* 76:44-48, 1993.

4. Sacks DB: Carbohydrates. In Burtis CA, Ashwood ER, editors: *Tietz textbook of clinical chemistry,* ed 2, Philadelphia, 1994, WB Saunders.

5. Service FJ, Dale AJD, Elveback LR, et al: Insulinoma: clinical and diagnostic features of 60 consecutive cases, *Mayo Clin Proc* 51:417-429, 1976.

DIAGNOSTIC INFORMATION	REMARKS

Values are consistently higher in plasma than in serum; thus serum is preferred. Compared with fasting values in nonobese nondiabetic individuals, insulin levels are higher in obese nondiabetic persons and lower in trained athletes. Although proinsulin cross-reacts in most competitive insulin assays, it does not contribute appreciably to insulin values except in certain situations (e.g., insulinomas). Proinsulin does not cross-react in two-site immunometric assays for intact insulin.[10,13] In most insulin assays, bovine and porcine insulin are indistinguishable from human insulin. Insulin antibodies develop in patients treated with bovine or porcine insulin and in some patients treated with human insulin. (See *Insulin Antibodies*.) These antibodies may interfere with immunoassays for insulin, even for months or years after discontinuation. In rare cases, these antibodies may interfere with the action of the administered insulin. To monitor insulin therapy, some investigators suggest measuring insulin after PEG precipitation of the insulin antibodies (see *Insulin, Free*) or measuring "total" insulin after acidification (to separate bound insulin) and PEG precipitation of insulin antibodies. The widespread use of human insulin, plus improvements in the purity of porcine and bovine insulin, has led to significant reduction in the production of interfering antibodies.

In pregnancy, there is a relative insulin resistance. A progressive decrease of plasma glucose, immunoreactive insulin, and C-peptide during sleeping hours from the second to third trimester of pregnancy has been claimed.[14]

The elevation of insulin in amniotic fluid >8 µU/mL [56 pmol/L] during the 34-38th weeks of gestation prevents the normal increase of the L/S ratio. The complete absence of insulin during the last trimester is associated with intrauterine death.	It has been suggested that amniotic fluid insulin is of fetal origin. In poorly controlled diabetic patients, amniotic fluid, umbilical cord, and newborn urinary levels of insulin are markedly increased (up to 27 times the normal level) and could perhaps be used to predict neonatal hypoglycemia and macrosomy.

6. Sobey WJ, Beer SF, Carrington CA, et al: Sensitive and specific two-site immunoradiometric assays for human insulin, proinsulin, 65-66 split and 32-33 split proinsulins, *Biochem J* 260:535-541, 1989.

7. Yalow R, Bauman WA: Plasma insulin in health and disease. In Ellenberg M, Rifkin H, editors: *Diabetes mellitus; theory and practice,* New York, 1983, Excerpta Medica.

8. Turkington RW, Weindling HD: Insulin secretion in the diagnosis of adult-onset diabetes mellitus, *JAMA* 240:833-836, 1978.

9. Fajans S, Floyd J: Fasting hypoglycemia in adults, *N Engl J Med* 294:766-772, 1976.

TEST NAME AND METHOD	SPECIMEN REQUIREMENTS	REFERENCE INTERVAL, CONVENTIONAL [INTERNATIONAL RECOMMENDED UNITS]				CHEMICAL INTERFERENCES AND IN VIVO EFFECTS

Insulin, Immunoreactive—CONT

10. Andersen S, Dinesen B, Jørgensen P, et al: Enzyme immunoassay for intact human insulin in serum or plasma, *Clin Chem* 39:578-582, 1993.

11. Kraft JR: Detection of diabetes mellitus in situ (occult diabetes), *Lab Med* 6:10-22, 1975.

12. Turkington RW, Weindling HD: Insulin secretion in the diagnosis of adult-onset diabetes mellitus, *JAMA* 240:833-836, 1978.

TEST NAME AND METHOD	SPECIMEN REQUIREMENTS	REFERENCE INTERVAL, CONVENTIONAL [INTERNATIONAL RECOMMENDED UNITS]				CHEMICAL INTERFERENCES AND IN VIVO EFFECTS
Insulin-like Growth Factor I (IGF-I, Growth Factor I, Somatomedin C)[1-7] *RIA, IRMA*[8,9] *ELISA (Filter Paper Blood Spots)*[10]	Serum. Freeze immediately. Stable 30 days frozen.		*ng/mL*[12]		*mg/L*	↓ V Estrogen administration (high dose). Androgenic progestins oppose the estrogen-induced IGFBP-1 increase.[13]
		1-2 yr				
		M:	31-160	× 1.0	[31-160]	
		F:	11-206		[11-206]	
		3-6 yr				
		M:	16-288		[16-288]	
		F:	70-316		[70-316]	
		7-10 yr				
		M:	136-385		[136-385]	
		F:	123-396		[123-396]	
		11-12 yr				
		M:	136-440		[136-440]	
		F:	191-462		[191-462]	
		13-14 yr				
		M:	165-616		[165-616]	
		F:	286-660		[286-660]	
		15-18 yr				
		M:	134-836		[134-836]	
		F:	152-660		[152-660]	
		19-25 yr				
		M:	202-433		[202-433]	
		F:	231-550		[231-550]	
		Adult, 26-85 yr:	135-449		[135-449]	
	Amniotic fluid[11]	<12 wk:	Undetectable			

1. Breier B, Gallaher B, Gluckman P: Radioimmunoassay for insulin-like growth factor-I: solutions to some potential problems and pitfalls, *J Endocrinol* 128:347-357, 1991.

13. Toivonen E, Hemmila I, Jorgensen P, et al: Two-site time-resolved immunofluorometric assay of human insulin, *Clin Chem* 32:637-640, 1986.

14. Cousins L, Rigg L, Hollinsworth D, et al: The 24-hour excretion and diurnal rhythm of glucose, insulin, and C-peptide in normal pregnancy, *Am J Obstet Gynecol* 136:483-488, 1980.

S ↑ Acromegaly

S ↓ Dwarfism, hypopituitarism, hypothyroidism, malnutrition (after refeeding, high levels of GH decrease and low levels of IGF-I increase), anorexia, emotional deprivation syndrome, Laron dwarfism (in the presence of elevated GH), cirrhosis of the liver, and other hepatocellular diseases

The primary source of circulating IGF-I is from liver, although many tissues synthesize IGF-I. Only ~1% of circulating IGF-I is present as free, uncomplexed molecules[8]; the remainder are bound to IGF-specific binding proteins (IGFBPs). Six of the IGFBPs have been identified.[14] IGFBP-3 is the most abundant IGFI binding protein, which forms a ternary complex with IGF-I and another protein, the acid labile subunit (ALS). The IGFBP-3 is tightly regulated by growth hormone.[15]

Blood concentrations of IGF-I are constant during the day and after eating. In acromegaly, the test may serve as an indicator of the severity of the disease; serial determinations may be used to monitor the efficacy of treatment. In dwarfism IGF-I may be used to determine the response to GH therapy. Concentrations of IGF-I increase during the first year of life, reaching the highest values in preadolescent or early adolescent years. Thereafter normal values tend to decline progressively until age 50 yr. In pregnancy values are progressively higher. Children with low levels of IGF-I may need provocative testing to establish a diagnosis of GH deficiency, especially if a child is well-nourished and no cause of growth failure is apparent.

The test is also useful in diagnosing patients with active acromegaly who have relatively low basal levels of GH and patients suspected of acromegaly who show suppression of GH to normal after glucose administration. This test also appears to be more sensitive than prealbumin, retinol-binding protein, or transferrin in evaluating the effectiveness of nutritional repletion.

Circulating IGF-I increases insulin sensitivity. Reduced levels of IFG-I are associated with insulin resistance or a risk for subsequent development of impaired glucose or type 2 diabetes.[16]

IGF-I is also associated with several types of tumors.[17-19] Plasma IGF has been proposed to be a predictor of prostate cancer.[20]

2. Clemmons DR, Van Wyk JJ, Ridgway EG, et al: Evaluation of acromegaly by radioimmunoassay of somatomedin C, *N Engl J Med* 301:1138-1142, 1979.

TEST NAME AND METHOD	SPECIMEN REQUIREMENTS	REFERENCE INTERVAL, CONVENTIONAL [INTERNATIONAL RECOMMENDED UNITS]		CHEMICAL INTERFERENCES AND IN VIVO EFFECTS

Insulin-like Growth Factor I—CONT

3. Mitchell M, Hermos R, Schoepfer P, et al: Reference ranges for insulin-like growth factor-I in healthy children and adolescents, determined with filter-paper blood specimens, *Clin Chem* 36:2138-2139, 1990.

4. Phillips LS, Vassilopoulous-Sellin R: Somatomedins (part I), *N Engl J Med* 302:371-380, 1980.

5. Phillips LS, Vassilopoulous-Sellin R: Somatomedins (part II), *N Engl J Med* 302:438-446, 1980.

6. Spencer EM: Anterior pituitary and somatomedins. II. Somatomedins. In Greenspan FS, Forsham PH, editors: *Basic and clinical endocrinology,* Los Altos, CA, 1983, Lange Medical Publications.

7. Whitley RJ, Meikle AW, Watts NB: Endocrinology. In Burtis CA, Ashwood ER, editors: *Tietz textbook of clinical chemistry,* ed 2, Philadelphia, 1994, WB Saunders.

8. Ranke MB, Feldt-Rasmussen U, Bang P, et al: How should insulin-like growth factor I be measured? A consensus statement, *Horm Res* 55(suppl 2):106-109, 2001.

9. Clemmons DR: Commercial assays available for insulin-like growth factor I and their use in diagnosing growth hormone deficiency, *Horm Res* 55(suppl 2):73-79, 2001.

10. Jones JS: Insulin-like growth factor I measurement on filter paper blood spots, *Horm Res* 55(suppl 2):80-83, 2001.

11. Tulchinsky D, Ryan KJ, editors: *Maternal-fetal endocrinology,* Philadelphia, 1980, WB Saunders.

12. Endocrine Sciences: *Pediatric laboratory services,* Tarzana, CA, 1992, Endocrine Sciences.

TEST NAME AND METHOD	SPECIMEN REQUIREMENTS	REFERENCE INTERVAL, CONVENTIONAL		[INTERNATIONAL RECOMMENDED UNITS]	CHEMICAL INTERFERENCES AND IN VIVO EFFECTS
Insulin-like Growth Factor II (IGF-II)[1-4]	Plasma, fasting (EDTA). Store frozen.	ng/mL^5		mg/L	None found.
		Child,			
		prepubertal:	334-642	$\times$ 1.0	[334-642]
		Child, pubertal:	245-737		[245-737]
RIA		Adult:	288-736		[288-736]
		GH deficiency:	51-299		[51-299]

1. Wilson JD, Foster DW, editors: *Williams textbook of endocrinology,* ed 8, Philadelphia, 1992, WB Saunders.

2. Blum W, Ranke M, Bierich RR: A specific radioimmunoassay for insulin-like growth factor II: the interference of IGF binding proteins can be blocked by excess IGF-I, *Acta Endocrinol* 118:374-380, 1988.

3. Daughaday WH, Trivedi B, Kapadia M: Measurement of IGF-II by a specific radioreceptor assay in serum of normal individuals, patients with abnormal GH secretion, and patients with tumor-assisted hypoglycemia, *J Clin Endocrinol Metab* 53:289-294, 1981.

4. Rudd B: Growth, growth hormone and the somatomedins: an historical perspective and current concepts, *Ann Clin Biochem* 28:542-555, 1991.

5. Endocrine Sciences: *Pediatric laboratory services,* Tarzana, CA, 1992, Endocrine Sciences.

6. Rosenfeld RG, Wilson DM, Lee PDK, et al: Insulin-like growth factors I and II in evaluation of growth retardation, *J Pediatr* 109:428-433, 1986.

7. Zaina S, Nilsson J: Insulin-like growth factor II and its receptors in atherosclerosis and in conditions predisposing to atherosclerosis, *Curr Opin Lipidol* 14:483-489, 2003.

DIAGNOSTIC INFORMATION	REMARKS

13. Campagnoli C, Abba C, Ambroggio S, et al: Differential effects of progestins on the circulating IGF-I system, *Maturitas* 46(suppl 1):S39-S44, 2003.

14. Hwa V, Oh Y, Rosenfeld RG: The insulin-like growth factor-binding protein (IGFBP) superfamily, *Endocr Rev* 20:761-787, 1999.

15. Leung KC, Ho KK: Measurement of growth hormone, insulin-like growth factor I and their binding proteins: the clinical aspects, *Clin Chim Acta* 313:119-123, 2001.

16. Dunger DB, Ong KK, Sandhu MS: Serum insulin-like growth factor-I levels and potential risk of type 2 diabetes, *Horm Res* 60(suppl 3):131-135, 2003.

17. Zumkeller W: IGFs and IGFBPs: surrogate markers for diagnosis and surveillance of tumour growth? *Mol Pathol* 54:285-288, 2001.

18. Druckmann R, Rohr UD: IGF-1 in gynaecology and obstetrics: update 2002, *Maturitas* 41(suppl 1):S65-S83, 2002.

19. LeRoith D, Roberts CT Jr: The insulin-like growth factor system and cancer, *Cancer Lett* 195:127-137, 2003.

20. Chan JM, Stampfer MJ, Giovannucci E, et al: Plasma insulin-like growth factor-I and prostate cancer risk: a prospective study, *Science* 279:563-566, 1998.

↑ Hypoglycemia associated with non–islet cell tumors, hepatoma, and Wilms' tumor

↓ Growth hormone deficiency

Like IGF-I, the plasma is the main source of plasma IGF-II released into the circulation.

IGF-I (somatomedin C) and IGF-II are structurally related to proinsulin. In its actions, IGF-I is more insulin-like than IGF-II.

Unlike IGF-I, IGF-II does not usually increase in acromegaly but does increase in tumor-related hypoglycemia. Eighty-two percent of growth hormone-deficient children have low levels of IGF-I, and 52% have low levels of IGF-II; 96% have decreased levels of either IGF-I or IGF-II, or both.[6]

IGF-II may be associated with atherosclerosis.[7]

TEST NAME AND METHOD	SPECIMEN REQUIREMENTS	REFERENCE INTERVAL, CONVENTIONAL [INTERNATIONAL RECOMMENDED UNITS]			CHEMICAL INTERFERENCES AND IN VIVO EFFECTS
Insulinoma-Associated-2 Autoantibody Insulinoma-associated islet tyrosine phosphatase autoantibody, protein-tyrosine phosphatase-2, protein kinase phosphatase-like molecule IA-2 (IA-2, IA-2A, ICA512) *Radioimmunoprecipitation assay [or radiobinding assay (RBA)]*	Serum	0.0-0.8 Kronus units/mL[1]			Unknown

1. Available at: http://www.aruplab.com/guides/ug/tests/0050202.jsp. Last accessed 1/31/04.
2. Schmidli RS, Colman PG, Cui L, et al: Antibodies to the protein tyrosine phosphatases IAR and IA-2 are associated with progression to insulin-dependent diabetes (IDDM) in first-degree relatives at-risk for IDDM, *Autoimmunity* 28:15-23, 1998.
3. Gorus FK, Goubert P, Semakula C, et al: IA-2-autoantibodies complement GAD65-autoantibodies in new-onset IDDM patients and help predict impending diabetes in their siblings. The Belgian Diabetes Registry, *Diabetologia* 40:95-99, 1997.

TEST NAME AND METHOD	SPECIMEN REQUIREMENTS	REFERENCE INTERVAL, CONVENTIONAL		[INTERNATIONAL RECOMMENDED UNITS]	CHEMICAL INTERFERENCES AND IN VIVO EFFECTS
Inter-α-Trypsin Inhibitor (IαTI)[1-4] *RID*[5]	Serum. Analyze fresh or store at 4° C for <72 hr. Stable frozen at −20° C for 6 mo or at −70° C indefinitely. Specimens without lipemia or hemolysis are preferred.	20-70 mg/dL (x̄: 55)	× 10	[200-700 mg/L] [x̄: 550]	None found.

1. Ritzmann SE, Tucker ES III: *Protein analysis in disease—current concepts. Workshop manual,* Chicago, 1979, American Society of Clinical Pathologists, Commission for Continuing Education.
2. Schwick H-G, Haupt H: Chemistry and function of human plasma proteins, *Angew Chem* 191:87-99, 1980.
3. Odum L, Hansen-Nord G, Byrjalsen I: Human inter-alpha-trypsin inhibitor and immunologically related inhibitors investigated by quantitative immunoelectrophoresis, *Clin Chim Acta* 162:189-198, 1987.
4. Chawla RK, Rausch DJ, Miller FW, et al: Abnormal profile of serum proteinase inhibitors in cancer patients, *Cancer Res* 44:2718-2723, 1984.
5. Chawla RK, Miller FW, Lawson DH, et al: Urinary cancer-related protein EDC1 and serum inter-alpha-trypsin inhibitor in breast cancer, *Tumour Biol* 5:351-363, 1984.

DIAGNOSTIC INFORMATION	REMARKS

I A-2 is a predictor to the future progression to overt type 1 diabetes.

Combination of IA-2 and GADA improves the sensitivity for predicting type 1 diabetes.

The IA-2 autoantigen is a member of the protein tyrosine phosphatase family of receptor-like and cytoplasmic signal-transducing enzymes that catalyze dephosphorylation of phosphotyrosines. It has a signal peptide, an extracellular domain, a transmembrane domain, and a cytoplasmic domain. ICA512 includes the transmembrane domain and the cytoplasmic domain of IA-2.

More than 60% of new-onset cases of type 1 diabetes are IA-2A positive compared with 2-3% of the general population.[2] The autoantibodies are also detected in individuals at increased risk of developing the disease.[3]

A combination of IA-2 antibodies and GADA autoantibodies has a higher sensitivity as a predictive marker for type 1 diabetes than ICA alone.[3]

↓ S Concentrations are decreased with cirrhosis, malignancies, and some inflammatory conditions.[3-5]

U Increased urinary concentrations of EDC1, a fragment of IαTI, can be found in patients with malignancies.[4,6]

The IαTI family consists of several serine protease inhibitors that are similar structurally.[7] Activity of human IαTI is against trypsin, chymotrypsin, cathepsin G, and leukocyte elastase.[8]

Proteolytic cleavage of IαTI releases its light chain (bikunin), which is excreted into the urine.[9] Bikunin has been shown to be an inhibitor of calcium oxalate crystal formation.[10]

MW: 220,000.

6. Rudman D, Chawla RK, Nixon DW: The specific proteinuria of cancer patients, *Trans Assoc Am Physicians* 91:229-241, 1978.
7. Martin-Vandelet N, Paris S, Bourguignon J, et al: Assembly and secretion of recombinant chains of human inter-alpha-trypsin inhibitor in COS-7 cells, *Eur J Biochem* 259:476-484, 1999.
8. Swaim MW, Pizzo SV: Modification of the tandem reactive centers of human inter-alpha-trypsin inhibitor with butane-dione and cis-dichlorodiammineplatinum (II), *Biochem J* 254:171-178, 1988.
9. Balduyck M, Piva F, Mizon C, et al: Human leukocyte elastase (HLE) preferentially cleaves the heavy chain H2 of inter-alpha-trypsin inhibitor (ITI), *Biol Chem Hoppe Seyler* 374:895-901, 1993.
10. Kobayashi H, Shibata K, Fujie M, et al: Identification of structural domains in inter-alpha-trypsin inhibitor involved in calcium oxalate crystallization, *Kidney Int* 53:1727-1735, 1998.

TEST NAME AND METHOD	SPECIMEN REQUIREMENTS	REFERENCE INTERVAL, CONVENTIONAL [INTERNATIONAL RECOMMENDED UNITS]		CHEMICAL INTERFERENCES AND IN VIVO EFFECTS
Intrinsic Factor (IF) Antibodies[1-3] *RIA*[4,5]	Serum or plasma (EDTA); avoid administration of vitamin B_{12} for 48 hr before drawing specimen. Stable 4 hr at room temperature or 3 days refrigerated. Store at $-20°$ C.	Negative		↑ Cyanocobalamin may give false-positive test.

1. Ward PC: Modern approaches to the investigation of vitamin B12 deficiency, *Clin Lab Med* 22:435-445, 2002.
2. Waters HM, Smith C, Howarth JE, et al: New enzyme immunoassay for detecting total, type I, and type II intrinsic factor antibodies, *J Clin Pathol* 42:307-312, 1989.
3. Shackleton PJ, Fish DI, Dawson DW: Intrinsic factor antibody tests, *J Clin Pathol* 42:210-212, 1989.
4. Gullberg R: Sensitive test for antibody type I to intrinsic factors, *Clin Exp Immunol* 9:833-838, 1871.
5. Fairbanks VF, Lennon VA, Kokmen E, et al: Tests for pernicious anemia: serum intrinsic factor blocking antibody, *Mayo Clin Proc* 58:203-204, 1983.
6. Mayo Medical Laboratories: *Interpretative handbook,* Rochester, MN, 2001, Mayo Medical Laboratories.
7. ARUP: *Reference manual,* Salt Lake City, UT, 2004, ARUP.

TEST NAME AND METHOD	SPECIMEN REQUIREMENTS		*mL/min** (2 SD)		*mL/sec* (2 SD)	CHEMICAL INTERFERENCES
Inulin Clearance (Exogenous)[1-4]	Serum. Draw at beginning and end of urine collection.	20-29 yr				↑ V Dopamine, methylprednisolone
Colorimetric	Urine. Have patient empty bladder 30 min after dose. Thereafter collect three 20-min samples. (Average the results.)	M:	90-174 (x̄: 132)	× 0.00963	[0.87-1.68] [x̄: 1.27]	↑ C Dextran, glucose
Dose: 25 mL of 10% solution, IV, followed by maintenance infusion of 500 mL of 1.5% solution (rate: 4 mL/min)		F:	84-156 (x̄: 119)		[0.81-1.50] [x̄: 1.15]	↓ V Diazoxide, nephrotoxic substances (Table I-6)
		30-39 yr				
		M:	88-168 (x̄: 128)		[0.85-1.62] [x̄: 1.23]	
		F:	82-150 (x̄: 116)		[0.79-1.44] [x̄: 1.12]	
		40-49 yr				
		M:	78-162 (x̄: 120)		[0.75-1.56] [x̄: 1.16]	
		F:	82-146 (x̄: 114)		[0.79-1.41] [x̄: 1.10]	

↑ In 50% of patients with PA, false-positive results are rare.

Pernicious anemia (PA) results from failure of the gastric mucosa to form IF and is invariably associated with severe gastric mucosal atrophy.

Much evidence supports the hypothesis that PA is an autoimmune disease. Sera of patients with PA commonly exhibit antibodies to gastric parietal cells and to IF. Detection of the IF antibodies is of diagnostic value because they are rarely encountered in other disorders (3-6% in persons with hyperthyroidism or insulin-dependent diabetes). Parietal cell antibodies are so commonly found in sera of persons who do not have (and do not develop) PA that tests for gastric parietal cell antibodies are not usually of diagnostic value.[6,7]

See also *Vitamin B$_{12}$ Intrinsic Factor* and *Vitamin B$_{12}$ Absorption Test.*

See *Glomerular Filtration Rate.*

Measurement of inulin clearance on a patient at rest may not reflect true "active" GFR. Edematous patients or those in renal failure may require several tests to attain a meaningful result. Inulin clearance is the most accurate measure of GFR, but methods for quantitating inulin are limited. Adequate hydration of the patient is essential. Children <2 yr and adults past middle age have reduced clearance rates.

The test traditionally has been the reference method for measuring GFR. However, it has not been used widely because it requires continuous infusion, is time-consuming, and has low precision. Isotope tests are now done with increasing frequency. See *Glomerular Filtration Rate.*

TEST NAME AND METHOD	SPECIMEN REQUIREMENTS	REFERENCE INTERVAL, CONVENTIONAL [INTERNATIONAL RECOMMENDED UNITS]		CHEMICAL INTERFERENCES AND IN VIVO EFFECTS

Inulin Clearance (Exogenous)—CONT

50-59 yr

M: 68-152 [0.65-1.46]
(x̄: 110) [x̄: 1.06]

F: 66-142 [0.63-1.37]
(x̄: 104) [x̄: 1.00]

60-69 yr

M: 57-137 × 0.00963 [0.55-1.32]
(x̄: 97) [x̄: 0.93]

F: 58-130 [0.56-1.25]
(x̄: 94) [x̄: 0.91]

70-79 yr

M: 42-122 [0.40-1.17]
(x̄: 82) [x̄: 0.79]

F: 45-121 [0.43-1.17]
(x̄: 83) [x̄: 0.80]

80-89 yr 39-105 [0.38-1.01]
(x̄: 67) [x̄: 0.65]

*Corrected to 1.73 m^2 body surface area.

1. Brown SS, Mitchell FL, Young DS, editors: *Chemical diagnosis of disease,* Amsterdam, 1979, Elsevier/North Holland Biomedical Press.

2. Henry JB, editor: *Clinical diagnosis and management by laboratory methods,* ed 18, Philadelphia, 1991, WB Saunders.

3. Henry RJ, Cannon DC, Winkelman JW, editors: *Clinical chemistry: principles and technics,* ed 2, Hagerstown, MD, 1974, Harper and Row.

4. Tietz NW, editor: *Fundamentals of clinical chemistry,* ed 3, Philadelphia, 1987, WB Saunders.

TEST NAME AND METHOD	SPECIMEN REQUIREMENTS	REFERENCE INTERVAL, CONVENTIONAL		CHEMICAL INTERFERENCES AND IN VIVO EFFECTS
Iron (Fe)[1,2] *Colorimetric, AAS*	Serum, morning specimen.[5] Draw blood before other specimens that require anticoagulated tubes. Reject hemolyzed samples.		*mcg/dL*	*μmol/L*	S ↑ V Chloramphenicol, cisplatin, estrogens, ethanol, iron dextran, lead, methotrexate, and oral contraceptives
		Newborn:	100-250 × 0.179	[17.9-44.8]	
		Infant:	40-100	[7.2-17.9]	
		Child:	50-120	[9.0-21.5]	
		Adult			
		M:	65-175	[11.6-31.3]	
		F:	50-170	[9.0-30.4]	S ↓ V Allopurinol, anabolic steroids, aspirin (large doses), corticotropin, cortisone, and metformin
		Intoxicated child[6]:	280-2550	[50.1-456.5]	
		Fatally poisoned child[6]:	>1800	[>322.2]	

DIAGNOSTIC INFORMATION	REMARKS

S ↑ Pernicious, aplastic, and hemolytic anemias; hemochromatosis, acute leukemia, lead poisoning, acute hepatitis, vitamin B_6 deficiency, thalassemia, excessive Fe therapy, repeated transfusions, acute Fe poisoning (children), and nephritis

S ↓ Iron-deficiency anemia, remission of PA; acute and chronic infection, carcinoma, nephrosis, hypothyroidism, postoperative state, and kwashiorkor

See also Table II-13.

AAS methods using diluted serum without protein precipitation give falsely high values owing to microhemolysis (Hb iron). Ferrous sulfate is frequently encountered as a cause of accidental childhood poisoning. Symptoms of Fe poisoning include abdominal pain, vomiting, bloody diarrhea, cyanosis, lethargy, and convulsions. Serum Fe diurnal variation is inconsistent; generally higher levels occur in the morning. Levels may vary widely for an individual within the same day or from day to day. Serum Fe tests on patients who have had blood transfusions should be delayed several days. Sleep deprivation or stress causes loss of diurnal variation (lower Fe levels). Newborns show a decline in Fe within a few hours of birth.

TEST NAME AND METHOD	SPECIMEN REQUIREMENTS	REFERENCE INTERVAL, CONVENTIONAL [INTERNATIONAL RECOMMENDED UNITS]			CHEMICAL INTERFERENCES AND IN VIVO EFFECTS
Iron—CONT					
	Urine. Acidify to pH 1; collect in metal-free container.	2-70 mcg/L[7] 3-98 mcg/day[7] Higher in premenopausal females.	× 0.0179	[0.04-1.3 μmol/L] [0.05-1.8 μmol/day]	S ↓ C *Color:* EDTA, fluoride-oxalate, and sodium citrate
	CSF.[1] Avoid contamination with blood.	23.0-52.0 mcg/dL	× 0.179	[4.1-9.3 μmol/L]	*Ferrochem*[8]: Pyrazinamide
Needle biopsy[3]	Liver, needle biopsy.[3] Refrigerate if assay is delayed 3 days.	*mcg/g dry wt.* 530-900	× 0.0179	*μmol/g dry wt.* [9.5-16.1]	
X-ray fluorescence spectrometry[4]	Bronchoalveolar lavage fluid	*ng/10³ macrophages* 0.3-20.4	× 17.9	*fol/macrophage* [5.4-365]	
		2.0-130 mg/L	× 0.0179	[0.04-2.33 mmol/L]	

1. Eastham RD: *Biochemical values in clinical medicine,* ed 7, Bristol, UK, 1985, John Wright and Sons Ltd.

2. Henry JB, editor: *Clinical diagnosis and management by laboratory methods,* ed 18, Philadelphia, 1991, WB Saunders.

3. Mayo Medical Laboratories: *Test catalog,* Rochester, MN, 1993, Mayo Medical Laboratories.

4. Maier EA, Rastegar F, Heimburger R, et al: Simultaneous determination of trace elements in lavage fluids from human bronchial alveoli by energy dispersive X-ray flourescence. 1: Technique and determination of the normal reference interval, *Clin Chem* 31:551-555, 1985.

5. Burtis CA, Ashwood ER, editors: *Tietz textbook of clinical chemistry,* ed 2, Philadelphia, 1994, WB Saunders.

6. Baselt RC: *Analytical procedures for therapeutic drug monitoring and emergency toxicology,* ed 2, Littleton, MA, 1987, PSG Publishing Co.

7. Schramel VP, Lill G, Hasse S: Mineral and trace elements in human urine, *J Clin Chem Clin Biochem* 23:293-301, 1985.

8. Alsever RN, Gotlin RW: *Handbook of endocrine tests in adults and children,* ed 2, Chicago, 1978, Year Book Medical Publishers Inc.

TEST NAME AND METHOD	SPECIMEN REQUIREMENTS		REFERENCE INTERVAL, CONVENTIONAL		[INTERNATIONAL RECOMMENDED UNITS]	CHEMICAL INTERFERENCES
Iron Saturation (% Transferrin Saturation)[1] *Colorimetric, AAS*	Serum.[2] Avoid hemolysis. See *Iron* and *Iron-Binding Capacity, Total.*	M: F:	*Percent saturation* 20-50 15-50	× 0.01	*Fraction saturation* [0.20-0.50] [0.15-0.50]	See *Iron* and *Iron-Binding Capacity, Total.*

1. Henry JB, editor: *Clinical diagnosis and management by laboratory methods,* ed 18, Philadelphia, 1991, WB Saunders.

2. Burtis CA, Ashwood ER, editors: *Tietz textbook of clinical chemistry,* ed 2, Philadelphia, 1994, WB Saunders.

See also *Ferritin; Iron-Binding Capacity, Total;* and *Iron Saturation.*

See Tables II-5 and II-6.

↑ Hemochromatosis, excessive iron intake, thalassemia, vitamin B_6 deficiency, and aplastic anemias

↓ Hypochromic anemias, malignancy of stomach and small intestine

See Table II-13.

Percent [fraction] saturation is a better index of iron stores than is serum iron alone.

Iron saturation can be calculated as follows:

$$\% \text{ Saturation} = \frac{\text{Serum Fe} \times 100}{\text{TIBC}}$$

$$\left[\text{Fraction saturation} = \frac{\text{Serum Fe}}{\text{TIBC}} \right]$$

Saturation <15% [<<0.15] represents iron deficiency.

TEST NAME AND METHOD	SPECIMEN REQUIREMENTS	REFERENCE INTERVAL, CONVENTIONAL [INTERNATIONAL RECOMMENDED UNITS]	CHEMICAL INTERFERENCES AND IN VIVO EFFECTS
Iron Stain (Prussian Blue Reaction, Perls' Stain)[1-3]	Blood or bone marrow films. Stable several years. May be stained for iron after other stains, e.g., Romanowsky stains, are applied.	Normally, about one third of the normoblasts in the marrow are sideroblasts. Storage iron is readily identifiable in macrophages in particles of marrow tissue on the marrow films. Siderocytes are rarely found in normal blood or marrow.	None found.
	Urine, random, freshly voided.	Negative	

1. Dacie JV, Lewis SM: *Practical haematology,* ed 7, Edinburgh, 1991, Churchill Livingstone.
2. Henry JB, editor: *Clinical diagnosis and management by laboratory methods,* ed 18, Philadelphia, 1991, WB Saunders.
3. Bessis M: *Blood smears reinterpreted,* Brecher G, translator. New York, 1976, Springer-Verlag.

TEST NAME AND METHOD	SPECIMEN REQUIREMENTS	REFERENCE INTERVAL, CONVENTIONAL			[INTERNATIONAL RECOMMENDED UNITS]		CHEMICAL INTERFERENCES AND IN VIVO EFFECTS
Iron-Binding Capacity, Total (TIBC)[1] *Colorimetric, AAS*	Serum or plasma (heparin). Avoid hemolysis. Stable 4 days at room temperature.		*mg/dL*[2]			*mmol/L*	↑ V Estrogens, oral contraceptives ↓ V Asparaginase, chloramphenicol, corticotropin, cortisone, and testosterone
		Infant:	100-400	× 0.179		[17.9-71.6]	
		Adult:	250-425			[44.8-76.1]	

1. Burtis CA, Ashwood ER, editors: *Tietz textbook of clinical chemistry,* ed 2, Philadelphia, 1994, WB Saunders.
2. Painter PC, Cope JY, Smith JL: Reference information for the clinical laboratory. In Burtis CA, Ashwood ER, editors: *Tietz textbook of clinical chemistry,* ed 3, Philadelphia, 1999, WB Saunders.

DIAGNOSTIC INFORMATION	REMARKS

↑ *Storage iron:* Hemochromatosis, hemolytic anemias, anemias resulting from decreased erythropoiesis (e.g., aplastic anemia), anemias with ineffective erythropoiesis (e.g., megaloblastic anemias, sideroblastic anemias), anemias of chronic disorders.

↑ *Sideroblasts:* Hemochromatosis, hemolytic anemias, anemias resulting from decreased erythropoiesis (e.g., aplastic anemia), anemias with ineffective erythropoiesis (e.g., megaloblastic anemias). In sideroblastic anemias, a large proportion of the normoblasts are ring sideroblasts.

↑ *Siderocytes (blood):* After splenectomy or in asplenia.

↓ *Storage iron:* Iron deficiency anemia, usually resulting from chronic blood loss (except in infancy, adolescence, and pregnancy).

↓ *Sideroblasts.* Iron deficiency anemias, anemia of chronic disorders.

The Prussian blue reaction stains iron in aggregated ferritin and hemosiderin blue but does not stain iron in heme. Storage iron, as ferritin and hemosiderin, is stained in macrophages of the bone marrow (and other reticuloendothelial organs). Normoblasts containing stainable iron granules are known as sideroblasts; erythrocytes containing them are siderocytes. Generally, the ratio of the serum iron concentration to total iron-binding capacity closely parallels the proportion of marrow normoblasts that are sideroblasts (in normal individuals, 1/3). Some sideroblastic granules in pathological conditions also appear as basophilic granules with Romanowsky stains; these are known as Pappenheimer bodies.

See *Ferritin* and *Iron-Binding Capacity, Total.*

U ↑ Stainable iron is present in epithelial cells (or as granules from degenerated epithelial cells) in urinary sediment in hemochromatosis or in intravascular hemolysis, especially PNH, PCH, transfusion reactions (after several days), and fragmentation hemolysis (resulting from microangiopathy or heart valve). (See also *Hemosiderin.*)

Hemosiderin is not detected in alkaline urine.[2]

↑ Hypochromic anemias, acute hepatitis, and late pregnancy

↓ Anemia (non–iron deficient), chronic infections, hemochromatosis, cirrhosis, neoplastic and renal disease, and thalassemia

See also Table II-13.

TIBC correlates with serum transferrin, but the relationship is not linear over a wide range of transferrin values and is disrupted in diseases affecting transferrin-binding capacity or other iron-binding proteins. Large analytical and within-subject biological variations have been observed for TIBC levels.

See also *Transferrin.*

TEST NAME AND METHOD	SPECIMEN REQUIREMENTS	REFERENCE INTERVAL, CONVENTIONAL [INTERNATIONAL RECOMMENDED UNITS]			CHEMICAL INTERFERENCES AND IN VIVO EFFECTS
Ischemia Modified Albumin (IMA)[1-8] *Colorimetric Albumin Cobalt Binding (ACB) Test*[1,2]	Serum, collected in serum separator tube. Plasma specimens and any specimens containing chelators unacceptable. Stable at room temperature after clot removal for 2.5 hr. Freeze at <20° C. Do not dilute samples.	35-98 yr	*95th percentile* 85 U/mL	*Cutoff for ischemia* 105 U/mL	ACB test should be interpreted with caution when total serum albumin is <2.0 g/dL or >5.5 g/dL. Increased lactate acid ammonia levels interfere with the assay. IMA levels may be increased in patient with cancer, bacterial or viral infections, end-stage renal disease, liver cirrhosis, brain ischemia, and gastrointestinal ischemia.[3] No known interference from drugs, bilirubin, lipemia (triglycerides 60 mg/dL and 779 mg/dL).

1. Bhagavan NV, Lai EM, Rios PA, et al: Evaluation of human serum albumin cobalt binding assay for the assessment of myocardial ischemia and myocardial infarction, *Clin Chem* 49:581-585, 2003.

2. Wu AH, Morris DL, Fletcher DR, et al: Analysis of the Albumin Cobalt Binding (ACB) test as an adjunct to cardiac troponin I for the early detection of acute myocardial infarction, *Cardiovasc Toxicol* 1:147-152, 2001.

3. Wu AHB, Crosby P, Fagan G, et al: Ischemia-modified albumin, free fatty acids, whole blood choline, B-type natriuretic peptide, glycogen phosphorylase BB, and cardiac troponin. In Wu AHB, editor: *Cardiac markers*, Totowa, NJ, 2003, Humana Press.

4. Roy D, Quiles J, Aldama G, et al: Ischemia modified albumin for the assessment of patients presenting to the emergency department with acute chest pain but normal or non-diagnostic 12-lead electrocardiograms and negative cardiac troponin T, *Int J Cardiol* 97:297-301, 2004.

5. Christenson RH, Duh SH, Sanhai W, et al: Characteristics of an albumin cobalt binding test for assessment of acute coronary syndrome patients: a multicenter study, *Clin Chem* 47:464-470, 2001.

6. Sinha MK, Roy D, Gaze DC, et al: Role of "Ischemia Modified Albumin," a new biochemical marker of myocardial ischaemia, in the early diagnosis of acute coronary syndromes, *Emerg Med J* 21:29-34, 2004.

7. Quiles J, Roy D, Gaze D, et al: Relation of ischemia-modified albumin (IMA) levels following elective angioplasty for stable angina pectoris to duration of balloon-induced myocardial ischemia, *Am J Cardiol* 92:322-324, 2003.

8. Sinha MK, Gaze DC, Tippins JR, et al: Ischemia modified albumin is a sensitive marker of myocardial ischemia after percutaneous coronary intervention, *Circulation* 107:2403-2405, 2003.

DIAGNOSTIC INFORMATION	REMARKS

The test is cleared by the FDA according to the following statement: "in patients with chest pain or equivalent symptoms suggestive of cardiac origin, with non-diagnostic ECG and normal troponin, a negative IMA can be used as an aid to rule out ACS in low risk patients."[4-6] The test is not FDA cleared as a biomarker for ischemia.

Serum albumin in patients with myocardial ischemia produces a lower metal binding capacity for cobalt than albumin in non-ischemic normal controls. This has been demonstrated in a coronary angioplasty model whereby myocardial ischemia without irreversible necrosis is induced by the inflation of the balloon.[7,8] The ACB test is a quantitative assay that measures ischemia modified albumin (IMA) in human serum. In principle, in serum of patients with ischemia, cobalt added to serum does not bind to the N-terminus of IMA, leaving more free cobalt to react with dithiothreitol and form a darker color. The absorbance is read at 500 nm. The total assay imprecision is <9% at the medical decision cutoff, a lower limit of detection at 14 U/mL, and linearity to 200 U/mL.

TEST NAME AND METHOD	SPECIMEN REQUIREMENTS	REFERENCE INTERVAL, CONVENTIONAL [INTERNATIONAL RECOMMENDED UNITS]	CHEMICAL INTERFERENCES AND IN VIVO EFFECTS
Isoagglutinins **(Normal,** **Expected),** (Anti-A, Anti-B)[1-7] *Agglutination of test red blood cells of known ABO group in slide, tube, gel, or microplate format.*	Serum or EDTA-anticoagulated plasma. Store at 4° C for 1 wk or up to 6 mo at–30° C. If sample has been collected in EDTA, plasma must be separated from cells before frozen storage.	The presence of anti-A and/or anti-B antibodies corresponds to the absence of the corresponding antigens. For example, type O persons have both anti-A and anti-B, whereas type A individuals have anti-B antibodies in their sera. The strength of the antibody reaction is not routinely reported. Range of titer is wide, with titer ≥1:8 expected.	Paraproteins, plasma expanders, unexpected antibodies, like cold-reactive autoantibodies or alloantibodies to non-ABO antigens. Passive transfer of isoagglutinins present in some intravenous immunoglobulin preparations may give discrepant results.

1. Brecher M, editor: *Technical manual,* ed 16, Bethesda, MD, 2005, AABB.
2. Chapman JF, Elliott C, Knowles SM, et al: Guidelines for compatibility procedures in blood transfusion laboratories, *Transfus Med* 14:59-73, 2004.
3. Issitt P, Anstee D: *Applied blood group serology,* ed 4, Durham, NC, 1998, Montgomery Scientific Publications.
4. Judd W: Red blood cell immunology and compatibility testing. In Simon T, Dzik W, Snyder E, et al, editors: *Rossi's principles of transfusion medicine,* Philadelphia, 2002, Lippincott Williams & Wilkins, pp. 69-88.
5. Mollison P, Engelfriet C, Contreras M: *Blood transfusion in clinical medicine,* ed 10, Oxford, 1997, Blackwell Scientific Publications.
6. Shulman IA, Downes KA, Sazama K, et al: Pretransfusion compatibility testing for red blood cell administration, *Curr Opin Hematol* 8:397-404, 2001.
7. Roitt I, Brostoff J, Male D: *Immunology,* ed 4, London, 1996, Mosby.
8. Koskela P, Nurmi T, Haiva VM: IgA, IgG and IgM anti-blood group A antibodies induced by pneumococcal vaccine, *Vaccine* 6:221-222, 1988.
9. Buchs JP, Maillard H, Nydegger U: [Anti-A/B-IgM/G immune response to accidental A-O transfusion and to Toxocara canis infestation], *Schweiz Med Wochenschr* 121:347-350, 1991.

TEST NAME AND METHOD	SPECIMEN REQUIREMENTS	REFERENCE INTERVAL, CONVENTIONAL [INTERNATIONAL RECOMMENDED UNITS]	CHEMICAL INTERFERENCES AND IN VIVO EFFECTS
Isocitrate **Dehydrogenase** (ICD; EC 1.1.1.42)[1] *340 nm, Ellis and Goldberg, 37° C[2]*	Serum or plasma (citrate). Avoid hemolysis and lipemia. Separate serum from cells immediately because platelets contain 700 times the ICD activity of serum.	*U/L* $\quad\quad\quad\quad$ $\mu Kat/L$ Adult: 1.2-7.0 × 0.017 [0.02-0.12] Cord blood: 2 × adult values Newborn: Increases to 4 × adult values 2 wk: Decreases to upper limit of adult range	S ↑ V Allopurinol, aminosalicylic acid, amodiaquine, amphotericin B, anabolic steroids, androgens, anesthetic agents, carbon tetra-
Colorimetric, Bell and Baron, 37° C[3]	Stable at room temperature for 6 hr, at 4° C for 2 wk. Unstable at −70° C.	*U/L* $\quad\quad\quad$ $\mu Kat/L$ Adult (n = 19): 3.0-8.5 × 0.017 [0.05-0.14]	chloride, chenodiol, chlorpromazine, clindamycin, ethanol, isoniazid, mechlorethamine, methotrexate, and phenylbutazone
Wolfson and Williams-Ashman, 25° C[4]		*nmol/hr/mL* $\quad\quad\quad$ *U/L* Newborn: 123-487 × 0.0167 [2.05-8.13] Adult: 50-260 [0.84-4.34]	S ↑ C Hemolysis, Mn^{2+}, Co^{2+}, and Mg^{2+}

DIAGNOSTIC INFORMATION	REMARKS

Test is usually performed as a component of ABO typing. In this situation, it is often referred to as "back-typing." Expected antibodies may be absent or decreased in concentration in immune deficiency (infancy, hypogammaglobulinemia, infection, neoplasia, immunosuppressive therapy, and old age).

Isoagglutinin titers may be helpful in following engraftment kinetics after hematopoietic stem cell transplantation.

Titer increases after exposure to antigens. Elevated titers may be observed after transfusion, pregnancy, vaccination,[8] and *Toxocara* infection.[9]

Weak subgroups of antigens may be associated with the presence of antibodies to antigens of the ABO system, e.g. anti-A_1 and anti-B in A_2 and B_{el} individuals, respectively.

Isoagglutinins include IgM and IgG classes of immunoglobulins.

S ↑ Viral, toxic, and chronic hepatitis; carcinoma metastatic to liver, hepatic hypoxia resulting from hemodynamic causes, bacterially infected hepatic lesions, cirrhosis, obstructive jaundice, infectious mononucleosis, acute inflammation of biliary tract, neonatal biliary duct atresia, kwashiorkor, preeclamptic toxemia, severe pulmonary infarct, myeloid leukemia, megaloblastic anemia, and hyperthyroidism

Serum values are normal in uncomplicated myocardial infarction and normal pregnancy.

Increase in ICD activity is a sensitive indicator of parenchymal liver disease. Measured activity in serum is the result of the cytoplasmic NADP-dependent enzyme from liver. In hyperthyroidism, ICD is increased out of proportion to ALT (compared with the greater increases in ALT in other forms of hepatic injury), perhaps because of ICD's centrilobular distribution.[5] Although the myocardium is rich in ICD activity, no elevation of serum ICD activity is found after a myocardial infarction; the released mitochondrial ICD activity is heat labile and is rapidly cleared.

TEST NAME AND METHOD	SPECIMEN REQUIREMENTS	REFERENCE INTERVAL, CONVENTIONAL [INTERNATIONAL RECOMMENDED UNITS]		CHEMICAL INTERFERENCES AND IN VIVO EFFECTS

Isocitrate Dehydrogenase—CONT

| | CSF[1] | $\leq$0.3 U/L | | S $\downarrow$ C EDTA, oxalate, fluoride, p-chloromercuribenzoate, iodoacetate, Ba^{2+}, Zn^{2+}, Ca^{2+}, CN^{-}, N-ethylmaleimide, NaCl, heavy metal ions, and isocitrate |

1. Burtis CA, Ashwood ER, editors: *Tietz textbook of clinical chemistry,* ed 2, Philadelphia, 1994, WB Saunders.
2. Goldberg DM, Ellis G: Isocitrate dehydrogenase. In Bergmeryer HU, editor: *Methods of enzymatic analysis, vol III,* ed 3, Weinheim, 1983, Verlag Chemie.
3. Bell JL, Baron DN: A colorimetric method for determination of isocitric dehydrogenase, *Clin Chim Acta* 5:740-747, 1960.
4. Wolfson SK Jr, Williams-Ashman HG: Isocitric and 6-phosphogluconic dehydrogenase in human blood serum, *Proc Soc Exp Biol Med* 96:231-234, 1957.
5. Chung Y, Jung S, Song B, et al: Plasma isocitrate dehydrogenase as a marker of centrilobular hepatic necrosis in patients with hyperthyroidism, *J Clin Gastroenterol* 33:118-122, 2001.

Isoleucine (Ile)[1-6]

Ion-exchange chromatography

	Plasma (heparin) or serum, fasting. Place blood in ice water immediately; separate and freeze within 1 hr of collection. Stable for 1 wk at $-20°$ C; for longer periods deproteinize and store at $-70°$ C.[7,8]		*mg/dL*		*mmol/L*[11]	P $\downarrow$V Alanine, glucose, histidine (after oral load), and oral contraceptives
		Premature, 1 day:	0.52 $\pm$ 0.26 (SD)	$\times$ 76.3	[40 $\pm$ 20]	
		Newborn, 1 day:	0.35-0.69		[27-53]	P $\uparrow$ V Ethanol
		1 day-1mo	0.34-1.19		[26-91][6]	
		1-3 mo:	0.77 $\pm$ 0.18 (SD)		[59 $\pm$ 14]	
		2-6 mo:	0.50-1.61		[38-123]	
		9 mo-2 yr:	0.34-1.23		[26-94]	
		3-10 yr:	0.37-1.10		[28-84]	
		6-18 yr:	0.50-1.24		[38-95][12]	
		Adult:	0.48-1.28		[37-98]	

	Urine, 24 hr. Add 10 mL of 6 mol/L HCl at start of collection. (Alternatively, refrigerate specimen during collection.) Store frozen at $-20°$ C.[9]		*mg/day*		*mmol/day*[11]	U $\uparrow$ V Ascorbic acid (after large intake)[15]
		10 days-7 wk:	<0.4	$\times$ 7.63	[<3]	
		3-12 yr:	2-7		[15-53]	
		Adult:	5-24		[38-183]	
			mg/g creatinine		*mmol/mol creatinine*	
		or	3 $\pm$ 1 (SD)	$\times$ 0.86	[2.6 $\pm$ 0.9]	

	CSF. Collect in sterile tubes; store frozen. Stable at $-20°$ C for 1 wk or at $-70°$ C for 2 mo.[10]		*mg/dL*	*µmol/L*	
		Neonate:	0.107 $\pm$ 0.047 (SEM) $\times$ 7.63	[8.2 $\pm$ 3.6][10]	
		3 mo-2 yr:	0.069 $\pm$ 0.016 (SD)	[5.3 $\pm$ 1.2][13]	
		2-10 yr:	0.047 $\pm$ 0.010	[3.6 $\pm$ 0.8][13]	
		Adult:	0.069 $\pm$ 0.007	[5.3 $\pm$ 0.5][11]	

DIAGNOSTIC INFORMATION	REMARKS

CSF ↑ Acute bacterial meningitis, vascular cerebral lesions, tumors primary or metastatic to cerebrospinal system.

P ↑ Branched-chain ketoaciduria (maple syrup urine disease), obesity, starvation, and viral hepatitis

P ↓ Carcinoid syndrome, kwashiorkor, acute hunger, hyperinsulinism, severely burned patients (day 4),[16] after abdominal surgery (day 1),[17] Huntington's chorea, and hepatic encephalopathy

High levels of leucine, valine, and alloisoleucine are also observed in maple syrup urine disease as a result of a defect in branched-chain ketoacid decarboxylase. In this autosomal recessive disorder of primary overflow aminoaciduria, there may be extreme acidosis, vomiting, CNS symptoms, mental retardation, respiratory failure, and death.

See also Table II-2A.

U ↑ Hartnup disease, maple syrup urine disease, generalized aminoaciduria, oasthouse disease, and hepatic failure

CSF ↑ Maple syrup urine disease, bacterial meningitis, meningoradiculitis, Garin-Bujadoux-Bannwarth, and carcinomatous meningitis[18]

Values in children (3 mo-10 yr) were measured using reversed-phase liquid chromatography.

TEST NAME AND METHOD	SPECIMEN REQUIREMENTS	REFERENCE INTERVAL, CONVENTIONAL [INTERNATIONAL RECOMMENDED UNITS]		CHEMICAL INTERFERENCES AND IN VIVO EFFECTS
Isoleucine—CONT				
Tandem mass spectrometry	Dried blood spot collected onto newborn screening filter paper. Allow to air dry before analysis.	Neonate: 1.98 ± 0.61	[151 ± 47][14]	Tandem mass spectrometry without LC separation does not differentiate between leucine and isoleucine. Reference interval is sum of both amino acids.

1. Friedman RB, Young DS: *Youngs effect on line,* 2006, American Association for Clinical Chemistry.
2. Scriver CR, Beaudet AL, Valle D, et al, editors: *The metabolic and molecular bases of inherited disease,* ed 8, New York, 2001, McGraw-Hill.
3. Young DS: *Effects of drugs on clinical laboratory tests,* ed 3, Washington, DC, 1990, American Association for Clinical Chemistry.
4. Bremer HJ, Duran M, Kamerling JP, et al: *Disturbances of amino acid metabolism: clinical chemistry and diagnosis,* Baltimore, 1981, Urban and Schwarzenburg.
5. Nyhan W, Sakait N: *Diagnostic recognition of genetic disease,* Philadelphia, 1987, Lea & Febiger.
6. Slocum RH, Cummings JD: Amino acid analysis of physiological samples. In Hommes FA, editor: *Techniques in diagnostic human biochemical genetics,* New York, 1991, Wiley-Liss.
7. Cummings JG: Routine amino acids analysis in the clinical laboratory, *Am Clin Prod Rev* Feb:20-25, 1988.
8. Schaefer A, Piquard F, Haberey P: Plasma amino acids analysis: effects of delayed samples preparation and of storage, *Clin Chim Acta* 164:163-169, 1987.
9. Pesce A, Kaplan L, editors: *Methods in clinical chemistry,* St. Louis, 1987, CV Mosby.
10. Heiblim DI, Evans HE, Glass L, et al: Amino acid concentrations in cerebrospinal fluid, *Arch Neurol* 35:765-768, 1978.
11. Shih V: *Laboratory techniques for the detection of hereditary metabolic disorders,* Boca Raton, FL, 1973, CRC Press.
12. Meites S, editor: *Pediatric clinical chemistry,* ed 3, Washington, DC, 1989, American Association for Clinical Chemistry.
13. Goldsmith RF, Earl JW, Cunningham AM: Determination of δ-aminobutyric acid and other amino acids in cerebrospinal fluid of pediatric patients by reversed-phase liquid chromatography, *Clin Chem* 33:1736-1740, 1987.
14. Chace DH, Hillman SL, Millington DS, et al: Rapid diagnosis of maple syrup urine disease in blood spots from newborns by tandem mass spectrometry, *Clin Chem* 41:62-68, 1995.
15. Tsao C, Muyashita K: Effects of large intake of ascorbic acid on the urinary excretion of amino acids and related compounds, *IRCS Med Sci* 13:855-856, 1985.
16. Cynober L, Dinh FN, Saizy R, et al: Plasma amino acid levels in the first few days after burn injury and their predictive value, *Intensive Care Med* 9:325-331, 1983.
17. Jain KM, Rush BF Jr, Seelig RF, et al: Changes in plasma amino acid profiles following abdominal operations, *Surg Gynecol Obstet* 152:302-306, 1981.
18. Schott KJ, Meier D: Free amino acid pattern of cerebrospinal fluid in meningeal pathology, *Acta Neurol Scand* 75:304-309, 1987.

DIAGNOSTIC INFORMATION	REMARKS

↑ Maple syrup urine disease, fasting ketosis, and liver disease   See also *Valine*.

TEST NAME AND METHOD	SPECIMEN REQUIREMENTS	REFERENCE INTERVAL, CONVENTIONAL [INTERNATIONAL RECOMMENDED UNITS]			CHEMICAL INTERFERENCES AND IN VIVO EFFECTS
Lactate Dehydrogenase (LD, LDH, L-Lactate: NAD$^+$ Oxidoreductase; EC 1.1.1.27)	Serum, plasma (heparin). Store at room temperature; do not refrigerate or freeze. Remove from clot and analyze promptly.	Neonate: 415-690 U/L Adult: 140-280 U/L Reference ranges are highly method dependent.			↑ V Acebutolol, anesthetic agents, azlocillin, cephalosporins, dicumarol, ethanol, filgrastim, fluorouracil, heparin, imipramine, interferons, isotretinoin, ketoconazole, labetalol, methotrexate, metoprolol, nitrofurantoin, NSAIDs (e.g., diflunisal, ketoprofen, piroxicam), penicillamine, piperacillin, plicamycin, propoxyphene, quinidine, sulfonamides, ticarcillin, tretinate, and valproic acid.
Pyruvate to lactate *30° C*[1] *SCE, 37° C*[2] *Lactate to pyruvate* *30° C*[3]	Red blood cells contain substantially greater amounts of LD than serum; thus hemolyzed specimens are not acceptable.	Adult: 208-378 U/L Adult: 35-100 U/L			
BMD LDH-L Tris, 37° C			*U/L*		↑ C Triamterene (fluor.); even minimal hemolysis (owing to the high LD activity in erythrocytes); *DuPont aca:* iron salts
		0-4 days:	290-775		
		4-10 days:	545-2000		
		10 days-24 mo:	180-430		
		24 mo-12 yr:	110-295		↓ C Oxalate and urea; *Seralyzer:* amikan, metronidazole; *colorimetric:* ketoprofen
		12-60 yr:	100-190		
		60-90 yr[5]:	110-210		
		>90 yr:	99-284		
	CSF. Store as for serum. Assay as soon as possible.	<20 U/L[1]			↓ V Clofibrate, fluoride (low doses) NADH forms a potent LD inhibitor on storage, accelerated by moisture; new lots of NADH must therefore be examined.[7]
ICSH, 37° C[4]	Hemolysate of washed erythrocytes. Submit whole blood (ACD, EDTA, or heparin). Stable 20 days at 4° C, 5 days at 25° C.	*U/g Hb* 200 ± 26.5 (SD) *U/10^{12} Ercs* 5800 ± 768 *U/mL Ercs* 68.0 ± 9.01 Slightly higher in newborns.[6] U/g Hb × 29 = U/10^{12} Ercs U/g Hb × 0.34 = U/mL Ercs† *Conversion factor based on MW of Hb of 64,500. †See Note, *Acetylcholinesterase.*	× 0.0645* × 10^{-3} × 1.0	*MU/mol Hb* [12.9 ± 1.7] *nU/Erc* [5.80 ± 0.77] *kU/L Ercs* [68.0 ± 9.01]	Some drugs and chemicals alter serum levels of this enzyme. The effect on erythrocyte levels has not been established.

| DIAGNOSTIC INFORMATION | REMARKS |

LD activity is found in most cells in the body. The highest activities are found in the heart, liver, muscle, kidney, lung, and red blood cells. Thus serum LD activity is increased in a variety of clinical pathologies.

Historically, LD has been monitored regarding tumor activity involving anemias and lung cancer, liver disease, renal disease, and after MI. The use of LD for MI detection has been replaced with cardiac troponins.

↑↑↑ Megaloblastic and pernicious anemia, extensive carcinomatosis, viral hepatitis, shock, hypoxia, and extreme hyperthermia

↑↑ Cirrhosis, obstructive jaundice, renal diseases of many types, skeletomuscular diseases, neoplastic diseases, and congestive heart failure

↑ Any cellular injury that results in loss of cytoplasm, myocardial or pulmonary infarction, leukemias, hemolytic anemias, hepatitis (nonviral), sickle cell disease, lymphoma, renal infarction, and acute pancreatitis.

↓ Genetic deficiency of H or M subunits

↑ Intracerebral meningeal deposits of carcinoma, leukemia, or lymphosarcoma; meningitis, subarachnoid hemorrhage, and cerebrovascular accident

Deficiency produces no known clinical effects.

The pyruvate-to-lactate reaction is preferred on theoretical grounds because the equilibrium constant (2.7×10^{11}) is so large.[7] The rates for any given amount of enzyme are 2-3 times faster for the pyruvate-to-lactate reaction; hence, smaller samples and shorter observation periods can be used.

Disadvantages of the pyruvate-to-lactate reaction include its earlier loss of linearity as compared with the lactate-to-pyruvate reaction and the greater substrate inhibition of the enzyme.

Values are slightly higher in young erythrocytes.[8]

TEST NAME AND METHOD	SPECIMEN REQUIREMENTS	REFERENCE INTERVAL, CONVENTIONAL [INTERNATIONAL RECOMMENDED UNITS]			CHEMICAL INTERFERENCES AND IN VIVO EFFECTS

Lactate Dehydrogenase—CONT

1. Vassault A: Lactate dehydrogenase—UV-method with pyruvate and NADH. In Bergmeyer HU, editor: *Methods of enzymatic analysis, vol III,* ed 3, Weinheim, 1983, Verlag Chemie.

2. Committee on Enzymes of the Scandinavian Society for Clinical Chemistry and Clinical Physiology: Recommended methods for the determination of four enzymes in blood, *Scand J Clin Lab Invest* 33:291-306, 1974.

3. Wahlefeld AW: UV-method with L-lactate and NAD. In Bergmeyer HU, editor: *Methods of enzymatic analysis, vol III,* ed 3, Weinheim, 1983, Verlag Chemie.

4. Beutler E: *Red cell metabolism: a manual of biochemical methods,* ed 3, New York, 1984, Grune & Stratton.

TEST NAME AND METHOD	SPECIMEN REQUIREMENTS	REFERENCE INTERVAL, CONVENTIONAL [INTERNATIONAL RECOMMENDED UNITS]			CHEMICAL INTERFERENCES AND IN VIVO EFFECTS
L-Lactate (Lactic Acid)[1-8] *Colorimetric*[4,5]	Whole blood (heparin). Protein precipitation should be performed immediately. Note whether sample is venous or arterial. See *Remarks* regarding use of tourniquet.	*mg/dL* Venous: 8.1-15.3 Arterial: <11.3 Patient should be at complete rest. Values may increase 20-50% after meals.	× 0.111	*mmol/L* [0.9-1.7] [<1.3]	B ↑ V Aspirin toxicity (late metabolic acidosis), epinephrine (particularly excessive doses), ethanol, fructose, glucose, isoniazid (with overdosage), metformin, methylprednisolone, nalidixic acid, phenformin, propylene glycol (diluent in injections), sodium bicarbonate (IV), sucrose, terbutaline, and tetracosactrin B ↓ V Methylene blue, morphine
Amperometric (Nova SP7)[9]	Plasma (heparin). Keep sample on ice; analyze immediately.	*mg/dL* 6.3-22.5		*mmol/L* [0.7-2.5]	B ↑ C Ascorbate (>10 mmol/L)
Enzymatic[4]	Plasma (fluoride/ oxalate tubes). Separate from cells within 15 min. Keep sample on ice; analyze promptly. Lactate in plasma is stable for up to 8 hr at room temperature and 14 days at 2-8° C. Avoid hemolysis. Note whether sample is venous or arterial.	*mg/dL* Venous: 4.5-19.8 Arterial: 4.5-14.4 Patient should be at complete rest. Lactate/pyruvate (L/P) ratio: 10/1	× 0.111	*mmol/L* [0.5-2.2] [0.5-1.6]	

DIAGNOSTIC INFORMATION   **REMARKS**

5. Tietz NW, Shuey DF, Wekstein DR: Laboratory values in fit aging individuals—sexagenarians through centenarians, *Clin Chem* 38:1167-1185, 1992.

6. Oski FA: Red cell metabolism in the newborn infant. V. Glycolytic intermediate and glycolytic enzymes, *Pediatrics* 44:84-91, 1969.

7. Howell BF, McGune S, Schaffer R: Lactate-to-pyruvate or pyruvate-to-lactate assay for lactate dehydrogenase: a re-examination, *Clin Chem* 25:269-272, 1979.

8. Beutler E: *Hemolytic anemia in disorders of red cell metabolism,* New York, 1978, Plenum Pub. Co.

B, P ↑ *Type I lactic acidosis* (increased lactic acid, no significant acidosis, normal L/P ratio): muscular exercise, hyperventilation, glucagon, glycogen storage disease, severe anemia, insulin infusions, and Reye's syndrome

Type IIA, hypoxia related (increased L/P ratio): any condition with inadequate oxygen delivery to tissues, acute hemorrhage, severe acute congestive heart failure or other causes of circulatory collapse, cyanotic heart disease or other causes of acute hypoxia, and extracorporeal circulation

Type IIB, idiopathic (increased L/P ratio): mild uremia, infections (especially pyelonephritis), cirrhosis, third trimester of pregnancy, severe vascular disease, leukemias, anemias, chronic alcoholism, subacute bacterial endocarditis, poliomyelitis, and diabetes (~50%)

Use of tourniquet or clenching of hands increases lactate. Lactate increases rapidly in improperly preserved samples and during exercise and hyperventilation. In McArdle's disease, sample drawn 1 min after initiation of exercise will show no increase in lactate. Lactic acidosis is suspected when the anion gap is >18 mmol/L in the absence of other causes, such as renal failure, salicylate ingestion, methanol poisoning, ethanol abuse, and significant ketonemia.

TEST NAME AND METHOD	SPECIMEN REQUIREMENTS	REFERENCE INTERVAL, CONVENTIONAL [INTERNATIONAL RECOMMENDED UNITS]		CHEMICAL INTERFERENCES AND IN VIVO EFFECTS

L-Lactate—CONT

Colorimetric	Urine, 24 hr.[5] Refrigerate.	*mg/day* 496-1982	× 0.0111	*mmol/day* [5.5-22.0]
	CSF.[3,5] Refrigerate.	*mg/dL*[3]		*mmol/L*
		Neonate: 10-60	× 0.111	[1.1-6.7]
		3-10 days: 10-40		[1.1-4.4]
		>10 days: 10-25		[1.1-2.8]
		Adult: 9-26		[1.0-2.9]
Qualitative	Gastric fluid[5]	Negative		

1. Burtis CA, Ashwood ER, editors: *Tietz textbook of clinical chemistry,* ed 2, Philadelphia, 1994, WB Saunders.
2. Eastham RD: *Biochemical values in clinical medicine,* ed 7, Bristol, UK, 1985, John Wright and Sons Ltd.
3. Henry JB, editor: *Clinical diagnosis and management by laboratory methods,* ed 20, Philadelphia, 2001, WB Saunders.
4. Jacobs DS, DeMott WR, De Mott WR, editors: *Laboratory test handbook,* ed 5, Stow, OH, 2001, Lexi-Comp, Inc.
5. Burtis CA, Ashwood ER, editors: *Tietz fundamentals of clinical chemistry,* ed 5, Philadelphia, 2000, WB Saunders.
6. Wallace J, editors: *Interpretation of diagnostic tests,* ed 7, Philadelphia, 2000, Lippincott.
7. Kasper DL, Hauser SL, Longo DL, et al, editors: *Harrison's principles of internal medicine,* ed 16, New York, 2005, McGraw-Hill.
8. Toffaletti JG: Blood lactate: biochemistry, laboratory methods, and clinical interpretation, *Crit Rev Clin Lab Sci* 28:253-268, 1991.
9. Toffaletti JG, Hammes ME, Gray R, et al: Lactate measured in diluted and undiluted whole blood and plasma: comparison of methods and effect of hematocrit, *Clin Chem* 38:2430-2434, 1992.
10. Controni G, Rodriguez WJ, Hicks JM, et al: Cerebrospinal fluid lactic acid levels in meningitis, *J Pediatr* 91:379-384. 1977.
11. Knight JA, Dudek SM, Hammond RE: Increased cerebral spinal fluid lactate and early diagnosis of bacterial meningitis, *Clin Chem* 25:809-810, 1979.

Lactate Dehydrogenase (LD, LDH) Isoenzymes (L-Lactate: NAD⁺ Oxidoreductase; EC 1.1.1.27)[1]	Serum. Store at room temperature.[6] LD-5 is least stable; in 48 hr, 13% is lost at room temperature, 18% at 4° C.	*Percent of total*		*Fraction of total activity*	↑ Hemolysis
		LD fraction			See *Lactate*
		1	18-33 × 0.01	[0.18-0.33]	*Dehydrogenase.*
		2	28-40	[0.28-0.40]	
		3	18-30	[0.18-0.30]	
		4	6-16	[0.06-0.16]	
		5	2-13	[0.02-0.13]	

EP, cellulose acetate[2]

EP, agarose[1]

	LD fraction		
	1	14-26	[0.14-0.26]
	2	29-39	[0.29-0.39]
	3	20-26	[0.20-0.26]
	4	8-16	[0.08-0.16]
	5	6-16	[0.06-0.16]

CSF ↑ Reduced cerebral blood flow or oxygenation, increased intracranial pressure, trauma, seizures, intracranial hemorrhage, brain abscess, multiple sclerosis, primary or metastatic CNS carcinoma, hypocapnia, and bacterial and tuberculous meningitis (see *Remarks*)

Recent reports indicate that the measurement of CSF lactate may be a useful screening test for CNS disease and an aid in distinguishing bacterial from viral meningitis. In essentially all bacterial and fungal meningitides, the value will exceed 35 mg/dL [3.9 mmol/L], whereas in viral meningitis the concentration is invariably <35 mg/dL [<3.9 mmol/L]. Measurement is of doubtful clinical value because culture of the organism gives the final answer. Increased levels of lactate in CSF following head injury suggest a poor prognosis.[10,11]

GF ↑ Carcinoma of stomach, pyloric obstruction

LD isoenzyme patterns cannot be interpreted without knowledge of the clinical history.

↑ LD-1 and/or LD-2 (LD-1/LD-2) "flip" can be present in patients after acute myocardial infarction; in pernicious, hemolytic, acute sickle cell or megaloblastic anemia; in acute renal cortical necrosis; or in cases of in vivo or in vitro hemolysis of any cause. The optimum decision threshold for the LD-1/LD-2 ratio is, by ROC-curve analysis, 0.92-0.94.[7,8]

↑ LD-1, particularly in germ cell tumors (e.g., teratoma, seminoma of testis, dysgerminoma of ovary); injury to skeletal muscle.

↑ LD-5, in injury to skeletal muscle, any inflammatory or degenerative diseases of skeletal muscle, many types of liver injury (cirrhosis, all types of hepatitis, and passive congestion of the liver), and cancer (insensitive and nonspecific finding).

Chemical inhibition methods using urea or lactate give unreliable results. Heat inactivation procedures in which LD-5 is destroyed are also of very limited use because all isoenzymes show some heat instability, and excellent temperature control is required to get reproducible results. Immunoinhibition methods detect changes in LD-1 only.[3] Minicolumn methods can separate LD-1 and LD-2 but include LD-3 to LD-5 in the first fraction.[9] Some minicolumn methods, however, may only separate LD-1.[10]

An additional LD isoenzyme, called LD-6, has been described cathodal to LD-5; it may be released from liver. It is seen only when prognosis is poor. LD-6 has provisionally been identified as alcohol dehydrogenase.

LD binding to IgA or IgG can produce a variety of additional or decreased LD zones or distorted LD patterns.

TEST NAME AND METHOD	SPECIMEN REQUIREMENTS	REFERENCE INTERVAL, CONVENTIONAL [INTERNATIONAL RECOMMENDED UNITS]			CHEMICAL INTERFERENCES AND IN VIVO EFFECTS
Lactate Dehydrogenase (LD, LDH) Isoenzymes—CONT					
LD-1 immunoinhibition assays[3]		LD-1:	37-50	[0.37-0.50]	
		LD-1:	<40	[<0.40]	
Isomune-LD (Roche)					
LD-1 Immuno (Seragen)					
LD-1 chemical inhibition assays[4,5]		LD-1:	23-39	[0.23-0.39]	
		LD-1:	<40	[<0.40]	
1,6-hexanediol[5]					
Sodium perchlorate[4,5]					

1. McKenzie D, Henderson AR: Electrophoresis of lactate dehydrogenase isoenzymes. In Cooper GR, editor: *Standard methods of clinical chemistry, vol 10,* Washington, DC, 1983, American Association for Clinical Chemistry.

2. Di Giorgio J: Determination of serum lactic dehydrogenase isoenzymes by use of the "Diagnostest" cellulose acetate electrophoresis system, *Clin Chem* 17:326-331, 1971.

3. Ranjan P, Karcher RE, Epstein E, et al: Electrophoresis and the Isomune-LD and LD-1 immuno methods compared for measurement of lactate dehydrogenase isoenzyme-1, *Clin Chem* 33:1884-1886, 1987.

4. Onigbinde TA, Wu AHB, Johnson M, et al: Clinical evaluation of an automated chemical inhibition assay for lactate dehydrogenase isoenzyme 1, *Clin Chem* 36:1819-1822, 1990.

5. Paz JM, Garcia A, Gonzales M, et al: Evaluation of determination of lactate dehydrogenase isoenzyme 1 by chemical inhibition with perchlorate or with 1,6-hexanediol, *Clin Chem* 36:355-358, 1990.

6. Kreutzer HH, Fennis WHS: Lactic dehydrogenase isoenzymes in blood serum after storage at different temperatures, *Clin Chim Acta* 9:64-68, 1964.

7. Leroux ML, Rabson J, Desjardin PRE: Clinical effectiveness of the DuPont aca measurement of creatine kinase MB in serum from patients in a coronary-care unit, *Clin Chem* 30:1552-1554, 1984.

8. Pellar TG, Leung FY, Henderson AR: A computer program for rapid generation of receiver operating characteristic curves and likelihood ratios in the evaluation of diagnostic tests, *Ann Clin Biochem* 25:411-416, 1988.

9. Mercer DW: Improved column method for separating lactate dehydrogenase isoenzymes 1 and 2, *Clin Chem* 24:480-482, 1978.

10. Morin LG, Barton EG: A "column batch" method for separating MB and LD$_1$ in a single fraction, *Clin Chem* 29:1741-1745, 1983.

11. Leung FY, Henderson AR: Influence of hemolysis on the serum lactate dehydrogenase-1/lactate dehydrogenase-2 ratio as determined by an accurate thin-layer agarose electrophoresis procedure, *Clin Chem* 27:1708-1711, 1981.

12. Kazmierczak SC, Castellani WJ, Van Lente F, et al: Effect of reticulocytosis on lactate dehydrogenase isoenzyme distribution in serum: in vivo and in vitro studies, *Clin Chem* 36:1638-1641, 1990.

13. Van Lente F, Marschand A, Galen RS: Diagnosis of hemolytic disease by electrophoresis of erythrocyte lactate dehydrogenase isoenzymes on cellulose acetate or agarose, *Clin Chem* 27:1453-1455, 1981.

14. Jaffe AS, Landt Y, Parvin CA, et al: Comparative sensitivity of cardiac troponin I and lactate dehydrogenase isoenzymes for diagnosing acute myocardial infarction, *Clin Chem* 42:1770-1776, 1996.

DIAGNOSTIC INFORMATION	REMARKS

The "isomorphic pattern," i.e., a normal-appearing pattern in the presence of an abnormal total LD in serum, is observed in many patients with cardiac, liver, skeletomuscular, neoplastic, and other disorders, including multisystem diseases.

Increases in the midzone fractions, i.e., LD-2, LD-3, and LD-4, are seen when there is massive platelet destruction (e.g., pulmonary embolism, after extensive blood transfusion) and in lymphatic system involvement such as infectious mononucleosis, lymphomas, and lymphocytic leukemias; injury to skeletal muscle.

Hemolysis may invalidate test, depending on the endogenous LD-1/LD-2 ratio of erythrocytes[11]; this ratio is likely to be elevated when reticulocytosis is markedly increased.[12] The ratio depends on method of separation; cellulose acetate more often gives a ratio >1, agarose a ratio <1.[13]

Chemical inhibition methods using either 1,6-hexanediol or sodium perchlorate are effective.[4,5]

The use of LD isoenzymes for detection of late-presenting MIs has been replaced with cardiac troponin monitoring.[14]

TEST NAME AND METHOD	SPECIMEN REQUIREMENTS	REFERENCE INTERVAL, CONVENTIONAL [INTERNATIONAL RECOMMENDED UNITS]			CHEMICAL INTERFERENCES AND IN VIVO EFFECTS
Lactose Tolerance Test[1,2] Dose: Lactose orally, 50 g or 2 g/kg body wt. (In water at room temperature.)	Serum. Draw samples at 0, 30, 45, 60, and 90 min.	Change in glucose from fasting value: Inconclusive: Abnormal:	*mg/dL* >30 20-30 <20	× 0.0555	*mmol/L* [>1.7] [1.1-1.7] [<<1.1]	See *Glucose*. Thirty percent false-normal rate because of tight glucose control.
	Breath[3]	H_2 < 12 ppm above baseline.			

1. Caraway WT, Watts NB: Carbohydrates. In Tietz NW, editor: *Textbook of clinical chemistry,* Philadelphia, 1986, WB Saunders.
2. Newcomer AD, McGill DB, Thomas PJ, et al: Prospective comparison of indirect methods for detecting lactase deficiency, *N Engl J Med* 293:1232-1236, 1975.
3. Newcomer AD, McGill DB, Thomas PJ, et al: Prospective comparison of indirect methods for detecting lactase deficiency, *N Engl J Med* 293:1232-1235, 1975.

Lamellar Body Count (LBC)[1]	Amniotic fluid, ≤500 µL. Sample should be mixed on a rocker for 2 min or with 20 gentle inversions of the collection tube. Do not centrifuge specimens. Samples collected from "free-flowing" vaginal pools are acceptable, but vaginal pool specimens containing obvious mucus should not be used.[2]	≥50,000/µL: Mature[2] >15,000/µL – <50,000/µL: Transitional ≤15,000/µL: Immature Reference ranges can vary based on type of instrument used for counting and whether samples are centrifuged (centrifugation is not recommended). Institutions performing LBC should determine reference values by performing clinical outcome studies and by comparing their method with a method used in an outcome study with paired amniotic fluid specimens.[3]			Samples with hematocrit >1% will produce a biphasic change in LBC, initially increasing counts because of platelets, then decreasing counts as clotting occurs.[1,4] Moderate meconium increases LBC by ~5000/µL.[1,2]

1. Dubin SB: Characterization of amniotic fluid lamellar bodies by resistive-pulse counting: relationship to measures of fetal lung maturity, *Clin Chem* 35:612-616, 1989.
2. Neerhof MG, Dohnal JC, Ashwood ER, et al: Lamellar body counts: a consensus on protocol, *Obstet Gynecol* 97:318-320, 2001.
3. Ashwood ER: Evaluation of the high risk pregnancy at term. In Sherwin JE, Ashwood ER, Geaghan S, et al, editors: *NACB LMPG (draft guidelines-version 2) maternal and fetal health risk assessment,* Washington, DC, 2003, National Academy of Clinical Biochemistry.
4. Ashwood ER, Palmer SE, Taylor JS, et al: Lamellar body counts for rapid fetal lung maturity testing, *Obstet Gynecol* 81:619-624, 1993.

DIAGNOSTIC INFORMATION	REMARKS
Impairment of carbohydrate absorption is caused by a deficiency of small bowel mucosal lactase. (See also *Disaccharide Absorption Tests.*)	Serum glucose must be quantitated using a method specific for glucose. To eliminate misinterpretation of test results, a glucose tolerance test and a galactose tolerance test may need to be performed to rule out monosaccharide malabsorption.
>20 ppm increase over baseline is diagnostic of lactose intolerance.

Positive in some cases of bacterial overgrowth of the small intestine. | 99% sensitive, 90% specific

A late increase in H_2 may occur if lactose reaches the large bowel. |
| The LBC has a slightly better specificity than the L/S ratio.[5] As with other FLM tests, LBC is a strong predictor of maturity but a weak predictor of immaturity.[6] | Lamellar bodies constitute the storage form of surfactant released into amniotic fluid by fetal breathing movements. Because of their size (0.2-2 μm), lamellar bodies can be enumerated using the platelet channel of an electronic cell counter. This is the basis for the LBC test.[1]

Advantages of LBC include a rapid result time (<20 min), low cost to perform, wide availability of instrumentation, and high intraassay precision.[7,8] |

5.   Wijnberger LD, Huisjes AJ, Voorbij HA, et al: The accuracy of lamellar body count and lecithin/sphingomyelin ratio in the prediction of neonatal respiratory distress syndrome: a meta-analysis, *BJOG* 108:583-588, 2001.

6.   Ashwood ER: Markers of fetal lung maturity. In Gronowski AM, editor: *Handbook of clinical laboratory testing during pregnancy,* Totowa, NJ, 2004, Humana Press Inc., pp. 55-70.

7.   Dubin SB: Assessment of fetal lung maturity. Practice parameter, *Am J Clin Pathol* 110:723-732, 1998.

8.   Szallasi A, Gronowski AM, Eby CS: Lamellar body count in amniotic fluid: a comparative study of four different hematology analyzers, *Clin Chem* 49:994-997, 2003.

TEST NAME AND METHOD	SPECIMEN REQUIREMENTS	REFERENCE INTERVAL, CONVENTIONAL [INTERNATIONAL RECOMMENDED UNITS]			CHEMICAL INTERFERENCES AND IN VIVO EFFECTS
Lead (Pb)[1-3] *Colorimetric, AAS*	Whole blood (EDTA). Collect in pretested metal-free container. Refrigerate.	Child[7]: Adult: Acceptable for industrial exposure: Toxic concentration[5]:	*mcg/dL* <10 <25 <50 $\geq$100	× 0.0483	μ*mol/L* [<0.48] [<1.21] [<2.42] [$\geq$4.83]	The addition to specimens of anticoagulants or preservatives other than heparin may cause reduced recoveries with flame AAS. Anticoagulants other than oxalate do not interfere with graphite furnace AAS.
	Urine, 24 hr.[2] Collect in acid-washed, metal-free container. Acidify to pH 2.0. Stable 1 wk at 4° C.	Acceptable for industrial exposure:	*mcg/L* <80 ($\bar{x}$: 21.5)[8] <120	× 0.00483	μ*mol/L* [<0.39] [$\bar{x}$: 0.10] [<0.58]	
	Hair[5]	Child: Adult:	*mcg/g dry wt.* <70 <155	× 0.00483	μ*mol/g dry wt.* [<0.34] [<0.75]	
ICP-MS	Whole blood.[6] Collect in pretested, metal-free container.	Child: Adult:	*mcg/dL* 0.0-9.9 0.0-24.9	× 0.0483	μ*mol/L* [0.0-0.48] [0.0-1.20]	
	Urine.[6] Collect in acid-washed, metal-free container.	0-23 mcg/L 0-31 mcg/day		× 0.00483	[0.0-0.11 μmol/L] [0-0-0.15 μmol/day]	
X-ray fluorescence spectrometry[4]	Bronchoalveolar lavage fluid	<0.23	*ng/10³ macrophages*	× 4.83	*fmol/macrophage* [<1.1]	

1. Henry JB, editor: *Clinical diagnosis and management by laboratory methods,* ed 18, Philadelphia, 1991, WB Saunders.
2. Tietz NW, editor: *Fundamentals of clinical chemistry,* ed 3, Philadelphia, 1987, WB Saunders.
3. Boeckx RL: Lead poisoning in children, *Anal Chem* 58:274A-288A, 1986.
4. Maier EA, Rastegar F, Heimburger R, et al: Simultaneous determination of trace elements in lavage fluids front human bronchial alveoli by energy dispersive X-ray florescence. 1: Technique and determination of the normal reference interval, *Clin Chem* 31:551-555, 1985.
5. Johnson HL, Sauberlich HE: Trace clement analysis in biological samples. In Prasad AS, editor: *Clinical, biochemical, and nutritional aspects of trace elements,* New York, 1982, Alan R. Liss, Inc.
6. Associated Regional & University Pathologists, Inc. web site (www.aruplab.com). Available at: http://www.aruplab.com/testing/user_guide.jsp. Last accessed 9/2004.
7. Centers for Disease Control and Prevention Screening Young Children for Lead Poisoning: *Guidance for state and local public health officials,* Atlanta, 1997, CDC.
8. Schramel VP, Lill G, Hasse S: Mineral and trace elements in human urine, *J Clin Chem Clin Biochem* 23:293-301, 1985.
9. Hu H, Aro A, Payton M, et al: The relationship fo bone and blood lead to hypertension. The normative aging study, *JAMA* 275:1171-1176, 1996.
10. Lin J-L, Lin-Tan D-T, Hsu K-H, et al: Environmental lead exposure and progression of chronic renal disease in patients without diabetes, *N Engl J Med* 348:277-286, 2003.

DIAGNOSTIC INFORMATION	REMARKS

↑ Industrial exposure, ingestion of Pb-containing paint, ceramic glazes, and so on.

Pb poisoning may result in anorexia, abdominal pain, vomiting, irritability, apathy, Pb encephalopathy, anemia, and peripheral neuropathy. Increased exposure to Pb results in an increased risk of hypertension[9] and accelerates progression of chronic renal disease.[10] Behavioral delays in puberty and neurological effects have been documented in subclinical lead poisoning of children.[11,12] High-risk children include those aged 3-12 yr who live in or visit old, dilapidated housing.

See also Table II-11 for classification of blood levels in children and OSHA action levels.[13,14]

Lead levels in blood may fluctuate in part because of specimen contamination during collection. If blood or random urine is analyzed, several specimens may be needed to rule out lead poisoning. The use of contamination-free specimens is extremely important. Urinary δ-aminolevulinic acid and coproporphyrin III and free erythrocyte protoporphyrin increase in Pb poisoning. Diagnostic sensitivity of ALA and protoporphyrin assays at threshold of 10 mcg/dL is poor.[15] Blood lead measurement is considered the best indicator of lead poisoning and is recommended by the CDC.

Pb poisoning can be confirmed with a mobilization test. See also δ-*Aminolevulinic Acid, Lead Mobilization Test,* and *Porphyrins.*

See also Tables II-6, II-9, and II-11.

11. Canfield RL, Henderson CR, Cory-Slechta DA, et al: Intellectual impairment in children with blood lead concentrations below 10 μg per deciliter, *N Engl J Med* 348:1517-1526, 2003.

12. Selevan SG, Rice DC, Hogan KA, et al: Blood lead concentrations and delayed puberty in girls, *N Engl J Med* 348:1527-1536, 2003.

13. National Institute of Occupational Safety: *Working with lead in the construction industry,* Washington, DC, 1991, U.S. Dept. of Labor, U.S. Department of Health and Human Services, OSHA 3126.

14. Roper WL: *Preventing lead poisoning in young children,* Atlanta, 1991, Centers for Disease Control, U.S. Department of Health and Human Services.

15. Parsons PJ, Reilly AA, Esernio-Jenssen D: Screening children exposed to lead: an assessment of the capillary blood fingerstick test, *Clin Chem* 43:302-311, 1997.

TEST NAME AND METHOD	SPECIMEN REQUIREMENTS	REFERENCE INTERVAL, CONVENTIONAL [INTERNATIONAL RECOMMENDED UNITS]	CHEMICAL INTERFERENCES AND IN VIVO EFFECTS
Lead Mobilization Test[1] *Colorimetric, AAS* Dose[1]: 50 mg of CaNa$_2$ EDTA/kg, parenterally	Urine collected in an acid-washed, metal-free container, 24 hr. Begin collection after dose.	Index value: <1 (Ratio = Pb mcg/24 hr divided by Ca EDTA in mg)	See *Lead.*

1. Henry JB, editor: *Clinical diagnosis and management by laboratory methods,* ed 18, Philadelphia, 1991, WB Saunders.

TEST NAME AND METHOD	SPECIMEN REQUIREMENTS	REFERENCE INTERVAL, CONVENTIONAL [INTERNATIONAL RECOMMENDED UNITS]	CHEMICAL INTERFERENCES AND IN VIVO EFFECTS
Lecithin: Cholesterol Acyltransferase (LCAT, EC 2.3.1.43)[1-12] *Radioenzymatic (activity)*[1,7,13,14]	Plasma (EDTA), serum, or HDL fraction. Stable at least 2 mo if frozen promptly at −20° C. Do not refreeze.	*Fractional Esterification Rate (HDL; mean ± SD)*[14]: F: 10.6 ± 3.6%/hr M: 16.8 ± 4.5%/hr Hypertensive F: 18.0 ± 6.4%/hr Hypertensive M: 28.6 ± 8.6%/hr Diabetic F: 26.3 ± 10.8%/hr Diabetic M: 35.3 ± 3.3%/hr Enzyme Activity (plasma)[7]: 25-35 nmol/hr/mL plasma is expected. However, assays vary considerably, and reference intervals must be established in-house. <2 nmol/hr/mL is consistent with LCAT deficiency or its variant, fish-eye disease. <20 nmol/hr/mL (or ~50% of normal) in a first-degree relative of a patient with LCAT deficiency is consistent with heterozygous LCAT deficiency states.	↑ V Prednisolone. ↓ C Poor sample storage. ↓ V Bezafibrate, indomethacin, lisinopril, propranolol, fish oils, weight loss in overweight individuals, and pregnancy.
RIA, ELISA (mass)[7,15,16]		*mcg/mL (mean ± SD)* *mg/L* M: 5.56 ± 0.91 × 1.0 [5.56 ± 0.91] F: 5.91 ± 1.02 [5.91 ± 1.02]	

1. Albers JJ, Segrest JP, editors: *Plasma lipoproteins, part b: characterization, cell biology, and metabolism. Method in enzymology, vol 129,* Orlando, FL, 1986, Academic Press.

2. Dobiasova M, Frohlich JJ: Advances in understanding of the role of lecithin cholesterol acyltransferase (LCAT) in cholesterol transport, *Clin Chim Acta* 286:257-271, 1999.

3. Henry JB, editor: *Clinical diagnosis and management by laboratory methods,* ed 19, Philadelphia, 1996, WB Saunders.

4. Jin W, Marchadier D, Rader DJ: Lipases and HDL metabolism, *Trends Endocrinol Metab* 13:174-178, 2002.

DIAGNOSTIC INFORMATION   REMARKS

↑ Lead intoxication (index value >1)

Test for Pb burden not poisoning should be reserved for asymptomatic patients.

↑ Hypertriglyceridemia.

↓ Familial LCAT deficiency, fish-eye disease, and hepatocellular disorders.

Patients with LCAT deficiency may develop renal disease, anemia, and corneal opacities, but premature CHD is rare.

LCAT activity represents the endogenous cholesterol esterification rate, which depends not only on the amount of functionally active enzyme present but also on the enzyme substrates, cofactors, and other constituents in the plasma. Use of an artificial substrate (lecithin-cholesterol liposomes containing apo A-I) allows more accurate measurement of the active enzyme in plasma.

Except in rare cases, LCAT mass is highly correlated with enzyme activity. Calculation of the cholesterol esterification rate (CER) is useful for differential diagnosis of fish-eye disease (LCAT activity is very low or absent, but CER is low normal).

The fractional esterification rate (FER) in HDL is proportional to the amount of small HDL particles in the circulation.

---

5. Kuivenhoven JA, Pritchard H, Hill J, et al: The molecular pathology of lecithin:cholesterol acyltransferase (LCAT) deficiency syndromes, *J Lipid Res* 38:191-205, 1997.

6. Rader DJ: Lipid disorders. In Topol EJ, editor: *Textbook of cardiovascular medicine,* ed 2, Philadelphia, 2002, Lippincott Williams & Wilkins.

7. Rifai N, Warnick GR, Dominiczak MH, editors: *Handbook of lipoprotein testing,* ed 2, Washington, DC, 2000, AACC Press.

TEST NAME AND METHOD	SPECIMEN REQUIREMENTS	REFERENCE INTERVAL, CONVENTIONAL [INTERNATIONAL RECOMMENDED UNITS]		CHEMICAL INTERFERENCES AND IN VIVO EFFECTS

Lecithin: Cholesterol Acyltransferase—CONT

8. Rye KA, Clay MA, Barter PJ: Remodelling of high density lipoproteins by plasma factors, *Atherosclerosis* 145:227-238, 1999.

9. Santamarina-Fojo S, Lambert G, Hoeg JM, et al: Lecithin-cholesterol acyltransferase: role in lipoprotein metabolism, reverse cholesterol transport and atherosclerosis, *Curr Opin Lipid* 11:267-275, 2000.

10. Williams PT, Albers JJ, Krauss RM, et al: Associations of lectithin:cholesterol acyltransferase (LCAT) mass concentrations with exercise, weight loss, and plasma lipoprotein subfraction concentrations in men, *Atherosclerosis* 82:53-58, 1990.

11. Young DS: *Effects of drugs on clinical laboratory tests,* ed 5, Washington, DC, 2000, AACC Press.

12. Young DS: *Effects of preanalytical variables on clinical laboratory tests,* ed 2, Washington, DC, 1997, AACC Press.

Leucine (Leu)[1-5]

Ion-exchange chromatography

Plasma (heparin) or serum, fasting. Place blood in ice water immediately; separate and freeze within 1 hr of collection. Stable for 1 wk at −20° C; for longer periods deproteinize and store at −70° C.[7,8]

	mg/dL	$\mu mol/L$[11]
Premature, 1 day:	0.92 ± 0.33 (SD) × 76.3	[70 ± 25]
Newborn, 1 day:	0.62-1.43	[47-109]
1 day-1 mo:	0.63-2.10	[48-160][12]
1-3 mo:	1.36 ± 0.39 (SD)	[104 ± 30]
9 mo-2 yr:	0.59-2.03	[45-155]
3-10 yr:	0.73-2.33	[56-178]
6-18 yr:	1.03-2.28	[79-174][13]
Adult:	0.98-2.29	[75-175]

P ↓ V Alanine, glucose, histidine (after oral load), and oral contraceptives

---

Urine, 24 hr. Add 10 mL of 6 mol/L HCl at start of collection. (Alternatively, refrigerate specimen during collection.) Store frozen at −20° C.[9]

	mg/day	$\mu mol/day$[11]
10 days-7 wk:	0.9-2.0 × 7.63	[7-15]
3-12 yr:	3.0-11.0	[23-84]
Adult:	2.6-8.1	[20-62]

	mg/g creatinine	*mmol/mol creatinine*
or	4 ± 2 (SD) × 0.86	[3.4 ± 1.7]

	$\mu mol/g$ creatinine[13]	mmol/mol creatinine
0-1 mo:	41-220 × 0.113	[4.63-24.9]
1-6 mo:	26-209	[2.94-23.6]
6 mo-1 yr:	31-183	[3.5-20.7]
1-2 yr:	28-136	[3.2-15.4]
2-3 yr:	34-217	[3.8-24.5]

U ↑ V Ascorbic acid (after large intake)[14]

CSF. Collect in sterile tubes; store frozen. Stable at −20° C for 1 wk or at −70° C for 2 mo.[10]

	mg/dL	$\mu mol/L$
Neonate:	0.278 ± 0.111 × 76.3 (SEM)	[21.2 ± 8.5][10]
3 mo-2 yr:	0.157 ± 0.030 (SD)	[12.0 ± 2.3][14]
2-10 yr:	0.119 ± 0.018	[9.1 ± 1.4][14]
Adult:	0.195 ± 0.014	[14.9 ± 1.1][11]

13. Dieplinger H, Kostner GM: The determination of lecithin:cholesterol acyltransferase in the clinical laboratory: a modified enzymatic procedure, *Clin Chim Acta* 106:319-324, 1980.

14. Ordovas JM, editor: *Lipoprotein protocols,* Totowa, NJ, 1998, Humana Press.

15. Albers JJ, Adolphson JL, Chen C: Radioimmunoassay of human plasma lecithin-cholesterol acyltransferase, *J Clin Invest* 67:141-148, 1981.

16. Albers JJ, Chen CH, Adolphson JL: Lecithin:cholesterol acyltransferase (LCAT) mass: its relationship to LCAT activity and cholesterol esterification rate, *J Lipid Res* 22:1206-1213, 1981.

P ↑ Branched-chain ketoaciduria (maple syrup urine disease), viral hepatitis, obesity, and starvation

P ↓ Kwashiorkor, acute hunger, hyperinsulinism, severely burned patients (day 4),[15] after abdominal surgery (day 1),[16] Huntington's chorea, and hepatic encephalopathy

High levels of isoleucine, valine, and alloisoleucine are also seen in maple syrup urine disease as a result of a defect in branched-chain ketoacid decarboxylase. In this autosomal recessive disorder of primary overflow aminoaciduria, there may be extreme acidosis, vomiting, CNS symptoms, mental retardation, respiratory failure, and death.

See also Table II-2A.

U ↑ Hartnup disease, maple syrup urine disease, first trimester of pregnancy (levels decrease thereafter), generalized aminoaciduria, burn patients,[17] oasthouse disease, starvation, and hepatic failure

CSF ↑ Maple syrup urine disease, bacterial meningitis, aseptic meningitis, meningoradiculitis, Garin-Bujadoux-Bannwarth, and carcinomatous meningitis.[18]

Values in children (3 mo-10 yr) were measured using reversed-phase liquid chromatography.

TEST NAME AND METHOD	SPECIMEN REQUIREMENTS	REFERENCE INTERVAL, CONVENTIONAL [INTERNATIONAL RECOMMENDED UNITS]		CHEMICAL INTERFERENCES AND IN VIVO EFFECTS
Leucine—CONT				
Tandem mass spectrometry[6]	Dried blood spot. Collect blood spot onto newborn screening filter paper. Allow to air dry before analysis.	Neonate: 1.98 ± 0.61	[151 ± 47]	Tandem mass spectrometry without LC separation does not differentiate between leucine and isoleucine. Reference interval is for sum of both amino acids.

1. Friedman RB, Young DS: *Youngs effect on line,* 2006, American Association for Clinical Chemistry.
2. Scriver CR, Beaudet AL, Valle D, et al, editors: *The metabolic and molecular bases of inherited disease,* ed 8, New York, 2001, McGraw-Hill.
3. Young DS: *Effects of drugs on clinical laboratory tests,* ed 3, Washington, DC, 1990, American Association for Clinical Chemistry.
4. Bremer HJ, Duran M, Kamerling JP, et al: *Disturbances of amino acid metabolism: clinical chemistry and diagnosis,* Baltimore, 1981, Urban and Schwarzenburg.
5. Nyhan W, Sakait N: *Diagnostic recognition of genetic disease,* Philadelphia, 1987, Lea & Febiger.
6. Schulze A, Lindner M, Kohlmoller D, et al: Expanded newborn screening for inborn errors of metabolism by electrospray ionization-tandem mass spectrometry: results, outcome, and implications, *Pediatrics* 111:1399-1406, 2003.
7. Cummings JG: Routine amino acids analysis in the clinical laboratory, *Am Clin Prod Rev* Feb:20-25, 1988.
8. Schaefer A, Piquard F, Haberey P: Plasma amino acids analysis: effects of delayed samples preparation and of storage, *Clin Chim Acta* 164:163-169, 1987.
9. Pesce A, Kaplan L, editors: *Methods in clinical chemistry,* St. Louis, 1987, CV Mosby.
10. Heiblim DI, Evans HE, Glass L, et al: Amino acid concentrations in cerebrospinal fluid, *Arch Neurol* 35:765-768, 1978.
11. Shih V: *Laboratory techniques for the detection of hereditary metabolic disorders,* Boca Raton, FL, 1973, CRC Press.
12. Slocum RH, Cummings JG: Amino acid analysis of physiological samples. In Hommes FA, editor: *Techniques in human biochemical genetics,* New York, 1991, Wiley-Liss, pp. 87-126.
13. Meites S, editor: *Pediatric clinical chemistry,* ed 3, Washington, DC, 1989, American Association for Clinical Chemistry.
14. Goldsmith RF, Earl JW, Cunningham AM: Determination of δ-aminobutyric acid and other amino acids in cerebrospinal fluid of pediatric patients by reversed-phase liquid chromatography, *Clin Chem* 33:1736-1740, 1987.
15. Cynober L, Dinh FN, Saizy R, et al: Plasma amino acid levels in the first few days after burn injury and their predictive value, *Intern Care Med* 9:325-331, 1983.
16. Jain KM, Rush BF Jr, Seelig RF, et al: Changes in plasma amino acid profiles following abdominal operations, *Surg Gynecol Obstet* 152:302-306, 1981.
17. Cynober L, Dinh FN, Blonde F, et al: Plasma and urinary amino acid pattern in severe burn patients: evolution throughout the healing period, *Am J Clin Nutr* 36:416-425, 1982.
18. Schott KJ, Meier D: Free amino acid pattern of cerebrospinal fluid in meningeal pathology, *Acta Neurol Scand* 75:304-309, 1987.

Leukocyte Acid Phosphatase (Cytochemical)	Fresh blood films (<1 wk old), bone marrow aspiration smears, and tissue imprints.	Acid phosphatase activity is demonstrable in almost all nucleated cells of the hematopoietic system.	None found.
Tartrate-inhibited acid phosphatase[1,2]			

DIAGNOSTIC INFORMATION   REMARKS

↑ Maple syrup urine disease, fasting ketosis, and liver disease   See also *Valine*.

In T-cell lymphoblastic leukemia, strong focal reaction in Golgi areas of leukemic cells is characteristic but not diagnostic.

Cell surface immunophenotyping is the best technique for the diagnosis of T-cell lymphoblastic leukemia.

See also Table II-14.

TEST NAME AND METHOD	SPECIMEN REQUIREMENTS	REFERENCE INTERVAL, CONVENTIONAL [INTERNATIONAL RECOMMENDED UNITS]	CHEMICAL INTERFERENCES AND IN VIVO EFFECTS

Leukocyte Acid Phosphatase—CONT

Tartrate-resistant acid phosphatase (TRAP)[1-4]

When the acid phosphatase reaction is carried out in the presence of L(+)-tartrate, normal cells do not show activity.

---

1. Beutler E, Lichtman MA, Coller B, editors: *Williams hematology,* ed 6, New York, 2000, McGraw-Hill.
2. Hayhoe FGJ, Quaglino D: *Haematological cytochemistry,* Edinburgh, 1980, Churchill Livingstone.
3. Brunning RD, McKenna RW: *Tumors of the bone marrow,* Washington, DC, 1994, Armed Forces Institute of Pathology.
4. Yam LT, Li CY, Lam KW: Tartrate-resistant acid phosphatase isoenzyme in the reticulum cells of leukemic reticuloendotheliosis, *N Engl J Med* 284:357-360, 1971.

TEST NAME AND METHOD	SPECIMEN REQUIREMENTS	REFERENCE INTERVAL, CONVENTIONAL $\times 10^3$ cells/mL	[INTERNATIONAL RECOMMENDED UNITS] $\times 10^9$ cells /L	CHEMICAL INTERFERENCES AND IN VIVO EFFECTS
Leukocyte Count (White Blood Cell Count, WBC Count)[1-3]	Whole blood (EDTA). Stable 24 hr at 23° C or 48 hr at 4° C. Do not use heparin.	Fetal,[4] 18-20 wk: 4.20 ± 0.83 (SD) × 1.0 21-22 wk: 4.19 ± 0.84 23-25 wk: 3.95 ± 0.69	[4.20 ± 0.83] [4.19 ± 0.84] [3.95 ± 0.69]	↑ C False increase in the presence of cryoproteins in stored blood
Electronic or hemocytometer	Fetal blood. Collect by percutaneous umbilical blood sampling (PUBS).	26-30 wk: 4.44 ± 0.85 Birth: (18.1) 9.0-30.0 12 hr: (22.8) 13.0-38.0 24 hr: (18.9) 9.4-34.0	[4.44 ± 0.85] [18.1] [9.0-30.0] [22.8] [13.0-38.0] [18.9] [9.4-34.0]	↓ C Chronic lymphocytic leukemia (some cases, when counts are performed on a Coulter counter, apparently because of fragility of cells), cold agglutinin disease, or
	CSF (see *Spinal Fluid White Cell Count*)	1 wk: (12.2) 5.0-21.0 2 wk: (11.4) 5.0-20.0 1 mo: (10.8) 5.0-19.5 6 mo: (11.9) 6.0-17.5 1 yr: (11.4) 6.0-17.5 2 yr: (10.6) 6.0-17.0 4 yr: (9.1) 5.5-15.5 6 yr: (8.5) 5.0-14.5 8 yr: (8.3) 4.5-13.5 10 yr: (8.1) 4.5-13.5 16 yr: (7.8) 4.5-13.0 21 yr: (7.4) 4.5-11.0	[12.2] [5.0-21.0] [11.4] [5.0-20.0] [10.8] [5.0-19.5] [11.9] [6.0-17.5] [11.4] [6.0-17.5] [10.6] [6.0-17.0] [9.1] [5.5-15.5] [8.5] [5.0-14.5] [8.3] [4.5-13.5] [8.1] [4.5-13.5] [7.8] [4.5-13.0] [7.4] [4.5-11.0]	monoclonal gammopathy (some cases, because of clumping of leukocytes) ↓ C Patients with untreated leukemia, with uremia, or on one of the following drugs may have lower counts if counts are performed on a Coulter counter: azathioprine, chlorambucil, cyclophosphamide, daunorubicin, hydroxyurea, melphalan, methortrexate, pred-
		Blacks[5]: 3.6-10.2 Data are insufficient for a reliable estimate for those aged <6 mo.[6,7]	[3.6-10.2]	nisone, and vincristine.[7,8] See Table II-18.

DIAGNOSTIC INFORMATION	REMARKS
↑ In hairy cell leukemia, the leukemic cells are usually strongly TRAP positive.	In hairy cell leukemia, TRAP is helpful in diagnosis, but it is not diagnostic. The diagnosis of hairy cell leukemia is made by integrating morphologic, cytochemical, and immunophenotypic findings. TRAP is also present in mast cells, osteoclasts, Gaucher cells, and in the leukemic cells of some cases of chronic lymphocytic leukemia.[3] See also Table II-14.
↑ Leukemia, leukemoid reaction, infection, acute hemolysis, after acute hemorrhage, immediately postsplenectomy,[9] and polycythemia vera *Physiological leukocytosis:* Exercise, emotional disturbance (fever, pain), menstruation, exposure to cold, anesthesia, obstetrical labor, paroxysmal tachycardia, sunlight, ultraviolet irradiation, convulsive seizures, nausea and vomiting, and electric shock *Pathological leukocytosis:* Infectious mononucleosis (variable), infectious lymphocytosis, mumps, chicken pox, German measles, viral hepatitis (variable), chronic infections; lymphomas, tissue necrosis; tumors involving peripheral blood, marrow, serous cavities, GI tract, liver; drug or metabolic intoxication, and hypersensitivity states ↓ (Leukopenia) *Certain infections:* Typhoid fever, paratyphoid fever, tularemia, brucellosis, influenza, measles, infectious hepatitis, psittacosis, infectious mononucleosis (unusual cases), rubella, scrub typhus, sand fly fever, dengue, relapsing fever, kala-azar, malaria, miliary tuberculosis, septicemia, and overwhelming bacterial infections *Hematopoietic disorders:* Pernicious anemia, some cases of acute leukemia and myelodysplasia, aplastic anemia, hypersplenism, Gaucher's disease, Felty's syndrome, Chédiak-Higashi syndrome, and paroxysmal nocturnal hemoglobunuria	According to extensive data collected since 1971 by the National Health and Nutrition Examination Surveys,[9] it is very probable that the leukocyte count in the U.S. population has declined between 4-10% in different population groups. Between ages 1 and 15 yr, males and females of both black and white races show a decrease in the leukocyte count, which then increases until age 20 yr, after which it has a downward trend. After age 30 yr, white males appear to have a somewhat higher leukocyte count than white females.[9] Leukocyte count is lower in persons of African and Asian ancestry than in Caucasians, owing entirely to lower concentrations of neutrophils. See Table II-18.[5,9,10]

TEST NAME AND METHOD	SPECIMEN REQUIREMENTS	REFERENCE INTERVAL, CONVENTIONAL [INTERNATIONAL RECOMMENDED UNITS]	CHEMICAL INTERFERENCES AND IN VIVO EFFECTS

Leukocyte Count—CONT

1. Henry JB, editor: *Clinical diagnosis and management by laboratory methods,* ed 20, Philadelphia, 2001, WB Saunders.
2. Beutler E, Lichtman MA, Coller B, editors: *Williams hematology,* ed 6, New York, 2000, McGraw-Hill.
3. Rudolph AM: *Pediatrics,* ed 18, Norwalk, CT, 1987, Appleton & Lange.
4. Forestier F, Daffos F, Galacteros F, et al: Hematologic values of 163 normal fetuses between 18 and 30 weeks of gestation, *Pediatr Res* 20:342-346, 1986.
5. Orfanakis NG, Ostlund RE, Bishop CR, et al: Normal blood leukocyte concentration values, *Am J Clin Pathol* 53:647-651, 1970.
6. Rudolph AM: *Pediatrics,* ed 18, Norwalk, CT, 1987, Appleton & Lange.
7. Koepke JA: Drug interference with leukocyte counting (spurious leukopenia), *Drug Ther* June:79-83, 1974.
8. Luke RG, Koepke JA, Siegel RR: The effects of immunosuppressive drugs and uremia on automated leukocyte counts, *Am J Clin Pathol* 56:503-507, 1971.
9. Yip R, Johnson C, Dallman PR: Age-related changes in laboratory values used in the diagnosis of anemia and iron deficiency, *Am J Clin Nutr* 39:427-436, 1984.
10. Van Assendelft OW: Reference values for the total differential leukocyte count, *Blood Cells* 11:77-96, 1985.
11. Saxena S, Wong ET: Heterogeneity of common hematologic parameters among racial, ethnic and gender subgroups, *Arch Pathol Lab Med* 114:715-719, 1990.

TEST NAME AND METHOD	SPECIMEN REQUIREMENTS	REFERENCE INTERVAL, CONVENTIONAL [INTERNATIONAL RECOMMENDED UNITS]	CHEMICAL INTERFERENCES AND IN VIVO EFFECTS
Leukocyte Differential Count (WBC Differential Count)[1,2] *Microscopy, Wright's or Wright's Giemsa stained smears*	Whole blood (EDTA). Stable for 24 hr at 23° C or 48 hr at 4° C. Do not use heparin.	See Table II-17.	See Table II-18.
Automated methods: *Electronic impedance, high-frequency current conductivity and laser light scatter: Coulter STKS, MAXM, GEN-S*			False-positive and false-negative detection of immature cells (blasts) is common, and frequency depends on the specific automated method in use.

DIAGNOSTIC INFORMATION	REMARKS

Physical agents: Ionizing radiation

Miscellaneous: Cachexia and inanition, anaphylactoid shock, and SLE

For differential diagnosis, refer to Table I-21.

See Table II-18.

Automated methods give higher relative and absolute monocyte counts than the manual method because of the tendency for larger monocytes to concentrate on the edge (uncounted area) of blood smears.

TEST NAME AND METHOD	SPECIMEN REQUIREMENTS	REFERENCE INTERVAL, CONVENTIONAL [INTERNATIONAL RECOMMENDED UNITS]	CHEMICAL INTERFERENCES AND IN VIVO EFFECTS
Leukocyte Differential Count—CONT			
Laser light scatter and peroxidase-based cyto-chemisty: Bayer Advia 1200			
Radiofrequency, direct current, and selective cell lysis: Sysmex SF-3000, SF-9000, and XE-2100			
Multiangle polar-ized scatter separa-tion: Abbott Cell-Dyn 3500R, 3700, 4000			

1. Rodak BF, editor: *Hematology; clinical principles and applications,* ed 2, Philadelphia, 2002, WB Saunders.
2. Esmon CT: The regulation of natural anticoagulant pathways, *Science* 235:1348-1351, 1987.

| **Leukocyte Esterases**

Naphthol AS-D chloroacetate, pH 7.0-7.6[1-6] | Blood or bone marrow films. If films are kept dry and in the dark, they are stable for 4 wk unfixed. Films are stable several months if fixed in buffered formalin/acetone. Histological sections from tissue fixed in buffered formalin are stable indefinitely. Decalcified acid-fixed tissues are unacceptable. | Positive: Neutrophilic series (strongest reaction in more mature cells), mast cells. Normal myeloblasts are negative, but leukemic myeloblasts may be positive.

Negative: Eosinophils, lymphocytes, plasma cells, normoblasts, megakaryocytes, and monocytes. | None found. |
| *α-Naphthyl acetate, pH 6.0-6.3[2-5]* | Blood or bone marrow films. If films are kept dry and in the dark, they are stable 1 wk unfixed. Histological sections cannot be used. | Positive: Monocytes (diffuse), macrophages, megakaryocytes, and platelets; variable in promyelocytes and in neutrophilic myelocytes; focal in plasma cells and some lymphocytes.

Negative: Myeloblasts, eosinophils, basophils, lymphocytes, and normoblasts. | |

DIAGNOSTIC INFORMATION	REMARKS

Positive: Blast cells of most cases of acute myeloid leukemia (AML)

Negative: Blast cells of acute lymphoid leukemia (ALL) and some AMLs (M5, M7)

Reaction parallels the reaction of Sudan black B and myeloperoxidase but is more consistently negative in monocytes. Sudan black B and peroxidase are more sensitive and reliable in neutrophilic series. This technique is useful in the subclassification of acute nonlymphocytic leukemia (ANLL).

See also Table II-14.

Positive: >20% of nonerythroid cells of M4 marrow, >80% of nonerythroid cells of M5 marrow, erythroid cells of M6 marrow, erythroid cells in megaloblastic anemia, leukemic cells in some cases of M3 and M7, and monocytes and monoblasts in myelodysplastic syndromes

Negative: Blast cells of M1, M2, M3, and most cases of ALL (focal cytoplasmic positivity in some cases of ALL)

Activity in monocytes, megakaryocytes, platelets, and plasma cells is inhibited by NaF, but it is not inhibited in lymphocytes and neutrophils. This method is useful in the subclassification of ANLL.

TEST NAME AND METHOD	SPECIMEN REQUIREMENTS	REFERENCE INTERVAL, CONVENTIONAL [INTERNATIONAL RECOMMENDED UNITS]	CHEMICAL INTERFERENCES AND IN VIVO EFFECTS
Leukocyte Esterases—CONT			
α-Naphthyl bu-tyrate, pH 6.0-6.3[2-5]		Positive: Monocytes (diffuse), macrophages, and some megakaryocytes (weak); focal in some lymphocytes.	
		Negative: Neutrophils, lymphocytes, and megakaryocytes.	

1. Rodak BF, editor: *Hematology; clinical principles and applications,* ed 2, Philadelphia, 2002, WB Saunders.
2. Beutler E, Lichtman MA, Coller B, editors: *Williams hematology,* ed 6, New York, 2000, McGraw-Hill.
3. Hayhoe FGJ, Quaglino D: *Haematological cytochemistry,* Edinburgh, 1980, Churchill Livingstone.
4. Li CY, Lam KW, Yam LT: Esterases in human leukocytes, *J Histochem Cytochem* 21:1-12, 1973.
5. Brunning RD, McKenna RW: *Tumors of the bone marrow,* Washington, DC, 1994, Armed Forces Institute of Pathology.
6. Jaffe ES, Harris NL, Stein H, et al, editors: *World Health Organization classification of tumours. Pathology and genetics of tumours of haematopoietic and lymphoid tissues,* Lyon, 2001, IARC Press.

TEST NAME AND METHOD	SPECIMEN REQUIREMENTS	REFERENCE INTERVAL, CONVENTIONAL [INTERNATIONAL RECOMMENDED UNITS]	CHEMICAL INTERFERENCES AND IN VIVO EFFECTS
Leukocyte Peroxidase (Myeloperoxi-dase)[1-3]	Freshly made films from blood or marrow. Process within 1 day or store in the dark no longer than 2 wk at room temperature. EDTA samples are satisfactory if films are made within 2 hr of collection.	Positive: Neutrophilic and eosinophilic granulocytes and precursors, monocytes (weaker, smaller granules), leukemic myeloblasts, and basophils (some methods)	None found.
Diaminobenzidine oxidation[1,4]		Negative: Early myeloblasts, lymphocytes, lymphoblasts, plasma cells, megakaryocytes, platelets, normoblasts, and basophils (most methods)	
p-Phenylene-diamine dihydrochloride[5]			
Flow cytometry (fluorescent-labeled myeloperoxidase antibody)[3,6]	Flow cytometry can be performed on EDTA or heparin anticoagulated blood or bone marrow stored at room temperature <24 hr or refrigerated <48 hr.		
Immunohisto-chemistry[3]			
	Immunohistochemical methods are available for frozen or paraffin-embedded tissue.		

1. Beutler E, Lichtman MA, Coller B, editors: *Williams hematology,* ed 6, New York, 2000, McGraw-Hill.
2. Brunning RD, McKenna RW: *Tumors of the bone marrow,* Washington, DC, 1994, Armed Forces Institute of Pathology.

DIAGNOSTIC INFORMATION	REMARKS

Positive: >20% of nonerythroid cells of M4 marrow, >80% of nonerythroid cells of M5 marrow, monocytes and monoblasts in myelodysplastic syndromes, and hairy cell leukemia (characteristic pattern)

Negative: Blast cells of M1, M2, M3, M7, and ALL

This reaction is less sensitive but more specific for monocytes than the α-naphthyl acetate method. Activity in monocytes is inhibited by NaF. A characteristic pattern of positivity (cytoplasmic granules and paranuclear crescents) is exhibited in a high proportion of cases of hairy cell leukemia.

Positive: In acute myeloid leukemia (AML; M1 through M6), ≥3% of blast cells (myeloblasts) are positive. Reaction is strongest in promyelocytic leukemia (M3); it is weak to negative in acute monocytic leukemia (M5).

Negative: Blast cells in acute lymphoid leukemia (ALL), M5 (usually), and M7. In hereditary myeloperoxidase deficiency, all neutrophils and monocytes are deficient, but eosinophils are positive.

See Table II-14.

Presence or absence of intracellular myeloperoxidase is used to distinguish AML from ALL. Myeloblasts that have no granules stainable with Wright's stain may be positive by cytochemical or immunostaining methods for peroxidase. Auer rods are positive. Peroxidase is demonstrable in the ultrastructure of platelets and in the nuclear envelope of megakaryocytes. A positive reaction may be used to define the megakaryoblasts of M7.

Peroxidase in mature neutrophils may be deficient in some mature neutrophils of myelodysplastic syndromes, in AML, and in severe infections.

Immunocytochemical methods are more sensitive for the detection of myeloperoxidase in the blasts of minimally differentiated acute myeloid leukemia (M0).[3,6]

Plasma levels of myeloperoxidase have been proposed to be an early predictor of myocardial infarction.

---

3.   Jaffe ES, Harris NL, Stein H, et al, editors: *World Health Organization classification of tumours. Pathology and genetics of tumours of haematopoietic and lymphoid tissues,* Lyon, 2001, IARC Press.

TEST NAME AND METHOD	SPECIMEN REQUIREMENTS	REFERENCE INTERVAL, CONVENTIONAL [INTERNATIONAL RECOMMENDED UNITS]				CHEMICAL INTERFERENCES AND IN VIVO EFFECTS

Leukocyte Peroxidase—CONT

4. Hayhoe FGJ, Quaglino D: *Haematological cytochemistry,* Edinburgh, 1980, Churchill Livingstone.
5. Rodak BF, editor: *Hematology; clinical principles and applications,* ed 2, Philadelphia, 2002, WB Saunders.

TEST NAME AND METHOD	SPECIMEN REQUIREMENTS					CHEMICAL INTERFERENCES AND IN VIVO EFFECTS
Light Chains, Free (L-Chains)[1-3] *Nephelometric,[4] immunofixation electrophoresis, RID, and Ouchterlony*	Serum or concentrated urine. Serum. Analyze fresh or stable at room temperature for 7 days. Store at 4° C for up to 4 wk, frozen at −20° C for 2 mo. Specimens without lipemia or hemolysis are preferred.	Kappa: Lambda: K/L Ratio:	*mg/dL[3]* 0.33-1.94 0.571-2.63 0.26-1.65	× 10	*mg/L* [3.3-19.4] [5.71-26.3]	β_2-microglobulin,[2] plasma expanders,[6] and other molecules can cause discreet bands in urine protein electrophoretic studies. These can be mistaken for a Bence Jones proteinuria if confirmatory immunochemical studies are not performed. Excessive turbidity can affect nephelometric methods.
	Urine. Analyze fresh, or store at 4° C for up to 4 wk. For prolonged storage, frozen at ≤−20° C.[4]	Kappa: Lambda: Ratio K/L:	*mg/dL[5]* 0.039-1.5 0.081-1.0 0.461-4.00	× 10	*mg/L* 0.39-15.1 0.81-10.1	

1. Knowles DM, editor: *Neoplastic hematopathology,* ed 2, Philadelphia, 2001, Lippincott Williams & Wilkins.
2. Handy B: Urinary beta-2 microglobulin masquerading as a Bence Jones protein, *Arch Pathol Lab Med* 125:555-557, 2001.
3. Tate JR, Gill D, Cobcroft R, et al: Practical considerations for the measurement of free light chains in serum, *Clin Chem* 49:1252-1257, 2003.
4. Katzmann JA, Clark RJ, Abraham RS, et al: Serum reference intervals and diagnostic ranges for free kappa and free lambda immunoglobulin light chains: relative sensitivity for detection of monoclonal light chains, *Clin Chem* 48:1437-1444, 2002.
5. *Package insert, FREELITE™ Reagent Kit, The Binding Site,* July 21, 2004, Birmingham, UK.
6. Summer R, Lapin A: Plasma expanders as a cause of paraproteinuria-like artifact, *Lancet* 337:499, 1991.
7. Cohen G: Immunoglobulin light chains in uremia, *Kidney Int* 84(suppl):S15-18, 2003.
8. Hopper JE, Sequeira W, Martellotto J, et al: Clinical relapse in systemic lupus erythematosus: correlation with antecedent elevation of urinary free light-chain immunoglobulin, *J Clin Immunol* 9:338-350, 1989.
9. Pritchard PH, Bergseth M, McLeod R, et al: Urinary proteins in a patient with Tangier disease, *Clin Biochem* 18:98-101, 1985.

6. Kaleem Z, Crawford E, Pathan MH, et a.: Flow cytometric analysis of acute leukemias, *Arch Pathol Lab Med* 127:42-48, 2003.

↑ S *Polyclonal:* Immunoglobulin free light chains undergo primarily renal catabolism, and renal dysfunction is associated with increased serum values.[7]

↑ S *Monoclonal:* Serum concentrations are also frequently increased with disorders associated with a monoclonal gammopathy.

↑ U *Polyclonal:* Increased urinary concentrations of polyclonal free light chains can be found with impaired renal protein reabsorption (tubular proteinuria) or with conditions involving B-lymphocyte activation such as systemic lupus erythematosus[8] and chronic infectious processes.[9] Despite their polyclonal nature, multiple, evenly spaced bands can be seen with urine immunofixation studies using concentrated urine samples,[10] This pattern can complicate the identification of/or be mistaken for the presence of a Bence Jones protein.[1]

↑ U *Monoclonal:* Monoclonal free light chains are characteristically found with malignant B-cell–derived disorders such as multiple myeloma, plasmacytomas, Waldenström's macroglobulinemia, and amyloidosis. They are also found with the benign monoclonal gammopathy of undetermined significance and in association with a wide variety of connective tissue, endocrine, hematologic, inflammatory, neurologic, and neoplastic conditions.[2]

Whole immunoglobulin molecules consist of two identical light chains joined to two identical heavy chains. Although there are five classes of heavy chains (μ, γ, α, δ, ϵ), there are only two types of light chains (κ, λ). Antigen recognition involves the variable regions of both the heavy and light chains.

Because they are produced in excess of immunoglobulin heavy chains, small quantities of free light chains are normally found in both serum and urine.[7] These exist as monomers, fragments, and polymers. Urine concentrations are also affected by adequacy of renal function.

Reagent strips and standard urine protein precipitation or dye-binding methods are not adequate for the detection of Bence Jones proteins. Protein electrophoresis of concentrated urine combined with immunofixation is currently recommended. Some monoclonal light chains, however, have "hidden determinates" and despite the use of polyclonal reagent antisera cannot be typed by immunofixation. In such cases, other techniques, such as immunoselection, have been used.[11]

MW: 23,000.

10. Harrison HH: The "ladder light chain" or "pseudo-oligoclonal" pattern in urinary immunofixation electrophoresis (IFE) studies: a distinctive IFE pattern and an explanatory hypothesis relating it to free polyclonal light chains, *Clin Chem* 37:1559-1564, 1991.

11. Netto D, Vladutiu AO: A simple technique for identification of "un-reactive" light chains of immunoglobulins, *Clin Chim Acta* 116:253-260, 1981.

TEST NAME AND METHOD	SPECIMEN REQUIREMENTS	REFERENCE INTERVAL, CONVENTIONAL [INTERNATIONAL RECOMMENDED UNITS]			CHEMICAL INTERFERENCES AND IN VIVO EFFECTS
Lipase (Triacylglycerol acyl-hydrolase; EC 3.1.1.3)[1] *pH-Stat titration, 37° C*[2]	Serum. Stable at room temperature for several days if bacterial contamination is avoided. Store refrigerated or frozen.	*U/L* <200 <160	× 0.017	*μKat/L* [>3.4] [<2.72]	↑ V Drugs causing spasm of the sphincter of Oddi (e.g., narcotic analgesics, bethanechol, secretin) or pancreatitis (see *Amylase* for list of drugs causing increase), and heparin (release of lipoprotein and hepatic lipases)
Fluorimetric Progen Conflulip (fluorescing glyceride-forming triglyceride		0-120 mU/L			↑ C Severe hemolysis interferes with visual endpoint titrations. ↓ V Protamine
[1-oleoyl-2, 3-diacetylglycerol])[3]		23-300 U/L		[0.4-5.0 μKat/L]	↓ C Diisopropyl fluorophosphate, EDTA, heavy metals, and quinine
Roche Cobas Integra (Mira, Hitachi) and Polymedico: Colorimetric [1,2-o-dilauryl-rac-glycero-3-glutaric acid-(6-methyl-resoruffin)]	Serum or lithium heparin.	13-60 U/L		[0.22-1.00 μKat/L]	↓ Gross lipemia (chemical effect) ↓ Aminoasalicylate
Roche Cobas Integra: Turbidimetric (Triolein; Colipase optimized)		<190 U/L		[<3.2 μKat/L]	
Pointe Scientific (1,2-diglyceride)		<60 U/L		[<1.00 μKat/L]	
Alpha Diagnostic International (ELISA: lipase AB)		26-150 U/L		[0.4-2.5 μKat/L]	

1. Tietz NW, Shuey DF: Lipase in serum—the elusive enzyme: an overview, *Clin Chem* 39:746-756, 1993.
2. Tietz NW, Huang WY, Rauh DF, et al: Laboratory tests in the differential diagnosis of hyperamylasemia, *Clin Chem* 32:301-307, 1986.
3. Mauck JC, Weaver MS, Stanton C: Development of a Kodak Ektachem clinical chemistry slide for lipase, *Clin Chem* 30:1058-1059, 1984.

DIAGNOSTIC INFORMATION	REMARKS

Ascitic fluid may have very high lipase activity in pancreatitis. Pleural transudates may contain lipase activity; the lipase rarely comes from a lung tumor.

Methods with substrates such as tributyrin, triacetin, methyl butyrate, β-naphthyl laurate, β-naphthyl palmitate, or β-nitrophenyl stearate should not be used because these compounds are true substrates for esterases, not lipase. Good clinical correlation with pancreatitis has been shown for methods employing emulsified vegetable oils (e.g., olive oil, corn oil) because lipase acts only at the interface of an oil-in-water emulsion.[2]

Two or more lipase isoforms may be present in serum.[1]

The Vitros method utilizes an unconventional substrate of questionable specificity for pancreatic lipase.[1]

4. Tietz NW: Support of the diagnosis of pancreatitis by enzyme tests—old problems, new techniques, *Clin Chim Acta* 257:85-98, 1997.
5. Yadav D, Agarwal N, Pitchumoni CS: A critical evaluation of laboratory tests in acute pancreatitis, *Am J Gastroenterol* 97:1309-1318, 2002.

TEST NAME AND METHOD	SPECIMEN REQUIREMENTS	REFERENCE INTERVAL, CONVENTIONAL [INTERNATIONAL RECOMMENDED UNITS]				CHEMICAL INTERFERENCES AND IN VIVO EFFECTS

Lipoprotein(a) [Lp(a)][1-19]
 	
Immunoassay[15,20,21]
 	
Electrophoresis[3,15,22-24]
 	
Chromatography (e.g., lectin affinity/lysine-sepharose)[3,13,25-27]
	Serum, plasma. Fasting is not required. Stable for 1 day at 4° C, progressive decrease in immunoreactive Lp(a) with freezing, especially at −20° C. It is best to assay fresh specimens as soon as possible after blood collection; freezing at −70° C is acceptable. Avoid repeated freezing and thawing.	*Lipoprotein(a):*
		
		        mg/dL[28]
		        5th-95th
		        Percentile
		African
		Americans
		F: 1.8-29.9
		M: 1.7-26.5
		Caucasian
		F: 0.7-22.2
		M: 0.5-21.3
		
		Recommended Cutpoint[12]*:*
		<30 mg/dL
		
		Lipoprotein(a) Cholesterol:
		        mg/dL[26]
		        5th-95th
		        Percentile
		F: 1.24-20.1
		M: 1.35-19.6
			× 0.01
			
			× 0.01
			
			× 0.01
				g/L
				5th-95th
				Percentile
				
				[0.018-0.299]
				[0.017-0.265]
				
				[0.007-0.222]
				[0.005-0.213]
				
				[<0.30 g/L]
				[<75 nmol/L]
				
				g/L
				5th-95th
				Percentile
				[0.012-0.201]
				[0.014-0.196]
						↑ V Hypothyroidism, types 1 and 2 diabetes, bisphosphonates, proteinuria, cigarette smoking, intense exercise, pregnancy, infection, and inflammation.
						
						↓ V Estrogens, tamoxifen, stanozolol, niacin, neomycin, aspirin, *N*-acetylcysteine, cyclosporine, thyroid hormone replacement, omega-3 fatty acids (fish oil), strict vegetarianism, acute myocardial infarction, stroke, and hospitalization for CABG.

1. Ariyo AA, Thach C, Tracy R, for the Cardiovascular Health Study Investigators: Lp(a) lipoprotein, vascular disease, and mortality in the elderly, *N Engl J Med* 349:2108-2115, 2003.

2. Bostom AG, Shemin D, Lapane KL, et al: Hyperhomocysteinemia, hyperfibrinogenemia, and lipoprotein(a) excess in maintenance dialysis patients: a matched case-control study, *Atherosclerosis* 125:91-101, 1996.

3. Bradley WA, Gianturco SH, Segrest JP, editors: *Plasma lipoproteins, part C: quantitation. Methods in enzymology, vol 263,* San Diego, CA, 1996, Academic Press.

4. Craig WY, Neveux LM, Palomaki GE, et al: Lipoprotein(a) as a risk factor for ischemic heart disease: metaanalysis of prospective studies, *Clin Chem* 44:2301-2306, 1998.

5. Danesh J, Collins R, Peto R: Lipoprotein(a) and coronary heart disease: meta-analysis of prospective studies, *Circulation* 102:1082-1085, 2000.

6. Hopkins PN, Wu LL, Hunt SC, et al: Lipoprotein(a) interactions with lipid and nonlipid risk factors in early familial coronary artery disease, *Arterioscl Thromb Vasc Biol* 17:2783-2792, 1997.

7. Kronenberg F, Kronenberg MF, Kiechl S, et al: Role of lipoprotein(a) and apolipoprotein(a) phenotype in atherogenesis: prospective results from the Bruneck Study, *Circulation* 100:1154-1160, 1999.

8. Kronenberg F, Lobentanz E-M, Konig P, et al: Effect of sample storage on the measurement of lipoprotein[a], apolipoproteins B and A-IV, total and high density lipoprotein cholesterol and triglycerides, *J Lipid Res* 35:1318-1328, 1994.

9. Laker MF, Evans K: Analysis of apolipoproteins, *Ann Clin Biochem* 33:5-22, 1996.

10. Lippi G, Guidi G: Lipoprotein(a): an emerging cardiovascular risk factor, *Crit Rev Clin Lab Sci* 40:1-42, 2003.

11. Marcovina SM, Albers JJ, Scanu AM, et al: Use of a reference material proposed by the International Federation of Clinical Chemistry and Laboratory Medicine to evaluate analytical methods for the determination of plasma lipoprotein(a), *Clin Chem* 46:1956-1967, 2000.

12. Marcovina SM, Koschinsky ML, Albers JJ, et al: Report of the National Heart, Lung, and Blood Institute workshop on lipoprotein(a) and cardiovascular disease: recent advances and future directions, *Clin Chem* 49:1785-1796, 2003.

DIAGNOSTIC INFORMATION	REMARKS

↑ Premature coronary artery disease, stenosis of cerebral arteries, uncontrolled diabetes, hypothyroidism, chronic renal failure, and nephrotic syndrome.

Increased serum Lp(a) concentrations are associated with increased risk of premature coronary artery disease and stroke. Because Lp(a) levels are highly heritable, Lp(a) may be an important marker for premature CHD, especially among Caucasians. Although Lp(a) levels are higher in African-Americans than in Caucasians, associated CHD risk appears to be less.

In view of standardization issues, it is important that each laboratory establish its own reference interval.

Intraindividual variability averages ~8-9%.

13. Nguyen TT, Ellefson RD, Hodge DO, et al: Predictive value of electrophoretically detected lipoprotein(a) for coronary heart disease and cerebrovascular disease in a community-based cohort of 9936 men and women, *Circulation* 96:1390-1397, 1997.

14. Rader DJ, Hoeg JM, Brewer HB: Quantitation of plasma apolipoproteins in the primary and secondary prevention of coronary artery disease, *Ann Intern Med* 120:1012-1025, 1994.

15. Rifai N, Warnick GR, Dominiczak MH, editors: *Handbook of lipoprotein testing,* ed 2, Washington, DC, 2000, AACC Press.

16. Scanu AM: Atherothrombogenicity of lipoprotein(a): the debate, *Am J Cardiol* 82:26Q-33Q, 1998.

17. Sgoutas DS, Tuten T: Effect of freezing and thawing of serum on the immunoassay of lipoprotein(a), *Clin Chem* 38:1873-1877, 1992.

18. Young DS: *Effects of drugs on clinical laboratory tests,* ed 5, Washington, DC, 2000, AACC Press.

19. Young DS: *Effects of preanalytical variables on clinical laboratory tests,* ed 2, Washington, DC, 1997, AACC Press.

20. Levine DM, Sloan BJ, Donner JE, et al: Automated measurement of lipoprotein(a) by immunoturbidimetric analysis, *Int J Clin Lab Res* 22:173-178, 1992.

21. Taddei-Peters WC, Butman BT, Jones GR, et al: Quantification of lipoprotein(a) particles containing various apolipoprotein(a) isoforms by a monoclonal anti-apo(a) capture antibody and a polyclonal anti-apolipoprotein B detection antibody sandwich enzyme immunoassay, *Clin Chem* 39:1382-1389, 1993.

22. Contois JH, Gillmor R, Moore R, et al: Quantitative determination of cholesterol in lipoprotein fractions by electrophoresis, *Clin Chim Acta* 282:1-14, 1999.

23. Lynch GJ, Arbuckle GB, Cowley DM, et al: Routine lipid screening by cholesterol staining electrophoresis including lipoprotein(a) cholesterol (Lp(a)-c), *Aust J Med Sci* 19:123-126, 1998.

24. Nauck M, Winkler K, Marz W, et al: Quantitative determination of high-, low-, and very-low density lipoproteins and lipoprotein(a) by agarose gel electrophoresis and enzymatic cholesterol staining, *Clin Chem* 41:1761-1767, 1995.

TEST NAME AND METHOD	SPECIMEN REQUIREMENTS	REFERENCE INTERVAL, CONVENTIONAL [INTERNATIONAL RECOMMENDED UNITS]	CHEMICAL INTERFERENCES AND IN VIVO EFFECTS

Lipoprotein(a)—CONT

25. Ordovas JM, editor: *Lipoprotein protocols,* Totowa, NJ, 1998, Humana Press.

26. Seman LJ, DeLuca C, Jenner JL, et al: Lipoprotein(a)-cholesterol and coronary heart disease in the Framingham Heart Study, *Clin Chem* 45:1039-1046, 1999.

27. Seman LJ, Jenner JL, McNamara JR, et al: Quantification of lipoprotein(a) in plasma by assaying cholesterol in lectin-bound plasma fraction, *Clin Chem* 40:400-403, 1994.

| **Lipoprotein Lipase** (LPL, EC 3.1.1.3)[1-13]

Radioenzymatic (activity)[1,7-10,14]

ELISA (mass)[1,7,9] | Plasma (EDTA or heparin), fasting. Draw 15-20 min after IV heparin injection (100 U/kg). Avoid hemolysis. Enzyme is unstable; process plasma and freeze if not assayed immediately. | LPL activity in postheparin plasma has been found to vary 10-fold between different laboratories. There are no representative reference ranges available. The following data are for illustrative purpose only.

mU/mL^9
Preheparin: 1.5 ± 1.0
Postheparin: 304 ± 108

ng/mL^9
Preheparin: 93.9 ± 37.2
Postheparin: 847 ± 289 | ↑ C Requires apo C-II as activator (serum or HDL), hemolysis.

↑ V Diets high in carbohydrates and polyunsaturated fats, ethanol, fibric acid derivative (e.g., clofibrate, gemfibrozil), niacin, and aerobic exercise.

↓ C Protamine sulfate, high salt concentrations, and apo C-III are inhibitors.

↓ V Acute ethanol ingestion, dietary fat restriction, and insulin treatment. |

1. Blades B, Vega GL, Grundy SM: Activities of lipoprotein lipase and hepatic triglyceride lipase in postheparin plasma of patients with low concentrations of HDL cholesterol, *Arterioscl Thromb* 13:1227-1235, 1993.

2. Bradley WA, Gianturco SH, Segrest JP, editors: *Plasma lipoproteins, part C: quantitation. Methods in enzymology, vol 263,* San Diego, CA, 1996, Academic Press.

3. Eckel RH: Lipoprotein lipase: a multifunctional enzyme relevant to common metabolic diseases, *N Engl J Med* 320:1060-1068, 1989.

4. Henry JB, editor: *Clinical diagnosis and management by laboratory methods,* ed 19, Philadelphia, 1996, WB Saunders.

5. Hokanson JE: Lipoprotein lipase gene variants and risk of coronary disease: a quantitative analysis of population-based studies, *Int J Clin Lab Res* 27:24-34, 1997.

6. Rader DJ: Lipid disorders. In Topol EJ, editor: *Textbook of cardiovascular medicine,* ed 2, Philadelphia, 2002, Lippincott Williams & Wilkins.

7. Rifai N, Warnick GR, Dominiczak MH, editors: *Handbook of lipoprotein testing,* ed 2, Washington, DC, 2000, AACC Press.

8. Tornvall P, Karpe F, Proudler A, et al: High-density lipoprotein: relations to metabolic parameters and severity of coronary artery disease, *Metabolism* 45:1375-1382, 1996.

9. Tornvall P, Olivecrona G, Karpe F, et al: Lipoprotein lipase mass and activity in plasma and their increase after heparin are separate parameters with different relations to plasma lipoproteins, *Arterioscler Thromb Vasc Biol* 15:1086-1093, 1995.

DIAGNOSTIC INFORMATION   **REMARKS**

28. Marcovina SM, Albers JJ, Jacobs DR, et al: Lipoprotein [a] concentrations and apolipoprotein [a] phenotypes in caucasians and African Americans: the CARDIA Study, *Arterioscl Thromb* 13:1037-1045, 1993.

↓ Hypertriglyceridemia (hyperchylomicronemia and increased VLDL), low HDL cholesterol. Associated with recurrent abdominal pain, pancreatitis, hepatosplenomegaly, eruptive xanthomas, and lipemia retinalis, obesity, diabetes, hypothyroidism, chronic renal failure, pancreatitis, alcoholism, and nephrotic syndrome.

LPL is synthesized in many tissues, but it is predominantly active in adipose tissue, skeletal muscle, and cardiac muscle. It is transferred to capillary endothelium where it hydrolyzes triglycerides from triglyceride-rich lipoproteins. Although LPL is frequently measured in adipose and muscle tissue, a simpler method involves measurement in plasma after an IV injection of heparin to release LPL and hepatic triglyceride lipase (HTGL) from the vascular endothelial surface into the blood. Unlike LPL, HTGL is resistant to protamine and salt and does not require apo C-II as a cofactor. Use of a specific inhibitor or antibody to LPL or HTGL allows the selective measurement of one of the two enzymes in postheparin plasma.

LPL mass can also be measured directly in plasma by ELISA. LPL mass is highly correlated with LPL activity in postheparin plasma. LPL measurement in postheparin plasma is assumed to reflect the LPL available at the endothelial surface.

LPL activity before and after heparin injection do not correlate, suggesting a lack of equilibrium between bound and circulating LPL levels.

10. Vilella E, Joven J, Fernandez M, et al: Lipoprotein lipase in human plasma is mainly inactive and associated with cholesterol-rich lipoproteins, *J Lipid Res* 34:1555-1564, 1993.

11. Young DS: *Effects of drugs on clinical laboratory tests,* ed 5, Washington, DC, 2000, AACC Press.

12. Young DS: *Effects of preanalytical variables on clinical laboratory tests,* ed 2, Washington, DC, 1997, AACC Press.

13. Zechner R: The tissue-specific expression of lipoprotein lipase: implications for energy and lipoprotein metabolism, *Curr Opin Lipid* 8:77-86, 1997.

14. Segrest JP, Albers JJ, editors: *Plasma lipoproteins, part A: preparation, structure, and molecular biology. Method in enzymology, vol 128,* Orlando, FL, 1986, Academic Press.

TEST NAME AND METHOD	SPECIMEN REQUIREMENTS	REFERENCE INTERVAL, CONVENTIONAL [INTERNATIONAL RECOMMENDED UNITS]	CHEMICAL INTERFERENCES AND IN VIVO EFFECTS
Lipoprotein-Associated Phospholipase A$_2$ (Lp-PLA$_2$)[1-4] *Immunoassay*[5]	EDTA plasma, serum. Separate plasma from cells within 4 hr. Stable up to 3 days at 4° C.	*ng/mL*[5] *5th-95th Percentile* 40-70 yr F: 120-342 M: 131-376	

1. Ballantyne CM, Hoogeveen RC, Bang H, et al: Lipoprotein-associated phospholipase A$_2$, high-sensitivity C-reactive protein, and risk for incident coronary heart disease in middle-aged men and women in the Atherosclerosis Risk in Communities (ARIC) Study, *Circulation* 109:837-842, 2004.

2. Blake GJ, Dada N, Fox JC, et al: A prospective evaluation of lipoprotein-associated phospholipase A$_2$ levels and the risk of future cardiovascular events in women, *J Am Coll Cardiol* 38:1302-1306, 2001.

3. Caslake MJ, Packard CJ, Suckling KE, et al: Lipoprotein-associated phospholipase A$_2$, platelet-activating factor acetylhydrolase: a potential new risk factor for coronary artery disease, *Atherosclerosis* 150:413-419, 2000.

4. Packard CJ, O'Reilly DSJ, Caslake MJ, et al: Lipoprotein-associated phospholipase A$_2$ as an independent predictor of coronary heart disease, *N Engl J Med* 343:1148-1155, 2000.

5. DiaDexus, Inc.: *PLAC test, enzyme immunoassay for the determination of Lp-PLA2 in human plasma,* South San Francisco, CA, 2004, DiaDexus, Inc.

Liver Kidney Microsome Type 1 Antibodies (LKM1) *Indirect immunofluorescence* *Solid phase EIA*	Serum, frozen or refrigerated is preferable.	Negative is normal. Sera reactive at a ≥1-20 dilution are positive. Negative: <20 U Equivocal: 20-25 U Positive: >25 U Results are expressed in arbitrary units. Interpretive reference intervals vary with reagent manufacturer. Results are semiquantitative.	None known.

1. Czaja AJ, Homburger HA: Autoantibodies in liver disease, *Gastroenterology* 120:239-249, 2001.

DIAGNOSTIC INFORMATION	REMARKS
An elevated Lp-PLA$_2$ concentration is associated with an increased risk of CHD.	Lp-PLA$_2$ (also known as platelet-activating factor acetylhydrolase) is a member of the phospholipase A$_2$ enzyme family, primarily secreted by macrophages. Lp-PLA$_2$ attaches to circulating LDL particles where it apparently contributes to atherogenesis by attacking oxidized LDL, generating lysophosphatidylcholine and oxidized fatty acids, which subsequently trigger the expression of adhesion molecules and inflammatory cytokines.
LKM1 antibodies are a serologic marker for autoimmune hepatitis type 2. Type 2 AIH patients tend to be young, female, and have a severe disease that responds well to treatment with immunosuppressive drugs,[1]	LKM1 antibodies react with cytochrome monooxygenase P450 2D6. LKM1 antibodies that react with different epitopes than in patients with AIH type 2 occur in some patients with chronic hepatitis C infection (1).

TEST NAME AND METHOD	SPECIMEN REQUIREMENTS	REFERENCE INTERVAL, CONVENTIONAL [INTERNATIONAL RECOMMENDED UNITS]		CHEMICAL INTERFERENCES AND IN VIVO EFFECTS
Low-Density Lipoprotein Cholesterol (LDL-C)[1-13] *Calculation*[11,14-19] Direct/homogeneous[11,20-23] *Ultracentrifugation/ β-quantification*[11,24-26] Lipoprotein precipitation[11,24] Electrophoresis[11,25,27,28] Chromatography[11,24,25]	Serum, plasma (EDTA or perhaps heparin, but not oxalate, fluoride, or citrate), fasting ≥12 hr is recommended; nonfasting specimen is acceptable for direct measurement of LDL-C if it is not part of a fasting lipid profile. Patient should be sitting for 5 min before blood draw; avoid prolonged tourniquet use. Stable 1-7 days at 4° C. Avoid repeated freezing and thawing.	*Recommended Cutpoints*[4,29] Adults: Optimal: <100 mg/dL × 0.0259 Near optimal: <130 mg/dL Borderline high: 130-159 mg/dL High: 160-189 mg/dL Very high: ≥190 *Children:* Acceptable: <110 mg/dL × 0.0259 Borderline: 110-129 mg/dL High: ≥130 mg/dL *Therapeutic goals*[4,5] (see *Remarks*) High risk (CHD or CHD risk equivalents): <100 mg/dL Moderately high risk (2+ risk factors; 10-yr risk 10-20%): <130 mg/dL Moderate risk (2+ risk factors; 10-yr risk <10%): <130 mg/dL Lower risk (0-1 risk factors): <160 mg/dL	[<2.85 mmol/L] [<3.37 mmol/L] [3.37-4.12 mmol/L] [4.14-4.90 mmol/L] [≥4.92 mmol/L] [<2.85 mmol/L] [2.85-3.34 mmol/L] [≥3.37 mmol/L] [<2.59 mmol/L] [<3.37 mmol/L] [<3.37 mmol/L] [4.14 mmol/L]	↑ V Androgens (including anabolic steroids), β-blockers, cyclosporine, danazol, diuretics, corticosteroids, high saturated fat and high cholesterol diet, progestins, and retinoids. ↓ V Aminosalicylic acid, cholestyramine, colestipol, cyproterone, acetate, doxazosin, estrogens, fibric acid derivatives (e.g., clofibrate, gemfibrozil), HMG CoA reductase inhibitors (statins), interferon, interleukin, ketoconazole, neomycin, niacin, prazosin, probucol, terazosin, thyroxine, low saturated fat and low cholesterol diet, high polyunsaturated fat diet, weight loss in overweight individuals, exercise, hospitalization for AMI, stroke, and cardiac catheterization.

	mg/dL[30] *5th-95th Percentile*		*mmol/L* *5th-95th Percentile*
Non-Hispanic black 12-19 yr			
M:	60-138	× 0.0259	[1.55-3.57]
F:	58-154		[1.50-3.99]
Non-Hispanic white 12-19 yr			
M:	48-152		[1.24-3.94]
F:	54-161		[1.40-4.17]
Mexican American 12-19 yr			
M:	56-135		[1.45-3.50]
F:	52-139		[1.35-3.60]

| DIAGNOSTIC INFORMATION | REMARKS |

↑ Familial hypercholesterolemia, familial combined hyperlipidemia, familial dysbetalipoproteinemia (type III), familial defective apo B-100, polygenic (sporadic) hypercholesterolemia, and coronary heart disease. Secondary elevation caused by hypothyroidism, nephrotic syndrome, obstructive liver disease, hepatocellular disorders, pregnancy, diabetes, chronic renal failure, and Cushing's syndrome.

↓ Hypobetalipoproteinemias, abetalipoproteinemia. Secondary decrease caused by hyperthyroidism, severe hepatocellular dysfunction, infection, inflammation, and malignancy.

There is a direct relationship between LDL-C and the incidence of coronary heart disease (CHD). Intervention to decrease LDL-C will decrease CHD risk.

The National Cholesterol Education Program (NCEP) recommends that all adults aged >20 yr be screened for CHD risk with measurement of total cholesterol, LDL-C, HDL-C, and triglyceride concentrations. Treatment decisions and therapeutic goals are also largely based on LDL-C concentrations.

Recent epidemiological studies have confirmed the efficacy of aggressive cholesterol-lowering therapy in high-risk patients. In high-risk individuals, the recommended LDL-C goal is <100 mg/dL, but when risk is very high, an optional goal is <70 mg/dL or a 30-40% reduction in LDL-C levels.

In clinical laboratories LDL-C is most often determined using the "Friedewald formula" using measured values for total cholesterol (TC), HDL-C, and triglyceride (TG):

$$LDL\text{-}C = (TC) - (HDL\text{-}C) - (VLDL\text{-}C)$$

where:

$$VLDL\text{-}C \ (mg/dL) = \frac{TG \ (mg/dL)}{5}$$

or:

$$VLDL\text{-}C \ (mmol/L) = \frac{TG \ (mmol/L)}{1.181}$$

This calculation is not valid for specimens having TG >400 mg/dL [>4.52 mmol/L], for patients with type III hyperlipoproteinemia or chylomicronemia, or nonfasting specimens. Alternative equations for LDL-C estimation based on apo B measurement are not subject to these same assumptions but are less well validated.

Intraindividual variability in LDL-C measurement averages 9.5%. Because of analytical and biological variability, at least two serial samples may be necessary for clinical decision making.

The goal for LDL-C determination, as defined by the Working Group on Lipoprotein Measurement of NCEP, is a total error ≤12%, consistent with a precision ≤4% CV and a bias ±4%.

TEST NAME AND METHOD	SPECIMEN REQUIREMENTS	REFERENCE INTERVAL, CONVENTIONAL [INTERNATIONAL RECOMMENDED UNITS]		CHEMICAL INTERFERENCES AND IN VIVO EFFECTS

Low-Density Lipoprotein Cholesterol—CONT

		mg/dL[31] *5th-95th Percentile*		*mmol/L* *5th-95th Percentile*
Black				
45-49 yr				
M:		79-201	× 0.0259	[2.05-5.21]
F:		71-202		[1.84-5.23]
50-54 yr				
M:		68-220		[1.76-5.70]
F:		74-215		[1.92-5.57]
55-59 yr				
M:		72-219		[1.86-5.67]
F:		77-218		[1.99-5.65]
60-64 yr				
M:		83-207		[2.15-5.36]
F:		85-221		[2.20-5.72]
White				
45-49 yr				
M:		79-199		[2.05-5.15]
F:		73-184		[1.89-4.77]
50-54 yr				
M:		85-202		[2.20-5.23]
F:		77-204		[1.99-5.28]
55-59 yr				
M:		84-202		[2.18-5.23]
F:		84-212		[2.18-5.49]
60-64 yr				
M:		81-196		[2.10-5.08]
F:		83-210		[2.15-5.44]

1. Bachorik PS, Ross JW: National Cholesterol Education Program recommendations for measurement of low-density lipoprotein cholesterol: executive summary. The National Cholesterol Education Program Working Group on Lipoprotein Measurement, *Clin Chem* 41:1414-1420, 1995.

2. Cohn JS, McNamara JR, Cohn SD, et al: Postprandial plasma lipoprotein changes in human subjects of different ages, *J Lipid Res* 29:469-479, 1988.

3. Cooper GR, Myers GL, Smith J, et al: Blood lipid measurements: variations and practical utility, *JAMA* 267:1652-1660, 1992.

4. Expert Panel on Detection, Evaluation, and Treatment of High Blood Cholesterol in Adults: Executive Summary of the Third Report of the National Cholesterol Education Program (NCEP) Expert Panel on Detection, Evaluation, and Treatment of High Blood Cholesterol in Adults (Adult Treatment Panel III), *JAMA* 285:2486-2497, 2001.

5. Grundy SM, Cleeman JI, Merz CN, et al: Implications of recent clinical trials for the National Cholesterol Education Program Adult Treatment Program III guidelines, *Circulation* 110:227-239, 2004.

6. Harris N, Neufeld EJ, Newburger JW, et al: Analytical performance and clinical utility of a direct LDL-cholesterol assay in a hyperlipidemic pediatric population, *Clin Chem* 42:1182-1188, 1996.

7. Henkin Y, Como JA, Oberman A: Secondary dyslipidemia: inadvertent effects of drugs in clinical practice, *JAMA* 267:961-968, 1992.

DIAGNOSTIC INFORMATION	REMARKS

8. Henry JB, editor: *Clinical diagnosis and management by laboratory methods,* ed 19, Philadelphia, 1996, WB Saunders.

9. Ockene IS, Chiriboga DE, Stanek EJ, et al: Seasonal variation in serum cholesterol levels, *Arch Intern Med* 164:863-870, 2004.

10. Rader DJ: Lipid disorders. In Topol EJ, editor: *Textbook of cardiovascular medicine,* ed 2, Philadelphia, 2002, Lippincott Williams & Wilkins.

11. Rifai N, Warnick GR, Dominiczak MH, editors: *Handbook of lipoprotein testing,* ed 2, Washington, DC, 2000, AACC Press.

12. Young DS: *Effects of drugs on clinical laboratory tests,* ed 5, Washington, DC, 2000, AACC Press.

13. Young DS: *Effects of preanalytical variables on clinical laboratory tests,* ed 2, Washington, DC, 1997, AACC Press.

14. Bairaktari E, Hatzidimou K, Tzallas C, et al: Estimation of LDL cholesterol based on the Friedewald formula and on apo B levels, *Clin Biochem* 33:549-555, 2000.

15. DeLong DM, DeLong ER, Wood PD, et al: A comparison of methods for the estimation of plasma low- and very low-density lipoprotein cholesterol: the Lipid Research Clinics Prevalence Study, *JAMA* 256:2372-2377, 1986.

16. Friedewald WT, Levy RI, Fredrickson DS: Estimation of the concentration of low-density lipoprotein cholesterol in plasma, without the use of the preparative ultracentrifuge, *Clin Chem* 18:499-502, 1972.

TEST NAME AND METHOD	SPECIMEN REQUIREMENTS	REFERENCE INTERVAL, CONVENTIONAL [INTERNATIONAL RECOMMENDED UNITS]	CHEMICAL INTERFERENCES AND IN VIVO EFFECTS

Low-Density Lipoprotein Cholesterol—CONT

17. McNamara JR, Cohn JS, Wilson PW, et al: Calculated values for low-density lipoprotein cholesterol in the assessment of lipid abnormalities and coronary heart disease risk, *Clin Chem* 36:36-42, 1990.

18. Planella T, Cortes M, Martinez-Bru C, et al: Calculation of LDL-cholesterol by using apolipoprotein B for classification of nonchylomicronemic dyslipidemia, *Clin Chem* 43:808-815, 1997.

19. Warnick GR, Knopp RH, Fitzpatrick V, et al: Estimating low-density lipoprotein cholesterol by the Friedewald equation is adequate for classifying patients on the basis of nationally recommended cutpoints, *Clin Chem* 36:15-19, 1990.

20. Fei H, Maeda S, Kirii H, et al: Evaluation of two different homogeneous assays for LDL-cholesterol in lipoprotein-X-positive serum, *Clin Chem* 46:1351-1356, 2000.

21. McNamara JR, Cole TG, Contois JH, et al: Immunoseparation method for measuring low-density lipoprotein cholesterol directly from serum evaluated, *Clin Chem* 41:232-240, 1995.

22. Rifai N, Iannotti E, DeAngelis K, et al: Analytical and clinical performance of a homogeneous enzymatic LDL-cholesterol assay compared with the ultracentrifugation-dextran sulfate-Mg^{2+} method, *Clin Chem* 44:1242-1250, 1998.

23. Sugiuchi H, Irie T, Uji Y, et al: Homogeneous assay for measuring low-density lipoprotein cholesterol in serum with tri-block copolymer and α-cyclodextrin sulfate, *Clin Chem* 44:522-531, 1998.

24. Albers JJ, Segrest JP, editors: *Plasma lipoproteins, part B: characterization, cell biology, and metabolism. Method in enzymology, vol 129,* Orlando, FL, 1986, Academic Press.

TEST NAME AND METHOD	SPECIMEN REQUIREMENTS	REFERENCE INTERVAL, CONVENTIONAL [INTERNATIONAL RECOMMENDED UNITS]	CHEMICAL INTERFERENCES AND IN VIVO EFFECTS

Low-Density Lipoprotein Subfractions (LDL subfractions)[1-14]
 	
 Gradient gel electrophoresis (GGE)[9,11,14-17]
 	
 Nuclear magnetic resonance (NMR) spectroscopy[12,18]
 	
 Ultracentrifugation[12,18]
 	
 HPLC[12,19,20]
	Serum, EDTA plasma. Fasting is preferred but not required. Stable for 5-6 days at 4° C. Freeze at −70° C for longer-term storage (EDTA plasma is preferable specimen for freezing). Do not refreeze.	Phenotype A:
		    Predominance of small, dense LDL particles
		    (diameter <255 Å)
		
		 Phenotype B:
		    Predominance of larger, buoyant LDL particles
		    (diameter >255 Å)
		
		 Note: Methods vary in the number of LDL subclasses determined and in the procedure used to classify phenotype. Up to seven LDL subclasses have been identified by GGE; most individuals have one to three subclasses present in serum or plasma. Phenotype can be defined as the most abundant subclass, or a "score" can be calculated based on a weighted mean of all subclasses present.
			A shift from small, dense LDL particles to larger, more buoyant LDL particles has been achieved through exercise, weight loss, dietary changes, and the use of estrogens, fibric acid derivatives, HMG CoA reductase inhibitors (statins), and niacin.

1. Austin M, Breslow J, Hennekens C, et al: Low-density-lipoprotein subclass patterns and risk of myocardial infarction, *JAMA* 260:1917-1921, 1988.

2. Austin M, King MC, Vranizan KM, et al: The atherogenic lipoprotein phenotype. A proposed genetic marker for coronary heart disease risk, *Circulation* 82:495-506, 1990.

3. Austin MA, Mykkanen L, Kuusisto J, et al: Prospective study of small LDLs as a risk factor for non-insulin-dependent diabetes mellitus in elderly men and women, *Circulation* 92:1770-1778, 1995.

4. Austin MA, Rodriguez BL, McKnight B, et al: Low-density lipoprotein particle size, triglycerides, and high-density lipoprotein cholesterol as risk factors for coronary heart disease in older Japanese-American men, *Am J Cardiol* 86:412-416, 2000.

5. Blake GJ, Albert MA, Rifai N, et al: Effect of pravastatin on LDL particle concentration as determined by NMR spectroscopy: a substudy of a randomized placebo controlled trial, *Eur Heart J* 24:1843-1847, 2003.

DIAGNOSTIC INFORMATION	REMARKS

25. Ordovas JM, editor: *Lipoprotein protocols,* Totowa, NJ, 1998, Humana Press.

26. Segrest JP, Albers JJ, editors: *Plasma lipoproteins, part A: preparation, structure, and molecular biology. Method in enzymology, vol 128,* Orlando, FL, 1986, Academic Press.

27. Contois JH, Gillmor R, Moore R, et al: Quantitative determination of cholesterol in lipoprotein fractions by electrophoresis, *Clin Chim Acta* 282:1-14, 1999.

28. Nauck M, Winkler K, Marz W, et al: Quantitative determination of high-, low-, and very-low density lipoproteins and lipoprotein(a) by agarose gel electrophoresis and enzymatic cholesterol staining, *Clin Chem* 41:1761-1767, 1995.

29. National Cholesterol Education Program (NCEP): Highlights of the Report of the Expert Panel on Blood Cholesterol Levels in Children and Adolescents, *Pediatrics* 89:495-501, 1992.

30. Hickman TB, Briefel RR, Carroll MD, et al: Distributions and trends of serum lipid levels among United States children and adolescents ages 4-19 years: data from the third National Health and Nutrition Examination Survey, *Prev Med* 27:879-890, 1998.

31. Brown SA, Hutchinson R, Morrisett J, et al: Plasma lipid, lipoprotein cholesterol, and apoprotein distributions in selected US communities: The Atherosclerosis Risk in Communities (ARIC) Study, *Arterioscl Thromb* 13:1139-1158, 1993.

LDL phenotype A is a component of the cluster of risk factors that comprise the metabolic syndrome and is associated with an increased risk of CHD.

Small, dense LDL particles are more atherogenic than larger particles. Prospective epidemiological studies have shown that smaller LDL particles are associated with an increased risk of coronary heart disease but suggest that LDL size is not independent of other risk factors.

6. Blake GJ, Otvos JD, Rifai N, et al: Low-density lipoprotein particle concentration and size as determined by nuclear magnetic resonance spectroscopy as predictors of cardiovascular disease in women, *Circulation* 106:1930-1937, 2002.

7. Kuller L, Arnold A, Tracy R, et al: Nuclear magnetic resonance spectroscopy of lipoproteins and risk of coronary heart disease in the cardiovascular health study, *Arterioscl Thromb Vasc Biol* 22:1175-1180, 2002.

8. Lamarche B, Tchernof A, Moorjani S, et al: Small, dense low-density lipoprotein particles as a predictor of risk of ischemic heart disease in men: prospective results from the Quebec Cardiovascular Study, *Circulation* 95:69-75, 1997.

9. McNamara JR, Campos H, Ordovas JM, et al: Effect of gender, age, and lipid status on low-density-lipoprotein subfraction distribution: results from the Framingham Offspring Study, *Arteriosclerosis* 7:483-490, 1987.

10. Mykkanen L, Kuusisto J, Haffner SM, et al: LDL size and risk of coronary heart disease in elderly men and women, *Arterioscl Thromb Vasc Biol* 19:2742-2748, 1999.

TEST NAME AND METHOD	SPECIMEN REQUIREMENTS	REFERENCE INTERVAL, CONVENTIONAL [INTERNATIONAL RECOMMENDED UNITS]	CHEMICAL INTERFERENCES AND IN VIVO EFFECTS

Low-Density Lipoprotein Subfractions—CONT

11. Rajman I, Kendall MJ, Cramb R, et al: Investigation of low density lipoprotein subfractions as a coronary risk factor in normotriglyceridaemic men, *Atherosclerosis* 125:231-242, 1996.

12. Rifai N, Warnick GR, Dominiczak MH, editors: *Handbook of lipoprotein testing,* ed 2, Washington, DC, 2000, AACC Press.

13. Skoglund-Andersson C, Tang R, Bond MG, et al: LDL particle size distribution is associated with carotid intima-media thickness in healthy 50-year-old men, *Arterioscler Thromb Vasc Biol* 19:2422-2430, 1999.

14. Stampfer MJ, Krauss RM, Ma J, et al: A prospective study of triglyceride level, low density lipoprotein particle diameter, and risk of myocardial infarction, *JAMA* 276:882-888, 1996.

15. Hoefner DM, Hodel SD, O'Brien JF, et al: Development of a rapid, quantitative method for LDL subfractionation with use of the Quantimetrix Lipoprint LDL system, *Clin Chem* 47:266-274, 2001.

16. Krauss RM, Burke DJ: Identification of multiple subclasses of plasma low density lipoproteins in normal humans, *J Lipid Res* 23:97-104, 1982.

L/S Ratio (Lecithin/Sphin- gomyelin Ratio) *1D-TLC*[1,2] (Com- mercially available with PG as Fetal Tek 200 from Helena, Beaumont, TX; see *Phos- phatidylglycerol*)	Amniotic fluid, 3-4 mL minimum, obtained by amniocentesis. Vaginal pool samples are ade- quate only when the fluid has been in the vagina for a short time and the fluid is chilled rapidly after collection.[3,4] Centrifuge samples gently (short duration at low speed).[5] If the test is delayed more than a few hours, refrigeration or freez- ing is recommended.[6]	*Ratio* *State of fetal maturity* <1.5: Immature 1.5-2.4 Transitional ≥2.5: Mature Values are based on densitometric (not concentra- tion) measurements of L to S. The above reference intervals are for methods omit- ting the acetone precipitation step found in the orig- inal procedure of Gluck et al.[2] If the acetone precip- itation step is utilized, the L/S ratio for a mature result is lowered to 2.0. Additionally, as TLC is technique dependent, institutions using this method should establish their own maturity criterion.[7]	Blood *(See Remarks)* and meconium produce vari- able results, either falsely increasing or decreasing the L/S ratio.[8,9] Debris from samples collected vaginally may also interfere.[9]

---

1. Ashwood ER: Clinical chemistry of pregnancy. In Burtis CA, Ashwood ER, editors: *Tietz textbook of clinical chemistry,* ed 3, Philadelphia, 1999, WB Saunders.

2. Gluck L, Kulovich MV, Borer RC, et al: Diagnosis of the respiratory distress syndrome by amniocentesis, *Am J Obstet Gynecol* 109:440-445, 1971.

3. Dombroski RA, MacKenna J, Brame RG: Comparison of amniotic fluid lung maturity profiles in paired vaginal and am- niocentesis specimens, *Am J Obstet Gynecol* 140:461-464, 1981.

4. Shaver DC, Spinnato JA, Whybrew D, et al: Comparison of phospholipids in vaginal and amniocentesis specimens of pa- tients with premature rupture of membranes, *Am J Obstet Gynecol* 156:454-457, 1987.

5. Ashwood ER: Markers of fetal lung maturity. In Gronowski AM, editor: *Handbook of clinical laboratory testing during pregnancy,* Totowa, NJ, 2004, Humana Press, Inc., pp. 55-70.

6. Schwartz DB, Engle MJ, Brown DJ, et al: The stability of phospholipids in amniotic fluid, *Am J Obstet Gynecol* 141:294-298, 1981.

7. Gluck L, Kulovich MV, Borer PC, et al: Diagnosis of the respiratory distress syndrome by amniocentesis, *Am J Obstet Gy- necol* 109:440-445, 1971.

17. Ordovas JM, editor: *Lipoprotein protocols,* Totowa, NJ, 1998, Humana Press.

18. Kulharni KR, Garber DW, Jones MK, et al: Identification and cholesterol quantification of low-density–lipoprotein subclasses in young adults by VAP-II methodology, *J Lipid Res* 36:2291-2302, 1995.

19. Scheffer PG, Bakker SJ, Heine RJ, et al: Measurement of low-density-lipoprotein particle size by high performance gel-filtration chromatography, *Clin Chem* 43:1904-1912, 1997.

20. Scheffer PG, Bakker SJ, Heine RJ, et al: Measurement of LDL particle size in whole plasma and serum by high performance gel-filtration chromatography using a fluorescent lipid probe, *Clin Chem* 44:2148-2151, 1998.

Sensitivity is ~95% with 65% specificity. The predictive value of an L/S ratio ≥2.5 (mature) is 97-98% at relatively advanced gestational ages (28-34 wk) but falls off sharply with decrease in gestational age and as the incidence of respiratory distress syndrome (RDS) increases. There is disagreement as to whether poorly controlled diabetes affects test results.[5]

Precision for the L/S ratio is poor, especially between laboratories.[10]

The L/S ratio of blood varies between 1.5 and 2.0. Thus values from blood-contaminated amniotic fluid specimens are pulled into that range. A very high L/S ratio, even in the presence of significant blood contamination, can be used to predict lung maturity. Similarly, blood-contaminated specimens with very low ratios can safely be used to predict immaturity. Borderline ratios cannot be interpreted.[1]

If a rapid FLM test is available, referral of L/S ratio requests to another laboratory is acceptable practice.[11]

L/S ratio can be combined with analysis for phosphatidylglycerol (PG) and phosphatidylinostol to produce a "lung profile," which has been reported to enhance the ability to detect RDS.[12-14] (See also *Phosphatidylglycerol.*)

8. Longo SA, Towers CV, Strauss A, et al: Meconium has no lecithin or sphingomyelin but affects the lecithin/sphingomyelin ratio, *Am J Obstet Gynecol* 179:1640-1642, 1998.

9. Brown LM, Duck-Chong CG: Methods of evaluating fetal lung maturity, *Crit Rev Clin Lab Sci* 16:85-159, 1982.

10. Dubin SB: Assessment of fetal lung maturity. Practice parameter, *Am J Clin Pathol* 110:723-732, 1998.

11. Ashwood ER: Evaluation of the high risk pregnancy at term. In Sherwin JE, Ashwood ER, Geaghan S, et al, editors: *NACB LMPG (draft guidelines-version 2) maternal and fetal health risk assessment,* Washington, DC, 2003, National Academy of Clinical Biochemistry.

12. Kulovich MV, Gluck L: The lung profile. II. Complicated pregnancy, *Am J Obstet Gynecol* 135:64-70, 1979.

13. Kulovich MV, Hallman MB, Gluck L: The lung profile. I. Normal pregnancy, *Am J Obstet Gynecol* 135:57-63, 1979.

14. Hallman M, Kulovich M, Kirkpatrick E, et al: Phosphatidylinositol and phosphatidylglycerol in amniotic fluid: indices of lung maturity, *Am J Obstet Gynecol* 125:613-617, 1976.

TEST NAME AND METHOD	SPECIMEN REQUIREMENTS	REFERENCE INTERVAL, CONVENTIONAL [INTERNATIONAL RECOMMENDED UNITS]	CHEMICAL INTERFERENCES AND IN VIVO EFFECTS
Lupus Anticoagulant (LA) Test[1-6] *Screening tests with diluted phospholipid: Tissue thromboplastin inhibition (TTI) dilute Russell viper venom time (dRVVT); dilute phospholipid APTT* *Confirmatory tests with increased phospholipid: Platelet neutralization; high phospholipid APTT*	Plasma for clot-based assays (blue top-citrate); place on ice and separate platelet-poor plasma by centrifugation at 4° C. Stable at 4° C for 4 hr, at 20° C for 2 mo. Serum for anticardiolipin (ELISA).	Clot-based assays: Negative results: Screening test(s) within normal range. Positive results: Screening test(s) prolonged; no correction with a 1:1 mixing study (patient plasma mixed with normal plasma). Confirmatory test(s): correction of inhibitor effect by excess phospholipid confirms the presence of LA. Various methods of providing excess phospholipids are available (hexagonal phospholipids, platelet neutralization procedure). If the excess phospholipid does not correct, other inhibitors may be present. Assays for acquired coagulation inhibitors (factor VIII inhibitor) and heparin should be performed. Immunoassays: Anticardiolipin antibody: <15 Note: Laboratory tests for antiphospholipid antibodies, including clot-based lupus anticoagulant assays and ELISAs for anticardiolipin antibodies, should be repeated at least twice (typically 6-8 wk apart) before making a diagnosis of antiphospholipid syndrome.	Heparin; hirudin, argatroban, and danaparoid False-positive results may be caused by specific factor inhibitors, factor deficiency, or oral anticoagulant therapy.

1. Lewis SM, Bain BJ, Bates I, editors: *Dacie and Lewis practical hematology,* ed 9, Edinburgh, 2001, Churchill Livingstone.
2. Jacobs DS, Demott WR, Oxley DK, editors: *Laboratory test handbook,* ed 5, Hudson, OH, 2001, Lexi-Comp, Inc.
3. Levine JS, Branch DW, Rauch J: The antiphospholipid syndrome, *N Engl J Med* 346:752-763, 2002.
4. Brandt JD, Berna LK, Triplett DA: Laboratory identification of lupus anticoagulant: results of the Second International Workshop for Identification of Lupus Anticoagulants, *Thromb Haemost* 74:1597-1603, 1995.

DIAGNOSTIC INFORMATION	REMARKS

Antiphospholipid antibody syndrome

LA may be identified in a variety of clinical conditions, including autoimmune disorders, rare cases of drug exposure, infection, and in otherwise healthy persons.

The antiphospholipid antibodies include the lupus anticoagulant, anticardiolipin antibodies (IgG, IgM, IgA), anti-B_2-glycoprotein I, and antiphosphatidylserine antibodies. These antibodies may be associated with thrombosis, autoimmune disorders (SLE), infections, and drugs, and may be further detected in otherwise healthy individuals.

The lupus anticoagulant is generally considered a "nonspecific" autoantibody that recognizes various combinations of phospholipids and/or phospholipid-binding proteins, and which clinically may result in hypercoagulability (antiphospholipid syndrome).

Current criteria for demonstration of a lupus anticoagulant require (1) prolongation of a phospholipid-dependent clot-based assay (e.g., screening APTT or dRVVT); (2) failure to correct the prolonged assay with a mixing study; (3) confirmation of the lupus anticoagulant by correction of the prolonged assay with excess phospholipids; and (4) rule-out of specific inhibitor.

Screening should be performed on assays with low phospholipid concentrations (e.g., dilute PT, dilute PTT, and dilute dRVVT). Ideally, these tests evaluate different portions of the coagulation cascade: dilute PTT for the intrinsic pathway, dilute dRVVT for the common pathway, and dilute PT (also known as tissue thromboplastin inhibition test) for the extrinsic pathway.

The anticardiolipin antibodies and anti-B_2-glycoprotein I and antiphosphatidylserine antibodies are detected by immunoassays (see separate section).

Multiple tests (clot-based, ELISA) should be performed because patients may be negative with one test and positive with another. Transient antiphospholipid antibodies may be associated with infections and drugs, particularly in the pediatric population.

5. Lopez LR: Anti-B2-glycoprotein I and antiphosphatidylserine antibodies are predictors of arterial thrombosis in patients with antiphospholipid syndrome, *Am J Clin Pathol* 121:142-149, 2004.

6. Favaloro EJ, Silvestrini R: Assessing usefulness of anticardiolipin antibody assays, *Am J Clin Pathol* 118:548-557, 2002.

TEST NAME AND METHOD	SPECIMEN REQUIREMENTS	REFERENCE INTERVAL, CONVENTIONAL [INTERNATIONAL RECOMMENDED UNITS]			CHEMICAL INTERFERENCES AND IN VIVO EFFECTS
Lutropin (Luteinizing Hormone, LH)[1-6] *Immunoassay*	Serum. Store refrigerated or frozen. Stable for 8 days at room temperature or for 14 days at 4° C.	*mU/mL*[8] *(WHO 1st IRP 68/40)**		*U/L*	S ↑ V Anticonvulsants, clomiphene, naloxone, and spironolactone
		Prepubertal child			
		Cord blood, M, F: 0.04-2.6	× 1.0	[0.04-2.6]	S ↓ V Digoxin,
		2-11 mo, M, F: 0.02-8.0		[0.02-8.0]	gonadotropin-releasing
		1-10 yr			hormone analogs (contin-
		M: 0.04-3.6		[0.04-3.6]	uous administration),
		F: 0.03-3.9		[0.03-3.9]	megestrol (suppresses
		Puberty			LH peak), norethindrone,
		Tanner stage			oral contraceptives, phe-
		1			nothiazines, progesterone
		M: 0.04-3.6		[0.04-3.6]	(suppresses LH peak), and
		F: 0.03-3.0		[0.03-3.0]	stanozolol
		2			
		M: 0.26-4.8		[0.26-4.8]	With estrogens (diethyl-
		F: 0.10-4.1		[0.10-4.1]	stilbestrol, ethinyl estra-
		3			diol, mestranol), effects
		M: 0.56-6.3		[0.56-6.3]	depend on dose and dura-
		F: 0.20-9.1		[0.20-9.1]	tion. Large doses decrease
		4-5			and small doses increase;
		M: 0.56-7.8		[0.56-7.8]	effects may last only a
		F: 0.50-15.0		[0.50-15.0]	few days.
		Adult			
		M: 1.24-7.8		[1.24-7.8]	
		F,			
		Follicular phase: 1.68-15		[1.68-15.0]	
		Ovulatory peak: 21.9-56.6		[21.9-56.6]	
		Luteal phase: 0.61-16.3		[0.61-16.3]	
		Postmenopausal: 14.2-52.3		[14.2-52.3]	
	Urine, 24 hr. Use no preservatives. Store frozen.	*U/day*[9] *(WHO 1st IRP 68/40)**			U ↑ V Clomiphene, estrogen (comments above apply)
		Prepubertal child (1-10 yr)			
		M: <1.0-5.6			
		F: 1.4-4.9			
		*World Health Organization, first International Reference Preparation 68/40 of LH.			
		U/day *(WHO 1st IRP 68/40)**			
		Puberty[10] Tanner stage			
		1			
		M: 1-5			
		F: 1-5			
		2			
		M: 1.5-11			
		F: 3-10			

DIAGNOSTIC INFORMATION	REMARKS

↑ Primary gonadal dysfunction, polycystic ovary syndrome (if LH is increased and FSH is normal or decreased, the LH/FSH ratio is abnormally high in ~60% of cases), post-menopause, and pituitary adenoma (rare).

↓ Pituitary or hypothalamic impairment, isolated gonadotropic deficiency associated with anosmia or hyposmia (Kallmann's syndrome), anorexia nervosa, isolated LH deficiency ("fertile eunuch"), severe stress, malnutrition, and severe illness. Delayed onset of the pubertal synthesis and release of LH and FSH characterizes the syndrome of constitutional delay in growth and sexual development.

Physiological variations in gonadotropin secretion include episodic secretion, diurnal variation, and cyclic secretion. Throughout puberty circulating gonadotropin levels are higher during sleep than during waking time. Episodic fluctuations in LH secretion are greater than for FSH. This means that multiple or pooled samples give more reliable information than a single blood sample.

Intact LH may cross-react with hCG in some radioimmunoassays such that LH estimations are invalid in pregnant or postpartum subjects and in individuals with hCG-secreting tumors. (LH and hCG show extensive similarities in the b-subunit with large regions of homology.) In some RIAs TSH also cross-reacts with LH to a small extent such that high levels of TSH in untreated hypothyroid patients can result in falsely elevated LH. The introduction of two-site immunometric assays has essentially overcome hCG and TSH interferences in LH assays.

Owing to variation in purity of standards, many assays express concentrations in terms of international units of either the World Health Organization's 1st International Reference Preparation (WHO 1st IRP) of LH or the 2nd International Reference Preparation of human menopausal gonadotropin (IRP-2-hMG). Recently, highly purified pituitary reference material has been used for assay standardization of LH assays (WHO 2nd International Standard 80/552).

Test is used to determine the preovulatory LH surge; test also provides an integrated picture of LH secretion throughout the day.[11,12]

Timed collections over a 3-hr period correlate with both 24-hr specimens and serum samples.

TEST NAME AND METHOD	SPECIMEN REQUIREMENTS	REFERENCE INTERVAL, CONVENTIONAL [INTERNATIONAL RECOMMENDED UNITS]	CHEMICAL INTERFERENCES AND IN VIVO EFFECTS
Lutropin—CONT			
	3		
	M:	2.5-13	
	F:	5-18	
	4		
	M:	5-16	
	F:	6-21	
	5		
	M:	4-28	
	F:	5-24	
	Adult		
	M:	9-23	
	F, non-midcycle:	4-30	

	Amniotic fluid[7]	mU/mL†		U/L
		Fetus-3 mo		
		M:	20 ± 16 (SD) × 1.0	[20 ± 16]
		F:	28 ± 13	[28 ± 13]
		3-6 mo		
		M:	69 ± 64	[69 ± 64]
		F:	214 ± 122	[214 ± 122]
		6-9 mo		
		M:	12 ± 3.2	[12 ± 3.2]
		F:	4.8 ± 3.0	[4.8 ± 3.0]

*World Health Organization, first International Reference Preparation 68/40 of LH.

†Second International Reference Preparation of human menopausal gonadotropin.

1. Ashby C: Lutropin assays: analytical and clinical expectations, *AACC Endo Metabolism In-Service Training Continuing Educ* 9:3-6, 1991.

2. Beastall G, Ferguson K, O'Reilly D, et al: Assays for follicle-stimulating hormone and luteinizing hormone: guidelines for the provision of a clinical biochemistry service, *Ann Clin Biochem* 24:246-262, 1987.

3. Thorner MO, Vance ML, Horvath E, et al: The anterior pituitary. In Wilson JD, Foster DW, editors: *Williams textbook of endocrinology,* ed 8, Philadelphia, 1992, WB Saunders.

4. Vermes I, Bonte H, Veer G, et al: Interpretations of five monoclonal immunoassays of lutropin and follitropin: effects of normalization with WHO standards, *Clin Chem* 37:415-421, 1991.

5. Whitley RJ, Meikle AW, Watts NB: Endocrinology. In Burtis CA, Ashwood ER, editors: *Tietz textbook of clinical chemistry,* ed 2, Philadelphia, 1994, WB Saunders.

6. Wiedemann G, Jonetz-Mentzel L, Panse R: Establishment of reference ranges for follitropin and lutropin in neonates, infants, children, and adolescents, *Eur Clin Chem Clin Biochem* 31:395-401, 1933.

7. Johnson TR, Moore WM, Jefferies JE: *Children are different: developmental physiology,* ed 2, Columbus, OH, 1978, Ross Laboratories.

DIAGNOSTIC INFORMATION	REMARKS

8. Nichols Institute Reference Laboratories: *Test catalog,* San Juan Capistrano, CA, 1993, Nichols Institute Reference Laboratories.

9. Endocrine Sciences: *Pediatric laboratory services,* Tarzana, CA, 1992, Endocrine Sciences.

10. Endocrine Sciences: *Pediatric laboratory services,* Tarzana, CA, 1988, Endocrine Sciences.

11. Beitins IZ, O'Loughlin K, Ostrea T, et al: Gonadotropin determinations in timed 3-hour urine collections during the menstrual cycle and LRH testing, *J Clin Endocrinol Metab* 43:46-55, 1976.

12. Kerin JF, Warnes GM, Crocker J, et al: 3-Hour urinary radioimmunoassay for luteinizing hormone to detect onset of preovulatory LH surge, *Lancet* 2:430-431, 1980.

TEST NAME AND METHOD	SPECIMEN REQUIREMENTS	REFERENCE INTERVAL, CONVENTIONAL [INTERNATIONAL RECOMMENDED UNITS]		CHEMICAL INTERFERENCES AND IN VIVO EFFECTS
Lysine (Lys)[1-5] *Ion-exchange chromatography*	Plasma (heparin) or serum, fasting. Place blood in ice water immediately; separate and freeze within 1 hr of collection. Stable for 1 wk at $-20°$ C; for longer periods deproteinize and store at $-70°$ C.[6,7]	*mg/dL* Premature, 1 day: $\quad$ 2.77 ± 0.88 (SD) Newborn, 1 day: $\quad$ 1.66-3.93 1 day-1 mo $\quad$ 1.34-4.74 1-3 mo: $\quad$ 1.50 ± 0.48 (SD) 9 mo-2 yr: $\quad$ 0.66-2.10 3-10 yr: $\quad$ 1.04-2.20 6-18 yr: $\quad$ 1.58-3.40 Adult: $\quad$ 1.21-3.47	$\mu mol/L$[10] × 68.5 $\quad$ [190 ± 60] [114-269] [92-325] [103 ± 33] [45-144] [71-151] [108-233][11] [83-238]	P ↑ V Histidine (after oral load)
	Urine, 24 hr. Add 10 mL of 6 mol/L HCl at start of collection. (Alternatively, refrigerate specimen during collection.) Store frozen at $-20°$ C.[8]	*mg/day* 10 days-7 wk: $\quad$ 5.7-10.9 3-12 yr: $\quad$ 9.3-93.7 Adult: $\quad$ 3.1-153.0 *mg/g creatinine* or $\quad$ 8 ± 2(SD) $\mu mol/g$ $creatinine$[10] 0-1 mo: $\quad$ 454-2313 1-6 mo: $\quad$ 284-1507 6 mo-1 yr: $\quad$ 391-1661 1-2 yr: $\quad$ 352-1083 2-3 yr: $\quad$ 279-1017	$\mu mol/day$[10] × 6.85 $\quad$ [39-75] [64-642] [21-1048] *mmol/mol creatinine* × 0.77 $\quad$ [6.2 ± 1.5] $mmol/mol$ $creatinine$ × 0.113 $\quad$ [51.3-261.4] [32.1-170.3] [44.2-187.7] [39.8-122.4] [31.5-114.9]	U ↑ V Cycloleucine
	CSF. Collect in sterile tubes; store frozen. Stable at $-20°$ C for 1 wk or at $-70°$ C for 2 mo.[9]	*mg/dL* Neonate: $\quad$ 0.360 ± 0.168 (SEM) 3 mo-2 yr: $\quad$ 0.196 ± 0.057 (SD) 2-10 yr: $\quad$ 0.197 ± 0.047 Adult: $\quad$ 0.425 ± 0.023	$\mu mol/L$ × 76.3 $\quad$ [24.7 ± 11.5][9] [13.4 ± 3.9][13] [13.5 ± 3.2][13] [29.1 ± 1.6][14]	

1. Scriver CR, Beaudet AL, Valle D, et al, editors: *The metabolic and molecular bases of inherited disease.* ed 8, New York, 2001, McGraw-Hill.

2. Bremer HJ, Duran M, Kamerling JP, et al: *Disturbances of amino acid metabolism: clinical chemistry and diagnosis,* Baltimore, 1981, Urban and Schwarzenburg.

3. Kruse T, Reiber H, Neuhoff V: Amino acid transport across the human blood-CSF barrier, *J Neurol Sci* 70:129-138, 1985.

4. Nyhan W, Sakait N: *Diagnostic recognition of genetic disease,* Philadelphia, 1987, Lea & Febiger.

5. Slocum RH, Cummings JG: Amino acid analysis in physiological samples. In Hommes FA, editor: *Techniques in human biochemical genetics,* New York, 1991, Wiley-Liss, pp. 87-126.

6. Cummings JG: Routine amino acids analysis in the clinical laboratory, *Am Clin Prod Rev* Feb:20-25, 1988.

7. Schaefer A, Piquard F, Haberey P: Plasma amino acids analysis: effects of delayed samples preparation and of storage, *Clin Chim Acta* 164:163-169, 1987.

8. Pesce A, Kaplan L, editors: *Methods in clinical chemistry,* St. Louis, 1987, CV Mosby.

9. Heiblim DI, Evans HE, Glass L, et al: Amino acid concentrations in cerebrospinal fluid, *Arch Neurol* 35:765-768, 1978.

DIAGNOSTIC INFORMATION	REMARKS
P ↑↑ Saccharopinuria	Arginine is also elevated in hyperlysinemia that is associated with hyperammonemia.
P ↑ Hyperlysinemia, hyperornithinemia, and glutaric academia type 2	See also Table II-2B.
P ↓ Carcinoid syndrome, 1-2 days after abdominal surgery Lysinuric protein intolerance	
U ↑↑ Saccharopinuria, dibasic aminoaciduria, lysinuric protein intolerance (LPI)[15]	Urinary excretion depends on age. Within the first half-year of life, a high excretion of lysine and cystine is frequently present (physiological cystinlysinuria). Slight cystinlysinuria may also occur in the second half of the first year and in toddlers. In addition to lysine, high levels of cystine, arginine, and ornithine are also seen in the cystinurias. In dibasic aminoaciduria, arginine and ornithine are also excreted in high amounts, but cystine excretion is normal.
U ↑ Cystinurias, hyperlysinemia, first trimester of pregnancy (levels decrease thereafter), and burn patients[16]	
CSF ↑ Hyperlysinemia, bacterial meningitis, meningoradiculitis, Garin-Bujadoux-Bannwarth, and carcinomatous meningitis[17]	Values in children (3 mo-10 yr) were measured using reversed-phase liquid chromatography.

10. Shih V: *Laboratory techniques for the detection of hereditary metabolic disorders,* Boca Raton, FL, 1973, CRC Press.

11. Meites S, editor: *Pediatric clinical chemistry,* ed 3, Washington, DC, 1989, American Association for Clinical Chemistry.

12. Mayo Medical Laboratories: *Test catalog,* Rochester, MN, 1993, Mayo Medical Laboratories.

13. Goldsmith RF, Earl JW, Cunningham AM: Determination of δ-aminobutyric acid and other amino acids in cerebrospinal fluid of pediatric patients by reversed-phase liquid chromatography, *Clin Chem* 33:1736-1740, 1987.

14. Shih V: *Laboratory techniques for the detection of hereditary metabolic disorders,* Boca Raton, FL, 1973, CRC Press.

15. Scriver CR, Beaudet AL, Valle D, et al, editors: *The metabolic and molecular bases of inherited disease,* ed 8, New York, 2001, McGraw-Hill Publishing Co.

16. Cynober L, Dinh FN, Blonde F, et al: Plasma and urinary amino acid pattern in severe burn patients: evolution throughout the healing period, *Am J Clin Nutr* 36:416-425, 1982.

17. Schott KJ, Meier D: Free amino acid pattern of cerebrospinal fluid in meningeal pathology, *Acta Neurol Scand* 75:304-309, 1987.

TEST NAME AND METHOD	SPECIMEN REQUIREMENTS	REFERENCE INTERVAL, CONVENTIONAL [INTERNATIONAL RECOMMENDED UNITS]		CHEMICAL INTERFERENCES AND IN VIVO EFFECTS
Lysolecithin Acyltransferase in Erythrocytes (EC 2.3.1.23)[1]	Not stated in published method.	1070 ± 260 nmol/10^{12} Ercs/min (37° C) [$\times 1.0 = 1070 \pm 260$ fU/Erc]		None found.

1. Pohl A, Bugajer-Gleitman HE, Lachmann D, et al: Glutathionreductasemangel mit Membrandefekt bei hereditärer hämolytischer Anämie, *Acta Haematol* 56:47-57, 1976.

TEST NAME AND METHOD	SPECIMEN REQUIREMENTS	*mcg/mL*	*μmol/L*	CHEMICAL INTERFERENCES
Lysozyme (Muramidase; EC 3.2.1.17)[1-6]	Serum or plasma (EDTA). Separate and freeze within 2 hr of collection. Serum lysozyme is stable for at least 1 mo at $-20°$ C.	4-15.6[1]	[0.28-1.1]	C ↓ Heparin
Turbidimetric		0.2-15.8[4]	[0.14-1.1]	
Radial immunodiffusion		9-17[1]	[0.63-1.2]	
Turbidimetric	Tears	1151-1383[1]	[80-96]	
Radial immunodiffusion	Urine, 3 mL aliquot from well-mixed random specimen. Use no preservative. Stable for 7 days at 2-8° C and for 3 mo when frozen ($-20°$ C).	<4 mcg/mL[3]	[<0.28 μmol/L]	

1. Pesce A, Kaplan L, editors: *Methods in clinical chemistry,* St. Louis, 1987, CV Mosby.
2. Williams WJ, Beutler E, Erslev AJ, et al, editors: *Hematology,* ed 4, New York, 1990, McGraw-Hill Publishing Co.
3. ARUP Laboratories: *2004 test catalog,* Salt Lake City, UT, 2004, ARUP Laboratories.
4. Mayo Clinic Laboratories: *2004 test catalog,* Rochester, MN, 2004, Mayo Clinic Laboratories.
5. Beutler E, Lichtman MA, Coller B, editors: *Williams hematology,* ed 6, New York, 2000, McGraw-Hill.
6. Brunning RD, McKenna RW: *Tumors of the bone marrow,* Washington, DC, 1994, Armed Forces Institute of Pathology.
7. Jaffe ES, Harris NL, Stein H, et al, editors: *World Health Organization classification of tumours. Pathology and genetics of tumours of haematopoietic and lymphoid tissues,* Lyon, 2001, IARC Press.

DIAGNOSTIC INFORMATION	REMARKS

Deficiency in rare congenital hemolytic anemia (autosomal dominant) reported in a single family.

S,U ↑↑↑ Acute monocytic or myelomonocytic leukemia

S,U ↑ Chronic myeloid leukemia, polycythemia vera, certain kidney diseases, chronic infections (especially tuberculosis), sarcoidosis, megaloblastic anemia, Crohn disease, ulcerative colitis, and acute bacterial infections

S,U ↓ Neutropenia with hypoplasia of bone marrow (but increased or normal if marrow is hypercellular and neutropenia is caused by peripheral cell destruction)

Sal. ↑ Sjögren's syndrome

U ↑↑ Patients with proximal renal tubular damage such as that caused by heavy metal intoxication (e.g., cadmium), renal allograft rejection, and acute thermal burns

The highly basic, carbohydrate-free, low-molecular-weight protein is synthesized by macrophages, neutrophils, and monocytes and is a normal constituent of plasma. It catalyzes the hydrolysis of bacterial cell walls by disrupting N-acetylglucosamine linkages. External secretions contain very high levels of lysozyme, which acts as a first line of defense against bacterial pathogens. At birth, levels are equivalent to those of adults. However, they decrease during the first months of life and gradually assume adult levels in much the same manner as do other plasma proteins. Electrophoretically the protein migrates at the cathodal limit of the slowest immunoglobulins and even beyond. Appearance of a discrete band can often be misleading and may suggest the presence of a small monoclonal immunoglobulin.

Serum and urine lysozyme may be useful as indicators of monocyte proliferation and, to a lesser extent, of neutrophil proliferation.[5] An elevated lysozyme concentration of >3 times normal is one of the criteria that can be used for the diagnosis of both acute monocytic leukemia (M5) and acute myelomonocytic leukemia (M4) in the modified French-American-British (FAB) classification of acute leukemia.[6,7]

MW: 14,000.

TEST NAME AND METHOD	SPECIMEN REQUIREMENTS	REFERENCE INTERVAL, CONVENTIONAL [INTERNATIONAL RECOMMENDED UNITS]	CHEMICAL INTERFERENCES AND IN VIVO EFFECTS
Macroamylase[1,2] *Chromatography, ultracentrifugation, EP, immunochemical, polyethylene glycol precipitation*[3,4]	Serum. Store at 4° C or −20° C.	Present in ~1% of healthy subjects with normal serum amylase activity and in 2.5% of patients with high activity.[1,2]	See *Amylase*.

1. Fridhandler L, Berk IE: Macroamylasemia, *Adv Clin Chem* 20:267-286, 1978.
2. Kleinman DS, O'Brien JF: Macroamylase, *Mayo Clin Proc* 61:669-670, 1986.
3. Fridhandler L, Berk JE, Ueda M: Macroamylasemia: rapid detection method, *Clin Chem* 17:423-426, 1971.
4. Levit, MD, Ellis CJ: A rapid and simple assay to determine if macroamylasemia is the cause of hyperamylasemia, *Gastroenterology* 83:378-382, 1982.
5. Oita T, Yamashiro A, Mizutani F, et al: Simultaneous presence of macroamylase and macrolipase in a patient with celiac disease, *Rinsho Byori* 54:974-977, 2003.
6. Absztyn A, Green PH, Berti I, et al: Macroamylasemia in patients with celiac disease, *Am J Gastroenterol* 96:1096-1100, 2001.
7. Dürr HK, Bode C, Krupinski R, et al: A comparison between naturally occurring macroamylasaemia and macroamylasaemia induced by hydroxyethyl-starch, *Eur J Clin Invest* 8:189-191, 1978.
8. Kazmierczak SC, Van Lente F, McHugh AM, et al: Macroamylasemia with a markedly increased amylase clearance ratio in a patient with a renal cell carcinoma, *Clin Chem* 34:435-438, 1988.

DIAGNOSTIC INFORMATION	REMARKS

There are three distinct types of macroamylasemia.[1]

Type I: Classic macroamylasemia characterized by high total serum amylase activity, large proportions in serum of enzymatically active macroamylase complex, and low amylase/creatinine clearance ratio (see *Amylase/Creatinine Clearance Ratio*).

Type II: Hyperamylasemia but lower proportion of macroamylase so that amylase/creatinine clearance ratio may not be diminished.

Type III: Normal activities of serum and urine amylase.

Macroamylasemia is usually a benign condition with few signs or symptoms, but it must be differentiated from other conditions that cause hyperamylasemia (see *Amylase*).

Has been reported in association with macrolipase.[5]

Macroamylasemia is more common in patients with celiac disease (16%). The rate is lower (7%) in treated celiac disease patients.[6]

Screening for macroamylasemia may use amylase/creatinine clearance ratio, polyethylene glycol precipitation followed by P-type isoamylase assay on the supernatant,[7] or gel-filtration chromatography. However, a single report[8] documents a high amylase/creatinine clearance ratio occurring in a case of macroamylasemia caused by a renal cell carcinoma secreting an S-type isoamylase. The authors suggest that an amylase/creatinine clearance ratio may not always be a suitable screening test.

Infusion of hydroxyethyl starch has produced macroamylasemia.[9] Macroamylase is considered an immune complex with circulating antibodies.

Macroamylase of types I and II causes elevated serum amylase without increased urine amylase.

On electrophoresis, macroamylase appears as a diffuse isoenyzme complex when stained for amylase activity.

Total amylase level may fluctuate widely over time when macroamylase is present.[10]

Macroamylases react differently with different substrates.[11]

9. Van Deun A, Cobbaert C, Van Orshoven A, et al: Comparison of some recent methods for the differentiation of elevated serum amylase and the detection of macroamylasaemia, *Ann Clin Biochem* 26:422-426, 1989.

10. Sachdeva CK, Bank S, Greenberg R, et al: Fluctuations in serum amylase in patients with macroamylasemia, *Am J Gastroenterol* 90:800-803, 1995.

11. Rosenblum JL, Hortin GL, Smith CH, et al: Macroamylases: differences in activity against various-sized substrates, *Clin Chem* 38:1725-1729, 1992.

TEST NAME AND METHOD	SPECIMEN REQUIREMENTS	REFERENCE INTERVAL, CONVENTIONAL [INTERNATIONAL RECOMMENDED UNITS]			CHEMICAL INTERFERENCES AND IN VIVO EFFECTS
α_2-**Macroglobulin** (α_2M)[1-4]	Serum. Stable at room temperature for 24 hr, 4° C for 7 days, and frozen for 3 mo.	*mg/dL* Adults: 66-265	× 0.01	*g/L* [0.66-2.65]	S ↑ V Estrogens, oral contraceptives.
Nephelometric		*mg/dL* M: 150-350 (x̄: 240)	× 0.01	*g/L* [1.50-3.50] [x̄: 2.40]	S ↓ V Dextran, streptokinase
RID[5]	Serum or plasma (EDTA). Stable for 2 days at 4° C and for 7 days at −20° C.	F: 175-420 (x̄: 290)		[1.75-4.20] [x̄: 2.90]	Excessive turbidity can affect nephelometric methods.
		Newborn: Values are 1.5 times those of adult males. They decrease in the teens and increase again >70 yr.			
EID[2]		*mg/dL* M: 108-297 F: 144-315	× 0.01	*g/L* [1.08-2.97] [1.44-3.15]	
ELISA,[5,6] *Nephelometric*[7]	CSF. Analyze fresh or store at 4° C for 14 days.	*mg/dL*[8] 0.11-0.45 Values can increase with increasing age.[7]	× 10	*mg/L* [1.1-4.5]	
IEP[8]	Amniotic fluid. Centrifuge before analysis. Analyze fresh or store at 4° C for <72 hr. Stable frozen at −20° C for 6 mo or at −70° C indefinitely. Specimens should not contain blood.	15-39 wk gestation: 0.10-0.15 mg/dL	× 10	[1.0-1.5 mg/L]	

1. Schwick H-G, Haupt H: Chemistry and function of human plasma proteins, *Angew Chem* 191:87-99, 1980.
2. Putnam FW, editor: *The plasma proteins: structure, functions and genetic control, vols 1-3,* ed 2, New York, 1977, Academic Press.
3. Ohtani H, Saito M, Koshiba K: Alpha-2-macroglobulin deficiency in patients with advanced prostate cancer, *Oncology* 42:341-344, 1985.
4. Ades EW, Hinson A, Chapuis-Cellier C, et al: Modulation of the immune response by plasma protease inhibitors, *Scand J Immunol* 15:109-113, 1982.
5. Ritzmann SE, Tucker ES III: *Protein analysis in disease—current concepts. Workshop manual,* Chicago, 1979, American Society of Clinical Pathologists, Commission for Continuing Education.
6. Kanoh Y, Ohtani H: Levels of interleukin-6, CRP, and alpha-2-macroglobulin in cerebrospinal fluid (CSF) and serum as indicator of blood-CSF barrier damage, *Biochem Mol Biol Int* 43:269-278, 1997.
7. Garton MJ, Keir G, Lakshmi MV, et al: Age-related changes in cerebrospinal fluid protein concentrations, *J Neurol Sci* 104:74-80, 1991.
8. Meucci G, Rossi G, Bettini R, et al: Laser nephelometric evaluation of albumin, IgG and alpha-2-macroglobulin: applications to the study of alterations in the blood-brain barrier, *J Neurol Sci* 118:73-78, 1993.

↑ Exogenous estrogen therapy, pregnancy, females (pre-menopausal) have higher overall values compared with males,[10] chronic liver disease,[3] diabetes, nephrotic syndrome is associated with markedly elevated levels secondary to renal loss of lower molecular weight proteins,[3,11] malignancies,[3] and psoriasis.[11]

↓ Acute pancreatitis,[12] cardiopulmonary bypass,[13] disseminated intravascular coagulation, multiple myeloma, prostate cancer and other malignancies,[3,14,15] preeclampsia, rheumatoid arthritis,[3,16] and hereditary deficiency.[3]

↑ CSF Bacterial and viral meningitis (less frequently seen with viral),[6] breakdown of the blood-brain barrier.[6]

α_2-Macroglobulin (α_2M) is a plasma protease inhibitor of high molecular weight. It is found in only small quantities in nonplasma body fluids because of its large size. The inhibitory spectrum of α_2M is broad, encompassing a variety of protease types to which it complexes and covalently binds. The subsequent alteration in its conformation promotes reticuloendothelial clearance. α_2M has a role in the regulation of the fibrinolytic/coagulation, kallikrein, and complement cascades, in addition to the transport of molecules such as growth hormone and divalent cations.[17,18] Studies have shown that it possesses immunosuppressive capabilities, including the capacity to inhibit cell-mediated cytotoxicity and lymphocyte proliferation.[3,4,19,20]

Although variants exist, no specific disorder resulting from hereditary α_2M deficiencies is known.

MW: 725,000.
$t_{1/2}$:   5 days

9.   van Kamp GJ, Calliauw J: Determination of α2-macroglobulin in amniotic fluid in diagnosis of neural tube defect, *Clin Chem* 26:1362-1363, 1980.

10. Ganrot PO, Schersten B: Serum alpha-2-macroglobulin concentration and its variation with age and sex, *Clin Chim Acta* 15:113-120, 1967.

11. Rocha-Pereira P, Santos-Silva A, Rebelo I, et al: The inflammatory response in mild and severe psoriasis, *Br J Dermatol* 150:917-928, 2004.

12. Lasson A, Ohlsson K: Consumptive coagulopathy, fibrinolysis and protease-antiprotease interactions during acute human pancreatitis, *Thromb Res* 41:167-183, 1986.

13. Siminelakis S, Bossinakou I, Antoniou F, et al: A study of the effects of extracorporeal circulation on the immunologic system of humans, *J Cardiothorac Vasc Anesth* 10:893-898, 1996.

14. Ohtani H, Hirasawa M: Serum glycoproteins in malignant neoplasms (in Japanese), *Physicochem Biol* 18:32-33, 1974.

15. Ohtani H, Koide A: Fluctuation of serum glycoproteins in malignancies-with special reference to alpha-2-macroglobulin (in Japanese), *Kitasato Med* 10:30-34, 1980.

16. Housley J: Alpha-2-macroglobulin levels in disease in man, *J Clin Pathol* 21:27-31, 1968.

TEST NAME AND METHOD	SPECIMEN REQUIREMENTS	REFERENCE INTERVAL, CONVENTIONAL [INTERNATIONAL RECOMMENDED UNITS]			CHEMICAL INTERFERENCES AND IN VIVO EFFECTS

α₂-Macroglobulin—CONT

17. Kratzsch J, Selisko T, Birkenmeier G: Identification of transformed alpha-2-macroglobulin as a growth hormone binding protein in human blood, *J Clin Endocrinol Metab* 80:585-590, 1995.

18. Pratt CW, Pizzo SV: The effect of zinc and other divalent cations on the structure and function of human alpha-2-macroglobulin, *Biochim Biophys Acta* 791:123-130, 1984.

TEST NAME AND METHOD	SPECIMEN REQUIREMENTS	REFERENCE INTERVAL, CONVENTIONAL [INTERNATIONAL RECOMMENDED UNITS]			CHEMICAL INTERFERENCES AND IN VIVO EFFECTS
Magnesium (Mg)[1,2]	Serum, fasting.[4] Collect in metal-free container. Separate red cells immediately. Avoid hemolysis and venous stasis. Stable for several days if refrigerated.	*mg/dL* Newborn: 1.5-2.2 ×0.4114 5 mo-6 yr: 1.7-2.3 6-12 yr: 1.7-2.1 12-20 yr: 1.7-2.2 Adult: 1.6-2.6 60-90 yr[7]: 1.6-2.4 >90 yr: 1.7-2.3 Higher in females during menses.		*mmol/L* [0.62-0.91] [0.70-0.95] [0.70-0.86] [0.70-0.91] [0.66-1.07] [0.66-0.99] [0.70-0.95]	↑ C *AAS:* Trichloroacetic acid ↓ C *Titan yellow:* Calcium gluconate (IV), citrates S ↑ V Aspirin (prolonged therapy), lithium, Mg products, medroxyprogesterone, progesterone, triamterene, and vitamin D (chronic renal failure)
Colorimetric, xylidyl blue[3]		1.26-2.10 mEq/L ×0.5 [0.63-1.05 mmol/L]			
AAS	Erythrocytes. Collect in metal-free container.	3.3-5.3 mEq/L ×0.5 [1.65-2.65 mmol/L]			S ↓ V Albuterol (salbutamol), aldosterone, aminoglycosides, ammonium chloride, amphotericin B, calcium salts, cisplatin, citrates (blood transfusion), cyclosporine, digoxin, diuretics (ethacrynic acid, furosemide, thiazide diuretics), ethanol, glucagon, insulin (large doses in diabetic coma), laxatives (chronic abuse), oral contraceptives, pentamidine, and phenytoin
	Urine, 24 hr.[5] Collect in metal-free container; use no preservative. Acidify to pH 1.0.	*mEq/day* Adults: 6.0-10.0 ×0.5 Random urine[8]:		*mmol/day* [3.00-5.00]	U ↑ V Cyclosporine
		mg/dL M <40 yr: 2.1-23.2 ×0.4114 ≥40 yr: 0.6-13.7		*mmol/L* [0.86-9.54] [0.25-5.63]	

DIAGNOSTIC INFORMATION	REMARKS

19. Ford WH, Caspary EA, Shenton B: Purification and properties of a lymphocyte inhibition factor from human serum, *Clin Exp Immunol* 15:169-179, 1973.

20. Goutner A, Simmler MC, Tapon J, et al: Modulation by alpha-2-macroglobulin of human lymphocyte proliferation in response to mitogens and antigen, *Differentiation* 5:171-173, 1976.

S ↑ Dehydration, renal insufficiency (acute and chronic), uncontrolled diabetes mellitus (rare), adrenocortical insufficiency, Addison's disease, tissue trauma, hypothyroidism, lupus erythematosus, and multiple myeloma. See also *Remarks*.

S ↓ Disorders associated with inadequate intake and/or impaired absorption of Mg (e.g., malabsorption syndrome, kwashiorkor, and diet low in proteins and calories); acute pancreatitis, hypoparathyroidism, chronic alcoholism, delirium tremens, disorders associated with increased Mg requirement and inadequate replacement of prolonged or severe loss of body fluids, chronic glomerulonephritis, disorders associated with impaired renal conservation of Mg such as hypercalcemia of any cause (e.g., hyperparathyroidism), hyperaldosteronism, diabetic acidosis, excessive lactation, inappropriate secretion of ADH; pregnancy (second and third trimester); some cases of hypomagnesemia are idiopathic.

Tetany may occur at Mg concentrations of 0.3-1.0 mEq/L [0.15-0.50 mmol/L] at normal pH and normal calcium concentrations.

Serum Mg levels may remain normal even when total body stores of Mg are depleted up to 20%. Phytate, fatty acids, and an excess of phosphate impair Mg absorption. Hypomagnesemia may impair secretion and the end-organ action of PTH. Symptoms of deficiency usually do not occur until serum levels are <1.0 mEq/L [<0.50 mmol/L]. Symptoms of severe depletion are weakness, irritability, tetany, EKG changes, delirium, and convulsions. An upright position causes an increase in Mg of ~4%. Inappropriate dosage of therapeutic agents (magnesium sulfate) or antacids causes hypermagnesemia. Hypermagnesemia potentiates the cardiac effect of hyperkalemia.

Effects of severe hypermagnesemia, 5.0-10.0 mEq/L [2.50-5.00 mmol/L]: Retards cardiac conduction system.

10-13.0 mEq/L [5.00-6.50 mmol/L]: Deep-tendon reflexes are lost.

15.0 mEq/L [7.50 mmol/L]: Respiratory paralysis occurs; general anesthesia may occur.

>25 mEq/L [>12.50 mmol/L]: Cardiac arrest occurs in diastole.

At least 65-70% of Mg is in an ionized state; ~35% of serum Mg is protein bound.

Serum concentrations are frequently paralleled in CSF and erythrocytes. Interference from mercurial diuretics can be removed by treating the sample with H_2S.

Accuracy of the colorimetric method is within 10%.

U ↑ Alcohol, diuretics, Bartter's syndrome, corticosteroids, and cisplatin therapy

Urinary excretion of Mg is diet dependent. See *Magnesium Load Test*.

TEST NAME AND METHOD	SPECIMEN REQUIREMENTS	REFERENCE INTERVAL, CONVENTIONAL [INTERNATIONAL RECOMMENDED UNITS]		CHEMICAL INTERFERENCES AND IN VIVO EFFECTS
Magnesium—CONT				
		F		
		<40 yr: 1.2-18.7	[0.49-7.69]	
		≥40 yr: 0.4-15.0	[0.16-6.17]	
		mg/g creatinine	*mmol/g creatinine*	
		M: 18-110 × 0.04114	[0.74-4.53]	
		F: 14-139	[0.58-5.72]	
Colorimetric, titan yellow	CSF.[6] Collect in metal-free container. Avoid contamination with blood.	*mEq/L* 2.0-2.7 × 0.5 2.2-3.0	*mmol/L* [1.00-1.35] [1.10-1.50]	
AAS	Mononucleated blood cells.[1] Separate over Ficoll Hypaque gradient.	*fg/cell* 70.7 ± 14.1 × 0.04114	*fmol/cell* [2.91 ± 0.58]	

1. Elin RJ: Assessment of magnesium status, *Clin Chem* 33:1965-1970, 1987.
2. Milne DB: Trace elements. In Burtis CA, Ashwood ER, editors: *Tietz textbook of clinical chemistry,* ed 3, Philadelphia, 1999, WB Saunders.
3. Duncanson GO, Worth GJ: Determination of reference intervals for serum magnesium, *Clin Chem* 36:756-758, 1990.
4. Alsever RN, Gotlin RW: *Handbook of endocrine tests in adults and children,* ed 2, Chicago, 1978, Year Book Medical Publishers Inc.
5. Burtis CA, Ashwood ER, editors: *Tietz fundamentals of clinical chemistry,* ed 5, Philadelphia, 2000, WB Saunders.
6. Tietz NW, editors: *Fundamentals of clinical chemistry,* ed 3, Philadelphia, 1987, WB Saunders.
7. Tietz NW, Shuey DF, Wekstein DR: Laboratory values in fit aging individuals—sexagenarians through centenarians, *Clin Chem* 38:1167-1185, 1992.
8. Bond LW, Garber C, Ottinger W, et al: Reference intervals for common analytes in random urine specimens, *Clin Chem* 55:submitted, 2005.

Magnesium (Mg) Load Test[1] Dose[2]: After a pretest urine sample, 30 mmol MgSO$_4$ in 1 L of NaCl (154 mmol) is given IV over 8 hr overnight. Urine is collected from the start for 24 hr.	Urine, 24 hr See *Magnesium.*	Dose recovered in 24 hr: 18-30 mmol Mg Magnesium deficiency: <18 nmol Mg/24 hr urine	See *Magnesium.* ↑ Drug therapy (cyclosporine and thiazide diuretics) enhances excretion.[3,4]

DIAGNOSTIC INFORMATION	REMARKS

CSF ↓ Meningitis, ischemic brain disease

↓ Malabsorption, acute and chronic alcoholism, and long-term parenteral therapy

See *Magnesium.*

↑ Chronic glomerulonephritis and aldosteronism[4]

TEST NAME AND METHOD	SPECIMEN REQUIREMENTS	REFERENCE INTERVAL, CONVENTIONAL [INTERNATIONAL RECOMMENDED UNITS]	CHEMICAL INTERFERENCES AND IN VIVO EFFECTS

Magnesium (Mg) Load Test—CONT

1. Elin RJ: Assessment of magnesium status, *Clin Chem* 33:1965-1970, 1987.
2. Eastham RD: *Biochemical values in clinical medicine,* ed 7, Bristol, UK, 1985, John Wright and Sons Ltd.

| **Malate Dehydrogenase (MDH, MD; EC 1.1.1.37)[1]** | Serum; avoid hemolysis. Assay immediately; stable at 4° C for 2 wk, at −70° C for 6 mo. | M: 5-40 U/L   × 0.017   [0.09-0.68 μKat/L] | ↑ C Hemolysis

↓ C Excess malate or oxaloacetate |

Malate, 340 nm, 37° C[1]

Malate, 340 nm, 37° C[2]		*U/L*	*μKat/L*
	M:	18.5 ± 11.1 (2 SD)	[0.31 ± 0.19]
	F:	17.4 ± 12.0 (2 SD)	[0.30 ± 0.20]

1. Smith AF: Malate dehydrogenase. In Bergmeyer HU, editor: *Methods of enzymatic analysis, vol III,* ed 3, Weinheim, 1983, Verlag Chemie.
2. Goldberg DM, Herraez-Domingues M, Wilcock AR: Assay of malate dehydrogenase activity with L-malate as substrate and its application to patients with myocardial infarction and liver disease. In Goldberg DM, Werner M, editors: *Selected topics in clinical enzymology, vol 1,* Berlin, 1983, Walter De Gruyter.
3. Kawai M, Hosaki S: Clinical usefulness of malate dehydrogenase and its mitochondrial isoenzyme in comparison with aspartate aminotransferase and its mitochondrial isoenzyme in sera of patients with liver disease, *Clin Biochem* 23:327-334, 1990.

Manganese (Mn)[1] *AAS[2]*	Whole blood.[4] Collect in metal-free container. Stable 7 days at room temperature.	10.9 ± 0.6 mcg/L × 18.2 [198 ± 11 nmol/L]	Sodium heparin anticoagulant may contaminate blood sample with Mn.[8]
	Plasma (Na₂ EDTA)[4]	0.9 ± 0.1 mcg/L [16.4 ± 2.0 nmol/L]	
	Hair.[5] Cut specimens close to scalp in 2- to 5-cm lengths. Wash in acetone solution, and digest in 70% ultrapure nitric acid.	*mcg/g dry wt.* *nmol/g dry wt.* 0.2-4.4 × 18.2 [3.6-80.1]	
AAS	Serum.[5] Collect in metal-free container.	0.59 ± 0.16 mcg/L × 18.2 [10.7 ± 3.0 nmol/L]	

DIAGNOSTIC INFORMATION	REMARKS

3. Goldman RD, Koren G: Amphotericin B nephrotoxicity in children, *J Pediatr Hematol Oncol* 26:421-426, 2004.
4. Mayo Medical Laboratories: *Interpretive handbook,* Rochester, MN, 2001, Mayo Medical Laboratories.

↑ Myocardial infarct, hemolytic diseases, megaloblastic anemias, sickle cell anemia, acute hepatic disease, generalized metastatic carcinoma, diseases of skeletal muscle, and trauma

Determinations of MDH and mitochondrial MDH are suggested to be more diagnostically sensitive indicators of severe hepatic disease than AST and mitochondrial AST,[3] particularly in hepatocellular carcinoma and in ischemic liver disease.

Controversy exists as to the stability of MDH activity. In general, MDH levels of activity follow those of lactate dehydrogenase (LDH). Because of the wide tissue distribution, serum determination of MDH lacks a high degree of diagnostic specificity. MDH exists as cytosolic and mitochondrial forms. The latter form is rarely present in serum unless organ damage is especially severe. The mitochondrial form can be determined by the ratio of activity using NAD versus thionicotinamide adenine dinucleotide (thio-NAD) as cofactor.[3]

↑ Acute hepatitis, industrial exposure, and myocardial infarction

↓ Seizure disorders, phenylketonuria

P ↑ Rheumatoid arthritis

Hair ↓ Diabetes (0.12 ± 0.07 mcg/g dry wt.; 2 ± 1 nmol/g dry wt.)

Chronic inhalation damages the basal ganglia of the brain, resulting in parkinsonian symptoms. Most manganese in blood is bound to hemoglobin in the erythrocytes. Manganese is excreted primarily in feces. Industrial exposure is seen in foundry workers and welders and in the manufacture of drugs, glass, varnish, feed additives, and ceramics.

Magnetic resonance imaging may be helpful in the diagnosis of chronic manganese intoxication.[9,10]

TEST NAME AND METHOD	SPECIMEN REQUIREMENTS	REFERENCE INTERVAL, CONVENTIONAL [INTERNATIONAL RECOMMENDED UNITS]		CHEMICAL INTERFERENCES AND IN VIVO EFFECTS
Manganese—CONT				
	Urine.[5] Collect in acid-washed, metal-free container.	0.5-9.8 mcg/L Toxic concentration: >10 mcg/L	[9.1-178 nmol/L] [>182 nmol/L]	
	Erythrocytes.[6] Collect whole blood (sodium heparin) in metal-free container.	*mcg/dL* M: 1.4 ± 0.3 × 182 F: 1.7 ± 0.6	*nmol/L* [255 ± 55] [309 ± 109]	
X-ray fluorescence spectrometry[3]	Bronchoalveolar lavage (BAL) fluid	*ng/10³ macrophages* <0.17 × 18.2	*fmol/macrophage* [<3.1]	
ICP-MS	Serum.[7] Collect in pretested, metal-free container.	*mcg/L* 0.0-2.0 × 18.2 4.2-16.5	*nmol/L* [0.0-36.4] [76.4-300.3]	
	Whole blood.[7]	0.0-2.0	[0.0-36.4]	
	Urine.[7] Collect in acid-washed, metal-free container. Refrigerate during and after collection.			

1. Milne DB: Trace elements. In Burtis CA, Ashwood ER, editors: *Tietz textbook of clinical chemistry,* ed 2, Philadelphia, 1994, WB Saunders.

2. Neve J, Leclercq N: Factors affecting determinations of manganese in serum by atomic absorption spectrometry, *Clin Chem* 37:723-728, 1991.

3. Maier EA, Rastegar F, Heimburger R, et al: Simultaneous determination of trace elements in lavage fluids front human bronchial alveoli by energy dispersive X-ray flourescence. 1: Technique and determination of the normal reference interval, *Clin Chem* 31:551-555, 1985.

4. Milne DB, Sims RL, Ralston NVC: Manganese content of the cellular components of blood, *Clin Chem* 36:450-452, 1990.

5. Iyengar GV, Woittiez J: Trace elements in human clinical specimens: evaluation of literature data to identify tolerence values, *Clin Chem* 34:474-481, 1988.

6. Versieck J, Barbier F, Speecke A, et al: Manganese, copper and zinc concentrations in serum and packed blood cells during acute hepatitis, chronic hepatitis and posthepatic cirrhosis, *Clin Chem* 20:1141-1145, 1974.

7. Associated Regional & University Pathologists, Inc. web site (www.aruplab.com): Available at: http://www.aruplab.com/testing/user_guide.jsp. Last accessed 9/2004.

8. Cornells R, Versieck J, Mees L, et al: The ultratrace element vanadium in human serum, *Biol Trace Elem Res* 3:257-263, 1981.

9. Arjona A, Bonet M: Diagnosis of chronic manganese intoxication by magnetic resonance imaging (to the editor), *N Engl J Med* 336:965, 1997.

10. Nelson K, Golnick J, Korn T, et al: Manganese encephalopathy: utility of early magnetic resonance imaging, *Br J Indust Med* 50:510-513, 1993.

DIAGNOSTIC INFORMATION   **REMARKS**

Ercs ↑ Rheumatoid arthritis

TEST NAME AND METHOD	SPECIMEN REQUIREMENTS	REFERENCE INTERVAL, CONVENTIONAL [INTERNATIONAL RECOMMENDED UNITS]			CHEMICAL INTERFERENCES AND IN VIVO EFFECTS
Matrix Metallo-proteinase-9 (gelatinase B, 92 kDa type IV collagenase, type V collagenase)[1-3]	Serum, heparinized plasma, and urine. Re-peated freeze-thaw cy-cles should be avoided.		*Active mcg/L*	*Total (active + inactive)*	Tubes containing EDTA and citrate cannot be used because uncomplexed zinc and calcium are required.
		Serum:	0-597	0-1463	
		Heparinized plasma:	0-107	35-221	
		Urine:	0-10.9	0-46	
Immunoassay[1]					

1. *Human active MMP-9 fluorescent assay. Package insert,* Minneapolis, MN, 2004, R & D Systems, Inc.
2. Jovanovic DV, Martel-Pelletier J, Di Battista JA, et al: Stimulation of 92-kd gelatinase (matrix metalloproteinase 9) produc-tion by interleukin-17 in human monocyte/macrophages: a possible role in rheumatoid arthritis, *Arthritis Rheum* 43:1134-1144, 2000.
3. Sundstrom J, Evans JC, Benjamin EJ, et al: Relations of plasma matrix metalloproteinase-9 to clinical cardiovascular risk factors and echocardiographic left ventricular measures: the Framingham Heart Study, *Circulation* 109:2850-2856, 2004.
4. Reynolds MA, Hirchick HJ, Dahlen JR, et al: Early biomarkers of stroke, *Clin Chem* 49:1733-1739, 2003.
5. Pellikainen JM, Roponnen KM, Kataja VV, et al: Expression of matrix metalloproteinase (MMP)-2 and MMP-9 in breast cancer with a special reference to activator protein-2, HER2, and prognosis, *Clin Cancer Res* 10:7621-7628, 2004.
6. Moran A, Iniesta P, Garcia-Aranda C, et al: Clinical relevance of MMP-9, MMP-2, TIMP-1 and TIMP-2 in colorectal can-cer, *Oncol Rep* 13:115-120, 2005.

Mean Cell Hemoglobin (MCH)[1-3]	Whole blood (EDTA). Stable 6 hr at 25° C, 24 hr at 4° C.	*pg/cell*		↑ C Lipemia, icterus, chy-lomicrons, and hyper-leukocytosis (WBC
		Fetal[4]		>100,000/μL). False ele-
		18-20 wk	43.14 ± 2.71 (SD)	vations may be found in
Electronic counter	Fetal blood. Collect by	21-22 wk:	41.39 ± 3.32	the presence of Hb C or
	percutaneous umbilical	23-25 wk:	40.48 ± 2.88	Hb S, advanced liver dis-
	blood sampling	26-30 wk:	37.94 ± 3.67	ease, and easily precipi-
	(PUBS).	Cord blood[5]:	31-37 (2 SD)	tated globulins, e.g., in
		0.5 mo[6]:	30-37	multiple myeloma or
		1 mo:	29-36	Waldenström's
		2 mo:	27-34	macroglobulinemia.
		4 mo:	25-32	
		6 mo:	24-30	
		9 mo:	25-30	↓ V Excess intake of
		12 mo:	24-30	alcohol
		1-2 yr[7]:	22-30 (95% range)	
		3-5 yr:	25-31	
		6-8 yr:	25-31	
		9-11 yr:	26-32	
		12-14 yr		
		M:	26-32	
		F:	26-32	
		15-17 yr		
		M:	27-32	
		F:	26-34	

DIAGNOSTIC INFORMATION	REMARKS
For research purposes, matrix metalloproteinases have been examined in a variety of clinical conditions, including arthritis,[2] acute coronary disease,[3] stroke,[4] and cancer.[5,6]	Matrix metalloproteinases (MMP-9) are a family of zinc and calcium-dependent endopeptidases that break down the extracellular matrix. MMP-9 is an 82-kDa enzyme with high specific activity for denatured collagens. It is produced by neutrophils, monocytes, macrophages, fibroblasts, osteoclasts, and endothelial and epithelial cells.

DIAGNOSTIC INFORMATION	REMARKS
The calculated value of MCH is not generally considered helpful in the classification of anemias.[8] See also *MCHC*.	Value in pg/cell is calculated from hemoglobin and erythrocyte (RBC) count: $$MCH = Hb\ (g/dL) \times 10/RBC\ count\ (\times 10^{12}/L)$$ See also *Hematocrit*.

TEST NAME AND METHOD	SPECIMEN REQUIREMENTS	REFERENCE INTERVAL, CONVENTIONAL [INTERNATIONAL RECOMMENDED UNITS]	CHEMICAL INTERFERENCES AND IN VIVO EFFECTS

Mean Cell Hemoglobin—CONT

18-44 yr		
M:	27-34	
F:	27-34	
45-64 yr		
M:	27-35	
F:	27-34	
65-74 yr		
M:	27-34	
F:	27-35	

1. Henry JB, editor: *Clinical diagnosis and management by laboratory methods,* ed 20, Philadelphia, 2001, WB Saunders.

2. Greer JP, Foerster J, Lukens JN, et al: *Wintrobe's clinical hematology,* ed 11, Philadelphia, 2003, Lippincott, Williams & Wilkins.

3. Beutler E, Lichtman MA, Coller B, editors: *Williams hematology,* ed 6, New York, 2000, McGraw-Hill.

4. Forestier F, Daffos F, Galacteros F, et al: Hematologic values of 163 normal fetuses between 18 and 30 weeks of gestation, *Pediatr Res* 20:342-346, 1986.

5. Nathan DG, Oski FA: *Hematology of infancy and childhood,* ed 3, Philadelphia, 1987, WB Saunders.

6. Saarinen UM, Siimes MA: Development changes in red blood cell counts and indices of infants after exclusion of iron deficiency by laboratory criteria and continuous iron supplementation, *J Pediatr* 92:412-416, 1978.

7. Yip R, Johnson C, Dallman PR: Age-related changes in laboratory values used in the diagnosis of anemia and iron deficiency, *Am J Clin Nutr* 39:427-436, 1984.

8. Rodak BF, editor: *Hematology; clinical principles and applications,* ed 2, Philadelphia, 2002, WB Saunders.

TEST NAME AND METHOD	SPECIMEN REQUIREMENTS	REFERENCE INTERVAL, CONVENTIONAL		CHEMICAL INTERFERENCES AND IN VIVO EFFECTS
Mean Cell Hemoglobin Concentration (MCHC)[1-4]	Whole blood (EDTA). Stable 6 hr at 25° C, 24 hr at 4° C.		*g Hb/dL Ercs*	*g Hb/L Ercs*	↑ C Cold agglutinins, lipemia, icterus, chylomicrons, and hyperleukocytosis (WBC >100,000/μL)
		Fetal[5]			
		18-20 wk:	32.0 ± 2.3 (SD)	[320 ± 24]	
		21-22 wk:	31.7 ± 2.78	[317 ± 28]	
Electronic counter	Fetal blood. Collect by	23-25 wk:	32.1 ± 3.20	[321 ± 32]	
	percutaneous umbilical	26-30 wk:	32.1 ± 3.60	[321 ± 36]	
	blood sampling	Cord blood[6]:	30-36 (2 SD)	[300-360]	
	(PUBS).	0.5 mo:	28-35	[280-350]	
		1 mo:	28-36	[280-360]	
		2 mo:	28-35	[280-350]	
		4 mo:	29-37	[290-370]	
		6-12 mo:	32-37	[320-370]	
		1-2 yr:	32-38 (95% range)	[320-380]	
		3-11 yr:	32-37	[320-370]	
		12-14 yr			
		M:	32-37	[320-370]	
		F:	32-36	[320-360]	
		15-17 yr			
		M:	32-36	[320-360]	
		F:	32-36	[320-360]	
		18-44 yr			
		M:	32-37	[320-370]	
		F:	32-36	[320-360]	

DIAGNOSTIC INFORMATION   **REMARKS**

↑ Spherocytosis (hereditary spherocytosis or immune hemolysis)

↓ Iron deficiency, thalassemia syndromes

Mean cell hemoglobin concentration (g/dL) is calculated from Hb and Hct:

$$MCHC = Hb\ (g/dL) \times 100/Hct\ (\%)$$

The value may be misleading in the presence of a dimorphic population of erythrocytes.

See also *Hematocrit.*

TEST NAME AND METHOD	SPECIMEN REQUIREMENTS	REFERENCE INTERVAL, CONVENTIONAL [INTERNATIONAL RECOMMENDED UNITS]		CHEMICAL INTERFERENCES AND IN VIVO EFFECTS

Mean Cell Hemoglobin Concentration—CONT

	45-64 yr		
	M:	32-36	[320-360]
	F:	31-36	[310-360]
	65-74 yr		
	M:	31-36	[310-360]
	F:	32-36	[320-360]

Capillary blood (heparin)		g Hb/dL Ercs	g Hb/L Ercs
	1 day[6]:	31.6 ± 1.9 (SD)	[316 ± 19]
	4 days:	32.6 ± 1.5	[326 ± 15]
	7 days:	32.0 ± 1.6	[320 ± 16]
	1-2 wk:	32.1 ± 2.9	[321 ± 29]
	3-4 wk:	33.5 ± 1.6	[335 ± 16]
	5-6 wk:	34.1 ± 2.9	[341 ± 29]
	7-8 wk:	33.7 ± 2.6	[337 ± 26]
	9-10 wk:	34.3 ± 2.9	[343 ± 29]
	11-12 wk:	34.8 ± 2.2	[348 ± 22]

1. Henry JB, editor: *Clinical diagnosis and management by laboratory methods,* ed 20, Philadelphia, 2001, WB Saunders.
2. Greer JP, Foerster J, Lukens JN, et al: *Wintrobe's clinical hematology,* ed 11, Philadelphia, 2003, Lippincott, Williams & Wilkins.
3. Beutler E, Lichtman MA, Coller B, editors: *Williams hematology,* ed 6, New York, 2000, McGraw-Hill.
4. Rodak BF, editor: *Hematology; clinical principles and applications,* ed 2, Philadelphia, 2002, WB Saunders.
5. Matoth Y, Zaizon R, Varsano I: Postnatal changes in some red cell parameters, *Acta Paediatr Scand* 60:317-323, 1971.
6. Nathan DG, Orkin SH, Ginsburg D, et al: *Hematology of infancy and childhood,* ed 6, Philadelphia, 2003, WB Saunders.

Mean Cell Volume (MCV)[1-3] *Electronic counter*	Whole blood (EDTA). Stable 6 hr at 25° C, 24 hr at 4° C. Fetal blood. Collect by percutaneous umbilical blood sampling (PUBS).	*fL*	↑ V Excess intake of alcohol, zidovudine
		Fetal[4]	
		18-20 wk: 133.9 ± 8.8 (SD)	
		21-22 wk: 130.1 ± 6.2	Drugs that cause mega-
		23-25 wk: 126.2 ± 6.2	loblastic anemia include
		26-30 wk: 118.2 ± 5.8	acyclovir, aminosalicylic
		Cord blood[5]: 98-118 (2 SD)	acid, anticonvulsants, aza-
		0.5 mo[6]: 88-140	thioprine, azauridine,
		1 mo: 91-112	colchicine, cycloserine,
		2 mo: 84-106	cytarabine, fluorouracil,
		4 mo: 76-97	glutethimide, hydroxy-
		6 mo: 68-85	urea, isoniazid, mefe-
		9 mo: 70-85	namic acid, mercapto-
		12 mo: 71-84	purine, metformin,
		0.5-2 yr[7]: 70-84 (95% range)	methotrexate, neomycin,

DIAGNOSTIC INFORMATION	REMARKS

↑ Megaloblastic anemias (e.g., vitamin B_{12} and folate deficiency), nonmegaloblastic macrocytosis (e.g., acute blood loss anemia, hemolytic anemias, aplastic anemias, hypothyroidism, liver disease, and disseminated malignant disease), smoking, alcohol consumption (in men, increasing age, smoking, and alcohol consumption have independent effects); women after menopause, with oral contraceptive use, and with increasing age.[10]

↓ Hypochromic and microcytic anemias, including iron deficiency, anemia of chronic disorders, thalassemias; some hemoglobinopathies, occasionally in hyperthyroidism.

The mean cell volume may not be reliable when a large number of abnormal erythrocytes (e.g., sickle cells) or a dimorphic population of erythrocytes is present. A large number of reticulocytes will elevate the MCV. Many automated cell counters directly measure the MCV. The value in femtoliters (fL) may also be calculated from the hematocrit and erythrocyte count:

$$MCV = Hct\ (\%) \times 10/RBC\ count\ (\times\ 10^{12}/L)$$

See also *Hematocrit*.

TEST NAME AND METHOD	SPECIMEN REQUIREMENTS	REFERENCE INTERVAL, CONVENTIONAL [INTERNATIONAL RECOMMENDED UNITS]	CHEMICAL INTERFERENCES AND IN VIVO EFFECTS
Mean Cell Volume—CONT			
		2-5 yr: 73-85	nitrofurans, oral contra-
		5-9 yr: 75-87	ceptives, pentamidine,
		9-12 yr: 76-90	phenacetin,
		12-14 yr	pyrimethamine, thiogua-
		M[8]: 77-94	nine, triamterene, and
		F: 73-95	trimethoprim.
		15-17 yr	
		M: 79-95	↑ C Cold agglutinins;
		F: 78-98	marked leukocytosis
		18-44 yr	(WBC>100×10^9/L with
		M: 80-99	automated cell counters);
		F: 81-100	prolonged fixation of red
		45-64 yr	cells in EDTA causes
		M: 81-101	them to swell and can
		F: 81-101	falsely increase the MCV.
		65-74 yr	
		M: 81-103	
		F: 81-102	
	Capillary blood (heparin)	1 day[9]: 119 ± 9.4 (SD)	
		4 days: 114 ± 7.5	
		7 days: 118 ± 11.2	
		1-2 wk: 112 ± 19.0	
		3-4 wk: 105 ± 7.5	
		5-6 wk: 102 ± 10.2	
		7-8 wk: 100 ± 13.0	
		9-10 wk: 91 ± 9.3	
		11-12 wk: 88 ± 7.9	

1. Henry JB, editor: *Clinical diagnosis and management by laboratory methods,* ed 20, Philadelphia, 2001, WB Saunders.
2. Greer JP, Foerster J, Lukens JN, et al: *Wintrobe's clinical hematology,* ed 11, Philadelphia, 2003, Lippincott, Williams & Wilkins.
3. Beutler E, Lichtman MA, Coller B, editors: *Williams hematology,* ed 6, New York, 2000, McGraw-Hill.
4. Forestier F, Daffos F, Galacteros F, et al: Hematologic values of 163 normal fetuses between 18 and 30 weeks of gestation, *Pediatr Res* 20:342-346, 1986.
5. Nathan DG, Orkin SH, Ginsburg D, et al: *Hematology of infancy and childhood,* ed 6, Philadelphia, 2003, WB Saunders.
6. Saarinen UM, Siimes MA: Development changes in red blood cell counts and indices of infants after exclusion of iron deficiency by laboratory criteria and continuous iron supplementation, *J Pediatr* 92:412-416, 1978.
7. Dallman PR, Siimes MA: Percentile curves for hemoglobin and red cell volume in infancy and childhood, *J Pediatr* 94:26-31, 1979.
8. Yip R, Johnson C, Dallman PR: Age-related changes in laboratory values used in the diagnosis of anemia and iron deficiency, *Am J Clin Nutr* 39:427-436, 1984.
9. Matoth Y, Zaizon R, Varsano I: Postnatal changes in some red cell parameters, *Acta Paediatr Scand* 60:317-323, 1971.
10. Chalmers DM, Levi AJ, Chanarin I, et al: Mean cell volume in a working population: the effects of age, smoking, alcohol, and oral contraceptives, *Br J Haematol* 43:631-636, 1979.

DIAGNOSTIC INFORMATION   REMARKS

11.   Osserman EF, Lawler DP: Serum and urinary lysozyme (muramidase) in monocytic and monomyelocytic leukemia, *J Exp Med* 124:921-951, 1966.

TEST NAME AND METHOD	SPECIMEN REQUIREMENTS	REFERENCE INTERVAL, CONVENTIONAL [INTERNATIONAL RECOMMENDED UNITS]			CHEMICAL INTERFERENCES AND IN VIVO EFFECTS
Mercury (Hg)[1,2] *Quantitative: AAS*	Whole blood (EDTA). Collect in pretested, metal-free container.[3]	0.6-59.0 mcg/L Values <5 mcg/L [<25 mmol/L] may be seen in individuals who do not consume fish.	× 4.99	[3.0-294.4 nmol/L]	↓ *AAS:* Gold, platinum, and organic solvents that absorb at 253.7 nm
AAS	Erythrocytes[4]	3.3-15.0 mcg/L	× 4.99	[16.5-74.9 nmol/L]	Gadolinium may interfere with analysis.
AAS, NAA	Plasma or serum[3]	1.0-5.8 mcg/L		[5.0-28.9 nmol/L]	

			mcg/L	*mmol/L*	
AAS, colorimetric (mercury dithizone)	Urine, 24 hr. Collect in acid-washed, metal-free bottles. Acidify to pH 2 with nitric acid. Stable at room temperature.	Adult (nonexposed)[3]: (occupational exposure)[6] Toxic concentration: Lethal concentration[7]: 150 mcg/L [0.75 μmol/L] indicates exposure to 0.05 mg Hg vapor/m³ of air (suggested maximum allowable concentration for industrial atmosphere).[8]	<20 × 0.00499 20-50 >150 >800	[<0.10] [0.10-0.25] [>0.75] [>4.00]	U ↑ V Dimercaprol and penicillamine when used to treat poisoning U ↓ Iodine-containing medication

	Hair, at least 1.0 g cut close to the scalp. Wash to remove surface contamination.	~300 times blood level[9]	*mcg/ g dry wt.*[10]	*nmol/ g dry wt.*	
		Child and adult: Persons consuming large amounts of Hg-contaminated fish:	<15 × 4.99 5-70	[<75] [25-349]	

AAS, NAA[3]	Liver	*mcg/kg dry wt.* 33-490	× 4.99	*nmol/kg dry wt.* [165-2445]	
ICP-MS	Whole blood.[5] Collect in pretested, metal-free container.	0.0-10.0 mcg/dL	× 4.99	[0.0-49.9 nmol/L]	
	Urine.[5] Collect in acid-washed, metal-free container. Refrigerate during and after collection.	0.0-10.0 mg/dL 0.0-35.0 mcg/g creatinine		[0.0-49.9 nmol/L] [0.0-35.0 nmol/g creatinine]	

1. Henry JB, editor: *Clinical diagnosis and management by laboratory methods,* ed 18, Philadelphia, 1991, WB Saunders.
2. Wyngaarden JB, Smith LH Jr, editors: *Cecil textbook of medicine,* ed 18, Philadelphia, 1988, WB Saunders.

DIAGNOSTIC INFORMATION	REMARKS

↑ Overexposure, excessive therapeutic intake

Acute poisoning is usually from oral ingestion of inorganic Hg, which has a corrosive effect on the GI tract and causes renal tubular damage. Chronic poisoning is from inhalation or ingestion of small amounts; it results in gingivitis, stomatitis, erethism, tremors, nephrotic syndrome, colitis, anemia, and acrodynia (in children). Organic Hg intoxication results in fatigue, headache, loss of memory, apathy, emotional instability, paresthesia, ataxia, deafness, dysarthria, progressive visual deterioration, and dysphagia, and may lead to coma and death. Transdermal absorption of very small quantities of dimethylmercury can be fatal.[11]

Hg compounds are found in some medications, fungicides, dental amalgam, and in industrial processes. Elevated blood Hg levels and symptomatic Hg poisoning have been reported in dental workers. More than 90% of whole blood Hg is associated with erythrocytes. Whole blood or erythrocytes are recommended specimens for measuring methyl mercury poisoning. Toenail Hg may be associated with increased risk for myocardial infarction.[12]

See Table II-6.

Urine is the recommended specimen for measuring inorganic Hg. Bacteria may convert mercury compounds into a volatile Hg form.

Investigations have shown that hair may represent a longitudinal record of Hg exposure.[9]

3. Iyengar GV, Woittiez J: Trace elements in human clinical specimens: evaluation of literature data to identify tolerence values, *Clin Chem* 34:474-481, 1988.

TEST NAME AND METHOD	SPECIMEN REQUIREMENTS	REFERENCE INTERVAL, CONVENTIONAL [INTERNATIONAL RECOMMENDED UNITS]	CHEMICAL INTERFERENCES AND IN VIVO EFFECTS

Mercury—CONT

4. Johnson HL, Sauberlich HE: Trace element analysis in biological samples. In Prasad AS, editor: *Clinical, biochemical, and nutritional aspects of trace elements,* New York, 1982, Alan R. Liss, Inc.

5. Associated Regional & University Pathologists, Inc. web site (www.aruplab.com): Available at: http://www.aruplab.com/testing/user_guide.jsp. Last accessed 9/2004.

6. Clarkson TW, Laszlo M, Meyers GJ: The toxicology of mercury—current exposures and clinical manifestations, *N Engl J Med* 349:1731-1737, 2003.

7. Baselt RC: *Biological monitoring methods for industrial chemicals,* Davis, CA, 1980, Biomedical Pub.

8. Henry JB, editor: *Clinical diagnosis and management by laboratory methods,* ed 18, Philadelphia, 1991, WB Saunders.

TEST NAME AND METHOD	SPECIMEN REQUIREMENTS	REFERENCE INTERVAL, CONVENTIONAL [INTERNATIONAL RECOMMENDED UNITS]	CHEMICAL INTERFERENCES AND IN VIVO EFFECTS
Metanephrines, Fractionated[1,2] *HPLC*[3,4]	Urine, 24 hr. Collect with 20 mL of HCl, 6 mol/L. Stable for several weeks at 4° C.	*Normetanephrine, free plus conjugated*[3]	U ↑ V Hydrazine derivatives, MAO inhibitors, tricyclic antidepressants, levodopa, and significant physical stress.

Normetanephrine, free plus conjugated[3]

	mcg/day		nmol/day
0-3 mo:	47-156	× 5.46	[257-852]
4-6 mo:	31-111		[171-607]
7-9 mo:	42-109		[230-595]
10-12 mo:	23-103		[127-562]
1-2 yr:	32-118		[175-647]
2-6 yr:	50-111		[274-604]
6-10 yr:	47-176		[255-964]
10-16 yr:	53-290		[289-1586]
>16 yr[8]			
M:	128-934		[700-5100]
F:	92-604		[500-3300]

	mcg/g creatinine		μmol/mol creatinine
0-3 mo:	1535-3355	× 0.617	[947-2070]
4-6 mo:	737-2194		[454-1354]
7-9 mo:	592-1046		[365-645]
10-12 mo:	271-1117		[167-689]
1-2 yr:	350-1275		[216-787]
2-6 yr:	104-609		[64-376]
6-10 yr:	103-452		[63-279]
10-16 yr:	96-411		[59-254]

Metanephrine, free plus conjugated,[3]

	mcg/day		nmol/day
0-3 mo:	5.9-37	× 5.07	[30-188]
4-6 mo:	6.1-42		[31-213]
7-9 mo:	12.0-41		[61-210]
10-12 mo:	8.5-101		[43-510]
1-2 yr:	6.7-52		[34-264]
2-6 yr:	11-99		[56-501]
6-10 yr:	54-138		[275-701]
10-16 yr:	39-243		[200-1231]
>16 yr[8]			
M:	59-394		[300-2000]
F:	39-256		[200-1300]

U ↑ C Buspirone

9. Hair analysis for mercury, *Lab Rep Phys* 2:85-87, 1980.
10. Johnson HL, Sauberlich HE: Trace element analysis in biological samples. In Prasad AS, editor: *Clinical, biochemical, and nutritional aspects of trace elements,* New York, 1982, Alan R. Liss, Inc.
11. Nordren RE, Chang MB, Siegler RW, et al: Delayed cerebellar disease and death after accidental exposure to dimethylmercury, *N Engl J Med* 338:1672-1676, 1998.
12. Guallar E, Sanz-Gallardo MI, van't Veer P, et al: Mercury, fish oils, and the risk of myocardial infarction, *N Engl J Med* 347:1747-1752, 2002.

↑ In catecholamine-secreting neurochromaffin tumors such as pheochromocytoma, paraganglioma, and neuroblastoma.

Test provides higher diagnostic sensitivity than assays for catecholamines. Radiographic studies are warranted when total metanephrine (normetanephrine + metanephrine) concentration is >1300 mcg/day.

Although this is a reliable screening test for pheochromocytoma, the recommended first line test is plasma-free metanephrines. Use of urine metanephrines is suggested to confirm elevated plasma results.

TEST NAME AND METHOD	SPECIMEN REQUIREMENTS	REFERENCE INTERVAL, CONVENTIONAL [INTERNATIONAL RECOMMENDED UNITS]		CHEMICAL INTERFERENCES AND IN VIVO EFFECTS

Metanephrines, Fractionated—CONT

		mcg/g creatinine		μmol/mol creatinine
	0-3 mo:	202-708	× 0.574	[116-407]
	4-6 mo:	156-572		[89-328]
	7-9 mo:	150-526		[86-302]
	10-12 mo:	148-651		[85-374]
	1-2 yr:	40-526		[23-302]
	2-6 yr:	74-504		[42-289]
	6-10 yr:	121-319		[69-183]
	10-16 yr:	46-307		[26-176]

LC-MS/MS[5]

Normetanephrine, free plus conjugated[9]

		mcg/day		nmol/day
Normotensive				
0-2 yr:	Not established			
3-8 yr				
M:		34-169	× 5.46	[186-923]
F:		29-145		[158-792]
9-12 yr				
M:		84-422		[459-2304]
F:		55-277		[300-1512]
13-17 yr				
M:		91-456		[497-2490]
F:		57-286		[311-1562]
18-29 yr:		103-390		[562-2129]
30-39 yr:		111-419		[606-2288]
40-49 yr:		119-451		[650-2462]
50-59 yr:		128-484		[699-2643]
60-69 yr:		138-521		[753-2845]
≥70 yr:		148-560		[808-3058]
Hypertensive		<900		[<4914]

	mcg/g creatinine		μmol/mol creatinine
0-2 yr:	121-946	× 0.617	[75-584]
3-8 yr:	92-718		[57-443]
9-12 yr:	53-413		[33-255]
13-17 yr:	37-286		[23-176]
18-29 yr			
M:	53-190		[33-117]
F:	81-330		[50-204]
30-39 yr			
M:	60-216		[37-133]
F:	93-379		[57-234]
40-49 yr			
M:	69-247		[43-152]
F:	107-436		[66-269]

TEST NAME AND METHOD	SPECIMEN REQUIREMENTS	REFERENCE INTERVAL, CONVENTIONAL [INTERNATIONAL RECOMMENDED UNITS]		CHEMICAL INTERFERENCES AND IN VIVO EFFECTS

Metanephrines, Fractionated—CONT

50-59 yr			
M:	78-282	[48-174]	
F:	122-500	[75-309]	
60-69 yr			
M:	89-322	[55-199]	
F:	141-574	[87-354]	
≥70 yr			
M:	102-367	[63-226]	
F:	161-659	[99-407]	

Metanephrine, free plus conjugated[9]

	mcg/day		nmol/day
Normotensive			
0-2 yr:	Not established		
3-8 yr			
M:	29-92	× 5.07	[147-466]
F:	18-144		[91-730]
9-12 yr			
M:	59-188		[299-953]
F:	43-122		[218-619]
13-17 yr			
M:	69-221		[350-1120]
F:	33-185		[167-938]
≥18 yr			
M:	44-261		[223-1323]
F:	30-180		[152-913]
Hypertensive	<400		[<2028]

	mcg/g creatinine		μmol/mol creatinine
0-2 yr:	82-418	× 0.574	[47-240]
3-8 yr:	65-332		[37-191]
9-12 yr:	41-209		[24-120]
13-17 yr:	30-154		[17-88]
≥18 yr:	29-158		[17-91]

TEST NAME AND METHOD	SPECIMEN REQUIREMENTS	REFERENCE INTERVAL, CONVENTIONAL [INTERNATIONAL RECOMMENDED UNITS]		CHEMICAL INTERFERENCES AND IN VIVO EFFECTS
HPLC[6] *LC-MS/MS*[7]	Plasma (EDTA). Maintain at 4° C, and centrifuge within 6 hr. Stable for 3 days at 4° C. Store at −20° C in plastic vial.[8] See also *Remarks*.	*Normetanephrine, free*[10] <165 pg/mL × 0.0054 [<0.9 nmol/L] *Metanephrine, free* <99 pg/mL × 0.0051 [<0.5 nmol/L]		P ↑ V MAO inhibitors, lidocaine, halothane, withdrawal from sedatives (ethanol, benzodiazepines), and opioids. P ↑ C Acetaminophen

Plasma metanephrines have high diagnostic sensitivity (99%) for detecting pheochromocytoma but have less diagnostic specificity than urine metanephrines.[6,10]

Interference by acetominophen can be eliminated by method modification.[11]

Epinephrine and epinephrine-like drugs should be discontinued for ≥1 wk before testing. Patients should be fasting for a minimum of 4 hr before collection.

TEST NAME AND METHOD	SPECIMEN REQUIREMENTS	REFERENCE INTERVAL, CONVENTIONAL [INTERNATIONAL RECOMMENDED UNITS]	CHEMICAL INTERFERENCES AND IN VIVO EFFECTS

Metanephrines, Fractionated—CONT

1. Rosano TG, Whitley RJ: Catecholamines and serotonin. In Burtis CA, Ashwood ER, editors: *Tietz textbook of clinical chemistry*, Philadelphia, 1999, WB Saunders.

2. Hernandez FC, Sanchez M, Alvarez A, et al: A five-year report on experience in the detection of pheochromocytoma, *Clin Biochem* 33:649-655, 2000.

3. Abeling N, van Gennip A, Overmars H, et al: Simultaneous determination of catecholamines and metanephrines in urine by HPLC with fluorometric detection, *Clin Chim Acta* 137:211-226, 1984.

4. Jouve J, Mariotte N, Sureau C, et al: High-performance liquid chromatography with electrochemical detection for the simultaneous determination of the methoxylated amines, normetanephrine, metanephrine and 3-methoxytyramine, in urine, *J Chromatogr* 274:53-62, 1983.

5. Taylor RL, Singh RJ: Validation of liquid chromatography-tandem mass spectrometry method for analysis of urinary conjugated metanephrine and normetanephrine for screening of pheochromocytoma, *Clin Chem* 48:533-539, 2002.

6. Lenders JW, Eisenhofer G, Armando I, et al: Determination of metanephrines in plasma by liquid chromatography with electrochemical detection, *Clin Chem* 39:97-103, 1993.

Methemalbumin (Fairley's pigment)[1-3]	Plasma or serum	Negative	None found.
	Amniotic fluid. Centrifuge to remove		
Schumm test, ether, and ammonium sulfide	turbidity.[2]		
EP	Serum		
Spectrophotometry (dithionite reduction)[3]	Plasma or serum		

1. Dacie JV, Lewis SM: *Practical haematology,* ed 8, Edinburgh, 1995, Churchill Livingstone.
2. Henry JB, editor: *Clinical diagnosis and management by laboratory methods,* ed 20, Philadelphia, 2001, WB Saunders.
3. Lee GR, Bithell TC, Foerster J, et al: *Wintrobe's clinical hematology,* ed 11, Philadelphia, 2003, Lea & Febiger.

Methemoglobin (MetHb, Hemiglobin)[1,2]	Whole blood (EDTA, heparin, or ACD). Stable 1 hr at room temperature.	0.06-0.24 g/dL × 155*	[9.3-37.2 mmol/L]	↑ V Aniline dyes, benzene derivatives (especially nitro compounds), benzocaine, chlorates, chloroquine,
Spectrophotometry[1,3]				dapsone, ionizing radiation, isoniazid, lidocaine, metoclopramide, nitrates,
Starch gel EP, pH 7.0[4]		*% of total Hb* 0.78 ± 0.37 × 0.01	*Mass fraction of total Hb* [0.008 ± 0.0037]	nitrites, nitroglycerin, phenacetin, phenazone, phenazopyridine, pri-

7. Lagerstedt SA, O'Kane DJ, Singh RJ: Measurement of plasma free metanephrine and normetanephrine by liquid chromatography-tandem mass spectrometry for diagnosis of pheochromocytoma, *Clin Chem* 50:603-611, 2004.

8. Kairisto V, Koskinen P, Mattila K, et al: Reference intervals for 24-h urinary normetanephrine, metanephrine, and 3-methoxy-4-hydroxymandelic acid in hypertensive patients, *Clin Chem* 38:416-420, 1992.

9. Mayo Medical Laboratories: *Test catalog,* Rochester, MN, 2004, Mayo Medical Laboratories.

10. Sawka AM, Jaeschke R, Singh RJ, et al: A comparison of biochemical tests for pheochromocytoma: measurement of fractionated plasma metanephrines compared with the combination of 24-hour urinary metanephrines and catecholamines, *J Clin Endocrinol Metab* 88:553-558, 2003.

11. Roden M, Raffesberg W, Raber W, et al: Quantification of unconjugated metanephrines in human plasma without interference by acetaminophen, *Clin Chem* 47:1061-1067, 2001.

↑ Intravascular hemolysis, e.g., paroxysmal nocturnal hemoglobinuria (PNH), paroxysmal cold hemoglobinuria (PCH), hemolytic disease of the newborn (HDN), hemolytic transfusion reaction, traumatic hemolytic anemia, and falciparum malaria; acute hemorrhagic pancreatitis.

Methemalbumin (hematin bound to serum albumin) is formed in plasma when haptoglobin is depleted after intravascular hemolysis; oxidized heme is bound to hemopexin or to albumin (methemalbumin). In hemorrhagic pancreatitis, however, haptoglobin is present, suggesting that the methemalbumin is not the result of intravascular hemolysis but caused by the entrance of already oxidized heme (hematin) into the circulation.

↑ *Acquired:* See *Interferences.*

↑ *Hereditary:*
Deficiency of NADH-MetHb reductase (cytochrome b5 reductase).
Structural hemoglobin variants, designated hemoglobin M (Hb M).

In methemoglobin, the heme iron has been oxidized to the ferric state, and it is incapable of combining with and transporting oxygen. MetHb levels of 1-2 g/dL [155-310 μmol/L] result in visible cyanosis. Administration of methylene blue facilitates the reduction of MetHb to Hb in the enzyme deficiency and ameliorates the cyanosis. Methylene blue has no effect in reducing Hb M variants or in relieving the cyanosis that they cause. Heinz bodies may be associated with some forms of toxic methemoglobinemia.

TEST NAME AND METHOD	SPECIMEN REQUIREMENTS	REFERENCE INTERVAL, CONVENTIONAL [INTERNATIONAL RECOMMENDED UNITS]	CHEMICAL INTERFERENCES AND IN VIVO EFFECTS

Methemoglobin—CONT

maquine, resorcinol, sulfasalazine, sulfonamides, sulfones, smoking, and trimethoprim.

↑ C Specimen too old

↓ Improper handling

*Conversion factor based on MW for Hb of 64,500.   (MetHb is unstable.)

1. Henry JB, editor: *Clinical diagnosis and management by laboratory methods,* ed 20, Philadelphia, 2001, WB Saunders.
2. Bunn HF, Forget BG: *Hemoglobin: molecular, genetic and clinical aspects,* Philadelphia, 1986, WB Saunders.
3. Burtis CA, Ashwood ER, editors: *Tietz textbook of clinical chemistry,* ed 3, Philadelphia, 1999, WB Saunders.
4. Huisman THJ: *The hemoglobinopathies. Methods in hematology, vol 15,* Edinburgh, 1986, Churchill Livingstone.

Methionine (Met)[1-6]

Ion-exchange chromatography

Plasma (heparin) or serum, fasting. Place blood in ice water immediately; separate and freeze within 1 hr of collection. Stable for 1 wk at −20° C; for longer periods deproteinize and store at −70° C.[7,8]

	mg/dL	*μmol/L*[11,12]
Premature		
1 day:	0.52 ± 0.07 (SD) × 67.1	[35 ± 5]
Newborn		
1 day:	0.13-0.61	[9-41]
1 day-1 mo:	0.15-0.89	[10-60]
1-3 mo:	0.31 ± 0.13 (SD)	[21 ± 9]
2-6 mo:	0.24-0.73	[16-49]
9 mo-2 yr:	0.04-0.43	[3-29]
3-10 yr:	0.16-0.24	[11-16]
6-18 yr:	0.24-0.55	[16-37][13]
Adult:	0.09-0.60	[6-40]

In many ion-exchange chromatography systems, methionine does not separate from homocitrulline. Homocitrulline is elevated in hyperornithinemia, hyperammonemia, homocitrullinemia (HHH) syndrome.

Urine, 24 hr. Add 10 mL of 6 mol/L HCl at start of collection. (Alternatively, refrigerate specimen during collection.) Store frozen at −20° C.[9]

	mg/day	*μmol/day*[11]
10 days-7 wk:	0.1-1.9 × 6.7	[1-13]
3-12 yr:	3.0-14.2	[20-95]
Adult:	<9.3	[<62]
	mg/g creatinine	*mmol/mol creatinine*
or	4.5 ± 2.5 (SD) × 0.76	[3.4 ± 1.9]

U ↑ V Amobarbital

CSF. Collect in sterile tubes; store frozen. Stable at −20° C for 1 wk or at −70° C for 2 mo.[10]

	mg/dL	*μmol/L*
Neonate:	0.101 ± 0.037 (SEM) × 67.1	[6.8 ± 2.5][10]
Adult:	0.037 ± 0.003 (SD)	[2.5 ± 0.2][11]

CSF ↓ V Levodopa

DIAGNOSTIC INFORMATION	REMARKS

Spectrophotometric quantitation of MetHb is unreliable for Hb M variants because of their abnormal ferrihemoglobin spectra. Hb M can be detected and quantified using EP. The two forms of congenital methemoglobinemia are distinguished by NADH-MetHb reductase (diaphorase) assay for the enzyme deficiency and by analysis of the ferrihemoglobin spectrum and starch gel electrophoresis at pH 7.0 for detection of Hb M.

P ↑ Septicemia,[14] carcinoid syndrome, homocystinuria (cystathionine β-synthetase deficiency), hypermethioninemia, tyrosinemia, methionine adenosyltransferase deficiency, transient hypermethioninemia, and severe liver disease.

P ↓ Homocystinuria (if caused by deficient 5-methyltetrahydrofolate-dependent homocysteine methylation), protein malnutrition.

See Table II-2, A and B.

U ↑ Cystinuria, homocystinuria, oasthouse disease, tyrosinosis, methionine malabsorption syndrome, and methionine adenosyl-transferase deficiency.

U ↓ Severely burned patients.[5]

CSF ↑ Bacterial meningitis,[16] homocystinuria.

TEST NAME AND METHOD	SPECIMEN REQUIREMENTS	REFERENCE INTERVAL, CONVENTIONAL [INTERNATIONAL RECOMMENDED UNITS]	CHEMICAL INTERFERENCES AND IN VIVO EFFECTS
Methionine—CONT			
Tandem mass spectrometry	Dried blood spot. Collect blood spot onto newborn screening card. Allow to air dry before analysis.	Neonate: 0.28 ± 0.12 mg/dL [19 ± 8 μmol/L]	

1. Burtis CA, Ashwood ER, editors: *Tietz textbook of clinical chemistry,* ed 2, Philadelphia, 1994, WB Saunders.
2. Friedman RB, Young DS: *Effects of disease on clinical laboratory tests,* ed 2, Washington, DC, 1989, American Association for Clinical Chemistry.
3. Scriver CR, Beaudet AL,Valle D, et al, editors: *The metabolic and molecular bases of inherited disease,* ed 8, New York, 2001, McGraw-Hill.
4. Young DS: *Effects of drugs on clinical laboratory tests,* ed 3, Washington, DC, 1990, American Association for Clinical Chemistry.
5. Bremer HJ, Duran M, Kamerling JP, et al: *Disturbances of amino acid metabolism: clinical chemistry and diagnosis,* Baltimore, 1981, Urban and Schwarzenburg.
6. Nyhan W, Sakait N: *Diagnostic recognition of genetic disease,* Philadelphia, 1987, Lea & Febiger.
7. Cummings JG: Routine amino acids analysis in the clinical laboratory, *Am Clin Prod Rev* Feb:20-25, 1988.
8. Schaefer A, Piquard F, Haberey P: Plasma amino acids analysis: effects of delayed samples preparation and of storage, *Clin Chim Acta* 164:163-169, 1987.
9. Pesce A, Kaplan L, editors: *Methods in clinical chemistry,* St. Louis, 1987, CV Mosby.
10. Heiblim DI, Evans HE, Glass L, et al: Amino acid concentrations in cerebrospinal fluid, *Arch Neurol* 35:765-768, 1978.
11. Shih V: *Laboratory techniques for the detection of hereditary metabolic disorders,* Boca Raton, FL, 1973, CRC Press.
12. Chace DH, Hillman SL, Millington DS, et al: Rapid diagnosis of homocystinuria and other hypermethioninemias from newborns blood spots by tandem mass spectrometry, *Clin Chem* 42:349-355, 1996.
13. Meites S, editor: *Pediatric clinical chemistry,* ed 3, Washington, DC, 1989, American Association for Clinical Chemistry.
14. Freund H, Atamian S, Holyroyde J, et al: Plasma amino acids as predictors of the severity and outcome of sepsis, *Ann Surg* Nov:571-576, 1979.
15. Mårtensson J, Larsson J, Norström H: Amino acid metabolism during the anabolic phase of severely burned patients: with special reference to sulfur amino acids, *Eur J Clin Invest* 17:130-135, 1987.
16. Schott KJ, Meier D: Free amino acid pattern of cerebrospinal fluid in meningeal pathology, *Acta Neurol Scand* 75:304-309, 1987.
17. Schulze A, Lindner M, Kohlmoller D, et al: Expanded newborn screening for inborn errors of metabolism by electrospray ionization-tandem mass spectrometry: results, outcome, and implications, *Pediatrics* 111:1399-1406, 2003.

| **3-Methoxy-4-hydroxyphenylglycol** (MHPG)[1] *HPLC*[2-4] | Plasma (heparin or EDTA). Separate from blood cells soon after collection. Store frozen. Stable for 1 yr at −70° C. | Free (unconjugated)[5]

      mcg/L (SD)
Adult
M: 3.57 ± 0.97   × 5.43*
F: 3.68 ± 0.90 | *nmol/L*

[19.4 ± 5.3]
[20.0 ± 4.9] | U ↑ V Ajmaline, disulfiram, methylphenidate, reserpine, and syrosingopine.

U ↓ V Brofaromine, dextroamphetamine, |

DIAGNOSTIC INFORMATION	REMARKS

Cutoff for positive newborn screen for homocystinuria
>65 μmol/L.[17]

↓ V Endogenous depression

MHPG is a major metabolite of norepinephrine and is used as a marker for depression, for diagnosing anxiety disorders, and for monitoring therapeutic responses.[7]

TEST NAME AND METHOD	SPECIMEN REQUIREMENTS	REFERENCE INTERVAL, CONVENTIONAL [INTERNATIONAL RECOMMENDED UNITS]	CHEMICAL INTERFERENCES AND IN VIVO EFFECTS
3-Methoxy-4-hydroxyphenylglycol—CONT			
	Urine, 24 hr. Preserve with 50% acetic acid added within 4 hr of collection. Store refrigerated at 4° C.	Total (free plus conjugated)[6] Adults: 0.9-3.5 mg/day × 5.43* [4.9-19.0 μmol/day] *Conversion factor based on MW of MHPG of 184.	imipramine, MAO inhibitors, methyldopa, moclobemide, reserpine (long-term administration), and verapamil.

1. Maas JW, editor: *MHPG: basic mechanisms and psychopathology,* New York, 1987, Academic Press.
2. Gupta R, Steiner M, Lew M: Determination of unconjugated 3-methoxy-4-hydroxyphenylglycol by liquid chromatography for monitoring inhibition of monoamine oxidase activity in plasma, *Clin Chem* 33:2078-2080, 1987.
3. Moleman P, Borstrok JJM: Analysis of urinary 3-methoxy-4-hydroxyphenylglycol by high performance liquid chromatography and electrochemical detection, *J Chromatogr* 227:391-405, 1983.
4. Julien C, Rodriguez C, Sacquet J, et al: Liquid-chromatographic determination of free and total 3,4-dihydroxyphenylglycol and 3-methoxy-4-hydroxyphenylglycol in urine, *Clin Chem* 34:966-969, 1988.
5. Hariharan M, VanNoord T, Cameron O, et al: Free 3-methoxy-4-hydroxyphenylglycol determined in plasma by liquid chromatography with coulometric detection, *Clin Chem* 35:202-205, 1989.
6. Mayo Medical Laboratories: *Test catalog,* Rochester, MN, 2004, Mayo Medical Laboratories.
7. Filser JG, Muller WE, Beckmann H: Should plasma or urinary MHPG be measured in psychiatric research? A critical comment, *Br J Psychiatry* 148:95-97, 1986.

TEST NAME AND METHOD	SPECIMEN REQUIREMENTS	REFERENCE INTERVAL, CONVENTIONAL			[INTERNATIONAL RECOMMENDED UNITS]	CHEMICAL INTERFERENCES AND IN VIVO EFFECTS
1-Methylhistidine [His (p Me)][1-3] *Ion-exchange chromatography*	Plasma (heparin) or serum, fasting. Place blood in ice water immediately; separate and freeze within 1 hr of collection. Stable for 1 wk at −20° C; for longer periods, deproteinize and store at −70° C.[4,5]	6 mo-3 yr: Adult: 2-17 yr:	*mg/dL* 0.08-0.56 <0.42 <0.57	× 59.2	*mmol/L*[7] [5-33] [<25] [<34][8]	None found.
	Urine, 24 hr. Add 20 mL of toluene at start of collection. (Alternatively, refrigerate specimen during collection.) Store frozen at −20° C.[6]	10 day-7 wk: 3-16 yr: Adult: or	*mg/day* 0.8-1.7 6.9-50.7 11.5-144 *mg/g creatinine* 26 ± 12 (SD)[9]	× 5.92 × 0.67	*mmol/day* [5-10][9] [41-300][10] [68-852][10] *mmol/mol creatinine* [17.4 ± 8.0]	

1. Pesce A, Kaplan L, editors: *Methods in clinical chemistry,* St. Louis, 1987, CV Mosby.
2. Scriver CR, Beaudet AL, Sly WS, et al, editors: *The metabolic basis of inherited disease,* ed 6, New York, 1989, McGraw-Hill Publishing Co.

DIAGNOSTIC INFORMATION	REMARKS

P ↑ Chronic renal failure

U ↑ High-meat diet

Occurs in the dipeptide anserine. Large amounts of anserine are found in the meat of poultry and cattle.

3. Bremer HJ, Duran M, Kamerling JP, et al: *Disturbances of amino acid metabolism: clinical chemistry and diagnosis,* Baltimore, 1981, Urban and Schwarzenburg.
4. Cummings JG: Routine amino acids analysis in the clinical laboratory, *Am Clin Prod Rev* Feb:20-25, 1988.

TEST NAME AND METHOD	SPECIMEN REQUIREMENTS	REFERENCE INTERVAL, CONVENTIONAL [INTERNATIONAL RECOMMENDED UNITS]		CHEMICAL INTERFERENCES AND IN VIVO EFFECTS

1-Methylhistidine—CONT

5. Schaefer A, Piquard F, Haberey P: Plasma amino acids analysis: effects of delayed samples preparation and of storage, *Clin Chim Acta* 164:163-169, 1987.

6. Pesce A, Kaplan L, editors: *Methods in clinical chemistry,* St. Louis, 1987, CV Mosby.

7. Meites S, editor: *Pediatric clinical chemistry,* ed 3, Washington, DC, 1989, American Association for Clinical Chemistry.

| **3-Methylhistidine** [His (τ Me)][1-4] *Ion-exchange chromatography* | Plasma (heparin) or serum, fasting. Place blood in ice water immediately; separate and freeze within 1 hr of collection. Stable for 1 wk at −20° C; for longer periods, deproteinize and store at −70° C.[5,6] | *mg/dL*
 2-17 yr: <0.03
 Adult: <0.10 | *mmol/L*[8]
 × 59.2 [<2]
 [<6] | None found. |
| | Urine, 24 hr. Add 20 mL of toluene at start of collection. (Alternatively, refrigerate specimen during collection.) Store frozen at −20° C.[7] | *mg/day*
 10 days-7 wk: 1.2-3.5
 3-16 yr: 7.1-22.8
 Adult: 10.8-54.0

 mg/g creatinine
 or 27 ± 6 (SD)[9] | *mmol/day*
 × 5.92 [7-21][9]
 [42-135][10]
 [64-320][10]

 mmol/mol creatinine
 × 0.67 [18.1 ± 4.0] | U ↑ V Ascorbic acid (after large intake)[11] |

1. Scriver CR, Beaudet AL, Sly WS, et al, editors: *The metabolic basis of inherited disease,* ed 6, New York, 1989, McGraw-Hill Publishing Co.

2. Young DS: *Effects of drugs on clinical laboratory tests,* ed 3, Washington, DC, 1990, American Association for Clinical Chemistry.

3. Bremer HJ, Duran M, Kamerling JP, et al: *Disturbances of amino acid metabolism: clinical chemistry and diagnosis,* Baltimore, 1981, Urban and Schwarzenburg.

4. Nyhan W, Sakait N: *Diagnostic recognition of genetic disease,* Philadelphia, 1987, Lea & Febiger.

5. Cummings JG: Routine amino acids analysis in the clinical laboratory, *Am Clin Prod Rev* Feb:20-25, 1988.

6. Schaefer A, Piquard F, Haberey P: Plasma amino acids analysis: effects of delayed samples preparation and of storage, *Clin Chim Acta* 164:163-169, 1987.

7. Pesce A, Kaplan L, editors: *Methods in clinical chemistry,* St. Louis, 1987, CV Mosby.

8. Baylor College of Medicine, Biochemical Genetics Laboratory: *Test catalog,* Houston, TX, 1992, Baylor College of Medicine, Biochemical Genetics Laboratory.

9. Mayo Medical Laboratories: *Test catalog,* Rochester, MN, 1993, Mayo Medical Laboratories.

10. Shih V: *Laboratory techniques for the detection of hereditary metabolic disorders,* Boca Raton, FL, 1973, CRC Press.

11. Tsao C, Muyashita K: Effects of large intake of ascorbic acid on the urinary excretion of amino acids and related compounds, *IRCS Med Sci* 13:855-856, 1985.

DIAGNOSTIC INFORMATION	REMARKS

8. Baylor College of Medicine, Biochemical Genetics Laboratory: *Test catalog,* Houston, TX, 1992, Baylor College of Medicine, Biochemical Genetics Laboratory.
9. Shih V: *Laboratory techniques for the detection of hereditary metabolic disorders,* Boca Raton, FL, 1973, CRC Press.
10. Mayo Medical Laboratories: *Test catalog,* Rochester, MN, 1994, Mayo Medical Laboratories.

P ↑ Chronic renal failure

U ↑ Severe burns, multiple trauma

U ↓ Malnutrition

TEST NAME AND METHOD	SPECIMEN REQUIREMENTS	REFERENCE INTERVAL, CONVENTIONAL [INTERNATIONAL RECOMMENDED UNITS]				CHEMICAL INTERFERENCES AND IN VIVO EFFECTS

Methylmalonic Acid (Indirect Test for Vitamin B_{12} status)[1,2]

GC-MS[1] *LC-tandem mass spectrometry*[2]	Serum, fasting. Analyze fresh or store at −70° C.		*µmol/L*		*mcg/dL*	↑ Succinate may interfere with tandem mass spectrometric methods.
		Newborn:	0.24-0.39	× 11.66	2.8-4.6	
		6 wk-6 mo:	0.36-1.51		4.2-17.8	
		1-10 yr:	0.11-0.17		1.3-2.0	
		10.5-15 yr:	0.13-0.22		1.5-2.6	
		15.5-19 yr:	0.12-0.18		1.4- 2.1	
		Adults:	<0.2		< 2.4	
	Urine, random. Collect second voided specimen after overnight fast. Store frozen.	*mg/g creatinine* <3.76		× 0.957	*mmol/mol creatinine*[3] [<3.6]	

1. Monsen AL, Refsum H, Markestad T, et al: Cobalamin status and its biochemical markers methylmalonic acid and homocysteine in different age groups from 4 days to 19 years, *Clin Chem* 49:2067-2075, 2003.
2. Magera MJ, Helgeston JK, Matern D, et al: Methylmalonicacid measurement in plasma and urine by stable isoptope dilution and electrospray tandem mass spectrometry, *Clin Chem* 46:1804-1810, 2000.
3. Norman EJ: Urine methylmalonic acid test may have greater value than the total homocysteine assay for screening elderly individuals for cobalamin deficiency, *Clin Chem* 50:1482-1483, 2004.
4. Metz J, McGrath K, Bennett MJ, et al: Biochemical indices of vitamin B12 nutrition in pregnant patients with subnormal serum vitamin B12 levels, *Am J Hematol* 48:251-255, 1995.

Methylmercury[1] *GC-ECD*[2]	Blood (heparin)	<0.02 mg/dL Toxic concentration: >0.2 mg Hg/L	× 4.34 × 4.99	[<0.09 µmol/L] [>1.00 µmol Hg/L]	None found.
AA[3]	Hair	Toxic content: >200 mg Hg/kg	× 4.99	[>998 µmol Hg/kg]	
	Urine	<0.01 mg/dL Toxic concentration: >0.09 mg Hg/L	× 4.34 × 4.99	[<0.04 µmol/L] [>0.45 µmol Hg/L]	

1. Baselt RC: *Biological monitoring methods for industrial chemicals,* Davis, CA, 1980, Biomedical Pub.
2. Goolvard L, Smith H: Determination of methylmercury in human blood, *Analyst* 105:726-729, 1980.
3. Richardson RA: Automated method for determination of mercury in urine, *Clin Chem* 22:1604-1607, 1976.

DIAGNOSTIC INFORMATION	REMARKS

$\uparrow$ Plasma: vitamin B_{12} deficiency, pregnancy.[4]

$\uparrow\uparrow$ Plasma and urine: cobalamin genetic defects

$\uparrow\uparrow\uparrow$ Plasma and urine: classical methylmalonic acidemia

Transdermal absorption of dimethylmercury can be fatal.[4] Major toxic effects on CNS especially brain, variable latent period, paresthesia, ataxia, dysarthria, constriction of visual fields, hearing loss, coma, and death.[5]

Mercury is converted to methylmercury by microflora in water; it is lipophilic and is concentrated by marine organisms. Conversion to methylmercury may also occur in the human GI tract.

About 95% of total mercury in blood is concentrated in erythrocytes, largely as methylmercury. (See *Mercury* for other effects.) About 1% per day is converted to inorganic divalent mercury.

Kinetic values
$t_{1/2}$:   70 days.

4. Nordren RE, Chang MB, Siegler RW, et al: Delayed cerebellar disease and death after accidental exposure to dimethylmercury, *N Engl J Med* 338:1672-1676, 1998.

5. Clarkson TW: The three modern faces of mercury, *Environ Health Perspect* 110(suppl):11-23, 2002.

TEST NAME AND METHOD	SPECIMEN REQUIREMENTS	REFERENCE INTERVAL, CONVENTIONAL [INTERNATIONAL RECOMMENDED UNITS]			CHEMICAL INTERFERENCES AND IN VIVO EFFECTS
Metyrapone (Metopyrone, Metopirone) Stimulation Test[1]	Serum	*After metyrapone* 11-Deoxycortisol: >7 mcg/dL	× 28.9	[>202 nmol/L]	↓ V Amitriptyline, chlordiazepoxide, estrogens, glucocorticoids, methysergide, oral contraceptives, phenobarbital, phenothiazines, phenytoin, progestogens, and rifampin. See also individual tests.
Standard oral multiple-dose test		Cortisol: <3 mcg/dL or <30% [<0.30] of the sum of cortisol and 11-deoxycortisol	× 27.6	[<83 mmol/L]	
Dose, adult[2]: 750 mg every 4 hr × 6	Urine, 24 hr	*After metyrapone* 17-OHCS: 2-4 times base level			
Child[3]: 15 mg/kg		17-KGS: 2.5- to 3-fold increase, but at least 10 mg/day × 3.47 [35 μmol/day]			
		17-KS[1]: >2 times base level			
Single-dose test[4] Dose: 30 mg/kg orally with milk or snack at midnight	Collect serum for 11-deoxycortisol, cortisol, and ACTH at 8:00 AM the following morning.	11-Deoxycortisol: >7 mcg/dL	× 28.9	[>202 nmol/L]	
		Cortisol: <3 mcg/dL	× 27.6	[<83 mmol/L]	
		ACTH: >150 pg/mL	× 0.22	[>33 pmol/L]	

1. Abboud CF, Laws ER Jr: Clinical endocrinological approach to hypothalamic-pituitary disease, *J Neurosurg* 51:271-291, 1979.

2. Orth D, Kovacs D, DeBold C: The adrenal cortex. In Wilson JH, Foster DW, editors: *Williams textbook of endocrinology,* ed 8, Philadelphia, 1992, WB Saunders.

3. Endocrine Sciences: *Pediatric laboratory services,* Tarzana, CA, 1988, Endocrine Sciences.

4. Crapo L: Cushing's syndrome: a review of diagnostic tests, *Metabolism* 28:955-977, 1979.

5. Meikle AW: Secretion and metabolism of the corticosteroids and adrenal function and testing. In DeGroot LJ, editor: *Endocrinology,* Philadelphia, 1989, WB Saunders.

		mg/dL (x)			*mg/L (x)*	
β₂-Microglobulin (β₂M, Thymotaxin)[1-5]	Serum. Analyze fresh or store at 4° C for <72 hr. Stable frozen at −20° C for 6 mo or at −70° C indefinitely. Specimens without lipemia or hemolysis are preferred.	Neonates: 0-59 yr: 60-69 yr: >70 yr:	0.30 0.19 0.21 0.24	× 10	[3.0] [1.9] [2.1] [2.4]	S ↑ V Cyclosporine, lithium, and radiographic contrast media
Nephelometry, IEMA, IRMA, RIA						Excessive turbidity can affect nephelometric methods.

DIAGNOSTIC INFORMATION	REMARKS

See *11-Deoxycortisol* (Compound S).

No or impaired response: Hypopituitarism, Cushing's syndrome caused by adrenal tumors or ectopic ACTH-secreting tumors.[2,5]

Exaggerated response: Pituitary Cushing's disease

See individual steroids. This test should not be performed if primary adrenal insufficiency is likely. A normal response to exogenous ACTH should be demonstrated before initiating this test. (See *Adrenocorticotropic Hormone Stimulation Test, Rapid.*)

To ensure accuracy of 24-hr urine collections and of metyrapone administration, and to monitor possible adverse effects, the standard test should be done on hospitalized patients.

Test is useful to distinguish normal persons from patients with secondary adrenal insufficiency. Single-dose test may be done on outpatients.

↑ Conditions associated with increased cell turnover or immune activation, including inflammatory conditions, autoimmune diseases, infections, chronic renal failure, graft rejection,[4,10,11] graft versus-host disease (acute and chronic),[12] lymphoproliferative, myeloproliferative, and myelodysplastic disorders.[13]

β_2-Microglobulin (β_2M) is a low-molecular-weight protein that is the light chain of the class I MHC antigens. Because it is present on all nucleated cells and is almost totally reabsorbed and catabolized by the proximal tubules,[15] it serves as a marker of immune activation and proximal tubular function. It is found in nearly all body fluids.

TEST NAME AND METHOD	SPECIMEN REQUIREMENTS	REFERENCE INTERVAL, CONVENTIONAL [INTERNATIONAL RECOMMENDED UNITS]			CHEMICAL INTERFERENCES AND IN VIVO EFFECTS

β₂-Microglobulin—CONT

| | Urine, 24 hr. Centrifuge and adjust to pH 7.0. Analyze fresh. Stable at 4° C for 14 days or frozen at −20° C for up to 1 yr. | 0.03-0.37 mg/day[6]

<0.03 mg/dL | ($\bar{x}$: 0.1)

× 10 | [<0.3 mg/L][7] | U ↑ V Aminoglycoside antibiotics, carboplatin, cisplatin, cyclosporine, nifedipine, and radiographic contrast media |
| | CSF. Centrifuge before analysis. Analyze fresh or store at 4° C for <72 hr. Stable frozen at −20° C for 6 mo or at −70° C indefinitely. Specimens should not contain blood. | 1.5 ± 0.2 mg/L (SE)[8,9] | | | |

1. Ritzmann SE, Daniels JC, editors: *Serum protein abnormalities, diagnostic and clinical aspects,* Boston, 1975, Little, Brown and Co.

2. Ritzmann SE, Tucker ES III: *Protein analysis in disease—current concepts. Workshop manual,* Chicago, 1979, American Society of Clinical Pathologists, Commission for Continuing Education.

3. Putnam FW, editors: *The plasma proteins: structure, functions and genetic control, vol 1-3,* ed 2, New York, 1977, Academic Press.

4. Vivarelli M, Smith HM, Naoumov NV, et al: Quantitative assessment of serum beta-2 microglobulin in liver transplant recipients and relation to liver graft rejection, *Eur J Gastroenterol Hepatol* 7:1215-1219, 1995.

5. Child JA, Kushwaha MR: Serum beta-2 microglobulin in lyphoproliferative and meloproliferative diseases, *Hematol Oncol* 2:391-401, 1984.

6. Pesce AJ, First MR: *Proteinuria—an integrated review,* New York, 1979, Marcel Dekker.

7. Specialty Laboratories Directory of Services on-line: Available at: http://www.specialtylabs.com/. Last accessed 9/28/04.

8. Lutz CT, Cornell SH, Goeken JA: Establishment of a reference interval for beta 2-microglobulin in cerebrospinal fluid with the use of two commercial assays, *Clin Chem* 37:104-107, 1991.

9. Mavligit G, Stuckey SE, Cabinillas FF, et al: Diagnosis of leukemia or lymphoma in the central nervous system by beta 2-microglobulin determination, *N Engl J Med* 303:718-722, 1980.

10. Teufelsbauer H, Prischl FC, Havel M, et al: Beta-2 microglobulin. A reliable parameter for differentiating between graft rejection and severe infection after cardiac transplantation, *Circulation* 80:1681-1688, 1989.

11. Korcakova L, Svobodova J, Sedlackova E, et al: Serum beta-2 microglobulin before and after renal and heart allotransplantation and in infection, *Czech Med* 12:158-161, 1989.

12. Norfolk DR, Forbes MA, Cooper EH, et al: Changes in plasma beta-2 microglobulin concentrations after allogeneic bone marrow transplantation, *J Clin Pathol* 40:657-662, 1987.

13. Meryhew N, Zoschke DC, Messner RP, et al: Anti-beta-2 microglobulin antibodies in systemic lupus erythematosus and ankylosing spondylitis: effects on in vitro lymphocyte function, *J Rheumatol* 13:83-89, 1986.

14. Par A, Falus A: Serum beta-2 microglobulin (beta 2m) and anti-beta 2m antibody in chronic hepatitis, *Acta Med Hung* 43:343-349, 1986.

15. Karlsson FA, Wibell L, Evrin PE: Beta-2 microglobulin in clinical medicine, *Scand J Clin Lab Invest* 40(suppl 154):27-37, 1980.

DIAGNOSTIC INFORMATION	REMARKS

Anti-β_2M antibodies have been identified in patients with SLE,[13] ankylosing spondylitis,[13] and chronic hepatitis.[14]

Because of its accumulation with renal dysfunction and its ability to become glycosylated, form fibrils, and deposit in tissues, β_2M is a cause of dialysis-associated amyloidosis.[16]

Serum β_2M values are elevated in many hematological malignancies. An association has been found between serum β_2M concentrations and tumor burden in some lymphoproliferative disorders, particularly multiple myeloma, making it a valuable prognostic marker in these conditions.[5]

CSF ↑ Central nervous system involvement with lymphoproliferative malignancy.

β_2M is not stable in urine with a pH <7.0 and is markedly affected at pH <6.0. Consequently, it is recommended that urine specimens are alkalinized at the time of voiding because a random urine with acid pH may not provide an accurate result.[17]

MW: 11,800.

16.   Winchester JF, Salsberg JA, Levin NW: Beta-2 microglobulin in ESRD: an in-depth review, *Adv Ren Replace Ther* 10:279-309, 2003.
17.   Donaldson MD, Chambers RE, Woolridge MW, et al: Stability of alpha 1-migroglobulin, beta-2 microglobulin and retinal binding protein in urine, *Clin Chim Acta* 179:73-77, 1989.

TEST NAME AND METHOD	SPECIMEN REQUIREMENTS	REFERENCE INTERVAL, CONVENTIONAL [INTERNATIONAL RECOMMENDED UNITS]			CHEMICAL INTERFERENCES AND IN VIVO EFFECTS
Mitochondrial Antibodies (AMA)	Serum, frozen or refrigerated is preferable.	Negative is normal. Sera reactive at a ≥1-20 dilution are positive.			None known.
Indirect immunofluorescence		Negative: <1.0 U			
		Positive: >1.0 U			
Solid-phase EIA		Results are expressed in arbitrary units. Interpretive ranges vary with reagent manufacturer. Results are semiquantitative.			

1. Van Norstrand MD, Hurwich D, Malinchoc M, et al: Quantitative measurement of autoantibodies to recombinant 2-oxo-acid dehydrogenase enzymes: relationship of autoantibody titers to disease progression in primary biliary cirrhosis, *Hepatology* 25:6-11, 1997.
2. Van de Water J, Cooper A, Surh CD, et al: Detection of autoantibodies to recombinant mitochondrial proteins in patients with primary biliary cirrhosis, *N Engl J Med* 320:1377-1380, 1989.

TEST NAME AND METHOD	SPECIMEN REQUIREMENTS	REFERENCE INTERVAL, CONVENTIONAL [INTERNATIONAL RECOMMENDED UNITS]			CHEMICAL INTERFERENCES AND IN VIVO EFFECTS
Molybdenum (Mo)[1,2]	Serum.[3,4] Collect in pretested, metal-free container.	*mcg/L* 0.1-3.0	× 10.42	*nmol/L* [1.0-31.3]	None found.
AAS					
NAA	Plasma (citrate).[5] Collect in pretested, metal-free container.	0.59 ± 0.23 (SD)		[6.1 ± 2.4]	
ES, NAA	Whole blood[4]	0.8-3.3		[8.3-34.4]	
ES	Urine[4]	8-34		[83-354]	
ES, NAA	Hair[4,6]	*mcg/kg dry wt.* 20-490	× 0.0104	*nmol/g dry wt.* [0.21-5.10]	

1. Behrman RE. Kliegman RM, Nelson WE, et al, editors: *Nelson textbook of pediatrics,* ed 14, Philadelphia, 1992, WB Saunders.
2. Milne DB: Trace elements. In Burtis CA, Ashwood ER, editors: *Tietz textbook of clinical chemistry,* ed 2, Philadelphia, 1994, WB Saunders.
3. Centers for Disease Control: *Preventing lead poisoning in young children,* Atlanta, 1985, U.S. Dept. of Health and Human Services.
4. Iyengar GV, Woittiez J: Trace elements in human clinical specimens: evaluation of literature data to identify tolerence values, *Clin Chem* 34:474-481, 1988.
5. Kasperek K, Iyengar GV, Kiem J, et al: Elemental composition of platelets. Part III. Determinations of Ag, Au, Cd, Co, Cr, Cs, Mo, Rb, Sb, and Se in normal human platelets by neutron activation analysis, *Clin Chem* 25:711-715, 1979.
6. Johnson HL, Sauberlich HE: Trace element analysis in biological samples. In Prasad AS, editor: *Clinical, biochemical, and nutritional aspects of trace elements,* New York, 1982, Alan R. Liss, Inc.
7. Vyskocil A, Viau C: Assessment of molybdenum toxicity in humans, *J Appl Toxicol* 19:185-192, 1999.

DIAGNOSTIC INFORMATION	REMARKS

Positive results for AMA are detectable in >90% of patients with primary biliary cirrhosis (PBC[1]). AMA is also highly specific for PBC. The titer or levels of AMA do not indicate disease activity or prognosis in patients with PBC.[1]

The mitochondrial antigens recognized by AMA have been designated M1-M9. AMA from patients with PBC recognize the M2 antigen complex, which comprises enzymes of the 2-oxoacid dehydrogenase complex, including pyruvate dehydrogenase (PDH-E2) and 2-oxoglutarate dehydrogenase.[2] Positive AMA results are found occasionally in patients with CREST syndrome and other autoimmune diseases.

One case of molybdenum deficiency reported in a patient on long term TPN showed decreases in serum and urine uric acid and sulfate, as well as increases in urine sulfite, oxypurine, xanthine, and hypoxanthine.

Molybdenum toxicity mimics copper deficiency. Treatment with copper reverses symptoms.[7]

Molybdenum is a component of a few metalloenzymes, including xanthine, aldehyde, and sulfite oxidases. It is readily absorbed from the intestine and is excreted chiefly in urine. The normal pattern of urinary sulfur excretion is altered in Mo deficiency. Toxicity has not been established in humans. Molybdenum-poisoned mammals show inhibition of ceruloplasmin and cytochrome (copper oxidase) enzymes, as well as decreased activities of glutaminase, cholinesterase, and sulfite oxidase. Individuals who are copper deficient may be at greater risk for Mo toxicity.[7] A high activity of xanthine oxidase caused by elevated Mo levels may result in high serum uric acid levels and a predisposition to gout.

TEST NAME AND METHOD	SPECIMEN REQUIREMENTS	REFERENCE INTERVAL, CONVENTIONAL [INTERNATIONAL RECOMMENDED UNITS]		CHEMICAL INTERFERENCES AND IN VIVO EFFECTS
Monophospho-glyceromutase (MPGM) in Erythrocytes (EC 2.7.5.3)[1] *ICSH, 37 ° C*[1,2]	Hemolysate of washed Ercs. Submit whole blood (ACD, EDTA, or heparin). Stable 20 days at 4° C, 5 days at 25° C.	*U/g Hb* 37.71 ± 5.56 (SD) *U/10^{12} Ercs* 1093.6 ± 161.2 *U/mL Ercs* 12.8 ± 1.89	× 0.0645* × 10^{-3} × 1.0	*MU/mol Hb* [2.43 ± 0.36] *nU/Erc* [1.09 ± 0.16] *kU/L Ercs* [12.8 ± 1.89] None found.

See *Acetylcholinesterase.*

*Conversion factor based on MW of Hb of 64,500.

1. Beutler E: *Red cell metabolism: a manual of biochemical methods,* ed 4, New York, 1986, Grune & Stratton.
2. Beutler E, Blume KG, Kaplan JC, et al: International committee for standardization in haematology: recommended methods for red-cell enzyme analysis, *Br J Haematol* 35:331-340, 1977.
3. Beutler E: Red cell enzyme defects as nondiseases and as disease, *Blood* 54:1-7, 1979.
4. Beutler E: *Hemolytic anemia in disorders of red cell metabolism,* New York, 1978, Plenum Pub. Co.

Mucopoly-saccharide (MPS, glycosaminogly-can)[1] *Quantitative analysis (Alcian blue)*[1]		*mg/mmol creatinine* 0-1 mo 18.8 ± 4.7 1-3 mo 16.6 ± 5.7 4-6 mo 11.6 ± 4.9 7-12 mo 9.9 ± 3.7 1-2 yr 7.9 ± 2.7 2-5 yr 6.2 ± 1.8 5-9 yr 4.4 ± 1.2 9-16 yr 3.1 ± 1.2 16-60 yr 1.6 ± 1.0	↑ Heparin, turbidity of urine, and polyphos-phates.
Qualitative analysis[1] *TLC, electrophoresis*		Normal pattern MPS I (Hurler/Scheie) MPS II (Hunter) MPS IIIA (SanfilippoA) MPS IIIB (Sanfilippo B) MPS IIIC (Sanfilippo C) MPS IIID (Sanfilippo D) MPS IV A (Morquio A) MPS IV B (Morquio B) MPS VI (Maroteaux-Lamy) MPS VII (Sly)	Chondroitin sulfate only Dermatan sulfate/heparan sulfate Dermatan sulfate/heparan sulfate Heparan sulfate Heparan sulfate Heparan sulfate Heparan sulfate Keratan sulfate/chondroitin sulfate Keratan sulfate Dermatan sulfate Dermatan sulfate/chondroitin sulfate

1. Dembure PP, Roesel RA: Screening for mucopolysaccharidoses by analysis of urinary glycosaminoglycans. In Hommes FA, editor: *Techniques in diagnostic human biochemical genetics,* New York, 1991, Wiley-Liss, pp. 77-86.

DIAGNOSTIC INFORMATION	REMARKS

Deficiency produces no known effects.[3]

Activity is higher in young erythrocytes and may require testing of reticulocyte-depleted samples if high reticulocyte count.[4]

$$U/g\ Hb \times 29 = U/10^{12}\ Ercs$$
$$U/g\ Hb \times 0.34 = U/mL\ Ercs*$$

*See Note, *Acetylcholinesterase.*

The mucopolysaccharidoses are a group of diseases involving the connective tissue and affecting vascular and joint tissue. Substantial amounts of chondroitin-6-sulfate, heparan sulfate, and keratan sulfate are excreted.

This test is now rarely used, owing to false-positive results. The most commonly used quaternary ammonium salts are cetylpyridinium chloride and cetyltrimethylammonium bromide. A reagent blank reduces the interference from urine turbidity. This test has been adapted to quantitate the individual mucopolysaccharides.

This is the most common test to screen urine for the presence of increased amounts of mucopolysaccharides. The assay has a high rate of false-positive results. Qualitative analysis of glycosaminoglycan species is preferred.

Observation of abnormal glycosaminoglycan profiles should be followed up by enzymatic analysis of white cells.

TEST NAME AND METHOD	SPECIMEN REQUIREMENTS	REFERENCE INTERVAL, CONVENTIONAL [INTERNATIONAL RECOMMENDED UNITS]			CHEMICAL INTERFERENCES AND IN VIVO EFFECTS
Myelin Basic Protein (MBP)[1,2] *RIA*[1] ELISA[8]	CSF. Centrifuge before analysis. Analyze fresh or store at 4° C for <72 hr. Stable frozen at −20° C for 6 mo or at −70° C indefinitely. Specimens should not contain blood.	<2.5 ng/mL	× 1.0	[<2.5 mcg/L]	None found.

1. Bates HM: Radioimmunoassay of myelin basic protein in cerebrospinal fluid, *Lab Manage* Nov:19-22, 1978.
2. Glasser L: Body fluids. III: Tapping the wealth of information in CSF, *Diagn Med* 4:23-33, 1981.
3. Matthieu J-M, Burgisser P: Radioimmunological determination of myelin basic protein in the CSF of neurological patients, *Protide Biol Fluids* 30:223-226, 1982.
4. Gaur A, Wiers B, Liu A, et al: Amelioration of autoimmune encephalopathy by myelin basic protein synthetic peptide-induced anergy, *Science* 258:1491-1494, 1992.
5. Carnegie PR, Weise MJ: Visna and myelin basic protein, *Nature* 329:294, 1987.
6. Tienari PJ, Wikstrom J, Sajantila A, et al: Genetic susceptibility to multiple sclerosis linked to myelin basic protein gene, *Lancet* 340:987-991, 1992.
7. Warren KG, Catz I: An extensive search for autoantibodies to myelin basic protein in cerebrospinal fluid of non-multiple-sclerosis patients: implications for the pathogenesis of multiple sclerosis, *Eur Neurol* 42:95-104, 1999.
8. Chamczuk AJ, Ursell M, O'Connor P, et al: A rapid ELISA-based serum assay for myelin basic protein in multiple sclerosis, *J Immunol Methods* 262:21-27, 2002.

TEST NAME AND METHOD	SPECIMEN REQUIREMENTS	REFERENCE INTERVAL, CONVENTIONAL [INTERNATIONAL RECOMMENDED UNITS]		CHEMICAL INTERFERENCES AND IN VIVO EFFECTS
Myeloperoxidase Antibodies (MPO) *Solid-phase EIA*	Serum, frozen or refrigerated is preferable. Plasma is acceptable for analysis.	<5 U: 5-15 U: >15 U:	Negative Borderline Positive Results are expressed in arbitrary units. Reference intervals may vary with reagent manufacturer.	None known.

1. Russel KA, Wiegert E, Schroeder DR, et al: Detection of anti-neutrophil cytoplasmic antibodies under actual clinical testing conditions, *Clin Immunol* 103:196-203, 2002.
2. Falk RL, Jennette JC: Anti-neutrophil cytoplasmic autoantibodies with specificity for myeloperoxidase in patients with systemic vasculitis and idiopathic necrotizing and crescentic glomerulonephritis, *N Engl J Med* 318:1651-1657, 1988.

DIAGNOSTIC INFORMATION	REMARKS

↑↑ CNS trauma, stroke, tumor, multiple sclerosis, subacute sclerosing panencephalitis, viral encephalitides, and other neurological conditions.[3]

MBP is released into the CSF whenever there is damage to neural tissue.[4] The discovery of an elevated CSF level is thus a nonspecific indicator of active disorders. Levels increase within days after an insult and reflect destruction of intact myelin sheaths.

There is some suggestion that MBP released into the CSF is not identical with that found in tissue.[3] In patients with MS, antibodies to MBP have been detected in the CSF.

Viruses have been found that possess homology with MBP and suggest a novel form of mimicry.[5,6]

Clinical sensitivities and specificities range from 77 to >90% and 95-98%, respectively.[7,8]

MW: 18,500.

MPO autoantibodies occur in patients with microscopic polyangiitis.[1] This disease is often accompanied by glomerulonephritis (pauci immune necrotizing glomerulonephritis). MPO autoantibodies also occur in patients with LE, Goodpasture's syndrome, and Churg-Strauss syndrome.

MPO autoantibodies may be involved in the pathogenesis of microscopic polyangiitis.[2]

TEST NAME AND METHOD	SPECIMEN REQUIREMENTS	REFERENCE INTERVAL, CONVENTIONAL [INTERNATIONAL RECOMMENDED UNITS]	CHEMICAL INTERFERENCES AND IN VIVO EFFECTS
Myocardial Antibodies *Indirect immuno-fluorescence*	Serum, frozen or refrigerated is preferable.	Negative is normal. Sera reactive at a dilution of ≥1-20 are positive. Sera that contain striated muscle antibodies may produce indeterminate results.	None known.

1. Twomey SL, Bernett GE: Immunofluorescence method for detecting anti-myocardial antibodies, and its use in diagnosing heart disease, *Clin Chem* 21:1903-1906, 1975.

Myoglobin[1-8] *Immunoassay*[1,2] *Point-of-care immunoassays assays also available*[3]	Serum and plasma collected with or without separating gels (see individual manufacturer's package inserts for acceptable anticoagulants) are acceptable specimens for immunoassays. Specimens are stable at 2-8° C for 1 wk and at −20° C for 3 mo.[1] Samples containing precipitates should be centrifuged before assaying.	*mcg/L* Beckman Access Heparin plasma and serum F: 14.3-65.8 M: 17.4-105.7 EDTA plasma F: 11.1-57.5 M: 15.2-91.2 Bayer Centaur <110 Ortho ECi All: <101 F: <61.5 M: <121 Biosite Triage <107 Reference intervals for serum myoglobin vary according to age, race, and sex. On the average, serum concentrations increase with age, men have higher concentrations than women, and blacks have higher concentrations than whites. For consistency with cardiac troponin and CK-MB, the 99th percentile of a reference population should be used as the reference cutoff. The normal range also varies by assay. An effort of standardizing myoglobin has been initiated.[5]	Assays are generally unaffected by icterus (bilirubin, <65 mg/dL), hemolysis (Hb, <1.5 g/dL, lipemia (intralipid, <2200 mg/dL), and rheumatoid factors (<1500 U/L). High concentrations of HAMAs or heterphile antibodies may cause interferences.

Testing for myocardial antibodies is useful in patients suspected of having a post–cardiotomy or post–myocardial infarction inflammatory syndrome or inflammatory cardiomyopathy.[1] Positive results occur in 30-70% of such cases.

Circulating myocardial antibodies become positive 2-3 wk after myocardial injury because of infarction or surgery.

Myoglobin is known for its excellent clinical sensitivity early after AMI; however, it has not become a widely used test in clinical or laboratory practice.[6-8] The majority of clinical and laboratory testing guidelines suggest a possible role for myoglobin for early myocardial detection and early monitoring. However, in general practice, the lack of tissue specificity has been its major obstacle for growth in clinical practice. The major advantage offered by myoglobin as a serum marker for early, myocardial injury is that it is released earlier from damaged cells than CK-MB and cardiac troponin, allowing for earlier detection of MI. Myoglobin is a very sensitive marker (90-100%) for AMI. Serum concentrations of myoglobin increase above the reference interval as early as 1 hr after MI, with peak sensitivity in the range of 2-12 hr, suggesting that serum myoglobin reflects the early course of myocardial necrosis. Myoglobin is rapidly cleared and thus has a substantially reduced clinical sensitivity after 12 hr. If myoglobin is to have a role in detecting AMI, it must be within the first 0-4 hr, the time period in which CK-MB and possibly cardiac troponin are still within its reference interval. The measurement of serum myoglobin has not been extensively utilized in clinical laboratories for the routine analysis in AMI because it has poor clinical specificity (60-95%), which is caused by the large quantities of myoglobin found in skeletal muscle. The best use of early serum myoglobin measurements after admission to emergency departments is as a negative predictor of AMI. If myoglobin concentrations remain unchanged and within the reference interval on multiple, early samplings within 2-6 hr after the onset of chest pain, there is almost 100% certainty (99% negative predictive value) that muscle (either cardiac or skeletal) injury has not occurred recently.

Myoglobin is an oxygen-binding protein of cardiac and skeletal muscle with a molecular mass of 17,800 Da. The protein's low molecular weight and cytoplasmic location probably account for its early appearance in the circulation after muscle (heart or skeletal) injury. There is no difference in the myoglobin protein localization in the heart versus skeletal muscle. Increases in serum myoglobin occur after trauma to either skeletal or cardiac muscle, as in crush injuries or MI. Serum myoglobin methods are unable to distinguish the tissue of origin because the proteins are identical. Even minor injury to skeletal muscle may result in elevated concentrations of serum myoglobin, which may lead to the misinterpretation for myocardial injury. Because myoglobin is cleared by the kidney, changes in GFR will cause increases. It has a very short half-life of 10 min in blood.

TEST NAME AND METHOD	SPECIMEN REQUIREMENTS	REFERENCE INTERVAL, CONVENTIONAL [INTERNATIONAL RECOMMENDED UNITS]	CHEMICAL INTERFERENCES AND IN VIVO EFFECTS

Myoglobin—CONT

Ammonium sulfate solubility (presumptive test); EP (paper, starch, cellulose acetate); IEF (polyacrylamide gel)	Urine, fresh or adjusted to pH 7.0 with 0.1 mol/L NaOH.[4] Freeze at $-25°$ C for 2 yr.	No myoglobin present.	U $\uparrow$ V Aminocaproic acid (high doses, 20-30 g/day), amphetamines (abuse, IV), amphotericin B, barbiturates (poisoning), carbenoxolone, carbon monoxide (poisoning), ethanol (alcoholism), licorice, and succinylcholine (IV, particularly children).

Colorimetric		A_{600}/A_{580} Myoglobin: >0.85 Hemoglobin: <0.8 Metmyoglobin: 0.90-0.96 Methemoglobin: 0.67-0.75	U $\uparrow$ V Hb C or E. In patients with Hb C or E in erythrocytes, hemoglobinuria, and myoglobinuria cannot be differentiated by the EP method because myoglobin in the urine has the same mobility as Hb C and E.
Ultrafiltration		The presence of heme protein in ultrafiltrate indicates myoglobin.	

1. Wu AH, Laios I, Green S, et al: Immunoassays for serum and urine myoglobin: myoglobin clearance assessed as a risk factor for acute renal failure, *Clin Chem* 40:796-802, 1994.

2. Zaninotto M, Pagani F, Altinier S, et al: Multicenter evaluation of five assays for myoglobin determination, *Clin Chem* 46:1631-1637, 2000.

3. Muller-Bardorff M, Sylven C, Rasmanis G, et al: Evaluation of a point-of-care system for quantitative determination of troponin T and myoglobin, *Clin Chem Lab Med* 38:567-574, 2000.

4. Chen-Levy Z, Wener MH, Toivola B, et al: Factors affecting urinary myoglobin stability in vitro, *Am J Clin Pathol* 123:432-438, 2005.

5. Panteghini M, Linsinger T, Wu AHB, et al: Standardization of immunoassays for measurement of myoglobin in serum. Phase I: evaluation of candidate secondary reference materials, *Clin Chim Acta* 341:65-72, 2004.

6. Newby LK, Storrow AB, Gibler WB, et al: Bedside multimarker testing for risk stratification in chest pain units: the chest pain evaluation by creatine kinase-MB, myoglobin, and troponin I (CHECKMATE) study, *Circulation* 103:1832-1837, 2001.

7. Collinson PO, Stubbs PJ, Kessler AC, et al: Multicentre Evaluation of Routine Immunoassay of Troponin T Study. Multicentre evaluation of the diagnostic value of cardiac troponin T, CK-MB mass, and myoglobin for assessing patients with suspected acute coronary syndromes in routine clinical practice, *Heart* 89:280-286, 2003.

8. Gibler WB, Gibler CD, Weinshenker E, et al: Myoglobin as an early indicator of acute myocardial infarction, *Ann Emerg Med* 16:851-856, 1987.

9. Laios I, Caruk R, Wu AHB: Myoglobin clearance as an early indicator for rhabdomyolysis-induced acute renal failure, *Ann Clin Lab Sci* 25:179-184, 1995.

U ↑ Injury to skeletal or cardiac muscle, secondary toxic myo-globinuria (Haff disease), severe electrical shock, thermal burns, and arterial occlusion with ischemia of large areas of muscle mass.

In the context of increased serum myoglobin, a ↓ myoglobin clearance indicates rhabdomyolysis that is at high risk for de-velopment of acute renal failure because of obstruction of renal tubules by myoglobin.[1,9]

Myoglobin is soluble in 80% saturated ammonium sulfate, but hemoglobin is not.

The EP method cannot be used to differentiate between hemo-globinemia and myoglobinemia because hemoglobin attached to haptoglobin has the same electrophoretic mobility as free myoglobin.

The isoelectric focusing method is useful for the detection of myoglobin when a patient has an abnormal hemoglobin variant in blood.

The colorimetric method is sensitive to a myoglobin concentra-tion of 30 mg/dL [300 mg/L].

$A_{600}/A_{580} < 0.8$ indicates the presence of hemoglobin only if the benzidine test indicates the presence of heme protein.

Myoglobin passes through a Millipore filter 8-12 nm in pore diameter; hemoglobin does not.

TEST NAME AND METHOD	SPECIMEN REQUIREMENTS	REFERENCE INTERVAL, CONVENTIONAL [INTERNATIONAL RECOMMENDED UNITS]		CHEMICAL INTERFERENCES AND IN VIVO EFFECTS
Myosin	Plasma. Stable at 4° C for 4 days or frozen for	Sedentary individuals:	$<60\ \mu U/L$	None.
Heavy chain	1 mo.	Athletes:	$<120\ \mu U/L$	
IRMA monoclonal antibody[1]				
Light chain	Serum. Stable at 4° C for 4 days or frozen for	x̄: 0.13 mcg/L		
EIA monoclonal antibody[2]	1 mo.	Cutoff value:	0.95 mcg/L (3 SD)	

1. Larue C, Calzolari C, Léger J, et al: Immunoradiometric assay of myosin heavy chain fragments in plasma for investigation of myocardial infarction, *Clin Chem* 37:78-83, 1991.
2. Niederwieser A, Curtius H-C: Tetrahydrobiopterin deficiencies in hyperphenylalaninemia. In Bickel H, Wachtel U, editors: *Inherited diseases of amino acid metabolism,* Stuttgart, 1985, Thieme, Inc.

NADH Methemo-globin Reductase (NADH Di-aphorase, Cy-tochrome b_5 Reductase) in Erythrocytes[1,2]	Hemolysate of washed Ercs. Submit whole blood (ACD, EDTA, or heparin). Stable 5 d at 25 ° C, >20 d at 4 ° C.	*U/g Hb* 19.21 ± 3.85 *U/10^{12} Ercs* 557.1 ± 111.7 *U/mL Ercs* 6.53 ± 1.31	× 0.0645* × 10^{-3} × 1.0	*MU/mol Hb* [1.24 ± 0.25] *nU/Erc* [0.56 ± 0.11] *kU/L Ercs* [6.53 ± 1.31]	None found
NADH ferricyanide reductase, 30° C[1]		See *Acetylcholinesterase.*		
Fluorimetric (dichloropheno-linophenol), 25° C (screening test)[1]	Hemolysate of washed Ercs. Submit whole blood (heparin or ACD).	No fluorescence after 30 min		
Ferrihemoglobin-ferrocyanide (screening test)[3]	Hemolysate of washed Ercs. Submit whole blood (EDTA or hep-arin) or capillary.	No color change within 8 min *Conversion factor based on MW of Hb of 64,500		

1. Beutler E: *Red cell metabolism: a manual of biochemical methods,* ed 4, New York, 1986, Grune & Stratton.
2. Beutler E, Blume KG, Kaplan JC, et al: International committee for standardization in haematology: recommended methods for red-cell enzyme analysis, *Br J Haematol* 35:331-340, 1977.
3. Rogers LE: Rapid method for detection of erythrocyte NADH-methemoglobin reductase deficiency, *Am J Clin Pathol* 57:186-187, 1972.
4. Mansouri A, Nandy I: NADH-methemoglobin reductase (cytochrome b5 reductase) levels in two groups of American blacks and whites, *J Investig Med* 46:82-86, 1998.

↑ Acute myocardial infarction (up to 40-fold the upper reference interval), cardiac surgery, cardiac trauma, acute and chronic myocarditis.

↓ Cardiac atrophy resulting from severe malnutrition and cachexia in far-advanced malignancy or AIDS.

Myosin is found in the thick filament of the myofibrillar sarcomere of muscle. After myocardial cell necrosis, myosin is released into serum as myosin light- and heavy-chain fragments. These chains are detectable from 2-10 days after onset of myocardial infarction. The assay of myosin chains is therefore useful for the retrospective detection of myocardial cell damage.

↓ Congenital methemoglobinemia (autosomal recessive), usually associated with mild cyanosis. Proportion of methemoglobin is usually 10-15% and is completely corrected by oral or intravenous administration of methylene blue.

↑ Heterozygous β-thalassemia [4]

The natural receptor is cytochrome b_5.

U/g Hb $\times$ 29 = U/10^{12} Ercs
U/g Hb $\times$ 0.34 = U/mL Ercs*

Enzyme is unstable at 37° C; assay is best performed at 25° C.

Procedure is not reliable for detection of heterozygotes.

*See Note, *Acetylcholinesterase.*

TEST NAME AND METHOD	SPECIMEN REQUIREMENTS	REFERENCE INTERVAL, CONVENTIONAL [INTERNATIONAL RECOMMENDED UNITS]	CHEMICAL INTERFERENCES AND IN VIVO EFFECTS

Neuromuscular, Autonomic, and Central Synaptic Autoimmunity: includes myasthenia gravis (MG), Lambert-Eaton syndrome (LES), acquired disorders of continuous muscle fiber activity (e.g., neuromyotonia), autoimmune autonomic neuropathies and miscellaneous autoimmune encephalomyeloneuropathies. All of these disorders can occur spontaneously or in a paraneoplastic context (usually with small-cell lung carcinoma or thymoma). The profile of muscle and neuronal autoantibodies revealed by comprehensive serological evaluation helps to formulate the neurological diagnosis and may predict the presence of a neoplasm. Serological evaluation is recommended for (1) confirming the autoimmune basis of a defect in neuromuscular, autonomic, and central nervous system transmission, (2) distinguishing LES from autoimmune forms of MG, (3) increasing the index of suspicion for thymoma or primary lung carcinoma, and (4) providing a quantitative autoantibody baseline for future comparisons in monitoring a patient's clinical course and response to immunomodulatory treatment or cancer therapy. The following tests are most pertinent:

TEST NAME AND METHOD	SPECIMEN REQUIREMENTS	REFERENCE INTERVAL, CONVENTIONAL [INTERNATIONAL RECOMMENDED UNITS]	CHEMICAL INTERFERENCES AND IN VIVO EFFECTS
Muscle Acetylcholine Receptor (AChR) Binding Ab[1-3] Radioimmunoassay; serum is added to detergent-solubilized skeletal muscle AChR complexed with ^{125}I-labeled α-bungarotoxin.	Serum. Refrigerate if not shipped same day. Serum stable up to 2 weeks.	≤0.02 nmol/L	A mixture of adult and fetal-type human muscle AChR antigens provides optimal sensitivity. Ab may disappear with immunosuppressant therapy; the neurological diagnosis is further confounded if steroid myopathy develops. Unexplainable positive muscle AChR or striational Ab values occur in 40% of patients with autoimmune liver disorders, ~10% of patients with lung cancer, and in patients with graft-versus-host disease and recipients of D-penicillamine.
Muscle AChR-Modulating Ab[1-3] ^{125}I-α-bungarotoxin detects AChR remaining on living muscle membranes.	Serum. Refrigerate if not shipped same day. Serum stable up to 2 weeks.	0-20% (reported as % loss of AChR)	Curare-like drugs used during general anesthesia can yield transient false-positive AChR-modulating Ab results. Multifactorial false-positive results also occur because this is a bioassay.
Muscle AChR-Blocking Ab[1-3] Radioimmunoassay; ^{125}I-α-bungarotoxin is added to detergent-solubilized muscle AChR after serum.	Serum. Refrigerate if not shipped same day. Serum stable up to 2 weeks.	0-25% (reported as % AChR blockade)	Curare-like drugs used during general anesthesia can yield transient false-positive AChR-blocking Ab results.

DIAGNOSTIC INFORMATION	REMARKS

Muscle AChR-binding Ab is found in 90% of adult patients with acquired myasthenia gravis (MG) who have generalized weakness, 80% with weakness restricted to extraocular muscles, and in 100% of nonimmunosuppressed MG patients who have thymoma.[1] The seroprevalence of muscle AChR Abs is lower in children with MG. Severity cannot be predicted by Ab titer, but Ab levels are generally high with severe weakness. Ab specific for an alternative muscle autoantigen, MuSK, accounts for approximately one third of "seronegative" patients with acquired MG. These patients have predominantly oculobulbar symptoms.[6] Muscle AChR binding or modulating Ab is detected in 10% of patients with Lambert-Eaton syndrome (LES) or autoimmune autonomic neuropathy, but calcium channel Abs are not found in patients with MG, nor with thymoma.[1-3]

The patient's autoAb profile is more informative than the result of any single test for supporting a diagnosis of MG or LES and for predicting the likelihood of thymoma or lung carcinoma.[1] Muscle AChR Abs are characteristic but not diagnostic of MG. AChR and striational Abs may be undetectable for 6-12 mo after MG symptom onset. Only ~5% of nonimmunosuppressed adult patients with generalized MG remain seronegative for muscle AChR and striational Abs beyond 12 mo.[1-3] All muscle AChR Abs can occur with neoplasia without evidence of a neuromuscular transmission defect.[4,7]

AChR-modulating Ab is usually found with generalized MG. AChR-modulating Ab activity tends to parallel weakness. A positive striational Ab result is most predictive of thymoma, or other neoplasm, when the AChR-modulating Ab value ≥90% AChR loss.[1-3]

AChR-blocking Ab is the least sensitive of muscle AChR Ab assays for diagnosis of MG and is never positive when the AChR-modulating Ab assay result is negative. Only 55% of adult patients with acquired MG are seropositive. High values of AChR-blocking Ab are generally accompanied by severe clinical signs of MG.

Testing for muscle AChR-blocking Ab is not indicated unless the AChR-modulating Ab result is positive. The result provides a baseline value for future comparison in the course of remission, exacerbation, or immunosuppressant therapy. All muscle AChR Abs may be positive in LES, but calcium channel Abs are not found in MG, except in the context of lung cancer (N-type).[1-3]

TEST NAME AND METHOD	SPECIMEN REQUIREMENTS	REFERENCE INTERVAL, CONVENTIONAL [INTERNATIONAL RECOMMENDED UNITS]	CHEMICAL INTERFERENCES AND IN VIVO EFFECTS
Striational (Striated Muscle) Ab[1,6,7] Indirect immunofluorescence; substrate of cryosectioned rodent muscle, or glycerinated myofibrils, pelleted by Cytospin.	Serum. Refrigerate if not shipped same day. Serum stable up to 2 weeks. Ship whole blood immediately. Negative at 1:60.	<1:60	Immunosuppressant and chemotoxic therapies may reduce the antibody level below detection limit.
ELISA using KCL extracted rodent sarcomeric proteins.	Negative at 1:60.		
Muscle-Specific Tyrosine Kinase (MuSK) Ab[4] Radioimmunoassay; antigen is ^{125}I-recombinant extracellular domain of MuSK.	Serum. Refrigerate if not shipped same day. Serum stable up to 2 weeks. Ship whole blood immediately.	Lab-dependent	Immunosuppressant therapies may reduce the Ab level below the detection limit.
Calcium Channel Binding Ab, P/Q-Type[1-3,5,8-10] Radioimmunoassay; antigen is detergent-solubilized brain VGCC complexed with ^{125}I-labeled ω-conotoxin-MVIIC.	Serum	≤20 pmol/L	High-dose intravenous IgG therapy may cause false-negative or lowering of values. Plasma specimens and monoclonal (myeloma M proteins) or polyclonal hypergammaglobulinemia can yield false-positive results.
Calcium Channel Binding Ab, N-Type[1-3,5,8-10] Radioimmunoassay; antigen is detergent-solubilized brain VGCC complexed with ^{125}I-labeled ω-conotoxin-GVIA.	Serum	≤20 pmol/L	High-dose intravenous IgG therapy may cause false-negative or lowering of values. N-type calcium channel binding Ab may become undetectable soon after commencing corticosteroid treatment.

Striational Ab seropositivity aids the diagnosis of thymoma, especially in patients with MG onset younger than age 45 yr, or with an AChR modulating Ab value $\geq$90% AChR loss.[1] This profile's predictive value for thymoma is greatest when accompanied by CRMP-5-IgG, GAD65 Ab, neuronal potassium channel Ab or ganglionic AChR Ab.[4] Seronegativity does not exclude a thymoma (24% are negative). Striational Ab seropositivity is useful as a confirmatory test for MG in older patients, especially when tests for muscle AChR Abs are negative. Serial measurements are useful in monitoring the efficacy of immunosuppressant treatment in patients with MG, and after treating thymoma. Striational Abs may be detected in patients with LES, small cell carcinoma of the lung, breast carcinoma, treated with D-penicillamine, autoimmune liver disorders, and bone marrow transplant recipients with graft-versus-host disease.[5]

AutoAbs that bind to the contractile elements of striated muscle (titin, actin, alpha-actinin, myosin, or rhyanodine receptor) are found in 30% of adult patients with MG and in 80% of those with thymoma. Striational Abs are detected in 21% of patients who have thymoma without clinical evidence of MG, 25% of rheumatoid arthritis (RA) patients treated with D-penicillamine, 4% of untreated RA patients, and 5% of patients with LES and/or small-cell lung carcinoma. The seroprevalence in healthy subjects is <1%. An increasing titer after removal of thymoma may indicate thymoma recurrence or a second neoplasm.[7]

MuSK Ab is detected in ~30% of patients with generalized MG who lack detectable AChR Abs.[6] A majority have a phenotype of bulbar MG, and are prone to respiratory failure. Thymectomy is not beneficial in treatment. Plasmapheresis and immunosuppressant therapies are effective, and acetylcholinesterase inhibitors sometimes help. No paraneoplastic case has been identified.

MuSK is a muscle endplate tyrosine kinase receptor for the neurotrophic factor agrin, secreted by motor neurons. It is essential for establishing and maintaining high-density clusters of AChR in the postsynaptic membrane. MuSK Ab rarely coexists with muscle AChR or striational Ab.

P/Q-type calcium channel Ab is detected in >90% of non-immunosuppressed patients who have LES (usually >100 pmol/L), and in 20% of patients who have encephalomyeloneuropathies related to carcinoma of lung, breast, or ovary.[1,7,10] Seropositivity also implicates autoimmunity as a pathogenic mechanism in patients with complex neurologic presentations, particularly in those with a history of cancer, or risk factors for cancer. Seropositivity can occur with limbic encephalitis, cerebellar ataxia, peripheral neuropathy or autonomic neuropathy.

P/Q-type calcium channels regulate neurotransmitter release at motor nerve terminals and are involved in central neurotransmission. AutoAbs directed against extracellular epitopes of P/Q-type calcium channels are implicated as the effectors of LES and possibly some cerebellar ataxias.[1-3] P/Q-type Ca^{2+} channel Ab commonly coexists with neuronal nuclear and cytoplasmic paraneoplastic autoAbs, except in patients whose LES is not accompanied by other paraneoplastic autoimmune neurologic disorders.[7]

N-type calcium channel binding Ab is more frequent in LES patients who have lung cancer (75%) than in those with other types of cancer or no cancer (36%). This Ab is also found in patients with paraneoplastic encephalomyeloneuropathies complicating lung, ovarian or breast carcinoma, and in some adults and children with acquired cerebellar ataxia or autonomic neuropathy, including gastrointestinal dysmotilities without evidence of a tumor. Neuroblastoma is sometimes found in seropositive children.[10]

N-type Ca^{2+} channel Ab commonly coexists with neuronal nuclear and cytoplasmic paraneoplastic autoAbs, except in patients whose LES is not accompanied by other paraneoplastic autoimmune neurologic disorders.[1,7]

TEST NAME AND METHOD	SPECIMEN REQUIREMENTS	REFERENCE INTERVAL, CONVENTIONAL [INTERNATIONAL RECOMMENDED UNITS]	CHEMICAL INTERFERENCES AND IN VIVO EFFECTS
Voltage-Gated Neuronal Potassium Channel Ab (VGKC)[11-15] Radioimmunoassay; antigen is detergent-solubilized brain VGKC complexed with ^{125}I-labeled α-dendrotoxin.	Serum	≤20 pmol/L	Immunosuppressant therapies may reduce the Ab level below detection limit.
Neuronal Ganglionic Acetylcholine (AChR) Binding Ab[16-19] Radioimmunoassay; antigen is ganglionic AChR solubilized from membranes of a human peripheral neuroblastoma and complexed with ^{125}I-epibatidine.	Serum	≤20 pmol/L	Immunosuppressant therapies may reduce the Ab level below detection limit.

1. Lennon VA: Serological profile of myasthenia gravis and distinction from the Lambert-Eaton myasthenic syndrome, *Neurology* 48(suppl 5):S23-S27, 1997.

2. Lennon VA, Kryzer TJ, Griesmann GE, et al: Calcium-channel antibodies in the Lambert-Eaton myasthenic syndrome and other paraneoplastic syndromes, *N Engl J Med* 332:1467-1474, 1995.

3. Harper CM, Lennon VA: Chapter: Lambert-Eaton syndrome. In Kaminski HJ, editor: *Current clinical neurology: myasthenia gravis and related disorders,* Totowa, NJ, 2002, Humana Press, pp. 269-291.

4. Vernino S, Lennon VA: Autoantibody profiles and neurological correlations of thymoma, *Clin Cancer Res* 10:7270-7275, 2004.

5. Cikes N, Momoi MY, Williams CL, et al: Striational autoantibodies: quantitative detection by enzyme immunoassay in myasthenia gravis, thymoma, and recipients of D-penicillamine or allogeneic bone marrow, *Mayo Clin Proc* 63:474-481, 1988.

6. Hoch W, McConville J, Helms S, et al: Auto-antibodies to the receptor tyrosine kinase MuSK in patients with myasthenia gravis without acetylcholine receptor antibodies, *Nat Med* 7:365-368, 2001.

7. Pittock SJ, Kryzer TJ, Lennon VA: Paraneoplastic antibodies often coexist and predict cancer not neurologic syndrome, *Ann Neurol* 56:715-719, 2004.

8. Lennon VA, Lambert EH: Autoantibodies bind solubilized calcium channel-omega-contotoxin complexes from small cell lung carcinoma: a diagnostic aid for Lambert-Eaton myasthenic syndrome, *Mayo Clin Proc* 64:1498-1504, 1989.

9. Vernino S, Lennon V: Muscle and neuronal autoantibody markers of thymoma: neurological correlations, *Ann NY Acad Sci* 998:359-361, 2003.

VGKC Ab is a marker of acquired neuromuscular hyperexcitability disorders (e.g. Isaacs disease, which is characterized electromyographically by high-frequency neuromyotonic discharges).[11,12] VGKC Ab also is found (usually at higher levels), in patients with limbic encephalitis. Patients with this inflammatory disorder of mesial temporal lobes present with subacute seizures, memory impairment, and personality change. It is reversible in early stages by a 5-day course of high dose i.v. methylprednisolone. Maintenance immunosuppression is recommended to prevent relapse.[13-15]

Ganglionic AChR Ab complements VGKC Ab as a marker of autoimmune neuromuscular hyperexcitability and limbic encephalitis. Both autoAbs accompany small cell carcinoma and thymoma and can coexist with other autoantibody markers of these neoplasms.[7]

Patients with subacute limbic encephalitis require thorough and repeated evaluation for neoplasia regardless of their Ab status.

Seropositivity distinguishes idiopathic and paraneoplastic autonomic neuropathy from other acquired forms of dysautonomia.[16,17] Seronegativity does not exclude the diagnosis of autoimmune autonomic neuropathy. Ganglionic AChR Ab is detected in 50% of patients with autoimmune autonomic neuropathy (AAN). Serum Ab levels correlate with the severity of autonomic dysfunction and fall or disappear with clinical improvement. Patients with isolated gastrointestinal dysmotility, postural tachycardia and "pure autonomic failure" are sometimes seropositive. Ganglionic AChR Ab, usually in relatively low titer, complements VGKC Ab as a marker of autoimmune neuromuscular hyperexcitability disorders. Detection of ganglionic AChR Ab warrants aggressive search for a lung carcinoma or thymoma.

Ganglionic AChR Ab, isolated from serum of AAN patients or ganglionic AChR-immunized rabbits, causes subacute dysautonomia when injected into mice.[18,19]

10. Lennon VA: Calcium channel and related paraneoplastic disease autoantibodies. In Peter JP, Schoenfeld Y, editors: *Textbook of autoantibodies,* Amsterdam, 1996, Elsevier Science Publishers, B.V., pp. 139-147.

11. Vernino S, Lennon VA: Ion channel and striational antibodies define a continuum of autoimmune neuromuscular hyperexcitability, *Muscle Nerve* 26:702-707, 2002.

12. Hart IK, Vincent A, Newland C, et al: Autoantibodies detected to expressed K^+ channels are implicated in neuromyotonia, *Ann Neurol* 41:238-246, 1997.

13. Buckley C, Oger J, Clover L, et al: Potassium channel antibodies in two patients with reversible limbic encephalitis, *Ann Neurol* 50:73-78, 2001.

14. Thieben MJ, Lennon VA, Boeve BF, et al: Potentially reversible autoimmune limbic encephalitis with neuronal potassium channel antibody, *Neurology* 62:1177-1182, 2004. Accompanying editorial: 62:1040-1041, 2004.

15. Pozo-Rosich P, Clover L, Saiz A, et al: Voltage-gated potassium channel antibodies in limbic encephalitis, *Ann Neurol* 54:530-533, 2003.

16. Vernino S, Low PA, Fealey RD, et al: Autoantibodies to ganglionic acetylcholine receptors in autoimmune autonomic neuropathies, *N Engl J Med* 343:847-855, 2000.

17. Vernino S, Adamski J, Kryzer TJ, et al: Neuronal nicotinic ACh receptor antibody in subacute autonomic neuropathy and cancer-related syndromes, *Neurology* 50:1806-1813, 1998.

18. Lennon VA, Ermilov LG, Szurszewski JH, et al: Immunization with neuronal nicotinic acetylcholine receptor induces neurological autoimmune disease, *J Clin Invest* 111:907-913, 2003.

19. Vernino S, Ermilov LG, Sha L, et al: Passive transfer of autoimmune autonomic neuropathy to mice, *J Neurosci* 24:7037-7042, 2004.

TEST NAME AND METHOD	SPECIMEN REQUIREMENTS	REFERENCE INTERVAL, CONVENTIONAL [INTERNATIONAL RECOMMENDED UNITS]	CHEMICAL INTERFERENCES AND IN VIVO EFFECTS
Neutrophil Alkaline Phosphatase (Leukocyte Alkaline Phosphatase, LAP)[1,2] *Kaplow, naphthol AS-BI phosphate (Sigma Chemical Co.), fast red-violet LB, pH 9.72*	Finger-stick blood preferred. Collect venous blood in heparin or oxalate. Do not use EDTA. Fix slides in formalin/methanol within 30 min or keep in desiccator until fixed.	Score: 40-130 Score is based on 0-4+ rating of 100 neutrophils. Reference interval must be determined for each laboratory.	↓ C EDTA (Enzyme activity diminishes rapidly with time.)

1. Henry JB, editor: *Clinical diagnosis and management by laboratory methods,* ed 20, Philadelphia, 2001, WB Saunders.
2. Williams WJ, Beutler E, Erslev AJ, et al, editors: *Hematology,* ed 4, New York, 1990, McGraw-Hill Publishing Co.
3. Miale JB: *Laboratory medicine: hematology,* ed 6, St. Louis, 1982, CV Mosby.

TEST NAME AND METHOD	SPECIMEN REQUIREMENTS	REFERENCE INTERVAL, CONVENTIONAL [INTERNATIONAL RECOMMENDED UNITS]	CHEMICAL INTERFERENCES AND IN VIVO EFFECTS
anti-Neutrophil Cytoplasmic Antibodies (ANCA): Includes cANCA and pANCA *Indirect immunofluorescence*	Serum, frozen or refrigerated, is preferable. Plasma specimens are acceptable for analysis.	Negative is normal. Sera reactive at a dilution of ≥1-4 are considered positive. Sera that produce the cANCA staining pattern are typically titered to endpoint. Sera that produce the pANCA staining pattern are often reported qualitatively as positive without an endpoint titer.	None known.

1. Specks U, Wheatley CL, McDonald TJ, et al: Anticytoplasmic autoantibodies in the diagnosis and follow-up of Wegener's granulomatosis, *Mayo Clin Proc* 64:28-36, 1989.
2. Falk RL, Jennette JC: Anti-neutrophil cytoplasmic autoantibodies with specificity for myeloperoxidase in patients with systemic vasculitis and idiopathic necrotizing and crescentic glomerulonephritis, *N Engl J Med* 318:1651-1657, 1988.
3. Russel KA, Wiegert E, Schroeder DR, et al: Detection of anti-neutrophil cytoplasmic antibodies under actual clinical testing conditions, *Clin Immunol* 103:196-203, 2002.

DIAGNOSTIC INFORMATION	REMARKS

↑ Polycythemia vera (highest values), leukemoid reactions, Down syndrome,[3] myeloproliferative disorders, stress, pregnancy, after administration of ACTH, acute lymphoblastic leukemia, Hodgkin's disease, agnogenic myeloid metaplasia, aplastic anemia, and bacterial infection.

↓ Chronic myelogenous leukemia, sideroblastic anemia, idiopathic thrombocytopenic purpura (ITP), paroxysmal noctural hemoglobinuria (PNH), collagen diseases, AML, acute monocytic leukemia, cirrhosis, congestive heart failure with passive congestion of the liver, diabetes mellitus, gout, pernicious anemia (increases after treatment), hereditary hypophosphatasia, and sarcoidosis.

The terms *neutrophil alkaline phosphatase* and *leukocyte alkaline phosphatase* (LAP) are interchangeable. LAP is principally of value in distinguishing chronic myeloid leukemia (CML) from leukemoid reactions and other myeloproliferative disorders. In remission of CML, the LAP may return to normal, and in the aggressive phase of CML, or blast crisis, the LAP may be elevated.

ANCA occur in patients with vasculitis, both systemic and localized. The cANCA pattern of staining occurs in ~85% of patients with active Wegener's granulomatosis (WG) (renal and pulmonary involvement), and the pANCA staining pattern occurs in patients with microscopic polyangiitis and pauci immune necrotizing glomerulonephritis.[1,2] A negative test for cANCA does not rule out WG, but false-positive results are rare. Positive results for pANCA may occur in patients with lupus erythematosus (LE) or Goodpasture's syndrome. In patients with documented WG, increasing titers of cANCA suggest relapse of disease and decreasing titers suggest successful treatment.

cANCA produce diffuse cytoplasmic staining of neutrophils and monocytes and are caused by antibodies to proteinase 3, a 29-kDa serine protease. pANCA produce perinuclear staining of ethanol-fixed neutrophils and are often specific for neutrophil enzymes, including myeloperoxidase (MPO). Testing for antibodies to PR3 and MPO by EIA is recommended to confirm the presence of autoantibodies in patients with positive cANCA or pANCA, respectively.[3] The pANCA staining pattern can also be seen in patients with nonvasculitic diseases, including ulcerative colitis. This reactivity is not because of anti-MPO antibodies but represents reactivity with various other neutrophil autoantigens.

TEST NAME AND METHOD	SPECIMEN REQUIREMENTS	REFERENCE INTERVAL, CONVENTIONAL [INTERNATIONAL RECOMMENDED UNITS]		CHEMICAL INTERFERENCES AND IN VIVO EFFECTS
Niacin (Nicotinic Acid) Metabolites[1-4] *N1-Methylnicotinamide* *Fluorimetric*[2,3]	Urine, 24 hr; acidify with HCl (1 vol%).	Adult, M and nonpregnant F: 2.4-6.4 mg/day × 7.30 [17.5-46.7 μmol/day]		↓ V Glibenclamide, isoniazid, and valproic acid
2-Pyridone *HPLC*[2,5-7]		Adult, M: 2-20 mg/day × 6.58 [13-132 μmol/day]		
N1-Methylnicotinamide *Fluorimetric*[3]	Urine, random; acidify with HCl.	*mg/g creatinine* Adult, M and non-pregnant F: 1.6-4.3	*mmol/g creatinine* × 7.30 [11.7-31.4]	
N1-Methylnicotinamide *HPLC*[7]	Plasma; deproteinized with 20% TCA.	*ng/mL* Adult: 3.0-36	*nmol/L* 0.41-4.9	

1. Brown ML, editor: *Present knowledge in nutrition,* ed 6, Washington DC, 1990, International Life Sciences Institute, Nutrition Foundation.

2. Jacob RA, Swendseid ME, McKee RW, et al: Biochemical markers for assessment of niacin status in young men: urinary and blood levels of niacin metabolites, *J Nutr* 119:591-598, 1989.

3. Sauberlich HE, Dowdy RP, Skala JH: *Laboratory tests for the assessment of nutritional status,* Boca Raton, FL, 1974, CRC Press Inc.

4. Shils ME, Olson JA, Shike M, editors: *Modern nutrition in health and disease,* ed 8, Philadelphia, 1994, Lea & Febiger.

5. Gillmor HA, Bolton CH, Hopton M, et al: Measurement of nicotinamide and N-methyl-2-pyridone-5-carboxamide in plasma by high performance liquid chromatography, *Biomed Chromatogr* 13:360-362, 1999.

DIAGNOSTIC INFORMATION	REMARKS

↓ Pellagra, alcoholism, carcinoid syndrome, anorexia nervosa, ulcerative cholitis, and Hartnup disease.

The diagnosis of Pellagra should be focused on three points "the 3Ds" (diarrhea, dermatitis, and dementia). Other findings may include anemia, hypoproteinemia, increased serum calcium, abnormal liver function tests, and increased serum porphyrins.[7] Advanced dermatitis includes the appearance of Casal's necklace. Mental changes include fatigue, insomnia, and apathy. These are followed by encephalopathy along with confusion, hallucination, loss of memory, and eventually frank organic psychoses.

Pellagra is the clinical syndrome resulting from severe niacin deficiency. Niacin functions primarily as the coenzyme forms NAD and NADP. Erythrocyte NAD is often reduced in niacin deficiency. Niacin is biosynthesized from the amino acid tryptophan so that 60 mg of dietary tryptophan = 1 mg of niacin intake = 1 niacin equivalent (NE). U.S. RDA (1989) = 6.6 NE per 1000 kcal. Excess niacin is methylated in the liver and excreted, principally as N1-methylnicotinamide and N1-methyl-2-pyridone-5-carboxamide (2-pyridone). Excretion of the two methylated metabolites provides the most reliable measure of niacin intake and body status. (In children, levels of urine niacin metabolites are dependent on age.) Diagnosis of niacin deficiency is often based on patient history and physical examination. When clinic information points to niacin deficiency, niacin replacement is started and diagnosis is made in part based on patient's response.[8] Neither blood nor urinary niacin levels are of value in assessing niacin nutritional status.

There is usually a concurrent deficiency of other B vitamins in pellagra. Niacin deficiency may be associated with anemia or, in the young, with a failure to grow.

A protein-rich diet can be used to treat niacin deficiency. Food sources of niacin include meat, poultry, fish, eggs, nuts, whole grain cereals, and legumes.[8,9]

Nicotinic acid given as a drug (1.0-3.0 g/day) improves lipoprotein abnormalities, reducing LDL cholesterol, triglyceride, and Lp(a), while increasing HDL. Immediate release, extended release, and long-acting fulmulations are available, and side effects vary depending on the formulation. Immediate release niacin is associated with flushing of the skin (face and hands), gastrointestinal symptoms, and elevations in blood glucose, whereas with long-acting time release niacin there is reduced flushing but increased risk of hepatotoxic effects. Rarer additional symptoms include hyperuricemia and gout, cardiac arrhythmias, hypotension, and acanthosis nigricans.[10]

6. Moore WP, Bolton CH, Downs L, et al: Measurement of N-methyl-2-pyridone-5-carboxamide in urine by high performance liquid chromatography, *Biomed Chromatogr* 14:69-71, 2000.

7. Musfeld, C, Biollaz J, Belaz N, et al: Validation of an HPLC method for the determination of urinary and plasma levels of N1-methylnicotinamide, an endogenous marker of renal cationic transport and plasma flow, *J Pharm Biomed Anal* 24:391-404, 2001.

8. Hegyi J, Schwartz RA, Hegyi V: Pellagra: dermatitis, dementia, and diarrhea, *Int J Dermatol* 43:1-5, 2004.

9. Karthikeyan K, Thappa DM: Pellagra and skin, *Int J Dermatol* 41:476-481, 2002.

10. McKenney J: New perspectives on the use of niacin in the treatment of lipid disorders, *Arch Intern Med* 164:697-705, 2004.

TEST NAME AND METHOD	SPECIMEN REQUIREMENTS	REFERENCE INTERVAL, CONVENTIONAL [INTERNATIONAL RECOMMENDED UNITS]			CHEMICAL INTERFERENCES AND IN VIVO EFFECTS
Nickel (Ni)[1] AAS	Whole blood. Collect in pretested, metal-free container.[3]	1.0-28.0 mcg/L × 17 0.6-1.8 mcg/L[8]		[17-476 nmol/L] [10-31 nmol/L]	↓ C *AAS* (slight): Cadmium 10 mcg/dL [1700 nmol/L] or gold 25 mcg/dL [4250 nmol/L].
	Serum or plasma.[4] Collect in pretested, metal-free tubes.	0.14-1.0 mcg/L Metal refinery workers[9]:	3-11 mcg/L	[2.4-17.0 nmol/L] [50-187 nmol/L]	
	Urine. Collect in acid-washed, metal-free container.	0.1-10 mcg/day × 17		[2-170 nmol/day]	
		mcg/L 0.1-8.0 × 0.017 Metal refinery workers[9]: 8-800 Nickel carbonyl poisoning[9]: 100-2500		*µmol/L* [0.002-0.136] [0.1-13.6] [1.7-42.5]	
	Feces.[5] Collect in acid-washed, metal-free container.	260 ± 120 mcg/ day (SD) × 0.017		[4.4 ± 2.0 µmol/day]	
	Hair.[6] Take proximal (scalp-end) sections for analysis. Wash to remove surface contamination.	*mcg/g dry wt.* 0.01-1.8 × 17		*nmol/g dry wt.* [0.2-30.6]	
X-ray fluorescence spectrometry[2]	Bronchoalveolar lavage (BAL) fluid	*ng/10[3] macrophages* <0.71 × 17		*fmol/macrophage* [<12.1]	
ICP-MS	Serum.[7] Collect in pretested, metal-free container.	0.6-7.5 mcg/L × 17 0.0-5.2 mcg/L		[10.2-127.5 nmol/L] [0.0-88.4 nmol/L]	
	Urine.[7] Collect in acid-washed, metal-free container. Refrigerate during and after collection.				

1. Milne DB: Trace elements. In Burtis CA, Ashwood ER, editors: *Tietz textbook of clinical chemistry,* ed 2, Philadelphia, 1994, WB Saunders.
2. Maier EA, Rastegar F, Heimburger R, et al: Simultaneous determination of trace elements in lavage fluids front human bronchial alveoli by energy dispersive X-ray flourescence. 1: Technique and determination of the normal reference interval, *Clin Chem* 31:551-555, 1985.
3. Iyengar GV, Woittiez J: Trace elements in human clinical specimens: evaluation of literature data to identify tolerence values, *Clin Chem* 34:474-481, 1988.

DIAGNOSTIC INFORMATION	REMARKS
↑ Industrial exposure, nickel carbonyl intoxication, acute myocardial infarction (early decrease followed by a sharp increase), acute stroke, extensive thermal burns, and dialysis patients. Disulfiram therapy.[10]	Serum and urine levels are useful indices of chronic environmental exposure and exposure from the manufacture of ink, magnets, spark plugs, paints, stainless steel (including welding), enamels, ceramics, batteries, glass, and alloys.
Inhalation of nickel compounds leads to malignancies of lungs and nasal sinuses.	One percent of soluble nickel in food is absorbed versus 25% in water after a 12-hr fast.[11]
↓ Hepatic and renal diseases	Chronic toxic effects are hypersensitivity (dermatitis) and carcinogenesis (respiratory). Nickel allergy affects 10-15% of the population and can develop from occupational exposure or exposure to nickel-containing jewelry or implanted prostheses and results in local or generalized dermatitis.
	Refinery dust and nickel subsulfide are classified as human carcinogens.

4. Nixon DE, Moyer TP: Determination of serum nickel by graphite furnace atomic absorption spectrometry with Zeeman-effect background correction: values in a normal population and a population undergoing dialysis, *Analyst* 114:1671-1674, 1989.

5. Brown SS, Mitchell FL, Young DS, editors: *Chemical diagnosis of disease,* Amsterdam, 1979, Elsevier/North Holland Biomedical Press.

6. Jacob RA: Hair as a biopsy material. In Williams DF, editor: *Systemic aspects of biocompatibility,* Boca Raton, FL, 1981, CRC Press, Inc.

TEST NAME AND METHOD	SPECIMEN REQUIREMENTS	REFERENCE INTERVAL, CONVENTIONAL [INTERNATIONAL RECOMMENDED UNITS]	CHEMICAL INTERFERENCES AND IN VIVO EFFECTS

Nickel—CONT

7. Associated Regional & University Pathologists, Inc. web site (www.aruplab.com): Available at: http://www.aruplab.com/testing/user_guide.jsp. Last accessed 9/2004.

8. Sunderman FW Jr, Crisostomo MC, Reid MC, et al: Rapid analysis of nickel in serum and whole blood by electrothermal atomic absorption spectrophotometry, *Ann Clin Lab Sci* 14:232-241, 1984.

9. Baselt RC: *Analytical procedures for therapeutic drug monitoring and emergency toxicology,* ed 2, Littleton, MA, 1987, PSG Publishing Co., Inc.

Nitrites[5] *Colorimetric, ion-selective electrode,*[1] *HPLC*[2]	Blood (heparin, oxalate, or EDTA)	See *Methemoglobin.* Toxic amount: Methemoglobin, 5% of total Hb [$\times$ 0.01 = 0.05 fraction of total Hb]	None found.
	Urine; first morning specimen is preferred.	Negative Toxic concentration: See *Remarks.*	

1. Choi KK, Fung FW: Determination of nitrate and nitrite in meat products by using a nitrate ion-selective electrode, *Analyst* 105:241-245, 1980.

2. Thayer JR, Huffaker RC: Determination of nitrate and nitrite by high-pressure liquid chromatography: comparison with other methods for nitrite determination, *Anal Biochem* 102:110-119, 1980.

3. Hall AH, Rumack BH: Clinical toxicology of cyanide, *Ann Emerg Med* 15:1067-1074, 1986.

Nitroblue Tetra-zolium Reduction (NBT)[1-3] *Spontaneous NBT test*[1]	Whole blood (heparin, EDTA; with Ficoll added later). Stable for 1 hr at 25° C.	Adult: (Higher in normal newborns)	*Percent positive cells* 3-10	*Number fraction positive cells* [0.03-0.10]	↑ V Indomethacin, oral contraceptives, and typhoid vaccine. ↓ V Antibiotics, glucocorticoids, phenylbutazone, and salicylates.
Stimulated NBT test (screening test for Chronic Granulomatous Disease [CGD])[2,3]	Single drop of blood.	Control:	>90	[>0.90]	

1. Lace JK, Tan JS, Watanakunakorn C: An appraisal of nitroblue tetrazolium reduction test, *Am J Med* 58:685-694, 1975.

2. Nathan DG, Orkin SH, Ginsburg D, et al: *Hematology of infancy and childhood,* ed 6, Philadelphia, 2003, WB Saunders.

DIAGNOSTIC INFORMATION	REMARKS

10. Hopfer SM, Linden JV, Rezuke WN, et al: Increased nickel concentrations in body fluids of patients with chronic alcoholism during disulfiram therapy, *Res Comm Chem Pathol Pharmacol* 55:101-109, 1987.

11. Sunderman FW Jr, Hopfer SM, Sweeney KR, et al: Nickel absorption and kinetics in human volunteers, *Proc Soc Exp Biol Med* 19:5-11, 1989.

These substances convert hemoglobin to methemoglobin and cause a decrease in the availability of oxygen to tissues. Prompt measurement of methemoglobin is a useful clinical test for nitrite toxicity. Toxicity is caused by uncontrolled vasodilation and/or methemoglobinemia.

Inorganic and organic nitrites are used therapeutically. When used therapeutically, all nitrite is completely metabolized. Sodium nitrite is used as an antidote for cyanide poisoning[3] and as a curing agent for processed meats. The nitrite ion disappears rapidly from plasma, but urinary concentrations can be used to assess exposure.

↑ Patients with bacterial tuberculosis; some viral, some parasitic, and some fungal infections; and lymphomas

Normal in some viral and bacterial infections.

↓ Chronic granulomatous disease (CGD), some other neutrophil enzymatic defects, some types of complement deficiency, and agammaglobulinemia

When stimulated to phagocytosis, neutrophils generate superoxides that reduce the nitroblue tetrazolium from a soluble, yellow compound to a blue precipitate. The spontaneous NBT test is not reliable in the differential diagnosis of bacterial infection and has no established use in clinical practice.

An alternative to the NBT slide test is the neutrophil oxidative burst assay (DHR), which is performed by flow cytometry.

↓ CGD carriers, 45-90% [0.45-0.90] positive cells

↓↓ CGD-positive cells

The stimulated NBT test is useful in screening for CGD, in which there is a defect in the ability of neutrophils to generate superoxide in response to phagocytosis. It is particularly useful in detecting the carrier state in families with one of the X-linked subtypes of CGD. Carriers show a mixture of NBT-positive and NBT-negative cells. Screening of fetal blood by the NBT slide test is problematic because of maternal blood contamination.

3. Segal AW: Nitroblue-tetrazolium, *Lancet* 2:1248-1252, 1974.

TEST NAME AND METHOD	SPECIMEN REQUIREMENTS	REFERENCE INTERVAL, CONVENTIONAL [INTERNATIONAL RECOMMENDED UNITS]	CHEMICAL INTERFERENCES AND IN VIVO EFFECTS
Nonesterified Fatty Acids (NEFA, Free fatty acids)[1] *Enzymatic*[1-5] *Colorimetric*[3,6-8]	Plasma (EDTA, citrate, oxalate, sodium fluoride) or serum. Heparin plasma is not acceptable. Patient must be fasting for at least 12 hr. Keep specimen on ice, and centrifuge as soon as possible. Freeze specimen if not assayed immediately.	*Expected values*[5]: 0.1-0.6 mmol/L (mEq/L) *Expected values*[6]: 0.2-0.8 mmol/L	↑ C Valproic acid (method-specific), bilirubin (method-specific), delay in separation of red cells, and improper storage of specimens. ↑ V Alcoholism, high blood pressure, fasting, obesity, pregnancy, stress, and cigarette smoking. ↓ C Isoproterenol, elevated norepinephrine, and long-term frozen storage. ↓ V Aspirin, atenolol, clofibrate, metoprolol, niacin, HMG-CoA reductase inhibitors (statins), and fish oils.

1. Rifai N, Warnick GR, Dominiczak MH, editors: *Handbook of lipoprotein testing,* ed 2, Washington, DC, 2000, AACC Press.
2. Miles J, Glasscock R, Aikens J, et al: A microfluorometric method for the determination of free fatty acids in plasma, *J Lipid Res* 24:96-99, 1983.
3. Mulder C, Schouten JA, Popp-Snijders C: Determination of free fatty acids: a comparative study of the enzymatic versus the gas chromatographic and the colorimetric method, *J Clin Chem Clin Biochem* 21:823-827, 1983.
4. Shimizu S, Inoue R, Tani Y, et al: Enzymatic determination of serum free fatty acids, *Anal Biochem* 98:341-345, 1979.
5. Wako Chemicals USA, Inc.: *NEFA C: ACS-ACOD method package insert,* Richmond, VA, 2004, Wako Chemicals USA, Inc.
6. Brunk SD, Swanson JR: Colorimetric method for free fatty acids in serum validated by comparison with gas chromatography, *Clin Chem* 27:924-926, 1981.
7. Duncombe WG: The colorimetric micro-determination of non-esterified fatty acids in plasma, *Clin Chim Acta* 9:122-125, 1964.
8. Itaya K, Ui M: Colorimetric determination of free fatty acids in biological fluids, *J Lipid Res* 6:16-20, 1965.

Non–High-Density Lipoprotein Cholesterol (NonHDL-C)[1-3] *Calculation*	Serum, plasma (EDTA or perhaps heparin, but not oxalate, fluoride, or citrate), fasting is not required.	*Therapeutic goals*[1] (See *Remarks.*) High risk (CHD or CHD risk equivalents): <130 mg/dL [<3.37 mmol/L] Moderate risk (2+ risk factors; 10 yr risk ≤20%): <160 mg/dL [<4.14 mmol/L] Lower risk (0-1 risk factors): <190 mg/dL [<4.92 mmol/L]	

DIAGNOSTIC INFORMATION	REMARKS

↑ An elevated NEFA concentration is associated with the cluster of risk factors that comprise the metabolic syndrome and are associated with increased CHD risk: obesity, type 2 diabetes, insulin resistance, low HDL, and hypertriglyceridemia.

NEFAs are essential components for the building and maintenance of cell membranes. They also form triglyceride and cholesteryl esters that form the core of lipoproteins to provide a means of delivering fatty acids to peripheral tissue to meet cellular energy needs.

Methods such as GC, HPLC, and MS are available to separate and identify specific fatty acid species; the methods described here measure total NEFA.

↑ An elevated non-HDL-C is associated with metabolic syndrome and increased coronary heart disease risk.

The National Cholesterol Education Program (NCEP) has identified non-HDL-C as a secondary target of therapy in individuals with elevated serum triglycerides (≥ 200 mg/dL). Non-HDL-C is calculated as:

$$\text{Non-HDL-C} = (\text{Total Cholesterol}) - (\text{HDL-Cholesterol})$$

Non-HDL-C reflects the sum of all potentially atherogenic particles: LDL, VLDL, IDL, and lipoprotein(a).

TEST NAME AND METHOD	SPECIMEN REQUIREMENTS	REFERENCE INTERVAL, CONVENTIONAL [INTERNATIONAL RECOMMENDED UNITS]			CHEMICAL INTERFERENCES AND IN VIVO EFFECTS

Non–High-Density Lipoprotein Cholesterol—CONT

		mg/dL^3 5th-95th Percentile		$mmol/L$ 5th-95th Percentile	
		Black			
		25+ yr			
		F:	83-230	× 0.0259	[2.15-5.96]
		M:	84-231		[2.18-5.98]
		Mexican American			
		25+ yr			
		F:	87-226		[2.25-5.85]
		M:	97-230		[2.51-5.96]
		White			
		25+ yr			
		F:	90-234		[2.33-6.06]
		M:	96-231		[2.49-5.98]
		All subjects			
		25-34 yr			
		F:	77-196		[1.99-5.08]
		M:	81-214		[2.10-5.54]
		35-44 yr			
		F:	89-205		[2.31-5.31]
		M:	95-231		[2.46-5.98]
		45-54 yr			
		F:	96-240		[2.49-6.22]
		M:	107-236		[2.77-6.11]
		55-64 yr			
		F:	109-262		[2.82-6.79]
		M:	104-238		[2.69-6.16]
		65-74 yr			
		F:	109-254		[2.82-6.58]
		M:	103-233		[2.67-6.03]
		75-84 yr			
		F:	104-260		[2.69-6.73]
		M:	104-228		[2.69-5.91]
		85+ yr			
		F:	103-235		[2.67-6.09]
		M:	92-210		[2.38-5.44]

1. Expert Panel on Detection, Evaluation, and Treatment of High Blood Cholesterol in Adults: Executive Summary of the Third Report of the National Cholesterol Education Program (NCEP) Expert Panel on Detection, Evaluation, and Treatment of High Blood Cholesterol in Adults (Adult Treatment Panel III), *JAMA* 285:2486-2497, 2001.

2. Frost PH, Havel RJ: Rationale for the use of non-high-density lipoprotein cholesterol rather than low-density lipoprotein cholesterol as a tool for lipoprotein cholesterol screening and assessment of risk and therapy, *Am J Cardiol* 81:26B-31B, 1998.

3. Gardner CD, Winkleby MA, Fortmann SP: Population frequency distribution of non-high-density lipoprotein cholesterol (Third National Health and Nutrition Examination Survey [NHANES III], 1988-1994, *Am J Cardiol* 86:299-304, 2000.

DIAGNOSTIC INFORMATION

REMARKS

TEST NAME AND METHOD	SPECIMEN REQUIREMENTS	REFERENCE INTERVAL, CONVENTIONAL [INTERNATIONAL RECOMMENDED UNITS]			CHEMICAL INTERFERENCES AND IN VIVO EFFECTS
Nonprotein Nitrogen (NPN) *Digestion and colorimetric (nesslerization),* [1,2] *pyrochemilumines-cence (Antek Instruments)* [3]	Whole blood, serum, or plasma (fluoride or oxalate)	Serum: Blood:	*mg/dL* <35 <50	× 0.714	*mmol/L* [<25.0] [<35.7]	S ↑ V Drugs causing nephrotoxicity (Table II-6) vitamin D. S ↑ C EDTA
	Urine, 24 hr		*g/day* 10-15	× 71.4	*mmol/day* [714-1071]	
	Feces, 72-hr sample.[2] Refrigerate or freeze until analysis.	Infant: Adult:	*g/day* 0.11-0.52 <2	× 71.4	*mmol/day* [7.9-37.1] [<142.8]	

1. Henry JB, editor: *Clinical diagnosis and management by laboratory methods,* ed 18, Philadelphia, 1991, WB Saunders.
2. Henry RJ, Cannon DC, Winkelman JW, editors: *Clinical chemistry: principles and technics,* ed 2, Hagerstown, MD, 1974, Harper and Row.
3. Ward MWN, Owens CWI, Rennie MJ: Nitrogen estimation in biological samples by use of chemilumines, *Clin Chem* 26:1336-1339, 1980.
4. Cerra F, Blackburn G, Hirsch J, et al: The effect of stress level, amino acid formula, and nitrogen dose on nitrogen retention in traumatic and septic stress, *Ann Surg* Mar:282-287, 1987.
5. Konstantinides FN: Nitrogen balance studies in clinical nutrition, *Nutr Clin Pract* 7:231-238, 1992.

TEST NAME AND METHOD	SPECIMEN REQUIREMENTS	REFERENCE INTERVAL, CONVENTIONAL [INTERNATIONAL RECOMMENDED UNITS]		CHEMICAL INTERFERENCES AND IN VIVO EFFECTS
NT-pro B-Type Natriuretic Peptide (NT-proBNP) *Immunoassay* [1,2] *Roche Dade Behring, Ortho Clinical Diagnostics, Inverness Medical (POCT)*	Serum, EDTA plasma collected. Samples stable for 24 hr at room temperature, 72 hr at 2-8° C, and >3 days at −20° C.[3,4]	*Cutoff concentration for HF:* <75 yr ≥75 yr *Cannot convert to pmol/L because the assay measures NT-proBNP and proBNP. There are several practical issues regarding the use of serum/plasma/whole blood monitoring of NT-proBNP. First, reference intervals vary, depending on which assay is used and the nature of the reference population tested. Second, a number of clinical factors affect the NT-proBNP concentrations, most importantly age, gender, and renal function. Significant differences are observed between men and women (higher) and with increasing concentrations with age by decades. Third, the relative importance of those factors in relation to the degree of left ventricular dysfunction remains to be debated.	*mcg/L** 125 450	Assays may differ in their susceptibility to analytical interferences. Interferences from rheumatoid factors or heterophilic antibodies may lead to false test results. Formulation of immunoassay kits remains very important in minimizing interference from heterophilic antibodies, and in some situations only addition of the non-immune serum from the animal species that was used to raise the antibodies is effective.

DIAGNOSTIC INFORMATION	REMARKS

S,B ↑ High-protein diet, late pregnancy; prerenal azotemia, intrinsic renal disease, and urinary tract obstruction.

Blood or serum NPN is rarely measured because it offers no more information than urea nitrogen.

S,B ↓ Severe hepatic insufficiency, hepatic necrosis.

See also *Urea Nitrogen.*

U ↑ Metabolic stress, postoperative stress sepsis.[4]

Urine NPN (total urinary nitrogen, TUN) is ~85% urea, 3% ammonia, 5% creatinine, and 1% uric acid. These figures vary in individual patients depending on clinical circumstances, especially in those receiving enteral and parenteral nutritional support.[5] For this reason, total urinary nitrogen is a more reliable indicator of nitrogen balance than urinary urea nitrogen in some patients.

↑ Severe diarrhea, steatorrhea, pancreatic disease, and gastrocolic fistula.

Output of fecal nitrogen is dependent on dietary intake; a standard diet (Schmidt or Nothman) is recommended.

The biochemistry and physiology specifically of NT-proBNP have been described.[6] In head-to-head comparisons, the clinical utility of NT-proBNP is similar to that of BNP.[7,8] However, results of NT-proBNP cannot be converted to equivalent BNP results.[9] See also *B-type Natriuretic Peptide.*

See *B-type Natriuretic Peptide.* NT-proBNP has been shown to be useful for diagnosis of heart failure in patients presenting with dyspnea,[10] staging, and risk stratification of patients with HF[11] and acute coronary artery disease.[12]

There is uncertainty whether proBNP is split in the myocyte or later in the plasma as corin, a circulating protease, cleaves proBNP into the N-terminal and the active BNP moiety. Circulating proBNP has been documented.[15] However, the major circulating forms are the resulting NT-proBNP, function unknown, and C-terminal BNP (physiologically active hormone). BNP is cleared via degradation by NEP (neutral endopeptidases), by receptor-mediated clearance, and perhaps a bit via the kidneys, which also can secrete BNP. The NT-proBNP is not cleared via receptor-mediated mechanisms, leading some to suggest that it will be more sensitive to changes in renal function.[9]

TEST NAME AND METHOD	SPECIMEN REQUIREMENTS	REFERENCE INTERVAL, CONVENTIONAL [INTERNATIONAL RECOMMENDED UNITS]	CHEMICAL INTERFERENCES AND IN VIVO EFFECTS

NT-pro B-Type Natriuretic Peptide (NT-proBNP)—CONT

Increased NT-proBNP concentrations >400 ng/L in the >60 yr population have demonstrated a high negative predictive value (NPV) in ruling out HF. There is an inverse relationship between values and body mass index.[5]

Antibody recognition:

Assay	Antigen	Capture Ab	Detection Ab
Roche	NT-proBNP a.a. 1-76	Roche (N-term)	Roche (central)
(Dade Behring)	Pro-BNP a,a, 1-108 truncated NT-proBNP		

↑ Icteric and hemolyzed samples may also be a problem in certain immunoassays with fluorimetric detection of the signal. Some analyzers may be particularly susceptible to the presence of particles (e.g., fibrin strands) or bubbles in the sample, thereby causing erroneous test results.

1. Prontera C, Emdin M, Zucchelli DC, et al: Analytical performance and diagnostic accuracy of a fully-automated electrochemiluminescent assay for the N-terminal fragment of pro-peptide of brain natriuretic peptide in patients with cardiomyopathy: comparison with immunoradiometric assay methods for brain natriuretic peptide and atrial natriuretic peptide, *Clin Chem Lab Med* 42:37-44, 2004.

2. Yeo KTJ, Wu AHB, Apple FS, et al: Multicenter evaluation of the Roche NT-proBNP assay and comparison to the Biosite Triage BNP assay, *Clin Chim Acta* 338:107-115, 2003.

3. van der Merwe D, Henley R, Lane G, et al: Effect of different sample types and stability after blood collection of N-terminal pro-b-type natriuretic peptide as measured with Roche Elecsys system, *Clin Chem* 50:779-780, 2004.

4. Nowatzke WL, Cole TG: Stability of N-terminal pro-brain natriuretic peptide after storage frozen for one year and after multiple freeze thaw cycles, *Clin Chem* 49:1560-1562, 2003.

5. Hermann-Arnhof KM, Hanush-Enserer U, Kaestenbauer T, et al: N-terminal pro-B-type natriuretic peptide as an indicator of possible cardiovascular disease in severely obese individuals: comparison with patients in different stages of heart failure, *Clin Chem* 51:138-143, 2005.

6. Hall C: Essential biochemistry and physiology of (NT-pro)BNP, *Eur J Heart Fail* 6:257-260, 2004.

7. Hammerer-Lercher A, Neubauer E, Muller S, et al: Head-to-head comparison of N-terminal pro-brain natriuretic peptide, brain natriuretic peptide and N-terminal pro-atrial natriuretic peptide in diagnosing left ventricular dysfunction, *Clin Chim Acta* 310:193-197, 2001.

8. Mueller T, Gegenhuber A, Poelz W, et al: Diagnostic accuracy of B type natriuretic peptide and amino terminal proBNP in the emergency diagnosis of heart failure, *Heart* 91:606-612, 2005.

9. Sykes E, Karcher RE, Eisenstadt J, et al: Analytical relationships among Biosite, Bayer, and Roche methods for BNP and NT-proBNP, *Am J Clin Pathol* 123:584-590, 2005.

10. Januzzi JL Jr, Camargo CA, Anwarrudin S, et al: The N-terminal Pro-BNP investigation of dyspnea in the emergency department (PRIDE) study, *Am J Cardiol* 95:948-954, 2005.

11. Poge U, Gerhardt TM, Woitas RP: N-terminal pro-B-type natriuretic peptide and mortality in coronary heart disease [comment], *N Engl J Med* 352:2025-2026, 2005.

12. Dokainish H, Zogbhi WA, Lakkis NM, et al: Incremental predictive power of B-type natriuretic peptide and tissue Doppler echocardiography in the prognosis of patients with congestive heart failure, *J Am Coll Cardiol* 45:1223-1226, 2005.

DIAGNOSTIC INFORMATION

REMARKS

TEST NAME AND METHOD	SPECIMEN REQUIREMENTS	REFERENCE INTERVAL, CONVENTIONAL [INTERNATIONAL RECOMMENDED UNITS]			CHEMICAL INTERFERENCES AND IN VIVO EFFECTS
Nuclear Matrix Protein 22 (NMP22)[1,2] *EIA*	Urine. Single void collected between midnight and noon. Must be stabilized immediately using NMP22 urine collection kit. Stabilized sample can remain at room temperature for 96 hr before centrifugation; for longer periods, store at 2-8° C. Processed samples are stable up to 1 wk at 2-8° C. For longer periods, store frozen, at −20° C for up to 8 wk, or −80° C for longer periods.	≤10 U/mL	× 1.0	[≤10 kU/L]	

1. Konety BR, Getzenberg RH: Urine based markers of urological malignancy, *J Urol* 165:600-611, 2001.
2. Fritsche HA: Bladder cancer and urine tumor marker tests. In Diamandis EP, Fritsche HA, Lilja H, et al, editors: *Tumor markers. Physiology, pathobiology, technology, and clinical applications,* Washington, DC, 2002, AACC Press.

TEST NAME AND METHOD	SPECIMEN REQUIREMENTS	REFERENCE INTERVAL, CONVENTIONAL [INTERNATIONAL RECOMMENDED UNITS]			CHEMICAL INTERFERENCES AND IN VIVO EFFECTS
5′-Nucleotidase (5′-NT; EC 3.1.3.5)[1-4] *Colorimetric*[1,2,4]	Serum or plasma (heparin). Stable at 4° C for 4 days; if frozen, stable for 4 mo.	2-17 U/L	× 0.017	[0.03-0.29 μKat/L]	↑ V Acetaminophen, anticonvulsants (especially phenytoin),[8] asparaginase, aspirin, carbenoxolone, drugs causing cholestasis (see Table II-5).
Kinetic, 30° C[5]		3.5-12.7 U/L		[0.06-0.22 μKat/L]	↑ C Hemolysis, Mg[2+]
Kinetic, 30° C[6]		5.4-9.8 U/L		[0.09-0.17 μKat/L]	
Radiometric (14C), 37° C[7]		0.24-0.67 mmol/hr/mL	× 16.7	[4-11 U/L]	↓ C Ni[2+], EDTA

1. Burtis CA, Ashwood ER, editors: *Tietz textbook of clinical chemistry,* ed 2, Philadelphia, 1994, WB Saunders.
2. Ellis G, Goldberg DM: An improved kinetic 5′-nucleotidase assay, *Anal Letters* 5:65-73, 1972.
3. Sunderman FW: The clinical biochemistry of 5′-nucleotidase, *Ann Clin Lab Sci* 20:123-139, 1990.
4. Van der Slik W, Persijn JP, Engelman E, et al: Serum 5′-nucleotidase, *Clin Biochem* 3:59-80, 1970.

DIAGNOSTIC INFORMATION   **REMARKS**

↑ Bladder cancer (transitional cell carcinoma). Assay has a sensitivity of 70.6% and a specificity of 78.0% for recurrence of disease and a sensitivity of 62.5% and a specificity of 78% for detection of disease in symptomatic or high-risk individuals. Elevations observed in healthy individuals after extreme exercise, interstitial cystitis, urinary tract infections, renal cancer, patients treated with chemotherapy for any malignancy, and total cystectomy patients. Tissue damage from cystoscopy or urethral catheterization may cause elevated values within 5 days of the procedure.

Nuclear matrix proteins (NMPs) make up the internal structural framework of the nucleus and function in DNA replication, RNA synthesis, hormone binding, and regulation and coordination of gene expression. The NMP22 assay measures the nuclear matrix protein NuMA, nuclear mitotic apparatus protein, which is found in all cells. NuMA is overexpressed in bladder cancer and released into the urine during cell death and with breakdown in the bladder wall as a result of bladder cancer.[1,2]

A quantitative EIA for NMP22 (Matritech, Inc., Newton, MA) in urine is indicated for the management of patients with transitional cell carcinoma (TCC) of the bladder, after surgical treatment to identify patients with occult or rapidly recurring TCC using an assay cutoff of >10 U/mL. The test is further indicated as an aid in the diagnosis of TCC of the bladder in patients with symptoms or risk factors in conjunction with standard diagnostic procedures with an assay cutoff of ≥7.5 U/mL. A qualitative, immunochromatographic, point of care NMP22 test (NMP22 BladderChek Test) is available as an aid in monitoring patients with a history of bladder cancer.

↑ Hepatobiliary disease with intrahepatic or extrahepatic biliary obstruction, hepatic carcinoma, early biliary cirrhosis, pregnancy (third trimester), preeclampsia,[9] graft-versus-host (GVH) disease, and inflammatory arthritis.[10]

5'-Nucleotidase levels parallel those of alkaline phosphatase in cholestatic hepatobiliary diseases but are not significantly increased in bone disease.[3,11] 5'-NT is a better test for secondary tumors and lymphomas of liver than is alkaline phosphatase.[12] Values are high in infants, decrease in adolescents, and increase again in elderly persons.[6,13]

5. Harvey MS, Van der Stoel AG, Backer ET: Determination of serum 5'-nucleotidase with a centrifugal analyzer, *Clin Chem* 25:918-923, 1979.

6. Moses GC, Tuckerman JF, Henderson AR: Biological variance of cholinesterase and 5'-nucleotidase in serum of healthy persons, *Clin Chem* 32:175-176, 1986.

TEST NAME AND METHOD	SPECIMEN REQUIREMENTS	REFERENCE INTERVAL, CONVENTIONAL [INTERNATIONAL RECOMMENDED UNITS]	CHEMICAL INTERFERENCES AND IN VIVO EFFECTS

5'-Nucleotidase—CONT

7. Chatterjee SK, Bhattacharya M, Barlow JJ: Evaluation of 5'-nucleotidase as an enzyme marker in ovarian carcinoma, *Cancer* 47:2648-2653, 1981.

8. Fortman CS, Witte DL: Serum 5'-nucleotidase in patients receiving antiepileptic drugs, *Am J Clin Pathol* 84:197-201, 1985.

9. Yoneyama Y, Suzuki S, Sawa R, et al: Plasma 5'-nucleotidase activities and uric acid levels in women with pre-eclampsia, *Gynecol Obstet Invest* 54:168-171, 2002.

10. Johnson S, Patel S, Bruckner F, et al: 5'-Nucleotidase as a marker of both general and local inflammation in rheumatoid arthritis patients, *Rheumatology* 38:391-396, 1999.

TEST NAME AND METHOD	SPECIMEN REQUIREMENTS	REFERENCE INTERVAL, CONVENTIONAL [INTERNATIONAL RECOMMENDED UNITS]	CHEMICAL INTERFERENCES AND IN VIVO EFFECTS
Occult Blood[1-3] *Quantitative:* ^{51}Cr[1,4]	Feces, random. See *Remarks* for chief restrictions.	<0.32* *Ratio of counts in stool to counts per mL of blood.	↑ V Drugs causing gastrointestinal bleeding, e.g., aspirin, corticosteroids, nonsteroidal antiinflammatory drugs (e.g., indomethacin, ibuprofen, sulindac); drugs causing colitis (e.g., methyldopa and a variety of antibiotics).
Heme-porphyrin		≤2.0 mg total hemoglobin/g feces[2]	
Qualitative: *Immunochemical*		Negative	
Peroxidase		Negative	↑ C Peroxidase-containing foods (see *Remarks*). ↓ C Ascorbic acid

11. Reichling JJ, Kaplan MM: Clinical use of serum enzymes in liver disease, *Dig Dis Sci* 33:1601-1614, 1988.
12. Deeble TJ, Goldberg DM: Assessment of biochemical tests for bone and liver involvement in malignant lymphoma patients, *Cancer* 45:1451-1457, 1980.
13. Belfield A, Goldberg DM: Normal ranges and diagnostic value of serum 5'-nucleotidase and alkaline phosphatase activities in infancy, *Arch Dis Child* 46:842-846, 1971.

↑ Peptic ulcers, gastritis (especially associated with alcohol, aspirin, or indomethacin), variceal bleeding, GI malignancies (especially of colon), diverticular disease, GI polyps, ischemic bowel disease, Mallory-Weiss tears, inflammatory lesions (e.g., ulcerative colitis, Crohn's disease, shigellosis, amebiasis, typhoid fever), trauma, bleeding diatheses (e.g., primary blood dyscrasias, Osler-Weber-Rendu disease, scurvy, pseudoxanthoma elasticum), vasculitis (e.g., polyarteritis nodosa, Henoch's purpura, Schönlein's purpura), amyloidosis, Turner's syndrome, uremia, intussusception, hiatal hernia, radiation, neurofibromatosis, Kaposi's sarcoma, and hematobilia.

Isotope tests are more specific than peroxidase tests but are impractical for large-scale screening[1] and should be used only for measuring trace amounts. Combination with other techniques can lead to location of the bleeding source.

Sensitivity: >5 mL blood/day

Fluorometric assay for porphyrins and heme. Vegetable peroxidases do not interfere; however, red meat and aspirin should be avoided before testing. Limited used because of laboratory-based analysis and high false-positive rate.[3] Available through reference laboratories as HemoQuant.

Immunochemical tests use antibodies to human intact hemoglobin and globin. Tests are unaffected by diet, animal hemoglobin, and medications. High sensitivity for colonic blood (0.3 mL). It is suited for screening for occult blood in the lower intestinal tract, but it is insensitive to upper GI bleeding. Tests require laboratory development and have limited acceptance and availability in the U.S.[3,5,6]

In peroxidase tests, peroxidase/pseudoperoxidase activity in the sample, such as from heme, turns guaic-impregnated slides blue with the addition of hydrogen peroxide in the developer solution. Hemoccult II Sensa, a more specific version of Hemoccult II, has sensitivity of 80% and a specificity of 94%. The reliability of the Hemoccult test is increased and the number of false-negative results obtained is reduced by performing the test on three separate days to account for intermittent neoplasm bleeding tests with the patient on a diet free from exogenous peroxidase activity (e.g., dietary Hb in red meat and fish, turnips, and horseradish) and vitamin C from supplements and citrus products (250 mg/day) 3 days before and during testing. Nonsteroidal antiinflammatory medications should also be avoided 7 days before and during testing. Rehydration of the test card is not recommended before developing. Small amounts of bright red blood on the stool surface are often because of hemorrhoids, anal fissures and fistulas, proctitis, or rectal polyps.[3,5-6] The American Cancer Society recommends

TEST NAME AND METHOD	SPECIMEN REQUIREMENTS	REFERENCE INTERVAL, CONVENTIONAL [INTERNATIONAL RECOMMENDED UNITS]		CHEMICAL INTERFERENCES AND IN VIVO EFFECTS

Occult Blood—CONT

1. Henry JB, editor: *Clinical diagnosis and management by laboratory methods,* ed 18, Philadelphia, 1991, WB Saunders.

2. Henderson AR, Rinker AD: Gastric, pancreatic, and intestinal function. In Burtis CA, Ashwood ER, editors: *Tietz textbook of clinical chemistry,* ed 3, Philadelphia, 1999, WB Saunders.

3. Rockey DC: Occult gastrointestinal bleeding, *N Engl J Med* 341:38-46, 1999.

4. Fall DJ, Kuiper DH, Pollard HM: Use of isotopes in determining occult blood, *Cancer* 28:135-136, 1971.

5. Ahlquist DA, Shuber AP: Stool screening for colorectal cancer: evolution from occult blood to molecular markers, *Clin Chim Acta* 315:157-168, 2002.

6. Levin B, Brooks D, Smith RA, et al: Emerging technologies in screening for colorectal cancer: DT colonography, immunochemical fecal occult blood tests, and stool screening using molecular markers, *CA Cancer J Clin* 53:44-55, 2003.

7. Young GP, St. John JB, Winanwer SJ, et al: Choice of fecal occult blood tests for colorectal cancer screening: recommendations based on performance characteristics in population studies, *Am J Gastroenterol* 97:2499-2507, 2002.

8. Smith RA, Cokkinides V, Eyre HJ: American cancer society guidelines for the early detection of cancer, 2004, *CA Cancer J Clin* 54:41-52, 2004.

Ornithine (Orn)[1-4]

Ion-exchange chromatography

Plasma (heparin) or serum, fasting. Place blood in ice water immediately; separate and freeze within 1 hr of collection. Stable for 1 wk at −20° C; for longer periods, deproteinize and store at −70° C.[5,6]

	mg/dL		*mmol/L*[9]
Premature			
1 day:	1.19 ± 0.26 (SD)	× 75.8	[90 ± 20]
Newborn			
1 day:	0.65-1.99		[49-151]
1-3 mo:	0.95 ± 0.30 (SD)		[72 ± 23]
9 mo-2 yr:	0.13-1.41		[10-107]
3-10 yr:	0.36-1.13		[27-86]
6-18 yr:	0.25-1.07		[19-81][10]
Adult:	0.40-1.40		[30-106]

P ↓ V Histidine (after oral load), progesterone (high doses)

Urine, 24 hr. Add 10 mL of 6 mol/L HCl at start of collection. (Alternatively, refrigerate specimen during collection.) Store frozen at −20° C.[7]

	mg/day		*mmol/day*[9]
10 days-7 wk:	2.2-2.8	× 7.58	[17-21]
3-12 yr:	<5.0		[<38]
Adult:	<7.0		[<53]

	mg/g creatinine		*mmol/mol creatinine*
or	1.3 ± 0.4 (SD)	× 0.86	[1.1 ± 0.3]

CSF. Collect in sterile tubes; store frozen. Stable at −20° C for 1 wk or at −70° C for 2 mo.[8]

	mg/dL		*μmol/L*
Neonate:	0.136 ± 0.067 (SEM)	× 75.8	[10.3 ± 5.1][8]
3 mo-2 yr:	0.079 ± 0.020 (SD)		[6.0 ± 1.5][11]
2-10 yr:	0.069 ± 0.017		[5.2 ± 1.3][11]
Adult:	0.065 ± 0.008		[4.9 ± 0.6][9]

| DIAGNOSTIC INFORMATION | REMARKS |

annual screening for the early detection of adenomatous polyps and colorectal cancer in adults over age 50 yr with average risk. Fecal occult blood testing is one of five options for screening. [8]

P ↑ Hyperornithinemia-hyperammonemia-homocitrullinuria (HHH) syndrome, gyrate atrophy of the choroid and retina, severe burns,[12] and hemolysis

See Table II-2B.

P ↓ Carcinoid syndrome, chronic renal failure, and after abdominal surgery[13]

U ↑ Cystinurias, dibasic aminoaciduria

High levels of cystine, lysine, and arginine are also seen in the cystinurias. Increased excretion of lysine and arginine is also found in dibasic aminoaciduria; cystine excretion is normal.

CSF ↑ Bacterial meningitis, meningoradiculitis, and Garin-Bujadoux-Bannwarth syndrome[9]

TEST NAME AND METHOD	SPECIMEN REQUIREMENTS	REFERENCE INTERVAL, CONVENTIONAL [INTERNATIONAL RECOMMENDED UNITS]	CHEMICAL INTERFERENCES AND IN VIVO EFFECTS

Ornithine—CONT

1. Scriver CR, Beaudet AL, Valle D, et al, editors: *The metabolic and molecular bases of inherited disease,* ed 8, New York, 2001, McGraw-Hill.

2. Young DS: *Effects of drugs on clinical laboratory tests,* ed 3, Washington, DC, 1990, American Association for Clinical Chemistry.

3. Bremer HJ, Duran M, Kamerling JP, et al: *Disturbances of amino acid metabolism: clinical chemistry and diagnosis,* Baltimore, 1981, Urban and Schwarzenburg.

4. Nyhan W, Sakait N: *Diagnostic recognition of genetic disease,* Philadelphia, 1987, Lea & Febiger.

5. Cummings JG: Routine amino acids analysis in the clinical laboratory, *Am Clin Prod Rev* Feb:20-25, 1988.

6. Schaefer A, Piquard F, Haberey P: Plasma amino acids analysis: effects of delayed samples preparation and of storage, *Clin Chim Acta* 164:163-169, 1987.

7. Pesce, A, Kaplan L, editors: *Methods in clinical chemistry,* St. Louis, 1987, CV Mosby.

Osmolal Gap (Millimole Discriminant, mmol-D)[1,2]	Serum	5-10 mOsm/kg H_2O* *In the SI, 5-10 mmol osmotically active particles/kg H_2O.	See *Osmolality.*

1. Burtis, CA, Ashwood ER, editors: *Tietz textbook of clinical chemistry,* ed 3, Philadelphia, 1999, WB Saunders.
2. Gennari FJ: Serum osmolality. Uses and limitations, *N Engl J Med* 310:102-105, 1984.

Osmolality Ratio, Urine/Serum[1]	Urine, serum	Random urine (average fluid intake): After 12-hr fluid restriction:	1.0-3.0 See *Osmolality.* 3.0-4.7

1. Burtis CA, Ashwood ER, editors: *Tietz textbook of clinical chemistry,* ed 3, Philadelphia, 1999, WB Saunders.

8. Heiblim DI, Evans HE, Glass L, et al: Amino acid concentrations in cerebrospinal fluid, *Arch Neurol* 35:765-768, 1978.

9. Shih V: *Laboratory techniques for the detection of hereditary metabolic disorders,* Boca Raton, FL, 1973, CRC Press.

10. Meites S, editor: *Pediatric clinical chemistry,* ed 3, Washington, DC, 1989, American Association for Clinical Chemistry.

11. Goldsmith RF, Earl JW, Cunningham AM: Determination of δ-aminobutyric acid and other amino acids in cerebrospinal fluid of pediatric patients by reversed-phase liquid chromatography, *Clin Chem* 33:1736-1740, 1987.

12. Schott KJ, Meier D: Free amino acid pattern of cerebrospinal fluid in meningeal pathology, *Acta Neurol Scand* 75:304-309, 1987.

13. Jain KM, Rush BF Jr, Seelig RF, et al: Changes in plasma amino acid profiles following abdominal operations, *Surg Gynecol Obstet* 152:302-306, 1981.

This test is used to detect low-molecular-weight toxins such as ethanol, methanol, isopropanol, ethylene glycol, and acetone.

Millimole discriminant is the difference between calculated and measured osmolality. Osmolality can be calculated as follows:

$$(\text{Na, mmol/L} \times 2) + \frac{\text{Urea N, mg/dL}}{2.8} + \frac{\text{glucose, mg/dL}}{18}$$

The osmolal gap may also be elevated with hyperlipidemia or hyperproteinemia. In these cases, the serum water content is significantly reduced. (See *Osmolality.*)

↓ In polyuria of diabetes insipidus: 0.2-0.7, even after fluid restriction; ratio also decreased in patients with renal tubular deficiency.

In diabetes insipidus, ratio may be >1.0 with marked dehydration (serum osmolality >320 mOsm/kg; in the SI, >320 mmol osmotically active particles/kg).

In polyuria of neurogenic origin, the ratio may be normal without fluid restriction and will increase after fluid restriction. After diuretics or in severe renal insufficiency, ratio is ~1.0; in water intoxication, it is ~0.5.

TEST NAME AND METHOD	SPECIMEN REQUIREMENTS	REFERENCE INTERVAL, CONVENTIONAL [INTERNATIONAL RECOMMENDED UNITS]		CHEMICAL INTERFERENCES AND IN VIVO EFFECTS
Osmolality[1-5] *Freezing-point depression* *Vapor pressure technique*	Serum or plasma (heparin). Stable up to 3 hr at room temperature.	Neonate: Child, adult: >60 yr:	$mOsm/kg* H_2O$[21] May be as low as 266 275-295 280-301	P ↑ C Glucose, urea P ↑ V Corticosteroids, glycerin, insulin (massive doses), mannitol, methoxyflurane (post-surgery), and urea P ↓ V Carbamazepine, chlorthalidone, cisplatin, cyclophosphamide, fluoxetine, lorcainide, and thiazides
	Urine, random[6]	50-1200 mOsm/kg* H_2O, depending on fluid intake. On average fluid intake: After 12-hr fluid restriction:	$mOsm/kg* H_2O$ 300-900 >850	U ↓ C Glucose, urea: Both osmotically active U ↑ V Anesthetic agents (during surgery), carbamazepine, chlorpropamide, cyclophosphamide, metolazone, and vincristine
	Urine, 24 hr. Stable up to 24 hr at 4° C.[6]	~300-900 mOsm/kg* H_2O *In the SI system, 1 mOsm/kg = 1 mmol osmotically active particles/kg H_2O.		U ↓ V Acetohexamide, demeclocycline, glyburide, lithium salts, tolazamide, muscular exercise, and starvation

1. Burtis CA, Ashwood ER, editors: *Tietz textbook of clinical chemistry,* ed 3, Philadelphia, 1999, WB Saunders.
2. Eastham RD: *Biochemical values in clinical medicine,* ed 7, Bristol, UK, 1985, John Wright and Sons Ltd.
3. Henry JB, editor: *Clinical diagnosis and management by laboratory methods,* ed 20, Philadelphia, 2001, WB Saunders.
4. Wallace J, editor: *Interpretation of diagnostic tests,* ed 7, Philadelphia, 2000, Lippincott.
5. Weisberg HF: Unraveling the laboratory model of a syndrome: the osmolality model. In Young DS, Hicks J, Nipper H, et al, editors: *Clinician and chemist. The relationship of the laboratory to the physician,* Washington, DC, 1979, American Association of Clinical Chemistry.
6. Burtis CA, Ashwood ER, editors: *Tietz textbook of clinical chemistry,* ed 2, Philadelphia, 1994, WB Saunders.

Osmotic Fragility (OF) Test [Erc (RBC) Fragility][1,2] *Direct, pH 7.4, 20° C*[1]	Whole blood (heparin) or defibrinated. Do not use oxalate or citrate.	Hemolysis begins at 0.50, w/v [5.0 g/L] NaCl, and is complete at 0.30, w/v [3.0 g/L] NaCl. Compare with normal curve.	Hemolytic organisms in the blood, such as malarial parasites, may cause hemolysis independent of the test.

NaCl, w/v		NaCl, g/L	% Hemolysis	Hemolyzed fraction
0.30	× 10	[3.0]	97-100	× 0.01 [0.97-1.00]
0.35		[3.5]	90-99	[0.90-0.99]

DIAGNOSTIC INFORMATION	REMARKS
S ↑ Water depletion, hyperosmolar nonketotic diabetic coma, diabetic ketoacidosis, hypernatremic ethanol intoxication, diabetes insipidus, hypercalcemia, and cerebral lesions; often with tube feeding	Precision of freezing-point depression method is ±2 mOsm/kg; the vapor pressure method is less precise.
S ↓ Adrenocortical insufficiency, panhypopituitarism, water intoxication, postoperative states (especially with excessive water replacement therapy), and syndrome of inappropriate ADH secretion	

U ↓ Diabetes insipidus, primary polydipsia	See *Water Deprivation Antidiuretic Hormone Stimulation Test* and *Water Loading Antidiuretic Hormone Suppression Test.*

↑ Hereditary spherocytosis (HS), spherocytosis associated with acquired immune hemolytic anemias, and hereditary stomatocytosis	Osmotic fragility (OF) indicates the ability of erythrocytes to take up water without lysing; this ability is determined by the ratio of their surface area to volume. Spherocytes have increased OF because of decreased surface volume, whereas cells with increased membrane redundancy (hypochromic cells and target cells) have decreased OF.
↓ Hypochromic, microcytic anemias (e.g., iron deficiency, thalassemias), and leptocytosis associated with asplenia or liver disease	

TEST NAME AND METHOD	SPECIMEN REQUIREMENTS	REFERENCE INTERVAL, CONVENTIONAL [INTERNATIONAL RECOMMENDED UNITS]		CHEMICAL INTERFERENCES AND IN VIVO EFFECTS

Osmotic Fragility (OF) Test—CONT

0.40	[4.0]	50-95	[0.50-0.95]
0.45	[4.5]	5-45	[0.05-0.45]
0.50	[5.0]	<6	[0.06]
0.55	[5.5]	0	[0.00]

After sterile incubation of blood at 37° C for 24 hr[1]

Compare with normal control. Hemolysis begins at 0.70 e/v [7.0 g/L] NaCl and is complete at 0.40-0.15 w/v [4.0-1.5 g/L] NaCl.

NaCl, w/v		*NaCl, g/L*	*% Hemolysis*		*Hemolyzed fraction*
0.20	× 10	[2.0]	95-100	× 0.01	[0.95-1.00]
0.30		[3.0]	85-100		[0.85-1.00]
0.35		[3.5]	75-100		[0.75-1.00]
0.40		[4.0]	65-100		[0.65-1.00]
0.45		[4.5]	55-95		[0.55-0.95]
0.50		[5.0]	40-85		[0.40-0.85]
0.55		[5.5]	15-70		[0.15-0.70]
0.60		[6.0]	<40		[<0.40]
0.65		[6.5]	<10		[<0.10]
0.70		[7.0]	<5		[<0.05]
0.85		[8.5]	0		[0.00]

1. Dacie JV, Lewis SM: *Practical haematology,* ed 8, Edinburgh, 1995, Churchill Livingstone.
2. Henry JB, editor: *Clinical diagnosis and management by laboratory methods,* ed 20, Philadelphia, 2001, WB Saunders.

TEST NAME AND METHOD	SPECIMEN REQUIREMENTS		ng/mL	µg/L	CHEMICAL INTERFERENCES
Osteocalcin (Bone Gla Protein, BGP)[1-14]	Serum, fasting. Separate within 1 hr and freeze.	Child			↑ V Anticonvulsants, 1,25-dihydroxyvitamin D, thyroid hormones, fluoride, and GH
		6-9.9 yr:	40.2-108	[40.2-108]	
IRMA[15]		10-13.9 yr:	35.8-166	[35.8-166]	
		14-17.9 yr:			↓ V Glucocorticoids, estrogens, bisphosphonates, and calcitonin
		M:	27.8-194	[27.8-194]	
		F:	16.3-68.7	[16.3-68.7]	
ICMA[16]		Adult			
		M:	11.3-35.4	[11.3-35.4]	
		F:	7.2-27.9	[7.2-27.9]	
		Adult			
		M:	1.1-7.2	[1.1-7.2]	
		F, premenopausal:	0.5-7.0	[0.5-7.0]	

Normal in secondary hemolytic anemia, PNH, and G6PD
deficiency

↑ *Hereditary spherocytosis:* An increase in incubated osmotic
fragility compared with that of control blood is characteristic
of HS and is greater than that in other hemolytic anemias, including autoimmune hemolytic anemia with spherocytes. OF
values may be increased in hereditary elliptocytosis and in severe pyruvate kinase deficiency. In mild HS, the unincubated
OF may be normal, with only the incubated OF showing
abnormalities.

↓ *Hypochromic microcytic anemias:* Thalassemia, liver disease, and iron deficiency anemia

Incubation of the blood sample for 24 hr at 37° C (incubated
osmotic fragility) may unmask abnormal OF in cases of mild
HS that have normal or slightly increased OF by standard testing. Normal erythrocytes (and Ercs in most other disorders)
swell during incubation causing them to become more spheri-
cal and hence demonstrate increased OF. Ercs in hereditary
spherocytosis show a greater increase in OF than do normal
cells or Ercs in other disorders, including autoimmune hemolysis with spherocytes.[2]

↑ High-turnover osteoporosis, Paget's disease, primary hyperparathyroidism, renal osteodystrophy, hyperthyroidism, osteomalacia, metastatic bone disease, acromegaly, recent fractures,
bone growth, exercise, lactation, menopause, and age

↓ Pregnancy, growth hormone deficiency, hypothyroidism, hypoparathyroidism, liver disease, and alcoholism

Osteocalcin (OC) is produced by the osteoblast and is a marker
of bone formation. It is the major noncollagenous protein in
bone comprising ~1% of total protein. This 49 amino acid protein contains three glutamyl residues that are converted to
γ-carboxyglutamyl (Gla) by a posttranslation, vitamin
K-dependent enzymatic carboxylation. OC is cleared by the
kidney and has a $t_{1/2}$, in vivo, of ~5 min. There is a marked diurnal variation in bone resorption/formation and serum OC levels, with a nocturnal peak, decreasing by as much as 50% to
the morning nadir.

For monitoring therapy, serial specimens should be collected at
the same time of the day. Serum bone alkaline phosphatase
shows less within-subject variability (see *Alkaline Phosphatase, Bone*). The response of OC to antiresorptive therapies
is delayed compared with resorption markers (see *Collagen
Telopeptides and Pyridinium Crosslinks*) reading a plateau at
6 to 12 months.

TEST NAME AND METHOD	SPECIMEN REQUIREMENTS	REFERENCE INTERVAL, CONVENTIONAL [INTERNATIONAL RECOMMENDED UNITS]	CHEMICAL INTERFERENCES AND IN VIVO EFFECTS
Osteocalcin—CONT			

1. Banfi G, Daverio R: In vitro stability of osteocalcin, *Clin Chem* 40:833-834, 1994.

2. Blumsohn A, Hannon R, Eastell R: Apparent instability of osteocalcin in serum as measured with different commercially available immunoassays, *Clin Chem* 41:318-319, 1995.

3. Calvo MS, Eyre DR, Gundberg CM: Molecular basis and clinical applications of biological markers of bone turnover, *Endocr Rev* 17:333-368, 1996.

4. Garnero P, Delmas PD: Measurements of biochemical markers: methods and limitations. In Bilezikian JP, Raisz LG, Rodan GA, editors: *Principles in bone biology,* San Diego, 1996, Academic Press, pp. 1277-1291.

5. Garnero P, Delmas PD: Biochemical markers of bone turnover in osteoporosis. In Marcus R, Feldman D, Kelsey J, editors: *Osteoporosis,* ed 2, San Diego, 2001, Academic Press, pp. 459-477.

6. Garnero P, Grimaux M, Seguin P, et al: Characterization of immunoreactive forms of human osteocalcin in vivo and in vitro, *J Bone Miner Res* 9:255-264, 1994.

7. Gundberg CM: Biochemical markers of bone formation, *Clin Lab Med* 20:489-501, 2000.

8. Gundberg CM: Osteocalcin. In Fastell R, Baumann M, Hoyle NR, et al, editors: *Bone markers: biochemical and clinical perspectives,* London, 2001, Martin Dunitz, pp. 65-72.

9. Lee AJ, Hodges S, Eastell R, et al: Measurement of osteocalcin, *Ann Clin Biochem* 37:432-446, 2000.

10. Power MJ, Fottrell PF: Osteocalcin: diagnostic methods and clinical applications, *Crit Rev Clin Lab Sci* 28:287-335, 1991.

11. Rosenquist C, Qvist P, Bjarnason N, et al: Measurement of a more stable region of osteocalcin in serum by ELISA with two monoclonal antibodies, *Clin Chem* 41:1439-1445, 1995.

12. Seibel MJ: Biochemical markers of bone remodeling, *Endocrinol Metabol Clin N Am* 32:83-113, 2003.

13. Seibel MJ, Robins SP, Bilezikian JP: Markers of bone metabolism. In Becker KL, editor: *Principles and practice of endocrinology and metabolism,* ed 3, Philadelphia, 2001, Lippincott, Williams & Wilkins, pp. 548-557.

14. Taylor AK, Lueken SA, Libanatic C, et al: Biochemical markers of bone turnover for the clinical assessment of bone metabolism, *Rheum Dis Clin North Am* 20:589-607, 1994.

DIAGNOSTIC INFORMATION	REMARKS

Many competitive and noncompetitive immunoassays have been developed for OC, including RIAs, EIAs, IRMAs, ELISAs, and ICMAs. As illustrated by the methods listed here, OC levels are method-specific and vary widely between methods. In vitro, intact OC is rapidly degraded to a large amino(N)-terminal fragment containing the N-terminal and mid-region amino acids, probably 1-43. Serum OC levels are more stable when measured with methods recognizing both intact OC and N-terminal fragments. Consequently, these methods are more reproducible and widely used than intact OC methods.

In normal individuals, serum OC levels are highest in children, higher in males than females, and increase with age in adults. The highest levels occur during periods of rapid bone growth. OC levels may not accurately reflect bone formation in several situations, including (1) patients treated with 1,25 dihydroxyvitamin D or abnormalities of this hormone because it regulates OC, (2) patients with impaired renal function, and (3) during bed rest.

15. Osteocalcin. In *Quest Diagnostics manual: endocrinology test selection and interpretation,* ed 3, San Juan Capistrano, CA, 2004, Quest-Nichols, p. 127.

16. *Nichols Advantage human osteocalcin direction insert,* San Clemente, CA, 2003, Nichols Institute Diagnostics, pp. 1-9.

TEST NAME AND METHOD	SPECIMEN REQUIREMENTS	REFERENCE INTERVAL, CONVENTIONAL [INTERNATIONAL RECOMMENDED UNITS]		CHEMICAL INTERFERENCES AND IN VIVO EFFECTS
Oxalate[1-8] *GC, GCMS, CZE, enzymatic, colorimetric*	Serum	*mg/L* 1.0-2.4 × 11.4 Ethylene glycol poisoning: >20	*μmol/L* [11-27] [>228]	S ↑ V Ascorbic acid (in dialysis patients), methoxyflurane
	Urine, 24 hr. Collect in a bottle containing 20 mL of HCl, 6 mol/L; final pH should be 1.5-2.0.	*mg/day* Adult M: 20-60 × 11.4 F: 20-55 *mg/L* Ethylene glycol poisoning: >150 × 11.4 Random urine[9]:	*μmol/day* [228-684] [228-627] *μmol/L* [>1710]	U ↑ V Ascorbic acid (large doses), ethylene glycol; ingestion of rhubarb, strawberries, spinach, and tomatoes; methoxyflurane anesthesia, oxalate poisoning, purines, gelatin, and calcium
		mg/dL M: <40 yr 0.7-6.1 × 11.4 ≥40 yr 0.3-4.5 F: <40 yr 0.30-8.95 ≥40 yr 0.30-6.05	*mmol/L* [8.0-69.5] [3.4-51.3] [3.4-102] [3.4-69.0]	U ↑ C Glucose (30 g/L; 166 mmol/L) and oxaloacetic acid (10 mg/L; 114 mmol/L) can interfere in the colorimetric assay. U ↓ V Nifedipine, pyridoxine
		mg/g creatinine M: 5.9-28.6 × 1.14 F: 9.2-45.4	*mmol/g creatinine* [6.7-32.6] [10.5-51.8]	

1. Eder AF, McGrath CM, Dowdy YG, et al: Ethylene glycol poisoning: toxicokinetic and analytical factors affecting laboratory diagnosis, *Clin Chem* 44:168-177, 1998.

2. Fraser AD: Clinical toxicologic implications of ethylene glycol and glycolic acid poisoning, *Ther Drug Monit* 24:232-238, 2002.

3. Harris AH, Freel RW, Hatch M: Serum oxalate in human beings and rats as determined with the use of ion chromatography, *J Lab Clin Med* 44:45-52, 2004.

4. Khan SR, Kok DJ: Modulators of urinary stone formation, *Front, Biosci* 9:1450-1482, 2004.

5. Milardovic S, Grabaric Z, Tkalcec M, et al: Determination of oxalate in urine, using an amperometric biosensor with oxalate oxidase immobilized on the surface of a chromium hexacyanoferrate-modified graphite electrode, *J AOAC Int* 83:1212-1217, 2000.

6. Pak CY, Heller HJ, Pearle MS, et al: Prevention of stone formation and bone loss in absorptive hypercalciuria by combined dietary and pharmacological interventions, *J Urol* 169:465-469, 2003.

7. Qi L, Danielson ND: Determination of lactate or oxalate using injected lactate oxidase and peroxidase by capillary electrophoresis with UV detection, *Electrophoresis* 24:2070-2075, 2003.

8. Sriboonlue P, Suwantrai S, Prasongwatana V: An indirect method for urinary oxalate estimation, *Clin Chim Acta* 273:59-68, 1998.

9. Bond LW, Garber C, Ottinger W, et al: Reference intervals for common analytes in random urine specimens, *Clin Chem* 55:submitted, 2005.

DIAGNOSTIC INFORMATION	REMARKS

Systemic poisoning is characterized by corrosive effects, renal damage, and a marked decrease in calcium levels with resulting shock, collapse, and convulsions. Primary hyperoxaluria is a genetic disorder resulting in increased serum and urine levels. Up to 99% of administered oxalic acid is excreted in urine within 36 hr.

Normally oxalate is derived from dietary oxalic acid ($\sim$10%) and the metabolism of ascorbic acid (35-50%) and glycine (40%). Oxalic acid and its salts are used in cleaning and bleaching agents.

U ↑ Primary hyperoxaluria (100-600 mg/day; 1110-6670 μmol/day), diabetes mellitus, cirrhosis, pyridoxine deficiency, sarcoidosis, steatorrhea caused by pancreatic insufficiency, celiac disease, bacterial overgrowth, ileal resection, jejunoileal shunt, biliary tract disease, bowel disease with excessive absorption, and small bowel disease

Urine samples from individuals taking megadoses of ascorbic acid when analyzed by ion chromatography may have increased levels of oxalate. The oxidation of ascorbic acid to oxalate in vitro can be avoided by using a diluent containing boric acid, 0.3 mol/L, instead of water.

There is an increased incidence of urolithiasis in workers heavily exposed to oxalic acid.

U ↓ Renal failure

See also *Glycolic Acid* and *Glyceric Acid*.

TEST NAME AND METHOD	SPECIMEN REQUIREMENTS	REFERENCE INTERVAL, CONVENTIONAL [INTERNATIONAL RECOMMENDED UNITS]		CHEMICAL INTERFERENCES AND IN VIVO EFFECTS
Oxygen, P₅₀ (PO_2[0.5], p50)[1] *Spectrophotometry, potentiometry*	Whole blood (heparin) See *Carbon Dioxide, Partial Pressure.*	Newborn: Adult, corrected to pH(P) 7.40:	*mm Hg* 18-24 × 0.133 25-29	*kPa* [2.39-3.19] [3.33-3.86]	None found.

1. Burtis CA, Ashwood ER, editors: *Tietz fundamentals of clinical chemistry,* ed 5, Philadelphia, 2000, WB Saunders.
2. Fairbanks VF: *Hemoglobinopathies and thalassemias,* New York, 1980, Thieme-Stratton.
3. Fairbanks VF, Maldonado JE, Charache S, et al: Familial erythrocytosis due to electrophoretically undetectable hemoglobin with impaired oxygen dissociation (Hemoglobin Malmo $\alpha_2 \beta_2^{97gin}$), *Mayo Clin Proc* 46:721-727, 1971.
4. Stamatoyannopoulos G, Parer JT, Finch CA: Physiologic implications of hemoglobin with decreased oxygen affinity (Hemoglobin Seattle), *N Engl J Med* 281:804-808, 1969.

TEST NAME AND METHOD	SPECIMEN REQUIREMENTS	REFERENCE INTERVAL, CONVENTIONAL [INTERNATIONAL RECOMMENDED UNITS]		CHEMICAL INTERFERENCES AND IN VIVO EFFECTS
Oxygen, Partial Pressure (PO_2, P(a)o_2, PO_2)[1-3] *Clarkoxygen Electrode*[4]	Collect arterial blood anaerobically in a well-sealed heparinized syringe. Place in ice water and send to the laboratory immediately. Do not use plastic syringe; loss of oxygen may occur (some new syringes are satisfactory). To avoid dilutional errors and pH changes, do not use excess liquid heparin.	Cord blood[5] Arterial: Venous: Birth[1]: 5-10 min: 30 min: 1 hr: 1 day: Thereafter: >60 yr[3]: >70 yr: >80 yr: >90 yr:	*mm Hg* 18.0 ± 6.2 (SD) × 0.133 29.2 ± 5.9 8-24 33-75 31-85 55-80 54-95 83-108 >80 >70 >60 >50	*kPa* [2.4 ± 0.8] [3.9 ± 0.8] [1.06-3.19] [4.39-9.96] [4.12-11.31] [7.32-10.64] [7.18-12.64] [11.04-14.36] [>10.64] [>9.31] [>7.98] [>6.65]	↓ V Drugs causing respiratory depression, e.g., barbiturates, diazepam, heroin, meperidine, and midazolam

When breathing
100% O_2: >500 mm Hg × 0.133 [>66.50 kPa]

Values decrease with age and high altitude.

$$P_{O_2} = (-0.27 \times age) + 104$$

DIAGNOSTIC INFORMATION	REMARKS

↑ Displacement of the O_2 curve to right (decreased affinity of Hb for O_2) is observed in hyperthermia, acidemia, and hypercapnia, increases in 2,3-DPG, presence of abnormal Hb (e.g., Hb Seattle), and pregnancy.

Po_2 at half saturation of the hemoglobin (Hb), Po_2 (0.5), is a measure of the affinity of Hb for oxygen, which, in turn, determines the delivery of oxygen to tissues. The value of Po_2 (0.5) is influenced by temperature, pH, 2,3-DPG concentration, and type of Hb.

↓ Displacement of O_2 curve to the left (increased affinity of Hb for O_2) may be caused by hypothermia, acute alkalemia, and hypocapnia, decreases in 2,3-DPG, abnormal Hb (e.g., Hb Yakima and Hb F), and preeclampsia.[2-4]

↑ Breathing O_2-enriched air, exercise, and in angiomas of brain (increased Po_2 found in jugular venous blood)

At 55 mm Hg [7.32 kPa] $P(a)o_2$ is the shoulder of the dissociation curve; below this level there is a precipitous decrease in oxygen content. With pure oxygen treatment, the arterial Po_2 may increase to ~640 mm Hg [85.12 kPa], depending on the degree of shunting of blood in the lungs.

↓ Hypoxemia (e.g., high altitude), decreased cardiac output, carbon monoxide exposure, anesthesia, and near drowning

Decreased alveolar gas exchange, e.g., respiratory distress syndrome in newborns, lymphangitic carcinomatosis, pulmonary adenomatosis, sarcoidosis, berylliosis, Hamman-Rich syndrome, and pulmonary hemosiderosis secondary to mitral stenosis; decreased alveolocapillary membrane surface, e.g., after resection or compression of the lung

The risk of admixture of blood from venules to capillary blood is especially pronounced in patients in shock, newborn infants in the first hours or even days after birth, newborn infants with respiratory distress syndrome, and patients receiving oxygen therapy.

Ventilation/perfusion inequalities: Bronchitis, asthma, emphysema, bronchiectasis, atelectasis, pneumoconiosis, granulomata, neoplasm, pulmonary infarction, pneumonia, mucoviscidosis, airway obstruction (i.e., by foreign body), croup, retained secretions, tumor, and shock

Capillary blood is not suitable for estimation of high arterial Po_2 values.

Po_2 values measured at 37° C must be corrected to the actual temperature of the patient.[4,6]

Generalized alveolar hypoventilation of peripheral origin: Suffocation, submersion, skeletal abnormalities (e.g., kyphoscoliosis, flail chest resulting from trauma), neuromuscular conditions affecting respiration (phrenic nerve paralysis, tetanus, acute poliomyelitis, and pickwickian syndrome)

Transcutaneous O_2 monitors and intraarterial optodes provide continuous real-time information.[7]

Of central origin: Depression of respiratory center by drugs like barbiturates or morphine, by head injury, or cerebrovascular incident

TEST NAME AND METHOD	SPECIMEN REQUIREMENTS	REFERENCE INTERVAL, CONVENTIONAL [INTERNATIONAL RECOMMENDED UNITS]	CHEMICAL INTERFERENCES AND IN VIVO EFFECTS

Oxygen, Partial Pressure—CONT

1. Henry JB, editor: *Clinical diagnosis and management by laboratory methods,* ed 20, Philadelphia, 2001, WB Saunders.
2. Burtis CA, Ashwood ER, editors: *Tietz fundamentals of clinical chemistry,* ed 5, Philadelphia, 2000, WB Saunders.
3. Wallace J, editor: *Interpretation of diagnostic tests,* ed 7, Philadelphia, 2000, Lippincott.
4. Ashwood ER, Kost G, Kenny M: Temperature correction of blood-gas and pH measurements [review], *Clin Chem* 29:1877-1885, 1983.
5. Yeomans ER, Hauth JC, Gilstrap LC III, et al: Umbilical cord pH, PCO_2, and bicarbonate following uncomplicated term vaginal deliveries, *Am J Obstet Gynecol* 151:798-800, 1985.
6. van Stekelenburg GJ: Temperature correction of blood pO_2 measurements [letter], *Clin Chem* 30:595, 1984.
7. Howanitz JH, Howanitz PJ, editors: *Laboratory medicine: test selection and interpretation,* New York, 1991, Churchill Livingstone.

Oxygen Saturation (SO_2)[1,2]

Spectrophotometry,[2] *pulse oximetry, transcutaneous monitoring, intraarterial optode*[3]

Anaerobically drawn whole blood, arterial (heparinized syringe). Place in ice water and send to the laboratory immediately.

	Percent saturation[2]		*Fraction saturation*	See *Oxygen, Partial Pressure.*
Newborn:	40-90	$\times 0.01$	[0.40-0.90]	
Thereafter:	94-98		[0.94-0.98]	

Values decrease with age.

1. Eastham RD: *Biochemical values in clinical medicine,* ed 7, Bristol, UK, 1985, John Wright and Sons Ltd.
2. Burtis CA, Ashwood ER, editors: *Tietz fundamentals of clinical chemistry,* ed 5, Philadelphia, 2000, WB Saunders.
3. Howanitz JH, Howanitz PJ, editors: *Laboratory medicine: test selection and interpretation,* New York, 1991, Churchill Livingstone.

DIAGNOSTIC INFORMATION	REMARKS

Right to left shunt: Intrapulmonary venoarterial shunting, congenital heart disease

More than one of these mechanisms may operate simultaneously.

Values <40 mm Hg [<5.32 kPa] indicate severe hypoxemia; values <20 mm Hg [<2.66 kPa] are frequently associated with death.

Measurement of oxygen saturation may be clinically useful in cyanosis and erythrocytosis. It may differentiate between diminished oxygenation of blood, as in pulmonary diseases, and admixture of venous blood, as in an arteriovenous shunt.

Estimation of oxygen saturation of samples obtained at various sites during cardiac catheterization is helpful when used in conjunction with intracardiac pressure measurements in the detection of intracardiac abnormalities.

Oxygen desaturation may occur after sedation for peritoneoscopy with resultant hypoxemia, hypercarbia, and acidosis.[4]

In Rh incompatibility caused by blocking antibodies, the oxygen-carrying capacity of Ercs is 10-15% less than normal.

The oxygen saturation is calculated as follows:

$$So_2 = \left(\frac{O_2\,Hb}{O_2\,Hb + HHB} \right) \times 100\%$$

The availability of oxygen to tissues is dependent not only on the So_2 but also on the affinity of O_2 to Hb.

See *Oxygen, P_{50}, and 2,3-Diphosphoglycerate in Erythrocytes.*

Pulse oximetry is most accurate between 80 and 100% O_2 saturation. Below 80% saturation accuracy decreases, but measurements reflect trend. Pulse oximetry may give inaccurate results in severe anemia, hypovolemia, hypotension, hypothermia, and arrhythmias, as well as in the presence of carboxy-, met-, and fetal hemoglobin and angiographic dyes.[3] Pulse oximetry cannot distinguish between Po_2 values of 100 or >100 mm Hg (13.3 kPa).

---

4.   Jacobs DS, DeMott WR, Oxley DK, editors: *Laboratory test handbook,* ed 5, Stow, OH, 2001, Lexi-Comp, Inc.

TEST NAME AND METHOD	SPECIMEN REQUIREMENTS	REFERENCE INTERVAL, CONVENTIONAL [INTERNATIONAL RECOMMENDED UNITS]			CHEMICAL INTERFERENCES AND IN VIVO EFFECTS
Oxytocin[1,2]	Plasma (EDTA). Freeze immediately. Signifi-		$\mu U/mL$ (SEM)	mU/L (SEM)	None found.
	cant deterioration oc-	M:	1.5 ± 0.2 × 1.0	[1.5 ± 0.2]	
RIA	curs with prolonged	F,			
	storage.	nonpregnant:	1.4 ± 0.2	[1.4 ± 0.2]	
		Second stage of			
		labor:	4.2 ± 1.1	[4.2 ± 1.1]	
		1 μU is equivalent to 2 pg synthetic oxytocin.			
	Amniotic fluid[3]		pg/mL (x)	ng/L (x)	
		Term:	275 × 1.0	[275]	
		During labor:	695	[695]	

1. Leake R, Weitzmon R, Glatz T, et al: Plasma oxytocin concentrations in men, nonpregnant women, and pregnant women before and during spontaneous labor, *J Clin Endocrinol Metab* 53:730-733, 1981.

2. Ludmir J, Alvarez JG, Mennutti M, et al: Cholesteryl palmitate as a predictor of fetal lung maturity, *Am J Obstet Gynecol* 157:84-88, 1987.

3. Tulchinsky D, Ryan KJ, editors: *Maternal-fetal endocrinology,* Philadelphia, 1980, WB Saunders.

TEST NAME AND METHOD	SPECIMEN REQUIREMENTS	REFERENCE INTERVAL, CONVENTIONAL [INTERNATIONAL RECOMMENDED UNITS]			CHEMICAL INTERFERENCES AND IN VIVO EFFECTS
P Component (C1t, α_1M-Glyco- protein, α_1M, amyloid P)[1-3]	Serum. Analyze fresh or store at 4° C for <72 hr. Stable frozen at −20° C for 6 mo or	3-8 mg/dL (x̄: 5.5)	× 10	[30-80 mg/L] [x̄: 55]	None found.
RID[1,4]	at −70° C indefinitely. Specimens without				
ELISA[5]	lipemia or hemolysis are preferred.				

1. Ritzmann SE, Tucker ES III: *Protein analysis in disease—current concepts. Workshop manual,* Chicago, 1979, American Society of Clinical Pathologists, Commission for Continuing Education.

2. Putnam FW, editors: *The plasma proteins: structure, functions and genetic control, vol 1-3,* ed 2, New York, 1977, Academic Press.

3. DuClos TW: The interaction of C-reactive protein and serum amyloid P component with nuclear antigens, *Mol Biol Rep* 23:253-260, 1996.

4. Hashimoto S, Katou M, Dong Y, et al: Effects of hormone replacement therapy on serum amyloid P component in postmenopausal women, *Maturitas* 26:113-119, 1997.

5. Saïle R, Kandoussi A, Deveaux M, et al: Quantification of serum amyloid P by enzyme-linked immunosorbent assay, *Clin Chem* 37:1742-1745, 1991.

6. Katz A, Weicker-Thorne J, Painter RH: The relationship of a serum protein, C1t, to a common nonfibrillar constituent of amyloid (P component) as revealed by immunohistochemical studies, *Am J Pathol* 88:679-698, 1977.

DIAGNOSTIC INFORMATION	REMARKS

↓ Stress and psychic factors (e.g., fright)

In females, oxytocin induces uterine contractions and stimulates the lactating mammary gland. Physiological effects are unknown in males. The origin of oxytocin in amniotic fluid is unknown.

P component is not an acute phase reacting protein.[3] Serum values increase with increasing age and may be higher in males compared with age-matched females.[4]

$\alpha_1 M$ is a member of the pentraxin family of proteins and is identical to C1t and amyloid P component.[6,7] No polymorphisms or deficiency states have been identified.[3] It can activate complement using the classical pathway and can opsonize microorganisms and other particles for phagocytosis by white blood cells.[3,8] As the precursor of the P component of tissue amyloid deposits, evidence suggests that serum amyloid P component may stabilize amyloid β-peptide fibrils.[9] It also binds to chromatin and appears to have a protective role against the development of autoimmunity.[3,10]

MW: 233,000-300,000.

---

7. Pinteric L, Assimeh SN, Kells DI, et al: The ultrastructure of C1t, a subcomponent of the first component of complement: an E.M. and ultracentrifuge study, *J Immunol* 117:79-83, 1976.

8. Dwaipayan B, Mold C, Markham E, et al: Serum amyloid P component binds to Fcg receptors and opsonizes particles for phagocytosis, *J Immunol* 166:6735-6741, 2001.

9. Holm Nielsen E, Nybo M, Junker K, et al: Localization of human serum amloid P component and heparin sulfate proteoglycan in in vitro-formed Abeta fibrils, *Scand J Immunol* 52:110-112, 2000.

10. Burlingame RW, Volzer MA, Harris J, et al: The effect of acute phase proteins on clearance of chromatin from the circulation of normal mice, *J Immunol* 156:4783, 1996.

TEST NAME AND METHOD	SPECIMEN REQUIREMENTS	REFERENCE INTERVAL, CONVENTIONAL [INTERNATIONAL RECOMMENDED UNITS]			CHEMICAL INTERFERENCES AND IN VIVO EFFECTS
PABA (***p*-Aminobenzoic Acid) Test** (NBT-PABA, Bentiromide Test)[1,2] *Colorimetric* Test Meal: Standard lunch meal with 666 mg of bentiromide in 300 mL of water	Serum, before test meal and 90 min thereafter	*mg/L* >2	× 7.3	*mmol/L* [>22]	
HPLC[3,4] Dose: NBT-PABA, 1 g	Plasma (heparin), 3 hr after test meal. Separate plasma immediately, and store at −20° C.	48 ± 9.5 mmol/L (SD)[3]			↑ C Procainamide-type local anesthetics[3]
CHYMEX[5] *Colorimetric* Dose, adult: 500 mg of bentiromide (contains 170 mg of PABA). Follow immediately with 250 mL of water. Give another 250 mL of water 2 hr postdose, then 500 mL of water between 2 and 6 hr postdose.[6] Child: 14 mg bentiromide/kg body weight	Urine. After overnight fast, patient should urinate before taking the drug. Collect all urine up to 6 hr after drug dose. Refrigerate specimen to retard microbial growth.[5]	≥50% excretion of PABA (See *Diagnostic Information.*)			↑ C Acetaminophen, benzocaine, chloramphenicol, furosemide, lidocaine, multivitamins, pancreatic enzymes, phenacetin, procainamide, procaine, some sun-absorbing skin lotions, sulfonamides, and thiazide diuretics may cause false-negative results. Apples, cranberries, plums, and prunes may interfere with urinary arylamine determinations by increasing the percent of PABA recovered.

The serum test has a greater specificity (88%), sensitivity (94%), and efficiency (91%) than the excretion ratio of PABA/14C-PABA.[2] Test is less sensitive in detecting slight or moderate forms of exocrine pancreatic insufficiency.[1]

↓ Chronic pancreatitis (<5 μmol/L), cystic fibrosis, and steatorrhea

HPLC is more specific than colorimetric assays.[3]

Under conditions of normal pancreatic, gastric, gut, and kidney function, >50% of PABA contained in CHYMEX (Savage Laboratories, Melville, NY) appears in the urine within 6 hr after administration of this agent.

The smaller the recovery of urinary arylamine, the greater the likelihood that there is diminished exocrine pancreatic function.[5]

U ↓ Malabsorption, impaired renal function (creatinine >1.5 mg/dL; 133 μmol/L), severe hepatic dysfunction, and gastric stasis.[5]

In testing diabetic patients, suitable adjustments in insulin may be needed to accommodate the fasting patient. In adults, oral pancreatic enzyme supplements should be discontinued 5 days before the administration of bentiromide. The time interval is reduced to 1 day in children with cystic fibrosis.[5] Some patients with documented pancreatic insufficiency may have normal results.[5]

TEST NAME AND METHOD	SPECIMEN REQUIREMENTS	REFERENCE INTERVAL, CONVENTIONAL [INTERNATIONAL RECOMMENDED UNITS]	CHEMICAL INTERFERENCES AND IN VIVO EFFECTS
PABA (*p*-Aminobenzoic Acid) Test—CONT			
HPLC[7] Dose: 1 g of bentiromide and 300 mg of *p*-aminosalicylic acid (PAS) with 25 g of casein in 400 mL of chocolate-flavored drink. Patient should drink 1 L of water during test.	Same as for CHYMEX test	PABA excretion index: 93% ± 12 (SD)[7]	None found.[8]

1. Henderson AR, Tietz NW, Rinker AD: Gastric, pancreatic, and intestinal function. In Burtis CA, Ashwood ER, editors: *Tietz textbook of clinical chemistry,* ed 2, Philadelphia, 1994, WB Saunders.

2. Tanner AR, Robinson DP: Pancreatic function testing—serum PABA measurement is a reliable and accurate measurement of exocrine function, *Gut* 29:1736-1740, 1988.

3. Lawson N, Berg JD, Chesner IM: Liquid-chromatographic determination of p-aminobenzoic acid in plasma and to evaluate exocrine pancreatic function, *Clin Chem* 31:1073-1075, 1985.

4. Yung-Jato LL, Durie PR, Soldin SJ: Liquid chromatographic measurement of p-aminobenzoic acid and its metabolites in serum, *Clin Chem* 34:2235-2238, 1988.

5. Adria Laboratories, Inc.: *CHYMEX, laboratory procedure for determining PABA in urine specimens,* Columbus, OH, 1983, Adria Laboratories, Inc.

6. Goldstein DE, Little RR, Wiedmeyer HM, et al: Glycated hemoglobin: methodologies and clinical applications, *Clin Chem* 32:B64-B70, 1986.

7. Berg JD, Chesner IM, Allen-Narker RAC, et al: Exocrine pancreatic function as determined in a same-day test with use of bentiromide and p-aminosalicylic acid, *Clin Chem* 32:1010-1012, 1986.

8. Berg JD, Chesner IM, Lawson N: Practical assessment of the NBT-PABA pancreatic function test using high performance liquid chromatography determination of p-aminobenzoic acid in urine, *Ann Clin Biochem* 22:586-590, 1985.

Patients with proven, severe chronic exocrine pancreatic dysfunction have index values of <5-26%.[6,7]

Use of combined preparations containing a fixed ratio of bentiromide to PAS avoids the need for precise calculation of dose based on body weight. This approach is convenient for children, for whom use of radioactivity (e.g., 14C-PABA) is undesirable.[7] The PABA excretion index is defined as PABA recovery/PAS recovery, where recovery means the part of administered dose accounted for.[7]

Pancreatic supplements should be stopped 48 hr before test. Analyze pretest urine to rule out any interferences.[8]

TEST NAME AND METHOD	SPECIMEN REQUIREMENTS	REFERENCE INTERVAL, CONVENTIONAL [INTERNATIONAL RECOMMENDED UNITS]			CHEMICAL INTERFERENCES AND IN VIVO EFFECTS
Pancreatic Polypeptide (PP)[1-6]	Plasma, fasting (EDTA). Freeze.		pg/mL^7	ng/L	None found.
		20-29 yr:	26-158	× 1.0	[26-158]
		30-39 yr:	55-284		[55-284]
RIA		40-49 yr:	64-243		[64-243]
		>50 yr:	51-326		[51-326]

1. Bloom SR, Polak JM: Gastrointestinal hormones in disease. In Mutt V, editor: *Advances in metabolic disorders,* Orlando, FL, 1985, Academic Press.

2. Buchanan KD: The gastrointestinal hormones: general concepts, *Clin Endocrinol Metab* 8:249-263, 1979.

3. Floyd JC, Fajans SS, Pek S, et al: A newly recognized pancreatic polypeptide; plasma levels in health and disease, *Recent Prog Horm Res* 33:519-570, 1977.

4. Friesen SR: Tumors of the endocrine pancreas, *N Engl J Med* 306:580-590, 1982.

5. Henderson AR, Tietz NW, Rinker AD: Gastric, pancreatic, and intestinal function. In Burtis CA, Ashwood ER, editors: *Tietz textbook of clinical chemistry,* ed 2, Philadelphia, 1994, WB Saunders.

6. Khakhaloud GM, editor: *Handbook of Physiology—Section b: The gastrointestinal system. Volume II: Neural and endocrine biopsy,* New York, Oxford University.

7. Burtis CA, Ashwood ER, editors: *Tietz textbook of clinical chemistry,* ed 3, Philadelphia, 1999, WB Saunders.

8. Service FJ, Koch MB, Jay JM, et al: Pancreatic polypeptide: a marker for lean non-insulin-dependent diabetes mellitus? *Diabetes Care* 8:349-353, 1985.

DIAGNOSTIC INFORMATION	REMARKS
↑ Benign or malignant functioning pancreatic endocrine tumors (e.g., gastrinomas, insulinomas, VIPomas, glucagonomas), some carcinoid tumors arising outside the pancreas, metastases of some islet cell tumors (in islet cell tumors very high plasma levels are more likely when primary and liver metastases are present); some adenocarcinomas of pancreas, stomach, colon, rectum; duodenal ulcer, diabetes mellitus, advancing age, renal failure; multiple endocrine neoplasia type I (MEN-1), medullary thyroid carcinoma; and Zollinger-Ellison syndrome	All ingested nutrients stimulate PP release; most potent is protein. PP release is mediated by vagal stimulation. Insulin-induced hypoglycemia also produces a large increase in PP concentrations. There are suggestions that PP can be a cause of watery diarrhea syndrome in islet cell tumors. Elevated PP levels may be characteristic of lean noninsulin-dependent diabetic (NIDDM) patients.[8]
↓ Chronic pancreatitis with exocrine insufficiency. (There is impaired response to hypoglycemia induced by insulin or a meal.)	

TEST NAME AND METHOD	SPECIMEN REQUIREMENTS	REFERENCE INTERVAL, CONVENTIONAL [INTERNATIONAL RECOMMENDED UNITS]		CHEMICAL INTERFERENCES AND IN VIVO EFFECTS
Pantothenic Acid (Vitamin B$_5$)[1-5]	Whole blood (sodium citrate) or serum	Total: 0.2-1.8 mcg/mL × 4.56	[0.9-8.2 μmol/L]	None found.
MB (T. pyriformis, L. plantarum, L. casei, or S. uvarum), RIA[6]	Urine, 24 hr; collect with volatile preservative (chlorobenzene, ethylene dichloride, 1-chlorobutane).[1]	1-15 mg/day × 4.56 (x̄: 4)	[5-68 μmol/day] [x̄: 18.2]	
		mg/g creatinine ≥2.0 × 0.516	mmol/mol creatinine [≥1.03]	

1. Baker H, Frank O: *Clinical vitaminology. Methods and interpretation,* New York, 1968, Interscience.

2. Brown ML, editor: *Present knowledge in nutrition,* ed 6, Washington, DC, 1990, International Life Sciences Institute, Nutrition Foundation.

3. Kinney JM, Jeejeebhoy KN, Hill GL, et al: *Nutrition and metabolism in patient care,* Philadelphia, 1988, WB Saunders.

4. Sauberlich HE, Dowdy RP, Skala JH: *Laboratory tests for the assessment of nutritional status,* Boca Raton, FL, 1974, CRC Press Inc.

5. Shils ME, Olson JA, Shike M, editors: *Modern nutrition in health and disease,* ed 8, Philadelphia, 1994, Lea & Febiger.

6. Wyese BW, Wittwer C, Hansen RG: Radioimmunoassay for pantothenic acid in blood and other tissues, *Clin Chem* 25:108-111, 1979.

7. Bender DA: Optimum nutrition: thiamin, biotin and pantothenate, *Proc Nutr Soc* 58:427-433, 1999.

8. McCormick DB, Greene HL: Vitamins. In Burtis CA, Ashwood ER, editors: *Tietz textbook of clinical chemistry,* ed 3, Philadelphia, 1999, WB Saunders, pp. 1029-1055.

9. Kaplan LA, Pesce AJ, editors: *Clinical chemistry: theory, analysis and correlation,* ed 2, St. Louis, 1989, CV Mosby.

10. Rychlik M: Quantification of free and bound pantothenic acid in foods and blood plasma by a stable isotope dilution assay, *J Agric Food Chem* 48:1175-1181, 2000.

11. Rychlik M: Pantothenic acid quantification by a stable isotope dilution assay based on liquid chromatography-tandem mass spectrometry, *Analyst* 128:832-837, 2003.

Pantothenate deficiency is associated with nutritional erythromelalgia (burning foot syndrome), abdominal distress, burning cramps, paresthesia of hands and feet, and impaired wound healing. Because uncomplicated pantothenate deficiency is rare, symptoms described above that have been attributed to pantothenic acid deficiency may have resulted for multi-B vitamin deficiency. People fed synthetic diets free of pantothenate developed postural hypotension, rapid heart rate on exertion, epigastric distress, numbness and tingling of hands and feet, and hyperactive deep tendon reflexes, and the eosinopenic response to adrenocorticotropic hormone was impaired.[7,8]

Pantothenic acid is ubiquitous in nature, being present in most foods, and as such, uncomplicated pantothenic acid deficiency is unlikely to occur except in experimental situations.[7]

Most (80%) pantothenic acid is converted to coenzyme A; it is also converted to acyl carrier protein. Pantothenate deficiency does not occur naturally; it can be caused either by antagonists or by a diet that is low in pantothenic acid. Toxicity is unknown; ingestion of 10-20 g of calcium pantothenate is associated with occasional diarrhea. Chronic alcoholics have increased excretion of pantothenic acid. Patients with circulatory, cardiovascular, and peptic ulcer diseases have reduced circulating pantothenic acid. Reduced levels and low urinary excretion of pantothenate have been reported in patients with chronic malnutrition and acute rheumatism.[9]

Stable isotope dilution methods based on gas chromatography-mass spectrometry[10] and liquid chromatography-mass spectrometry[11] have been developed for measurement of pantothenic acid in pharmaceuticals and foods.

TEST NAME AND METHOD	SPECIMEN REQUIREMENTS	REFERENCE INTERVAL, CONVENTIONAL [INTERNATIONAL RECOMMENDED UNITS]	CHEMICAL INTERFERENCES AND IN VIVO EFFECTS

Paraneoplastic Autoantibody Evaluation is useful for (1) Investigating a subacute multifocal neurological disorder without obvious cause, especially in a patient with past or family history of cancer or smoking history, (2) directing a focused search for cancer, (3) investigating neurological symptoms that appear in the course or wake of cancer therapy and are not explainable by metastasis, (4) differentiating autoimmune neuropathies from neurotoxic effects of chemotherapy, (5) monitoring the immune response of seropositive patients in the course of cancer therapy, and (6) detecting early evidence of cancer recurrence in previously seropositive patients (Fig. II-7).

TEST NAME AND METHOD	SPECIMEN REQUIREMENTS	REFERENCE INTERVAL, CONVENTIONAL [INTERNATIONAL RECOMMENDED UNITS]	CHEMICAL INTERFERENCES AND IN VIVO EFFECTS
Anti-Neuronal Nuclear Antibody (Ab), Type 1 (ANNA-1); anti-Hu[1-3] Indirect immuno-fluorescence; composite mouse tissue substrate. IgG binds to nucleus and cytoplasm of all neurons (CNS and PNS). Western blot; native CNS protein (35, 37, 38, and 40 kD bands) or recombinant antigen	Draw blood in a plain, red-top tube(s) or serum gel tube(s). Spin down and send 3.0 mL of serum refrigerated.	Negative at 1:120 Negative	Immunosuppressant and chemotoxic therapies may reduce the antibody level below detection limit. Applies to all antibodies in this section.
Anti-Neuronal Nuclear Ab, Type 2 (ANNA-2); anti-Ri[3,4] Indirect immuno-fluorescence; composite mouse tissue substrate. IgG binding restricted to CNS neurons. Western blot; native CNS protein (50, 52, and 70 kD) or recombinant antigen	Draw blood in a plain, red-top tube(s) or serum gel tube(s). Spin down and send 3.0 mL of serum refrigerated.	Negative at 1:120 Negative	

DIAGNOSTIC INFORMATION	REMARKS

Neurologic accompaniments of ANNA-1 are subacute in onset and usually multifocal[1]; 66% of cases are female. Most frequent are neuropathies (pure sensory, mixed sensorimotor, predominantly autonomic, and rarely motor), limbic encephalitis, subacute cerebellar degeneration, myelopathy, or radiculopathy. Intestinal dysmotility (commonly gastroparesis or pseudoobstruction) occurs in 30% of ANNA-1-positive patients, gut dysautonomia is sometimes the sole paraneoplastic presentation.[2] Small cell lung carcinoma or extrapulmonary small cell carcinoma is almost always present but usually limited in spread and difficult to find. Rarely, thymoma is present. In most cases ANNA-1 detection precedes cancer diagnosis, new or recurrent.[1] Children presenting with intestinal dysmotility, cerebellar ataxia, brainstem encephalitis, or encephalomyeloneuropathy are sometimes positive for ANNA-1, with and without evidence of cancer (neuroblastoma).

Most ANNA-1-positive patients have a history of tobacco use, social/occupational exposure to carcinogen, or family history of lung cancer. PET scanning and magnetic resonance imaging of the chest may reveal malignant adenopathy when CT is negative. SCLC is confirmed in 83% of ANNA-1-positive patients with adequate follow-up evaluation. In 15% of these patients, the search for cancer reveals an unrelated but more obvious primary malignancy; surveillance for small cell carcinoma must continue. Thorough evaluation of serum and CSF is advised when a paraneoplastic disorder is suspected. The individual patient's profile of autoAbs predicts the underlying cancer but does not necessarily predict a specific neurological syndrome. One or more other paraneoplastic autoantibodies coexist with ANNA-1 in 43% of seropositive patients, all predicting small cell carcinoma or, rarely, thymoma.[3]

Neurologic accompaniments of ANNA-2 are subacute in onset and usually multifocal; 70% of cases are female. Neurologic signs, in decreasing frequency: brainstem syndrome (majority opsoclonus/myoclonus; also cranial neuropathy), cerebellar syndrome, myelopathy, neuropathy (sensorimotor > polyradiculopathy > cauda equina syndrome), movement disorder, encephalopathy, Lambert-Eaton myasthenic syndrome, seizures, laryngospasm, and trismus. A positive result has 80% predictive value for small cell lung carcinoma or breast adenocarcinoma.[4]

ANNA-2 is less common than ANNA-1 (1:20),[3] but in 35% of seropositive patients, one or more autoAbs coexist with ANNA-2 (e.g., ANNA-1, ion channel, etc.).[4] Thorough evaluation of serum and CSF is advised when a paraneoplastic disorder is suspected. The individual patient's profile of autoAbs predicts the underlying cancer (lung or breast carcinoma) but not necessarily a specific neurological syndrome.

TEST NAME AND METHOD	SPECIMEN REQUIREMENTS	REFERENCE INTERVAL, CONVENTIONAL [INTERNATIONAL RECOMMENDED UNITS]	CHEMICAL INTERFERENCES AND IN VIVO EFFECTS
Paraneoplastic Autoantibody Evaluation—CONT			
Anti-Neuronal Nuclear Ab, Type 3 (ANNA-3)[3,5] Indirect immuno-fluorescence; composite mouse tissue substrate. IgG binds to nuclei only, and only in a subset of CNS neurons (cerebellar Purkinje > Golgi = dentate > molecular) and renal glomerular podocytes. Western blot; native CNS protein (170 kD) or recombinant antigen	Draw blood in a plain, red-top tube(s) or serum gel tube(s). Spin down and send 3.0 mL of serum refrigerated.	Negative at 1:120 Negative	
Anti-Neuronal Nuclear Ab, Type Ma2; Anti-Ma/Ta[6] Punctate immuno-staining of nuclei in brainstem neurons has been reported. Western blot; re-combinant Ma2 protein	Serum. Refrigerate if not shipped same day. Serum stable up to 3 days. Ship whole blood immediately.	Negative	
Purkinje Cell Cytoplasmic Ab, Type 1 (PCA-1) or anti-Yo[3,7,8] Indirect immuno-fluorescence; composite substrate of mouse tissues. IgG binds to perikaryon	Draw blood in a plain, red-top tube(s) or serum gel tube(s). Spin down and send 3.0 mL of serum refrigerated.	Negative at 1:120 Negative	

DIAGNOSTIC INFORMATION	REMARKS

Neurologic accompaniments of ANNA-3 are subacute and usually multifocal; 64% of cases are female. Neurological presentations include sensory and sensorimotor neuropathies, cerebellar ataxia, myelopathy, brainstem, and limbic encephalopathy.[5] A positive result has 90% predictive value for an aerodigestive carcinoma, usually small cell lung carcinoma that is new or recurrent and confined to the chest.[5] A coexisting unrelated cancer is found in 15% of seropositive patients.

ANNA-3 is a very rare autoAb.[3,5] Forty percent of seropositive patients have a coexisting paraneoplastic autoAb, all predicting small cell carcinoma.[3]

Ma2 Ab has been reported with subacute paraneoplastic limbic and brainstem encephalitis associated with testicular cancer.[6] Seropositive female patients have been reported with several other neoplasms. The frequency of Ma2 detection has not been reported.

Scrotal ultrasound is advised for men who present with unexplained subacute rhomboencephalitis. A minority of Ma2-positive patients exhibit narcolepsy (with low CSF hypocretin), presumably reflecting autoimmune hypothalamitis.[24]

PCA-1 Ab is found in serum and CSF of patients with paraneoplastic cerebellar ataxia associated with gynecologic or breast carcinoma. PCA-1 Ab is rare in male patients (1%; associated with intraabdominal adenocarcinoma). In 10% of PCA-1-positive patients, the presentation is sensorimotor, motor, or autonomic neuropathy, thus far all with gynecologic cancer.[3,7] Cancer, new or recurrent, is identified in 91% of PCA-1-positive patients, usually after the neurologic presentation.[3] The associated cancers are typically limited in metastatic spread, may not be detected by imaging procedures,[8] and

PCA-1 Ab is not found in healthy subjects. It is rare in patients with gynecologic cancer without neurologic dysfunction (<2%) and not found with primary lung cancer. PCA-1 is readily distinguished from PCA-Tr (a marker of Hodgkin's lymphoma) and PCA-2 (a marker of small cell lung carcinoma) by immunostaining criteria. PCA-1 is remarkable for its lack of coexisting neuronal nuclear or cytoplasmic paraneoplastic autoAbs.[3]

TEST NAME AND METHOD	SPECIMEN REQUIREMENTS	REFERENCE INTERVAL, CONVENTIONAL [INTERNATIONAL RECOMMENDED UNITS]	CHEMICAL INTERFERENCES AND IN VIVO EFFECTS

Paraneoplastic Autoantibody Evaluation—CONT

of large neurons in the CNS and PNS.

Western blot using native CNS protein (53-57 kD) or recombinant antigen

Purkinje Cell Cytoplasmic Ab, Type 2 (PCA-2)[3,9] Indirect immunofluorescence; composite mouse tissue substrate. IgG binds to perikaryon and dendrites of CNS neurons and peripheral autonomic neurons. Western blot using native CNS protein (280 kD)	Draw blood in a plain, red-top tube(s) or serum gel tube(s). Spin down and send 3.0 mL of serum refrigerated.	Negative at 1:120 Negative	
Purkinje Cell Cytoplasmic Ab, Type Tr[10,11] Indirect immunofluorescence; composite mouse tissue substrate. IgG binds in coarse punctate pattern to perikaryon of Purkinje neurons and dendritic spines in molecular layer of cerebellar cortex. No Western blot correlate.	Draw blood in a plain, red-top tube(s) or serum gel tube(s). Spin down and send 3.0 mL of serum refrigerated.	Negative at 1:120	

DIAGNOSTIC INFORMATION	REMARKS

serum antigen markers (e.g., CA125) may be negative. If mammography is negative, exploratory laparotomy is advised (as for a "second look" in management of ovarian carcinoma). Breast carcinoma may coexist with a mullerian cancer.

Neurologic accompaniments of PCA-2 are subacute in onset, usually multifocal, and include brainstem or limbic encephalitis, cerebellar ataxia, Lambert-Eaton myasthenic syndrome, and autonomic and motor neuropathy.[9] Fifty-five percent of cases are female. Small cell lung carcinoma is detected in 80% of PCA-2-positive patients.	One or more coexisting paraneoplastic autoAbs are found in 63% of PCA-2-positive patients. All predict small cell carcinoma.[3]
PCA-Tr is a marker of paraneoplastic cerebellar degeneration associated with Hodgkin's lymphoma.[10,11] Unlike other paraneoplastic autoimmune neurological disorders, a diagnosis of neoplasia (Hodgkin's lymphoma) usually precedes the neurologic presentation in PCA-Tr-positive patients.	This autoAb is the rarest of all paraneoplastic autoAbs recognized to date.

TEST NAME AND METHOD	SPECIMEN REQUIREMENTS	REFERENCE INTERVAL, CONVENTIONAL [INTERNATIONAL RECOMMENDED UNITS]	CHEMICAL INTERFERENCES AND IN VIVO EFFECTS
Paraneoplastic Autoantibody Evaluation—CONT			
Amphiphysin Ab[3,12-14] Indirect immuno-fluorescence; composite mouse tissue substrate. IgG binds intensely to synapses in molecular and granular layers of cerebellar cortex and midbrain, cytoplasm, and synaptic elements of enteric neurons. Western blot using native CNS protein (115 kD) or recombinant antigen	Draw blood in a plain, red-top tube(s) or serum gel tube(s). Spin down and send 3.0 mL of serum refrigerated.	Negative at 1:120 Negative	
Collapsin Response-Mediator Protein (CRMP)-5 IgG; anti-CV2[3,15,16] Indirect immuno-fluorescence; composite mouse tissue substrate. IgG binds in a similar distribution to amphiphysin, but the pattern is fuzzy and bleached out. Western blot using native CNS protein (62 kD) or recombinant antigen	Draw blood in a plain, red-top tube(s) or serum gel tube(s). Spin down and send 3.0 mL of serum refrigerated.	Negative at 1:120 Negative	

Only a minority of amphiphysin Ab-positive women (~40%) and men (~10%) present with encephalomyelitis with rigidity (stiff-man phenomena). Very few patients fulfill neurologic criteria for diagnosis of stiff-man (Moersch-Woltmann) syndrome.[12] Neurologic presentations are usually multifocal and include, in decreasing frequency, peripheral neuropathy, encephalopathy, myelopathy, encephalomyelitis with rigidity, cerebellar syndrome, Lambert-Eaton syndrome, myoclonus, focal pain, optic neuritis, and pruritis.

Amphiphysin IgG is associated with small cell lung carcinoma (SCLC) more commonly than breast carcinoma. Melanoma is sometimes found.[12-14]

One or more coexisting paraneoplastic autoAbs are found in 38% of amphiphysin-IgG-positive patients. The autoAb profile predicts small cell carcinoma or breast carcinoma.[3] Many of the neurologic manifestations are attributable to targeting of autoantigens identified by coexisting autoAb markers (e.g., ANNA-1 in sensory neuronopathies, K^+ channel Ab in limbic encephalitis and neuromyotonia, P/Q-type Ca^{2+} channel Ab in Lambert-Eaton syndrome, and CRMP-5-IgG in optic neuritis and radicular pain).[3,11]

Neurologic accompaniments of CRMP-5-IgG are subacute and multifocal and may mimic vascular disease or multiple sclerosis. Basal ganglionitis (particularly chorea), cranial neuropathies (particularly loss of vision and smell/taste), myelopathy, and radiculoplexopathy are considered "syndromic" because of their remarkably high frequency with CRMP-5-IgG. Most common are limbic manifestations, peripheral neuropathy, autonomic neuropathy, cerebellar ataxia, and neuromuscular junction disorders.

Small cell lung carcinoma (usually limited) is found in 80% of patients, and thymoma in 7%; rarely is thyroid carcinoma found.[15,16] When accompanied by muscle AChR binding Ab, a high level of AChR-modulating Ab, and striational Abs, a thymoma is usually identified.

CRMP-5-IgG is as common as ANNA-1. Approximately 30% of CRMP-5-IgG-positive patients have a coexisting antineuronal nuclear or neuronal cytoplasmic autoAb, and 30% have a coexisting ion channel or striational Ab.[3] Thromboembolic phenomena and systemic symptoms and signs suggestive of vasculitis are documented in ~10% of patients before lung cancer is found. Neurologic symptoms usually precede cancer diagnosis.

TEST NAME AND METHOD	SPECIMEN REQUIREMENTS	REFERENCE INTERVAL, CONVENTIONAL [INTERNATIONAL RECOMMENDED UNITS]	CHEMICAL INTERFERENCES AND IN VIVO EFFECTS
Paraneoplastic Autoantibody Evaluation—CONT			
Recoverin IgG; Cancer Associated Retinopathy [CAR] Ab[17-19] Western blot using native retinal proteins (23 kD) or recombinant recoverin	Serum. Refrigerate if not shipped same day. Serum stable up to 3 days. Ship whole blood immediately.	Negative	
Glutamic Acid Decarboxylase (GAD65) Ab[20-22] Immunoprecipitation RIA; ^{125}I-labeled recombinant human antigen	Draw blood in a plain, red-top tube(s) or a serum gel tube(s). Spin down and send 1.0 mL of serum refrigerated.	≤0.02 nmol/L	

1. Lucchinetti CF, Kimmel DW, Lennon VA: Paraneoplastic and oncological and profiles of patients seropositive for type 1 antineuronal nuclear autoantibodies, *Neurology* 50:652-657, 1998.

2. Lucchinetti CF, Camilleri M, Lennon VA: Gastrointestinal dysmotility spectrum in patients seropositive for paraneoplastic type 1 anti-neuronal nuclear autoantibodies, *Clin Auton Res* 4:206, 1994.

3. Pittock SJ, Kryzer TJ, Lennon VA: Paraneoplastic antibodies often coexist and predict cancer not neurologic syndrome, *Ann Neurol* 56:715-719, 2004.

4. Pittock SJ, Lucchinetti CF, Lennon VA: Anti-neuronal nuclear autoantibody-type 2 (ANNA-2): paraneoplastic accompaniments, *Ann Neurol* 54:580-587, 2003.

5. Chan KH, Vernino S, Lennon VA: ANNA-3 anti-neuronal nuclear antibody: marker of lung cancer-related autoimmunity, *Ann Neurol* 50:301-311, 2001.

6. Voltz R, Gultekin SH, Rosenfeld MR, et al: A serologic marker of paraneoplastic limbic and brain-stem encephalitis in patients with testicular cancer, *N Engl J Med* 340:1788-1795, 1999.

7. Peterson K, Rosenblum MK, Kotanides H, et al: Paraneoplastic cerebellar degeneration. I. A clinical analysis of 55 anti-Yo antibody-positive patients, *Neurology* 42:1931-1937, 1992.

DIAGNOSTIC INFORMATION	REMARKS

Cancer-associated retinopathy is characterized by painless and progressive vision loss.[17-19] Electroretinography demonstrates loss of rod and cone function. Small cell lung carcinoma is the associated neoplasm. CRMP-5-IgG is a far more common marker of paraneoplastic autoimmune vision loss related to small cell lung carcinoma. Its ophthalmologic presentation is a combination of optic neuritis and retinitis.[23]

The "CAR" autoantigen, recoverin, is a retinal photoreceptor calcium-binding protein that regulates rhodopsin phosphorylation and is involved in light and dark adaptation. Case reports have linked paraneoplastic retinopathy to endometrial, cervical, ovarian, and breast carcinomas and melanoma.[17,18]

GAD65 Ab is an important serological marker of predisposition to type 1(insulin-dependent) diabetes. Its detection distinguishes type 1 from type 2 diabetes, but seronegativity does not exclude a diagnosis of type 1 diabetes. Eighty percent of type 1 diabetic patients are seropositive. GAD65 Ab also serves as a marker of predisposition to autoimmune diseases that frequently coexist with type 1 diabetes, e.g., Graves' disease, Hashimoto's thyroiditis, pernicious anemia, premature ovarian failure, Addison's disease (idiopathic adrenocortical failure), and vitiligo.[21]

GAD is a neuronal enzyme involved in the synthesis of the neurotransmitter γ-aminobutyric acid (GABA) and is a major pancreatic islet cell and neuronal autoantigen. The serum level of GAD65 Ab in patients who have type 1 diabetes without a polyendocrine or autoimmune neurologic syndrome is generally <20 nmol/L and in those with polyendocrine disorders is generally ≥20 nmol/L. A second islet cell Ab (IA-2) is more predictive for development of type 1 diabetes, but the IA-2 Ab assay is less sensitive than the GAD65 Ab assay. Assays for gastric parietal cell Ab, thyroglobulin Ab, and thyroid peroxidase Ab complement GAD65 and IA-2 Abs in the serological evaluation of type 1 diabetes susceptibility.

GAD65 Ab prevalence is heightened in all autoimmune neurologic disorders (e.g., myasthenia gravis, Lambert-Eaton syndrome, neuromyotonia). Serum levels are highest in classic stiff-man syndrome (93% positive) and in acquired cerebellar ataxia, sporadic epilepsy, and nonparaneoplastic encephalomyelopathies. GAD65 Ab is the most recently recognized marker of thymoma-related neurological autoimmunity.[22]

About 8% of healthy subjects have low positive values. These are not "false-positives." Values ≥0.03 nmol/L are consistent with susceptibility to autoimmune (type 1) diabetes and related endocrine disorders (thyroiditis and pernicious anemia).

8. Hetzel DJ, Stanhope CR, O'Neill BP, et al: Gynecologic cancer in patients with subacute cerebellar degeneration predicted by anti-Purkinje cell antibodies and limited in metastatic volume, *Mayo Clin Proc* 65:1558-1563, 1990.

9. Vernino S, Lennon VA: New Purkinje cell antibody (PCA-2): marker of lung cancer-related neurological autoimmunity, *Ann Neurol* 47:297-305, 2000.

10. Trotter JL, Hendin BA, Osterland CK: Cerebellar degeneration with Hodgkin disease. An immunological study, *Arch Neurol* 33:660-661, 1976.

11. Graus F, Gultekin SH, Ferrer I, et al: Localization of the neuronal antigen recognized by anti-Tr antibodies from patients with paraneoplastic cerebellar degeneration and Hodgkin's disease in the rat nervous system, *Acta Neuropathol (Berl)* 96:1-7, 1998.

12. Pittock SJ, Stephan CL, Lucchinetti CF, et al: Amphiphysin autoantibody: paraneoplastic accompaniments in 60 patients, *Neurology* 62 (suppl 5):A263-A264.

13. De Camilli P, Thomas A, Cofiell R, et al: The synaptic vesicle-associated protein amphiphysin is the 128-kD autoantigen of stiff-man syndrome with breast cancer, *J Exp Med* 178:2219-2223, 1993.

TEST NAME AND METHOD	SPECIMEN REQUIREMENTS	REFERENCE INTERVAL, CONVENTIONAL [INTERNATIONAL RECOMMENDED UNITS]	CHEMICAL INTERFERENCES AND IN VIVO EFFECTS

Paraneoplastic Autoantibody Evaluation—CONT

14. Folli F, Solimena M, Cofiell R, et al: Autoantibodies to a 128-kd synaptic protein in three women with the stiff-man syndrome and breast cancer, *N Engl J Med* 328:546-551, 1993.

15. Yu Z, Kryzer TJ, Griesmann GE, et al: CRMP-5 neuronal autoantibody: marker of lung cancer and thymoma-related autoimmunity, *Ann Neurol* 49:146-154, 2001.

16. Vernino S, Tuite P, Adler CH, et al: Paraneoplastic chorea associated with CRMP-5 neuronal antibody and lung carcinoma, *Ann Neurol* 51:625-630, 2002.

17. Sawyer RA, Selhorst JB, Zimmerman LE, et al: Blindness caused by photoreceptor degeneration as a remote effect of cancer, *Am J Ophthalmol* 81:606-613, 1976.

18. Thirkill CE, Roth AM, Keltner JL: Cancer-associated retinopathy, *Arch Ophthalmol* 105:372-375, 1987.

19. Thirkill CE, FitzGerald P, Sergott RC, et al: Cancer-associated retinopathy (CAR syndrome) with antibodies reacting with retinal, optic-nerve, and cancer cells, *N Engl J Med* 321:1589-1594, 1989.

Paraquat[1-3] *Colorimetric, GC-MS,*[4] *HPLC*[5]	Whole blood (EDTA)	Negative			None found.
			mg/L	*μmol/L*	
		Toxic concentration:	>0.2 × 3.89	[>0.8]	
	Urine	Occupational exposure:	>0.9	[>3.5]	

1. Baselt RC: *Analytical procedures for therapeutic drug monitoring and emergency toxicology,* ed 2, Littleton, MA, 1987, PSG Publishing Co., Inc.

2. Baselt RC: *Biological monitoring methods for industrial chemicals,* Davis, CA, 1980, Biomedical Pub.

3. Winchester JF, Gelfand MC, Knepshield JH, et al: Dialysis and hemoperfusion of poisons and drugs—update, *Trans Am Soc Artif Intern Organs* 23:762-842, 1977.

4. Draffan GH, Clare RA, Davies G, et al: Quantitative determination of the herbicide paraquat in human plasma by gas chromatographic and mass spectrometric methods, *J Chromatogr* 139:311-320, 1977.

5. Miller JJ, Sanders E, Webb D: Measurement of paraquat in serum by high-performance liquid chromatography, *J Anal Toxicol* 3:1-3, 1979.

6. Suntres ZE: Role of antioxidants in paraquat toxicity, *Toxicology* 180:65-77, 2002.

7. Shintani S: Paraquat (treatment protocol/overview). In *POISINDEX information system, vol 78,* Denver, CO, 1993, Micromedex, Inc.

DIAGNOSTIC INFORMATION	REMARKS

20. Walikonis JE, Lennon VA: Radioimmunoassay for glutamic acid decarboxylase (GAD65) autoantibodies as a diagnostic aid for stiff-man syndrome and a correlate of susceptibility to type 1 diabetes mellitus, *Mayo Clin Proc* 73:1161-1166, 1998.

21. Saiz A, Arpa J, Sagasta A, et al: Autoantibodies to glutamic acid decarboxylase in three patients with cerebellar ataxia, late-onset insulin-dependent diabetes mellitus and polyendocrine autoimmunity, *Neurology* 49:1026-1030, 1997.

22. Vernino S, Lennon VA: Autoantibody profiles and neurological correlations of thymoma, *Clin Cancer Res* 10:7270-7275, 2004.

23. Cross SA, Salomao DR, Parisi JE, et al: Paraneoplastic autoimmune optic neuritis with retinitis defined by CRMP-5-IgG, *Ann Neurol* 54:38-50, 2003.

24. Overeem S, Dalmau J, Bataller L, et al: Hypocretin-1 CSF levels in anti-Ma2 associated encephalitis, *Neurology* 61:138-140, 2004.

Toxic effects of topical exposure include skin eruptions and epistaxis on contact. Ingestion leads to epigastric pain, vomiting, dysuria, and jaundice. The major target organ is the lung, where oxidative damage to the alveolar epithelium leads to fibrosis.[6]

Paraquat is a quaternary nitrogen herbicide used for broadleaf weed control. Toxicity in humans is associated with the generation of superoxide anion, which generates additional reactive oxygen species.[6] Paraquat is not significantly biotransformed in humans. Elimination is mainly by the kidneys.

The chromophore formed in the colorimetric method is unstable.

Nearly all paraquat adsorbed on treated marijuana plants is pyrolyzed to dipyridyl as the leaves burn. Paraquat treatment of leaves is not likely to increase the adverse effects of natural marijuana smoke on the lungs.[7]

TEST NAME AND METHOD	SPECIMEN REQUIREMENTS	REFERENCE INTERVAL, CONVENTIONAL [INTERNATIONAL RECOMMENDED UNITS]	CHEMICAL INTERFERENCES AND IN VIVO EFFECTS
Parathyroid Hormone (Parathyrin, PTH)[1-7]	Serum or plasma (EDTA). Fasting morning specimen preferred. Place on ice; refrigerate during centrifugation, and freeze immediately. Store at −20 to −70° C. Simultaneous determinations of total serum calcium, ionized calcium, and phosphorus are recommended.		↑ V Anticonvulsants, corticosteroids, isoniazid, lithium, phosphates (up to 125% increase at 1 hr after 1 g orally), rifampin ↓ V Cimetidine, pindolol, and propranolol

C-terminal and midmolecule *RIA*		Serum 1-16 yr: Adults: Plasma (EDTA): <50 μLEq/mL	*pg/mL*[10] 51-217 50-330	*ng/L* × 1.0 [51-217] [50-330] × 1.0 [<50 mLEq/L][11]

N-terminal *RIA*	Serum	2-13 yr: Adult:	*pg/mL*[10] 14-21 8-24	*ng/L* × 1.0 [14-21] [8-24]
Bioassay (adenylate cyclase stimulation)	Plasma (EDTA)	<6.1 pmol/L[11]		

Intact molecule (bioactive, biointact)[8,9] *ICMA*	Serum	Cord: 2-20 yr: Adults:	*pg/mL*[10] ≤3 9-52 10-65	*ng/L* × 1.0 [≤3] [9-52] [10-65]
IRMA	Plasma (EDTA)	1.0-5.0 pmol/L[11]		

| DIAGNOSTIC INFORMATION | REMARKS |

↑ Primary hyperparathyroidism; secondary hyperparathyroidism [e.g., chronic renal disease (up to 10 times the upper limit), pseudohypoparathyroidism, hereditary vitamin D dependency types I and II, vitamin D deficiency], Z-E syndrome, fluorosis, spinal cord trauma, pseudogout, familial medullary thyroid carcinoma, and MEN types I, IIa, IIb

↓ Autoimmune hypoparathyroidism; in surgical hypoparathyroidism associated with thyroidectomy (condition probably transient if PTH is detectable by RIA), sarcoidosis (even in the presence of renal failure), nonparathyroid hypercalcemia in the absence of renal failure, hyperthyroidism, hypomagnesemia, transient neonatal hypocalcemia, and DiGeorge syndrome

In normal individuals, intact "whole" PTH (amino acids 1-84) has a circulating half-life of ~5 min. Inactive carboxyl-terminal and midmolecule fragments (e.g., amino acids 53-84, 44-68, 35-64) make up ~90% of total circulating PTH. These fragments are cleared exclusively by the kidney and have half-lives of ~1-2 hr. A circulating amino-terminal fragment (amino acids 1-34) has an estimated half-life of 1-2 min; it is present in very small concentrations in blood. Only the intact PTH 1-84 and N-terminal PTH 1-34 possess biological activity. In addition to renal excretion, intact and N-terminal PTH is also removed from plasma by other mechanisms. Patients with chronic renal failure will have very high C-terminal/midmolecule PTH values even if parathyroid disease is absent.

PTH is detectable in infancy and increases in the early postnatal period. Circadian rhythm is observed with highest values at 2:00-4:00 PM, declining to baseline at 8:00 AM. Values in plasma are reported to be 5-10% lower than in serum. In humans, lowering of the plasma Ca by 1.5 mg/dL [0.38 mmol/L] may increase plasma PTH as much as 400%.

The C-terminal/midmolecule test measures the whole (intact) PTH molecule and carboxyl-terminal and midmolecule fragments.[12] The assay does not detect N-terminal fragments. In both normal and hyperparathyroid individuals, C-terminal and midmolecule fragments predominate. The test is ~85% sensitive and 95% specific for detecting hyperparathyroidism. For each assay system, PTH results must be used in conjunction with serum calcium data for meaningful clinical interpretation. Figure II-3 illustrates such data.

The N-terminal test measures both intact PTH molecule and amino-terminal fragments; it does not measure C-terminal and midmolecule fragments. The test is used mainly for evaluating patients with renal failure and patients with normal or equivocal results of other PTH assays. The bioassay is reported to be 75% sensitive for detection of primary hyperparathyroidism.

Most first-generation intact molecule assays are prone to falsely elevated results because of the presence of large PTH fragments in blood.[8,9] These larger fragments of PTH include the N-terminal truncated (7-84) and the amino-PTH. The amino-PTH is formed from posttranslational modification of the PTH that makes it functionally inactive. The N-terminal truncated PTH is reported to act as a PTH antagonist with no biological activity. The clinical significance of the amino-PTH has not been determined. The second- and third-generation intact PTH assays are less prone to interference from these large PTH frag-

TEST NAME AND METHOD	SPECIMEN REQUIREMENTS	REFERENCE INTERVAL, CONVENTIONAL [INTERNATIONAL RECOMMENDED UNITS]	CHEMICAL INTERFERENCES AND IN VIVO EFFECTS
Parathyroid Hormone—CONT			

1. Burtis CA, Ashwood ER, editors: *Tietz textbook of clinical chemistry,* ed 2, Philadelphia, 1994, WB Saunders.

2. Armitage EK: Parathyrin (parathyroid hormone): metabolism and methods for assay, *Clin Chem* 32:418-424, 1986.

3. Barzel US: Primary hyperparathyroidism: problems in management, *Hosp Pract* 27:165-176, 1992.

4. Bilezikian JP: Primary hyperparathyroidism, *Trends Endocrinol Metab* 1:3-6, 1989.

5. Grant FD, Conlin PR, Brown EM: Rate and concentration dependence of parathyroid hormone dynamics during stepwise changes in serum ionized calcium in normal humans, *J Clin Endocrinol Metab* 71:370-378, 1990.

6. Klee GC, Preissner CM, Schryver PG, et al: Multisite immunochemiluminometric assay for simultaneously measuring whole-molecule and amino-terminal fragments of human parathyrin, *Clin Chem* 38:628-635, 1992.

7. Klee GG, Kao PC, Heath H III: Hypercalcemia, *Endocrinol Metab Clin North Am* 17:573-600, 1988.

8. Lepage R, Roy L, Brossard JH, et al: A non-(1-84) circulating parathyroid hormone (PTH) fragment interferes significantly with intact PTH commercial assay measurements in uremic patients, *Clin Chem* 44:805-809, 1998.

9. Savoca R, Bock A, Kraenzlin ME, et al: An automated 'bio-intact' PTH assay: a step towards standardization and improved correlation with parathyroid function in renal disease, *Clin Chim Acta* 343:167-171, 2004.

10. Nichols Institute Reference Laboratories: *Test catalog,* San Juan Capistrano, CA, 1993, Nichols Institute Reference Laboratories.

11. Mayo Medical Laboratories: *Test catalog,* Rochester, MN, 1993, Mayo Medical Laboratories.

12. Ashby JP, Thakkar H: Diagnostic limitations of region-specific parathyroid hormone assays in the investigation of hypercalcaemia, *Ann Clin Biochem* 25:275-279, 1988.

13. Endres DB, Villanueva R, Sharp CF, et al: Immunochemiluminometric and immunoradiometric determination of intact and total immunoreactive parathyrin: performance in the differential diagnosis of hypercalcemia and hypo-parathyroidism, *Clin Chem* 37:162-168, 1991.

TEST NAME AND METHOD	SPECIMEN REQUIREMENTS	REFERENCE INTERVAL, CONVENTIONAL [INTERNATIONAL RECOMMENDED UNITS]	CHEMICAL INTERFERENCES AND IN VIVO EFFECTS
Parathyroid Hormone-Related Protein (PTH-RP)[1-5] *IRMA*	Plasma (heparin). Collect in tubes that contain protease inhibitors, aprotinin, and leupeptin. Chill specimens immediately in ice water. Plasma should be separated in a refrigerated centrifuge and then frozen immediately at −20° C in plastic vials.	Adult[6]: <1.5 pmol/L	

DIAGNOSTIC INFORMATION	REMARKS

ments, and the enhanced assays measure only the biologically intact PTH molecule.[9] Patients with chronic renal failure and renal bone disease are prone to present with higher levels of these large fragments. Clear distinction of primary hyperparathyroidism from hypercalcemia of malignancy is claimed. A good correlation with bone status in secondary hyperparathyroidism is reported. Most intact assays can also differentiate normal subjects from patients with hypoparathyroidism.[13]

↑ Humoral hypercalcemia of malignancy, lymphomas, squamous cell cancer, and breast cancer

Measurement of PTH-RP is useful clinically in differentiating primary hyperparathyroidism from hypercalcemia related to malignancy. The test is also useful as a marker in the management of patients with tumor-associated hypercalcemia.

Production of PTH-RP by the fetoplacental unit can cause transient increase during pregnancy, especially in the third trimester.[7]

TEST NAME AND METHOD	SPECIMEN REQUIREMENTS	REFERENCE INTERVAL, CONVENTIONAL [INTERNATIONAL RECOMMENDED UNITS]	CHEMICAL INTERFERENCES AND IN VIVO EFFECTS

Parathyroid Hormone-Related Protein—CONT

1. Burtis WJ: Parathyroid hormone-related protein: structure, function, and measurement, *Clin Chem* 38:2171-2183, 1992.
2. Burtis WJ, Brady TG, Orloff JJ, et al: Immunochemical characterization of circulating parathyroid hormone-related protein in patients with humoral hypercalcemia of cancer, *N Engl J Med* 322:1106-1112, 1990.
3. Goltzman D, Hendy G, Banville D: Parathyroid hormone-like peptide: molecular characterization and biological properties, *Trends Endocrinol Metab* 1:39-44, 1989.
4. Heath DA: Parathyroid hormone-related protein, *Clin Endocrinol* 38:135-136, 1993.

Parietal Cell Antibodies (PCA)[1-3] *IIF*	Serum. Stable for 12 mo at −20° C.	Negative: <1:20 Weakly positive: 1:20-1:40 Positive: ≥1:80	None found.

1. Ungar B, Whittingham S, Francis CM: Pernicious anaemia: incidence and significance of circulating antibodies to intrinsic factor and parietal cells, *Aust Ann Med* 16:226-229, 1967.
2. Snow CF: Laboratory diagnosis of vitamin B12 and folate deficiency: a guide for the primary care physician, *Arch Intern Med* 159:1289-1298, 1999.
3. Kraft SC, Kirsner JB: Immunology in gastroenterology. In Berk JE, Haubrich WS, Kalser MH, et al, editors: *Bockus gastroenterology, vol 7,* ed 4, Philadelphia, 1985, WB Saunders, pp. 4490-4491.
4. Oh R, Brown DL: Vitamin B12 deficiency, *Am Fam Phys* 67:979-986, 2003.

Pemphigoid and Pemphigus Antibodies, IgG Isotype *Indirect immunofluorescence, on monkey esophagus or human skin*	Serum, frozen or refrigerated is preferable.	Negative is normal. Sera that produce positive staining are reported at endpoint titer and with a pattern.	None known.

1. Beutner EH, Chorzelski TP, Kumar V, editors: In *Immunopathology of the skin,* ed 3, New York, 1987, Wiley Medical Publication.
2. Gammon WR, Briggaman RA, Inman AO III, et al: Differentiating anti-lamina lucida and anti-sublamina densa anti-BMZ antibodies by indirect immunofluorescence on 1.0 M sodium chloride-separated skin, *J Invest Dermatol* 82:139-144, 1984.

| DIAGNOSTIC INFORMATION | REMARKS |

5. Martin TJ: Properties of parathyroid hormone-related protein and its role in malignant hypercalcemia, *Q J Med* 76:771-786, 1990.
6. Pandian MR, Morgan CH, Carlton E, et al: Modified immunoradiometric assay of parathyroid hormone-related protein: clinical application in the differential diagnosis of hypercalcemia, *Clin Chem* 38:282-288, 1992.
7. Hirota Y, Anai T, Miyakawa I: Parathyroid hormone-related protein levels in maternal and cord blood, *Am J Obstet Gyncol* 177:702-706, 1997.

Parietal cell antibodies are present in ~90% of patients with pernicious anemia, in up to 50% of patients with atrophic gastritis without pernicious anemia, and in 33% of patients with thyroiditis. PCA also occurs with lower frequency in patients with Addison's disease, myasthenia gravis, juvenile diabetes mellitus, gastric ulcer, iron deficiency anemia, and Sjögren's syndrome.

This assay detects the microsomal and cell surface parietal cell autoantibodies. Fifty to 60% of patients with pernicious anemia also have intrinsic factor blocking antibodies. The PCA assay is more sensitive but less specific than intrinsic factor-blocking antibodies for pernicious anemia.[4]

This test is useful for confirming a diagnosis of pemphigoid, pemphigus, epidermolysis bullosa acquisita, or bullous LE. Anti-cell surface (CS) antibodies occur in pemphigus, and anti-basement zone (BMZ) antibodies occur in bullous pemphigoid, epidermilysis bullosa acquisita (EBA), or bullous LE.[1,2]

Indirect immunofluorescence testing for IgG antibodies may be diagnostic when conventional histologic or direct immunofluorescence testing of skin biopsies is inconclusive. Low titer antibodies (20 or 40) are not diagnostic.

TEST NAME AND METHOD	SPECIMEN REQUIREMENTS	REFERENCE INTERVAL, CONVENTIONAL [INTERNATIONAL RECOMMENDED UNITS]			CHEMICAL INTERFERENCES AND IN VIVO EFFECTS
Pentachlorophe-nol *(CAS 87-86-5)*	Plasma (EDTA)	mg/L^5 <1	× 3.75	$\mu mol/L$ [<4]	
GLC,[1] *spectrophotometry,*[2] *GC-ECD*[3]	Occupational exposure:	<20 >30		[<75] [>113]	
NCI-MS[4]					
	Urine	*mg/L* <0.6	× 3.75	*µmol/L* [<2]	
	Occupational exposure:	<4 >4		[<15] [>15]	

1. Baselt RC: *Analytical procedures for therapeutic drug monitoring and emergency toxicology,* ed 2, Littleton, MA, 1987, PSG Publishing Co., Inc.
2. Clayton GD, Clayton FE, editors: *Patty's industrial hygiene and toxicology, vol 2A, Toxicology,* ed 3, New York, 1981, John Wiley and Sons.
3. Benevue A, Emerson ML, Casarette LJ, et al: A sensitive gas chromatographic method for the determination of pentachlorophenol in human blood, *J Chromatogr* 38:467-472, 1968.
4. Kuehl DW, Dougherty RC: Pentachlorophenol in the environment. Evidence for its origin from commercial pentachlorophenol by negative chemical ionization mass spectrometry, *Environ Sci Tech* 14:447-449, 1980.
5. Ewers U, Krause C, Schulz C, et al: Reference values and human biological monitoring values for environmental toxins. Report of the work and recommendations of the Commission on Human Biological Monitoring of the German Federal Environmental Agency, *Int. Arch Occup Environ Health* 72:255-260, 1999.
6. Baselt RC: *Biological monitoring methods for industrial chemicals,* Davis, CA, 1980, Biomedical Pub.
7. Kalman DA, Horstman SW: Persistence of tetrachlorophenol and pentachlorophenol in exposed woodworkers, *J Toxicol Clin Toxicol* 20:343-352, 1983.

Pentoses[1-3]	Urine, 24 hr. Store at −20° C. Stable for >6 mo.	Total pentoses, Fruit-free diet:			↑ V Morphine, antipyretics, cortisone, thyroid hormones; ingestion of cherries, plums, grapes, and prunes
Colorimetric[3]		2-5 mg/kg/day Slightly higher in children	× 6.66	[13-33 µmol/kg/day]	
			mg/day	*µmol/day*	↑ V *Xylulose:* Administration of glucuronic acid, drugs generating glucuronic acid (e.g., menthol)
		L-Xylulose:	<60 × 6.66	[<400]	
		D-Ribose:	<15	[<100]	
		D-Ribulose:	Traces		

DIAGNOSTIC INFORMATION	REMARKS

Chronic respiratory exposure can cause inflammation of the upper respiratory tract. Dermal exposure can cause dermatitis. There are limited data on oral exposure in humans, but animal studies indicate that pentachlorophenol affects liver, kidney, CNS, endocrine, and immune function.

Pentachlorophenol toxicity is due, in part, to the uncoupling of oxidative phosphorylation.

Pentachlorophenol is used as a wood preservative in utility poles, railroad ties, and wharf pilings, and human exposure to this chemical usually is in the industrial setting. Plasma contains 99% of pentachlorophenol in whole blood. PCP is oxidized to tetrachlorohydroquinone, which is an inhibitor of glucuronidase.

Conjugates must be hydrolyzed by hot acidic solutions before urine extraction.[6]

The elimination half-life may be up to 20 days in chronically exposed persons.[7]

Kinetic values
$t_{1/2}$:   3-5 days[6]
V_d: 0.35 L/kg
PB: 99%

U ↑↑ Essential pentosuria

U ↑ Fever, allergy, and cirrhosis

U ↑ *Arabinose and xylose:* Alimentary pentosuria (<100 mg/day; <666 μmol/day)

U ↑ *Xylulose:* Essential pentosuria (1.0-4.0 g/day; 7-27 μmol/day), cirrhosis

---

U ↑ *Ribose:* Muscular dystrophy (<30 mg/day; <100 μmol/day)

Pentoses are reducing sugars. Their presence can be confirmed with Tollen's or Bial's test. Identification is obtained by TLC.

TEST NAME AND METHOD	SPECIMEN REQUIREMENTS	REFERENCE INTERVAL, CONVENTIONAL [INTERNATIONAL RECOMMENDED UNITS]	CHEMICAL INTERFERENCES AND IN VIVO EFFECTS

Pentoses—CONT

| | Serum. Store at −20° C. | L-Xylulose: <2 mg/dL   × 66.6   [<133 μmol/L] | |

1. Henry JB, editor: *Clinical diagnosis and management by laboratory methods,* ed 18, Philadelphia, 1991, WB Saunders.
2. Henry RJ, Cannon DC, Winkelman JW, editors: *Clinical chemistry: principles and technics,* ed 2, Hagerstown, MD, 1974, Harper and Row.
3. Scriver CR, Beaudet AL, Sly WS, et al, editors: *The metabolic basis of inherited disease,* ed 6, New York, 1989, McGraw-Hill Publishing Co.

Pepsinogen I (PG I)[1-6]

RIA[1,8]

ELISA

Serum, fasting. Freeze.

None found.

	ng/mL[9]		mcg/L
Premature:	22 ± 2 (SEM)	× 1.0	[22 ± 2]
Cord:	26 ± 2		[26 ± 2]
Child			
<1 yr:	77 ± 5		[77 ± 5]
1-2 yr:	98 ± 8		[98 ± 8]
3-6 yr:	92 ± 12		[92 ± 12]
7-10 yr:	95 ± 8		[95 ± 8]
11-14 yr:	107 ± 11		[107 ± 11]
Adult:	133 ± 9		[133 ± 9]

Adult[10]:   28-100 ng/mL   × 1.0   [28-100 mcg/L]

1. Hirschowitz BI: Pepsinogen, *Postgrad Med J* 60:743-750, 1984.
2. Ichinose M, Miki K, Furihate C, et al: Radioimmunoassay of serum group I and group II pepsinogens in normal controls and patients with various disorders, *Clin Chim Acta* 126:183-191, 1982.
3. Nomura AM, Stemmermann GN, Samloff IM: Serum pepsinogen I as a predictor of stomach cancer, *Ann Intern Med* 93:537-540, 1980.
4. Samloff IM: Pepsinogens I and II: purification from gastric mucosa and radioimmunoassay in serum, *Gastroenterology* 82:26-33, 1982.
5. Samloff IM: Peptic ulcer. The many proteinases of aggression, *Gastroenterology* 96:586-595, 1989.

DIAGNOSTIC INFORMATION	REMARKS

↑ In states with hypergastrinemia, increased gastric acid output, and related increased parietal mass; Z-E syndrome; also in some patients with duodenal ulcer (30-50%); acute gastritis

Values for pepsinogen I and II increase with renal retention.

↓ *Hypergastrinemia from other causes:* Atrophic gastritis; gastric carcinoma; patients with myxedema, Addison's disease, and hypopituitarism; pernicious anemia

Seven fractions of pepsinogen in blood have been identified: five are called group I pepsinogens (PG I) and are found only in chief and mucous neck cells; two are called group II pepsinogens (PG II) and are found in other glands.

The secretion level of pepsinogens into the lumen of the stomach is related to the chief cell mass and controlled by the hormone gastrin. In diseases associated with increased gastric output, high serum levels of PG I may be expected. Conversely, low serum PG I levels may be expected in diseases associated with decreased chief cell mass. Low gastrin and pepsinogen levels are claimed to be 100% specific for atrophic gastritis. High PG I levels are reported in siblings of probands with duodenal ulcer. An elevated serum PG I level is inherited as an autosomal dominant trait and may serve as a subclinical marker of the ulcer tendency. For establishing a diagnosis of ulcers, gastritis, or gastric cancer, endoscopy is easier and more definitive than measuring serum PG I.

This test is rarely used.

See *Pepsinogen II.*

6. Samloff IM, Stemmermann GN, Heilbrun LK, et al: Elevated serum pepsinogen I and II levels differ as risk factors for duodenal ulcer and gastric ulcer, *Gastroenterology* 90:570-576, 1986.

7. Broughton A: Pepsinogen I and gastrin radioimmunoassay in the diagnosis of gastric pathology, *Lab Man* 18:46-48, 1980.

8. Plebani M, Di Mario F, Vianello F, et al: Pepsinogen group I radioimmunoassay and total serum pepsinogen colorimetric determination: a comparative study in normal subjects and in peptic ulcer patients, *Clin Biochem* 16:20-22, 1983.

9. Waldum HL, Straume BK, Burhol PG, et al: Serum group I pepsinogens in children, *Acta Paediatr Scand* 69:215-218, 1980.

10. InterScience Institute: *Current unique and rare endocrine assays. Patient and specimen requirements,* Inglewood, CA, 1988, InterScience Institute.

TEST NAME AND METHOD	SPECIMEN REQUIREMENTS	REFERENCE INTERVAL, CONVENTIONAL [INTERNATIONAL RECOMMENDED UNITS]			CHEMICAL INTERFERENCES AND IN VIVO EFFECTS
Pepsinogen II (PG II)[1-3]	Serum (fasting); separate from cells as soon as possible. Store frozen.	3-19 ng/mL[4,5]	× 1.0	[3-19 mcg/L]	↑ V Omeprazole
RIA					
ELISA					
Ratio of PGI:PGII		Normally > 3.0			

1. Hirschowitz BI: Pepsinogen, *Postgrad Med J* 60:743-750, 1984.
2. Matsukura N, Onda M, Tokunaga A, et al: Significance of serum markers pepsinogen I and II for chronic atrophic gastritis, peptic ulcer, and gastric cancer, *J Clin Gastroenterol* 17(suppl 1):S146-S150, 1993.
3. Samloff IM, Stemmermann GN, Heilbrun LK, et al: Elevated serum pepsingogen I and II levels differ as risk factors for duodenal ulcer and gastric ulcer, *Gastroenterology* 90:570-576, 1986.
4. Samloff IM: Pepsinogens I and II: purification from gastric mucosa and radioimmunoassay in serum, *Gastroenterology* 82:26-33, 1982.
5. Walsh JH: Gastrointestinal hormones. In Johnson LR, editor: *Physiology of the gastrointestinal tract,* ed 2, New York, 1987, Raven Press.
6. Henderson AR, Tietz NW, Rinker AD: Gastric, pancreatic, and intestinal function. In Burtis CA, Ashwood ER, editors: *Tietz textbook of clinical chemistry,* ed 2, Philadelphia, 1994, WB Saunders.
7. Howanitz JH, Howanitz PJ, editors: *Laboratory medicine: test selection and interpretation,* New York, 1991, Churchill Livingstone.
8. Kitahara F, Kobayashi K, Sato T: Accuracy of screening for gastric cancer using serum pepsinogen concentrations, *Gut* 44:693-697, 1999.

Perchlorate Discharge (Flush) Test[1,2]	Perform standard uptake test at 1 hr; then give oral dose of 500 mg of liquid KClO₄ and repeat ¹³¹I-uptake 1 hr later.	Discharge should not exceed 10% [× 0.01 = >0.10-0.15, fraction discharge] of 1-hr uptake; i.e., 85-90% [0.85-0.90, fraction discharge] of the ¹³¹I should be incorporated organically and not discharged by the perchlorate.	See *Thyroid Uptake of Radioactive Iodine,* ¹³¹*I or* ¹²³*I.*
Dose: 5 μCi ¹³¹I orally			

↑ Gastric and duodenal ulcers, Z-E syndrome, and acute and chronic superficial gastritis[6]

↓ Gastrectomy, gastritis, gastric neoplasia, gastric resection, Addison's disease, and myxedema[7]

Decreases with eradication of *H. pylori*[8]

Only PG II is found in the gastric antrum and proximal duodenum, Brunner's glands, and pyloric glands. Both PG I and PG II are found in serum, but PG II is not found in urine. Whereas an increased PG II level is a risk factor for gastric ulcer, a high level of PG I is a major risk factor for duodenal ulcer. In contrast to the low or undetectable levels of PG I seen in pernicious anemia, PG II levels in PA are normal. However, cheaper and more specific tests than the pepsinogens are available for identifying PA and Z-E syndrome, and endoscopy is preferred for diagnosing ulcers.

Pepsinogen levels exhibit a diurnal pattern.[7]

See *Pepsinogen I.*

Ratio < 3.0 in gastric CA and chronic gastritis.[8]

This test is used to expose organification defects in patients who are euthyroid or hypothyroid and have an elevated radioactive iodine uptake test. Excessive discharge (loss) of accumulated radioactive iodine by perchlorate is seen in patients with inherited defects of organification of iodine and in those with Hashimoto's thyroiditis.

In the normal thyroid, iodide is trapped by an active transport mechanism and bound to thyroglobulin (Tg). Perchlorate selectively inhibits iodide trapping and releases (discharges) unbound iodide. The normal gland organifies most ^{131}I, and only 10-15% of the accumulated radioactive iodine is lost after administration of perchlorate.

The most common cause of an organification defect is Hashimoto's thyroiditis.

TEST NAME AND METHOD	SPECIMEN REQUIREMENTS	REFERENCE INTERVAL, CONVENTIONAL [INTERNATIONAL RECOMMENDED UNITS]	CHEMICAL INTERFERENCES AND IN VIVO EFFECTS

Perchlorate Discharge (Flush) Test—CONT

1. Wolff S: Perchlorate and the thyroid gland, *Pharmacol Rev* 50:89-105, 1998.
2. Larsen PR, Davies TF, Schlumberger MJ, et al: Thyroid physiology and diagnostic evaluation of patients with thyroid disorders. In *Williams textbook of endocrinology,* ed 10, Philadelphia, 2003, WB Saunders.

TEST NAME AND METHOD	SPECIMEN REQUIREMENTS	REFERENCE INTERVAL, CONVENTIONAL [INTERNATIONAL RECOMMENDED UNITS]	CHEMICAL INTERFERENCES AND IN VIVO EFFECTS
Periodic Acid Schiff Stain (PAS)[1-5]	Whole blood or bone marrow. Freshly made films are preferred, but PAS staining is satisfactory on air-dried films or Romanowsky-stained films after several years. Heparin is unsatisfactory as an anticoagulant.	Stains: Granulocytes (beginning at the promyelocyte stage, staining intensity increases with maturity), megakaryocytes, and platelets Does not stain: Most normal lymphocytes, myeloblasts, normoblasts, and megakaryoblasts Intermediate staining: Monocytes, promegakaryocytes, and lymphocytes (a small proportion of normal lymphocytes contain fine PAS-positive granules)	None found.

1. Beutler E, Lichtman MA, Coller B, editors: *Williams hematology,* ed 6, New York, 2000, McGraw-Hill.
2. Brunning RD: Morphologic alterations in nucleated blood and marrow cells in genetic disorders, *Hum Pathol* 1:99-124, 1970.
3. Hayhoe FGJ: Cytochemistry of the acute leukaemias, *Histochem J* 16:1051-1059, 1984.
4. Brunning RD, McKenna RW: *Tumors of the bone marrow,* Washington, DC, 1994, Armed Forces Institute of Pathology.
5. Jaffe ES, Harris NL, Stein H, et al, editors: *World Health Organization Classification of tumours. Pathology and genetics of tumours of haematopoietic and lymphoid tissues,* Lyon, 2001, IARC Press.

TEST NAME AND METHOD	SPECIMEN REQUIREMENTS	REFERENCE INTERVAL, CONVENTIONAL [INTERNATIONAL RECOMMENDED UNITS]		CHEMICAL INTERFERENCES AND IN VIVO EFFECTS
pH (37° C)[1-3] *Potentiometry*[1]	Whole blood, arterial (heparinized syringe); place on ice and send to the laboratory immediately. Do not ask patient to clench fist. To avoid dilutional errors and pH changes, do not use excess liquid heparin.	Cord blood[9] Arterial: Venous: Newborn Premature, 48 hr: Full term Birth: 5-10 min: 30 min: 1 hr: 1 day:	7.28 ± 0.05 (SD) 7.35 ± 0.05 7.35-7.50 7.11-7.36 7.09-7.30 7.21-7.38 7.26-7.49 7.29-7.45	↑ V Acetates, antacids, aspirin (initially respiratory alkalosis), carbenicillin, carbenoxolone, citrates, diuretics (e.g., bumetanide, ethacrynic acid, furosemide, thiazides), glutamic acid, glycyrrhiza (licorice), lactate, laxatives (chronic use), mafenide (respira-

DIAGNOSTIC INFORMATION	REMARKS

Positive: Lymphoblasts of ~67% of cases of acute lymphoid leukemia (ALL, FAB L1 and L2), coarse granules or blocks of PAS-positive material, acute monocytic leukemia (FAB M5, discrete granules in blasts of some cases), erythroblasts of some cases of erythroleukemia (FAB M6) and some cases of myelodysplastic syndrome, lymphocytes of Sezary syndrome, hairy cells of hairy cell leukemia, lymphocytes of glycogenosis type II (Pompe's disease), and Dutcher bodies in plasmacytoid lymphoma

Less positive: Erythroblasts of some cases of iron deficiency and thalassemia, lymphocytes of some cases of chronic lymphocytic leukemia (CLL), Hodgkin's disease, non-Hodgkin's lymphoma, and infectious mononucleosis

Negative: Lymphoblasts of ALL (FAB L3 or Burkitt lymphoma), megaloblasts of nutritional megaloblastic anemia (although a minority opinion holds that megaloblasts of pernicious anemia are positive)

PAS stains intracellular glycogen, polysaccharides, mucoproteins, and glycoproteins. Except for pigment in macrophages largely derived from cell debris, the PAS-positive material in blood and marrow cells is predominantly glycogen. Glycogen does not stain with PAS after treating the slides with amylase. The PAS reaction cannot be used to distinguish between ALL and acute myeloid leukemia (AML) or between benign and malignant lymphocytic disorders.

B, P ↑ *Metabolic alkalosis* (plasma bicarbonate excess)

Excessive alkali administration (see *Interferences*) *Loss of gastric HCl or gastric aspiration*

Potassium depletion: Gastrointestinal loss (e.g., chronic diarrhea), lack of potassium intake (e.g., anorexia nervosa, IV fluids without potassium supplements for treatment of vomiting or postoperatively), diuresis (see *Interferences*), excess of adrenal steroids (e.g., primary aldosteronism, Cushing's disease) or administration of steroids, large amounts of licorice, glycogen

pH compatible with life is 6.80-7.80. The arteriovenous pH difference is 0.01-0.03 but is greater in patients with congestive heart failure and in shock. Arterialized capillary blood has been recommended as a suitable substitute for arterial blood. However, in decreased cardiac output when the systolic pressure is <95 mm Hg [<12.64 kPa] or when there is vasoconstriction, capillary blood yields unreliable data. Special care must be taken not to expose the sample to air. The pH of freshly drawn blood decreases on standing at a rate of 0.04 to 0.08 pH unit/hr at 37° C, by ~0.03 pH unit/hr at 25° C, but by only 0.008 pH unit/hr at 4° C. Changes are greater in leukemia.

TEST NAME AND METHOD	SPECIMEN REQUIREMENTS	REFERENCE INTERVAL, CONVENTIONAL [INTERNATIONAL RECOMMENDED UNITS]		CHEMICAL INTERFERENCES AND IN VIVO EFFECTS
pH—CONT				
		Children, adults		tory alkalosis), phenylbu-
		Arterial:	7.35-7.45	tazone, triamcinolone,
		Venous:	7.32-7.43	tromethamine, and
		Adults		tubocurarine (low doses)
		60-90 yr:	7.31-7.42[10]	
		>90 yr:	7.26-7.43	↓ V Acetazolamide, ace-
				tone, aminobenzoic acid,
		or H$^+$ concentration:	36-45 nmol/L	aminosalicylic acid, am-
				monium chloride, arigi-
				nine, aspirin (late effect),
				calcium chloride, capto-
				pril, cholestyramine, cotri-
				moxazole, cyclosporine,
				dimercaprol, ethanol,
				ether, ethylene glycol
				(poisoning), fluorides
				(poisoning), ifosfamide,
				isoniazid (large doses),
				mafenide (systemic acido-
				sis), methanol, metho-
				cyflurane, nalidixic acid,
				paraldehyde, phenformin,
				sprionolactone, tetracy-
				cline, trimethadione, and
				tubocurarine
				↓ C Citrates, oxalates,
				and edetic acid if these
				substances used as
				anticoagulants
pH electrode,	Urine, fresh random.[3]	Newborn:	5-7	↑ V Acetazolamide, aldos-
reagent strip	Perform test immedi-	Thereafter:	4.5-8	terone, amiloride, ampho-
(Miles Inc.	ately; otherwise, store	Average:	5-6	tericin B, carbenoxolone,
Hema-Combistix,	filled container and re-			epinephrine, mafenide,
Combistix,	frigerate. Mix well af-			niacinamide, phenacetin,
Multistix,	ter storage; do not			potassium citrate, and
Bili-Labstix,	centrifuge.			sodium bicarbonate
Labstix[4]*; BMC*				
Chemstrips)[1,5-7]				↓ V Acid phosphate, am-
				monium chloride, ascor-
				bic acid, corticotropin, di-
				azoxide, methenamine

DIAGNOSTIC INFORMATION	REMARKS

deposition, chronic alkalosis, and potassium-losing nephropathy

Respiratory alkalosis (decreased dissolved CO_2): Hysteria; stimulation of the respiratory center by increased intracranial pressure or brainstem lesions with normal lung function; stimulation of the respiratory center by hypoxia with normal overall alveolar diffusion of CO_2, fever, salicylate poisoning (early); and excessive artificial ventilation

B, P ↓ *Metabolic* (bicarbonate deficit)
Increased formation of acids: Ketosis (e.g., diabetes mellitus, starvation, hyperthyroidism, high-fat and low-carbohydrate diet, after trauma), cellular hypoxia including lactic acidosis

Decreased excretion of H^+: Renal failure (prerenal, renal, postrenal), renal tubular acidosis, Faconi's syndrome, aquired (drugs, hypercalcemia), inherited (cystinosis, Wilson's disease), ureterocolic anastomosis, Addison's disease

Increased acid intake (e.g., ion-exchange resins, salicylates, ammonium chloride)

Increased loss of alkaline body fluids: Intestine (e.g., diarrhea, fistulas, aspiration of contents), biliary (biliary and pancreatic fluids), renal (carbonic anhydrase inhibitors), and secondary to other metabolic disorders (excess potassium)

Respiratory acidosis: Acute, caused by decreased alveolar centilation (emphysema, pneumonia, pulmonary edema, bronchoconstriction, plugs, drugs depressing the respiratory center); congestive heart failure; chronic (with bicarbonate increase) obstructive or restrictive pulmonary disease

If the analysis is to be performed on plasma, the blood must be warmed to 37° C before separation of red cells from plasma by centrifugation, or else falsely high pH values are obtained. pH values decrease with increase in body temperature and vice versa. Corrections must be made. See nomogram, Fig. II-2. The bicarbonate concentration can be calculated from the P_{CO_2} and pH (see Fig. II-1).

U ↑ Diet high in fruits and vegetables, especially citrus fruits; metabolic alkalosis without potassium depletion, prolonged vomiting or gastric suction, respiratory alkalosis, urinary tract infection with urea-splitting organisms (e.g., *Proteus* or *Pseudomonas*), after meals (alkaline tide), renal tubular acidosis,[12] Fanconi's and Milkman's syndrome (increased loss of HCO_3^-), and alkali therapy[8]

U ↓ Diet high in meat protein or cranberries, metabolic acidosis (e.g., diabetic), metabolic alkalosis resulting from potassium depletion, respiratory acidosis, starvation diets, and severe diarrhea

On standing, pH tends to increase because of formation of ammonia by microorganisms. Urine containing glucose may have decreasing pH as microorganisms metabolize the glucose. Therefore "standing" renders the sample unacceptable for pH measurement. pH of 9 is associated with improperly preserved samples.[7]

Bacterial infections can alter the pH in either direction, depending on the end products of bacterial metabolism. Persistently acid urine may indicate a predisposition to uric acid calculi.

TEST NAME AND METHOD	SPECIMEN REQUIREMENTS	REFERENCE INTERVAL, CONVENTIONAL [INTERNATIONAL RECOMMENDED UNITS]	CHEMICAL INTERFERENCES AND IN VIVO EFFECTS
pH—CONT			
			hippurate and mandelate, and methionine
			↑ C *False-positive (Combistix):* Serenium, Azo Gantrisin, pyridium, nitrofurantoin, and riboflavin
Potentiometry	Serous fluids (pleural, pericardial, ascitic)[8]	6.8-7.6	
	Pleural fluid[8]	Transudates: 7.4-7.5 Exudates: 7.35-7.45	
	Synovial fluid[8]	Parallels serum	
	CSF[8]	7.35-7.40	
	Semen[8]	7.2-8.0	
	Feces	7.0-7.5[8]	
		Newborns/neonates: 5.0-7.0 Bottle-fed infants: neutral or slightly alkaline[11] Breast-fed infants: slightly acidic[11]	

1. Burtis CA, Ashwood ER, editors: *Tietz textbook of clinical chemistry,* ed 3, Philadelphia, 1999, WB Saunders.
2. Henry JB, editor: *Clinical diagnosis and management by laboratory methods,* ed 20, Philadelphia, 2001, WB Saunders.
3. Burtis CA, Ashwood ER, editors: *Tietz fundamentals of clinical chemistry,* ed 5, Philadelphia, 2000, WB Saunders.
4. Miles Inc., Diagnostics Division: *Multistix package insert,* Elkhart, IN, 1992, Miles Inc., Diagnostics Division.
5. Roche Diagnostics: *Chemstrip 10 UA package insert,* Indianapolis, IN, 1999, Roche Diagnostics.
6. Free HM, editor: *Modern urine chemistry,* Elkhart, IN, 1991, Miles Inc., Diagnostics Division.
7. Strasinger SK: *Urinalysis and body fluids: a self-instructional text,* ed 2, Philadelphia, 1991, FA Davis.
8. Wallach J, editor: *Interpretation of diagnostic tests,* ed 7, Philadelphia, 2000, Lippincott.
9. Yeomans ER, Hauth JC, Gilstrap LC III, et al: Umbilical cord pH, PCO$_2$, and bicarbonate following uncomplicated term vaginal deliveries, *Am J Obstet Gynecol* 151:798-800, 1985.
10. Tietz NW, Shuey DF, Wekstein DR: Laboratory values in fit aging individuals—sexagenarians through centenarians, *Clin Chem* 38:1167-1185, 1992.
11. Jacobs DS, DeMott WR, Oxley DK, editors: *Laboratory test handbook,* ed 5, Stow, OH, 2001, Lexi-Comp, Inc.
12. Narins RG, Emmett M: Simple and mixed acid-base disorders. A practical approach, *Medicine* 59:161-187, 1980.
13. Jacobs DS, Kasten BL, DeMott WR, et al, editors: *Laboratory test handbook,* ed 2, Stow, OH, 1990, LexiComp, Inc.
14. Ringsrud KM, Linné JJ, editors: *Urinalysis and body fluids, a color text and atlas,* ed 1, St. Louis, 1995, Mosby.

DIAGNOSTIC INFORMATION	REMARKS

pH values are lowest after overnight fast and highest after meals.

Persistent pH 7-8 suggests urinary tract infection (UTI).
pH <7 may suggest an idiopathic constitutional predisposition to uric acid calculi.[7]

Urine pH may be measured in patients at risk for urinary stone formation to see that alkalinizing agents are being taken (monitor compliance) and also to adjust dose of these agents.[14]

F ↑ Increased protein breakdown,[13] secretory diarrhea without food intake, colitis, and villous adenoma

F ↓ Intestinal lactase deficiency, high lactose intake, decreased absorption of carbohydrates,[1] and decreased fat absorption[12]

TEST NAME AND METHOD	SPECIMEN REQUIREMENTS	REFERENCE INTERVAL, CONVENTIONAL [INTERNATIONAL RECOMMENDED UNITS]		CHEMICAL INTERFERENCES AND IN VIVO EFFECTS
Phenols *(Phenol, CAS 108-95-2; cresols, CAS 1319-77-3)* *Colorimetric, GC-FID*[1]	Urine		*mg/L* Phenol: <10 Toxic concentration: >10 p-Cresol: 20-200 Toxic concentration: >200 o-Cresol, Toxic concentration: >2 m-Cresol, Toxic concentration: >2	*μmol/L* × 10.6 [<106] [>106] × 9.25 [185-1850] [>1850] [>19] [>19]	U ↑ V Benzene

1. Nomoto Y, Fujita T, Kitani Y: Serum and urine levels of phenol following phenol blocks, *Can J Anesth* 34:307-310, 1987.

TEST NAME AND METHOD	SPECIMEN REQUIREMENTS	REFERENCE INTERVAL, CONVENTIONAL [INTERNATIONAL RECOMMENDED UNITS]		CHEMICAL INTERFERENCES AND IN VIVO EFFECTS
Phenylalanine (Phe)[1-6] *Fluorimetry*	Plasma (heparin) or serum, fasting. Place blood in ice water immediately; separate and freeze within 1 hr of collection. Stable for 1 wk at −20° C; for longer periods deproteinize and store at −70° C.[7,8]	*mg/dL*[1] Newborn Full-term and normal-weight: 1.2-3.4 Low-birth-weight or premature: 2.0-7.5 Phenylketonuric, 2-3 days after birth: >4.5 Untreated, at 10 days: 15-30 Adult: 0.8-1.8	*μmol/L* × 60.5 [73-206] [121-454] [>272] [907-1815] [48-109]	
Ion-exchange chromatography		*mg/dL* Premature: 1.49 ± 0.33 (SD) Newborn, 1 day: 0.69-1.82 1-3 mo: 0.86 ± 0.23 (SD) 2-6 mo: 0.86-1.60 9 mo-2 yr: 0.38-1.14 3-10 yr: 0.43-1.01 6-18 yr: 0.64-1.26 Adult: 0.61-1.45	*μmol/L*[10] × 60.5 [90 ± 20] [42-110] [52 ± 14] [52-97] [23-69] [26-61] [39-76][11] [37-88]	P ↑ C Ampicillin P ↑ V Aspartame, cotrimoxazole P ↓ V Ascorbic acid (premature infants), glucose, histidine (after oral load), and progesterone (high doses)
	Urine, 24 hr. Add 10 mL of 6 mol/L HCl at start of collection. (Alternatively, refrigerate specimen during collection.) Store frozen at −20° C.[4]	*mg/day* 10 days-7 wk: 1.2-1.7 3-12 yr: 4.0-17.5 Adult: <16.5 *mg/g creatinine* or 6 ± 2 (SD)	*μmol/day*[11] × 6.05 [7-10] [24-106] [<100] *mmol/mol creatinine* × 0.68 [4.1 ± 1.4]	U ↑ V Ascorbic acid (after large intake),[15] progesterone

DIAGNOSTIC INFORMATION	REMARKS

Toxic effects include headache, dizziness, hyperpnea, weakness, and pulmonary, hepatic, or renal effects.

These substances are corrosive and are widely used in cleaning solutions as disinfectants. Absorption may occur by inhalation or by skin contact.

o-Cresol and *m*-cresol are normally not present in urine. Any detectable amount indicates exposure.

Colorimetric methods are nonspecific.

Kinetic values
TLV: 5 ppm (19 mg/m^3)

Cord blood cannot be used for analysis. Two days of protein feeding are recommended before specimens are obtained. False-negative results are seen if protein intake is inadequate. False-positive results are seen in premature infants as a result of liver immaturity. Antibiotics will interfere in the assay, and results cannot be interpreted. All positive results must be confirmed with a quantitative chemical test or chromatography.

P ↑ Hyperphenylalaninemias, sepsis, severe burns,[16] transient tyrosinemia of the newborn, transient hyperphenylalaninemia of the newborn, phlebotomus fever, viral hepatitis, and hepatic encephalopathy. Immature liver particularly in premature newborn

In normal newborns, a diurnal variation of Phe is seen; highest levels occur at 7:00 PM and lowest levels occur at 7:00 AM.

Hyperphenylalaninemia can result from a deficiency of phenylalanine hydroxylase (classic PKU) or from defects associated with the enzyme cofactor tetrahydrobiopterin (BH$_4$). BH$_4$ defects can be caused by a deficiency of dihydropteridine reductase (DHPR) or by a defect in biopterin biosynthesis. BH$_4$ defects account for 1-3% of patients with hyperphenylalaninemia.

Specimens for measuring DHPR in blood and pteridines in urine are obtained if elevated phenylalanine levels are found. See *Dihydropteridine Reductase.*

See also Table II-2A.

U ↑ Hyperphenylalaninemias, Hartnup disease, first trimester of pregnancy (levels decrease thereafter), oasthouse disease, cystinosis, and hepatolenticular degeneration

TEST NAME AND METHOD	SPECIMEN REQUIREMENTS	REFERENCE INTERVAL, CONVENTIONAL [INTERNATIONAL RECOMMENDED UNITS]		CHEMICAL INTERFERENCES AND IN VIVO EFFECTS

Phenylalanine—CONT

		mmol/g creatinine[13]		*mmol/mol creatinine*	
		0-1 mo:	62-220	× 0.113	[7.01-24.86]
		1-6 mo:	49-391		[5.54-44.18]
		6 mo-1 yr:	107-367		[12.09-41.47]
		1-2 yr:	57-314		[6.44-35.48]
		2-3 yr:	80-306		[9.04-34.58]

			mg/dL	*μmol/L*
	CSF. Collect in sterile tubes; store frozen. Stable at −20° C for 1 wk or at −70° C for 2 mo.[9]	Neonate:	0.385 ± 0.124 (SEM) × 60.5	[23.3 ± 7.5][11]
		3 mo-2 yr:	0.142 ± 0.030 (SD)	[8.6 ± 1.8][13]
		2-10 yr:	0.111 ± 0.021	[6.7 ± 1.3][13]
		Adult:	0.157 ± 0.012	[9.5 ± 0.7][10]

			mg/dL	*μmol/L*
Tandem mass spectrometry	Whole blood on filter paper. See above.	neonate	<2	<120
		ratio phenylalanine/tyrosine[14]		
		2.5		

1. Burtis CA, Ashwood ER, Bruns DE, editors: *Tietz textbook of clinical chemistry and molecular bases,* ed 4, Philadelphia, 2005, WB Saunders.

2. Friedman RB, Young DS: *Effects of disease on clinical laboratory tests,* ed 2, Washington, DC, 1989, American Association for Clinical Chemistry.

3. Pesce A, Kaplan L, editors: *Methods in clinical chemistry,* St. Louis, 1987, CV Mosby.

4. Scriver CR, Beaudet AL, Valle D, et al, editors: *The metabolic and molecular bases of inherited disease,* ed 8, New York, 2001, McGraw-Hill.

5. Bremer HJ, Duran M, Kamerling JP, et al: *Disturbances of amino acid metabolism: clinical chemistry and diagnosis,* Baltimore, 1981, Urban and Schwarzenburg.

6. Nyhan W, Sakait N: *Diagnostic recognition of genetic disease,* Philadelphia, 1987, Lea & Febiger.

7. Cummings JG: Routine amino acids analysis in the clinical laboratory, *Am Clin Prod Rev* Feb:20-25, 1988.

8. Schaefer A, Piquard F, Haberey P: Plasma amino acids analysis: effects of delayed samples preparation and of storage, *Clin Chim Acta* 164:163-169, 1987.

9. Heiblim DI, Evans HE, Glass L, et al: Amino acid concentrations in cerebrospinal fluid, *Arch Neurol* 35:765-768, 1978.

10. Shih V: *Laboratory techniques for the detection of hereditary metabolic disorders,* Boca Raton, FL, 1973, CRC Press.

11. Meites S, editor: *Pediatric clinical chemistry,* ed 3, Washington, DC, 1989, American Association for Clinical Chemistry.

12. Mayo Medical Laboratories: *Test catalog,* Rochester, MN, 2005, Mayo Medical Laboratories.

13. Goldsmith RF, Earl JW, Cunningham AM: Determination of δ-aminobutyric acid and other amino acids in cerebrospinal fluid of pediatric patients by reversed-phase liquid chromatography, *Clin Chem* 33:1736-1740, 1987.

14. Chace DH, Sherwin JE, Hillman SL, et al: Use of phenylalanine to tyrosine ratio determined by tandem mass spectrometry to improve newborn screening for phenylketonuria of early discharge specimens collected in the first 24 hours, *Clin Chem* 44:2405-2409, 1998.

15. Tsao C, Muyashita K: Effects of large intake of ascorbic acid on the urinary excretion of amino acids and related compounds, *IRCS Med Sci* 13:855-856, 1985.

DIAGNOSTIC INFORMATION	REMARKS

CSF ↑ Hyperphenylalaninemia, bacterial meningitis, aseptic meningitis, meningoradiculitis, Garin-Bujadoux-Bannwarth, and carcinomatous meningitis

Values in children (3 mo-10 yr) were measured using reversed-phase liquid chromatography.

↑ PKU, hyperphenylalaninemias, and immature liver of prematurity. Other genetic liver diseases including tyrosinemia.

↑ Ratio of phenylalanine to tyrosine more specific for genetic hyperphenylalaninemias.

16. Cynober L, Dinh FN, Blonde F, et al: Plasma and urinary amino acid pattern in severe burn patients: evolution throughout the healing period, *Am J Clin Nutr* 36:416-425, 1982.

TEST NAME AND METHOD	SPECIMEN REQUIREMENTS	REFERENCE INTERVAL, CONVENTIONAL [INTERNATIONAL RECOMMENDED UNITS]	CHEMICAL INTERFERENCES AND IN VIVO EFFECTS
Phosphatidyl-ethanol (PEth)[1,2] *Chromatographic methods*	Whole blood[3]	Undetectable, heparinized[3,4]	↑ Phenytoin; carba-mazepine

1. Laposata M: Assessment of ethanol intake. Current tests and new assays on the horizon, *Am J Clin Pathol* 112:443-450, 1999.
2. Musshoff F: Chromatographic methods for the determination of markers of chronic and acute alcohol consumption, *J Chromatogr B Analyt Technol Biomed Life Sci* 781:457-480, 2002.
3. Hansson P, Caron M, Johnson G, et al: Blood phosphatidylethanol as a marker of alcohol abuse: levels in alcoholic males during withdrawal, *Alcohol Clin Exp Res* 21:108-110, 1997.
4. Gunnarsson T, Karlsson A, Hansson P: Determination of phosphatidylethanol in blood from alcoholic males using high-performance liquid chromatography and evaporative light scattering or electrospray mass spectrometric detection, *J Chromatogr B Biomed Sci Appl* 705:243-249, 1998.

TEST NAME AND METHOD	SPECIMEN REQUIREMENTS	REFERENCE INTERVAL, CONVENTIONAL [INTERNATIONAL RECOMMENDED UNITS]		CHEMICAL INTERFERENCES AND IN VIVO EFFECTS
Phosphatidylglyc-erol (PG) *1D-TLC*[1] (Commercially available with L/S ratio as Fetal Tek 200 from Helena, Beaumont, TX; see *L/S ratio*.)	Amniotic fluid, 3-4 mL minimum. (See *L/S ratio* for additional information.)	Absent: Present:	Fetal lung immaturity Fetal lung maturity	↑ C Excessive meconium contamination (>3%) can mimic the presence of PG by some methods.[5,6] Vaginal pool specimens may contain PG-producing flora.[7-10]
Slide agglutina-tion (Amnio-Stat-FLM)[2,3]	Amniotic fluid, 0.025 mL. Excessive centrifugation may sediment PG and lead to falsely lowered results.[4] (See *L/S ratio* for additional information.)	High-positive: Low-positive: Negative:	*mg/L* >2.0[3] >0.5 <0.5	None found.

DIAGNOSTIC INFORMATION	REMARKS

↑ Ethanol intake

Phosphatidylethanol (PE) is an aberrant phospholipid formed within cell membrane only in the presence of ethanol. The formation of PE is catalyzed by phospholipase D, which normally catalyzes the hydrolysis of phospholipids to phosphatidic acid.

The rate of degradation of PE is slower than that of formation, with a half-life of ~4 days. Because of the high specificity and prolonged elimination, PE has been suggested as a long-term marker of alcohol intake.

High values of PG are reliable indicators of lung maturity even in samples with an immature L/S ratio. The absence of PG or presence of low levels cannot dependably predict the presence or absence of RDS.[1] By densitometry the cutoff point for maturity is PG = 2-3% of total phospholipid.[11] Because TLC methods for PG differ in sensitivity, laboratories should use this quantitative measure to guide qualitative assessment of PG.[12,13]

Diabetes, regardless of glucose control, delays PG production. Many diabetic patients will deliver term infants with mature surfactant status before PG is detected.[14,15]

PG and phosphatidylinositol (PI) serve to stabilize surfactant, although PG-deficient surfactant can have normal properties. The concentration of PG increases significantly after ~34 wk gestational age.[1]

Measurement of PG is an especially valuable marker of fetal lung maturity when amniotic fluid samples are contaminated with moderate amounts of blood or <3% meconium. These substances will not cause interference in the majority of methods for detection of PG but will interfere in most other tests for fetal lung maturity.[19]

This test is often combined with the L/S ratio and phosphatidylinositol (PI) to produce a "lung profile."[7,11,20] (See also *L/S Ratio.*)

A high-positive result (PG >2 mg/L) is reported to correlate 100% with the absence of RDS.[16] A low-positive result (PG >0.5 mg/L) also has a high correlation with fetal lung maturity.[17] The predictive value of this test for maturity is 98-100%, but the test is a very poor predictor for immaturity (40%).[18]

The test uses an antibody to PG. Advantages include rapid turnaround time, no interference from blood, meconium, and bilirubin, and the small volume of sample required.

TEST NAME AND METHOD	SPECIMEN REQUIREMENTS	REFERENCE INTERVAL, CONVENTIONAL [INTERNATIONAL RECOMMENDED UNITS]				CHEMICAL INTERFERENCES AND IN VIVO EFFECTS

Phosphatidylglycerol—CONT

1. Brown LM, Duck-Chong CG: Methods of evaluating fetal lung maturity, *Crit Rev Clin Lab Sci* 16:85-159, 1982.

2. Garite TJ, Yabusaki KK, Moberg LJ, et al: A new rapid slide agglutination test for amniotic fluid phosphatidylglycerol: laboratory and clinical correlation, *Am J Obstet Gynecol* 147:681-686, 1983.

3. Irvine Scientific: *AmnioStat-FLM,* Santa Ana, CA, 2002, Irvine Scientific.

4. Oulton M: The role of centrifugation in the measurement of surfactant in amniotic fluid, *Am J Obstet Gynecol* 135:337-343, 1979.

5. Schmidt-Sommerfeld E, Litmeyer H, Penn D: A rapid qualitative method for detecting phosphatidylglycerol in amniotic fluid, *Clin Chim Acta* 119:243-247, 1982.

6. Tsao FH, Zachman RD: Determination of phosphatidylglycerol in amniotic fluid by a simple one-dimensional thin-layer chromatography method, *Clin Chim Acta* 118:109-120, 1982.

7. Hallman M, Kulovich M, Kirkpatrick E, et al: Phosphatidylinositol and phosphatidylglycerol in amniotic fluid: indices of lung maturity, *Am J Obstet Gynecol* 125:613-617, 1976.

8. Lambers DS, Brady K, Leist PA, et al: Ability of normal vaginal flora to produce detectable phosphatidylglycerol in amniotic fluid in vitro, *Obstet Gynecol* 85:651-655, 1995.

9. Pastorek JG, Letellier RL, Gebbia K: Production of a phosphatidylglycerol-like substance by genital flora bacteria, *Am J Obstet Gynecol* 159:199-202, 1988.

10. Schumacher RE, Parisi VM, Steady HM, et al: Bacteria causing false positive test for phosphatidylglycerol in amniotic fluid, *Am J Obstet Gynecol* 151:1067-1068, 1985.

Phospho-ethanolamine (PEA)[1-6] *Ion-exchange chromatography*	Plasma. Separate plasma within 1 hr. Store at −20° C until analysis.[6]		*mg/dL*	×70.87	*μmol/L*	U ↑ V Ascorbic acid (after large intake)[9]
		Premature	0.07-0.49		[5-35]	
		1 day-1 mo	0.04-0.38		[3-27]	
		1-24 mo	0-0.08		[0-6]	
		2 yr-Adult	0-0.97		[0-69]	
	Urine, 24 hr. Add 10 mL of 6 mol/L HCl at start of collection. (Alternatively, refrigerate specimen during collection.) Store frozen at −20° C.[7]		*mg/day*	×7.09	*μmol/day*[8]	
		0-4 mo:	0-9.9		[0-70]	
		4 mo-2 yr:	0-17.6		[0-125]	
		12 yr-Adult:	0-27.8		[0-197]	
			μmol/g creatinine[8]		*mmol/mol creatinine*	
		0-21 days:	0-590	×0.113	[0-67]	
		21-90 days:	0-284		[0-32]	
		3 mo-3 yr:	0-697		[0-79]	
		3-12 yr:	0-430		[0-49]	

1. Friedman RB, Young DS: *Effects of disease on clinical laboratory tests,* ed 2, Washington, DC, 1989, American Association for Clinical Chemistry.

2. Scriver CR, Beaudet AL, Valle D, et al, editors: *The metabolic and molecular bases of inherited disease,* ed 8, New York, 2001, McGraw-Hill.

3. Young DS: *Effects of drugs on clinical laboratory tests,* ed 3, Washington, DC, 1990, American Association for Clinical Chemistry.

4. Bremer HJ, Duran M, Kamerling JP, et al: *Disturbances of amino acid metabolism: clinical chemistry and diagnosis,* Baltimore, 1981, Urban and Schwarzenburg.

5. Nyhan W, Sakait N: *Diagnostic recognition of genetic disease,* Philadelphia, 1987, Lea & Febiger.

11. Kulovich MV, Hallman MB, Gluck L: The lung profile. I. Normal pregnancy, *Am J Obstet Gynecol* 135:57-63, 1979.

12. Spillman T, Cotton DB, Golunski E: Detection frequency by thin-layer chromatography of phosphatidylglycerol in amniotic fluid with clinically functional pulmonary surfactant, *Clin Chem* 34:1976-1982, 1988.

13. Spillman T, Cotton DB: Current perspectives in assessment of fetal pulmonary surfactant status with amniotic fluid, *Crit Rev Clin Lab Sci* 27:341-389, 1989.

14. Tsai MY, Shultz EK, Nelson JA: Amniotic fluid phosphatidylglycerol in diabetic and control pregnant patients at different gestational lengths, *Am J Obstet Gynecol* 149:388-392, 1984.

15. Moore TR: A comparison of amniotic fluid fetal pulmonary phospholipids in normal and diabetic pregnancy, *Am J Obstet Gynecol* 186:641-650, 2002.

16. Garite TJ, Yabusaki KK, Moberg LJ, et al: A new rapid slide agglutination test for amniotic fluid phosphatidylglycerol: laboratory and clinical correlation, *Am J Obstet Gynecol* 147:681-686, 1983.

17. Gupta R, Steiner M, Lew M: Determination of unconjugated 3-methoxy-4-hydroxyphenylglycol by liquid chromatography for monitoring inhibition of monoamine oxidase activity in plasma, *Clin Chem* 33:2078-2080, 1987.

18. Lockitch G, Whittman BK, Mara SM, et al: Evaluation of the Amniostat-FLM assay for assessment of fetal lung maturity, *Clin Chem* 30:1233-1237, 1984.

19. Dubin SB: Assessment of fetal lung maturity. Practice parameter, *Am J Clin Pathol* 110:723-732, 1998.

20. Kulovich MV, Gluck L: The lung profile. II. Complicated pregnancy, *Am J Obstet Gynecol* 135:64-70, 1979.

P, U ↑ Hypophosphatasia

U ↑ Hypertension, metabolic bone disorders

Urinary PEA levels are diet dependent and follow a circadian rhythm.[2]

6. Slocum RH, Cummings JG: Amino acid analysis of physiological samples. In *Techniques in human biochemical genetics,* New York, 1991, Wiley-Liss, pp. 87-126.

7. Pesce A, Kaplan L, editors: *Methods in clinical chemistry,* St. Louis, 1987, CV Mosby.

8. University of Minnesota Clinical Laboratories: *Outreach program catalog,* Minneapolis, MN, 1992, University of Minnesota Clinical Laboratories.

9. Tsao C, Muyashita K: Effects of large intake of ascorbic acid on the urinary excretion of amino acids and related compounds, *IRCS Med Sci* 13:855-856, 1985.

TEST NAME AND METHOD	SPECIMEN REQUIREMENTS	REFERENCE INTERVAL, CONVENTIONAL [INTERNATIONAL RECOMMENDED UNITS]		CHEMICAL INTERFERENCES AND IN VIVO EFFECTS
Phosphofructoki-nase (PFK) in Erythrocytes (EC 2.7.1.11)[1-3]	Hemolysate of washed Ercs. Submit whole blood (ACD, EDTA, or heparin). Stable 6 days at 4° C in EDTA or	*U/g Hb* 9.05 ± 1.89 (SD) *U/10¹² Ercs*	× 0.0645*	*MU/mol Hb* [0.58 ± 0.12] *nU/Erc*	↓ In the presence of copper unless EDTA (400 mmol/L) is also present
		262 ± 55	× 10⁻³	[0.26 ± 0.05]	
ICSH, 37° C[4]	heparin, 20 days in ACD; stable 2 days at 25° C in ACD, 1 day in	*U/mL Ercs* 3.08 ± 0.64	× 1.0	*kU/L Ercs* [3.08 ± 0.64]	
		Levels lower in newborns.			
Oxidation of NADH, 37° C[2]	EDTA or heparin.	*U/g Hb* 11.01 ± 2.33 (SD) *U/10¹² Ercs*	× 0.0645*	*MU/mol Hb* [0.7 ± 0.2] *nU/Erc*	
		319.3 ± 67.6	× 10⁻³	[0.32 ± 0.07]	
		U/mL Ercs 3.74 ± 0.79	× 1.0	*kU/L Ercs* [3.74 ± 0.79]	

See *Acetylcholinesterase.*

*Conversion factor based on MW of Hb of 64,500.

1. Beutler E: *Hemolytic anemia in disorders of red cell metabolism,* New York, 1978, Plenum Pub. Co.
2. Beutler E: *Red cell metabolism: a manual of biochemical methods,* ed 4, New York, 1986, Grune & Stratton.
3. Williams JJ, Beutler E, Ersley JJ, et al, editors: *Manual of hematology,* ed 6, New York, 2003, McGraw-Hill Publishing Co.
4. Beutler E, Blume KG, Kaplan JC, et al: International committee for standardization in haematology: recommended methods for red-cell enzyme analysis, *Br J Haematol* 35:331-340, 1977.
5. Nakajima H, Raben N, Hamaguchi T, et al: Phosphofructokinase deficiency; past, present and future, *Curr Mol Med* 2:197-212, 2002.

TEST NAME AND METHOD	SPECIMEN REQUIREMENTS	REFERENCE INTERVAL, CONVENTIONAL [INTERNATIONAL RECOMMENDED UNITS]		CHEMICAL INTERFERENCES AND IN VIVO EFFECTS
Phosphoglucomu-tase (PGM) in Erythrocytes (EC 2.7.5.1)[1,2]	Hemolysate of washed Ercs. Submit whole blood (ACD, EDTA, or heparin). Stable	*U/g Hb* 5.5 ± 0.62 (SD) *U/10¹² Ercs*	× 0.0645*	*MU/mol Hb* [0.35 ± 0.04] *nU/Erc*	None found.
		160 ± 18	× 10⁻³	[0.16 ± 0.02]	
ICSH, 37° C	>20 days at 4° C, >5 days at 25° C.	*U/mL Ercs* 1.87 ± 0.21	× 1.0	*kU/L Ercs* [1.87 ± 0.21]	
		Levels higher in infants.			

See *Acetylcholinesterase.*

*Conversion factor based on MW of Hb of 64,500.

1. Beutler E: *Hemolytic anemia in disorders of red cell metabolism,* New York, 1978, Plenum Pub. Co.
2. Beutler E: *Red cell metabolism: a manual of biochemical methods,* ed 4, New York, 1986, Grune & Stratton.

DIAGNOSTIC INFORMATION	REMARKS
↓ May be associated with severe muscle dysfunction (type VII glycogen storage disease).[3] Deficiency causes mild congenital hemolytic disorder and is commonly associated with mild myopathy.[5]	Activity is normal or increased in young erythrocytes, and reticulocyte-depleted samples may be necessary if active hemolysis with increased reticulocytes is occurring. U/g Hb × 29 = U/10^{12} Ercs U/g Hb × 0.34 = U/mL Ercs* *See Note, *Acetylcholinesterase.*
Deficiency of PGM has no known clinical effect. Rare cases reported.	U/g Hb × 29 = U/10^{12} Ercs U/g Hb × 0.34 = U/mL Ercs* *See Note, *Acetylcholinesterase.*

TEST NAME AND METHOD	SPECIMEN REQUIREMENTS	REFERENCE INTERVAL, CONVENTIONAL [INTERNATIONAL RECOMMENDED UNITS]		CHEMICAL INTERFERENCES AND IN VIVO EFFECTS
6-Phosphoglu-conate Dehydroge-nase (6-PGD) in Erythrocytes (EC 1.1.1.43)[1-3] *Glock and McLean (UV), 37° C; ICSH, 37° C*[2]	Hemolysate of washed Ercs. Submit whole blood (ACD, EDTA, or heparin). Stable for >20 days at 4° C, 5 days at 25° C.	*U/g Hb* 8.78 ± 0.78 (SD) $\times$ 0.0645* *U/10^{12} Ercs* 255 ± 22.6 $\times$ 10^{-3} *U/mL Ercs* 2.99 ± 0.27 $\times$ 1.0 See *Acetylcholinesterase.* *Conversion factor based on MW of Hb of 64,500.	*MU/mol Hb* [0.57 ± 0.05] *nU/Erc* [0.25 ± 0.02] *kU/L Ercs* [2.99 ± 0.27]	None found.

1. Beutler E: *Hemolytic anemia in disorders of red cell metabolism,* New York, 1978, Plenum Pub. Co.
2. Beutler E: *Red cell metabolism: a manual of biochemical methods,* ed 4, New York, 1986, Grune & Stratton.
3. Williams JJ, Beutler E, Ersley JJ, et al, editors: *Manual of hematology,* ed 6, New York, 2003, McGraw-Hill Publishing Co.
4. Caprari P, Caforio MP, Cianciulli P, et al: 6-Phosphogluconate dehydrogenase deficiency in an Italian family, *Ann Hematol* 80:41-44, 2001.
5. Vives Corrons JL, Colomer D, Pujades A, et al: Congenital 6-phosphogluconate dehydrogenase (6PGD) deficiency associated with chronic hemolytic anemia in a Spanish family, *Am J Hematol* 53:221-227, 1996.
6. Miwa S, Fujii H: Molecular basis of erythroenzymopathies associated with hereditary hemolytic anemia: tabulation of mutant enzymes, *Am J Hematol* 51:122-132, 1996.

TEST NAME AND METHOD	SPECIMEN REQUIREMENTS	REFERENCE INTERVAL, CONVENTIONAL [INTERNATIONAL RECOMMENDED UNITS]		CHEMICAL INTERFERENCES AND IN VIVO EFFECTS
Phosphoglycerate Kinase (PGK) in Erythrocytes (EC 2.7.2.3)[1-3] *ICSH, 37° C*	Hemolysate of washed Ercs. Submit whole blood (ACD, EDTA, or heparin). Stable for 20 days at 4° C, 5 days at 25° C.	*U/g Hb* 320 ± 36.1 (SD) $\times$ 0.0645* *U/10^{12} Ercs* 9280 ± 1047 $\times$ 10^{-3} *U/mL Ercs* 109 ± 12.3 $\times$ 1.0 See *Acetylcholinesterase.* *Conversion factor based on MW of Hb of 64,500.	*MU/mol Hb* [20.64 ± 2.33] *nU/Erc* [9.28 ± 1.05] *kU/L Ercs* [1.09 ± 12.3]	↓ In the presence of copper unless EDTA (400 μmol/L) is also present

1. Beutler E: *Hemolytic anemia in disorders of red cell metabolism,* New York, 1978, Plenum Pub. Co.
2. Beutler E: *Red cell metabolism: a manual of biochemical methods,* ed 4, New York, 1986, Grune & Stratton.
3. Williams JJ, Beutler E, Ersley JJ, et al, editors: *Manual of hematology,* ed 6, New York, 2003, McGraw-Hill Publishing Co.

TEST NAME AND METHOD	SPECIMEN REQUIREMENTS	REFERENCE INTERVAL, CONVENTIONAL [INTERNATIONAL RECOMMENDED UNITS]	CHEMICAL INTERFERENCES AND IN VIVO EFFECTS
Phospholipids, Total (PL)[1] *Enzymatic*[1-3] *Fluorometric*[4]	Plasma (EDTA, heparin, citrate, oxalate, sodium fluoride) or serum. Stable at least 7 days at 4° C. Avoid repeated freezing and thawing.	*Expected values:* 150-250 mg/dL	↑ C Free choline ↑ V Alcoholism, high fat meal, obesity, pregnancy, and estrogens ↓ C Ascorbic acid

DIAGNOSTIC INFORMATION	REMARKS
Deficiency of 6-PGD has been associated with episodic and chronic nonspherocytic hemolysis in rare cases.[4-6]	Activity is higher in young erythrocytes.[1] $U/g\ Hb \times 29 = U/10^{12}\ Ercs$ $U/g\ Hb \times 0.34 = U/mL\ Ercs*$ *See Note, *Acetylcholinesterase.*
X-chromosome-linked enzyme deficiency may be associated with neurological disturbances and congenital hemolytic anemia. CNS tissue may also lack PGK.[12]	Activity is similar in all erythrocytes including reticulocytes.[1] $U/g\ Hb \times 29 = U/10^{12}\ Ercs$ $U/g\ Hb \times 0.34 = U/mL\ Ercs*$ *See Note, *Acetylcholinesterase.*
↑ An elevated PL concentration is associated with various hyperlipidemias, cholestatic liver disease, Schistosomiasis infection, and trauma. ↓ A decreased PL concentration is associated with hematologic cancers, cerebrovascular disease.	PL, essential components of cell membranes and lipoproteins, comprise several subclasses, including phosphatidyl choline (PC), lysophosphatidyl choline, phosphatidyl ethanolamine, phosphatidyl serine, and phosphatidyl inositol. In addition to serving as structural components of lipoproteins, PLs are also substrates for several plasma enzymes, such as LCAT, lipoprotein lipase, and hepatic triglyceride lipase.

TEST NAME AND METHOD	SPECIMEN REQUIREMENTS	REFERENCE INTERVAL, CONVENTIONAL [INTERNATIONAL RECOMMENDED UNITS]				CHEMICAL INTERFERENCES AND IN VIVO EFFECTS

Phospholipids, Total—CONT

Colorimetric[5,6]

↓ V Weight loss in over-weight individuals, medroxyprogesterone, niacin, HMG-CoA reductase inhibitors (statins), and fibric acid derivatives

1. Rifai N, Warnick GR, Dominiczak MH, editors: *Handbook of lipoprotein testing,* ed 2, Washington, DC, 2000, AACC Press.
2. Blaton V, DeBuyzere M, Spincemaille J, et al: Enzymic assay for phosphatidylcholine and sphingomyelin in serum, *Clin Chem* 29:806-809, 1996.
3. Cham BE, Mahon M, Kostner K, et al: Phospholipids in EDTA-treated plasma and serum, *Clin Chem* 39:2347-2348, 1993.
4. Jouanel P, Motta C, Delattre J, et al: A rapid and sensitive fluorometric assay of serum phospholipid, *Clin Chim Acta* 105:173-181, 1980.
5. Sandhu RS: Serum phospholipids determined without acid digestion, *Clin Chem* 22:1973-1975, 1976.
6. Stewart JCM: Colorimetric determination of phospholipids with ammonium ferrothiocyanate, *Anal Biochem* 104:10-14, 1980.

TEST NAME AND METHOD	SPECIMEN REQUIREMENTS	REFERENCE INTERVAL, CONVENTIONAL			[INTERNATIONAL RECOMMENDED UNITS]	CHEMICAL INTERFERENCES AND IN VIVO EFFECTS
Phosphorus, Inorganic (P_i)[1-4] *Colorimetric, phosphomolybdate*	Serum, fasting. Avoid hemolysis and venous stasis. Separate from erythrocytes within 1 hr after collection. Stable at 4° C for several days or frozen for several months.	0-9 days: 10 days-2 yr: 3-9 yr: 10-15 yr: 16-59 yr: 60-89 yr M: F: >89 yr M: F:	*mg/dL* 4.5-9.0 4.0-6.5 3.2-5.8 3.3-5.4 2.4-4.4 2.3-3.7 2.8-4.0 2.2-3.9 2.5-4.2	× 0.323	*mmol/L* [1.45-2.91] [1.29-2.10] [1.03-1.87] [1.07-1.74] [0.78-1.42] [0.74-1.20] [0.90-1.26] [0.71-1.26] [0.81-1.36]	S ↑ V Anabolic steroids, androgens, β-adrenergic blockers (e.g., acebutolol, pindolol), ethanol, ergocalciferol, furosemide, growth hormone, hydrochlorothiazide, methicillin (occurs with nephrotoxicity), phosphates, sodium etidronate, tetracycline (occurs with nephrotoxicity), and vitamin D S ↑ C Bilirubin, detergents (contaminated glassware), fat emulsions, hemoglobin, lipemia, and methotrexate S ↓ V Acetazolamide, albuterol, aluminum-containing antacids, amino acids, anesthetic agents, calcitonin, carbamazepine, epinephrine,

DIAGNOSTIC INFORMATION	REMARKS

The measurement of total PL takes advantage of the fact that all PL contain a lipid-bound phosphate group. The most common enzymatic method uses phospholipase D to hydrolyze PC to free choline. The method is specific for PC, which accounts for ~95% of the total PL in plasma. This method does not require lipid extraction and is easily automated.

S ↑ Osteolytic metastatic bone tumors, myelogenous leukemia, sarcoidosis, milk-alkali syndrome, vitamin D intoxication, healing fractures, renal failure, hypoparathyroidism, pseudohypoparathyroidism, diabetes mellitus with ketosis, malignant hyperpyrexia following anesthesia, acromegaly, portal cirrhosis, pulmonary embolism, lactic acidosis, and respiratory acidosis

S ↓ Osteomalacia, steatorrhea, renal tubular acidosis, growth hormone deficiency, acute alcoholism, gram-negative bacterial septicemia, hypokalemia, familial hypophosphatemic rickets, vitamin D deficiency, severe malnutrition, malabsorption, severe diarrhea, vomiting, nasogastric suction, primary hyperparathyroidism, PTH-producing tumors, familial hypocalciuric hypercalcemia, severe hypercalemia of any cause, acute gout, salicylate poisoning, respiratory infections, treatment of diabetes mellitus (hyperinsulinemia), respiratory alkalosis, osteoblastic metastases of cancer, renal tubular defects (e.g., Fanconi's syndrome), and diuretic phase of severe burns

Serum phosphorus concentrations have a circadian rhythm (highest level in late morning, lowest in evening) and are subject to rapid change secondary to environmental factors such as diet (carbohydrate), phosphate-binding antacids, and fluctuations in growth hormone, insulin, and renal function. There is a seasonal variation with maximum levels in May and June (lowest levels in winter). During first decade of menopause values increase ~0.2 mg/dL [~0.06 mmol/L]. Bed rest causes increase up to 0.5 mg/dL [0.16 mmol/L]. Ingestion of food may cause a transient decrease in blood levels. Low values are also seen during menstruation.

Serum or plasma should be separated from erythrocytes soon after the specimen is collected; otherwise, the phosphatase and inorganic phosphates present in the red cells will interfere and give falsely high values.

Hypophosphatemia is found in about half of the cases of primary hyperparathyroidism. The measurement of TRP (tubular reabsorption of phosphate) has been suggested as an adjunct test for diagnosis of 1° hyperparathyroidism.[8] (See *Tubular Reabsorption of Phosphate.*)

TEST NAME AND METHOD	SPECIMEN REQUIREMENTS	REFERENCE INTERVAL, CONVENTIONAL [INTERNATIONAL RECOMMENDED UNITS]		CHEMICAL INTERFERENCES AND IN VIVO EFFECTS

Phosphorus, Inorganic—CONT

esramustine, estrogens, fructose, glucocorticoids, glucose, hydrochlorothiazide (prolonged treatment), ifosfamide, insulin, isoniazid, oral contraceptives, phenytoin, and sucralfate

S ↓ C Citrates, mannitol, oxalate, tartrates (all decrease color development); phenothiazines

Urine, 24 hr. Collect in acid-washed, detergent-free container; acidify with HCl after collection (pH <3); stable for 6 mo.[5]

		g/day		mmol/day
Constant daily diet:*		<1.0	× 32.3	[<32.3]
Nonrestricted diet:		0.4-1.3[6]		[12.9-42.0]
Random urine[7]:				

		mg/dL		mmol/L
Adult				
M:		5-189	× 0.323	[1.6-61]
F:		7-148		[2.3-48]

		mg/g creatinine		mmol/g creatinine
M				
<40 yr:		36-1770	× 0.032	[1.16-57.2]
≥40 yr:		54-860		[1.74-27.8]
F				
<40 yr:		111-927		[3.58-29.9]
≥40 yr:		[105-1081]		[3.39-34.9]

*Constant daily diet, 0.9-1.5 g P [29-48 mmol P] and 10 mg Ca/kg [0.25 mmol Ca/kg].

U ↑ V Acetazolamide, L-alanine, asparaginase, aspirin, bicarbonate, bismuth salts, calcitonin, corticosteroids, dihydrotachysterol, hydrochlorothiazide, metolazone, phosphates, PTH, tryptophan, valine, and vitamin D

U ↓ V Alanine (fasting, obese subjects), aluminum-containing antacids

U ↓ C Mannitol (complexes molybdate, decreases color development)

1. Burtis CA, Ashwood ER, editors: *Tietz textbook of clinical chemistry,* ed 3, Philadelphia, 1999, WB Saunders.
2. Jacobs DS, Kasten BL Jr, DeMott WR, et al, editors: *Laboratory test handbook,* Stow, OH/St. Louis, 1988, LexiComp/Mosby.
3. Wallach J, editor: *Interpretation of diagnostic tests,* ed 5, Boston, 1992, Little, Brown and Co.
4. Juan D: The causes and consequences of hypophosphatemia, *Surg Gynecol Obstet* 153:589-597, 1981.
5. Kaplan LA, Pesce AJ, editors: *Clinical chemistry: theory, analysis, and correlation,* St. Louis, 1984, CV Mosby.
6. A.B. Chandler Medical Center Clinical Laboratories: *Reference ranges and general information,* Lexington, KY, 2003, University of Kentucky; values used and partially established at the University of Kentucky Medical Center.

DIAGNOSTIC INFORMATION	REMARKS

U ↑ Hyperparathyroidism, vitamin D–resistant rickets, immobilization after paraplegia or a fracture, vitamin D intoxication, renal tubular damage (e.g., Fanconi's syndrome), familial hypophosphatemia, and nonrenal acidosis (increased phosphate excretion as a urine buffer)

U ↓ Hypoparathyroidism, pseudohypoparathyroidism, and parathyroidectomy

There is a significant diurnal variation in the excretion of P_i in urine, with values in the afternoon being highest. The output varies widely, depending on diet. Measurement of phosphaturia is not useful in detecting osteomalacia. All tests involving urinary Ca and phosphate excretion require a creatinine clearance >40-50 mL/min for valid interpretation.

7. Bond LW, Garber C, Ottinger W, et al: Reference intervals for common analytes in random urine specimens, *Clin Chem* 55:submitted, 2005.

8. Bringhurst FR, Demay MB, Kronenberg HM: Hormones and disorders of mineral metabolism. In Larsen PR, Kroneberg HM, Melmed S, et al, editors: *Williams textbook of endocrinology,* ed 10, Philadelphia, 2003, WB Saunders.

TEST NAME AND METHOD	SPECIMEN REQUIREMENTS	REFERENCE INTERVAL, CONVENTIONAL [INTERNATIONAL RECOMMENDED UNITS]			CHEMICAL INTERFERENCES AND IN VIVO EFFECTS
Phytanic Acid[1,2] *GLC*[2]	Serum		*% of total serum fatty acids*	*Fraction of total serum fatty acids*	None found.
		Normal:	<0.3 × 0.01	[<0.003]	
		Borderline:	0.3-0.5	[0.003-0.005]	
		Suggestive of disease:	>0.5	[>0.005]	
Gas chromatography mass spectrometry[3]	Serum	*Age*			
		0-4 mo:	≤5.28 μmol/L		
		5-8 mo:	≤5.70 μmol/L		
		9-12 mo:	≤4.40 μmol/L		
		13-23 mo:	≤8.62 μmol/L		
		≥24 mo:	≤9.88 μmol/L		

1. Mayo Medical Laboratories: *Test catalog,* Rochester, MN, 1993, Mayo Medical Laboratories.

2. Nelson GJ, editor: *Blood lipids and lipoproteins: quantitation, composition and metabolism,* New York, 1972, Wiley-Interscience.

3. Lagerstedt SA, Hinrichs DR, Batt SM, et al: Quantitative determination of plasma c8-c26 total fatty acids for the biochemical diagnosis of nutritional and metabolic disorders, *Mol Genet Metab* 73:38-45, 2001.

4. Wanders RJA, Jakobs C, Skjeldal OH: In Scriver SC, Beaudet AL, Sly WS, et al, editors: *The metabolic & molecular bases of inherited disease,* ed 8, New York, 2001, McGraw-Hill, pp. 3303-3321.

5. Jansen GA, Waterham HR, Wanders RJ: Molecular basis of Refsum disease: sequence variations in phytanoyl-CoA hydroxylase (PHYH) and the PTS2 receptor (PEX7), *Hum Mutat* 23:209-218, 2004.

TEST NAME AND METHOD	SPECIMEN REQUIREMENTS	REFERENCE INTERVAL, CONVENTIONAL [INTERNATIONAL RECOMMENDED UNITS]		CHEMICAL INTERFERENCES AND IN VIVO EFFECTS
Pituitary Glycoprotein Hormones, α-Subunit (α-PGH)[1,2] *Immunoassay*	Serum. Stable 3 days at 4° C; for longer periods store frozen.	*Adult*[3] M: F: Premenopausal: Postmenopausal:	*ng/L* 70-450 50-460 290-1500	None found.

1. Demura R, Jibiki K, Kubo O, et al: The significance of α-subunit as a tumor marker for gonadotropin-producing adenomas, *J Clin Endocrinol Metab* 63:564-569, 1986.

2. Ishibashi M, Yamaji T, Takaku F, et al: Secretion of glycoprotein α-subunit by pituitary tumors, *J Clin Endocrinol Metab* 64:1187-1193, 1987.

3. Oppenheim D, Kana A, Sangha J, et al: Prevalence of α-subunit hypersecretion in patients with pituitary tumors: clinically nonfunctioning and somatotroph adenomas, *J Clin Endocrinol Metab* 70:859-864, 1990.

DIAGNOSTIC INFORMATION	REMARKS
↑ Refsum's disease, Zellweger syndrome, neonatal adrenoleukodystrophy, infantile Refsum's disease (a peroxisome biogenesis disorder), and rhizomelic chondrodysplasia punctata type I	Phytanic acid in serum is elevated in Refsum's disease as a result of a deficiency of phytanic acid α-oxidation. The enzymes involved have been discovered recently and include an acyl-CoA synthetase, phytanoyl-CoA hydroxylase, 2-hydroxyphytanoyl-CoA lyase, and an aldehyde dehydrogenase.[4,5] The molecular basis of Refsum's disease has been ascribed to sequence variations in two genes: phytanoyl-CoA hydroxylase and the PTS2 receptor.[5]
↑ Pituitary adenomas, choriocarcinoma, hydatidiform mole, pregnancy, and primary hypothyroidism	Test detects α-subunits of LH, FSH, TSH, and hCG. Intact hormones show little cross-reactivity. Measurement of free α-subunit may be useful in postoperative monitoring for tumor recurrence. Test may also be useful as a marker of tumor response to therapy.

TEST NAME AND METHOD	SPECIMEN REQUIREMENTS	REFERENCE INTERVAL, CONVENTIONAL [INTERNATIONAL RECOMMENDED UNITS]	CHEMICAL INTERFERENCES AND IN VIVO EFFECTS
Placental Alkaline Phosphatase (PLAP)[1] *IEMA*	Serum. Stable up to 4 wk at 2-8° C. For longer periods, freeze at −20° C or colder.	0-1.85 mcg/mL[2] × 1.0 [0-1.85 mg/L] (Values may be higher in smokers.)	

1. Millan JL, Stighrand T: Sandwich enzyme immunoassay for placental alkaline phosphalase, *Clin Chem* 27:2014-2018, 1981.
2. Lang PH, Millan JL, Stighrand T, et al: Placental alkaline phosphatase as a tumor marker for seminoma, *Cancer Res* 43:3244-3247, 1982.

TEST NAME AND METHOD	SPECIMEN REQUIREMENTS	REFERENCE INTERVAL, CONVENTIONAL [INTERNATIONAL RECOMMENDED UNITS]	CHEMICAL INTERFERENCES AND IN VIVO EFFECTS
Placental Lactogen (PL; Chorionic Somatomammotropin, CS)[1-4] *RIA*	Serum. Freeze immediately.	Male and nonpregnant female: Not detected Pregnancy, 5-38 wk: 0.5-11 mcg/Ml[6] [× 46.30 = 23-509 nmol/L]	None found.
	Amniotic fluid[5]		

	mcg/mL (x)		nmol/L (x)
<20 wk:	0.3-0.4	× 46.30	[14-18]
36-40 wk:	0.4-0.6		[18-28]

1. Ahmed M, Cemerikic B, Agbas A: Properties and functions of human placental opioid system, *Life Sci* 50:83-97, 1992.
2. Ashwood ER: Clinical chemistry of pregnancy. In Burtis CA, Ashwood ER, editors: *Tietz textbook of clinical chemistry,* ed 2, Philadelphia, 1994, WB Saunders.
3. Handwerger S: Clinical counterpoint: the physiology of placental lactogen in human pregnancy, *Endocr Rev* 12:329-336, 1991.
4. Zhang WY, Yen GL: Serum SP1, hPL, and beta-hCG levels in trophoblastic disease, *Clin Med J* 104:995-998, 1991.
5. Tulchinsky D, Ryan KJ, editors: *Maternal-fetal endocrinology,* Philadelphia, 1980, WB Saunders.
6. Specialty Laboratories, Inc.: *Test catalog,* Los Angeles, CA, 1988, Specialty Laboratories, Inc.
7. Cunningham FG, McDonald PC, Gant NF, editors: *Williams obstetrics,* ed 18, Norwalk, CT, 1989, Appleton & Lange.

DIAGNOSTIC INFORMATION	REMARKS

↑ 20% of women with breast or ovarian cancer. It has been proposed as an excellent marker to monitor patients with seminomas; elevations are seen in >50% of these patients.[1,2]

PLAP is the heat-stable, placental isoenzyme of alkaline phosphatase. The enzyme can be measured during pregnancy from the 12th wk of gestation. PLAP has an MW of 120,000 and is synthesized in the placental trophoblast.

S ↑ Trophoblastic tumors

S ↓ Hypertensive toxemia (decrease precedes abortion); low PL with normal or elevated urinary hCG after 8 wk of pregnancy is pathognomonic of molar pregnancy; <4 mcg/mL [<4 mg/L] after 30 wk indicates risk for the fetus; choriocarcinoma.

Higher values exist in multiple pregnancies, in diabetic patients, and in Rh incompatibility. Levels are related to placental and fetal weight. In the past, PL was used to evaluate fetal well-being, but currently the clinical value of PL is questionable.[7] (See *Estriol, Free;* and *Estriol, Total.*) PL is also produced by trophoblastic tumors; the greater the degree of malignancy, the lower the PL value in relation to hCG. For monitoring treatment, β-hCG is clearly superior.

AF ↑ Severe erythroblastosis fetalis (some reports)

PL amniotic fluid levels are 15-20-fold lower than those in maternal serum but are considerably higher than those found in umbilical cord blood. Although PL is known to be produced solely by the placenta, its route of entry into the amniotic fluid is unknown.

See also *Chorionic Gonadotropin, β-Subunit.*

TEST NAME AND METHOD	SPECIMEN REQUIREMENTS	REFERENCE INTERVAL, CONVENTIONAL [INTERNATIONAL RECOMMENDED UNITS]	CHEMICAL INTERFERENCES AND IN VIVO EFFECTS
Plasma Volume (PV)[1,2] *Most methods are based on dilution analysis of tracer molecules in the intravascular compartment. The gold standard method uses radiolabeled proteins, mostly [125]I- or ^{131}I-human serum albumin (HSA).*	*[125]I- or ^{131}I-Albumin method* After 15-min rest, sterilely collect whole blood using heparin anticoagulation. Add radiolabeled albumin to separated plasma and reinject. Take IV blood sample (heparin, EDTA) 10, 20, and 30 min after injection, and measure radioactivity.	40-50 mL/kg[1]	↑ *Plasma Volume* Anesthetic agents: Carbon dioxide, chloroform, halothane, morphine, spinal anesthesia (midthoracic), and thiopental; vasodilators ↓ *Plasma Volume* Vasoconstrictors
Methods using unlabeled colloids or small molecules, such as T-1824 (Evan's blue dye), that specifically and tightly bind to intravascular macromolecules are available. A rapid method that does not require blood sampling has also been described.[4]	*T-1824 (Evan's blue dye) method* Take blood sample (heparin, EDTA) 10 min after IV injection of a measured amount of T-1824; determine dye concentration in plasma.		

1. Lewis S, Bain B, Bates I, et al, editors: *Practical haematology,* ed 9, Edinburgh, 2001, Churchill Livingstone.
2. International Committee for Standardization in Haematology: Recommended methods for measurement of red-cell and plasma volume, *J Nucl Med* 21:793-800, 1980.
3. Margarson MP, Soni NC: Plasma volume measurement in septic patients using an albumin dilution technique: comparison with the standard radio-labelled albumin method, *Intensive Care Med* 31:289-295, 2005.
4. Haruna M, Kumon K, Yahagi N, et al: Blood volume measurement at the bedside using ICG pulse spectrophotometry, *Anesthesiology* 89:1322-1328, 1998.

TEST NAME AND METHOD	SPECIMEN REQUIREMENTS	REFERENCE INTERVAL, CONVENTIONAL [INTERNATIONAL RECOMMENDED UNITS]	CHEMICAL INTERFERENCES AND IN VIVO EFFECTS
Plasminogen[1,2]	Plasma (blue top-citrate); stable at room temperature for 8 hr. Typically a send-out test (submit frozen) to reference laboratory.	Functional (activity): 80-160% Immunoassay (antigen): <20 mg/dL Newborn levels are decreased compared with adult levels.	Bilirubinemia (in chromogenic substrate assay) ↓ V Alteplase (t-PA), streptokinase, and urokinase

DIAGNOSTIC INFORMATION	REMARKS

↑ Anemia, polycythemia, splenomegaly, emphysema, macroglobulinemia, myeloma (some), cardiac failure, cirrhosis, acidosis, thyrotoxicosis, vasodilation, overhydration, renal insufficiency, pregnancy (peak of 165% of normal in third trimester), and recumbency

↓ Smoking (probably includes stress erythrocytosis, spurious polycythemia), dehydration resulting from salt loss, preeclampsia, acute hemorrhage, chronic infection, vomiting, diarrhea, diabetes, old age, radiation, A-V fistula, tissue hypoxia, upright position (~10%), and confinement to bed (change greater in edematous than in normal subjects)

Both radiolabeled albumin and dye methods estimate plasma volume satisfactorily in healthy persons but overestimate it in many diseases because of loss of albumin from the vascular system. More variation occurs in reference values for PV in different series than for red cell volume, probably because PV is labile and varies with posture and because the quality of albumin used is not consistent.[2]

Recipients of [125]I- or ^{131}I-albumin should receive nonradioactive iodine to block uptake of radioactive iodine by the thyroid gland.

Unlabeled colloid or dye methods are preferred when the use of radioactive materials may not be justified.

↑ Acute phase reactant (infection, trauma, malignant disease, myocardial infarction); pregnancy (peak of 165% of normal level in third trimester)

↓ Rare cases of hereditary deficiency; thrombolytic therapy with streptokinase or urokinase; DIC; and severe liver disease

Plasminogen is a precursor of plasmin and a major component of the physiologic fibrinolytic system.

Heterozygous plasminogen deficiency has been reported in patients with thrombosis; the nature of this association is unclear; therefore routine evaluation of plasminogen for thrombosis is not recommended. Homozygous deficiency of plasminogen has been associated with ligneous conjunctivitis.

TEST NAME AND METHOD	SPECIMEN REQUIREMENTS	REFERENCE INTERVAL, CONVENTIONAL [INTERNATIONAL RECOMMENDED UNITS]	CHEMICAL INTERFERENCES AND IN VIVO EFFECTS
Plasminogen—CONT			

1. Lewis SM, Bain BJ, Bates I, editors: *Dacie and Lewis practical hematology,* ed 9, Edinburgh, 2001, Churchill Livingstone.
2. Brandt JT: Plasminogen and tissue-type plasminogen activator deficiency as risk factors for thromboembolic disease, *Arch Pathol Lab Med* 126:1376-1381, 2002.

TEST NAME AND METHOD	SPECIMEN REQUIREMENTS	REFERENCE INTERVAL, CONVENTIONAL [INTERNATIONAL RECOMMENDED UNITS]	CHEMICAL INTERFERENCES AND IN VIVO EFFECTS
Plasminogen Activator Inhibitor (PAI-1)[1,2]	Plasma (citrate). Centrifuge rapidly at 4° C to obtain platelet-poor plasma (platelets are a rich source of PAI-1). Stable at 4° C for 6 hr, at −20° C for 3 mo.	Reference intervals have been difficult to establish for the functional and antigenic assays. Each laboratory should establish its own range. Large diurnal variations of PAI-1 activity have been reported, morning values being about twofold higher than afternoon values. Functional: usually <15 IU/mL* × 1.0 [<15 kIU/L] Antigenic: generally 11-69 ng/mL *One International Unit (IU) of PAI-1 is defined as the amount that inhibits one unit of human t-PA international standard.	Antifibrinolytic agents: aprotinin and ε-aminocaproic acid Bilirubinemia (in chromogenic substrate assay), platelet contamination of plasma (in immunoassay)

1. Lewis SM, Bain BJ, Bates I, editors: *Dacie and Lewis practical hematology,* ed 9, Edinburgh, 2001, Churchill Livingstone.
2. Francis CW: Plasminogen activator inhibitor-1 levels and polymorphisms, *Arch Pathol Lab Med* 126:1401-1403, 2002.

TEST NAME AND METHOD	SPECIMEN REQUIREMENTS	REFERENCE INTERVAL, CONVENTIONAL [INTERNATIONAL RECOMMENDED UNITS]	CHEMICAL INTERFERENCES AND IN VIVO EFFECTS
Platelet Aggregation[1,2]	Platelet-rich plasma. Draw whole blood (citrate) into a plastic tube. Do not refrigerate. Obtain platelet-rich plasma by centrifuging at 100*g* for 10-15 min. Stable for 2 hr at room	Full aggregation (generally >60%) in response to ADP, collagen, epinephrine, thrombin, ristocetin, and arachidonic acid. The response may be biphasic (primary and secondary waves) or single phase, depending on different doses used for agonists (e.g., 0.5 μm, 2.5 μm, or 5 μm for ADP).	↑ Heparin, hemolysis, lipemia, and nicotine ↓ V Aspirin, azlocillin, captopril, carbamate, carbenicillin, chloroquine, chlorpromazine, clofibrate, cyproheptadine,

DIAGNOSTIC INFORMATION	REMARKS
	Plasminogen can be measured with a functional assay or antigenic (immunologic) assay. The functional (activity) is typically a chromogenic assay. A qualitative deficiency will not be detected with an antigenic assay.
↑ Acute phase reactant, myocardial infarction, deep vein thrombosis, sepsis, malignancy, hyperlipoproteinemia, hypertriglyceridemia, and pregnancy (in third trimester) ↓ Rare bleeding disorder resulting from hyperfibrinolysis secondary to PAI-1 deficiency	Plasminogen activator inhibitor-1 (PAI-1) is a glycoprotein in the normal fibrinolytic system. It is a potent inhibitor of tissue-plasminogen activator (t-PA) and urokinase plasminogen activator (u-PA). A deficiency or excess of PAI-1 has been associated with either bleeding or thrombosis, respectively. The predictive value of a high PAI-1 is uncertain, and there are insufficient data to recommend PAI-1 in evaluating thrombophilia. PAI-1 is a rarely performed test for investigation of the fibrinolytic system. PAI-1 *activity* is measured by a functional chromogenic test. The PAI-1 *antigen* is measured by ELISA. Because PAI-1 may be free or t-PA bound, reference ranges have been difficult to establish.
An abnormal platelet aggregation study may be associated with hereditary and acquired disorders of platelet adhesion, activation, and aggregation. Interpretation of an abnormal profile should be done with caution since several factors (e.g., aspirin, garlic) may interfere with this test. *Glanzmann's thrombasthenia:* Lack of glycoprotein IIb/IIIa; absent aggregation with ADP, collagen, epinephrine, and thrombin; normal agglutination with ristocetin	Platelet aggregation studies evaluate qualitative (functional) platelet disorders. These may include hereditary or acquired disorders of platelet adhesion, activation/release, or aggregation and are generally associated with variable degrees of bleeding. This study is usually performed after screening tests for bleeding disorders (PT, PTT, platelet count, vWD workup) are normal.

TEST NAME AND METHOD	SPECIMEN REQUIREMENTS	REFERENCE INTERVAL, CONVENTIONAL [INTERNATIONAL RECOMMENDED UNITS]	CHEMICAL INTERFERENCES AND IN VIVO EFFECTS
Platelet Aggregation—CONT	temperature. Must perform as soon as possible. A specimen received on ice or more than 2 hr after collection is inadequate.		dextran, dipyridamole, diuretics, flufenamic acid, hydroxychloroquine, isosorbide dinitrate, mezlocillin, moxalactam, nifedipine, nitofurantoin, nonsteroidal antiinflammatory agents (e.g., diclofenac, fenoprofen, ibuprofen, indomethacin, ketoprofen, meclofenamate, mefenamic acid, naproxen, phenylbutazone, piroxicam, sulindac, tolmetin, zomepirac), penicillin, phentolamine, piperacillin, promethazine, propranolol, prostaglandin E_1, pyridinol, sulfinpyrazone, ticarcillin, tricyclic antidepressants, and volatile general anesthetics (e.g., methoxyflurane, halothane, nitrous oxide); thrombocytopenia

1. Lewis SM, Bain BJ, Bates I, editors: *Dacie and Lewis practical hematology,* ed 9, Edinburgh, 2001, Churchill Livingstone.
2. Jacobs DS, Demott WR, Oxley DK, editors: *Laboratory test handbook,* ed 5, Hudson, OH, 2001, Lexi-Comp, Inc.

TEST NAME AND METHOD	SPECIMEN REQUIREMENTS	REFERENCE INTERVAL, CONVENTIONAL [INTERNATIONAL RECOMMENDED UNITS]	CHEMICAL INTERFERENCES AND IN VIVO EFFECTS
Platelet Antibodies[1-4]	Dependent on methodology. Generally whole blood at room temperature. Do not separate plasma or freeze.	Depending on methodology used.	Samples from patients with platelet counts <10,000/µL may be difficult to process.

DIAGNOSTIC INFORMATION	REMARKS

Bernard-Soulier syndrome: Lack of glycopretein Ib; normal aggregation with ADP, collagen, and epinephrine; lack of agglutination with ristocetin. Unlike von Willebrand's disease, agglutination with ristocetin is not corrected on addition of normal plasma.

Storage pool deficiency (Chédiak-Higashi syndrome, glycogen storage disease type I, gray platelet syndrome, Hemansky-Pudlak syndrome, TAR syndrome, Wiskott-Aldrich syndrome): Platelet aggregation may be abnormal with variable-decreased epinephrine and ADP (frequently because of absence or decrease in secondary ADP release).

Cyclooxygenase deficiency: Abnormal platelet aggregation caused by the inability to activate prostaglandin pathway; aspirin-like defect.

von Willebrand's disease: Normal aggregation with ADP, collagen, and epinephrine; absent or reduced agglutination with ristocetin (except in type IIB where abnormal agglutination with a low concentration of ristocetin occurs).

Acquired disorders of platelets also affect the platelet aggregation studies: uremia, paraproteinemia, and DIC, collagen-vascular disorders (Marfan's syndrome, osteogenesis imperfecta), and myeloproliferative disorders (essential thrombocythemia, polycythemia vera, CML).

Functional platelet disorders can be differentiated by the use of several aggregating agents, typically epinephrine, ADP, arachidonic acid, collagen, and ristocetin. Because aggregation is dependent on platelet count, the platelet count should be >100,000.

Drugs, typically aspirin, nonsteroidal antiinflammatory drugs, and platelet-inhibiting medications, are the most common cause of an abnormal platelet aggregation study: the patient should refrain from taking aspirin within 7-10 days of the test.

Interpretation of a platelet aggregation study is difficult and should always be interpreted in the context of the patient's clinical history. Otherwise normal individuals may have "abnormal" profiles (e.g., some individual's platelets do not aggregate with epinephrine).

Electron microscopy may be necessary for assessment of granular content. Newer methods for assessment of platelet function are also available, including the PFA-100, an automated whole blood platelet function analyzer, and flow cytometry.

Autoantibodies measured as IgG occur in >90% of patients with chronic ITP.

Note: Patients with nonimmune thrombocytopenias may have false-positive results.

Platelet antibodies may be alloimmune or autoimmune. Clinically significant platelet alloantibodies include those associated with neonatal immune thrombocytopenia, posttransfusion purpura, and platelet refractoriness caused by HLA antibodies. Idiopathic thrombocytopenic purpura (ITP) is associated with autoimmune platelet antibodies.

Alloantibodies are most commonly directed at the human platelet antigen referred to as HPA-1a (also known as PI^{A1}). In contrast, ITP autoantibodies typically target platelet glycoproteins IIb/IIIa (CD41) or less commonly Ib/IX (CD42).

Several methods with variable sensitivity and specificity are available, and no method detects all antibodies. Routine use of

TEST NAME AND METHOD	SPECIMEN REQUIREMENTS	REFERENCE INTERVAL, CONVENTIONAL [INTERNATIONAL RECOMMENDED UNITS]	CHEMICAL INTERFERENCES AND IN VIVO EFFECTS
Platelet Antibodies—CONT			

1. Lewis SM, Bain BJ, Bates I, editors: *Dacie and Lewis practical hematology,* ed 9, Edinburgh, 2001, Churchill Livingstone.
2. Cines DB, Blanchette VS: Immune thombocytopenic purpura, *N Engl J Med* 346:995-1008, 2002.
3. Guidelines for the investigation and management of idiopathic thrombocytopenia purpura in adults, children, and in pregnancy, *Br J Haematol* 120:574-596, 2003.
4. Fabris F, Scandellari R, Ruzzon E, et al: Platelet-associated autoantibodies as detected by a solid-phase modified antigen capture ELISA test (MACE) are a useful prognostic factor in idiopathic thrombocytopenic purpura, *Blood* 103:4562-4564, 2004.

TEST NAME AND METHOD	SPECIMEN REQUIREMENTS	REFERENCE INTERVAL, CONVENTIONAL [INTERNATIONAL RECOMMENDED UNITS]	CHEMICAL INTERFERENCES AND IN VIVO EFFECTS
Platelet Function Analyzer (PFA-100 Analyzer)[1]	Whole blood sample (citrate)	Results reported as *closure time (CT)*. Each laboratory should determine its own reference interval. Reference interval with collagen-epinephrine test cartridges: 80-169 sec Reference interval with collagen-ADP test cartridges: 58-119 sec	Any medication capable of interacting with platelet aggregation (see platelet aggregation section).

1. Fressinaud E, Veyradier A, Truchaud F, et al: Screening for von Willebrand disease with a new analyzer using high shear stress: a study of 60 cases, *Blood* 91:1325-1331, 1998.

DIAGNOSTIC INFORMATION	REMARKS

these platelet antibody assays is generally not recommended; in selected cases (i.e., refractory ITP) these studies may be of value.

A direct assay for the measurement of platelet-bound antibodies is more informative than detection of unbound plasma antibody. A combination of a sensitive binding assay such as a platelet immunofluorescence test (PIFT) along with an antigen capture immunoassay is recommended. The PIFT can be measured by fluorescence microscopy or flow cytometry and will detect platelet-associated immunoglobulins (commonly IgG in autoimmune thrombocytopenia). An antigen capture immunoassay (monoclonal antibody immobilization of platelet antigens) may differentiate between platelet-specific antibodies (anti-HPA) and HLA antibodies or detect platelet-specific glycoproteins. ELISA kits are also available that will detect specific antibodies against platelet glycoproteins or HLA class I antigens.

Molecular genotyping by PCR analysis is also available for identifying polymorphism of platelet glycoproteins.

↑ von Willebrand disease (except type 2N); other hereditary or acquired platelet function disorders

The PFA-100 test system allows for a rapid and simple assessment of platelet function in primary hemostasis.

The system comprises disposable test cartridges and an analyzer. An aliquot of whole blood is aspirated into a capillary system under high shear stress, simulating a damaged blood vessel wall. The system measures the ability of platelets to occlude an aperture in a biologically active membrane treated with collagen and ADP or collagen and epinephrine.

The PFA-100 is a more sensitive test than the bleeding time for the screening of patients with vWD.

TEST NAME AND METHOD	SPECIMEN REQUIREMENTS	REFERENCE INTERVAL, CONVENTIONAL [INTERNATIONAL RECOMMENDED UNITS]	CHEMICAL INTERFERENCES AND IN VIVO EFFECTS
Platelet Genotyping (Platelet-specific Antigen or Human Platelet Antigen [HPA] Genotyping)[1-4] Polymerase chain reaction (PCR)-based tests	Whole blood (EDTA). Transport at 2-8° C.	Not applicable.	PCR inhibition by anticoagulants (heparin, EDTA)

1. Davoren A, Curtis BP, Aster RH, et al: Human platelet antigen-specific alloantibodies implicated in 1162 cases of neonatal alloimmune thrombocytopenia, *Transfusion* 44:1220-1225, 2004.
2. Goldman M, Trudel E, Richard L: Report on the Eleventh International Society of Blood Transfusion Platelet Genotyping and Serology Workshop, *Vox Sang* 85:149-155, 2003.
3. Hurd CM, Cavanagh G, Schuh A, et al: Genotyping for platelet-specific antigens: techniques for the detection of single nucleotide polymorphisms, *Vox Sang* 83:1-12, 2002.
4. Randen I, Sorensen K, Killie MK, et al: Rapid and reliable genotyping of human platelet antigen (HPA)-1, -2, -3, -4, and -5 a/b and Gov a/b by melting curve analysis, *Transfusion* 43:445-450, 2003.

Pleural Effusion (PE) Analysis[1,2]	Aspirate. Collect 5 mL in EDTA tube for cell counts and remainder in heparin tube for microbiology and chemistry.					Traumatic tap

		Transudate	*Exudate*	*Transudate*	*Exudate*
Clarity		Clear	Cloudy		
Color		Straw	Yellow or red		
Cell counts					
WBC (/μL)		<1000	>1000	×0.001 [<1 × 10^9/L]	[>1 × 10^9/L]
RBC (/μL)		<1000	>100,000	×0.001 [<1 × 10^9/L]	[>100 × 10^9/L]
Chemistry					
Protein (PE/serum)		≤0.5	>0.5	×100 [≤50%]	[>50%]
LDH (PE/serum)		≤0.45	>0.45	×100 [≤45%]	[>45%]
Chol. (mg/dL)		≤45	>45	×0.026 [≤1.2 mmol/L]	[>1.2 mmol/L]

ULN, Upper limit of normal for serum; *LDH,* lactate dehydrogenase.

1. Clarke W, Palmer-Toy DE: Clinical chemistry of urine, pleural effusions, and ascites. In Lewandrowski KB, editor: *Clinical chemistry,* Philadelphia, 2002, Lippincott Williams & Wilkins, pp. 849-864.
2. Light RW, Macgregor MI, Luchsinger PC, et al: Pleural effusions: the diagnostic separation of transudates and exudates, *Ann Intern Med* 77:507-513, 1972.

DIAGNOSTIC INFORMATION	REMARKS
Determination of human platelet antigen genotype offers a reliable alternative to serologic phenotyping. The test is most widely used in the evaluation of neonatal alloimmune thrombocytopenia. Other indications are posttransfusion purpura and platelet refractoriness caused by antibodies directed against platelet-specific antigens.	Platelet genotyping has largely replaced determination of platelet antigens by serological methods. Advantages of genotyping methods are that they can be readily performed in situations where serotyping cannot be used or is of limited utility, such as in typing for HPAs for which reliable serotyping reagents are rare, in thrombocytopenic states, in the presence of HLA class I antibodies, and in prenatal testing.

Alternative Criteria for Exudates:
1. LDH $>0.45\times$ ULN or PE LDH/serum LDH >0.6 or PE protein/serum protein >0.5
2. LDH $>0.45\times$ ULN or chol. >0.45 mg/dL
3. LDH $>0.45\times$ ULN or chol. >0.45 mg/dL or protein >2.9 g/dL

Any combination above has sensitivity $\cong 97\%$ and specificity $\cong 70\%$.[3]

Primary goal to distinguish exudates (e.g., infectious, malignant, drug reactions) from transudates (e.g., congestive heart failure, cirrhosis, atelectasis, nephrotic syndrome).

Etiology can be determined in 75% of cases. Diagnosing infectious etiology is most important.

pH <7.2 warrants urgent drainage of infectious effusion.

---

3. Heffner JE, Brown LK, Barbieri CA: Diagnostic value of tests that discriminate between exudative and transudative pleural effusions, *Chest* 11:970-980, 1997.

TEST NAME AND METHOD	SPECIMEN REQUIREMENTS	REFERENCE INTERVAL, CONVENTIONAL [INTERNATIONAL RECOMMENDED UNITS]		CHEMICAL INTERFERENCES AND IN VIVO EFFECTS
Polybrominated Biphenyls (PBB) and Polybrominated Diphenyl Esters (PBDE)[1]	Serum	Negative	*mg/L*	None found.
		Michigan residents, 1977:	<0.1	
		After exposure:	<1.5	
GC-ECD,[2] *GC-MS*[3]	Adipose tissue	Negative	*mg/kg*	
		Urban Michigan residents, 1975:	0.226	
		Rural Michigan residents, nonquarantined, 1975:	0.516	
		Rural Michigan residents, quarantined, 1975:	2.0	

1. Baselt RC: *Biological monitoring methods for industrial chemicals,* Davis, CA, 1980, Biomedical Pub.
2. Burse VM, Needham LL, Liddle JA: Interlaboratory comparison for results of analyses for polybrominated biphenyls in human serum, *J Anal Toxicol* 4:22-26, 1980.
3. Lewis RG, Sovocool GW: Identification of polybrominated biphenyls in the adipose tissues of the general population of the United States, *J Anal Toxicol* 6:196-198, 1982.
4. Darnerud PO, Eriksen GS, Johannesson T, et al: Polybrominated diphenyl ethers: occurrence, dietary exposure, and toxicology, *Environ Health Perspect* 109(suppl 1):49-68, 2001.

Polychlorinated Biphenyls (PCB)[1]	Plasma	<0.029 mg/L	Other organochlorine compounds may interfere.
		Toxic concentration[4]: >0.2 mg/L	Most interference can be removed by Florisil col-
GC-ECD,[2] *GC-MS*[3]	Adipose tissue	<2 mg/kg	umn chromatography.

1. Baselt RC, Cravey RH: *Disposition of toxic drugs and chemicals in man,* ed 3, Chicago, 1989, Year Book Medical Publishers, Inc., pp. 702-703.
2. Chen PH, Gaw JM, Wong CK, et al: Levels of gas chromatographic patterns of polychlorinated biphenyls in the blood of patients after PCB poisoning in Taiwan, *Bull Environ Contam Toxicol* 25:325-329, 1980.
3. Biros FJ, Walker AC, Medbery A: Polychlorinated biphenyls in human adipose tissue, *Bull Environ Contam Toxicol* 5:317-323, 1970.
4. Lauwerys RR: *Industrial chemical exposure. Guidelines for biological monitoring,* Davis, CA, 1983, Biomedical Pub.

DIAGNOSTIC INFORMATION	REMARKS

Toxic exposure may cause fatigue, joint pain, dizziness, and skin eruptions. Serum concentrations >0.001 mg/L are associated with a 14% incidence of increased ALT (SGPT). Increased urinary porphyrin excretion has also been correlated with elevated serum PBBs.

Four epidemiologic studies have been conducted on workers at facilities where flame-retardant polymers were extruded. The workers were potentially exposed to brominated flame retardants, including PBDEs. These studies found no adverse effects attributable to exposure to these chemicals.[4]

PBBs are highly lipophilic. Excretion is slow (0.1% in urine and 6.6% in feces over 42 days). PBBs and PBDEs are fire retardants. Widespread contamination occurred in Michigan in 1975.

Toxic exposure causes local skin irritation leading to chloracne and neurological manifestations, including headache, nervousness, fatigue, and dizziness. Elevation in AST (SGOT) has been reported. PCBs accumulate in fish.

PCBs are highly lipophilic. The rate of elimination is a function of the metabolic rate, which in turn depends on the extent of chlorination. Highly chlorinated derivatives are extremely long lived. PCBs were formerly widely used in industry as coolant and insulator fluids, but their manufacture in the U.S. was halted in 1977. Electrical devices manufactured before 1977 may contain PCBs, and the compounds are a common environmental contaminant because of historically heavy industrial usage.

TEST NAME AND METHOD	SPECIMEN REQUIREMENTS	REFERENCE INTERVAL, CONVENTIONAL [INTERNATIONAL RECOMMENDED UNITS]			CHEMICAL INTERFERENCES AND IN VIVO EFFECTS
Porphobilinogen (PBG) *Colorimetric (Watson-Schwartz)*[1,2] *(qual.)*	Urine, fresh random. Collect during or immediately after episode of abdominal pain. Stable at 4° C for 1-2 wk, and at −20° C for several weeks.	Negative			↑ V Drugs that precipitate acute porphyria, see Table I-10.[11] ↑ C Urobilinogen, and phenazopyridine HCl if test not properly performed ↓ V Cisplatin (high dose)
Hoesch (qual.)[3]		Negative			↓ C Indolic compounds (indole, indican, 5-hydroxyindoleacetic acid), methyldopa, and phenazopyridine HCl ↓ V Cisplatin (high dose)
Spectrophotometry (quant.)[4,5]	Urine, 24 hr. Collect in dark container with 5 g of Na_2CO_3. Refrigerate. Specimen is also suited for porphyrias. If no Na_2CO_3 is added, urine can also be used for ALA determination.	<2.0 mg/L[7] <2.7 mg/day[8]	× 4.42	[<8.8 μmol/L] [<15.0 μmol/day] <11.0 μmol/day[9]	↑ C Phenothiazines ↓ V Cisplatin (high dose)
Liquid chromatography tandem mass spectrometry (LC-MS/MS) (quant.)[6]	Urine, fresh random. Or 24 hr collected in dark container with 5 g of Na_2CO_3. Stable at −20° C for several weeks.	≤0.5 mg/g creatinine[10] ≤0.5 mg/24 hr[6,10]		[≤2.2 μmol/24 hr]	

1. Watson CJ, Schwartz S: A simple test for urinary porphobilinogen, *Proc Soc Exp Biol Med* 47:393, 1941.

2. Watson CJ, Taddeini L, Bossenmaier I: Present status of the Erlich aldehyde reaction for urinary porphobilinogen, *JAMA* 190:501, 1964.

3. Lamon J, With TK, Redeker AG: The Hoesch test: bedside screening for urinary porphobilinogen in patients with suspected porphyria, *Clin Chem* 20:1438-1440, 1974.

4. Buttery JE, Chamberlain BR, Beng CG: Assessment of two anion-exchange resins for direct use in the screening method for urinary porphobilinogen, *Clin Chem* 36:584, 1990.

5. Buttery JE, Stuart S: Measurement of porphobilinogen in urine by a simple resin method with use of a surrogate standard, *Clin Chem* 37:2133-2136, 1991.

6. Ford RE, Magera MJ, Kloke KM, et al: Quantitative measurement of porphobilinogen in urine by stable-isotope dilution liquid chromatography-tandem mass spectrometry, *Clin Chem* 47:1627-1632, 2001.

7. Laboratory Corporation of America: *Test catalog,* Burlington, NC, 2003, Laboratory Corporation of America.

DIAGNOSTIC INFORMATION	REMARKS

↑ During crisis in acute hepatic porphyrias (acute intermittent, variegate, and hereditary coproporphyria), may be slightly elevated in porphyria cutanea tarda.

See Table II-9.

Porphobilinogen (PBG) excretion in urine increases in acute porphyric attacks, and the measurement of PBG is particularly important in diagnosing the acute porphyrias (acute intermittent porphyria, hereditary coproporphyria, and variegate porphyria) during the acute stage. Markedly increased urine PBG is diagnostic for acute porphyria.[6] A qualitative test on random urine during the attack is the most common test used for diagnosis. However, the qualitative test should be confirmed with the quantitative test, performed on 24 hr urine, and by measuring porphyrins. If the diagnosis of acute porphyria remains a possibility, the quantitative test should be performed even in face of a negative qualitative test.

Porphobilinogen quantitation by LC-MS/MS is both sensitive and specific. Mild PBG elevations can be detected between acute events in AIP. Mild PBG elevations (3.0-15 mg/24 hr) can be observed in affected yet asymptomatic (never had symptoms) postpubertal family members of patients with diagnosed AIP. This test has become very useful in family studies, identifying asymptomatic individuals who can be counseled to avoid substances/conditions known to precipitate acute episodes.

8. Nichols Institute Reference Laboratories/Quest Diagnostics: *Test catalog,* San Juan Capistrano, CA, 2004, Nichols Institute Reference Laboratories/Quest Diagnostics.

9. ARUP: *Test catalog,* Salt Lake City, UT, 2004, ARUP.

10. Mayo Medical Laboratories: *Test catalog,* Rochester, MN, 2004, Mayo Medical Laboratories.

11. Kappas A, Sassa S, Galbrait RA, et al: The porphyrias. In Scriver CR, Beaudet AL, Sly WS, et al, editors: *The metabolic basis of inherited disease,* ed 6, New York, 1989, McGraw-Hill, Inc.

TEST NAME AND METHOD	SPECIMEN REQUIREMENTS	REFERENCE INTERVAL, CONVENTIONAL [INTERNATIONAL RECOMMENDED UNITS]		CHEMICAL INTERFERENCES AND IN VIVO EFFECTS
Porphobilinogen (PBG) Deaminase (PBG Uroporphyrinogen I synthase, Hydroxymethylbilane synthase; EC 4.3.1.8)[1-3] *Fluorimetric*[4-6]	Erythrocytes. Collect whole blood (heparin; avoid potassium oxalate). Erythrocytes should be washed three times with cold saline, volume recorded, and shipped frozen. A control may be requested.	$\geq$7.0 nmol/sec/L 0.080-0.238 nmol/hr/mg protein or $\approx$100% control sample activity *nmol/hr/mL* 20.9-42.2 30.0-73.7	$\times$ 0.278	*nmol/sec/L* [5.8-11.7] [8.3-20.5]	$\downarrow$ C In vitro: Lead, mercury

1. Batlle A: Porphobilinogen deaminase: accumulation and detection of tetrapyrrole intermediates using enzyme immobilization, *Methods Enzymol* 354:368-380, 2002.
2. Ellefson RD: Porphyrinogens, porphyrins, and the porphyrias, *Mayo Clin Proc* 57:454-458, 1982.
3. Anderson KE, Sassa S, Bishop DF, et al: Disorders of heme biosynthesis: X-linked sideroblastic anemia and the porphyrias. In Scriver SC, Beaudet AL, Sly WS, et al, editors: *The metabolic & molecular bases of inherited disease,* ed 8, New York, 2001, McGraw-Hill, pp. 2991-3062.
4. Ford RE, Ou CN, Ellefson RD: Assay for erythrocyte uroporphyrinogen I synthase activity, with porphobilinogen as substrate, *Clin Chem* 26:1182-1185, 1980.
5. Hsiao KJ, Lee FY, Wu SJ, et al: Determination of erythrocyte porphobilinogen deaminase activity using porphobilinogen as substrate, *Clin Chim Acta* 168:257-258, 1987.
6. Erlandsen EJ, Jorgensen PE, Markussen S, et al: Determination of porphobilinogen deaminase activity in human erythrocytes: pertinent factors in obtaining optimal conditions for measurements, *Scand J Clin Lab Invest* 60:627-634, 2000.

Porphyrins[1-4] *Fluorimetric (qual.)*	Urine, fresh random.[6] Collect in dark container and store at 4-8° C.	Negative or trace	$\uparrow$ V The most common cause of increased urine porphyrin concentration is coproporphyrinuria, which occurs secondary to liver dysfunction, ethanol intake, drug therapy, heavy metal intoxication, and a number of other miscellaneous conditions.[1] Drugs that precipitate acute porphyrias[2] can also increase porphyrins in unaffected individuals. (Table II-10).
	Feces, pea-sized solid sample.[5,6] Protect from light.	Negative or trace	
	Plasma (heparin).[7] Separate from cells; avoid hemolysis.	No emission peak at 626 nm, with excitation at 405 nm.	

DIAGNOSTIC INFORMATION	REMARKS

↓ Acute intermittent porphyria (AIP)

See also Table II-9.

AIP is an autosomal dominant acute hepatic porphyria that results from 50% decrease in activity of the PBG-D enzyme. Approximately 5% of patients with AIP will have normal PBG-D activity. The PBG deaminase assay can be used to confirm the diagnosis of AIP based on biochemical findings and to differentiate AIP from other acute porphyrias (variegate and hereditary coproporphyria). There is genetic heterogeneity in AIP mutations, but most appear to lead to decreased erythrocyte PBG deaminase activity and similar clinical presentations. The assay can be used to identify family members with genetic defect and latent symptoms (for genetic counseling and avoidance of precipitating drugs); however, young erythrocytes (accelerated hematopoiesis) have higher enzyme activity that could mask the diagnosis.

There are · 170 different mutations in the PBGD gene. Molecular testing may be performed on families in which a diagnosis of AIP has been confirmed.

The porphyrias are uncommon disorders of the heme biosynthesis. However, because the clinical features of the porphyrias are wide and variable, they are included in the differential diagnosis of many diseases. Therefore acute care hospital laboratories should have available simple and reliable methods to exclude the porphyrias and to identify individuals who need more specialized methods for investigation of porphyria.[1] Please also refer to the sections on porphobilinogen and aminolevulinic acid testing. See Table II-9.

Use of qualitative porphyrin tests for urine and feces is not recommended because of their inaccuracies and the simplicity of quantitative fluorometric screening tests (see below).[5,8]

Screening plasma specimens fluorimetrically for protoporphyrin-protein complexes can be helpful in differentiating variegate porphyria (VP) from other porphyrias.[2] The complex of variegate porphyria, excited at 405 nm, has an emission peak at 626 nm. Plasma fluorescence seen in porphyria cutanea tarda (PCT), acute intermittent porphyria (AIP), and hereditary coproporphyria (HCP), excited at 398 nm, has an emission peak at 619 nm; plasma fluorescence in protoporphyria, excited at 409 nm, has a peak at 634 nm.

TEST NAME AND METHOD	SPECIMEN REQUIREMENTS	REFERENCE INTERVAL, CONVENTIONAL [INTERNATIONAL RECOMMENDED UNITS]			CHEMICAL INTERFERENCES AND IN VIVO EFFECTS

Porphyrins—CONT

TEST NAME AND METHOD	SPECIMEN REQUIREMENTS	REFERENCE INTERVAL, CONVENTIONAL [INTERNATIONAL RECOMMENDED UNITS]			CHEMICAL INTERFERENCES AND IN VIVO EFFECTS
Spectrophotometry or fluorimetry (quant.) "Screening" or "First-line" tests[5]	Urine, 24 hr.[5,9,10] Collect in dark container with 5 g of Na_2CO_3. Refrigerate.	Total porphyrins: 20-320 nmol/L[5] Uroporphyrin fraction: <33 mcg/day 17-52 mcg/day	× 1.2	[<40 nmol/day][5,6] [20-62 nmol/day][10]	↑ C For possible technical interferences with each method, see Elder et al.[5]
		Coproporphyrin fraction: <183 mcg/day <204 mcg/day 52-163 mcg/day	× 1.53	[<280 nmol/day][5] [<450 nmol/day][6] [80-250 nmol/day][10]	↓ C If specimen is not extracted into acid or has been diluted.[5] U ↓ V Cisplatin (high dose)
	Feces, fresh random, 5-10 g.[11] Should not be liquid. Stable for 36 hr at 25° C and for several months frozen.	Total porphyrins: <200 nmol/g dry weight[11]			
	Whole blood (heparin or EDTA).[5,12] Stable at 4° C for up to 5 days.	0.4-1.7 mmol/L[5] <1.0 μmol/L[6] Total porphyrins: <60 mcg/dL[12]	× 10	[<600 mcg/L]	
	Plasma (heparin).[4] Store frozen, protected from light.	Total plasma porphyrins: <1 mcg/dL	× 10	[<10 mcg/L]	
Fluorimetric, HPLC (quant.)[5]	Urine, 24 hr.[13,14] Collect in dark container with 5 g of Na_2CO_3. Refrigerate.	Uroporphyrins: *Octacarboxyl* <20 mcg/L 3-25 mcg/day	× 1.2	[<24 nmol/L][5] [4-30 nmol/day][4]	↓ C Loss of analyte because of adhesion to precipitates in acid urine[15] or caused by pH and matrix problems[16] has been reported for HPLC methods
		Heptacarboxyl <3 mcg/L 0-7 mcg/day	× 1.27	[<4 nmol/L][5] [0-9 nmol/day][4]	
		Hexacarboxyl <2 mcg/L 0-6 mcg/day	× 1.34	[<3 nmol/L][5] [0-8 nmol/day][4]	
		Pentacarboxyl <3 mcg/L 0-7 mcg/day	× 1.43	[<5 nmol/L][6] [0-10 nmol/day][4]	
		Coproporphyrin: *Tetracarboxyl* 15-75 mg/L M: 25-150 mcg/day F: 8-110 mcg/day	× 1.53	[23-115 nmol/L][5] [38-229 nmol/day][4] [12-168 nmol/day]	

DIAGNOSTIC INFORMATION	REMARKS

See Table II-9.

"First-line" screening tests for porphyrins are generally quantitative, but they do not identify individual porphyrin species or isomers. There are numerous published methods, and some of the most commonly used ones are referenced. All are rapid and convenient. However, because there is never a need to determine porphyrins urgently, as there is for porphobilinogen in the acute porphyrias (see *Porphobilinogen*), an argument can be made that fractionation and quantitation of individual porphyrin species with HPLC methods is the best way to "screen" for disorders in porphyrin metabolism (see below).

For whole blood, the determination of total porphyrin includes both Zn-protoporphyrin (Zn-PP) and nonchelated or "free" protoporphyrin within the erythrocytes. If the total is elevated, then the gentler ethanol extraction method[17] differentiates Zn-PP from protoporphyrin IX. This will allow diagnosis of protoporphyria (no increase in Zn-PP). HPLC fractionation of protoporphyrins from washed Ercs can also be performed[4] to quantitate free and zinc protoporphyrin.

See Table II-9.

The interpretation of porphyrin elevations in urine and stool is complex. Patients with symptoms suggestive of the clinical porphyrias should be referred to an expert to avoid misdiagnosis, which is very common. Generally the porphyrias show marked elevations of particular heme precursors in particular fluids or tissues; the pattern and character of these elevations can aid in reaching a correct diagnosis. Minor elevations in urinary or stool porphyrins are usually nonspecific findings but often cause physicians who are not expert to label their difficult patients with a diagnosis of one of the rare porphyrias. Although reference intervals are cited, the degree of porphyrin elevation varies considerably.

Quantitative analysis of fecal porphyrins may be particularly helpful if porphyrin isomers are separated and separately quantitated.[3] Fecal porphyrin analysis in this manner can distinguish between the acute porphyrias, with values being normal to mildly elevated in AIP, whereas HCP has elevated coproporphyrins with and increased coproporphyrin III to copropoprhyrin I ratio (ratio 10-20:1 with normal ratio <1.2:1), and VP with increased coproporphyrins and protoporphyrins (protoporphryin exceeding coproporphyrin) and an elevated coproporphyrin III:1 ratio (ratio 5-10:1).

TEST NAME AND METHOD	SPECIMEN REQUIREMENTS	REFERENCE INTERVAL, CONVENTIONAL [INTERNATIONAL RECOMMENDED UNITS]	CHEMICAL INTERFERENCES AND IN VIVO EFFECTS

Porphyrins—CONT

| | Feces, 24 hr.[11,14] Weigh and homogenize. Ship aliquot frozen. | Uroporphyrins: Uroporphryin I
 <120 mcg/day   × 1.2   [<144 nmol/day][4]
 Uroporphyrin III
 <50 mcg/day   [<60 nmol/day]
 <2% of total porphyrins
 (10-200 nmol/g dry wt.)[5]

 Coproporphyrins:
 Coproporphyrin I
 <500 mcg/day   × 1.53   [<765 nmol/day][4]
 Coproporphyrin III
 <400 mcg/day   [<612 nmol/day]
 2-33% of total porphyrins[5]

 Protoporphyrins:
 Protoporphyrin IX
 <1500 mcg/day   × 1.78   [<2670 nmol/day][4]
 60-98% of total porphyrins[5] | |

1. Deacon AC, Elder GH: ACP Best Practice No. 165: front line tests for the investigation of suspected porphyria, *J Clin Pathol* 54:500-507, 2001.

2. Anderson KE, Sussa S, Bishop DF, et al: Disorders of heme biosynthesis: X-linked sideroblastic anemia and the porphyrias. In Scriver SC, Beaudet AL, Sly WS, et al, editors: *The metabolic & molecular bases of inherited disease,* ed 8, New York, 2001, McGraw-Hill, pp. 2991-3062.

3. Kauppinen R: Porphyrias, *Lancet* 365:241-252, 2005.

4. Mayo Medical Laboratories: *Test catalog,* Rochester, MN, 2005, Mayo Medical Laboratories.

5. Elder GH, Smith SG, Smyth SJ: Laboratory investigation of the porphyrias, *Ann Clin Biochem* 27:395-412, 1990.

6. Moore MR, Smith SG, Smyth SJ, et al: Laboratory investigation of the porphyrias. In *Disorders of porphyrin metabolism. Topics in hematology series,* New York, 1987, Plenum Press.

7. Poh-Fitzpatrick MB: A plasma porphyrin fluorescence marker for variegate porphyria, *Arch Dermatol* 116:543-547, 1980.

8. Deacon AC: Performance of screening tests for porphyria, *Ann Clin Biochem* 24:392-397, 1988.

9. Valcarcel M, Gomez Hens A, Rubio S, et al: Direct quantification of coproporphyrins and uroporphyrins in urine by derivative synchronous fluorescence spectroscopy, *Clin Chem* 33:1826-1831, 1987.

10. Westerlund J, Pudek M, Schreiber WE: A rapid and accurate spectrofluorometric method for quantification and screening of urinary porphyrins, *Clin Chem* 34:345-351, 1988.

11. Lockwood WH, Poulos V, Rossi E, et al: Rapid procedure for fecal porphyrin assay, *Clin Chem* 31:1163-1167, 1985.

12. Piomelli S: Free erythrocyte porphyrins in the detection of undue absorption of Pb and of Fe deficiency, *Clin Chem* 23:264-269, 1977.

13. Johnson PM, Perkins SL, Kennedy SW: A high speed liquid-chromatographic method for measuring urinary porphyrins, *Clin Chem* 34:103-105, 1988.

14. Lim CK, Peters TJ: Urine and faecal porphyrin profiles by reversed-phase high-performance liquid chromatography in the porphyrias, *Clin Chim Acta* 139:55-62, 1984.

15. Hill RH, Bailey SL: Loss of coproporphyrin by centrifuging urine samples before liquid-chromatography, *Clin Chem* 32:377-378, 1986.

DIAGNOSTIC INFORMATION	REMARKS

16. Perkins SL, Johnson PM: Loss of porphyrins from solution during analysis: effect of sample pH and matrix on porphyrin quantification in urine by "high-performance" liquid chromatography, *Clin Chem* 35:1508-1512, 1989.

17. Garden JS, Mitchell DG, Jackson KW, et al: Improved ethanol extraction procedure for determining zinc protoporphyrin in whole blood, *Clin Chem* 23:1585-1589, 1977.

TEST NAME AND METHOD	SPECIMEN REQUIREMENTS	REFERENCE INTERVAL, CONVENTIONAL [INTERNATIONAL RECOMMENDED UNITS]			CHEMICAL INTERFERENCES AND IN VIVO EFFECTS
Potassium (K)[1-4] *FES, AAS, ISE, kinetic, spectrophotometry*[5-7]	Serum. Separate from cells as soon as possible. Avoid hemolysis.	Premature, cord: Premature, 48 hr: Newborn, cord: Newborn: Infant: Child: Thereafter:	*mEq/L*[4] 5.0-10.2 3.0-6.0 5.6-12.0 3.7-5.9 4.1-5.3 3.4-4.7 3.5-5.1	× 1.0	*mmol/L* [5.0-10.2] [3.0-6.0] [5.6-12.0] [3.7-5.9] [4.1-5.3] [3.4-4.7] [3.5-5.1]	P, S ↑ V β-Adrenergic blockers (rare), amiloride, aminocaproic acid, angiotensin-converting enzyme (ACE) inhibitors, antineoplastic agents (e.g., cyclophosphamide, vincristine), arginine, cephaloridine, cyclosporine, digoxin (toxicity), epinephrine (initial effect), foscarnet sodium, heparin, histamine (IV), isoniazid, lithium, mannitol, methicillin, nonsteroidal antiinflammatory agents, penicillin (if potassium salt), phenformin (lactic acidosis), salt substitutes, spironolactone, succinylcholine, tetracycline, triamterene, and tromethamine
	Plasma (lithium heparin) is the preferred specimen. Remove from cells promptly. Do not use plasma from blood that has been stored in ice water.[8] Do not use ammonium heparin with ISEs.[9]	M: F:	3.5-4.5 3.4-4.4		[3.5-4.5] [3.4-4.4]	
	Whole blood, with use of direct ISEs.					P, S ↑ C *Ion-selective potentiometry:* Procainamide S ↑ C *Seralyzer:* Ascorbic acid (high doses), levodopa, and lithium P, S ↓ C β-Adrenergic agonists (e.g., salbutamol, terbutaline), albuterol, aminoglycosides, *p*-aminosalicylate, aminosalicylic acid (rare), amphotercin, azlocillin, bisacodyl, capreomycin, carbenicillin, carbenoxolone, cholestyramine, cisplatin, clopamide, corticosteroid, corticotropin,

DIAGNOSTIC INFORMATION	REMARKS

S, P ↑ *Increased supply of potassium:* Rapid K infusion, failure to stop K therapy when depletion has been corrected

Redistribution of potassium in the body [gain of K by extracellular fluid (ECF) from cells]: Massive hemolysis, severe tissue damage, severe acute starvation (as in anorexia nervosa), hyperkinetic activity (as in status epilepticus), malignant hyperpyrexia after anesthesia, hyperkalemic periodic paralysis (attacks occur especially 30-40 min after exercise), acidosis, and dehydration

Reduced renal excretion of potassium: Any cause of acute renal failure with oliguria or anuria and acidosis, end stage of chronic renal failure with oliguria (GFR <3-5 mL/min), Addison's disease, hypofunction of renin-angiotensin-aldosterone system, pseudohypoaldosteronism, other states with sodium depletion, after severe exercise (especially in individuals taking β-blockers), in shock, in presence of severe hemolysis, and in tissue ischemia

S, P ↓ *Reduced potassium intake:* Chronic starvation, dilution of extracellular K during prolonged administration of potassium-poor fluids when no additional K salts or potassium-containing foods are being taken by mouth (e.g., postoperative states)

Loss of potassium from the body

In intestinal secretions: Prolonged vomiting, diarrhea, loss because of intestinal fistulas, villous adenoma of the intestine

In urine: Renal tubular acidosis, renal tubular failure, Fanconi's syndrome, primary and secondary aldosteronism, Cushing's syndrome, Bartter's syndrome, osmotic diuresis (e.g., of hyperglycemia), alkalosis, in diabetic ketosis during gluconeogenesis; during administration of ACTH, cortisone, or testosterone

In sweat: Cystic fibrosis

S, P ↓ *Redistribution in the body (loss into cells):* Glucose and insulin therapy, familial periodic paralysis, loss of K from ECF by more than one route (into cells and urine in alkalosis and

Spuriously elevated serum K levels may be obtained in the following circumstances: Exercise of arm with occlusive cuff in place (may result in an increase of plasma K levels of 10-20%); hemolysis of blood sample or delayed separation of plasma from erythrocytes (hemolysis of 0.5% of the erythrocytes can increase serum K^+ level by 0.5 mmol/L); release of K from platelets during clotting if serum is used; chronic lymphatic leukemia with very high leukocyte counts if the blood sample is left at room temperature, thrombocytosis ($>1000 \times 10^9$/L), and leukemia.

There is a diurnal variation in serum K level (minimum at ~10:00 PM, maximum at 8:00 AM). Normal adults when deprived of a normal K intake continue to excrete 20-30 mmol of K/day for 4 days before the excretion rate decreases. Administration of NaCl to potassium-depleted patients will cause a further loss of K in the urine. In metabolic alkalosis with good renal function, plasma K concentrations are usually decreased; in metabolic alkalosis with poor renal function there is K deficiency, but the plasma K level is normal or elevated.

Clinical symptoms of hypokalemia (tiredness, weakness, hyporeflexia, and finally ventricular fibrillation) may occur at <2.0 mmol/L, especially if the decrease in K concentration is sudden. Hyperkalemia results in muscular irritability. ECG shows peaked T waves, and concentrations >7.0 mmol/L may be dangerous.

A calculation of the trans-tubular potassium gradient (TTKG) is useful for diagnosing the cause of hyperkalemia[17]:

$$TTKG = \frac{urine_K}{plasma_K} \div \frac{urine_{osm}}{plasma_{osm}}$$

The TTKG in a normal person on a normal diet is 8-9. With a high potassium intake, more potassium is excreted and the TTKG is >10. During low potassium intake and hypokalemia, the TTKG should normally be reduced to <3. A TTKG <7 during hyperkalemia may indicate a mineralocorticoid deficiency, especially if accompanied by hyponatremia and hypernatriuria.

TEST NAME AND METHOD	SPECIMEN REQUIREMENTS	REFERENCE INTERVAL, CONVENTIONAL [INTERNATIONAL RECOMMENDED UNITS]		CHEMICAL INTERFERENCES AND IN VIVO EFFECTS

Potassium—CONT

cyanocobalamin, dextrose anhydride, diclofenamide, diuretics (including acetazolamide, bumetanide, chlorthalidone, ethacrynic acid, furosemide, metolazone, quinethazone, thiazides), EDTA, enoxolone, fluconazole, glucagons, glucose, ifosfamide, insulin, levodopa, licorice, mezlocillin, nafcillin, penicillin G (sodium salt), phenolphthalein, piperacillin, polymyxin B, salicylates, sodium bicarbonate, sodium chloride, ticarcillin, and theophyline

S ↓ C *Seralyzer:* Aspirin

Urine, 24 hr.

	mEq/day		*mmol/day*
6-10 yr			
M:	17-54[11]	× 1.0	[17-54]
F:	8-37		[8-37]
10-14 yr			
M:	22-57		[22-57]
F:	18-58		[18-58]
Adult:	25-125[4]		[25-125]
	Level varies with diet.		

Random urine[12]:

	mEq/L		*mmol/L*
M			
<40 yr:	11-80	× 1.0	[11-80]
≥40 yr:	17-99		[17-99]
F			
<40 yr:	17-145		[17-145]
≥40 yr:	22-164		[22-164]

	mEq/g creatinine	*mmol/g creatinine*
M:	13-116	[13-116]
F:	8-129	[8-129]

U ↑ V Amphotericin, corticosteroids, corticotropin, desoxycorticosterone, calcitonin, carbenicillin, carbenoxolone, gentamicin, glycyrrhiza, levodopa, mafenide, nafcillin, penicillin, streptozotocin, sulfates, ticarcillin, and diuretics (see examples under plasma interferences)

U ↓ V Alanine (in fasting obese), amiloride, clopamide, diazoxide, epinephrine, general anesthetic agents, growth hormone, indomethacin, and levarterenol

DIAGNOSTIC INFORMATION	REMARKS

into cells, urine, and intestine in pyloric stenosis with alkalosis)

Miscellaneous: Hypothermia, loss from draining wounds or burns, treatment of megaloblastic anemia with vitamin B12 or folic acid, pancreatic islet cell tumor that produces vasoactive intestinal polypeptide >200 pg/mL [>200 ng/L], and bulimia

---

U ↑ Onset of starvation (later decreases to ~10 mmol/day), Cushing's syndrome, primary and secondary aldosteronism, primary renal diseases (renal tubular syndromes, during recovery phase of acute tubular necrosis, metabolic acidosis, metabolic alkalosis), Albright type of renal tubular diseases; during treatment with ACTH, hydrocortisone, and cortisone

U ↓ In chronic K deficiency states, Addison's disease, and renal diseases with decreased urine flow (severe glomerulonephritis, pyelonephritis, nephrosclerosis)

Spectrophotometric methods are not suitable because of ammonia interference.

Urine K^+ values <20 nmol/L are associated with nonrenal conditions, values >20 nmol/L with renal causes.

TEST NAME AND METHOD	SPECIMEN REQUIREMENTS	REFERENCE INTERVAL, CONVENTIONAL [INTERNATIONAL RECOMMENDED UNITS]	CHEMICAL INTERFERENCES AND IN VIVO EFFECTS
Potassium—CONT			
	CSF[10]	70% of plasma level × 0.01 [0.70, fraction of plasma level]	
		2.5-3.2 mEq/L × 1.0 [2.5-3.2 mmol/L] Level increases with plasma hyperosmolality.	
	Feces, 24 hr.	~5 mEq/day[1] × 1.0 [~5 mmol/day] 18.2 ± 2.5 mEq/ day (SEM) [18.2 ± 2.5 mmol/day][13]	
	Gastric juices[10]	~10 mEq/L × 1.0 [~10 mmol/L] Parietal and nonparietal juices have the same concentration.	
	Erythrocytes	96-109 mEq/L[1,4] × 1.0 [96-109 mmol/L] 84 ± 10 mEq/L [84 ± 10 mmol/L][14]	
	Saliva[4]	*mEq/L* *mmol/L* Without stimulation: 19-23 × 1.0 [19-23] With stimulation: 18-19 [18-19]	
	Sweat[4]	M: 4.4-9.7[10] [4.4-9.7] F: 7.6-15.6 [7.6-15.6] In cystic fibrosis: 14-30 ($\bar{x}$ = 23)[15] [14-30]	
	Platelets	4.5 ± 1.5 µEq/10^8 cells [× 1.0 = 4.5 ± 1.5 mmol/10^8 cells][16]	

1. Eastham RD: *Biochemical values in clinical medicine,* ed 7, Bristol, UK, 1985, John Wright and Sons Ltd.

2. Burtis CA, Ashwood ER, editors: *Tietz fundamentals of clinical chemistry,* ed 5, Philadelphia, 2000, WB Saunders.

3. Young DS: *Effects of drugs on clinical laboratory tests,* ed 5, Washington, DC, 2000, American Association for Clinical Chemistry.

4. Scott MG, Heusel JW, LeGrys VA, et al: Electrolyte, and blood gases. In Burtis CA, Ashwood ER, editors: *Tietz textbook of clinical chemistry,* ed 3, Philadelphia, 1999, WB Saunders.

5. Berry MN, Mazzachi RD, Pejakovic M, et al: Enzymatic determination of potassium in serum, *Clin Chem* 35:817-820, 1988.

6. Kimura S, Asari S, Hayashi S, et al: New enzymatic method with tryptophanase for determining potassium in serum, *Clin Chem* 38:44-47, 1992.

7. Kumar A, Chapoteau E, Czech BP, et al: Chromogenic ionophore-based methods for spectrophotometric assay of sodium and potassium in serum and plasma, *Clin Chem* 34:1709-1712, 1988.

8. Moran RF: Effects of icing whole-blood samples in plastic go beyond PO_2 alone [letter], *Clin Chem* 39:162, 1993.

9. Pesce A, Kaplan L, editors: *Methods in clinical chemistry,* St. Louis, 1987, CV Mosby.

10. Willing SK, Gamlen TR: Sweat osmolality values in normal adults, *Clin Chem* 33:612-613, 1987.

11. Liappis N, Reimnitz R: Referenzwerte her natrium-, kalium- kalzium-, chlorid-, und anorganischen phosphat—Ausscheidung im 24h-urin gesunder kinder, *Klin Padiatr* 196:367-369, 1984.

DIAGNOSTIC INFORMATION	REMARKS
F ↑ Severe diarrhea, ≥60 mmol/day; villous tumors of colon and rectum	Measurement of fecal K is used only in metabolic balance studies.
Gast ↑ In damage to gastric muscosal membrane	
Ercs ↑ Congestive heart failure	
Ercs ↓ Longstanding diuretic therapy, hyperaldosteronism	
Sal ↑ Cystic fibrosis (less reliable than sweat)	
Sw ↑ Cystic fibrosis, hyperadrenalism, and congestive heart failure	

12. Bond LW, Garber C, Ottinger W, et al: Reference intervals for common analytes in random urine specimens, *Clin Chem* 55:submitted, 2005.
13. Cuprilli R, Sopranzi N, Colaperi O, et al: Salt-losing diarrhea in idiopathic proctocolitis, *Scand J Gastroenterol* 13:331-335, 1979.
14. Touyz RM, Milne FJ: A method for determining total magnesium, calcium, and potassium contents of human platelets, *Miner Electrol Metab* 17:173-178, 1991.
15. Wallach J, editor: *Interpretation of diagnostic tests,* ed 5, Boston, 1992, Little, Brown and Co.
16. Touyz RM, Milne FJ: A method for determining the total magnesium, calcium, sodium and potassium contents of human platelets, *Miner Electrolyte Metab* 17:173-178, 1991.
17. http://en.wikipedia.org/wiki/Trans-tubular_potassium_gradient. Accessed 12/31/05.

TEST NAME AND METHOD	SPECIMEN REQUIREMENTS	REFERENCE INTERVAL, CONVENTIONAL [INTERNATIONAL RECOMMENDED UNITS]	CHEMICAL INTERFERENCES AND IN VIVO EFFECTS
α_2-**Pregnancy-Associated Glycoprotein** (α_2-PAG, SP$_3$, Pregnancy Zone Protein, PZP)[1-4] *RID*[2]	Serum. Analyze fresh or store at 4° C for <72 hr. Stable frozen at −20° C for 6 mo or at −70° C indefinitely. Specimens without lipemia or hemolysis are preferred.	Maternal: <180 mg/dL × 0.01 [<1.80 g/L] Values increase with gestational age (with considerable individual variations). Increase begins in 8-12th gestational wk and reaches an average of 100 mg/dL [1.00 g/L] in the third trimester. 6 wk postpartum: <10 mg/dL × 0.01 [<0.10 g/L]	S ↑ V Estrogens, oral contraceptives

1. Berne BH: Pregnancy-associated alpha 2-glycoprotein levels in pregnancy, oral contraception and choriocarcinoma. In Peeters H, editor: *Protides of the biological fluids, Proceedings of the 24th Colloquium, vol 24,* Oxford, 1976, Pergamon Press.

2. Bohn H, Dati F: Placental and pregnancy proteins. In Ritzmann SE, editor: *Protein abnormalities, vol 1. Physiology of immunoglobulins: diagnostic and clinical aspects,* New York, 1982, Alan R. Liss, Inc.

3. Ritzmann SE, Tucker ES III: *Protein analysis in disease—current concepts. Workshop manual,* Chicago, 1979, American Society of Clinical Pathologists, Commission for Continuing Education.

Pregnancy-Associated Plasma Protein A (PAPP-A)[1-3] *RID, EID*[2]	Serum. Analyze fresh or store at 4° C for <72 hr. Stable frozen at −20° C for 6 mo or at −70° C indefinitely. Specimens without lipemia or hemolysis are preferred.	*mU/L* 3.8-10.4 Male and nonpregnant female Pregnancy[4,5] Weeks of gestation	

		Weeks of gestation	
		8	90-7000
		9	<10-5800
		10	140-7000
		11	575-7250
		12	900-9000
		13	550-11,500
		14	2200-39,500

Values decrease rapidly postpartum; they become undetectable within a few days to 3-5 wk.

	Amniotic fluid	Weeks of gestation	
		8	<10-64
		9	<10-22.5
		10	<10-210
		11	<10-16.5
		12	<10-15
		13	<10-23
		14	<10-110
		17	<10-2135

DIAGNOSTIC INFORMATION	REMARKS

↑ This protein is the major pregnancy-associated serum protein. Levels increase 20- to 100-fold during a normal gestation and are detectably increased within a few weeks of conception. Levels of 100 mg/dL [1 g/L] are not uncommon in late pregnancy. Serum levels also increase in both men and women during administration of estrogen. Increases have also been reported in patients with a variety of neoplastic and immunological disorders; however, because alterations in normal estrogen metabolism also may occur as a result of malignancy or therapy, the meaning of these increases is uncertain.

↓ A level of PZP below the expected value for the end of the first and the second trimester is often associated with a fetus at risk.

This large globulin is synthesized in the liver; it is also found to be synthesized in certain nonhepatoma neoplastic cell lines in vitro and in hepatitis B virus infections.[5] Tissue localization has identified the protein in the syncytiotrophoblast and on the surface of B lymphocytes and monocytes. The function of PZP is uncertain, but there is good evidence that its function is to clear proteinases from the circulation by the formation of complexes. PZP may also be an acute phase reactant. The protein exhibits considerable homology with α_2-macroglobulin.

MW: 360,000.

4. von Schoultz B: A quantitative study of the pregnancy zone protein in the sera of pregnant and puerperal women, *Am J Obstet Gynecol* 119:792-797, 1974.

5. Zarzur JA, Aldao M, Seleoni S, et al: Serum pregnancy-associated α_2-glycoprotein levels in the evolution of hepatitis B virus infection, *J Clin Lab Anal* 3:73-77, 1989.

↑ Acute coronary syndrome (unstable angina, myocardial infarction)[5]

↓ Down syndrome and used as a marker for maternal screening of Down syndrome during first or early second trimesters.[6-8]

PAPP-A is a 200 kDa metalloproteinase. During pregnancy, placenta secretes PAPP-A, and the levels elevate with gestational age. In addition to placenta, PAPP-A is also produced by a variety of tissues at much lower levels. Circulating PAPP-A is a heterotetrameric protein complex composed of two 200-250-kDa subunits disulfide-linked to two molecules of the proform of eosinophil major basic protein. Pregnancy serum or plasma contains traces (<1%) of uncomplexed PAPP-A.[9-12]

The association of PAPP-A levels with pregnancy complications remains to be determined.

PAPP-A is expressed within unstable or ruptured coronary artery plaques but not stable plaques. The release pattern is highly variable for patients with acute coronary syndrome.[5]

TEST NAME AND METHOD	SPECIMEN REQUIREMENTS	REFERENCE INTERVAL, CONVENTIONAL [INTERNATIONAL RECOMMENDED UNITS]	CHEMICAL INTERFERENCES AND IN VIVO EFFECTS

Pregnancy-Associated Plasma Protein A—CONT

1. Bohn H, Dati F: Placental and pregnancy proteins. In Ritzmann SE, editor: *Protein abnormalities, vol 1. Physiology of immunoglobulins: diagnostic and clinical aspects,* New York, 1982, Alan R. Liss, Inc.

2. Lin TM, Halbert SP: Immunological comparison of various human pregnancy-associated plasma proteins, *Int Arch Allergy Appl Immunol* 48:101-115, 1975.

3. Stabile I, Grudzinskas JG, Chard T: Clinical applications of pregnancy protein estimations with particular reference to pregnancy-associated plasma protein A (PAPP-A), *Obstet Gynecol Surv* 43:73-82, 1988.

4. Iles RK, Wathen NC, Sharma KB, et al: Pregnancy-associated plasma protein A levels in maternal serum, extraembryonic coelomic and amniotic fluids in the first trimester, *Placenta* 15:693-699, 1994.

5. Bayes-Genis A, Conover CA, Overgaard MT, et al: Pregnancy-associated plasma protein A as a marker of acute coronary syndromes, *N Engl J Med* 345:1022-1029, 2001.

6. Knight GJ, Palomaki GE, Haddow JE, et al: Pregnancy-associated plasma protein A as a marker for Down syndrome in the second trimester of pregnancy, *Prenat Diagn* 13:222-223, 1993.

7. Wald N, Stone R, Cuckle HS, et al: First trimester concentrations of pregnancy associated plasma protein A and placenta protein 14 in Down's syndrome, *BMJ* 305:24, 1992.

Pregnanediol[1,2]

GLC

Urine, 24 hr. Preserve with boric acid.

	mg/day[4]		*μmol/day*
Child			
<2 yr:	<0.1	× 3.12	[<0.3]
3-5 yr:	<0.3		[<0.9]
6-9 yr:	<0.5		[<1.6]
10-15 yr			
M:	0.01-0.7		[0.3-2.2]
F:	0.1-1.2		[0.3-3.7]
Adult			
M:	0-1.9		[0-5.9]
F, follicular[1]:	<2.6		[<8]
Luteal:	2.6-10.6		[8-33]

	mg/day		*μmol/day*
Pregnancy[1]			
First trimester:	10-35	× 3.12	[31-109]
Second trimester:	35-70		[109-218]
Third trimester:	70-100		[218-312]

↑ V Corticotropin, gonadotropins

↓ V Ampicillin, estrogens, medroxyprogesterone, oral contraceptives, and phenothiazines

↑ C *Colorimetric:* Phenazopyridine

RIA

Amniotic fluid[3]

Term, x̄: 145 ng/mL × 3.12 [452 nmol/L]

1. Eastham RD: *Biochemical values in clinical medicine,* ed 7, Bristol, UK, 1985, John Wright and Sons Ltd.

2. Loraine JA, Bell ET: *Hormone assays and their clinical application,* New York, 1976, Churchill Livingstone.

3. Tulchinsky D, Ryan KJ, editors: *Maternal-fetal endocrinology,* Philadelphia, 1980, WB Saunders.

4. Mayo Medical Laboratories: *Test catalog,* Rochester, MN, 1993, Mayo Medical Laboratories.

DIAGNOSTIC INFORMATION	REMARKS

8. Christiansen M, Jaliashvili I: Total pregnancy-associated plasma protein A—a first trimester maternal serum marker for Down's syndrome: clinical and technical assessment of a poly-monoclonal enzyme immunoassay, *Scand J Clin Lab Invest* 63:407-415, 2003.

9. Oxvig C, Sand O, Kristensen T, et al: Circulating human pregnancy-associated plasma protein-A is disulfide-bridged to the proform of eosinophil major basic protein, *J Biol Chem* 268:12243-12246, 1993.

10. Overgaard MT, Haaning J, Boldt HB, et al: Expression of recombinant human pregnancy-associated plasma protein-A and identification of the proform of eosinophil major basic protein as its physiological inhibitor, *J Biol Chem* 275:31128-31133, 2000.

11. Bersinger NA, Altermatt HJ, Birkhauser MH, et al: Non-placental production of pregnancy-associated plasma protein A (PAPP-A): old and new evidence, *Early Pregnancy* 3:96-101, 1997.

12. Beguin Y: Soluble transferrin receptor for the evaluation of erythropoiesis and iron status, *Clin Chim Acta* 329:9-22, 2003.

↑ In precocious puberty of girls, adult levels with normal menses suggest isosexual precocity; if menses are absent or irregular, an hCG-secreting tumor may be suspected.

↑ Chorioepithelioma (8-15 mg/day [25-47 μmol/day] has been reported), congenital adrenal hyperplasia caused by 17α-hydroxylase and 11β-hydroxylase deficiency, granulosa theca cell tumors of ovary, luteal cyst of ovary, and arrhenoblastoma of ovary

↓ Placental insufficiency, fetal death (if values are <5 mg/day [<16 μmol/day], abortion is inevitable), amenorrhea, preeclamptic toxemia, essential hypertension in pregnancy, threatened and habitual abortion, chronic nephritis in pregnancy, and ovarian failure

Pregnanediol levels in normally menstruating women remain relatively constant from one subject to another during the follicular phase but vary greatly in the luteal phase. Values increase markedly after successful artificial insemination. Excretion gradually increases as pregnancy advances, with values decreasing sharply before the onset of labor and after delivery. In anovular menstruation, a cyclic pattern of pregnanediol output is not observed, and there is no increase during the luteal phase. Serial determinations of urinary pregnanediol may be used for monitoring progesterone production during pregnancy.

Urinary pregnanediol assays are no longer used as an index of progesterone secretion. See *Progesterone.*

There is a sharp increase in amniotic fluid pregnanediol after 40 wk of gestation. This may perhaps help in the diagnosis of postmaturity.

TEST NAME AND METHOD	SPECIMEN REQUIREMENTS	REFERENCE INTERVAL, CONVENTIONAL [INTERNATIONAL RECOMMENDED UNITS]			CHEMICAL INTERFERENCES AND IN VIVO EFFECTS
Pregnanetriol[1]	Urine, 24 hr. Collect with 25 mL of acetic	*mg/day*		*μmol/day*	↑ V Gonadotropin
GLC	acid, 8.5 mol/L. Store refrigerated.	Child[2]			
		0-5 yr:	<0.1 × 2.97	[<0.3]	
		6-9 yr:	<0.3	[<0.9]	
		10-15 yr			
		M:	0.2-0.6	[0.6-1.8]	
		F:	0.1-0.6	[0.3-1.8]	
		Adult[3]			
		M:	0.4-2.5	[1.2-7.5]	
		F, Follicular phase:	0.1-1.8	[0.3-5.3]	
		Luteal phase:	0.9-2.2	[2.7-6.5]	

1. Loraine JA, Bell ET: *Hormone assays and their clinical application,* New York, 1976, Churchill Livingstone.
2. Mayo Medical Laboratories: *Test catalog,* Rochester, MN, 1993, Mayo Medical Laboratories.
3. Eastham RD: *Biochemical values in clinical medicine,* ed 7, Bristol, UK, 1985, John Wright and Sons Ltd.
4. Orth D, Kovacs D, DeBold C: The adrenal cortex. In Wilson JH, Foster DW, editors: *Williams textbook of endocrinology,* ed 8, Philadelphia, 1992, WB Saunders.

TEST NAME AND METHOD	SPECIMEN REQUIREMENTS	REFERENCE INTERVAL, CONVENTIONAL [INTERNATIONAL RECOMMENDED UNITS]			CHEMICAL INTERFERENCES AND IN VIVO EFFECTS
Pregnenolone[1]	Serum. Freeze and store at −20° C.	*ng/dL*[4]		*nmol/L*	↑ Metoclopramide
RIA[2]		Cord blood:	900-4000 × 0.0316	[28.4-126.4]	
		Newborn (1-7 days):	150-2000	[4.7-63.2]	
		Infants and prepubertal children:	21-110	[0.7-3.5]	
		Puberty (11-16 yr):	50-126	[1.6-4.0]	
		Adults:	46-225	[1.5-7.1]	
	Urine, 24 hr.[3] Use no preservatives.	*mg/day*		*μmol/day*	
		M:	<0.5 × 3.16	[<1.6]	
		F:	<4.0	[<12.6]	

1. McKenna TJ, Miller RB, Liddle GW: Plasma pregnenolone and 17-OH pregnenolone in patients with adrenal tumors, ACTH excess, or idiopathic hirsutism, *J Clin Endocrinol Metab* 44:231-236, 1977.
2. Abraham GE, Manlimos FS, Garza K: Radioimmunoassay of steroids. In Abraham GE, editor: *Handbook of radioimmunoassay,* New York, 1977, Marcel Dekker.
3. InterScience Institute: *Current unique and rare endocrine assays,* Inglewood, CA, 1987, InterScience Institute.
4. Endocrine Sciences: *Pediatric laboratory services,* Tarzana, CA, 1992, Endocrine Sciences.

DIAGNOSTIC INFORMATION	REMARKS

↑ Congenital adrenal hyperplasia caused by 21-hydroxylase defect (values are as high as 15.4-27.3 mg/day; 45.8-81.1 μmol/day), 11β-hydroxylase deficiency syndrome, Stein-Leventhal syndrome, and ovarian and adrenal tumors

↓ 17a-Hydroxylase deficiency syndrome (rare), ovarian failure

Muscular exercise increases values. Pregnanetriol is a urinary metabolite of 17-hydroxyprogesterone. Currently diagnosis of 21-hydroxylase (P-450$_{C21}$) deficiency is largely based on demonstrating increased basal or ACTH-stimulated serum 17-hydroxyprogesterone concentration.[4] Measurements of urinary adrenal androgens (17-ketosteroids) or pregnanetriol are used infrequently.

↑ Hirsutism, adrenal carcinoma, 3β-hydroxysteroid dehydrogenase deficiency, Cushing's syndrome caused by ACTH-secreting pituitary adenoma or ectopic ACTH-secreting tumor, after ACTH administration in normal adults and children.

Pregnenolone levels decrease after birth and are within the prepubertal range by 3 mo.

TEST NAME AND METHOD	SPECIMEN REQUIREMENTS	REFERENCE INTERVAL, CONVENTIONAL [INTERNATIONAL RECOMMENDED UNITS]		CHEMICAL INTERFERENCES AND IN VIVO EFFECTS
Pregnenolone **Sulfate**[1,2] *RIA*	Plasma. Store frozen.	mg/dL^3 Cord: 109 ± 49 (SD) 2-10 days: 54 ± 32 Adult: 5.3 ± 2.6	$\mu mol/L$ $\times 0.0242$ [2.64 $\pm$ 1.19] [1.31 $\pm$ 0.78] [0.13 $\pm$ 0.06]	None found.

1. Boizel R, de Peretti E, Cathiard AM, et al: Pattern of plasma levels of cortisol, dehydroepiandrosterone, and pregnenolone sulfate in normal subjects and in patients with homozygous familial hypercholesterolemia during ACTH infusion, *Clin Endocrinol* 25:363-371, 1986.
2. de Peretti E, Forest MG, Loras B, et al: Usefulness of plasma pregnenolone sulfate in testing pituitary-adrenal function in children, *Acta Endocrinol* 279(suppl):259-263, 1986.
3. de Peretti E, Mappus E: Pattern of plasma pregnenolone sulfate levels in humans from birth to adulthood, *J Clin Endocrinol Metab* 57:550-556, 1983.
4. Tagawa1 N, Tamanaka J, Fujinami A, et al: Serum dehydroepiandrosterone, dehydroepiandrosterone sulfate, and pregnenolone sulfate concentrations in patients with hyperthyroidism and hypothyroidism, *Clin Chem* 46:523-528, 2000.

TEST NAME AND METHOD	SPECIMEN REQUIREMENTS	REFERENCE INTERVAL, CONVENTIONAL [INTERNATIONAL RECOMMENDED UNITS]	CHEMICAL INTERFERENCES AND IN VIVO EFFECTS
Prekallikrein (Fletcher Factor)[1,2]	Plasma (blue top-citrate). Stable for 4 hr at room temperature.	Prekallikrein factor assay: ~50-150%. This test is similar to other APTT-based factor assays; for prekallikrein, the patient plasma is incubated with prekallikrein-deficient plasma. A screening test is also available: patient's sample is preincubated to allow prolonged contact activation with a kaolin-like activator; a correction of the PTT after incubation is suggestive of prekallikrein deficiency.	See *Activated Partial Thromboplastin Time.*

1. Jacobs DS, Demott WR, Oxley DK, editors: *Laboratory test handbook,* ed 5, Hudson, OH, 2001, Lexi-Comp, Inc.
2. Roberts HR, Escobar MA: Less common congenital disorders of hemostasis. In Kitchens CS, Alving BM, Kessler CM, editors: *Consultative hemostasis and thrombosis,* Philadelphia, 2002, WB Saunders, pp. 57-74.

DIAGNOSTIC INFORMATION	REMARKS
↑ 21-Hydroxylase deficiency	
↑ Hyperthyroidism[4]	
↓ Adrenal insufficiency in children, familial hypercholesterolemia	
↓ Hypothyroidism[4]	
↓ Hereditary deficiency, severe liver and renal disease	Similar to deficiencies of factor XII and high-molecular kininogen, prekallikrein deficiency may cause a prolonged PTT but no bleeding.
	A deficiency of prekallikrein can be initially suspected with a mixing study: a correction of APTT would support a factor deficiency. If there is no history of bleeding, a factor XII assay will be commonly performed in most laboratories. If factor XII is normal, prekallikrein and HMW kininogen assays should be ordered (these are usually send-out tests done in a few reference laboratories). A chromogenic assay is also available.

TEST NAME AND METHOD	SPECIMEN REQUIREMENTS	REFERENCE INTERVAL, CONVENTIONAL [INTERNATIONAL RECOMMENDED UNITS]			CHEMICAL INTERFERENCES AND IN VIVO EFFECTS
Progesterone (P4)[1-3]	Serum. Stable 7 days at 4° C, 3 mo at −20° C.		ng/dL^6	$nmol/L$	↑ V Clomiphene (increase over normal in luteal phase)
		Cord blood:	8000-56,000 $\times 0.0318$	[254-1780]	
RIA		Premature:	84-1360	[2.7-43.2]	
		Prepubertal child			↑ C Corticosterone,
		(1-10 yr):	7-52	[0.2-1.7]	11-deoxycortisol, 11-deoxycorticosterone,
			ng/dL^6	$nmol/L$	dihydroprogesterone, hydroxyprogesterone, and
		Puberty, Tanner stage 1			pregnanedione crossreact.
		M:	<10-33 $\times 0.0318$	[<0.3-1.0]	↓ V Ampicillin, dinoprost
		F:	<10-33	[<0.3-1.0]	tromethamine ($PGF_{2\alpha}$),
		2			ethinyl estradiol, and oral
		M:	<10-33	[<0.3-1.0]	contraceptives
		F:	<10-55	[<0.3-1.7]	
		3			
		M:	<10-48	[<0.3-1.5]	
		F:	<10-450	[<0.3-14.3]	
		4			
		M:	<10-108	[<0.3-30.2]	
		F:	<10-1300	[<0.3-41.3]	
		5			
		M:	21-82	[0.7-2.6]	
		F:	10-950	[0.3-30.2]	
		Adult			
		M:	13-97	[0.4-3.1]	
		F			
		Follicular:	15-70	[0.5-2.2]	
		Luteal:	200-2500	[6.4-79.5]	
		Pregnancy[7]			
		First trimester:	1025-4400	[32.6-139.9]	
		Second trimester:	1950-8250	[62.0-262.4]	
		Third trimester:	6500-22,900	[206.7-728.2]	
CPB assay[4]	Urine		mg/g creatinine (SD)	$\mu mol/mol$ creatinine	
		M:	0.12 ± 0.10 $\times 0.359$	[0.04 ± 0.04]	
		F			
		Follicular:	1.4 ± 1.1	[0.50 ± 0.39]	
		Luteal:	7.7 ± 4.6	[2.76 ± 1.65]	

Pregnancy: Values increase by 1.5-25.7 mg/g creatinine (0.54-9.23 μmol/mol creatinine) above normal.

DIAGNOSTIC INFORMATION	REMARKS

↑ Congenital adrenal hyperplasia caused by 21-hydroxylase, 17α-hydroxylase, and 11β-hydroxylase deficiency (as much as 10-fold normal), lipoid ovarian tumor, theca lutein cyst, molar pregnancy, and chorioepithelioma of ovary

↓ Threatened abortion, primary or secondary hypogonadism, and short luteal phase syndrome

The diagnostic value of this test lies in its detection of ovulation and in the evaluation of the function of the corpus luteum. Serial sampling during the menstrual cycle is required. Levels increase sharply during the luteal phase, reaching a maximum 5-10 days after the LH peak at midcycle. During pregnancy a gradual increase in blood progesterone is observed from 9-32 wk (may increase 10-100 times). Levels of progesterone in twin pregnancy are higher than in single pregnancy. Test is useful for monitoring patients having ovulation during induction with hCG, hMG, FSH/LH-RH, or clomiphene; for monitoring progesterone replacement therapy; and to evaluate patients at risk for early abortion. For diagnosis of short luteal phase syndrome, some authorities recommend correlation with endometrial biopsy.

Sensitivity of the assay is 0.24 mg/L urine [0.76 nmol/L].

TEST NAME AND METHOD	SPECIMEN REQUIREMENTS	REFERENCE INTERVAL, CONVENTIONAL [INTERNATIONAL RECOMMENDED UNITS]	CHEMICAL INTERFERENCES AND IN VIVO EFFECTS
Progesterone—CONT			
	Amniotic fluid[5]	Pregnancy, 10-20 wk: 3000-6000 ng/dL, with a gradual decrease thereafter [× 0.0318 = 95-191 nmol/L (highest value)]	

1. Wallach J, editor: *Interpretation of diagnostic tests,* ed 5, Boston, 1992, Little, Brown and Co.

2. Demetriou J: Progesterone. In Pesce A, Kaplan LA, editors: *Methods in clinical chemistry,* St. Louis, 1987, CV Mosby.

3. Wood P, Groom G, Moore A, et al: Progesterone assays: guidelines for the provision of a clinical biochemistry service, *Ann Clin Biochem* 22:1-24, 1985.

4. Schon VF, Hackenberg K, Paar D, et al: Die Bestimmung von Progesteron im Harn mit der kompetitiven Protein-bindungsmethode, *J Clin Chem Clin Biochem* 18:355-361, 1980.

5. Tulchinsky D, Ryan KJ, editors: *Maternal-fetal endocrinology,* Philadelphia, 1980, WB Saunders.

6. Endocrine Sciences: *Pediatric laboratory services,* Tarzana, CA, 1992, Endocrine Sciences.

7. Nichols Institute Reference Laboratories: *Test catalog,* San Juan Capistrano, CA, 1993, Nichols Institute Reference Laboratories.

TEST NAME AND METHOD	SPECIMEN REQUIREMENTS	REFERENCE INTERVAL, CONVENTIONAL [INTERNATIONAL RECOMMENDED UNITS]	CHEMICAL INTERFERENCES AND IN VIVO EFFECTS
Progesterone (Progestin) Receptor Protein (PRP)[1-3] *Immunohisto-chemistry*	Tissue, frozen or formalin-fixed paraffin-embedded. Tumor and biopsy, including core and fine-needle aspirates, specimens acceptable.	Subjective interpretation dependent on intensity of staining and number of positive cells. Only the staining of the cell nuclei is considered positive. Reported as positive or negative or as percent of positive cells. Favorable response >20% of cells stain; borderline, 11-20%; unfavorable, <10%.	In fine-needle aspirates, false-negative results are caused by air-drying artifacts or inadequate nuclei.
Ligand binding: dextran-coated charcoal method (DCC)[4]	Tissue, 0.1-1 g. Tissue must be dissected to be free of fat and normal tissue, cut into small pieces, placed in a plastic tube, and snap frozen in liquid nitrogen within 30 min of surgical removal. Store at −70° C. Frozen tissue is stable for several months.	*fmol/mg cytosol protein* / *nmol/kg cytosol protein* Negative: <6 × 1.0 [<6] Borderline: 6-10 (or inhibition <60% by unlabeled hormone) Positive: >10 [>10] (with K_d >5 × 10^{-9} mol/L)	↓ V Endogenous estrogens saturating receptor sites. Potentially falsely low results in fibrotic tumors, samples with low protein concentrations, and from degradation of thermolabile receptor proteins.
EIA		*fmol/mg cytosol protein* / *nmol/kg cytosol protein* Negative: <15 × 1.0 [<15] Positive: >15 [>15]	

DIAGNOSTIC INFORMATION	REMARKS

The pattern of the decrease of AF progesterone toward the end of pregnancy is contrary to its continued increase in maternal and fetal serum. Nonimmunologic techniques give much higher values.

Test is used primarily for identifying patients with breast cancers likely to respond to either additive or ablative hormone therapies.

Patients positive for PRP and estrogen receptor protein (ERP, see also *Estrogen Receptor Protein*) have a higher percentage (75-80%) response to hormonal therapy than do women positive for either ERP or PRP alone. Only 40-50% of ERP-positive, PRP-negative patients respond; 25-30% of ERP-negative, PRP-positive show a response. Response is observed in only ≤10% of patients who are negative for both ERP and PRP. The percentage of positive specimens is greater in postmenopausal women than in those who are premenopausal. Receptor status is also influenced by age.

Patients who are hormone-receptor positive have a better prognosis for disease-free survival and overall survival than those who are receptor negative. The definition of positive or negative may vary from one laboratory to the next. Results can vary because of tissue and antibody treatment and antibody specificity.[3,5]

Estrogen receptors are a part of the nuclear steroid hormone receptor family and play a role in hormone-directed transcriptional activation. Similar to estrogen receptors, progesterone receptors also consist of two separate receptors; however, in contrast to the estrogen receptors, the progesterone isoforms are transcribed from the same gene.[1-3,5]

Estrogen and progesterone receptors can be measured by quantitative ligand binding assays (DCC) and immunoassays and semiquantitative/qualitative immunocytochemical assays.

IHC measures receptors in the invasive carcinoma cells and not intraductal carcinoma or normal breast tissue in contrast to ligand binding methods and are not influenced by the presence of estrogens, antiestrogens, or steroid-binding proteins.

Although clinical data and guidelines for the use of estrogen and progesterone receptors were primarily developed using older techniques such as DCC, immunhistochemistry is considered equivalent or superior and is the preferred method in clinical practice.[3,6,7]

The American Society for Clincal Oncology, among other groups, recommends measurement of estrogen and progesterone receptors in primary breast cancers.[5,6]

TEST NAME AND METHOD	SPECIMEN REQUIREMENTS	REFERENCE INTERVAL, CONVENTIONAL [INTERNATIONAL RECOMMENDED UNITS]	CHEMICAL INTERFERENCES AND IN VIVO EFFECTS

Progesterone (Progestin) Receptor Protein—CONT

1. Chan DW, Sell S: Tumor markers. In Burtis CA, Ashwood ER, editors: *Tietz textbook of clinical chemistry,* ed 3, Philadelphia, 1999, WB Saunders.

2. Spyratos F: Prognostic and predictive markers for breast cancer. In Diamandis EP, Fritsche HA, Lilja H, et al, editors: *Tumor markers. Physiology, pathobiology, technology, and clinical applications,* Washington, DC, 2002, AACC Press.

3. Elledge RM, Allred DC: Clinical aspects of estrogen and progesterone receptors. In Harris JR, Lippman ME, Morrow M, et al, editors: *Diseases of the breast,* ed 3, Philadelphia, 2004, Lippincott Williams & Wilkins.

4. Menendez-Botet CJ, Schwartz MK: A review of methodology for estrogen and progesterone receptor protein analysis, *J Int Fed Clin Chem* 4:94-99, 1992.

Proinsulin, Immunoreactive[1-6] *RIA*	Serum, fasting. Store frozen at −20° C. Stable for at least 3 mo at −70° C.	2.0-2.6 pmol/L[7]	Rosiglitazone, a thiazolidinedione insulin sensitizer, reduces circulating proinsulin and the proinsulin:insulin ratio in type 2 diabetes. Sulfonylurea glyburide increases plasma proinsulin and the proinsulin:insulin ratio.[8]

1. Cibull M, Whitley R: Boy with thick lips. In Tietz NW, editor: *Applied laboratory medicine,* Philadelphia, 1992, WB Saunders.

2. Deacon CF, Conlon JM: Measurement of circulating human proinsulin concentrations using a proinsulin-specific antiserum, *Diabetes* 34:491-497, 1985.

3. Gerbitz KD, Spelsberg F, Bach S, et al: Pancreatic β-cell peptides as parameters for diagnosis and localization of hormone-secretin tumors, *J Clin Chem Clin Biochem* 23:377-380, 1985.

4. Robbins DC, Tager HS, Rubenstein AH: Biologic and clinical importance of proinsulin, *N Engl J Med* 310:1165-1175, 1984.

5. Sacks DB: Carbohydrates. In Burtis CA, Ashwood ER, editors: *Tietz textbook of clinical chemistry,* ed 2, Philadelphia, 1994, WB Saunders.

6. Ward WK, Paquette TL, Frank BH, et al: A sensitive radioinimunoassay for human proinsulin with sequential use of antisera to C-peptide and insulin, *Clin Chem* 21:728-733, 1986.

7. Sobey WJ, Beer SF, Carrington CA, et al: Sensitive and specific two-site immunoradiometric assays for human insulin, proinsulin, 65-66 split and 32-33 split proinsulins, *Biochem J* 260:535-541, 1989.

8. Smith SA, Porter LE, Biswas N, et al: Rosiglitazone, but not glyburide, reduces circulating proinsulin and the proinsulin:insulin ratio in type 2 diabetes, *J Clin Endocrinol Metab* 89:6048-6053, 2004.

DIAGNOSTIC INFORMATION	REMARKS

5. Fleisher M, Dnistrian AM, Sturgeon CM, et al: Practice guidelines and recommendations for use of tumor markers in the clinic. In Diamandis EP, Fritsche HA, Lilja H, et al, editors: *Tumor markers. Physiology, pathobiology, technology, and clinical applications,* Washington, DC, 2002, AACC Press.

6. Bast RC, Ravdin P, Hayes DF, et al: 2000 update of recommendations for the use of tumor markers in breast and colorectal cancer: clinical practice guidelines of the American Society of Clinical Oncology, *J Clin Oncol* 19:1865-1878, 2001.

7. Harvey JM, Clark GM, Osborne CK, et al: Estrogen receptor status by immunohistochemistry is superior to the ligand-binding assay for predicting response to adjuvant endocrine therapy in breast cancer, *J Clin Oncol* 17:1474-1481, 1999.

↑ Familial hyperproinsulinemia, pancreatic β-cell tumors (insulinomas), islet β-cell secretory defects, chronic renal failure, hyperthyroidism, cirrhosis, severe hypoglycemic hyperinsulinemia, and independent risk factors for death and morbidity of coronary heart disease in nondiabetic persons.[9]

Elevation of the proinsulin:insulin ratio has been used as an indirect marker of β-cell function.[10,11] The elevation of the ratio correlates with a decreased acute illness response to glucose in type 2 diabetic patients.[10] The increased ratio is also predictive of the development of type 2 diabetes.[12-14]

Proinsulin ($t_{1/2}$, 17 min) is cleared from plasma much more slowly than insulin ($t_{1/2}$, 5 min). In the fasting state, proinsulin-like immunoreactivity in peripheral blood accounts for ~10-20% of the total immunoreactive insulin on a molar basis.[7] In the pancreatic islet cells, the amount of proinsulin is <5% that of insulin.

Proinsulin immunoassays using proinsulin-specific polyclonal and monoclonal antibodies and biosynthetic human standards are available. Cross-reactivities of these antibodies with insulin or C-peptide are claimed to be low (<1%). However, substantial cross-reactivities with proinsulin conversion intermediates occur in many assays, and caution should be used in interpreting results.

9.   Zethelius B, Byberg L, Hales CN, et al: Proinsulin is an independent predictor of coronary heart disease: report from a 27-year follow-up study, *Circulation* 105:2153-2158, 2002.

10. Roder ME, Porte D Jr, Schwartz RS, et al: Disproportionately elevated proinsulin levels reflect the degree of impaired B cell secretory capacity in patients with noninsulin-dependent diabetes mellitus, *J Clin Endocrinol Metab* 83:604-608, 1998.

11. Choi CS, Kim CH, Lee WJ, et al: Elevated plasma proinsulin/insulin ratio is a marker of reduced insulin secretory capacity in healthy young men, *Horm Metab Res* 31:267-270, 1999.

12. Kahn SE, Leonetti DL, Prigeon RL, et al: Relationship of proinsulin and insulin with noninsulin-dependent diabetes mellitus and coronary heart disease in Japanese-American men: impact of obesity—clinical research center study, *J Clin Endocrinol Metab* 80:1399-1406, 1995.

13. Nijpels G, Popp-Snijders C, Kostense PJ, et al: Fasting proinsulin and 2-h post-load glucose levels predict the conversion to NIDDM in subjects with impaired glucose tolerance: the Hoorn Study, *Diabetologia* 39:113-118, 1996.

14. Haffner SM, Gonzalez C, Mykkanen L, et al: Total immunoreactive proinsulin, immunoreactive insulin and specific insulin in relation to conversion to NIDDM: the Mexico City Diabetes Study, *Diabetologia* 40:830-837, 1997.

TEST NAME AND METHOD	SPECIMEN REQUIREMENTS	REFERENCE INTERVAL, CONVENTIONAL [INTERNATIONAL RECOMMENDED UNITS]			CHEMICAL INTERFERENCES AND IN VIVO EFFECTS
Prolactin	Serum. Collect 3-4 hr after patient has awakened. Specimen may be stored at 4° C for 24 hr. Freeze for long-term stability.		ng/mL^{10}	mg/L	↑ Antihistamines, antipsychotics (e.g., haloperidol,
(PRL)[1-7]		Cord blood:	45-539 × 1.0	[45-539]	loxapine, molindone, phe-
		Newborn,			nothiazines, pimozide,
Immunometric		1-7 days[11]:	30-495	[30-495]	sulpiride, thiothixene),
assay		Children			arginine, beer, benser-
		Tanner stage			azide, carbidopa, estro-
		1			gens, histamine antago-
		M:	<10	[<10]	nists (e.g., cimetidine),
		F:	3.6-12	[3.6-12]	labetalol, metoclo-
		2-3			pramide, monoamine oxi-
		M:	<6.1	[<6.1]	dase inhibitors, opiates,
		F:	2.6-18	[2.6-18]	oral contraceptives, reser-
		4-5			pine, TRH, tricyclic anti-
		M:	2.8-11.0	[2.8-11.0]	depressants, and
		F:	3.2-20	[3.2-20]	verapamil
		Adult			
		M:	3.0-14.7	[3.0-14.7]	
		F:	3.8-23.2	[3.8-23.2]	↓ V Clonidine, dopamine,
		Pregnancy,			ergot alkaloids (includes
		third trimester:	95-473	[95-473]	bromocriptine), levodopa,
	Amniotic fluid[8-9]	Low before 12 wk; increases rapidly to peak levels of 2000-3000 ng/mL [× 0.001 = 2-3 mg/L] between 15-20 wk and decreases gradually in the last trimester.			and pergolide mesylate

1. Ashby D: Prolactin. In Pesce A, Kaplan LA, editors: *Methods in clinical chemistry,* St. Louis, 1987, CV Mosby.

2. Cowden EA, Ratcliffe WA, Beastall GH, et al: Laboratory assessment of prolactin status, *Ann Clin Biochem* 16:113-121, 1979.

3. Flückiger E, delPozo E, von Werder K: *Prolactin: physiology, pharmacology, and clinical findings,* Berlin, 1982, Springer-Verlag.

4. Franks S, Jacobs HS: Hyperprolactinemia, *Clin Endocrinol Metab* 12:648-668, 1983.

5. Jeffcoate S, Bacon R, Beastall G, et al: Assays for prolactin: guidelines for the provision of a clinical biochemistry service, *Ann Clin Biochem* 23:638-651, 1986.

6. Molitch ME, Reichlin S: Hyperprolactinemic disorders, *Dis Mon* 28:1-58, 1982.

7. Wiedemann G, Jonetz-Mentzel L, Panse R: Establishment of reference ranges for follitropin and lutropin in neonates, infants, children, and adolescents, *Eur Clin Chem Clin Biochem* 31:395-401, 1933.

8. Ismail AA: *Biochemical investigations in endocrinology,* London, 1981, Academic Press.

9. Tulchinsky D, Ryan KJ, editors: *Maternal-fetal endocrinology,* Philadelphia, 1980, WB Saunders.

10. Nichols Institute Reference Laboratories: *Test catalog,* San Juan Capistrano, CA, 1993, Nichols Institute Reference Laboratories.

11. Endocrine Sciences: *Pediatric laboratory services,* Tarzana, CA, 1992, Endocrine Sciences.

DIAGNOSTIC INFORMATION	REMARKS

S ↑ Prolactin-secreting pituitary tumors (macroadenomas, PRL frequently >1000 ng/mL [>1000 mcg/L]; in microadenoma, PRL >150 ng/mL [>150 mcg/L]); three quarters of patients with amenorrhea and/or galactorrhea, Chiari-Frommel and Argonz Del Castillo syndromes; various types of hypothalamic-pituitary diseases (e.g., sarcoidosis, granulomatous diseases, craniopharyngioma, metastatic cancer, empty sella syndrome), primary hypothyroidism, anorexia nervosa, polycystic ovary syndrome, renal failure, insulin-induced hypoglycemia, chest wall injury, adrenal insufficiency, and surgery (e.g., pituitary stalk section)

S ↓ Pituitary apoplexy (Sheehan's syndrome)

Physiologic elevations are found in the fetus and newborn; in adults during sleep (peak in early morning hours), stress, and exercise; and in females during pregnancy, after coitus, and while nursing. Measurement of PRL is useful in assessing completeness of hypophysectomy.

Stimulation and suppression tests may help assess prolactin reserve and abnormal prolactin secretion by the pituitary. (See *Prolactin Stimulation Test [after TRH], Prolactin Stimulation Test [after Chlorpromazine],* and *Prolactin Suppression Test [after L-dopa].*) These tests provide supporting information only and may not be helpful in diagnosing patients with persistent mild elevation of PRL and no evidence of pituitary tumor.

AF ↓ Hydramnios secondary to Rh isoimmunization

Throughout gestation the mean amniotic fluid PRL levels are 10- to 100-fold higher than those in the maternal and fetal blood, where a continuous increase of concentration is also observed. The origin of amniotic fluid PRL is maternal decidua. PRL is considered to have osmoregulating effects on amniotic fluid volume.

TEST NAME AND METHOD	SPECIMEN REQUIREMENTS	REFERENCE INTERVAL, CONVENTIONAL [INTERNATIONAL RECOMMENDED UNITS]		CHEMICAL INTERFERENCES AND IN VIVO EFFECTS
Prolactin Stimulation Test (after Chlorpromazine)[1-3]	Serum. Draw at 0, 60, 90, 120, and 180 min after stimulation. Obtain samples through an indwelling needle.	Prolactin M: F:	2- to 3-fold increase over baseline 2- to 5-fold increase over baseline	L-dopa prevents stimulation. See also *Prolactin.*
Dose, adult: 25-50 mg chlorpromazine, IM				
Child: Chlorpromazine, 0.4 mg/kg, orally				

1. Alsever RN, Gotlin RW: *Handbook of endocrine tests in adults and children,* ed 2, Chicago, 1978, Year Book Medical Publishers Inc.
2. Loraine JA, Bell ET: *Hormone assays and their clinical application,* New York, 1976, Churchill Livingstone.
3. Thorner MO, Vance ML, Horvath E, et al: The anterior pituitary. In Wilson JD, Foster DW, editors: *Williams textbook of endocrinology,* ed 8, Philadelphia, 1992, WB Saunders.
4. Miller RE, Ngai B: *Manual of endocrine diagnostic tests,* ed 4, Lexington, KY, 1991, Department of Medicine, University of Kentucky.

TEST NAME AND METHOD	SPECIMEN REQUIREMENTS	REFERENCE INTERVAL, CONVENTIONAL [INTERNATIONAL RECOMMENDED UNITS]		CHEMICAL INTERFERENCES AND IN VIVO EFFECTS
Prolactin Stimulation Test (after TRH)[1-6]	Serum. Draw at 0, 15, and 30 min after stimulation.	Prolactin M and child: F:	3- to 5-fold increase over baseline 6- to 20-fold increase over baseline	↓ V L-dopa, dopamine, glucocorticoids, and thyroxine
Dose, adult: 100 mcg TRH, IV				↑ V Cyproheptadine, estrogens
Child: 1 mcg/kg TRH, IV				See also *Prolactin.*

1. Alsever RN, Gotlin RW: *Handbook of endocrine tests in adults and children,* ed 2, Chicago, 1978, Year Book Medical Publishers Inc.
2. Burtis CA, Ashwood ER, editors: *Tietz textbook of clinical chemistry,* ed 2, Philadelphia, 1994, WB Saunders.
3. Wilson JD, Foster DW, editors: *Williams textbook of endocrinology,* ed 8, Philadelphia, 1992, WB Saunders.
4. Abboud CF, Laws ER Jr: Clinical endocrinological approach to hypothalamic-pituitary disease, *J Neurosurg* 51:271-291, 1979.
5. Lechan RM: Update on thyrotropin-releasing hormone, *Thyroid Today* XVI(1), 1993.
6. Loraine JA, Bell ET: *Hormone assays and their clinical application,* New York, 1976, Churchill Livingstone.
7. Endocrine Sciences: *Pediatric laboratory services,* Tarzana, CA, 1992, Endocrine Sciences.

DIAGNOSTIC INFORMATION	REMARKS

There is no response in hypothalamic disease and in some patients with PRL-secreting tumors.

This test is used to assess pituitary PRL reserve. In healthy individuals, chlorpromazine increases PRL secretion by competitive inhibition of dopamine receptors in the hypothalamus and pituitary.[4] Risks include hypotension, dizziness, and idiosyncratic drug reaction. Alternative agents with similar action include metoclopramide, sulpiride, and apomorphine.

Hyperprolactinemia related to pituitary tumor: 90% of patients with prolactinoma have less than twofold increase above baseline; a blunted response is usually seen regardless of the cause of hyperprolactinemia. Subjects with hypopituitarism will have a low baseline and a blunted increase after TRH. Patients with hypothalamic disease usually have a delayed hyperresponse.

Responses vary with age, sex, and PRL base level. In postpubertal females, a maximum response is seen during the luteal phase of the menstrual cycle and postpartum. Renal failure and thyrotoxicosis may suppress prolactin response to TRH; hypothyroidism and hepatic failure may exaggerate the response. Basal prolactin levels increase during sleep or with stress.[7]

A reduced or absent PRL response to TRH stimulation is consistent with, but not diagnostic of, a prolactinoma. The presence of a PRL response to TRH does not exclude a prolactinoma, nor does an exaggerated PRL response signify a hypothalamic origin of the hyperprolactinemia.[8]

8. Whitley RJ: Thyrotropin-releasing hormone (TRH) stimulation test, *AACC Endo Metab In-Service Training Cont Educ* 11:207-209, 1993.

TEST NAME AND METHOD	SPECIMEN REQUIREMENTS	REFERENCE INTERVAL, CONVENTIONAL [INTERNATIONAL RECOMMENDED UNITS]	CHEMICAL INTERFERENCES AND IN VIVO EFFECTS
Prolactin Suppression Test (after L-dopa)[1-4] Dose: Patient >70 lb, 500 mg L-dopa orally; 30-70 lb, 250 mg; 125 mg	Serum. Draw at 0, 30, 60, 90, 120, and 180 min after L-dopa.	Prolactin, >50% decrease in mass concentration at 1, 2, or 3 hr [× 0.01 = >0.50, fraction decrease in mass concentration]	Antipsychotic drugs prevent L-dopa suppression. See also *Prolactin*.

1. Alsever RN, Gotlin RW: *Handbook of endocrine tests in adults and children,* ed 2, Chicago, 1978, Year Book Medical Publishers Inc.

2. Abboud CF, Laws ER Jr: Clinical endocrinological approach to hypothalamic-pituitary disease, *J Neurosurg* 51:271-291, 1979.

3. Kryston LJ: *Endocrine disorders: focus on clinical disorders,* Garden City, NY, 1981, Medical Examination Publishing Co.

4. Loraine JA, Bell ET: *Hormone assays and their clinical application,* New York, 1976, Churchill Livingstone.

TEST NAME AND METHOD	SPECIMEN REQUIREMENTS	REFERENCE INTERVAL, CONVENTIONAL [INTERNATIONAL RECOMMENDED UNITS]			CHEMICAL INTERFERENCES AND IN VIVO EFFECTS
Proline (Pro)[1-4] *Ion-exchange chromatography*	Plasma (heparin) or serum, fasting. Place blood in ice water immediately; separate and freeze within 1 hr of collection. Stable for 1 wk at −20° C; for longer periods, deproteinize and store at −70° C.[5,6]		*mg/dL*	$\mu mol/L^9$	P ↑ V Levodopa, testosterone P ↓ V Oral contraceptives
		Premature, 1 day:	2.64 ± 0.86 (SD) × 86.9	[230 ± 75]	
		Newborn, 1 day:	1.23-3.18	[107-277]	
		1-3 mo:	2.31 ± 0.71 (SD)	[201 ± 62]	
		9 mo-2 yr:	0.59-2.13	[51-185]	
		3-10 yr:	0.78-1.70	[68-148]	
		6-18 yr:	0.67-3.72	$[58-324]^{10}$	
		Adult:	1.17-3.86	[102-336]	
	Urine, 24 hr. Add 10 mL of 6 mol/L HCl at start of collection. (Alternatively, refrigerate specimen during collection.) Store frozen at −20° C.[7]	10 days-7 wk:	3.2-11.0 × 8.69 mg/day	[28-96 $\mu mol/day]^9$	
		3-12 yr:	Trace		
		Adult:	Trace		
			$\mu mol/g$ creatinine[11]	*mmol/mol creatinine*	
		0-1 mo:	70-2300 × 0.113	[7.91-259.9]	
		1-6 mo:	<600	[<67.8]	
		6 mo-1 yr:	<300	[<33.9]	
		1-2 yr:	<270	[<30.5]	
		2-3 yr:	<220	[<24.9]	

DIAGNOSTIC INFORMATION	REMARKS
PRL-secreting tumors may not respond.	Failure to respond to L-dopa suggests autonomous function of the pituitary prolactin cells. Test may not differentiate PRL-secreting tumors from functional hyperprolactinemia. Normal suppression has been observed in many patients with documented PRL-secreting tumors, i.e., false-negative results are common.
P ↑ Hyperprolinemia type I (proline oxidase deficiency), hyperprolinemia type II [Δ^1-pyrroline-5-carboxylate (P-5-c) dehydrogenase deficiency], lysinuric protein intolerance, protein malnutrition in infants, 1 day after severe burn.[13]	In ~5% of normal individuals there is a mild hyperprolinemia. Proline levels are elevated only 3-5 times of normal in type I hyperprolinemia, whereas they are 10-15 times greater in type II hyperprolinemia.
P ↓ After abdominal surgery,[14] 4 days after severe burn,[13] Huntington's chorea	High levels of hydroxyproline and glycine are also seen in the iminoglycinurias.

See also Table II-2A. |
| U ↑ type I and type II hyperprolinemias, Joseph's syndrome (severe prolinuria), carcinoid syndrome, iminoglycinurias, and hepatolenticular degeneration | |

TEST NAME AND METHOD	SPECIMEN REQUIREMENTS	REFERENCE INTERVAL, CONVENTIONAL [INTERNATIONAL RECOMMENDED UNITS]		CHEMICAL INTERFERENCES AND IN VIVO EFFECTS

Proline—CONT

| | CSF. Collect in sterile tubes; store frozen. Stable at $-20°$ C for 1 wk or at $-70°$ C for 2 mo.[8] | *mg/dL*
 Neonate: 0.77 ± 0.020 (SEM)
 Adult: 0.044 ± 0.006 (SD) | *μmol/L*
 $\times 86.9$ $[6.7 \pm 1.7]^{8}$
 $[3.8 \pm 0.50]^{12}$ | |

1. Friedman RB, Young DS: *Effects of disease on clinical laboratory tests,* ed 2, Washington, DC, 1989, American Association for Clinical Chemistry.

2. Scriver CR, Beaudet AL, Valle D, et al, editors: *The metabolic and molecular bases of inherited disease,* ed 8, New York, 2001, McGraw-Hill.

3. Bremer HJ, Duran M, Kamerling JP, et al: *Disturbances of amino acid metabolism: clinical chemistry and diagnosis,* Baltimore, 1981, Urban and Schwarzenburg.

4. Nyhan W, Sakait N: *Diagnostic recognition of genetic disease,* Philadelphia, 1987, Lea & Febiger.

5. Cummings JG: Routine amino acids analysis in the clinical laboratory, *Am Clin Prod Rev* Feb:20-25, 1988.

6. Schaefer A, Piquard F, Haberey P: Plasma amino acids analysis: effects of delayed samples preparation and of storage, *Clin Chim Acta* 164:163-169, 1987.

7. Pesce A, Kaplan L, editors: *Methods in clinical chemistry,* St. Louis, 1987, CV Mosby.

8. Heiblim DI, Evans HE, Glass L, et al: Amino acid concentrations in cerebrospinal fluid, *Arch Neurol* 35:765-768, 1978.

9. Shih V: *Laboratory techniques for the detection of hereditary metabolic disorders,* Boca Raton, FL, 1973, CRC Press.

10. Meites S, editor: *Pediatric clinical chemistry,* ed 3, Washington, DC, 1989, American Association for Clinical Chemistry.

11. Mayo Medical Laboratories: *Test catalog,* Rochester, MN, 2005, Mayo Medical Laboratories.

12. Kruse T, Reiber H, Neuhoff V: Amino acid transport across the human blood-CSF barrier, *J Neurol Sci* 70:129-138, 1985.

13. Cynober L, Dinh FN, Saizy R, et al: Plasma amino acid levels in the first few days after burn injury and their predictive value, *Intensive Care Med* 9:325-331, 1983.

14. Jain KM, Rush BF Jr, Seelig RF, et al: Changes in plasma amino acid profiles following abdominal operations, *Surg Gynecol Obstet* 152:302-306, 1981.

15. Schott KJ, Meier D: Free amino acid pattern of cerebrospinal fluid in meningeal pathology, *Acta Neurol Scand* 75:304-309, 1987.

| **Prostate-specific Antigen** (PSA)[1-4]

 Immunoassay | Serum. Stable up to 24 hr at 2-8° C. For longer periods, store frozen at $-20°$ C or colder. For extended periods store frozen at $-70°$ C. | *ng/mL*
 <4.0 | $\times 1.0$ | *mcg/L*
 <4.0 | S ↓ V Finasteride (average 50%), surgical or medical castration

 S ↑ V Digital rectal examination (DRE), needle biopsy, transurethral resection of the prostate (TURP), ejaculation, cystoscopy, and exercise. Prostate manipulations such as DRE may not result in clinically significant increases in PSA.[5] |

DIAGNOSTIC INFORMATION	REMARKS

CSF ↑ Bacterial meningitis, aseptic meningitis, meningoradiculitis Garin-Bujadoux-Bannwarth, and carcinomatous meningitis[15]

↑ Prostatic cancer, benign prostatic hyperplasia (BPH), and prostatitis.

PSA correlates in general with tumor volume and clinical and pathologic tumor stage but cannot accurately predict pathologic stage in an individual. One approach to improve accuracy is the use of nomograms and predictive algorithms such as the Partin Tables.[6] The Partin Tables use preoperative PSA, clinical TNM stage, and biopsy Gleason score to provide likelihood of pathologic stage at radical retropubic prostatectomy.[1,2,6]

Post-radical prostatectomy treatment values are expected to be undetectable. Biochemical recurrence is typically defined at a cutpoint of 0.2 ng/mL, although cutpoints from 0.1-0.4 are

PSA is a glycoprotein and has a physiological function as a serine protease as part of the kallikrein family and as such is also termed hk3. PSA is produced by epithelial cells in the prostatic acini and ducts and is secreted into the seminal fluid where it liquefies the seminal coagulum to increase sperm motility.

PSA is prostate tissue specific, not prostate cancer specific, and is produced by normal, hyperplastic, and neoplastic prostate tissue. Architectural changes in epithelial cells in prostate cancer results in greater PSA concentrations in the circulation per gram of tissue compared with BPH. PSA is present in serum in a free, unbound form ($\sim$<30%) and bound to protease inhibitors ($\sim$>70%), primarily α_1-antichymotrypsin (ACT) and

TEST NAME AND METHOD	SPECIMEN REQUIREMENTS	REFERENCE INTERVAL, CONVENTIONAL [INTERNATIONAL RECOMMENDED UNITS]	CHEMICAL INTERFERENCES AND IN VIVO EFFECTS

Prostate-specific Antigen—CONT

1. Polascik TJ, Oesterling JE, Partin AW: Prostate specific antigen: a decade of discovery—what we have learned and where we are going, *J Urol* 162:293-306, 1999.

2. Prostate-specific antigen (PSA) best practice policy. American Urological Association (AUA), *Oncology* 14:267-286, 2000.

3. Partin AW, Hanks GE, Klein EA, et al: Prostate-specific antigen as a marker of disease activity in prostate cancer, *Oncology* 16:1024-1042, 2002.

4. Haese A, Becker C, Diamandis EP, et al: Adenocarcinoma of the prostate. In Diamandis EP, Fritsche HA, Lilja H, et al, editors: *Tumor markers. Physiology, pathobiology, technology, and clinical applications,* Washington, DC, 2002, AACC Press.

5. Price CP, Allard J, Davies G, et al: Pre- and post-analytical factors that may influence use of serum prostate specific antigen and its isoforms in a screening programme for prostate cancer, *Ann Clin Biochem* 38:188-216, 2001.

6. Partin AW, Mangold LA, Lamm DM, et al: Contemporary update of prostate cancer staging (Partin Tables) for the new millennium, *Urology* 58:843-848, 2001.

7. Freedland SJ, Sutter ME, Dorey F, et al: Defining the ideal cutpoint for determining PSA recurrence after radical prostatectomy, *Urology* 61:365-369, 2003.

8. Fleisher M, Dnistrian AM, Sturgeon CM, et al: Practice guidelines and recommendations for use of tumor markers in the clinic. In Diamandis EP, Fritsche HA, Lilja H, et al, editors: *Tumor markers. Physiology, pathobiology, technology, and clinical applications,* Washington, DC, 2002, AACC Press.

9. Smith RA, Cokkinides V, Eyre HJ: American cancer society guidelines for the early detection of cancer, 2004, *CA Cancer J Clin* 54:41-52, 2004.

used. Ultrasensative PSA assays have been developed with limits of detection of ≤ 0.01 ng/mL. PSA doubling time can be used to predict risk of and time to recurrence.[3,7]

The acceptable PSA concentration is less clear after radiation therapy, where values may not reach undetectable concentrations. With a nadir <0.5 ng/mL, relapse is not likely with 5 yr of treatment. Biochemical recurrence has been defined by the American Society for Therapeutic Radiation and Oncology (ASTRO) as three consecutive increases in PSA above the nadir.[2,3,7]

α_2-macroglobulin (A2M). PSA assays measure free and complexed forms of PSA, exclusive of PSA-A2M. The differing proportions of free PSA in specimens from patients with cancer and benign prostatic diseases have been exploited to increase the specificity of PSA for cancer detection in the 4-10 ng/mL total PSA diagnostic gray zone.[1-4]

PSA values increase with age, and there is intraindividual variation from day to day. Lack of consensus exists among physician groups in the use of PSA for population-based screening for prostate cancer.[8]

PSA has been recommended by the American Cancer Society for use in conjunction with a DRE for the early detection of prostate cancer starting at age 50 yr for men with at least a 10-yr life expectancy. Men at high risk, such as those of African descent or with a family history of the disease (first-degree relative[s] diagnosed <65 yr) may begin testing at an earlier age.[9] The test is of greatest value as a marker of therapeutic response after definitive treatments including surgery (radical prostatectomy), radiation, and hormonal (antiandrogen) therapy.[2,3]

It is recommended that the same assay method be used for longitudinal monitoring.

TEST NAME AND METHOD	SPECIMEN REQUIREMENTS	REFERENCE INTERVAL, CONVENTIONAL [INTERNATIONAL RECOMMENDED UNITS]			CHEMICAL INTERFERENCES AND IN VIVO EFFECTS
Prostate-specific Antigen, Complexed (cPSA)[1,2] *Immunoassay*[3]	Serum. Stable up to 48 hr at 2-8° C. For longer periods, store frozen at −20° C or colder. For extended periods, store frozen at −70° C.	*ng/mL* <3.2	× 1.0	*mcg/L* <3.2	S ↓ V Antiandrogens, LHRH agonists and antagonists, and finasteride S ↑ V Prostate manipulation (digital rectal examination, needle biopsy, cystoscopy), although cPSA may be less affected than free PSA.[2]

1. Parsons JK, Partin AW: Applying complexed prostate-specific antigen to clinical practice, *Urology* 63:815-818, 2004.
2. Haese A, Becker C, Diamandis EP, et al: Adenocarcinoma of the prostate. In Diamandis EP, Fritsche HA, Lilja H, et al, editors: *Tumor markers. Physiology, pathobiology, technology, and clinical applications,* Washington, DC, 2002, AACC Press.
3. Allard WJ, Zhou Z, Yeung KK: Novel immunoassay for the measurement of complexed prostate-specific antigen in serum, *Clin Chem* 44:1216-1223, 1998.
4. Partin AW, Brawer MK, Bartsch G, et al: Complexed prostate specific antigen improves specificity for prostate cancer detection: results of a prospective multicenter clinical trial, *Urology* 170:1787-1791, 2003.
5. Parsons JK, Brawer MK, Cheli CD, et al: Complexed prostate specific antigen (PSA) reduces unnecessary prostate biopsies in the 2.6-4.0 ng/mL range of total PSA, *BJU Int* 94:47-50, 2004.
6. Allard WJ, Cheli CD, Morris DL, et al: Multicenter evaluation of the performance and clinical utility in longitudinal monitoring of the Bayer Immuno 1 complexed PSA assay, *Int J Biol Markers* 14:73-83, 1999.
7. Sokoll LJ, Mangold LA, Partin AW, et al: Complexed prostate-specific antigen as a staging tool for prostate cancer: a prospective study in 420 men, *Urology* 60(Suppl 1):18-23, 2002.

TEST NAME AND METHOD	SPECIMEN REQUIREMENTS	REFERENCE INTERVAL, CONVENTIONAL [INTERNATIONAL RECOMMENDED UNITS]		CHEMICAL INTERFERENCES AND IN VIVO EFFECTS
Prostate-specific Antigen (PSA), Free Percentage[1,2] *Immunoassay*	Serum. Centrifuge and refrigerate within 3 hr of blood draw. Stable up to 24 hr at 2-8° C. For longer periods, store frozen at −20° C or colder. For extended periods, store frozen at −70° C.	*Single cutoff*[3] *Individual risk assessment*[3] *Percent free PSA* 0-10% 10-15% 15-20% 20-25% >25%	>25% *Probability of prostate cancer* 56% 28% 20% 16% 8%	S ↓ V Finasteride (average 50%) for free and total PSA, no effect %free PSA S ↑ V Free PSA and %free PSA: digital rectal examination (DRE), needle biopsy, ejaculation,

↑ Prostatic cancer, benign prostatic hyperplasia (BPH), and prostatitis.

The majority of studies, including a recent multicenter clinical trial,[4] have shown similar sensitivity for cancer detection for cPSA compared with total PSA with increased specificity in the clinically relevant PSA range of 2-20 ng/mL.[1,2] Increased specificity for cPSA has been particularly observed for total PSA concentrations <4 ng/mL.[5] There is not agreement, however, comparing the diagnostic performance of cPSA with %free PSA.

cPSA correlated with total PSA in the longitudinal monitoring of prostate cancer patients[6] and was equivalent to PSA in predicting organ-confined disease and favorable pathologic features. However, neither cPSA nor total PSA individually was a reliable predictor of final pathologic stage.[7]

PSA is present in serum in a free, unbound form (~<30%) and bound to protease inhibitors (~>70%), primarily α_1-antichymotrypsin (ACT) and α_2-macroglobulin (A2M). Total PSA assays measure free and complexed forms of PSA, exclusive of PSA-A2M. Proportions of free and complexed forms of PSA differ among men with prostate cancer and normal men or men with benign prostatic diseases. Men with prostate cancer have higher percentages of circulating complexed forms of PSA compared with men without cancer.

An assay for complexed PSA (cPSA) has been developed by Bayer HealthCare (Tarrytown, NY) that measures only serum PSA-ACT and other minor PSA complexes because free PSA is blocked with a free PSA-specific antibody and rendered nonreactive in the assay.[3] Assays are available on automated platforms and in a microtiter plate ELISA format. The FDA-indicated uses for the cPSA assay include detection of prostate cancer (in men ≥50 yr in conjunction with DRE) and monitoring of disease and treatment in prostate cancer patients. A cPSA concentration of 3.2 ng/mL is equivalent to a PSA cutoff of 4.0 ng/mL, the standard cutoff for biopsy consideration. The proposed lower PSA threshold of 2.5 ng/mL corresponds to a cPSA concentration of 2.2 ng/mL.[1,4]

Percent free PSA results can be interpreted using a single cutoff or a continuum of values to determine the relative risk of prostate cancer in individual men. In biopsies from men with a total PSA between 4 and 10 ng/mL and a DRE nonsuspicious for cancer, sensitivity for cancer detection was 95% using a %free PSA cutoff of ≤25%. Using this same cutoff (>25%), 20% of men who underwent biopsy with benign disease could be spared from biopsy.[3] Percent free PSA may also be beneficial in men with a total PSA between 4 and 10 ng/mL with a previous negative biopsy.[1]

PSA is a glycoprotein and has a physiological function as a serine protease as part of the kallikrein family and as such is also termed hk3. PSA is present in serum in a free, unbound form (~<30%) and bound to protease inhibitors (~>70%), primarily α_1-antichymotrypsin (ACT) and α_2-macroglobulin (A2M). Total PSA assays measure free and complexed forms of PSA, exclusive of PSA-A2M.[1,2]

TEST NAME AND METHOD	SPECIMEN REQUIREMENTS	REFERENCE INTERVAL, CONVENTIONAL [INTERNATIONAL RECOMMENDED UNITS]	CHEMICAL INTERFERENCES AND IN VIVO EFFECTS

Prostate-specific Antigen (PSA), Free Percentage—CONT

Reference ranges are assay specific.

cystoscopy, and lower urinary tract symptoms.[4]

1. Polascik TJ, Oesterling JE, Partin AW: Prostate specific antigen: a decade of discovery—what we have learned and where we are going, *J Urol* 162:293-306, 1999.
2. Haese A, Becker C, Diamandis EP, et al: Adenocarcinoma of the prostate. In Diamandis EP, Fritsche HA, Lilja H, et al, editors: *Tumor markers. Physiology, pathobiology, technology, and clinical applications,* Washington, DC, 2002, AACC Press.
3. Catalona WJ, Partin AW, Slawin KM, et al: Use of the percentage of free prostate-specific antigen to enhance differentiation of prostate cancer from benign prostatic disease: prospective multicenter clinical trial, *JAMA* 20:1542-1547, 1998.
4. Price CP, Allard J, Davies G, et al: Pre- and post-analytical factors that may influence use of serum prostate specific antigen and its isoforms in a screening programme for prostate cancer, *Ann Clin Biochem* 38:188-216, 2001.

TEST NAME AND METHOD	SPECIMEN REQUIREMENTS	REFERENCE INTERVAL, CONVENTIONAL		[INTERNATIONAL RECOMMENDED UNITS]	CHEMICAL INTERFERENCES AND IN VIVO EFFECTS
Prostatic Acid Phosphatase (PAP, *o*-Phosphoric monoester phosphohydrolase; EC 3.1.3.2)[1] *Tartrate inhibition (phenyl phosphate, a-naphthyl phosphate), 37° C[2]* *Thymolphthalein monophosphate, 37° C[3]*	Serum. Avoid hemolysis. Separate serum and analyze immediately or add citrate buffer or acetic acid to attain a pH of 5.4-6.2; otherwise, rapid loss in activity occurs. Store at 4 or −20° C; avoid repeated freezing and thawing.	0-0.8 U/L	× 1.0	[0-0.8 U/L]	↑ Moderate hemolysis (trace hemolysis without effect); goserelin (transient effect early in treatment) ↑ V Alglucerase (values should decrease with treatment), androgens (females), and clofibrate ↑ C Fluoride, oxalate, heparin: Tartrate and ethanol inhibit the prostatic fraction; formalin inhibition of nonprostatic fraction probably accounts for excellent histologic staining of prostatic fraction ↓ V Ketoconazole (in prostatic carcinoma)

DIAGNOSTIC INFORMATION	REMARKS

One approach to improve the specificity of PSA for prostate cancer detection to distinguish cancer from benign prostatic diseases, particularly in the 4-10 ng/mL total PSA diagnostic gray zone, is the measurement of free PSA. Free PSA is not used alone but is most useful expressed in a ratio with total PSA (%free PSA = free PSA/total PSA $\times$ 100). Patients with benign conditions have a higher proportion of free PSA compared with men with prostate cancer.

Total and free PSA measurements should be made from the same specimen in parallel using assays from the same manufacturer.

S ↑ Prostatic cancer (especially, but not always, with metastases),[6] Gaucher's disease and Niemann-Pick disease, for 1-2 days after prostatic surgery or biopsy, after prostatic manipulation or catheterization, benign prostatic hypertrophy (BPH), prostatitis, and prostate infarct[1,7]

Elevations in 80% of individuals with metastatic prostate cancer are related to the stage. PAP is not elevated in early stage prostate disease.[6] Currently, PAP has little role in the early detection and management of prostate cancer, having been replaced by the more sensitive PSA test. PAP may have utility in limited cases. A high preoperative PAP in a patient with clinically localized prostate cancer suggests pathologically advanced stage disease, and this patient may not be a good candidate for surgical cure. PAP may also be used to monitor disease in very rare cases where a tumor does not produce PSA.[8]

Immunochemical methods are specific for prostatic acid phosphatase and more sensitive, although their use does not offer any advantages.[8]

Acid phosphatase is a lysosomal enzyme. The prostatic enzyme is found in lysosomes of the prostate epithelium and is a glycoprotein with an MW of 100,000. The biological $t_{1/2}$ is 1.1-2.6 hr.

The greatest activity per gram of tissue of total acid phosphatase and PAP is found in the prostate gland. Lesser activities of nonprostate-specific acid phosphatase are found in liver, spleen, erythrocytes, platelets, and bone marrow (with negligible quantities of PAP). Total serum acid phosphatase in males consists of approximately one half prostatic and the rest from liver and disintegrating platelets and erythrocytes. In females, the serum activity is presumably from liver, erythrocytes, and platelets.

TEST NAME AND METHOD	SPECIMEN REQUIREMENTS	REFERENCE INTERVAL, CONVENTIONAL [INTERNATIONAL RECOMMENDED UNITS]			CHEMICAL INTERFERENCES AND IN VIVO EFFECTS

Prostatic Acid Phosphatase—CONT

Immunoassay[4]	Serum. Stable up to 24 hr at 2-8° C. For longer periods, store frozen at −20° C or colder.	<2.5 ng/mL	× 1.0	[<2.5 mcg/L]	
4-Nitrophenyl-phosphate (with tartrate inhibition), 37° C[5]	Semen or seminal plasma. Treat like serum.	~50,000 U/L			
	Place swab with vaginal fluid in 1 mL NaCl, 0.155 mol/L, and keep frozen until assay.	<2 U/L			

1. Rubinstein M, Guinam PO, McKiel CF, et al: Review of acid phosphatase in the diagnosis and prognosis of prostatic cancers, *Clin Physiol Biochem* 6:241-252, 1988.
2. Saw D, Schwartz MK, Smith C, et al: Comparison of assays for prostatic and total acid phosphatase, *Clin Biochem* 23:505-508, 1990.
3. Roy A, Brower ME, Hayden JE: Sodium thymolphthalein monophosphate: a new acid phosphatase substrate with greater specificity for the prostatic enzyme in serum, *Clin Chem* 17:1093-1102, 1971.
4. Henderson AR, Nealon DA: Enzyme measurements by mass: an interim review of the clinical efficacy of some mass measurements of prostatic acid phosphate and the isoenzymes of creatine kinase, *Clin Chim Acta* 115:9-32, 1981.
5. Gohara WF: Rate of decrease of glutamyltransferase and acid phosphatase activities in the human vagina after coitus, *Clin Chem* 26:254-257, 1980.
6. Heller JE: Prostatic acid phosphatase: its current clinical status, *J Urol* 137:1091-1103, 1987.
7. Schwartz MK: Enzymes in cancer, *Clin Lab Med* 9:757-765, 1989.
8. Haese A, Becker C, Diamandis EP, et al: Adenocarcinoma of the prostate. In Diamandis EP, Fritsche HA, Lilja H, et al, editors: *Tumor markers. Physiology, pathobiology, technology, and clinical applications,* Washington, DC, 2002, AACC Press.

Protamine Neutralization Assay[1]	Plasma (citrate). Stable for 7 days at room temperature or for 23 days at 4° C.	A prolonged thrombin time should become normal when all the heparin in the plasma has been neutralized with protamine sulfate.	Elevated FDP level may give false-positive result.

1. Olson J, Arkin CF, Brandt JT, et al: College of American Pathologists Conference XXXI on Laboratory Monitoring of Anticoagulant Therapy. Laboratory monitoring of unfractionated heparin therapy, *Arch Pathol Lab Med* 122:782-798, 1998.

DIAGNOSTIC INFORMATION	REMARKS

↑ Vaginal swabs from rape victims[5]

Used to calculate the dose of protamine sulfate necessary to neutralize circulating heparin.

Protamine neutralizes the anticoagulant effect of heparin. The protamine neutralization assay is most commonly used to calculate the dose of protamine necessary to neutralize heparin after cardiac surgery or hemodialysis. It may also be used to monitor unfractionated heparin.

The test is dependent on heparin concentration. High concentration of heparin requires more protamine to shorten thrombin time.

These assays are not readily automated because of the need for several dilutions and therefore are not used for routine monitoring.

TEST NAME AND METHOD	SPECIMEN REQUIREMENTS	REFERENCE INTERVAL, CONVENTIONAL [INTERNATIONAL RECOMMENDED UNITS]			CHEMICAL INTERFERENCES AND IN VIVO EFFECTS
Protein, Total (TP)[1-5] *Refractometry, biuret*	Serum. Analyze fresh or store at 4° C for <72 hr. Stable frozen at −20° C for 6 mo or at −70° C indefinitely. Specimens without lipemia or hemolysis are preferred.	Cord: Premature: Newborn: 1 wk: 7 mo-1 yr: 1-2 yr: ≥3 yr: Adult, Ambulatory: Recumbent: >60 yr:	*g/dL*[1] 4.8-8.0 3.6-6.0 4.6-7.0 4.4-7.6 5.1-7.3 5.6-7.5 6.0-8.0 6.4-8.3 6.0-7.8 Lower by ~0.2	× 10	*g/L* [48-80] [36-60] [46-70] [44-76] [51-73] [56-75] [60-80] [64-83] [60-78] [~2.0]	S ↑ C Dextran (biuret) S ↑ V Anabolic steroids, androgens, clofibrate, corticosteroids, corticotropin, epinephrine, insulin, progesterone, and thyroid preparations S ↓ C Dextran, sulfasalazine S ↓ V Allopurinol, estrogens
Turbidimetry, nephelometry	Urine, 24 hr. Use no preservatives. Centrifuge and adjust to pH 7.0. Analyze fresh. Stable frozen at −20° C for up to 1 yr.	1-14 mg/dL[9] At rest: 50-80 mg/day After intense exercise: Random urine[10]: *g/dL* M: 1-16 F: 0-16 M: 16-138 F: 14-134	× 10 <250 mg/day × 10 × 10	[10-140 mg/L] *g/L* [10-160] [0-160] [160-1380] [140-1340]	U ↑ C Aminosalicylic acid, aspirin, chlorpromazine, gentamicin, nafcillin, penicillin, phenolphthalein, promazine, radiographic contrast media, and sodium bicarbonate U ↑ V Acetaminophen, aminoglycosides, amphotericin B, bacitracin, bismuth salts, capreomycin, captopril, chloropropamide, colistin, corti-

DIAGNOSTIC INFORMATION	REMARKS

S ↑ Hyperimmunoglobulinemia caused by polyclonal or monoclonal gammopathies, acute phase response[1]

Pseudohyperproteinemia: Hemoconcentration caused by dehydration (in vivo), sample desiccation (in vitro)

S ↓ *Protein loss:* Protein-losing gastroenteropathies, acute burns, and nephrotic syndrome

Decreases caused by decreased synthesis of proteins: Severe protein deficiency, chronic liver disease, malabsorption syndrome, malnutrition, and agammaglobulinemia

Insulin and IGF-I decrease protein degradation, whereas growth hormone stimulates protein synthesis.[5]

Prolonged application of a tourniquet increases concentrations of all proteins in the blood sample. Sample obtained above an IV infusion site can show erroneously low values as a result of local hemodilution.[13] Erroneously increased protein concentrations can be caused by evaporation of serum samples in the laboratory. Inadequate mixing of thawed samples may cause values in error by 10-200% of true values.

Upright posture for several hours after rising increases concentrations of all macromolecular analytes.[14] Significantly over levels are found early in the day. Even 1 hr of ambulation after overnight recumbent posture results in a demonstrable increase. Serum total protein for bedridden patients is lower by ~0.3 g/dL [~3 g/L] than expected for the same age.

Serum total protein decreases in the third trimester of pregnancy. During overnight recumbency values decrease 1.0-1.3 g/dL [10-13 g/L]; they decrease still farther with prolonged bed rest. IV infusions substantial enough to cause hemodilution will decrease serum total protein levels. Venous stasis resulting from occlusion caused by disease processes or peripheral vascular collapse can elevate levels.

Refractometric determination of total protein can be affected by hyperglycemia when glucose accounts for a large proportion of total blood solutes; total protein concentration appears to be greater than it actually is. Severe hyperlipidemia, hyperbilirubinemia, or hemolysis has the same effect. Results of the biuret method may be falsely elevated by lipemia, icterus, and hemolysis; reliable procedures incorporate corrections to minimize these effects. Refractometric and biuret methods give comparable results on clean, clear serum samples.

U ↑ Nephrotic syndrome, diabetic nephropathy, monoclonal gammopathies such as multiple myeloma and other myeloproliferative or lymphoproliferative disorders, abnormal renal tubular absorption (e.g., Fanconi syndrome, heavy metal poisoning, sarcoidosis, and sickle cell disease), urinary tract malignancies, and inflammatory, degenerative, and irritative conditions of the lower urinary tract. After exercise (levels vary with type of exercise, 22-340 mg/day).

False-negative results may occur with highly alkaline urine. Total urine protein by precipitation methods cannot be relied on to quantify urinary immunoglobulin light chains. Some samples will remain fully soluble after precipitation of all other species. Turbidimetric and dye-binding based methodologies may not have equal sensitivity or specificity for all proteins and may underestimate low-molecular-weight proteins and immunoglobulin light chains.[1]

TEST NAME AND METHOD	SPECIMEN REQUIREMENTS	REFERENCE INTERVAL, CONVENTIONAL [INTERNATIONAL RECOMMENDED UNITS]		CHEMICAL INTERFERENCES AND IN VIVO EFFECTS

Protein, Total—CONT

costeroids, cortimoxazole, cyclosporin, enalapril, gold, griseofulvin, hydralazine, interferon, isoniazid, lithium, mitomycin, nonsteroidal antiinflammatory drugs, pencillamine, penicillins, polymyxin, rifampin, sulfonamides, sulfones, tetracycline, and tolbutamide metabolites[12]

U ↓ V Indomethacin (in patients with nephrotic syndrome)

U ↓ C Highly alkaline urine[12]

	CSF. Centrifuge before analysis. Analyze fresh or store at 4° C for <72 hr. Stable frozen at −20° C for 6 mo or at −70° C indefinitely. Specimens should not contain blood.	mg/dL^{11}		mg/L	↑ C Aspirin, chlorpromazine, imipramine, lidocaine, methicillin, methotrexate, morphine, penicillin, phenacetin, procaine, streptomycin, and tyrosine
		Premature:	15-130 ×10	[150-1300]	
		Full-term newborn:	40-120	[400-1200]	
		<1 mo:	20-80	[200-800]	
		>1 mo:	15-40	[150-400]	
$Column^6$			mg/dL	mg/L	↑ V Ibuprofen, sulindac
		Adult Lumbar:	8-32	[80-320]	
$Turbidimetry, biuret^7$		Lumbar fluid:	15-45	[150-450]	
		Cisternal fluid:	15-25	[150-250]	
		Ventricular fluid:	5-15	[50-150]	
$Biuret^8$	Amniotic fluid. Centrifuge before analysis. Analyze fresh or store at 4° C for <72 hr. Stable frozen at −20° C for 6 mo or at −70° C indefinitely. Specimens should not contain blood.	g/dL		g/L	
		Early pregnancy:	0.2-1.7 ×10	[2.0-17.0]	
		Late pregnancy:	0.175-0.705	[1.8-7.1]	
			($\bar{x}$: 0.24)	[$\bar{x}$: 2.4]	

DIAGNOSTIC INFORMATION	REMARKS

CSF ↑ In diseases leading to the "influx syndrome" (i.e., breakdown of the blood-CNS barrier), such as meningitis, encephalomyelitis

Excessive concentrations of total CSF proteins are seen in Froin's syndrome (protein >500 mg/dL; >5000 g/L), clotted CSF specimens, xanthochromia, or in the presence of free blood.

In premature infants, values >130 mg/dL [>1300 mg/L] may occasionally be observed.

TEST NAME AND METHOD	SPECIMEN REQUIREMENTS	REFERENCE INTERVAL, CONVENTIONAL [INTERNATIONAL RECOMMENDED UNITS]		CHEMICAL INTERFERENCES AND IN VIVO EFFECTS

Protein, Total—CONT

Turbidimetry, biuret	Transudate fluid (e.g., bronchial fluid).[7] Centrifuge before analysis. Analyze fresh or store at 4° C for <72 hr. Stable frozen at −20° C for 6 mo or at −70° C indefinitely. Specimens should not contain blood.	<2.0 g/dL	× 10	<20 g/L
	Exudate fluid.[7] Centrifuge before analysis. Analyze fresh or store at 4° C for <72 hr. Stable frozen at −20° C for 6 mo or at −70° C indefinitely. Specimens should not contain blood.	>2.0 g/dL		>20 g/L

1. Tietz NW, editor: *Textbook of clinical chemistry,* Philadelphia, 1999, WB Saunders.
2. Ritzmann SE, Daniels JC, editors: *Serum protein abnormalities, diagnostic and clinical aspects,* Boston, 1975, Little, Brown and Co.
3. Ritzmann SE, Tucker ES III: *Protein analysis in disease—current concepts. Workshop manual,* Chicago, 1979, American Society of Clinical Pathologists, Commission for Continuing Education.
4. Behrman RE, Vaughan VC III, editors: *Nelson textbook of pediatrics,* ed 13, Philadelphia, 1987, WB Saunders.
5. Liu Z, Barrett EJ: Human protein metabolism: its measurement and regulation, *Am J Physiol Endocrinol Metab* 283:E1105-E1112, 2002.
6. Beeson PB, McDermott W, Wyngaarden JB, editors: *Cecil textbook of medicine,* ed 15, Philadelphia, 1979, WB Saunders.
7. Brown SS, Mitchell FL, Young DS, editors: *Chemical diagnosis of disease,* Amsterdam, 1979, Elsevier/North Holland Biomedical Press.
8. Natelson S, Scommegna A, Epstein MB, editors: *Amniotic fluid,* New York, 1974, John Wiley & Sons.
9. Pesce AJ, First MR: *Proteinuria—an integrated review,* New York, 1979, Marcel Dekker.
10. Bond LW, Garber C, Ottinger W, et al: Reference intervals for common analytes in random urine specimens, *Clin Chem* 55:submitted, 2005.
11. Meites S, editor: *Pediatric clinical chemistry,* ed 2, Washington, DC, 1981, American Association for Clinical Chemistry.
12. Strasinger SK: *Urinalysis and body fluids: a self-instructional text,* ed 2, Philadelphia, 1991, FA Davis.
13. Read DC, Viera H, Arkin C: Effect of drawing blood specimens proximal to an in-place but discontinuous intravenous solution, *Am J Clin Pathol* 90:702-706, 1988.
14. Miller M, Bachorick PS, Cloey TA: Normal variation of plasma lipoproteins: postural effects on plasma concentrations of lipids, lipoproteins and apolipoproteins, *Clin Chem* 38:569-574, 1992.

TEST NAME AND METHOD	SPECIMEN REQUIREMENTS	REFERENCE INTERVAL, CONVENTIONAL [INTERNATIONAL RECOMMENDED UNITS]		CHEMICAL INTERFERENCES AND IN VIVO EFFECTS
Protein C Assay[1-3]	Plasma (citrate). Stable at room temperature for 8 hr, at −20° C for 1 mo.	Approximately 70-140%. There may be an overlap between normal and heterozygous individuals. Laboratory reference ranges should be established. Protein C levels are physiologically low in neonates and infants because of liver immaturity.		↓ Oral anticoagulant therapy, L-asparaginase ↑ V Oral contraceptives, stanozolol

1. Lewis SM, Bain BJ, Bates I, editors: *Dacie and Lewis practical hematology,* ed 9, Edinburgh, 2001, Churchill Livingstone.
2. Jacobs DS, Demott WR, Oxley DK, editors: *Laboratory test handbook,* ed 5, Hudson, OH, 2001, Lexi-Comp, Inc.
3. Kottke-Marchant K, Comp P: Laboratory issues in diagnosing abnormalities of protein C, thrombomodulin, and endothelial cell protein C receptor, *Arch Pathol Lab Med* 126:1337-1348, 2002.

Protein Electrophoresis[1-4]	Serum. Analyze fresh or store at 4° C for <72 hr. Stable frozen at −20° C for 6 mo or at −70° C indefinitely. Specimens without lipemia or hemolysis are preferred.	g/dL[3,5]		g/L	Chylous or hemolyzed sample, plasma, and sample containing visible precipitates
		Cellulose acetate			
Albumin		Adult:	3.5-5.0[1] 3.2-5.5[6,7]	× 10	[35-50] [32-55]	See *Albumin.*
		Agarose				
		0-15 days:	3.0-3.9		[30-39]	
		15 days-1 yr	2.2-4.8		[22-48]	
		1-16 yr	3.6-5.2		[36-52]	
		>16 yr	3.9-5.1		[39-51]	
α₁-*Globulin*		*Cellulose acetate*				S ↑ V Testosterone
		Adult:	0.1-0.3		[1-3]	
		Agarose				
		<1 yr:	0.1-0.3		[1-3]	
		1-16 yr:	0.1-0.4		[1-4]	
		>16 yr:	0.2-0.4		[2-4]	

DIAGNOSTIC INFORMATION	REMARKS

↓ *Congenital deficiency:* Type I protein C deficiency with low activity and low antigen level; type II with low activity but normal antigen level.

Acquired deficiency is observed in: liver disorders; during warfarin therapy; vitamin K deficiency; consumptive coagulopathies; renal insufficiency; acute thrombosis; postoperative state; and plasma exchange.

Heterozygous protein C deficiency is associated with an increased risk of venous thrombosis. Homozygous protein C deficiency is rare, but it is associated with neonatal venous thrombosis, usually presenting as purpura fulminans neonatorum.

Laboratory evaluation of protein C includes antigenic and functional assays. The antigenic assays include ELISA, electroimmunoassay, and radioimmunoassay. The functional assays are clot-based or chromogenic, the latter usually favored because of less interferences. In general, a chromogenic assay is recommended for initial testing.

The diagnosis of protein C deficiency should only be established after acquired causes of protein C deficiency are excluded.

Measurement of protein C levels is not advised during acute illness/acute thrombotic event due to consumption of protein C and in patients receiving oral anticoagulant because warfarin will decrease protein C levels. Repeat testing is recommended once patients are off oral anticoagulation (best done 30 days after cessation). Correlation with family studies is also recommended.

See *CSF,* below.

See *Albumin, serum.*

See *Albumin, Serum.*

S ↑ α_1-Antitrypsin is an acute phase reacting protein. Concentrations increase with inflammation, infection, trauma, malignancies, and some hepatic disorders.

S ↓ Hereditary α_1-antitrypsin deficiency, Tangier disease (α_1-lipoprotein)

The α_1-fraction primarily consists of α_1-antitrypsin, α_1-lipoprotein, and α_1-acid glycoprotein.

TEST NAME AND METHOD	SPECIMEN REQUIREMENTS	REFERENCE INTERVAL, CONVENTIONAL [INTERNATIONAL RECOMMENDED UNITS]		CHEMICAL INTERFERENCES AND IN VIVO EFFECTS
Protein Electrophoresis—CONT				
α_2-*Globulin*	*Cellulose acetate*			S ↑ V Estrogens, oral contraceptives, and phenytoin
	Adult:	0.6-1.0	[6-10]	
	Higher in children	<15 yr		S ↓ V Asparaginase
	Agarose			
	0-15 days:	0.3-0.6	[3-6]	
	15 days-1 yr:	0.5-0.9	[5-9]	
	1-16 yr:	0.5-1.2	[5-12]	
	>16 yr:	0.4-0.8	[4-8]	
β-*Globulin*	*Cellulose acetate*			S ↑ V Estrogens, oral contraceptives
	Adult:	0.7-1.1	[7-11]	
	Agarose			S ↓ V Asparaginase
	0-15 days:	0.4-0.6	[4-6]	
	15 days-1 yr:	0.5-0.9	[5-9]	
	1-16 yr:	0.5-1.1	[5-11]	
	>16 yr:	0.5-1.0	[5-10]	
γ-*Globulin*	*Cellulose acetate*			
	Adult:	0.8-1.6	[8-16]	
	Agarose			
	0-15 days:	0.7-1.4	[7-14]	
	15 days-1 yr:	0.5-1.3	[5-13]	
	1-16 yr:	0.5-1.7	[5-17]	
	>16 yr:	0.6-1.2	[6-12]	

DIAGNOSTIC INFORMATION	REMARKS
S ↑ Nephrotic syndrome, subacute and chronic inflammatory disorders, and tumors S ↓ Hemolysis, pancreatitis	The α_2-fraction contains α_2-macroglobulin, haptoglobin, and apolipoprotein B. α_2-Macroglobulin is the component that increases markedly with nephrotic syndrome.
S ↑ Primary or secondary hyperlipoproteinemias (especially type II), monoclonal gammopathies S ↓ Hypo-β-lipoproteinemias, IgA deficiency	The β-fraction contains transferrin (increases with iron deficiency), hemopexin, complement factors, antithrombin III, and immunoglobulins. In fresh serum, the β-globulin region is often split. The smaller β_2-fraction mainly contains lipoproteins. With specimen degradation, the β_2-band becomes diminished and may no longer be visible, particularly with samples older than 3 days.[4] Monoclonal proteins of the IgA type frequently migrate within the beta region or near the β-γ junction. Consequently, these may be missed if obscured by the β-bands.
S ↑ *Polyclonal gammopathies:* Chronic inflammatory conditions, chronic infections, autoimmune disease, and liver disease (may be associated with β-γ bridging) *Oligoclonal gammopathies:* Response to infection, autoimmune disorders, circulating immune complexes, and previous immunosuppressive therapy *Monoclonal gammopathies:* Plasma cell dyscrasias/lymphoproliferative disorders (e.g., multiple myeloma, Waldenstroms macroglobulinemia, amyloidosis, lymphoma, chronic lymphocytic leukemia), monoclonal gammopathy of undetermined significance S ↓ Immune deficiency or suppression, lymphoproliferative disorder	The γ-fraction contains immunoglobulins G, A, M, D, and E. Spikes suspected to be caused by M-proteins within the γ-, β-, or α-globulin regions require immunofixation electrophoresis for confirmation and characterization. Fibrinogen migrates within the γ region, near the β-γ junction. It may be present if a plasma sample (rather than serum) is used, the patient has received anticoagulant therapy or has a coagulopathy, or if the specimen was not allowed to clot sufficiently. C-reactive protein (CRP) also migrates within the γ-fraction and like fibrinogen, can appear as a small band if sufficiently increased. Both fibrinogen and CRP can be mistaken for the presence of an M-protein if immunofixation electrophoresis is not performed. Monoclonal cryoglobulins (most frequently IgM) may precipitate at room temperature, resulting in falsely low quantitation of the M-protein peak. When their presence is suspected, the specimen should be warmed to 37° C immediately before electrophoresis. Monoclonal immunoglobulins may polymerize (most often IgM, less often IgA), inhibiting optimal migration. Sample pretreatment with a reducing agent such as 2-mercaptoethanol may be required.[4]

TEST NAME AND METHOD	SPECIMEN REQUIREMENTS	REFERENCE INTERVAL, CONVENTIONAL [INTERNATIONAL RECOMMENDED UNITS]		CHEMICAL INTERFERENCES AND IN VIVO EFFECTS

Protein Electrophoresis—CONT

Cellulose acetate, agarose	CSF. Centrifuge before analysis. Analyze fresh or store at 4° C for <72 hr. Stable frozen at −20° C for 6 mo or at −70° C indefinitely. Specimens should not contain blood.	*Percent of total protein*[6]	*As a fraction of total protein*	
		Prealbumin: 2-7	× 0.01 [0.02-0.07]	
		Albumin: 56-76	[0.56-0.76]	
		α_1-Globulin: 2-7	[0.02-0.07]	
		α_2-Globulin: 4-12	[0.04-0.12]	
		β-Globulin: 8-18	[0.08-0.18]	
		γ-Globulin: 3-12	[0.03-0.12]	

1. Tietz NW, editor: *Textbook of clinical chemistry,* Philadelphia, 1999, WB Saunders.
2. Ritzmann SE, Daniels JC, editors: *Serum protein abnormalities, diagnostic and clinical aspects,* Boston, 1975, Little, Brown and Co.
3. Ritzmann SE, Tucker ES III: *Protein analysis in disease—current concepts. Workshop manual,* Chicago, 1979, American Society of Clinical Pathologists, Commission for Continuing Education.
4. Janik B: *Electrophoresis and immunofixation of the proteins of serum, urine and cerebrospinal fluid: a brief guide,* Norcross, GA, 2001, Sebia, Inc.
5. AB Chandler Medical Center Clinical Laboratories: *Reference ranges and general information,* Lexington, KY, 1993, University of Kentucky; values partially established at the University of Kentucky Medical Center.
6. Glasser L: Body fluids. III: Tapping the wealth of information in CSF, *Diagn Med* 4:23-33, 1981.

Protein S Assay[1]	Plasma (citrate). Stable at room temperature for 8 hr, at −20° C for 1 mo.	Total protein S: 65-140%	Decreased protein S levels may be caused by acute phase reaction or hormonal effect (oral contraceptives, hormone replacement therapy, pregnancy).
		Protein S levels are lower in neonates and infants but generally increase to adult levels by 6-12 mo.	
			Increased protein S: the lupus anticoagulant may interfere with the functional assay.

1. Goodwin AJ, Rosendaal FR, Kottke-Marchant K, et al: A review of the technical, diagnostic, and epidemiologic considerations for protein S assays, *Arch Pathol Lab Med* 126:1349-1366, 2002.

DIAGNOSTIC INFORMATION	REMARKS

CSF ↓ *Physiological:* In infants of 3-4 mo of age, congenital hypo- or agammaglobulinemia

High-resolution agarose electrophoresis of CSF is useful when assessing for the presence of oligoclonal bands. The CSF electrophoretic pattern should be compared with that of a simultaneously collected serum sample. The use of silver staining can be used to increase sensitivity. CSF oligoclonal bands in the γ region are found in the majority of patients with multiple sclerosis. They can also be present with other conditions involving the CNS such as neurosyphilis, subacute sclerosing panencephalitis, progressive rubella panencephalitis, and other infections, as well as metastatic and primary CNS malignancies.

↓ *Hereditary deficiency:* Type I—activity and antigen (free and total) levels are decreased; type II—activity decreased and antigen (free and total) normal; type III—low activity, low free, normal total.

Acquired deficiency: Acute thrombotic events, DIC, surgery; liver disorders; oral anticoagulant treatment (repeat at least 30 days after cessation of warfarin therapy); L-asparaginase treatment; acute phase reactant (the in vivo increase of C_{4b}-binding protein [C4b-BP] may contribute to increased binding of protein S and result in decreased free and functional protein S levels).

Protein S is a vitamin K–dependent protein synthesized in the liver. It enhances the anticoagulant action of activated protein C as a cofactor. In normal human plasma, protein S exists in two forms: free (~40%) and bound to C4b-BP (~60%). Only the free form of protein S expresses biological activity, whereas the bound one is functionally inactive.

Protein S assays are technically challenging. Protein S can be tested by functional (activity) and immunologic (antigen) assays. Current ELISA tests can measure free and bound PS antigen. Measurement of free PS may be more useful than total PS. A functional test is generally recommended for initial screening.

Protein levels vary with age, sex, and hormonal status. It is preferable not to test for PS deficiency during an acute thrombotic event (although a normal PS level would essentially exclude PS deficiency).

TEST NAME AND METHOD	SPECIMEN REQUIREMENTS	REFERENCE INTERVAL, CONVENTIONAL [INTERNATIONAL RECOMMENDED UNITS]	CHEMICAL INTERFERENCES AND IN VIVO EFFECTS
Proteinase 3 Antibodies (PR3) *Solid-phase EIA*	Serum, frozen or refrigerated is preferable. Plasma is acceptable for analysis.	<5 U: Negative 5-15 U: Borderline >15 U: Positive Results are expressed in arbitrary units. Reference ranges may vary with reagent manufacturer.	None known.

1. Russel KA, Wiegert E, Schroeder DR, et al: Detection of anti-neutrophil cytoplasmic antibodies under actual clinical testing conditions, *Clin Immunol* 103:196-203, 2002.

TEST NAME AND METHOD	SPECIMEN REQUIREMENTS	REFERENCE INTERVAL, CONVENTIONAL [INTERNATIONAL RECOMMENDED UNITS]	CHEMICAL INTERFERENCES AND IN VIVO EFFECTS
Prothrombin Time[1-4]	Plasma (blue top-citrate). Stable for 24 hr at room temperature.	Reference values will vary with the type of thromboplastin. Each laboratory should determine its own reference range. In general: 11-16 sec Newborn: Prolonged, reaches adult levels by 6 mo Monitoring warfarin[4]: *INR** generally 2.0-3.0 *INR = [Patient PT/Normal mean PT]^{ISI†} †ISI = International Sensitivity Index of thromboplastin. The manufacturer assigns an ISI for each thromboplastin reagent.	↑ V Acetaminophen (poisoning), acetohexamide, aminosalicylic acid, anabolic steroids, anistreplase, asparaginase, aspirin (large-dose effect), carbenicillin, cephalosporins (particularly cefamandole, cefmetazole, cefoperazone, cefotetan, moxalactam), cholestyramine (rare), cholestipol (rare), cyclophosphamide, ethanol (large quantities, alcoholism), halothane, heparin (concentration-related effect, more likely with intermittent doses), hetastarch (transient), interferon α-2b, laxatives, methotrexate, niacin, oral anticoagulants, plicamycin, pyrazinamide, quinidine, quinine, thiazides, ticarcillin, tolazamide, and tolbutamide. The drugs listed above may produce an additive effect to oral anticoagulants. Other drugs that may interact with the oral anticoagulant to enhance its action include allopurinol, amiodarone, chloral hydrate (initial effect),

DIAGNOSTIC INFORMATION	REMARKS

PR3 autoantibodies are detectable in >80% of patients with active WG and have a high positive predictive value for WG.[1]

PR3 is a 29 kDa serine protease that exists as a protein triplet in human neutrophils. PR3 autoantibodies may be involved in the pathogenesis of WG.

↑ Oral anticoagulant drugs (warfarin); liver disease; vitamin K deficiency; DIC; hereditary deficiency of factors VII, X, V, and II; afibrinogenemia, hypofibrinogenemia, and dysfibrinogenemia; a circulating anticoagulant affecting the PT system (rarely lupus anticoagulant).

The prothrombin time (PT) is the most widely performed coagulation assay. The PT evaluates the extrinsic and common coagulation pathways and may be prolonged with low plasma levels of factors II, V, VII, X, and fibrinogen. The sensitivity of the PT test to factor deficiencies varies among the reagent thromboplastins available from different manufacturers. The thromboplastin reagents may be from a human, rabbit, or bovine source.

The PT is the most commonly used test for monitoring oral anticoagulant therapy (warfarin). In addition to results reported in seconds, the International Normalized Ratio (INR) is calculated. The INR was introduced in 1983 to improve PT reporting and enhance standardization. An International Sensitivity Index (ISI) is assigned to each thromboplastin by the reagent manufacturer. The ISI is a measure of a reagent's responsiveness to low levels of Vitamin-K–dependent coagulation factors compared with the primary WHO International Reference Preparation.

Despite the improvement with INR reporting, significant variation in INR results between laboratories persists. These differences in INR reflect local variables (i.e., reagent and/or instrument system used in the local laboratory). A high-sensitivity, low ISI thromboplastin reagent (e.g., recombinant thromboplastins) is recommended to improve precision and accuracy of the INR, resulting in better anticoagulation control.[3]

International consensus with regard to optimal INR ranges for prophylaxis and treatment of venous and arterial thromboembolism has been recently established.[4]

TEST NAME AND METHOD	SPECIMEN REQUIREMENTS	REFERENCE INTERVAL, CONVENTIONAL [INTERNATIONAL RECOMMENDED UNITS]	CHEMICAL INTERFERENCES AND IN VIVO EFFECTS
Prothrombin Time—CONT			chloramphenicol (inhibits metabolism), cimetidine, clofibrate, disulfiram, erythromycin, ethacrynic acid, glucagons, mefenamic acid, metronidazole, miconazole, nalidixic acid, oxyphenbutazone, phenyramidol, phenytoin (transient initial effect), sulfinpyrazone, sulfonamides, tamoxifen, thyroxine, and phenylbutazone.
			↓ V Alcohol (chronic abuse), aspirin (small doses), menadiol, mercaptopurine, phytonadione, and oral contraceptives
			Other drugs that may interact with oral anticoagulants to decrease their effect include aminoglutethimide, barbiturates, carbamazepine, corticosteroids, ethanol, ethchlorvynol, glutethimide, phenytoin (chronic use), griseofulvin, rifampin, cholestyramine (impairs absorption), and chlorinated hydrocarbon insecticides.
			↓ High level of antithrombin
			List not all-inclusive

1. Lewis SM, Bain BJ, Bates I, editors: *Dacie and Lewis practical hematology,* ed 9, Edinburgh, 2001, Churchill Livingstone.
2. Jacobs DS, Demott WR, Oxley DK, editors: *Laboratory test handbook,* ed 5, Hudson, OH, 2001, Lexi-Comp, Inc.
3. Ansell J, Hirsh J, Poller L, et al: The pharmacology and management of the vitamin K antagonists, *Chest* 126:2045-2335, 2004.
4. Adcock DM, Brien WF, Duff SL, et al: Procedures for validation of INR and local calibration of PT/INR systems: approved guidelines, *Clinical and Laboratory Standards Institute.*

DIAGNOSTIC INFORMATION   **REMARKS**

TEST NAME AND METHOD	SPECIMEN REQUIREMENTS	REFERENCE INTERVAL, CONVENTIONAL [INTERNATIONAL RECOMMENDED UNITS]	CHEMICAL INTERFERENCES AND IN VIVO EFFECTS
PT, aPTT Mixing Studies (Inhibitor Screen)[1,2]	Plasma (blue top tube-citrate). Stable for 1 hr at 4° C, 4 hr on ice, or for 28 days if frozen.	Three patterns seen: 1. PTT of mixture normal immediate and after 2-hr incubation (correction pattern): consistent with factor deficiency. No evidence of an inhibitor. 2. PTT of mixture prolonged at immediate and after 2-hr incubation: consistent with an inhibitor, most commonly a lupus anticoagulant. Of note, some specific inhibitors may not be time dependent (e.g., factors IX, XI, or XII) and will show a similar mixing study pattern to a lupus anticoagulant. 3. PTT of mixture is initially normal but prolonged at 2-hr incubation: consistent with a specific factor VIII inhibitor. A rare factor V inhibitor may have a similar pattern. Same considerations with a *PT* mixing study. Patients on warfarin will show a "correction pattern" consistent with factor deficiency(ies).	↑ Heparin, hirudin, and argatroban

1. Lewis SM, Bain BJ, Bates I, editors: *Dacie and Lewis practical hematology,* ed 9, Edinburgh, 2001, Churchill Livingstone.
2. Jacobs DS, Demott WR, Oxley DK, editors: *Laboratory test handbook,* ed 5, Hudson, OH, 2001, Lexi-Comp, Inc.

TEST NAME AND METHOD	SPECIMEN REQUIREMENTS	REFERENCE INTERVAL, CONVENTIONAL [INTERNATIONAL RECOMMENDED UNITS]	CHEMICAL INTERFERENCES AND IN VIVO EFFECTS
4-Pyridoxic Acid[1,2] *Ion-exchange chromatography, fluorimetry*[1]	Urine, 24 hr; preserve with toluene. Stable if stored at 0° C.	0.5-1.3 mg/day × 5.46 [2.7-7.1 μmol/day] See *Vitamin B₆*.	

1. Leklem JE: Vitamin B-6: a status report, *J Nutr* 120(11S):1503-1507, 1990.
2. Shils ME, Olson JA, Shike M, editors: *Modern nutrition in health and disease,* ed 8, Philadelphia, 1994, Lea & Febiger.

DIAGNOSTIC INFORMATION   **REMARKS**

Mixing studies are typically performed when there is an unexplained prolonged aPTT or PT. If there is a factor deficiency (e.g., hemophilia), normal plasma (1:1 mixture) will correct an abnormally prolonged aPTT or PT. If there is a nonspecific inhibitor such as a lupus anticoagulant, normal plasma will generally not correct the aPTT.

Specific (e.g., factor VIII inhibitor) or nonspecific inhibitors (e.g., lupus anticoagulant) affecting the aPTT or PT may be immediately acting or time dependent. To detect both types of inhibitors, a mixing study is tested immediately after mixing and after incubation at 2 hr. A factor VIII inhibitor may only be detected after 2-hr incubation.

The test is based on the evaluation of aPTT or PT in a 50:50 mixture of patient's plasma with normal plasma. Normal plasma and the patient's plasma are also tested immediately and at 2 hr as controls.

↓ B6 deficiency

4-Pyridoxic acid is the major metabolite of vitamin B_6, and its excretion may reflect recent dietary intake of vitamin B_6 rather than functional tissue status. Measurement of urine metabolites and xanthurenic acid (or cystathionine) after tryptophan (or methionine) oral loads can provide an indirect measure of functional vitamin B_6 deficiency.[1] These tests of urine metabolites are not widely used but can provide confirmation of vitamin B_6 deficiency. See *Vitamin B_6*.

TEST NAME AND METHOD	SPECIMEN REQUIREMENTS	REFERENCE INTERVAL, CONVENTIONAL [INTERNATIONAL RECOMMENDED UNITS]			CHEMICAL INTERFERENCES AND IN VIVO EFFECTS
Pyrimidine-5'-Nucleotidase (P-5'-NT, Pyrimidine-5'-Nucleotide Nucleosidase; EC 3.2.2.10) in Erythrocytes[1-4]	Hemolysate of washed Ercs. Submit whole blood (heparin, EDTA, or ACD).	*mU/g Hb* 152.2 ± 17.2 (SD) *U/10^{12} Ercs* 4.41 ± 0.50 *mU/mL Ercs* 51.7 ± 5.85	× 0.0645* × 1.0 × 1.0	*kU/mol Hb* [9.81 ± 1.11] *pU/Erc* [4.4 ± 0.50] *U/L Ercs* [51.7 ± 5.85]	↓ C Lead[7] ↓ V Lead
Radiometric (^{14}C-CMP)[5]		*Conversion factor based on MW of Hb of 64,500.			
Phosphate release[6]	Hemolysate of washed Ercs. Submit whole blood (heparin or EDTA). Hemolysates are stable 6 days at 4° C if mercaptoethanol is added at the time of assay.	*mU/g Hb* 148 ± 18.3 (SD) or: *Substratemmol* UMP†: UMP and MCE‡: CMP§: CMP and MCE: In patients with ↑ reticulocytes: UMP: UMP and MCE: CMP: CMP and MCE: See *Acetylcholinesterase.*	× 0.0645* *P$_i$/hr/g Hb (SD)* 6.6 ± 2.0 7.3 5.5 ± 1.4 6.2 14.1 ± 6.6 15.1 ± 7.5 10.8 ± 4.2 12.2 ± 5.1	*kU/mol Hb* [9.55 ± 1.18] *kU/mol Hb* × 1.075 [7.1 ± 2.2] [7.8] [5.9 ± 1.5] [6.7] [15.2 ± 7.1] [16.2 ± 8.1] [11.6 ± 4.5] [13.1 ± 5.5]	
Screening test	Hemolysate of washed Ercs. Submit whole blood (ACD, EDTA, or heparin). Extract purines and pyrimidines from erythrocytes into 0.16 mol/L perchloric acid (caution: explosive).	Absorbance at 257 nm (from purines) much higher than absorbance at 270 nm (from pyrimidines). *Conversion factor based on MW of Hb of 64,500. †*UMP*, Uridine monophosphate. ‡*MCE*, Mercaptoethanol. §*CMP*, Cytidine monophosphate.			

1. Beutler E: *Hemolytic anemia in disorders of red cell metabolism,* New York, 1978, Plenum Pub. Co.
2. Williams JJ, Beutler E, Ersley JJ, et al, editors: *Manual of hematology,* ed 6, New York, 2003, McGraw-Hill Publishing Co.
3. Henze T, Neuner M, Michaelis HC: Determination of erythrocyte-bound acetylcholinesterase activity for monitoring pyridostigmine therapy in myasthenia gravis, *J Neurol* 238:225-229, 1991.
4. Weatherall DJ: ABC of clinical haematology. The hereditary anaemias, *BMJ* 314:492-496, 1197.
5. Torrance J, West C, Beutler E: A simple rapid radiometric assay for pyrimidine-5'-nucleotidase, *J Lab Clin Med* 90:563-568, 1977.

DIAGNOSTIC INFORMATION	REMARKS

↓ Hemolytic anemia (autosomal recessive; many cases have been reported), pyrimidine-5′-nucleotidase deficiency, severe lead poisoning,[7] occupational lead exposure,[8] β-thalassemia,[9] or hemoglobin.[8]

Deficiency is characterized by intracellular accumulations of pyrimidine-containing nucleotides, marked basophilic stippling, splenomegaly, and hemolysis. Deficiency is the most common abnormality of nucleotide metabolism.[10]

Epiphenomenal findings are elevated cellular GSH and phosphoribosyl-1-pyrophosphate synthetase (PRPP synthetase).[11,12]

mU/g Hb $\times$ 29 = mU/10^{12} Ercs

mU/g Hb $\times$ 0.34 = mU/mL Ercs*

*See Note, *Acetylcholinesterase.*

Total nucleotides in affected persons are 3-6 times normal; 80% contain pyrimidine.[12] Procedure is dependent on Mg^{2+} concentration.[6] CMP is less affected by inhibitory substances and storage time; the use of MCE reduces the effect of stimulation and inhibition.[6]

P-5′-NT is the lymphocyte differentiation marker CD73.

Red cells will show characteristic coarse basophilic stippling.

In cases of pyrimidine-5′-nucleotidase deficiency, extract exhibits high pyrimidine absorbance peak at 270 nm, much lower purine absorbance at 257 nm.

---

6. Paglia DE, Valentine WN: Characteristics of a pyrimidine-specific 5′-nucleotidase in human erythrocytes, *J Biol Chem* 250:7973-7979, 1979.

7. Miwa S, Fujii H: Molecular basis of erythroenzymopathies associated with hereditary hemolytic anemia: tabulation of mutant enzymes, *Am J Hematol* 51:122-132, 1996.

8. Paglia DE, Renner SW, Bhambhani K: Differential effects of low-level lead exposure on the natural isozymes of erythrocyte 5′-nucleotidase, *Clin Biochem* 32:193-199, 1999.

9. Vives Corrons JL, Miguel-Garcia A, Pujades MA, et al: Increased susceptibility of microcytic red blood cells to in vitro oxidative stress, *Eur J Haematol* 55:327-331, 1995.

TEST NAME AND METHOD	SPECIMEN REQUIREMENTS	REFERENCE INTERVAL, CONVENTIONAL [INTERNATIONAL RECOMMENDED UNITS]	CHEMICAL INTERFERENCES AND IN VIVO EFFECTS

Pyrimidine-5′-Nucleotidase (P-5′-NT, Pyrimidine-5′-Nucleotide Nucleosidase; EC 3.2.2.10) in Erythrocytes—CONT

10. Rees DC, Duley JA, Marinaki AM: Pyrimidine 5′ nucleotidase deficiency, *Br J Haematol* 120:375-383, 2003.

11. Paglia DE, Valentine WN, Dahlgren JG: Effects of low level lead exposure on pyrimidine-5′-nucleotidase and other erythrocyte enzymes, *J Clin Invest* 56:1164-1169, 1979.

TEST NAME AND METHOD	SPECIMEN REQUIREMENTS	REFERENCE INTERVAL, CONVENTIONAL [INTERNATIONAL RECOMMENDED UNITS]				CHEMICAL INTERFERENCES AND IN VIVO EFFECTS
Pyruvate (Pyruvic Acid)[1-5] *Colorimetric*[6,7] *Enzymatic*[1]	Whole blood. Specify whether sample is venous or arterial. Note: Protein precipitation should be performed immediately. See *L-Lactate, Remarks* for special precautions.	Fasting venous blood: Arterial blood:	*mg/dL* 0.3-0.9 0.02-0.08	× 114	*μmol/L* [34-103] [2-9]	None reported for properly collected samples.
	CSF[7]	0.5-1.7 mg/day	× 11.4	[6-19 μmol/day]		

1. Burtis CA, Ashwood ER, editors: *Tietz textbook of clinical chemistry,* ed 2, Philadelphia, 1994, WB Saunders.

2. Eastham RD: *Biochemical values in clinical medicine,* ed 7, Bristol, UK, 1985, John Wright and Sons Ltd.

3. Henry JB, editor: *Clinical diagnosis and management by laboratory methods,* ed 18, Philadelphia, 1991, WB Saunders.

4. Kaplan LA, Pesce AJ, editors: *Clinical chemistry: theory, analysis and correlation,* ed 2, St. Louis, 1989, CV Mosby.

5. Pesce A, Kaplan L, editors: *Methods in clinical chemistry,* St. Louis, 1987, CV Mosby.

6. Henry RJ, Cannon DC, Winkelman JW, editors: *Clinical chemistry: principles and technics,* ed 2, Hagerstown, MD, 1974, Harper and Row.

7. Tietz NW, editor: *Fundamentals of clinical chemistry,* ed 3, Philadelphia, 1987, WB Saunders.

8. Wallach J, editor: *Interpretation of diagnostic tests,* ed 5, Boston, 1992, Little, Brown and Co.

9. Friedman RB, Anderson RE, Entine SM, et al: Effects of diseases on clinical laboratory tests, *Clin Chem* 26: supplementary issue, 1980.

10. Schiavello R, Cavaliere F, Sollazzi L, et al: Changes of serum pyruvate and lactate in open-heart surgery, *Resuscitation* 11:35-45, 1984.

TEST NAME AND METHOD	SPECIMEN REQUIREMENTS	REFERENCE INTERVAL, CONVENTIONAL [INTERNATIONAL RECOMMENDED UNITS]	CHEMICAL INTERFERENCES AND IN VIVO EFFECTS
Rapid Platelet Function Assay (RPFA-ASA)[1] *Accumetrics Ultegra Analyzer*	Whole blood (3.2% citrate). Samples should be collected 2-30 hr after ingestion of aspirin. Perform between 30 min after collection up to 4 hr. Do not refrigerate or freeze sample.	Results reported as Aspirin Reaction Units (ARUs). <550 ARU: Aspirin working (platelet dysfunction detected) >550 ARU: Aspirin is not working (no platelet dysfunction detected)	Dipyridamole, clopidogrel, ticlopidine, Aggrenox, NSAIDs, glycoprotein IIb/IIIa inhibitors (Reo-Pro), and thrombolytic agents (streptokinase).

1. Coleman JL, Wang JC, Simon DI: Determination of individual response to aspirin therapy using the Accumetrics *Ultegra* RFPA-ASA system, *Point Care* 3:77-82, 2004.

12. Valentine WN, Fink K, Paglia DE, et al: Hereditary hemolytic anemia with human erythrocyte pyrimidine-5'-nucleotidase deficiency, *J Clin Invest* 54: 866-879, 1974.

B ↑ Acute advanced beriberi, advanced liver disease, severe cardiac failure, uremia, heavy metal poisoning (arsenic, antimony, gold, mercury), insulin-sensitive diabetes mellitus, diabetic ketosis, hepatolenticular degeneration, thiamine deficiency,[8] and von Gierke's disease,[9] malignant hyperthermia, and Reye's syndrome

B ↓ Open heart surgery[10]

This test is principally used to calculate the lactate/pyruvate ratio and, in conjunction with lactate and glucose determinations, to diagnose malignant hyperthermia. See *L-Lactate, lactate/pyruvate ratio.*

Pyruvate decreases in the sample after 1 min if it is not drawn into a protein precipitant such as metaphosphoric acid (preferred).

Patient must be fasting and at rest. In McArdle's syndrome, there is no increase in blood pyruvate after exercise.

↑ Aspirin resistance

The effect of hereditary platelet function disorders (e.g., von Willebrand disease) is unknown.

Aspirin resistance refers to patients who while on aspirin do not display an adequate degree of platelet inhibition. The RPFA-ASA point of care assay may identify patients who are resistant to aspirin therapy.

The test is based on the patient's activated platelets binding to fibrinogen-coated beads, with subsequent platelet aggregation measured by a turbidimetric-based optical detection system.

TEST NAME AND METHOD	SPECIMEN REQUIREMENTS	REFERENCE INTERVAL, CONVENTIONAL [INTERNATIONAL RECOMMENDED UNITS]	CHEMICAL INTERFERENCES AND IN VIVO EFFECTS
Red Blood Cell (RBC) Antigen Genotyping[1-4] *Polymerase chain reaction (PCR)–based methods*	Fetal genotype: Amniotic cells or fluid or chorionic villus sample. Recently cell-free fetal DNA in maternal plasma has been explored as source material for fetal genotyping.[5] Parental genotype: Whole blood (EDTA). It is preferable to test the biological mother and father concurrently.	Not applicable.	PCR inhibition by sample contaminants (heparin, EDTA). Similar to other genetic tests, RBC genotype analysis for some blood group systems may need to be specifically validated for specific racial or ethnic groups; otherwise, the interpretations may be misleading.

1. Flegel WA, Wagner FF, Muller TH, et al: Rh phenotype prediction by DNA typing and its application to practice, *Transfus Med* 8:281-302, 1998.
2. van der Schoot CE, Tax GH, Rijnders RJ, et al: Prenatal typing of Rh and Kell blood group system antigens: the edge of a watershed, *Transfus Med Rev* 17:31-44, 2003.
3. Daniels G: Molecular blood grouping, *Vox Sang* 87(suppl 1):63-66, 2004.
4. Reid ME: Applications of DNA-based assays in blood group antigen and antibody identification, *Transfusion* 43:1748-1757, 2003.
5. Rijnders RJ, Christiaens GC, Bossers B, et al: Clinical applications of cell-free fetal DNA from maternal plasma, *Obstet Gynecol* 103:157-164, 2004.
6. Castilho L, Rios M, Bianco C, et al: DNA-based typing of blood groups for the management of multiply-transfused sickle cell disease patients, *Transfusion* 42:232-238, 2002.
7. Montalvo L, Walker P, Wen L, et al: Clinical investigation of posttransfusion Kidd blood group typing using a rapid normalized quantitative polymerase chain reaction, *Transfusion* 44:694-702, 2004.

TEST NAME AND METHOD	SPECIMEN REQUIREMENTS	REFERENCE INTERVAL, CONVENTIONAL	[INTERNATIONAL RECOMMENDED UNITS]	CHEMICAL INTERFERENCES AND IN VIVO EFFECTS
Red Cell Distribution of Width (RDW)*[1-4] *Electronic counter* *Reported as RDW-CV on Sysmex instruments.	Whole blood (EDTA). Stable 6 hr at 25° C, 24 hr at 4° C.	*Percent* 11.5-14.5%	*Number fraction* 0.115-0.145	↑ C Cold agglutinins; chronic lymphocytic leukemia (high leukocyte count); hyperglycemia ↑ V Post–red cell transfusion; marked red cell fragmentation

DIAGNOSTIC INFORMATION	REMARKS

RBC antigen genotyping allows inference of the RBC phenotype in situations where standard serological testing cannot be used (hemolytic disease of the newborn) or is unreliable (multiply[6] or recently transfused patients[7]). DNA-based assays for blood group antigens are superior to agglutination tests for typing patients with weakly expressed or variant antigens (e.g., D variants) or with a positive DAT. Other applications include resolution of complex serological problems, RHD zygosity determination of the father, and forensic and paternity testing.[3,4]

Blood group genotyping as a means to predict phenotypic expression of RBC antigens is still being developed. Genotyping results may on occasion differ from RBC phenotype by conventional serological testing. Clinical decisions should therefore not be made on genotyping results alone.

↑ Anemias with heterogeneous red cell size including nutritional, myelodysplastic, megaloblastic, myelopthistic, and sideroblastic types; homozygous thalassemias and some homozygous hemoglobinopathies. Marked reticulocytosis can increase RDW.

Normal in anemias with homogeneous red cell size including anemia of chronic disease, acute blood loss, aplastic anemia, thalassemia trait, hereditary spherocytosis, and hemoglobin E trait and disease.

Automated instruments calculate and report the RDW. It may also be calculated from the standard deviation of the red cell volume and the MCV:

$$\text{RDW \%} = \frac{\text{Standard deviation of red cell volume (fL)}}{\text{MCV (fL)}} \times 100$$

The Sysmex NE-series instruments report RDW-CV, which is the coefficient of variation of red cell volume (%) and correlates with the Coulter and Bayer instrument RDW. The Sysmex instruments also report an RDW-SD, which is the standard deviation of red cell volume (fL).

TEST NAME AND METHOD	SPECIMEN REQUIREMENTS	REFERENCE INTERVAL, CONVENTIONAL [INTERNATIONAL RECOMMENDED UNITS]	CHEMICAL INTERFERENCES AND IN VIVO EFFECTS

Red Cell Distribution of Width—CONT

1. Rodak BF, editor: *Hematology; clinical principles and applications,* ed 2, Philadelphia, 2002, WB Saunders.
2. Kjeldsberg C, Elenitoba-Johnson K, Foucar K, et al, editors: *Practical diagnosis of hematologic disorders,* ed 3, Chicago, 2000, ASCP Press.
3. Bessman JD: *Automated blood counts and differentials,* ed 2, Baltimore, 1988, The Johns Hopkins University Press.
4. Bessman JD, Ridgway G, Gardner FH: Improved classification of anemias by MCV and RDW, *Am J Clin Pathol* 80:322-326, 1988.

TEST NAME AND METHOD	SPECIMEN REQUIREMENTS	REFERENCE INTERVAL, CONVENTIONAL [INTERNATIONAL RECOMMENDED UNITS]	CHEMICAL INTERFERENCES AND IN VIVO EFFECTS
Red Cell (Erythrocyte) Mass (RCM)[1-4] $^{51}Chromium\ (^{51}Cr)$ $^{99m}Technetium$ (^{99m}Tc) $^{32}Phosphorus\ (^{32}P)$ $^{125}Iodine\ (^{125}I)$	Sterile whole blood (heparin or EDTA) after 15-min rest. Label red cells and reinject. Take samples of whole blood (heparin or EDTA) 10 and 20 min after injection to measure radioactivity.	mL/kg^3 M: 20.0-39.7 F: 17.2-32.3	↓ C Ascorbic acid and antibiotics impair the labeling process when chromium-51 is used. ↓ V Obesity can cause spurious low values because RBC is related to lean body mass.[5]

DIAGNOSTIC INFORMATION	REMARKS

There is no known pathologic cause of a decreased RDW.

See Table II-15.

Some authors recommend using RDW in conjunction with the mean cell volume (MCV) for improved classification of anemias. For differential diagnosis, refer to Table II-15.

See also *Mean Cell Volume (MCV)*.

↑ *Primary Polycythemia (Polycythemia vera)*

↑ *Secondary polycythemia caused by tissue hypoxia:* Pulmonary disease, right to left cardiac shunt, congenital cardiac abnormalities, methemoglobinemia, carboxyhemoglobinemia (especially smoking), high-affinity hemoglobinopathy, and high altitude

↑ *Secondary polycythemia caused by excess erythropoietin or steroid production:* Renal cell carcinoma, hepatoma, cerebellar hemangioma, large uterine leiomyomas, polycystic kidney disease, hydronephrosis, adrenal cortical hyperplasia, and newborn infants

An elevated red cell mass is seen in primary and secondary polycythemia but not in relative polycythemia as a result of decreased plasma volume.

↓ Anemia, acute and chronic hemorrhage, bed rest, old age, pheochromocytoma, chronic infection, radiation, starvation, chronic azotemia, and obesity (fat is relatively avascular).

Red cell volume (RCV) is the actual measured parameter from which RCM is calculated. ^{99m}Tc is considered to be slightly less accurate than ^{51}Cr but has lower radioactivity. Red cell mass is calculated from red cell volume as follows:

$$\text{RCM, mL/kg} = \frac{\text{RCV (mL)}}{\text{patient weight (kg)}}$$

At hematocrit values between 20 and 55% [0.20 and 0.55], a linear relationship exists between Hct and RCV. If Hct >55% [0.55], RCV increases disproportionately to Hct; i.e., Hct underestimates RCV. When RCV is related to total body water or lean body mass (instead of body weight), there is no difference between the values of obese and lean persons and between those of males and females.

Recently published data suggest that the ^{125}I method is simpler and less expensive with equivalent results as compared with ^{51}C.

TEST NAME AND METHOD	SPECIMEN REQUIREMENTS	REFERENCE INTERVAL, CONVENTIONAL [INTERNATIONAL RECOMMENDED UNITS]	CHEMICAL INTERFERENCES AND IN VIVO EFFECTS

Red Cell (Erythrocyte) Mass—CONT

1. Greer JP, Foerster J, Lukens JN, et al: *Wintrobe's clinical hematology,* ed 11, Philadelphia, 2003, Lippincott, Williams & Wilkins.

2. Beutler E, Lichtman MA, Coller B, editors: *Williams hematology,* ed 6, New York, 2000, McGraw-Hill.

3. Fairbanks VF, Klee GG, Wiseman GA, et al: Measurement of blood volume and red cell mass: re-examination of ^{51}Cr and ^{125}I methods, *Blood Cell Mol Dis* 22:169-186, 1986.

Reducing Substances[1-3] *Reagent tablet (Bayer Corporation Clinitest)*[4,5]	Urine, fresh random specimen. Refrigerate if test cannot be performed immediately.	Negative	↑ V Aminosalicylic acid, corticosteroids, EDTA, glucuronic acid and conjugated glucuronides, lithium, nicotinic acid (high doses), nucleoproteins, oxalates, phenolic substances, phenothiazines (long-term use), phenylpyruvate (PKU), rhubarb, thiazides, and D-thyroxine.[1,4,6,7] ↑ C *Clinitest tablets:* Ascorbic acid (urinary levels >250 mg/dL; >13.9 mmol/L), first-generation cephalosporins, diatrizoates (black color),[1] fructose, galactose, hemogentisic acid, isoniazid, lactose, levodopa, maltose, nalidixic acid, pentose, probenecid, and salicylates.

1. Eastham RD: *Biochemical values in clinical medicine,* ed 7, Bristol, UK, 1985, John Wright and Sons Ltd.

2. Henry JB, editor: *Clinical diagnosis and management by laboratory methods,* ed 18, Philadelphia, 1991, WB Saunders.

3. Newall RG, editor: *Clinical urinalysis,* Buckinghamshire, UK, 1990, Ames Division, Miles Ltd.

4. Wallach J, editor: *Interpretation of diagnostic tests,* ed 5, Boston, 1992, Little, Brown and Co.

5. Bayer Corporation: *Clinitest package insert,* Elkhart, IN, 1995, Bayer Corporation.

6. Tietz NW, editor: *Fundamentals of clinical chemistry,* ed 3, Philadelphia, 1987, WB Saunders.

7. Sonnenwirth AC, Jarrett L, editors: *Gradwohl's clinical laboratory methods and diagnosis,* ed 8, St. Louis, 1980, CV Mosby.

| DIAGNOSTIC INFORMATION | REMARKS |

4. International Committee for Standardization in Haematology (ICSH): Recommended methods for measurement of red-cell and plasma volume, *J Nucl Med* 21:793-800, 1980.
5. Alving BM: The antiphospholipid syndrome: clinical presentation, diagnosis, and patient management. In Kitchens CS, Alving BM, Kessler CM, editors: *Consultative hemostasis and thrombosis,* Philadelphia, 2002, WB Saunders, pp. 269-278.

↑ Any cause of glycosuria (see *Glucose*), normal late pregnancy and lactation (lactose), galactosemia (galactose), essential pentosuria (pentoses), muscular dystrophy (ribose), and infants on artificial diets

Lower limit of detection for the Clinitest procedure (5-drop method) is 250 mg/dL [13.9 mmol/L], as glucose. Comparison of results from copper reduction tests and glucose oxidase reagent strips differentiates glucose from other reducing substances.

Urines with low specific gravity show enhanced positive results. X-ray contrast media (HYPAQUE Meglumine) cause reduced reactivity and possible false-negative results.[5]

Clinitest tablets should be used when screening infants and young pediatric patients because glucose oxidase strips will not detect galactose and other sugars of potential importance.[3] Healthy neonates (10-14 days old) may show positive reaction because of excretion of glucose, galactose, fructose, and lactose. Normal pregnant and postpartum women may show positive Clinitest results because of lactose in urine.[2]

The 2-drop Clinitest method was devised to detect very high levels (5 g/dL; 278 mmol/L) of reducing sugars that might otherwise be missed (false negative) on the 5-drop method. Pass-through phenomenon refers to the color change from orange back to blue to blue-green, which occurs when very high concentrations of glucose are encountered. This phenomenon causes false-negative results unless the reaction is monitored constantly until it is complete.

TEST NAME AND METHOD	SPECIMEN REQUIREMENTS	REFERENCE INTERVAL, CONVENTIONAL [INTERNATIONAL RECOMMENDED UNITS]	CHEMICAL INTERFERENCES AND IN VIVO EFFECTS
Reinsch Test *Qualitative:* *Copper strip or* *copper spiral*[1]	Urine, vomitus, gastric lavage, and tissue homogenate. Collect in acid-washed, metal-free container. Specimen preparation depends on particular modification of Reinsch test.	No deposit on copper strip. If 100 mL of urine and 10 mL of concentrated HCl are used, no deposit on copper strip indicates: $\qquad\qquad$ *mcg/L* $\qquad\qquad$ *μmol/L* Arsenic: $\quad$ <25 $\quad$ × 0.0133 $\quad$ [<0.33] Mercury: $\quad$ <50 $\quad$ × 0.00499 $\quad$ [<0.25] Selenium: $\quad$ <50 $\quad$ × 0.0127 $\quad$ [<0.64] Gray-to-black deposit: positive for arsenic (dull black), selenium, antimony (purple sheen), bismuth (shiny black), tellurium, or some sulfur compounds Light gray-to-silver deposit and strip become shiny on rubbing: positive for mercury	None found.

1. Tietz NW, editor: *Textbook of clinical chemistry,* Philadelphia, 1986, WB Saunders.

		mg/dL[6] 5th-95th Percentile	mmol/L 5th-95th Percentile	
Remnant Lipoproteins (RLP)[1-3] *Immunoaffinity gel/enzymatic*[3-5]	Serum, EDTA, or heparin plasma. Separate plasma or serum from cells within 4 hr. Stable up to 1 wk at 4° C. Specimens with triglycerides <400 mg/dL can be stored at −70° C for up to 3 mo; otherwise, do not freeze. Do not refreeze.	RLP Cholesterol: All ages $\quad$ F: $\quad$ M: 30-39 yr $\quad$ F: $\quad$ M: 40-49 yr $\quad$ F: $\quad$ M: 50-59 yr $\quad$ F: $\quad$ M: 60-69 yr $\quad$ F: $\quad$ M: 70-79 yr $\quad$ F: $\quad$ M: RLP Triglyceride: All ages $\quad$ F: $\quad$ M: 30-39 yr $\quad$ F: $\quad$ M:	 4.9-10.9 5.0-15.9 4.5-8.1 4.9-15.3 4.7-9.7 5.0-15.3 5.2-11.9 5.2-16.7 5.2-12.4 5.1-15.7 5.2-9.3 4.9-22.0 6.8-44.0 7.9-77.9 5.6-25.2 7.2-77.9	 [0.127-0.282] [0.129-0.411] [0.116-0.210] [0.127-0.396] [0.122-0.251] [0.129-0.396] [0.135-0.308] [0.135-0.432] [0.135-0.321] [0.132-0.406] [0.135-0.241] [0.127-0.569] [0.077-0.497] [0.089-0.880] [0.063-0.285] [0.081-0.880]
				↑ C Freezing may cause an increase in RLP-C, especially if TG >400 mg/dL. Specimens with TG ≥800 mg/dL may give inaccurate results.

DIAGNOSTIC INFORMATION	REMARKS

This test is obsolete and nonspecific for listed metals. Quantitative tests for specific metals are more accurate for diagnosis. 0.5 mL of potassium cyanide will dissolve a deposit caused by arsenic, selenium, tellurium, and/or sulfur; 1 mL of nitric acid, 2.25 mol/L, will selectively dissolve a deposit caused by bismuth. See specific metal for quantitative methods.

↑ An elevated RLP-C concentration is associated with an increased risk of CHD.

An elevated RLP-C/TG ratio is associated with type III hyperlipoproteinemia.

Chylomicron and VLDL remnants are formed by the removal of triglycerides and phospholipids by lipolysis. The accumulation of these remnant particles is atherogenic.

Measurement of RLP cholesterol is useful for CHD risk assessment and for the diagnosis of type III hyperlipoproteinemia.

TEST NAME AND METHOD	SPECIMEN REQUIREMENTS	REFERENCE INTERVAL, CONVENTIONAL [INTERNATIONAL RECOMMENDED UNITS]		CHEMICAL INTERFERENCES AND IN VIVO EFFECTS

Remnant Lipoproteins—CONT

40-49 yr
F:	6.8-41.0	[0.077-0.463]
M:	7.4-77.1	[0.084-0.871]

50-59 yr
F:	7.0-55.0	[0.079-0.621]
M:	8.6-81.1	[0.097-0.916]

60-69 yr
F:	7.1-56.4	[0.080-0.637]
M:	7.9-72.3	[0.089-0.817]

70-79 yr
F:	8.6-28.0	[0.097-0.316]
M:	8.8-108.2	[0.099-1.223]

Recommended Cutpoints[5]
RLP Cholesterol:
Fasting:	<6.6 mg/dL	[<0.17 mmol/L]
Nonfasting:	<8.8 mg/dL	[<0.23 mmol/L]

RLP cholesterol/triglyceride ratio ≥0.10 (if both measured in mg/dL) or ≥0.23 (if both measured in mmol/L) is consistent with type III hyperlipoproteinemia.

1. Gianturco SH, Bradley WA: Pathophysiology of triglyceride-rich lipoproteins in atherothrombosis: cellular aspects, *Clin Cardiol* 22(suppl):II7-14, 1999.
2. Kugiyama K, Doi H, Takazoe K, et al: Remnant lipoprotein levels in fasting serum predict coronary events in patients with coronary artery disease, *Circulation* 99:2858-2860, 1999.
3. Rifai N, Warnick GR, Dominiczak MH, editors: *Handbook of lipoprotein testing,* ed 2, Washington, DC, 2000, AACC Press.
4. Nakajima K, Saito T, Tamura A, et al: Cholesterol in remnant-like lipoproteins in human serum using monoclonal anti apoB-100 and anti apoA-I immunoaffinity mixed gels, *Clin Chim Acta* 223:53-71, 1993.
5. Polymedco, Inc.: *RLP-Cholesterol Assay package insert,* Cortlandt Manor, NY, 2002, Polymedco, Inc.
6. McNamara JR, Shah PK, Nakajima K, et al: Remnant lipoprotein cholesterol and triglyceride reference ranges from the Framingham Heart Study, *Clin Chem* 44:1224-1232, 1998.

TEST NAME AND METHOD	SPECIMEN REQUIREMENTS	REFERENCE INTERVAL, CONVENTIONAL		[INTERNATIONAL RECOMMENDED UNITS]	CHEMICAL INTERFERENCES AND IN VIVO EFFECTS
Renin Activity, Plasma (PRA)[1,2] *RIA*	Plasma (Na₂EDTA). Place in ice water, and centrifuge at 4° C. Separate plasma and freeze promptly at −20° C. Stable for up to 1 yr.		*ng AI*/ mL/hr*[3]	*mg AI* × hr⁻¹ × L⁻¹*	↑ V Captopril, chlor-propamide, diazoxide, enalapril, estrogens, guanethidine (in sodium-depleted patients), hy-dralazine, lisinopril, mi-noxidil, nifedipine (young patients), nitroprusside, oral contraceptives, potassium-sparing diuretics (e.g., amiloride,
		Cord blood:	4.0-32.0 × 1.0	[4.0-32.0]	
		Newborn (1-7 days):	2.0-35.0	[2.0-35.0]	
		Child, Normal sodium diet, supine			
		1-12 mo:	2.4-37.0	[2.4-37.0]	
		1-3 yr:	1.7-11.2	[1.7-11.2]	
		3-5 yr:	1.0-6.5	[1.0-6.5]	

DIAGNOSTIC INFORMATION	REMARKS

↑ *With consequent secondary aldosteronism*

Hypertensive states: Malignant or severe hypertension, unilateral renal disease with malignant or severe hypertension, high-renin forms of hypertension, renal parenchymal diseases, renin-secreting tumors, oral contraceptive-induced hypertension, and pheochromocytoma

Edematous normotensive states: Cirrhosis, hepatitis, nephrosis, and congestive heart failure

Hypokalemic normotensive states: Juxtaglomerular cell hyperplasia (Bartter's syndrome), other nephropathies with Na^+ or K^+ wastage, and alimentary disorders with electrolyte loss

Renin activity is measured indirectly by the ability of the patient's plasma to generate angiotensin.[4] Normal values depend on the laboratory and the patient's prevailing Na^+ and K^+, status of hydration, and posture. (Low-sodium diets, upright posture, and diuretics, e.g., increase renin levels.) Only stimulated values (e.g., after furosemide stimulation) are of practical value in evaluating hypertensive patients. Simultaneous measurements of 24-hr urine Na^+ and creatinine and plasma K^+, Na^+, and creatinine are recommended. PRA decreases gradually with age in men and women and is slightly lower in women than in men. In older subjects the responses of PRA to

TEST NAME AND METHOD	SPECIMEN REQUIREMENTS	REFERENCE INTERVAL, CONVENTIONAL [INTERNATIONAL RECOMMENDED UNITS]			CHEMICAL INTERFERENCES AND IN VIVO EFFECTS

Renin Activity, Plasma—CONT

	5-10 yr:	0.5-5.9		[0.5-5.9]	spironolactone, tri-
	10-15 yr:	0.5-3.3		[0.5-3.3]	amterene), and thiazide
	Adult,				diuretics (e.g., ben-
	Normal				droflumethiazide,
	sodium diet				chlorthalidone)
	Supine:	0.2-1.6		[0.2-1.6]	
	Standing (4 hr):	0.7-3.3		[0.7-3.3]	↓ V β-Adrenergic-
					blocking agents (e.g., pro-
	AI, Angiotensin I.				pranolol), angiotensin

(when given IV), aspirin, carbenoxolone, clonidine, deoxycorticosterone, guanethidine (in patients with normal sodium), indomethacin, licorice, methyldopa, potassium administration, prazosin, and reserpine

1. Kaplan N: Endocrine hypertension. In Wilson JH, Foster DW, editors: *Williams textbook of endocrinology,* ed 8, Philadelphia, 1992, WB Saunders.
2. Sealey J: Plasma renin activity and plasma prorenin assays, *Clin Chem* 37:1811-1819, 1991.
3. Endocrine Sciences: *Pediatric laboratory services,* Tarzana, CA, 1992, Endocrine Sciences.
4. Sealey J, Campbell G, Preibisz J: Hormone assays: renin, aldosterone, peripheral vein, and urinary assays. In Laragh J, Brenner B, editors: *Hypertension: pathophysiology, diagnosis, and management,* New York, 1990, Raven Press.

Renin, Direct[1]	See *Renin Activity, Plasma.*	*mU/L*[4]		*mU/L*	See *Renin Activity, Plasma.*
IRMA[2]		Adults			
		Supine: 12-79	× 1.0	[12-79]	
		Upright: 13-114		[13-114]	
ICMA[3]					
		Upright: 5.7-116	× 1.0	[5.7-116]	
		Supine: ~30% lower than upright reference interval			

1. Sealey J, Campbell G, Preibisz J: Hormone assays: renin, aldosterone, peripheral vein, and urinary assays. In Laragh J, Brenner B, editors: *Hypertension: pathophysiology, diagnosis, and management,* New York, 1990, Raven Press.
2. Simon D, Hartmann D, Badouaille G, et al: Two-site direct immunoassay for active renin, *Clin Chem* 38:1959-1962, 1992.

DIAGNOSTIC INFORMATION	REMARKS

↑ *Without consequent secondary aldosteronism*
Adrenocortical insufficiency, potassium depletion state (alimentary)

↓ *With adrenocortical disease*
Hypertensive states: Primary aldosteronism because of adrenal adenoma, pseudoprimary or idiopathic aldosteronism (usually bilateral adrenocortical hyperplasia), glucocorticoid-suppressible aldosteronism, adrenal carcinoma with mineralocorticoid excess, and adrenal enzyme defects with oversecretion of other mineralocorticoids

↓ *Without adrenocortical disease*
Hypertensive states: Low-renin essential hypertension; in certain patients with renal parenchymal diseases, Liddle's syndrome (pseudohyperaldosteronism), and licorice or mineralocorticoid ingestion
Normotensive states: Renal parenchymal diseases, autonomic disorders with postural hypotension, uninephrectomized subjects, and drug-induced adrenergic blockade, hyperkalemia

the administration of furosemide, dietary Na^+ restriction, or upright posture are significantly less than in younger subjects. In females, renin concentration is low during the follicular phase, increases just before ovulation, and remains high during the luteal phase. PRA is also increased during pregnancy.

PRA is useful in assessing mineralocorticoid therapy and patient compliance.

Some methods use an exogenous renin substrate rather than the angiotensinogen present in the test plasma; this type of assay is generally known as a plasma renin concentration assay.

Newer so-called "direct renin" IRMA and ICMA sandwich assays directly measure the mass concentration of renin in human plasma and are independent of the plasma renin substrate (See *Renin, Direct*).

See *Renin Activity, Plasma*

The IRMA and ICMA sandwich assays directly measure the mass concentration of active renin in human plasma and are independent of the plasma renin substrate. See *Renin Activity, Plasma.*

3. Perschel FH, Schemer R, Seiler L, et al: Rapid screening test for primary hyperaldosteronism: ratio of plasma aldosterone to renin concentration determined by fully automated chemiluminescence immunoassays, *Clin Chem* 50:1650-1655, 2004.

4. Nichols Institute Reference Laboratories: *Test catalog,* San Juan Capistrano, CA, 1993, Nichols Institute Reference Laboratories.

TEST NAME AND METHOD	SPECIMEN REQUIREMENTS	REFERENCE INTERVAL, CONVENTIONAL [INTERNATIONAL RECOMMENDED UNITS]	CHEMICAL INTERFERENCES AND IN VIVO EFFECTS
Renin (PRA), Renal Veins[1]	Plasma for renin from both renal veins. See *Renin Activity, Plasma.*	Renin activity from both veins within the reference interval. See *Renin Activity, Plasma.*	See *Renin Activity, Plasma;* and *Remarks.*

1. Kaplan N: Endocrine hypertension. In Wilson JH, Foster DW, editors: *Williams textbook of endocrinology,* ed 8, Philadelphia, 1992, WB Saunders.
2. Vaughan E, Buhler F, Laragh J: Renovascular hypertension: renin measurements to indicate hypersecretion and contralateral suppression, estimate renal plasma flow, and score for surgical curability, *Am J Med* 55:402-414, 1973.

TEST NAME AND METHOD	SPECIMEN REQUIREMENTS	REFERENCE INTERVAL, CONVENTIONAL [INTERNATIONAL RECOMMENDED UNITS]	CHEMICAL INTERFERENCES AND IN VIVO EFFECTS
Reptilase Time[1-3]	Plasma (blue top-citrate). Stable for 4 hr at 4° C or for 28 days if frozen.	Approximately 18-22 sec	↑ Anistreplase (plasminogen-streptokinase activator complex), paraproteins

1. Lewis SM, Bain BJ, Bates I, editors: *Dacie and Lewis practical hematology,* ed 9, Edinburgh, 2001, Churchill Livingstone.
2. Jacobs DS, Demott WR, Oxley DK, editors: *Laboratory test handbook,* ed 5, Hudson, OH, 2001, Lexi-Comp, Inc.

TEST NAME AND METHOD	SPECIMEN REQUIREMENTS	REFERENCE INTERVAL, CONVENTIONAL [INTERNATIONAL RECOMMENDED UNITS]	CHEMICAL INTERFERENCES AND IN VIVO EFFECTS
Reticulin Antibodies[1,2] *IgA, IgG* *IFA*	Serum. Stable 1 wk at room temperature, 2 wk at 4° C, and 1 yr frozen.	Normal: Negative	Testing in children is not as useful because celiac disease antibodies may not have developed. May be negative in patients taking gluten-free diets. 2.6% of patients will be negative because of selective IgA deficiency. A

DIAGNOSTIC INFORMATION	REMARKS
↑ In hypertension related to renal artery stenosis or unilateral renal parenchymal disease	This is a test for determining the functional significance of a stenotic renal arterial lesion; it is also useful for determining whether unilateral renal parenchymal disease may be responsible for hypertension.[2] It is used only rarely to evaluate the presence of a renin-secreting tumor.
A functionally significant stenotic lesion is inferred if the absolute renin activities are elevated and if the PRA on the stenotic side is increased >1.5 times that of the contralateral side. In some patients, this may be apparent only after furosemide administration.	The patient should not receive drugs that inhibit renin (propranolol, methyldopa, guanethidine, or clonidine) for 1 wk before the test.
↑ Hereditary: Decreased or abnormal fibrinogen (hereditary afibrinogenemia, hypofibrinogenemia, or dysfibrinogenemia)	Reptilase is an enzyme derived from the venom of the snake, *Bothrops atrox*. The reptilase time is essentially similar to the thrombin time. The snake venom used as the reagent is, in contrast to the thrombin reagent used in the thrombin time, not inhibited by heparin.
Acquired: Liver disease, paraproteinemia (multiple myeloma, Waldenström's macroglobulinemia, primary systemic amyloidosis)	The reptilase test, together with the thrombin time, is generally performed together in evaluation of a qualitative fibrinogen disorder (dysfibrinogenemia); the reptilase time is generally more affected than the thrombin time by dysfibrinogenemia.
In celiac disease, the IgA assay is 60% sensitive and 60% specific. In dermatitis herpetiformis, the sensitivity is 25%.	See *Tissue Transglutaminase Antibody, Endomyosial Antibody,* and *Gliadin Antibody.*
The IgG assay is positive in other diseases (Crohn's, bullous dermatosis) and normal subjects.	Celiac disease is an immune disorder found in 1% of the NA population that is stimulated by gluten. It is characterized by typical GI symptoms and a variety of less common symptoms.
	Small bowel biopsy is needed for definitive diagnosis.
	More than 97% of people with celiac disease have DQ2 and/or DQ8 HLA haplotypes compared with 40% of the population.

TEST NAME AND METHOD	SPECIMEN REQUIREMENTS	REFERENCE INTERVAL, CONVENTIONAL [INTERNATIONAL RECOMMENDED UNITS]	CHEMICAL INTERFERENCES AND IN VIVO EFFECTS

Reticulin Antibodies—CONT

serum IgA should be carried out and, if abnormal, IgG-based testing carried out.

1. Wong RC, Steele RH, Reeves GE, et al: Antibody and genetic testing in coeliac disease, *Pathology* 35:285-304, 2003.
2. Devlin SM, Andrews CN, Beck PL: Celiac disease: CME update for family physicians, *Can Fam Physician* 50:719-725, 2004.

Reticulocyte Count[1-3]

Whole blood (EDTA) or capillary blood with direct dilution. Stable 24 hr at room temperature. Stable 72 hr at 4° C.

Manual, supravital stain (new methylene blue)

	Percent*	*Number fraction reticulocytes*
Newborn:	3-7	[0.03-0.07]
1 day:	3-7	[0.03-0.07]
3 days:	1-3	[0.01-0.03]
7 days[6]:	0-1	[0.00-0.01]
1 mo:	0.2-2	[0.002-0.02]
1.5 mo:	0.3-3.5	[0.003-0.035]
2 mo:	0.4-4.8	[0.004-0.048]
2.5 mo:	0.3-4.2	[0.003-0.042]
3 mo:	0.3-3.6	[0.003-0.036]
4-12 mo[7]:	0.2-2.8	[0.002-0.028]
Adult:	0.5-1.5	[0.005-0.015]

Adult: 24-84 $\times 10^3/\mu L \times 10^6$ [24-84 $\times 10^9$/L]

*Expressed as percentage of erythrocytes.

By flow cytometry[8]

	Percent	*Absolute count*
0-14 days:	1.61-8.28	238.9-404.1 $\times 10^9$/L
14 days-1 yr:	1.09-3.00 $\times 0.01$	45.8-137.8 $\times 10^9$/L
1-3 yr:	1.11-5.00 $\times 0.01$	50.2-141.0 $\times 10^9$/L
3-8 yr:	0.95-4.03 $\times 0.01$	45.4-163.1 $\times 10^9$/L
8-12 yr:	1.18-3.78 $\times 0.01$	54.8-154.4 $\times 10^9$/L

$\downarrow$ V Drugs causing aplastic anemia, as listed in Table II-4.

$\uparrow$ V In the recovery phase after drug-induced aplastic anemia; drugs causing hemolysis (in G6PD deficiency or immune reactions), as listed in Table II-4.

Automated, flow cytometry for optical scatter or fluorescence after treatment with fluorescent dyes or supravital stains[3-5]

Whole blood (EDTA). Stable 24 hr at room temperature. Stable 72 hr at 4° C.

12 yr-Adult: 1.32-4.91 $\times 0.01$ 58.6-146.2 $\times 10^9$/L

$\uparrow$ C The presence of red cell inclusions that stain with supravital stains or fluorescent dyes, such as Howell-Jolly bodies, may interfere depending on the instrumentation used. Falsely increased reticulocyte counts measured by

DIAGNOSTIC INFORMATION	REMARKS

↑ Increased erythropoiesis as in hemolytic anemias, blood loss anemia (before development of iron deficiency), and anemias under specific treatment (iron deficiency, megaloblastic anemia)

The use of inserts in microscope ocular lenses is recommended to reduce counting error in manual counts.

A reticulocyte production index (RPI) is calculated by correcting the count for anemia and for the shift of immature reticulocytes prematurely from marrow into blood. RPI is a good estimate of erythrocyte production. Failure of RPI to increase 2-3 times normal in an anemic patient indicates hypoproliferative anemia.

↓ Red cell aplasia (including transient erythroblastopenia of childhood), aplastic anemia (including drugs causing aplastic anemia, Table II-4), renal disease, endocrine disease, and marrow replacement

↓ *Disorders of maturation:* Iron deficiency anemia, anemia of chronic disease, sideroblastic anemias, and megaloblastic anemias

$$\text{RPI} = \% \text{ reticulocytes} \times \left(\frac{\text{patient Hct}}{\text{normal Hct}}\right) \times \left(\frac{1}{\text{maturation time}}\right)$$

Correction is made for maturation time of reticulocytes prematurely released into blood if large polychromatophilic cells or nucleated erythrocytes are noted on the blood film. RPI varies with Hct as follows:

Hct	Maturation time (day)
45% [0.45]	1.0
35% [0.35]	1.5
25% [0.25]	2.0
15% [0.15]	2.5

Automated flow cytometric counting of large numbers of cells significantly enhances precision. Automated methods may be practical and useful in a laboratory that has >60 reticulocyte counts per day. Newer automated flow cytometric systems may provide additional data by analyzing the stages of reticulocyte maturation present in a sample.[10,11]

TEST NAME AND METHOD	SPECIMEN REQUIREMENTS	REFERENCE INTERVAL, CONVENTIONAL [INTERNATIONAL RECOMMENDED UNITS]			CHEMICAL INTERFERENCES AND IN VIVO EFFECTS

Reticulocyte Count—CONT

					automated flow cytometry resulting from intracellular parasites such as malaria and babesia have been reported with some analyzers.[9]

1. Henry JB, editor: *Clinical diagnosis and management by laboratory methods,* ed 20, Philadelphia, 2001, WB Saunders.
2. Beutler E, Lichtman MA, Coller B, editors: *Williams hematology,* ed 6, New York, 2000, McGraw-Hill.
3. Rodak BF, editor: *Hematology; clinical principles and applications,* ed 2, Philadelphia, 2002, WB Saunders.
4. Greer JP, Foerster J, Lukens JN, et al: *Wintrobe's clinical hematology,* ed 11, Philadelphia, 2003, Lippincott, Williams & Wilkins.
5. Metzger DK, Charache S: Flow cytometric reticulocyte counting with thioflavin T in a clinical hematology laboratory, *Arch Pathol Lab Med* 111:540-544, 1987.
6. Rudolph AM: *Pediatrics,* ed 18, Norwalk, CT, 1987, Appleton & Lange.
7. Hoffman R, Benz EJ, Shattil SJ, et al, editors: *Hematology basic principles and practice,* ed 3, New York, 2000, Churchill Livingstone.
8. Laurencet FM, Martinix T, Beris P: Spurious extreme reticulocytosis with an automated reticulocyte analyzer, *N Engl J Med* 337:1922-1923, 1997.
9. Simson E, Relopez J: *Absolute cell counts: reporting for today's technology,* McGaw Park, IL, 1992, Baxter Diagnostics Inc.
10. Nathan DG, Orkin SH, Ginsburg D, et al: *Hematology of infancy and childhood,* ed 6, Philadelphia, 2003, WB Saunders.
11. Temporin V, Toffolo L: Five fully automated methods for performing immature reticulocyte fraction; comparison in diagnosis of bone marrow aplasia, *Am J Clin Pathol* 117:871-879, 2002.

TEST NAME AND METHOD	SPECIMEN REQUIREMENTS	REFERENCE INTERVAL, CONVENTIONAL		[INTERNATIONAL RECOMMENDED UNITS]	CHEMICAL INTERFERENCES AND IN VIVO EFFECTS
Retinol-Binding Protein (RBP)[1,2] *RID*[3]	Serum, plasma (EDTA, heparin, or citrate). Analyze fresh or store at 4° C for <72 hr. Stable frozen at −20° C for 6 mo, or at −70° C indefinitely. Specimens without lipemia or hemolysis are preferred.	3-6 mg/dL (x̄: 4.0)	× 10	[30-60 mg/L] [x̄: 40]	S ↑ Estrogens, oral contraceptives,[8] and some anticonvulsants.[9]
Nephelometric[4] *ELISA*[5]	Serum. Analyze fresh or store at 4° C for 1 wk. Stable frozen at −20° C for 3 mo. Specimens without lipemia or hemolysis are preferred.	mg/dL[4] 1.5-6.7 x̄: 4.3[5]	× 10	mg/L [15-67] [43]	Excessive turbidity can affect nephelometric methods.

DIAGNOSTIC INFORMATION	REMARKS

↓ Vitamin A deficiency, protein-energy malnutrition, or protein deficiency states[10] (restoration of dietary protein can return RBP concentrations to normal levels even in the absence of vitamin A supplementation), hepatic disease,[1] cystic fibrosis,[11] and zinc deficiency[12]

↑ Chronic renal failure[1]

Retinol-binding protein circulates bound to transthyretin in the form of a macromolecular complex. Typically 90% saturated with retinol, RBP is the specific carrier protein of the hydrophobic retinol molecule. The RBP-transthyretin complex transports retinol from the liver to downstream target tissues and also avoids urinary loss by glomerular filtration of the otherwise low molecular weight RBP.[2] Formation of the complex functions to stabilize the binding of retinol to RBP. Specific receptors for retinol/retinol-RBP are present on target cells.[14]

RBP is nearly completely reabsorbed (99.97%) by the renal tubules, and elevated urine concentrations are indicators of tubular dysfunction.[13,15]

Plasma RBP concentrations correlate with those of vitamin A.

MW: 20,960.

TEST NAME AND METHOD	SPECIMEN REQUIREMENTS	REFERENCE INTERVAL, CONVENTIONAL [INTERNATIONAL RECOMMENDED UNITS]	CHEMICAL INTERFERENCES AND IN VIVO EFFECTS

Retinol-Binding Protein—CONT

RID[6,7]	Urine, 24 hr. Centrifuge and adjust to pH 7.0.	x̄: 0.1 mg/day	
ELISA[5]	Analyze fresh. Stable frozen at −20° C for up to 1 yr.	x̄: 101 mcg/g creatinine	

1. Goodman DS: Plasma retinol binding protein, *Ann NY Acad Sci* 348:378-390, 1980.

2. Bellovino D, Apreda M, Gragnoli S, et al: Vitamin A transport: in vitro models for the study of RBP secretion, *Mol Aspects Med* 24:411-420, 2003.

3. Ritzmann SE, Tucker ES III: *Protein analysis in disease—current concepts, Workshop manual,* Chicago, 1979, American Society of Clinical Pathologists, Commission for Continuing Education.

4. Quest Diagnostics Directory of Services online: Available at: http://www.questdiagnostics.com/. Last accessed 9/29/04.

5. Lucertini S, Valcavi P, Mutti A, et al: Enzyme-linked immunosorbent assay of retinol-binding protein in serum and urine, *Clin Chem* 30:149-151, 1984.

6. Cheung CK, Swaminathan R: Automated immunoturbidimetric methods for the determination of retinol binding protein, prealbumin and transferrin in urine, *Clin Biochem* 22:425-427, 1989.

7. Scarpioni L, Dall'aglio PO, Poisetti PG, et al: Retinol binding protein in serum and in urine of glomerular and tubular nephropathies, *Clin Chim Acta* 68:107-113, 1976.

8. Anonymous: The effect of oral contraceptives on blood vitamin A levels and the role of sex hormones, *Nutr Rev* 37:346-348, 1979.

9. Kozlowski BW, Taylor ML, Baer MT, et al: Anticonvulsant medication use and circulating levels of total thyroxine, retinol binding protein, and vitamin A in children with delayed cognitive development, *Am J Clin Nutr* 46:360-368, 1987.

10. Ingenbleek Y, Van Den Schrieck HG, DeNayer P, et al: The role of retinol binding protein in protein-calorie malnutrition, *Metabolism* 24:633-641, 1975.

11. James DR, Owen G, Campbell IA, et al: Vitamin A absorption in cystic fibrosis: risk of hypervitaminosis A, *Gut* 33:707-710, 1992.

12. Honkanen V, Konttinen YT, Mussalo-Rauhamaa H: Vitamins A and E, retinol binding protein and zinc in rheumatoid arthritis, *Clin Exp Rheumatol* 7:465-469, 1989.

13. Pereira AB, Nishida SK, Vieira JG, et al: Monoclonal antibody-based immunoenzymometric assays of retinol binding protein, *Clin Chem* 39:472-476, 1993.

14. Anonymous: Cell-surface receptors for retinol binding protein, *Nutr Rev* 49:218-221, 1991.

15. Smith GC, Winterborn MH, Taylor CM, et al: Assessment of retinol binding protein excretion in normal children, *Pediatr Nephrol* 8:148-150, 1994.

TEST NAME AND METHOD	SPECIMEN REQUIREMENTS	REFERENCE INTERVAL, CONVENTIONAL *ng/dL*[8]			[INTERNATIONAL RECOMMENDED UNITS] *nmol/L*	CHEMICAL INTERFERENCES AND IN VIVO EFFECTS
Reverse Triiodothyronine (rT₃)[1-5]	Serum.[1] Stable for 7 days at room temperature, but storage at 4° C preferred. Stable for at least 30 days frozen.	Cord:	130-300	× 0.0154	[2.00-4.62]	↑ V Amiodarone, gluco-corticoids (high dose),
		1 day:	83-194		[1.28-2.99]	methylthiouracil, oral
		2 days:	107-209		[1.65-3.22]	cholecystographic agents
RIA		3 days:	102-166		[1.57-2.56]	(ipodate and iopanoic
		1 mo-20 yr:	10-35		[0.15-0.54]	acid), propranolol, and
		Adult:	10-40		[0.15-0.61]	propylthiouracil

DIAGNOSTIC INFORMATION	REMARKS

U ↑ Renal tubular dysfunction[13]

---

rT_3 is elevated with acute medical or surgical stress, starvation, some severe systemic diseases, hepatic diseases, treatment of obesity by starvation, advancing age, postpartum women, and moderate or severe chronic (nonthyroidal) illness.[2]

This test is useful to differentiate true hypothyroidism from nonthyroidal illness.

Essentially 80% of rT_3 production is accounted for by peripheral deiodination of T_4 rather than by direct secretion by the thyroid gland. rT_3 is metabolically inactive.[9] In listed conditions, diversion of T_4 metabolism takes place to rT_3 rather than T_3, so that the T_3/rT_3 ratio decreases (T_3 level decreases, rT_3 increases); the ratio of serum T_3 to T_4 is likewise reduced; the T_4 level usually remains unchanged.

TEST NAME AND METHOD	SPECIMEN REQUIREMENTS	REFERENCE INTERVAL, CONVENTIONAL [INTERNATIONAL RECOMMENDED UNITS]		CHEMICAL INTERFERENCES AND IN VIVO EFFECTS

Reverse Triiodothyronine—CONT

| | Maternal serum[6] | 15-40 wk: | 11-33 | [0.17-0.51] | |

	Amniotic fluid.[7] Centrifuge at 900g. Stable for 1 day at 4° C, up to 3 mo frozen. Do not use hemolyzed specimens.		*ng/dL*		*nmol/L*
		<17 wk:	130-159	× 0.0154	[2.00-9.22]
		17-22 wk:	163-599		[2.51-9.22]
		35-42 wk:	15-98		[0.23-1.51]

1. Cavallo L, Margiotta W, Kerncamp C, et al: Serum levels of thyrotropin, thyroxine, 3, 3′, 5-triiodothyronine and 3, 3′,5′-triiodothyronine (reverse Ts) in the first six days of life, *Acta Paediatr Scand* 69:43-47, 1980.

2. Chopra IJ, Solomon DH, Hepner GW, et al: Misleadingly low free thyroxine index and usefulness of reverse triiodothyronine measurement in nonthyroidal illness, *Ann Intern Med* 90:905-912, 1979.

3. Kaplan MM: Clinical and laboratory assessment of thyroid abnormalities, *Med Clin N Am* 69:863-880, 1985.

4. Larsen PR, Davies TF: The thyroid gland. In Larsen PR, Kronenberg HM, Melmed S, et al, editors: *Williams textbook of endocrinology,* ed 10, Philadelphia, 2003, WB Saunders.

5. Tulchinsky D, Ryan KJ, editors: *Maternal-fetal endocrinology,* Philadelphia, 1980, WB Saunders.

6. Cooper E, Aickin CM, Burke CW: Serum concentrations of 3, 3′, 5-triiodothyronine (reverse T_3) in normal pregnancy, *Clin Chim Acta* 106:347-349, 1980.

7. Cooper E, Anderson A, Bennett MJ, et al: Radioimmunoassay of thyroxine and 3, 3′, 5-triiodothyronine (reverse T_3) in human amniotic fluid, *Clin Chim Acta* 118:57-66, 1982.

8. Nichols Institute Reference Laboratories: *Test catalog,* San Juan Capistrano, CA, 2001, Nichols Institute Reference Laboratories.

9. Demers LM, Spencer C: The thyroid. In Burtis CA, Ashwood ER, editors: *Tietz textbook of clinical chemistry,* ed 4, Philadelphia, 2006, WB Saunders.

| **Rheumatoid Factor** (RF)[1-4] *Agglutination of latex particles coated with human IgG*[4] | Fresh serum. Store for 24 hr at 2-8° C. If test cannot be done within 24 hr, freeze serum at −20° C. Do not refreeze. Do not use plasma. | Negative | | Lipemia, cryoglobulins, incomplete heat inactivation of serum, and circulating immune complexes ↑ V Methyldopa |

DIAGNOSTIC INFORMATION	REMARKS

Increased rT_3 with low T_3 (and sometimes low T_4) suggests sick euthyroid syndrome rather than true hypothyroidism. Sensitive TSH, however, is probably better for this differential diagnosis. (See *Thyroid-Stimulating Hormone Stimulation Test*.)

rT_3 is increased several fold in sick euthyroid syndrome.

AF ↑ Diabetes mellitus (overlap with normal interval), very sick and anemic fetuses

The correlation of rT_3 concentrations in amniotic fluid with those in fetal serum suggests the possibility of monitoring fetal thyroid status. rT_3 concentrations decrease with increasing gestational age, correlating significantly with the L/S ratio. There is no correlation with subsequent Apgar scores.

Rheumatoid factor is found in rheumatoid arthritis, Sjögren's syndrome, scleroderma, dermatomyositis, Waldenström's disease, sarcoidosis, and SLE. Only ~75% of patients with rheumatoid arthritis have detectable RF of the IgM class. In rheumatoid arthritis, the highest titers are seen in severe, active, chronic disease with vasculitis and subcutaneous nodules.

Eighty to 90% of patients with Sjögren's syndrome will have high titers of RF.[2]

Rheumatoid factor (RF) consists of autoantibodies that will react with autologous IgG and that are usually of the IgM class, although ~15% of patients with rheumatoid arthritis have IgG-class RF.[2] Most methods detect only IgM-class RF.

Titers ≤1:80 are questionable and can be seen in infectious mononucleosis, acute inflammation, and elderly persons. Standardization with reference serum is mandatory. The latex agglutination test is more sensitive [75% positive in rheumatoid arthritis (RA)] but less specific than the sheep cell test (75% true-positive in RA). Positive results should be confirmed.

TEST NAME AND METHOD	SPECIMEN REQUIREMENTS	REFERENCE INTERVAL, CONVENTIONAL [INTERNATIONAL RECOMMENDED UNITS]			CHEMICAL INTERFERENCES AND IN VIVO EFFECTS
Rheumatoid Factor—CONT					
Sheep cell aggluti-nation test (SCAT)		Negative (<1:17)			Circulating immune complexes
Nephelometric[3]		<30 U/mL	× 1.0	[<30 kU/L]	Severe lipemia
RIA[2]		Negative			None found.

1. Isselbacher KJ, Adams RD, editors: *Harrison's principles of internal medicine: update 4,* New York, 1983, McGraw-Hill Book Co.
2. Rose NR, Friedman H, Fahey JL, editors: *Manual of clinical laboratory immunology,* ed 3, Washington, DC, 1986, American Society for Microbiology.
3. Finley PR, Hicks MJ, Williams RJ, et al: Rate nephelometric measurement of rheumatoid factor in serum, *Clin Chem* 25:1909-1914, 1979.
4. Hanson SL, Mazer FD, Klinefelter HF: A clinical evaluation of a card agglutination test for rheumatoid factor, *Am J Clin Pathol* 73:110-113, 1980.

TEST NAME AND METHOD	SPECIMEN REQUIREMENTS	REFERENCE INTERVAL, CONVENTIONAL [INTERNATIONAL RECOMMENDED UNITS]			CHEMICAL INTERFERENCES AND IN VIVO EFFECTS
Riboflavin (Vitamin B$_2$)[1,2] *Fluorimetric*[3,4]	Erythrocytes; protect from light. Stable at −20° C.	10-50 mcg/dL	× 26.6	[266-1330 nmol/L]	
Fluorimetric[5] *HPLC*[6-8]	Serum or plasma (EDTA, heparin), fast-ing; protect from light. Stable at −20° C.	4-24 mcg/dL		[106-638 nmol/L]	
HPLC[6,8]	Urine, 24 hr; protect from light. Stable at −4° C.	>100 mcg/day	× 2.66	[>266 nmol/day]	U ↑ V Antibiotics, barbiturates, and phenothiazines
Fluorimetric[9]	Urine, fasting (ran-dom); protect from light.	*mcg/g creatinine* >80	× 0.3	*μmol/mol creatinine* [>24]	

DIAGNOSTIC INFORMATION	REMARKS

Negative results have been observed in the presence of rheumatoid disease. SCAT is less sensitive than the latex procedure. The test is relatively specific when positive (90% true-positive in RA) but less sensitive than the latex test (50-60% positive in RA).

Thirty to 50 U/mL [30-50 kU/L] is considered weakly positive in the nephelometric reaction.

↓ Alcoholism, hypothyroidism, liver disease, anorexia, malabsorption (tropical sprue, celiac disease, malignancy, small bowel resection, GI and biliary obstruction, diarrhea, infectious enteritis, irritable bowel syndrome), phototherapy of infants with jaundice, oculourogenital syndrome, angular cheilitis, atrophic glossitis (magenta tongue), conjunctivitis, genital hyperpigmentation (resembling zinc deficiency), and seborrheic dermatitis around the nose, eyes, and ears

Vitamin B_2, in the form of riboflavin-5′-phosphate, serves as a component of prosthetic units (FAD and FMN) of the flavoproteins that function as hydrogen carriers in biologic oxidation-reduction processes.[1]

Ariboflavinosis (dietary deficiency of riboflavin) occurs almost invariably in combination with other water-soluble vitamin deficiencies. Deficiency causes a syndrome characterized by sore throat, hyperemia and edema of the pharyngeal and oral mucous membranes, cheilitis, angular stomatitis, glossitis, corneal vascularization, dyssebacia with dermatitis, and normochromic, normocytic anemia.

Severe deficiency of vitamin B_2 can diminish conversion of vitamin B6 to its active "coenzyme" form and curtail conversion of tryptophan to niacin.

During recent years, deficiencies of riboflavin and vitamin B_6 have been suggested as potentiating factors for chronic progressive nerve compression disorders, such as carpal tunnel syndrome.[2]

TEST NAME AND METHOD	SPECIMEN REQUIREMENTS	REFERENCE INTERVAL, CONVENTIONAL [INTERNATIONAL RECOMMENDED UNITS]	CHEMICAL INTERFERENCES AND IN VIVO EFFECTS
Riboflavin—CONT			

1. Fishman SM, Christian P, Wesk KP: The role of vitamins in the prevention and control of anemia, *Public Health Nutr* 3:125-150, 2000.

2. Folkers K, Ellis J: Successful therapy with vitamin B6 and vitamin B2 of the carpal tunnel syndrome and need for determination of RDAs for vitamins B6 and B2 for disease states, *Ann NY Acad Sci* 585:295-301, 1990.

3. Knobloch E, Hodr R, Houdkova V: Spectrofluorimetric determination of FAD, FMN and free riboflavin in the blood, *Cesk Farm* 37:108-111, 1988.

4. Knobloch E, Hodr R, Janda J, et al: Spectrofluorimetric micromethod for determining riboflavin in the blood of new-born babies and their mothers, *Int J Vitam Nutr Res* 49:144-151, 1997.

5. Hustad S, Ueland PM, Schneede J: Quantification of riboflavin, flavin mononucleotide, and flavin adenine dinucleotide in human plasma by capillary electrophoresis and laser-induced fluorescence detection, *Clin Chem* 45:862-868, 1999.

6. Li Y, Brown PR: The optimization of HPLC-UV conditions for use with FTIR detection in the analysis of B vitamins, *J Chromatogr Sci* 41:96-99, 2003.

7. Capo-chichi CD, Gueant JL, Feillet F, et al: Analysis of riboflavin and riboflavin cofactor levels in plasma by high-performance liquid chromatography, *J Chromatogr B Biomed Sci Appl* 739:219-224, 2000.

8. Lopez-Anaya A, Mayersohn M: Quantification of riboflavin, riboflavin 5'-phosphate and flavin adenine dinucleotide in plasma and urine by high-performance liquid chromatography, *J Chromatogr* 423:105-113, 1987.

9. Su AK, Lin CH: Determination of riboflavin in urine by capillary electrophoresis-blue light emitting diode-induced fluorescence detection combined with a stacking technique, *J Chromatogr B Analyt Technol Biomed Life Sci* 785:39-46, 2003.

TEST NAME AND METHOD	SPECIMEN REQUIREMENTS	REFERENCE INTERVAL, CONVENTIONAL		[INTERNATIONAL RECOMMENDED UNITS]	CHEMICAL INTERFERENCES AND IN VIVO EFFECTS
Rubidium (Rb) *NAA, AAS*	Serum.[2] Collect in metal-free container.	80-560 mg/L	× 0.0117	[0.9-6.5 μmol/L]	None found.
	Packed blood cells.[3] Collect in metal-free container.	*mg/kg wet wt.* 4.28 ± 0.98 (SD)	× 11.7	*μmol/kg wet wt.* [50 ± 11]	
	Urine.[2] Collect in metal-free container.	1-3 mg/day	× 11.7	[11.7-35.1 μmol/day]	
	Hair.[2,4] Cut close to scalp and analyze proximal segments.	*mcg/g dry wt.* 0.1-2.0	× 11.7	*nmol/g dry wt.* [1.2-23.4]	

Neither blood nor urine levels of B_2 are as sensitive indicators of riboflavin status as is the stimulation of erythrocyte glutathione reductase activity by FAD (coenzyme form of B_2). Urine concentration reflects recent dietary intake and can be artificially increased in negative nitrogen balance and after surgery or prolonged fasting. There is little body storage of B_2, and toxicity is unknown. See *Glutathione Reductase in Erythrocytes.*

Rubidium is nonessential for humans and animals. Toxicity has not been observed in humans.

TEST NAME AND METHOD	SPECIMEN REQUIREMENTS	REFERENCE INTERVAL, CONVENTIONAL [INTERNATIONAL RECOMMENDED UNITS]	CHEMICAL INTERFERENCES AND IN VIVO EFFECTS
Rubidium—CONT			
X-ray fluorescence spectrometry[1]	Bronchoalveolar lavage (BAL) fluid	$ng/10^3$ *macrophages* <0.13 × 11.7	*fmol/macrophage* [<1.5]

1. Maier EA, Rastegar F, Heimburger R, et al: Simultaneous determination of trace elements in lavage fluids front human bronchial alveoli by energy dispersive X-ray flourescence. 1: Technique and determination of the normal reference interval, *Clin Chem* 31:551-555, 1985.

2. Iyengar GV, Woittiez J: Trace elements in human clinical specimens: evaluation of literature data to identify tolerence values, *Clin Chem* 34:474-481, 1988.

3. Versieck J, Hoste J, Barbier F, et al: Simultaneous determination of iron, selenium, rubidium, and cesium in serum and packed blood cells by neutron activation analysis, *Clin Chem* 23:1301-1305, 1977.

4. Iyengar GV, Kollmer WE, Bowen HJM: *The elemental composition of human tissues and body fluids,* Weinheim, 1978, Verlag Chemie.

TEST NAME AND METHOD	SPECIMEN REQUIREMENTS	REFERENCE INTERVAL, CONVENTIONAL [INTERNATIONAL RECOMMENDED UNITS]	CHEMICAL INTERFERENCES AND IN VIVO EFFECTS
S100β Protein[1-8] *Immunoassay*[1]	Serum, heparinized plasma or cerebrospinal fluid. Citrated plasma can be used if 5 mmol/L calcium is added. Otherwise, results of citrate or EDTA of plasma are lower.[1]	*mcg/L* Serum: 0.021[2] Spinal fluid[3]: M 20-39 yr: 2.2 40-59 yr: 2.5 60-89 yr: 3.1 F 20-39 yr: 2.2 40-59 yr: 2.4 60-89 yr: 2.3	

1. Takahashi M, Chamczuk A, Hong Y, et al: Rapid and sensitive immunoassay for the measurement of serum S100B using isoform-specific monoclonal antibody, *Clin Chem* 45:1307-1311, 1999.

2. Mokuno K, Kato K, Kawai K, et al: Neuron-specific enolase and S-100 protein levels in cerebrospinal fluid of patients with various neurological diseases, *J Neurol Sci* 60:443-451, 1983.

3. Persson L, Hardemark HG, Gustafsson J, et al: S-100 protein and neuron-specific enolase in cerebrospinal fluid and serum: markers of cell damage in human central nervous system, *Stroke* 18:911-918, 1987.

4. Fassbender K, Schmidt R, Schreiner A, et al: Leakage of brain-originated proteins in peripheral blood: temporal profile and diagnostic value in early ischemic stroke, *J Neurol Sci* 148:101-105, 1997.

5. Missler U, Wiesmann M, Friedrich C, et al: S-100 protein and neuron-specific enolase concentrations in blood as indicators of infarction volume and prognosis in acute ischemic stroke, *Stroke* 28:1956-1960, 1997.

6. Kanner AA, Marchi N, Fazio V, et al: Serum S100β. A noninvasive marker of blood-brain barrier function and brain lesions, *Cancer* 97:2806-2813, 2003.

7. Buttner T, Lack B, Jager M, et al: Serum levels of neuron-specific enolase and s-100 protein after single tonic-clonic seizures, *J Neurol* 246:459-461, 1999.

8. Michetti F, Gazzolo D: S-100B protein in biological fluids: a tool for perinatal medicine, *Clin Chem* 48:2097-2104, 2002.

DIAGNOSTIC INFORMATION   **REMARKS**

S100β has been suggested as a marker for stroke. S100β be-gins to increase within the first 8 hr after the onset of stroke and remains increased for 72 hr.[4] The concentration of S100β correlates to the infarct volume and neurological out-comes.[5] S100β is also increased in other neurological disorders associated with the breakdown of the blood-brain barrier[6] and seizures.[7]

S100 is a family of acidic calcium binding proteins. It has solu-bility in 100% ammonium sulfate. There are some 20 isoforms of S100, mostly found in free cytosolic pools. The αα isoform is found in cardiac myocytes, αβ in glial cells, and ββ in astro-cytes and Schwann cells of the brain.[8] The S100β is 21 kDa, which may facilitate appearance of this marker into blood from the cerebrospinal fluid. The biological half-life in blood is ~2 hr.

TEST NAME AND METHOD	SPECIMEN REQUIREMENTS	REFERENCE INTERVAL, CONVENTIONAL [INTERNATIONAL RECOMMENDED UNITS]	CHEMICAL INTERFERENCES AND IN VIVO EFFECTS
Saccharomyces cerevisiae **Antibodies (ASCA), IgA and IgG** *Solid-phase EIA*	Serum, frozen or refrigerated is preferable.	IgA or IgG Isotype <25 U: Negative 25-35 U: Equivocal >35 U: Positive The reference intervals cited above may vary with reagent manufacturer.	None known.

1. Sandborn WJ, Loftus EV Jr, Homburger HA, et al: Evaluation of serological disease markers in a population-based cohort of patients with ulcerative colitis and Crohn's disease, *Inflamm Bowel Dis* 7:192-201, 2001.
2. Vidrich A, Lee J, Janes E: Segregation of pANCA antigenic recognition by DNase treatment of neutrophils: ulcerative colitis, type 1 autoimmune hepatitis, and primary sclerosing cholangitis, *J Clin Immunol* 15:293-299, 1995.

| **Secretin**[1-5]

 RIA | Plasma, fasting. Collect blood in heparin-Trasylol. Plasma should be separated in a refrigerated centrifuge within 30 min of collection and then frozen immediately. Keep frozen until assayed. | 12-75 pg/mL | ↓ V Cimetidine, somatostatin |

1. Kaplan LA, Pesce AJ, editors: *Clinical chemistry: theory, analysis, and correlation,* St. Louis, 1984, CV Mosby.
2. InterScience Institute: *Current unique and rare endocrine assays,* Inglewood, CA, 1987, InterScience Institute.
3. Languish PG: Function tests in the diagnosis of chronic pancreatitis. Critical evaluation, *Int J Pancreatol* 14:9-20, 1993.
4. Rayford PL, Hejtmancik L, Thompson JC: Radioimmunoassay of gastrointestinal hormones, *World J Surg* 3:423-431, 1979.
5. Walsh JH: Gastrointestinal hormones. In Johnson LR, editor: *Physiology of the gastrointestinal tract,* ed 2, New York, 1987, Raven Press.
6. Chey WY, Chang TM: Secretin, 100 years later, *J Gastroenterol* 38:1025-1035, 2003.

DIAGNOSTIC INFORMATION	**REMARKS**

ASCAs occur in patients with inflammatory bowel diseases, especially Crohn's disease.[1] Positive results for both IgA and IgG ASCA occur in ~40% of patients with Crohn's disease with a positive predictive value that approaches 90%. ASCAs occur less commonly in other inflammatory intestinal diseases, including ulcerative colitis and celiac disease.

Testing for ASCA is often performed along with the test for pANCA. Patients with ulcerative colitis often test positive for pANCA and do not usually have elevated levels of ASCA,[2] whereas patients with Crohn's disease test negative for pANCA. These two patterns of results (ASCA positive, pANCA negative, and vice versa) have high predictive values for Crohn's disease and ulcerative colitis, respectively, but occur in <50% of patients with inflammatory bowel disease. The test for ASCA is not appropriate for screening patients with intestinal symptoms for inflammatory bowel disease.

↑ Intraduodenal acidification (50-fold over fasting). Gastric acid hypersecretion (e.g., gastrinomas or Zollinger-Ellison syndrome), duodenal ulcers, starvation, diabetes mellitus, and chronic renal failure

↓ Celiac disease (gluten-sensitive enteropathy), pernicious anemia, and achlorhydria

Antacid medications or medications affecting intestinal motility should be discontinued 48 hr before testing. Wide variations in reference intervals have been reported, depending on the method of measurement. Plasma levels increase rapidly after acid stimulation, peaking at 3 min, and then decreasing to basal levels in 60 min.

In patients with Zollinger-Ellison syndrome, secretin infusion causes an increase in serum gastrin (see *Gastrin Stimulation Test [after Secretin]*).

TEST NAME AND METHOD	SPECIMEN REQUIREMENTS	REFERENCE INTERVAL, CONVENTIONAL [INTERNATIONAL RECOMMENDED UNITS]	CHEMICAL INTERFERENCES AND IN VIVO EFFECTS
Sediment, Urinary[1-14]	Urine, fresh random; first morning specimen preferred. Examine immediately. If preservation is required, add 1 crystal thymol/ 10-15 mL or formalin (40% v/v), 1 drop/10 mL.	Values differ with method and concentration of specimen.	Thymol will interfere with the acid precipitation test for protein if carried out on same specimen.
Casts *Hyaline casts*		Occasional (0-1) casts/hpf	↑ V Amphotericin, cephaloridine, ethacrynic acid, and furosemide
RBC (Erc) casts		Not seen	
WBC (Lkc) casts		Not seen	
Granular casts		Not seen	↑ V Amphotericin, bismuth salts, calcitonin, cephaloridine, indomethacin, and kanamycin
Waxy casts		Not seen	
Epithelial casts		Tubular epithelial: Not seen Transitional and squamous epithelial: Not seen	

DIAGNOSTIC INFORMATION	REMARKS
The type and number of formed elements may give valuable diagnostic information about the presence, type, and localization of pathological processes within the urinary tract (see below). Casts form only in the renal tubule and thus reflect disease within the renal parenchyma, generally high in the nephron.	Optimal preservation is achieved in acid, hypertonic urine. Refrigerate if examination is not performed within 2 hr. Approximately 50% of the cells are lost after 2-3 hr standing at room temperature. RBC (Erc) lysis occurs at a specific gravity <1.010.[4] A combined cytocentrifugation and Papanicolaou staining method has been used to evaluate renal allograft recipients; a standard slide procedure (the KOVA system) is also available and is more reproducible than conventional bright-field microscopy.
↑ All renal diseases that cause glomerular proteinuria; also seen with fever, strenuous exercise, diuretic therapy, hypertension, acute pyelonephritis, and congestive heart failure The presence of particulate or cellular inclusions increases the likelihood of intrinsic renal disease. The presence of hyaline casts is a relatively sensitive indicator of intrinsic renal disease but is very nonspecific.	Increased acidity and electrolyte concentration enhance the precipitation of casts. Hyaline casts dissolve rapidly in alkaline urine; excessive excretion of hyaline and lightly granular casts can continue for decades in treated essential hypertension, gouty nephropathy, nonprogressive glomerulonephritis, and other inactive diseases.[17] Casts reflect the shape and diameter of the lumina of origin.
The presence of RBC casts usually indicates glomerular pathology ↑↑ Acute poststreptococcal and rapidly progressive glomerulonephritis; present in other forms of glomerulonephritis, polyarteritis, subacute bacterial endocarditis, Goodpasture's syndrome, renal infarction, renal vein thrombosis, and malignant hypertension; very rarely in tubulointerstitial disease	RBC casts have greater diagnostic significance than any other variety. Their presence helps differentiate hematuria caused by glomerular disease from other sources of urinary tract bleeding.
The presence of WBC casts reflects tubulointerstitial disease, most notably pyelonephritis; these casts are also seen with lupus nephritis but are uncommon with glomerular disease and noninfectious interstitial nephritis.	WBC casts may be the only clue to pyelonephritis. When present they may greatly aid in the differentiation of pyelonephritis from cystitis.
Granular casts may be present in active glomerulonephritis, diabetic nephropathy, pyelonephritis, viral disease, lead intoxication, amyloidosis, malignant hypertension, acute allograft rejection (intermittent), strenuous exercise, fever, and pure carbohydrate diet. The presence of granular casts is indicative of pathology but is nonspecific.	There is no clinical difference between coarse and fine granular casts. Their presence in a resting, afebrile subject is indicative of renal disease. Bile-stained granular casts are excreted in large numbers in obstructive jaundice, often without any other evidence of renal disease.[17]
Waxy casts are observed most frequently in patients with chronic renal failure; they are also found in amyloidosis and occasionally in allograft rejection.	Broad, waxy casts ("renal failure casts") generally suggest severe, chronic renal disease.
These casts may be present in acute tubular necrosis, viral disease (e.g., CMV), heavy metal poisoning, ethylene glycol or salicylate intoxication, acute allograft rejection, or amyloidosis.	Epithelial casts are the rarest of casts. Their presence after the third postoperative day constitutes one of the most reliable indicators of acute allograft rejection.[14]

TEST NAME AND METHOD	SPECIMEN REQUIREMENTS	REFERENCE INTERVAL, CONVENTIONAL [INTERNATIONAL RECOMMENDED UNITS]	CHEMICAL INTERFERENCES AND IN VIVO EFFECTS
Sediment, Urinary—CONT			
Fatty casts		Not seen	
Mixed casts		Not seen	
Crystal casts		Not seen	
Cells *Red blood cells (RBC, Ercs)*		0-2/hpf	↑ V Allopurinol, amphotericin, anticoagulants, aspirin, colchicine, cyclophosphamide, gold, indomethacin, levodopa, methenamine, oxyphenbutazone, penicillins, phenols, phenylbutazone, radiographic agents, sulfonamides, and turpentine
White blood cells (WBC, Lkcs)		M: 0-3/hpf F child: 0-5/hpf	↑ V Allopurinol, ampicillin, aspirin, capreomycin, heroin (in addicts), ipodate, iron salts, kanamycin, L-dopa, and methicillin
Tubular epithelial cells		Few; more frequent in newborn	↑ V Acetaminophen, bismuth salts, caffeine, calcitonin, castor oil, cortisone, phenacetin, salicylates, and thallium

DIAGNOSTIC INFORMATION	REMARKS

Fatty casts are associated with nephrotic syndrome and major skeletal trauma.

The presence of mixed casts suggests tubulointerstitial disease or any of the above, depending on composition.

See *Crystals,* below.

Erythrocytes are present in renal disease (e.g., glomerulonephritis), lupus nephritis, focal glomerulitis (Berger's disease [IgA nephropathy], Alport's syndrome, benign familial recurrent hematuria), calculus, tumor, infection, tuberculosis, infarction, renal vein thrombosis, trauma, hydronephrosis, polycystic kidney, analgesic nephropathy and occasionally acute tubular necrosis and malignant nephrosclerosis, urinary tract disease (including inflammation), infection, calculus, tumor, obstruction, prostatitis, and systemic febrile disease (including malaria, yellow fever, blackwater fever)

Various extrarenal diseases (e.g., appendicitis, salpingitis, diverticulitis); tumors of the colon, rectum, and pelvis; gout, scurvy, subacute bacterial endocarditis, polyarteritis nodosa, malignant hypertension, infectious mononucleosis, hemoglobinopathies, coagulation disorders, and heart failure

Drugs and toxins: See *Interferences.*

Others: Radiation, exercise, lordosis, smoking,[4] and hypercatabolic states

RBC (Ercs) may originate from any point along the genitourinary tract and may indicate hematological, neoplastic, or other genitourinary disease. Hence, their presence is relatively nonspecific. The most common causes of isolated hematuria are urinary tract stones and neoplasms, tuberculosis, trauma, cystitis, and prostatitis, whereas the most common cause of recurrent hematuria of glomerular origin is Berger's disease (IgA nephropathy). RBCs, in conjunction with RBC casts, suggest an intrarenal source, whereas the absence of casts or proteinuria suggests a source distal to the kidney. Hematuria may be one of the earliest signs of inadequate anticoagulant control.

↑ Almost all renal disease and diseases of the genitourinary tract (especially tubulointerstitial nephritis, lupus nephritis, pyelonephritis, urinary tract infections), renal transplant rejections, fever, and exercise

Values >50 WBC (Lkcs)/hpf are strongly suggestive of acute infection.

Phosphaturia, not pyuria, is the most common cause of cloudy urine. Number and appearance of WBC (Lkcs) are influenced by urine pH, osmolality, temperature, associated proteinuria and bacteriuria, and the interval between voiding and examination. Repeated sterile cultures in the presence of 50 WBC/hpf may indicate tuberculosis or lupus nephritis, whereas gross pyuria may reflect rupture of a renal or urinary tract abscess. Concomitant presence of casts implicates renal origin.

Acute tubular damage: Pyelonephritis, necrotizing papillitis, acute tubular necrosis, various drugs and toxins (especially salicylate intoxication, heavy metal or ethylene glycol poisoning), malignant nephrosclerosis, and acute renal allograft rejection

It is often difficult to distinguish renal epithelial cells from other cells within the sediment; values >15 cells/hpf seen 3 days after transplantation provide strong evidence of impending allograft rejection.[4] Tubular cells that have absorbed lipids (oval fat bodies) may result in fatty casts, suggestive of the nephrotic syndrome.

TEST NAME AND METHOD	SPECIMEN REQUIREMENTS	REFERENCE INTERVAL, CONVENTIONAL [INTERNATIONAL RECOMMENDED UNITS]		CHEMICAL INTERFERENCES AND IN VIVO EFFECTS
Sediment, Urinary—CONT				
Transitional or squamous epithelial cells				Excessive numbers of squamous epithelial cells increase the possibility of contamination of the urine by vaginal fluids.
Bacteria[12,15]	Specimen bottle should be new plastic or sterilized glass. Analyze urine quickly because bacteria multiply rapidly. See also *Specimen Requirements*.	Unspun:	No organisms/oil immersion field	
		Spun:	<20 organisms/hpf	
Ova and Parasites (see *Section IV, Ova and Parasite Examination*)				
Yeast (Candida)				

DIAGNOSTIC INFORMATION	REMARKS
Transitional cell carcinoma may show clumps or sheets of transitional epithelial cells.	Normal desquamation may lead to the presence of a few transitional cells. Squamous cells have little diagnostic significance.
↑ Urinary tract infections	Significant infections are usually associated with counts $>10^5$ organisms/mL [$>10^8$ organisms/L] of a clean-catch midvoid specimen. A bacteriological loop represents $\sim$10 mL. If bacteria are seen in a smear of a loopful, this is probably significant bacteriuria. The presence of many squamous epithelial cells and mixed vaginal-type flora indicates contamination and the need for a repeat specimen, regardless of the count. Low counts may be the result of dilution in a well-hydrated patient. Marked pyuria can mask bacteria in the sediment; obscuring crystals may be dissolved by warming the specimen. Bacteria are no longer present in the urine 24-48 hr after an appropriate antimicrobial treatment. Most urinary tract infections are ascending and involved gram-negative enteric organisms. Eighty percent of infections not associated with voiding defects involve *Escherichia coli;* 95% of all recurrent infections arise from an external rather than an internal port of entry. Only $\sim$50% of patients with significant bacteriuria ($>10^5$ organisms/mL [$>10^8$ organisms/L]) have accompanying pyuria. Several types of chemical screening tests for bacteriuria exist. See *Bacteria Screen.* Screening procedures for positive urine cultures yield a sensitivity of 92% and specificity of 81% using the Bac T-Screen (Vitek Systems Inc., Hazelwood, MO). Addition of the leukocyte esterase dipstick improves the specificity of the combined tests to 99% but results in a sensitivity of only 73%.[15]
See *Remarks.*	Yeast may represent a harmless saprophyte or a significant pathogen, particularly in the immunocompromised or diabetic patient. Generally microscopic or gross pyuria accompanies *Candida* infection.

TEST NAME AND METHOD	SPECIMEN REQUIREMENTS	REFERENCE INTERVAL, CONVENTIONAL [INTERNATIONAL RECOMMENDED UNITS]	CHEMICAL INTERFERENCES AND IN VIVO EFFECTS
Sediment, Urinary—CONT			
Tumor cells (Papanicolaou method)[16]			
Crystals		See *Remarks.*	A number of drugs may form crystals in the urine, particularly at extreme pH values.

1. Boehringer Mannheim Corp.: *Urinalysis today,* Indianapolis, IN, 1986, Boehringer Mannheim Corp.

2. Conn RB, editor: *Current diagnosis,* ed 7, Philadelphia, 1985, WB Saunders.

3. DeGowin EL, DeGowin RL: *Bedside diagnostic examination,* ed 5, New York, 1987, Macmillan Pub Co.

4. Henry JB, editor: *Clinical diagnosis and management by laboratory methods,* ed 18, Philadelphia, 1991, WB Saunders.

5. Miale JB: *Laboratory medicine: hematology,* ed 6, St. Louis, 1982, CV Mosby.

6. Miles Inc., Diagnostics Division: *Modern urine chemistry,* Elkhart, IN, 1991, Miles Inc., Diagnostics Division.

7. Tietz NW, editor: *Fundamentals of clinical chemistry,* ed 3, Philadelphia, 1987, WB Saunders.

8. Wilson JD, Braunwald E, Isselbacher KJ, et al, editors: *Harrison's principles of internal medicine,* ed 12, New York, 1991, McGraw-Hill Publishing Co.

9. Wyngaarden JB, Smith LH Jr, Bennett JC, editors: *Cecil textbook of medicine,* ed 19, Philadelphia, 1992, WB Saunders.

10. Free A, Free H: *Urinalysis in clinical laboratory practice,* Cleveland, 1975, CRC Press.

11. Graff L: *A handbook of routine urinalysis,* Philadelphia, 1983, JB Lippincott.

12. Kunin CM: *Detection, prevention and management of urinary tract infections,* ed 4, Philadelphia, 1987, Lea & Febiger.

13. Schumann GS, Friedman SK: *Wet urinalysis: interpretations, correlations and implications,* Chicago, 2003, ASCP Press.

14. Schumann GB, Harris S, Henry JB: An improved technic for examining urinary casts and a review of their significance, *Am J Clin Pathol* 69:18-23, 1978.

15. Madan E, Quittner H, Blackwell J: Urine screening: an alternative to urine cultures, *Ann Clin Lab Sci* 18:116-119, 1988.

DIAGNOSTIC INFORMATION	REMARKS
See *Remarks*.	Demonstration of tumor cells provides an important mechanism for recognizing cancer of the kidney, ureters, or bladder. False-negative results are much more common than false-positive results. Multiple specimen examination improves accuracy. Automated staining with the Cyto-Tek (Miles, Inc., Diagnostic Division, Elkhart, IN) is available. The UROCYTE System (Dianon Systems, Inc., Stratford, CT) determines DNA aneuploidy and is effective in monitoring bladder cancer patients.
Triple phosphate: Increased amounts of fruit in diet	Most crystals have little clinical significance. Phosphates, urates, and oxalates are especially common in normal urine. Knowledge of urine pH is a prerequisite to identification. Amorphous urates are seen in acid urine, whereas amorphous phosphates appear in alkaline urine. Cystine crystals are among the most important crystals found; renograffin crystals frequently appear after radiographic examinations of the urinary tract High doses of ampicillin, sulfonamides, 6-mercaptopurine, or primidone may result in crystal formation.
Calcium oxalate: Increased amounts of cabbage, asparagus, rhubarb in diet,[7] severe chronic renal disease, ethylene glycol and methoxyflurane toxicity, and small bowel resection	
Cystine: Present in cystinuria, homocystinuria	
Leucine and tyrosine: May be present in severe liver disease	
Cholesterol: May be seen in severe urinary tract infections, nephritis, rupture of lymphatic vessels into the renal pelvis	
Uric acid: Increased in 16% of gout patients,[13] malignant lymphoma, and leukemia	

16. Free A, Free H: *Urinalysis in clinical laboratory practice,* Cleveland, 1975, CRC Press.
17. Wyngaarden JB, Smith LH Jr, Bennett JC, editors: *Cecil textbook of medicine,* ed 19, Philadelphia, 1992, WB Saunders.

TEST NAME AND METHOD	SPECIMEN REQUIREMENTS	REFERENCE INTERVAL, CONVENTIONAL [INTERNATIONAL RECOMMENDED UNITS]			CHEMICAL INTERFERENCES AND IN VIVO EFFECTS
Selenium (Se)[1] *Fluorimetric, AAS, NAA*	Whole blood (heparin, EDTA).[2] Collect in pretested, metal-free container.	58-234 mcg/L × 0.0127 [0.74-2.97 μmol/L] Serum values are ~20% lower. Toxic concentration: >500 mcg/L [>6.35 μmol/L]			↑ Indapamide, ascorbic acid ↓ Carbamazepine, phenytoin, and valproic acid
	Serum.[2] Collect in pretested, metal-free container.	46-143 mcg/L		[0.58-1.82 μmol/L]	
	Erythrocytes.[2] Collect in pretested, metal-free container.	75-240 mcg/kg × 0.0127 [0.95-3.05 μmol/kg]			
NAA	Platelets (pure).[3] Collect in metal-free container.	*ng/g wet wt.* 782 ± 127 (SD) × 0.0127		*μmol/kg wet wt.* [9.9 ± 1.6]	
	Hair.[2] Cut close to scalp and analyze proximal segments.	*mcg/g dry wt.* 0.2-1.4 × 12.7		*nmol/g dry wt.* [2.5-17.8]	Hair ↑ C Selenium-containing dandruff shampoos
AAS	Urine, 24 hr.[2] Collect in acid-washed, metal-free container. Use no preservative.	7-160 mcg/L × 0.0127 [0.09-2.03 μmol/L] Toxic concentration: >400 mcg/L [>5.08 μmol/L]			
ICP-MS	Serum.[4] Collect in pretested, metal-free container.	23-190 mcg/L × 0.0127 [0.29-2.41 nmol/L]			
	Urine.[4] Collect in acid-washed, metal-free container. Refrigerate during and after collection.	0-200 mcg/L		[0.00-2.54 nmol/L]	

1. Milne DB: Trace elements. In Burtis CA, Ashwood ER, editors: *Tietz textbook of clinical chemistry,* ed 2, Philadelphia, 1994, WB Saunders.

2. Iyengar GV, Woittiez J: Trace elements in human clinical specimens: evaluation of literature data to identify tolerence values, *Clin Chem* 34:474-481, 1988.

3. Kasperek K, Iyengar GV, Kiem J, et al: Elemental composition of platelets. Part III. Determinations of Ag, Au, Cd, Co, Cr, Cs, Mo, Rb, Sb, and Se in normal human platelets by neutron activation analysis, *Clin Chem* 25:711-715, 1979.

4. Associated Regional & University Pathologists, Inc. web site (www.aruplab.com): Available at: http://www.aruplab.com/testing/user_guide.jsp.

5. Cirelli A, Ciardi M, De Simone C, et al: Serum selenium concentration and disease progress in patients with HIV infection, *Clin Biochem* 24:211-214, 1991.

6. Arthur JR: The role of selenium in thyroid hormone metabolism, *Can J Physiol Pharmacol* 69:1648-1652, 1991.

DIAGNOSTIC INFORMATION	REMARKS

B ↑ Reticuloendothelial neoplasia, industrial toxicity

B ↓ GI cancer, malnutrition, TPN, pregnancy, cirrhosis, hepatitis, cardiomyopathy (Keshan's disease, an endemic cardiomyopathy), and HIV[5]

Selenium is an essential metal for human glutathione peroxidase and iodothyronine deiodinase. Erythrocyte GSH-Px is a useful functional index of Se status. See *Glutathione Peroxidase in Erythrocytes.*

Exposure to selenium results in garlic smell in breath and urine, metallic taste, headaches, nausea, vomiting, numbness, convulsions, pneumonia, pulmonary edema, and circulatory collapse.

Human deficiency has been observed as endemic cretinism,[6,7] Balkan nephropathy,[8] Keshan's disease,[9] and Kashin-Back disease.[10] Selenium is metabolized to dimethyl selenide, which is excreted by the lungs. Industrial exposure to selenium occurs in the manufacture of glass pigments, paints, dyes, electronic equipment, fungicides, rubber, and semiconductors.

Depending on the environment, selenium concentrations in foods, body tissues, and body fluids vary widely. Twenty-four–hour urine specimens should be used to assess toxicity.

7. Contempre B, Vanderpas J, Dumont JE: Cretinism, thyroid hormones and selenium, *Mol Cell Endocrinol* 81:C193-195, 1991.

8. Maksimovic ZJ: Selenium deficiency and Balkin endemic nephropathy, *Kidney Int Suppl* 34:12-14, 1991.

9. Lockitch G, Taylor GP, Wong LTK, et al: Cardiomyopathy associated with nonendemic selenium deficiency in a Caucasian adolescent, *Am J Clin Nutr* 52:572-577, 1990.

10. Levander OA: A global view of human selenium nutrition, *Ann Rev Nutr* 7:227-250, 1987.

TEST NAME AND METHOD	SPECIMEN REQUIREMENTS	REFERENCE INTERVAL, CONVENTIONAL [INTERNATIONAL RECOMMENDED UNITS]	CHEMICAL INTERFERENCES AND IN VIVO EFFECTS
Semen Analysis (Sperm Count)[1]	Ejaculate. Specimen should be maintained at ~37° C during transport to the laboratory and examined within 3 hr of collection. For the collection, follow physician's instructions.	See analysis table below.	↓ Azathioprine, cimetidine, cyclophosphamide, estrogens, fluoxymesterone, ketoconazole, methotrexate, methyltestosterone, nitrofurantoin (effect probably transient), nitrogen mustard, procarbazine, sulfasalazine, testicular radiation, and vincristine

ANALYSIS TABLE[2,3]

	Normal	Pathological		Normal	Pathological
Volume, mL:	2-6	<1.5	×0.001	[0.002-0.006 L]	[<0.0015 L]
Sperm density ×10^6/mL:	>20	<10	×10^3	[>20 × 10^9/L]	[<10 ×10^9]
Total number of spermatozoa (×10^6/ejaculate):	>80	<20		[>80]	[<20]
Progressive motility score*:	3-4	0-1		[3-4]	[0-1]

	Percent of total			Fraction of total	
Live spermatozoa:	≥50 <35	×0.01		[≥0.50] [<0.35]	
1 hr after ejaculation:	≥70			[≥0.70]	
2 hr after ejaculation:	≥60			[≥0.60]	
4 hr after ejaculation:	>50 <35			[>0.50] [<0.35]	
Normal spermatozoa:	≥60 <35			[≥0.60] [<0.35]	
Defective heads:	<35 >60			[<0.35] [>0.60]	
Defective midpieces:	≤20 <25			[≤0.20] [<0.25]	
Defective tails:	≤20 >25			[≤0.20] [>0.25]	
Immature forms:	<4			[<0.04]	

*Evaluated 2-4 hr after ejaculation.

ANALYSIS TABLE[2,3]

Coagulation:	Specimen coagulates		
Liquefaction:	Complete in 10-30 min		
Leukocyte count/mL:			
≤2000	× 106	[≤2 × 10^9/L]	
pH:	7.2-7.8		
Fructose:			
150-600 mg/dL	× 0.0555	[8.33-33.30 mmol/L]	

1. Griffin JE, Wilson JD: Disorders of the testes and male reproductive tract. In Wilson JD, Foster DW, editors: *Williams textbook of endocrinology*, ed 8, Philadelphia, 1992, WB Saunders.
2. Glasser L: Seminal fluid and sub fertility, *Diagn Med* July/Aug:28-45, 1981.
3. Seamark RF: *Semen analysis. The Royal College of Pathologists of Australia, broadsheet no. 20,* 1979, Surry Hills, New South Wales, Australia, The Royal College of Pathologists of Australia.
4. Gunalp S, Onculoglu C, Gurgan T, et al: A study of semen parameters with emphasis on sperm morphology in a fertile population: an attempt to develop clinical thresholds, *Hum Reprod* 16:110-114, 2001.

DIAGNOSTIC INFORMATION	REMARKS

↓ Cryptorchidism, primary and secondary testicular failure, idiopathic oligospermia, obstruction of ejaculatory system, hyperpyrexia, and postvasectomy

Aggregates of >10 spermatozoa in a well-mixed specimen are found in some patients with prostatitis. Good initial but rapidly declining motility (as opposed to bad initial motility) may be caused by a genital infection and/or prostatic dysfunction that is treatable.

Normal fructose levels confirm vas deferens patency

There is marked variation in sperm concentration; therefore three or more samples should be examined during a 2-3-mo period. In the majority of infertile men with oligospermia the cause is unknown.

The estimations of motility and morphology of spermatozoa are most closely correlated with fertility.

Motility is graded as: 0 = none, 1 = poor, 2 = moderate, 3 = good, and 4 = excellent.

As an initial screen for infertility, the following combination had a 90% negative predictive value[4]:

Normal morphology >5%

Motility >30% (>14% progressive)

Sperm density $>9 \times 10^6$/mL

TEST NAME AND METHOD	SPECIMEN REQUIREMENTS	REFERENCE INTERVAL, CONVENTIONAL [INTERNATIONAL RECOMMENDED UNITS]		CHEMICAL INTERFERENCES AND IN VIVO EFFECTS
Serine (Ser)[1-6] *Ion-exchange chromatography*	Plasma (heparin) or serum, fasting. Place blood in ice water immediately; separate and freeze within 1 hr of collection. Stable for 1 wk at $-20°$ C; for longer periods, deproteinize and store at $-70°$ C.[7,8]	*mg/dL* Newborn 1 day: 0.99-2.55 1-3 mo: 1.20 ± 0.20 (SD) 9 mo-2 yr: 0.35-1.34 3-10 yr: 0.83-1.18 6-18 yr: 0.75-1.90 Adult: 0.68-2.03	$\mu mol/L$[11] × 95.2 [94-243] [114 ± 19] [33-128] [79-112] [71-181][12] [65-193]	P ↑ V Glycine, histidine (after oral load)
	Urine, 24 hr. Add 10 mL of 6 mol/L HCl at start of collection. (Alternatively, refrigerate specimen during collection.) Store frozen at $-20°$ C.[9]	*mg/day* 10 days-7 wk: 6.2-24.7 3-12 yr: 16.3-56.7 Adult: 13.6-145.7 *mg/g creatinine* or 23 ± 12 (SD) $\mu mol/g$ *creatinine*[13] 0-1 mo: 287-3844 1-6 mo: 382-2778 6 mo-1 yr: 342-2117 1-2 yr: 379-1565 2-3 yr: 338-1202	$\mu mol/day$[11] × 9.52 [59-235] [155-540] [129-1387] *mmol/mol creatinine* × 1.08 [24.8 ± 13.0] *mmol/mol creatinine* × 0.113 [32-434] [43-314] [39-239] [43-177] [38-136]	U ↑ V Glycine U ↓ V Ascorbic acid (after large intake)[15]
	CSF. Collect in sterile tubes; store frozen. Stable at $-20°$ C for 1 wk or at $-70°$ C for 2 mo.[10]	*mg/dL* Neonate: 0.838 ± 0.246 (SEM) 3 mo-2 yr: 0.283 ± 0.058 (SD) 2-10 yr: 0.215 ± 0.044 Adult: 0.247 ± 0.013	$\mu mol/L$ × 95.2 [79.8 ± 23.4][10] [26.9 ± 5.5][14] [20.5 ± 4.2][14] [23.5 ± 1.2][11]	

1. Friedman RB, Young DS: *Effects of disease on clinical laboratory tests,* ed 2, Washington, DC, 1989, American Association for Clinical Chemistry.

2. Pesce A, Kaplan L, editors: *Methods in clinical chemistry,* St. Louis, 1987, CV Mosby.

3. Scriver CR, Beaudet AL, Valle D, et al, editors: *The metabolic and molecular bases of inherited disease,* ed 8, New York, 2001, McGraw-Hill.

4. Young DS: *Effects of drugs on clinical laboratory tests,* ed 3, Washington, DC, 1990, American Association for Clinical Chemistry.

5. Bremer HJ, Duran M, Kamerling JP, et al: *Disturbances of amino acid metabolism: clinical chemistry and diagnosis,* Baltimore, 1981, Urban and Schwarzenburg.

6. Nyhan W, Sakait N: *Diagnostic recognition of genetic disease,* Philadelphia, 1987, Lea & Febiger.

7. Cummings JG: Routine amino acids analysis in the clinical laboratory, *Am Clin Prod Rev* Feb:20-25, 1988.

8. Schaefer A, Piquard F, Haberey P: Plasma amino acids analysis: effects of delayed samples preparation and of storage, *Clin Chim Acta* 164:163-169, 1987.

DIAGNOSTIC INFORMATION	REMARKS
P ↑ Lysinuric protein intolerance (LPI)	
P ↓ Gout, phosphoglycerate dehydrogenase deficiency[17]	
U ↑ Burn patients,[16] Hartnup disease	Ingestion of poultry (especially white meat) may increase urinary excretion of serine, carnosine, and 1-methylhistidine.
	Values in children (3 mo-10 yr) were measured using reversed-phase liquid chromatography.

9. Pesce A, Kaplan L, editors: *Methods in clinical chemistry,* St. Louis, 1987, CV Mosby.

10. Heiblim DI, Evans HE, Glass L, et al: Amino acid concentrations in cerebrospinal fluid, *Arch Neurol* 35:765-768, 1978.

11. Shih V: *Laboratory techniques for the detection of hereditary metabolic disorders,* Boca Raton, FL, 1973, CRC Press.

12. Meites S, editor: *Pediatric clinical chemistry,* ed 3, Washington, DC, 1989, American Association for Clinical Chemistry.

13. Mayo Medical Laboratories: *Test catalog,* Rochester, MN, 1993, Mayo Medical Laboratories.

14. Goldsmith RF, Earl JW, Cunningham AM: Determination of δ-aminobutyric acid and other amino acids in cerebrospinal fluid of pediatric patients by reversed-phase liquid chromatography, *Clin Chem* 33:1736-1740, 1987.

15. Tsao C, Muyashita K: Effects of large intake of ascorbic acid on the urinary excretion of amino acids and related compounds, *IRCS Med Sci* 13:855-856, 1985.

16. Cynober L, Dinh FN, Blonde F, et al: Plasma and urinary amino acid pattern in severe burn patients: evolution throughout the healing period, *Am J Clin Nutr* 36:416-425, 1982.

17. Jaeken J, Detheux M, Van Maldergem L, et al: 3-Phosphoglycerate kinase deficiency: an inborn of serine biosynthesis, *Arch Dis Child* 74:542-545, 1996.

TEST NAME AND METHOD	SPECIMEN REQUIREMENTS	REFERENCE INTERVAL, CONVENTIONAL [INTERNATIONAL RECOMMENDED UNITS]		CHEMICAL INTERFERENCES AND IN VIVO EFFECTS
Serotonin (5-OH Tryptamine)[1,2] *HPLC*	Whole blood, preserved with 10 mg of EDTA and 75 mg of ascorbic acid. Freeze immediately.	ng/mL^2 50-200 $\times$ 0.00568	$\mu mol/L$ [0.28-1.14]	Reserpine and methyldopa deplete serotonin from tissue stores. MAO inhibitors promote retention of amine and expansion of amine stores in a variety
	Plasma, collect in ice, freeze immediately.	ng/mL^1 0.6 $\pm$ 0.11 $\times$ 0.00568	$\mu mol/L$ [0.002 $\pm$ 0.00055]	of tissues. Lithium can either increase or decrease turnover rate of serotonin
HPLC	Platelets. Collect blood in EDTA. Promptly prepare the platelet-rich plasma (PRP) by centrifugation at 150g for 20 min at 4° C. Prepare platelet pellets from the PRP, and store on dry ice until assayed.	$ng/10^9 platelets^2$ 125-500 $\times$ 0.00568	$\mu mol/platelet$ [0.7-2.8]	in various areas of the brain. Morphine seems to affect serotonin synthesis and metabolism.

1. Lee MS, Cheng FC, Yeh HZ, et al: Determination of plasma serotonin and 5-hydroxyindole acetic acid in healthy subjects and cancer patients, *Clin Chem* 46:422-423, 2000.
2. Shultz A: Serotonin. In Pesce A, Kaplan LA, editors: *Methods in clinical chemistry,* St. Louis, 1987, CV Mosby.

TEST NAME AND METHOD	SPECIMEN REQUIREMENTS	REFERENCE INTERVAL, CONVENTIONAL [INTERNATIONAL RECOMMENDED UNITS]		CHEMICAL INTERFERENCES AND IN VIVO EFFECTS
Sex Hormone– Binding Globulin (SHBG)[1-7] *Binding capacity*[8]	Serum. Store frozen at −20° C. Stable for at least 8 mo.	*mcg/dL* * Cord blood: 0.6-1.7 $\times$ 34.7 1 mo-2 yr: 1.5-6.3 Prepubertal child: 1.8-5.5 Puberty M: 0.4-2.5 F: 0.9-3.2 Adult M: 0.5-1.5 F: 1.0-3.0	*nmol/L* [20.8-58.9] [52.0-218.6] [62.4-190.7] [13.9-86.8] [31.2-111.0] [17.4-52.1] [34.7-104.0]	S $\uparrow$ V Anticonvulsants S $\downarrow$ V Danazol, stanozolol, and testosterone
Immunoassay[9]		*mg/L* Adult, M: 0.59-4.72 $\times$ 16.9† F, Nonpregnant: 1.18-7.67 Pregnancy[10] 10-15 wk: 2.70-9.91 20-25 wk: 10.15-15.28 35-40 wk: 19.00-26.90	*nmol/L* [10-80] [20-130] [52-168] [172-260] [321-456]	

DIAGNOSTIC INFORMATION	REMARKS

B ↑ Metastasizing abdominal carcinoid tumor, if carcinoid syndrome is present, >400 ng/mL [>2.3 mmol/L]

Slight increase in dumping syndrome, acute intestinal obstruction, cystic fibrosis, acute myocardial infarction, and nontropical sprue

B ↓ Down syndrome, untreated phenylketonuria, Parkinson's disease, and severe depression

Some benign cystic teratomas or dermoids may contain serotonin, as may some tumors producing atypical carcinoid syndrome (oat cell, islet cell, and medullary thyroid tumors).

Blood serotonin is unstable and must be preserved. The most commonly used test for diagnosing carcinoid tumors is urinary 5-hydroxyindoleacetic acid (5-HIAA). Blood levels of serotonin are most appropriate when normal or borderline increases in 5-HIAA are found in a patient with clinical evidence of carcinoid syndrome. (See also *5-Hydroxyindoleacetic Acid* and *Substance P.*)

↑ Hyperthyroidism, excess estrogens, thyroid hormone administration, anorexia nervosa, pregnancy, and liver cirrhosis

↓ Hypothyroidism, excess testosterone, hirsutism, obesity, and polycystic ovary syndrome

Gonadal hormones such as testosterone and estrogens are bound to circulating SHBG. This protein is also referred to as testosterone-estradiol-binding globulin (TeBG). Binding capacity is expressed as mg testosterone bound/dL serum.

Variation in circulating levels of total androgen or estrogen hormones is affected by abnormalities in steroid hormone production or changes in SHBG concentration or affinity. SHBG levels in both sexes increase gradually with age. Before menopause, parous women have higher levels than nulliparous women. Married women also have higher levels than single women.

In hirsute females, SHBG levels may be low, thereby increasing the free androgen fraction with no significant change in total androgen concentration.

In males with Klinefelter's syndrome, SHBG concentrations may be normal.

TEST NAME AND METHOD	SPECIMEN REQUIREMENTS	REFERENCE INTERVAL, CONVENTIONAL [INTERNATIONAL RECOMMENDED UNITS]		CHEMICAL INTERFERENCES AND IN VIVO EFFECTS

Sex Hormone–Binding Globulin—CONT

| | Amniotic fluid[10] | 0.71 ± 0.24 mg/L | $\times$ 16.9 | $[12 \pm 4$ nmol/L$]$ |

*µg testosterone bound/dL serum.
†Conversion is based on 1 steroid binding site per dimeric polypeptide molecule, MW 59,000.[11]

1. Cunningham SK, Loughlin T, Culliton M, et al: The relationship between sex steroids and sex hormone-binding globulin in plasma in physiological and pathological conditions, *Ann Clin Biochem* 22:489-497, 1985.

2. de Mayer PM, Lambot MP, Desmons MC, et al: Sex hormone-binding protein in hyperthyroxinemic patients: a discriminator for thyroid status in thyroid hormone resistance and familial dysalbuminemic hyperthyroxinemia, *J Clin Endocrinol Metab* 62:1309-1312, 1986.

3. Dowsett M, Attree SL, Virdee SS, et al: Oestrogen-related changes in sex hormone-binding levels during normal and gonadotrophin-stimulated menstrual cycles, *Clin Endocrinol* 23:303-312, 1985.

4. Maruyama Y, Aoki N, Suzuki Y, et al: Variations with age in the levels of sex steroid-binding plasma protein as determined by radioimmunoassay, *Acta Endocrinol* 106:428-432, 1984.

5. Plymate SR, Paulsen A, Smith ML: The value of sex hormone-binding globulin in clinical medicine, *Ligand Rev* 3:7-11, 1981.

6. Rosner W: Measurement of TeBG in biological fluids: evolution and problems. In Forest M, Pugear M, editors: *Binding proteins of steroid hormones, Colloque INSERM/J Libby Eurotext,* 149:207-214, 1986.

7. Selby C: Sex hormone-binding globulin: origin, function and clinical significance, *Ann Clin Biochem* 27:532-541, 1990.

8. Endocrine Sciences: *Pediatric laboratory services,* Tarzana, CA, 1992, Endocrine Sciences.

9. Mayo Medical Laboratories: *Test catalog,* Rochester, MN, 1993, Mayo Medical Laboratories.

10. Chang CY, Bardin CW, Musto NA, et al: Radioimmunoassay of testosterone-estradiol-binding globulin in humans: a reassessment of normal values, *J Clin Endocrinol Metab* 56:68-75, 1983.

Sham Feeding Test (Confirmation of Complete Vagotomy)[1,2]	After 12-hr fast, collect gastric secretions for 15-min intervals for 1 hr to establish BAO. Then measure acid output for 30 min during and 30 min after sham feeding (SAO). Measure acid output after pentagastrin stimulation (PAO).	SAO/PAO: Complete vagotomy:	>0.10[1] ≤ 0.10	Swallowing of large amounts of food may falsely increase or decrease SAO.[3]
Test meal: Serve sirloin steak, French fries, and water. Patient should chew, not swallow, and expectorate chewed food.				
6 mg/kg pentagastrin, SC, to determine PAO				

DIAGNOSTIC INFORMATION	REMARKS
	In euthyroid hyperthyroxinemic states (i.e., thyroid hormone resistance and familial dysalbuminemic hyperthyroxinemia), SHBG levels are normal, thus providing an index of tissue (end-organ) responsiveness.

11. Petra PH: The serum sex steroid–binding protein: precipitation, characterization, and immunologic properties of the human and rabbit proteins, *J Steroid Biochem* 11:245-252, 1979.

After adequate vagotomy, sham feeding does not stimulate acid secretion. SAO/PAO ≤ 0.10 suggests complete vagotomy with 95% confidence.[3,4] If PAO is close to zero, use of SAO/PAO ratio may be misleading.[1] Therefore in patients with a PAO <5 mmol/hr, the results must be interpreted with caution. If BAO/PAO >0.10, SAO/PAO will be within the normal range even if SAO is not higher than BAO. Thus in a postoperative patient with a recurrent ulcer and a BAO $>10\%$ of PAO, it may be unnecessary to carry out a sham feeding test.	This test is rarely performed today because vagotomy has declined significantly. Basal acid output (BAO) and sham feeding-stimulated acid output (SAO) are defined as the sum of four consecutive 15-min outputs during the basal and sham feeding hours, respectively. Peak acid output (PAO) represents the two highest consecutive 15-min outputs after pentagastrin; their sum is multiplied by 2 to express results in mmol/hr.[3] Sham feeding stimulates as much acid secretion as an IV insulin challenge of 0.1 U/kg.[5]

TEST NAME AND METHOD	SPECIMEN REQUIREMENTS	REFERENCE INTERVAL, CONVENTIONAL [INTERNATIONAL RECOMMENDED UNITS]	CHEMICAL INTERFERENCES AND IN VIVO EFFECTS

Sham Feeding Test—CONT

1. Feldman M, Richardson CT, Fordtran JS: Effect of sham feeding on gastric acid secretion in healthy subjects and duodenal ulcer patients and evidence for increased basal vagal tone in some ulcer patients, *Gastroenterology* 79:796-800, 1980.

2. Sleisenger MH, Fordtran JS, editors: *Gastrointestinal disease: pathophysiology, diagnosis, management,* ed 4, Philadelphia, 1989, WB Saunders.

3. Feldman M, Richardson CT, Fordtran JS: Experience with sham feeding as a test for vagotomy, *Gastroenterology* 79:792-795, 1980.

TEST NAME AND METHOD	SPECIMEN REQUIREMENTS	REFERENCE INTERVAL, CONVENTIONAL [INTERNATIONAL RECOMMENDED UNITS]	CHEMICAL INTERFERENCES AND IN VIVO EFFECTS
Sialic Acid, Total (TSA)[1,2] *Colorimetric assays, fluorescence assays, enzymatic assay, chromatographic methods, immunoassay*	Serum.	1.58-2.22 mmol/L or 0.52-0.73 g/L	Hexoses, pentoses, and uronic acid interfere with orcinol colorimetric method.

		Total sialic acid,[3] mmol/mol creatinine	Free sialic acid, mmol/mol creatinine
Urine.	3 mo	105.1-302.7	24.3-139.9
	6 mo	78.3-225.7	18.6-110.8
	1 yr	67.5-201.5	16.9-94.1
	2 yr	60.1-128.3	8.2-76.4
	3 yr	47.5-119.7	13.0-69.0
	4 yr	51.8-118.0	14.8-58.8
	5 yr	45.7-104.9	11.2-49.6
	6 yr	36.5-103.5	10.9-50.9
	7 yr	41.1-114.5	10.4-53.2
	8 yr	27.4-81.4	8.2-34.4
	9 yr	27.0-81.4	12.0-40.6
	10 yr	26.4-78.2	11.8-33.0
	11-12 yr	26.6-68.6	7.7-29.7
	13-15 yr	26.6-71.6	10.1-35.1
	16-19 yr	16.9-62.3	9.0-27.8
	20-29 yr	10.5-44.9	3.9-20.3
	30-39 yr	20.1-56.5	9.0-32.2
	40-49 yr	28.8-76.2	11.0-34.2
	50-59 yr	23.3-69.9	13.8-36.6
	60-69 yr	23.4-66.2	12.9-30.9

1. Sillanaukee P, Ponnio M, Jaaskelainen IP: Occurrence of sialic acids in healthy humans and different disorders, *Eur J Clin Invest* 29:413-425, 1999.

2. Waters PJ, Lewry E, Pennock CA: Measurement of sialic acid in serum and urine: clinical applications and limitations, *Ann Clin Biochem* 29:625-637, 1992.

3. Fang-Kircher SG: Comparison of sialic acids excretion in spot urines and 24-hour-urines of children and adults, *Eur J Clin Chem Clin Biochem* 35:47-52, 1997.

DIAGNOSTIC INFORMATION	REMARKS

4. Kronborg O, Anderson D: Acid response to sham feeding as a test for completeness of vagotomy, *Scand J Gastroenterol* 75:119-121, 1980.

5. Stenquist B, Knutson U, Olbe L: Gastric acid responses to adequate and modified sham feeding and to insulin hypoglycemia in duodenal ulcer patients, *Scand J Gastroenterol* 13:357-362, 1978.

S ↑ Cancer, inflammatory disorders, acute-phase reactions, coronary heart disease, atherosclerosis, diabetes, sialidosis (Salla's disease and infantile sialic acid storage disease), sialyloligosaccharides (neuraminidase deficiency), alcohol consumption, chronic glomerulonephritis, chronic renal failure, chronic liver disease, pneumonia, chronic cadmium exposure, teratospermia, sympathetic ophthalmitis, and idiopathic acute iridocyclitis.

U, Bound ↑ Sialidosis, galactosialidosis, mucolipidosis II, mucolipidosis III, and Kanzaki disease.

U, Free ↑ Infantile sialic acid storage disease, Salla disease, and sialuria.

Sialic acid (SA) is a generic name for a group of compounds derived from the 9 carbon sugar neuraminic acid. SAs are generally found as terminal sugar residues on oligosaccharides of both glycoproteins and glycolipids. Their functions include stabilization of glycoprotein conformational states, protease resistance, cell-surface receptor components, antigenic determinants, cell-cell interaction, and developmental regulation. The most common sialic acid found on human plasma glycoproteins and glycolipids is 5-*n*-acetylneuraminic acid, frequently linked to galactose. *O*-acetylated derivatives are not normally found in the plasma of healthy human.

TEST NAME AND METHOD	SPECIMEN REQUIREMENTS	REFERENCE INTERVAL, CONVENTIONAL [INTERNATIONAL RECOMMENDED UNITS]		CHEMICAL INTERFERENCES AND IN VIVO EFFECTS
Sickle Cell Tests[1-3] *Sickling test* (*sodium metabisulfite; sickle cell prep.*)	Whole blood (EDTA, heparin, or oxalate) or capillary blood. Stable up to 20 days at 4° C.	Negative		↓ V Low concentration of cells containing Hb S (after transfusion, infancy), low proportion of Hb S per cell (coexisting α-thalassemia, iron deficiency), and high concentration of Hb F
				↓ C Deterioration of reducing agent (not freshly prepared)
Solubility test (*dithionite or hydrosulfite tube test*)	Whole blood (EDTA, heparin, or citrate) or capillary blood. Stable 20 days at 4° C.	Negative		↑ V Unstable hemoglobin disorders (postsplenectomy), hyperglobulinemia, and extremely lipemic blood
				↓ V Low concentration of cells containing Hb S, low proportion of Hb S per cell, high concentration of Hb F, and total Hb <80 g/L [<8 g/dL]
				↓ C Deterioration of reducing agent
Immunoassay (*monoclonal Ab directed against specific mutant amino acid sequence in Hb S*)[3]				None found.

1. Hall R, Malia RG: *Medical laboratory haematology,* ed 2, London, 1991, Butterworths.
2. Henry JB, editor: *Clinical diagnosis and management by laboratory methods,* ed 20, Philadelphia, 2001, WB Saunders.
3. Isolab Inc.: *Hemocard hemoglobin S package insert,* Akron, OH, 1992, Isolab Inc.

| **Silver** (Ag) *NAA*[1] | Serum. Collect in metal-free container. | *mcg/L* 2.1 ± 1.5 (SD) | × 9.27 | *nmol/L* [19.5 ± 13.9] | S ↑ Silver sulfadiazine (used topically in burn patients) |
| | Plasma (citrate). Collect in metal-free container. | 0.68 ± 0.63 (SD) | | [6.3 ± 5.8] | |

DIAGNOSTIC INFORMATION	REMARKS

Test is positive in the presence of Hb S or other rare sickling hemoglobins, e.g., Hb C-Harlem. Disorders with Hb S include sickle cell anemia, sickle trait, and combinations of the Hb S gene with other disorders: α-thalassemia, β-thalassemia, α-chain structural hemoglobin variants, and β-chain structural hemoglobin variants.[3]

The sickling test detects Hb S in concentrations of >25% [>0.25] Hb S. The test has largely been replaced by solubility tests.

A positive sickling or solubility test does not distinguish reliably between sickle trait and sickle cell anemia, nor does it provide information about other coexisting hemoglobin abnormalities. Additional studies are required for diagnosis. (See *Hemoglobin Electrophoresis.*)

The solubility test is unreliable in severe anemia, Hb <8 g/dL [<80 g/L], or in polycythemia unless adjustments are made in technique, such as using washed erythrocytes or using hemolysates with a standard hemoglobin concentration.[1]

Test is positive in the presence of Hb S and Hb C-Harlem, a rare sickling hemoglobin variant that has the identical valine for glutamic acid substitution.

The immunoassay can detect even very small amounts of Hb S and should not be used to distinguish between sickle trait and any of the sickling disorders. (See *Hemoglobin Electrophoresis.*)

Clinical findings of argyria are (irreversible) discolorations (gray to blue-black) of the skin, mucous membranes, and nails. Argyrosis refers to ocular silver deposition, with findings of limbic rings resembling Kayser-Fleischer rings.

Silver salts are used as antiseptic and bacteriostatic agents. Ingestion or inhalation of silver or Ag salts can cause argyria or argyrosis.

In normal individuals, silver slowly accumulates in body tissues with age but causes no apparent harm.

TEST NAME AND METHOD	SPECIMEN REQUIREMENTS	REFERENCE INTERVAL, CONVENTIONAL [INTERNATIONAL RECOMMENDED UNITS]			CHEMICAL INTERFERENCES AND IN VIVO EFFECTS
Silver—CONT					
	Platelets (pure). Collect in metal-free container.	*ng/g wet wt.* 29 ± 18 (SD)	× 9.27	*nmol/kg wet wt.* [269 ± 167]	
AAS[2]	Urine, 24 hr. Collect in metal-free bottles. Add 20 mL of 6 N HNO_3 at start of urine collection.	<1 mcg/day	× 9.27	[<9.3 nmol/day]	
FES, NAA	Hair.[3] Cut close to scalp and analyze proximal segments.	*mg/g dry wt.* 0.02-1.00	× 9.27	*nmol/g dry wt.* [0.2-9.3]	

1. Kasperek K, Iyengar GV, Kiem J, et al: Elemental composition of platelets. Part III. Determinations of Ag, Au, Cd, Co, Cr, Cs, Mo, Rb, Sb, and Se in normal human platelets by neutron activation analysis, *Clin Chem* 25:711-715, 1979.

2. Mayo Medical Laboratories: *Test catalog,* Rochester, MN, 1993, Mayo Medical Laboratories.

3. Iyengar GV, Woittiez J: Trace elements in human clinical specimens: evaluation of literature data to identify tolerence values, *Clin Chem* 34:474-481, 1988.

4. Nordberg GF, Gerhardsson L: Silver. In Seiler HG, Sigel H, editors: *Handbook on toxicity of inorganic compounds,* New York, 1988, Marcel Dekker, pp. 619-623.

Smooth Muscle Antibodies[1]	Serum. Store at −20° C.	Negative			↑ V Nitrofurantoin
IIF					

1. Biggazi PE, Burek CL, Rose NR: Antibodies to tissue-specific endocrine, gastrointestinal and surface receptor antigens. In Rose NR, Friedman H, Fahey JL, editors: *Manual of clinical laboratory immunology,* ed 4, Washington, DC, 1992, American Society for Microbiology.

2. Czaja A, Freese D: Diagnosis and treatment of autoimmune hepatitis, *Hepatology* 36:479-497, 2002.

3. Czaja A, Cassani F, Cataleta M, et al: Frequency and significance of antibodies to actin in type 1 autoimmune hepatitis, *Hepatology* 24:1068-1073, 1996.

Accidental ingestion of silver nitrate causes corrosive damage to GI tract, abdominal pain, diarrhea, vomiting, shock, convulsions, and death.

Silver dose required to induce argyria is >1 g for soluble silver salts.[4]

Primarily excreted in the feces.

See Table II-6.

These antibodies are present in up to 70% of patients with type 1 chronic active hepatitis.[2] Lower titers may be present in other disorders, including primary biliary cirrhosis, viral hepatitis, infectious mononucleosis, neoplasia, and occasionally in normal individuals.

Substrate for IIF is usually tissue containing smooth muscle of human or animal origin. Antibodies to actin, the major antigen in smooth muscle detected by the antibodies, are increasingly being detected by ELISA methods instead of smooth muscle antibodies.[3]

TEST NAME AND METHOD	SPECIMEN REQUIREMENTS	REFERENCE INTERVAL, CONVENTIONAL [INTERNATIONAL RECOMMENDED UNITS]			CHEMICAL INTERFERENCES AND IN VIVO EFFECTS
Sodium (Na)[1-4] *Flame emission photometry, AAS, ISE, kinetic, spectrophotometry*[5,6]	Serum or plasma (lithium or ammonium heparin)[7]; centrifuge blood as soon as possible. Avoid hemolysis.		*mEq/L*[7]	*mmol/L*	S, P ↑ V ACTH, anabolic steroids, androgens, carbenicillin, carbenoxolone, clonidine, corticosteroids, diazoxide, enoxolone, estrogens, guanethidine analogs, lactulose, licorice, methoxyflurane, methyldopa, oral contraceptives, oxyphenbutazone, phenylbutazone, reserpine, and sodium bicarbonate
		Premature, Cord:	116-140 × 1.0	[116-140]	
		Premature, 48 hr:	128-148	[128-148]	
		Newborn, Cord:	126-166	[126-166]	
		Full-term:	133-146	[133-146]	
		Infant:	139-146	[139-146]	
		Child:	138-145	[138-145]	
		Thereafter:	136-145	[136-145]	
		>90 yr[8]:	132-146	[132-146]	

S ↑ C Sodium-containing anticoagulants, ethanol (Vitros)

S ↓ PV Aminoglutethimide, aminoglycosides, ammonium chloride, amphotericin B, angiotensin-converting enzyme (ACE) inhibitors, captopril, carbamazepine, carboplatin, chloroporpamide, cholestyramine, cisplatin, clofibrate, cyclophosphamide, desmopressin, diuretics (including acid, furosemide, metolazone, mannitol, quinethazone, spironolactone, thiazides, triamterene, urea), fluoxetine, glucose (hypertonic solution), haloperidol, heparin, indomethacin, ketoconazole, lithium, lorcainide, miconazole, nonsteroidal antiinflammatory agents (NSAIDs), oxytocin, phenothiazines, tienilic acid, tolbutamide, tricyclic antidepressants (e.g., amitriptyline), vasopressin, vinblastine, and vincristine

S, P ↓ C *ISE:* Heparin

S ↑ Conditions with water loss in excess of salt loss through skin (profuse sweating), lungs (prolonged hyperpnea), GI tract (severe vomiting or diarrhea of several etiologies), and kidneys (in polyuric states, e.g., diabetes insipidus, diabetic acidosis); increased renal sodium conservation in hyperaldosteronism, Cushing's syndrome or disease; inadequate water intake because of inadequate thirst mechanism (e.g., coma, hypothalamic disease); dehydration; and excessive saline therapy.

S ↓ Low sodium intake; sodium losses (depletional hyponatremia) caused by vomiting, diarrhea, excessive sweating with adequate water and inadequate salt replacement, diuretics abuse (most common clinical cause), or salt-losing nephropathy (polycystic and medullary cystic renal disease, chronic pyelonephritis, renal tubular acidosis); osmotic diuresis; metabolic acidosis (with increased excretion of cations); primary and secondary adrenocortical insufficiency; congenital adrenal hyperplasia (CAH) with 21-hydroxylase deficiency (most common) and other forms of CAH with salt wastage, isolated hypoaldosteronism, pseudohypoaldosteronism (unresponsiveness of renal tubule to aldosterone); dilutional hyponatremia with edema, ascites in chronic cardiac failure, diabetes mellitus, hepatic cirrhosis, hepatic failure, nephrotic syndrome, interstitial nephritis, malnutrition, or fluid intoxication; hypothyroidism; hyperosmolality; SIADH, which may relate to carcinoma of lung, pancreas, CNS disease, lung infections; acute intermittent porphyria; psychogenic polydipsia; artifactual hyponatremia in extremely marked hypertriglyceridemia or hyperproteinemia; and hyperglycemia

Excessive ADH production

Ratio of plasma Na to osmolality is 0.43-0.50. The ratio is decreased when there is an increase in osmotically active substances (e.g., salicylate poisoning, uremia, diabetes). Sodium decreases ~1.5-3.0 mmol/L for each 100-mg/dL increase of blood glucose. The combination of hyponatremia with urine osmolality consistently higher than plasma osmolality suggests the possibility of inappropriate ADH secretion. Na <120 mmol/L results in weakness; <110 mmol/L results in bulbar or pseudobulbar palsy; 90-105 mmol/L results in severe neurological signs and symptoms. Concentrations >155 mmol/L may produce cardiovascular and renal symptoms, especially if accompanied by plasma volume depletion. Values >160 mmol/L are potentially hazardous.

Methods using ion-selective electrodes measure ion activity, not concentration. Corrections are generally calculated by the instrument.

Changes in methodologies, mainly to ISEs, require a reevaluation of the reference interval. For sera from patients with hyperlipemia or severe hyperproteinemia, the solvent exclusion effect will affect the results differently, depending on the specific method used, e.g., direct or indirect potentiometry. Therefore the reference interval may be higher or lower than that given here.

Direct ISE measurements do not give the volume displacement error in specimens with high lipid or protein content, as indirect ISE and flame measurements do.

TEST NAME AND METHOD	SPECIMEN REQUIREMENTS	REFERENCE INTERVAL, CONVENTIONAL [INTERNATIONAL RECOMMENDED UNITS]		CHEMICAL INTERFERENCES AND IN VIVO EFFECTS

Sodium—CONT

| | Erythrocytes | *mEq/L*
 7.3 ± 1.0 (2 SD)[1]
 10.4 ± 1.8 (2 SD)[9] | × 1.0 | *mmol/L*
 $[7.3 \pm 1.0]$
 $[10.4 \pm 1.8]$ | |

| | Platelets | *μEq/10⁸ cells*
 1.55 ± 0.6 (2 SD) | × 1.0 | *μmol/10⁸ cells*
 $[1.55 \pm 0.6]$[9] | |

Urine, 24 hr

		mEq/day		*mmol/day*	U ↑ V Caffeine, calcitonin, captopril, carbonic anhydrase inhibitors, cisplatin, diuretics, dopamine, heparin, lithium (initial transient effect), niacin, progesterone (high doses), sulfates, tetracycline, and vincristine
	6-10 yr				
	M:	41-115[10]	× 1.0	[41-115]	
	F:	20-69		[20-69]	
	10-14 yr				
	M:	63-177		[63-177]	
	F:	48-168		[48-168]	
	Adult:	40-220[7]		[40-220]	
		27-287[11]		[27-287]	

Full-term, 7-14-day-old neonates have sodium clearance of ~20% of adult values.[1]

U ↓ V Corticosteroids, diazoxide, epinephrine, levarterenol, and propranolol

Random urine[12]:

		mEq/L		*mmol/L*
M:				
	<40 yr	25-301	× 1.0	[25-301]
	≥40 yr	18-214		[18-214]
F:				
	<40 yr	15-267		[15-267]
	≥40 yr	15-237		[15-237]

	mEq/g creatinine		*mmol/g creatinine*
M:	23-229	× 1.0	[23-229]
F:	26-297		[26-297]

Colorimetric, coulometric, ISE	Sweat (iontophoresis)[4]		*mEq/L*		*mmol/L*
	Child and adult:		10-40	× 1.0	[10-40]
	Child, x̄:		27		[27]
	Adult, x̄:		33		[33]
	Cystic fibrosis:		70-190		[70-190]

	Saliva[3]	Without stimulation: (varies with flow rate)	6.5-21.7 (?)	[6.5-21.7]
		After stimulation:	43-46	[43-46]

	Feces	<10 mEq/day[1]	× 1.0	[<10 mmol/day]
		7.8 ± 2 mEq/day[13]		$[7.8 \pm 2$ mmol/day]

Ercs ↑ Stomatocytosis (with reduced red cell potassium), hyperthyroidism

U ↑ Increased sodium intake, postmenstrual diuresis (physiological states), adrenal failure (primary and secondary) Na >10 mmol/L, salt-losing nephritis Na >10 mmol/L, tubulointerstitial disease, renal tubular acidosis (Lightwood type), diuretic therapy, diabetes mellitus, Bartter's syndrome, SIADH of different etiology, any form of alkalosis and other conditions in which the urine is alkaline

The renal threshold for sodium is 110-130 mmol/L. The rate of sodium excretion during the night is one fifth of the peak rate during the day, indicating a large diurnal variation.

Excretion of urinary sodium is highly dependent on dietary intake and state of hydration.

Sodium values <15 mmol/L are seen in prerenal acidosis; much higher values in acute tubular necrosis.[14]

U ↓ Low sodium intake, premenstrual sodium and water retention (physiological), extrarenal sodium loss with adequate water intake (Na <10 mmol), first 24-48 hr after operations (stress syndrome diuretics), adrenocortical hyperfunctions, states with reduced glomerular filtration rate (e.g., congestive heart failure); acute oliguria and prerenal azotemia (Na <10 mmol/L), as opposed to acute tubular necrosis with oliguria (where Na >30 mmol/L), diarrhea, and excessive sweating

Sw ↑ Cystic fibrosis, Addison's disease, familial hypoparathyroidism, familial ectodermal dysplasia with sensorineural deafness, hereditary nephrogenic diabetes insipidus, and hypoparathyroidism

Sw ↓ Adrenocortical hyperfunction

Falsely low results may be observed in salt depletion; high values may be seen in meconium ileus, ectodermal dysplasia, mucopolysaccharidosis, fucosidosis, hereditary nephrogenic diabetes, G6PD deficiency, alcoholic pancreatitis, papillatonia hyporeflexia, familial cholestasis, malnutrition, and some cases of renal disease.[15]

Sal ↑ Cystic fibrosis, overlap with normals; rheumatoid arthritis

Sal ↓ Congestive heart failure, adrenal hyperfunction

TEST NAME AND METHOD	SPECIMEN REQUIREMENTS	REFERENCE INTERVAL, CONVENTIONAL [INTERNATIONAL RECOMMENDED UNITS]		CHEMICAL INTERFERENCES AND IN VIVO EFFECTS
Sodium—CONT				
	CSF	*mEq/L* 136-150 142-150[13]	× 1.0	*mmol/L* [136-150] [142-150]
	Amniotic fluid	28 wk: 48 wk:	124-148 115-139	[124-148] [115-139]

1. Eastham RD: *Biochemical values in clinical medicine,* ed 7, Bristol, UK, 1985, John Wright and Sons Ltd.

2. Friedman RB, Anderson RE, Entine SM, et al: Effects of diseases on clinical laboratory tests, *Clin Chem* 26:1D-474D, 1980.

3. Tietz NW, editor: *Fundamentals of clinical chemistry,* ed 2, Philadelphia, 1976, WB Saunders.

4. Scott MG, Heusel JW, Legrys VA, et al: Electrolyte, and blood gases. In Burtis CA, Ashwood ER, editors: *Tietz textbook of clinical chemistry,* ed 3, Philadelphia, 1999, WB Saunders.

5. Berry MN, Mazzachi RD, Pejakovic M, et al: Enzymatic determination of sodium in serum, *Clin Chem* 34:2295-2298, 1988.

6. Kumar A, Chapoteau E, Czech BP, et al: Chromogenic ionophore-based methods for spectrophotometric assay of sodium and potassium in serum and plasma, *Clin Chem* 34:1709-1712, 1988.

7. Chandler Medical Center Clinical Laboratories: *Reference ranges and general information,* Lexington, KY, 2003, University of Kentucky.

8. Tietz NW, Schreg DF, Wekstein DR: Laboratory values in fit aging individuals—sexagenarians through centenarians, *Clin Chem* 38:1167-1185, 1992.

9. Touyz RM, Milne FJ: A method for determining the total magnesium, calcium, sodium and potassium contents of human platelets, *Miner Electrolyte Metab* 17:173-178, 1991.

10. Liappis N, Reimnitz P: Referenzwerte der Natrium-, Kalium-, Kalzium-, Chlorid-, und anorganischen Phosphat-Ausscheidung im 24 h-urin gesunder Kinder, *Klin Padiatr* 196:367-369, 1984.

11. Jacobs DS, Kasten BL, DeMott WR, et al, editors: *Laboratory test handbook,* ed 2, Stow, OH, 1990, LexiComp, Inc.

12. Bond LW, Garber C, Ottinger W, et al: Reference intervals for common analytes in random urine specimens, *Clin Chem* 55:submitted, 2005.

13. Wallach J, editor: *Interpretation of diagnostic tests,* ed 5, Boston, 1992, Little, Brown and Co.

14. Kamel KS, Ethier JH, Richardson RMA, et al: Urine electrolytes and osmolality: when and how to use them, *Am J Nephrol* 10:89-102, 1990.

15. Shwachman H, Mahmoodian A: The sweat test and cystic fibrosis, *Diagn Med* June:61-77, 1982.

Somatostatin (SS)[1-6] RIA	Plasma (EDTA), fasting. Patient should not be on antacid medications or medications affecting intestinal motility. Collect blood in prechilled tubes containing Trasylol. Cen-	<25 pg/mL[7]	× 1.0	[<25 ng/L]　↓ C Theophylline

DIAGNOSTIC INFORMATION	REMARKS
F ↑ Diarrhea (may exceed 60 mmol/L)	Fecal sodium estimations are performed only in metabolic balance studies.

↑ Somatostatin-producing tumor (somatostatinoma), medullary thyroid carcinoma, pheochromocytoma, duodenal ulcer, active ulcerative colitis, irritable bowel syndrome, alcoholic liver disease, and acromegaly (fasting somatostatin, mainly SS-14, levels).[8] ↓ After vagotomy	Somatostatin is a 14-amino acid peptide found in the hypothalamus, pancreas, gastric mucosa, and intestine. It is a potent inhibitor of pituitary, pancreatic, and GI hormones but possesses other nonendocrine functions as well. Somatostatin is rapidly degraded in blood and has a very short half-life (1-4 min). Some tumors are associated with elevated plasma somatostatin levels; others such as carcinoid tumors, small cell carcinomas of the lung, retinoblastomas, and endocrine tumors of the pancreas and gut have also been shown to contain varying numbers of somatostatin-positive cells.

TEST NAME AND METHOD	SPECIMEN REQUIREMENTS	REFERENCE INTERVAL, CONVENTIONAL [INTERNATIONAL RECOMMENDED UNITS]		CHEMICAL INTERFERENCES AND IN VIVO EFFECTS

Somatostatin (SS)—CONT

trifuge immediately at 4° C and freeze. Store at −20° C.

1. Binimelis J, Webb SM, Monés J, et al: Circulating immunoreactive somatostatin in gastrointestinal diseases, *Scand J Gastroenterol* 22:931-937, 1987.

2. Conlon JM, McCulloch AJ, Alberti KGMM: Circulating somatostatin concentrations in healthy and non-insulin-dependent (type II) diabetic subjects, *Diabetes* 32:723-729, 1983.

3. Henderson AR, Tietz NW, Rinker AD: Gastric, pancreatic, and intestinal function. In Burtis CA, Ashwood ER, editors: *Tietz textbook of clinical chemistry,* ed 2, Philadelphia, 1994, WB Saunders.

4. Patel YC, Tannenbaum GS, editors: *Somatostatin,* New York, 1985, Plenum Press.

5. Reichlin S: Neuroendocrinology. In Wilson JD, Foster DW, editors: *Williams textbook of endocrinology,* ed 8, Philadelphia, 1992, WB Saunders.

6. Saito H: Radioimmunoassay of plasma somatostatin: methods and levels in normal and pathological states, *Ligand Rev* 2:17-22, 1980.

7. Interscience Institute: Current unique and rare endocrine assays: patient and specimen requirements, Inglewood, CA, 1988.

8. Arosio M, Porretti S, Epaminonda P, et al: Elevated circulating somatostatin levels in acromegaly, *J Endocrinol Invest* 26:499-502, 2003.

9. Koshimizu T, Ohyama Y, Yokota Y, et al: Peripheral plasma concentrations of somatostatin-like immunoreactivity in newborns and infants, *J Clin Endocrinol Metab* 61:78-82, 1985.

10. Holst N, Jenssen TG, Burhol PG: Plasma concentrations of motilin and somatostatin are increased in late pregnancy and postpartum, *Br J Obstet Gynaecol* 99:338-341, 1992.

TEST NAME AND METHOD	SPECIMEN REQUIREMENTS	REFERENCE INTERVAL, CONVENTIONAL		[INTERNATIONAL RECOMMENDED UNITS]	CHEMICAL INTERFERENCES AND IN VIVO EFFECTS
Sorbitol Dehydrogenase (SDH, Iditol Dehydrogenase; EC 1.1.1.14)[1-3] *Kinetic*	Serum, plasma (heparin). Enzyme is very unstable; freeze immediately.	25° C[1]: 30° C[4]: 37° C[5]:	*U/L* <1.5 1-3 0-2.6	× 0.017	*μKat/L* [<0.03] [0.02-0.05] [0.00-0.04]	↓ V Phenothiazines ↓ C Ag$^+$, borate, CN$^-$, cysteine, dimercaptoethanol,[1,2] EDTA, glutathione, Hg^{2+}, and monoiodoacetate

1. Gerlach U: Sorbitol dehydrogenase. In Bergmeyer HU, editor: *Methods of enzymatic analysis, vol III,* ed 3, Weinheim, 1983, Verlag Chemie.

2. Guilbault GG: *Handbook of enzymatic methods of analysis,* New York, 1976, Marcel Dekker.

3. Wolf PL, Williams D, Von der Muehll E: *Practical clinical enzymology: techniques and interpretations and biochemical profiling,* New York, 1973, John Wiley and Sons.

4. Dooley JF, Turnquist LJ, Racich L: Kinetic determination of serum sorbitol dehydrogenase activity with centrifugal analyzer, *Clin Chem* 25:2026-2029, 1979.

5. Rose CI, Henderson AR: Reaction-rate assay of serum sorbitol dehydrogenase activity at 37 °C, *Clin Chem* 21:1619-1626, 1975.

DIAGNOSTIC INFORMATION	REMARKS
	Neonates have elevated levels of circulating somatostatin for the first 10 mo. The elevation peaks at the age of 3 mo.[9] Elevated levels are also found during pregnancy, especially during the late phases.[10]

↑ Acute infectious hepatitis, toxic hepatitis, hypoxic liver damage, cirrhosis, and primary or secondary neoplastic or infectious disease in the liver	Generally SDH levels are not detectable or are barely detectable in normal serum. The appearance of any measurable activity indicates the presence of parenchymal cell damage.

TEST NAME AND METHOD	SPECIMEN REQUIREMENTS	REFERENCE INTERVAL, CONVENTIONAL [INTERNATIONAL RECOMMENDED UNITS]		CHEMICAL INTERFERENCES AND IN VIVO EFFECTS
Specific Gravity[1-4] *Urinometer, reflectometer*[2,4]	Urine, random or timed fresh sample. Do not refrigerate sample.	Newborn: Infant: Adult: After 12-hr fluid restriction: Urine, 24 hr:	1.012 1.002-1.006 1.002-1.030 >1.025 1.015-1.025	↑ C Dextran, radiographic contrast media (e.g., diatrizoate), and sucrose ↑ V Isotretinoin ↓ V Aminoglycosides, carbenoxolone, colistin, cyclosporine, lithium, and methoxyflurane
Reagent strips (Bayer Corporation Multistix SG[5]; *BMCChemstrips)*				↑ Protein levels 100-750 mg/dL [1.0-7.5 g/L] ↓ C Alkaline urines (pH >6.5)[6]

1. Free HM, editor: *Modern urine chemistry,* Elkhart, IN, 1991, Miles Inc., Diagnostics Division.
2. Henry JB, editor: *Clinical diagnosis and management by laboratory methods,* ed 18, Philadelphia, 1991, WB Saunders.
3. Strasinger SK: *Urinalysis and body fluids: a self-instructional text,* ed 2, Philadelphia, 1991, FA Davis.
4. Tietz NW, editor: *Fundamentals of clinical chemistry,* ed 3, Philadelphia, 1987, WB Saunders.
5. Boehringer Mannheim Corp.: *Chemstrip 10 UA package insert,* Indianapolis, IN, 1992, Boehringer Mannheim Corp.
6. Bayer Corporation: *Multistix package insert,* Elkhart, IN, 1992, Bayer Corporation, Diagnostics Division.
7. Newall RG, editor: *Clinical urinalysis,* Buckinghamshire, UK, 1990, Ames Division, Miles Ltd..
8. Boehringer Mannheim Corp.: *Urinalysis today,* Indianapolis, IN, 1991, Boehringer Mannheim Corp.

Squamous Cell Carcinoma Antigen (SCC)[1,2] *MEIA*	Serum or plasma (EDTA or heparin). Separate and freeze immediately. Store at −20° C or lower.	<2.0 ng/mL	× 1.0	[<2.0 mcg/L]	None found.

↑ States with decreased renal perfusion but intact concentrating mechanism, inappropriate antidiuretic hormone secretion (SIADH), uncontrolled diabetes mellitus, proteinuria, glomerulonephritis, obstructive uropathy, toxemia of pregnancy, congestive heart failure, and acute febrile states

↓ Renal tubular damage, chronic renal insufficiency, nephrogenic or idiopathic diabetes insipidus, psychogenic diabetes insipidus, malignant hypertension; antidiuretic hormone (ADH) resistance as seen with hypercalcemia, hypokalemia, lithium toxicity, and renal tubular dysfunction caused by rare inborn or acquired defects[7]

Specific gravity varies greatly with fluid intake and state of hydration. Refrigeration of samples may cause moderate increase in specific gravity. Inaccuracy may arise from unclean glassware, uncalibrated urinometers, or temperature variations in samples. Urine specific gravity should be corrected for protein and glucose; protein increases specific gravity by 0.001 for each 0.4 g/dL [4 g/L]. Each 10 g/L of sugar in the urine increases the specific gravity by 0.004 units.

Specific gravity >1.040 suggests radiopaque contrast media in the urine.

To correct for alkaline pH, add 0.05 to manual reading if pH is ≤6.5 on Multistix or 7.0 on Chemstrip.

Range of detection: Multistix: 1.005-1.030
                       Chemstrip: 1.111-1.030

Glucose and urea concentration of >1% may cause lowered Chemstrip specific gravity results relative to other methods. Ketoacidosis may increase specific gravity readings with Chemstrip.[8]

The measurement of specific gravity is useful in monitoring fluid intake of patients at risk for developing urinary stone formation.[7]

See also *Adulteration (toxicology)*.

↑ Squamous cell carcinomas; some patients with adenocarcinomas, renal impairment, and some women with benign gynecological disease.

SCC antigen is a subfraction of TA-4, a tumor-associated antigen obtained from liver metastases of patients with squamous cell carcinoma of the cervix. It has an MW of 42,000 and relatively low carbohydrate content (0.6%). SCC is probably related functionally to cytokeratins. The assay does not have FDA approval for clinical use. Commercial assay by Abbott Diagnostics.

TEST NAME AND METHOD	SPECIMEN REQUIREMENTS	REFERENCE INTERVAL, CONVENTIONAL [INTERNATIONAL RECOMMENDED UNITS]			CHEMICAL INTERFERENCES AND IN VIVO EFFECTS

Squamous Cell Carcinoma Antigen—CONT

1. Kato H, Tongoe T: Radioimmunoassay for tumor antigen of human cervical squamous cell carcinoma, *Cancer* 40:1621-1628, 1977.
2. Torre GC: SCC antigen in malignant and nonmalignant squamous lesions, *Tumor Biol* 19:517-526, 1998.
3. Kato H, Morcoka H, Aranaki S, et al: Prognostic significance of the tumor antigen TA-4 in squamous cell carcinoma of the uterine cervix, *Am J Obstet Gynecol* 145:350-354, 1983.

Substance P[1,2] *Immunoassay*	Plasma, fasting (EDTA). Collect blood into prechilled tubes; plasma should be separated from the cells and frozen immediately.	<240 pg/mL[3]	× 1.0	[<240 ng/L]	None found.

1. Kvols LK, Moertel CG, O'Connell MJ, et al: Treatment of the malignant carcinoid syndrome, *N Engl J Med* 315:663-666, 1986.
2. Lavin N: *Manual of endocrinology and metabolism,* Boston, 1986, Little, Brown and Co.
3. Hicks JM, Young DS: *DORA '92-'93: directory of rare analyses,* Washington, DC, 1992, AACC Press.

Sucrose Hemolysis and Sugar-water Tests for Paroxysmal Nocturnal Hemoglobinuria (PNH)[1-3] *Sugar-water test at 23° C*	Whole blood (citrate or oxalate). Do not use EDTA or defibrinated blood.	Negative: Questionable: Positive:	No visible hemolysis Trace of hemolysis Obvious or marked hemolysis		None found.

DIAGNOSTIC INFORMATION	REMARKS

There is a correlation between SCC and stage and extent of tumor in squamous cell carcinoma of lung, cervix, and head and neck. Test is useful in monitoring response to therapy in these cancers and in patients with metastatic disease. Elevations may also be of prognostic significance.

↑ Carcinoid tumors, chronic leukemia, and medullary carcinoma of the thyroid

It is suggested that substance P may be responsible for clinical symptoms in some patients with carcinoid tumors. Substance P may be measured in initial workups for carcinoid tumors and used for monitoring if elevated. Measurements of substance P in specific venous return sites of various organs obtained through selective catheterization may be useful in localizing carcinoid tumors.

The sugar-water test is positive in PNH; it is questionable in occasional anemic non-PNH patients.

False-negative tests may occur in the sugar-water test if blood is collected in EDTA or heparin or, in the sucrose hemolysis test, if serum lacks complement. False-positive tests may occur with defibrinated blood in anemic patients and if sugar solution is not fresh.

Values in the questionable range may occur in myeloproliferative diseases, megaloblastic anemia, or immune hemolytic anemia, but the acidified serum test is negative in these patients. A single negative sucrose hemolysis test does not rule out PNH; the pro-

TEST NAME AND METHOD	SPECIMEN REQUIREMENTS	REFERENCE INTERVAL, CONVENTIONAL [INTERNATIONAL RECOMMENDED UNITS]		CHEMICAL INTERFERENCES AND IN VIVO EFFECTS

Sucrose Hemolysis and Sugar-water Tests for Paroxysmal Nocturnal Hemoglobinuria—CONT

Sucrose hemolysis test	Washed erythrocytes; fresh, normal, and ABO-compatible serum	*Percent lysis*	*Number fraction lysed*	
		Negative: ≤5 × 0.01	[≤0.05]	
		Questionable: 6-10	[0.06-0.10]	
		Positive: >10	[>0.10]	

1. Dacie JV, Lewis SM: *Practical haematology,* ed 8, Edinburgh, 1995, Churchill Livingstone.
2. Williams WJ, Beutler E, Erslev AJ, et al, editors: *Hematology,* ed 4, New York, 1990, McGraw-Hill Publishing Co.
3. Krauss JS: Laboratory diagnosis of paroxysmal nocturnal hemoglobinuria, *Ann Clin Lab Sci* 33:401-406, 2003.

Sudan Black B Stain (for distinguishing among acute leukemias)[1-4]	Blood or bone marrow films. Stable several years.	Strongly positive: Neutrophilic and eosinophilic granulocytes and precursors, increasing with progressive maturity	None found.
		Weakly positive: Monocytes, megakaryocytes, and platelets	
		Negative: Lymphocytes, plasma cells, and normoblasts	

1. Beutler E, Lichtman MA, Coller B, editors: *Williams hematology,* ed 6, New York, 2000, McGraw-Hill.
2. Brunning RD, McKenna RW: *Tumors of the bone marrow,* Washington, DC, 1994, Armed Forces Institute of Pathology.
3. Jaffe ES, Harris NL, Stein H, et al, editors: *World Health Organization classification of tumours. Pathology and genetics of tumours of haematopoietic and lymphoid tissues,* Lyon, 2001, IARC Press.
4. Hayhoe FGJ, Quaglino D: *Haematological cytochemistry,* Edinburgh, 1980, Churchill Livingstone.

Sulfhemoglobin[1-4] *Spectrophotometry*	Whole blood (EDTA, heparin, or ACD), fresh	*Percent of total Hb* <1.0 × 0.01	*Mass fraction, total Hb* [<0.010]	↑ V Oxidant drugs, e.g., acetanilid, aniline dyes, aspirin, benzene derivatives, nitrates, nitrites, phenacetin, sulfides, sulfonamides, and sulfones
		Sulfhemoglobin is not measured by the cyanmethemoglobin or oxyhemoglobin methods for determining total Hb.		

1. Lee GR, Foerster J, Lukens J, et al: *Wintrobe's clinical hematology,* ed 10, Philadelphia, 1998, Williams & Wilkins.
2. Burtis CA, Ashwood ER, editors: *Tietz textbook of clinical chemistry,* ed 3, Philadelphia, 1999, WB Saunders.

DIAGNOSTIC INFORMATION	REMARKS

Positive in PNH

portion of PNH cells may be low, and most of the PNH produced may have been destroyed in the circulation.

Both tests are screening tests. The acidified serum test is considered the confirmatory test for PNH.

Positive: In acute myeloid leukemia (AML, M1-M6), $\geq$3% of blast cells (myeloblasts) are positive. Reaction is strongest in promyelocytic leukemia (M3) and is weak to negative in acute monocytic leukemia (M5).

Negative: Blast cells in acute lymphoid leukemia (ALL) and in acute megakaryocytic leukemia (M7).

See also Table II-14.

Sudan black B (SBB) stain has been traditionally used to distinguish AML from ALL. The stain has affinity for sterols and phospholipids. Staining rather closely parallels the peroxidase reaction and may be slightly more sensitive, but rare SBB-positive cases of ALL have been reported. Myeloblasts that have no stainable granules with Wright's stain may be positive with Sudan black B (and peroxidase).

↑ Chronic constipation, purging

Sulfhemoglobin is an impure, green monochrome formed by oxidative sulfation of one or two of the four heme groups of hemoglobin.[3] It cannot be reduced to Hb but may be oxidized further and will contribute to Heinz body formation in some instances. Generally it is very stable in blood and is lost from the circulation only with the breakdown of erythrocytes. It is incapable of carrying oxygen and shifts the P50 to the right. Sulfhemoglobinemia is characterized by cyanosis. Symptoms are not usually present.[1]

---

3. Jandl JH: *Blood: textbook of hematology,* ed 2, Boston, 1996, Little, Brown and Co.

4. Nathan DG, Oski FA: *Hematology of infancy and childhood,* ed 3, Philadelphia, 1987, WB Saunders.

TEST NAME AND METHOD	SPECIMEN REQUIREMENTS	REFERENCE INTERVAL, CONVENTIONAL [INTERNATIONAL RECOMMENDED UNITS]		CHEMICAL INTERFERENCES AND IN VIVO EFFECTS

Synovial Fluid Analysis[1]

Aspirate. Ideally 15 mL divided into two sodium heparin tubes and one sterile tube without additives. Collect 2-5 mL in the sodium heparin tubes for microbiology (including Gram stain) and microscopy and the remainder in the plain tube for clot analysis and chemistry.

See analysis table.

Li heparin or EDTA-anticoagulated tubes can produce crystalline artifacts.

	Normal	*Pathological*		*Normal*	*Pathological*
Volume, mL (knee):	<4	≥4	×0.001	[<0.004 L]	[≥0.004 L]
Viscosity					
String test	+ (high)	− (low)			
Mucin clot	Firm	Friable			
Clarity	Clear	Cloudy			
Color	Straw	Red			

Cell counts					
WBC (/μL)	<200	>2000	×0.001	[<0.2 × 10⁹/L]	[>2 × 10⁹/L]

	Percent of total			*Fraction of total*	
PMN	<25	>75	×0.01	[<0.25]	[>0.75]
RBC	<2	>50	×0.01	[<0.02]	[>0.50]

Chemistry					
Total protein (g/dL)	1.2-3.0	>4.0	×10	[12-30 g/L]	[>40 g/L]
Glucose (mg/dL)	Serum level	<60	0.056	Serum level	[<3.4 mmol/L]

1. Curry JL, Hesham MA, Theil KS: Synovial, pleural, and peritoneal fluids. In McClatchey KD, editor: *Clinical laboratory medicine,* 2002, pp. 501-514.

Taurine
(2-Aminoethane-sulfonic acid, Tau)[1-4]

Ion-exchange chromatography

Plasma (heparin) or serum, fasting. Place blood in ice water immediately; separate and freeze within 1 hr of collection. Stable for 1 wk at −20° C; for longer periods, deproteinize and store at −70° C.[5,6]

	mg/dL	*μmol/L*[9]	P ↑ V Histidine (after oral load)
Premature, 1 day:	2.25 ± 0.94 (SD) ×80.0	[180 ± 75]	
Newborn, 1 day:	0.93-2.70	[74-216]	P ↓ V Tranylcypromine
1-3 mo:	0.31 ± 0.18 (SD)	[25 ± 14]	
2-6 mo:	0.58-1.08	[46-86]	
9 mo-2 yr:	0.24-1.14	[19-91]	
3-10 yr:	0.71-1.44	[57-115]	
2-17 yr:	0.08-2.01	[6-161][10]	
Adult:	0.34-2.10	[27-168][9]	

DIAGNOSTIC INFORMATION	REMARKS

Normal: low vol.; high visc.; firm clot; ~100 WBC/mm^3; few PMN; no crystals; glucose ≈ serum glucose.

Mucin clot produced on addition of acetic acid.

Noninflammatory: ↑ vol.; ↑ visc.; firm clot; ↑ WBC.

Microbiology and microscopy can be diagnostic, but gross and chemical findings are generally nonspecific.

Inflammatory: ↑ vol.; ↓ visc.; cloudy; friable clot; ↑↑ WBC w/ ↑ PMN.

Uric acid is best measured in serum, which parallels synovial fluid levels.

Septic: ↑ vol.; ↑ visc.; cloudy; friable clot; ↑↑↑ WBC w/ ↑PMN; ↓ glucose.

Elevated protein levels occur in inflammation, but this is insensitive and nonspecific.

Crystal: ↑ vol.; friable clot; cloudy; ↑↑ WBC w/ ↑ PMN; ↓ glucose.

Very low glucose levels can occur in septic arthritis, but there is considerable overlap with other inflammatory processes.

Hemorrhagic: ↑ vol.; red. ↑ RBC; hemosiderin; hematoidin crystals

P ↑ Sulfite oxidase deficiency, sepsis[13]

Contamination with leukocytes and thrombocytes will falsely elevate plasma values.

P ↓ Manic depressive disorder, depressive neurosis, and after abdominal surgery (day 4)[14]

TEST NAME AND METHOD	SPECIMEN REQUIREMENTS	REFERENCE INTERVAL, CONVENTIONAL [INTERNATIONAL RECOMMENDED UNITS]		CHEMICAL INTERFERENCES AND IN VIVO EFFECTS

Taurine—CONT

	Urine, 24 hr. Add 10 mL of 6 mol/L HCl at start of collection. (Alternatively, refrigerate specimen during collection.) Store frozen at $-20°$ C.[7]	*mg/day*	*μmol/day*	U ↑ V Progesterone
		10 days-7 wk: 3.3-19.6 $\times$ 8.0	[26-157][9]	
		3-12 yr: 7.9-12.1	[63-97][9]	U ↓ V Aspirin and
		Adult: 19.0-168.0[11]	[152-1344]	phenylbutazone both reduce elevated levels in patients with rheumatoid arthritis.
		mg/g creatinine	*mmol/mol creatinine*	
		or 55 ± 41 (SD)[9] $\times$ 0.90	[49.5 ± 36.9]	

	CSF. Collect in sterile tubes; store frozen. Stable at $-20°$ C for 1 wk or at $-70°$ C for 2 mo.[8]	*mg/dL*	*μmol/L*	
		Neonate: 0.216 ± 0.071 (SEM) $\times$ 80.0	[17.3 ± 5.7][8]	
		3 mo-2 yr: 0.058 ± 0.005 (SD)	[4.6 ± 0.4][12]	
		2-10 yr: 0.056 ± 0.009	[4.5 ± 0.7][12]	
		Adult: 0.080 ± 0.006	[6.4 ± 0.5][9]	

1. Scriver CR, Beaudet AL, Valle D, et al, editors: *The metabolic and molecular bases of inherited disease,* ed 8, New York, 2001, McGraw-Hill.

2. Young DS: *Effects of drugs on clinical laboratory tests,* ed 3, Washington, DC, 1990, American Association for Clinical Chemistry.

3. Bremer HJ, Duran M, Kamerling JP, et al: *Disturbances of amino acid metabolism: clinical chemistry and diagnosis,* Baltimore, 1981, Urban and Schwarzenburg.

4. Nyhan W, Sakait N: *Diagnostic recognition of genetic disease,* Philadelphia, 1987, Lea & Febiger.

5. Cummings JG: Routine amino acids analysis in the clinical laboratory, *Am Clin Prod Rev* Feb:20-25, 1988.

6. Schaefer A, Piquard F, Haberey P: Plasma amino acids analysis: effects of delayed samples preparation and of storage, *Clin Chim Acta* 164:163-169, 1987.

7. Pesce A, Kaplan L, editors: *Methods in clinical chemistry,* St. Louis, 1987, CV Mosby.

8. Heiblim DI, Evans HE, Glass L, et al: Amino acid concentrations in cerebrospinal fluid, *Arch Neurol* 35:765-768, 1978.

9. Shih V: *Laboratory techniques for the detection of hereditary metabolic disorders,* Boca Raton, FL, 1973, CRC Press.

10. Baylor College of Medicine, Biochemical Genetics Laboratory: *Test catalog,* Houston, TX, 1992, Baylor College of Medicine, Biochemical Genetics Laboratory.

11. Ghossein RA, Ross DG, Salomon RN, et al: Rapid detection and species identification of mycobacteria in paraffin-embedded tissues by polymerase chain reaction, *Diag Mol Patrol* 1:115-191, 1992.

12. Goldsmith RF, Earl JW, Cunningham AM: Determination of δ-aminobutyric acid and other amino acids in cerebrospinal fluid of pediatric patients by reversed-phase liquid chromatography, *Clin Chem* 33:1736-1740, 1987.

13. Freund H, Atamian S, Holyroyde J, et al: Plasma amino acids as predictors of the severity and outcome of sepsis, *Ann Surg* 190:571-576, 1979.

14. Jain KM, Rush BF Jr, Seelig RF, et al: Changes in plasma amino acid profiles following abdominal operations, *Surg Gynecol Obstet* 152:302-306, 1981.

15. Mårtensson J, Larsson J, Norström H: Amino acid metabolism during the anabolic phase of severely burned patients: with special reference to sulfur amino acids, *Eur J Clin Invest* 17:130-135, 1987.

16. Schott KJ, Meier D: Free amino acid pattern of cerebrospinal fluid in meningeal pathology, *Acta Neurol Scand* 75:304-309, 1987.

DIAGNOSTIC INFORMATION	REMARKS
U ↑ Pernicious anemia, folic acid deficiency, hyper-b-alaninemia, in first trimester of pregnancy (levels decrease thereafter), sulfite oxidase deficiency, and severely burned patients[15]	Increased excretion may follow ingestion of shellfish.
CSF ↑ Bacterial meningitis, carcinomatous meningitis[16]	Values in children (3 mo-10 yr) were measured using reversed-phase liquid chromatography.

TEST NAME AND METHOD	SPECIMEN REQUIREMENTS	REFERENCE INTERVAL, CONVENTIONAL [INTERNATIONAL RECOMMENDED UNITS]		CHEMICAL INTERFERENCES AND IN VIVO EFFECTS

Testosterone, Bioavailable[1-5]

Ammonium sulfate precipitation[6]

Serum. Stable for 2 days refrigerated and for 2 mo at −20° C.

		ng/dL		*nmol/L*
	Adults[7]			
	M:	66-417	× 0.0347	[2.29-14.5]
	F:	0.6-5.0		[0.02-0.129]

		% of total		*Fraction of total*
	Adults			
	M:	12.3-63.0	× 0.01	[0.123-0.630]
	F:	2.4-12.9		[0.24-0.129]

1. Barini A, Liberale I, Menini E: Simultaneous determination of free testosterone and testosterone bound to non-sex-hormone-binding globulin by equilibrium dialysis, *Clin Chem* 39:936-941, 1993.

2. Blight LF, Judd SJ, White GH: Relative diagnostic value of serum non-SHBG-bound testosterone, free androgen index and free testosterone in the assessment of mild to moderate hirsutism, *Ann Clin Biochem* 26:311-316, 1989.

3. Carter GD, Holland SM, Alaghband-Zadeh J, et al: Investigation of hirsutism: testosterone is not enough, *Ann Clin Biochem* 20:262-263, 1983.

4. Gumming DC, Wall SR: Non-sex hormone-binding globulin-bound testosterone as a marker for hyperandrogenism, *J Clin Endocrinol Metab* 61:873-876, 1985.

5. Pearce S, Dowsett M, Jeffcoate S: Three methods for estimating the fraction of testosterone and estradiol not bound to sex-hormone binding globulin, *Clin Chem* 35:632-635, 1989.

6. O'Connor S, Baker H, Dulmans A, et al: The measurement of sex steroid binding globulin by differential ammonium sulphate precipitation, *J Steroid Biochem* 4:331-339, 1973.

7. Nichols Institute Reference Laboratories: *Test catalog,* San Juan Capistrano, CA, 1993, Nichols Institute Reference Laboratories.

Testosterone, Free[1-6]

RIA (equilibrium tracer dialysis)

Serum. Stable for 2 days refrigerated and for 2 mo at −20° C.

S ↑ V Danazol

See also *Testosterone, Total.*

		pg/mL[7]		*pmol/L*	*% of total*		*Fraction of total*
	Cord						
	M:	5-22	× 3.47	[17.2-76.3]	2.0-4.4	× 0.01	[0.02-0.04]
	F:	4-16		[13.9-55.5]	2.0-3.9		[0.02-0.04]
	Newborn (1-15 days)						
	M:	1.5-31.0		[5.2-107.5]	0.9-1.7		[0.01-0.017]
	F:	0.5-2.5		[1.7-8.7]	0.8-1.5		[0.008-0.015]
	1-3 mo						
	M:	3.3-8.0		[11.5-62.5]	0.4-0.8		[0.004-0.008]
	F:	0.1-1.3		[0.3-4.5]	0.1-1.1		[0.004-0.11]

DIAGNOSTIC INFORMATION	**REMARKS**

↑ Hirsutism, hyperandrogenism

The assay measures the non-SHBG-bound testosterone (free plus albumin-bound testosterone).

Testosterone circulates in three forms: non-protein-bound or free, a weakly bound or albumin bound, and tightly bound to SHBG. SHBG-bound testosterone is not biologically active. In females, 1-2% of testosterone is free and 25-65% is weakly bound to albumin. The remainder is tightly bound to SHBG.

Bioavailable testosterone is independent of SHBG concentrations. In obesity, SHBG and total testosterone are low, but bioavailable testosterone is within the reference intervals. In hirsutism, SHBG levels may be low and total testosterone may not be elevated. Bioavailable testosterone is an apparent marker for androgen activity.

↑ Hirsutism, adrenal virilizing tumor, polycystic ovary syndrome, and androgen resistance

↓ Hypogonadism, P-450$_{C17}$ enzyme deficiency

An increase in concentration of sex hormone-binding globulin (SHBG) and a decrease in plasma-free testosterone are reported in old age in men.

See *Testosterone, Total; Testosterone, Bioavailable;* and *Sex Hormone-Binding Globulin.*

Free (non-protein-bound) testosterone is independent of changes in concentrations of the principal testosterone transport protein, sex hormone-binding globulin. In those situations in which SHBG is frequently increased (e.g., hyperthyroidism, hyperestrogenic states such as pregnancy or oral contraceptive use, and administration of antiepileptic drugs) or decreased (e.g., hypothyroidism, androgen excess, and obesity), measurements of free testosterone may be more appropriate than measurements of total testosterone.

Values for free testosterone performed by equilibrium tracer dialysis compare favorably with those performed by membrane ultrafiltration and gel filtration methods. Alternative assessments of free testosterone include bioavailable testosterone (an estimation of free and weakly bound testosterone); analog

TEST NAME AND METHOD	SPECIMEN REQUIREMENTS	REFERENCE INTERVAL, CONVENTIONAL [INTERNATIONAL RECOMMENDED UNITS]			CHEMICAL INTERFERENCES AND IN VIVO EFFECTS

Testosterone, Free—CONT

	3-5 mo				
	M:	0.7-14.0	[2.4-48.6]	0.4-1.1	[0.004-0.11]
	F:	0.3-1.1	[1.0-3.8]	0.5-1.0	[0.005-0.01]
	5-7 mo				
	M:	0.4-4.8	[1.4-16.6]	0.4-1.0	[0.004-0.01]
	F:	0.2-0.6	[0.7-2.1]	0.5-0.8	[0.005-0.008]
	Children[8]				
	6-9 yr				
	M:	0.1-3.2	[0.3-1.1]	0.9-1.7	[0.009-0.017]
	F:	0.1-0.9	[0.3-3.1]	0.9-1.4	[0.009-0.014]
	10-11 yr				
	M:	0.6-5.7	[2.1-19.8]	1.0-1.9	[0.010-0.019]
	F:	1.0-5.2	[3.5-18.0]	1.0-1.9	[0.010-0.019]
	12-14 yr				
	M:	1.4-156	[4.9-541]	1.3-3.0	[0.013-0.030]
	F:	1.5-5.2	[3.5-18.0]	1.0-1.9	[0.010-0.019]
	15-17 yr				
	M:	80-159	[278-552]	1.8-2.7	[0.018-0.027]
	F:	1.0-5.2	[3.5-18.0]	1.0-1.9	[0.010-0.019]
	Adult[7]				
	M:	50-210	[174-729]	1.0-2.7	[0.010-0.027]
	F:	1.0-8.5	[3.2-29.5]	0.5-1.8	[0.005-0.018]

1. Blight LE, Judd SJ, White GH: Relative diagnostic value of serum non-SHBG-bound testosterone, free androgen index and free testosterone in the assessment of mild to moderate hirsutism, *Ann Clin Biochem* 26:311-316, 1989.

2. Nanjes MN, Wheeler MJ: Plasma free testosterone—is an index sufficient? *Ann Clin Biochem* 22:387-390, 1985.

3. Paulson JD, Keller DW, Wiest WG, et al: Free testosterone concentration in serum: elevation is the hallmark of hirsutism, *Am J Obstet Gynecol* 128:851-857, 1977.

4. Smith S: Free testosterone, *AACC Endo Metab In-Service Training Cont Educ* 11:59-62, 1993.

5. Whitley RJ, Meikle AW, Watts NB: Endocrinology. In Burtis CA, Ashwood ER, editors: *Tietz textbook of clinical chemistry,* ed 2, Philadelphia, 1994, WB Saunders.

6. Wilke TJ, Utley DJ: Total testosterone, free-androgen index, calculated free testosterone, and free testosterone by analog RIA compared in hirsute women and in otherwise normal women with altered binding of sex hormone-binding globulin, *Clin Chem* 33:1372-1375, 1987.

7. Endocrine Sciences: *Pediatric laboratory services,* Tarzana, CA, 1992, Endocrine Sciences.

8. Nichols Institute Reference Laboratories: *Test catalog,* San Juan Capistrano, CA, 1993, Nichols Institute Reference Laboratories.

9. Ekins R: Hirsutism: free and bound testosterone, *Ann Clin Biochem* 27:91-93, 1990.

10. Said El Shami A, Ito T, Durham A: First solid-phase radioimmunoassay for free testosterone by the analog method, *Clin Chem* 31:910, 1985.

DIAGNOSTIC INFORMATION   **REMARKS**

tracer RIA[9,10]; free androgen index (a measure of testosterone corrected for abnormalities in sex hormone-binding globulin); and calculated free testosterone using values for testosterone, SHBG, albumin, and mass action equations.

TEST NAME AND METHOD	SPECIMEN REQUIREMENTS	REFERENCE INTERVAL, CONVENTIONAL [INTERNATIONAL RECOMMENDED UNITS]			CHEMICAL INTERFERENCES AND IN VIVO EFFECTS
Testosterone, Total[1-5]	Serum. Stable for 1 wk refrigerated and for 6 mo at −20° C.		*ng/dL*	*nmol/L*	S ↑ V Anticonvulsants, barbiturates, clomiphene,
		Cord[7]			estrogens, gonadotropin
		M:	13-55 × 0.0347	[0.45-1.91]	(males), and oral
RIA		F:	5-45	[0.17-1.56]	contraceptives
		Premature[7]			
		M:	37-198	[1.28-6.87]	
		F:	5-22	[0.17-0.76]	S ↓ V Androgens, cyprot-
		Newborn[7]			erone, dexamethasone, di-
		M:	75-400	[2.6-13.9]	ethylstilbestrol (≥1 mg),
		F:	20-64	[0.69-2.22]	digitalis, digoxin (males),
		Prepubertal child[8]			ethanol (male alcoholics),
		1-5 mo			glucocorticoids,[9] glucose,
		M:	1-177	[0.03-6.14]	gonadotropin-releasing
		F:	1-5	[0.03-0.17]	hormone analogs (contin-
		6-11 mo			uous administration),[10]
		M:	2-7	[0.07-0.24]	halothane, ketoconazole,
		F:	2-5	[0.07-0.17]	metoprolol, metyrapone,
		1-5 yr			phenothiazines, spirono-
		M:	2-25	[0.07-0.87]	lactone, and tetracycline
		F:	2-10	[0.07-0.35]	
		6-9 yr			
		M:	3-30	[0.10-1.04]	
		F:	2-20	[0.07-0.69]	
		Puberty[8]			
		Tanner stage			
		1			
		M:	2-23	[0.07-0.80]	
		F:	2-10	[0.07-0.35]	
		2			
		M:	5-70	[0.17-2.43]	
		F:	5-30	[0.17-1.04]	
		3			
		M:	15-280	[0.52-9.72]	
		F:	10-30	[0.35-1.04]	
		4			
		M:	105-545	[3.64-18.91]	
		F:	15-40	[0.52-1.39]	
		5			
		M:	265-800	[9.19-27.76]	
		F:	10-40	[0.35-1.39]	
			ng/dL	*nmol/L*	
		Adult[8]			
		M:	280-1100 × 0.0347	[0.52-38.17]	
		F:	15-70	[0.52-2.43]	
		(higher at midcycle peak)			
		Pregnancy:	3-4 × adult level		
		Postmenopause:	8-35	[0.28-1.22]	

↑ Idiopathic sexual precocity and adrenal hyperplasia in boys (values may be within adult range), some adrenocortical tumors, extragonadal tumors producing gonadotropin in men, trophoblastic disease during pregnancy, testicular feminization, idiopathic hirsutism, virilizing ovarian tumors, arrhenoblastoma, hilar cell tumor, and virilizing luteoma

↓ Down syndrome, uremia, myotonic dystrophy, hepatic insufficiency, cryptorchidism, primary and secondary hypogonadism, and delayed puberty in boys

This test is a measure of total circulating testosterone, both protein-bound and free. In boys, a sharp increase in serum testosterone occurs during pubertal (Tanner) stages 3 and 4. Subsequently the testosterone level remains relatively constant. In adult men, serum testosterone levels peak in the early morning, decreasing 25% to the evening minimum; levels increase after exercise and decrease after immobilization and after glucose load; progessive decreases begin after age 50 yr.

In women, values are lower than in men, showing a cyclic pattern of elevation for 1-2 days at midcycle. In virilizing conditions, values are usually >200 ng/dL [>6.94 nmol/L]; slight elevations are seen in idiopathic hirsutism and in a majority of patients with polycystic ovary syndrome.

Secretion is episodic, with peak about 7:00 AM and minimum about 8:00 PM; multiple or pooled samples give more reliable information than a single sample.

TEST NAME AND METHOD	SPECIMEN REQUIREMENTS	REFERENCE INTERVAL, CONVENTIONAL [INTERNATIONAL RECOMMENDED UNITS]		CHEMICAL INTERFERENCES AND IN VIVO EFFECTS

Testosterone, Total—CONT

	Urine, 24 hr	Pubertal child (4-10 yr): 0.2-2.3 mcg/day × 3.47 [0.7-8 nmol/day]		U ↑ V Clomiphene, corticotropin, and gonadotropin
		mcg/kg body weight/day, $\bar{x}$	*nmol/kg body weight/day, $\bar{x}$*	U ↓ V Dexamethasone (females)
		Prepubertal stage		
		1		
		M: 0.25 × 3.47	[0.87]	
		F: 0.16	[0.56]	
		2		
		M: 0.34	[1.18]	
		F: 0.16	[0.56]	
		3		
		M: 0.37	[1.28]	
		F: 0.16	[0.56]	
		4		
		M: 0.49	[1.70]	
		F: 0.16	[0.56]	
		5		
		M: 0.57	[1.90]	
		F: 0.16	[0.56]	
		mcg/day	*nmol/day*	
		20-50 yr		
		M: 50-135 × 3.47	[173.5-468.5]	
		F: 2-12	[6.9-41.6]	
		>50 yr		
		M: 40-60	[138.8-208.2]	
		F: 2-8	[6.9-27.8]	
	Amniotic fluid[6]	*ng/dL*	*nmol/L*	
		Fetal age		
		9-12 wk		
		M: 2.0-72.6 × 0.0347	[0.07-2.52]	
		Median: 5.0	[0.17]	
		F: 1.3-4.0	[0.05-0.14]	
		Median: 2.7	[0.09]	
		12-16 wk		
		M: 7.0-72.4	[0.24-2.51]	
		Median: 25.0	[0.87]	
		F: 1.3-10.0	[0.05-0.35]	
		Median: 2.6	[0.09]	
		16-19 wk		
		M: 8.4-29.0	[0.29-1.0]	
		Median: 19.3	[0.67]	
		F: 1.0-9.0	[0.03-0.31]	
		Median: 2.9	[0.10]	

DIAGNOSTIC INFORMATION   **REMARKS**

Values represent normative data for unconjugated testosterone.
Values for conjugated testosterone in AF are available.[11]

TEST NAME AND METHOD	SPECIMEN REQUIREMENTS	REFERENCE INTERVAL, CONVENTIONAL [INTERNATIONAL RECOMMENDED UNITS]		CHEMICAL INTERFERENCES AND IN VIVO EFFECTS
Testosterone, Total—CONT				
		28-34 wk		
		M: 8.4-26.4	[0.29-0.92]	
		Median: 12.3	[0.43]	
		34-40 wk		
		M: 2.0-16.0	[0.07-0.56]	
		Median: 18.0	[0.62]	
		F: 2.2-10.2	[0.08-0.35]	
		Median: 3.4	[0.12]	

1. Endocrine Sciences: *Pediatric laboratory services,* Tarzana, CA, 1992, Endocrine Sciences.
2. Nichols Institute Reference Laboratories: *Test catalog,* San Juan Capistrano, CA, 1993, Nichols Institute Reference Laboratories.
3. Blight LF, Judd SJ, White GH: Relative diagnostic value of serum non-SHBG-bound testosterone, free androgen index and free testosterone in the assessment of mild to moderate hirsutism, *Ann Clin Biochem* 26:311-316, 1989.
4. Smith S: Free testosterone, *AACC Endo Metab In-Service Training Cont Educ* 11:59-62, 1993.
5. Whitley RJ, Meikle AW, Watts NB: Endocrinology. In Burtis CA, Ashwood ER, editors: *Tietz textbook of clinical chemistry,* ed 2, Philadelphia, 1994, WB Saunders.
6. Warne GL, Faiman C, Reyes FI, et al: Studies on human sexual development. V. Concentrations of testosterone, 17-hydroxyprogesterone and progesterone in human amniotic fluid throughout gestation, *J Clin Endocrinol Metab* 44:934-938, 1977.
7. Said El Shami A, Ito T, Durham A: First solid-phase radioimmunoassay for free testosterone by the analog method, *Clin Chem* 31:910, 1985.
8. Ekins R: Hirsutism: free and bound testosterone, *Ann Clin Biochem* 27:91-93, 1990.
9. MacAdams MR, White RH, Chipps BE: Reduction of serum testosterone levels during chronic glucocorticoid therapy, *Ann Intern Med* 104:648-651, 1986.
10. Cutler GB Jr, moderator: Therapeutic applications of luteinizing hormone-releasing hormone and its analogs, *Ann Intern Med* 102:643-657, 1985.
11. Tulchinsky D, Ryan KJ, editors: *Maternal-fetal endocrinology,* Philadelphia, 1980, WB Saunders.

TEST NAME AND METHOD	SPECIMEN REQUIREMENTS	REFERENCE INTERVAL, CONVENTIONAL		[INTERNATIONAL RECOMMENDED UNITS]	CHEMICAL INTERFERENCES AND IN VIVO EFFECTS
Tetrahydrocortisol (Tetrahydro F, THF)[1] *RIA*	Urine, 24 hr. Refrigerate during collection. Aliquot and freeze immediately.	0.5-1.5 mg/day	× 2.72	[1.4-4.1 μmol/day]	See *Cortisol, Total;* and *17-Hydroxycorticosteroids.*

1. Alsever RN, Gotlin RW: *Handbook of endocrine tests in adults and children,* ed 2, Chicago, 1978, Year Book Medical Publishers Inc.

DIAGNOSTIC INFORMATION	REMARKS

↑ Cushing's (pituitary) disease, adrenal adenoma, and carcinoma

↑↑ Ectopic ACTH syndrome

↓ Addison's disease, congenital adrenal hyperplasia (adrenogenital syndromes), and hypopituitarism (need for functional tests)

There is a diurnal variation in THF excretion with the maximum in the early morning (about 7:00 AM).

THF is one of the major liver metabolites of cortisol. It is also known as urocortisol.

TEST NAME AND METHOD	SPECIMEN REQUIREMENTS	REFERENCE INTERVAL, CONVENTIONAL [INTERNATIONAL RECOMMENDED UNITS]			CHEMICAL INTERFERENCES AND IN VIVO EFFECTS
Tetrahydrodeoxy-cortisol (Tetrahydro-11-deoxycortisol, TetrahydroCompound S, THS)[1,2] *RIA*	Urine, 24 hr. Preserve with 1 g of boric acid.	20-130 mcg/day[3]	× 0.00285	[0.1-0.4 μmol/day]	See *11-Deoxycortisol*.

1. White PC, New MI, Dupont B: Congenital adrenal hyperplasia. Part 1, *N Engl J Med* 316:1519-1524, 1987.
2. White PC, New MI, Dupont B: Congenital adrenal hyperplasia. Part 2, *N Engl J Med* 316:1580-1586, 1987.
3. Hicks JM, Young DS: *DORA '90-'91: directory of rare analyses,* Washington, DC, 1990, AACC Press.

TEST NAME AND METHOD	SPECIMEN REQUIREMENTS	REFERENCE INTERVAL, CONVENTIONAL [INTERNATIONAL RECOMMENDED UNITS]			CHEMICAL INTERFERENCES AND IN VIVO EFFECTS
Thallium (Tl)[1,2] *AAS*	Whole blood (sodium heparin).[3] Collect in pretested, metal-free container.	<0.5 mcg/dL Clinical intoxication: 10-800 mcg/dL	× 48.9 × 0.0489	[<24.5 nmol/L] [0.5-39.1 μmol/L]	The use of EDTA as an anticoagulant may slightly reduce recovery.
	Urine, 24 hr.[4] Collect in acid-washed, metal-free container. Stable for 7 days at room temperature.	<2.0 mcg/L Clinical intoxication: 1.0-20.0 mg/L	× 4.89 × 4.89	[<9.8 nmol/L] [4.9-97.8 μmol/L]	
ICP-MS	Whole blood.[4] Collect in pretested, metal-free container.	0-10 mcg/L	× 4.89	[0.0-48.9 nmol/L]	
	Urine.[4] Collect in acid-washed, metal-free container. Refrigerate during and after collection.				

1. Wyngaarden JB, Smith LH Jr, editors: *Cecil textbook of medicine,* ed 18, Philadelphia, 1988, WB Saunders.
2. Klaasen CD, Amdur MO, Doull J, editors: *Casarett and Doull's toxicology. The basic science of poisons,* ed 3, New York, 1986, Macmillan Pub. Co., Inc.
3. Baselt RC: *Analytical procedures for therapeutic drug monitoring and emergency toxicology,* ed 2, Littleton, MA, 1987, PSG Publishing Co., Inc.
4. Associated Regional & University Pathologists, Inc. web site (www.aruplab.com): Available at: http://www.aruplab.com/testing/user_guide.jsp.
5. Moeschlin S: Thallium poisoning, *Clin Toxicol* 17:133-146, 1980.
6. Mercurio M, Hoffman RS: In Goldfrank LR, Flomenbaum NE, Lewin NA, et al, editors: *Thallium. Goldfrank's toxicologic emergencies,* ed 6, Stamford, CT, 1998, Appleton and Lange, pp. 1349-1357.

DIAGNOSTIC INFORMATION	REMARKS
↑ Congenital adrenal hyperplasia caused by 11β-hydroxylase deficiency; pancreatitis, eclampsia, and other forms of severe stress	Measurement of THS is also useful in determining pituitary reserve with the metyrapone test. See *Metyrapone Stimulation Test*.
↓ Addison's disease, hypopituitarism	After metyrapone administration, there is normally a 10-fold increase over baseline THS.

Symptoms of poisoning include alopecia (unique sign), ataxia, choreiform movements, pulmonary edema, vomiting, abdominal pain, GI bleeding, diarrhea, restlessness, delirium, and eventually coma. Poisoning results in optic neuropathy, blindness, facial paralysis, paresthesias, peripheral neuropathy, respiratory paralysis and liver and renal damage.	Thallium salts (sulfate and acetate) are used in medications, cosmetics, and pesticides. Tl salts burn with a bright green flame. Trace amounts of ^{201}Tl are used in radiological procedures. Tl poisoning occurs from ingestion or from absorption through intact skin and mucous membranes. Average lethal dose is 10-15 mg Tl/kg.[5] Tl accumulates in liver, kidney, bone, and muscle tissue. Elimination half-life after poisoning is <2 days.[6]

See Table II-6. |

TEST NAME AND METHOD	SPECIMEN REQUIREMENTS	REFERENCE INTERVAL, CONVENTIONAL [INTERNATIONAL RECOMMENDED UNITS]		CHEMICAL INTERFERENCES AND IN VIVO EFFECTS
Thiamine (Vitamin B_1) *HPLC, Thiochromefluori-metric*[1]	Whole blood (heparin). Stable for 7 mo if frozen ($-70°$ C).	275-675 ng/g hemoglobin[1]	[0.65-1.59 nmol/g hemoglobin]	S ↓ V Barbiturates S ↓ V Barbiturates
HPLC, Thiochromefluori-metric[2,3]	Serum or plasma. Stable for 1 mo if frozen ($-20°$ C).	0.32 ± 0.11 mcg/dL $\times$ 29.6* [9.5 ± 3.3 nmol/L] *Conversion factor based on the molecular mass of thiamine hydrochloride (337.28).		
HPLC, Thiochromefluori-metric[4]	Erythrocyte hemolysate; collect whole blood (heparin). Freeze hemolysate if assay is delayed.	4.5-10.3 mcg/dL[4] $\times$ 23.57† [106-242 nmol/L] (thiamine pyrophosphate) †Conversion factor based on the molecular mass of thiamine pyrophosphate (424.31).		

1. Talwar D, Davidson H, Cooney J, et al: Vitamin B(1) status assessed by direct measurement of thiamine pyrophosphate in erythrocytes or whole blood by HPLC: comparison with erythrocyte transketolase activation assay, *Clin Chem* 46:704-710, 2000.

2. Tallaksen CM, Bohmer T, Karlsen J, et al: Determination of thiamine and its phosphate esters in human blood, plasma, and urine, *Methods Enzymol* 279:67-74, 1997.

DIAGNOSTIC INFORMATION	REMARKS

S, B ↑ Leukemia, polycythemia vera, and Hodgkin's disease

S, B ↓ Alcoholism with and without liver disease, deficient diet, excessive consumption of raw fish (which contains a microbial thiaminase) and tea (which contains an antithiamine factor), chronic febrile infections, prolonged diarrhea, diabetes, cancer, and chronic illness

Thiamine-responsive inborn errors: Megaloblastic anemia of unknown origin, impaired pyruvate carboxylase, impaired ketoacid dehydrogenase, and subacute necrotizing encephalopathy

Wet beriberi: Symptoms are (or include) high-output left ventricular heart failure, tachycardia, increased central venous pressure, sodium retention, and edema. In acute deficiency, there is severe dyspnea, increased thirst, cardiac failure, glove-stocking cyanosis, marked cardiomegaly, and hepatomegaly.

Dry beriberi (Wernicke-Korsakoff syndrome): Progression of symptoms includes symmetrical motor and sensory dysfunction, nystagmus, ophthalmoplegia, ataxia, confusion, coma, and death. Impaired memory and cognition may persist after treatment.

Thiamine deficiency causes an increase in serum level of lactate, α-ketoglutarate, pyruvate, and glyoxylate.

Thiamine (vitamin B_1) is a coenzyme for transketolase and the $E_1\alpha$ subunit of the enzymes, pyruvate dehydrogenase, α-ketoglutarate dehydrogenase, and branched chain α-ketoacid dehydrogenase complexes.[5,6] The average total thiamine pool in adults is ~30 mg, and an intake of 0.5 mg/1000 kcal/day is needed to maintain this pool.[5,7] Thiamine deficiency most commonly occurs in elderly persons and in individuals with chronic gastrointestinal problems, on cancer treatment, or on long-term treatment with diuretics.[5,7,8] Because of its short storage time in vivo, marginal thiamine deficiency can occur within 10 days and more severe deficiency within 21 days if dietary intake is inadequate.[9] Severe thiamine deficiency results in cardiac failure (beriberi) or neurological manifestations (Wernicke's encephalopathy).[5] Subclinical insufficiency may affect intellectual performance and general well-being without overt clinical symptoms.[5] Because the symptoms associated with thiamine deficiency are nonspecific and could be observed in a variety of clinical settings, determination of a patient's thiamine status is frequently requested in diverse clinical situations.

Thiamine diphosphate (TDP) is the physiologically active form of thiamine, and TDP is the predominant form present in erythrocytes. Several authors have suggested that thiamine status is best determined by measurement of TDP in whole blood or erythrocyte blood by high-performance liquid chromatography (HPLC).[4,7,10] Blood TDP measurement may be a more sensitive indicator of thiamine status than the transketolase activation assay.[1,11] Further studies are needed to confirm this.

Free thiamine is the predominant form in plasma, which contains no appreciable amount of TDP. Thiamine has a relatively short half-life in plasma. The utility of measurement of plasma thiamine to assess thiamine nutritive status needs further study.

Determination of urinary thiamine in a timed collection may be helpful in differentiating extremes of thiamine deficiency; however, excretion can be influenced by dietary intake, absorption, and other factors.[12]

Toxicity to thiamine only occurs when it is given parenterally in doses several hundredfold in excess of requirements. See *Transketolase.*

3. Weber W, Kewitz H: Determination of thiamine in human plasma and its pharmacokinetics, *Eur J Clin Pharmacol* 28:213-219, 1985.
4. Lynch PL, Trimble ER, Young IS: High-performance liquid chromatographic determination of thiamine diphosphate in erythrocytes using internal standard methodology, *J Chromatogr B Biomed Sci Appl* 701:120-123, 1997.

TEST NAME AND METHOD	SPECIMEN REQUIREMENTS	REFERENCE INTERVAL, CONVENTIONAL [INTERNATIONAL RECOMMENDED UNITS]		CHEMICAL INTERFERENCES AND IN VIVO EFFECTS

Thiamine—CONT

5. Gubler C: Thiamin. In Machlin L, editor: *Handbook of vitamins,* ed 2, New York, 1991, Marcel Dekker, Inc., pp. 233-281.

6. Robinson B: Lactic acidemia: disorders of pyruvate carboxylase and pyruvate dehydrogenase. In: Scriver C, Beaudet A, Sly W, et al, editors: *The metabolic and molecular basis of inherited disease,* ed 8, New York, 2001, McGraw-Hill, pp. 2275-2295.

7. Lynch PL, Young IS: Determination of thiamine by high-performance liquid chromatography, *J Chromatogr A* 881:267-284, 2000.

8. Rieck J, Halkin H, Almog S, et al: Urinary loss of thiamine is increased by low doses of furosemide in healthy volunteers, *J Lab Clin Med* 134:238-243, 1999.

TEST NAME AND METHOD	SPECIMEN REQUIREMENTS	REFERENCE INTERVAL, CONVENTIONAL [INTERNATIONAL RECOMMENDED UNITS]			CHEMICAL INTERFERENCES AND IN VIVO EFFECTS
Thiocyanate[1-4] *Colorimetric*	Plasma (EDTA), serum		*mg/L*	*μmol/L*	Some antibiotics (i.e., penicillin, cloxacillin, cephalothin) interfere. Avoid by washing column with ammonium chloride before elution.
		Nonsmokers:	1-4 × 17.2	[17-69]	
		Smokers:	3-12	[52-206]	
		Nitroprusside infusion:	6-29	[103-499]	
	Urine		*mg/day*	*μmol/day*	
		Nonsmokers:	1-4	[17-69]	↑ V Nitroprusside
		Smokers:	7-17	[120-292]	

1. Baselt RC: *Analytical procedures for therapeutic drug monitoring and emergency toxicology,* ed 2, Littleton, MA, 1987, PSG Publishing Co., Inc.

2. Bruggeman IM, Temmink JHM, van Bladeren PJ: Glutathione- and cysteine-mediated cytotoxicity of allyl and benzyl isothiocyanate, *Toxicol Appl Pharmacol* 83:349-359, 1986.

3. Schulz V, Bonn R, Kindler J: Kinetics of elimination of thiocyanate in 7 healthy subjects and in 8 subjects with renal failure, *Klin Wochenschr* 57:243-247, 1979.

4. Sollmann TH: *A manual of pharmacology and its applications to therapeutics and toxicology,* ed 8, Philadelphia, 1957, WB Saunders.

5. Leuoker RV, Pechacek TF, Murray DM, et al: Saliva thiocyanate: a chemical indicator of cigarette smoking in adolescents, *Am J Public Health* 71:1320-1324, 1981.

TEST NAME AND METHOD	SPECIMEN REQUIREMENTS	REFERENCE INTERVAL, CONVENTIONAL [INTERNATIONAL RECOMMENDED UNITS]			CHEMICAL INTERFERENCES AND IN VIVO EFFECTS
Threonine (Thr)[1-5] *Ion-exchange chromatography*	Plasma (heparin) or serum, fasting. Place blood in ice water immediately; separate and freeze within 1 hr of collection. Stable for 1 wk at −20° C; for longer periods, deproteinize and store at −70° C.[6,7]		*mg/dL*	*μmol/L*[10,11]	P ↑ V Histidine (after oral load) P ↓ V Glucose, progesterone (high doses)
		Premature, 1 day:	2.56 ± 0.71 (SD) × 84.0	[215 ± 60]	
		Newborn, 1 day:	1.36-3.99	[114-335]	
		1-3 mo:	1.71 ± 0.48 (SD)	[144 ± 40]	
		2-6 mo:	2.27-4.33	[191-364]	
		1-24 mo:	0.29-2.07	[24-174][11]	
		3-10 yr:	0.50-1.13	[42-95]	
		6-18 yr:	0.88-2.40	[74-202][12]	
		Adult:	0.94-2.30	[79-193]	

DIAGNOSTIC INFORMATION	REMARKS

9. Brin M: Erythrocyte as biopsy tissue for functional evaluation of thiamine adequacy, *JAMA* 187:762-766, 1964.

10. Baines M: Improved high performance liquid chromatographic determination of thiamine diphosphate in erythrocytes, *Clin Chim Acta* 153:43-48, 1985.

11. Warnock LG, Prudhomme CR, Wagner C: The determination of thiamine pyrophosphate in blood and other tissues, and its correlation with erythrocyte transketolase activity, *J Nutr* 108:421-427, 1978.

12. McCormick DB, Greene HL: Vitamins. In Burtis CA, Ashwood ER, editors: *Tietz textbook of clinical chemistry,* ed 3, Philadelphia, 1999, WB Saunders, pp. 999-1028.

See also *Cyanide.*

Thiocyanate may be used to determine smoking habits, especially in children.[5]

Thiocyanate measurements in serum are used to monitor nitroprusside therapy.

A metabolite of cyanide, thiocyanate is primarily of interest in the study of the toxicity of cyanide and its derivatives.

P ↓ Phlebotomus fever, chronic renal failure

TEST NAME AND METHOD	SPECIMEN REQUIREMENTS	REFERENCE INTERVAL, CONVENTIONAL [INTERNATIONAL RECOMMENDED UNITS]		CHEMICAL INTERFERENCES AND IN VIVO EFFECTS

Threonine—CONT

	Urine, 24 hr. Add 10 mL of 6 mol/L HCl at start of collection. (Alternatively, refrigerate specimen during collection.) Store frozen at −20° C.[8]	*mg/day*	$\mu mol/day$[10]	U ↑ V Tetracycline, ascorbic acid (after large intake)[15]
		10 days-7 wk: 1.5-11.9 × 8.4	[13-100]	
		3-12 yr: 10.1-29.6	[85-249]	
		Adult: 14.3-46.7	[120-392]	
		mg/g creatinine	*mmol/mol creatinine*	
		or 14 ± 7 (SD) × 0.95	[13.3 ± 6.7]	
		$\mu mol/g$ creatinine[13]	*mmol/mol creatinine*	
		0-1 mo: 218-1486 × 0.113	[25-168]	
		1-6 mo: 254-1379	[29-156]	
		6 mo-1 yr: 206-1146	[23-129]	
		1-2 yr: 170-976	[19-110]	
		2-3 yr: 149-810	[17-92]	

	CSF. Collect in sterile tubes; store frozen. Stable at −20° C for 1 wk or at −70° C for 2 mo.[9]	*mg/dL*	$\mu mol/dL$	
		Neonate: 0.726 ± 0.261 (SEM) × 84.0	[61.0 ± 21.9][9]	
		3 mo-2 yr: 0.208 ± 0.050 (SD)	[17.5 ± 4.2][14]	
		2-10 yr: 0.189 ± 0.038 (SD)	[15.9 ± 3.2][14]	
		Adult: 0.375 ± 0.018 (SD)	[31.5 ± 1.5][10]	

1. Friedman RB, Young DS: *Effects of disease on clinical laboratory tests,* ed 2, Washington, DC, 1989, American Association for Clinical Chemistry.

2. Scriver CR, Beaudet AL, Valle D, et al, editors: *The metabolic and molecular bases of inherited disease,* ed 8, New York, 2001, McGraw-Hill.

3. Young DS: *Effects of drugs on clinical laboratory tests,* ed 3, Washington, DC, 1990, American Association for Clinical Chemistry.

4. Bremer HJ, Duran M, Kamerling JP, et al: *Disturbances of amino acid metabolism: clinical chemistry and diagnosis,* Baltimore, 1981, Urban and Schwarzenburg.

5. Nyhan W, Sakait N: *Diagnostic recognition of genetic disease,* Philadelphia, 1987, Lea & Febiger.

6. Cummings JG: Routine amino acids analysis in the clinical laboratory, *Am Clin Prod Rev* Feb:20-25, 1988.

7. Schaefer A, Piquard F, Haberey P: Plasma amino acids analysis: effects of delayed samples preparation and of storage, *Clin Chim Acta* 164:163-169, 1987.

8. Pesce A, Kaplan L, editors: *Methods in clinical chemistry,* St. Louis, 1987, CV Mosby.

9. Heiblim DI, Evans HE, Glass L, et al: Amino acid concentrations in cerebrospinal fluid, *Arch Neurol* 35:765-768, 1978.

10. Shih V: *Laboratory techniques for the detection of hereditary metabolic disorders,* Boca Raton, FL, 1973, CRC Press.

11. Slocum RH, Cummings JG: Amino acid analysis of physiological samples. In Hommes FA, editor: *Techniques in human biochemical genetics,* New York, 1991, Wiley-Liss, pp. 87-126.

12. Meites S, editor: *Pediatric clinical chemistry,* ed 3, Washington, DC, 1989, American Association for Clinical Chemistry.

13. Mayo Medical Laboratories: *Test catalog,* Rochester, MN, 2003, Mayo Medical Laboratories.

14. Goldsmith RF, Earl JW, Cunningham AM: Determination of δ-aminobutyric acid and other amino acids in cerebrospinal fluid of pediatric patients by reversed-phase liquid chromatography, *Clin Chem* 33:1736-1740, 1987.

DIAGNOSTIC INFORMATION	REMARKS

U ↑ Hartnup disease, pregnancy, burn patients,[16] and hepato-lenticular degeneration

U ↓ Rheumatoid arthritis

Values in children (3 mo-10 yr) were measured using reversed-phase liquid chromatography.

15. Tsao C, Muyashita K: Effects of large intake of ascorbic acid on the urinary excretion of amino acids and related compounds, *IRCS Med Sci* 13:855-856, 1985.

16. Cynober L, Dinh FN, Blonde F, et al: Plasma and urinary amino acid pattern in severe burn patients: evolution throughout the healing period, *Am J Clin Nutr* 36:416-425, 1982.

TEST NAME AND METHOD	SPECIMEN REQUIREMENTS	REFERENCE INTERVAL, CONVENTIONAL [INTERNATIONAL RECOMMENDED UNITS]			CHEMICAL INTERFERENCES AND IN VIVO EFFECTS
Thrombin Time **(TT)**[1,2]	Plasma (blue top-citrate). Stable for 4 hr on ice or store frozen.	Variable depending on reagent-instruments used, 17-23 sec.			↑ V Heparin, hirudin, argatroban, anistreplase, asparaginase, fibrinogen, or fibrin degradation products. LMWH may produce a mild prolongation of the TT.

1. Lewis SM, Bain BJ, Bates I, editors: *Dacie and Lewis practical hematology,* ed 9, Edinburgh, 2001, Churchill Livingstone.
2. Jacobs DS, Demott WR, Oxley DK, editors: *Laboratory test handbook,* ed 5, Hudson, OH, 2001, Lexi-Comp, Inc.

β-Thromboglobu-lin (βTG)[1]	Plasma. Collect whole blood (Na citrate). Cool at 4° C. Add prostaglandin E1 and theophylline to Na citrate anticoagulant. Stable for 2 hr at 4° C. Specimens without lipemia and hemolysis are preferred.	12-80 ng/mL	× 1.0	[12-80 mcg/L]	None found.

1. Kaplan KL, Owen J: Plasma levels of beta-thromboglobulin and platelet factor 4 as indices of platelet activation in vivo, *Blood* 57:199-202, 1981.

DIAGNOSTIC INFORMATION	REMARKS

↑ Hereditary: Decreased or abnormal fibrinogen (hereditary afibrinogenemia, hypofibrinogenemia, or dysfibrinogenemia)

Acquired: Heparin, DIC, liver disease, increased FDP, and hypoalbuminemia

The thrombin time (TT) is a clot-based assay that measures the conversion of fibrinogen to fibrin. The TT is therefore affected by the level of fibrinogen and the presence of FDPs. Because it bypasses all other coagulation reactions, it is not influenced by deficiencies of other coagulation factors.

The TT is very sensitive to heparin and has been used to monitor unfractionated heparin. However, other tests have replaced the TT for heparin monitoring; when used for this purpose, a recalcified TT assay is recommended. A modification of the TT, the high-dose TT, has been used for monitoring high doses (>1.5 U/mL) of heparin.

A common cause of a significantly prolonged TT is heparin; if heparin effect is suspected, heparin neutralization or a Reptilase time can be performed (Reptilase time not affected by heparin). Heparin neutralization has replaced the need for a TT for evaluation of heparin contamination in many laboratories.

↑ In vivo activation of platelets; renal failure, diabetes mellitus, deep-vein thrombosis, after acute myocardial infarction, and in preeclampsia

β-Thromboglobulin (β-TG) is rarely performed for evaluating platelet "hyperreactivity" and activation. β-TG is a heparin-binding protein found on platelet alpha granules and released on platelet activation.

β-TG can be measured by immunoassays (ELISA or RIA). The test is subject to in vitro platelet β-TG release and therefore may have falsely high values.

TEST NAME AND METHOD	SPECIMEN REQUIREMENTS	REFERENCE INTERVAL, CONVENTIONAL [INTERNATIONAL RECOMMENDED UNITS]			CHEMICAL INTERFERENCES AND IN VIVO EFFECTS
Thyroglobulin (Tg)[1-5] *Immunoassay*	Serum. Stable up to 2 days at 2-8° C. For longer periods, store frozen at −70° C; avoid repeated freezing and thawing.	3-40 ng/mL[1]* *Reference intervals are assay dependent.	× 1.0	[3-40 mcg/L]	

1. Baloch Z, Carayon P, Conte-Devolx B, et al: Laboratory medicine practice guidelines. Laboratory support for the diagnosis and monitoring of thyroid disease, *Thyroid* 13:3-126, 2003.

2. Ringel MD, Ladenson PW: Controversies in the follow-up and management of well-differentiated thyroid cancer, *Endocr Relat Cancer* 11:97-116, 2004.

3. Whitley RJ, Ain KB: Thyroglobulin: a specific serum marker for the management of thyroid carcinoma, *Clin Lab Med* 24:29-47, 2004.

4. Demers LM, Spencer C: The thyroid. In Burtis CA, Ashwood ER, Bruns DE, editors: *Tietz textbook of clinical chemistry,* ed 4, Philadelphia, 2006, WB Saunders.

5. Spencer CA, Wang C-C: Thyroglobulin measurement. Techniques, clinical benefits, and pitfalls, *Endocrinol Metab Clin North Am* 24:841-863, 1995.

TEST NAME AND METHOD	SPECIMEN REQUIREMENTS	REFERENCE INTERVAL, CONVENTIONAL [INTERNATIONAL RECOMMENDED UNITS]				CHEMICAL INTERFERENCES AND IN VIVO EFFECTS
Thyroid Hormone-Binding Ratio (THBR)[1-4]	Serum. Store at 4° C if test is not performed in 24 hr. Stable for at least 30 days frozen.	*THBR*[5] Cord:	0.75-1.05 (x̄: 0.90)	× 1.0	*AU** [0.75-1.05] [x̄: 0.90]	↑ V Androgens, asparaginase, barbiturates, bishydroxycoumarin, corticosteroids, danazol, phenylbutazone, salicylates, and valproic acid
		1-3 days:	0.90-1.40 (x̄: 1.15)		[0.90-1.40] [x̄: 1.15]	
		1-2 wk:	0.85-1.15 (x̄: 1.00)		[0.85-1.15] [x̄: 1.00]	
		1-4 mo:	0.75-1.05 (x̄: 0.90)		[0.75-1.05] [x̄: 0.90]	↓ V Estrogens, methadone, and oral contraceptives
		1-15 yr:	0.88-1.12 (x̄: 1.00)		[0.88-1.12] [x̄: 1.00]	

DIAGNOSTIC INFORMATION	REMARKS

Thyroglobulin (Tg) is a tumor marker for monitoring the status of patients with well-differentiated (papillary or follicular) thyroid cancer. It is used for the determination of residual thyroid tissue or recurrent disease, not for the diagnosis of thyroid cancer. Sensitivity for detecting recurrence can be improved with TSH stimulation of Tg concentrations after either thyroxine withdrawal or recombinant TSH administration. In this setting, Tg may be used in conjunction with whole body ^{131}I scans. Validation of use of Tg as a tumor marker postoperatively can be confirmed by preoperative measurements where two thirds of patients have elevated Tg concentrations.[2,3]

The majority of patients with elevated Tg concentrations have benign thyroid conditions because Tg is a nonspecific indicator of thyroid dysfunction. Concentrations can be elevated in Hashimoto's thyroiditis, Graves' disease, thyroid adenoma, and subacute thyroiditis. Serum Tg measurements may also aid in diagnosing thyrotoxicosis factitia, characterized by a low serum Tg, and investigating the etiology of congenital hypothyroidism in infants.[1,4]

Tg is a 660-kDa dimeric glycoprotein synthesized in the follicular colloid of the thyroid gland and regulated by TSH. Tg is the precursor protein for thyroid hormone synthesis. Most normal euthyroid individuals have detectable serum Tg concentrations. Tg concentrations and therefore reference intervals can be affected by iodine intake influenced by geographic location.[1,3]

Assays for Tg include both RIA and immunometric (IMA) formats, and several methods are available on automated platforms. Both assay formats can be affected by interference from Tg autoantibodies present in ~20% of thyroid cancer patients and 10% of normal subjects. IMA assays are more likely to be affected by Tg autoantibodies, causing an underestimation in Tg concentrations. Therefore the Tg autoantibody status of patients should be determined when measuring Tg.[1,3,5]

↑ Hyperthyroidism, states with decreased TBG (e.g., androgen treatment, chronic liver disease), protein loss (renal, gastrointestinal) or genetically low TBG, and thyrotoxicosis factitia

↓ Hypothyroidism, states with increased TBG (e.g., estrogen treatment, pregnancy, acute hepatitis, genetically high TBG)

Concordant variance of T_4 and THBR tests suggests altered thyroid function; discordant variance suggests primary change in TBG in a euthyroid state (e.g., pregnancy). In pregnancy, the FT_4I (THBR × T_4) should be within the reference interval. (See also *Free Thyroxine Index*.)

The THBR is derived from a version of the T_3 or T_4 uptake test. In the isotopic T uptake test, resin (or other solid-phase binding material) and radioactive T_3 or T_4 are added to a patient's serum, and the proportion of tracer bound by the solid matrix (the "uptake") is measured. In most nonisotopic assays, the binder is a T_4 antibody.

The result for the patient's serum is divided by that for a reference serum to give a ratio. The ratio is proportional to the free fraction of T_4 or T_3 in serum and is properly known as the THBR:

$$THBR = \frac{\% \text{ T uptake (patient serum)}}{\% \text{ T uptake (reference serum)}}$$

TEST NAME AND METHOD	SPECIMEN REQUIREMENTS	REFERENCE INTERVAL, CONVENTIONAL [INTERNATIONAL RECOMMENDED UNITS]	CHEMICAL INTERFERENCES AND IN VIVO EFFECTS
Thyroid Hormone-Binding Ratio—CONT			
		Adult[6]	↓ C Triidothyronine autoantibodies
		20-49 yr: 0.85-1.14 [0.85-1.14]	
		50-90 yr: 0.78-1.15 [0.78-1.15]	
		Pregnancy	
		(last 5 mo): 0.68-0.87 [0.68-0.87]	
		*AU, Arbitrary units.	

1. Alsever RN, Gotlin RW: *Handbook of endocrine tests in adults and children,* ed 2, Chicago, 1978, Year Book Medical Publishers, Inc.

2. Committee on Nomenclature of the American Thyroid Association: Revised nomenclature for tests of thyroid hormones and thyroid-related proteins in serum, *J Clin Endocrinol Metab* 64:1089-1094, 1987.

3. Hay ID, Bayer MF, Kaplan MK, et al: American Thyroid Association assessment of current free thyroid hormone and thyrotropin measurement and guidelines for future clinical assays, *Clin Chem* 37:2002-2008, 1991.

4. Demers LM, Spencer C: The thyroid. In Burtis CA, Ashwood ER, Bruns DE, editors: *Tietz textbook of clinical chemistry,* ed 4, Philadelphia, 2006, WB Saunders.

5. Hung W, August GP, Glasgow AM: *Pediatric endocrinology,* New Hyde Park, NY, 1983, Medical Examination Publishing Co.

6. Nichols Institute Reference Laboratories: *Test catalog,* San Juan Capistrano, CA, 1993, Nichols Institute Reference Laboratories.

Thyroid Microsomal Antibodies[1,2]	Serum. Inactivate at 56° C for 30 min. Freeze if test not performed within 24 hr.	Undetectable	None found.
Hemagglutination			
Complement-fixation antibody[3]		<1:100	

DIAGNOSTIC INFORMATION	REMARKS

A THBR >1.15 indicates reduced availability of TBG binding sites for T_4, whereas a THBR <0.85 indicates an increased availability of TBG binding sites for T_4.

Although centered on a ratio of 1.0, reference values may differ with laboratory and method. THBR replaces the T_3 resin uptake test.

In pregnancy, the THBR gradually decreases (as early as 3-6 wk after conception) until the end of the first trimester and then remains relatively constant. It returns to normal 12-13 wk postpartum, but in certain cases of habitual threatened abortion and in pregnancy complicated by hyperthyroidism decreases are not observed.

The THBR test is useful in differentiating T_3 and T_4 changes in primary thyroidal disorders from changes in total T_3 and T_4 as a result of primary changes in TBG.

THBR is not acceptable as an independent and isolated test because it correlates poorly with the concentration of T_4 in serum and with the clinical status of the patient, largely because of the variability of the concentration of TBG in health and disease. THBR is only useful when combined with total T_4 to calculate the FT_4 index. (See *Free Thyroxine Index; Thyroxine, Free;* and *Thyroxine-Binding Globulin.*)

Low titers have been detected in 5-10% of normal individuals with no symptoms of disease.

This test is more sensitive for Hashimoto's thyroiditis than the thyroglobulin antibodies assay but not better than the thyroid peroxidase antibody test for assessing thyroid antibodies. See *Thyroglobulin Antibodies and Anti-TPO.*

An agglutination test positive at a 1:2500 dilution is equivalent to histological proof of Hashimoto's disease. There is no greater frequency of detection in multinodular goiter and thyroid adenomas or carcinomas than in normal subjects.

Frequency of positive results in thyroid autoimmune disease is higher than in the thyroglobulin antibodies test, especially in people aged <20 yr but about the same for anti-TPO.

Titers decrease progressively during pregnancy and increase transiently postpartum.

Positive: Hashimoto's thyroiditis (up to 8% give negative results), thyroid carcinoma (positive in $<10\%$ of cases), early hypothyroidism (positive in 99% of cases), pernicious anemia (in $>5\%$ of cases, low titers); also detectable in some patients with Graves' disease.

Positive titer in conjunction with the presence of thyroglobulin antibodies is highly indicative of Hashimoto's thyroiditis. Complement-fixing microsomal antibodies are often not found in proven cases of thyroiditis, suggesting a lack of sensitivity of the technique. Any positive test should be accepted as significant.

TEST NAME AND METHOD	SPECIMEN REQUIREMENTS	REFERENCE INTERVAL, CONVENTIONAL [INTERNATIONAL RECOMMENDED UNITS]	CHEMICAL INTERFERENCES AND IN VIVO EFFECTS
Thyroid Microsomal Antibodies—CONT			
CPB radioassay[4,5]	Serum. Patient should not have received therapeutic amounts of radioactive material for 1 mo before test.	Adult, child: $\leq$25 U/mL[7] × 1.0 [$\leq$25 kU/L]	
IRMA[6]	Serum. Store at −20° C.	280 ± 60 U/mL (SEM) × 1.0 [280 ± 60 kU/L]	

1. Baker BA, Gharib H, Markowitz H: Correlation of thyroid antibodies and cytologic features in suspected autoimmune thyroid disease, *Am J Med* 74:941-944, 1983.
2. Mathé G, editor: *A symposium on physiological levels of calcitonin in man,* New York, 1984, Masson Publishing USA.
3. Alsever RN, Gotlin RW: *Handbook of endocrine tests in adults and children,* ed 2, Chicago, 1978, Year Book Medical Publishers, Inc.
4. Nichols Institute Reference Laboratories: *Test catalog,* San Juan Capistrano, CA, 2001, Nichols Institute Reference Laboratories.
5. Mori T, Kriss JP: Measurements by competitive-binding radioassay of serum anti-thyroglobulin antibodies in Graves' disease and other thyroid disorders, *J Clin Endocrinol Metab* 33:688-698, 1971.
6. Massart C, Guilhem I, Gibassier J, et al: Comparison of thyroperoxidase and microsomal antibody assays in sera from patients with Graves' disease, *Clin Chem* 37:1777-1780, 1991.
7. Ng M, Rajna A, Khalid B: Enzyme immunoassay for simultaneous measurement of autoantibodies against thyroglobulin and thyroid microsome in serum, *Clin Chem* 33:2286-2288, 1987.

TEST NAME AND METHOD	SPECIMEN REQUIREMENTS	REFERENCE INTERVAL, CONVENTIONAL [INTERNATIONAL RECOMMENDED UNITS]	CHEMICAL INTERFERENCES AND IN VIVO EFFECTS
Thyroid Peroxidase (TPO) Antibodies[1-3] *Immunometric assay*[4]	Serum. Store at −20° C.	69 ± 15 U/mL (SEM)[3] × 1.0 [69 ± 15 kU/L]	None found.

DIAGNOSTIC INFORMATION	**REMARKS**
	Sensitivity: 20 U/mL [20 kU/L]; abnormal values with this method may exceed 500,000 U/mL [500,000 kU/L]. It is claimed that the CPB method gives high results in 80-90% of patients with Hashimoto's thyroiditis and is elevated in all patients with Graves' disease. [131]I treatment of Graves' disease increases the levels ~15-fold.
Values >400 U/mL [>400 kU/L] have been observed in Graves' disease (77% of cases, median value being 8100 U/mL [8100 kU/L]).[6]	IRMA and ELISA[7] techniques are more sensitive and specific than hemagglutination assays for the detection of thyroid autoantibodies and are now the methods of choice for determining thyroid autoantibodies. In addition, measurement of antibodies to thyroid peroxidase (anti-TPO) has essentially replaced the measurement of antimicrosomal antibody titers for assessing thyroid autoantibodies in patients with thyroid disease. See also *Thyroid Peroxidase Antibodies*.
Autoimmune thyroid disease (Hashimoto's thyroiditis, idiopathic myxedema, Graves' disease) Positive titers are found in >50% of patients with Graves' disease, >80% of patients with autoimmune thyroiditis, and ~40% of patients with insulin-dependent diabetes mellitus. Approximately 14% of pregnant women have a positive titer for anti-TPO.	TPO is the principal and possibly only autoantigenic component of thyroid microsomes. ELISA-based assays for anti-TPO antibodies provide greater sensitivity and specificity than hemagglutination assays for microsomal antibodies for detecting and monitoring autoimmune thyroid disorders.[2]

TEST NAME AND METHOD	SPECIMEN REQUIREMENTS	REFERENCE INTERVAL, CONVENTIONAL [INTERNATIONAL RECOMMENDED UNITS]	CHEMICAL INTERFERENCES AND IN VIVO EFFECTS
Thyroid Peroxidase (TPO) Antibodies—CONT			

1. Endres D: Antithyroid peroxidase antibodies (antimicrosomal antibodies) in thyroid disease, *AACC Endo Metab In-Service Training Cont Educ* 10:3-5, 1991.
2. Demers LM, Spencer C: The thyroid. In Burtis CA, Ashwood ER, Bruns DE, editors: *Tietz textbook of clinical chemistry,* ed 4, Philadelphia, 2006, WB Saunders.
3. Massart C, Guilhem I, Gibassier J, et al: Comparison of thyroperoxidase and microsomal antibody assays in sera from patients with Graves' disease, *Clin Chem* 37:1777-1780, 1991.
4. Ruf J, Czarnocka B, Ferrand M, et al: Novel routine assay of thyroperoxidase autoantibodies, *Clin Chem* 34:2231-2234, 1988.

TEST NAME AND METHOD	SPECIMEN REQUIREMENTS	REFERENCE INTERVAL, CONVENTIONAL [INTERNATIONAL RECOMMENDED UNITS]	CHEMICAL INTERFERENCES AND IN VIVO EFFECTS
Thyroid Scan with Radioactive Iodine[1-5] Dose, adult: 100-300 μCi ^{123}I orally Child: ^{123}I, age-adjusted dose	Scintiscan of the thyroid region is obtained 24 hr after the administration of radioiodine.	Homogeneous pattern with symmetrical lobes. The right lobe is slightly larger and ~0.5 cm [5 mm] higher than the left. In adults, the right lobe measures 5.1 ± 0.8 cm [51 ± 8 mm] and the left 4.6 ± 0.8 cm [46 ± 8 mm]. The width of each lobe is 2.6 ± 0.2 cm [26 ± 2 mm]. The margins may be slightly lobulated. The isthmus is ~2 cm [20 mm] in width. The finding of a pyramidal lobe suggests thyroid disease.	See *Thyroid Uptake of Radioactive Iodine,* ^{131}*I* or ^{123}*I.*

1. Alsever RN, Gotlin RW: *Handbook of endocrine tests in adults and children,* ed 2, Chicago, 1978, Year Book Medical Publishers, Inc.
2. DeGroot LJ, Larsen PJ, Refetoff S, et al: *The thyroid and its diseases,* ed 5, New York, 1984, John Wiley and Sons.
3. Larsen PR, Davies TF, Schlumberger MJ, et al: The thyroid gland. In Larsen PR, Kronenberg HM, Melmed S, et al, editors: *Williams textbook of endocrinology,* ed 10, Philadelphia, 2003, WB Saunders.
4. Miller RE, Ngai B: *Manual of endocrine diagnostic tests,* ed 4, Lexington, KY, 1991, Department of Medicine, University of Kentucky.
5. Wartofsky L, Ingbar SH: Diseases of the thyroid. In Wilson JD, Braunwald E, Isselbacher KJ, et al, editors: *Harrison's principles of internal medicine,* ed 12, New York, 1991, McGraw-Hill Inc.

DIAGNOSTIC INFORMATION	REMARKS

In nonimmune thyroid disease, the frequency of detectable anti-TPO antibodies is similar to that observed in normal individuals.

Antibodies to thyroid peroxidase are found in 8-27% of the normal population.

In Graves' disease, hyperfunctioning enlarged thyroid tissue usually delineates the entire gland; in toxic nodular goiter, only hyperfunctioning adenomas are visible on the scan; subacute thyroiditis fails to portray the thyroid gland when the inflammation is bilateral. The presence of a single "cold" nodule increases suspicion of malignancy. A "hot" nodule is considered benign in 99.8% of cases with ^{123}I scans and in 98% with ^{99m}Tc scans. (See *Technetium Scan Procedure.*)

Indications for thyroid scan: Detection of ectopic thyroid tissue in thyroid agenesis; evaluation of extraglandular, functioning thyroid carcinoma after ablation of the normal gland; and evaluation of glands in patients with previous neck irradiation (of tonsils, thymus, and acne).

Cold nodules on ^{123}I (or ^{131}I) scans are rarely hot on ^{99m}Tc scans. For children the thyroid scan has limited indications. Because technetium scans may be produced in a matter of minutes, they are generally preferred over ^{123}I for children, except for those rare instances that require definition of the kinetics of iodine metabolism, e.g., familial goiter resulting from enzyme defect. (See also *Perchlorate Discharge Test.*)

A significantly larger dose of radioactive iodine is needed for a scan than for an uptake test. Unless specific information regarding distribution of function is desired, one should not request a radioactive iodine scan as part of a routine thyroid workup. ^{123}I is preferred over ^{131}I for routine scanning because radiation exposure and half-life are less.

TEST NAME AND METHOD	SPECIMEN REQUIREMENTS	REFERENCE INTERVAL, CONVENTIONAL [INTERNATIONAL RECOMMENDED UNITS]			CHEMICAL INTERFERENCES AND IN VIVO EFFECTS
Thyroid Uptake of Radioactive Iodine, ^{131}I or ^{123}I (RAIU)[1-3] Dose: 2-15 μCi ^{131}I or 100-350 μCi ^{123}I, usually orally	Count activity over thyroid gland at intervals between 20 min and 24 hr.[1]		*%* 2 hr: <6 × 0.01 6 hr: 3-20 24 hr: 8-30 24-hr uptake of ^{131}I averages 70% [fractional uptake, 0.70] during the first 3 days of life and then decreases rapidly; normal values for infants and children tend to be higher than those for adults.[4]	*Fractional uptake* [<0.06] [0.03-0.20] [0.08-0.30]	↑ V Lithium ↓ V Aminosalicylic acid (PAS), antithyroid drugs (propylthiouracil, methimazole), clofibrate, corticosteroids, corticotropin, oxyphenylbutazone, phenylbutazone, sulfonylureas, and vitamin A (retinol) Intake of preparations containing iodine can cause a decrease in RAIU, e.g., cough syrups and lozenges, gargles, cod liver oil products, multivitamin products, salt substitutes, toothpaste, asthma medications, radiographic contrast media, potassium iodide (large doses), and Lugol's solution. ↓ C Anti-T_3

1. Eastham RD: *Biochemical values in clinical medicine,* ed 7, Bristol, UK, 1985, John Wright and Sons Ltd.
2. Wilson JD, Braunwald E, Isselbacher KJ, et al, editors: *Harrison's principles of internal medicine,* ed 12, New York, 1991, McGraw-Hill Publishing Co.
3. Miller RE, Ngai B: *Manual of endocrine diagnostic tests,* ed 4, Lexington, KY, 1991, Department of Medicine, University of Kentucky.
4. Gardner LI, editor: *Endocrine and genetic diseases of childhood and adolescence,* Philadelphia, 1975, WB Saunders.

Thyroid-Stimulating Hormone (TSH) Stimulation Test[1-3] Dose, adult: 10 U Thyrotropin (Thytropar), IM, daily for 1-3 days	Day 1: Give 2-15 μCi ^{131}I. Day 2: Measure 24-hr ^{131}I-uptake and give 10 U TSH, IM. Days 3-4: Give 10 U TSH on days 3 and 4.	Normal thyroid glands increase ^{131}I-uptake into the slightly hyperthyroid range, and the second ^{131}I-uptake should be higher than the first by 10-20%. Subjects with "low normal" uptake show increase to "high normal."	See *Thyroid Uptake of Radioactive Iodine,* ^{131}I or ^{123}I.

DIAGNOSTIC INFORMATION	REMARKS

↑ Hyperthyroidism with rapid release: 2 hr, >40% [>0.40]; 6 hr, >30% [>0.30]; and 24 hr, >55% [>0.55]. Compensatory hyperactivity without thyrotoxicosis (endemic goiter) caused by low iodide intake with slow release; gigantism and acromegaly (if basal metabolic rate is increased); after withdrawal of thyroid-suppressing drug; after excessive thyroxine loss in urine in some cases of nephrosis; and acute renal failure.

↓ Hypothyroidism, hypopituitarism, chronic renal failure; in early phase of subacute thyroiditis at 24-hr activity decreased to 0-1% [0.0-0.01] unless the disease is still unilateral; thyrotoxicosis factitia; and iodine-induced hyperthyroidism.

Identify hot and cold spots of iodine uptake directly to establish the diagnosis of thyroid adenoma or thyroid cancer.

The only direct test of thyroid function uses a radioactive isotope of iodine. ^{123}I is preferred because of lower radiation dose. Reference interval varies with geographical location and is inversely related to the intake. The test is falsely low in individuals with expanded total iodine pool and falsely increased in patients with contracted iodine pool. Thirty to 70% of hyperthyroid patients with rapid iodine turnover in the thyroid give normal results (24-hr values); 6-hr values often demonstrate the thyroid's increased affinity for iodine.

False elevations may be seen in some euthyroid patients with Hashimoto's thyroiditis or congenital organification defects.

Test is less reliable in hypothyroidism. In children, RAIU is limited to rare instances that require definition of the kinetics of iodine metabolism, e.g., familial goiter resulting from enzyme defect (see *Perchlorate Discharge Test*). See also *Technetium Uptake*.

Test used less frequently than in the past because of improvements in indirect methods for assessing thyroid status and the widespread increase in dietary iodine intake in most countries.

Positive response in secondary hypothyroidism; no response in primary hypothyroidism or diminished thyroid reserve.

Other important uses of the test include determining whether nonfunctioning areas of the thyroid (as indicated by scanning methods) are actually capable of function; determining thyroid reserve in patients taking thyroid hormone replacement; and determining whether the thyroid is capable of function after ablation of thyroid adenomas.

The 3-day test is preferred; nausea, vomiting, local painful reactions at the site of the injection, and hypersensitivity have been reported.

The normal thyroid gland responds to exogenous TSH stimulation by increasing the rate of iodine accumulation. In primary hypothyroidism, the failing thyroid gland is maximally stimulated by endogenous TSH and does not respond to further stimulation. Availability of sensitive TSH assays and the TRH test has markedly reduced the use of this test in clinical practice.

TEST NAME AND METHOD	SPECIMEN REQUIREMENTS	REFERENCE INTERVAL, CONVENTIONAL [INTERNATIONAL RECOMMENDED UNITS]				CHEMICAL INTERFERENCES AND IN VIVO EFFECTS

Thyroid-Stimulating Hormone (TSH) Stimulation Test—CONT

Child: 5 U Thytropar	On day 4, count neck background and give tracer dose [131]I.
	Day 5: Measure 24-hr ^{131}I-uptake (correct for background).

1. Alsever RN, Gotlin RW: *Handbook of endocrine tests in adults and children,* ed 2, Chicago, 1978, Year Book Medical Publishers, Inc.
2. Kaplan S, editor: *Clinical pediatric and adolescent endocrinology,* Philadelphia, 1982, WB Saunders.
3. Larsen PR, Ingbar SH: The thyroid gland. In Wilson JH, Foster DW, editors: *Williams textbook of endocrinology,* ed 8, Philadelphia, 1992, WB Saunders.

TEST NAME AND METHOD	SPECIMEN REQUIREMENTS	REFERENCE INTERVAL				CHEMICAL INTERFERENCES
Thyrotropin (Thyroid-Stimulating Hormone, TSH)	Serum. Stable for 7 days at 4° C and for at least 1 mo frozen.		$\mu U/mL$[10]		mU/L	↑ V Amiodarone, benserazide, clomiphene, decrease in serum-binding proteins, haloperidol, iodides, lithium, methimazole, metoclopramide, morphine, oral radiographic dyes, phenothiazines, propylthiouracil, and TRH
		Premature infants (28-36 wk gestation):				
		1-4 days:	0.7-27	× 1.0	[0.7-27]	
Immunometric assay (third generation)[1-8]		2-20 wk:	1.0-39		[1.0-39]	
		5 mo-20 yr:	1.7-9.1		[1.7-9.1]	
		Adults	0.7-6.4		[0.7-6.4]	
		21-54 yr:	0.4-4.2		[0.4-4.2]	
		55-87 yr:	0.5-8.9		[0.5-8.9]	
		Pregnancy				↑ C TSH autoantibodies (polyclonal assays)
		First trimester:	0.3-4.5		[0.3-4.5]	
		Second trimester:	0.5-4.6		[0.5-4.6]	
		Third trimester:	0.8-5.2		[0.8-5.2]	↓ V Bromocriptine, carbamazepine, corticosteroids, cyproheptadine, dopamine, heparin (IV administration; amounts in hemodialysis fluid sufficient to cause effect), levodopa, metergoline, phentolamine, somatostatin, and triiodothyronine
	Whole blood (heel puncture). Collect 3-7 days after birth.	Newborn screen[11]:	<20		[<20]	
Immunoassay	Amniotic fluid[9]	Trimester				
		Second:	≤1.7		[≤1.7]	↓ C TSH autoantibodies (monoclonal assays)
		Third:	≤0.55		[≤0.55]	

DIAGNOSTIC INFORMATION	REMARKS

↑ Primary hypothyroidism (3-100 times normal), Hashimoto's thyroiditis with clinical hypothyroidism and 33% of patients with Hashimoto's thyroiditis who are clinically euthyroid, ectopic TSH secretion (lung, breast tumors), subacute thyroiditis (recovery phase), nonthyroidal illness (recovery phase), and thyroid hormone resistance

TSH has diurnal rhythm, peaks at 2:00-4:00 AM, and has lowest level at 5:00-6:00 PM with ultradian variations (periods shorter than circadian). Moderately high TSH is often found in euthyroid patients during treatment for hyperthyroidism. In treated hyperthyroid patients, TSH may remain low for 4-6 wk after euthyroid state is achieved.

↓ Primary hyperthyroidism, secondary hypothyroidism (pituitary), tertiary hypothyroidism (hypothalamic), subclinical hyperthyroidism (e.g., toxic multinodular goiter, autonomous thyroid hormone secretion, exogenous thyroid hormone therapy, treated Graves' disease, ophthalmopathy of euthyroid Graves' disease), and euthyroid sick syndrome

TSH surges with birth, peaking at 30 min at 25-160 μU/mL [25-160 mU/L], declining back to cord blood levels by 3 days, and reaching adult values in the first week of life.

TSH measurements with sufficient sensitivity to distinguish low (suppressed) levels from normal have become the preferred first-line test for hyperthyroidism and hypothyroidism. The high-sensitivity test appears to be especially useful in distinguishing sick euthyroid patients; in differentiating mild, subclinical hyperthyroidism from overt Graves' disease; in monitoring thyroid cancer patients on thyroxine; and in monitoring the adequacy of thyroid hormone replacement in hypothyroid patients. If basal serum TSH levels are detectable by a sensitive assay, then no diagnostic benefit is gained by performing a TRH stimulation test.

Immunometric assays including chemiluminescence-based assay sensitivity: 0.01 μU/mL [0.01 mU/L]. Sensitive TSH test is considered by some to be the preferred screening test for evaluation of all thyrometabolic states. Reference ranges and diagnostic utility should be developed for each assay. Some endocrinologists have suggested that the upper reference limit for adults should be reduced to 2.5 mU/L.

Reference ranges for newborn screening should be determined by each laboratory providing screening; significant numbers of samples must be screened to determine sensitivity and specificity for tests provided by that laboratory.

TEST NAME AND METHOD	SPECIMEN REQUIREMENTS	REFERENCE INTERVAL, CONVENTIONAL [INTERNATIONAL RECOMMENDED UNITS]	CHEMICAL INTERFERENCES AND IN VIVO EFFECTS

Thyrotropin—CONT

1. Brabant G, Brabant A, Ranft U, et al: Circadian and pulsatile thyrotropin secretion in euthyroid man under the influence of thyroid hormone and glucocorticoid administration, *J Clin Endocrinol Metab* 65:83-88, 1987.

2. Hay ID, Bayer MF, Kaplan MM, et al: American Thyroid Association assessment of current free thyroid hormone and thyrotropin measurement and guidelines for future clinical assays, *Clin Chem* 37:2002-2008, 1991.

3. Klee GG, Hay ID: Assessment of sensitive thyrotropin assays for an expanded role in thyroid functions testing: proposed criteria for analytic performance and clinical utility, *J Clin Endocrinol Metab* 64:461-471, 1987.

4. Larsen PR, Davies TF, Schlumberger MJ, et al: Thyroid physiology and diagnostic evaluation of patients with thyroid disorders. In Larsen PR, Kronenberg HM, Melmed S, et al, editors: *Williams textbook of endocrinology,* ed 10, Philadelphia, 2003, WB Saunders.

5. Liewendahl K: Thyroid function tests: performance and limitations of current methodologies, *Scand J Clin Lab Invest* 52:435-445, 1992.

6. Nicoloff JT, Spencer CA: The use and misuse of sensitive thyrotropin assays [clinical review 12], *J Clin Endocrinol Metab* 71:553-558, 1990.

TEST NAME AND METHOD	SPECIMEN REQUIREMENTS	REFERENCE INTERVAL, CONVENTIONAL [INTERNATIONAL RECOMMENDED UNITS]	CHEMICAL INTERFERENCES AND IN VIVO EFFECTS
Thyrotropin Autoantibodies (Anti-TSH)[1] *RBA*	Serum or plasma. Stable 4 days at room temperature, 30 days at 4° C.	Negative[2]	None found.

1. Davies TF, Larsen PR: Thyrotoxicosis. In Larsen PR, Kronenberg HM, Melmed S, et al, editors: *Williams textbook of endocrinology,* ed 10, Philadelphia, 2003, WB Saunders.

2. Nichols Institute Reference Laboratories: *Test catalog,* San Juan Capistrano, CA, 2001, Nichols Institute Reference Laboratories.

TEST NAME AND METHOD	SPECIMEN REQUIREMENTS	REFERENCE INTERVAL, CONVENTIONAL [INTERNATIONAL RECOMMENDED UNITS]	CHEMICAL INTERFERENCES AND IN VIVO EFFECTS
Thyrotropin- (TSH-) Receptor Antibodies[1-8] *In vitro adenyl cyclase stimulation assay*	Serum. Store frozen.	<130% of basal activity[9] [× 0.01 = <1.30, basal activity fraction]	None found.

7. Ross DS, Ardisson LG, Meskell MJ: Measurement of thyrotropin in clinical and subclinical hyperthyroidism using a chemiluminescent assay, *J Clin Endocrinol Metab* 69:684-688, 1989.

8. Demers LM, Spencer C: Laboratory medicine practice guidelines: laboratory support for thyroid testing, *Thyroid* 13:4-104, 2003.

9. Kourides IA, Heath CV, Ginsberg-Fellner F: Measurement of thyroid-stimulating hormone in human amniotic fluid, *J Clin Endocrinol Metab* 54:635-637, 1982.

10. Nichols Institute Reference Laboratories: *Test catalog,* San Juan Capistrano, CA, 1993, Nichols Institute Reference Laboratories.

11. Quest diagnostics, Nichols Institute reference manual, 2001, Quest Laboratories.

Autoantibodies to thyrotropin have been described in rare patients with hypopituitarism and spuriously high serum TSH.

Thyrotropin autoantibodies can interfere with immunoassay measurements of TSH; their presence should be considered whenever TSH results are incongruous with the clinical state. See *Thyroxine Autoantibodies.*

Values between 1.3 and 2.0 are seen in 10% of patients with thyroid diseases other than Graves' disease. Values >2.8 have been found only in patients with Graves' disease. High levels of TSI (thyroid-stimulating immunoglobulins) in pregnancy have some predictive value for neonatal thyrotoxicosis. High titers do not necessarily mean high risk to the fetus, but low titers indicate low risk. Test is also useful for predicting relapse or remission in hyperthyroid patients.[7]

Thyrotropin-receptor antibodies are generally used to (1) confirm clinical diagnosis of Graves' disease; (2) evaluate euthyroid patient with bilateral exophthalmos; and (3) determine prognosis of patients with Graves' disease treated with antithyroid agents.

Thyrotropin-receptor antibodies are a group of related heterogeneous IgG immunoglobulins that bind to thyroid cell membranes at or near the TSH-receptor site. Their effects on thyroid function are variable.

Two types of tests are usually used for the detection of thyrotropin-receptor antibodies. The first test (TBII) determines the capacity of patient serum or IgG to inhibit binding of ^{125}I-labeled TSH-to-TSH receptors from thyroid membrane preparations.

The second test, also called TSI or TSAb (thyroid-stimulating antibodies), assesses the capacity of patient serum or IgG to stimulate adenylate cyclase or to enhance thyroid hormone or Tg secretion or iodine uptake in isolated thyroid epithelial cells. Routine use of this test has been improved by the use of cloned, functioning rat thyroid follicular cells (FRTL-5); human thyroid cells were used previously. The usefulness of the TSI test is limited because it detects stimulating antibodies only.

TEST NAME AND METHOD	SPECIMEN REQUIREMENTS	REFERENCE INTERVAL, CONVENTIONAL [INTERNATIONAL RECOMMENDED UNITS]	CHEMICAL INTERFERENCES AND IN VIVO EFFECTS
Thyrotropin- (TSH-) Receptor Antibodies—CONT			
Binding inhibition assay		<10% inhibition[10] [× 0.01 = <0.10 fraction inhibition]	
In vitro radiobioassay		<130% of basal activity[11] [× 0.01 = <1.30, basal activity fraction]	

1. Arikawa K, Ichikawa Y, Yoshida T, et al: Blocking antithyrotropin receptor antibody in patients with nongoitrous hypothyroidism: its incidence and characteristics of action, *J Clin Endocrinol Metab* 60:953-959, 1985.

2. Autoimmune thyroid disease, *Lab Rep Physicians* 7:26-31, 1985.

3. Davies TF, Larsen PR: Thyrotoxicosis. In Larsen PR, Kronenberg HM, Melmed S, et al, editors: *Williams textbook of endocrinology,* ed 10, Philadelphia, 2003, WB Saunders.

4. Drexhage HA: Immunoglobulins affecting thyroid growth, *Thyroid Today* 8:1-5, 1985.

5. Konishi J, Iida Y, Kasagi K, et al: Primary myxedema with thyrotropin-binding inhibitor immunoglobulins, *Ann Intern Med* 103:26-31, 1985.

6. Kraiem Z, Glaser B, Yigla M, et al: Toxic multinodular goiter: a variant of autoimmune hyperthyroidism, *J Clin Endocrinol Metab* 65:659-664, 1987.

7. Morris J, Hay I, Nelson R, et al: Clinical utility of thyrotropin-receptor antibody assays: comparison of radioreceptor and bioassay methods, *Mayo Clin Proc* 63:707-717, 1988.

8. Van Der Gagg RG, Drexhage HA, Wiersinga WM, et al: Further studies on thyroid growth-stimulating immunoglobulins in euthyroid nonendemic goiter, *J Clin Endocrinol Metab* 60:972-979, 1985.

9. Mayo Medical Laboratories: *Test catalog,* Rochester, MN, 2004, Mayo Medical Laboratories.

10. Nichols Institute Reference Laboratories: *Test catalog,* San Juan Capistrano, CA, 2001, Nichols Institute Reference Laboratories.

11. Fisher DA, Pandian M, Carlton E: *Thyroid growth stimulating immunoglobulin. Assay report from Nichols Institute,* San Juan Capistrano, CA, Nichols Institute Reference Laboratories.

12. Massart C, Hody B, Mouchel L, et al: Assays for thyrotropin-receptor binding and thyroid-stimulating antibodies in sera from patients with Graves' disease, *Clin Chem* 32:1332-1335, 1986.

Assay detects TSH-receptor antibodies in >85% of patients with Graves' disease, treated or untreated.[12] Test is of some use in following the course of therapy, predicting remission or relapse, and predicting neonatal thyroid disease secondary to maternal disease.

The TBII (thyroid-binding inhibiting immunoglobulins) test detects all TSH-receptor antibodies (stimulating, neutral, and inhibiting antibodies) but gives no information regarding functions of the antibodies. TBII is more definitive than TSI for suspected acute toxic goiter, and the frequency of positive results in patients with active disease is ~90%.

↑ Graves' disease, autoimmune thyroiditis, and nonspecific goiter

Further clinical correlation is needed, but presently test is most useful in identifying a possible cause for unexplained goiter (e.g., no TSI or TBII detected).

Test is also called TGI (thyroid-growth immunoglobulins). TGI stimulates labeled thymidine uptake (DNA synthesis) causing follicle cell growth, independent of TSI. However, test has limited clinical usefulness.

In active thyrotoxicosis, TGI is detected only in the presence of thyroid enlargement. In simple goiters, TGI is present but has 10 times less potency

TEST NAME AND METHOD	SPECIMEN REQUIREMENTS	REFERENCE INTERVAL, CONVENTIONAL [INTERNATIONAL RECOMMENDED UNITS]			CHEMICAL INTERFERENCES AND IN VIVO EFFECTS
Thyroxine Autoantibodies (Anti-T$_4$)[1-6] *RBA*	Serum or plasma. Stable 4 days at room temperature, 30 days at 4° C.	Negative[7]			None found.

1. Allan DJ, Murphy F, Needham CA, et al: Sensitive test for thyroid hormone autoantibodies in serum, *Lancet* 2:824, 1982.
2. Beck-Peccoz P, Romelli PB, Cattaneo MG, et al: Evaluation of free thyroxine methods in the presence of iodothyronine-binding autoantibodies, *J Clin Endocrinol Metab* 58:736-739, 1984.
3. DeGroot LJ, Larsen PJ, Refetoff S, et al: *The thyroid and its diseases,* ed 5, New York, 1984, John Wiley and Sons.
4. Karlsson FA, Wibell L, Wide L: Hypothyroidism due to thyroid hormone binding antibodies, *N Engl J Med* 296:1146-1148, 1977.
5. Larsen PR, Davies TF, Schlumberger MJ, et al: The thyroid gland. In Larsen PR, Kronenberg HM, Melmed S, et al, editors: *Williams textbook of endocrinology,* ed 10, Philadelphia, 2003, WB Saunders.
6. Sakata S, Nakamura S, Miura K: Autoantibodies against thyroid hormones or iodothyronine, *Ann Intern Med* 103:579-589, 1985.
7. Nichols Institute Reference Laboratories: *Test catalog,* San Juan Capistrano, CA, 1993, Nichols Institute Reference Laboratories.
8. Hay ID, Bayer MF, Kaplan MK, et al: American Thyroid Association assessment of current free thyroid hormone and thyrotropin measurement and guidelines for future clinical assays, *Clin Chem* 37:2002-2008, 1991.

TEST NAME AND METHOD	SPECIMEN REQUIREMENTS	REFERENCE INTERVAL, CONVENTIONAL			[INTERNATIONAL RECOMMENDED UNITS]	CHEMICAL INTERFERENCES AND IN VIVO EFFECTS
Thyroxine, Free (FT$_4$)[1-5] *Equilibrium dialysis (direct)*[6,7]	Serum. Stable for 7 days at room temperature, but storage at 4° C is preferred. Stable for at least 30 days frozen.	Newborn (1-4 days): Child (2 wk-20 yr): Adult (21-87 yr): Pregnancy First trimester: Second and third trimesters:	*ng/dL*[10] 2.2-5.3 0.8-2.0 0.8-2.7 0.7-2.0 0.5-1.6	× 12.9	*pmol/L* [28-68] [10-26] [10-35] [9-26] [6-21]	↑ V Amiodarone, aspirin, danazol, iopanoic acid, and propranolol ↓ V Anticonvulsants (carbamazepine, phenytoin), methadone, and rifampicin
Equilibrium dialysis (tracer)[4]		Cord: Newborn: Adult:	1.7-4.0[11] 2.6-6.3 0.8-2.3		[22-52] [34-81] [10-30]	↑ C Diflunisal, furosemide, heparin (equilibrium dialysis), and meclofenamic acid
Immunoassays (direct two-step and one-step)[8,9]			0.7-2.0[12]		[9-26]	↓ C Heparin (in analog assays)

DIAGNOSTIC INFORMATION	REMARKS

Thyroxine autoantibodies are present in Hashimoto's thyroiditis and primary hypothyroidism (54%), Graves' disease (26%), nodular or diffuse goiter (9%), and thyroid cancer (1%); role in pathogenesis is unclear.[6]

The presence of thyroxine autoantibodies is relatively rare but when present can interfere with RIA for total and free (direct-analog) thyroid hormone assays. This interference produces either low or high results, depending on the separation method.[6] The calculated FT_4 index may also be abnormally high when T_4 autoantibodies are present.[8] The presence of autoantibodies should be considered when T_4 test results are discordant with the clinical state. Autoantibodies to thyroid hormones are a rare cause of hypothyroidism. They usually do not interfere with thyroid function.

FT_4 methods are still valid if the tracer does not come into contact with plasma proteins during the assay procedure.

↑ Hyperthyroidism; hypothyroidism treated with thyroxine

FT_4 is 0.02-0.04% of total T_4.

↓ Hypothyroidism; hypothyroidism treated with triiodothyronine; and late pregnancy

FT_4 assays based on direct equilibrium dialysis (or ultrafiltration) are considered reference methods. These procedures separate free hormone from protein-bound hormone before direct measurement of the free fraction with a sensitive T_4 immunoassay. All other methods for assessing FT_4 concentrations are estimates: FT_4E is being used to denote FT_4 estimate. FT_4 derived from equilibrium tracer dialysis; direct, including two-step and one-step (analog), immunoassays; and the calculated FT_4 index.

Fluctuations in FT_4 level may occur in euthyroid patients during acute or chronic nonthyroidal illnesses.

Used in conjunction with sensitive TSH result except in patients with known pituitary failure.

FT_4 results obtained by dialysis or reference methods are independent of abnormal binding proteins. FT_4 estimate methods give results comparable with reference methods in healthy subjects, hyperthyroid and hypothyroid patients, and patients with only mild binding protein abnormalities. FT_4 estimate methods, particularly the FT_4 index and one-step methods, are unreliable in euthyroid patients with dysalbuminemic hyperthy-

TEST NAME AND METHOD	SPECIMEN REQUIREMENTS	REFERENCE INTERVAL, CONVENTIONAL [INTERNATIONAL RECOMMENDED UNITS]	CHEMICAL INTERFERENCES AND IN VIVO EFFECTS
Thyroxine, Free—CONT			

1. Demers LM, Spencer C: Laboratory medicine practice guidelines: laboratory support for thyroid testing, *Thyroid* 13:4-104, 2003.
2. Larsen PR, Davies TF, Schlumberger MJ, et al: The thyroid gland. In Larsen PR, Kronenberg HM, Melmed S, et al, editors: *Williams textbook of endocrinology,* ed 10, Philadelphia, 2003, WB Saunders.
3. Pearce CJ, Byfield PGH: Free thyroid hormone assays and thyroid function, *Ann Clin Biochem* 23:230-237, 1986.
4. Whitley RJ, Meikle AW, Watts NB: Endocrinology. In Burtis CA, Ashwood ER, editors: *Tietz textbook of clinical chemistry,* ed 2, Philadelphia, 1994, WB Saunders.
5. Wilke TJ: Estimation of free thyroid hormone concentrations in the clinical laboratory [review], *Clin Chem* 32:585-592, 1986.
6. Nelson J, Tomei R: Direct determination of free thyroxin in undiluted serum by equilibrium dialysis/radioimmunoassay, *Clin Chem* 34:1737-1744, 1988.
7. Tikanoja S, Liewendahl R: New ultrafiltration method for free thyroxin compared with equilibrium dialysis in patients with thyroid dysfunction and nonthyroidal illness, *Clin Chem* 36:800-804, 1990.
8. Ekins R: Measurement of free hormones in blood, *Endocr Rev* 11:5-46, 1990.
9. Liewendahl K: Thyroid function tests: performance and limitations of current methodologies, *Scand J Clin Lab Invest* 52:435-445, 1992.
10. Nichols Institute Reference Laboratories: *Test catalog,* San Juan Capistrano, CA, 2001, Nichols Institute Reference Laboratories.
11. Endocrine Sciences: *Pediatric laboratory services,* Tarzana, CA, 1992, Endocrine Sciences.
12. Mayo Medical Laboratories: *Test catalog,* Rochester, MN, 2004, Mayo Medical Laboratories.

TEST NAME AND METHOD	SPECIMEN REQUIREMENTS	REFERENCE INTERVAL, CONVENTIONAL [INTERNATIONAL RECOMMENDED UNITS]	CHEMICAL INTERFERENCES AND IN VIVO EFFECTS
Thyroxine Suppression Test[1,2] Dose: 3 mg of L-thyroxine orally (single dose)	^{131}I-uptake measured before and 1 wk after thyroxine administration.	>50% decrease of ^{131}I-uptake at 24 hr in second measurement	See *Thyroid Uptake of Radioactive Iodine,* [131]*I or* [123]*I.*

roidism, congenital TBG excess or deficiency, nonthyroidal illnesses, and patients with circulating T_4 antibodies. In these situations, FT_4 by direct dialysis or two-step immunoassay methods (see also *Free Thyroxine Index*) better reflect the true free hormone concentration.

FT_4 estimates derived from equilibrium tracer dialysis once served as the accepted reference method; however, results have been found to vary substantially among laboratories, probably because of the presence of impurities in the tracer, variations in the temperature and duration of dialysis, or in vitro generation of free fatty acids.

See *Triiodothyronine Suppression Test.*

This test is better tolerated by most patients than the triiodothyronine suppression test. The thyroxine suppression test may precipitate hyperthyroid crisis in patients with underlying heart disease. Test has limited usefulness.

Administration of a single dose of hormone eliminates the problem, often seen in the triiodothyronine suppression test, of spurious nonsuppression caused by patient noncompliance.

TEST NAME AND METHOD	SPECIMEN REQUIREMENTS	REFERENCE INTERVAL, CONVENTIONAL [INTERNATIONAL RECOMMENDED UNITS]	CHEMICAL INTERFERENCES AND IN VIVO EFFECTS

Thyroxine Suppression Test—CONT

1. Alsever RN, Gotlin RW: *Handbook of endocrine tests in adults and children,* ed 2, Chicago, 1978, Year Book Medical Publishers Inc.

Thyroxine/TBG Ratio[1-5]	Serum. (See *Thyroxine-Binding Globulin.*)	T_4 (mcg/dL)/TBG (mg/dL) = 3-5 [$\times$ 0.065* = 0.19-0.32 (mole ratio)] *Conversion factor based on a molecular weight for TBG of ~50,000.	See *Thyroxine, Total;* and *Thyroxine-Binding Globulin.*

1. Eastham RD: *Biochemical values in clinical medicine,* ed 7, Bristol, UK, 1985, John Wright and Sons Ltd.

2. Burr WA, Ramsden DB, Evans SE, et al: Concentration of thyroxine-binding globulin: value of direct assay, *BMJ* 1:485-488, 1977.

3. Larsen PR, Davies TF, Schlumberger MJ, et al: The thyroid gland. In Larsen PR, Kronenberg HM, Melmed S, et al, editors: *Williams textbook of endocrinology,* ed 10, Philadelphia, 2003, WB Saunders.

4. Demers LM, Spencer C: The thyroid. In Burtis CA, Ashwood ER, Bruns DE, editors: *Tietz textbook of clinical chemistry,* ed 4, Philadelphia, 2006, WB Saunders.

5. Wilke TJ: Free thyroid hormone index, thyroid hormone/thyroxine-binding globulin ratio, triiodothyronine uptake and thyroxine-binding globulin compared for diagnostic value regarding thyroid function, *Clin Chem* 29:74-79, 1983.

6. Attwood EC, Atkin GE: The T4:TBG ratio: a re-evaluation with particular reference to low and high serum TBG levels, *Ann Clin Biochem* 19:101-103, 1982.

TEST NAME AND METHOD	SPECIMEN REQUIREMENTS	REFERENCE INTERVAL, CONVENTIONAL			[INTERNATIONAL RECOMMENDED UNITS]	CHEMICAL INTERFERENCES AND IN VIVO EFFECTS
Thyroxine (T_4), Total[1-5] *Immunoassay*	Serum; refrigerate immediately. Stable for 7 days at room temperature, but storage at 4° C is preferred. Stable for at least 30 days frozen. Do not use lipemic specimens.	Cord:	*mcg/dL*[6] 7.4-13.0	$\times$ 12.9	*nmol/L* [95-168]	S ↑ V Amiodarone, amphetamines, dextrothyroxine (D-T_4), dinoprost
		1-3 days:	11.8-22.6		[152-292]	tromethamine ($PGF_{2\alpha}$),
		1-2 wk:	9.8-16.6		[126-214]	estrogens, heroin,
		1-4 mo:	7.2-14.4		[93-186]	levarterenol, levodopa,
		4-12 mo:	7.8-16.5		[101-213]	methadone, oral cholecystographic agents (iopanoic
		1-5 yr:	7.3-15.0		[94-194]	acid, ipodate), oral contraceptives, propranolol, thyroid preparations, thyrotropin, and TRH
		5-10 yr:	6.4-13.3		[83-172]	
		10-15 yr:	5.6-11.7		[72-151]	
		Adult				
		M:	4.6-10.5		[59-135]	
		F:	5.5-11.0		[71-142]	↑ C Anti-T_4 (double-antibody technique),
		>60 yr:	5.0-10.7		[65-138]	heparin
		Maternal serum[7]				
		15-40 wk:	9.1-14.0		[117-181]	

DIAGNOSTIC INFORMATION	REMARKS

2. Larsen PR, Davies TF, Schlumberger MJ, et al: The thyroid gland. In Larsen PR, Kronenberg HM, Melmed S, et al, editors: *Williams textbook of endocrinology,* ed 10, Philadelphia, 2003, WB Saunders.

↑ Hyperthyroidism, familial dysalbuminemic hyperthyroxinemia, and congenital TBG excess

↓ Hypothyroidism (values overlap with euthyroid patient), third trimester of pregnancy, and congenital TBG deficiency

In primary increases of TBG, both T_4 and TBG will increase and the ratio will remain essentially unaltered. In primary decreases of TBG, both T_4 and TBG will decrease and the ratio will also remain unaltered. Higher than expected ratios have been observed with very low TBG levels and vice versa.[6]

The thyroxine/TBG ratio correlates variably with FT_4I but is particularly useful in cases with mildly altered TBG concentrations. The ratio represents an approximation to free thyroxine (FT_4) concentration.

See also *Free Thyroxine Index* and *Thyroid Hormone-Binding Ratio.*

S ↑ Hyperthyroidism, states with increased TBG (e.g., pregnancy, oral contraceptives, genetically determined increases in TBG, acute intermittent porphyria, primary biliary cirrhosis), thyrotoxicosis factitia, some cases of acute thyroiditis, hepatitis (by 4 wk), obesity, acute psychiatric illnesses, and hyperemesis gravidarum

T_4 may also be elevated in euthyroid patients because of familial dysalbuminemic hyperthyroxinemia, increased T_4 binding by TBPA, or T_4 autoantibodies; T_3 will be normal in these cases.

S ↓ Hypothyroidism, states with decreased TBG (e.g., nephrotic syndrome, chronic liver disease, GI protein loss, genetically decreased TBG, malnutrition), panhypopituitarism, and strenuous exercise

Sensitive TSH measurements are now used as the initial test of thyroid function (see *Thyrotropin*). T_4 testing is more commonly used to confirm abnormal TSH results when TSH levels are abnormally high or low.[10]

By itself, the serum total T_4 does not provide adequate clinical information. A free thyroxine estimate, such as free T_4 by immunoassay or a calculated FT_4 index, should be reported with every total T_4 measurement (see also *FT_4 Free Thyroxine Index* and *Thyroid Hormone-Binding Ratio*).

T_4 levels are lower in cord blood from preterm than from full-term infants[11] and correlate positively with birthweight in term neonates.[12] T_4 values are higher in the neonate because of elevated TBG; FT_4 is near adult levels. Values increase abruptly in the first few hours after birth and decline gradually until the age of 5 yr. Males experience a gradual decline in T_4 as they mature sexually; females do not.

TEST NAME AND METHOD	SPECIMEN REQUIREMENTS	REFERENCE INTERVAL, CONVENTIONAL [INTERNATIONAL RECOMMENDED UNITS]				CHEMICAL INTERFERENCES AND IN VIVO EFFECTS

Thyroxine (T$_4$), Total—CONT

						S ↓ V Aminoglutethimide, aminosalicylic acid, amiodarone (rare), androgens, anticonvulsants (phenytoin, valproic acid), asparaginase, aspirin, corticosteroids, corticotropin, danazol, ethionamide, furosemide (large doses), growth hormone (slight), iodides, isotretinoin, lithium, methimazole, oxyphenbutazone, penicillin, phenylbutazone, propylthiouracil, reserpine, rifampicin, somatotropin, sulfonamides, and triiodothyronine
Whole blood (heel or cord). Collect 48 hr after birth. Avoid touching the filter paper or exposing to extreme heat or light.	Newborn screen[8] 1-5 days: >6 days:	*mcg/dL* >7.5 >6.5	× 12.9	*nmol/L* [>97] [>84]		
						↓ C Anti-T$_4$ (single-antibody technique), hemolysis
Amniotic fluid	<17 wk: 17-22 wk: 35-42 wk:	*mcg/dL* 0.06-0.35 0.08-1.16 0.08-0.65		*nmol/L*[9] [0.8-4.5] [1.0-15.0] [1.0-8.4]		AF ↓ Maternal intake of iodides, radioactive iodine, propylthiouracil, and methimazole is likely to decrease T$_3$ and T$_4$.

1. Eastham RD: *Biochemical values in clinical medicine,* ed 7, Bristol, UK, 1985, John Wright and Sons Ltd.
2. Dussault JH, Morissette J, Laberge C: Blood thyroxine concentrations are lower in low-birth-weight infants, *Clin Chem* 25:2047-2049, 1979.
3. Klein AH, Murphy BEP, Artal R, et al: Amniotic fluid thyroid hormone concentrations during human gestation, *Am J Obstet Gynecol* 136:626-630, 1980.
4. Larsen PR, Davies TF, Schlumberger MJ, et al: The thyroid gland. In Larsen PR, Kronenberg HM, Melmed S, et al, editors: *Williams textbook of endocrinology,* ed 10, Philadelphia, 2003, WB Saunders.
5. Demers LM, Spencer C: The thyroid. In Burtis CA, Ashwood ER, Bruns DE, editors: *Tietz textbook of clinical chemistry,* ed 4, Philadelphia, 2006, WB Saunders.
6. Hung W, August GP, Glasgow AM: *Pediatric endocrinology,* New Hyde Park, NY, 1983, Medical Examination Publishing Co.
7. Cooper E, Aickin CM, Burke CW: Serum concentrations of 3, 3′, 5′-triiodothyronine (reverse T$_3$) in normal pregnancy, *Clin Chim Acta* 106:347-349, 1980.
8. Quest Clinical Laboratories: *Quest diagnostic reference manual,* Atlanta, GA, 2001, SmithKline Beecham Clinical Laboratories.
9. Cooper E, Anderson A, Bennett MJ, et al: Radioimmunoassay of thyroxine and 3, 3′, 5′-triiodothyronine (reverse T$_3$) in human amniotic fluid, *Clin Chim Acta* 118:57-66, 1982.

DIAGNOSTIC INFORMATION	REMARKS

In hypothyroidism, total serum T_4 decreases before T_3. Elevated T_4 and FT_4 levels with thyroxine replacement do not necessarily indicate overtreatment; normal T_3 confirms euthyroid state.

Test is useful for monitoring propylthiouracil therapy. It is not affected by organic dyes and inorganic iodine compounds. Radioactive materials like ^{131}I or ^{99m}Tc may interfere when given in mCi amounts and serum specimen is obtained within 2-3 days. If patient is on thyroid therapy, stop treatment for 1 mo to obtain true baseline.

Reference intervals for newborn screening should be developed by each laboratory providing screening for neonatal hypothyroidism; significant numbers of samples must be screened to determine sensitivity and specificity for that laboratory. Cutoff values for detection of congenital disease are usually set to preclude false-negative results.[13]

Levels are unaltered with increasing gestational age and do not correlate with Apgar scores.[3]

Amniotic fluid T_4 levels increase from weeks 10-30 and then decrease to term.[3]

10. Klee GG, Hay ID: Assessment of sensitive thyrotropin assays for an expanded role in thyroid functions testing: proposed criteria for analytic performance and clinical utility, *J Clin Endocrinol Metab* 64:461-471, 1987.

11. Delange F, Bourdoux P, Ermans A-M: Transient disorders of thyroid function and regulation in preterm infants, *Pediatr Adolesc Endocrinol* 14:369-393, 1985.

12. Franklin RC, Carpenter LM, O'Grady CM: Neonatal thyroid function: influence of perinatal factors, *Arch Dis Child* 60:141-144, 1985.

13. Jewell S, Slazyk W, Smith S, et al: Sources of imprecision in laboratories screening for congenital hypothyroidism: analysis of nine years of performance data, *Clin Chem* 35:1701-1705, 1989.

TEST NAME AND METHOD	SPECIMEN REQUIREMENTS	REFERENCE INTERVAL, CONVENTIONAL [INTERNATIONAL RECOMMENDED UNITS]			CHEMICAL INTERFERENCES AND IN VIVO EFFECTS
Thyroxine-Binding Globulin (TBG)[1-6]	Serum. Refrigerate immediately.		mg/dL^8	mg/L	↑ V Estrogens, methadone, oral contra-
		Cord:	3.6-9.6 × 10	[36-96]	ceptives, and tamoxifen
			(x̄: 5.9)	[x̄: 59]	
		1-3 days:	(x̄: 5.0)	[x̄: 50]	
Immunoassay		4-12 mo:	3.1-5.6	[31-56]	↓ V Anabolic steroids, an-
			(x̄: 4.4)	[x̄: 44]	drogens, asparaginase,
		1-5 yr:	2.9-5.4	[29-54]	corticosteroids, corti-
			(x̄: 4.2)	[x̄: 42]	cotropin, danazol, phenyt-
		5-10 yr:	2.5-5.0	[25-50]	oin, and propranolol
			(x̄: 3.8)	[x̄: 38]	
		10-15 yr:	2.1-4.6	[21-46]	
			(x̄: 3.3)	[x̄: 33]	
		Adult[9]			
		M:	1.2-2.5	[12-25]	
		F:	1.4-3.0	[14-30]	
		F on oral contraceptive:	1.5-5.5	[15-55]	
		Pregnancy, third trimester[10]:	5.3 ± 0.6 (SD)	[53.0 ± 6.0]	
		As T4-binding capacity[8]: 16-24 mcg/dL × 12.9		[206-309 nmol/L]	
	Amniotic fluid[7]	0.3 ± 0.04 mg/dL (SD) × 10		[3 ± 0.4 mg/L]	

1. Eastham RD: *Biochemical values in clinical medicine,* ed 7, Bristol, UK, 1985, John Wright and Sons Ltd.
2. Bristow A, Gaines-Das R, Buttress N: The international standard for thyroxine binding globulin, *Clin Endocrinol* 38:361-366, 1993.
3. Hesch R-D, Gatz J, Jüppner H, et al: TBG-dependency of age-related variations of thyroxine and triiodothyronine, *Hum Metab Res* 9:141-146, 1977.
4. Keane PM, Walker WH, Thornton G, et al: Studies of thyroxine binding to plasma proteins in health and disease, *Clin Biochem* 19:52-57, 1986.
5. Demers LM, Spencer C: Laboratory medicine practice guidelines: laboratory support for the diagnosis and monitoring of thyroid disease, *Thyroid* 13:4-104, 2003.
6. Nelson J, Linarelli L, Pandian M: Discordant RIA results for thyroxin-binding globulin (TBG): a new indicator of variant TBG molecules with decrease affinity for thyroxin, *Clin Chem* 35:1257-1258, 1989.
7. Alsever RN, Gotlin RW: *Handbook of endocrine tests in adults and children,* ed 2, Chicago, 1978, Year Book Medical Publishers Inc.
8. Hung W, August GP, Glasgow AM: *Pediatric endocrinology,* New Hyde Park, NY, 1983, Medical Examination Publishing Co.
9. Mayo Medical Laboratories: *Test catalog,* Rochester, MN, 2004, Mayo Medical Laboratories.
10. Maberly G, Waite K, Ma G, et al: Binding characteristics of thyroxin-binding globulin in serum of normal, pregnant, and severely ill euthyroid patients, *Clin Chem* 32:616-620, 1986.
11. Refetoff S: Inherited thyroxine-binding globulin abnormalities in man, *Endo Rev* 10:275-293, 1989.
12. Murata Y, Takamatsu J, Refetoff S: Inherited abnormality of thyroxine-binding globulin with no demonstrable thyroxine binding activity and high serum levels of denatured thyroxine binding globulin, *N Engl J Med* 314:694-699, 1986.

DIAGNOSTIC INFORMATION	REMARKS

S ↑ Infectious hepatitis, acute intermittent porphyria, genetically determined high TBG,[11] hypothyroidism (some cases), and pregnancy

This glycoprotein is the principal carrier for T_3 and T_4. The balance of these hormones is carried by transthyretin (prealbumin) and albumin.

S ↓ Major illness, surgical stress, protein malnutrition, malabsorption resulting from various causes, protein-losing enteropathy, nephrotic syndrome, active acromegaly, ovarian hypofunction, and genetically determined low TBG

TBG declines with age in parallel with total and free T_4 and T_3. The latter changes are accompanied by an increase in rT_3 and rT_3 index, suggesting a decrease in peripheral conversion of T_4 and T_3 rather than a change in the secretory behavior of the thyroid gland itself. With the availability of better free thyroid hormone tests, the determination of TBG is rarely used to assess thyroid hormone binding status. The TBG test was used to differentiate total T_3 and T_4 changes in primary thyroidal disorders from changes in total T_3 and T_4 as a result of primary changes in TBG.

Molecular variants of TBG with low avidity for T_3 and T_4 are not uncommon, especially in certain ethnic groups such as the Australian aborigines.[12-14]

13.   Pearce CJ, Byfield PGH: Free thyroid hormone assays and thyroid function, *Ann Clin Biochem* 23:230-237, 1986.
14.   Takamatsu J, Refetoff S, Charbonneau M, et al: Two new inherited defects of the thyroxine-binding globulin (TBG) molecule presenting as partial TBG deficiency, *J Clin Invest* 79:833-840, 1987.

TEST NAME AND METHOD	SPECIMEN REQUIREMENTS	REFERENCE INTERVAL, CONVENTIONAL [INTERNATIONAL RECOMMENDED UNITS]			CHEMICAL INTERFERENCES AND IN VIVO EFFECTS
Tin (Sn)[1] *NAA*[2]	Serum. Collect in pretested, metal-free container using polypropylene cannula.	0.40-0.64 mcg/L	× 8.4	[3.4-5.4 nmol/L]	
Colorimetric[3]	Whole blood. Collect in metal-free container.	x̄: 140 mcg/L	× 8.4	[x̄: 1176 nmol/L]	
	Urine, 24 hr. Collect in acid-washed, metal-free container.	<40 mcg/L (x̄: 23)	× 8.4	[<337 nmol/L] [x̄: 194]	U ↑ C High concentration of other metals U ↓ C High concentration of anions

1. Milne DB: Tin. In Frieden E, editor: *Biochemistry of the essential ultratrace elements,* New York, 1984, Plenum Press.
2. Versieck J, Vanballenberghe L: Determination of tin in human blood serum by radiochemical neutron activation analysis, *Anal Chem* 63:1143-1146, 1991.
3. Baselt RC: *Biological monitoring methods for industrial chemicals,* ed 2, Littleton, MA, 1988, PSG Publishing Co., Inc.

TEST NAME AND METHOD	SPECIMEN REQUIREMENTS	REFERENCE INTERVAL, CONVENTIONAL [INTERNATIONAL RECOMMENDED UNITS]			CHEMICAL INTERFERENCES AND IN VIVO EFFECTS
Tissue Plasminogen Activator (tPA)[1,2]	Functional assay: To prevent tPA inhibition, collect blood either into ice-cold vacutainer containing Na citrate and immediately mix 500 mL of blood with 250 mL of Na acetate, 1 mol/L, or use Stabilyte blood collection tube (American Diagnostica, Inc.). Centrifuge blood and mix 200 mL of plasma with 10 mL of 20% acetic acid to destroy antiplasmin.	Basal level: 0-0.04 U/mL After venous occlusion: 1.4-14 U/mL	× 1000 × 1.0	[<40 U/L] [1.4-14 kU/L]	Plasminogen activator inhibitors (PAI), α₂-antiplasmin
	ELISA: Plasma (citrate or EDTA).	3-10 ng/mL	× 1.0	[3-10 mg/L]	

1. Lewis SM, Bain BJ, Bates I, editors: *Dacie and Lewis practical hematology,* ed 9, Edinburgh, 2001, Churchill Livingstone.
2. Brant JT: Plasminogen and tissue-type plasminogen activator deficiency as risk factors for thromboembolic disease, *Arch Pathol Lab Med* 126:1376-1381, 2002.
3. Lijnen HR, Collen D: Congenital and acquired deficiencies of components of the fibrinolytic system and their relation to bleeding or thrombosis, *Fibrinolysis* 3:67-77, 1989.

Information is limited concerning the toxicity of tin in humans. Inorganic tin is not readily absorbed. The ingestion of soluble salts or large doses of metallic tin from nonlacquered or corroded cans may result in gastric irritation. Acute exposure to tin oxide results in mild irritation to eyes, skin, and mucous membranes. Chronic inhalation of tin dust in industrial settings causes stannosis, a benign form of pneumoconiosis.

Tin is used in the manufacture of alloys. Tin plating is used for food containers, and tin salts are used in calico printing. Organic tin compounds are found in polyvinyl plastics, chlorinated rubber paints, fungicides, insecticides, and antihelmintics.

Increased levels in DVT, after venous occlusion, stress, exercise, desmopressin (DDAVP) infusion; also in a rare hereditary disorder associated with bleeding.[3]

Reduced levels have been documented as a familial defect associated with thrombotic manifestations.[3]

Tissue plasminogen activator (tPA) is a major component of the fibrinolytic system. Deficiency of tPA has been proposed to be associated with thromboembolic disease.

In light of the fact that there is no conclusive evidence that tPA deficiency contributes to the risk of thrombosis, a 2002 consensus conference on thrombophilia stated that routine evaluation of tPA in patients with apparent thrombophilia is not recommended.[2]

tPA can be measured by functional (activity) and/or immunologic (antigenic) assays. The presence of plasminogen activator inhibitors (PAI-1) and antiplasmin interferes with functional tPA assays but not with the determination of tPA antigen.

TEST NAME AND METHOD	SPECIMEN REQUIREMENTS	REFERENCE INTERVAL, CONVENTIONAL [INTERNATIONAL RECOMMENDED UNITS]	CHEMICAL INTERFERENCES AND IN VIVO EFFECTS
Tissue Transglutaminase Antibody[1,2] *IgA, IgG* *ELISA*	Serum. Stable 1 wk at room temperature, 2 wk at 4° C, and 1 yr frozen.	Normal: Negative	Testing in children is not as useful because celiac disease antibodies may not have developed. May be negative in patients taking gluten-free diets. 2.6% of patients will be negative because of selective IgA deficiency. A serum IgA should be carried out, and, if abnormal, IgG-based testing carried out.

1. Wong RC, Steele RH, Reeves GE, et al: Antibody and genetic testing in coeliac disease, *Pathology* 35:285-304, 2003.
2. Devlin SM, Andrews CN, Beck PL: Celiac disease: CME update for family physicians, *Can Fam Physician* 50:719-725, 2004.

Toluene[1,2]

(Methyl benzene; CAS 108-88-3)

GLC,[3]*colorimetric (hippuric acid),*[3] *GC-FID,*[4] *GC-MS*[5]

Serum — Negative

	mg/L		μmol/L
Occupational exposure:	<2	× 10.9	[<22]
Toxic concentration:	>2		[>22]
Possibly lethal:	>10		[>109]

Urine[6]

	g/g creatinine		mol/mol creatinine
As hippuric acid:	<1.5	× 0.631	[<0.95]
At TLV (threshold limit value):	2.8		[1.77]

Breath[7]

Occupational exposure: <100 ppm × 10.9 [<1090 μmol/L]

None found.

1. Baselt RC: *Biological monitoring methods for industrial chemicals,* Davis, CA, 1980, Biomedical Pub.
2. Baselt RC, Cravey RH: *Disposition of toxic drugs and chemicals in man,* ed 3, Chicago, 1989, Year Book Medical Publishers, Inc., pp. 812-813.
3. Tomokuni K, Ogata M: Direct colorimetric determination of hippuric acid in urine, *Clin Chem* 18:349-351, 1972.
4. Garriott JC, Foerster E, Juarez L: Measurement of toluene in blood and breath in cases of solvent abuse, *Clin Toxicol* 18:411-479, 1981.

DIAGNOSTIC INFORMATION	REMARKS

In celiac disease, it is 90-98% sensitive and 94-97% specific.

It is 70% positive in dermatitis herpetiformis.

See *Reticulin Antibody, Endomyosial Antibody,* and *Gliadin Antibody.*

Celiac disease is an immune disorder found in 1% of the NA population that is stimulated by gluten. It is characterized by typical GI symptoms and a variety of less common symptoms.

TTG is the antigen for endomyosial antibodies.

Small bowel biopsy is needed for definitive diagnosis.

More than 97% of people with celiac disease have DQ2 and/or DQ8 HLA haplotypes compared with 40% of the population.

Toxic effects include headache, nausea, lassitude, impairment of coordination, and loss of memory. Chronic abuse causes permanent changes to brain structure, including loss of gray and white matter differentiation; and cerebral, cerebellar, and brainstem atrophy.

Toluene is a product of petroleum distillation and has many commercial uses, including aerosols, paints and paint thinners, lacquer, adhesives, and industrial solvents. Most toxic exposures are occupationals or the result of abuse by inhalation. Eighty percent of absorbed toluene is metabolized to benzoic acid, which is excreted conjugated with glucuronide or glycine (hippuric acid). Urinary hippuric acid (normally 1.4 mg/L [7.81 μmol/L]) is increased with exposure to toluene. Twenty percent of toluene is eliminated in breath.[6]

Kinetic values
$t_{1/2}$: 7.5 hr

5. Bellanca JA, Davis PL, Donnelly B, et al: Detection and quantitation of multiple volatile compounds in tissues by GC and GC/MS, *J Anal Toxicol* 6:238-240, 1982.

6. Lauwerys RR: *Industrial chemical exposure. Guidelines for biological monitoring,* Davis, CA, 1983, Biomedical Pub.

7. Moffat AC: *Clarke's isolation and identification of drugs,* London, 1986, The Pharmaceutical Press.

TEST NAME AND METHOD	SPECIMEN REQUIREMENTS	REFERENCE INTERVAL, CONVENTIONAL [INTERNATIONAL RECOMMENDED UNITS]		CHEMICAL INTERFERENCES AND IN VIVO EFFECTS
TPS (Tissue Polypeptide-Specific Antigen)[1,2] *Immunoassay*	Serum. Stable up to 24 hr at 2-8° C. For longer periods, freeze at −20° C or colder. Avoid repeated freeze-thaw cycles.	<80 U/L[3] (95% of healthy individuals)	× 1.0 [<80 U/L]	None found.

1. Barak V, Goike H, Panaretakis KW, et al: Clinical utility of cytokeratins as tumor markers, *Clin Biochem* 37:529-540, 2004.
2. Chan DW, Sell S: Tumor markers. In Burtis CA, Ashwood ER, editors: *Tietz textbook of clinical chemistry,* ed 3, Philadelphia, 1999, WB Saunders.
3. Available at: www.idl.se. Last accessed 12/15/04.

Transcobalamin II (TC II)[1-4] *RIA,*[5-7] *ELISA*[8] *(HoloTC)*	Serum. Analyze fresh or store at 4° C for <72 hr. Stable frozen at −20° C for 6 mo or at −70° C indefinitely. Specimens without lipemia or hemolysis are preferred.	37-171 pmol/L[11]	None found.
ELISA (total TC)[9]		600-1500 pmol/L[9]	
Cobalamin (Cbl) binding level (ApoTC)[10]		400-930 pmol/L[10]	

DIAGNOSTIC INFORMATION	REMARKS

TPS is a useful indicator of progressive disease in most forms of epithelial-cell carcinoma. It can be used to monitor therapy and predict recurrence of disease in patients with breast, prostate, gynecological, gastrointestinal, lung, and bladder cancers. The marker indicates tumor activity and not tumor burden. Values may be increased in pregnancy and inflammatory disease.[1-3]

TPA (tissue polypeptide antigen) is a cytokeratin marker measuring cytokeratins 8, 18, and 19. TPA is a more specific assay detecting a defined epitope on cytokeratin 18 using the M3 monoclonal antibody. TPS is reported to be an indicator of cell proliferation. It is produced during the S and G_2 phase of the cell cycle and is released immediately after mitosis. Impaired liver or kidney function, as well as infection and various inflammatory disorders, may cause increased values. These elevations are transient and can be identified by repeated assays.[1-3] TPS immunoassays are available from IDL Biotech AB (Bromma, Sweden) and on the IMMULITE platform (Diagnostic Products Corporation). This test does not have FDA approval for clinical use.

↑ TC-II: Myeloproliferative disorders (not in leukemoid reactions), monocyte-macrophage neoplasia, lymphoproliferative disorders, and autoimmune diseases.[10]

↓ TC-II: Infants with severe megaloblastic anemia, TC II congenital deficiency, and TC II functional deficiency

↓ HoloTC: Vitamin B_{12} deficiency

Transcobalamin II (TC II) binds and transports vitamin B_{12} in plasma. Other cobalamin binders are haptocorrin in plasma and intrinsic factor in the intestine. Intrinsic factor is needed for vitamin B_{12} uptake in the intestine, and transcobalamin II ensures internalization of the vitamin into all cells of the body. Haptocorrin carries most of the vitamin B_{12} in plasma, but its function is unknown.

Holotranscobalamin (holoTC) represents the biologically active fraction of vitamin B_{12} that can be delivered into DNA-synthesizing cells.[4] It has therefore been suggested that holoTC may be a sensitive marker of vitamin B_{12} deficiency.

Laboratory support for the diagnosis and management of vitamin B deficiency is controversial and somewhat problematic.[12] Plasma vitamin B_{12} concentration does not readily rule out vitamin B_{12} deficiency.[4] The use of methylmalonic acid (MMA) and homocysteine (HCY) measurement has been helpful, but the specificities of these tests has been debated because renal insufficiency may also cause elevation of MMA and HCY.[4]

More work needs to be done to determine the best diagnostic strategy for assessment of vitamin B status.

MW: 53,900.

TEST NAME AND METHOD	SPECIMEN REQUIREMENTS	REFERENCE INTERVAL, CONVENTIONAL [INTERNATIONAL RECOMMENDED UNITS]	CHEMICAL INTERFERENCES AND IN VIVO EFFECTS

Transcobalamin II—CONT

1. Bor MV, Nexo E, Hvas AM: Holo-transcobalamin concentration and transcobalamin saturation reflect recent vitamin B12 absorption better than does serum vitamin B12, *Clin Chem* 50:1043-1049, 2004.

2. Lloyd-Wright Z, Hvas AM, Moller J, et al: Holotranscobalamin as an indicator of dietary vitamin B12 deficiency, *Clin Chem* 49:2076-2078, 2003.

3. Lindgren A, Kilander A, Bagge E, et al: Holotranscobalamin—a sensitive marker of cobalamin malabsorption, *Eur J Clin Invest* 29:321-329, 1999.

4. Hvas AM, Nexo E: Holotranscobalamin—a first choice assay for diagnosing early vitamin B deficiency? *J Intern Med* 257:289-298, 2005.

5. Hvas AM, Nexo E: Holotranscobalamin as a predictor of vitamin B12 status, *Clin Chem Lab Med* 41:1489-1492, 2003.

6. Loikas S, Pelliniemi TT, Koskinen P: No bias between the first and the new version of radioimmunoassay for serum holo-transcobalamin by Axis-Shield, *Clin Chem Lab Med* 42:569-570, 2004.

TEST NAME AND METHOD	SPECIMEN REQUIREMENTS	REFERENCE INTERVAL, CONVENTIONAL [INTERNATIONAL RECOMMENDED UNITS]			CHEMICAL INTERFERENCES AND IN VIVO EFFECTS
Transferrin (Siderophilin, Tf)[1]	Serum. Analyze fresh or store at 4° C for <72 hr. Stable frozen at −20° C for 6 mo, or at −70° C indefinitely. Specimens without lipemia or hemolysis are preferred.		*mg/dL*	*g/L*	S ↑ V Estrogens, oral contraceptives
		0-4 days:	130-275 × 0.01	[1.30-2.75]	
		3 mo-16 yr:	203-360	[2.03-3.60]	
Nephelometric		16-60 yr			S ↓ V Asparaginase, dextran, corticotropin, corticosteroids, and testosterone
		M:	215-365	[2.15-3.65]	
		F:	250-380	[2.50-3.80]	
		60-90 yr:[2]	190-375	[1.90-3.75]	
		>90 yr:	186-347	[1.86-3.47]	
		Maternal (at term), $\bar{x}$[3,4]:	305	[3.05]	Extreme turbidity may affect nephelometric methods.
		Adult levels are reached by 9 mo.			
RID	Urine, 24 hr. Centrifuge and adjust to pH 7.0.	0.68 mg/day			
EID	Analyze fresh. Stable frozen at −20° C for up to 1 yr.	0.04-0.45 mg/day ($\bar{x}$: 0.17)			
		Values are based on the Reference Preparation for Serum Proteins (RPSP) obtained from the College of American Pathologists, Skokie, IL.[5]			

7. Ulleland M, Eilertsen I, Quadros EV, et al: Direct assay for cobalamin bound to transcobalamin (holo-transcobalamin) in serum, *Clin Chem* 48:526-532, 2002.

8. Nexo E, Christensen AL, Hvas AM, et al: Quantification of holo-transcobalamin, a marker of vitamin B12 deficiency, *Clin Chem* 48:561-562, 2002.

9. Nexo E, Christensen AL, Petersen TE, et al: Measurement of transcobalamin by ELISA, *Clin Chem* 46:1643-1649, 2000.

10. Gimsing P, Nexo E: Cobalamin-binding capacity of haptocorrin and transcobalamin: age-correlated reference intervals and values from patients, *Clin Chem* 35:1447-1451, 1989.

11. Loikas S, Lopponen M, Suominen P, et al: RIA for serum holo-transcobalamin: method evaluation in the clinical laboratory and reference interval, *Clin Chem* 49:455-462, 2003.

12. Klee GG: Cobalamin and folate evaluation: measurement of methylmalonic acid and homocysteine vs vitamin B(12) and folate, *Clin Chem* 46:1277-1283, 2000.

↑ Estrogen (e.g., pregnancy, oral contraceptives), iron deficiency (elevated levels often precede the appearance of anemia by days to months)

Serum ferritin levels decrease with iron deficiency and with generalized malnutrition but remain normal in the presence of inflammation and iron deficiency. The combination of ferritin and transferrin levels is therefore useful in differentiating these disorders.[6,7] See also *Ferritin*.

↓ Inherited atransferrinemia (rare)[8]; in any disorder associated with inflammation or necrosis; chronic inflammation or malignancy, especially of the lower intestinal tract (↓↓); generalized malnutrition; in the nephrotic syndrome; and in conditions with increased oncotic pressure (multiple myeloma, hepatocellular disease).[1] Serum transferrin levels decrease with evolving iron overload states, including multiple transfusion and hereditary hemochromatosis.

Indications for quantitation include screening for nutritional status and differential diagnosis of anemia. To control the effects of estrogens and acute phase responses, other acute phase proteins should be assayed at the same time. Iron deficiency and iron overload are best diagnosed using assays of serum levels of iron, transferrin, and ferritin in combination.[8]

Transferrin is the major plasma transport protein for iron. Only a small amount of transferrin is required for normal homeostasis. A level >0.15 g/L is associated with nearly normal erythrocyte production in patients with congenital atransferrinemia.[7]

The presence of moderate amounts of unsaturated transferrin may be important in control of infections and infestations by iron-requiring organisms.[9] As a result, anemia in the face of severe infection or parasitic infestation should probably be treated by transfusion rather than supplementation with iron (if indeed treatment of the anemia is essential) until the infection is controlled.

Immunochemical assays of transferrin are more accurate than chemical assays of total iron-binding capacity.[10] Assuming a molecular weight for transferrin of 89,000, 1 mg of transferrin binds 1.25 mcg of iron. Therefore a serum transferrin level of 300 mcg/dL [3.0 g/L] is equal to a total iron-binding capacity of 300 × 1.25 or 375 mcg/dL [3.75 g/L].

Transferrin in CSF appears in its desialated form, the Tau protein (β_2-transferrin). This form can be identified electrophoretically by immunofixation with antitransferrin antibody. The clinical application for identification of the Tau protein is the investigation of rhinorrhea or otorrhea, where the presence of the Tau protein confirms the source being cerebrospinal leakage through a fracture or operative or traumatic site.[11,12] Partly desialated transferrin is also found to be a marker of heavy alcohol ingestion.[13,14]

TEST NAME AND METHOD	SPECIMEN REQUIREMENTS	REFERENCE INTERVAL, CONVENTIONAL [INTERNATIONAL RECOMMENDED UNITS]	CHEMICAL INTERFERENCES AND IN VIVO EFFECTS
Transferrin—CONT			

1. Putnam FW: Transferrin. In Putnam FW, editor: *The plasma proteins, vol 1,* ed 2, New York, 1975, Academic Press.
2. Tietz NW, Schreg DF, Wekstein DR: Laboratory values in fit aging individuals—sexagenarians through centenarians, *Clin Chem* 38:1167-1185, 1982.
3. Cederqvist LL, Eddey G, Abdel-Latif N, et al: The effect of smoking during pregnancy on cord blood and maternal serum immunoglobulin levels, *Am J Obstet Gynecol* 148:1123-1126, 1984.
4. Maroulis GB, Buckley RH, Younger JB: Serum immunoglobulin concentrations during normal pregnancy, *Am J Obstet Gynecol* 109:971-976, 1971.
5. Reimer CB, Smith SJ, Wells TW, et al: Collaborative calibration of the U.S. National and the College of American Pathologists reference preparations for specific serum proteins, *Am J Clin Pathol* 77:12-19, 1982.
6. Finch CA, Huebers H: Perspectives in iron metabolism, *N Engl J Med* 306:1520-1528, 1982.
7. Lipschitz DA, Cook JD, Finch CA: A clinical evaluation of serum ferritin as an index of iron stores, *N Engl J Med* 290:1213-1216, 1982.
8. Goya N, Miyazaki S, Kodate S, et al: A family of congenital atransferrinemia, *Blood* 40:239-245, 1972.
9. Weinberg ED: Infection and iron metabolism, *Am J Clin Nutr* 30:1485-1490, 1977.
10. Beilby J, Olynyk J, Ching S, et al: Transform index: an alternative method for calculating the iron saturation of transferrin, *Clin Chem* 38:2078-2081, 1992.
11. Porter MJ, Brookes GB, Zeman AZ, et al: Use of protein electrophoresis in the diagnosis of cerebrospinal fluid rhinorrhoea, *J Laryngol Otol* 106:504-506, 1992.
12. Zaret DL, Morrison N, Gulbranson R, et al: Immunofixation to quantify β_2-transferrin in cerebrospinal fluid to detect leakage of cerebrospinal fluid from skull injury, *Clin Chem* 38:1909-1912, 1992.
13. Storey EL, Anderson GJ, Mack U, et al: Desialylated transferrin as a serological marker of chronic excessive alcohol ingestion, *Lancet* 1:1292-1293, 1987.
14. Storey EL, Mack U, Powell EW, et al: Use of chromalofocusing to detect a transferrin in serum of alcoholic subjects, *Clin Chem* 31:1543-1545, 1985.

TEST NAME AND METHOD	SPECIMEN REQUIREMENTS	REFERENCE INTERVAL, CONVENTIONAL [INTERNATIONAL RECOMMENDED UNITS]		CHEMICAL INTERFERENCES AND IN VIVO EFFECTS
β_2-Transferrin (t fraction)	Serum, CSF, nasal or ear drainage fluid. Freeze specimen if not analyzed within 24 hr.	CSF:	Positive	None found.
		Serum:	Negative	
$EP,$[1] *immunofixation,*[2] *Western blot,*[3] *semiquantitative*		Nasal fluid:	Negative	
		Middle ear fluid:	Negative	
		Inner ear perilymph[3]:	Positive	
		Saliva:	Negative	
		Sputum:	Negative	

1. Zaret DL, Morrison N, Gulbranson R, et al: Immunofixation to quantify β_2-transferrin in cerebrospinal fluid to detect leakage of cerebrospinal fluid from skull injury, *Clin Chem* 38:1909-1912, 1992.
2. Rouah E, Rogers BB, Buffone G: Transferrin analysis by immunofixation as an aid in the diagnosis of cerebrospinal fluid otorrhea, *Arch Pathol Lab Med* 111:756-757, 1987.

DIAGNOSTIC INFORMATION	REMARKS
	See Table II-13 for transferrin saturation in clinical disease.
	MW: 89,000
	$t_{1/2}$: 8-12 days

Present in nasal or ear drainage (or related fluids) when CSF leak or perilymphatic fistula has occurred.	β_2-Transferrin is the desialated form of transferrin. Desialation occurs only in the CNS, ocular humors, and inner ear. Presence of β_2-T in serum, nasal fluid, middle ear fluid, saliva, or sputum indicates leakage from cerebrospinal or inner ear perilymphatic spaces or from aqueous or vitreous humor.

3.   Bassiouny M, Hirsch B, Kelly RH, et al: Beta$_2$-transferrin application in otology, *Am J Otol* 13:552-555, 1992.

TEST NAME AND METHOD	SPECIMEN REQUIREMENTS	REFERENCE INTERVAL, CONVENTIONAL [INTERNATIONAL RECOMMENDED UNITS]			CHEMICAL INTERFERENCES AND IN VIVO EFFECTS
Transferrin Receptor, Serum (soluble transferrin receptor, sTfR)[1-5] *Immunoassay*	Serum. Analyze fresh or store at 4° C for 1 wk, −20° C for 1 mo, or at −70° C for 1 yr. Specimens without lipemia, bilirubin, or hemolysis are preferred.[6,7]	Adult[6,8]*: Infants Age 1 yr[9]: Prepubertal male Age 11-12 yr *Determined by Ramco Human TfR Assay Kit (Ramco Laboratories, Houston, TX).	*mg/L* 2.9-3.8 4.5-11.1 4.7-9.2	× 0.001	*g/L* [0.0029-0.0038] [0.0045-0.0111] [0.0047-0.0092]	S ↑ V Physical activity, EDTA (certain assay kits)

1. Beguin Y: Soluble transferrin receptor for the evaluation of erythropoiesis and iron status, *Clin Chim Acta* 329:9-22, 2003.
2. Feelders RA, Kuiper-Kramer EP, van Eijk HG: Structure, function and clinical significance of transferrin receptors, *Clin Chem Lab Med* 37:1-10, 1999.
3. Voss HF: Saliva as a fluid for measurement of estriol levels, *Am J Obstet Gynecol* 180:S226-S231, 1999.
4. Nuttall KL, Klee GG: Analytes of hemoglobin metabolism—porphyrin, iron, and bilirubin. In Burtis CA, Ashwood ER, editors: *Fundamentals of clinical chemistry,* ed 5, Philadelphia, 2001, WB Saunders.
5. Iles RK, Wathen NC, Sharma KB, et al: Pregnancy-associated plasma protein A levels in maternal serum, extraembryonic coelomic and amniotic fluids in the first trimester, *Placenta* 15:693-699, 1994.
6. Worwood M: Serum transferrin receptor assays and their application, *Ann Clin Biochem* 39:221-230, 2002.

DIAGNOSTIC INFORMATION	REMARKS

↑ With elevated erythroid proliferation or with iron deficiency such as thalassemias, hemolytic anemias, and polycythemias

↓ Aplastic anemia, posttransplantational anemia, and chronic renal failure

Transferrin receptor (TfR) is a transferrin-specific membrane receptor, which mediates the uptake of iron into a cell. TfR binds diferric transferrin to form a complex; the transferrin-TfR complex is internalized; and the iron is released into the cytosol. Almost all cells, except mature red cells, have TfR on their surface, but are highly expressed on immature erythroids, placental tissue, liver, and actively dividing cells.

TfR is a disulfide-linked dimer of two identical 95-kDa subunits. Each subunit consists of a 61-amino acid N-terminal cytoplasmic domain, a transmembrance region, and a large extracellular domain. The extracellular domain is subject to protealytic cleavage and released into circulation primarily as a truncated 74-kDa monomoer.

The major serum TfR (sTfR) is the cleaved extracellular monomer that is complexed with transferrin. The sTfR levels are proportional to the estimated total body mass of cellular transferrin receptor and reflect the number of bone marrow-nucleated erythroids for patients with adequate iron stores. About 80% of sTfR is contained within erythroid marrow.

In the absence of iron deficiency, the level of sTfR provides a quantitative measure of total erythropoiesis that is more sensitive and less invasive than bone marrow examination.

The sTfR is a more reliable marker than ferritin to distinguish iron deficiency anemia from the anemia of chronic disease. Plasma transferrin levels are usually normal or elevated for patients with iron deficiency who have coexisting anemia of chronic diseases. However, sTfR levels are usually not elevated unless iron supply of the bone marrow is limited.

The sTfR levels determined by different assay systems cannot be directly compared because reference intervals differ.

MW: 190,000 (membranous dimer), 95,000 (membranous monomer), and 85,000 (soluble or serum monomer).

7.   Raya G, Henny J, Steinmetz J, et al: Soluble transferrin receptor (sTfR): biological variations and reference limits, *Clin Chem Lab Med* 39:1162-1168, 2001.

8.   Wians FH Jr, Urban JE, Kroft SH, et al: Soluble transferrin receptor (sTfR) concentration quantified using two sTfR kits: analytical and clinical performance characteristics, *Clin Chim Acta* 303:75-81, 2001.

9.   Virtanen MA, Viinikka LU, Virtanen MK, et al: Higher concentrations of serum transferrin receptor in children than in adults, *Am J Clin Nutr* 69:256-260, 1999.

TEST NAME AND METHOD	SPECIMEN REQUIREMENTS	REFERENCE INTERVAL, CONVENTIONAL [INTERNATIONAL RECOMMENDED UNITS]	CHEMICAL INTERFERENCES AND IN VIVO EFFECTS
Transketolase (Functional Test for Thiamine)[1] *Ribose/sedoheptulose (EC 2.2.1.1), 580 and 670 nm, 37° C*[2]	Whole blood hemolysate; collect whole blood (heparin). Hemolyze in phosphate buffer containing sodium chloride and magnesium sulfate.	9-12 μmol/hr/mL whole blood [× 16.67 = 150-200 U/L whole blood]	None found.
NADH-dependent, 340 nm, 37° C Manual[3] *or semi-automated*[4,5]	Erythrocyte hemolysate; collect whole blood (heparin). Hemolysate is stable for at least 4 wk if frozen.	*U/L Ercs (SD)*[6] M: 172 ± 30 F: 160 ± 36 0.75-1.30 U/g Hb[7] [× 64.52 = 48.39-83.9 kU/mol Hb] % TPP* stimulation: 0-15%[2] × 0.01 [Fractional increase: 0-0.15] *TPP, Thiamine pyrophosphate.	

1. Shils ME, Olson JA, Shike M, editors: *Modern nutrition in health and disease,* ed 8, Philadelphia, 1994, Lea & Febiger.
2. Tietz NW, editor: *Fundamentals of clinical chemistry,* ed 2, Philadelphia, 1976, WB Saunders.
3. Bayoumi RA, Rosalki SB: Evaluation of methods of coenzyme activation of erythrocyte enzymes for detection of deficiency of vitamins B_1, B_2, and B_6, *Clin Chem* 22:327-335, 1976.
4. Vuilleumier JP, Keller HE, Keck E: Clinical chemical methods for the routine assessment of the vitamin status in human populations. 3. The apoenzymic stimulation tests for vitamin-B_1, vitamin-B_2, and vitamin-B_6 adapted to the Cobas-Bio analyzer, *Int J Vit Nutr Res* 60:126-135, 1990.
5. Waring PP, Fisher D, McDonnell J, et al: A continuous-flow (Auto Analyzer II) procedure for measuring erythrocyte transketolase activity, *Clin Chem* 28:831-833, 1982.
6. Herbeth B, Zittoun J, Miravet L, et al: Reference intervals for vitamins B_1, B_2, E, D, retinol, beta-carotene, and folate in blood: usefulness of dietary selection criteria, *Clin Chem* 32:1756-1759, 1986.
7. SmithKline Beecham Clinical Laboratories: *The SmithKline Beecham Laboratories handbook,* ed 14, Van Nuys, CA, 1987, SmithKline Beecham Clinical Laboratories.
8. Gans DA, Harper AE: Thiamin status of incarcerated and nonincarcerated adolescent males: dietary intake and thiamin pyrophosphate response, *Am J Clin Nutr* 53:1471-1475, 1991.
9. Talwar D, Davidson H, Cooney J, et al: Vitamin B(1) status assessed by direct measurement of thiamin pyrophosphate in erythrocytes or whole blood by HPLC: comparison with erythrocyte transketolase activation assay, *Clin Chem* 46:704-710, 2000.
10. Warnock, LG, Prudhomme CR, Wagner C: The determination of thiamin pyrophosphate in blood and other tissues, and its correlation with erythrocyte transketolase activity, *J Nutr* 108:421-427, 1978.

DIAGNOSTIC INFORMATION	REMARKS

B ↑ Pernicious anemia. See also *Thiamine*.

B ↓ Diabetes mellitus, polyneuritis

Repeated freezing and thawing significantly decreases ETK activity.

If anemia is present, erythrocyte transketolase (ETK) activity should be expressed per unit of hemoglobin.

Ercs ↑ Thiamine deficiency (≥25%); 15-24% indicates marginal deficiency, but this criterion is not wholly reliable when used as the sole index of thiamine status.[8]

$$\% \text{ TPP stimulation} = \frac{\text{ETK with TPP} - \text{ETK without TPP}}{\text{ETK without TPP}} \times 100$$

The TPP stimulation test indicates thiamine deficiency when addition of TPP to the reaction mixture enhances transketolase activity >25% over the unstimulated activity. Blood TDP measurement may be a more sensitive indicator of thiamine status than the transketolase activation assay.[9,10]

See *Thiamine*.

TEST NAME AND METHOD	SPECIMEN REQUIREMENTS	REFERENCE INTERVAL, CONVENTIONAL [INTERNATIONAL RECOMMENDED UNITS]				CHEMICAL INTERFERENCES AND IN VIVO EFFECTS
Transthyretin (Prealbumin, PA, Tryptophan-Rich Prealbumin, Thyroxine-Binding Prealbumin, TBPA)[1-3] *RID, nephelometric, turbidimetric*[4,5]	Serum. Analyze fresh or store at 4° C for <72 hr. Stable frozen at −20° C for 6 mo, or at −70° C indefinitely. Specimens without lipemia or hemolysis are preferred.	Cord: *mg/dL*[2]	13	× 10	*mg/L* [130]	S ↑ V Anabolic steroids/androgens, corticosteroids
		0-5 days: *mg/dL*[6]	6.0-21.0		*mg/L* [60-210]	S ↓ V Estrogens, some oral contraceptives
		1-5 yr:	14.0-30.0		[140-300]	
		6-9 yr:	15.0-33.0		[150-330]	Excessive turbidity can affect nephelometric methods.
		10-13 yr:	20.0-36.0		[200-360]	
		14-19 yr:	22.0-45.0		[220-450]	
		Adult: *mg/dL*	18-45		*mg/L* [180-450]	
	Urine, 24 hr. Centrifuge and adjust to pH 7.0. Analyze fresh. Stable frozen at −20° C for up to 1 yr.	0.017-0.047 mg/day[7]			($\bar{x}$: 0.026)	
	CSF. Centrifuge before analysis. Analyze fresh or store at 4° C for <72 hr. Stable frozen at −20° C for 6 mo, or at −70° C indefinitely. Specimens should not contain blood.	~2% [× 0.01 = ~0.02, mass fraction] of total CSF protein				

1. Henry JB, editor: *Clinical diagnosis and management by laboratory methods,* ed 20, Philadelphia, 2001, WB Saunders.
2. Putnam FW, editor: *The plasma proteins: structure, functions and genetic control, vol 1,* ed 2, New York, 1977, Academic Press.
3. Ingenbleek Y, Young V: Transthyretin (prealbumin) in health and disease: nutritional implications, *Ann Rev Nutr* 14:495-533, 1994.
4. Coore J, Ambler J: Potential problems with standardization of prealbumin (transthyretin) results in immunoturbidimetry, *Clin Chem* 37:58, 1991.
5. Pressac M, Vignoli L, Aymard P: Immunoturbidimetric assay of transthyretin by random-access analysis, *Clin Chem* 34:176, 1988.
6. Soldin SJ, Brugnara C, Wong EC, editors: *Pediatric reference ranges,* ed 4, Washington, DC, 2003, AACC Press.
7. Poortmans J, Jeanloz RW: Quantitative immunological determination of 12 plasma proteins excreted in human urine collected before and after exercise, *J Clin Invest* 47:386-393, 1968.
8. Cano NJ: Metabolism and clinical interest of serum transthyretin (pralbumin) in dialysis patients, *Clin Chem Lab Med* 40:1313-1319, 2002.
9. Raguso CA, Genton L, Dupertuis YM, et al: Assessment of nutritional status in organ transplant: is transthyretin a reliable indicator? *Clin Chem Lab Med* 40:1325-1328, 2002.
10. Miller SR, Sekijima Y, Kelly JW: Native state stabilization by NSAIDs inhibits transthyretin amyloidogenesis from the most common familial disease variants, *Lab Invest* 84:545-552, 2004.

DIAGNOSTIC INFORMATION	REMARKS

↑ Chronic renal failure,[8] high concentrations of corticosteroids, and Hodgkin's disease

↓ Inflammation, hepatic dysfunction, protein deficiency states, cancer, cystic fibrosis, and chronic illness

Transthyretin (prealbumin) is a homotetrameric unglycosylated protein that transports the thyroid hormones T_3 and T_4, as well as retinol (with retinol-binding protein). Because its hepatic synthesis is highly dependent on the availability of sufficient energy and protein stores, in addition to its comparatively short half-life, this protein has been used as a surrogate marker of nutritional status.[3] Transthyretin is also a negative acute-phase reacting protein; consequently levels decrease rapidly in inflammatory states, despite adequate nutritional stores.[9] Consequently it has been suggested that simultaneous measurement of an inflammatory marker such as CRP may be helpful in the assessment of changes in transthyretin levels.[8]

Approximately 38 variants are currently known, and many are associated with dissociation of the tetrameric protein, formation of insoluble fibrils, and amyloid deposition (familial). All are the result of single amino acid substitutions caused by single point mutations.[3] Amyloid disease caused by deposition of fibrils containing wild-type protein (senile systemic amyloidosis) also occurs. Onset of disease is typically at an earlier age with the familial forms. Nonsteroidal antiinflammatory medications can inhibit amyloid fibril formation.[10]

MW: 54,980
$t_{1/2}$: 1-2 days

TEST NAME AND METHOD	SPECIMEN REQUIREMENTS	REFERENCE INTERVAL, CONVENTIONAL [INTERNATIONAL RECOMMENDED UNITS]	CHEMICAL INTERFERENCES AND IN VIVO EFFECTS
TRH (Thyrotropin-Releasing Hormone) Stimulation Test[1-6]	Serum collected at baseline and 30 and 60 min after intravenous TRH	TSH: A normal response is a threefold increase in TSH above baseline. A typical normal response is an increase of 2-25 μU/mL (2-25 mU/L) above baseline ranges.	↑ V Amiodarone, overtreatment with antithyroid drugs, cimetidine, domperidone, haloperidol, lithium, metoclopramide, mor-
RIA		For baseline, see *Thyrotropin*.	phine, oral cholecystographic agents (iopanoic acid, ipodate), phenothiazines, and theophylline (IV)
Dose, adult: 500 mcg TRH (Thypinone), IV, rapid			
Child: 7 mcg/kg, IV, over 15-30 sec			↓ V Alcoholism, aspirin,[7] corticosteroids, dopamine, estrogens, fenclofenac, indomethacin,[7] levodopa, somatostatin, and thyroid hormones

1. Alsever RN, Gotlin RW: *Handbook of endocrine tests in adults and children,* ed 2, Chicago, 1978, Year Book Medical Publishers, Inc.

2. Eastham RD: *Biochemical values in clinical medicine,* ed 7, Bristol, UK, 1985, John Wright and Sons Ltd.

3. Wallach J, editor: *Interpretation of diagnostic tests,* ed 5, Boston, 1992, Little, Brown and Co.

4. Hershman JM: Clinical application of thyrotropin-releasing hormone, *N Engl J Med* 290:886-890, 1974.

5. Lechan RM: Update on thyrotropin-releasing hormone, *Thyroid Today* XVI(1), 1993.

6. Snyder PJ, Utiger RD: Response to thyrotropin releasing-hormone in normal man, *J Clin Endocrinol Metab* 34:380-385, 1972.

7. Ramey JN, Burrow GN, Spaulding SW, et al: The effect of aspirin and indomethacin on the TRH response in man, *J Clin Endocrinol Metab* 43:107-114, 1976.

8. Liewendahl K: Thyroid function tests: performance and limitations of current methodologies, *Scand J Clin Lab Invest* 52:435-445, 1992.

9. Extein I, Gold MS: Psychiatric applications of thyroid tests, *J Clin Psychiatry* 47(suppl 1):13-16, 1986.

10. Whitley RJ: Thyrotropin-releasing hormone (TRH) stimulation test, *AACC Endo Metab In-Service Training Cont Educ* 11:207-209, 1993.

11. Demers LM, Spencer C: Laboratory medicine practice guidelines: laboratory support for the diagnosis and monitoring of thyroid disease, *Thyroid* 13:14-104, 2003.

12. Spencer CA, Schwarzbein D, Guttler RB, et al: Thyrotropin (TSH)-releasing hormone stimulation test responses employing third and fourth generation TSH assays, *J Clin Endocrinol Metab* 76:494-498, 1993.

Exaggerated response, >35 μU/mL [>35 mU/L], observed in primary hypothyroidism and with thyroid hormone resistance. Inadequate or no response found in hypothyroidism caused by pituitary deficiency (secondary) and in primary hyperthyroidism (except with TSH-producing tumors). In hypothyroidism secondary to hypothalamic disorders (tertiary), response of normal magnitude is seen, but peak may be delayed (>60 min). These responses are not seen consistently, and differentiation of pituitary and hypothalamic hypothyroidism often requires other tests of thyroid and pituitary function.[8] Patients with nonthyroidal illnesses have a normal response.

Hormonal responses to TRH are also useful in the diagnosis and treatment of hypothalamic-pituitary disorders (e.g., increased ACTH in Cushing's disease, increased GH in acromegaly, increased FSH and LH in gonadotropin-secreting pituitary adenomas).[5]

In major depressive disorders, TSH blunting, ≤7.0 μU/mL [≤7.0 mU/L], is seen in 25% of patients. Failure of the response to normalize after antidepressant or electroconvulsant therapy is associated with a higher rate of relapse. The test may help differentiate mania from schizophrenia.[9]

Test essentially amplifies basal TSH levels. With the advent of high-sensitivity TSH assays, test has become less useful.[10]

Test should always be performed in the morning because of nyctohumeral rhythmicity in TSH secretion.

The magnitude of TSH release is proportional to the dose of TRH (up to a dose of 200-300 mcg of TRH) and the age and sex of the subject; responses decline with increasing age in men aged >40 yr but not in women. Response is increased in pregnancy. Side effects of IV TRH include mild nausea, flushing, dizziness, peculiar taste, an increase in arterial blood pressure, and an urge to urinate. These effects last only a few minutes and may be lessened by slow injection.

Because dopamine and glucocorticoids suppress TSH production, use of these agents is contraindicated for this test.

With the introduction of third-generation TSH assays, TRH stimulatory testing is now rarely needed (1) to differentiate mild (subclinical) hyperthyroidism from Graves' disease; (2) to distinguish sick hyperthyroidism from sick euthyroid patients; (3) to adjust T_4 replacement therapy in hypothyroid patients; and (4) to monitor T_4 suppressive therapy in patients with thyroid carcinoma.[11,12]

TEST NAME AND METHOD	SPECIMEN REQUIREMENTS	REFERENCE INTERVAL, CONVENTIONAL [INTERNATIONAL RECOMMENDED UNITS]			CHEMICAL INTERFERENCES AND IN VIVO EFFECTS
Triglycerides (TG)[1-18] *Enzymatic*[15,16,19,20]	Serum, EDTA plasma, but not heparin, oxalate, fluoride, or citrate. Heparin may cause artifactual reduction in TG by activating lipases. Fasting ≥12 hr is required. Stable for 4-7 days at 4° C. Avoid repeated freezing and thawing.		*Recommended cutpoints, mg/dL*[5]	*mmol/L*	↑ C Ascorbic acid, free glycerol (method-specific)
		Normal:	<150	× 0.0113 [<1.70]	↑ V Amiodarone, β-blockers, bile acid sequestrants (resins, e.g., cholestyramine, colestipol), corticosteroids, diuretics (especially thiazides), estrogens, ethanol, retinoids, interferons, HIV protease inhibitors, high energy (caloric) or carbohydrate diet, cigarette smoking, and alcohol consumption
		Borderline high:	150-199	[1.70-2.25]	
		High:	200-499	[2.26-5.64]	
		Very high:	≥500	[≥5.65]	
			(5th-95th Percentile) mg/dL[21]	*(5th-95th Percentile) mmol/L*	
		Non-Hispanic black 12-19 yr:	35-126	[0.40-1.42]	
		Non-Hispanic white 12-19 yr, M:	39-216	[0.44-2.44]	
		Mexican-American 12-19 yr, M:	42-205	[0.47-2.32]	
			(5th-95th Percentile) mg/dL[22]	*(5th-95th Percentile) mmol/L*	↓ C Bilirubin (method-specific)
		Black 45-49 yr			↓ V Ascorbic acid (high doses), aminosalicylic acid, asparaginase, fibric acid derivatives (e.g., clofibrate, gemfibrozil, fenofibrate), HMG CoA reductase inhibitors (statins), heparin, niacin, omega-3 fatty acids (fish oil), exercise, and weight reduction in overweight individuals
		M:	45-235	× 0.0113 [0.51-2.66]	
		F:	45-164	[0.51-1.85]	
		50-54 yr			
		M:	48-249	[0.54-2.81]	
		F:	48-203	[0.54-2.29]	
		55-59 yr			
		M:	46-244	[0.52-2.76]	
		F:	53-215	[0.60-2.43]	
		60-64 yr			
		M:	52-215	[0.59-2.43]	
		F:	55-226	[0.62-2.55]	
		White 45-49 yr			
		M:	56-326	[0.63-3.68]	
		F:	49-229	[0.55-2.59]	
		50-54 yr			
		M:	54-298	[0.61-3.37]	
		F:	53-287	[0.60-3.24]	
		55-59 yr			
		M:	59-309	[0.67-3.49]	
		F:	58-273	[0.66-3.08]	
		60-64 yr			
		M:	59-312	[0.67-3.53]	
		F:	58-295	[0.66-3.33]	

DIAGNOSTIC INFORMATION	REMARKS

↑ Familial hypertriglyceridemia, familial combined hyperlipidemia, familial dysbetalipoproteinemia, severe hypertriglyceridemia (type V, TG >1000 mg/dL), pancreatitis, familial lipoprotein lipase deficiency, apolipoprotein C-II deficiency, eruptive or planar xanthomas, and lipemia retinalis

The following primary disease states or conditions are associated with elevation of TG: obesity, impaired glucose tolerance, type 2 diabetes, hyperuricemia, viral hepatitis, alcoholism, biliary cirrhosis, extrahepatic biliary obstruction, nephrotic syndrome, chronic renal failure, Cushing's syndrome, pregnancy, infection, inflammation, certain glycogen storage diseases, and stress.

↓ Abetalipoproteinemia, hypobetalipoproteinemia. The following primary disease states can lead to secondary decrease of TG: malnutrition, malabsorption,

Metaanalysis of recent epidemiological studies indicate that an elevated TG is an independent risk factor for CHD, especially in women. TG is also important in the diagnosis and treatment of certain hyperlipidemias, in the assessment of abdominal pain and pancreatitis, and in the estimation of LDL cholesterol with the Friedewald equation. In clinical practice, an elevated TG is often a component of metabolic syndrome.

The National Education Program (NCEP) recommends that all adults aged >20 yr be screened with measurement of total cholesterol, HDL-C, and LDL-C and triglyceride concentrations. Fasting TG can vary by as much as 40% over ≥1 mo in some individuals. Because of biological and analytical variation, at least two serial samples may be necessary for clinical decision-making.

In the clinical laboratory, TG is almost always measured by enzymatic methods. Goals for TG measurement as defined by the Working Group on Lipoprotein Measurement of NCEP are a total error ≤15%, consistent with a bias ±5% and a total variability ≤5% CV. Most laboratories do not correct for endogenous glycerol, which typically accounts for an ~10 mg/dL overestimation of TG, although free glycerol can be markedly elevated as a result of strenuous exercise, liver damage, diabetes, hemodialysis, parenteral nutrition, IV medications containing glycerol, and stress.

TEST NAME AND METHOD	SPECIMEN REQUIREMENTS	REFERENCE INTERVAL, CONVENTIONAL [INTERNATIONAL RECOMMENDED UNITS]			CHEMICAL INTERFERENCES AND IN VIVO EFFECTS

Triglycerides—CONT

1. Austin MA: Plasma triglyceride and coronary heart disease, *Arterioscler Thromb* 11:2-14, 1991.

2. Cohn JS, McNamara JR, Cohn SD, et al: Postprandial plasma lipoprotein changes in human subjects of different ages, *J Lipid Res* 29:469-479, 1988.

3. Cooper GR, Myers GL, Smith J, et al: Blood lipid measurements: variations and practical utility, *JAMA* 267:1652-1660, 1992.

4. Durrington PN: Triglycerides are more important in atherosclerosis than epidemiology has suggested, *Atherosclerosis* 141(suppl 1):S57-S62, 1998.

5. Expert Panel on Detection, Evaluation, and Treatment of High Blood Cholesterol in Adults: Executive Summary of the Third Report of the National Cholesterol Education Program (NCEP) Expert Panel on Detection, Evaluation, and Treatment of High Blood Cholesterol in Adults (Adult Treatment Panel III), *JAMA* 285:2486-2497, 2001.

6. Friedewald WT, Levy RI, Frederickson DS: Estimation of the concentration of low-density lipoprotein cholesterol in plasma, without the use of the preparative ultracentrifuge, *Clin Chem* 18:499-502, 1972.

7. Henkin Y, Como JA, Oberman A: Secondary dyslipidemia: inadvertent effects of drugs in clinical practice, *JAMA* 267:961-968, 1992.

8. Hokanson JE, Austin MA: Plasma triglyceride level as a risk factor for cardiovascular disease independent of high-density lipoprotein cholesterol level: a meta-analysis of population-based prospective studies, *J Cardiovasc Risk* 1996:312-319, 1996.

9. Hortin GL, Cole TG, Gibson DW, et al: Decreased stability of triglycerides and increased free glycerol in serum for heparin-treated patients, *Clin Chem* 34:1847-1849, 1988.

10. Klotzsch SG, McNamara JR: Triglyceride measurements: a review of methods and interferences, *Clin Chem* 36:1605-1613, 1990.

11. Miller M, Seidler A, Moalemi A, et al: Normal triglyceride levels and coronary artery disease events: the Baltimore Coronary Observational Long-Term Study, *J Am Coll Cardiol* 31:1252-1257, 1998.

TEST NAME AND METHOD	SPECIMEN REQUIREMENTS	REFERENCE INTERVAL, CONVENTIONAL		[INTERNATIONAL RECOMMENDED UNITS]	CHEMICAL INTERFERENCES AND IN VIVO EFFECTS
Triiodothyronine, Free (FT$_3$)[1-4] *Equilibrium dialysis (tracer)*	Serum. Stable for 7 days at room temperature, but storage at 4° C is preferred. Stable for at least 30 days frozen.	*pg/dL*[5] Cord blood (>37 wk): Child and adult: Pregnancy First trimester: Second and third trimester:	15-391 260-480 211-383 196-338	*pmol/L* × 0.0154 [0.2-6.0] [4.0-7.4] [3.2-5.9] [3.0-5.2]	↑ V Dextrothyroxine (D-T$_4$) ↓ V Amiodarone, oral cholecystographic agents (iopanoic acid, ipodate), phenytoin, propranolol, and valproic acid ↑ C Fenoprofen (Amerlex kit) ↓ C *Amerlex kit:* heparin, phenytoin

1. Larsen PR, Davies TF, Schlumberger MJ, et al: The thyroid gland. In Larsen PR, Kronenberg HM, Melmed S, et al, editors: *Williams textbook of endocrinology,* ed 10, Philadelphia, 2003, WB Saunders.

2. Pearce CJ, Byfield PGH: Free thyroid hormone assays and thyroid function, *Ann Clin Biochem* 23:230-237, 1986.

3. Demers LM, Spencer C: The thyroid. In Burtis CA, Ashwood ER, Bruns DR, editors: *Tietz textbook of clinical chemistry,* ed 4, Philadelphia, 2006, WB Saunders.

12. Ockene IS, Chiriboga DE, Stanek EJ, et al: Seasonal variation in serum cholesterol levels, *Arch Intern Med* 164:863-870, 2004.

13. Ooi TC, Ooi DS: The atherogenic significance of an elevated plasma triglyceride level, *Crit Rev Clin Lab Sci* 35:489-516, 1998.

14. Rader DJ: Lipid disorders. In Topol EJ, editor: *Textbook of cardiovascular medicine,* ed 2, Philadelphia, PA, 2002, Lippincott Williams & Wilkins.

15. Rifai N, Warnick GR, Dominiczak MH, editors: *Handbook of lipoprotein testing,* ed 2, Washington, DC, 2000, AACC Press.

16. Stein EA, Myers GL: National Cholesterol Education Program recommendations for triglyceride measurement: executive summary. The National Cholesterol Education Program Working Group on Lipoprotein Measurement, *Clin Chem* 41:1421-1426, 1995.

17. Young DS: *Effects of drugs on clinical laboratory tests,* ed 5, Washington, DC, 2000, AACC Press.

18. Young DS: *Effects of preanalytical variables on clinical laboratory tests,* ed 2, Washington, DC, 1997, AACC Press.

19. Artiss JD, Strandbergh DR, Zak B: Elimination of glycerol interference in a colorimetric enzymic triglyceride assay, *Clin Chim Acta* 182:109-116, 1989.

20. Witte DL, Brown LF, Feld RD: Enzymatic analysis of serum cholesterol and triglycerides: a brief review, *Lab Med* 9:39-44, 1978.

21. Hickman TB, Briefel RR, Carroll MD, et al: Distributions and trends of serum lipid levels among United States children and adolescents ages 4-19 years: data from the third National Health and Nutrition Examination Survey, *Prev Med* 27:879-890, 1998.

22. Brown SA, Hutchinson R, Morrisett J, et al: Plasma lipid, lipoprotein cholesterol, and apoprotein distributions in selected US communities: the Atherosclerosis Risk in Communities (ARIC) Study, *Arterioscl Thromb* 13:1139-1158, 1993.

↑ Hyperthyroidism, T_3 toxicosis, peripheral resistance syndrome, and high altitude

↓ Hypothyroidism, third trimester of pregnancy

In nonthyroidal illness, a low FT_3 is a nonspecific finding.

See also *Triiodothyronine, Total.*

Neither FT_3 nor FT_4 has demonstrated a clear advantage over the other in analyzing thyrotoxicosis. FT_3 by tracer dialysis is an indirect estimate of the free hormone and is determined by multiplying the fraction of T_3 (measured by equilibrium tracer dialysis) by the total T_3 concentration (measured separately by immunoassay). Measuring FT_3 is mainly of value in diagnosing T_3 toxicosis, in determining the T_3 response to therapy, and in clarifying protein binding abnormalities. FT_3 can also be of use in the early progression of subclinical hyperthyroidism to overt thyrotoxicosis when FT_4 is normal and TSH is suppressed. In this setting, FT_3 is often the first to be increased.

FT_3 is ~0.2-0.5% of total T_3.

Triiodothyronine autoantibodies produce erroneous results unless serum is pretreated with PEG.[6]

FT_3 can be measured by a two-step immunoassay method using chemiluminescence.[3]

4. Wilke TJ: Estimation of free thyroid hormone concentrations in the clinical laboratory [review], *Clin Chem* 32:585-592, 1986.

5. Nichols Institute Reference Laboratories: *Test catalog,* San Juan Capistrano, CA, 1993, Nichols Institute Reference Laboratories.

6. Sakata S, Komaki T, Nakamura S, et al: Measurement of free triiodothyronine in serum in the presence of autoantibodies to it [letter], *Clin Chem* 31:1252-1253, 1985.

TEST NAME AND METHOD	SPECIMEN REQUIREMENTS	REFERENCE INTERVAL, CONVENTIONAL [INTERNATIONAL RECOMMENDED UNITS]			CHEMICAL INTERFERENCES AND IN VIVO EFFECTS
Triiodothyronine (T$_3$), Total[1-5] *RIA*[6] *Immunoassay*[7]	Serum. Stable for 7 days at room temperature, but storage at 4° C is preferred. Stable for at least 30 days at −20° C.	*ng/dL*[7] Cord (>37 wk): 1-3 days: 1-11 mo: 1-5 yr: 6-10 yr: 11-15 yr: 16-20 yr: Adult 20-50 yr: 50-90 yr: Pregnancy (last 5 mo):	5-141 × 0.0154 100-740 105-245 105-269 94-241 82-213 80-210 70-204 40-181 116-247	*nmol/L* [0.08-2.17] [1.54-11.40] [1.62-3.77] [1.62-4.14] [1.45-3.71] [1.26-3.28] [1.23-3.23] [1.08-3.14] [0.62-2.79] [1.79-3.80]	↑ V Amiodarone (rare), dextrothyroxine (D-T$_4$), dinoprost tromethamine (PGF$_{2\alpha}$), estrogens, heroin, high altitude, methadone, oral contraceptives, and terbutaline ↑ C Anti-T$_3$ (double-antibody technique), fenoprofen (Amerlex kit) ↓ V Amiodarone, androgens, anticonvulsants (carbamazepine, phenytoin), asparaginase, cimetidine, dexamethasone, iodides, isotretinoin, lithium, oral cholecystographic agents (iopanoic acid, ipodate), propranolol, propylthiouracil, and salicylates (large doses) ↓ C Anti-T$_3$ (single-antibody technique)

1. Alsever RN, Gotlin RW: *Handbook of endocrine tests in adults and children,* ed 2, Chicago, 1978, Year Book Medical Publishers, Inc.

2. Chen JJS, Ladenson PW: Discordant hypothyroxinemia and hypertriiodothyroninemia in treated patients with hyperthyroid Graves' disease, *J Clin Endocrinol Metab* 63:102-106, 1986.

3. Larsen PR, Davies TF, Schlumberger MJ, et al: The thyroid gland. In Larsen PR, Kronenberg HM, Melmed S, et al, editors: *Williams textbook of endocrinology,* ed 10, Philadelphia, 2003, WB Saunders.

4. Nystrom E, Bengtsson C, Lindquist O, et al: Serum triiodothyronine and hyperthyroidism in a population sample of women, *Clin Endocrinol* 20:31-42, 1981.

5. Takamatsu J, Kuma K, Mozai T: Serum triiodothyronine to thyroxine ratio: a newly recognized predictor of the outcome of hyperthyroidism due to Graves' disease, *J Clin Endocrinol Metab* 62:980-983, 1986.

6. Witherspoon L, Shuler S, Baird F, et al: Measurement of triiodothyronine (T$_3$) by RIA compared to automated systems, *Clin Chem* 38:954, 1992.

7. Demers LM, Spencer C: The thyroid. In Burtis CA, Ashwood ER, Bruns DR, editors: *Tietz textbook of clinical chemistry,* ed 4, Philadelphia, 2006, WB Saunders.

8. Nichols Institute Reference Laboratories: *Test catalog,* San Juan Capistrano, CA, 1993, Nichols Institute Reference Laboratories.

DIAGNOSTIC INFORMATION	REMARKS

↑ Hyperthyroidism, T_3 thyrotoxicosis, treated hyperthyroidism, early thyroid failure, iodine deficiency goiter, states with increased TBG, thyrotoxicosis factitia, and pregnancy

↓ Hypothyroidism, states with decreased TBG, and acute and subacute nonthyroidal illnesses

In early or mild primary hypothyroidism, T_4 is reduced more than T_3 (high T_3/T_4 ratio). In sick euthyroid syndrome, a reduced T_3 is often the first change observed.

At least 80% of circulating T_3 is derived from monodeiodination of T_4 in peripheral tissues. T_3 has 10- to 15-fold lower affinity for TBG than T_4 but has 15-fold higher affinity for thyroid receptor. T_3 is 4-5 times more potent in biological systems than T_4. Even though serum T_3 levels are 100-fold lower than T_4 concentrations, most T_3 immunoassays have negligible cross-reactivity with T_4. Because T_3 levels fluctuate rapidly in response to stress and other nonthyroidal factors, measurement of T_3 is not a good general test of thyroid status.[8]

T_3 toxicosis is uncommon in the early stages of thyrotoxicosis. There is a state of "compensated hypothyroidism" (after surgery or treatment with radioactive iodine or antithyroid drugs) in which serum T_4 is high, T_3 is high or normal, and TSH is high.

Serum T_3 values decrease with age even in healthy individuals.

TEST NAME AND METHOD	SPECIMEN REQUIREMENTS	REFERENCE INTERVAL, CONVENTIONAL [INTERNATIONAL RECOMMENDED UNITS]	CHEMICAL INTERFERENCES AND IN VIVO EFFECTS
Triiodothyronine Suppression Test (Werner Test)[1-3] Dose, adult: 70-100 mcg of triiodothyronine (Cytomel) orally in divided doses, 3 × daily for 7-10 days Child and adolescent: 50-75 mcg/day	Measure initial 2-hr (or 4- or 6-hr) and 24-hr ^{131}I-uptake, and then give Cytomel. At end of test period, perform second measure of ^{131}I-uptake. T$_4$ and TSH levels may also be measured at the start and end of T$_3$ administration.	^{131}I-uptake at 2 and 24 hr decreases after suppression to <50% of baseline. (If the baseline for RAIU is >40%, it should decrease to <20%. If the baseline for RAIU is <40%, it should decrease by >50%.) T$_4$ level should decrease below the reference interval or to less than half of baseline. If TSH levels are high initially, they usually approach reference interval by the end of 1 wk. When interpreting test results of second uptake test, correct for residual radioactivity. For baseline, see *Thyroid Uptake of Radioactive Iodine, ^{131}I or ^{123}I.*	See *Thyroid Uptake of Radioactive Iodine, ^{131}I or ^{123}I; Thyroxine, Total;* and *Thyrotropin.*

1. Alsever RN, Gotlin RW: *Handbook of endocrine tests in adults and children,* ed 2, Chicago, 1978, Year Book Medical Publishers, Inc.
2. Eastham RD: *Biochemical values in clinical medicine,* ed 7, Bristol, UK, 1985, John Wright and Sons Ltd.
3. Larsen PR, Ingbar SH: The thyroid gland. In Wilson JH, Foster DW, editors: *Williams textbook of endocrinology,* ed 8, Philadelphia, 1992, WB Saunders.

TEST NAME AND METHOD	SPECIMEN REQUIREMENTS					CHEMICAL INTERFERENCES AND IN VIVO EFFECTS
Triiodothyronine Uptake Test (T$_3$U)[1-3]	Serum. Refrigerate up to 7 days. Store at −20° C for longer periods. Do not use plasma (T$_3$U levels are lower).		%	× 1.0	*AU* [25-37]	See *Thyroid Hormone-Binding Ratio.*
		Newborn:	25-37		[25-37]	
		Adult:	24-34		[24-34]	
		>60 yr				
		M:	24-32		[24-32]	
		F:	22-32		[22-32]	

*AU, Arbitrary units.

1. Alsever RN, Gotlin RW: *Handbook of endocrine tests in adults and children,* ed 2, Chicago, 1978, Year Book Medical Publishers, Inc.
2. Committee on Nomenclature of the American Thyroid Association: Revised nomenclature for tests of thyroid hormones and thyroid-related proteins in serum, *J Clin Endocrinol Metab* 64:1089-1094, 1987.
3. Lavin N: *Manual of endocrinology and metabolism,* Boston, 1986, Little, Brown and Co.

DIAGNOSTIC INFORMATION   **REMARKS**

No response or inadequate response is consistent with hyperthyroidism and subclinical Graves' disease. Normal suppression excludes the diagnosis of hyperthyroidism. Normal suppression is also seen in goiter (in iodine deficiency) and in congenital and acquired defects in hormone synthesis.

Test assesses the integrity of a normal thyroid-pituitary feedback. Test is used to detect thyroid gland autonomy or the presence of an abnormal stimulator. This test is rarely used in clinical practice because a suppressed basal TSH level or an absent TSH response to TRH provides the same information (see *Thyrotropin* and *TRH Stimulation Test*).

Test should be used with caution in elderly patients with heart disease, hypertension, or other vascular problems. T_3 may precipitate atrial fibrillation, angina, or heart failure. Test is infrequently used. In very young children or in patients with heart failure or general debility, a dose of 25-50 mcg T_3/day is recommended.

This test was designed to correct for variability in protein binding of thyroid hormone when used in conjunction with total thyroid hormone measurements.

This test should be replaced with the thyroid hormone-binding ratio test in those few instances where direct free hormone measurements are not useful.

See *Thyroid Hormone-Binding Ratio.*

TEST NAME AND METHOD	SPECIMEN REQUIREMENTS	REFERENCE INTERVAL, CONVENTIONAL [INTERNATIONAL RECOMMENDED UNITS]	CHEMICAL INTERFERENCES AND IN VIVO EFFECTS
Tropomyosin[1] *RIA*[1]	Serum. Stable at 30° C for up to 1 yr.	1-3 mcg/L	S ↑ V Skeletal muscle tropomyosin after very severe exercise and rhabdomyolysis.[2]

1. Cummins P, McGurk B, Littler WA: Radioimmunoassay of human cardiac tropomyosin in acute myocardia infarction, *Clin Sci* 60:251-259, 1981.
2. Cummins P, Young A, Auckland ML, et al: Comparison of serum cardiac specific troponin-I with creatine kinase creatine kinase-MB isoenzyme, tropomyosin, myoglobin and C-reactive protein release in marathon runners: cardiac or skeletal muscle trauma? *Eur J lin Invest* 17:317-324, 1987.

TEST NAME AND METHOD	SPECIMEN REQUIREMENTS	REFERENCE INTERVAL, CONVENTIONAL [INTERNATIONAL RECOMMENDED UNITS]	CHEMICAL INTERFERENCES AND IN VIVO EFFECTS
Troponin-I, Cardiac (cTnI)[1-21] *Immunoassay*[1,2] *Point-of-care immunoassays also available*[3]	Serum, heparin plasma, and EDTA plasma For all point-of-care assays anticoagulated whole blood (EDTA, heparin). Heparin plasma should not be used interchangeably with serum because some assays measure cTn at 5-20% lower.[4] If analysis is not to be performed within 4-6 hr, specimens should be stored refrigerated for up to 24 hr. Stable −20 to −80° C for 6 mo to several years when freeze/thaw cycles are avoided. Limited information is available on serum and plasma tubes (glass and plastic) containing separator gels.	*Assay*[5] LLD 99th 10% CV Abbott AxSYM (n) 0.14 0.5 0.8 Bayer Centaur (s) 0.02 0.1 0.35 Beckman Access (p) 0.01 0.04 0.06 Dade-Behring Dimension (s) 0.04 0.07 0.14 DPC Immulite (s) 0.20 0.20 0.60 Ortho Vitros ECi (p) 0.02 0.08 0.12 Tosoh AIA 600II (b) 0.06 <0.06 0.06 All results in mcg/L. Specimen types as indicated in the manufacturer's package inserts used for determination of 99th percentile reference ranges: s = serum, p = heparin plasma, b = both, n = not specified. All concentrations >99th limit are designated as irreversible myocardial injury. In the presence of the clinical setting of ischemia, an increased cTn >99th percentile indicative of acute myocardial infarction (MI).	Fibrin or cellular matter, turbid serum or plasma, ↑ bilirubin, and moderate-gross hemolysis cause interferences in most assays.[7] Although most assays are configured with sufficient IgG to block human anti-mouse antibodies (HAMAs), rheumatoid factors (RFs), and heterophile antibodies, these interferents may cause false-positive results in patients without myocardial injury.[8] Immunoglobulin can cause falsely low cTn MI patients. Whenever inconsistent serial increasing or decreasing patterns are observed, these types of interferents should be considered. Reassaying of suspected false-positive specimens by an alternate cTn assay recommended.[9,10] No underlying skeletal muscle

DIAGNOSTIC INFORMATION	REMARKS

↑↑ Myocardial infarction, severe muscle damage caused by trauma, viral and bacterial infections, alcohol, cocaine, or ischemia. A myopathy may increase serum tropomyosin; neurogenic atrophy of skeletal muscle will not.

Serum tropomyosin increases 2-6 hr after infarction and can remain elevated for up to 12 days.[1]

Antibody generated against α-tropomyosin from cardiac muscle is contaminated with minor quantities of the β-form and may give false-positive results with the test. In addition, both α- and β-forms are found in skeletal muscle. Thus false-positive results may occur after muscle damage such as observed during very severe exercise.[1,2]

To assist in differentiating patients with AMI from non-AMI, the ESC/ACC has redefined AMI, predicated on biomarkers, specifically cTnI or cTnT: (1) a maximal concentration of cTnI or cTnI >99% of a reference group, on at least one occasion during the first 24 hr after the event; (2) a maximal value of CK-MB mass >99% of a reference group on two successive samples or a maximal value >2× reference limit during the first hour after the event (although the consensus document states values for CK-MB should increase and decrease, either a increasing or decreasing pattern should be considered diagnostic; however, values that remain increased without change are rarely due to MI; and (3) in the absence of availability of a cTn or CK-MB assay, total creatine kinase (CK) >2× the upper reference limit.[12,13]

Also, the ACC/AHA guidelines for management of unstable angina recommend monitoring cTn in ACS patients for differentiating unstable angina (defined as when cTn within the 99% limit) and non–ST-segment-elevation MI (NSTEMI, defined as when cTn > the 99th percentile limit). Blood should be obtained for testing at admission (0 hr), 6-9 hr, and 12-24 hr if the earlier specimens are normal and the clinical index of suspicion is high.[14]

For patients in need of an early diagnosis, that will parallel a rapid triage protocol, a rapidly appearing biomarker has been suggested along with serial cTn. Some studies suggest a role for multimarker testing, including myoglobin, for risk stratification in chest pain units and for exclusion of MI.[15] The early release kinetics of cTn are similar to those of CK-MB after

Increased cTn is predicative of adverse outcomes in acute coronary syndrome (ACS). From 26 studies, odds ratios (ORs) for both short-term (30 days) and long-term (5 mo-3 yr) outcomes (endpoint death or nonfatal MI) in patients with and without ST-segment elevation and in UA patients for 6000 patients studied was 8.4.[20] Because cTnI offers powerful risk assessment, cTn monitoring should be included in practice guidelines, not only regarding diagnosis and management of ACS patients but also for risk stratification.

The timing of sampling is critical for cardiac marker because results from a single draw at presentation may conflict with findings based on serial draws 24 hr after presentation. Two samples are recommended for cTn on ACS patients who do not rule in for AMI; at presentation and ≥6-9 hr after.[21] To allow for an increase in cTn above baseline in a patient presenting with a recent acute coronary lesion. However, a normal cardiac cTn does not remove all risk. cTn results should be reported within 30-60 min (from the time blood is drawn to results reported to the physician), either using POC testing or the central laboratory.

The contractile proteins of the myofibril include troponin C (Ca-binding), I (inhibitory), and T (tropomyosin-binding). Subunits exist in as isoforms, distributed between cardiac muscle and slow and fast twitch skeletal muscle. Only two major isoforms of troponin C are found in human heart and skeletal muscle, characteristic of slow and fast twitch muscle. The heart isoform is identical with the slow twitch skeletal muscle isoform. Isoforms of cTnT and cTnI are products of unique genes.

TEST NAME AND METHOD	SPECIMEN REQUIREMENTS	REFERENCE INTERVAL, CONVENTIONAL [INTERNATIONAL RECOMMENDED UNITS]	CHEMICAL INTERFERENCES AND IN VIVO EFFECTS

Troponin-I, Cardiac (cTnI)—CONT

Reference range at the 99th percentile

Assay	All	M	F	White	Black	Hispanic	Asian
AxSYM	0.8	0.8	0.7	0.8	0.5	0.5	1.1
Centaur	0.15	0.17	0.14	0.17	0.17	0.00	0.09
Access	0.08	0.10	0.04	0.07	0.08	0.02	0.10
Dimension	0.06	0.06	0.06	0.04	0.03	0.01	0.09
Immulite	0.21	0.21	<0.2	0.21	<0.2	<0.2	<0.2
Vitros ECi	0.10	0.11	0.09	0.11	0.10	0.02	0.07
AIA 600II	0.07	0.07	<0.05	<0.06	0.17	<0.06	0.07

disease or end-stage renal disease cause falsely increased cTn concentrations; and increased cTn concentrations should be considered real when measured on these patient groups.[11]

A standard reference material for troponin I is available.[6]

1. Pagani F, Stefini F, Micca G, et al: Multicenter evaluation of the TOSOH AIA-pack second-generation cardiac troponin I assay, *Clin Chem* 50:1707-1709, 2004.

2. Uettwiller-Geiger D, Wu AHB, Apple FS, et al: Multicenter evaluation of an automated assay for troponin I, *Clin Chem* 48:869-876, 2002.

3. Apple FS, Murakami MM, Jesse RL, et al: Near-bedside whole-blood cardiac troponin I assay for risk assessment of patients with acute coronary syndromes, *Clin Chem* 48:1784-1787, 2002.

4. Gerhardt W, Nordin G, Herbert AK, et al: Troponin T and I assays show decreased concentrations in heparin plasma compared with serum: lower recoveries in early than in late phases of myocardial injury, *Clin Chem* 46:817-821, 2000.

5. Apple FS, Wu AHB, Jaffe AS: European Society of Trial Cardiology and American College of Cardiology guidelines for redefinition of myocardial infarction: how to use existing assays clinically and for clinical trials, *Am Heart J* 144:981-986, 2002.

6. Christenson RH, Duh SH, Apple FS, et al: Standardization of cardiac troponin I assays: round Robin of ten candidate reference materials, *Clin Chem* 47:431-437, 2001.

AMI with increases above the upper reference limit seen at 2-6 hr. The initial increase is caused by the 3-6% cytoplasmic fraction of cTn (CK-MB is 100% cytoplasmic). Second, cTn can remain increased up to 4-14 days after AMI because of ongoing release from the 94-97% myofibril-bound fraction. Third, the very low to undetectable cTn in healthy patients allows lower cutoffs than CK-MB for myocardial injury. Finally, cardiac tissue specificity of cTn eliminates false clinical impression of AMI in patients with increased CK-MB concentrations following skeletal muscle injuries.

Troponin is localized primarily in the myofibrils (94-97%), with a smaller cytoplasmic fraction (3-6%). cTnT and cTnI have different amino acid.[16]

Human cTnI has an additional posttranslational 31-amino acid residue on the N-terminal end compared with skeletal muscle TnI, giving cardiac specificity and 1 isoform. cTnI is not expressed in normal, regenerating, or diseased human or animal skeletal muscle. Troponin T is also encoded for by a different gene than encodes for skeletal muscle isoforms. An 11-amino acid amino terminal residue gives this marker unique cardiac specificity. However, during human fetal development, in regenerating rat skeletal muscle, and in diseased human skeletal muscle, small amounts of cTnT are expressed as one of four identified isoforms in skeletal muscle. In humans, cTnT isoform expression has been demonstrated in skeletal muscle specimens obtained from patients with muscular dystrophy, polymyositis, dermatomyositis, and end-stage renal disease.[17] cTnI is part of the T-I-C ternary complex as a structural and regulatory component of the myofibril. Following myocardial injury or because of genetic disposition, multiple forms are expressed in tissue and in blood including T-I-C, IC, free I, and multiple modifications of these, including oxidation, reduction, phosphorylation and dephosphorylation, and C- and N-terminal degradation. Detection of seven different cTnI forms in an injured human heart can appear depending on the antibodies used.[18] Different antibodies can lead to a substantially different recognition patterns. Assays should use antibodies that recognize epitopes in the stable region of cTnI and demonstrate an equimolar response to the different cTnI forms in blood.[19]

7. Krahn J, Parry DM, Leroux M, et al: High percentage of false-positive cardiac troponin I results in patients with rheumatoid factor, *Clin Biochem* 32:477-480, 1999.

8. Fitzmaurice T, Brown C, Rifai N, et al: False increase of cardiac troponin I with heterophilic antibodies, *Clin Chem* 44:2212-2214, 1998.

9. Bohner J, Pape K, Hannes W, et al: False-negative immunoassay results for cardiac troponin I probably due to circulating troponin I autoantibodies, *Clin Chem* 42:2046, 1996.

10. Eriksson S, Junikka M, Laitinen P, et al: Negative interference in cardiac troponin I immunoassays from a frequently occurring serum and plasma component, *Clin Chem* 49:1095-1104, 2003.

11. Apple FS, Murakami MM, Pearce LA, et al: Multi-biomarker risk stratification on N-terminal pro-B-type natriuretic peptide, high-sensitivity C-reactive protein, and cardiac troponin T and I in end-stage renal disease for all-cause death, *Clin Chem* 50:1-7, 2004.

12. Jaffe AS, Ravkilde J, Roberts R, et al: It's time for a change to a troponin standard, *Circulation* 102:1216-1220, 2000.

TEST NAME AND METHOD	SPECIMEN REQUIREMENTS	REFERENCE INTERVAL, CONVENTIONAL [INTERNATIONAL RECOMMENDED UNITS]	CHEMICAL INTERFERENCES AND IN VIVO EFFECTS

Troponin-I, Cardiac (cTnI)—CONT

13. Joint European Society of Cardiology/American College of Cardiology Committee: Myocardial infarction defined–a consensus document of the joint European Society of Cardiology/American College of Cardiology Committee for the redefinition of myocardial infarction, *J Am Coll Cardiol* 36:959-969, 2000.

14. Braunwald E, Antman EM, Beasley JW, et al: ACC/AHA guidelines for the management of patients with unstable angina and non-ST-segment elevation myocardial infarction, *J Am Coll Cardiol* 36:970-1062, 2000.

15. Newby LK, Storrow AB, Gibler WB, et al: Bedside multimarker testing for risk stratification in chest pain units: the chest pain evaluation by creatine kinase-MB, myoglobin, and troponin I (CHECKMATE) study, *Circulation* 103:1832-1837, 2001.

16. Wu AH, Feng YJ, Moore R, et al: Characterization of cardiac troponin subunit release into serum after acute myocardial infarction and comparison of assays for troponin T and I, *Clin Chem* 44:1198-1208, 1998.

TEST NAME AND METHOD	SPECIMEN REQUIREMENTS	REFERENCE INTERVAL, CONVENTIONAL [INTERNATIONAL RECOMMENDED UNITS]	CHEMICAL INTERFERENCES AND IN VIVO EFFECTS
Troponin-T, Cardiac (cTnT) *Immunoassay*[1] *Point-of-care immunoassays assays also available.*[2]	Serum, and EDTA plasma For all point-of-care assays, anticoagulated whole blood (EDTA, heparin). Heparin plasma should not be used interchangeably with serum because heparin plasma can measure cTnT at 5-20% lower.[3] If analysis is not to be performed within 4-6 hr, specimens should be stored refrigerated for up to 24 hr; otherwise, −20-80° C. Stable for 6 mo to several years, when freeze/thaw cycles are avoided.[4] Limited information is available on serum and plasma tubes (glass and plastic) containing separator gels.	*Upper reference limit for third-generation assay*[5]: 0.01 mcg/L (limit of detection) 0.01 mcg/L (99th percentile) 0.03 mcg/L (10% CV cutpoint) All concentrations >99th limit are designated as irreversible myocardial injury. In the presence of the clinical setting of ischemia, an increased cTn >99th percentile is indicative of acute myocardial infarction (MI).	See *Troponin-I, Cardiac.*

17. Apple FS: Tissue specificity of cardiac troponin I, cardiac troponin T, and creatine kinase MB, *Clin Chim Acta* 284:151-159, 1999.
18. Katrukha A, Bereznikova A, Filatov V, et al: Biochemical factors influencing measurement of cardiac troponin I in serum, *Clin Chem Lab Med* 37:1091-1095, 1999.
19. Panteghini M, Gerhardt W, Apple FS, et al: Quality specifications for cardiac troponin assays, *Clin Chem Lab Med* 39:175-179, 2001.
20. Heidenreich PA, Alloggiamento T, Melsop K., et al: The prognostic value of troponin in patients with non-ST elevation acute coronary syndromes: a meta-analysis, *J Am Coll Cardiol* 38:478-485, 2001.
21. Wu AH, Apple FS, Gibler WB, et al: National Academy of Clinical Biochemistry Standards of Laboratory Practice: recommendations for the use of cardiac markers in coronary artery diseases, *Clin Chem* 45:1104-1121, 1999.

See *Troponin-I, Cardiac* for a discussion of the clinical significance of cardiac troponin. In renal failure, increased cardiac troponin T and I are associated with an increased incidence of cardiac death at 2 yr. There is a considerably higher incidence of positive results for cTnT than cTnI at any cutoff (99th percentile, 10% CV, or receiver-operator characteristic curve cutoff).[6]

See *Troponin-I, Cardiac.*

TEST NAME AND METHOD	SPECIMEN REQUIREMENTS	REFERENCE INTERVAL, CONVENTIONAL [INTERNATIONAL RECOMMENDED UNITS]	CHEMICAL INTERFERENCES AND IN VIVO EFFECTS

Troponin-T, Cardiac (cTnT)—CONT

1. Wu AH, Valdes R Jr, Apple FS, et al: Cardiac troponin-T immunoassay for diagnosis of acute myocardial infarction, *Clin Chem* 40:900-907, 1994.

2. Muller-Bardorff M, Sylven C, Rasmanis G, et al: Evaluation of a point-of-care system for quantitative determination of troponin T and myoglobin, *Clin Chem Lab Med* 38:567-574, 2000.

3. Gerhardt W, Nordin G, Herbert AK, et al: Troponin T and I assays show decreased concentrations in heparin plasma compared with serum: lower recoveries in early than in late phases of myocardial injury, *Clin Chem* 46:817-821, 2000.

Trypsin (EC 3.4.21.4)[1] *p-Toluene-sulfonyl-L-arginine methyl ester (TAME)*[1]	Feces, fresh	*mcg trypsin/g stool* Child and adult: 40-760 Pancreatic insufficiency: 0-33 Fibrocystic child: <20	↑ Oral enzyme preparations; do not administer for 3 days before test. Proteolytic bacteria in stool (or from urine contamination) may augment or reduce trypsin catalytic activity.
Immunoreactive trypsin (cationic trypsin) *RIA*	Serum or plasma (EDTA, heparin; avoid citrate and oxalate). Store at 4° C or −20° C.	Method dependent	S ↑ V After endoscopic retrograde pancreatography or use of pancreatic stimulants (cholecystokinin, bombesin, secretin, or cerulein); after food
	Whole blood spotted on filter paper >4 mm diameter for each single assay. Stable for 8 days at 4° C,[2] but cystic fibrosis cases may still be detected after 7 yr at 4° C.[3] Avoid light.		Variability in extraction depending on type of filter paper used and characteristics of eluting fluid (e.g., pH, ionic strength, presence or absence of detergent)

4. Price A, Burgin C, Cruise M: Stability of cardiac troponins and CK-MB mass isoenzyme, *Clin Chem Lab Med* 38:1159-1160, 2000.
5. Hallermayer K, Klenner D, Vogel R: Use of recombinant human cardiac Troponin T for standardization of third generation Troponin T methods, *Scand J Clin Lab Investig Suppl* 230:128-131, 1999.
6. Apple FS, Murakami MM, Pearce LA, et al: Predictive value of cardiac troponin I and T for subsequent death in end-stage renal disease, *Circulation* 106:2941-2945, 2002.

Inadequate trypsin secretion can lead to malabsorption, flatus, and abdominal discomfort.

This test will probably be replaced by fecal elastase.

F ↓ Loss of >85% of pancreatic exocrine function; cystic fibrosis (feces and duodenal fluid)

Absent in stool but present in duodenal aspirate in neonatal intestinal obstruction.[4]

S ↑ Acute pancreatitis (particularly alcohol induced), chronic renal failure, liver disease, occasionally in peptic ulcer and gallstones, and in cystic fibrosis (cord blood)

S ↓ Chronic pancreatitis (especially if steatorrhea is present), pancreatic cancer (Some cases may have increased or normal values.)

Both low and high values occur in β-thalassemia. High values occur in acute malnutrition, and low values occur in chronic malnutrition.

Diabetes: Both juvenile and maturity-onset show depressed levels.

Viral infections: Serum levels are increased when silent invasion of pancreas has occurred.

Trypsin levels have diurnal variation, with higher values in the late evening.[11] Serum trypsin must be measured by mass (as a protein) rather than by its activity (as an enzyme) because the antiproteases in serum inhibit enzyme activity. Problems of standardization and different specificities of antisera to the various forms of trypsin (trypsinogen, trypsin bound to α_1-antitrypsin or to α_2-macroglobulin, and free trypsin) have been reported and account for major differences in assays with the two most common antisera (Sorin and Behringwerke). Measurement of trypsin in duodenal fluid after hormonal stimulation is very specialized, and results are too variable to define reference values.

Increases are highly sensitive. In pancreatitis it offers no diagnostic advantage over standard testing, and the specificity is low.[2]

High values are found in neonates with cystic fibrosis, readily distinguishing these infants from normal; values decrease with disease progression. Test has been incorporated into neonatal screening programs in some centers with promising results.[5-8] Test should be performed in the first month of life.

A two-step testing protocol has been proposed.[9] Using the CIS assay, 1-4-day-old infants with ≥140 mg/L are retested at 2-8 wk of age. If the value is ≥80 mg/L, a sweat test is performed. Another protocol retests, by direct gene analysis, all 4-5-day-old infants in the highest 1% of population.[10]

Not recommended for screening or diagnosis of CF.

TEST NAME AND METHOD	SPECIMEN REQUIREMENTS	REFERENCE INTERVAL, CONVENTIONAL [INTERNATIONAL RECOMMENDED UNITS]		CHEMICAL INTERFERENCES AND IN VIVO EFFECTS

Trypsin—CONT

1. Burtis CA, Ashwood ER, editors: *Tietz textbook of clinical chemistry,* ed 2, Philadelphia, 1994, WB Saunders.

2. Bourguignon JP, Deby-Dupoint G, Reuter A, et al: Variations in dried blood spot immunoreactive trypsin in relation to gestational age and during the first week of life, *Eur J Pediatr* 144:547-549, 1986.

3. Crossley JR, Smith PA, Edgar BW, et al: Neonatal screening for cystic fibrosis, using immunoreactive trypsin assay in dried blood spots, *Clin Chim Acta* 113:111-121, 1981.

4. Meisheri IV, Sawant VV, Gangal S, et al: Trypsin activity in stool and duodenal aspirate of neonates for differential diagnosis of intestinal obstruction, *Pediatr Surg Int* 18:104-106, 2002.

5. Canadian Task Force on the Periodic Health Examination: Periodic health examination, 1991. Update 4. Screening for cystic fibrosis, *CMAJ* 145:629-635, 1991.

6. Cassio A, Bernardi F, Piazzi S, et al: Neonatal screening for cystic fibrosis by dried blood spot trypsin assay. Results in 47,127 newborn infants from a homogeneous population, *Acta Paediatr Scand* 73:554-558, 1984.

Tryptophan (Trp)[1-5]

HPLC, fluorescence detection[6]

Ion-exchange chromatography

Plasma (heparin) or serum, fasting. Place blood in ice water immediately; separate and freeze within 1 hr of collection. Stable for 1 wk at $-20°$ C; for longer periods, deproteinize and store at $-70°$ C.[7,8]

TRP is bound in the circulation to albumin. Care should be taken to ensure complete deproteinization.

	mg/dL		*μmol/L*	P ↓ V Alclofenac, aspirin,
1-16 yr:	0.49-1.61	× 49.0	24-79	indomethacin, and
>16 yr:	0.41-1.94		20-95	glucose

	mg/dL	*mmol/L*[5]
Premature		
0-6 wk:	0.57-2.78	28-136
Newborn		
0-1 mo:	0-1.22	0-60
1-24 mo:	0.47-1.45	23-71
2-18 yr:	0-1.61	0-79
Adult	0.20-2.86	10-140

Urine, 24 hr. Add 10 mL of 6 mol/L HCl at start of collection. (Alternatively, refrigerate specimen during collection.) Store frozen at $-20°$ C.[9]

Adult: 5-39 mg/day[11]   × 4.90   [25-191 mmol/day]   U ↑ V Tetracycline

	mg/g creatinine		*mmol/mol creatinine*
or:	<30	× 0.55	[<16.5]

CSF. Collect in sterile tubes; store frozen. Stable at $-20°$ C for 1 wk or at $-70°$ C for 2 mo.[10]

	mg/dL (SD)		*μmol/L (SD)*
3 mo-2 yr:	0.053 ± 0.010	× 49.0	[2.6 ± 0.5][12]
2-10 yr:	0.043 ± 0.008		[2.1 ± 0.4][12]
Adult:	0.047 ± 0.014		[2.3 ± 0.7][13]

1. Friedman RB, Young DS: *Effects of disease on clinical laboratory tests,* ed 2, Washington, DC, 1989, American Association for Clinical Chemistry.

DIAGNOSTIC INFORMATION	REMARKS

7. Wilcken B, Brown ARD, Urwin R, et al: Cystic fibrosis screening by dried blood spot trypsin assay: results in 75,000 newborn infants, *J Pediatr* 102:383-387, 1983.

8. Southern K: Newborn screening for cystic fibrosis: the practical implications, *J R Soc Med* 15(suppl 44):707-712, 2003.

9. Hammond KB, Abman SH, Sokil RJ, et al: Efficacy of statewide neonatal screening for cystic fibrosis by assay of trypsinogen concentrations, *N Engl J Med* 525:769-774, 1991.

10. Ranieria E, Ryall RG, Morris CP, et al: Neonatal screening strategy for cystic fibrosis using immunoreactive trypsinogen and direct gene analysis, *BMJ* 302:1237-1240, 1991.

11. Florholmen J, Burhol PG, Jorde R: Postprandial response and diurnal variation of serum cationic trypsin-like immunoreactivity in man, *Scand J Gastroenterol* 19:622-625, 1984.

12. Yadav D, Agarwal N, Pitchumoni CS: A critical evaluation of laboratory tests in acute pancreatitis, *Am J Gastroenterol* 97:1309-1318, 2002.

P ↑ Hypertryptophanemia, sepsis,[14] and hepatic encephalopathy	Falsely low values are found when EDTA is used as anticoagulant.[18]
P ↓ Carcinoid syndrome, Hartnup disease, hypothermia, 1-2 days after abdominal surgery,[15] and regional enteritis	
P ↓↓ Pellagra (particularly in children),[16] protein-calorie malnutrition (kwashiorkor)	

U ↑ Hartnup disease

CSF ↑ Bacterial meningitis,[17] carcinomatous meningitis, hepatic encephalopathy, and cirrhosis	Values in children (3 mo-10 yr) were measured using reversed-phase liquid chromatography.
CSF ↓ Multiple sclerosis	

2. Scriver CR, Beaudet AL, Valle D, et al, editors: *The metabolic and molecular bases of inherited disease,* ed 8, New York, 2001, McGraw-Hill.

TEST NAME AND METHOD	SPECIMEN REQUIREMENTS	REFERENCE INTERVAL, CONVENTIONAL [INTERNATIONAL RECOMMENDED UNITS]	CHEMICAL INTERFERENCES AND IN VIVO EFFECTS

Tryptophan—CONT

3. Bremer HJ, Duran M, Kamerling JP, et al: *Disturbances of amino acid metabolism: clinical chemistry and diagnosis,* Baltimore, 1981, Urban and Schwarzenburg.

4. Nyhan W, Sakait N: *Diagnostic recognition of genetic disease,* Philadelphia, 1987, Lea & Febiger.

5. Slocum RH, Cummings JG: Amino acid analysis of physiological samples. In Hommes FA, editor: *Techniques in human biochemical genetics,* New York, 1991, Wiley-Liss, pp. 87-126.

6. Nichols Institute Reference Laboratories: *Test catalog,* San Juan Capistrano, CA, 1991, Nichols Institute Reference Laboratories.

7. Cummings JG: Routine amino acids analysis in the clinical laboratory, *Am Clin Prod Rev* Feb:20-25, 1988.

8. Schaefer A, Piquard F, Haberey P: Plasma amino acids analysis: effects of delayed samples preparation and of storage, *Clin Chim Acta* 164:163-169, 1987.

9. Pesce A, Kaplan L, editors: *Methods in clinical chemistry,* St. Louis, 1987, CV Mosby.

10. Heiblim DI, Evans HE, Glass L, et al: Amino acid concentrations in cerebrospinal fluid, *Arch Neurol* 35:765-768, 1978.

TEST NAME AND METHOD	SPECIMEN REQUIREMENTS	REFERENCE INTERVAL, CONVENTIONAL [INTERNATIONAL RECOMMENDED UNITS]	CHEMICAL INTERFERENCES AND IN VIVO EFFECTS
Tubular Reabsorption of Phosphate (TRP)[1,2]	Urine. Collect morning specimen over 2-4 hr for phosphate and creatinine.	82-95% × 0.01 *Fraction reabsorbed* [0.82-0.95] On average phosphorus intake in patients with normal renal function.[1]	See individual tests.
Patient consumes only water after midnight to maintain urine flow at 150-200 mL/hr. Patient receives normal Ca and P diet for at least 5 days before test.	Serum or plasma. Collect at midpoint of test period for phosphate and creatinine.		

1. Aurbach GD, Marx SJ, Spiegel AM: Parathyroid hormone, calcitonin, and the calciferols. In Wilson JD, Foster DW, editors: *Williams textbook of endocrinology,* ed 8, Philadelphia, 1992, WB Saunders.

2. McMurray JF, editor: *Manual of endocrine diagnostic tests,* ed 3, Lexington, KY, 1983, Division of Endocrinology, University of Kentucky Medical Center.

3. Walton RJ, Bijvoet OLM: Nomogram for derivation of renal threshold phosphate concentration, *Lancet* 2:309-310, 1975.

DIAGNOSTIC INFORMATION	REMARKS

11. Meites S, editor: *Pediatric clinical chemistry,* ed 3, Washington, DC, 1989, American Association for Clinical Chemistry.

12. Goldsmith RF, Earl JW, Cunningham AM: Determination of δ-aminobutyric acid and other amino acids in cerebrospinal fluid of pediatric patients by reversed-phase liquid chromatography, *Clin Chem* 33:1736-1740, 1987.

13. Kruse T, Reiber H, Neuhoff V: Amino acid transport across the human blood-CSF barrier, *J Neurol Sci* 70:129-138, 1985.

14. Freund H, Atamian S, Holyroyde J, et al: Plasma amino acids as predictors of the severity and outcome of sepsis, *Ann Surg* 190:571-576, 1979.

15. Jain KM, Rush BF Jr, Seelig RF, et al: Changes in plasma amino acid profiles following abdominal operations, *Surg Gynecol Obstet* 152:302-306, 1981.

16. Wallach J, editor: *Interpretation of diagnostic tests,* ed 5, Boston, 1992, Little, Brown and Co.

17. Schott KJ, Meier D: Free amino acid pattern of cerebrospinal fluid in meningeal pathology, *Acta Neurol Scand* 75:304-309, 1987.

18. Upton JD, Hindmarsh P: More pitfalls in human plasma amino acid analysis, *Clin Chem* 36:157-158, 1990.

↑ Hypoparathyroidism, pseudohypoparathyroidism

↓ Hyperparathyroidism (false-negative results may occur in 25% of cases)

$$TRP\% = 100 \times \left[1 - \left(\frac{P_u \times Cr_s}{Cr_u \times P_s} \right) \right]$$

P_u = urine phosphate in mg/dL
P_s = serum phosphate in mg/dL
Cr_u = urine creatinine in mg/dL
Cr_s = serum creatinine in mg/dL

Any degree of renal insufficiency increases excretion of phosphate relative to creatinine and invalidates the test. Serial measurements on consecutive days are recommended.

Using calculated TRP and measured serum phosphate, the renal phosphate threshold concentration can also be estimated with a nomogram.[3]

TRP reflects the role of PTH in regulating renal clearance of phosphate. However, determination of TRP does not replace direct measurements of PTH itself (see *Parathyroid Hormone*).

TEST NAME AND METHOD	SPECIMEN REQUIREMENTS	REFERENCE INTERVAL, CONVENTIONAL [INTERNATIONAL RECOMMENDED UNITS]		CHEMICAL INTERFERENCES AND IN VIVO EFFECTS
Tyrosine (Tyr)[1-6] *Fluorimetry* ——— *Ion-exchange chromatography*	Plasma (heparin) or serum, fasting. Place blood in ice water immediately; separate and freeze within 1 hr of collection. Stable for 1 wk at $-20°$ C; for longer periods, deproteinize and store at $-70°$ C.[7,8]	*mg/dL* Premature: 7.0-24.0 Newborn: 1.6-3.7 Adult: 0.8-1.3 *mg/dL* Premature 1 day: 2.17 ± 1.81 (SD) *mg/dL* Newborn 1 day: 0.76-1.79 1 day-1 mo: 1.00-2.66 1-3 mo: 1.48 ± 0.47 (SD) 2-6 mo: 1.30-3.91 9 mo-2 yr: 0.20-2.21 3-10 yr: 0.56-1.29 6-18 yr: 0.78-1.59 Adult: 0.40-1.58	$\times$ 55.2	$\mu mol/L$[11] [386-1325] [88-204] [44-72] $\mu mol/L$[6,12] [120 ± 100] $\mu mol/L$[12] [42-99] [55-147][6] [82 ± 26] [72-216] [11-122] [31-71] [43-88][13] [22-87]	P ↑ V Triiodothyronine P ↑ C Fluorimetric *assay:* 4-hydroxyphenylacetate, hydroxyphenylpyruvate, 5-hydroxytryptophan, tryptophan, and tyramine P ↓ V Androgens, ascorbic acid (premature infants), epinephrine, estrogens, glucagon, glucose, histidine, hydrocortisone, and testosterone
	Urine, 24 hr. Add 10 mL of 6 mol/L HCl at start of collection.[6] (Alternatively, refrigerate specimen during collection.) Store frozen at $-20°$ C.[9]	*mg/day* 10 day-7 wk: 4.0-7.2 3-12 yr: 7.2-30.4 Adult: 12.0-55.1[13] *mg/g creatinine* or 11 ± 6 (SD) 112 $\mu mol/g$ *creatinine*[14] 0-1 mo: 83-401 1-6 mo: 103-690 6 mo-1 yr: 103-944 1-2 yr: 96-542 2-3 yr: 111-591	$\times$ 5.52 $\times$ 0.62 $\times$ 0.113	*mmol/day* [22-40][12] [40-168][12] [66-304] *mmol/mol creatinine* [6.8 ± 3.7] *mmol/mol creatinine* [9-45] [12-78] [12-107] [11-61] [12-67]	U ↓ V Estrogens (males)
	CSF. Collect in sterile tubes; store frozen. Stable at $-20°$ C for 1 wk or at $-70°$ C for 2 mo.[10]	*mg/dL* Neonate: 0.556 ± 0.254 (SEM) 3 mo-2 yr: 0.179 ± 0.042 (SD) 2-10 yr: 0.145 ± 0.033 Adult: 0.163 ± 0.014	$\times$ 55.2	$\mu mol/L$ [30.7 ± 14.0][10] [9.9 ± 2.3][14] [8.0 ± 1.8][14] [9.0 ± 0.8][12]	
Tandem mass spectrometry	Dried blood spot. Collect blood spot onto newborn screening card. Allow to air dry before analysis.	*mg/dL* Neonate: 0.65-3.77	$\times$ 55.2	$\mu mol/L$ [36-208][15]	

DIAGNOSTIC INFORMATION	REMARKS

P ↑ Tyrosinemia, hepatic dysfunction of infectious or metabolic origin, prematurity (immature hepatic metabolism), and hyperthyroidism[16]

See Table II-2A.

P ↓ Polycystic kidney disease, hypothermia, phenylketonuria, chronic renal failure, carcinoid syndrome, myxedema, hypothyroidism, Huntington's chorea, rheumatoid arthritis, and phlebotomus fever

U ↑ Tyrosinemia, hepatic dysfunction, in first trimester of pregnancy (levels decrease thereafter), hyperthyroidism, burn patients,[16] oasthouse disease, Hartnup disease, and galactosemia

In acute type I hypertyrosinemia, a generalized overflow aminoaciduria is seen.

CSF ↑ Tyrosinemia,[6] bacterial meningitis, and carcinomatous meningitis[17]

Values in children (3 mo-10 yr) were measured using reversed-phase liquid chromatography.

DBS ↑ Tyrosinemia, premature neonate, and hepatic dysfunction

DBS ↓ PKU

TEST NAME AND METHOD	SPECIMEN REQUIREMENTS	REFERENCE INTERVAL, CONVENTIONAL [INTERNATIONAL RECOMMENDED UNITS]	CHEMICAL INTERFERENCES AND IN VIVO EFFECTS

Tyrosine—CONT

1. Friedman RB, Young DS: *Effects of disease on clinical laboratory tests,* ed 2, Washington, DC, 1989, American Association for Clinical Chemistry.

2. Scriver CR, Beaudet AL, Valle D, et al, editors: *The metabolic and molecular bases of inherited disease,* ed 8, New York, 2001, McGraw-Hill.

3. Young DS: *Effects of drugs on clinical laboratory tests,* ed 3, Washington, DC, 1990, American Association for Clinical Chemistry.

4. Bremer HJ, Duran M, Kamerling JP, et al: *Disturbances of amino acid metabolism: clinical chemistry and diagnosis,* Baltimore, 1981, Urban and Schwarzenburg.

5. Nyhan W, Sakait N: *Diagnostic recognition of genetic disease,* Philadelphia, 1987, Lea & Febiger.

6. Slocum RH, Cummings JG: Amino acid analysis of physiological samples. In Hommes FA, editor: *Techniques in human biochemical genetics,* New York, 1991, Wiley-Liss, pp. 87-126.

7. Cummings JG: Routine amino acids analysis in the clinical laboratory, *Am Clin Prod Rev* Feb:20-25, 1988.

8. Schaefer A, Piquard F, Haberey P: Plasma amino acids analysis: effects of delayed samples preparation and of storage, *Clin Chim Acta* 164:163-169, 1987.

Urea Nitrogen[1-5]

Colorimetric,[6] *enzymatic, conductimetric*

Serum or plasma. Avoid high concentration of Na fluoride because this inhibits urease. Ammonium heparin cannot be used when the conductimetric method is used. Stable up to 24 hr at room temperature, for several days at 4-6° C, and for at least 2-3 mo when frozen.

	Urea N, mg/dL		*Carbamide (urea), mmol/L*
Cord:	21-40	× 0.357	[7.5-14.3]
Premature			
1 wk:	3-25		[1.1-8.9]
<1 yr[4]:	4-19		[1.4-6.8]
Infant/child:	5-18		[1.8-6.4]
18-60 yr[7]:	6-20		[2.1-7.1]
60-90 yr:	8-23		[2.9-8.2]
>90 yr:	10-31		[3.6-11.1]

S ↑ V Corticosteroids, drugs causing nephrotoxicity frequently increase urea nitrogen (Table I-6), tetracyclines, and excess thyroxine

S ↓ V Growth hormone

S ↓ C *Urease method:* sodium citrate, sodium fluoride (high concentrations); *color:* chloramphenicol, streptomycin

Urine, 24 hr. Stable at 4-8° C for 4 days or preserve with thymol to avoid bacterial action.

12-20 g/day	× 0.0357	[0.43-0.71 mol/day]

Random urine[7]:

	mg/dL		*mmol/L*
M:	145-1542	× 0.357	[51.8-550]
F:	132-1629		[47.1-581]

	mg/g creatinine		*mmol/g creatinine*
M:	2864-9851	× 0.0357	[102-352]
F:	3129-11,639		[112-416]

U ↓ V Administration of growth hormone, testosterone, and insulin

1. Brown SS, Mitchell FL, Young DS, editors: *Chemical diagnosis of disease,* Amsterdam, 1979, Elsevier/North Holland Biomedical Press.

2. Eastham RD: *Biochemical values in clinical medicine,* ed 7, Bristol, UK, 1985, John Wright and Sons Ltd.

3. Henry JB, editor: *Clinical diagnosis and management by laboratory methods,* ed 18, Philadelphia, 1991, WB Saunders.

4. Jacobs DS, Kasten BL, DeMott WR, et al, editors: *Laboratory test handbook,* ed 2, Stow, OH, 1990, LexiComp, Inc.

5. Wallach J, editor: *Interpretation of diagnostic tests,* ed 5, Boston, 1992, Little, Brown and Co.

9. Pesce A, Kaplan L, editors: *Methods in clinical chemistry,* St. Louis, 1987, CV Mosby.

10. Heiblim DI, Evans HE, Glass L, et al: Amino acid concentrations in cerebrospinal fluid, *Arch Neurol* 35:765-768, 1978.

11. Tietz NW, editor: *Fundamentals of clinical chemistry,* ed 3, Philadelphia, 1987, WB Saunders.

12. Shih V: *Laboratory techniques for the detection of hereditary metabolic disorders,* Boca Raton, FL, 1973, CRC Press.

13. Meites S, editor: *Pediatric clinical chemistry,* ed 3, Washington, DC, 1989, American Association for Clinical Chemistry.

14. Mayo Medical Laboratories: *Test catalog,* Rochester, MN, 2005, Mayo Medical Laboratories.

15. Chace DH, Sherwin JE, Hillman SL, et al: Use of phenylalanine to tyrosine ratio determined by tandem mass spectrometry to improve newborn screening for phenylketonuria of early discharge specimens in the first 24 hours, *Clin Chem* 44:2405-2409, 1998.

16. Freund H, Atamian S, Holyroyde J, et al: Plasma amino acids as predictors of the severity and outcome of sepsis, *Ann Surg* Nov:571-576, 1979.

17. Cynober L, Dinh FN, Blonde F, et al: Plasma and urinary amino acid pattern in severe burn patients: evolution throughout the healing period, *Am J Clin Nutr* 36:416-425, 1982.

S ↑ *Impaired kidney function:* (1) Decreased renal perfusion as in congestive heart failure, salt and water depletion caused by vomiting, diarrhea, diuresis, or sweating; shock; in combination with increased protein catabolism, as in hemorrhage into GI tract, acute MI, stress, and burns; (2) acute or chronic intrinsic renal disease; (3) postrenal obstruction to urine flow; and (4) high-protein diet

Urea nitrogen concentrations increase with age and protein content of diet. Ammonium ions can interfere with urease methods but not with the diacetyl reaction.

The preferred methods are the conductimetric and the urease/GLDH procedures.

S ↓ Low-protein and high-carbohydrate diets, increased utilization of proteins for synthesis, late pregnancy, infancy, acromegaly, IV feedings only, severe liver damage, drug poisoning, and impaired absorption (celiac disease)

U ↑ Increased dietary protein, hyperthyroidism, and postoperatively

U ↓ Normal growing children and infants, pregnancy, low-protein and high-carbohydrate diets, convalescence, liver disease, toxemia, and renal damage and insufficiency from any cause.

6. Tietz NW, editor: *Fundamentals of clinical chemistry,* ed 3, Philadelphia, 1987, WB Saunders.

7. Tietz NW, Shuey WF, Wekstein DR: Laboratory values in fit aging individuals—sexagenarians through centenarians, *Clin Chem* 38:1167-1185, 1982.

8. Bond LW, Garber C, Ottinger W, et al: Reference intervals for common analytes in random urine specimens, *Clin Chem* 55:submitted, 2005.

TEST NAME AND METHOD	SPECIMEN REQUIREMENTS	REFERENCE INTERVAL, CONVENTIONAL [INTERNATIONAL RECOMMENDED UNITS]			CHEMICAL INTERFERENCES AND IN VIVO EFFECTS
Urea Nitrogen/ Creatinine Ratio (Calculated)[1-3]	See *Urea Nitrogen* and *Creatinine.*	*Mass ratio* 12:1 to 20:1 × 4.04	*Urea (carbamide):creatinine mole ratio* [48.5:1 to 80.8:1]		See *Urea Nitrogen* and *Creatinine.*

1. Henry JB, editor: *Clinical diagnosis and management by laboratory methods,* ed 18, Philadelphia, 1991, WB Saunders.
2. Jacobs DS, Kasten BL, DeMott WR, et al, editors: *Laboratory test handbook,* ed 2, Stow, OH, 1990, LexiComp, Inc.
3. Tietz NW, editor: *Fundamentals of clinical chemistry,* ed 3, Philadelphia, 1987, WB Saunders.
4. Wallach J, editor: *Interpretation of diagnostic tests,* ed 5, Boston, 1992, Little, Brown and Co.

TEST NAME AND METHOD	SPECIMEN REQUIREMENTS	REFERENCE INTERVAL, CONVENTIONAL [INTERNATIONAL RECOMMENDED UNITS]			CHEMICAL INTERFERENCES AND IN VIVO EFFECTS
Uric Acid[1-4] *Phosphotungstate*	Serum; separate from cells. Stable 3-5 days at 4° C, 6 mo at −20° C. Do not use oxalate for phosphotungstate method or EDTA or fluoride for uricase method.		*mg/dL*	*μmol/L*	↑ V β-Adrenergic blockers (e.g., atenolol, propranolol, nadolol, timolol), cisplatin, corticosteroids (in acute leukemias), cyclosporine, diazoxide, didanosine, diuretics (i.e., acetazolamide, chlorthalidone, ethacrynic acid [oral], furosemide [oral], quinethazone, thiazides, triamterene), epinephrine, ethanol, ethambutol, filgrastim, fructose (IV), nicotinic acid (large doses), norepinephrine, pyrazinamide, salicylates (small doses), some antineoplastic agents (e.g., fludarabine, hydroxyurea, idarubicin, mechlorethamine), and theophylline (IV)
		Child <12 yr:	2.0-5.5 × 59.48	[119-327]	
		Adult[6] M:	4.4-7.6	[262-452]	
		F:	2.3-6.6	[137-393]	
		60-90 yr M:	4.2-8.0	[250-476]	
		F:	3.5-7.3	[208-434]	
		>90 yr M:	3.5-8.3	[208-494]	
		F:	2.2-7.7	[131-458]	
Uricase		Child:	2.0-5.5	[119-327]	
			Higher in newborn		
		M:	3.5-7.2[1]	[208-428]	
		F:	2.6-6.0	[155-357]	
			Lower during pregnancy		
	CSF[5]		*mcg/dL*	*μmol/L*	
		Infants and adults:	85-932 × 0.059 (n = 9)	[5-55]	
	Urine, 24 hr; do not refrigerate. Add NaOH to keep urine alkaline.	*Diet* Average: Purine-free	*mg/day* 250-750 × 0.0059	*mmol/day* [1.48-4.43]	↑ C *Phosphotungstate method:* Acetaminophen, ascorbic acid (large amounts), cysteine, cystine, glucose, glutathione,
		M:	<420	[<2.48]	
		F:	Slightly lower		

DIAGNOSTIC INFORMATION	REMARKS

↑ Reduced renal perfusion (e.g., dehydration, hypovolemic shock, congestive heart failure); also may be seen in obstructive uropathy, implantation of ureter in colon or ileum, high-protein diet, high catabolic state, frontal lobe trauma, and occasionally with glomerular diseases or corticosteroid therapy[3]

↓ Acute renal tubular necrosis

Variation in dietary protein levels and muscle mass may cause significant fluctuations in results. Ratio is affected by specificity of creatinine method and by liver function.

S ↑ Gout, renal failure, leukemia, multiple myeloma, polycythemia, lymphoma, other disseminated neoplasms, toxemia of pregnancy, psoriasis, glycogenosis type I, Lesch-Nyhan syndrome, Down syndrome, polycystic kidney disease, and chronic lead nephropathy

In association with hyperlipidemia, obesity, hypertension, arteriosclerosis, diabetes mellitus, ethanol consumption, hypoparathyroidism, acromegaly, sarcoidosis, and liver disease; after gross tissue destruction (increased nucleoprotein breakdown), and in excessive nucleoprotein turnover (e.g., myeloid leukemia, pernicious anemia, and strychnine poisoning)

Acute (sometimes dangerous) elevation follows treatment of leukemia with cytotoxic drugs.

S ↓ Wilson's disease, Fanconi's syndrome, some malignancies (e.g., Hodgkin's disease, multiple myeloma, bronchogenic carcinoma), xanthinuria, SIADH, deficiencies of adenosine deaminase, purine, and nucleoside phosphorylase; low-purine diet

A purine-rich diet (liver, kidney, sweetbread), as well as severe exercise, increases uric acid values.

Rapid degradation of uric acid occurs at room temperature in the plasma of patients with tumor lysis syndrome who are treated with rasburicase (recombinant urate oxidase). Blood should be collected in prechilled tubes containing heparin, immediately immersed in an ice-water bath, centrifuged in a precooled centrifuge (4° C), and the separated plasma maintained in an ice-water bath and analyzed within 4 hr of collection.

U ↑ Leukemia, gout, Lesch-Nyhan syndrome, Wilson's disease, cystinosis, viral hepatitis, polycythemia vera, and sickle cell anemia

U ↓ Xanthinuria, folic acid deficiency, and lead toxicity

TEST NAME AND METHOD	SPECIMEN REQUIREMENTS	REFERENCE INTERVAL, CONVENTIONAL [INTERNATIONAL RECOMMENDED UNITS]	CHEMICAL INTERFERENCES AND IN VIVO EFFECTS

Uric Acid—CONT

		Diet	*mg/day*		*mmol/day*	L-dopa (and metabolites),
		Low-purine				methyldopa, methyluric
		M:	<480		[<2.83]	acid, metabolites of caf-
		F:	<400		[<2.36]	feine or theophylline, phe-
		High-purine:	<1000		[<5.90]	nols, tryptophan, and tyro-
		Random urine[7]:				sine; *Uricase method:*
						Aspirin

	mg/dL		*mmol/L*	
M				↓ V Acetohexamide, al-
<40 yr:	9-63	× 0.059	[0.53-3.7]	lopurinol, azathioprine,
≥40 yr:	6-114		[0.35-6.7]	bishydroxycoumarin,
F				chlorprothixene, clofi-
<40 yr:	6-71		[0.35-4.2]	brate, contrast media (i.e.,
≥40 yr:	4-93		[0.24-5.5]	diatrizoate, iodipamide,

	mg/g creatinine		*mmol/g creatinine*	iopanoic acid, ipodate),
				ethacrynic acid (IV),
M:	104-593	× 0.0059	[0.61-3.5]	fenofibrate, fenoprofen,
F:	95-741		[0.56-4.4]	furosemide (IV), guaifen-

esin, halofenate, phenylbutazone (weak effect), probenecid, salicylates (large doses), tienilic acid, and urate oxidase (rasburicase)

1. Tietz NW, editor: *Textbook of clinical chemistry,* Philadelphia, 1986, WB Saunders.

2. Wallach J, editor: *Interpretation of diagnostic tests,* ed 5, Boston, 1992, Little, Brown and Co..

3. Chonko AM, Grantham JJ: Disorders of urate metabolism and excretion. In Brenner BM, Rector FC, editors: *The kidney,* ed 4, Philadelphia, WB Saunders.

4. Faller J, Fox IH: Ethanol-induced hyperglycemia: evidence for increased urate production by activation of adenine nucleotide turnover, *N Engl J Med* 307:1598-1602, 1982.

5. Harkness RA, Lund RJ: Cerebrospinal fluid concentration of hypoxanthine, xanthine, uridine, and inosine: high concentrations of the ATP metabolite, hypoxanthine, after hypoxia, *J Clin Pathol* 36:1-8, 1983.

6. Tietz NW, Shuey DF, Wekstein DR: Laboratory values in fit aging individuals—sexagenarians through centenarians, *Clin Chem* 38:1167-1185, 1992.

7. Bond LW, Garber C, Ottinger W, et al: Reference intervals for common analytes in random urine specimens, *Clin Chem* 55:submitted, 2005.

DIAGNOSTIC INFORMATION	REMARKS

TEST NAME AND METHOD	SPECIMEN REQUIREMENTS	REFERENCE INTERVAL, CONVENTIONAL [INTERNATIONAL RECOMMENDED UNITS]			CHEMICAL INTERFERENCES AND IN VIVO EFFECTS
Urine Volume[1-5]	Urine, 24 hr		*mL/24 hr*	*mL/day*	↑ V Caffeine, diltiazem, diuretics (e.g., thiazides,
		Newborn			bumetanide, furosemide,
		1-2 days:	30-60 ×1.0	[30-60]	ethacrynic acid),
		Infant			dopamine (low to moder-
		3-10 days:	100-300	[100-300]	ate doses), ethanol,
		10-60 days:	250-450	[250-450]	lithium, demeclocycline,
		2 mo-1 yr:	400-500	[400-500]	methoxyflurane, pheny-
		Child			toin, propoxyphene, as-
		1-3 yr:	500-600	[500-600]	pirin, bumetanide, oral
		3-5 yr:	600-700	[600-700]	hypoglycemic agents,
		5-8 yr:	650-1000	[650-1000]	chlorpromazine, and
		8-14 yr:	800-1400	[800-1400]	digitalis[1,5]
		Adult			
		M:	800-1800	[800-1800]	
		F:	600-1600	[600-1600]	↓ V Drugs causing
		>60 yr:	250-2400	[250-2400]	nephrotoxicity (see Table I-6); bacitracin, carba-

Average output: 1200-1500 mL/day; values may be modified by fluid intake, sweating, outside temperature, vomiting, and diarrhea.

mazepine, corticotropin, disopyramide, in-domethacin, kanamycin, morphine, neomycin, phenylbutazone, and somatostatin

DIAGNOSTIC INFORMATION	REMARKS

↑ *Diabetes insipidus*[4]

Central: Pituitary pathology

Nephrogenic: Acquired renal disease [especially pyelonephritis, analgesic nephropathy, multiple myeloma, amyloidosis, obstructive uropathy, sarcoidosis, hypercalcemic or hypokalemic nephropathy (including primary aldosteronism and hyperparathyroidism), Sjögren's syndrome, sickle cell anemia, renal transplantation, renal artery stenosis, postobstructive diuresis, diuretic phase of acute tubular necrosis, medullary cystic disease, and sodium wasting in tubular damage]

Drug-induced: See *Interferences*

Excessive fluid intake: Psychogenic polydipsia, hypothalamic disease (postencephalitic, histiocytosis X), drug-induced polyuria (anticholinergic effect, especially thioridazine, chlorpromazine), and iatrogenic overhydration

Osmotic diuresis: Diabetes mellitus (glucosuria), high-protein diet or tube feedings, IV or hyperalimentation therapy (with Na^+, amino acids, and/or glucose), excessive salt intake, urea or mannitol infusion, radiographic contrast media, chronic renal failure, adrenal insufficiency, and drugs (see *Interferences*)

Others[6]: Last trimester of pregnancy, protein malnutrition, hyperthyroidism, altitude,[5] postmenstruation,[5] psychogenic polydipsia, and hypothalamic disease

↓ *Prerenal perfusion impairment:* Dehydration, blood loss, shock, congestive heart failure, cirrhosis, "third space" fluid losses (e.g., edema, peritonitis, bowel obstruction), nephritic syndrome, and acute arterial or renal vein obstruction

Obstructive uropathy

Renal parenchymal disease: Acute tubular necrosis, glomerulonephritis, acute vasculitis (SLE, periarteritis nodosa, dermatomyositis, Wegener's granulomatosis, hypersensitivity angiitis), DIC (sepsis, transfusion reaction), urate, hypercalcemic or analgesic nephropathy, chronic renal failure, and drug- or toxin-induced (see *Interferences*)

Postrenal obstruction, e.g., missing or poorly functioning kidney, renal calculi, cysts, and obstruction of ureter by tumors or calculi

Under ordinary physiological conditions, the chief determinant of urine volume is water intake. Patients cannot always distinguish urinary frequency from polyuria. Polyuria must be substantiated by 24-hr urine collection.

In oliguria, urinary output is between 50-400 mL/day. In anuria, the urinary output is 0-50 mL/day.

Some common laboratory tests can be used to differentiate prerenal from renal or postrenal oliguria, although the methods listed are not infallible. Generally in prerenal oliguria, urinary Na^+ is <20 mmol/L; urine/plasma (U/P) creatinine ratio is >40; U/P osmolality >1.2; and the fractional excretion of Na^+ is <1. In renal or postrenal oliguria, the urinary Na^+ is >40 mmol/L; U/P creatinine ratio is <20; U/P osmolality <1.2; and the fractional excretion of Na^+ is >1. The fractional excretion of Na^+ is most reliable.

TEST NAME AND METHOD	SPECIMEN REQUIREMENTS	REFERENCE INTERVAL, CONVENTIONAL [INTERNATIONAL RECOMMENDED UNITS]	CHEMICAL INTERFERENCES AND IN VIVO EFFECTS
Urine Volume—CONT			

1. Braunwald E, Isselbacher KJ, Petersdorf RG, et al, editors: *Harrison's principles of internal medicine,* ed 11, New York, 1987, McGraw-Hill Book Co.
2. DeGowin EL, DeGowin RL: *Bedside diagnostic examination,* ed 5, New York, 1987, Macmillan Pub. Co.
3. Henry JB, editor: *Clinical diagnosis and management by laboratory methods,* ed 18, Philadelphia, 1991, WB Saunders.
4. Wyngaarden JB, Smith LH Jr, Bennett JC, editors: *Cecil textbook of medicine,* ed 19, Philadelphia, 1992, WB Saunders.
5. Young DS: *Effects of drugs on clinical laboratory tests,* ed 3, Washington, DC, 1990, American Association for Clinical Chemistry.
6. Young DS, Friedman RB: *Effects of disease on clinical laboratory tests,* ed 4, vol 1, Washington DC, 2001, AACC Press, p. 819.

TEST NAME AND METHOD	SPECIMEN REQUIREMENTS	REFERENCE INTERVAL, CONVENTIONAL [INTERNATIONAL RECOMMENDED UNITS]	CHEMICAL INTERFERENCES AND IN VIVO EFFECTS
Uroporphyrinogen Decarboxylase (URO-D, UPGD; EC 4.1.1.37)[1-3] *HPLC*[1]	Erythrocytes. Collect whole blood (heparin; avoid potassium oxalate). Ercs should be washed three times with cold saline, volume recorded, and shipped frozen.[1]	1.0-3.0 relative units (normal) 0.80-0.99 relative units (marginal) <0.80 relative units (porphyria cutanea tarda or hepatoerythropoietic porphyria [HEP])[1]	

1. Mayo Medical Laboratories: *Test catalog,* Rochester, MN, 2004, Mayo Medical Laboratories.
2. Tavazzi D, Martinez di Montemuros F, Fargion S, et al: Levels of uroporphyrinogen decarboxylase (URO-D) in erythrocytes of Italian porphyria cutanea tarda patients, *Cell Mol Biol* 48:27-32, 2002.
3. Phillips JD, Parker TL, Schubert HL, et al: Functional consequences of naturally occurring mutations in human uroporphyrinogen decarboxylase, *Blood* 98:3179-3185, 2001.

DIAGNOSTIC INFORMATION	REMARKS

Others: Infections (pyelonephritis, septicemia, epidemic hemorrhagic fever, cholera, dysentery, typhus, Rocky Mountain spotted fever, malaria), sarcoidosis, crush injuries, protein malnutrition, sickle cell crisis, acute cortical crisis, and drugs (see *Interferences*)

↓ Porphyria cutanea tarda (PCT) type II (familial autosomal dominant), hepatoerythropoietic porphyria (HEP)

Porphyria cutanea tarda (PCT), the most prevalent form of porphyria, and the rare hepatoerythropoietic porphyria (HEP) are caused by deficiency of URO-D activity with accumulation of uroporphyrins and hepta-, hexa-, and pentacarboxyl porphyrins in skin, subcutaneous tissues, and liver.

In both PCT and HEP, photosensitivity with vesicular and bullous lesions on exposed surfaces of hands, arms, face, and legs, and fragility of the skin in relation to physical trauma. Other characteristics may include hypertrichosis, hyperpigmentation, and hyperkeratosis. The problems of PCT present mainly in adulthood; however, rare cases of PCT have been reported in childhood. HEP presents in early childhood.

PCT type I (sporadic) and PCT type III (familial rare, with hepatic URO-D deficiency) will have normal erythrocyte URO-D activity. Erythrocyte URO-D will be decreased in PCT type II (familial URO-D deficiency), which accounts for ~20% of PCT patients. The erythrocyte URO-D method is useful in distinguishing sporadic versus inherited PCT.

TEST NAME AND METHOD	SPECIMEN REQUIREMENTS	REFERENCE INTERVAL, CONVENTIONAL [INTERNATIONAL RECOMMENDED UNITS]		CHEMICAL INTERFERENCES AND IN VIVO EFFECTS
Uroporphyrinogen III (Co-) Synthase (URO-S, UPGC; EC 4.2.1.75)[1-3] *HPLC*[1]	Erythrocytes. Collect whole blood (heparin; avoid potassium oxalate). Ercs should be washed three times with cold saline, volume recorded, and shipped frozen.[1]	<75 relative units[1]		↑ V Erythrocyte transfusion can result in false-negative results. UPGC in the infused erythrocytes will be measured in the assay, normalizing enzyme activity of an affected individual.

1. Mayo Medical Laboratories: *Test catalog,* Rochester, MN, 2004, Mayo Medical Laboratories.
2. Ellefson RD: Porphyrinogens, porphyrins, and the porphyrias, *Mayo Clin Proc* 57:454-458, 1982.
3. Anderson KE, Sassa S, Bishop DF, et al: Disorders of heme biosynthesis: X-linked sideroblastic anemia and the porphyrias. In Scriver CR, Beaudet AL, Sly WS, et al, editors: *The metabolic basis of inherited disease,* ed 8, New York, 2001, McGraw-Hill Medical Publishing Division, pp. 2991-3062.
4. Mayo Medical Laboratories: *Interpretative handbook,* Rochester, MN, 2001, Mayo Medical Laboratories.

| **Valine** (Val)[1-6]

 Ion-exchange chromatography | Plasma (heparin) or serum, fasting. Place blood in ice water immediately; separate and freeze within 1 hr of collection. Stable for 1 wk at $-20°$ C; for longer periods, deproteinize and store at $-70°$ C.[8,9] | *mg/dL*
 Premature
 1 day:
 Newborn
 1 day:
 1 day-1 mo:
 1-3 mo:
 9 mo-2 yr:
 3-10 yr:
 6-18 yr:
 Adult: |

 1.52 ± 0.59 (SD)

 0.94-2.88
 1.00-2.22
 2.27 ± 0.57 (SD)
 0.67-3.07
 1.50-3.31
 1.83-3.37
 1.65-3.71 | $\mu mol/L$[12]

 $\times 85.5$ [130 ± 50]

 [80-246]
 [86-190][6]
 [194 ± 49]
 [57-262]
 [128-283]
 [156-288][13]
 [141-317] | P ↓ V Alanine, glucose, histidine (after oral load), oral contraceptives, and progesterone (high doses) |

| Urine, 24 hr. Add 10 mL of 6 mol/L HCl at start of collection.[6] (Alternatively, refrigerate specimen during collection.) Store frozen at $-20°$ C.[10] | *mg/day*
 10 day-7 wk: 1.4-3.2
 3-12 yr: 1.8-6.0
 Adult: 2.5-11.9

 mg/g creatinine
 or   4 ± 1 (SD) | $\mu mol/day$[12]
 $\times 8.55$ [12-27]
 [15-51]
 [21-102]

 mmol/mol creatinine
 $\times 0.97$ [3.9 ± 1.0] | U ↓ V Ascorbic acid (after large intake)[14] |

DIAGNOSTIC INFORMATION	REMARKS

↓ Congenital erythropoietic porphyria (CEP)

Values for UROS <75 relative units are suggestive of a biochemical diagnosis of CEP. This test does not reliably distinguish between individuals with heterozygous UROS deficiency and normal subjects.

Congenital erythropoietic porphyria (CEP) is an extremely rare and severe porphyria with a typical onset during early infancy. In most cases, the disorder has been suggested during the first few days or weeks of life by pink, violet, or brown urinary staining of diapers. A few cases of adult-onset CEP have been reported. Dermatological signs include skin photosensitivity, scarring and blistering, red or pink-brown dental discoloration, and hypertrichosis. Growth and cognitive developmental delays are commonly observed in individuals with CEP. CEP is inherited as an autosomal recessive trait.

Circulating red cells normally contain high levels of activity of UROS, and the diminished activity associated with CEP is readily demonstrable by incubation of red cells from an affected person.[4]

P ↑ Branched-chain ketoaciduria (maple syrup urine disease), ketosis, and hypervalinemia

P ↓ Protein malnutrition (kwashiorkor), carcinoid syndrome, acute hunger, hyperinsulinism, after severe burn (day 4),[15] Huntington's chorea, and hepatic encephalopathy

High levels of leucine, isoleucine, and alloisoleucine are also seen in maple syrup urine disease as a result of a defect in branched-chain ketoacid decarboxylase. In this autosomal recessive disorder of metabolism, there may be extreme acidosis, vomiting and CNS symptoms, mental retardation, respiratory failure, and death. In ketosis, leucine and isoleucine are elevated, but alloisoleucine is not present.

See Table II-2B.

Renal Fanconi syndromes may include other metabolic diseases, including hepatorenal tyrosinemia, galactosemia, and Lowe syndrome.

U ↑ Maple syrup urine disease, Hartnup disease, first trimester of pregnancy (levels decrease thereafter), hypervalinemia, burn patients,[16] and generalized aminoaciduria-renal Fanconi syndromes

TEST NAME AND METHOD	SPECIMEN REQUIREMENTS	REFERENCE INTERVAL, CONVENTIONAL [INTERNATIONAL RECOMMENDED UNITS]		CHEMICAL INTERFERENCES AND IN VIVO EFFECTS
Valine—CONT				
	CSF. Collect in sterile tubes; store frozen. Stable at $-20°$ C for 1 wk or at $-70°$ C for 2 mo.[11]	*mg/dL* Neonate: 0.395 ± 0.120 (SEM) Adult: 0.244 ± 0.019 (SD)	$\mu mol/L$ $\times 85.5$ [33.8 ± 10.3][11] [20.9 ± 1.6][12]	
Tandem mass spectrometry[7]	Dried blood spot. Collect blood spot onto newborn screening card. Allow to air dry before analysis.	*mg/dL* Neonate: 1.53 ± 0.68	$\mu mol/L$ 131 ± 58[7]	

1. Friedman RB, Young DS: *Effects of disease on clinical laboratory tests,* ed 2, Washington, DC, 1989, American Association for Clinical Chemistry.
2. Scriver CR, Beaudet AL, Valle D, et al, editors: *The metabolic and molecular bases of inherited disease,* ed 8, New York, 2001, McGraw-Hill.
3. Young DS: *Effects of drugs on clinical laboratory tests,* ed 3, Washington, DC, 1990, American Association for Clinical Chemistry.
4. Bremer HJ, Duran M, Kamerling JP, et al: *Disturbances of amino acid metabolism: clinical chemistry and diagnosis,* Baltimore, 1981, Urban and Schwarzenburg.
5. Nyhan W, Sakait N: *Diagnostic recognition of genetic disease,* Philadelphia, 1987, Lea & Febiger.
6. Hommes FA, editor: *Techniques in diagnostic human biochemical genetics,* New York, 1991, Wiley-Liss.
7. Chace DH, Hillman SL, Millington DS, et al: Rapid diagnosis of maple syrup urine disease in blood spots from newborns by tandem mass spectrometry, *Clin Chem* 42:349-355, 1996.
8. Cummings JG: Routine amino acids analysis in the clinical laboratory, *Am Clin Prod Rev* Feb:20-25, 1988.
9. Schaefer A, Piquard F, Haberey P: Plasma amino acids analysis: effects of delayed samples preparation and of storage, *Clin Chim Acta* 164:163-169, 1987.
10. Pesce A, Kaplan L, editors: *Methods in clinical chemistry,* St. Louis, 1987, CV Mosby.
11. Heiblim DI, Evans HE, Glass L, et al: Amino acid concentrations in cerebrospinal fluid, *Arch Neurol* 35:765-768, 1978.
12. Shih V: *Laboratory techniques for the detection of hereditary metabolic disorders,* Boca Raton, FL, 1973, CRC Press.
13. Meites S, editor: *Pediatric clinical chemistry,* ed 3, Washington, DC, 1989, American Association for Clinical Chemistry.
14. Tsao C, Muyashita K: Effects of large intake of ascorbic acid on the urinary excretion of amino acids and related compounds, *IRCS Med Sci* 13:855-856, 1985.
15. Cynober L, Dinh FN, Saizy R, et al: Plasma amino acid levels in the first few days after burn injury and their predictive value, *Intensive Care Med* 9:325-331, 1983.
16. Cynober L, Dinh FN, Blonde F, et al: Plasma and urinary amino acid pattern in severe burn patients: evolution throughout the healing period, *Am J Clin Nutr* 36:416-425, 1982.
17. Schott KJ, Meier D: Free amino acid pattern of cerebrospinal fluid in meningeal pathology, *Acta Neurol Scand* 75:304-309, 1987.

CSF ↑ Bacterial meningitis, aseptic meningitis, meningoradiculitis, Garin-Bujadoux-Bannwarth, and carcinomatous
meningitis.[17]

TEST NAME AND METHOD	SPECIMEN REQUIREMENTS	REFERENCE INTERVAL, CONVENTIONAL [INTERNATIONAL RECOMMENDED UNITS]		CHEMICAL INTERFERENCES AND IN VIVO EFFECTS
Vanadium (V)[1,2] *NAA*	Serum.[4,5] Collect in pretested, metal-free container.	0.014-0.230 mcg/L × 19.6	[0.27-4.51 nmol/L]	None found.
AAS[3]	Whole blood. Collect in pretested, metal-free container.	0.06-0.87 mcg/L × 19.6	[1.2-17.1 nmol/L]	
	Serum.	0.24 ± 0.21 mcg/L × 19.6	[4.7 ± 4.1 nmol/L]	
	Urine, 24 hr. Collect in acid-washed, metal-free container.	<0.08-0.24 mcg/L × 19.6	[<1.6-4.7 nmol/L]	
	Hair.[6] Cut close to scalp and analyze proximal segments.	*mcg/g dry wt.* 0.09-0.16 × 19.6	*nmol/g dry wt.* [1.8-3.1]	

1. Nechay BR, Nanninga LB, Nechay PSE, et al: Role of vanadium in biology, *Fed Proc* 45:123-132, 1986.
2. Nielson FH, Uthus E: The essentiality and metabolism of vanadium. In Chasteen ND, editor: *Vanadium in biological systems,* Amsterdam, 1990, Kluwer Academic Publishers.
3. Ishida O, Kihira K, Tsukamoto Y, et al: Improved determination of vanadium in biological fluids by electrothermal atomic absorption spectrometry, *Clin Chem* 35:127-130, 1989.
4. Byrne AR, Versieck J: Vanadium determination at the ultratrace level in biological reference materials and serum by radiochemical neutron activation analysis, *Biol Trace Elem Res* 26-27:529-540, 1990.
5. Cornells R, Versieck J, Mees L, et al: The ultratrace element vanadium in human serum, *Biol Trace Elem Res* 3:257-263, 1981.
6. Iyengar GV, Woittiez J: Trace elements in human clinical specimens: evaluation of literature data to identify tolerence values, *Clin Chem* 34:474-481, 1988.
7. Jacobs JJ: More on reaction to a foreign body after hip replacement, *N Engl J Med* 335:1690-1691, 1996.

Vanillylmandelic Acid (3-Methoxy-4-hydroxymandelic acid, VMA)[1,2] *HPLC[3-6]* *GC[7,8]* *GC-MS[9]* *LC-MS/MS[10]*	Urine, 24 hr. Preserve with 20 mL of HCl, 6 mol/L, and refrigerate. Stable for at least 2 wk.		*mg/day*[11]		*μmol/day*	↑ V Ajmaline, epinephrine, glucagon, guanethidine (initial doses), histamine, insulin (after insulin shock or high doses, none with normal dose), levodopa (small increase), rauwolfia alkaloids (e.g., reserpine, initial doses)
		3-6 yr:	1.0-2.6	× 5.05	[5-13]	
		6-10 yr:	2.0-3.2		[10-16]	
		10-16 yr:	2.3-5.2		[12-26]	
		16-83 yr[12]:	1.4-6.5		[7-33]	
			mcg/mg[13] *creatinine*		*mmol/mol creatinine*	
		0-3 mo:	5.9-37.0	× 0.571	[3.4-21.0]	
		3-12 mo:	8.4-43.8		[4.8-25.0]	
		1-2 yr:	7.9-23.0		[4.5-13.1]	
		2-5 yr:	2.9-23.0		[1.7-13.1]	↓ V Chlorpromazaine, clonidine (dose-dependent effect), debrisoquine, disulfiram, guanethidine,
		5-10 yr:	5.8-18.7		[3.3-10.7]	
		10-15 yr:	1.6-10.6		[1.0-6.1]	
		>15 yr:	2.8-8.3		[1.6-4.7]	

DIAGNOSTIC INFORMATION	REMARKS

Vanadium toxicity in humans is almost always associated with industrial processes. Major effects of vanadium toxicity include irritation to the mucous membranes of the eyes, nose, throat, and respiratory tract; bronchitis; GI distress; fatigue; cardiac palpitation; kidney damage; and other physiological disturbances of the CNS and cardiovascular system.[1] A clinical presentation of V toxicity may be green discoloration of the tongue.

Vanadium is used extensively in the steel industry and to a lesser degree in photography and in the manufacture of insecticides, dyes, inks, paints, and varnish. Vanadium is a component of some orthopedic prostheses. Vanadium particles have been observed in periprosthetic tissues, liver, and spleen.[7]

↑ In pheochromocytoma, paraganglioma, and neuroblastoma.

VMA is the major metabolite of the catecholamines and historically has been used to screen for pheochromocytoma. The current recommended test is now fractionated plasma-free metanephrines (See *Metanephrines, Fractionated.*)

Urinary VMA is elevated in ≥90% of patients with neuroblastoma, but concentrations within the reference interval do not exclude the diagnosis. Increased concentrations are consistent with pheochromocytoma but are not diagnostic. Additional tests for neuroblastoma includes HVA (See *Homovanillic Acid*).

In patients with neuroblastoma, a HVA/VMA ratio <1 or >2 had an unfavorable prognosis.[14]

TEST NAME AND METHOD	SPECIMEN REQUIREMENTS	REFERENCE INTERVAL, CONVENTIONAL [INTERNATIONAL RECOMMENDED UNITS]	CHEMICAL INTERFERENCES AND IN VIVO EFFECTS
Vanillylmandelic Acid—CONT			hydrazine derivatives, imipramine, MAO inhibitors, morphine; radiographic agents compete for excretion after IV pyelography; and rauwolfia alkaloids, e.g., reserpine (chronic)

1. Thomasson C, Blijenberg BG, Eilers G, et al: A comparative study of five different methods for the determination of 3-methoxy-4-hydroxymandelic acid in urine, *J Clin Chem Clin Biochem* 21:417-427, 1983.

2. Rosano TG, Whitley RJ: Catecholamines and serotonin. In Burtis CA, Ashwood ER, editors: *Tietz textbook of clinical chemistry,* Philadelphia, 1999, WB Saunders.

3. Moleman P, Borstrok JJM: Determination of urinary vanillylmandelic acid by liquid chromatography with electrochemical detection, *Clin Chem* 29:878-881, 1983.

4. Kinoshita Y, Yamada S, Haraguchi K, et al: Determination of vanillylmandelic acid, vanillactic acid, and homovanillic acid in dried urine on filter-paper discs by high-performance liquid chromatography with coulometric electrochemical detection for neuroblastoma screening, *Clin Chem* 34:2228-2230, 1988.

5. Fujita K, Maruta K, Ito S, et al: Urinary 4-hydroxy-3-methoxymandelic (vanillylmandelic) acid, 4-hydroxy-3-methoxyphenylacetic (homovanillic) acid, and 5-hydroxy-3-indoleacetic acid determined by liquid chromatography with electrochemical detection, *Clin Chem* 29:876-878, 1983.

6. Gironi A, Seghieri G, Niccolai M, et al: Simultaneous liquid-chromatographic determination of urinary vanillylmandelic acid, homovanillic acid, and 5-hydroxyindoleacetic acid, *Clin Chem* 34:2504-2506, 1988.

7. Brewster MA, Berry DH, Moriarty M: Urinary 3-methoxy-4-hydroxyphenylacetic (homovanillic) and 3-methoxy-4-hydroxymandelic (vanillylmandelic) acids: gas-liquid chromatographic methods and experience with 13 cases of neuroblastoma, *Clin Chem* 23:2247-2249, 1977.

8. Tuchman M, Crippin PJ, Krivit W: Capillary gas chromatographic determination of urinary homovanillic acid and vanillylmandelic acid, *Clin Chem* 29:828-831, 1983.

9. Fauler G, Leis HJ, Huber E, et al: Determination of homovanillic acid and vanillylmandelic acid in neuroblastoma screening by stable isotope dilution GC-MS, *J Mass Spectrom* 32:507-514, 1997.

10. Magera MJ, Thompson AL, Matern D, et al: Liquid chromatography-tandem mass spectrometry method for the determination of vanillylmandelic acid in urine, *Clin Chem* 49:825-826, 2003.

11. Prémel-Cabic A, Turcant A, Allain P: Normal reference intervals for free catecholamines and then acid metabolites in 24-h urines from children, as determined by liquid chromatography with amperometric detection, *Clin Chem* 32:1585-1587, 1986.

12. Gerlo A, Malfait R: High-performance liquid chromatographic assay of free norepinephrine, epinephrine, dopamine, vanillylmandelic acid and homovanillic acid, *J Chromatogr* 343:9-20, 1985.

13. Tuchman M, Morris C, Ramnaraine M, et al: Value of random urinary homovanillic acid and vanillylmandelic acid in the diagnosis and management of patients with neuroblastoma: comparison with 24-h urine collections, *Pediatrics* 75:324-328, 1985.

14. Nishi M, Miyake H, Takeda T, et al: The relationship between homovanillic/vanillylmandelic acid ratios and prognosis in neuroblastoma, *Oncol Rep* 5:631-633, 1998.

DIAGNOSTIC INFORMATION   **REMARKS**

Because chromatographic methods are not prone to interferences seen with older photometric methods, dietary restrictions during urine collection are not required.

Reference intervals may vary slightly according to methodology.

TEST NAME AND METHOD	SPECIMEN REQUIREMENTS	REFERENCE INTERVAL, CONVENTIONAL [INTERNATIONAL RECOMMENDED UNITS]	CHEMICAL INTERFERENCES AND IN VIVO EFFECTS
Vasoactive Intestinal Polypeptide (VIP)[1-4] *RIA*	Plasma (EDTA), fasting. Freeze.	Child and adult[5]: <50 pg/mL × 1.0 [<50 ng/L] Increases in the elderly.	None found.

1. Buchanan KD: The gastrointestinal hormones: general concepts, *Clin Endocrinol Metab* 8:249-263, 1979.
2. Henderson AR, Tietz NW, Rinker AD, et al: Gastric, pancreatic, and intestinal function. In Burtis CA, Ashwood ER, editors: *Tietz textbook of clinical chemistry,* ed 2, Philadelphia, 1994, WB Saunders.
3. Morgan LM, Marks VL: The gastrointestinal hormones. In Pennington GW, Naik S, editors: *Hormone analysis: methodology and clinical interpretation, vol 2,* Boca Raton, FL, 1981, CRC Press.
4. Said SI, editor: *Vasoactive intestinal peptide,* New York, 1982, Raven Press.
5. Nichols Institute Reference Laboratories: *Test catalog,* San Juan Capistrano, CA, 1993, Nichols Institute Reference Laboratories.
6. Lucia P, Caiola S, Coppola A, et al: Vasoactive intestinal peptide (VIP): a new neuroendocrine marker of clinical progression in chronic heart failure? *Clin Endocrinol (Oxf)* 59:723-727, 2003.

TEST NAME AND METHOD	SPECIMEN REQUIREMENTS	REFERENCE INTERVAL, CONVENTIONAL [INTERNATIONAL RECOMMENDED UNITS]	CHEMICAL INTERFERENCES AND IN VIVO EFFECTS
Vinyl Chloride[1] *(Chloroethene; chloroethylene; ethylene monochloride; CAS 75-01-4)* *GC-FID,*[2,3] *GC-MS*[4]	Breath Urine[5]	Occupational exposure:* <0.6 ppm × 16.0 [<10 μmol/L] As thiodiglycolic acid, Occupational exposure: *mg/g creatinine* *mmol/mol creatinine* <2 × 0.753 [<1.5] *After 8-hr exposure to 25 ppm [400 mmol/L].	None found.

1. Baselt RC: *Biological monitoring methods for industrial chemicals,* Davis, CA, 1980, Biomedical Pub.
2. Chen ZY, Gu XR, Lui MZ, et al: Sensitive flame-photometric detector analysis of thiodiglycolic acid in urine as a biological monitor of vinyl chloride, *Int Arch Occup Environ Health* 52:281-284, 1983.

DIAGNOSTIC INFORMATION	REMARKS

↑ Pancreatic VIP-secreting tumors (VIPomas), neural crest tumors in children (e.g., ganglioneuroblastoma, ganglioneuroma, and neuroblastoma), pancreatic islet cell hyperplasia, liver disease, MEN syndrome type I, pheochromocytoma, medullary thyroid carcinoma, bronchogenic carcinoma, retroperitoneal histiocytoma, and congestive heart failure.[6]

VIP is a member of the secretin-glucagon family; highest concentrations are found in the gut and nervous system. Measurement of VIP concentrations is useful to screen for VIP-secreting tumors, to detect occult metastases, and to evaluate the success of surgical or drug therapies.

Hypersecretion of VIP is believed to result in the Verner-Morrison syndrome (also called pancreatic cholera syndrome or WDHA [watery diarrhea with hypokalemia and achlorhydria] syndrome). However, VIP does not appear to be the sole mediator of the WDHA syndrome. Levels of VIP in CSF are ~10 times higher than in plasma. In Crohn's disease, there is a reported increase of 100% in the VIP content of the bowel.

Long term exposure to vinyl chloride is associated with hepatotoxicity and angiosarcoma.

Studies of workers who have developed "vinyl chloride disease," a syndrome consisting of Raynaud's phenomenon, acroosteolysis, joint and muscle pain, enhanced collagen deposition, stiffness of the hands, and scleroderma-like skin changes, indicate that this disease may have an immunologic basis.[6]

Vinyl chloride is an intermediate in the synthesis of polyvinyl chloride and has been used as an aerosol propellant. Industrial exposure is by inhalation. Blood concentrations are not helpful in monitoring exposure. A major urinary metabolite of vinyl chloride is thiodiglycolic acid.

Vinyl chloride in the breath of exposed workers declines slowly after removal from the source of exposure. Concentrations in the breath have been reported from 0.6 to 3.0 ppm [10-48 μmol/L].

Thiodiglycolic acid concentrations in urine of unexposed workers average 0.5-0.7 mg/L, whereas in workers exposed to 1-7 ppm [16-112 μmol/L] of vinyl chloride, thiodiglycolic acid concentration can range up to 4 mg/L.[7]

3. Zuccato E, Marcucci F, Fanelli R, et al: Headspace gas chromatographic analysis of vinyl chloride monomer in rat blood and tissues, *Xenobiotica* 9:27-31, 1979.

TEST NAME AND METHOD	SPECIMEN REQUIREMENTS	REFERENCE INTERVAL, CONVENTIONAL [INTERNATIONAL RECOMMENDED UNITS]		CHEMICAL INTERFERENCES AND IN VIVO EFFECTS

Vinyl Chloride—CONT

4. Muller G, Norpoth K, Wickramasinghe RH: An analytical method, using GC-MS, for the quantitative determination of urinary thiodiglycolic acid, *Int Arch Occup Environ Health* 44:185-191, 1979.

5. Klaassen CD, Amdur MO, Doull J: *Casarett and Doull's toxicology: the basic science of poisons,* ed 3, New York, 1986, Macmillan Pub. Co.

Viscosity[1]	Whole blood (heparin).	Cord blood[3]		None found.
Microviscometer	Reject clotted or hemolyzed specimens.	Shear rate, 11.5/sec: <11.8 cP	($\bar{x}$: 8.5)	
		Shear rate, 46/sec: <7.0 cP	($\bar{x}$: 6.0)	
Macroviscometer	Serum.[2] Stable for at least 4 days at 2-8° C.	1.00-1.24 cP	(relative to water at 37° C)	

1. Crawford J, Cohen HJ: Disorders of hyperviscosity. In Ritzmann SE, editor: *Protein abnormalities, vol 2,* New York, 1982, Alan R. Liss, Inc.

2. Robertson DA, Simpson FG, Losowsky MS: Blood viscosity after splenectomy *BMJ* 283:573-575, 1981.

3. Danish EH: Neonatal polycythemia, *Prog Hematol* 14:55-98, 1986.

4. Jacobs DS, Kasten BL, DeMott WR, et al, editors: *Laboratory test handbook,* ed 2, Stow, OH, 1990, LexiComp, Inc.

5. Williams WJ, Beutler E, Erslev AJ, et al, editors: *Hematology,* ed 4, New York, 1990, McGraw-Hill Publishing Co.

Vitamin A	Serum or plasma (heparin), fasting. Avoid		*mcg/dL*		*μmol/L*	↑ V Alcohol (moderate in-
(Retinol)[1,2]		1-6 yr:	20-43	× 0.0349	[0.70-1.50]	take), oral contraceptives
	hemolysis; protect from	7-12 yr:	26-49		[0.91-1.71]	
	light. Stable for 4 wk at	13-19 yr:	26-72		[0.91-2.51]	↓ V Alcohol (alcoholics),
	4° C, 2 yr at −20° C,	Adult:	30-80		[1.05-2.80]	allopurinol, cholestyr-
	or 5 yr at −20° C when					amine, colestipol, mineral
	vitamin A is extracted					oil, and neomycin
	in the presence of					
Fluorimetric,[9]	ascorbic acid. Do not					↑ C *HPLC:* Probucol
HPLC,[3-7] *LC-MS*[8]	ingest alcohol 24 hr before blood draw.					

DIAGNOSTIC INFORMATION	REMARKS

6. Available at: http://www.atsdr.cdc.gov/toxprofiles/tp20-c2.pdf. Last accessed 2/1/06.
7. Muller G, Norpoth K, Kusters E: Determination of thiodiglycolic acid in urine specimens of vinyl chloride-exposed workers, *Int Arch Occup Environ Health* 41:199-205, 1978.

B ↑ Polycythemia, rouleau formation, postsplenectomy[1,2,4]; altered shape of erythrocytes, and antibody-mediated erythrocyte membrane damage; also conditions listed below under serum

Measurement of whole blood viscosity is of limited clinical usefulness because of the differences in shear rates between instrumentation and in vivo conditions. Reference intervals are dependent on viscometer shear rates.[5]

In healthy infants, there is a direct relationship between the hematocrit and the log of blood viscosity, at shear rates of 11.5 and 46/sec (when the hematocrit is determined with the standard microhematocrit method).

Factors influencing globulin viscosity include concentration, intrinsic viscosity (IgM > IgA > IgE > IgG), aggregation (IgM, IgG$_3$), polymer formation (IgA), molecular asymmetry, cryoprecipitability, immune complex formation, and interaction with other plasma proteins.[1]

S ↑ Increased leukocyte count, thrombocytosis, hyperlipoproteinemia, hyperfibrinogenemia, hypercryofibrinogenemia, macroglobulinemia (such as Waldenström's), myeloma, amyloidosis, polyclonal hyperviscosity syndrome,[1,3] Sjögren's syndrome, SLE, lymphoproliferative disorders, hyperglobulinemia associated with cirrhosis, chronic active hepatitis, or acute thermal burns

There is less than ideal correlation between viscosity and clinical symptoms.[3]

The relative viscosity is expressed as a ratio of plasma (serum) flow time to water flow time.

↑ Idiopathic hypercalcemia in infants, hypervitaminosis, toxicity, chronic kidney disease, glucocorticoids, and oral contraceptives

↓ Night blindness, infantile blindness, hypothyroidism, sterility and teratogenesis; liver, GI, or pancreatic diseases; xerosis, chronic infections, pyrexia; disseminated tuberculosis, carcinoid syndrome, protein malnutrition and zinc deficiency resulting in decreased retinol-binding protein (RBP) levels; abetalipoproteinemia, cystic fibrosis

Other biologically active forms of vitamin A (retinal and retinoic acid) are present in plasma at very low concentrations (<1 mcg/dL; <10 mcg/L); retinyl esters usually comprise ~5% of the total vitamin A (3-5 mcg/dL; 30-50 mcg/L). Usual vitamin A supplemental intakes (5000-10,000 U/day) do not alter plasma levels of retinol but do cause a twofold increase in retinyl ester levels. In acute hypervitaminosis A (>50,000 U/day), retinyl esters can constitute >30% of the total vitamin A (1800 mcg/dL; 18 mg/L), and in severe toxicity

TEST NAME AND METHOD	SPECIMEN REQUIREMENTS	REFERENCE INTERVAL, CONVENTIONAL [INTERNATIONAL RECOMMENDED UNITS]	CHEMICAL INTERFERENCES AND IN VIVO EFFECTS
Vitamin A—CONT			↓ C Plastic tubing

Phytofluene must be removed or corrected for when using fluorimetric method (tomatoes contain significant quantities); contact with rubber materials should be avoided. |

1. Gillespie C, Ballew C, Bowman BA, et al: Intraindividual variation in serum retinol concentrations among participants in the third National Health and Nutrition Examination Survey, 1988-1994, *Am J Clin Nutr* 79:625-632, 2004.

2. Furr H: Analysis of retinoids and carotenoids: problems resolved and unsolved, *J Nutr* 134:281S-285S, 2004.

3. Quesada JM, Mata-Granados JM, Luque DeCastro MD: Automated method for the determination of fat-soluble vitamins in serum, *J Steroid Biochem Mol Biol* 89-90:473-477, 2004.

4. Lee BL, New AL, Ong CN: Simultaneous determination of tocotrienols, tocopherols, retinol, and major carotenoids in human plasma, *Clin Chem* 49:2056-2066, 2003.

5. Taibi G, Nicotra CM: Development and validation of a fast and sensitive chromatographic assay for all-trans-retinol and tocopherols in human serum and plasma using liquid-liquid extraction, *J Chromatogr B Analyt Technol Biomed Life Sci* 780:261-277, 2002.

6. Hartmann S, Froescheis O, Ringenbach F, et al: Determination of retinol and retinyl esters in human plasma by high-performance liquid chromatography with automated column switching and ultraviolet detection, *J Chromatogr B Biomed Sci Appl* 751:265-275, 2001.

Serum retinol, because of homeostatic control exerted by the liver, is not a good general indicator of body vitamin A stores. Values >20 mcg/dL [>0.70 μmol/L] represent adequate liver stores, whereas values <10 mcg/dL [<0.35 μmol/L] indicate severe deficiency and depletion of liver stores.

Children show an age-related increase in serum retinol, and the values are lower before puberty. Levels in adults increase slightly with age. Premenopausal females have slightly lower values than males; after menopause, values are similar.

the level of retinyl esters can be >1500 mcg/dL [>15 mg/L].[10] Symptoms of toxicity appear to occur only when the amount of plasma vitamin A exceeds the capacity of RBP to bind to it. Normal molar ratios of A:RBP are ~0.8-1.0.

Clinical manifestations of acute hypervitaminosis A include bulging fontanelles in infants, headache in adults, nausea, vomiting, and occasionally fever, vertigo, visual disorientation, and peeling of the skin. These symptoms are generally transient and do not result in permanent adverse effects. Chronic hypervitaminosis A is more common and is associated with anorexia, dry itchy skin, hair loss, increased intracranial pressure, hepatomegaly, and fatigue. Vitamin A toxicity is rarely associated with causing congenital abnormalities and death. Water-miscible preparations of vitamin A are more toxic than oil-based formulations. Toxicity is best assessed by measuring plasma retinyl ester levels rather than the concentration of vitamin A.

Diseases and conditions that impair the conversion of carotene to vitamin A or reduce the levels of RBP can contribute to the development of vitamin A deficiency. Symptoms of deficiency include bronchopulmonary dysplasia in prematures, night blindness, xerophthalmia, keratomalacia, Bitot spots, follicular hyperkeratosis, and photophobia. Ocular changes can be further documented by a dark adaptation test and electroretinography.

Further understanding of cellular retinol-metabolizing enzymes/proteins like lecithin-retinol acyltransferase and cellular retinol binding protein and their interaction with retinol and its metabolites will provide insights into better dietary management of vitamin A status.[11] See *Retinol-Binding Protein*.

See Table II-5.

7. Alvarez JC, De Mazancourt P: Rapid and sensitive high-performance liquid chromatographic method for simultaneous determination of retinol, alpha-tocopherol, 25-hydroxyvitamin D3 and 25-hydroxyvitamin D2 in human plasma with photodiode-array ultraviolet detection, *J Chromatogr B Biomed Sci Appl* 755:129-135, 2001.

8. Van Breemen RB, Huang CR: High-performance liquid chromatography-electrospray mass spectrometry of retinoids, *FASEB J* 10:1098-1101, 1996.

9. Driskell WJ, Hewett JS, Bashor MM: Evaluation of a direct fluorescence method for determination of serum retinol, *Clin Chem* 32:867-869, 1986.

10. Bendich A, Langseth L: Safety of vitamin A, *Am J Clin Nutr* 49:358-371, 1989.

11. Ross AC, Zolfaghari R: Regulation of hepatic retinol metabolism: perspectives from studies on vitamin A status, *J Nutr* 134:269S-275S, 2004.

TEST NAME AND METHOD	SPECIMEN REQUIREMENTS	REFERENCE INTERVAL, CONVENTIONAL [INTERNATIONAL RECOMMENDED UNITS]	CHEMICAL INTERFERENCES AND IN VIVO EFFECTS
Vitamin A Relative Dose-Response (RDR) Test[1,2] Dose: Retinyl palmitate is given either as a water-miscible solution of 1000 mcg administered IV over 30 min or as 450 mcg diluted in corn oil and administered orally. Fluids may be consumed during test period.	Serum or plasma; see *Vitamin A.* Fasting specimen drawn before dose and at 5 hr.	RDR: $<10\%$ $RDR = \dfrac{A_5 - A_o}{A_5} \times 100$ A_5 = Plasma vitamin A 5 hr after dose A_o = Plasma vitamin A just before dose	See *Vitamin A.*
Modified dose[2]: 3,4-didehy-droretinyl acetate (DRA) administered orally in graded standard doses 5.3 μmol/kg <6 yr 7.0 μmol/kg 6-12 yr 8.8 μmol/kg >12 yr	Modified: Serum or plasma; single measure 4-6 hr after dosing.	Modified: Ratio DRA/retinol[3] >0.06: Suggestive of deficiency 0.04-0.06: Intermediate ≤ 0.03: Satisfactory	

1. Underwood BA: Methods for assessment of vitamin A status, *J Nutr* 120:1459-1463, 1990.
2. Tanumihardjo SA, Cheng JC, Permaesih D, et al: Refinement of the modified-relative-dose-response test as a method for assessing vitamin A status in a field setting: experience with Indonesian children, *Am J Clin Nutr* 64:966-971, 1996.
3. Tanumihardjo SA, Suharno D, Permaesih D, et al: Application of the modified relative dose response test to pregnant Indonesian women for assessing vitamin A status, *Eur J Clin Nutr* 49:897-903, 1995.
4. Tanumihardjo SA: Assessing vitamin A status: past, present and future, *J Nutr* 134:290S-293S, 2004.

TEST NAME AND METHOD	SPECIMEN REQUIREMENTS	REFERENCE INTERVAL, CONVENTIONAL [INTERNATIONAL RECOMMENDED UNITS]				CHEMICAL INTERFERENCES AND IN VIVO EFFECTS
Vitamin B$_6$ (Pyridoxal Phosphate, PLP)[1] *Enzymatic, radiometric,*[2] *HPLC*[3-5]	Plasma (EDTA, heparin, or Na citrate) or serum, fasting; freeze. Protect from light. Plasma is stable for 12 mo at $-80°$ C[4] (50% loss in 7 days at $-20°$ C). Avoid repeated freezing and thawing.	Deficiency:	*ng/mL* 5-50 <5	$\times 4.046$	*nmol/L* [20-202][6] [<20]	$\downarrow$ V Amiodarone, anticonvulsants (e.g., carbamazepine, phenobarbital, phenytoin, primidone), cycloserine, disulfiram, ethanol (alcoholics), hydralazine, isoniazid, levodopa, oral contraceptives (plasma levels only), penicillamine, pyrazinoic acid, and theophylline

DIAGNOSTIC INFORMATION	REMARKS

↓ Malabsorption, cirrhosis, chronic cholestasis, hepatocellular disease, protein-calorie malnutrition, and zinc deficiency

RDR values >20% indicate depleted liver vitamin A stores.

The oral dose test is subject to the limitations of other absorption tests. In the absence of malabsorption or when the RDR is done with an IV dose, results of the RDR correlate well with liver stores of vitamin A and with dark adaptation. Plasma levels of vitamin A are maintained at normal concentrations until hepatic stores are almost depleted (<20 mcg/g; <0.07 μmol/g).

Modified:
Circulating concentration of DRA is relatively low, allowing a single measurement at 4-6 hr after a given oral dose. DRA is being made available to researchers through the University of Wisconsin-Madison, Department of Nutritional Sciences.[4] See *Vitamin A.*

↓ Chronic alcoholism, malnutrition, uremia, neonatal seizures, malabsorption, industrial exposure to hydrazine compounds, normal pregnancies, gestational diabetes, pellagra, lactation, renal dialysis, asthma, carpal tunnel syndrome, smoking, preeclamptic edema, and acute myocardial infarction.[7]

↑ Hypophosphatasia[8]

Plasma contains several forms of vitamin B_6, but PLP is quantitatively and biologically the most important. Plasma PLP levels are high in infants but decrease with age. Deficiency usually occurs in association with other nutrient deficiencies. Vitamin B_6 deficiency is associated with symptoms of irritability, weakness, depression, dizziness, peripheral neuropathy, dermatitis, cheilosis, glossitis, and seizures. Deficiencies in pediatrics have been characterized by diarrhea, anemia, seizures, and failure to thrive. Both erythrocyte and plasma transaminase activities are diminished in conjunction with vitamin B_6 deficiency.

TEST NAME AND METHOD	SPECIMEN REQUIREMENTS	REFERENCE INTERVAL, CONVENTIONAL [INTERNATIONAL RECOMMENDED UNITS]	CHEMICAL INTERFERENCES AND IN VIVO EFFECTS
Vitamin B$_6$—CONT			

1. Leklem JE: Vitamin B$_6$. In Machlin LJ, editor: *Handbook of vitamins,* New York, 1991, Marcel Dekker, p. 341.

2. Camp VM, Chipponi J, Faraj BA: Radioenzymatic assay for direct measurement of plasma pyridoxal 5'-phosphate, *Clin Chem* 29:642-644, 1983.

3. Kimura M, Kanehira K, Yokoi K: Highly sensitive and simple liquid chromatographic determination in plasma of B$_6$ vitamins, especially pyridoxal 5'-phosphate, *J Chromatogr A* 22:296-301, 1996.

4. Talwar D, Quasim T, McMillan DC, et al: Optimisation and validation of a sensitive high-performance liquid chromatography assay for routine measurement of pyridoxal 5-phosphate in human plasma and red cells using pre-column semicarbazide derivatisation, *J Chromatogr B Analyt Technol Biomed Life Sci* 792:333-343, 2003.

5. Deitrick CL, Katholi RE, Huddleston DJ, et al: Clinical adaptation of a high-performance liquid chromatographic method for the assay of pyridoxal 5'-phosphate in human plasma, *J Chromatogr B Biomed Sci Appl* 751:383-387, 2001.

6. Mayo Medical Laboratories: *Test catalog,* Rochester, MN, 2005, Mayo Medical Laboratories.

7. Serfontein WJ, Ubbink JB, De Villiers LS, et al: Plasma pyridoxal-5-phosphate level as risk index for coronary artery disease, *Atherosclerosis* 55:357-361, 1985.

8. Iqbal SJ, Brain A, Holland S, et al: Raised serum pyridoxal-5-phosphate levels in hypophosphatasia, *Proc ACB Natl Meet* 69, 1995.

TEST NAME AND METHOD	SPECIMEN REQUIREMENTS	REFERENCE INTERVAL, CONVENTIONAL [INTERNATIONAL RECOMMENDED UNITS]	CHEMICAL INTERFERENCES AND IN VIVO EFFECTS

Vitamin B$_6$ Functional Test (EALT,* EAST Index†)[1-3]	Erythrocyte hemolysate; collect whole blood (EDTA). Stable for several weeks at $-20°$ C and for 10 wk at $-70°$ C. Avoid repeated freezing and thawing.	EAST* index† as an indication of vitamin B$_6$ status:
		  Acceptable: <1.5
		  Vitamin B$_6$ deficiency: >1.5
		
		EAST, Erythrocyte aspartate aminotransferase.
		†Ratio of EAST activities measured in erythrocyte hemolysate after and before stimulation with pyridoxal phosphate (25 mcg/mL [0.1 µmol/mL] for 20 min).[3]
			See *Vitamin B$_6$.*

DIAGNOSTIC INFORMATION	REMARKS

Vitamin B_6 has very low toxicity, but very high doses can cause peripheral neuropathy. Urine measurements of vitamin B_6 are of limited diagnostic value.

Markedly elevated PLP is observed in cases of hypophosphatasia, a disorder characterized by low levels of alkaline phosphatase and a range of skeletal abnormalities.

See also *Vitamin B_6 Functional Test.*

↑ Vitamin B_6 deficiency

The index represents the functional availability of erythrocyte vitamin B_6 in its coenzyme form, and its value *increases* with vitamin B_6 deficiency. The EALT* (erythrocyte alanine aminotransferase) index can also be used as a functional measure of vitamin B_6 status.[3] Values for both EGOT and EGPT indices, as well as criteria for interpreting results, vary with the amount of pyridoxal phosphate added and with the method.

See also *Vitamin B_6.*

*Erythrocyte alanine aminotransferase
†Erythrocyte aspartate aminotransferase

TEST NAME AND METHOD	SPECIMEN REQUIREMENTS	REFERENCE INTERVAL, CONVENTIONAL [INTERNATIONAL RECOMMENDED UNITS]			CHEMICAL INTERFERENCES AND IN VIVO EFFECTS

Vitamin B$_6$ Functional Test—CONT

1. Bayoumi RA, Rosalki SB: Evaluation of methods of coenzyme activation of erythrocyte enzymes for detection of deficiency of vitamins B$_1$, B$_2$, and B$_6$, *Clin Chem* 22:327-335, 1976.

2. Hafkenscheid JCM, van Dijk CMCE: Influence of substrate concentration on the activation of transketolase, aspartate aminotransferase, and glutathione reductase by coenzymes, *Clin Chem* 30:143-144, 1984.

Test name and method	Specimen requirements	Reference interval conventional				Chemical interferences
Vitamin B$_{12}$[1-4] *CPB radioassay*	Serum, fasting; avoid heparin, ascorbic acid, fluoride, and hemolysis. Protect from light.	Newborn: Adult: 60-90 yr:	*pg/mL* 160-1300 200-835 110-770	× 0.738	*pmol/L* [118-959] [148-616] [81-568]	↓ V Alcohol (heavy intake >2 wk), aminoglycosides, aminosalicylic acid, antibiotics (e.g., neomycin), anticonvulsants (phenytoin, phenobarbital, primidone), cholestyramine, cimetidine, cobalt irradiation of small bowel, colchicine, extended-release potassium preparations, metformin, oral contraceptives, pentamidine, phenformin, ranitidine, and triamterene
MB, Lactobacillus leichmannii[5]	Specimens are stable overnight at 8° C and for 8 wk at −20° C. Avoid repeated freezing and thawing. When ruling out malabsorption, draw sample before Schilling test.		200-900		[148-664]	
Chemiluminescence (automated)[6]	Serum or plasma (EDTA, heparin, citrate). Freeze if assay delayed >8 hr. Protect from light.	250-1100 pg/mL		× 0.738	[185-812 pmol/L]	↓ C Methotrexate, pyrimethamine, and most antibiotics inhibit microbiological assays.

3. Leklem JE: Vitamin B-6: a status report, *J Nutr* 120(11S):1503-1507, 1990.

S ↑ Chronic renal failure, severe congestive heart failure, diabetes, increased levels of transcobalamin, acute and chronic myelogenous leukemia, about one third of cases of chronic lymphatic leukemia, some cases of monocytic leukemia; leukocytosis, polycythemia vera, some carcinomas (especially with liver metastases), liver disease (acute and chronic hepatitis, cirrhosis, hepatic coma), drug-induced cholestasis, erythroleukemia, and protein malnutrition

---

S ↓ Untreated vitamin B_{12} deficiency usually resulting in megaloblastic anemia. Causes: Lack of IF (PA, total or partial gastrectomy, atrophic gastritis, intrinsic factor antibody); malabsorption (e.g., regional ileitis, resected bowel, sprue, celiac disease, pancreatic insufficiency, small bowel bacterial overgrowth, achlorhydria); loss of ingested vitamin B_{12} (fish tapeworm); dietary deficiency (vegetarians); congenital disorders (orotic aciduria, transcobalamin deficiency, Immerslund-Grösbeck syndrome); progressive decrease during pregnancy sometimes to below normal levels in the last trimester (normal serum B_{12} in megaloblastic anemia of pregnancy)

B_{12} values obtained by CPB radioassay can be invalidated if the patient has previously received radioisotopes.

Vitamin B_{12} deficiency frequently causes macrocytic anemia, glossitis, peripheral neuropathy, weakness, hyperreflexia, ataxia, loss of proprioception, poor coordination, and affective behavioral changes. These manifestations may occur in any combination; many patients have the neurologic defects without macrocytic anemia.[7]

Serum levels of vitamin B_{12} are a better indicator of B_{12} status than are erythrocyte levels. However, the lower limit indicating frank deficiency is not well defined. Serum levels can be low in the absence of either anemia or macrocytosis (e.g., patients with myeloma or aplastic anemia). Conversely, elevated transcobalamin II can result in normal or elevated serum vitamin B_{12} levels despite deficient liver stores. Diagnosis of vitamin B_{12} deficiency is supported by evidence of blood and bone marrow megaloblasts and evaluation of histamine-fast achlorhydria and achylia. However, subclinical or early detection of cobalamin deficiency may be missed, and other factors may induce a megaloblastic anemia.[8] Newly developed test methods and new testing algorithms have been proposed for the assessment of vitamin B_{12} deficiency.[9] An algorithm using B_{12}, MMA, IF blocking antibody and serum gastrin analysis has been developed and is being utilized at the Mayo Clinic, which may allow more reliable assessment of vitamin B_{12} status.[7,10]

Another test that shows promise for the assessment of vitamin B_{12} deficiency is holotranscobalamin (holoTC). HoloTC represents the biologically active fraction of vitamin B_{12} that can be delivered into DNA synthesizing cells.[11] It has therefore been suggested that holoTC may be a sensitive marker of vitamin B_{12} deficiency.

Inadequate intake is rarely the cause of deficiency but occurs most commonly when there is damage to the stomach, ileum, or pancreas or the enterohepatic circulation of vitamin B_{12} is impaired. In some patients (e.g., gastrectomy), severe iron deficiency may also be present. Manifestations of vitamin B_{12} deficiency usually require several years to develop. Few infants develop deficiency, but it is frequently found in elderly persons. The latter may exhibit only neurological symptoms. Vitamin B_{12} deficiency may contribute to osteopenia of aging. Low serum vitamin B_{12} levels often occur in folate deficiency, and

TEST NAME AND METHOD	SPECIMEN REQUIREMENTS	REFERENCE INTERVAL, CONVENTIONAL [INTERNATIONAL RECOMMENDED UNITS]	CHEMICAL INTERFERENCES AND IN VIVO EFFECTS
Vitamin B$_{12}$—CONT			

1. Fairbanks VF, Elvebeck LR: Tests for pernicious anemia: serum vitamin B$_{12}$ assay, *Mayo Clin Proc* 58:135-137, 1983.

2. Kinney JM, Jeejeebhoy KN, Hill GL, et al: *Nutrition and metabolism in patient care,* Philadelphia, 1988, WB Saunders.

3. Sheridan BL, Pearce LC: Vitamin B$_{12}$ assays compared by use of patients' sera with low vitamin B$_{12}$ content, *Clin Chem* 31:734-736, 1985.

4. Shils ME, Olson JA, Shike M, editors: *Modern nutrition in health and disease,* ed 8, Philadelphia, 1994, Lea & Febiger.

5. Kelleher BP, Walshe KG, Scott JM, et al: Microbiological assay for vitamin B$_{12}$ with use of a colistin-sulfate-resistant organism, *Clin Chem* 33:52-54, 1987.

6. Ciba-Corning Diagnostics Corp.: *Automated chemiluminescence system,* Medfield, MA, 1993, Ciba-Corning Diagnostics Corp.

7. Mayo Medical Laboratories: *Test catalog,* Rochester, MN, 2005, Mayo Medical Laboratories.

8. Snow CF: Laboratory diagnosis of vitamin B$_{12}$ and folate deficiency: a guide for the primary care physician, *Arch Intern Med* 159:1289-1298, 1999.

9. Ward PC: Modern approaches to the investigation of vitamin B$_{12}$ deficiency, *Clin Lab Med* 22:435-445, 2002.

10. Klee GG: Cobalamin and folate evaluation: measurement of methylmalonic acid and homocysteine vs vitamin B(12) and folate, *Clin Chem* 46:1277-1283, 2000.

11. Hvas AM, Nexo E: Holotranscobalamin—a first choice assay for diagnosing early vitamin B deficiency? *J Intern Med* 257:289-298, 2005.

12. Ermens AA, Vlasveld LT, Lindemans J: Significance of elevated cobalamin (vitamin B$_{12}$) levels in blood, *Clin Biochem* 36:585-590, 2003.

B_{12} deficiency can be masked by folate therapy. Deficiency of vitamin B_{12}, but not folate, results in increased methylmalonic acid in urine and serum (see *Methylmalonic Acid*). Usual therapy is to administer vitamin B_{12} parenterally.

Elevated levels of cobalamin can be a sign of serious or even life-threatening disease.[12] Hematologic disorders like chronic myelogenous leukemia, promyelocytic leukemia, and polycythemia vera may result in high serum vitamin B_{12}. The cobalamin elevation is likely caused by the increased concentrations of the cobalamin binding protein haptocorrin, which are associated with these conditions.[12] In addition, several liver disorders, including acute hepatitis, cirrhosis, and hepatocellular carcinoma, may result in high serum vitamin B_{12} concentration. This may be the result of cobalamin release during hepatic cytolysis and/or decreased cobalamin clearance by the liver. Even though a toxicity to vitamin B_{12} has not been reported, an isolated observation of an elevated serum vitamin B_{12} may warrant further diagnostic workup to assess the presence of disease.[12]

See also *Transcobalamin* and *Vitamin B_{12} Adsorption Test*.

TEST NAME AND METHOD	SPECIMEN REQUIREMENTS	REFERENCE INTERVAL, CONVENTIONAL [INTERNATIONAL RECOMMENDED UNITS]		CHEMICAL INTERFERENCES AND IN VIVO EFFECTS
Vitamin B$_{12}$ Absorption Test (Schilling Test)[1-4] Dose: 0.5 or 1.0 μCi ^{57}Co-B$_{12}$ given to fasting subjects orally and "flushing" dose of 1.0 mg of unlabeled B$_{12}$, IM, given simultaneously or within 2 hr of oral dose.	Urine, 24 hr	*% of dose excreted* >7.5[8] × 0.01 >8[9] >9[4] If first 24-hr excretion is low, collect second 24-hr specimen to compensate for possible renal retention.[4]	*Fraction of dose excreted* [>0.075] [>0.080] [>0.090]	↓ V Barbiturate anticonvulsant (e.g., phenobarbital) can decrease absorption of ^{57}Co-cobalamin; aminosalicylic acid, neomycin, phenformin, and ranitidine ↑ V Cimetidine See also *Vitamin B$_{12}$*.
	Stool. Collect until <1% of the oral dose appears in 2 consecutive days of collection.[5]	*Administered dose excreted* ≤50%	*Fraction of dose excreted* [≤0.50]	
Dose as above; flushing dose not required	Plasma (oxalate). Collect 8 hr after oral dose.[6]	*Administered radioactivity/L of plasma* 1.4-4.1% (x̄: 2.3%)	*Fraction of administered radioactivity* [0.014-0.041/L plasma] [x̄: 0.023/L]	
Dose as above; flushing dose not required	External counting over liver after 1 wk.[7]	Significant counts		

1. Jacobs DS, Kasten BL, DeMott WR, et al, editors: *Laboratory test handbook,* ed 2, Stow, OH, 1990, LexiComp, Inc.

2. Wyngaarden JB, Smith LH Jr, editors: *Cecil textbook of medicine,* ed 18, Philadelphia, 1988, WB Saunders.

3. Henderson AR, Tietz NW, Rinker AD: Gastric, pancreatic, and intestinal function. In Burtis CA, Ashwood ER, editors: *Tietz textbook of clinical chemistry,* ed 2, Philadelphia, 1994, WB Saunders.

4. Nickoloff E: Schilling test: physiologic basis for and use as a diagnostic test, *CRC Crit Rev Clin Lab Sci* 26:263-276, 1988.

5. Silver S: *Radioactive nuclides in medicine and biology, vol 2,* ed 3, Philadelphia, 1968, Lea & Febiger.

6. Beck WS: The megaloblastic anemias. In Williams WJ, Beutler E, Erslev AJ, et al, editors: *Hematology,* ed 3, New York, 1983, McGraw-Hill Book Co.

7. Glass GB, Boyd LJ, Gellin GA, et al: Uptake of radioactive vitamin B$_{12}$ by the liver in humans: test for the measurement of intestinal absorption of vitamin B$_{12}$ and intrinsic factor activity, *Arch Biochem Biophys* 51:251-257, 1954.

8. Tietz NW, editor: *Fundamentals of clinical chemistry,* ed 3, Philadelphia, 1987, WB Saunders.

9. Wyngaarden JB, Smith LH Jr, editors: *Cecil textbook of medicine,* ed 18, Philadelphia, 1988, WB Saunders.

DIAGNOSTIC INFORMATION	REMARKS

U $\downarrow$ After resection of terminal ileum, extensive and severe ileal disease, bacterial overgrowth, PA (in urine, 0-2.5% of administered dose is excreted), after total gastrectomy, sometimes with pancreatic insufficiency, defective ileal mucosal cell receptors for B_{12} (rare), gluten-sensitive enteropathy, anatomical abnormalities of the small gut, chronic pancreatitis, cystic fibrosis, giardiasis, radiotherapy, Crohn's disease, myxedema, liver disease, and presence of antibodies to intrinsic factor in gastric juice

The Schilling test is useful for confirming PA and determining whether vitamin B_{12} deficiency is caused by malabsorption; it is unreliable in the presence of renal impairment. (If creatinine clearance is <60 mL/min, 48-hr urine collection is necessary to compensate for decreased renal function.) Reproducibility is not good in the presence of intestinal disease. The 1-mg flushing dose is an effective treatment in malabsorption. Therefore bone marrow examination for megaloblastic changes should be carried out before the Schilling test, and the reticulocyte response must be followed as usual for anemic patients. After a partial gastrectomy, a B_{12} deficiency may not be detected by the Schilling test.

F $\uparrow$ PA (85-100%) and in conditions listed above

If PA is suspected, the Schilling test may be repeated after 5 days with an additional 60-mg active hog intrinsic factor (IF) given orally. A normal result indicates IF deficiency. Simultaneous administration of ^{57}Co-B_{12} and ^{60}Co-B_{12}-IF (or ^{57}Co-B_{12}-IF and ^{58}Co-B_{12}) has been suggested as a routine method for differentiating B_{12} deficiency because of lack of IF from other causes of malabsorption.[4]

P $\downarrow$ PA (0-0.6%, $\bar{x}$: 0.2%) and in conditions listed above

The Schilling test is being utilized less frequently in the assessment of pernicious anemia. New testing algorithms have been developed using B_{12}, MMA, IF blocking antibody, and serum gastrin analysis have been developed that may ultimately replace the Schilling test.[10] However, there is still controversy with this strategy that must be borne out with further research.[11,12] See also *Vitamin B_{12} Intrinsic Factor.*

L $\downarrow$ PA (counts near zero) and in conditions listed above

External counting over liver is especially useful for outpatients. Results are valid in the presence of renal disease. Daily counting over the liver and abdomen has been suggested as a method for monitoring bowel function throughout the test. Liver counts should be 2.5-4 times higher than abdominal counts.

10. Klee GG: Cobalamin and folate evaluation: measurement of methylmalonic acid and homocysteine vs vitamin B(12) and folate, *Clin Chem* 46:1277-1283, 2000.

11. Ward PC: Modern approaches to the investigation of vitamin B_{12} deficiency, *Clin Lab Med* 22:435-445, 2002.

12. Snow CF: Laboratory diagnosis of vitamin B_{12} and folate deficiency: a guide for the primary care physician, *Arch Intern Med* 159:1289-1298, 1999.

TEST NAME AND METHOD	SPECIMEN REQUIREMENTS	REFERENCE INTERVAL, CONVENTIONAL [INTERNATIONAL RECOMMENDED UNITS]	CHEMICAL INTERFERENCES AND IN VIVO EFFECTS

Vitamin B$_{12}$ Therapeutic Response Test
 	
Dose[1]: 1-5 mcg vitamin B$_{12}$/day orally
 	
Dose[2]: 1-5 mcg vitamin B$_{12}$/day parenterally
	Draw respective baseline specimens before dose, other specimens as indicated to monitor hematological response. Bone marrow, smears prepared at bedside; serum (for iron); whole blood, EDTA (for Erc, Lkc, platelet, and reticulocyte counts). See individual tests for more information.	B$_{12}$ deficiency is indicated by favorable hematological response, such as:
		   Disappearance of megaloblastic changes in bone marrow
		   Decrease in serum iron level within 24-48 hr
		   Onset of reticulocytosis within 2-4 days, peaking at 7 days
		   Increase in Erc, Lkc, and platelet counts
		
		There is an increase in reticulocyte count on day 5, 6, or 7; peak occurs at ~30% [~0.30, number fraction] when Erc count <1.5 million/μL [<1.5 × 10^{12}/L] and at ~10% [~0.10, number fraction] when Erc count >2.5 million/μL [>2.5 × 10^{12}/L]. Erc count should increase to 3 million/μL [3 × 10^{12}/L] in the third week; higher levels of B$_{12}$ are required to establish a positive response in mildly anemic patients.
			See *Vitamin B$_{12}$.*

1. Conn RB, editor: *Current diagnosis,* ed 7, Philadelphia, 1985, WB Saunders.
2. Brown SS, Mitchell FL, Young DS, editors: *Chemical diagnosis of disease,* Amsterdam, 1979, Elsevier/North Holland Biomedical Press.

Vitamin C (Ascorbic Acid)[1,2] *Colorimetric*[1,3]; *HPLC (electrochemical detection)*[4-6]; *(ultraviolet detection)*[1,5] *enzymatic*[7]	Plasma (heparin or oxalate); avoid hemolysis. Stable ~3 hr in refrigerated whole blood, in plasma at −70° C for 10 days.[1,2] Deproteinize plasma or serum promptly with metaphosphoric acid (5 g/dL) or tricholoroacetic acid (10 g/dL). Supernatants stable at −20° C for 2 mo.	Deficiency:	*mg/dL* 0.4-2.0 <0.2	× 56.78	*μmol/L* [23-114] [<11]	P ↓ V Aminopyrine, aspirin, barbiturates, estrogens, heavy metals, oral contraceptives, nitrosamines, and paraldehyde P ↓ C EDTA[1,2]
Colorimetric,[7,8] *HPLC*[5,7,8]	Leukocyte-platelet (buffy coat); collect whole blood (EDTA or heparin). Avoid erythrocyte contamination; assay promptly.	Deficiency:	*mcg/10^7 Lkcs* 20-53 <10	× 0.0568	*fmol/Lkc* [1.14-3.01] [<0.57]	Lkcs ↓ Tetracycline

DIAGNOSTIC INFORMATION	REMARKS

An unequivocal response to therapy is the definitive sign for establishing vitamin B_{12} deficiency. The oral dose is used for diagnosing dietary deficiency of B_{12}.

The parenteral dose is used for determining B_{12} deficiency in megaloblastic anemia. The patient should be monitored for several days before test to rule out spontaneous reticulocytosis.

See also *Vitamin B_{12}*.

P ↓ Scurvy, hemodialysis, anemia, pregnancy, smoking,[1] steatorrhea, alcoholism, malabsorption, hyperthyroidism, rheumatoid disease, cancer, chronic renal failure, and Crohn's disease

Vitamin C is essential for enzymatic amidation of neuropeptides, production of adrenal cortical steroid hormones, promotion of the conversion of tropocollagen to collagen, and of the metabolism of tyrosine and of folate. Vitamin C is involved in activation of detoxifying enzymes in liver, antioxidation, interception, and destruction of free radicals, preservation and restoration of antioxidant potential of vitamin E, and blockade of the formation of carcinogenic nitrosamines. In addition, it appears to function in a variety of other metabolic processes in which its role has not been fully characterized.

Oral vitamin C supplementation will increase plasma levels; large doses (gram quantities) can result in transient plasma values of >2.0 mg/dL [113 μmol/L]. The renal threshold for vitamin C is ~1.0 mg/dL [57μmol/L] with urine being the major excretory route. During periods of inadequate ascorbate consumption, plasma levels decrease before leukocyte levels (the latter reflect general tissue storage).

Lkcs ↓ Scurvy, peptic ulcer, gastroduodenal disorders, and postoperative state

Results may be misleading when either leukocyte or platelet count is abnormal.

Many benefits have been ascribed to megadose therapy, but such claims remain unproved. Megadose intakes of vitamin C are believed to be nontoxic but may result in diarrhea. Induc-

TEST NAME AND METHOD	SPECIMEN REQUIREMENTS	REFERENCE INTERVAL, CONVENTIONAL [INTERNATIONAL RECOMMENDED UNITS]	CHEMICAL INTERFERENCES AND IN VIVO EFFECTS
Vitamin C—CONT			

1. Chung WY, Chung JK, Szeto YT, et al: Plasma ascorbic acid: measurement, stability and clinical utility revisited, *Clin Biochem* 34:623-627, 2001.

2. Terzuoli L, Pagani R, Frosi B, et al: Stability of serum and plasma ascorbic acid, *J Lab Clin Med* 143:67, 2004.

3. Janaszewska A, Bartosz G: Assay of total antioxidant capacity: comparison of four methods as applied to human blood plasma, *Scand J Clin Lab Invest* 62:231-236, 2002.

4. Bode AM, Rose RC: Analysis of water-soluble antioxidants by high-performance liquid chromatography with electrochemical detection, *Methods Enzymol* 299:77-83, 1999.

5. Pappa-Louisi A, Pascalidou S: Optimal conditions for the simultaneous ion-pairing HPLC determination of L-ascorbic, dehydro-L-ascorbic, D-ascorbic, and uric acids with on-line ultraviolet absorbance and electrochemical detection, *Anal Biochem* 263:176-182, 1998.

6. Lykkesfeldt J: Determination of ascorbic acid and dehydroascorbic acid in biological samples by high-performance liquid chromatography using subtraction methods: reliable reduction with tris [2-carboxyethyl] phosphine hydrochloride, *Anal Biochem* 282:89-93, 2000.

7. Washko PW, Welch RW, Dhariwal KR, et al: Ascorbic acid and dehydroascorbic acid analyses in biological samples, *Anal Biochem* 204:1-14, 1992.

8. Washko PW, Wang Y, Levine M: Ascorbic acid recycling in human neutrophils, *J Biol Chem* 268:15531-15535, 1993.

9. Baxmann AC, De O G Mendonca C, Heilberg IP: Effect of vitamin C supplements on urinary oxalate and pH in calcium stone-forming patients, *Kidney Int* 63:1066-1071, 2003.

tion of hyperoxaluria and oxalate kidney stones has been suggested, but the contribution of ascorbate to oxalate stone formation is controversial and has not been proven.[9] Anorexia is the major cause of inadequate ascorbate intake in patients, and scurvy will develop after 80-120 days of deficiency. Infantile scurvy can occur if the neonate receives little or no dietary vitamin C. Symptoms include impaired bone growth, irritability, retrobulbar hemorrhage, epistaxis, hematuria, and purpura. Adult scurvy is characterized by petechiae, ecchymoses, coiled hairs, gum changes, hyperkeratosis, congested follicles, Sjögren's syndrome, dyspnea, arthralgia, joint effusions, femoral neuropathy, and edema. Common complaints include weakness, lethargy, and aching of the legs. Urine measurements are of limited diagnostic value.

TEST NAME AND METHOD	SPECIMEN REQUIREMENTS	REFERENCE INTERVAL, CONVENTIONAL [INTERNATIONAL RECOMMENDED UNITS]			CHEMICAL INTERFERENCES AND IN VIVO EFFECTS
Vitamin D, 1,25-Dihydroxy [Calciferol, 1,25-Dihydroxy; 1,25(OH)$_2$ Calciferol][1-5] *RIA,*[6,7] *CPB*[3]	Serum or plasma (heparin); store frozen. Stable at room temperature for 72 hr or indefinitely at $-20°$ C.	16-65 pg/mL Maternal concentrations are twofold higher.	× 2.6	[42-169 pmol/L]	↓ Increased blood lead levels

1. Zerwekh JE: The measurement of vitamin D: analytical aspects, *Ann Clin Biochem* 41:272-281, 2004.
2. Holick MF: The use and interpretation of assays for vitamin D and its metabolites, *J Nutr* 120(suppl 11):1464-1469, 1990.
3. Carter GD, Carter CR, Gunter E, et al: Measurement of vitamin D metabolites: an international perspective on methodology and clinical interpretation, *J Steroid Biochem Mol Biol* 89-90:467-471, 2004.
4. Endres DB, Rude RK: Vitamin D and its metabolites. In Burtis CA, Ashwood ER, editors: *Tietz textbook of clinical chemistry,* ed 3, Philadelphia, 1999, WB Saunders, pp. 1417-1423.
5. Bringhurst FR, Demay MB, Kronenberg HM: Vitamin D (calciferols): metabolism of vitamin D. In Wilson JD, Foster DW, Kronenberg HM, et al, editors: *Williams textbook of endocrinology,* ed 9, Philadelphia, 1998, WB Saunders, pp. 1166-1169.
6. Fraser WD, Durham BH, Berry JL, et al: Measurement of plasma 1,25 dihydroxyvitamin D using a novel immunoextraction technique and immunoassay with iodine labelled vitamin D tracer, *Ann Clin Biochem* 34:632-637, 1997.
7. Bouillon R: Radiochemical assays for vitamin D metabolites: technical possibilities and clinical applications, *J Steroid Biochem* 19:921-927, 1983.

DIAGNOSTIC INFORMATION	REMARKS

↑ Tumoral calcinosis, primary hyperparathyroidism, idiopathic hypercalciuria, sarcoidosis, tuberculosis, lymphoma (some patients), normal growing children, and pregnant and lactating females

↓ Azotemic chronic renal failure, hypoparathyroidism, pseudo-hypoparathyroidism, vitamin D–dependent rickets, vitamin D–resistant rickets (familial hypophosphatemia), post-menopausal osteoporosis, tumor-induced osteomalacia, and adolescents with insulin-requiring diabetes mellitus

1,25-Dihydroxy vitamin D [1,25(OH)$_2$D] is not detectable in anephric patients.

Hydroxylation of 25(OH)D takes place in the kidney where 1-α hydroxylase, under the control of parathyroid hormone, hydroxylates 25(OH)D to yield 1,25(OH)$_2$D. 1,25(OH)$_2$D, the most active form of vitamin D. It enhances Ca absorption and mobilization, and its synthesis is influenced by the calcium and phosphorus content of the diet, PTH, and 1,25(OH)$_2$D. It is often useful to measure PTH in conjunction with 1,25(OH)$_2$D. 1,25(OH)$_2$D is a hormone and the direct antirachitic factor. Lack of 1,25(OH)$_2$D results in hypocalcemia, osteomalacia, and related disorders. Levels can increase to 200-300 pg/mL [480-720 pmol/L] during treatment of osteomalacia with physiological doses of vitamin D.

Measurement of 1,25(OH)$_2$D is not a good measure of overall vitamin D status but is useful in differentiating primary hyperparathyroidism from hypercalcemia of cancer, distinguishing between vitamin D–dependent and vitamin D–resistant rickets, monitoring the vitamin D status of patients with chronic renal failure, and assessing compliance of 1,25(OH)$_2$D therapy.

Most methods for 1,25(OH)$_2$D combine column chromatography with a radioreceptor assay. Vitamin D receptor from thymus is preferred and recognizes D$_2$ and D$_3$ equivalently.

See also *Vitamin D, 25-Hydroxy.*

TEST NAME AND METHOD	SPECIMEN REQUIREMENTS	REFERENCE INTERVAL, CONVENTIONAL [INTERNATIONAL RECOMMENDED UNITS]			CHEMICAL INTERFERENCES AND IN VIVO EFFECTS
Vitamin D Binding Protein (VDBP or DB Group-Specific Component, Gc-Globulin) *Immunonephelometric (automated)*[1,2]	Serum. Analyze fresh or store at 4° C for <72 hr. Stable frozen at −20° C for 6 mo or at −70° C indefinitely. Specimens without lipemia or hemolysis are preferred.	Liver disease: Pregnancy:	*g/L* 0.32-0.46 0.12-0.33 0.51-0.70	*mg/L* [320-460][2] [120-330][2] [510-700][2]	
Immunoturbidometric[3,4]		Nonpregnant females: M: Pregnancy:	*mcg/dL* 236-322 221-309 315-429	*mg/L* [236-322][4] [221-309][4] [315-429][4]	

1. Wians FH Jr, Lin W, Brown LP, et al: Immunonephelometric quantification of group-specific component protein in patients with acute liver failure, *Liver Transpl Surg* 3:28-33, 1997.
2. Haughton MA, Mason RS: Immunonephelometric assay of vitamin D-binding protein, *Clin Chem* 38:1796-1801, 1992.
3. Hamashima Y, Kanazawa T, Hirata A, et al: Measurement of vitamin D-binding protein in pleural fluids and sera by means of a turbidimetric immunoassay measuring system, *Clin Chim Acta* 321:23-28, 2002.
4. Tillmans LS, Heser DW, Khosla S, et al: Development of a vitamin D binding protein assay on the Hitachi 912 chemistry analyzer, *Clin Chem* 50:A68(B-109), 2004.
5. Schiodt FV, Ott P, Bondesen S, et al: Reduced serum Gc-globulin concentrations in patients with fulminant hepatic failure: association with multiple organ failure, *Crit Care Med* 25:1366-1370, 1997.
6. White P, Cooke, N: The multifunctional properties and characteristics of vitamin D-binding protein, *Trends Endocrinol Metab* 11:320-327, 2000.
7. Gomme PT, Bertolini J: Therapeutic potential of vitamin D-binding protein, *Trends Biotechnol* 22:340-345, 2004.

TEST NAME AND METHOD	SPECIMEN REQUIREMENTS	REFERENCE INTERVAL, CONVENTIONAL [INTERNATIONAL RECOMMENDED UNITS]			CHEMICAL INTERFERENCES AND IN VIVO EFFECTS
Vitamin D, 25-Hydroxy [Calciferol, 25-Hydroxy; 25(OH) Calciferol][1-5] *HPLC,*[6,7] *CPB,*[6,8] *RIA*[6,9]	Serum or plasma (heparin); store frozen. Stable at room temperature for 72 hr or indefinitely at −20° C.	14-60 ng/mL	× 2.496	[35-150 nmol/L]	↑ V Etidronate disodium (oral) ↓ V Aluminum hydroxide, anticonvulsants (e.g., carbamazepine, phenobarbital, phenytoin, primidone), cholestyramine, colestipol, etidronate disodium (IV), glucocorticoids, isoniazid, mineral oil, and rifampin

DIAGNOSTIC INFORMATION	REMARKS

↑ Estrogen excess (including oral contraceptives); levels double during the third trimester of pregnancy

↓ Severe hepatocellular disease, probably secondary to turnover related to actin binding, hepatic encephalopathy[5]

Vitamin D binding protein (VDBP), also known as Gc-globulin, is produced in the liver, has significant homology with albumin and α-fetoprotein, and functions in the binding and transport of vitamin D and its hydroxylated derivatives in plasma. Other VDBP functions are thought to include the transport of fatty acids and endotoxins, control of bone development, and the scavenging of actin from the circulation.[6,7] VDBP may also play a role in facilitating chemotaxis of neutrophils and monocytes in inflammation. VDBP concentrations in pregnant females are higher than in males or nonpregnant females.

VDBP is not routinely utilized for clinical assessment of patients, but its multiple functions suggest it may be useful in a number of settings. Further understanding of the activity and clinical utility of VDBP will require accurate and precise methods for measurement, yet few commercially available assays exist.

MW. 50,800.

↑ Vitamin D intoxication, excessive exposure to sunlight

↓ Malabsorption, dietary osteomalacia, steatorrhea, biliary and portal cirrhosis, anticonvulsant osteomalacia, some cases of renal osteodystrophy, osteitis fibrosa cystica, thyrotoxicosis, pancreatic insufficiency, celiac disease, inflammatory bowel disease, bowel resection, rickets, and Alzheimer's disease[11]

Hypoparathyroidism: <3 ng/mL [<7.5 nmol/L]; primary hyperparathyroidism: 2.5-11.0 ng/mL [6.2-27.5 nmol/L]; chronic renal failure: 0.5-1.5 ng/mL [1.2-3.7 nmol/L]

25(OH)D [25(OH) calciferol], the major circulating form of vitamin D, has only modest biological activity. Its measurement is, however, the best indicator of vitamin D status. 25(OH)D represents the main body reservoir and transport form of vitamin D, being stored in adipose tissue and tightly bound by a transport protein while in circulation. A fraction of circulating 25(OH)D is converted to its active metabolites 1,25-dihydroxy vitamin D_2 and D_3 (1,25(OH)D), mainly by the kidneys. This process is regulated by parathyroid hormone (PTH), which increases 1,25(OH)D synthesis at the expense of the alternative, biologically inactive hydroxylation product 24,25(OH)D.

TEST NAME AND METHOD	SPECIMEN REQUIREMENTS	REFERENCE INTERVAL, CONVENTIONAL [INTERNATIONAL RECOMMENDED UNITS]		CHEMICAL INTERFERENCES AND IN VIVO EFFECTS
Vitamin D, 25-Hydroxy—CONT				
Liquid chromatography tandem mass spectrometry (LC-MS/MS)[10]		<10 ng/mL (severe deficiency)	[<25 nmol/L]	
		10-24 ng/mL (mild-moderate deficiency)	[25-60 nmol/L]	
		25-80 ng/mL (optimal level)	[61-200 nmol/L]	
		>80 ng/mL (toxicity possible)	[>200 nmol/L]	

1. Zerwekh JE: The measurement of vitamin D: analytical aspects, *Ann Clin Biochem* 41:272-281, 2004.

2. Holick MF: The use and interpretation of assays for vitamin D and its metabolites, *J Nutr* 120(suppl 11):1464-1469, 1990.

3. Carter GD, Carter CR, Gunter E, et al: Measurement of vitamin D metabolites: an international perspective on methodology and clinical interpretation, *J Steroid Biochem Mol Biol* 89-90:467-471, 2004.

4. Endres DB, Rude RK: Vitamin D and its metabolites. In Burtis CA, Ashwood ER, editors: *Tietz textbook of clinical chemistry,* ed 3, Philadelphia, 1999, WB Saunders, pp. 1417-1423.

5. Bringhurst FR, Demay MB, Kronenberg HM: Vitamin D (calciferols): metabolism of vitamin D. In Wilson JD, Foster DW, Kronenberg HM, et al, editors: *Williams textbook of endocrinology,* ed 9, Philadelphia, 1998, WB Saunders, pp. 1166-1169.

6. Glendenning P, Noble JM, Taranto M, et al: Issues of methodology, standardization and metabolite recognition for 25-hydroxyvitamin D when comparing the DiaSorin radioimmunoassay and the Nichols Advantage automated chemiluminescence protein-binding assay in hip fracture cases, *Ann Clin Biochem* 40:546-551, 2003.

DIAGNOSTIC INFORMATION	REMARKS

Deficiency manifests as rickets in children and as osteomalacia in adults. Both are characterized by decreased plasma calcium and phosphorus and increased alkaline phosphatase; deficiency of 25(OH) calciferol is similar in presentation to hyperparathyroidism, which may develop secondarily along with decreased citrate levels. Biochemical workup of suspected cases of rickets and osteomalacia should include measurement of serum calcium, phosphorus, PTH, and 25-OH-VitD. When testing is not completely consistent with the suspected diagnosis, particularly if serum 25-OH-VitD levels are >10 ng/mL. Consideration should be given to an alternative cause for impaired mineralization. Possible differential diagnosis includes partly treated vitamin D deficiency, extremely poor calcium intake, vitamin D–resistant rickets, renal failure, renal tubular mineral loss with or without renal tubular acidosis, hypophosphatemic disorders (e.g., X-linked or autosomal dominant hypophosphatemic rickets), congenital hypoparathyroidism, activating calcium sensing receptor mutations, and osteopetrosis. Measurement of serum urea, creatinine, magnesium, and 1,25-OH-VitD is recommended as additional workup for these patients.[10]

Vitamin D toxicity (25(OH)D >150 ng/mL [>375 nmol/L]) is more common in infants and children than adults. Doses up to 2370 U/day have no detrimental effect on growth, but 4000 U/day is associated with mild idiopathic hypercalcemia. Large doses (50,000-100,000 U/day) can cause hypercalcemia, hyperphosphatemia, hypercalciuria, increased citrate levels, soft-tissue calcification, vomiting, constipation, anorexia, nausea, and growth and mental retardation. Toxicity can be treated with calcitonin and glucocorticoids. Hypoparathyroid patients receiving physiological doses of vitamin D can have 25(OH)D levels as high as 1250 ng/mL [3120 nmol/L].[12] 25(OH)D is the drug of choice for treating cholestatic liver disease and osteomalacia. See also *Vitamin D, 1,25-Dihydroxy.*

Population reference intervals for 25(OH)D vary widely depending on ethnic background, age, geographic location of the studied populations, and the sampling season.[10]

For routine clinical purposes, 25(OH)D assays should measure 25(OH)D$_2$ and 25(OH)D$_3$. Competitive binding assays measure both D$_2$ and D$_3$. Measurement of 25(OH)D by RIA is now possible because of the availability of antisera that cross-reacts with D$_2$ and D$_3$ on an equimolar basis. HPLC methods allow separate measurement of D$_2$ and D$_3$, but independent determination is complicated and does not appear to be clinically useful.

An Lc-MS/MS method has been developed that measures both 25(OH)D$_2$ and 25(OH)D$_3$. Reference intervals have been established.[10]

7. Mata-Granados JM, Luque De Castro MD, Quesada JM: Fully automated method for the determination of 24,25(OH)2 and 25(OH) D3 hydroxyvitamins, and vitamins A and E in human serum by HPLC, *J Pharm Biomed Anal* 35:575-582, 2004.

8. Wei S, Tanaka H, Kubo T, et al: A multiple assay for vitamin D metabolites without high-performance liquid chromatography, *Anal Biochem* 222:359-365, 1994.

9. Bouillon R: Radiochemical assays for vitamin D metabolites: technical possibilities and clinical applications, *J Steroid Biochem* 19:921-927, 1983.

10. Mayo Medical Laboratories: *Test catalog,* Rochester, MN, 2005, Mayo Medical Laboratories.

11. Sato Y, Asoh T, Oizumi K: High prevalence of vitamin D deficiency and reduced bone mass in elderly women with Alzheimer's disease, *Bone* 23:555-557, 1998.

12. Gray TK, McAdoo T: Radioimmunoassay for 1,25-dihydroxycholecalciferol, *Clin Chem* 29:196-200, 1993.

TEST NAME AND METHOD	SPECIMEN REQUIREMENTS	REFERENCE INTERVAL, CONVENTIONAL [INTERNATIONAL RECOMMENDED UNITS]		CHEMICAL INTERFERENCES AND IN VIVO EFFECTS
Vitamin E (α-Tocopherol, α-T) *HPLC*[1-3]	Serum or plasma (heparin), fasting; avoid vitamin supplementation for 24 hr before draw; protect from light. Avoid lipemia. Stable at 4° C for 4 wk and at −20 or −70° C for 1 yr.	*mg/L* Premature neonate: 2.5-3.7 1-12 yr: 3.0-9.0 13-19 yr: 6.0-10.0 Adult: 5.5-18.0 Values that indicate need for supplementation[6]: Premature: <2 mg/L Neonate: <2 mg/L Child (3 mo): <3 mg/L Child (2 yr): <4 mg/L Adult: <4 mg/L Values that indicate significant excess: Adult: >40 mg/L	× 2.322 *μmol/L* [6-9] [7-21] [14-23] [12-42]	↓ V Anticonvulsants (e.g., carbamazepine, phenobarbital, phenytoin), cholestyramine, ethanol, and mineral oil ↑ Lipemia Exogenous tocopheryl acetate taken as a supplement will interfere with HPLC assays that use this vitamin as an internal standard.
HPLC[4,5]	Platelets, fasting; isolate from EDTA blood, wash with isotonic saline and count.[5]	*mcg/10⁹ cells* Adult M: 10.35 ± 0.01 (SE)	*nmol/10⁹ cells* × 2.322 [0.82 ± 0.03]	

DIAGNOSTIC INFORMATION	REMARKS

↑ Hyperlipidemia (obstructive liver disease); α-T levels can be normal or elevated, despite deficient tissue levels.

↓ Malabsorptive states (steatorrhea, biliary atresia, cirrhosis, cystic fibrosis, chronic pancreatitis, pancreatic carcinoma, gluten enteropathy, regional enteritis, and chronic cholestasis, intestinal lymphangiectasia), premature infants (hemolytic anemia, encephalomalacia, retrolental fibroplasia and bronchopulmonary dysplasia), and abetalipoproteinemia

Deficiency may be associated with platelet hyperaggregation, ceroid deposition in smooth muscle, decreased erythrocyte survival, and increased susceptibility to hemolysis. Neurological degeneration can occur. When plasma vitamin E levels are low, an assessment of total lipids should be made. Normal ratios of α-tocopherol to total lipid are >0.6 mg α-T/g total lipid in children and >0.8 mg α-T/g total lipid in adults.

Vitamin E contributes to the normal maintenance of biomembranes, the vascular system, and the nervous systems and provides antioxidant protection for vitamin A. The level of vitamin E in the plasma or serum after a 12-14-hr fast reflects the individual's reserve status.[6]

Deficiency of vitamin E in children leads to reversible motor and sensory neuropathies; this problem has been suspected in adults also. Premature infants who require an oxygen-enriched atmosphere are at increased risk for bronchopulmonary dysplasia and retrolental fibroplasia; supplementation with vitamin E has been shown to lessen the severity of and may even prevent those problems.[6]

Vitamin E deficiency caused by inadequate dietary intake is not known to occur. Colorimetric and fluorometric assays measure total plasma tocopherols rather than α-tocopherol, which usually constitutes ~90% of the total vitamin E and is the most active form biologically. Appreciable amounts of γ-tocopherol can be present. Serum α-T levels correlate directly with total lipids and β-lipoprotein levels. Very low blood levels of vitamin E may be associated with abetalipoproteinemia, presumably as a result of a lack of the ability to form very low-density lipoproteins and chylomicrons in the intestinal absorptive cells of affected persons.

Vitamin E deficiency caused by malabsorption can generally be treated with water-miscible α-tocopheryl acetate preparations, whereas patients with biliary atresia and abetalipoproteinemia may require parenteral (IM) supplementation. Megadoses of vitamin E (100-800 mg/day) may significantly impair the absorption of vitamins D and K. Therefore beginning vitamin E supplementation in patients who are receiving oral anticoagulation therapy can result in overanticoagulation and increased bleeding risk. Such levels of supplementation have not been documented to have any health benefits except perhaps to alleviate intermittent claudication. Combined results from trials suggest that vitamin E supplementation does not beneficially or adversely affect cardiovascular outcomes.[7] Vitamin E toxicity has not been established clearly. Chronically excessive ingestion has been implicated as a cause of thrombophlebitis; however, the implied relationship lacks verification.

Platelet tocopherol is suggested to be a better measure of vitamin E nutritional status than plasma tocopherol because it is more sensitive to vitamin E intake and is not dependent on circulating lipid levels.[5]

TEST NAME AND METHOD	SPECIMEN REQUIREMENTS	REFERENCE INTERVAL, CONVENTIONAL [INTERNATIONAL RECOMMENDED UNITS]	CHEMICAL INTERFERENCES AND IN VIVO EFFECTS

Vitamin E—CONT

1. Taibi G, Nicotra CM: Development and validation of a fast and sensitive chromatographic assay for all-trans-retinol and to-copherols in human serum and plasma using liquid-liquid extraction, *J Chromatogr B Analyt Technol Biomed Life Sci* 780:261-267, 2002.

2. Gueguen S, Herbeth B, Siest G, et al: An isocratic liquid chromatographic method with diode-array detection for the simultaneous determination of alpha-tocopherol, retinol, and five carotenoids in human serum, *J Chromatogr Sci* 40:69-76, 2002.

3. Weinmann AR, Oliveira MS, Jorge SM, et al: Simultaneous high-performance liquid chromatographic determination of retinol by fluorometry and of tocopherol by ultraviolet absorbance in the serum of newborns, *J Chromatogr B Biomed Sci Appl* 729:231-236, 1999.

TEST NAME AND METHOD	SPECIMEN REQUIREMENTS	REFERENCE INTERVAL, CONVENTIONAL [INTERNATIONAL RECOMMENDED UNITS]	CHEMICAL INTERFERENCES AND IN VIVO EFFECTS
Vitamin K (Phylloquinone) *HPLC*[1,2]	Serum or plasma, fasting. Stable at $-20°$ C for 2 mo. Avoid freeze/thaw cycles and exposure to ultraviolet light.	0.10-2.20 ng/mL × 2.22 [0.22-4.88 nmol/L][3]	↓ V Antibiotics, anticoagulants, cholestyramine, and mineral oil See *Prothrombin Time.*

1. Wakabayashi H, Onodera K, Yamato S, et al: Simultaneous determination of vitamin K analogs in human serum by sensitive and selective high performance liquid chromatography with electrochemical detection, *Nutrition* 19:661-665, 2003.

2. Cham BE, Roeser HP, Kamst TW: Simultaneous liquid-chromatographic determination of vitamin K1 and vitamin E in serum, *Clin Chem* 35:2285-2289, 1989.

3. ARUP: *Reference manual,* Salt Lake City, UT, 2004, ARUP.

4. Kowdley KV, Emond MJ, Sadowski JA, et al: Plasma vitamin K1 level is decreased in primary biliary cirrhosis, *Am J Gastroenterol* 92:2059-2061, 1997.

5. Phillips JR, Angulo P, Petterson T, et al: Fat-soluble vitamin levels in patients with primary biliary cirrhosis, *Am J Gastroenterol* 96:2745-2750, 2001.

6. McCormick DB, Greene HL: Vitamins. In Burtis CA, Ashwood AR, editors: *Tietz textbook of clinical chemistry,* Philadelphia, 1999, WB Saunders, pp. 999-1028.

DIAGNOSTIC INFORMATION	REMARKS

4. Leray C, Andriamampandry M, Gutbier G, et al: Quantitative analysis of vitamin E, cholesterol and phospholipid fatty acids in a single aliquot of human platelets and cultured endothelial cells, *J Chromatogr B Biomed Sci Appl* 696:33-42, 1997.

5. Vatassery GT, Smith WE: Determination of alpha-tocopherolquinone (vitamin E quinone) in human serum, platelets, and red cell membrane samples, *Anal Biochem* 167:411-417, 1987.

6. Mayo Medical Laboratories: *Interpretative handbook,* Rochester, MN, 2005, Mayo Medical Laboratories.

7. Shekelle PG, Morton SC, Jungvig LK, et al: Effect of supplemental vitamin E for the prevention and treatment of cardiovascular disease, *J Gen Intern Med* 19:380-389, 2004.

↓ Primary biliary cirrhosis,[4,5] hemorrhagic disease of the newborn, infants with diarrhea (particularly those who are breast-fed), hypoprothrombinemia, GI disease, pancreatic disease, cystic fibrosis, chronic fat malabsorption, celiac disease, obstructive jaundice, and nutritional deficiency

Assessment of vitamin K status is readily achieved by the prothrombin time test. Vitamin K is an essential cofactor for the clotting factors II, VII, IX, X, protein C, and proteins. Thus a decrease in serum vitamin K results in a prolonged prothrombin clotting time. Reported signs of vitamin K deficiency include nosebleeds, bleeding peptic ulcers, urinary tract bleeding, cerebral hemorrhage, and ecchymoses resulting from minor bruising. Dietary deficiency in adults is rare, found typically in cases with chronic fat malabsorption, or during long-term administration of antibiotics or anticoagulants treatments.[6]

Large doses of vitamin K may result in hyperbilirubinemia and kernicterus in premature infants and G6PD-deficient newborns. Synthetic vitamin K (menadione) is more toxic than phylloquinone or menaquinone.

Plasma levels correlate with concentrations of triglyceride and α-tocopherol.

See *Prothrombin Time.*

TEST NAME AND METHOD	SPECIMEN REQUIREMENTS	REFERENCE INTERVAL, CONVENTIONAL [INTERNATIONAL RECOMMENDED UNITS]	CHEMICAL INTERFERENCES AND IN VIVO EFFECTS
von Willebrand Factor (vWF)[1,2] *Ristocetin Cofactor Functional qualitative assay based on ristocetin agglutination of normal platelets* *Antigen Enzyme-linked immunosorbent assay (ELISA)*	Plasma (blue top-citrate). Stable for 4 hr at room temperature. Can store frozen.	Vary according to blood type: blood type O 50-150 U/dL; blood type non-O 90-200 U/dL	See *Platelet Aggregation* and *Remarks.*

1. Marlar RA, Adcock DM, Arkin CF, et al: *Assays of von Willebrand antigen and ristocetin cofactor activity, approved guideline, NCCLS H51-A vol. 22 no. 20.*
2. Budde U, Drewke E, Mainusch K, et al: Laboratory diagnosis of congenital von Willebrand disease, *Semin Thromb Hemost* 28:173-189, 2002.

TEST NAME AND METHOD	SPECIMEN REQUIREMENTS	REFERENCE INTERVAL, CONVENTIONAL [INTERNATIONAL RECOMMENDED UNITS]	CHEMICAL INTERFERENCES AND IN VIVO EFFECTS
Water Deprivation Antidiuretic Hormone Stimulation Test[1-4]	Serum, at 6:00 AM for osmolality measurement. Collect urine hourly for specific gravity and osmolality. Order total fluid restriction from 6:00 AM; patient's bladder should be emptied, and patient should be weighed. When urine osmolality levels off in two consecutive samples (<30 mOsm/kg change), measure serum osmolality and ADH. Weigh patient, and administer 5 units	After fluid restriction, Urine flow: <0.5 mL/min Urine osmolality: Increase to >400 mOsm/kg* Serum osmolality: <300 mOsm/kg* Plasma ADH: Appropriate for serum osmolality (See reference interval under *Antidiuretic Hormone.*) Weight loss: ≤3% After ADH, Urine osmolality: No further increase *In the SI system, 1 mOsm/kg = 1 mmol osmotically active particles/kg.	See *Antidiuretic Hormone.*

DIAGNOSTIC INFORMATION	REMARKS

↓ All cases of hereditary or acquired von Willebrand's disease

However, in the rare type II von Willebrand's disease, the antigen may be normal, although the function is impaired.

For types of von Willebrand's disease, see Table I-24.

The von Willebrand factor is a multimeric plasma protein with two important functions in hemostasis: (1) promoting platelet adhesion at the site of injury; and (2) transporting and stabilizing factor VIII in plasma.

von Willebrand disease (vWD) is caused by hereditary quantitative or qualitative defects of the vWF. The diagnosis of vWD is challenging because of the many variables that may affect the results. Repeat testing is recommended for confirmation. Acquired vWD can occur but is rare.

Screening tests for vWD (bleeding time, platelet count, PT, and PTT) are typically followed by the diagnostic tests, R:CoF (functional assay) and vWFAg (antigenic assay). Further tests to distinguish among the subtypes of vWD include a factor VIII assay, a factor VIII binding capacity, platelet aggregation studies (low-dose ristocetin), and multimer analysis (crossed immunoelectrophoresis).

Newer tests that may be used in association with the established tests include the collagen-binding assay (ELISA) and the platelet function analyzer (PFA-100).

Decreased renal tubular function: Specific gravity is <1.020.

In severe renal tubular impairment: Specific gravity approaches 1.010.[5]

Impairment of renal concentration ability:
  Minimal: 600-800 mOsm/kg
  Moderate: 400-600 mOsm/kg
  Severe: <400 mOsm/kg
  These values are lower in hospitalized patients.

The ability to concentrate urine decreases with age.

In central diabetes insipidus (also called hypothalamic or neurogenic diabetes insipidus): There is no significant increase in urine osmolality or urine specific gravity after water deprivation but a >10% increase in urine osmolality after ADH administration; serum osmolality and serum sodium are seen to

Fluid restriction starts at midnight if psychogenic water drinking is suspected or if polyuria is absent. Observe high-risk patients for >3% weight loss and cardiovascular problems. This test is unreliable in the presence of any severe water and electrolyte imbalance, low-protein or low-salt diet, chronic liver disease, or pregnancy. Fluid deprivation is dangerous in renal failure and obligatory polyuria, poorly compensated renal damage, or extrarenal uremia.

In patients with associated adrenal insufficiency, corticoid administration may unmask subclinical diabetes insipidus by altering both the GFR and the osmotic threshold. The effect of glucocorticoids on the test results for normal subjects is not known.

Some investigators prefer to test renal concentration ability using vasopressin without fluid restriction.[6,7]

TEST NAME AND METHOD	SPECIMEN REQUIREMENTS	REFERENCE INTERVAL, CONVENTIONAL [INTERNATIONAL RECOMMENDED UNITS]	CHEMICAL INTERFERENCES AND IN VIVO EFFECTS

Water Deprivation Antidiuretic Hormone Stimulation Test—CONT

| | aqueous vasopressin subcutaneously. After 1 hr determine final urine osmolality. | | |

1. Alsever RN, Gotlin RW: *Handbook of endocrine tests in adults and children,* ed 2, Chicago, 1978, Year Book Medical Publishers Inc.
2. Abboud CF, Laws ER Jr: Clinical endocrinological approach to hypothalamic-pituitary disease, *J Neurosurg* 51:271-291, 1979.
3. Reeves W, Andreoli T: The posterior pituitary and water metabolism. In Wilson JD, Foster DW, editors: *Williams textbook of endocrinology,* ed 8, Philadelphia, 1992, WB Saunders.
4. Whitley RJ, Meikle AW, Watts NB: Endocrinology. In Burtis CA, Ashwood ER, editors: *Tietz textbook of clinical chemistry,* ed 2, Philadelphia, 1994, WB Saunders.
5. Wallach J, editor: *Interpretation of diagnostic tests,* ed 5, Boston, 1992, Little, Brown and Co.
6. Tryding N, Berg B, Ekman S, et al: DDAVP test for renal concentration capacity, *Scand J Urol Nephrol* 22:141-145, 1988.
7. Tryding N, Sterner G, Berg B, et al: Subcutaneous and intranasal administration of 1-deamino-8-d-argine vasopressin in the assessment of renal concentration capacity, *Nephron* 45:27-30, 1987.

TEST NAME AND METHOD	SPECIMEN REQUIREMENTS	REFERENCE INTERVAL, CONVENTIONAL [INTERNATIONAL RECOMMENDED UNITS]	CHEMICAL INTERFERENCES AND IN VIVO EFFECTS
Water Loading Antidiuretic Hormone Suppression Test[1,2]	After overnight fast patient should empty bladder. Tap water, 20 mL/kg, should be administered orally within 15-30 min. Keep patient in recumbent position. Collect urine specimens at hourly intervals for 4 hr after water ingestion for measurements of urine volume, specific gravity, and osmolality. Collect hourly speci-	Excretion of >90% [>0.9, volume fraction] of water load within 4 hr Urine osmolality decreases to <100 mOsm/kg*, and urine specific gravity decreases to 1.003. The maximum ratio of urine flow will exceed 2-3 mL/min. Serum osmolality should decrease by ≥5 mOsm/kg.* Plasma ADH should be appropriate for the serum osmolality. (See reference interval under *Antidiuretic Hormone.*)	The following drugs may produce a urine-diluting effect and will exaggerate test results: demeclocycline, lithium carbonate, and methoxyflurane. The following drugs may produce a urine-concentrating effect and thus diminish the magnitude of the test results: chlorpropamide, clofibrate, cyclophosphamide, diuretics, and diazoxide.

increase after fluid restriction, but plasma ADH values will be inappropriately low for the degree of hyperosmolality.

In nephrogenic diabetes insipidus: There is no significant increase in urine osmolality after water deprivation or after ADH administration.

In psychogenic polydipsia: Normal urine osmolality is usually seen after water deprivation. If the ratio of urine to plasma osmolality is <1.5 at the end of the test, primary polydipsia is unlikely. Measuring ADH in response to hypertonic saline may be needed if diagnosis is unclear.

Muscular exercise and starvation decrease urine osmolality. See *Osmolality.*

In decreased renal function, <80% of fluid intake is excreted and specific gravity may not decrease to <1.010; inadequate response is observed in adrenocortical insufficiency. Impaired diuresis is also observed in malabsorption syndrome, edema, ascites, obesity, hypothyroidism, dehydration, congestive heart failure, cirrhosis, and chlorpropamide therapy.

Syndromes with excessive ADH secretion (SIADH) give inadequate response: <90% of water load is excreted within 4 hr, and urine osmolality remains >100 mOsm/kg [>100 mmol osmotically active particles/kg]. Plasma ADH measured at 90 or 120 min after water loading confirms the diagnosis of SIADH.

Muscular exercise or starvation decreases urine-concentrating ability.

If diuresis does not occur in patients with adrenal insufficiency, diuretic function can be restored by steroid administration (50 mg cortisone acetate orally).

Risks: In patients with hypoosmolality or impaired ability to excrete a water load, seizures and fatal hyponatremia can occur.

TEST NAME AND METHOD	SPECIMEN REQUIREMENTS	REFERENCE INTERVAL, CONVENTIONAL [INTERNATIONAL RECOMMENDED UNITS]	CHEMICAL INTERFERENCES AND IN VIVO EFFECTS

Water Loading Antidiuretic Hormone Suppression Test—CONT

| | mens for serum osmo-lality and plasma ADH determinations. | *In the SI system, 1 mOsm/kg = 1 mmol osmotically active particles/kg. | |

1. Miller RE, Ngai B: *Manual of endocrine diagnostic tests,* ed 4, Lexington, KY, 1991, Department of Medicine, University of Kentucky.
2. Whitley RJ, Meikle AW, Watts NB: Endocrinology. In Burtis CA, Ashwood ER, editors: *Tietz textbook of clinical chemistry,* ed 2, Philadelphia, 1994, WB Saunders.

Test Name	Specimen	Reference			Chemical
Xylene	Blood (fluoride/oxalate)	Negative			None found.
			mg/L	*µmol/L*	
(Dimethylbenzene; methyltoluene; CAS 1330-20-7)		Occupational exposure:	<1.1 × 9.42	[<10.4]	
		Toxic concentration:	>3	[>28.3]	
GC,[1] *GC-MS,*[2] *LC*[3,4]	Urine	Negative			

1. Morin M, Chambon P, Chambon R, et al: Measurement of exposure to xylene by separate determination of m- and p-methylhippuric acid in urine, *J Chromatogr* 210:346-349, 1981.
2. Bellanca JA, Davis PL, Donnelly B, et al: Detection and quantitation of multiple volatile compounds in tissues by GC and GC/MS, *J Anal Toxicol* 6:238-240, 1982.
3. Ogata M, Tomokuni K, Takatsuta Y: Urinary excretion of hippuric acid and m- or p-methylhippuric acid in urine of persons exposed to vapours of toluene and m- or p-xylene as a test of exposure, *Br J Ind Med* 27:43-50, 1970.
4. Ogata M, Yamazaki Y, Sugihara R: Quantitation of urinary o-xylene metabolites of rats and human beings by high-performance liquid chromatography, *Int Arch Occup Environ Health* 46:127-139, 1980.
5. Available at: http://www.atsdr.cdc.gov/MHMI/mmg71.html. Last accessed 2/1/06.
6. Baselt RC, Cravey RH: *Disposition of toxic drugs and chemicals in man,* ed 3, Chicago, 1989, Year Book Medical Publishers, Inc., pp. 855-856.

Test Name	Specimen	Reference			Chemical
Xylose Absorption Test (D-Xylose Absorption Test)[1-5]	Whole blood (NaF/oxalate) Adults: before dose and 2 hr	*mg/dL* Child, 1 hr: Adult, 2 hr,	>30 × 0.0666	*mmol/L* [>2.0]	B ↓ V Aminosalicylic acid, arsenicals, colchicine, digitalis,
	Children: before dose and 1 hr	25-g dose:	>25	[>1.7]	ethionamide, gold, indomethacin, isocarboxazid, kanamycin, MAO
Dose, adult: D-Xylose, 25 g in 250 mL of H$_2$O,					inhibitors, metformin,

DIAGNOSTIC INFORMATION	REMARKS

Symptoms of acute exposure are typical of hydrocarbons and include headache, lightheadedness, dizziness, confusion, nausea, impaired gait, and blurred vision; excessive exposure can lead to tremors, rapid respiration, paralysis, loss of consciousness, coma, and death.

Chronic exposure is associated with the development of permanent neuropsychiatric abnormalities, sometimes diagnosed as "chronic toxic encephalopathy."[1]

Exposures are most often occupational or the result of solvent inhalation abuse.

Xylene exists as three isomers—ortho, meta, and para—and all three isomers are used as solvents, often as a mixture. Xylenes are rapidly metabolized to the corresponding o-, m-, or p-toluic acid (72%); 5% is excreted unchanged in breath and 0.01% in urine.[2]

Kinetic values
$t_{1/2}$: 20-30 hr

B ↓ Intestinal malabsorption (but normal in malabsorption caused by pancreatic insufficiency), bacterial overgrowth in the small intestine, vomiting, ascites, delayed gastric emptying, and Whipple's disease

This test is used in the diagnosis of malabsorption states and evaluates carbohydrate absorption by the mucosa of the proximal small intestine. Validity of the test is increased if blood and urine measurements are performed simultaneously to rule out renal retention. In patients with renal deficiency, rely on the serum test only; in functionally anephric patients, the test is unreliable.[6] Twenty-four hr before test, subjects should not eat

TEST NAME AND METHOD	SPECIMEN REQUIREMENTS	REFERENCE INTERVAL, CONVENTIONAL [INTERNATIONAL RECOMMENDED UNITS]	CHEMICAL INTERFERENCES AND IN VIVO EFFECTS

Xylose Absorption Test—CONT

orally, patient fasting ≥ 8 hr

Child: D-Xylose, 0.5 g/kg as

			nalidixic acid, neomycin, opium alkaloids, phenelzine, phenformin, and atropine
5% solution in H_2O, orally, maximum 25 g, patient fasting ≥ 4 hr	Urine, 5 hr. Collect in dark bottle; refrigerate.	Child: 16-40% of ingested dose [× 0.01 = 0.16-0.40, fraction of ingested dose]	U ↑ V Ethanol

$$\begin{array}{llll} & & g/5\ hr^1 & mmol/5\ hr \\ \text{Adult,} & & & \\ \text{25-g dose:} & >4.0 & & [>26.64] \\ \text{>65 yr:} & >3.5 & & [>23.31] \end{array}$$

U ↓ V Aspirin; see also blood interferences, above.

1. Burtis CA, Ashwood ER, editors: *Tietz textbook of clinical chemistry,* ed 2, Philadelphia, 1994, WB Saunders.
2. Henry RJ, Cannon DC, Winkelman JW, editors: *Clinical chemistry: principles and technics,* ed 2, Hagerstown, MD, 1974, Harper and Row.
3. Tietz NW, editor: *Fundamentals of clinical chemistry,* ed 3, Philadelphia, 1987, WB Saunders.
4. Sonnenwirth AC, Jarrett L, editors: *Gradwohl's clinical laboratory methods and diagnosis,* ed 8, St. Louis, 1980, CV Mosby.
5. Craig RM, Ehrenpreis ED: D-Xylose testing, *J Clin Gastroenterol* 29:143-150, 1999.
6. Craig RM, Atkinson AJ Jr: D-Xylose testing: a review, *Gastroenterology* 95:223-231, 1988.

^{14}C-D-Xylose Breath Test Dose: 10 μCi ^{14}C-D-xylose and 1 g unlabeled xylose in 250 mL of water, followed by another 250 mL of water.[1]	Breath. Fast 8 hr before dose and during 5 hr immediately after administration. Take breath specimen every 30 min. Express as percent ^{14}C-D-xylose, expired as ^{14}CO$_2$/mmol CO$_2$.	Expired breath ^{14}CO$_2$: $<44 \times 10^{-4}$ percent of dose/mmol CO$_2$ per hour at peak [$<44 \times 10^{-6}$, fraction of dose][2] Result is abnormal if the ^{14}CO$_2$ concentration at 30 min $>0.0013\%$ [13×10^{-6}, fraction of dose] of the administered dose per mmol CO$_2$.[3]	None found.

1. King CE, Toskes PP, Spivey JC, et al: Detection of small intestine bacterial overgrowth by means of a ^{14}C-D-xylose breath test, *Gastroenterology* 77:75-82, 1979.
2. Schneider A, Novis B, Chen V, et al: Value of the ^{14}C-D-xylose breath test in patients with intestinal bacterial overgrowth, *Digestion* 32:86-91, 1985.
3. Wright TL, Heyworth MF: Maldigestion and malabsorption. In Sleisenger MH, Fordtran JS, editors: *Gastrointestinal disease: pathophysiology, diagnosis, management,* ed 4, Philadelphia, 1989, WB Saunders.

DIAGNOSTIC INFORMATION	REMARKS

foods containing high levels of pentose (a sugar similar to D-xylose), including fruits, jams, jellies, and pastries.

U ↓ Intestinal malabsorption (but normal in malabsorption caused by pancreatic insufficiency), impaired renal function, hypothyroidism, ascites, bacterial overgrowth in the small intestine, vomiting, delayed gastric emptying, and Whipple's disease

Increased $^{14}CO_2$ levels appear within the first 60 min of the test in the breath of 85% of patients with increased small-intestinal bacterial overgrowth.[3]

False-positive results may be caused by rapid small intestinal transit time. Severe GI motor dysfunction may cause false-negative results at the usual timing.

In delayed gastric emptying, values may increase after 3 hr.

Xylose is catabolized by gram-negative aerobic bacteria.[3] It is absorbed predominantly in the proximal small bowel as contrasted to the predominant ileal absorption of bile salts, leading to virtually no "dumping" of xylose into the colon. Xylose is metabolized substantially less than other proximally absorbed substrates such as glucose. Comparison with the bile acid breath test in a series of patients with culture-proven overgrowth demonstrated no false-negative results with the ^{14}C-D-xylose breath test.[4] Regarded as more sensitive and specific compared with the bile acid breath test.[5]

4. King CE, Toskes PP, Guilarte TR, et al: Comparison of the one-gram α-[^{14}C] xylose breath test to the [^{14}C] bile acid breath test in patients with small-intestine bacterial growth, *Dig Dis Sci* 25:53-58, 1980.

5. Chang CS, Chan GH, Kao CH, et al: Increased accuracy of the carbon-14-D-xylose breath test in detecting small-intestinal bacterial overgrowth by correlation with the gastric emptying rate, *Eur J Nucl Med* 22:1118-1122, 1995.

TEST NAME AND METHOD	SPECIMEN REQUIREMENTS	REFERENCE INTERVAL, CONVENTIONAL [INTERNATIONAL RECOMMENDED UNITS]		CHEMICAL INTERFERENCES AND IN VIVO EFFECTS
Zinc (Zn)[1,2] *AAS*	Serum or plasma, fasting morning specimen. Use pretested, metal-free tubes. Avoid contact with rubber stopper. Separate from cells within 45 min.	70-120 mcg/dL × 0.153 Fasting AM values <70 mcg/dL [10.7 μmol/L] represent deficient Zn status.	[10.7-18.4 μmol/L]	S ↓ V Cisplatin, corticosteroids, estrogens, interferon, oral contraceptives, carbamazepine, valproic acid, phenytoin, and thiazides (long-term use) S ↑ V Chlorthalidone, penicillamine, and zurzuofin
	Erythrocytes.[1] See *Serum.*	10-16 mcg/mL × 15.3	[153-245 μmol/L]	
	Urine, 24 hr.[4,5] Collect in acid-washed, metal-free container. Acidify to pH 2.0 with HCl. Stable at room temperature.	180-850 mcg/L× 0.0153 [2.8-13.0 μmol/L] 150-1200 mcg/day × 0.0153 [2.3-18.4 μmol/day] Toxic concentration: >1200 mcg/day[>18.4 μmol/day]		U ↑ V Cisplatin, loop diuretics (e.g., ethacrynic acid) and furosemide given IV cause a brief increase in excretion; naproxen, sodium chloride (isotonic), and thiazide diuretics.
	Hair.[1] Cut specimens close to scalp in 2- to 5-cm lengths.	*mcg/g dry wt.* 124-320 × 0.0153	*μmol/g dry wt.* [1.9-4.9]	Hair ↑ C Some antidandruff shampoos
	Liver[1]	*mg/kg dry wt.* 32-70 × 15.3	*μmol/kg dry wt.* [490-1071]	
X-ray fluorescence spectrometry[3]	Bronchoalveolar lavage (BAL) fluid	*ng/10³ macrophages* 0.03-2.85 × 15.3	*fmol/macrophage* [0.46-43.60]	
ICP-MS	Serum.[6] Collect in pretested, metal-free container.	M: 75-291 mcg/dL × 0.153 [11.48-44.52 μmol/L] F: 65-256 mcg/dL [9.95-39.17 μmol/L]		
	Urine.[6] Collect in acid-washed, metal-free container.	150-1200 mcg/L [22.95-183.60 nmol/L]		

| DIAGNOSTIC INFORMATION | REMARKS |

S ↑ Primary osteosarcoma of bone, coronary heart disease, arteriosclerosis, and anemia

S ↓ Acrodermatitis enteropathica (Danbolt's disease), typhoid fever, pulmonary tuberculosis, metastatic carcinoma to liver, celiac sprue, and other GI diseases, thalassemia major, acute myocardial infarction, severe hepatocellular disease, acute infections, hypogonadal dwarfism, leukemias, lymphomas, PA, renal disease, and pregnancy; impaired smell, taste, and wound healing; various dermatological conditions, alopecia, and skin lesions; hypoalbuminemia, acute stress

Ercs ↓ Sickle cell anemia (SCA)

U ↑ Hyperparathyroidism, alcoholism, sickle cell anemia, hepatic cirrhosis, viral hepatitis, SCA, postsurgery, and TPN

U ↓ Hypogonadal dwarfism

Hair ↓ Diabetes [126 ± 49 mcg/g (SD); 1.9 ± 0.75 μmol/g]; celiac disease, protein malnutrition

Seventy-five to 88% of the total Zn in whole blood is in the erythrocytes. The serum concentration of Zn undergoes circadian variations that appear to peak around 9:00 AM and again around 6:00 PM.[7] Serum Zn levels decrease postprandially.

Protein precipitation methods with AAS give higher results for serum or plasma than do direct dilution techniques.

Elevated serum zinc may occur in patients undergoing hemodialysis against a dialysate containing a large amount of zinc. Exposure to the fumes of zinc salts can irritate the skin and the respiratory and GI tracts. Oral poisoning (uncommon) is caused by drinking from galvanized cans and produces fever and gastrointestinal distress. Zinc is important for wound healing, immune function, and fetal development. Zinc deficiency retards growth and sexual development and produces dermatitis, reduced taste acuity, anemia, and enlargement of the liver and spleen. Clinical signs of acute zinc deficiency will not usually be found until values decrease to <65 mcg/dL [10 μmol/L]. Skin rash, abdominal pain, diarrhea, and loss of appetite and of the senses of taste and smell are likely when levels remain <33 mcg/dL [5 μmol/L]. Human zinc deficiency is often associated with diets low in animal-derived protein but high in cereals (phytates) that bind zinc. Iatrogenic causes of zinc deficiency include treatment with anabolic or metal-chelating drugs (corticosteroids, penicillamine) and synthetic diet therapies (TPN).

Long-term zinc supplementation may induce Cu deficiency.

Reduced levels of zinc in hair have been shown to accompany body zinc deficiency, but hair zinc, because of exogenous contamination and other factors, is not a reliable measure. (Zinc is a component of some antidandruff shampoos.)

TEST NAME AND METHOD	SPECIMEN REQUIREMENTS	REFERENCE INTERVAL, CONVENTIONAL [INTERNATIONAL RECOMMENDED UNITS]		CHEMICAL INTERFERENCES AND IN VIVO EFFECTS

Zinc—CONT

1. Iyengar GV, Woittiez J: Trace elements in human clinical specimens: evaluation of literature data to identify tolerence values, *Clin Chem* 34:474-481, 1988.

2. Milne DB: Trace elements. In Burtis CA, Ashwood ER, editors: *Tietz textbook of clinical chemistry,* ed 2, Philadelphia, 1994, WB Saunders.

3. Maier EA, Rastegar F, Heimburger R, et al: Simultaneous determination of trace elements in lavage fluids front human bronchial alveoli by energy dispersive X-ray fluorescence. 1: Technique and determination of the normal reference interval, *Clin Chem* 31:551-555, 1985.

TEST NAME AND METHOD	SPECIMEN REQUIREMENTS	REFERENCE INTERVAL, CONVENTIONAL	[INTERNATIONAL RECOMMENDED UNITS]	CHEMICAL INTERFERENCES AND IN VIVO EFFECTS
Zinc α_2**-Glycoprotein** $(Zn-\alpha_2)^{1-3}$ *RID*	Serum.[1] Analyze fresh or store at 4° C for <72 hr. Stable frozen at −20° C for 6 mo or at −70° C indefinitely. Specimens without lipemia or hemolysis are preferred.	>1 yr: 2-15 mg/dL ($\bar{x}$: 5) Levels are lower at birth.	× 10	[0.02-0.15 g/L] [$\bar{x}$: 50] None found.

1. Ritzmann SE, Tucker ES III: *Protein analysis in disease—current concepts. Workshop manual,* Chicago, 1979, American Society of Clinical Pathologists, Commission for Continuing Education.

2. Poortmans JR, Schmid K: The level of Zn-alpha 2-glycoprotein in normal human body fluids and kidney extract, *J Lab Clin Med* 71:807-811, 1968.

3. Hale L, Price D, Sanchez L, et al: Zinc-α_2–glycoprotein is expressed by malignant prostatic epithelium and may serve as a potential serum marker for prostate cancer, *Clin Cancer Res* 7:846-853, 2001.

4. Lei G, Arany I, Selvanayagam P, et al: Detection and cloning of epidermal zinc-α_2–glycoprotein cDNA and expression in normal human skin and in tumors, *J Cell Biochem* 67:216-222, 1997.

5. Diez-Itza I, Sanchez L, Allende MT, et al: Zn-α_2–glycoprotein levels in breast cancer cytosols and correlation with clinical, histological and biochemical parameters, *Eur J Cancer* 29A:1256-1260, 1993.

6. Lei G, Arany I, Tyring S, et al: Zinc-α_2–glycoprotein has ribonuclease activity, *Arch Biochem Biophys* 355:160-164, 1998.

7. Todorov P, McDevitt T, Meyer D, et al: Purification and characterization of lipid-mobilizing factor, *Cancer Res* 58:2353-2358, 1998.

TEST NAME AND METHOD	SPECIMEN REQUIREMENTS	REFERENCE INTERVAL, CONVENTIONAL	[INTERNATIONAL RECOMMENDED UNITS]	CHEMICAL INTERFERENCES AND IN VIVO EFFECTS
Zinc Protoporphyrin (ZPP, Zn-PROTO, Zn-PP)$^{1-3}$ *Hematofluorimetric*^{2,4}	Whole blood (heparin or EDTA). Store at 4° C; avoid hemolysis.	17-77 mcg/dL 30-70 µmol ZPP/mol heme	× 0.0160	[0.27-1.23 µmol/L][2] ↑ C Elevated bilirubin, digitalis, hemolysis, and riboflavin. Interferences in plasma can be removed by washing erythrocytes.[9]

DIAGNOSTIC INFORMATION	REMARKS

4. Baselt RC: *Biological monitoring methods for industrial chemicals,* ed 2, Littleton, MA, 1988, PSG Publishing Co., Inc.
5. Schramel VP, Lill G, Hasse S: Mineral and trace elements in human urine, *J Clin Chem Clin Biochem* 23:293-301, 1985.
6. Associated Regional & University Pathologists, Inc. web site (www.aruplab.com): Available at: http://www.aruplab.com/testing/user_guide.jsp. Last accessed 9/2004.
7. Guillard O, Pirious A, Gomben J, et al: Diurnal variation of zinc, copper and magnesium in the serum of normal fasting adults, *Biomed* 31:193-194, 1979.

Studies indicate that Zn-α_2 may serve as a marker of differentiation in breast carcinomas, prostate carcinomas, and stratified epithelium.[3-5]

Zn-α_2 is a soluble protein that is found in many body fluids.[4] Its primary function is not yet completely known.[4] It has been found to have RNase activity and has substantial structural homology with major histocompatibility complex (MHC) class I antigens.[4,6] Evidence suggests that it may increase lipid catabolism in cancer-related cachexia.[7]

MW: 41,000.

↑ Fe deficiency, chronic lead poisoning, β-thalassemia,[10] sideroblastic anemia, anemia of chronic disease,[11] and the mild iron-deficient erythropoiesis seen with inflammation or accelerated erythropoiesis.

ZPP concentration by hematofluorometry was once widely used to screen for lead exposure in children; but ZPP is not reliable at Pb concentrations of <250 mcg/L [0.40 μmol/L] and should no longer be used for this application. However, it may be cost effective for screening of iron status.

TEST NAME AND METHOD	SPECIMEN REQUIREMENTS	REFERENCE INTERVAL, CONVENTIONAL [INTERNATIONAL RECOMMENDED UNITS]	CHEMICAL INTERFERENCES AND IN VIVO EFFECTS
Zinc Protoporphyrin—CONT			
HPLC[5-7]	Erythrocytes. Collect whole blood (heparin; avoid potassium oxalate). Ercs should be washed three times with cold saline, volume recorded, and shipped frozen.	10-38 mcg/dL packed cells[8] [0.16-0.61 μmol/L packed cells]	

1. Soldin OP, Pezzullo JC, Hanak B, et al: Changing trends in the epidemiology of pediatric lead exposure: interrelationship of blood lead and ZPP concentrations and a comparison to the US population, *Ther Drug Monit* 25:415-420, 2003.

2. Blumberg WE, Eisinger J, Lamola AA, et al: The hematofluorometer, *Clin Chem* 23:270-274, 1977.

3. Labbe RF, Vreman HJ, Stevenson DK: Zinc protoporphyrin: a metabolite with a mission, *Clin Chem* 45:2060-2072, 1999.

4. Louro MO, Tutor JC: Hematofluorometric determination of erythrocyte zinc protoporphyrin: oxygenation and derivatization of hemoglobin compared, *Clin Chem* 40:369-372, 1994.

5. Hart D, Piomelli S: Simultaneous quantitation of zinc protoporphyrin and free protoporphyrin in erythrocytes by acetone extraction, *Clin Chem* 27:220-222, 1981.

6. Ford RE, Ellefson RD: Quantitation of erythrocyte protoporphyrins and zinc protoporphyrin by high-pressure liquid chromatography, *Clin Chem* 30:972, 1984.

7. Bailey GG, Needham LL: Simultaneous quantification of erythrocyte zinc protoporphyrin and protoporphyrin IX by liquid chromatography, *Clin Chem* 32:2137-2142, 1986.

8. Mayo Medical Laboratories: *Test catalog,* Rochester, MN, 2005, Mayo Medical Laboratories.

9. Hastka J, Lasserre JJ, Schwarzbeck A, et al: Washing erythrocytes to remove interferents in measurements of zinc protoporphyrin by front-face hematofluorometry, *Clin Chem* 38:2184-2189, 1992.

10. Graham EA, Felgenhauer J, Detter JC, et al: Elevated zinc protoporphyrin associated with thallemia trait and hemoglobin E, *J Pediatr* 129:105-110, 1996.

11. Sherwood RA, Pippard MJ, Peters TJ: Iron homeostasis and the assessment of iron status, *Ann Clin Biochem* 35:693-708, 1998.

DIAGNOSTIC INFORMATION	REMARKS

TABLE II-1 SUMMARY CHART OF BLOOD COMPONENTS

COMPONENT/ PRODUCT	COMPOSITION	VOLUME	INDICATIONS
Whole blood	RBCs (Hct ~40%), plasma, WBCs, platelets	500 mL	Increase both red cell mass and plasma volume (WBCs and platelets not functional, plasma deficient in labile clotting factors V and VIII)
RBCs	RBCs (Hct ~75%), reduced plasma, WBCs, platelets	250 mL	Increase red cell mass in symptomatic anemia (WBCs and platelets not functional)
RBCs, adenine-saline added	RBCs (Hct ~60%), reduced plasma, WBCs, and platelets; 100 mL of additive solution	330 mL	Increase red cell mass in symptomatic anemia (WBCs and platelets not functional)
RBCs, WBCs reduced (prepared by filtration)	>85% original volume of RBCs, <5 x 106 WBCs, few platelets, minimal plasma	225 mL	Increase red cell mass, <5 x 10^6 WBCs to decrease the likelihood of febrile reactions, immunization to leukocytes (HLA antigens) or CMV transmission

COMPONENT/ PRODUCT	COMPOSITION	VOLUME	INDICATIONS
RBCs washed	RBCs (Hct ~75%), $<5 \times 10^8$ WBCs, no plasma	180 mL	Increase red cell mass, reduce risk of allergic reactions to plasma proteins
RBCs frozen; RBCs deglycerolized	RBCs (Hct ~75%), 5×10^8 WBCs, no platelets, no plasma	180 mL	Increase red cell mass, minimize febrile or allergic transfusion reactions, use for prolonged RBC blood storage
Granulocytes pheresis	Granulocytes ($>1.0 \times 10^{10}$ PMNs/unit), lymphocytes, platelets ($>2.0 \times 10^{11}$/unit), some RBCs	220 mL	Provide granulocytes for selected patients with sepsis and severe neutropenia (<500 PMNs/μL)
Platelets	Platelets (5.5×10^{10}/unit), RBCs, WBCs, plasma	50 mL	Bleeding caused by thrombocytopenia or thrombocytopathy

TABLE II-1 SUMMARY CHART OF BLOOD COMPONENTS—CONTINUED

COMPONENT/ PRODUCT	COMPOSITION	VOLUME	INDICATIONS
Platelets, pheresis	Platelets (>3 x 10^{11}/unit), <5 x 10^6 WBCs per final dose of pooled platelets	300 mL	Same as platelets, sometimes HLA matched
Platelets WBCs reduced	Platelets (as above), <5 x 10^6 WBCs per final dose of pooled platelets	300 mL	Same as platelets; <5 x 10^6 WBCs to decrease the likelihood of febrile reactions, alloimmunization to WBCs (HLA antigens), or CMV transmission
FFP; donor retested plasma; thawed plasma	FFP, donor retested plasma, all coagulation factors, thawed plasma has reduced factors V and VIII	220 mL	Treatment of some coagulation disorders

COMPONENT/ PRODUCT	COMPOSITION	VOLUME	INDICATIONS
Cryoprecipitated AHF	Fibrinogen, factors VIII and XIII, von Willebrand factor	15 mL	Deficiency of fibrinogen, factor XIII, second choice in treatment of hemophilia A, von Willebrand disease, topical fibrin sealant
Factor VIII (concentrates; recombinant human factor VIII)	Factor VIII, trace amount of other plasma proteins (products vary in purity)	Usually 10 mL	Hemophilia A (factor VIII deficiency), von Willebrand disease (off-label use for selected products only)
Factor IX (concentrates; recombinant human factor IX)	Factor IX, trace amount of other plasma proteins (products vary in purity)	Usually 10 mL	Hemophilia B (factor IX deficiency)

TABLE II-1 ## SUMMARY CHART OF BLOOD COMPONENTS—CONTINUED

COMPONENT/ PRODUCT	COMPOSITION	VOLUME	INDICATIONS
Albumin/PPF	Albumin, some α-, β-globulins	5% 25%	Volume expansion
Immune globulin	IgG antibodies, preparations for IV and/or IM use	Varies	Treatment of hypogammaglobulinemia or agammaglobulinemia, disease prophylaxis, autoimmune thrombocytopenia (IV only)
Rh immune globulin	IgG anti-D, preparations for IV and/or IM use	1 mL	Prevention of hemolytic disease of the newborn caused by D antigen, treatment of autoimmune thrombocytopenia

COMPONENT/ PRODUCT	COMPOSITION	VOLUME	INDICATIONS
Antithrombin	Antithrombin, trace amount of other plasma proteins	10 mL	Treatment of antithrombin deficiency
Activated protein C (recombinant)	Activated protein C		Severe sepsis
Factor VIIa (recombinant)	Factor VIIa	2.2 mL (1.2 mg)/8.5 mL (4.8 mg)	Bleeding episodes for hemophilia A or B with inhibitors, off-label use for uncontrolled bleeding in various clinical settings

RBC, Red blood cell; Hct, hemotocrit; WBC, white blood cell; CMV, cytomegalovirus; PMN, polymorphonuclear leukocyte; FFP, fresh frozen plasma; IV, intravenous; IM, intramuscular.
Adapted from Triulzi DJ, editor: *Blood transfusion therapy: a physician's handbook,* ed 7, Bethesda, MD, 2002, AABB, p 5. Modified with permission from the AABB.

TABLE 11-2 PRIMARY AND SECONDARY AMINO ACID DISORDERS[1]

A. PRIMARY OVERFLOW AMINOACIDURIAS (AUTOSOMAL RECESSIVE DISORDERS)

DISORDER	PREVALENCE	ABNORMAL ENZYME(S) (OR OTHER DEFECTS)	EXCESS IN BLOOD	EXCESSES IN URINE
Hyperphenylalaninemia				
Type I (Classic PKU)	1:10,000	Phenylalanine hydroxylase total deficiency	Phenylalanine	Phenylalanine and its metabolites (phenylpyruvate, phenyllactate, phenylacetate) when untreated
Type II (Variant PKU)	1:14,000	Phenylalanine hydroxylase partial deficiency	Phenylalanine	Variable
Type III (Transient neonatal)	1:30,000	Immature phenylalanine hydroxylase	Phenylalanine	Phenylalanine metabolites usually not found
Tetrahydrobiopterin defects	Rare	Dihydropteridine reductase deficiency GTP cyclohydrolase I deficiency, 6-pyruvoyl-tetrahydropterin synthase deficiency Pterin 4α-carbinolamine dehydratase deficiency	Phenylalanine Absent CSF neurotransmitters	Variable
Hypertyrosinemia				
Type I (Hepatorenal)	1:100,000 (1:16,000 in Quebec)	Fumarylacetoacetate hydrolase deficiency	Tyrosine	Tyrosine and its metabolites (PHPPA, PHPLA, PHPAA); generalized aminoaciduria
Type II (Oculocutaneous)	Rare	Tyrosine aminotransferase deficiency	Tyrosine	Tyrosine and its metabolites
Type III	Rare	4-hydroxyphenylpyruvic acid dioxygenase deficiency	Tyrosine	Tyrosine and its metabolites

Continued

DISORDER	PREVALENCE	ABNORMAL ENZYME(S) (OR OTHER DEFECTS)	EXCESS IN BLOOD	EXCESSES IN URINE
Transient neonatal	Full term, 1:10; premature, 1:3	Liver immaturity	Tyrosine; phenylalanine	Tyrosine and its metabolites
Alkaptonuria	1:250,000	Homogentisic acid oxidase deficiency	Homogentisic acid (slight)	Homogentisic acid
Homocystinuria	1:200,000	Cystathionine β-synthase deficiency	Homocysteine, methionine	Homocystine, methionine and its sulfoxide
	Total deficiency is rare	Methylenetetrahydrofolate reductase deficiency	Homocysteine, normal or low methionine	As in blood
	Rare	Cobalamin defects	Homocysteine, methyl-malonic acid	Homocystine, methylmalonic acid (organic acid)
Histidinemia	1:12,000	Histidase	Histidine	Imidazole pyruvic acid (organic acid)
Branched-chain ketoaciduria (maple syrup urine disease)	1:200,000	Branched-chain ketoacid decarboxylase	Leucine, isoleucine, alloisoleucine, valine, and corresponding 2-ketoacids	Amino acids as in blood
Nonketotic hyperglycinemia	1:150,000	Glycine cleavage enzyme	Glycine (CSF)	Glycine not always elevated
Propionic acidemia	1:50,000	Propionyl CoA carboxylase	Glycine, propionic acid	Glycine, propionate, 3-hydroxypropionate, and methylcitrate (organic acids)
Methylmalonic acidemia	1:20,000	Methylmalonyl CoA mutase	Glycine, methylmalonic acid	Glycine, methylmalonic acid (organic acid)
Cystathioninuria	1:70,000	γ-Cystathionase	Cystathionine	Cystathionine
Carnosinemia	1:500,000	Carnosinase	Carnosine	Carnosine, homocarnosine

Continued

TABLE II-2 PRIMARY AND SECONDARY AMINO ACID DISORDERS—CONTINUED

A. PRIMARY OVERFLOW AMINOACIDURIAS (AUTOSOMAL RECESSIVE DISORDERS)—CONTINUED

DISORDER	PREVALENCE	ABNORMAL ENZYME(S) (OR OTHER DEFECTS)	EXCESS IN BLOOD	EXCESSES IN URINE
Hyperprolinemia I and II	1:300,000	Type I: Proline oxidase Type II: D5-Pyrroline-5-carboxylic acid dehydrogenase	Proline	Proline, hydroxyproline, and glycine Pyrroline-5-carboxylic acid (organic acid)
UREA CYCLE DISORDERS				
Citrullinemia	1:100,000	Argininosuccinate synthetase	Citrulline, ammonia	Citrulline, orotic acid (organic acid)
Argininosuccinic aciduria	1:75,000	Argininosuccinate lyase	Argininosuccinic acid, citrulline, and ammonia	Argininosuccinic acid and its anhydride, citrulline, and orotic acid
Argininemia	Rare	Arginase	Arginine, ammonia after meals	Normal or excess arginine
Hyperornithinemia with gyrate atrophy of choroids	Rare	Ornithine aminotransferase (OAT)	Ornithine, glutamine, and homocitrulline (HHH) ammonia after meals	Ornithine
Hyperornithinemia/hyperammonemia/ homocitrullinemia (HHH)	Rare	Mitochondrial ornithine transporter (ORNT1)	Ammonia, glutamine	Ornithine, homocitrulline, and orotic acid (HHH)
Ornithine transcarbamylase deficiency X-linked	Most common urea cycle disorder	Ornithine transcarbamylase	Ammonia, glycine, and glutamine	Orotic acid, uridine, and uracil
Carbamoylphosphate synthetase defects	Rare	Carbamoylphosphate synthetase/ N-acetylglutamate synthase	Normal or excess arginine	Glutamine

1. Silverman LM, Christenson RH, Grant GH: Amino acids and proteins. In Tietz NW, editor: *Textbook of clinical chemistry*, Philadelphia, 1986, WB Saunders (modified).

TABLE II-2 PRIMARY AND SECONDARY AMINO ACID DISORDERS—CONTINUED

B. PRIMARY RENAL AMINOACIDURIAS (AUTOSOMAL RECESSIVE DISORDERS)

DISORDER	PREVALENCE	EXCESS AMINO ACIDS IN URINE
Cystinuria, classic	1:13,000	Lysine, ornithine, arginine, and cystine
Hypercystinuria	Rare	Cystine
Dibasic aminoaciduria and lysinuric protein intolerance	Rare	Lysine, ornithine, and arginine
Hartnup disease	1:18,000	All neutral amino acids
Iminoglycinuria	1:12,000	Glycine, proline, and hydroxyproline, free
Dicarboxylic aminoaciduria	Rare	Glutamic acid, aspartic acid
Methionine malabsorption	Rare	Methionine; also tyrosine, phenylalanine, and branched-chain amino acids, α-hydroxybutyric acid, and urinary odor

1. Silverman LM, Christenson RH, Grant GH: Amino acids and proteins. In Tietz NW, editor: *Textbook of clinical chemistry,* Philadelphia, 1986, WB Saunders (modified).

TABLE II-2   PRIMARY AND SECONDARY AMINOACIDURIAS

DISORDER	AMINO ACIDS INCREASED IN URINE

C.   SECONDARY AMINOACIDURIAS DUE TO PRIMARY INHERITED DISORDERS

Cystinosis	Generalized aminoaciduria
Fanconi syndrome	Generalized aminoaciduria
Hereditary fructose intolerance	Generalized aminoaciduria
Galactosemia	Generalized aminoaciduria
Glycogen storage disease type I (rarely)	Generalized aminoaciduria
Lowe's syndrome	Generalized aminoaciduria
Tyrosinemia type 1	Generalized aminoaciduria
Wilson's disease	Generalized aminoaciduria

D.   NONINHERITED, TRANSIENT, AND ACQUIRED DISORDERS

Aminoaciduria of normal newborns	Generalized
Body irradiation	Generalized
Connective tissue disorders	Hydroxyproline
Heavy metal toxicity	Generalized
Hepatic dysfunction	Tyrosine, methionine, and phenylalanine
Homocitrullinemia (nutritional)	Homocitrulline
Hyperparathyroidism	Hydroxyproline
Hyperthyroidism	Hydroxyproline
Malnutrition/ketosis	Leucine, valine, and isoleucine alanine
Neurosecretory tumors	Cystathionine
Nephrotic syndrome	Generalized
Outdated tetracycline ingestion	Generalized
Pregnancy	Generalized
Renal transplantation reaction	Generalized
Salicylate toxicity	Generalized
Steroid therapy	Generalized
Thermal burn	Cystathionine
Vitamin B deficiency	Generalized
Vitamin C deficiency	Generalized
Vitamin D deficiency	

TABLE II-3 INTERPRETATION OF ACYLCARNITINE PROFILES

ACYLCARNITINE	DISORDER
C0-free carnitine	↑ Free to acylcarnitine ratio in CPT 1A deficiency
C2-Acetyl-	↑ In ketosis
C3-Propionyl-	↑ PA, MMA
C3-DCA	↑ MCD
C4-Butyryl-/Isobutyryl-	↑ SCAD, isobutyryl-CoA dehydrogenase deficiency
C4-OH (hydroxyl C4)	↑ SCHAD, possibly elevated in ketosis
C4-DCA	↑ MMA (succinyl-carnitine has same mass)
C5-Isovaleryl, 2-methylbutyryl-	↑ IVA, 2-methylbutyryl-CoA dehydrogenase deficiency
C5-OH 3-hydroxyisovaleryl-	↑ MCC
C5-DCA glutaryl-	↑ GA I, GA II
C6-Hexanoyl-	↑ MCAD, GA II
C6-DCA methylglutaric-	↑ HMG-CoA lyase
C8-Octanoyl-	↑ MCAD, GA II
C10-Decanoyl-	↑ MCAD, GA II
C10:1-Decenoyl	↑ MCAD, GA II
C14:0	↑ VLCAD, CACT, and GA II
C14:1	↑ VLCAD, CACT
C14:2	↑ VLCAD, CACT
C14 OH	↑ LCHAD, TFP
C16:0	↑ CPT 2, VLCAD (minor), CACT, and GA II
C16:1	↑ CPT 2, VLCAD (minor), and CACT
C16:2	↑ CPT 2, VLCAD (minor), and CACT
C16-OH	↑ LCHAD, TFP
C18-OH	↑ LCHAD, TFP
C18:1-OH	↑ LCHAD, TFP
C18:2-OH	↑ LCHAD, TFP

CPT1A, Carnitine palmitoyltransferase 1A(hepatic) deficiency; *PA*, propionic acidemia; *MMA*, methylmalonic acidemia; *MCD*, malonyl-CoA decarboxylase deficiency; *SCAD*, short-chain acyl-CoA dehydrogenase deficiency; *SCHAD*, short/medium-chain 3-hydroxyacyl-CoA dehydrogenase deficiency; *IVA*, isovaleric acidemia; *MCC*, 3-methylcrotonyl-CoA carboxylase deficiency; *GA I*, glutaric acidemia type 1; *GA II*, glutaric acidemia type 2 (multiple acyl-CoA dehydrogenation defects MADD); *MCAD*, medium-chain acyl-CoA dehydrogenase deficiency; *HMG*, 3-hydroxy-3-methylglutaryl-CoA; *VLCAD*, very-long-chain acyl-CoA dehydrogenase deficiency; *CACT*, carnitine:acylcarnitine translocase deficiency; *LCHAD*, long-chain 3-hydroxyacyl-CoA dehydrogenase deficiency; *TFP*, mitochondrial trifunctional protein deficiency.

TABLE II-4 DRUGS CAUSING APLASTIC ANEMIA AND HEMOLYSIS

		HEMOLYSIS	
DRUG	**APLASTIC ANEMIA**	**G6PD DEFICIENCY**	**IMMUNE REACTION**
ANTINEOPLASTIC			
Azathioprine	x		
Busulfan	x		
Cyclophosphamide	x		
Cytarabine	x		
Daunorubicin	x		
Doxorubicin	x		
Fluorouracil	x		
Melphalan	x		x
Mercaptopurine	x		
Methotrexate	x		x
Nitrogen mustard	x		
Thioguanine	x		
Vinblastine	x		
Vincristine	x		
ANTIMICROBIAL			
Amphotericin B	x		x
Cephaloridine			x
Cephalothin			x
Chloramphenicol	x	x	
Penicillins	x		x
Ristocetin	x		
Streptomycin	x		
Sulfonamides	x	x	x
Tetracyclines	x		
ANALGESIC			
Aspirin	x	x	
Ibuprofen			x
Indomethacin	x		
Mefenamic acid			x
Phenacetin	x	x	x
Phenylbutazone	x		
Oxyphenbutazone	x		

Continued

TABLE II-4   DRUGS CAUSING APLASTIC ANEMIA AND HEMOLYSIS—CONTINUED

		HEMOLYSIS	
DRUG	**APLASTIC ANEMIA**	**G6PD DEFICIENCY**	**IMMUNE REACTION**
ANTICONVULSANT			
Carbamazepine	x		x
Mephenytoin	x		
Primidone	x		
Trimethadione	x		
METALS			
Arsenicals (organic)	x	x	
Bismuth	x		
Gold compounds	x		
Mercury	x		
Silver (colloidal)	x		
PSYCHOTROPIC			
Chlordiazepoxide	x		
Chlorpromazine	x		x
Meprobamate	x		
Promazine	x		
Trifluoperazine	x		
CINCHONA ALKALOIDS			
Quinidine			x
Quinine			x
ANTIMALARIAL			
Chloroquine		x	
Primaquine		x	
Pyrimethamine	x	x	
Quinacrine	x	x	
ANTIHYPERTENSIVE			
Captopril	x	x	
Procainamide			x

Continued

TABLE II-4 DRUGS CAUSING APLASTIC ANEMIA AND HEMOLYSIS—CONTINUED

| | | HEMOLYSIS | |
| | APLASTIC | G6PD | IMMUNE |
DRUG	ANEMIA	DEFICIENCY	REACTION
ORAL HYPOGLYCEMIC			
Carbutamide	x		x
Chlorpropamide	x		x
Tolbutamide	x		x
ANTITHYROIDS			
Carbimazole	x		
Methimazole	x		
Perchlorate	x		
Propylthiouracil	x		
Thiocyanate	x		
DIURETIC			
Acetazolamide	x		
Chlorothiazide	x		
Triamterene	x		
ANTIHISTAMINE			
Chlorpheniramine	x		
Tripelennamine	x		
SULFONES			
Dapsone		x	
Solapsone		x	
NITROFURANS			
Furazolidone		x	
Nitrofurantoin		x	
Nitrofurazone		x	

Continued

TABLE II-4 DRUGS CAUSING APLASTIC ANEMIA AND HEMOLYSIS—CONTINUED

| | | HEMOLYSIS | |
DRUG	APLASTIC ANEMIA	G6PD DEFICIENCY	IMMUNE REACTION
OTHERS			
Ascorbic acid (high dose)	x		x
p-Aminosalicylic acid	x		
Cinetidine	x		
Colchicine			
Dimercaprol		x	
Dinitrophenol	x		
Insulin			x
Isoniazid			x
Levodopa			x
Methyldopa			x
Methylene blue		x	
Nalidixic acid		x	
Penicillamine	x		
Phenazopyridine		x	
Probenecid		x	
Rifampin			x
Stibophen			x

TABLE II-5 HEPATOTOXIC DRUGS

DRUGS CAUSING CHOLESTASIS

Aminosalicylic acid	Erythromycin	Penicillamine
Amitriptyline	Estrogens	Penicillins
Anabolic steroids	Ethionamide	Phenothiazines
Androgens	Glyburide (glibenclamide)	Phenylbutazone
Azathioprine	Gold salts	Progestins
Benzodiazepines	Imipramine	Propoxyphene
Carbamazepine	Mercaptopurine	Sulfonamides
Carbarsone	Methimazole	Sulfones
Chlorothiazide	Mitoxantrone	Sulindac
Chlorpropamide	Nicotinic acid	Tamoxifen
Clavulanic acid	Nitrofurantoin	Tolbutamide
Dapsone	Oral contraceptives	

DRUGS CAUSING HEPATOCELLULAR INJURY

Acetaminophen	Estrogens	Paramethadione
Allopurinol	Ethanol (excess)	Perhexiline
Aminosalicylic acid	Ethionamide	Phenazopyridine
Amiodarone	Etretinate	Phenindione
Amitriptyline	Fluconazole	Phenobarbital
Anabolic steroids	Halothane	Phenylbutazone
Androgens	HMG-CoA reductase inhibitors	Phenytoin
Asparaginase	Ibuprofen	Plicamycin (mithramycin)
Aspirin	Imipramine	Probenecid
Azathioprine	Indomethacin	Procainamide
Carbamazepine	Iron salts (overdose)	Propylthiouracil
Chenodiol	Isoniazid	Pyrazinamide
Chlorambucil	Ketoconazole	Quinidine
Chloramphenicol (occasional)	MAO inhibitors	Rifampin
Chlorpropamide	Mercaptopurine	Salicylates
Cimetidine	Methotrexate	Sulfasalazine
Cyclosporine	Methoxyflurane	Sulfonamides
Danazol	Methyldopa	Tamoxifen
Dantrolene	Naproxen	Tetracyclines
Dapsone	Nicotinic acid	Trimethadione
Diclofenac	Nitrofurantoin	Valproic acid
Dicoumarol (rare)	Oral contraceptives	Vitamin A
Disulfiram	Papaverine	Warfarin (rare)

TABLE II-6 NEPHROTOXIC SUBSTANCES

METALS

Antimony
Arsenic
Bismuth
Cadmium
Copper
Gold
Iron
Lead
Lithium
Mercurials
Silver
Thallium
Uranium

ANALGESIC DRUGS

Acetaminophen (overdose)
Aminopyrine
Nonsteroidal anti-inflammatory drugs
(e.g., ibuprofen, indomethacin, naproxen, fenoprofen)
Phenacetin
Phenylbutazone
Salicylates

ANTIMICROBIAL AGENTS

Aminoglycosides (e.g., amikacin, gentamicin,
kanamycin, neomycin, streptomycin, tobramycin)
Amphotericin B
Capreomycin
Cephalosporins
(primarily cephaloridine and cephalothin)
Colistin
Cotrimoxazole
Foscarnet
Penicillins (e.g., ampicillin, methicillin, oxacillin)
Polymyxin B
Rifampin
Sulfonamides
Tetracyclines
Vancomycin

ANTINEOPLASTIC DRUGS

Carboplatin
Cisplatin
Cyclophosphamide
Ifosfamide
Methotrexate (high dose)
Mitomycin
Nitrosoureas (e.g., lomustine, semustine)
Plicamycin (mithramycin)
Streptozocin

ORGANIC SOLVENTS

Benzene
Carbon tetrachloride
Ethylene glycol
Tetrachloroethylene

OTHER DRUGS

Acetazolamide
ε-Aminocaproic acid
Aminosalicylic acid
Boric acid
Captopril
Cyclosporine
Dextran (low molecular weight)
Furosemide
Mannitol
Methoxyflurane
d-Penicillamine
Pentamidine
Phenindione
Quinine
Radiographic contrast media
Thiazide diuretics
Triamterene
Zoxazolamine

TABLE II-7 HEPATITIS TESTING

PURPOSE	MARKERS	ADDITIONAL TESTING INDICATED
Diagnosis of acute hepatitis	IgM-anti-HA Hb$_s$Ag IgM-anti-HB$_c$ Anti-HCV	
Diagnosis of chronic hepatitis	Hb$_s$Ag	**If negative but still suspect HBV:** Anti-HB$_s$, anti-HB$_c$, and HBV-DNA (optional) **If positive:** HB$_e$Ag, anti-HB$_e$, anti-HD, and HDAg (optional) **To assess therapy of HBV:** HB$_e$Ag, anti-HB$_e$, and HBV-DNA
	Anti-HCV	**If negative but still suspect HCV:** HCV-RNA
Determine efficacy of B vaccine	Anti-HB$_s$	
Determine natural immunity HBV	Anti-HB$_c$	

TABLE II-8 SPHINGOLIPIDOSES*†

DISEASE	NUMBER OF SUBTYPES	SPECIMEN USED FOR ENZYME ASSAY	ENZYME DEFICIENCY	LIPID ACCUMULATED
Gaucher's disease	3	Leukocytes, cultured skin fibroblasts	Cerebroside β-glucosidase (β-glucosidase, EC 3.2.1.21)	Glucosyl ceramide
Metachromatic leukodystrophy	4	Leukocytes, cultured skin fibroblasts, and serum	Arylsulfatase A (EC 3.1.6.1)	Sulfatide
Tay-Sachs disease (G$_{M2}$ gangliosidosis)	1	Leukocytes, cultured skin fibroblasts, and serum	Hexosaminidase A (N-acetyl-β-D-glucosaminidase, EC 3.2.1.30)	Ganglioside, GM2
Sandhoff disease (G$_{M2}$ gangliosidosis)	2	Leukocytes, cultured skin fibroblasts, and serum	Hexosaminidase A and B (N-acetyl-β-D-glucosaminidase, EC 3.2.1.30), G$_{M2}$ activator protein	Ganglioside, GM2, and globoside
G$_{M1}$ gangliosidosis	2	Leukocytes, cultured skin fibroblasts	Acid β-galactosidase (EC 3.2.1.23)	Ganglioside, GM1
Fabry's disease	1	Leukocytes, cultured skin fibroblasts, and serum	α-Galactosidase A (EC 3.2.1.22)	Trihexosyl ceramide
Niemann-Pick disease types A and B	2	Leukocytes, cultured skin fibroblasts, and serum	Sphingomyelinase (sphingomyelin phosphodiesterase, EC 3.1.4.12)	Sphingomyelin
Krabbe's disease (globoid cell leukodystrophy)	2	Leukocytes, cultured skin fibroblasts, and serum	Cerebroside β-galactosidase (β-galactosidase, EC 3.2.1.23)	Galactosyl ceramide
Farber's disease	7	Leukocytes, cultured skin fibroblasts, serum, and amniocytes	Acid ceramidase (acylsphingosine deacylase, EC 3.5.1.23)	Ceramide
Fucosidosis	2	Leukocytes	α-Fucosidase (EC 3.2.1.51)	H-antigen glycolipid
Schindler disease	3	Leukocytes, cultured skin fibroblasts, and amniocytes	α-N-Acetylgalactosaminidase	Glycopeptides

*All listed sphingolipidoses are autosomal recessive except Fabry's disease, which is X-linked. Prenatal diagnosis of homozygotes and identification of heterozygous carriers are available for the listed disorders.
†At present, diagnosis of Farber's disease is confirmed by biopsy and histological examination of subcutaneous nodules rather than by determination of enzyme activity.

TABLE II-9 INFORMATIVE BIOCHEMICAL FINDINGS IN PORPHYRIA

TYPE OF PORPHYRIA	DEFICIENT ENZYME	ENZYME ASSAY AVAILABLE
Porphyria cutanea tarda (PCT)	Uroporphyrinogen decarboxylase	Y
Hepatoerythropoietic porphyria (HEP)	Uroporphyrinogen decarboxylase	Y
Congenital erythropoietic porphyria (CEP)	Uroporphyrinogen cosynthase	Y
Erythropoietic protoporphyria (EPP)	Ferrochelatase	N
ALA dehydratase deficiency (ALAD)	ALA dehydratase	Y
Acute intermittent porphyria (AIP)	Porphobilinogen deaminase	Y
Hereditary coproporphyria (HCP)	Coproporphyrinogen oxidase	N
Variegate porphyria (VP)	Protoporphyrinogen oxidase	N

*Sometimes.

| BIOCHEMICAL FINDINGS | | | |
URINE	FECES	ERYTHROCYTES	PLASMA
Uroporphyrin, heptacarboxylporphyrin	Isocoproporphyrin, heptacarboxylporphyrin III		Uroporphyrin
Uroporphyrin, heptacarboxylporphyrin	Isocoproporphyrin, heptacarboxylporphyrin III	Zinc protoporphyrin	Uroporphyrin
Uroporphyrin, coproporphyrin	Uroporphyrin I, coproporphyrin I	Uroporphyrin, coproporphyrin, and zinc protoporphyrin	Uroporphyrin I, coproporphyrin I
	Protoporphyrin	Free protoporphyrin	Protoporphyrin[+]
ALA			
ALA, PBG, uroporphyrin, and coproporphyrin*	Uroporphyrin,* coproporphyrin*		Increased porphyrins and precursors during acute episodes
Coproporphyrin, ALA, and PBG	Coproporphyrin

↑ Coproporphyrin III/coproporphyrin I ratio | | Coproporphyrin |
| Coproporphyrin, PBG, and ALA | Protoporphyrin > coproporphyrin

↑ Coproporphyrin III/coproporphyrin I ratio | | |

TABLE II-10 REPORTED DRUG EXPERIENCE IN ACUTE PORPHYRIAS[1]

UNSAFE

ACE inhibitors (especially
  enalapril)
Antipyrine (phenazone)
Aminopyrine (amidopyrine)
Aminoglutethimide
Barbiturates
Calcium channel blockers
  (especially nifedipine)
Carbamazepine
Carisoprodol
Chlorpropamide
Danazol
Dapsone
Diclofenac
Diphenylhydantoin
Ergot preparations
Ethchlorvynol
Ethinamate
Ethosuximide
Glutethimide
Griseofulvin
Isopropylmeprobamate
Ketoconazole
Lamotrigine
Mephenytoin
Meprobamate
Methyprylon
Metoclopramide
N-Butylscopolammonium
  bromide
Nefazodone
Novobiocin
Pargyline
Phenylbutazone
Primidone
Progesterone and progestins
Pyrazolone preparations
Rifampin
Succinimides
Sulfasalazine
Sulfonamide antibiotics
Sulfonethylmethane
Sulfonmethane
Sulfonylureas
Synthetic estrogens, progestins

Tolazamide
Tolbutamide
Tranylcypromine
Trimethadione
Valproic acid

POTENTIALLY UNSAFE

Alfadolone acetate
Alfaxolone
Alkylating agents
Altretamine (hexamethylmel-
  amine)
2-Allyloxy-
  3-methylbenzamide
Amitriptyline
Bemegride
Benzodiazepines
Busulphan
Captopril
Cephalosporins
Chlorambucil
Chlordiazepoxide
Clonidine
Chloroform
Colistin
Cyclosporin
Dacarbazine
Diazepam
Diltiazem
Diphenhydramine
EDTA
Estrogens (synthetic)
Etomidate
Erythromycin
S-fluorouracil
Fluroxine
Food additives
Gold compounds
Heavy metals
Hydralazine
Hyoscine
Ifosfamide
Imipramine
Iron chelators (DFO < EDTA)
Ketamine

Lisinopril
Mefenamic acid
Melphalan
Methyldopa
Metyrapone
Mifepristone (RU-486)
Nalidixic acid
Nikethamide
Nitrazepam
Nitrofurantoin
Nortriptyline
Pentazocine
Pentylenetetrazol
Phenoxybenzamine
Pyrazinamide
Spironolactone
Theophylline
Tiagabine
Tolazamide
Tramadol
Tricyclic antidepressants

PROBABLY SAFE

Adrenaline
Azathioprine
Chloramphenicol
Chloroquine
Cisapride
Colchicine
Cytarabine
Daunorubicin
Dicoumerol
Digoxin
Doxazosin
Estrogens (natural/endoge-
  nous)
Ibuprofen
Indomethacin
Labetalol
Lithium
Losartan
Mandelamine
Methylphenidate
Naproxen
Neostigmine

Nitrous oxide
Penicillamine
Procaine
Propanidid
Propofol
Propoxyphene
Prostigmine
Rauwolfia alkaloids
6-Thioguanine
Thiouracil
Thyroxine
Tubocurarine
Vigabatrin
Vitamin B group
Vitamin C

SAFE

Acetaminophen (paracetamol)
Acetazolamide
Allopurinol
Amiloride
Aspirin
Atropine
Bethanidine
Bumetanidine
Bromides
Chloral hydrate
Cimetidine
Corticosteroids
Coumarins
Ether
Fluoxetine
Gabapentin
Gentamycin
Glucocorticoids
Guanethidine
Insulin
Narcotic analgesics
Ofloxacin
Penicillin and derivatives
Phenothiazines
Propranolol
Streptomycin
Succinylcholine
Tetracycline

1. Andersen KE, Sassa S, Bishop DF, et al: Disorders of heme biosynthesis: X-linked sideroblastic anemia and the porphyrias. In Scriver CR, Beaudet AL, Sly WS, editors: *The metabolic basis of inherited disease,* ed 8, New York, McGraw-Hill.

TABLE II-11   CDC CLASSIFICATION OF BLOOD LEAD LEVELS IN CHILDREN

CLASS	BLOOD LEAD*	ACTION
I	<10 mcg/dL	None (not lead poisoned)
IIA	10-14 mcg/dL	Educational intervention, rescreen within 3 mo
IIB	15-19 mcg/dL	Educational, possible social intervention, rescreen within 2 mo†
III	20-44 mcg/dL	Provide case and clinical management, environmental investigation, and consider chelation therapy
IV	45-69 mcg/dL	Initiate case and clinical management, environmental investigation, and lead hazard control within 48 hr; start chelation therapy
V	>69 mcg/dL	A medical emergency, hospitalize child, initiate case and clinical management, environmental management, and lead hazard control immediately

*Owing to possible contamination during collection, elevated levels should be confirmed with a second specimen before action is instituted.
†If two venous BLLs collected 3 mo apart are ≥15-19 mcg/dL, proceed with action for BLLs 20-44 mcg/dL.

TABLE II-12 OSHA-RECOMMENDED ACTION LEVELS FOR WORKERS EXPOSED TO CADMIUM[1]

LABORATORY FINDINGS	MCG/L	MCG/G CREATININE*	ACTION
LEVEL A			
Cadmium, whole blood†	≤5		Monitor annually, biennial medical examination, no
Cadmium, urine‡		≤3	action required
β₂-Microglobulin, urine§		≤300	
LEVEL B			
Cadmium, whole blood	>5	≤10	Monitor semiannually, annual medical examination,
Cadmium, urine	>3	≤7	discretionary removal from source of exposure‖
β₂-Microglobulin, urine	>300	≤750	
LEVEL C			
Cadmium, whole blood	>15	>10	Monitor quarterly, semiannual medical examination,
Cadmium, urine	>15	>7	mandatory removal from source of exposure
β₂-Microglobulin, urine	>1500	>750	

1. *Cadmium action levels beginning January 1999,* Federal Register 1999, Std CFR, Part 1910, 1027 Appendix A.
*Blood cadmium estimates current Cd exposure.
†Urine creatinine value.
‡Urine cadmium estimates Cd body burden.
§Urine β₂-microglobulin is an early marker of irreversible kidney damage and disease.
‖The determination of discretionary or mandatory removal is made by the examining physician consistent with the medical surveillance specifications in the Federal Register, 42456-42463.

TABLE II-13   SERUM IRON, TIBC, AND TRANSFERRIN SATURATION*

	SERUM IRON	TIBC	TRANSFERRIN SATURATION
Ingestion of medicinal iron†	↑	N	↑
Parenteral iron administration‡	↑	↑	Var
Iron deficiency states			
Chronic blood loss	↓N	↑N	↓N
Acute blood loss	N↓	N	N↓
Post-subtotal gastrectomy	N↓	↑N	↓N
Dietary deficiency (infants and children)	N↓	↑N	↓N
Polycythemia vera	↓N	↑N	↓N
Kwashiorkor	↓	↓	Var
Pregnancy (without Fe supplement)	↓N	↑N	↓N
Iron overload states			
Acute iron poisoning	↑	N	↑
Chronic iron overload (hemosiderosis, hemochromatosis, thalassemia major, sideroblastic anemias, other chronic anemias after numerous transfusions)	↑	N↓	↑
Chronic disorders			
Chronic infections	↓N	↓N	N↓
Rheumatoid arthritis	↓N	↓N	N↓
Malignancies	↓N	↓N	N↓
Laennec's cirrhosis	↓N	↓N	N↓
Acute disorders			
Acute infections	↓	N	↓
Myocardial infarction	↓	N	↓
Hepatitis or hepatic necrosis§	↑	↑N	Var
Physiological variations			
Diurnal rhythm			
Morning	N	N	N
Evening	↓	N	↓
Menstruation	↓	N	↓
Premenstrual interval	↑	N	N
Contraceptives (except when bleeding)	↑	↑	N
Pregnancy (with Fe supplement)	↑	↑	N
Miscellaneous			
Pernicious anemia			
Untreated	↑	N↓	↑
Early treatment (first week)	↓	N↓	↓N
Treated	N	N	N
Congenital atransferrinemia (*very* rare)	↓	↓	↑
Acquired atransferrinemia (from nephrotic syndrome)	↓	↓	↑
Hemolytic anemias	Var	Var	Var

*For each entry in this table, the most characteristic change is indicated first.

†The ingestion of a single tablet or capsule of an iron-containing medicinal can increase the serum iron concentration by 300-500 mcg/dL, an effect that often masks iron deficiency. Peak serum iron concentration occurs a few hours after ingestion; the effect is most pronounced in iron-deficient subjects.

‡Increased serum iron concentration may be observed for weeks after an injection of iron dextran. The mechanism of this has not been determined; most likely it reflects iron dextran in plasma. The increase in TIBC characteristically observed with automated methods probably does not reflect increased transferrin but a methodological artifact (additional release of iron from iron dextran as a result of the procedure?) because the unsaturated iron-binding capacity is normal in this situation.

§Increased iron concentrations are the result of extreme hyperferritinemia consequent to hepatocellular injury. The increase in TIBC characteristically observed with automated methods probably does not reflect increased transferrin but a methodological artifact (additional iron release from ferritin as a result of the procedure?).

TABLE II-14 IMMUNOPHENOTYPE AND CYTOCHEMISTRY OF ACUTE LEUKEMIAS[1-6]

	MO	M1/M2	M3	M4	M5A	M5B	M6	M7	E PB-ALL	C PB-ALL	PT-ALL
CD34	+	+	+/−	+/−	−	+/−	+	+	+	+	−
HLA-DR	+	+	−	+	+	+	+	+	+	+	−
CD13	+	+	+	+	+	+	+	+	−	−	−
CD33	+	+	+	+	+	+	+	+	+/−	+/−	−
CD14	−	−	−	+	−	+	−	−	NA	NA	NA
CD15	+/−	+/−	+/−	+	+	+	+/−	+/−	NA	NA	NA
CD41	+/−	+/−	+/−	+/−	+	+/−	+/−	NA	NA	NA	NA
CD61	−	+/−	−	+/−	−	+/−	−	+	NA	NA	NA
CD56	+/−	+/−	−	+/−	+	+	−	+/−	NA	NA	NA
CD64	−	+/−	−	+/−	+	+	−	−	NA	NA	NA
CD117	+	+	+	+	+	−	+	+	−	−	−
Cyt CD79a	−	−	NA	NA	NA	NA	NA	NA	+	+	−
CD10	−	−	−	−	−	−	−	−	−	+	+/−
CD19	+/−	+/−	−	−	−	−	−	−	+	+	−
CD20	−	−	−	+/−	+	+	−	−	+/−	+/−	−

1. Brunning RD, McKenna RW: *Tumors of the bone marrow,* Washington, DC, 1994, Armed Forces Institute of Pathology.

2. Jaffe ES, Harris NL, Stein H, et al, editors: *World Health Organization classification of tumours. Pathology and genetics of tumours of haematopoietic and lymphoid tissues,* Lyon, 2001, IARC Press.

3. Kaleem Z, Crawford E, Pathan MH, et al: Flow cytometric analysis of acute leukemias, *Arch Pathol Lab Med* 127:42-48, 2003.

4. Knowles DM, editor: *Neoplastic hematopathology,* ed 2, Baltimore, 2000, Lippincott Williams & Wilkins.

5. Khalidi HS, Medeiros LJ, Chang KL, et al: The immunophenotype of adult acute myeloid leukemia, *Am J Clin Pathol* 109:211-220, 1998.

6. Legrand O, Perrot J-Y, Baudard M, et al: The immunophenotype of 177 adults with acute myeloid leukemia, *Blood* 96:870-877, 2000.

TABLE II-14   IMMUNOPHENOTYPE AND CYTOCHEMISTRY OF ACUTE LEUKEMIAS—CONTINUED

	M0	M1/M2	M3	M4	M5A	M5B	M6	M7	E PB-ALL	C PB-ALL	PT-ALL
CD1	−	−	−	−	−	−	NA	−	−	−	+/−
CD2	+/−	−	+/−	+/−	−	+/−	−	−	−	−	+
sCD3	−	−	−	−	+/−	+/−	−	−	−	−	+/−
Cyt CD3	−	−	NA	NA	NA	NA	NA	NA	NA	−	+
CD4	+/−	+/−	−	+	−	+	−	−	−	−	+/−
CD5	−	−	−	−	+	+/−	−	−	−	−	+
CD7	+/−	+/−	−	+/−	−	+/−	+/−	+/−	−	−	+
CD8	−	−	−	−	−	−	NA	−	−	−	+/−
Gly A	−	−	−	−	−	−	+	−	NA	NA	NA
TdT	+	−	−	−	−	−	−	−	+	+	+
MPO flow cytometric	+	+	+	+	+/−	+/−	+/−	−	−	−	NA
MPO cytochem	−	+	+	+	−	+/−	+/−	−	−	−	−
NSE cytochem	−	−	−	+	+	+	−	−	−	−	−
SBB cytochem	−	+	+	+	−	+/−	+/−	−	−	−	−

+, Expressed by the blasts in >50% cases; +/−, expressed in 10-50% of cases; −, expressed in <10% of cases; *MPO*, myeloperoxidase; *NSE*, leukocyte nonspecific esterase; *M0, M1/M2, M3, M4, M5, M6, M7*, subtypes of acute myeloid leukemia (AML) in the FAB classification of AML[1]; *E p-B*, early precursor B-cell acute lymphoblastic leukemia (ALL); *C p-B*, common precursor B-cell ALL; *pT*, precursor T-cell ALL.[2]

TABLE II-15   DIFFERENTIAL DIAGNOSIS OF ANEMIAS BASED ON RED CELL DISTRIBUTION OF WIDTH (RDW) AND MEAN CELL VOLUME (MCV)[1-3]

	MCV LOW	MCV NORMAL	MCV HIGH
RDW increased	Iron deficiency, homozygous β-thalassemia, hemoglobin H disease, S-β thalassemia, sideroblastic anemia, and hemoglobin SC disease	Early iron deficiency, mixed nutritional deficiencies, hemoglobin S disease, hemoglobin SC disease, and sideroblastic anemia	Megaloblastic anemias, sideroblastic anemia, and marked reticulocytosis
Normal RDW	Anemia of chronic disease, hemoglobin E trait and disease, β-thalassemia minor, and α-thalassemia minor	Anemia of chronic disease, acute blood loss, and hereditary spherocytosis	Aplastic anemia

1. Bessman JD: *Automated blood counts and differentials,* ed 2, Baltimore, 1988, The Johns Hopkins University Press.
2. Bessman JD, Ridgway G, Gardner FH: Improved classification of anemias by MCV and RDW, *Am J Clin Pathol* 80:322-326, 1988.
3. Rodak BF, editor: *Hematology: clinical principles and applications,* ed 2, Philadelphia, 2002, WB Saunders.

TABLE II-16 CHARACTERISTIC IMMUNOPHENOTYPES OF SELECT CHRONIC (MATURE) LYMPHOPROLIFERATIVE DISORDERS[1-5]

B-CELL LYMPHOPROLIFERATIVE DISORDERS*

DISORDER	SIG	CD19	CD20	CD22	CD23	CD25	CD5	CD11C	CD10	CD79B	CD103	FMC7
CLL	dim	+	dim	dim	+	−	+	dim	−	−	−	−
PLL	+	+	+	+	−	−	+/−	−	−	+	−	+
HCL	+	+	+	+	−	+	−	+	−	−	+	+
MCL	+	+	+	+	−	−	+	−	−	+	−	+
MZL	+	+	+	+	−	−	−	+/−	−	+	−	+
FCC	+	+	+	+	−	−	−	−	+	+	−	+

1. Brunning RD, McKenna RW: *Tumors of the bone marrow,* Washington, DC, 1994, Armed Forces Institute of Pathology.
2. Foucar K: Chronic lymphoid leukemias and lymphoproliferative disorders, *Mod Pathol* 12:141-150, 1999.
3. DiGiuseppe JA, Borowitz MJ: Clinical utility of flow cytometry in the chronic lymphoid leukemias, *Semin Oncol* 25:6-10, 1998.
4. Turner JJ, Hughes AM, Kricker A, et al: Use of the WHO lymphoma classification in a population-based epidemiological study, *Ann Oncol* 15:631-637, 2004.5. Matutes E, Owusu-Ankomah K, Morilla R, et al: The immunological profile of B-cell disorders and proposal of a scoring system for the diagnosis of CLL, *Leukemia* 8:1640-1645, 1994.

+, Positive; +/−, variable; −, negative; *CLL,* chronic lymphocytic leukemia; *PLL,* prolymphocytic leukemia; *HCL,* hairy cell leukemia; *MCL,* mantle cell lymphoma/leukemia; *MZL,* marginal zone lymphoma; *FCC,* small cleaved follicular center-cell lymphoma.
*These are the "classic" immunophenotypes. Variations exist, some of which have prognostic significance.

T-CELL LYMPHOPROLIFERATIVE DISORDERS†

DISORDER	CD2	CD3	CD4	CD5	CD7	CD8	CD16	CD25	CD56	CD57
PLL	+	+	+	+	+	−	−	+/−	−	+/−
LGL	+	+	−	+	+/−	+	+	−	−	+
ATLL	+	+	+	+	−	−	−	+	−	NA
MF/SS	+	+	+	+	−	−	−	−	−	NA

+, Positive; +/−, variable; −, negative; *NA,* not available; *PLL,* prolymphocytic leukemia; *LGL,* large granular lymphocyte leukemia; *ATLL,* adult T-cell leukemia/lymphoma; *MF/SS,* mycosis fungoides/Sezary syndrome.
†These are the "classic" immunophenotypes. Variations exist, some of which have prognostic significance.

TABLE II-17 LEUKOCYTE DIFFERENTIAL COUNT IN BLOOD: REFERENCE RANGES[1-6]*

AGE	NEUTROPHILS	EOSINOPHILS	BASOPHILS	LYMPHOCYTES	MONOCYTES
Birth	6.0-26.0	0.02-0.85	0-0.64	2.0-11.0	0.4-3.1
12 hr	6.0-28.0			2.0-11.0	
24 hr	5.0-21.0			2.0-11.5	
1 wk	1.5-10.0	0.07-1.1	0-0.25	2.0-17.0	0.3-2.7
2 wk	1.0-9.5	0.07-1.0	0-0.23	2.0-17.0	0.2-2.4
1 mo	1.0-9.0	0.3		2.5-16.5	0.7
6 mo	1.0-8.5	0.3		4.0-13.5	0.6
1 yr	1.5-8.5	0.3		4.0-10.5	0.6
2 yr	1.5-8.5	0.3		3.0-9.5	0.5
4 yr	1.5-8.5	0.3		2.0-8.0	0.5
6 yr	1.5-8.0	0.2		1.5-7.0	0.4
8 yr	1.5-8.0	0.2		1.5-6.8	0.4
10 yr	1.8-8.0	0.2		1.5-6.5	0.4
16 yr	1.8-8.0	0.2		1.2-5.2	0.4
21 yr	1.8-7.7	0.2		1.0-4.8	0.3

| TABLE II-17 | LEUKOCYTE DIFFERENTIAL COUNT IN BLOOD: REFERENCE RANGES—CONTINUED | | | | |

AGE	NEUTROPHILS	EOSINOPHILS	BASOPHILS	LYMPHOCYTES	MONOCYTES
ADULTS					
Males					
White	1.51-7.07	0.00-0.42	0.00-0.16	0.65-2.80	0.00-0.51
Black	1.11-6.77	0.00-0.47	0.00-0.16	0.97-3.30	0.02-0.83
Females					
White	2.023-7.46	0.00-0.52	0.00-0.16	1.01-3.38	0.00-0.82
Black	1.5-8.14	0.00-0.46	0.00-0.20	1.05-3.48	0.02-0.72

1. Rodak BF, editor: *Hematology: clinical principles and applications,* ed 2, Philadelphia, 2002, WB Saunders.

2. Saxena S, Wong ET: Heterogeneity of common hematologic parameters among racial, ethnic and gender subgroups, *Arch Pathol Lab Med* 114:715-719, 1990.

3. Kjeldsberg C, Elenitoba-Johnson K, Foucar K, et al, editors: *Practical diagnosis of hematologic disorders,* ed 3, Chicago, 2000, ASCP Press.

4. Greer JP, Foerster J, Lukens JN, et al: *Wintrobe's clinical hematology,* ed 11, Philadelphia, 2003, Lippincott Williams & Wilkins.

5. Beutler E, Lichtman MA, Coller B, editors: *Williams hematology,* ed 6, New York, 2000, McGraw-Hill.

6. Nathan DG, Orkin SH, Ginsburg D, et al: *Hematology of infancy and childhood,* ed 6, Philadelphia, 2003, WB Saunders.

*Values are given as cell counts in thousands per microliter: 10^3 cells/μL (10^6 cells/L). These values are calculated by multiplying the percent (%) of each type of cell by the total leukocyte count. The ranges are derived from several sources with an emphasis on the most recent sources, which include automated counts. Mean values are given where range is not available. A racial difference exists in neutrophil counts. Healthy black males and Asian and black females have lower absolute neutrophil counts than do white persons. White women have higher segmented neutrophil counts than white men until age 45 yr and then the reverse holds.

TABLE II-18A LEUKOCYTE DIFFERENTIAL COUNT: DIAGNOSTIC INFORMATION AND INTERFERENCES

NEUTROPHILIC SERIES[1-3]

↑ NEUTROPHILS (NEUTROPHILIA)	↓ NEUTROPHILS (NEUTROPENIA)	INTERFERENCES
Infections: Bacterial, mycotic, spirochetal, some viral, rickettsial, parasitic *Inflammatory disorders or tissue necrosis:* Rheumatic fever, rheumatoid arthritis, tissue damage (e.g., after surgery), ischemic necrosis (e.g., myocardial infarction), gout, drug sensitivity, smoking, colitis, pancreatitis, nephritis, myositis, thyroiditis, dermatitis, peritonitis, hepatic necrosis *Endocrinologic or metabolic disorders:* Diabetes mellitus, uremia, eclampsia, hyperthyroidism, overproduction of ACTH *Hematological disorders:* Myeloproliferative disorders (including chronic myeloid leukemia, polycythemia vera, myelofibrosis with myeloid metaplasia), some types of acute myeloid and lymphoid leukemias, postsplenectomy, hemolytic anemias, hemorrhage, chronic idiopathic leukocytosis, rebound or recovery from bone marrow aplasia or nutritional deficiency *Physical and emotional stimuli:* Cold, heat, exercise, pain, burns, labor, pregnancy, trauma, nausea and vomiting, electric shock, anoxia, fear, anger, joy, severe depression *Malignant neoplasms:* A variety of neoplasms, especially bronchogenic carcinoma *Hereditary conditions:* Down syndrome	*Infections:* Bacterial (typhoid, paratyphoid, brucellosis), viral (influenza, measles, rubella, infectious hepatitis, chickenpox, Colorado tick fever, dengue, yellow fever), rickettsial (typhus, rickettsial pox, Rocky Mountain spotted fever), protozoal (malaria, kala-azar), overwhelming infections of any type (especially in elderly or debilitated individuals) *Hematological disorders:* Aplastic anemia, some acute leukemias and myelodysplastic syndromes, idiopathic neutropenia, hypersplenism, megaloblastic anemia, myelophthisic anemia (marrow replacement), paroxysmal nocturnal hemoglobinuria, some cases of T-cell large granular lymphocytic leukemia *Miscellaneous:* Anaphylactoid shock, hypothyroidism, thyrotoxicosis, hypopituitarism, cirrhosis of the liver, cyclic neutropenia, congenital neutropenias, Chédiak-Higashi syndrome, autoimmune	↑ V Pharmacologic granulocyte colony stimulating factors (G-CSF, GM-CSF), epinephrine, etiochonanolone, endotoxin, insect venoms, glucocorticoids, smoking tobacco, vaccines, lithium ↓ V Agents affecting occasional subjects because of individual sensitivity: *analgesics:* acetaminophen, aminopyrine, dipyrone, nonsteroidal antiinflammatory agents (e.g., ibuprofen, indomethacin, phenylbutazone, oxyphenbutazone); *anticonvulsants:* carbamazepine, ethosuximide, mephenytoin, phenytoin, trimethadione, valproic acid; *antihistamines:* methaphenilene, tripelennamine, brompheneramine; *antimicrobial agents:* cephalosporins, chloramphenicol, clindamycin, cotrimoxazole, gentamicin, imipenem, isoniazid, metronidazole, nitrofurantoin, novobiocin, *p*-aminobenzoic acid, penicillins, streptomycin, sulfonamides, tetracyclines, trimethoprim, vancomycin; *antithyroid agents:* carbimazole, methimazole, propylthiouracil, thiouracil; *antiviral agents:* ganciclovir, zidovudine; *cardiovascular agents:* ajmaline, amiodarone, aprindine, captopril, enalapril, quinidine, rauwolfia, tocainide; *diuretics:* acetazolamide, chlorthalidone, ethacrynic acid, spironolactone, thiazides; *hypoglycemic agents:* carbutamide, chlorpropamide, tolbutamide; *psychotropic agents:* antidepressants (e.g., amitriptyline, desipramine, imipramine, mianserin), barbiturates, benzodiazepines, clozapine, meprobamate, phenothiazines (e.g., chlorpromazine, prochlorperazine, thioridazine); *other agents:* aminoglutethimide,

Continued

TABLE II-18A	LEUKOCYTE DIFFERENTIAL COUNT: DIAGNOSTIC INFORMATION AND INTERFERENCES—CONTINUED

NEUTROPHILIC SERIES[1-3]

↑ NEUTROPHILS (NEUTROPHILIA)	↓ NEUTROPHILS (NEUTROPENIA)	INTERFERENCES
		antimony, cimetidine, cinophen, dapsone, DDT, diethazine, dinitrophenol, gold salts, imatinib mesylate, α- and γ-interferons, methazolamide, mycophenolate mofetil, omeprazole, penicillamine, phenindione, plasmochin, procainamide, pyrithyldione, quinine, ranitidine, tamoxifen, thioglycolic acid, ticlopidine
		↓ V Agents affecting all subjects if given in sufficient dosage: *antineoplastic drugs:* actinomycin D, amsacrine, asparaginase, azathioprine, busulfan, carboplatin, chlorambucil, cisplatin, cyclophosphamide, cytarabine, daunorubicin, dacarbazine, doxorubicin, epirubicin, etoposide, fluorouracil, melphalan, mechlorethamine, mercaptopurine, methotrexate, mitomycin, mitoxantrone, nitrosoureas, plicamycin, thioguanine, vincristine, vinblastine; *other agents:* ethanol

1. Greer JP, Foerster J, Lukens JN, et al: *Wintrobe's clinical hematology,* ed 11, Philadelphia, 2003, Lippincott Williams & Wilkins.

2. Beutler E, Lichtman MA, Coller B, editors: *Williams hematology,* ed 6, New York, 2000, McGraw-Hill.

3. Kjeldsberg C, Elenitoba-Johnson K, Foucar K, et al, editors: *Practical diagnosis of hematologic disorders,* ed 3, Chicago, 2000, ASCP Press.

TABLE II-18B LEUKOCYTE DIFFERENTIAL COUNT: DIAGNOSTIC INFORMATION AND INTERFERENCES

EOSINOPHILIC SERIES[1-3]		
↑ EOSINOPHILS (EOSINOPHILIA)	↓ EOSINOPHILS (EOSINOPENIA)	INTERFERENCES
Allergic disorders: Bronchial asthma, urticaria, angioneurotic edema, hay fever, some instances of drug sensitivity	Infections, labor, eclampsia, major surgery or shock associated with high levels of glucocorticoids	Eosinophilia is a frequent finding with allergic reactions to drugs such as anticonvulsants (e.g., carbamazepine, phenytoin), antimicrobials (cephalosporins,
Skin diseases (especially pemphigus and dermatitis herpetiformis): exfoliative dermatitis, eczema	Bone marrow aplasia	chloramphenicol, erythromycins, penicillins, sulfonamides, tetracyclines, vancomycin), antitubercular drugs, and phenothiazines
Parasitic infestations: Especially parasites that invade the tissues (e.g., trichinosis, echinococcus disease), less regularly in intestinal parasitism		↑ V IL-2 therapy
Infections: Scarlet fever, allergic bronchopulmonary aspergillosis, tuberculosis, coccidioidomycosis; in convalescent phase of other infections		↓ V Corticotropin, epinephrine, glucocorticoids, methysergide, niacin, procainamide
Hematological disorders: Chronic myeloid leukemia, polycythemia vera, Hodgkin lymphoma, after splenectomy, hypereosinophilic syndrome (Loeffler's syndrome), chronic idiopathic myelofibrosis, myelodysplastic syndromes, and acute myeloid leukemias associated with chromosomal abnormalities involving the CBF-β portion of chromosome 16.		
Malignant neoplasms: Especially with metastases or necrosis involving the liver		
Miscellaneous: Eosinophilic myalgia syndrome, pulmonary infiltration with eosinophilia (PIE syndrome), tropical eosinophilia, irradiation, periarteritis nodosa, rheumatoid arthritis, sarcoidosis, certain poisons, smoking, after radiation, contrast media, atheroembolic renal disease, as an inherited anomaly		

1. Greer JP, Foerster J, Lukens JN, et al: *Wintrobe's clinical hematology,* ed 11, Philadelphia, 2003, Lippincott Williams & Wilkins.
2. Beutler E, Lichtman MA, Coller B, editors: *Williams hematology,* ed 6, New York, 2000, McGraw-Hill.
3. Kjeldsberg C, Elenitoba-Johnson K, Foucar K, et al, editors: *Practical diagnosis of hematologic disorders,* ed 3, Chicago, 2000, ASCP Press.

| TABLE II-18C | LEUKOCYTE DIFFERENTIAL COUNT: DIAGNOSTIC INFORMATION AND INTERFERENCES |

BASOPHILIC SERIES[1-3]

↑ BASOPHILS (BASOPHILIA)	↓ BASOPHILS (BASOPENIA)	INTERFERENCES
Allergic or inflammatory disorders: Drug, food or inhalant hypersensitivity, ulcerative colitis, urticaria, juvenile rheumatoid arthritis	Hyperthyroidism, high levels of gluco-corticoids, bone marrow aplasia, ovulation, hypersensitivity reactions	↑ V Estrogens, antithyroid drugs, desipramine
Infections: Chickenpox, influenza, smallpox, tuberculosis		↓ V Corticotropin, glucocorticoids, radiation, procainamide
Endocrine: Diabetes mellitus, estrogen administration, hypothyroidism		↑ C Artifactual increase in measured fraction of basophils when poorly mixed whole blood specimen is analyzed on automatic counter
Hematological disorders: Chronic myeloproliferative disorders (chronic myeloid leukemia, polycythemia vera, essential thrombocythemia, chronic idiopathic myelofibrosis), myelodysplastic/myeloproliferative disorders (chronic myelomonocytic leukemia), acute basophilic leukemia, 5q minus syndrome		
Malignant neoplasms: Rare carcinomas		
Miscellaneous: Renal insufficiency, exposure to ionizing radiation, severe iron deficiency		

1. Greer JP, Foerster J, Lukens JN, et al: *Wintrobe's clinical hematology,* ed 11, Philadelphia, 2003, Lippincott Williams & Wilkins.
2. Beutler E, Lichtman MA, Coller B, editors: *Williams hematology,* ed 6, New York, 2000, McGraw-Hill.
3. Kjeldsberg C, Elenitoba-Johnson K, Foucar K, et al, editors: *Practical diagnosis of hematologic disorders,* ed 3, Chicago, 2000, ASCP Press.

TABLE II-18D LEUKOCYTE DIFFERENTIAL COUNT: DIAGNOSTIC INFORMATION AND INTERFERENCES

LYMPHOCYTIC SERIES[1-3]

↑ LYMPHOCYTES (LYMPHOCYTOSIS)	↓ LYMPHOCYTES (LYMPHOPENIA)	INTERFERENCES
Infections: Mononucleosis-like syndromes (EBV, CMV, acute HIV, HSV II, VZV, toxoplasmosis, adenovirus, acute hepatitis, rubella, roseola, mumps, HHV-6), Bordatella pertussis	*Congenital:* Congenital immunodeficiency syndromes, ataxia telangiectasia, Wiskott-Aldrich syndrome	↑ V Dilantin, smoking tobacco, tetrachlorethane poisoning, organic arsenicals
Drug reactions: Dilantin, PAS, sulfones	*Infections:* HIV/AIDS, influenza, HHV-8, tuberculosis, typhoid fever, sepsis	↓ V Corticotropin, glucocorticoids, radiation, immunosuppressive drugs
Hematological disorders: Chronic lymphoproliferative disorders, lymphomas involving the blood	*Nutritional:* Protein malnutrition, zinc deficiency, vitamin B12 deficiency, folate deficiency	
Malignant neoplasms: Rare carcinomas	*Autoimmune disorders:* Rheumatoid arthritis, systemic lupus erythematosus, myasthenia gravis	
Miscellaneous: Autoimmune disorders, cigarette smoking, chronic inflammation, hyposplenism, sarcoidosis, thymoma, Wegener's granulomatosis, acute stress lymphocytosis (transiently after resuscitated cardiac arrest, septic shock, major surgery, status epilepticus, sickle cell crisis, trauma)	*Iatrogenic:* Immunosuppressive drugs, glucocorticoids, PUVA, cytotoxic chemotherapy	
	Hematologic malignancies: Hodgkin and non-Hodgkin lymphoma	
	Malignant neoplasms: Rare carcinomas	
	Miscellaneous: Renal failure, sarcoidosis, thermal injury, protein-losing enteropathy, radiation exposure	

1. Greer JP, Foerster J, Lukens JN, et al: *Wintrobe's clinical hematology,* ed 11, Philadelphia, 2000, Lippincott Williams & Wilkins.
2. Beutler E, Lichtman MA, Coller B, editors: *Williams hematology,* ed 6, New York, 2000, McGraw-Hill.
3. Kjeldsberg C, Elenitoba-Johnson K, Foucar K, et al, editors: *Practical diagnosis of hematologic disorders,* ed 3, Chicago, 2000, ASCP Press.

TABLE II-18E LEUKOCYTE DIFFERENTIAL COUNT: DIAGNOSTIC INFORMATION AND INTERFERENCES

MONOCYTIC SERIES[1-3]

↑ MONOCYTES (MONOCYTOSIS)	↓ MONOCYTES (MONOPENIA)	INTERFERENCES
Infections: Subacute bacterial endocarditis, during recovery from acute infections, viral, mycotic, rickettsial, and protozoal infections	Bone marrow aplasia, low-grade B-cell lymphoproliferative disorders such as hairy cell leukemia	↑ V GM-CSF, carbon disulfide (poisoning), tetrachlorethane (poisoning), phosphorous (poisoning), griseofulvin, haloperidol, mephenytoin, methsuximide
Granulomatous diseases: Tuberculosis (especially active), syphilis, brucellosis, sarcoidosis, ulcerative colitis		↓ V Glucocorticoids, radiation
Hematological disorders: Acute monocytic leukemia, acute myelomonocytic leukemia, chronic myelomonocytic leukemia, juvenile myelomonocytic leukemia, monosomy 7 syndrome, malignant histiocytosis, myeloproliferative disorders, multiple myeloma, Hodgkin lymphoma and non-Hodgkin lymphomas, neutropenias of various causes, during recovery from aplastic anemia		↑ C Automated differential counting has a higher normal range than manual differential counting
Collagen vascular disease: Lupus erythematosus, rheumatoid arthritis, polyarteritis nodosa, fever of unknown origin		

1. Greer JP, Foerster J, Lukens JN, et al: *Wintrobe's clinical hematology,* ed 11, Philadelphia, 2003, Lippincott Williams & Wilkins.
2. Beutler E, Lichtman MA, Coller B, editors: *Williams hematology,* ed 6, New York, 2000, McGraw-Hill.
3. Kjeldsberg C, Elenitoba-Johnson K, Foucar K, et al, editors: *Practical diagnosis of hematologic disorders,* ed 3, Chicago, 2000, ASCP Press.

TABLE II-19 PLATELET COUNT: INTERFERENCES[1-4]

↑ C Cytoplasmic fragments of leukemic cells in blood counted as platelets, dust in diluent fluid, concentration of EDTA anticoagulant too high (>>2 mg/mL)

↓ C Platelet satellitism (EDTA dependent), platelet agglutination (usually EDTA dependent), platelet clumping caused by activation and incipient clotting in sample, cold agglutinins, abciximab (antiplatelet glycoprotein antibody used in cardiac revascularization), old specimen (platelets swell and degenerate with prolonged exposure to EDTA)

↑ V Acyclovir, alglucerase, aztreonam, cefotetan, ceftazidime, daptomycin, enoxacin, epinephrine, erythropoietin (high dose), metoprolol, miconazole, ofloxacin, penicillamine, propranolol, rifapentine, ticlopidine, vincristine

↓ V The following agents, if given in sufficient dose, affect all subjects

Antineoplastic agents: Actinomycin D, alemtuzumab, asparaginase, azathioprine, busulfan, chlorambucil, cisplatin, cyclophosphamide, cytarabine, dacarbazine, daunorubicin, doxorubicin, epirubicin, etoposide, fludaribine, imatinib, lomustine, mechlorethamine, mercaptopurine, methotrexate, nitrosoureas, plicamycin, procarbazine, thioguanine, vincristine (rare), vinblastine

↓ V The following agents affect only some subjects because of individual sensitivity

Analgesics: Acetaminophen, antipyrine, aspirin, codeine, meperidine, morphine, nonsteroidal antiinflammatory drugs (e.g., ibuprofen, indomethacin, naproxen), oxyphenbutazone, phenacetin, phenylbutazone, sodium salicylate

Antineoplastic agents: Efalizumab, gemcitabine, bortezomib, oxaliplatin, ibritumomab, α-interferon, levamisol, rituximab, tositumomab, tamoxifen

Anticoagulants: Unfractionated heparin, low molecular weight heparins and heparinoids

Anticonvulsants: Carbamazepine, divalproex, ethosuximide, mephenytoin, paramethadione, phenytoin, trimethadione, valproic acid

Antihistamines: Chlorpheniramine, diphenhydramine

Antimicrobial agents: p-Aminosalicylic acid, amphotericin B, azithromycin, cephalosporins, chloramphenicol, clindamycin, cotrimoxazole, erythromycin, gemfloxacin, isoniazid, linzolid, novobiocin, organic arsenicals, penicillin, pyrazinamide, rifampicin, stibophen (Faudin), streptomycin, sulfonamides, tetracyclines, vancomycin, voriconazole

Antithyroid agents: Methimazole, propylthiouracil, thiouracil

Cardiovascular agents: Abciximab, alprenolol, amiodarone, amrinone, captopril, digitoxin, mexiletine, nitroglycerin, oxprenolol, quinidine, reserpine, tocainide

Diuretics: Acetazolamide, bumetanide, diazoxide, furosemide, mercurial diuretics, thiazides, triamterene

Heavy metals: Bismuth, copper, gold compounds, silver

Hypoglycemic agents: Carbutamide, chlorpropamide, glibenclamide, insulin, tolbutamine

Psychotropic agents: Antidepressants (e.g., amitriptyline, desipramine), barbiturates, meprobamate, phenothiazines (e.g., chlorpromazine, trifluoperazine)

Other agents: Alcohol, allopurinol, azathioprin, chloroquine, cimetidine, colchicine, cyclosporin, dextroamphetamine, dinitrophenol, ergot, estrogens, ganciclovir, heparin, hydroxychloroquine, methyldopa, mycophenolate mofetil, penicillamine, potassium iodide, prednisone, procaine, quinine, ranitidine, saquinavir, sirolimus, ticlopidine, valgancyclovir, vitamin K

1. Rodak BF, editor: *Hematology: clinical principles and applications,* ed 2, Philadelphia, 2002, WB Saunders.
2. Kjeldsberg C, Elenitoba-Johnson K, Foucar K, et al, editors: *Practical diagnosis of hematologic disorders,* ed 3, Chicago, 2000, ASCP Press.
3. Legrand O, Perrot J-Y, Baudard M, et al: The immunophenotype of 177 adults with acute myeloid leukemia, *Blood* 96:870-877, 2000.
4. RxList, LLC: Available at: http://www.rxlist.com.

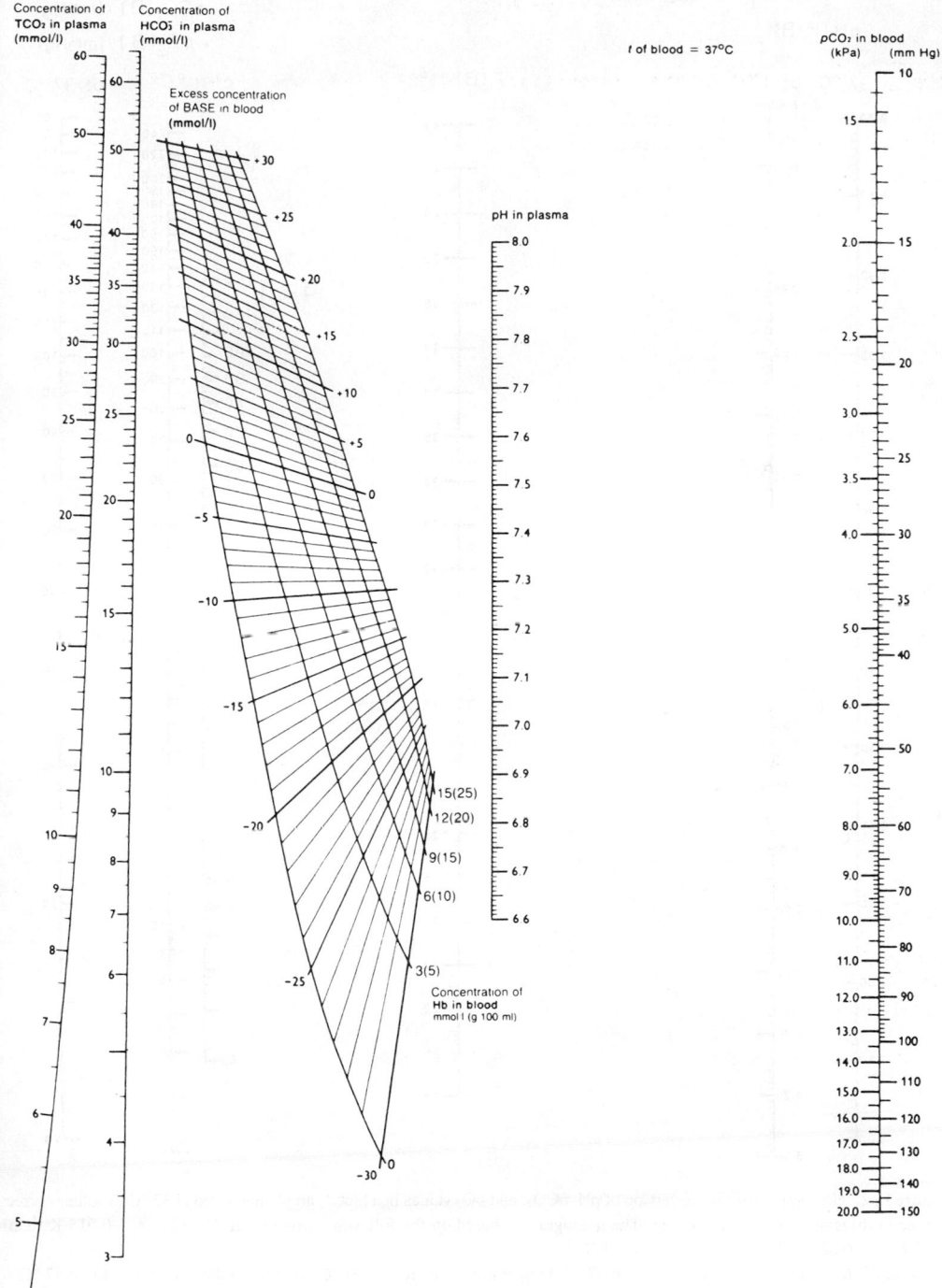

Figure II-1. The Siggard-Andersen alignment nomogram for the calculation of acid-base parameters. Modified from Radiometer A/S, Copenhagen, Demark.

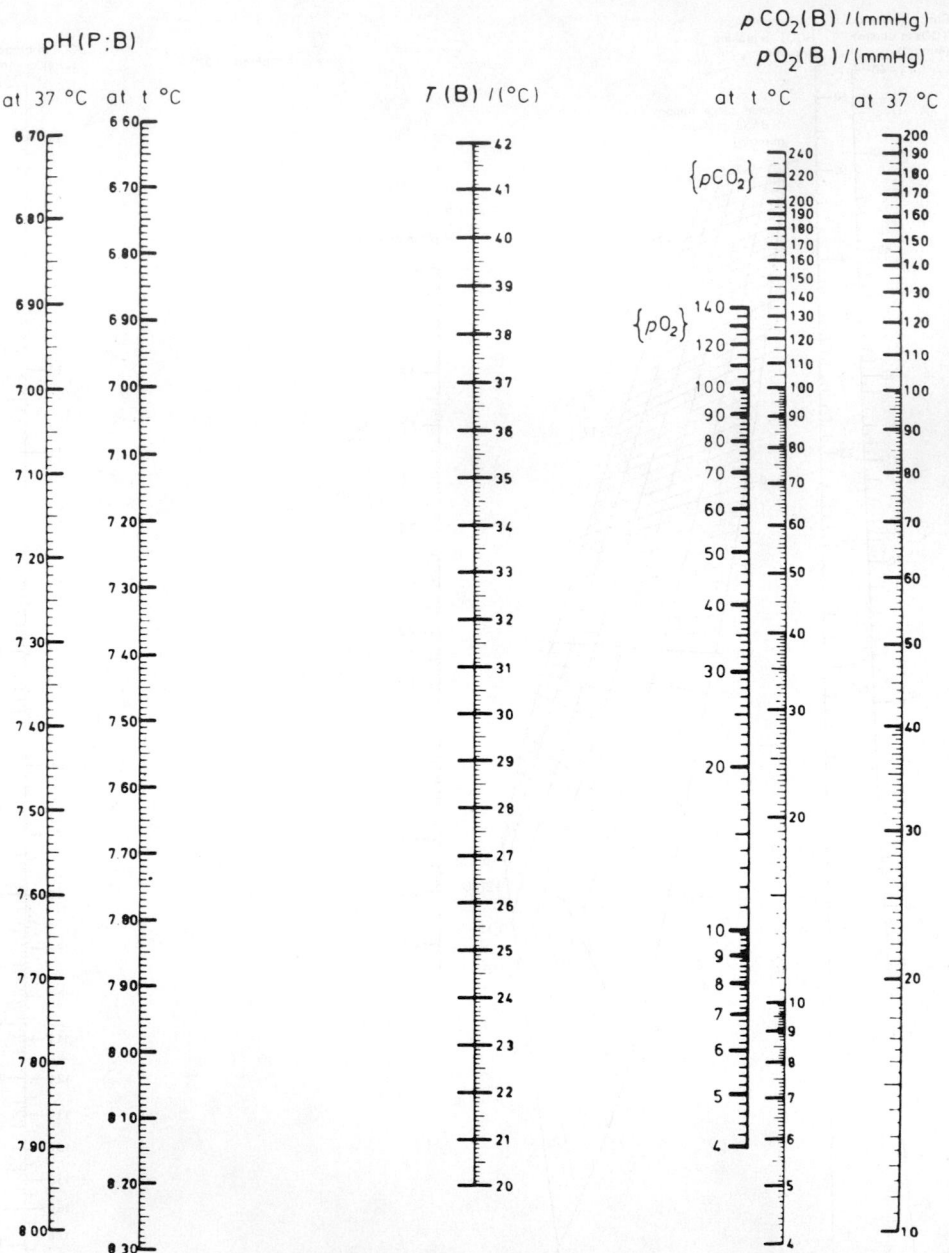

Figure II-2. Nomogram for the conversion of pH, pCO_2, and pO_2 values in a blood sample measured at 37 °C to values corrected for the body temperature of the patient. The nomogram is based on the following formulas: $\Delta pH(P)/\Delta T = -0.015 \text{ K}^{-1}$; $\Delta \log pCO_2/\Delta T = 0.021 \text{ K}^{-1}$; $\Delta \log pO_2/\Delta T = 0.031 \text{ K}^{-1}$.

Example: Measured $pCO_2 = 60$ mm Hg at 37 °C, temperature of patient = 31 °C. Find 60 on the scale for pCO_2 at 37 °C.

Find 31 on the temperature scale. Place line between the two points and read pCO_2 on the scale for pCO_2 at t °C (here 45 mm Hg). The procedure is similar for pO_2 and pH.

From Siggaard-Andersen O: Titratable acid or base of body fluids. Ann. N.Y. Acad. Sci., *133:* 41-58, 1966.

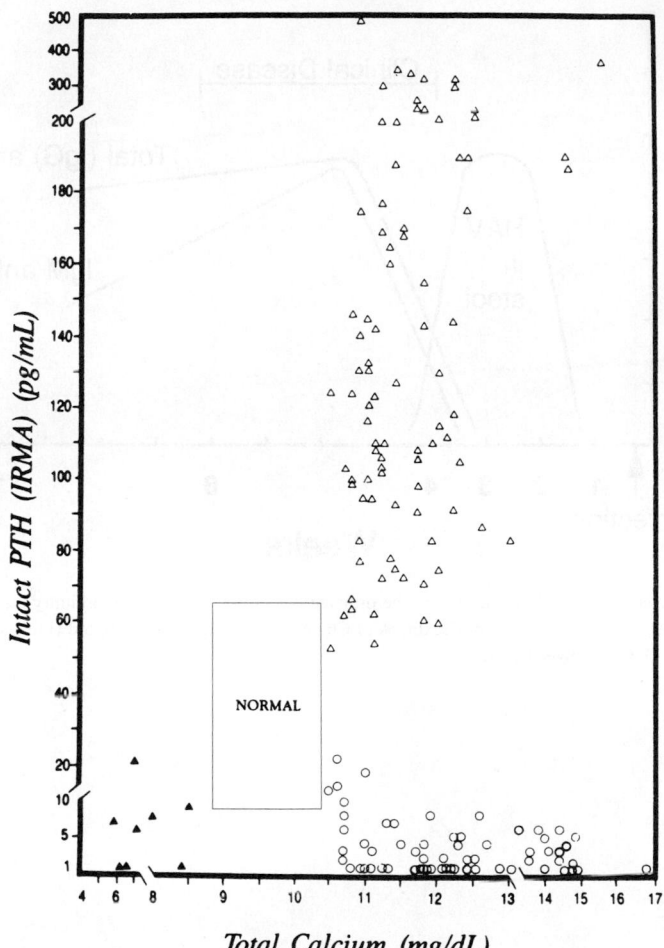

Figure II-3. Analysis of intact PTH (IRMA) vs. total calcium in various disease states. Reproduced with permission from: Pandian, M.R., Lavigne, J.R., Carlton, E.I., et al: Immunoradiometric Assay for Intact PTH: A New Generation of PTH Assay for Assessment of Parathyroid Function. San Juan Capistrano, CA, Nichols Institute Reference Laboratories, 1989.

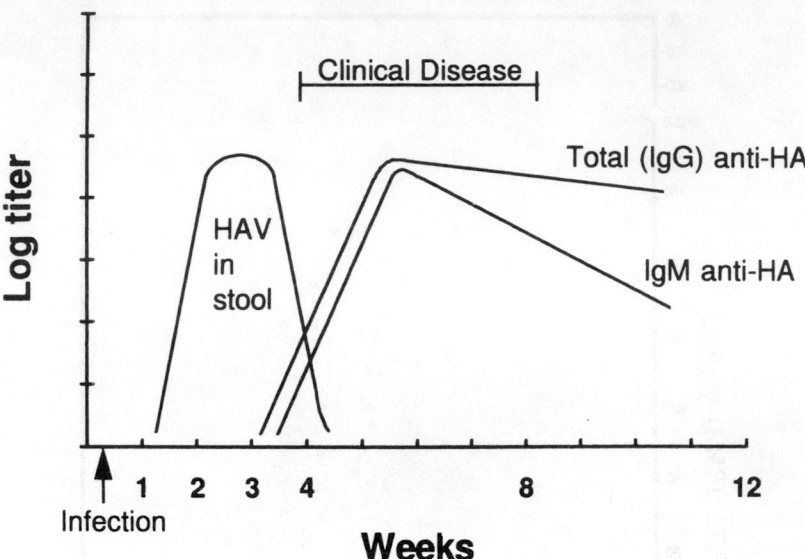

Figure II-4. Schematic course of an HAV infection. The ordinate is a logarithmic scale of arbitrary units. From McIntyre, N., Benhamou, J.-P., Bircher, J., et al. (Eds.): Oxford Textbook of Clinical Hepatology, Vol. 1. Oxford University Press, 1991. Reproduced by permission of Oxford University Press.

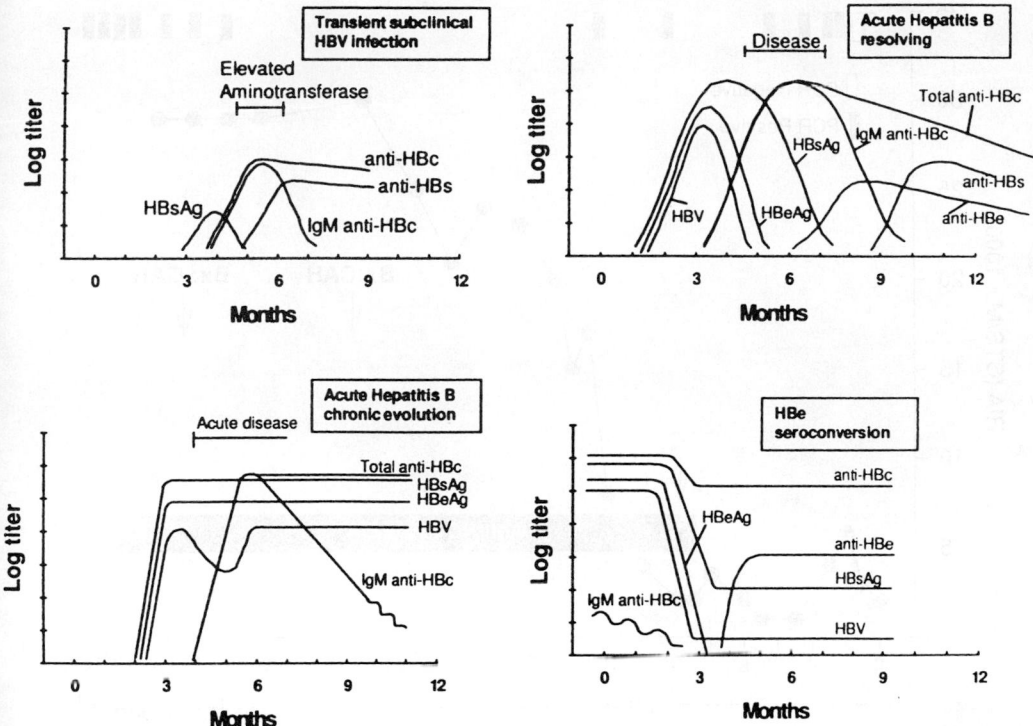

Figure II-5. Schematic serological profiles of HBV infections. The magnitude of the serological parameters is given in arbitrary units. From McIntyre, N., Benhamou, J.-P., Bircher, J., et al. (Eds.): Oxford Textbook of Clinical Hepatology, Vol. 1. Oxford, Oxford University Press, 1991. Reproduced by permission of Oxford University Press.

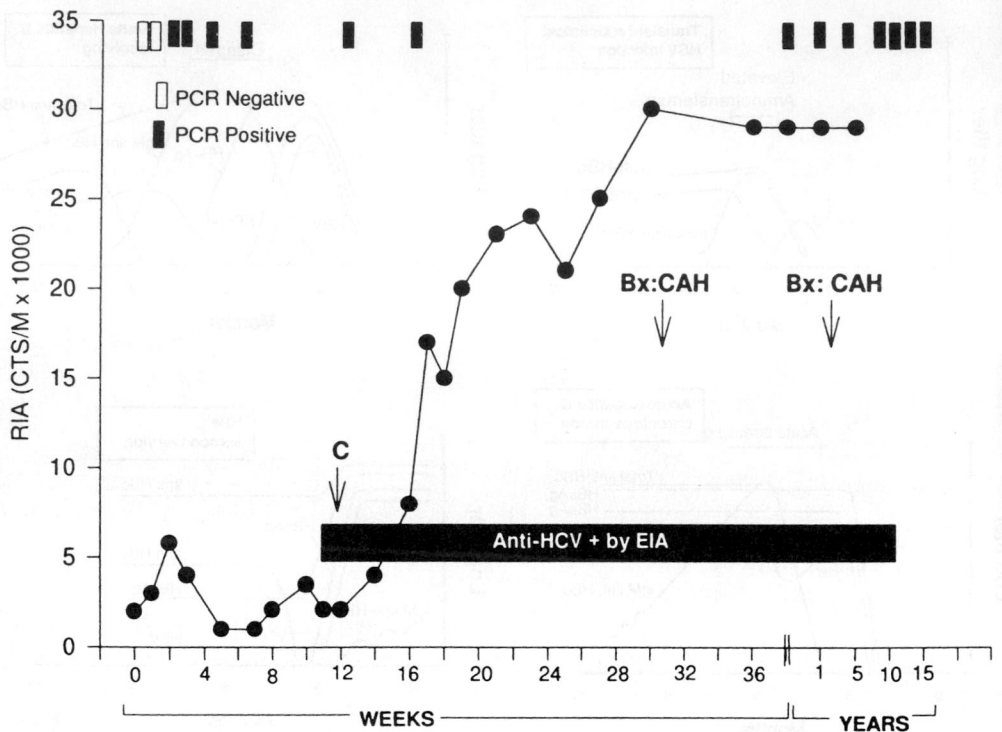

Figure II-6. Sequence of events in a patient with post-transfusion hepatitis C virus infection. The patient had the transfusion at time zero. Clinical hepatitis occurred from weeks 9 to 22. The solid circles indicate the onset and duration of antibody to the hepatitis C virus *(anti-HCV)* as measured by radioimmunoassay *(RIA)*. The horizontal bar indicates the onset and duration of anti-HCV as measured by enzyme immunoassay *(EIA)*. Polymerase chain reactivity *(PCR)* was noted 2 weeks after exposure and 9 weeks before the first appearance of anti-HCV. (C = infectivity established by chimp inoculation; Bx = liver biopsy; CAH = chronic active hepatitis.) Reproduced with permission and modified from Alter, H.J.: Descartes before the horse: I clone, therefore I am: The hepatitis C virus in current perspective. Ann. Intern. Med., *115:* 644-649, 1991.

SECTION III
MOLECULAR DIAGNOSTICS

PART A: MOLECULAR METHODS

TEST METHOD	SPECIMEN AND SPECIAL REQUIREMENTS	CLINICAL COMMENTS AND REMARKS
Fluorescence In Situ Hybridization (FISH)[1]	Interphase FISH: Fixed tissue sections, exfoliated cells (smears or cytospin preparations). Samples must adhere to glass microscopic slides.	FISH localizes identified targets at the cellular or chromosome level. Traditional metaphase FISH is performed on chromosome spreads created from synchronizing cells in culture. Interphase FISH can be applied to routinely fixed histological and cytological specimens and to archived paraffin-embedded tissue samples.
	Metaphase FISH: Chromosome spreads.	Test time: 2-7 days

1. Levsky JM, Singer RH: Fluorescence in situ hybridization: past, present, and future, *J Cell Sci* 116:2833-2838, 2003.

Forensic/Criminal Identity Testing *PCR, Southern blot, RFLP*	Body fluids, tissue. Store all body fluids at 4° C and all tissue at ≤−20° C until nucleic acids are isolated. Store isolated nucleic acids at ≤−20° C.	DNA testing supersedes traditional genotyping because of increased discriminatory power, application to a variety of biologic sources, and DNA resistance to environmental factors. Most techniques assay for variable number tandem repeat (VNTR) loci.[1,4-8]
Paternity Testing[1] *Southern blot, PCR*	Whole blood (ACD or EDTA), chorionic villi, and amniocytes. Store all body fluids at 4° C and cells at ≤−20° C until nucleic acids are isolated. Store isolated nucleic acids at ≤−20° C.	Multilocus probing provides unique individual identification and is more informative than single locus probing. A variety of probes have been used for both multilocus and single-locus probing.
Tissue Typing[1-3] *PCR*		HLA class II genes (HLA-DR, -DQ, and -DP) are highly polymorphic, and subtyping is readily achieved.

1. Devlin B, Rische N: Ethnic differentiation at VNTR loci, with special reference to forensic applications, *Am J Hum Genet* 51:534-548, 1993.

2. Mies C: Molecular pathology of paraffin-embedded tissue: current clinical applications, *Diagn Mol Pathol* 1:206-211, 1992.

3. Wilson LJ, Horvat RT, Tilzer L, et al: Identification of donor melanoma in a renal transplant recipient, *Diagn Mol Pathol* 1:266-271, 1992.

4. Comey CT, Budowle B, Adams DE, et al: PCR amplification and typing of the HDL Dqa gene in forensic samples, *J Forensic Sci* 38:230-249, 1993.

5. Hagleberg E, Gray IC, Jeffreys AJ: Identification of the skeletal remains of a murder victim by DNA analysis, *Nature* 252:427-429, 1991.

6. Harding RM, Boyce AJ, Clegg JB: The evolution of tandemly repetitive DNA: recombinational rules, *Genetics* 132:847-859, 1992.

7. Honma M, Yoshii T, Ishiyama I, et al: Individual identification from semen by the deoxyribonucleic acid (DNA) fingerprint technique, *J Forensic Sci* 34:222-227, 1989.

8. Tsongalis GJ, Coleman WB, Esch GL, et al: Identification of human DNA in complex biological samples using the Alu polymerase chain reaction, *J Forensic Sci* 38:961-967, 1993.

TEST METHOD	SPECIMEN AND SPECIAL REQUIREMENTS	CLINICAL COMMENTS AND REMARKS
In Situ Hybridization (ISH)[1]	Fixed tissue sections, exfoliated cells (smears or cytospin preparations). Samples must adhere to glass microscopic slides. Chromogenic detection of target sequences.	Because ISH occurs localized at the cellular level, it allows direct correlation of molecular data with a pathological process. Another advantage is its applicability to routinely fixed histological and cytological specimens and to archived paraffin-embedded tissue samples. However, compared with other molecular techniques, ISH has low sensitivity. ISH is most useful for detecting targets such as viruses in infected cells, which are present in high copy numbers. Test time: 3-7 days

1.   Qian X, Lloyd RV: Recent developments in signal amplification methods for in situ hybridization, *Diagn Mol Pathol* 12:1-13, 2003.

TEST METHOD	SPECIMEN AND SPECIAL REQUIREMENTS	CLINICAL COMMENTS AND REMARKS

In Vitro Amplification
 	
I. Sequence Amplification
  1. Polymerase chain reaction (PCR)[1]
  2. Transcription-mediated amplification (TMA)[2]
  3. Nucleic acid sequence based amplification (NASBA)[3]
  4. Strand displacement amplification (SDA)[4]
  5. Real-time PCR[5]
II. Signal Amplification
  Branched-chain DNA (bDNA)[6]
  Hybrid capture (HC)[7]
  Invader[8]
	Isolated nucleic acids (DNA or RNA). Crude cell lysates, serum, and whole blood may be used directly. Avoid anticoagulants. Nucleic acids should be stored frozen at $\leq -20°$ C.
	
	Heparin and heme are strong inhibitors of enzymatic reactions; citrate and EDTA are acceptable anticoagulants.
		Although traditional PCR was the first in vitro amplification technology to become widely used, many modifications to the PCR have been developed. The most common of these has become the real-time PCR or kinetic amplification technologies. Other in vitro amplification technologies have also been developed and have been applied to specific test types using specific instrumentation.
		
		Test time: 1-6 hr

1.   Baumforth KRN, Nelson PN, Digby JE, et al: The polymerase chain reaction, *J Clin Pathol Mol Pathol* 52:1-10, 1999.

2.   Gorrin G, Friesenhahn M, Lin P, et al: Performance evaluation of the VERSANT HCV RNA qualitative assay by using transcription mediated amplification, *J Clin Microbiol* 41:310-317, 2003.

3.   Deiman B, van Aarle P, Sillekens P: Characteristics and applications of nucleic acid sequence-based amplification (NASBA), *Mol Biotechnol* 20:163-180, 2002.

4.   Hellyer TJ, Nadeau JG: Strand displacement amplification: a versatile tool for molecular diagnostics, *Expert Rev Mol Diagn* 4:251-261, 2004.

5.   Wilhelm J, Pingoud A: Real-time polymerase chain reaction, *Chem Biochem* 4:1120-1128, 2003.

6.   Dewar RL, Highbarger HC, Sarmiento MD, et al: Application of branched DNA signal amplification to monitor human immunodeficiency virus type 1 burden in human plasma, *J Infect Dis* 170:1172-1179, 1994.

7.   Hubbard RA: Human papillomavirus testing methods, *Arch Pathol Lab Med* 127:940-945, 2003.

8.   de Arruda M, Lyamichev VI, Eis PS, et al: Invader technology for DNA and RNA analysis: principles and applications, *Expert Rev Mol Diagn* 2:487-496, 2002.

TEST METHOD	SPECIMEN AND SPECIAL REQUIREMENTS	CLINICAL COMMENTS AND REMARKS
Laser Capture Microdissection (LCM)[1,2]	Frozen or fixed tissue sections, cytology smears, or cytospin preparations.	LCM allows for the isolation of specific cell types from complex tissues or mixtures of cells. Once captured, the specimen can be used for isolation of nucleic acids or proteins. Test time: within 1 hr

1. Fend F, Raffeld M: Laser capture microdissection in pathology, *J Clin Pathol* 53:666-672, 2000.
2. Best CJ, Emmert-Buck MR: Molecular profiling of tissue samples using laser capture microdissection, *Expert Rev Mol Diagn* 1:53-60, 2001.

TEST METHOD	SPECIMEN AND SPECIAL REQUIREMENTS	CLINICAL COMMENTS AND REMARKS
Line Probe Assays (LiPA)[1,2]	This detection method is typically preceded by a PCR-based amplification of target sequences.	LiPA has become a routine detection method of PCR products for use in genotyping. Currently the most common application of this technology is for cystic fibrosis genotyping and hepatitis C virus genotyping. The method is designed as a reverse hybridization whereby probes are immobilized to a membrane and denatured PCR products are applied. Test time: 1-4 hr

1. Podzorski RP: Molecular testing in the diagnosis and management of hepatitis C virus infection, *Arch Pathol Lab Med* 126:285-290, 2002.
2. Lewis MJ, Lewis EH, Amos JA, et al: Cystic fibrosis, *Am J Clin Pathol* 120:S3-S13, 2003.

TEST METHOD	SPECIMEN AND SPECIAL REQUIREMENTS	CLINICAL COMMENTS AND REMARKS
Northern Blot	RNA isolated from tissue, cells, or RNA viruses	Test time: 5-7 days The Northern blot technique is preferentially utilized to determine gene expression levels by quantifying mRNA levels. Use extreme caution when isolating and examining RNA because RNAses are extremely stable and so resist many chemical treatments used in the extraction.

TEST METHOD	SPECIMEN AND SPECIAL REQUIREMENTS	CLINICAL COMMENTS AND REMARKS
Paternity Testing[1] *Southern blot, PCR*	Whole blood (ACD or EDTA), chorionic villi, and amniocytes. Store all body fluids at 4° C and cells at ≤−20° C until nucleic acids are isolated. Store isolated nucleic acids at ≤−20° C.	Multilocus probing provides unique individual identification and is more informative than single-locus probing. A variety of probes have been used for both multilocus and single-locus probing.

1. Devlin B, Risch N: Ethnic differences at VNTR loci, with special reference to forensic applications, *Am J Hum Genet* 51:534-548, 1992.

TEST METHOD	SPECIMEN AND SPECIAL REQUIREMENTS	CLINICAL COMMENTS AND REMARKS
Polymerase Chain Reaction (PCR)	Isolated nucleic acids (DNA or RNA). Crude cell lysates, serum, and whole blood may be used directly. Avoid anticoagulants. Nucleic acids should be stored frozen at $\leq -20°$ C. Heparin and heme are strong inhibitors of PCR; citrate and EDTA are acceptable anticoagulants.	Test time: 4-6 hr PCR allows amplification of specific sequences of DNA or RNA, thus making possible the identification and quantification of the sequences, for instance, as they occur in infectious agents or mRNA. PCR has the greatest sensitivity of current molecular techniques and is easily performed. Great caution is required to eliminate risk of contamination with extraneous DNA or RNA so that factitious amplification is avoided. Oligonucleotide (primer) synthesis is only possible if the DNA sequence is known and available.
Restriction Fragment Length Polymorphism (RFLP)[1]	DNA isolated from tissue or cells	RFLP analysis is easily performed and provides direct analysis of DNA for polymorphisms or mutations that alter restriction enzyme recognition sites. Mutations and polymorphisms arise from single base changes and also from deletions or insertions of DNA. This type of analysis is dependent on a known gene sequence, known alteration, and known restriction enzyme recognition site. RFLP analysis can also be used for genetic linkage studies to establish carrier (heterozygous) status in kindreds of individuals known to be afflicted with specific genetic disorders. Test time: 1-2 days

1.   Todd R, Donoff RB, Kim Y, et al: From the chromosome to DNA: restriction fragment length polymorphism analysis and its clinical application, *J Oral Maxillofac Surg* 59:660-667, 2001.

Sequencing[1,2]	DNA resulting from an in vitro amplification method or reverse-transcriptase polymerase chain reaction.	DNA sequencing typically was used for the confirmation of genetic alterations identified by other molecular methods. The advent of highly automated capillary electrophoretic systems and the changes in sequencing chemistries have resulted in this technology becoming mainstream. Direct sequencing approaches can be found in applications to genetic diseases, oncology, and infectious diseases. Test time: 2-8 days

1.   Marziali A, Akeson M: New DNA sequencing methods, *Annu Rev Biomed Eng* 3:195-223, 2001.

2.   Kim Y, Donoff RB, Wong DTW, et al: The nucleotide: DNA sequencing and its clinical application, *J Oral Maxillofac Surg* 60:924-930, 2002.

TEST METHOD	SPECIMEN AND SPECIAL REQUIREMENTS	CLINICAL COMMENTS AND REMARKS
Southern Blot[1,2]	DNA isolated from tissues or cells	The Southern blot technique is used to detect the presence of DNA sequences in total isolated DNA. It requires digestion with specific restriction enzymes. Mutations such as deletions and insertions, as well as mutations that alter the recognition site for the restriction enzyme, can be detected. The technique also allows distinction of integrated from episomal DNA. It is used to establish presence of specific gene rearrangements within or between chromosomes as occurs in clones of malignant cells. Test time: 4-8 days

1. Borst M, Miller DM: DNA isolation and Southern analysis: a clinician's view, *Am J Med Sci* 299:356-360, 1990.
2. Southern EM: Detection of specific sequences among DNA fragments separated by gel electrophoresis, *J Mol Biol* 95:503-517, 1975.

TEST METHOD	SPECIMEN AND SPECIAL REQUIREMENTS	CLINICAL COMMENTS AND REMARKS
Tissue Typing for Identity Testing[1-3] *PCR*	Whole blood (ACD or EDTA), tissue. Store all body fluids at 4° C and cells at $\leq -20°$ C until nucleic acids are isolated. Store isolated nucleic acids at $\leq -20°$ C.	HLA class II genes (HLD-DR, -DQ, and -DP) are highly polymorphic, and subtyping is readily achieved.

1. Devlin B, Risch N: Ethnic differences at VNTR loci, with special reference to forensic applications, *Am J Hum Genet* 51:534-548, 1992.
2. Mies C: Molecular pathology of paraffin-embedded tissue: current clinical applications, *Diagn Mol Pathol* 1:206-211, 1992.
3. Wilson LJ, Horvat RT, Tilzer L, et al: Identification of donor melanoma in a renal transplant recipient, *Diagn Mol Pathol* 1:266-271, 1992.

PART B: MOLECULAR TESTS

DISORDER	SPECIMEN AND SPECIAL REQUIREMENTS	CLINICAL COMMENTS AND REMARKS
Adenovirus, Enteric (EA)[1,2] *PCR, Real-time PCR, RFLP, Southern blot*	Serum, stool, eye swab, and respiratory tract specimens. Store all body fluids at 4° C; store tissue at $\leq -20°$ C.	The serotype determines the extent of disease. Pathology includes gastroenteritis, upper and lower respiratory infections, and conjunctivitis. The virus has oncogenic potential. Target: Hexon gene

1. McDonough M, Kew O, Hierholzer J: PCR detection of human adenoviruses. In Persing DH, Smith TF, Tenover FC, et al, editors: *Diagnostic molecular microbiology: principles and applications,* Washington, DC, 1993, ASM Press. pp. 389-393.
2. Wilhelmi I, Roman E, Sanchez-Fauquier A: Viruses causing gastroenteritis, *Clin Microbiol Infect* 9:247-262, 2003.

DISORDER	SPECIMEN AND SPECIAL REQUIREMENTS	CLINICAL COMMENTS AND REMARKS
Angelman Syndrome[1] *Chromosome 15q-q13 (γ-aminobutyric acid receptor subunit genes), ubiquitin-protein ligase E3A (UBE3A) gene*	Whole blood (ACD or EDTA), tissue. Store whole blood at room temperature or 4° C; store tissue frozen at $\leq -20°$ C if nucleic acids cannot be immediately extracted.	Approximately 70% of patients show a deletion involving the maternally inherited chromosome 15q11-q13, whereas others show either chromosome 15 paternal uniparental disomy, mutations in the imprinting center, or intragenic mutations of the ubiquitin-protein ligase E3A (UBE3A) gene.

1. Guerrini R, Carrozzo R, Rinaldi R, et al: Angelman syndrome: etiology, clinical features, diagnosis, and management of symptoms, *Paediatr Drugs* 5:647-661, 2003.

DISORDER	SPECIMEN AND SPECIAL REQUIREMENTS	CLINICAL COMMENTS AND REMARKS
α_1-Antitrypsin (α_1-AT, AAT) Deficiency[1,2] *PCR, Real-time PCR, RFLP, Southern blot*	Whole blood (ACD or EDTA), tissue. Store whole blood at room temperature or 4° C; store tissue frozen at $\leq -20°$ C if nucleic acids cannot be immediately extracted.	The Z mutation in the α_1-antitrypsin gene accounts for the vast majority of symptomatic disease. A primary screen for the disease can be performed with the quantitative AAT protein test in plasma or serum.

1. DeMeo DL, Silverman EK: Alpha1-antitrypsin deficiency. 2: Genetic aspects of alpha(1)-antitrypsin deficiency: phenotypes and genetic modifiers of emphysema risk, *Thorax* 59:259-264, 2004.
2. Lomas DA, Parfrey H: Alpha1-antitrypsin deficiency. 4: Molecular pathophysiology, *Thorax* 59:529-535, 2004.

DISORDER	SPECIMEN AND SPECIAL REQUIREMENTS	CLINICAL COMMENTS AND REMARKS
Astrocytoma[1] *FISH, Comparative genomic hybridization, PCR, Southern blot*	Tissue (fresh, frozen, or paraffin-embedded)	The most common genetic abnormality in astrocytoma is a gain of chromosome 7 copy number. This may result in overexpression of platelet-derived growth factor A (PDGFA). Target: Chromosome 7 (aneuploidy)

1. Shapiro JR: Genetic alterations associated with adult diffuse astrocytic tumors, *Am J Med Genet* 115:194-201, 2002.

Ataxia[1,2] *Southern blot, PCR, Sequencing*	Whole blood (ACD or EDTA), tissue. Store whole blood at room temperature or 4° C; store tissue frozen at $\leq-20°$ C if nucleic acids cannot be immediately extracted.	The spinocerebellar ataxias (SCAs) are hereditary neurodegenerative disorders. The ataxias, characterized by mutations in the genes listed above, all exhibit an autosomal dominant mode of inheritance except Friedreich ataxia (autosomal recessive). Target: SCA1, SCA2, SCA3, SCA6, SCA7, SCA8, SCA12, SCA17, Friedreich ataxia, and dentatorubral-pallidoluysian atrophy (DRPLA)

1. Schols L, Bauer P, Schmidt T, et al: Autosomal dominant cerebellar ataxias: clinical features, genetics, and pathogenesis, *Lancet Neurol* 3:291-304, 2004.
2. Pandolfo M: Friedreich ataxia, *Semin Pediatr Neurol* 10:163-172, 2003.

Bacteria, Molecular Typing[1,2] *Pulsed field gel electrophoresis, repPCR*	Cultured organisms	This form of testing is used to assess nosocomial infections, epidemiologic tracking of infections, and recurrence of infection in the same patient. Target: bacterial DNA fingerprinting

1. Tenover FC, Arbeit RD, Goering RV: How to select and interpret molecular strain typing methods for epidemiological studies of bacterial infections: a review for healthcare epidemiologists. Molecular Typing Working Group of the Society for Healthcare Epidemiology of America, *Infect Control Hosp Epidemiol* 18:426-439, 1997.
2. Zaidi N, Konstatinou K, Zervos M: The role of molecular biology and nucleic acid technology in the study of human infection and epidemiology, *Arch Pathol Lab Med* 127:1098-1105, 2003.

DISORDER	SPECIMEN AND SPECIAL REQUIREMENTS	CLINICAL COMMENTS AND REMARKS
BK Virus[1,2] *PCR, Real-time PCR*	CSF, plasma, urine, and tissue (brain or kidney; fresh, frozen, or paraffin-embedded). Store all body fluids at 4° C; store tissue at ≤−20° C.	BKV persists in latent form and activated in immunocompromised hosts. Responsible mostly for genitourinary tract symptoms. Target: small and large T region

1. Pahari A, Rees L: BK virus-associated renal problems: clinical implications, *Pediatr Nephrol* 18:743-748, 2003.
2. Behzad-Behbahani A, Klapper PE, Vallely PJ, et al: Detection of BK virus and JC virus DNA in urine samples from immunocompromised (HIV-infected) and immunocompetent (HIV-non-infected) patients using polymerase chain reaction and microplate hybridization, *J Clin Virol* 29:224-229, 2004.

DISORDER	SPECIMEN AND SPECIAL REQUIREMENTS	CLINICAL COMMENTS AND REMARKS
Bladder Cancer[1,2] *Methods: FISH, PCR, Sequencing* *UroVysion*	Tissue (fresh, frozen, or paraffin-embedded), liquid cytology specimens	Many abnormalities have been identified in the development of bladder cancer. These include chromosome abnormalities and mutations in numerous proto-oncogenes and tumor suppressor genes. MTS1 is an oncogene located on chromosome 9 and is associated with point mutations and allelic loss in pancreatic and esophageal cancers as well. Targets: P16/CDKN2A/MTSI (LOH), P53/TP53

1. Al-Sukhun S, Hussain M: Molecular biology of transitional cell carcinoma, *Crit Rev Oncol Hematol* 47:181-193, 2003.
2. Bubendorf L, Grilli B, Sauter G, et al: Multiprobe FISH for enhanced detection of bladder cancer in voided urine specimens and bladder washings, *Am J Clin Pathol* 116:79-86, 2001.

DISORDER	SPECIMEN AND SPECIAL REQUIREMENTS	CLINICAL COMMENTS AND REMARKS
Bloom Syndrome[1,2] *PCR, Sequencing*	Whole blood (ACD or EDTA), tissue. Store whole blood at room temperature or 4° C; store tissue frozen at ≤−20° C if nucleic acids cannot be immediately extracted.	Approximately 98% of Bloom syndrome patients have the 2281del6bp/ins7bp mutations in the BLM gene. Target: BLM (DNA helicase RecQ protein-like 3)

1. Kaneko H, Kondo N: Clinical features of Bloom syndrome and function of the causative gene, BLM helicase, *Expert Rev Mol Diagn* 4:393-401, 2004.
2. Hickson ID: RecQ helicases: caretakers of the genome, *Nat Rev Cancer* 3:169-178, 2003.

DISORDER	SPECIMEN AND SPECIAL REQUIREMENTS	CLINICAL COMMENTS AND REMARKS
Bordetella pertussis[1-3] PCR, *Real-time PCR,* *Blotting*	Nasopharyngeal aspirates or secretions	*Bordetella pertussis* is the organism responsible for whooping cough. Real-time PCR assays can provide a rapid turnaround time with increased sensitivity and specificity. Target: IS481

1. Parton R: Review of the biology of Bordetella pertussis, *Biologicals* 27:71-76, 1999.
2. Dragsted DM, Dohn B, Madsen J, et al: Comparison of culture and PCR for detection of Bordetella pertussis and Bordetella parapertussis under routine laboratory conditions, *J Med Microbiol* 53:749-754, 2004.
3. Fry NK, Tziyra O, Li YT, et al: Laboratory diagnosis of pertussis infections: the role of PCR and serology, *J Med Microbiol* 53:519-525, 2004.

DISORDER	SPECIMEN AND SPECIAL REQUIREMENTS	CLINICAL COMMENTS AND REMARKS
Borrelia burgdorferi[1-3] PCR, *Probe hybridization,* *Real-time PCR*	Whole blood, joint fluid, urine, and ticks	*Borrelia burgdorferi* is the organism associated with Lyme disease. Various tick vectors have been identified since the initial findings in deer ticks. Other tick-borne diseases may also be detected in a similar fashion. Target: groEL, recA, fla ospA

1. Parola P, Raoult D: Ticks and tickborne bacterial diseases in humans: an emerging infectious threat, *Clin Infect Dis* 32:897-928, 2001.
2. Park HS, Lee JH, Jeong EJ, et al: Rapid identification of Borrelia burgdorferi Sensu Alto by PCR-restriction fragment length polymorphism analysis of groEL gene, *Microbiol Immunol* 48:893-897, 2004.
3. Exner MM, Lewinski MA: Isolation and detection of Borrelia burgdorferi DNA from cerebral spinal fluid, synovial fluid, blood, urine, and ticks using the Roche MagNA Pure system and real time PCR, *Diagn Microbiol Infect Dis* 46:235-239, 2003.

DISORDER	SPECIMEN AND SPECIAL REQUIREMENTS	CLINICAL COMMENTS AND REMARKS
Breast Cancer[1,2] *FISH, Immunohisto-* *chemistry*	Tissue (frozen or paraffin-embedded).	Of the many abnormalities that have been identified in the development of breast cancer, only a small number have made it into the clinical laboratory. Gene patents for hereditary and sporadic cancers have limited laboratory testing opportunities. New laboratory testing may evolve from the need to identify therapeutic targets. Targets: HER2/neu (ERBB2), c-Myc, cyclin D1/CCND1/PRAD1, E-cadherin

1. Popescu NC, Zimonjic DB: Chromosome and gene alterations in breast cancer as markers for diagnosis and prognosis as well as pathogenetic targets for therapy, *Am J Med Genet* 115:142-149, 2002.
2. Ross JS, Fletcher JA, Bloom KJ, et al: HER-2/neu testing in breast cancer, *Am J Clin Pathol* 120:S53-S71, 2003.

DISORDER	SPECIMEN AND SPECIAL REQUIREMENTS	CLINICAL COMMENTS AND REMARKS
Burkitt's Lymphoma[1,2] *PCR, FISH, Southern blot*	Whole blood, bone marrow, and tissue (fresh, frozen, or paraffin-embedded).	In this form of cancer, the c-Myc proto-oncogene on chromosome 8 is juxtaposed proximal to the immunoglobulin enhancer sequences. This results in constitutive expression of the c-Myc. Targets: c-Myc, t(8;14), Epstein-Barr virus (EBV)

1. Campo E: Genetic and molecular genetic studies in the diagnosis of B-cell lymphomas I: Mantle cell lymphoma, follicular lymphoma, and Burkitt's lymphoma, *Hum Pathol* 34:330-335, 2003.
2. Kuppers R: B cells under influence: transformation of B cells by Epstein-Barr virus, *Nat Rev Immunol* 3:801-812, 2003.

DISORDER	SPECIMEN AND SPECIAL REQUIREMENTS	CLINICAL COMMENTS AND REMARKS
Canavan Disease[1] *PCR, Sequencing*	Whole blood (ACD or EDTA), tissue. Store whole blood at room temperature or 4° C; store tissue frozen at $\leq -20°$ C if nucleic acids cannot be immediately extracted.	This is a progressive CNS disorder for which carrier screening is highly recommended if one person of a couple is of Ashkenazi Jewish ancestry. Two founder mutations account for a 1/40 carrier frequency Target: Aspartoacylase (APA)

1. Surendran S, Michals-Matalon K, Quast MJ, et al: Canavan disease: a monogenic trait with complex genomic interaction, *Mol Genet Metab* 80:74-80, 2003.

DISORDER	SPECIMEN AND SPECIAL REQUIREMENTS	CLINICAL COMMENTS AND REMARKS
Cervical and Endometrial Tumors[1-4] *PCR, Southern blot, FISH, Immunohistochemistry*	Tissue (fresh, frozen, or paraffin-embedded). Liquid cytology specimens.	Human papillomavirus (HPV) has been implicated as having oncogenic potential because of its role in tumorigenesis when accompanied by alterations in other host cell genes. Numerous other proto-oncogenes, such as Ha-ras, c-myc, c-fos, c-jun, and int, have also been shown to be mutated in these tumors. Targets: E-cadherin, HER2/neu, human papillomavirus (HPV), mismatch repair genes (MLH1, MSH2, MSH6/GTBP), P53

1. Hubbard RA: Human papillomavirus testing methods, *Arch Pathol Lab Med* 127:940-945, 2003.
2. Inoue M: Current molecular aspects of the carcinogenesis of the uterine endometrium, *Int J Gynecol Cancer* 11:339-348, 2001.
3. Miturski R, Bogusiewicz M, Ciotta C, et al: Mismatch repair genes and microsatellite instability as molecular markers for gynecological cancer detection, *Exp Biol Med (Maywood)* 227:579-586, 2002.
4. Wolf JK, Ramirez PT: The molecular biology of cervical cancer, *Cancer Invest* 19:621-629, 2001.

DISORDER	SPECIMEN AND SPECIAL REQUIREMENTS	CLINICAL COMMENTS AND REMARKS
Charcot-Marie-Tooth Disease (CMT)[1,2] *PCR, Sequencing*	Whole blood (ACD or EDTA), tissue. Store whole blood at room temperature or 4° C; store tissue frozen at ≤−20° C if nucleic acids cannot be immediately extracted.	Charcot-Marie-Tooth disease (CMT) is the most common inherited disease of the peripheral nervous system. CMT, the hereditary motor and sensory neuropathies, is a clinically and genetically heterogeneous group of disorders, including demyelinating forms (CMT1, CMT3, and CMT4) and axonal forms (CMT2). Target: myelin protein zero (MPZ) gene

1. Kochanski A: Mutations in the Myelin Protein Zero result in a spectrum of Charcot-Marie-Tooth phenotypes, *Acta Myol* 23:6-9, 2004.
2. Berger P, Young P, Suter U: Molecular cell biology of Charcot-Marie-Tooth disease, *Neurogenetics* 4:1-15, 2002.

DISORDER	SPECIMEN AND SPECIAL REQUIREMENTS	CLINICAL COMMENTS AND REMARKS
Chlamydia trachomatis[1,2] *Hybrid capture, LCR, PCR, Probe hybridization, SDA, TMA*	Endocervical swab, urine, and intraurethral swab	The prevalence of *Chlamydia trachomatis* varies greatly. Laboratories must establish testing algorithms for repeat testing of positive samples and reporting. Target: cryptic plasmid, 23s rRNA, 16s rRNA

1. Johnson RE, Newhall WJ, Papp JR, et al: Screening tests to detect Chlamydia trachomatis and Neisseria gonorrhoeae infections—2002, *MMWR Recomm Rep* 51:1-38, 2002.
2. Peipert JF: Genital chlamydial infections, *N Engl J Med* 349:2424-2430, 2003.

DISORDER	SPECIMEN AND SPECIAL REQUIREMENTS	CLINICAL COMMENTS AND REMARKS
Colorectal Cancer: Adenocarcinoma, Familial Adenomatous Polyposis coli (FAP), Hereditary Nonpolyposis Colon Cancer (HNPCC)[1-3] *FISH, Immunohistochemistry, PCR and LOH analysis, Southern blot, Sequencing*	Tissue (fresh, frozen, or paraffin-embedded). Whole blood (ACD or EDTA). Store all body fluids at 4° C and all tissue at ≤−20° C until nucleic acids are isolated. Store isolated nucleic acids at ≤−20° C.	Although FAP and HNPCC remain the two most common forms of hereditary colon cancer, multiple molecular events have now been associated with tumor development and progression, including deletions of the DCC (deleted in colon cancer) and APC (adenomatous polyposis coli) genes. Point mutations have also been described in numerous proto-oncogenes and tumor suppressor genes. The MCC (mutated in colon cancer) gene has been implicated in the development of sporadic colon cancers along with numerous mutations in other proto-oncogenes. Targets: DCC, DPC4, mismatch repair genes (MLH1, MSH2, MSH6/GTBP)

1. Bendardaf R, Lamlum H, Pyrhonen S: Prognostic and predictive molecular markers in colorectal carcinoma, *Anticancer Res* 24:2519-2530, 2004.
2. Lynch HT, de la Chapelle A: Hereditary colorectal cancer, *N Engl J Med* 348:919-932, 2003.
3. Muller O: Identification of colon cancer patients by molecular diagnosis, *Dig Dis* 21:315-319, 2003.

DISORDER	SPECIMEN AND SPECIAL REQUIREMENTS	CLINICAL COMMENTS AND REMARKS
Coronavirus (Severe Acute Respiratory Syndrome, SARS) (SARS-CoV)[1,2] *Reverse-transcriptase (RT) PCR, Real-time RT-PCR*	Blood, urine, nasopharyngeal aspirates, and stool. Store all body fluids at 4° C.	Severe acute respiratory syndrome (SARS) is recognized as an emerging infectious disease. Coronaviruses are enveloped RNA viruses that currently have the largest RNA genomes. Target: polymerase gene, nucleocapsid region

1. Ziebuhr J: Molecular biology of severe acute respiratory syndrome coronavirus, *Curr Opin Microbiol* 7:412-419, 2004.
2. Hui DS, Wong PC, Wang C: SARS: clinical features and diagnosis, *Respirology* 8:S20-S24, 2003.

DISORDER	SPECIMEN AND SPECIAL REQUIREMENTS	CLINICAL COMMENTS AND REMARKS
Coxsackievirus[1,2] *Reverse-transcriptase (RT) PCR, Real-time RT-PCR, ISH*	Tissue (myocardium), whole blood, and CSF. Store all body fluids at 4° C and all tissue at $\leq -20°$ C.	Human enteroviruses are nonenveloped RNA viruses of the family *Picornaviridae* and include the following five groups: polioviruses, coxsackieviruses A and B, echoviruses, and enteroviruses. Coxsackievirus B is mostly associated with myocarditis. Target: 5'-nontranslated region

1. Smalling TW, Sefers SE, Li H, et al: Molecular approaches to detecting herpes simplex virus and enteroviruses in the central nervous system, *J Clin Microbiol* 40:2317-2322, 2003.
2. Baboonian C, Davies MJ, Booth JC, et al: Coxsackie B viruses and human heart disease, *Curr Top Microbiol Immunol* 223:31-52, 1997.

DISORDER	SPECIMEN AND SPECIAL REQUIREMENTS	CLINICAL COMMENTS AND REMARKS
Cystic Fibrosis (CF)[1-3] *PCR, RFLP, LiPA, OLA, Microarray, Bead array*	Whole blood (ACD or EDTA), tissue. Store whole blood at room temperature or 4° C; store tissue frozen at $\leq -20°$ C if nucleic acids cannot be immediately extracted.	Common mutations in the cystic fibrosis transmembrane regulator (CFTR) gene can be used to detect 75-80% of mutant alleles; other mutations are associated with different ethnic background or unusual clinical phenotype, such as patients with mild cystic fibrosis and pancreatic sufficiency or normal sweat chloride. Laboratory practice guidelines exist for diagnostic and screening applications for CFTR mutation analysis. Target: CFTR

1. Lewis MJ, Lewis EH, Amos JA, et al: Cystic fibrosis, *Am J Clin Pathol* 120(suppl 1):S3-S13, 2003.
2. Consortium, TCFGA: Cystic fibrosis mutation database, Available at: http://www.genet.sickkids.on.ca/cftr/. Last accessed 2/1/06.
3. ACOG: *Preconception and prenatal carrier screening for cystic fibrosis: clinical laboratory guidelines,* Washington, DC, 2001, American College of Obstetricians and Gynecologists.

DISORDER	SPECIMEN AND SPECIAL REQUIREMENTS	CLINICAL COMMENTS AND REMARKS
Cytomegalovirus (CMV)[1,2] *PCR, Real-time PCR, ISH*	Tissue, whole blood, and plasma. Store all body fluids at 4° C and all tissue at ≤−20° C.	Qualitative PCR for the detection of CMV is highly sensitive but may not be able to differentiate between latent and active infection. Quantitative detection may be used to predict severity of disease and to monitor therapy. Target: polymerase *(pol)* gene, glycoprotein *(gB)* gene

1. Nitsche A, Steuer N, Schmidt CA, et al: Different real-time PCR formats compared for quantitative detection of human cytomegalovirus DNA, *Clin Chem* 45:1932-1937, 1999.
2. Landolfo S, Gariglio M, Gribaudo G, et al: The human cytomegalovirus, *Pharmacol Ther* 98:269-297, 2003.

DISORDER	SPECIMEN AND SPECIAL REQUIREMENTS	CLINICAL COMMENTS AND REMARKS
Duchenne/Becker Muscular Dystrophy (DMD, BMD)[1,2] *PCR, RFLP, Southern blot, Sequencing*	Whole blood (ACD or EDTA), tissue. Store whole blood at room temperature or 4° C; store tissue frozen at ≤−20° C if nucleic acids cannot be immediately extracted.	The majority of DMD cases are caused by deletions within the dystrophin gene. In-frame versus out-of-frame deletions are used to discriminate between Becker and Duchenne muscular dystrophies. Target: dystrophin gene

1. Emery AE: Muscular dystrophy into the new millennium, *Neuromuscul Disord* 12:343-349, 2002.
2. Emery AE: The muscular dystrophies, *Lancet* 359:687-695, 2002.

DISORDER	SPECIMEN AND SPECIAL REQUIREMENTS	CLINICAL COMMENTS AND REMARKS
Enterovirus[1,2] *Reverse-transcriptase (RT) PCR, Real-time RT-PCR*	Tissue (myocardium), whole blood, and CSF. Store all body fluids at 4° C and all tissue at ≤−20° C.	Human enteroviruses are nonenveloped RNA viruses of the family *Picornaviridae* and include the following five groups: polioviruses, coxsackieviruses A and B, echoviruses, and enteroviruses. Coxsackievirus B is mostly associated with myocarditis. Target: 5′-nontranslated region

1. Stalkup JR, Chilukuri S: Enterovirus infections: a review of clinical presentation, diagnosis, and treatment, *Dermatol Clin* 20:217-223, 2002.
2. Smalling TW, Sefers SE, Li H, et al: Molecular approaches to detecting herpes simplex virus and enteroviruses in the central nervous system, *J Clin Microbiol* 40:2317-2322, 2002.

DISORDER	SPECIMEN AND SPECIAL REQUIREMENTS	CLINICAL COMMENTS AND REMARKS
Epstein-Barr Virus (EBV)[1,2] *PCR, Real-time RT-PCR, ISH, Southern blot*	Tissue (myocardium), whole blood, CSF, and saliva. Store all body fluids at 4° C and all tissue at $\leq -20°$ C.	The organism is associated with lymphoproliferative disorders (infectious mononucleosis, Hodgkin's disease, Burkitt's lymphoma) and nasopharyngeal carcinoma. Target: gp220, EBNA.2, EBER, BamHI-W

1. Thompson MP, Kurzrock R: Epstein-Barr virus and cancer, *Clin Cancer Res* 10:803-821, 2004.
2. Niesters HGM: Molecular diagnostic clinical virology in real time, *Clin Microbiol Infect* 10:5-11, 2004.

DISORDER	SPECIMEN AND SPECIAL REQUIREMENTS	CLINICAL COMMENTS AND REMARKS
Factor V Leiden[1] *PCR, Invader*	Whole blood (ACD or EDTA), tissue. Store whole blood at room temperature or 4° C; store tissue frozen at $\leq -20°$ C if nucleic acids cannot be immediately extracted.	This single mutation is the most common cause of hereditary thrombophilia. It has an incidence of ~2-8% in the general Caucasian population. Heterozygotes have a sevenfold increased risk for thrombosis and homozygotes an 80-fold increased risk. Target: Factor V gene

1. Caprini JA, Glase CJ, Anderson CB, et al: Laboratory markers in the diagnosis of venous thromboembolism, *Circulation* 109(suppl 1):I4-8, 2004.

DISORDER	SPECIMEN AND SPECIAL REQUIREMENTS	CLINICAL COMMENTS AND REMARKS
Familial Cancer *PCR, Southern blot, Immunohistochemistry, FISH* *Breast Cancer*	Tumor tissue, whole blood (ACD or EDTA). Store body fluids at 4° C; store fresh tissue at 4° C for 24 hr. However, it is preferred that tissue be frozen at $\leq -20°$ C if nucleic acids cannot be extracted immediately. Paraffin-embedded tissue may also be used.	Breast tumors are associated with *neu*/HER-2 (*erb*B-2) gene amplification and overexpression. Hereditary breast cancer is associated with the BRCA1 and BRCA2 genes.
Familial Polyposis coli		The gene is localized on the long arm of chromosome 5; linkage is available within families known to have multiple polyps leading to colon cancer. See *Colorectal Tumors.*
Li-Fraummeni Syndrome		The families who define the questionable inheritance pattern of this syndrome have had various types of cancer, among them breast cancer and sarcoma. The p53 tumor suppressor gene has been implicated as a cancer susceptibility gene.
Neurofibromatosis Type 1 and type 2		The target for neurofibromatosis is inactivating mutations in the neurofibromatosis-1 gene, a tumor suppressor gene on chromosome 17.

TEST METHOD	SPECIMEN AND SPECIAL REQUIREMENTS	CLINICAL COMMENTS AND REMARKS

Familial Cancer—CONT

Retinoblastoma
Rb-1

The retinoblastoma (Rb) gene is located at chromosome region 13q14 and encodes for a 105-kDa protein important in controlling the cell cycle. Other targets include p16/cyclin D1/CDK4/Rb.

Wilms' Tumor
(Nephroblastoma)
WT-1

Allele loss occurs at one or two separate loci on chromosome 11. WT-1 is a transcription factor.

Familial Dysautonomia[1,2]

PCR, Sequencing

Whole blood (ACD or EDTA), tissue. Store whole blood at room temperature or 4° C; store tissue frozen at $\leq -20°$ C if nucleic acids cannot be immediately extracted.

This is a progressive neurodegenerative condition. Mutations result in tissue-specific expression of mutant IκB kinase-associated protein (IKAP).

Target: IKBKAP, IKK complex-associated protein

---

1.   Axelrod FB: Familial dysautonomia, *Muscle Nerve* 29:352-363, 2004.
2.   Vallance H, Ford J: Carrier testing for autosomal-recessive disorders, *Crit Rev Clin Lab Sci* 40:473-497, 2003.

Fanconi's Anemia[1,2]

PCR, Sequencing

Whole blood (ACD or EDTA), tissue. Store whole blood at room temperature or 4° C; store tissue frozen at $\leq -20°$ C if nucleic acids cannot be immediately extracted.

Fanconi's anemia (FA) is an autosomal recessive chromosomal instability disorder, which is characterized by congenital abnormalities, defective hemopoiesis, and a high risk of developing acute myeloid leukemia and certain solid tumors. It can be caused by mutations in at least eight different genes responsible for the various complementation groups (A, B, C, D1, D2, E, F, G).

Target: Complementation group genes (FANC A, B, C, D1, D2, E, F, G)

---

1.   Tischkowitz M, Dokal I: Fanconi anaemia and leukaemia—clinical and molecular aspects, *Br J Haematol* 126:176-191, 2004.
2.   Tischkowitz MD, Hodgson SV: Fanconi anaemia, *J Med Genet* 40:1-10, 2003.

DISORDER	SPECIMEN AND SPECIAL REQUIREMENTS	CLINICAL COMMENTS AND REMARKS
Fragile X Syndrome (FRAX)[1,2] *PCR, Southern blot*	Whole blood (ACD or EDTA). Store whole blood at room temperature or 4° C.	This is the most common form of inherited mental retardation with a frequency of ~1/1000 males and 1/1400 females (or greater). The most common mutation of FMR-1 is a CGG trinucleotide repeat expansion upstream of the FMR-1 coding sequence. Target: FMR-1

1.   Willemsen R, Oostra BA, Bassell GJ, et al: The fragile X syndrome: from molecular genetics to neurobiology, *Ment Retard Dev Disabil Res Rev* 10:60-67, 2004.
2.   Oostra BA, Willemsen R: Diagnostic tests for fragile X syndrome, *Expert Rev Mol Diagn* 1:226-232, 2001.

DISORDER	SPECIMEN AND SPECIAL REQUIREMENTS	CLINICAL COMMENTS AND REMARKS
Gastrointestinal Cancer[1,2] *Methods: Immunohisto-chemistry, PCR, Sequencing*	Tissue (fresh, frozen, or paraffin-embedded). Store tissue at ≤−20° C until nucleic acids are isolated. Store isolated nucleic acids at 20° C.	c-kit is a proto-oncogene growth factor receptor that links the effect of growth factors and intracellular signal pathways. E-cadherin is a cell-to-cell adhesion molecule that has also been evaluated for detection of brain metastases.[3] The epidermal growth factor receptor and vascular endothelial growth factors are related to tumor growth. Targets: c-kit, E-cadherin, EGFR, P53, VEGF

1.   Kyrlagkitsis I, Karamanolis DG: Genes and gastric cancer, *Hepatogastroenterology* 51:320-327, 2004.
2.   Scartozzi M, Galizia E, Freddari F, et al: Molecular biology of sporadic gastric cancer: prognostic indicators and novel therapeutic approaches, *Cancer Treatment Rev* 30:451-459, 2004.
3.   Berx G, Becker KF, Hofler H, et al: Mutations of the human E-cadherin (CDH1) gene, *Hum Mutat* 12:226-237, 1998.

DISORDER	SPECIMEN AND SPECIAL REQUIREMENTS	CLINICAL COMMENTS AND REMARKS
Gaucher Disease[1,2] *PCR, Sequencing*	Whole blood (ACD or EDTA), tissue. Store whole blood at room temperature or 4° C; store tissue frozen at ≤−20° C if nucleic acids cannot be immediately extracted.	More than 150 mutations have been described in this gene. Common mutations account for >90% of cases in the Ashkenazi Jewish population. Carrier screening is recommended for couples in which one individual is of Ashkenazi ancestry. Target: acid-β gucosidase, glucocerbrosidase (GBA).

1.   Germain DP: Gaucher's disease: a paradigm for interventional genetics, *Clin Genet* 65:77-86, 2004.
2.   Elstein D, Abrahamov A, Dweck A, et al: Gaucher disease: pediatric concerns, *Paediatr Drugs* 4:417-426, 2002.

DISORDER	SPECIMEN AND SPECIAL REQUIREMENTS	CLINICAL COMMENTS AND REMARKS
Glioblastoma[1,2] *FISH, PCR fragment sizing*	Specimen: Tissue (fresh, frozen, or paraffin-embedded). Store tissue at $\leq -20°$ C until nucleic acids are isolated. Store isolated nucleic acids at $\leq -20°$ C.	Overexpression of epidermal growth factor receptors occurs in a variety of tumors, including breast, endometrial, and ovarian cancers. Targets: EGFR, P15, P16/CDKN2A/MTS1, P53, RB1

1. Hayashi Y, Yamashita J, Watanabe T: Molecular genetic analysis of deep-seated glioblastomas, *Cancer Genet Cytogenet* 153:64-68, 2004.
2. Mischel PS, Nelson SF, Cloughesy TF: Molecular analysis of glioblastoma: pathway profiling and its implications for patient therapy, *Cancer Biol Ther* 2:242-247, 2003.

DISORDER	SPECIMEN AND SPECIAL REQUIREMENTS	CLINICAL COMMENTS AND REMARKS
Head and Neck Cancer[1,2] *FISH, PCR*	Specimen: Tissue (fresh, frozen, or paraffin-embedded). Store tissue at $\leq -20°$ C until nucleic acids are isolated. Store isolated nucleic acids at $\leq -20°$ C.	The cyclins activate protein kinases. The D1 isoform is involved in transformation and tumor progression. PRAD is an oncogene found on chromosome 11. RET is a transmembrane receptor tyrosine kinase. Targets: Cyclin D1/CCND1/PRAD1, EGFR/RET

1. El-Rayes BF, LoRusso PM: Targeting the epidermal growth factor receptor, *Br J Cancer* 91:418-424, 2004.
2. Kim DS, McCabe CJ, Buchanan MA, et al: Oncogenes in thyroid cancer, *Clin Otolaryngol* 28:386-395, 2003.

DISORDER	SPECIMEN AND SPECIAL REQUIREMENTS	CLINICAL COMMENTS AND REMARKS
Hemoglobinopathies (sickle cell anemia, α-thalassemia, β-thalassemia)[1] *PCR, Southern blot, Sequencing*	Whole blood (ACD or EDTA), amniocytes, and chorionic villi. Store whole blood at 4° C; store cells at $\leq -20°$ C if nucleic acids cannot be extracted immediately.	Hemoglobin electrophoresis is the screening method of choice; the advantage of the DNA test is discrimination of compound heterozygotes. In sickle cell anemia, variability of clinical manifestations and benefits of early therapeutic intervention are cause for molecular genetic evaluation. Molecular analyses detect abnormalities in the hemoglobin gene. Ninety-five percent of α-thalassemia cases are caused by defective α-globin synthesis and deletions of one or both α-globin genes. Diagnosis of α-thalassemia trait requires quantitative PCR to detect reduced numbers of α-globin genes. β-thalassemia is caused by defective production of β-globin chains. When one β-globin gene is nonfunctional, then mild hematological abnormalities occur. β-thalassemia major or Cooley's anemia occurs when both β-globin genes are defective.

TEST METHOD	SPECIMEN AND SPECIAL REQUIREMENTS	CLINICAL COMMENTS AND REMARKS

Hemoglobinopathies (sickle cell anemia, α-thalassemia, β-thalassemia)—CONT

They are characterized by varying clinical severity and deletions or insertions within the β-globin gene.

Targets: hemoglobin, α-globin, β-globin

1.   Clark BE, Thein SL: Molecular diagnosis of haemoglobin disorders, *Clin Lab Haematol* 26:159-176, 2004.

Hemophilia A and B[1]

PCR, Real-time PCR, RFLP, Southern blot

Whole blood (ACD or EDTA), tissue. Store whole blood at room temperature or 4° C.

Coagulation studies (factor VIII) can be used for carrier risk estimate; most mutations are family-specific. Hemophilia A is caused by defective factor VIII. Deletions, insertions, and point mutations have all been detected in the factor VIII gene. Hemophilia B is caused by abnormal factor IX. One third of cases result from a point mutation in the factor IX gene.

Target: Factor VIII, factor IX genes

1.   Bolton-Maggs PH, Pasi KJ: Haemophilias A and B, *Lancet* 361:1801-1809, 2003.

Hepatitis B Virus (HBV)[1,2]

PCR, ISH, Southern blot

Tissue, whole blood, urine. Store all body fluids at 4° C and all tissue at ≤ −20° C.

Molecular diagnostic assays are not typically required to make a diagnosis of HBV infection in most instances. These assays are very useful in determining viral load or replicating virus.

Target: HBV surface and core antigen genes

1.   Servoss JC, Friedman LS: Serologic and molecular diagnosis of hepatitis B virus, *Clin Liver Dis* 8:267-281, 2004.
2.   Ganem D, Prince AM: Hepatitis B virus infection: natural history and clinical consequences, *N Engl J Med* 350:1118-1129, 2004.

DISORDER	SPECIMEN AND SPECIAL REQUIREMENTS	CLINICAL COMMENTS AND REMARKS
Hepatitis C Virus (HCV) **(Qualitative, Quantitative, Genotyping)**[1-3] *bDNA, TMA, RT-PCR, ISH, LiPA, Sequencing*	Tissue, plasma, and serum. Store all body fluids at 4° C and all tissue at ≤−20° C.	Qualitative assays for the detection of HCV are useful for confirmation of positive serologic tests and have in many institutions replaced RIBA testing. Quantitative or viral load testing for HCV has also become a standard of practice to monitor response to therapy. Genotyping to identify the HCV subtype is also performed routinely to determine potential response to therapy. Target: HCV 5'-noncoding region

1. Poynard T, Yuen MF, Ratziu V, et al: Viral hepatitis C, *Lancet* 362:2095-2100, 2003.
2. Richter SS: Laboratory assays for the diagnosis and management of hepatitis C virus infection, *J Clin Microbiol* 40:4407-4412, 2002.
3. Podzorski RP: Molecular testing in the diagnosis and management of hepatitis C virus infection, *Arch Pathol Lab Med* 126:285-290, 2002.

DISORDER	SPECIMEN AND SPECIAL REQUIREMENTS	CLINICAL COMMENTS AND REMARKS
Hepatocellular Carcinoma *PCR, Southern blot*	Tumor tissue. Store fresh tissue at 4° C for 24 hr. However, it is preferred that tissue be frozen at ≤−20° C if nucleic acids cannot be extracted immediately. Paraffin-embedded tissue may also be used.	Point mutations in the ras gene family and p53 tumor suppressor gene, as well as point mutations in numerous other genes, are common. Targets: P53, Ras

1. Suriawinata A, Xu R: An update on the molecular genetics of hepatocellular carcinoma, *Semin Liver Dis* 24:77-88, 2004.
2. Kim JW, Wang XW: Gene expression profiling of preneoplastic liver disease and liver cancer: a new era for improved early detection and treatment of these deadly diseases, *Carcinogenesis* 24:363-369, 2003.

DISORDER	SPECIMEN AND SPECIAL REQUIREMENTS	CLINICAL COMMENTS AND REMARKS
Hereditary Deafness[1,2] *PCR, Sequencing*	Whole blood, amniocytes	Mutations in the Connexin 26 gene account for ~80% of nonsyndromic recessive deafness. Target: Connexin 26 (GJB2), Connexin 30 (GJB6)

1. Nance WE: The genetics of deafness, *Ment Retard Dev Disabil Res Rev* 9:109-119, 2003.
2. Hone SW, Smith RJ: Genetics of hearing impairment, *Semin Neonatol* 6:531-541, 2001.

DISORDER	SPECIMEN AND SPECIAL REQUIREMENTS	CLINICAL COMMENTS AND REMARKS
Hereditary Hemochromatosis[1] *PCR, Invader*	Whole blood (ACD or EDTA), tissue. Store whole blood at room temperature or 4° C; store tissue frozen at $\leq -20°$ C if nucleic acids cannot be immediately extracted.	Hereditary hemochromatosis is characterized by a high absorption of iron in the gastrointestinal tract. One mutation (C282Y) and two polymorphisms (H63D, S65C) account for the majority of alleles associated with this disease. Target: HFE

1. Pietrangelo A: Hereditary hemochromatosis—a new look at an old disease, *N Engl J Med* 350:2383-2397, 2004.

DISORDER	SPECIMEN AND SPECIAL REQUIREMENTS	CLINICAL COMMENTS AND REMARKS
Herpes Simplex Virus (HSV)[1,2] *PCR, Real-time PCR, Hybridization*	Skin lesions (biopsies), tissue, liquid cytology specimens, vitreous humor, CSF, and serum. Store all body fluids at $-70°$ C and all tissue at $\leq -20°$ C.	Qualitative assays for the detection of HSV are critical to the diagnosis of viral encephalitis. Target: DNA *pol, gB, gD*

1. Stellrecht KA: Nucleic acid amplification technology for the diagnosis of genital herpes infection, *Expert Rev Mol Diagn* 4:485-493, 2004.
2. Waggoner-Fountain LA, Grossman LB: Herpes simplex virus, *Pediatr Rev* 25:86-92, 2004.

DISORDER	SPECIMEN AND SPECIAL REQUIREMENTS	CLINICAL COMMENTS AND REMARKS
Human Herpes Virus 8 (IIIIV8)[1-3] *PCR, Real-time PCR, Hybridization*	Tissue, whole blood, bone marrow, and urine. Store all body fluids at $-70°$ C and all tissue at $\leq -20°$ C.	HHV8 belongs to the subfamily of γ-herpes virus. Its linear genome has a central unique gene region flanked by several repetitive DNA sequences. HHV8 is found in all forms of Kaposi's sarcoma. Target: ORF26

1. Watzinger F, Suda M, Preuner S, et al: Real-time quantitative PCR assays for detection and monitoring of pathogenic human viruses in immunosuppressed pediatric patients, *J Clin Microbiol* 42:5189-5198, 2004.
2. Cathomas G: Human herpes virus 8: a new virus discloses its face, *Virchows Arch* 436:195-206, 2000.
3. Hengge UR, Ruzicka T, Tyring SK, et al: Update on Kaposi's sarcoma and other HHV8 associated diseases. Part 2: pathogenesis, Castleman's disease, and pleural effusion lymphoma, *Lancet* 2:344-352, 2002.

DISORDER	SPECIMEN AND SPECIAL REQUIREMENTS	CLINICAL COMMENTS AND REMARKS
Human Immunodeficiency Virus I (HIV-1) (Qualitative, Quantitative, Genotyping)[1,2] *bDNA, TMA, NASBA, Reverse-transcriptase (RT) PCR, Real-time RT-PCR, LipA, Sequencing*	Tissue, whole blood, plasma, and serum. Store all body fluids at $-70°$ C and all tissue at $\leq -20°$ C.	HIV causes acquired immunodeficiency syndrome (AIDS). Although HIV-1 is an RNA virus, early diagnosis in newborns can be performed by detection of HIV-1 reverse-transcribed cDNA. The majority of HIV-1 testing is performed as a quantitative assay to monitor therapy. HIV-1 genotyping is performed to detect viral mutations associated with resistance to antiretroviral therapies. Target: *env, gag, pol*

1. Zhang M, Versalovic J: HIV update. Diagnostic tests and markers of disease progression and response to therapy, *Am J Clin Pathol* 118:S26-S32, 2002.
2. Harrigan PR, Cote CF: Clinical utility of testing human immunodeficiency virus for drug resistance, *Clin Infect Dis* 30:S117-S122, 2002.

DISORDER	SPECIMEN AND SPECIAL REQUIREMENTS	CLINICAL COMMENTS AND REMARKS
Human Papillomavirus (HPV)[1] *Hybrid capture, PCR, LiPA, Other blotting techniques*	Liquid cytology specimens, cervical smears, biopsies, or scrapings; anogenital tissues. Various storage conditions apply depending on collection device. Store all body fluids at $-70°$ C and all tissue at $\leq -20°$ C. Paraffin-embedded tissues may also be used for testing.	DNA analysis for HPV testing has gone through several versions of guidelines and clinical indications. Clearly the majority of this testing is being performed on liquid cytology specimens for the detection of high-risk HPV types. Target: L1, E6, E7 genes

1. Hubbard RA: Human papillomavirus testing methods, *Arch Pathol Lab Med* 127:940-945, 2003.

DISORDER	SPECIMEN AND SPECIAL REQUIREMENTS	CLINICAL COMMENTS AND REMARKS
Huntington's Disease (HD)[1,2] *PCR, Southern blot, Sequencing*	Whole blood (ACD or EDTA). Store whole blood at $4°$ C.	Huntington's disease is a late-onset, autosomal-dominant neuropsychiatric disorder caused by the expansion of the trinucleotide repeat CAG within IT 15. Target: IT 15 (huntingtin)

1. Gardian G, Vecsei L: Huntington's disease: pathomechanism and therapeutic perspectives, *J Neural Transm* 111:1485-1494, 2004.
2. Margolis RL, Ross CA: Diagnosis of Huntington disease, *Clin Chem* 49:1726-1732, 2003.

DISORDER	SPECIMEN AND SPECIAL REQUIREMENTS	CLINICAL COMMENTS AND REMARKS
Influenza Virus A and B[1,2] *Real-time PCR*	Nasopharyngeal swab, wash, or aspirate	Molecular assays have proven more sensitive and specific but do not offer the turnaround time of more traditional rapid assays. Target: M gene, M1 gene, HA gene

1. Ward CL, Dempsey MH, Ring CJ, et al: Design and performance testing of quantitative real time PCR assays for influenza A and B viral load measurement, *J Clin Virol* 29:179-188, 2004.
2. Watzinger F, Suda M, Preuner S, et al: Real-time quantitative PCR assays for detection and monitoring of pathogenic human viruses in immunosuppressed pediatric patients, *J Clin Microbiol* 42:5189-5198, 2004.

DISORDER	SPECIMEN AND SPECIAL REQUIREMENTS	CLINICAL COMMENTS AND REMARKS
JC Virus[1,2] *PCR, Real-time PCR, Blotting techniques*	CSF, plasma, urine, and tissue (brain; fresh, frozen, or paraffin-embedded). Store all body fluids at 4° C; store tissue at ≤−20° C.	JCV persists in latent form and is activated in immunocompromised hosts. It is a member of the polyoma virus family, which also includes BKV and SV40. Target: small and large T region, late mRNA gene

1. Watzinger F, Suda M, Preuner S, et al: Real-time quantitative PCR assays for detection and monitoring of pathogenic human viruses in immunosuppressed pediatric patients, *J Clin Microbiol* 42:5189-5198, 2004.
2. Behzad-Behbahani A, Klapper PE, Vallely PJ, et al: Detection of BK virus and JC virus DNA in urine samples from immunocompromised (HIV-infected) and immunocompetent (HIV-non-infected) patients using polymerase chain reaction and microplate hybridization, *J Clin Virol* 29:224-229, 2004.

DISORDER	SPECIMEN AND SPECIAL REQUIREMENTS	CLINICAL COMMENTS AND REMARKS
Kennedy Disease/Spinal and Bulbar Muscular Atrophy (SBMA)[1] *PCR, Southern blot, Sequencing*	Whole blood (ACD or EDTA), tissue. Store whole blood at room temperature or 4° C; store tissue frozen at ≤−20° C if nucleic acids cannot be immediately extracted.	This is a degenerative neuromuscular disorder. Familial and sporadic cases are caused by expansion of a CAG trinucleotide repeat in exon 1 of this gene. Target: androgen receptor gene

1. Walcott JL, Merry DE: Trinucleotide repeat disease. The androgen receptor in spinal and bulbar muscular atrophy, *Vitam Horm* 65:127-147, 2002.

DISORDER	SPECIMEN AND SPECIAL REQUIREMENTS	CLINICAL COMMENTS AND REMARKS
Legionella pneumophila[1,2] *Hybrid capture, LCR, PCR,* *Probe hybridization, SDA,* *TMA*	Lung tissue, water sputum, bronchoalveolar lavage, and other respiratory fluids	The entire genome of *Legionella pneumophila* has been sequenced. Various genomic targets and amplification strategies have been used in its detection. Target: mip, dnaJ, 16S rRNA

1. Liu H, Li Y, Huang X, et al: Use of the dnaJ gene for the detection and identification of all Legionella pneumophila serogroups and description of the primers used to detect 16S rDNA gene sequences of major members of the genus Legionella, *Microbiol Immunol* 47:859-869, 2003.
2. Templeton KE, Scheltinga SA, Sillekens P, et al: Development and clinical evaluation of an internally controlled, single-tube multiplex real-time PCR assay for detection of Legionella pneumophila and other Legionella species, *J Clin Microbiol* 41:4016-4021, 2003.

DISORDER	SPECIMEN AND SPECIAL REQUIREMENTS	CLINICAL COMMENTS AND REMARKS
Leukemia[1] *Methods: FISH, PCR,* *Southern blot*	Bone marrow, whole blood (ACD or EDTA). Store all body fluids at 4° C and all tissue at $\leq -20°$ C until nucleic acids are isolated. Store isolated nucleic acids at $\leq -20°$ C.	Many leukemias are associated with specific chromosomal translocations and gene rearrangements, which can be detected by fluorescence in situ hybridization and Southern blot analysis.
Chronic Myeloid Leukemia (CML)		Target: t(9;22), bcr/abl (Philadelphia chromosome)
Acute Lymphoblastic Leukemia (ALL; L1, L2, L3)		Targets: IgH gene rearrangement, TCR gene rearrangement, t(1;19), pbx1/E2A, t(9;22)
Acute Myeloid Leukemia (AML)		Targets: t(8;21), aml1/eto, t(3;21), EAP, MDS1, or evil/aml1, t(9;11), mll/AF-9, t(11;16), mll/CBP
Acute Promyelocytic Leukemia (APL; M3)		Targets: Retinoic acid receptor, t(15;17), PML/RARα

1. Guttmacher AE, Collins FS: Molecular diagnosis of the hematologic cancers, *N Engl J Med* 348:1777-1785, 2003.

DISORDER	SPECIMEN AND SPECIAL REQUIREMENTS	CLINICAL COMMENTS AND REMARKS
Long-QT Syndrome[1] *PCR, Sequencing*	Whole blood (ACD or EDTA), tissue. Store whole blood at room temperature or 4° C; store tissue frozen at $\leq -20°$ C if nucleic acids cannot be immediately extracted.	The congenital form of long QT syndrome (LQTS) is characterized by QT prolongation in the electrocardiogram (ECG) and a polymorphic ventricular tachycardia. The LQT1, LQT2, and LQT3 forms of LQTS account for ~90% of LQTS patients. Target: LQT1, LQT2, LQT3, LQT5, LQT6

1. Shimizu W: Genotype-specific clinical manifestation in long QT syndrome, *Expert Rev Cardiovasc Ther* 1:401-409, 2003.

DISORDER	SPECIMEN AND SPECIAL REQUIREMENTS	CLINICAL COMMENTS AND REMARKS
Lung Tumors[1,2] *FISH, Immunohisto-* *chemistry, PCR,* *Sequencing, Southern blot*	Tumor tissue. Store fresh tissue at 4° C for 24 hr. However, it is preferred that tissue be frozen at $\leq -20°$ C if nucleic acids cannot be extracted immediately. Paraffin-embedded tissue may also be used.	Many proto-oncogenes (ras, myc, jun, *erb*B-1, *erb*B-2 [*neu*/HER 2]) and tumor suppressor genes (RB, p53) have been implicated in the development and progression of these tumors. Targets: c-Myc, EGFR, FHIT, P53

1. Fong KM, Sekido Y, Gazdar AF, et al: Lung cancer 9: molecular biology of lung cancer: clinical implications, *Thorax* 58:892-900, 2003.
2. Kim DW, Choy H: Potential role for epidermal growth factor receptor inhibitors in combined modality therapy for non-small cell lung cancer, *Int J Radiat Oncol Biol Phys* 59:11-20, 2004.

DISORDER	SPECIMEN AND SPECIAL REQUIREMENTS	CLINICAL COMMENTS AND REMARKS
Lymphoma[1,2] *Methods: FISH, PCR,* *Southern blot*	Tissue, bone marrow, and whole blood (ACD or EDTA). Store all body fluids at 4° C and all tissue at $\leq -20°$ C until nucleic acids are isolated. Store isolated nucleic acids at $\leq -20°$ C.	Many leukemias are associated with specific chromosomal translocations and gene rearrangements, which can be detected by fluorescence in situ hybridization and Southern blot analysis.
B-cell Lymphoma		Targets: Immunoglobulin gene rearrangements
Burkitt's Lymphoma		Targets: t(8;14)(q24;q32), c-Myc/IgH
Diffuse Large B-cell Lymphoma		Targets: Bcl-6, t(3;14) t(2;3), t(3;22)
Follicular Lymphoma		Targets: t(14;18)(q32q21), bcl-2/IgH
Mantle Cell Lymphoma		Targets: t(11;14)(q13;q32), Bcl-1/IgH
T-cell Lymphoma		Targets: T-cell receptor gene rearrangements
Anaplastic Large Cell Lymphoma		Targets: t(2;5)(p23;q35), ALK/NPM

1. Campo E: Genetic and molecular genetic studies in the diagnosis of B-cell lymphomas I: mantle cell lymphoma, follicular lymphoma, and Burkitt's lymphoma, *Hum Pathol* 34:330-335, 2003.
2. Guttmacher AE, Collins FS: Molecular diagnosis of the hematologic cancers, *N Engl J Med* 348:1777-1785, 2003.

DISORDER	SPECIMEN AND SPECIAL REQUIREMENTS	CLINICAL COMMENTS AND REMARKS
Melanoma[1,2] *FISH, PCR*	Tissue, whole blood (ACD or EDTA). Store all body fluids at 4° C and all tissue at ≤ −20° C until nucleic acids are isolated. Store isolated nucleic acids at ≤ −20° C.	A mutation in p16 is also seen in non–small cell lung cancer. Levels of the cell-dependent protein kinase CDK2 increase progressively from benign to primary to metastatic melanoma. This does not occur for the other cell cycle regulators (CDK1 or CDK4). The oncogene MTS1 is also seen in esophageal, biliary tract, and pancreatic cancer and is caused by an allelic loss in chromosome 9 and point mutations. Targets: P16/CDKN2A/MTS1

1. Flaherty KT: New molecular targets in melanomas, *Curr Opin Oncol* 16:150-154, 2004.
2. Sandberg AA, Bridge JA: Updates on cytogenetics and molecular genetics of bone and soft tissue tumors: clear cell sarcoma (malignant melanoma of soft parts), *Cancer Genet Cytogenet* 130:1-7, 2001.

DISORDER	SPECIMEN AND SPECIAL REQUIREMENTS	CLINICAL COMMENTS AND REMARKS
(Human) Metapneumovirus[1,2] *PCR, Real-time PCR*	Nasopharyngeal swab, wash, or aspirate	Molecular assays can be multiplexed to screen for multiple targets while maintaining increased sensitivity and specificity over traditional assays. Target: N (nucleoprotein) gene

1. Alto WA: Human metapneumovirus: a newly described respiratory tract pathogen, *J Am Board Fam Pract* 17:466-469, 2004.
2. Konig B, Konig W, Arnold R, et al: Prospective study of human metapneumovirus infection in children less than 3 years of age, *J Clin Microbiol* 42:4632-4635, 2004.

DISORDER	SPECIMEN AND SPECIAL REQUIREMENTS	CLINICAL COMMENTS AND REMARKS
Methylenetetrahydrofolate Reductase (MTHFR)[1] *PCR, Sequencing, Invader*	Whole blood (ACD or EDTA), tissue. Store whole blood at room temperature or 4° C; store tissue frozen at ≤ −20° C if nucleic acids cannot be immediately extracted.	5,10-Methylenetetrahydrofolate reductase (MTHFR) plays a key role in folate metabolism. MTHFR enzyme deficiency leads to hyperhomocysteinemia and homocystinuria, characterized by damage to the nervous and vascular systems. Two frequent polymorphisms in the human MTHFR gene, C677T and A1298C, result in moderate impairment of MTHFR activity. Target: Methylenetetrahydrofolate reductase (MTHFR) gene

1. Schwahn B, Rozen R: Polymorphisms in the methylenetetrahydrofolate reductase gene: clinical consequences, *Am J Pharmacogen* 1:189-201, 2001.

TEST METHOD	SPECIMEN AND SPECIAL REQUIREMENTS	CLINICAL COMMENTS AND REMARKS
Multiple Endocrine[1] **Neoplasia 2A/2B** *PCR, Sequencing*	Tissue, whole blood (ACD or EDTA). Store all body fluids at 4° C and all tissue at $\leq -20°$ C until nucleic acids are isolated. Store isolated nucleic acids at $\leq -20°$ C.	The RET oncogene is also a target in papillary thyroid cancer and pheochromocytoma. Target: RET

1. Eng C: Multiple endocrine neoplasia type 2 and the practice of molecular medicine, *Rev Endocr Metab Disord* 1:283-290, 2000.

Mycobacterium ***tuberculosis* (TB)**[1,2] *PCR, Real-time PCR,* *Probe Hybridization, TMA*	Lung tissue, respiratory fluids, and urine	Traditional identification by microscopy (AFB stain) has very low sensitivity, and culture times are long. Molecular assays are rapid, specific, and sensitive diagnostic tools. Amplification followed by oligonucleotide probe hybridization or restriction fragment length analysis can determine resistance. Target: 16S rRNA, IS6110

1. Garcia de Viedma D: Rapid detection of resistance in Mycobacterium tuberculosis: a review discussing molecular approaches, *Clin Microbiol Infect* 9:349-359, 2003.
2. Huggett JF, McHugh TD, Zumla A: Tuberculosis: amplification-based clinical diagnostic techniques, *Int J Biochem Cell Biol* 35:1407-1412, 2003.

Mycoplasma ***pneumoniae***[1,2] *PCR, Real-time PCR,* *Probe hybridization*	Sputum, bronchoalveolar lavage (BAL), nasopharyngeal and throat swabs, other respiratory fluids, and lung tissue. Store fluids at 4° C; store isolated nucleic acids and tissues at $-80°$ C.	*M. pneumoniae* is responsible for ~20% of community-acquired pneumonia. Amplification technologies offer rapid turnaround times and increased sensitivity and specificity. Target: P1, 16S rRNA, tuf, ATPase operon

1. Loens K, Ursi D, Goossens H, et al: Molecular diagnosis of Mycoplasma pneumoniae respiratory tract infections, *J Clin Microbiol* 41:4915-4923, 2003.

DISORDER	SPECIMEN AND SPECIAL REQUIREMENTS	CLINICAL COMMENTS AND REMARKS
Myotonic Dystrophy (MD)[1] *PCR, Southern blot, Sequencing*	Whole blood (ACD or EDTA). Store whole blood at 4° C.	The most common mutation associated with DM1 is expansion of the trinucleotide repeat CTG in the DMPK gene and for DM2, expansion of the CCTG repeat in the PROMM gene. Both diseases share some common clinical features. Target: DM1 or dystrophia myotonica protein kinase gene (DMPK), DM2 or proximal myotonic myopathy (PROMM) gene

1. Ranum LP, Day JW: Myotonic dystrophy: RNA pathogenesis comes into focus, *Am J Hum Genet* 74:793-804, 2004.

DISORDER	SPECIMEN AND SPECIAL REQUIREMENTS	CLINICAL COMMENTS AND REMARKS
Neisseria gonorrhoeae[1,2] *Hybrid capture, LCR, PCR, Probe hybridization, SDA, TMA*	Endocervical swab, urine, and intraurethral swab	*N. gonorrhoeae* is currently the second most common sexually transmitted microbe in the U.S. Targets: Opa, pilin, cryptic plasmid, 16S rRNA, cytosine methyltransferase

1. Johnson RE, Newhall WJ, Papp JR, et al: Screening tests to detect Chlamydia trachomatis and Neisseria gonorrhoeae infections—2002, *MMWR Recomm Rep* 51:1-38, 2002.
2. Morse SA: New tests for bacterial sexually transmitted diseases, *Curr Opin Infect Dis* 14:45-51, 2001.

DISORDER	SPECIMEN AND SPECIAL REQUIREMENTS	CLINICAL COMMENTS AND REMARKS
Neuroblastoma[1] *FISH, PCR*	Tissue, bone marrow (ACD or EDTA). Store all body fluids at 4° C and all tissue at $\leq -20°$ C until nucleic acids are isolated. Store isolated nucleic acids at $\leq -20°$ C.	The N-myc is part of a proto-oncogene family that includes c-myc and l-myc. N-myc is also a target in breast cancer. Target: N-myc

1. Riley RD, Heney D, Jones DR, et al: A systematic review of molecular and biological tumor markers in neuroblastoma, *Clin Cancer Res* 10:4-12, 2004.

DISORDER	SPECIMEN AND SPECIAL REQUIREMENTS	CLINICAL COMMENTS AND REMARKS
Neurofibromatosis (NF): von Recklinghausen's Disease (NF1) and Bilateral Acoustic NF (NF2)[1,2] *PCR, Southern blot*	Whole blood (ACD or EDTA), tumor tissue. Store whole blood at 4° C; store tissue at ≤−20° C if nucleic acids cannot be extracted immediately.	von Recklinghausen's NF is one of the most common genetic disorders of humans (1:3500). The NF1 gene is located at chromosomal region 17q11.2 and codes for the neurofibromin protein. Mutations in the merlin gene are responsible for NF2. This disorder is primarily characterized by bilateral vestibular schwannomas. Targets: NF1 gene, merlin

1.   Stephens K: Genetics of neurofibromatosis 1-associated peripheral nerve sheath tumors, *Cancer Invest* 2:897-914, 2003.
2.   Uppal S, Coatesworth AP: Neurofibromatosis type 2, *Int J Clin Pract* 57:698-703, 2003.

Niemann Pick Disease (Type A)[1,2] *PCR, Sequencing*	Whole blood (ACD or EDTA), tissue. Store whole blood at room temperature or 4° C; store tissue frozen at ≤−20° C if nucleic acids cannot be immediately extracted.	Three mutations account for >94% of cases that result in severe neurological disease in infancy and childhood. Target: acid sphingomyelinase (SMPD1)

1.   Kolodny EH: Niemann-Pick disease, *Curr Opin Hematol* 7:48-52, 2000.
2.   Schuchman EH, Miranda SR: Niemann-Pick disease: mutation update, genotype/phenotype correlations, and prospects for genetic testing, *Genet Test* 1:13-19, 1997.

Ovarian Tumors[1,2] *Immunohistochemistry, PCR*	Tumor tissue. Store fresh tissue at 4° C for 24 hr. However, it is preferred that tissue be frozen at ≤−20° C if nucleic acids cannot be extracted immediately. Paraffin-embedded tissue may also be used.	Point mutations in the ras gene family and p53 tumor suppressor gene, as well as point mutations in numerous other genes, are common. Targets: MSH2, P53

1.   Shih IM, Kurman RJ: Ovarian tumorigenesis: a proposed model based on morphological and molecular genetic analysis, *Am J Pathol* 164:1511-1518, 2004.
2.   Sherbert GV, Patil D: Genetic abnormalities of cell proliferation, invasion and metastasis, with special reference to gynaecological cancers, *Anticancer Res* 23:1357-1371, 2003.

DISORDER	SPECIMEN AND SPECIAL REQUIREMENTS	CLINICAL COMMENTS AND REMARKS
Pancreatic Cancer[1,2] *FISH, PCR, Sequencing, Immunohistochemistry*	Tumor tissue. Store tissue frozen at $\leq -20°$ C if nucleic acids cannot be extracted immediately. Paraffin-embedded tissue may also be used.	Point mutations in the ras gene family and p53 tumor suppressor gene, as well as point mutations in numerous other genes, are common. MTS1 is an oncogene located on chromosome 9 and is associated with point mutations and allelic loss in gastrointestinal and esophageal cancers as well. Targets: DPC4, HER2, K-ras, P16/CDKN2A/MTS1, P53

1. Safioleas MC, Moulakakis KG: Pancreatic cancer today, *Hepatogastroenterology* 51:862-868, 2004.
2. Li D, Xie K, Wolff R, et al: Pancreatic cancer, *Lancet* 363:1049-1057, 2004.

DISORDER	SPECIMEN AND SPECIAL REQUIREMENTS	CLINICAL COMMENTS AND REMARKS
Parvovirus B19[1-3] *PCR, Real-time PCR*	Whole blood, bone marrow, buffey coat, plasma, and tissue. Store all body fluids at 4° C; store tissues at $\leq -20°$ C.	Parvovirus B19 is the etiological agent in a variety of conditions, including asymptomatic infection, erythema infectiosum or "fifth disease," acute arthropathy, aplastic crisis in patients with underlying hemolytic disorders, and hydrops fetalis. In acquired or congenital immunocompromised states, persistent parvovirus B19 is a cause of chronic anemia and red cell aplasia. Target: VP2

1. Young NS, Brown KE: Parvovirus B19, *N Engl J Med* 350:586-597, 2004.
2. Watzinger F, Suda M, Preuner S, et al: Real-time quantitative PCR assays for detection and monitoring of pathogenic human viruses in immunosuppressed pediatric patients, *J Clin Microbiol* 42:5189-5198, 2004.
3. Patou G, Pillay D, Myint S, et al: Characterization of a nested polymerase chain reaction assay for the detection of Parvovirus B19, *J Clin Microbiol* 31:540-546, 1993.

DISORDER	SPECIMEN AND SPECIAL REQUIREMENTS	CLINICAL COMMENTS AND REMARKS
Phenylketonuria (PKU)[1] *PCR, Southern blot*	Whole blood (ACD or EDTA); store at 4° C; newborn screening cards, blotting paper.	The severity of the disease correlates with extent of mutation of the phenylalanine hydroxylase (PAH) gene. PAH activity determines type of replacement therapy. Target: PAH (phenylalanine hydroxylase) gene

1. Waters PJ: How PAH gene mutations cause hyper-phenylalaninemia and why mechanism matters: insights from in vitro expression, *Hum Mutat* 21:357-369, 2003.

DISORDER	SPECIMEN AND SPECIAL REQUIREMENTS	CLINICAL COMMENTS AND REMARKS
Prader-Willi Syndrome[1] *Southern blot, PCR, FISH, Sequencing*	Whole blood (ACD or EDTA), tissue. Store whole blood at room temperature or 4° C; store tissue frozen at ≤−20° C if nucleic acids cannot be immediately extracted.	Approximately 70% of patients show a deletion involving the paternally inherited chromosome 15q11-q13, whereas others may show chromosome 15 maternal uniparental disomy. Targets: SNRPN, Chromosome 15q11

1. Goldstone AP: Prader-Willi syndrome: advances in genetics, pathophysiology and treatment, *Trends Endocrinol Metab* 15:12-20, 2004.

DISORDER	SPECIMEN AND SPECIAL REQUIREMENTS	CLINICAL COMMENTS AND REMARKS
Prostate Cancer[1,2] *PCR, Immunohisto-chemistry*	Tumor tissue. Store tissue at ≤−20° C if nucleic acids cannot be extracted immediately. Paraffin-embedded tissue may also be used.	Point mutations in the ras gene family and p53 tumor suppressor gene, as well as point mutations in numerous other genes, are common, such as cadherin, a calcium-dependent transmembrane glycoprotein that stimulates cell-to-cell adhesion. Targets: DPC4, E-cadherin, PSA, P53

1. Canto EI, Shariat SF, Slawin KM: Molecular diagnosis of prostate cancer, *Curr Urol Rep* 5:203-211, 2004.
2. Chin JL, Reiter RE: Genetic alterations in prostate cancer, *Curr Urol Rep* 5:157-165, 2004.

DISORDER	SPECIMEN AND SPECIAL REQUIREMENTS	CLINICAL COMMENTS AND REMARKS
Prothrombin (Factor II)[1] *Southern blot, PCR, Invader*	Whole blood (ACD or EDTA), tissue. Store whole blood at room temperature or 4° C; store tissue frozen at ≤−20° C if nucleic acids cannot be immediately extracted.	Prothrombin is the precursor of thrombin in the coagulation cascade. A single nucleotide polymorphism has been described that is responsible for increased plasma prothrombin levels. Target: Factor II gene

1. Caprini JA, Glase CJ, Anderson CB, et al: Laboratory markers in the diagnosis of venous thromboembolism, *Circulation* 109(12 suppl 1):I4-8, 2004.

DISORDER	SPECIMEN AND SPECIAL REQUIREMENTS	CLINICAL COMMENTS AND REMARKS
Renal Tumors[1,2] *FISH, PCR, Sequencing*	Tumor tissue, whole blood (ACD or EDTA). Store all body fluids at 4° C; store fresh tissue at ≤ −20° C if nucleic acids cannot be extracted immediately. Paraffin-embedded tissue may also be used.	l-myc can be used as a predictor of poor prognosis. Other gene mutations have been described. Fragile histidine triad (FHIT) is located at chromosome 3p14.2 and is deleted in many solid tumors.[3] Targets: c-Met, FHIT, WT-1, VHL-1

1. Linehan WM, Walther MM, Zbar B: The genetic basis of cancer of the kidney, *J Urol* 170:2163-2172, 2003.
2. Ruteshouser EC, Huff V: Familial Wilms tumor, *Am J Med Genet* 129C:29-34, 2004.
3. Toledo G, Sola JJ, Lozano MD, et al: Loss of FHIT protein expression is related to high proliferation, low apoptosis and worse prognosis in non-small-cell lung cancer, *Mod Pathol* 17:440-448, 2004.

DISORDER	SPECIMEN AND SPECIAL REQUIREMENTS	CLINICAL COMMENTS AND REMARKS
Respiratory Syncytial Virus (RSV)[1,2] *Real-time PCR*	Nasopharyngeal swab, wash, or aspirate.	Molecular assays have proven more sensitive and specific than traditional laboratory testing. Target: N gene

1. Gruteke P, Glas AS, Dierdorp M, et al: Practical implications of a multiplex PCR for acute respiratory tract infections in children, *J Clin Microbiol* 42:5596-5603, 2004.
2. Watzinger F, Suda M, Preuner S, et al: Real-time quantitative PCR assays for detection and monitoring of pathogenic human viruses in immunosuppressed pediatric patients, *J Clin Microbiol* 42:5189-5198, 2004.

DISORDER	SPECIMEN AND SPECIAL REQUIREMENTS	CLINICAL COMMENTS AND REMARKS
Rotavirus[1] *RT-PCR, Real-time RT-PCR, Blotting techniques*	Specimen: Stool. Store at 4° C.	Group A rotaviruses are responsible for most pediatric gastroenteritis cases. The difficulty in culturing rotaviruses makes molecular analyses more practical and clinically relevant. Targets: vp7, vp4

1. Ramig RF: Pathogenesis of intestinal and systemic rotavirus infection, *J Virol* 78:10213-10220, 2004.

DISORDER	SPECIMEN AND SPECIAL REQUIREMENTS	CLINICAL COMMENTS AND REMARKS
Sarcomas[1,2] *FISH, PCR, Sequencing*	Tumor tissue. Store fresh tissue at $\leq -20°$ C if nucleic acids cannot be extracted immediately. Paraffin-embedded tissue may also be used.	Many leukemias are associated with specific chromosomal translocations and gene rearrangements that can be detected by fluorescence in situ hybridization and Southern blot analysis.

		Targets:	*Tumor type:*
		EWS-CHOP, t(12;22)	Myxoid, liposarcoma
		EWS-EIAF, t(17;22)	Ewing's
		EWS-ERG, t(21;22)	Ewing's
		EWS-ETV1, t(7;22)	Ewing's
		EWS-FEV, t(2;22)	Ewing's
		EWS-FLI1, t(11;22)	Ewing's
		EWS-WT1, t(11;22)	Desmoplastic small round cell
		FUS-CHOP, t(12;16)	Myxoid, liposarcoma
		PAX3-FKHR, t(2;13)	Alveolar rhabdomyosarcoma
		PAX7-FKHR, t(1;13)	Alveolar rhabdomyosarcoma
		SYT-SSX1, t(X;18)	Synovial
		SYT-SSX2, t(X;18)	Synovial

1. Cormier JN, Pollock RE: Soft tissue sarcomas, *CA Cancer J Clin* 54:94-109, 2004.
2. Helman LJ, Meltzer P: Mechanisms of sarcoma development, *Nat Rev Cancer* 3:685-694, 2003.

DISORDER	SPECIMEN AND SPECIAL REQUIREMENTS	CLINICAL COMMENTS AND REMARKS
***Staphylococcus aureus,* Methicillin Resistance**[1,2] *PCR, Real-time PCR, Probe hybridization*	Nasal swab, tissues, and other body fluids	Multiplex assays have been developed to distinguish between *Staphyloccocus aureus* and coagulase-negative *S. aureus* in primary samples. Resistance testing can also be performed in a multiplex reaction. Targets: mecA, SCCmec, orfX, 16S rRNA, nuc, mupA

1. Huletsky A, Giroux R, Rossbach V, et al: New real-time PCR assay for rapid detection of methicillin-resistant Staphylococcus aureus directly from specimens containing a mixture of staphylococci, *J Clin Microbiol* 42:1875-1884, 2004.
2. Warren DK, Liao RS, Merz LR, et al: Detection of methicillin-resistant staphylococcus aureus directly from nasal swab specimens by a real-time PCR assay, *J Clin Microbiol* 42:5578-5581, 2004.

DISORDER	SPECIMEN AND SPECIAL REQUIREMENTS	CLINICAL COMMENTS AND REMARKS
***Streptococcus agalactiae,* Group B (GBS)**[1,2] *PCR, Real-time PCR, Probe hybridization*	Vaginal/anal swab, whole blood	The FDA has approved real-time PCR assays for GBS. On major issue in providing this type of testing is laboratory staffing so that testing can be available 24/7. Targets: cfb, 16S rRNA

DISORDER	SPECIMEN AND SPECIAL REQUIREMENTS	CLINICAL COMMENTS AND REMARKS

Streptococcus agalactiae, **Group B (GBS)**—CONT

1. Davies HD, Miller MA, Faro S, et al: Multicenter study of a rapid molecular-based assay for the diagnosis of group B Streptococcus colonization in pregnant women, *Clin Infect Dis* 39:1129-1135, 2004.
2. Golden SM, Stamilio DM, Faux BM, et al: Evaluation of a real-time fluorescent PCR assay for rapid detection of Group B Streptococci in neonatal blood, *Diagn Microbiol Infect Dis* 50:7-13, 2004.

Tay-Sachs Disease[1] *PCR, Sequencing*	Whole blood (ACD or EDTA), tissue. Store whole blood at room temperature or 4° C; store tissue frozen at ≤−20° C if nucleic acids cannot be immediately extracted.	Tay-Sachs disease is an autosomal recessive disease caused by a deficiency of β-hexosaminidase A. Mutations in the α-subunit of hexosaminidase A are responsible for the enzyme deficiency. More than 75 mutations of the α-subunit gene have been described. Target: HEXA gene

1. Fernandes Filho JA, Shapiro BE: Tay-Sachs disease, *Arch Neurol* 61:1466-1468, 2004.

Enterococcus, **Vancomycin Resistance**[1,2] *PCR, Real-time PCR*	Perianal swab	Real-time PCR-based assays are considerably more sensitive than traditional culture methods. Targets: van A, van B, van C-1, van C-2

1. Diekema DJ, Dodgson KJ, Sigurdardottir B, et al: Rapid detection of antimicrobial-resistant organism carriage: an unmet clinical need, *J Clin Microbiol* 42:2879-2883, 2004.
2. Sloan LM, Uhl JR, Vetter EA, et al: Comparison of the Roche Lightcycler vanA/vanB detection assay and culture for detection of vancomycin-resistant Enterococci from perianal swabs, *J Clin Microbiol* 42:2636-2643, 2004.

Varicella-Zoster Virus (VZV)[1] *PCR, Real-time PCR, Blotting techniques, ISH*	Whole blood, skin lesions, tissue, and CSF. Store all body fluids at 4° C; store tissues at ≤−20° C.	Viral cultures have a longer turnaround time and low specificity. Both sensitivity and specificity are increased using molecular tests. Target: ORF38

1. Watzinger F, Suda M, Preuner S, et al: Real-time quantitative PCR assays for detection and monitoring of pathogenic human viruses in immunosuppressed pediatric patients, *J Clin Microbiol* 42:5189-5198, 2004.

SECTION IV
THERAPEUTIC DRUGS
AND DRUGS OF ABUSE

INTRODUCTION

Measurement of drug concentrations in biological fluids for the detection of drug overdose and the development of therapeutic drug-dosing regimens are important parts of patient care. Laboratories engaged in the measurement of drug concentrations for therapeutic monitoring must take into account a range of practical and methodological issues. Analytical techniques, proper sample collection and storage, and knowledge of concurrent pathological and therapeutic conditions of the patient are particularly important. Effective monitoring is dependent on correct sample collection and time of last drug dose, appropriate laboratory analysis, and appropriate interpretation of data. It is our purpose to provide practical information in these areas.

An understanding of the capabilities and limitations of the analytical methods is important to ensure meaningful results. The ideal analytical procedure chosen should be accurate and precise, easy to perform, readily automated, and inexpensive. For the quantitation of drug concentrations, it is important to use procedures with adequate sensitivity and specificity with regard to endogenous compounds, other drugs, and accumulated metabolites. Analytical procedures lacking sensitivity and specificity have generally been excluded from the section, or when such procedures have been included, appropriate comments have been made under the *Interferences* or *Remarks* column. Because of rapid advances in drug analysis, identification of all potential analytical problems for the various drug methodologies is clearly beyond the scope of this section. It is essential that each assay be thoroughly evaluated for specificity, with particular emphasis on the drug's metabolites and other drugs frequently coadministered. Laboratory personnel should keep current with new drug entities and their potential interference with existing drug assays.

Reference ranges listed in this section are those generally accepted in the literature and are believed to be most consistent with the current state of the art. Discrepancies in the literature are common, and additional experience is required before well-established values will be available. Commonly given mean peak plasma concentrations are reported for drugs without documented ranges. It is important to realize that these values are for **reference only because age, other physiological conditions, disease states, concomitant medications, and dialysis procedures may alter drug disposition significantly.** The use of these reference ranges to interpret drug and chemical concentrations in postmortem specimens may not be appropriate because factors affecting drug and chemical concentrations in living patients are frequently altered after death.

TEST NAME AND METHOD	SPECIMEN	REFERENCE (THERAPEUTIC) INTERVAL, CONVENTIONAL [INTERNATIONAL RECOMMENDED UNITS]			KINETIC VALUES	
Acetaminophen **(Tylenol,** **paracetamol)**[1-7] *GC, HPLC,* *GC-MS, LC-MS,* *IA, CZE* *MW: 151.17*	Serum, plasma (heparin, EDTA)	Therapeutic concentration: Toxic concentration: Adults, 4 hr postingestion Adults, 12 hr postingestion Pediatrics, 2 hr postingestion (liquid)	*mcg/mL* 10-20 >150 >40 >225	× 6.61	*μmol/L* [66-132] [>992] [>264] [>1487]	$t_{1/2}$: V_d: Cl_T: PB: F:	1-3 hr 0.8-1.0 L/kg 5.0 mL/min/kg ~25% at therapeutic dose <20% at toxic doses 25%

1. Anderson BJ, Holford NH, Armishaw JC, et al: Predicting concentrations in children presenting with acetaminophen overdose, *J Pediatr* 135:290-295, 1999.

2. Bessems JG, Vermeulen NP: Paracetamol (acetaminophen)-induced toxicity: molecular and biochemical mechanisms, analogues and protective approaches, *Crit Rev Toxicol* 31:55-138, 2001.

3. Hardman JG, Limbird LE, Molinoff PB, et al: *Goodman and Gilman's the pharmacological basis of therapeutics,* ed 9, New York, 1996, McGraw-Hill.

4. Jensen LS, Valentine J, Milne RW, et al: The quantification of paracetamol, paracetamol glucuronide and paracetamol sulphate in plasma and urine using a single high-performance liquid chromatography assay, *J Pharm Biomed Anal* 34:585-593, 2004.

5. Tanaka E, Yamazaki K, Misawa S: Update: the clinical importance of acetaminophen hepatoxocity in non-alcoholic and alcoholic subjects, *J Clin Pharm Ther* 25:325-332, 2000.

6. Vassallo S, Khan A, Howland MA: Use of the Rumack-Matthew nomogram in cases of extended-release acetaminophen toxicity, *Ann Intern Med* 125:940, 1996.

7. White S, Wong SHY: Standards of laboratory practice: analgesic drug monitoring, *Clin Chem* 44:1110-1123, 1998.

TEST NAME AND METHOD	SPECIMEN	REFERENCE (THERAPEUTIC) INTERVAL			KINETIC VALUES	
Acetohexamide **(Dymelor)**[1-6] *HPLC, GC, CZE,* *MEKC* *MW: 324.4*	Serum (note: therapeutic concentrations based on peak collection ~3-5 hr postdose)	Therapeutic concentration: Toxic concentration:	*mcg/mL* 21-56 >500	× 3.08	*μmol/L* [65-172] [>1540]	$t_{1/2}$: V_d: Cl_T: PB: F: T_{max}:	Acetohexamide: ~1.3 hr Hydroxyhexamide (active metabolite): 5-6 hr 0.2 L/kg NA 65-90% [× 0.01 = 0.65-0.90, protein-bound mole fraction] NA 3-5 hr

FACTORS INFLUENCING DRUG DISPOSITION	REMARKS AND INTERFERENCES

Metabolism
 Hepatic (CYP2E1, 1A2, 3A4, 2A6, 2D6)
Excretion
 Renal
Disease
 Hepatic: $t_{1/2}\uparrow$, $V_d\rightarrow$, $Cl_T\downarrow$
 Hyperthyroidism: $t_{1/2}\downarrow$, $V_d\rightarrow$, $Cl_T\uparrow$
 Obesity: $t_{1/2}\rightarrow$, $Cl_T\uparrow$
Age
 Neonates: $t_{1/2}\uparrow$
Dialysis
 Hemodialysis (+)
 Peritoneal (−)

Acetaminophen is commonly used for its antipyretic and analgesic effects. It is available in numerous forms, including extended-release formulas and in combination with other drugs such as codeine and diphenhydramine. Serum concentrations, used for toxicological evaluations, should be interpreted in conjunction with the time of ingestion. The potential for toxicity can be estimated using the Rumack-Matthew nomogram or by determining the half-life. Levels should be measured every 4-6 hr postingestion and treatment initiated if a level exceeds the lower limit defined on the nomogram or if the calculated $t_{1/2}$ is >4 hr.

The metabolite *N*-acetyl-p-benzoquinone (NAPQI) is responsible for the hepatotoxicity described. Renal toxicity is related to NAPQI and other reactive glutathione metabolites such as aminophenol-S-conjugates. Toxic effects include renal tubular necrosis, hypoglycemia, and thrombocytopenia. Toxicity has been reported with therapeutic doses, especially if the drug is taken over a prolonged period or with ethanol. Dose-dependent elimination is observed when doses are >2 g [13.23 mmol]. Antidote: *N*-acetylcysteine

See Tables II-5 and II-6.

Metabolism
 Hepatic
Excretion
 Renal

Acetohexamide is a sulfonylurea oral hypoglycemic agent used in treating type 2 diabetes. The hypoglycemic activity occurs when the drug binds to ATP-sensitive receptors or the pancreatic islet cells and induces insulin secretion. Extrapancreatic actions contribute and include reduced hepatic glucose production and increased peripheral sensitivity to insulin. The prolonged hypoglycemic effects are related to the production of an active metabolite, hydroxyhexamide. Adverse effects include transient leukopenia, thrombocytopenia, hemolytic anemia, pancytopenia, gastrointestinal disturbances, headache, tinnitus, photosensitivity, allergic skin reactions, and intolerance to alcohol. More serious side effects include hypoglycemia (may progress to coma and death) and hepatic dysfunction.

TEST NAME AND METHOD	SPECIMEN	REFERENCE (THERAPEUTIC) INTERVAL, CONVENTIONAL [INTERNATIONAL RECOMMENDED UNITS]		KINETIC VALUES	

Acetohexamide (Dymelor)—CONT

1. Baselt C: *Disposition of toxic drugs and chemicals in man,* ed 7, Foster City, CA, 2004, Biomedical Publications.
2. Ellenhorn MJ: *Ellenhorn's medical toxicology,* ed 2, Philadelphia, 1997, Williams and Wilkins, electronic.
3. Ku YR, Chag LY, Ho LK, et al: Analysis of synthetic antidiabetic drugs in adulterated traditional Chinese medicines by high-performance capillary electrophoresis, *J Pharm Biomed Anal* 33:329-339, 2003.
4. Nunez M, Ferguson JE, Machacek D, et al: Detection of hypoglycemic drugs in human urine using micellar electrokinetic chromatography, *Anal Chem* 67:3668-3675, 1995.

TEST NAME AND METHOD	SPECIMEN	REFERENCE (THERAPEUTIC) INTERVAL, CONVENTIONAL [INTERNATIONAL RECOMMENDED UNITS]			KINETIC VALUES	
N-Acetyl-procainamide (NAPA)[1-5] *HPLC, GLC, EIA, FPIA, FIA* *MW: 277*	Serum, plasma (heparin, EDTA, oxalate). Stable for ~6 mo at −20° C. Collect at trough concentration for assay of pro-cainamide and *N*-acetyl-procainamide. For determination of acetylator status, collect pro-cainamide/NAPA sample 3 hr after last dose.	*mcg/mL* Therapeutic concentration*: 10-20 Toxic concentration: >40 *NAPA should be analyzed in conjunction with procainamide concentrations.	× 3.61[6,7]	μ*mol/L* [>144]	PK[4,5]: $t_{1/2}$: V_d: Cl_T: PB: F:	5.5-6.2 hr 1.38 L/kg 3.1 ± 0.4 mL/min/kg 10% 85%

1. Valdes R Jr, Jortani SA, Gheorghiade M: Standards of laboratory practice: cardiac drug monitoring, *Clin Chem* 44:1096-1109, 1998.
2. Lexi-Comp Inc: *Up-to-date online 12.2, drug information,* Hudson, OH, 2004, Lexi-Comp, Inc.
3. Jurgens G, Graudal NA, Kampmann JP: Therapeutic drug monitoring of antiarrhythmic drugs, *Clin Pharmacokinet* 42:647-663, 2003.
4. Hardman JG, Limbird LE, Gilman AG, et al: *Goodman & Gilman's the pharmacological basis of therapeutics,* ed 10. New York, 2001, McGraw-Hill.
5. Baselt RC: *Disposition of toxic drugs and chemicals in man,* ed 7, Foster City, CA, 2004, Chemical Toxicology Institute.
6. Harmening DM: *Clinical hematology and fundamentals of hemostasis,* ed 2, Philadelphia, 1992, FA Davis.
7. Thomson JM, editor: *Blood coagulation and haemostasis,* ed 3, New York, 1985, Churchill Livingstone.
8. Niederweiser A, Matasovic A, Leumaun EP: Glycolic acid in urine: a colorimetric method with values in normal adult controls and in patients with primary hyperoxaluria, *Clin Chim Acta* 89:13-18, 1978.

TEST NAME AND METHOD	SPECIMEN	REFERENCE (THERAPEUTIC) INTERVAL		KINETIC VALUES	
Acyclovir (Zovirax) *HPLC[1,2]* *MB* *MW: 225.21*	Serum, plasma (heparin). Stable at 12° C for 7 days.[3]	Therapeutic concentration: Not defined Toxic concentration: Not defined		PK[4-6]: $t_{1/2}$: V_d: Cl_T: PB: F:	2-3 hr 0.69 ± 0.19 L/kg 4.66 ± 0.57 mL/min/kg 9-33% 15-30%

FACTORS INFLUENCING
DRUG DISPOSITION   REMARKS AND INTERFERENCES

5. Schulz M, Schmoldt A: Therapeutic and toxic blood concentrations of more than 800 drugs and other xenobiotics, *Pharmazie* 58:447-474, 2003.
6. Sheldon J, Anderson J, Stoner L: Serum concentration and urinary excretion of oral sulfonylurea compounds, *Diabetes* 14:362-367, 1965.

Metabolism
  None
Excretion
  Urine
Disease
  Renal: $t_{1/2}\uparrow$, ~40 hr; $V_d\rightarrow$, $Cl_T\downarrow$
  Coronary artery disease: $t_{1/2}\uparrow$, $V_d\rightarrow$, $Cl_T\downarrow$
  Obesity: $Cl_T\downarrow$
Age
  Elderly: $t_{1/2}\uparrow$, $Vd\rightarrow$, $Cl_1\downarrow$
Dialysis
  Hemodialysis (+)

Therapeutic and toxic concentrations are not well defined. *N*-Acetylprocainamide (NAPA), an active metabolite of the antiarrhythmic procainamide, is rapidly hydrolyzed in vitro to procainamide at a low pH. (See *Procainamide.*) NAPA concentrations should be evaluated in conjunction with procainamide concentrations. When the sum of NAPA and procainamide concentrations is >25-30 mg/L, the risk of toxicity is increased.[8]

Interferences: Heparin (FPIA). Hemolysis and lipemia interfere with all methods except GC and HPLC.

Metabolism
  Viral and cellular enzymes
Excretion
  Urine (primary)
Disease[7]
  Renal: $t_{1/2}\uparrow$, $V_d\rightarrow$, $Cl_T\downarrow$

This drug is a selective antiherpes viral agent available in topical, oral, and intravenous forms. Systemic absorption from the skin is limited. The bioavailability of acyclovir appears to decrease with increasing dosage. Mean peak acyclovir concentrations after multiple intravenous doses of 2.5, 5, 10, and 15 mg/kg [× 4.44 = 11.1, 22.2, 44.4, and 66.6 μmol/kg] every 8 hr were 5.2, 9.9, 20.7, and 23.6 mg/mL [× 4.44 = 23, 44, 92, and 105 μmol/L], respectively. Acyclovir appears to possess a wide therapeutic index.

TEST NAME AND METHOD	SPECIMEN	REFERENCE (THERAPEUTIC) INTERVAL, CONVENTIONAL [INTERNATIONAL RECOMMENDED UNITS]	KINETIC VALUES

Acyclovir (Zovirax)—CONT

1. Land G, Bye A: Simple high-performance liquid chromatographic method for the analysis of 9-(2-hydroxyethoxymethyl) guanine (acyclovir) in human plasma and urine, *J Chromatogr* 224:51-58, 1981.

2. Bangaru RA, Bansal YK, Rao AR, et al: Rapid, simple and sensitive high-performance liquid chromatographic method for detection and determination of acyclovir in human plasma and its use in bioavailability studies, *J Chromatogr B* 739:231-237, 2000.

3. Salamoun J, Sprta V, Sladek T, et al: Determination of acyclovir in plasma by column liquid chromatography with fluorescence detection, *J Chromatogr* 420:197-202, 1987.

4. Lexi-Comp, Inc.: *Up-to-date online 12.2, drug information,* Hudson, OH, 2004, Lexi-Comp, Inc.

5. Gilman A, Hardman J, Limbird L: *The pharmacological basis of therapeutics,* ed 10, New York, 2001, Pergamon Press, Inc.

6. Laskin OL: Clinical pharmacokinetics of acyclovir, *Clin Pharmacokinet* 8:187-201, 1983.

7. Bennett WM, Aronoff GR, Golper TA, et al: *Drug prescribing in renal failure,* ed 3, Philadelphia, 1994, American College of Physicians.

8. Micromedex: *Micromedex Healthcare series 2004,* Greenwood Village, CO, 2004, Thomson Micromedex.

(Urine) Adulteration[1-6]	Urine, random. Witnessed or unwitnessed	Adulterated:[4] <3 or ≥11 Invalid result: ≥3 and <4 or ≥10 and <11	NA
pH			

pH electrode
Colorimetric assay

Creatinine and Specific Gravity		creatinine, mg/dL	specific gravity
	Substituted[4]:	<2	≤1.001
Colorimetric assay	Substituted:	<2	≥1.020
and refractometry	Diluted:	≥2	<1.003
	Invalid:	≥2	1.000
	Invalid:	≥2 and <20	≥1.020

Nitrite[5]		mg/L
	Adulterated[4]:	≥500
Colorimetric assay	Invalid:	≥200 and <500

FACTORS INFLUENCING DRUG DISPOSITION	REMARKS AND INTERFERENCES

Age
  Neonate: $t_{1/2}\uparrow$, $V_d\downarrow$, $Cl_T\downarrow$
Dialysis
  Hemodialysis (+)

Drug interactions: Probenecid decreases renal clearance of acyclovir, presumably by inhibiting its tubular secretion. Acyclovir can decrease varicella vaccine effectiveness when used concurrently.[8]

Side effects of parenteral acyclovir include phlebitis, inflammation or pain at the site of injection, transient increases in blood urea nitrogen and serum creatinine, and acute renal failure. Encephalopathic changes may occur rarely with parenteral administration of acyclovir, but a causal relationship has not been established. Headache and gastrointestinal disturbances are the most common adverse effects seen with oral acyclovir.

Bioassay lacks sensitivity and accuracy at concentrations <2.3 mcg/mL [× 4.44 = <10 μmol/L].

Interferes with immunoassays and GC/MS confirmation assays for drugs of abuse.

Urine pH outside pH 3 and 11 is not compatible with normal physiologic or pathologic values and therefore suggests purposeful adulteration. Values between 3 and 4 and 10 and 11 may be the result of analytical inaccuracies and not adulteration.[1]

The use of saline will produce a low creatinine with a normal specific gravity.

Creatinine and specific gravity measure the concentrating capability of the kidneys. Low values suggest excess water intake, with the purpose of diluting drug concentrations to below their respective cutoffs. Very low values suggest substitution with a non–urine-based fluid.

Oxidizes certain drugs of abuse (tetrahydrocannabinol and opiates).

Nitrite concentrations exceeding the adulteration limit cannot be achieved by normal physiologic or pathologic processes and indicate purposeful adulteration.

TEST NAME AND METHOD	SPECIMEN	REFERENCE (THERAPEUTIC) INTERVAL, CONVENTIONAL [INTERNATIONAL RECOMMENDED UNITS]	KINETIC VALUES

(Urine) Adulteration—CONT

Chromium (VI)[3]

Ion
chromatography

≥Drug testing laboratory's limit of detection for this analyte.[4]

Aldehyde[6]

Colorimetric assay

≥Drug testing laboratory's limit of detection for this analyte.[4]

Halogen

Colorimetric assay

≥Drug testing laboratory's limit of detection for this analyte.[4]

Surfactant[1]

Colorimetric assay

≥Drug testing laboratory's limit of detection for this analyte.[4]

Pyridine[3]

Gas
chromatography

≥Drug testing laboratory's limit of detection for this analyte.[4]

1. Wu AHB: Integrity of urine specimens submitted for toxicologic analysis: adulteration, mechanisms of action, and laboratory detection, *Forensic Sci Rev* 10:47-65, 1999.
2. Wu AHB: Urine adulteration and substitution prior to drugs of abuse testing, *J Clin Ligand Assay* 26:11-18, 2003.
3. Wu AHB, Sexton K, Cassella G, et al: Adulteration of urine by "Urine Luck," *Clin Chem* 45:1051-1057, 1999.
4. Department of Health and Human Services. Substance Abuse and Mental Health Services Administration: Mandatory guidelines for federal workplace drug testing programs, *Fed Red* 66:43876-43882, 2001.
5. Tsai JSC, ElSohly MA, Tsai SF, et al: Investigation of nitrite adulteration on the immunoassay and GC-MS analysis of cannabinoids in urine specimens, *J Anal Toxicol* 24:708-714, 2000.
6. George S, Braithwaite RA: The effect of glutaraldehyde adulteration of urine specimens on Syva EMIT II drugs-of-abuse assays, *J Anal Toxicol* 20:195-196, 1996.

		mg/L		*mmol/L*		
Alprazolam	Serum, plasma				$t_{1/2}$:	6-20 hr
(Xanax)[1-14]		Therapeutic			V_d/F:	0.9-1.3 L/kg
		concentration:	10-50 × 3.24	[32-162]	Cl_T/F:	0.74 ± 0.14 mL/min/kg
GC, HPLC, LC-MS		Toxic			PB:	80%
		concentration:	>100	[>324]		[× 0.01 = 0.80, protein-
MW: 308.8						bound mole fraction]
IA, GC-MS	Urine					

FACTORS INFLUENCING DRUG DISPOSITION	REMARKS AND INTERFERENCES
Oxidizes certain drugs of abuse (tetrahydro-cannabinol and opiates).	
Interferes with immunoassays for drugs of abuse.	Aldehyde concentrations such as glutaraldehyde above the sensitivity are indicative of purposeful adulteration.
Oxidizes certain drugs of abuse (tetrahydro-cannabinol and opiates).	Halogen concentrations (e.g., fluoride, bromide) above the sensitivity are indicative of purposeful adulteration.
Interferes with immunoassays for drugs of abuse.	Surfactants such as dodecyclobenzene sulfonate concentrations above the sensitivity are indicative of purposeful adulteration.
When used with pyridinium chlorochromate, oxidizes certain drugs of abuse (tetrahydro-cannabinol and opiates).	Pyridine concentrations above the sensitivity are indicative of purposeful adulteration.

Metabolism
  Hepatic, CYP3A
Excretion
  Renal
Disease
  Cirrhosis: $t_{1/2}\uparrow, V_d\rightarrow, Cl_T\downarrow$
  Obesity: $t_{1/2}\uparrow, V_d\rightarrow, Cl_T\downarrow$
Age
  Elderly,
  M: $t_{1/2}\uparrow, V_d\rightarrow, Cl_T\downarrow$
  F: $t_{1/2}\rightarrow, V_d\rightarrow, Cl_T\rightarrow$

Alprazolam, a triazolobenzodiazepine derivative, is used for treatment of anxiety disorder, panic disorder, and anxiety associated with depression. Symptoms of overdose include somnolence, confusion, coma, and diminished reflexes. Its major pathway of metabolism is oxidation (hydroxylation) to α-hydroxyalprazolam and 4-hydroxyalprazolam.

TEST NAME AND METHOD	SPECIMEN	REFERENCE (THERAPEUTIC) INTERVAL, CONVENTIONAL [INTERNATIONAL RECOMMENDED UNITS]	KINETIC VALUES

Alprazolam (Xanax)—CONT

1. Baselt R: *Disposition of toxic drugs and chemicals in man,* ed 7, Foster City, CA, 2004, Biomedical Publications.
2. Schulz M, Schmoldt A: Therapeutic and toxic blood concentrations of more than 800 drugs and other xenobiotics, *Pharmazie* 58:447-474, 2003.
3. Hardman JG, Limbird LE, Gilman AG: *Goodman and Gilman's the pharmacological basis of therapeutics,* ed 10, New York, 2001, McGraw-Hill.
4. *Physicians desk reference,* ed 58, Montvale, NJ, 2004, Thomson PDR.
5. Greenblatt DJ, Divoll M, Abernethy DR, et al: Clinical pharmacokinetics of the newer benzodiazepines, *Clin Pharmacokinet* 8:233-252, 1983.
6. Clarke EGC: *Clarke's isolation and identification of drugs in pharmaceuticals, body fluids, and post-mortem material,* London, 1986, The Pharmaceutical Press.
7. Greenblatt DJ, Javaid JI, Cocniskar A, et al: Gas chromatography analysis of alprazolam in plasma: replicability, stability and specificity, *J Chromatogr* 534:202-207, 1990.
8. ACP's PIER: *Physicians' information and education resource (online version),* Philadelphia, 2004, American College of Physicians.
9. Goldfrank LR, editor: *Goldfrank's toxicological emergencies,* ed 7, (online version), New York, 2002, The McGraw-Hill Companies Inc.
10. Kratzsch C, Tenberken O, Peters FT, et al: Screening, library-assisted identification and validated quantification of 23 benzodiazepines, flumazenil, zaleplone, zolpidem and zopiclone in plasma by liquid chromatography/mass spectrometry with atmospheric pressure chemical ionization, *J Mass Spectrom* 39:856-872, 2004.
11. Borrey D, Meyer E, Lambert W, et al: Simultaneous determination of fifteen low-dosed benzodiazepines in human urine by solid-phase extraction and gas chromatography-mass spectrometry, *J Chromatogr B Biomed Sci Appl* 765:187-197, 2001.
12. Akerman KK, Jolkkonen J, Parviainen M, et al: Analysis of low-dose benzodiazepines by HPLC with automated solid-phase extraction, *Clin Chem* 42:1412-1416, 1996.
13. Reubsaet KJ, Ragnar NH, Hemmersbach P, et al: Determination of benzodiazepines in human urine and plasma with solvent modified solid phase micro extraction and gas chromatography; rationalization of method development using experimental design strategies, *J Pharma Biomed Anal* 18:667-680, 1998.
14. Rasanen I, Ojanpera I, Vuori E: Quantitative screening for benzodiazepines in blood by dual-column gas chromatography and comparison of the results with urine immunoassay, *J Anal Toxicol* 24:46-51, 2000.

Amantadine **(Symmetrel)** *GC-FI*[1] *MW: 918*	Serum, plasma (heparin).	Therapeutic concentration: >300 mg/L[3] [× 0.00661 = 1.98 µmol/L] (Influenza A prophylaxis)	PK[4-6]: $t_{1/2}$: 16 ± 6 hr V_d: 1.5–6.1 L/kg Cl_T: 2.5–10.5 L/hr PB: 67%
GC-MS,[2] GC-FI[1]	Urine. Store at −20° C.[2]		

FACTORS INFLUENCING DRUG DISPOSITION	REMARKS AND INTERFERENCES

Drug interactions: CYP3A4 inducers may decrease levels/effects of alprazolam, and CYP3A4 inhibitors may increase its levels/effects.

Metabolism
  Hepatic
Excretion
  Urine
Disease or condition
  Renal dysfunction: $t_{1/2}\uparrow$
Age
  Elderly: $t_{1/2}\uparrow$, $Cl_R\downarrow$
Dialysis
  Hemodialysis $(-)$
  Peritoneal $(-)$

Amantadine is an antiviral agent. In young healthy adults, a dose of 200 mg/day is associated with a trough plasma concentration of ~300 mg/mL at steady state. There may be an inverse relationship between Vd and dose. Depression, detachment, inability to concentrate, difficulty remembering, and drowsiness may be dose-related adverse effects. Other adverse effects may include insomnia, jitteriness, orthostatic hypotension, and dyspepsia. Concentrations >1000 mcg/L [6.61 μmol/L] may be associated with psychosis.

TEST NAME AND METHOD	SPECIMEN	REFERENCE (THERAPEUTIC) INTERVAL, CONVENTIONAL [INTERNATIONAL RECOMMENDED UNITS]			KINETIC VALUES

Amantadine (Symmetrel)—CONT

1. Belanger PM, Grech-Belanger O: Gas-liquid chromatographic determination of plasma and urinary levels of amantadine in man, *J Chromatogr* 228:327-332, 1982.

2. Koppel C, Tenczer J: A revision of the metabolic disposition of amantadine, *Biomed Mass Spectrom* 12:499-501, 1985.

3. Brenner M, Haass A, Jacobi P, et al: Amantadine sulphate in treating Parkinson's disease: clinical effects, psychometric tests, and serum concentrations, *J Neurol* 236:153-156, 1989.

4. Aoki FY, Sitar DS: Clinical pharmacokinetics of amantadine hydrochloride, *Clin Pharmacokinet* 14:35-51, 1988.

5. Somani SK, Degelau J, Cooper SL, et al: Comparison of pharmacokinetic and safety profiles of amantadine 50- and 100-mg daily doses in elderly nursing home residents, *Pharmacotherapy* 11:460-466, 1991.

6. Lexi-Comp, Inc: *Up-to-date online 12.2, drug information,* Hudson, OH, 2004, Lexi-Comp, Inc.

TEST NAME AND METHOD	SPECIMEN	REFERENCE (THERAPEUTIC) INTERVAL, CONVENTIONAL [INTERNATIONAL RECOMMENDED UNITS]			KINETIC VALUES	
Amikacin[1] **(Amikin)** *HPLC, GLC, REA, FPIA, EIA, FIA* *MW: 585.61*	Serum, plasma (EDTA). For patients taking penicillin or its derivatives, freeze sample if not analyzed within 4-6 hr. Routine collection of specimen should be at trough (within 30 min before the dose) and peak concentration (end of a 1-hr constant infusion, 30 min after the end of a 30-min constant infusion, or 1 hr after an IM dose).		*mcg/mL*	*μmol/L*	PK[2-4]: t_{1/2}	
		Therapeutic concentration			Neonate:	2-9 hr
		Peak:	25-35 × 1.71	[43-60]	Child:	0.5-2.5 hr
		Trough Less severe			Adult:	2-3 hr
		infection:	1-4	[2-7]	V_d:	0.26 L/kg
		Life-threatening			Cl_T:	1.3 mL/min/kg
		infection:	4-8	[7-14]	PB:	4-11%
		Toxic concentration				
		Peak:	>35-40	[>60-68]		
		Trough (nephrotoxicity):	>10-15	[>17-26]		

FACTORS INFLUENCING DRUG DISPOSITION	REMARKS AND INTERFERENCES

Drug interactions: The hydrochlorothiazide-triamterene combination increases plasma amantadine concentrations. Amantadine may decrease the V_d of acetaminophen. Benztropine and trihexyphenidyl, as well as agents with anticholinergic activity such as quinidine, tricyclics, and antihistamines, may potentiate CNS side effects of amantadine.[6]

Metabolism
  None
Excretion
  Urine
Disease
  Renal: $t_{1/2}\uparrow$, $Cl_T\downarrow$
  Burns: $t_{1/2}\downarrow$, $Cl_T\uparrow$
  Cystic fibrosis: $t_{1/2}\downarrow$, $Cl_T\uparrow$
  Obesity: $t_{1/2}\rightarrow$, $V_d\uparrow$ (based on IBW), $Cl_T\uparrow$
  (based on IBW)
Age
  Newborn: $t_{1/2}\uparrow$, $V_d\uparrow$, $Cl_T\downarrow$
  Child: $t_{1/2}\downarrow$, $V_d\uparrow$, $Cl_T\uparrow$
Dialysis
  Hemodialysis (+)
  Peritoneal (+)[5]

Drug interactions: Indomethacin IV, amphotericin, loop diuretics, vancomycin, enflurane, and methoxyflurane can increase toxicity of amikacin. Administration of amikacin can increase the effect of neuromuscular-blocking agents and polypeptide antibiotics.[6]

Amikacin is an aminoglycoside antibiotic. Therapeutic and toxic concentrations should be considered highly variable and individualized for the patient's condition. Penicillin and its derivatives inactivate amikacin in vivo and in vitro. Amikacin may be less sensitive than other aminoglycosides to this inactivation. A definitive cause-and-effect relationship between the trough concentration and the incidence of nephrotoxicity has not been established. Cl_T and $t_{1/2}$ are strongly correlated with glomerular filtration rate. Side effects include vestibular and auditory dysfunction (principally auditory), nephrotoxicity, and neuromuscular blockade.

Interferences: When a patient is also taking antibiotics (i.e., penicillins, cephalosporins, tetracyclines, clindamycin, chloramphenicol), the MB method may lack specificity. Penicillins and cephalosporins can be inactivated with a commercially available β-lactamase to minimize this interference.

See Table II-6.

TEST NAME AND METHOD	SPECIMEN	REFERENCE (THERAPEUTIC) INTERVAL, CONVENTIONAL [INTERNATIONAL RECOMMENDED UNITS]	KINETIC VALUES

Amikacin—CONT

1. Baselt RC: *Disposition of toxic drugs and chemicals in man,* ed 7, Foster City, CA, 2004, Chemical Toxicology Institute.
2. Pechere JC, Dugal R: Clinical pharmacokinetics of aminoglycoside antibiotics, *Clin Pharmacokinet* 4:170-199, 1979.
3. Evans WE, Schentag JJ, Jusko WJ: *Applied pharmacokinetics—principles of therapeutic drug monitoring,* ed 3, Vancouver, WA, 1992, Applied Therapeutics, Inc.

Aminocaproic Acid (Amicar)[1-4]

HPLC, GC

MW: 131.2

Serum, plasma (heparin, EDTA). Collect at trough concentration.

	mcg/mL		μ*mol/L*		
Therapeutic concentration:	100-400	× 7.62	[0.76-3.05]	$t_{1/2}$:	1-2 hr
				V_d:	0.4 L/kg
				Cl_T:	169 mL/min/kg
Toxic concentration:	Not well defined			PB:	Negligible

1. Adams RF, Schmidt GJ, Vandemark FL: Determination of ε-aminocaproic acid in serum by reversed-phase chromatography with fluorescence detection, *Clin Chem* 23:1226-1229, 1977.
2. Bennett-Guarrero E, Sorohan JG, Canada AT, et al: epsilon-Aminocaproic acid plasma levels during cardiopulmonary bypass, *Anesth Analg* 85:248-251, 1997.
3. Budris WA, Roxe DM, Duvel JM: High anion gap metabolic acidosis associated with aminocaproic acid, *Ann Pharmacother* 33:308-311, 1999.
4. Seymour BD, Rubinger M: Rhabdomyolysis induced by epsilon-aminocaproic acid, *Ann Pharmacother* 31:56-58, 1997.

Amiodarone[1,2] **(Cordarone)**

HPLC

MW: 645.33

Serum, plasma (EDTA). Stable for at least 6 mo at 20° C.[3]

	mg/mL		*mmol/L*	PK[2,4-6]:	
Therapeutic concentration:	0.5-2.0	× 1.55	[0.8-3.1]	$t_{1/2}$ Single IV dose:	3-80 hr
Toxic concentration:	>2.5		[>3.9]	Chronic PO therapy:	25-105 days
				V_d:	18-148 L/kg
				Cl_T:	1.9 ± 0.4 mL/min/kg
				PB:	~95%
				F:	~35%

| FACTORS INFLUENCING DRUG DISPOSITION | REMARKS AND INTERFERENCES |

4. Micromedex: *Micromedex Healthcare series 2004,* Greenwood Village, CO, 2004, Thomson Micromedex.
5. Chow-Tung E, Lau AH, Vidyasagar D, et al: Effect of peritoneal dialysis on serum concentrations of three drugs commonly used in pediatric patients, *Dev Pharmacol Ther* 8:85-95, 1985.
6. Lexi-Comp, Inc.: *Up-to-date online 12.2, drug information,* Hudson, OH, 2004, Lexi-Comp, Inc.

Metabolism
  Hepatic
Excretion
  Renal
Disease
  Renal: $t_{1/2}\uparrow$, $Cl_T\downarrow$
  Hemodialysis (+)
  Peritoneal dialysis (+)

Aminocaproic acid is used to treat excessive bleeding caused by hyperfibrinolysis. Its mechanism of action occurs primarily through the inhibition of plasminogen activators. Serum concentrations of 200-400 mcg/mL [1.52-3.05 mmol/L] correlate well with streptokinase clot lysis times of 36-48 hr.

Most significant adverse effects include thromboembolic complications, rhabdomyolysis, and metabolic acidosis. Other reactions include nasal stuffiness, abdominal discomfort, nausea, vomiting, diarrhea, hypotension, itching, and erythemia. There have been reports of increased serum potassium concentrations and metabolic acidosis (with high anion gap) in patients with renal disease.

Metabolism
  Hepatic
  Active metabolite: *N*-desethyl-amiodarone
Excretion
  Feces (primary)
  Urine (secondary)
Dialysis
  Hemodialysis (−)

Drug interactions: Amiodarone is a major substrate of CYP2C8/9 and minor substrate of CYP1A2, CYP2C19, CYP2D6, and CYP3A4. It is a strong inhibitor of CYP1A2, moderate inhibitor of CYP2A6, CYP2C8/9, CYP2D6, and CYP3A4, and a weak inhibitor of CYP2B6 and CYP2C19.[7] Because of the long half-life of amiodarone, drug interactions may take ≥1 week to develop. Amiodarone potentiates warfarin anticoagulation, probably through

This is a class III antiarrhythmic and an iodinated benzofuran derivative. Its therapeutic range is not well defined. A delay of as long as 28 days between the initiation of the amiodarone therapy and the antiarrhythmic effect is expected if no loading dose is administered. Side effects may not manifest until after >1 yr of therapy. Reported side effects include elevations of serum aminotransferases and alkaline phosphatase, jaundice, corneal microdeposits, facial pigmentation, thyroid dysfunction, and pulmonary toxicity. Because of its delayed onset of action, complex dosing schedule, and potential serious side effects, amidorone is used only when other agents are ineffective or cannot be tolerated.

Interferences: Some HPLC methods lack specificity for the parent compound and also measure desethylamiodarone (DEA), a major metabolite.

See Table II-5.

TEST NAME AND METHOD	SPECIMEN	REFERENCE (THERAPEUTIC) INTERVAL, CONVENTIONAL [INTERNATIONAL RECOMMENDED UNITS]	KINETIC VALUES

Amiodarone—CONT

1. Valdes R Jr, Jortani SA, Gheorghiade M: Standards of laboratory practice: cardiac drug monitoring, *Clin Chem* 44:1096-1109, 1998.

2. Baselt RC: *Disposition of toxic drugs and chemicals in man,* ed 7, Foster City, CA, 2004, Chemical Toxicology Institute.

3. Storey GC, Holt DW, Holt P, et al: High-performance liquid chromatographic measurement of amiodarone and its desmethyl metabolite: methodology and preliminary observations, *Ther Drug Monit* 4:385-388, 1982.

4. Gillis AM, Kates RE: Clinical pharmacokinetics of the newer antiarrhythmic agents, *Clin Pharmacokinet* 9:375-403, 1984.

5. Latini R, Tognoni G, Kates RE: Clinical pharmacokinetics of amiodarone, *Clin Pharmacokinet* 9:136-156, 1984.

6. McGovern B, Geer VR, LaRaia PJ, et al: Possible interaction between amiodarone and phenytoin, *Ann Intern Med* 101:650-651, 1984.

7. Lexi-Comp, Inc: *Up-to-date online 12.2, drug information,* Hudson, OH, 2004, Lexi-Comp, Inc.

TEST NAME AND METHOD	SPECIMEN					KINETIC VALUES
Amobarbital (Amytal)[1-12]	Serum, plasma		*mg/L*		*mmol/L*	$t_{1/2}$: 15-30 hr
		Therapeutic concentration:	1-5	× 4.42	[4-22]	V_d: 0.9-1.4 L/kg
Colorimetric, GC, HPLC, IA, CE		Toxic concentration:	>6		[>26.5]	PB: 58.5 ± 1.1% [× 0.01 = 0.59 ± 0.01, protein-bound mole fraction]
MW: 226.3						

1. Baselt R: *Disposition of toxic drugs and chemicals in man,* ed 7, Foster City, CA, 2004, Biomedical Publications.

2. Schulz M, Schmoldt A: Therapeutic and toxic blood concentrations of more than 800 drugs and other xenobiotics, *Pharmazie* 58:447-474, 2003.

3. Hardman JG, Limbird LE, Gilman AG: *Goodman and Gilman's the pharmacological basis of therapeutics,* ed 10, New York, 2001, McGraw-Hill.

4. *Physicians desk reference,* ed 58, Montvale, NJ, 2004, Thomson PDR.

FACTORS INFLUENCING DRUG DISPOSITION	REMARKS AND INTERFERENCES

inhibition of metabolism. Amiodarone also has been reported to cause an increase in plasma concentrations of quinidine, procainamide, flecainide, digoxin, and phenytoin, probably by inhibiting metabolism and decreasing clearance. Amiodarone may cause potentiation of bradycardia, sinus arrest, and atrioventricular block when used with β-adrenergic or calcium channel-blocking agents.

Metabolism
  Hepatic (primary), CYP2A6
  Major metabolites 3'-hydroxyamobarbital and N-glucosylamobarbital
Dialysis
  Hemodialysis (+)
  Hemoperfusion (+)
  Peritoneal (−)

Drug interactions: Amobarbital is a CYP2A6 inducer and may decrease the levels of CYP2A6 substrates. MAO inhibitors and valproic acid may inhibit metabolism of barbiturates increasing the clinical effect or toxicity.

Amobarbital is an intermediate-acting barbiturate used in short-term treatment of insomnia, to reduce anxiety and provide sedation preoperatively. It produces the following effects as dosage is increased: hypnosis, sedation, coma, respiratory arrest, and death. Toxicity is intensified when the drug is combined with ethanol or other CNS depressants.

5. Meatherall R: GC/MS confirmation of barbiturates in blood and urine, *J Forensic Sci* 42:1160-1170, 1997.
6. ACP's PIER: *Physicians' information and education resource (online version),* Philadelphia, 2004, American College of Physicians.
7. McEvoy GK, editor: *AHFS drug information (online version),* Bethesda, MD, 2004, American Society of Health-System Pharmacists Inc.
8. *USP DI drug information for the health care professional,* ed 24, (online version), Taunton, MA, 2004, Micromedex Inc.

TEST NAME AND METHOD	SPECIMEN	REFERENCE (THERAPEUTIC) INTERVAL, CONVENTIONAL [INTERNATIONAL RECOMMENDED UNITS]	KINETIC VALUES

Amobarbital—CONT

9. Tanaka E, Terada M, Tanno K, et al: Forensic analysis of 10 barbiturates in human biological samples using a new reversed-phase chromatographic column packed with 2-micrometre porous microspherical silica-gel, *Forensic Sci Int* 85:73-82, 1997.

10. Quinones-Torrelo C, Martin-Biosca Y, Sagrado S, et al: Determination of amobarbital and secobarbital in plasma samples using micellar liquid chromatography, *Biomed Chromatogr* 14:287-292, 2000.

Amoxapine (Asendin)[1-5]

HPLC, GC-MS, GC

MW: 313.8

Serum

Therapeutic concentration: sum of amoxapine and 8-OH amoxapine   *mcg/mL* 0.18-0.6

Toxic concentration: >3

$t_{1/2}$:
Parent:	8 hr
7-OH	4-6.5 hr
8-OH	30 hr
V_d:	91 L/kg
Cl_T:	3.2-114 L/kg
PB:	~90%
F:	18-54%
T_{max}:	1-2 hr

1. Baker DE: *Drugdex drug evaluations: amoxapine,* Greenwood Village, CO, 2004, Thomson Micromedex.

2. Baselt C: *Disposition of toxic drugs and chemicals in man,* ed 7, Foster City, CA, 2004, Biomedical Publications.

3. Hue B, Palomba B, Giacardy-Paty M, et al: Concurrent high-performance liquid chromatographic measurement of loxapine and amoxapine and of their hydroxylated metabolites in plasma, *Ther Drug Monit* 20:335-339, 1998.

4. Mazzola CD, Miron S, Jenkins AJ: Loxapine intoxication: case report and literature review, *J Anal Toxicol* 24:638-641, 2000.

5. Schulz M, Schmoldt A: Therapeutic and toxic blood concentrations of more than 800 drugs and other xenobiotics, *Pharmazie* 58:447-474, 2003.

Amphetamine[1-20] **(Adderall)**

GC, fluorimetric, colorimetric, GC-MS, IA, CE, LC-MS-MS

MW: 135.2

Serum, plasma

	ng/mL		*nmol/L*
Therapeutic concentration:	20-100	× 7.4	[148-740]
Toxic concentration:	200 ng/mL		[1480]

$t_{1/2}$: 4-8 hr (acidic urine) 12 hr (uncontrolled urine pH)
V_d: 3-5 L/kg
PB: 15-40%
[× 0.01 = 0.15-0.40, protein-bound mole fraction]

Urine   Negative

Alternative matrices: oral fluid, sweat, and hair   Negative

FACTORS INFLUENCING DRUG DISPOSITION	REMARKS AND INTERFERENCES

11. Ferslew KE, Hagardorn AN, McCormick WF: Application of micellar electrokinetic capillary chromatography to forensic analysis of barbiturates in biological fluids, *J Forensic Sci* 40:245-249, 1995.

12. Baselt RC: *Analytical procedures for therapeutic drug monitoring and emergency toxicology,* ed 2, Davis, CA, 1987, Biomedical Publications.

Metabolism
Hepatic, Active metabolites:
7-hydroxyamoxapine,
8-hydroxyamoxapine
Excretion
Renal, fecal

Amoxapine is an antidepressant. Common side effects include anorexia, blurred vision, drowsiness, tachycardia, and weight gain. More serious adverse effects include arrhythmias, palpitations, hemotological dyscrasias, and jaundice.

Metabolism
Hepatic, CYP2D6
Excretion
Renal

Drug interactions: CYP2D6 inhibitors may increase levels/effects of amphetamine. Amphetamine is itself a weak CYP2D6 inhibitor. Acidification of the urine will enhance the renal excretion of amphetamine, whereas alkalinization will reduce it.

Legal indications for the use of amphetamine include narcolepsy and adjunct treatment of attention deficit disorder with hyperactivity. Adderall contains d- and l-amphetamine salts in the ratio of 3:1. Chronic abuse of amphetamine may lead to emotional liability, loss of appetite, somnolence, and mental impairment. Symptoms of acute toxicity with amphetamine include pallor, flushing, palpitation, tachypnea, tremor, hypertension or hypotension, chest pain, heart block, cardiac arrhythmias, seizures, coma, and cardiovascular collapse.

Sympathomimetic amines may be distinguished from amphetamine and methamphetamine in urine by GC-MS.

For workplace drug testing, the widely accepted immunoassay cutoff concentration to separate positive and negative specimens is 1000 ng/mL [7400 nmol/L]; for GC-MS confirmation, 500 ng/mL [3700 nmol/L] (mandated by SAMHSA, formerly NIDA). At these cutoff concentrations, amphetamine may generally be detected in urine for 1-3 days following use.

Alternative matrices used for nonfederally regulated workplace drug testing and being considered for regulated testing include hair, oral fluid, and sweat.

TEST NAME AND METHOD	SPECIMEN	REFERENCE (THERAPEUTIC) INTERVAL, CONVENTIONAL [INTERNATIONAL RECOMMENDED UNITS]	KINETIC VALUES

Amphetamine—CONT

1. Soares ME, Carvalho M, Carmo H, et al: Simultaneous determination of amphetamine derivatives in human urine after SPE extraction and HPLC-UV analysis, *Biomed Chromatogr* 18125-18131, 2004.

2. Jenkins KM, Young MS, Mallet CR, et al: Mixed-mode solid-phase extraction procedures for the determination of MDMA and metabolites in urine using LC-MS, LC-UV, or GC-NPD, *J Anal Toxicol* 28:50-58, 2004.

3. Paul BD, Jemionek J, Lesser D, et al: Enantiomeric separation and quantitation of (+/−)-amphetamine, (+/−)-methamphetamine, (+/−)-MDA, (+/−)-MDMA, and (+/−)-MDEA in urine specimens by GC-EI-MS after derivatization with (R)-(−) or (S)-(+)-alpha-methoxy-alpha-(trifluoromethy)phenylacetyl chloride (MTPA), *J Anal Toxicol* 28:449-455, 2004.

4. Furesz J, Kocsis G, Gachalyi A, et al: Mass selective detection of amphetamine, methamphetamine, and related compounds in urine, *J Chromatogr Sci* 42:259-262, 2004.

5. Baselt RC: *Analytical procedures for therapeutic drug monitoring and emergency toxicology,* ed 2, Davis, CA, 1987, Biomedical Publications.

6. Jacob P III, Tisdale EC, Panganiban K, et al: Gas chromatographic determination of methamphetamine and its metabolite amphetamine in human plasma and urine following conversion to N-propyl derivatives, *J Chromatogr B Biomed Appl* 664:449-457, 1995.

7. Al-Dirbashi OY, Wada M, Kuroda N, et al: Achiral and chiral quantification of methamphetamine and amphetamine in human urine by semi-micro column high-performance liquid chromatography and fluorescence detection, *J Forensic Sci* 45:708-714, 2000.

8. Stout PR, Klette KL, Wiegand R: Comparison and evaluation of DRI methamphetamine, DRI ecstasy, Abuscreen ONLINE amphetamine, and a modified Abuscreen Online amphetamine screening immunoassays for the detection of amphetamine, methamphetamine, 3,4-methylenedioxyamphetamine, and 3,4-methylenedioxymethamphetamine in human urine, *J Anal Toxicol* 27:265-269, 2003.

9. Wood M, De Boeck G, Samyn N, et al: Development of a rapid and sensitive method for the quantitation of amphetamines in human plasma and oral fluid by LC-MS-MS, *J Anal Toxicol* 27:78-87, 2003.

10. Stout PR, Horn CK, Klette KL: Rapid simultaneous determination of amphetamine, methamphetamine, 3,4-methylenedioxyamphetamine, 3,4-methylenedioxymethamphetamine, and 3,4-methylenedioxyethylamphetamine in urine by solid-phase extraction and GC-MS: a method optimized for high-volume laboratories, *J Anal Toxicol* 26:253-261, 2002.

11. Mortier KA, Dams R, Lambert WE, et al: Determination of paramethoxyamphetamine and other amphetamine-related designer drugs by liquid chromatography/sonic spray ionization mass spectrometry, *Rapid Commun Mass Spectrom* 16:865-870, 2002.

12. Peters FT, Kraemer T, Maurer HH: Drug testing in blood: validated negative-ion chemical ionization gas chromatographic-mass spectrometric assay for determination of amphetamine and methamphetamine enantiomers and its application to toxicology cases, *Clin Chem* 48:1472-1485, 2002.

13. Ramseier A: Stereoselective screening for and confirmation of urinary enantiomers of amphetamine, methamphetamine, designer drugs, methadone and selected metabolites by capillary electrophoresis, *Electrophoresis* 20:2726-2738, 1999.

14. Nishida M, Namera A, Yashiki M, et al: On-column derivatization for determination of amphetamine and methamphetamine in human blood by gas chromatography-mass spectrometry, *Forensic Sci Int* 125:156-162, 2002.

15. Stanaszek R, Piekoszewski W: Simultaneous determination of eight underivatized amphetamines in hair by high-performance liquid chromatography-atmospheric pressure chemical ionization mass spectrometry (HPLC-APCI-MS), *J Anal Toxicol* 28:77-85, 2004.

FACTORS INFLUENCING DRUG DISPOSITION	REMARKS AND INTERFERENCES

See *Phenethylamines and Methamphetamine.*

Interferences: Nonprescription decongestants and diet aids containing ephedrine and phenylpropanolamine and prescription drugs including selegiline, benzphetamine, fenfluramine, mephentermine, phenmetrazine, and phentermine may cause positive IA results.

16. Nakashima K, Kaddoumi A, Ishida Y, et al: Determination of methamphetamine and amphetamine in abusers' plasma and hair samples with HPLC-FL, *Biomed Chromatogr* 17:471-476, 2003.

17. Musshoff F, Junker HP, Lachenmeier DW, et al: Fully automated determination of amphetamines and synthetic designer drugs in hair samples using headspace solid-phase microextraction and gas chromatography-mass spectrometry. *J Chromatogr Sci* 40:359-364, 2002.

18. Skender L, Karacic V, Brcic I, et al: Quantitative determination of amphetamines, cocaine, and opiates in human hair by gas chromatography/mass spectrometry, *Forensic Sci Int* 125:120-126, 2002.

19. Yonamine M, Tawil N, Moreau RL, et al: Solid-phase micro-extraction-gas chromatography-mass spectrometry and headspace-gas chromatography of tetrahydrocannabinol, amphetamine, methamphetamine, cocaine and ethanol in saliva samples, *J Chromatogr B Analyt Technol Biomed Life Sci* 789:73-78, 2003.

20. *Fed Register,* 53:11963, April 11, 1988; *Fed Register,* 62:51118, September 30, 1997; *Fed Register,* 69:19673, April 13, 2004.

TEST NAME AND METHOD	SPECIMEN	REFERENCE (THERAPEUTIC) INTERVAL, CONVENTIONAL [INTERNATIONAL RECOMMENDED UNITS]		KINETIC VALUES		

		mcg/mL	μmol/L	$t_{1/2}$ (hr)	V_d (L/kg)	PB (%)
Anesthetics, Inhalation[1-7]	Blood (fluoride/ oxalate).	Anesthesia				
		Chloroform: 20-230 × 8.4	[168-1932]	1.5	2.6	71-88
GC, GCMS	Refrigerate, 4° C.	Cyclopropane: 80-180 × 23.8	[1904-4284]	NA	NA	NA
		Desflurane: ~300 × 5.95	[1785]	23 (fat)	0.6	NA
		Diethyl ether: 500-1500 × 13.5	[6750-20250]	NA	NA	NA
		Enflurane: 50-100 × 5.4	[270-540]	36	NA	NA
		Halothane: 80-260 × 5.1	[408-1326]	43	1.0	NA
		Isoflurane: Not determined		58	NA	NA
		Methoxy-		NA	NA	NA
		flurane: 125-200 × 6.1	[763-1220]	1.8-3.8	0.5-0.7	NA
		Sevoflurane:	[12-90 μM (fluoride)]	30-38	NA	NA
		Trichlo- roethylene: 30-90 × 0.0076	[0.23-0.68]			

Toxic concentration for all above:
Anesthetic levels without life support.

1. Accorsi A, Barbieri A, Raffi GB, et al: Biomonitoring of exposure to nitrous oxide, sevoflurane, isoflurane, and halothane by automated GC/MS headspace urinalysis, *Int Arch Occup Environ Health* 74:541-548, 2001.

2. Baselt C: *Disposition of toxic drugs and chemicals in man,* ed 7, Foster City, CA, 2004, Biomedical Publications.

3. Baselt RC: *Analytical procedures for therapeutic drug monitoring and emergency toxicology,* Davis, CA, 1980, Biomedical Publications.

4. Behne M, Wilke HJ, Harder S: Clinical pharmacokinetics of sevoflurane, *Clin Pharmacokinet* 36:13-26, 1999.

5. Kojima T, Ishii A, Watanabe-Suzuki K: Sensitive determination of four general anaesthetics in human whole blood by capillary gas chromatography with cryogenic oven trapping, *J Chromatogr B Biomed Sci Appl* 762:103-108, 2001.

6. Watanabe K, Seno H, Ishii A: Capillary gas chromatography with cryogenic oven temperature for headspace samples: analysis of chloroform or methylene chloride in whole blood, *Anal Chem* 69:5178-5181, 1997.

7. Yag NC, Hwang KL, Shen CH, et al: Simultaneous determination of fluorinated inhalation anesthetics in blood by gas chromatography–mass spectrometry combined with a headspace autosampler, *J Chromatogr B Biomed Sci Appl* 759:307-318, 2001.

		mcg/mL	μmol/L	$t_{1/2}$ (hr)	V_d (L/kg)	PB (%)
Anesthetics, Local[1-3]	Serum	Therapeutic concentration				
	(therapeutic con-					
GC, HPLC, LCMS	centration based on	Bupivacaine: 0.25-1.5 × 3.46	[0.87-5.2]	1.3-2.8	0.4-1.0	92
	peak collections)	Lidocaine: 0.1-4.1 × 4.27	[0.47-17.5]	0.7-1.8	1.3	55-79
		Mepivacaine: 0.4-4.0 × 4.06	[1.6-16]	1.9	1.2	77
		Prilocaine: 0.06-5 × 4.54	[0.27-23]	0.5-2.5	0.7-4.4	55
		Procaine: 0.2-10 × 4.24	[0.85-43]	7-8 min	0.3-0.8	5
		Ropivacaine: 0.75-3.0 × 3.64	[2.7-10.9]	1.8-4.2	0.5-0.7	94

FACTORS INFLUENCING DRUG DISPOSITION	REMARKS AND INTERFERENCES

Metabolism
  Hepatic
Excretion
  Expired air, renal

Isoflurane, enflurane, halothane, sevoflurane, and desflurane are most commonly used. Cyclopropane and diethyl ether are seldom used because of their flammability. Chloroform and trichloroethylene are no longer used because of toxicities (cardiac arrhythmias, hepatotoxicity, and nephrotoxicity). The etiology of halothane-induced hepatitis is unknown but occurs more frequently in women >40 yr undergoing lengthy abdominal surgery. Enflurane can cause seizures, hepatic dysfunction, and nephrotoxicity (mild, reversible, decreased glomerular filtration rate). Methoxyflurane can cause hepatic dysfunction and nephrotoxicity.

Metabolism
  Hepatic
Excretion
  Renal

Local anesthetics are used in a number of settings to control pain by blocking the action potentials of nerve conduction. The duration of the effect is dependent on the drug's pKa, lipid solubility and molecular size. Adverse effects include nausea, headache, muscular rigidity, bradycardia, arrhythmias, hypotension, and convulsions.

Therapeutic and toxic ranges are not well defined for some of these agents.

TEST NAME AND METHOD	SPECIMEN	REFERENCE (THERAPEUTIC) INTERVAL, CONVENTIONAL [INTERNATIONAL RECOMMENDED UNITS]	KINETIC VALUES

Anesthetics, Local—CONT

		Toxic concentration	
		Bupivacaine: >2 mg/mL	[>6.9]
		Lidocaine: >6 mcg/mL	[>26]
		Mepivacaine: >5	[>20]
		Prilocaine: >5	[>23]
		Procaine: >15	[>64]
		Ropivacaine: >3	[>11]

1. Baselt C: *Disposition of toxic drugs and chemicals in man,* ed 7, Foster City, CA, 2004, Biomedical Publications.
2. Emanuelsson BK, Zaric D, Nydahl P, et al: Pharmacokinetics of ropivacaine and bupivacaine during 21 h of continuous epidural infusion in healthy male volunteers, *Anesth Analg* 81:1163-1168, 1995.
3. Wantanabe T, Namera A, Yashiki M, et al: Simple analysis of local anaesthetics in human blood using headspace solid-phase microextraction and gas chromatography-mass spectrometry-electron impact ionization selected ion monitoring, *J Chromatogr B Biomed Sci Appl* 709:225-232, 1998.

Antidepressants, Bicyclic[1-7]	Serum		*mcg/mL*		*μmol/L*	$t_{1/2}$:	4-6 days
		Therapeutic concentration:				V_d:	12-42 L/kg
						Cl_T:	2.7-16.5 mL/min/kg
Fluoxetine (Prozac)[1-7]		Fluoxetine	0.03-0.5	× 3.23	[0.1-1.62]	PB:	95% (albumin, α_1 acid glycoprotein)
		Norfluoxetine	0.02-0.47				
		Toxic				F:	100%
HPLC, GC-MS, GC		concentration:	>1		[>3.23]	T_{max}:	6-8 hr

MW: 309.8

1. Baselt R: *Disposition of toxic drugs and chemicals in man,* ed 7, Foster City, CA, 2004, Biomedical Publications.
2. Frahnert C, Rao ML, Grasmader K: Analysis of eighteen antidepressants, four atypical antipsychotics and active metabolites in serum by liquid chromatography: a simple tool for therapeutic drug monitoring, *J Chromatogr B Analyt Technol Biomed Life Sci* 794:35-47, 2003.
3. Hemeryck A, Belpaire FM: Selective serotonin reuptake inhibitors and cytochrome P-450 mediated drug-drug interactions: an update, *Curr Drug Metab* 3:13-37, 2002.
4. Isbister GK, Bowe SJ, Dawson A, et al: Relative toxicity of selective serotonin reuptake inhibitors (SSRIs) in overdose, *J Toxicol Clin Toxicol* 42:277-285, 2004.

FACTORS INFLUENCING DRUG DISPOSITION	REMARKS AND INTERFERENCES

Metabolism
  Hepatic, CYP2D6, CYP3A4, CYP2C9, and CYP2C19
  Active metabolite: norfluoxetine
Excretion
  Renal
Dialysis
  Hemodialysis (−)

Drug interactions: Fluoxetine is an inhibitor of CYP2D6, CYP3A4, CYP2C9, and CYP2C19. Numerous interactions are reported, including with desipramine, methadone, alprazolam, triazolam, carbamazepine, throphylline, clozapine, and warfarin. The metabolites contribute to the reported interactions.

Fluoxetine belongs to the group of antidepressants that act by selectively inhibiting neuronal reuptake of serotonin. It is used to treat other psychiatric disorders, including obsessive compulsive disorder, posttraumatic stress disorder, premenstrual dysphoric disorder, and anxiety disorders. The S- and R-enantiomers exhibit equivalent pharmacological activity. The enantiomers are metabolized to active S- and R-norfluoxetine, which have half-lives of 4-16 days.

5. Lacassie E, Gaulier JM, Marquet P, et al: Methods for the determination of seven selective serotonin reuptake inhibitors and three active metabolites in human serum using high-performance liquid chromatography and gas chromatography, *J Chromatogr B Biomed Sci Appl* 742:229-238, 2000.

6. Schulz M, Schmoldt A: Therapeutic and toxic blood concentrations of more than 800 drugs and other xenobiotics, *Pharmazie* 58:447-474, 2003.

7. Tournel G, Houdret N, Hedouin V, et al: High-performance liquid chromatographic method to screen and quantitate seven selective serotonin reuptake inhibitors in human serum, *J Chromatogr B Biomed Sci Appl* 761:147-158, 2001.

TEST NAME AND METHOD	SPECIMEN	REFERENCE (THERAPEUTIC) INTERVAL, CONVENTIONAL [INTERNATIONAL RECOMMENDED UNITS]		KINETIC VALUES	
Antidepressants, Heterocyclic	Serum		*mcg/mL*	$t_{1/2}$:	
		Therapeutic concentration: sum of amoxapine and 8-OH		Parent:	8 hr
				7-OH:	4-6.5 hr
Amoxapine		amoxapine	0.18-0.6	8-OH:	30 hr
(Asendin)[1-5]				V_d:	Unknown
		Toxic concentration:	>3	Cl_T:	3.2-114 L/kg
HPLC, GC-MS, GC				PB:	~90%
				F:	18-54%
MW: 313.8				T_{max}:	1-2 hr
Paroxetine	Serum, plasma		*mcg/mL*	*μmol/L*	$t_{1/2}$: 15-22 hr
(Paxil)[5-10]		Therapeutic			V_d: 8.7 L/kg
		concentration: <0.01-0.05 × 3.04 [0.03-0.15]			Cl_T: 0.5-1 L/kg
HPLC, GC-MS, GC					PB: 95%
		Toxic			F: NA
MW: 329.4		concentration: >0.35		[>1.06]	T_{max}: 1-2 hr
Sertraline	Serum, plasma		*mcg/mL*	*μmol/L*	$t_{1/2}$: 24-26 hr
(Zoloft)[4,6,7,10-13]		Therapeutic			V_d: 20 L/kg
		concentration: 0.05-0.25 × 3.26 [0.163-0.82]			Cl_T: 96 mL/min
HPLC, GC-MS, GC					PB: 99%
		Toxic			F: 100%
MW: 306.7		concentration: >0.3		[>0.98]	T_{max}: 4-8 hr
Trazodone	Serum, plasma		*mcg/mL*	*μmol/L*	$t_{1/2}$: 6.3-13 hr
(Desyrel)[5,14-25]		Therapeutic			V_d: 0.8-1.5 L/kg
		concentration: 0.5-2.5 × 2.69 [1.3-6.7]			PB: 89-95%
HPLC, GC, Voltammetry					F: 70-90%
		Toxic			
		concentration: >4.0		[10.8]	
MW: 371.9					
TLC	Urine				

FACTORS INFLUENCING DRUG DISPOSITION	REMARKS AND INTERFERENCES
Metabolism Hepatic, Active metabolites: 7-hydroxyamoxapine, 8-hydroxyamoxapine *Excretion* Renal, fecal	Amoxapine is an antidepressant. Common side effects include anorexia, blurred vision, drowsiness, tachycardia, and weight gain. More serious adverse effects include arrhythmias, palpitations, hemotological dyscrasias, and jaundice.
Metabolism Hepatic, CYP2D6 Saturatable kinetics *Excretion* Renal, fecal **Drug interactions:** Paroxetine is a potent inhibitor of CYP2D6 (the same CYP responsible for its metabolism) and possibly CYP3A4. Multiple drug interactions are possible.	Paroxetine belongs to the group of antidepressants that act by selectively inhibiting the reuptake of serotonin. Of this group, it is the most potent but least selective in its interaction with serotonin inhibition. It also exhibits an affinity for the muscarinic acetylcholine receptors similar to that of the tricyclic antidepressants. Paroxetine is also used to treat other psychiatric diorders such as obsessive-compulsive disorders, panic disorders, posttraumatic stress disorders, anxiety, and premenstrual dysphoric disorder. Common side effects include anorexia, gastrointestinal disturbances, insomnia, sweating, blurred vision, drowsiness, tachycardia, and weight gain. More serious adverse effects reported include suicide, hyponatremia, and seizures. Potentially lethal events include the development of serotonin syndrome and the syndrome of inappropriate antidiuretic hormone secretion.
Metabolism Hepatic, Active (weakly) metabolite: desmethylsertraline **Drug interactions:** Sertraline is known to inhibit CYP2D6 and CYP2C9 giving rise to possible drug interactions.	Sertraline is an antidepressant also used to treat other psychiatric disorders such as obsessive-compulsive disorder. The drug acts by selectively inhibiting the reuptake of serotonin. Common adverse effects reported include nausea, diarrhea, tremor, sweating, and sexual dysfunction. More serious adverse effects reported include suicidal ideologies, seizures, and hyponatremia. SSRIs should not be abruptly stopped but tapered. Increased transaminases have been observed during the first 9 wk of treatment. Trazodone, a serotonin reuptake inhibitor/antagonist, is used for treatment of major depressive episodes and has been used for treatment of chronic pain. Side effects include dizziness, syncope, drowsiness, lethargy, dry mouth, constipation, vomiting, blurred vision, skin rashes, and urinary hesitancy.
Metabolism Hepatic, CYP3A4 (major); CYP2D6 (minor) Active metabolite: 1-*m*-chorophenylpiperazine (MCPP) *Dialysis* Hemodialysis ($-$) **Drug interactions:** Trazadone may increase the levels/effects of CYP2D6 substrates and may decrease the levels/effects of CYP2D6 prodrug substrates. Trazadone levels/effects may be decreased by CYP3A4 inducers and increased by CYP3A4 inhibitors.	

TEST NAME AND METHOD	SPECIMEN	REFERENCE (THERAPEUTIC) INTERVAL, CONVENTIONAL [INTERNATIONAL RECOMMENDED UNITS]	KINETIC VALUES

Antidepressants, Heterocyclic—CONT

1. Baker DE: *Drugdex drug evaluations: amoxapine,* Greenwood Village, CO, 2004, Thomson Micromedex.
2. Baselt R: *Disposition of toxic drugs and chemicals in man,* ed 7, Foster City, CA, 2004, Biomedical Publications.
3. Hue B, Palomba B, Giacardy-Paty M, et al: Concurrent high-performance liquid chromatographic measurement of loxapine and amoxapine and of their hydroxylated metabolites in plasma, *Ther Drug Monit* 20:335-339, 1998.
4. Mazzola CD, Miron S, Jenkins AJ: Loxapine intoxication: case report and literature review, *J Anal Toxicol* 24:638-641, 2000.
5. Schulz M, Schmoldt A: Therapeutic and toxic blood concentrations of more than 800 drugs and other xenobiotics, *Pharmazie* 58:447-474, 2003.
6. Isbister GK, Bowe SJ, Dawson A, et al: Relative toxicity of selective serotonin reuptake inhibitors (SSRIs) in overdose, *J Toxicol Clin Toxicol* 42:277-285, 2004.
7. Lacassie E, Gaulier JM, Marquet P, et al: Methods for the determination of seven selective serotonin reuptake inhibitors and three active metabolites in human serum using high-performance liquid chromatography and gas chromatography, *J Chromatogr B Biomed Sci Appl* 742:229-238, 2000.
8. Richelson E: Pharmacokinetic drug interactions of new antidepressants: a review of the effects on the metabolism of other drugs, *Mayo Clin Proc* 72:835-847, 1997.
9. Tournel G, Houdret N, Hedouin V, et al: High-performance liquid chromatographic method to screen and quantitate seven selective serotonin reuptake inhibitors in human serum, *J Chromatogr B Biomed Sci Appl* 761:147-158, 2001.
10. ACP's PIER: *Physicians' information and education resource (online version),* Philadelphia, 2004, American College of Physicians.
11. Frahnert C, Rao ML, Grasmader K: Analysis of eighteen antidepressants, four atypical antipsychotics and active metabolites in serum by liquid chromatography: a simple tool for therapeutic drug monitoring, *J Chromatogr B Analyt Technol Biomed Life Sci* 794:35-47, 2003.
12. Hemeryck A, Belpaire FM: Selective serotonin reuptake inhibitors and cytochrome P-450 mediated drug-drug interactions: an update, *Curr Drug Metab* 3:13-37, 2002.
13. Rogowsky D, Marr M, Long G, et al: Determination of sertraline and desmethylsertraline in human serum using copolymeric bonded-phase extraction, liquid chromatography and gas chromatography-mass spectrometry. *J Chromatogr B Biomed Appl* 655:138-141, 1994.

Antidepressants, Tetracyclic	Serum, plasma		*mcg/mL*		*µmol/L*	$t_{1/2}$:	20-60 hr
		Therapeutic				V_d:	22.6 L/kg
		concentration:	0.1-0.25	× 3.60	[0.36-0.9]	PB:	88%
Maprotiline		Toxic				F:	100%
(Ludiomil)[1-6]		concentration:	>0.3		[>1.08]	T_{max}:	12 hr

GC, GC-MS, HPLC

MW: 277.4

1. Baselt R: *Disposition of toxic drugs and chemicals in man,* ed 7, Foster City, CA, 2004, Biomedical Publications.
2. Crome P, Ali C: Clinical features and management of self-poisoning with newer antidepressants, *Med Toxicol* 1:411-420, 1986.

FACTORS INFLUENCING
DRUG DISPOSITION

REMARKS AND INTERFERENCES

14. Hardman JG, Limbird LE, Gilman AG: *Goodman and Gilman's the pharmacological basis of therapeutics,* Ed 10, New York, 2001, McGraw-Hill.

15. Toney G, Ereshefsky L: The pharmacokinetics of cyclic antidepressants and their relationship to therapeutic drug monitoring, *AACC Inservice Training Contin Educ* 12:9-20, 1990.

16. DeVane CL: Pharmacokinetics of the selective serotonin reuptake inhibitors, *J Clin Psychiatry* 53:13-20, 1992.

17. *Physicians desk reference,* ed 58, Montvale, NJ, 2004, Thomson PDR.

18. Clarke EGC: *Clarke's isolation and identification of drugs in pharmaceuticals, body fluids, and post-mortem material,* London, 1986, The Pharmaceutical Press.

19. McEvoy GK, editor: *AHFS drug information (online version),* Bethesda, MD, 2004, American Society of Health-System Pharmacists Inc.

20. *USP DI drug information for the health care professional,* ed 24, (online version), Taunton, MA, 2004, Micromedex Inc.

21. Martinez MA, Sanchez de la Torre C, Almarza E: A comparative solid-phase extraction study for the simultaneous determination of fluoxetine, amitriptyline, nortriptyline, trimipramine, maprotiline, clomipramine, and trazodone in whole blood by capillary gas-liquid chromatography with nitrogen-phosphorus detection, *J Anal Toxicol* 27:353-358, 2003.

22. Waschgler R, Hubmann MR, Conca A, et al: Simultaneous quantification of citalopram, cozapine, fluoxetine, norfluoxetine, maprotiline, desmethylmaprotiline and trazodone in human serum by HPLC analysis, *Int J Clin Pharma Ther* 40:554-559, 2002.

23. Vatassery GT, Holden LA, Hazel DK, et al: Determination of trazodone and its metabolite, 1-m-chlorophenyl-piperazine, in human plasma and red blood cells by HPLC, *Clin Biochem* 30:149-153, 1997.

24. El-Enany N, Belal F, Rizk M: Voltammetric analysis of trazodone HCL in pharmaceuticals and biological fluids, *J Pharma Biomed Anal* 30:219-226, 2002.

25. Baselt RC: *Analytical procedures for therapeutic drug monitoring and emergency toxicology,* ed 2, Davis, CA, 1987, Biomedical Publications.

Metabolism
  Hepatic, CYP2D6
  Active metabolites: desmethylmaprotiline, maprotiline-*N*-oxide
Excretion
  Renal (minimal)
Age
  Elderly: $t_{1/2}\downarrow$

Drug interactions: Cisapride, monoamine oxidase inhibitors, in addition to those related to inhibition or induction of CYP2D6.

Maprotiline is a tetracyclic antidepressant. Adverse effects include hypotension, tachycardia, gastrointestinal distress, and tremor. In overdose, more serious effects encountered include seizures, respiratory arrest and severe tachycardia, arrhythmias, and hypotension.

3. Martinez MA, Sanchez de la Torre C, Almarza E: A comparative solid-phase extraction study for the simultaneous determination of fluoxetine, amitriptyline, nortriptyline, trimipramine, maprotiline, clomipramine, and trazodone in whole blood by capillary gas-liquid chromatography with nitrogen-phosphorus detection, *J Anal Toxicol* 27:353-358, 2003.

TEST NAME AND METHOD	SPECIMEN	REFERENCE (THERAPEUTIC) INTERVAL, CONVENTIONAL [INTERNATIONAL RECOMMENDED UNITS]			KINETIC VALUES	

Antidepressants, Tetracyclic—CONT

4. Namera A, Watanabe T, Yashiki M, et al: Simple analysis of tetracyclic antidepressants in blood using headspace-solid-phase microextraction and GC-MS, *J Anal Toxicol* 22:396-400, 1998.

5. Schulz M, Schmoldt A: Therapeutic and toxic blood concentrations of more than 800 drugs and other xenobiotics, *Pharmazie* 58:447-474, 2003.

Antidepressants,	Serum, plasma		*ng/mL*		*nmol/L*	$t_{1/2}$:	30-50 hr
Tricyclic (TCA)[1-19]		Therapeutic				V_d:	12-18 L/kg
		concentration:	100-250*	× 3.61	[361-903]	Cl_T:	6.1 ± 1.7 mL/min/kg
Amitriptyline		Toxic				PB:	95%
(Elavil)		concentration:	>500*		[>1805]		[× 0.01 = 0.95, protein-bound mole fraction]
HPLC, GC,		*Amitriptyline plus nortriptyline.				F:	56-70%
GC-MS, IA							[× 0.01 = 0.56-0.70, bioavailable mole fraction]
MW: 277.4							

Clomipramine	Serum, plasma, and		*ng/mL*		*nmol/L*	$t_{1/2}$:	12-36 hr
(Anafranil)	whole blood	Therapeutic				$t_{1/2}$:	21-65 hr (metabolite)
		concentration:	100-250	× 3.18	[318-794]	V_d:	9-25 L/kg
HPLC, GC,			ng/mL			Cl_T:	23-122 L/hr
GC-MS, IA		Toxic				PB:	96-97%
		concentration:	>400		[>1272]	F:	36-62%
MW: 314.9							
IA, HPLC	Urine						

Desipramine	Serum, plasma		*ng/mL*		*nmol/L*	$t_{1/2}$:	15-25 hr
(Norpramin)		Therapeutic				V_d:	24-60 L/kg
		concentration:	50-300	× 3.75	[187-1125]	Cl_T:	18-40 mL/min/kg
HPLC, GC, GC-MS		Toxic				PB:	90-92%
		concentration:	>400		[>1500]		[× 0.01 = 0.90-0.92, protein-bound mole fraction]
MW: 266.4						F:	33-51%
							[× 0.01 = 0.33-0.51, bioavailable mole fraction]

| FACTORS INFLUENCING DRUG DISPOSITION | REMARKS AND INTERFERENCES |

6. Frahnert C, Rao ML, Grasmader K: Analysis of eighteen antidepressants, four atypical antipsychotics and active metabolites in serum by liquid chromatography: a simple tool for therapeutic drug monitoring, *J Chromatogr B Analyt Technol Biomed Life Sci* 794:35-47, 2003.

Metabolism
  Hepatic, CYP2D6 (major); CYP1A2,
  CYP2B6, CYP2C8/9, CYP2C19, and
  CYP3A4 (all minor)
Disease
  Hyperlipoproteinemia: PB↑
Age
  Elderly: $t_{1/2}$↑, V_d↑, Cl_T→, PB→
Dialysis
  Hemodialysis (−)
  Peritoneal (−)

Drug interactions: CYP2D6 inhibitors may increase the levels/effects of amitriptyline. Amitriptyline is a weak inhibitor of the following enzyme systems: CYP1A2, CYP2C8/9, CYP2C19, CYP2D6, and CYP2E1.

Amitriptyline is metabolized to two active metabolites (nortriptyline and 10-hydroxynortriptyline). The metabolism is highly variable among patients. Side effects include dry mouth, epigastric distress, constipation, palpitations, blurred vision, urinary retention, tachycardia, hypotension, and arrhythmias.

See Table II-5.

Metabolism
  Hepatic, CYP2D6, CYP2C19, and CYP1A2
  (all major); CYP3A4 (minor)
Age
  Elderly: $t_{1/2}$↑, C_{max}↑
Dialysis
  Hemodialysis (−)
  Hemoperfusion (−)
  Peritoneal (−)

Drug interactions: CYP1A2, CYP2C19, and CYP2D6 inducers may decrease the levels/effects of clomipramine, and inhibitors may increase its levels/effects.

Clomipramine is used for treatment of obsessive-compulsive disorder (OCD). It is metabolized to the active metabolite desmethylclomipramine and two other metabolites that may be active: 8-hydroxyclomipramine and 8-hydroxy-desmethylclomipramine. Side effects include dry mouth, blurred vision, urinary retention, constipation, hypotension, and arrhythmias. Adverse effects occurring more often with clomipramine than with other TCAs include sexual dysfunction, seizures, nausea, and vomiting.

Metabolism
  Hepatic, CYP2D6 (major), and CYP1A2
  (minor)
Dialysis
  Hemodialysis (−)
  Peritoneal (−)

Drug interactions: Desipramine is a moderate inhibitor of the following enzyme systems: CYP3A4, CYP2A6, CYP2B6, and CYP2D6

Desipramine causes less sedation and anticholinergic effects than with amitriptyline or imipramine. It is metabolized to the active metabolite 2-hydroxydesipramine. Side effects include dry mouth, epigastric distress, constipation, tachycardia, palpitations, blurred vision, urinary retention, hypotension, arrhythmias, manic excitement, tremor, and sedation.

See also *Imipramine.*

TEST NAME AND METHOD	SPECIMEN	REFERENCE (THERAPEUTIC) INTERVAL, CONVENTIONAL [INTERNATIONAL RECOMMENDED UNITS]		KINETIC VALUES	

Antidepressants, Tricyclic—CONT

Dothiepin (*Prothiaden*)	Serum, plasma	Therapeutic concentration:	*ng/mL* 20-100 × 3.39	*nmol/L* [68-339]	$t_{1/2}$: 11-40 hr V_d: 20-92 L/kg PB: 85%
HPLC, GC, GC-MS		Toxic concentration:	>800	[2712]	Cl_T: 1.4-3.8 L/kg/hr F: 30%
MW: 331.9					
Doxepin (*Sinequan, Adapin*)	Serum, plasma	Therapeutic concentration:	*ng/mL* 110-250 × 3.58	*nmol/L* [537-895]	$t_{1/2}$: 8-25 hr V_d: 9-33 L/kg Cl_T: 14 ± 3 mL/min/kg
HPLC, GC, GC-MS, IA		Toxic concentration:	>500	[>1790]	PB: 80-85% [× 0.01 = 0.80-0.85, protein-bound mole fraction]
MW: 279.4					F: 27 ± 10% [× 0.01 = 0.27 ± 0.10, bioavailable mole fraction]
Imipramine (*Tofranil*)	Serum, plasma	Therapeutic concentration:	*ng/mL* 150-250 × 3.57	*nmol/L* [536- 893]	$t_{1/2}$: 6-24 hr
HPLC, GC, GC-MS, IA		Toxic concentration:	>500	[>1785]	V_d: 15 ± 6 L/kg Cl_T: 10-24 mL/min/kg PB: 89-95%
MW: 280.4					[× 0.01 = 0.89-0.95, protein-bound mole fraction]
					F: 29-79% [× 0.01 = 0.29-0.79, bioavailable mole fraction]

FACTORS INFLUENCING DRUG DISPOSITION	REMARKS AND INTERFERENCES

and a weak inhibitor of CYP2E1, and may increase the levels/effects of substrates of these systems. Inhibitors of CYP2D6 substrates may increase the levels/effects of desipramine.

Metabolism
  Hepatic
Age
  Elderly: $t_{1/2}\uparrow$, $V_d\downarrow$, $Cl_T\downarrow$

Dothiepin is metabolized to dothiepin-S-oxide, northiepin, and northiaden-S-oxide, all of which may be active. Side effects include dry mouth, drowsiness, constipation, nausea, vomiting, diarrhea, dizziness, tremor, sweating, insomnia, blurred vision, weight gain, palpitations, hypotension, headache, and arrhythmias.

Metabolism
  Hepatic, CYP1A2, CYP2D6, and CYP3A4
Dialysis
  Hemodialysis $(-)$
  Peritoneal $(-)$

Drug interactions: Inducers of CYP1A2, CYP2D6, and CYP3A4 may decrease levels/effects of doxepin, and inhibitors may increase the levels/effects.

Doxepin is metabolized to the active metabolite desmethyldoxepin, which has a much longer plasma $t_{1/2}$ (51 ± 11 hr). Therapeutic and toxic concentrations include the concentration of desmethyldoxepin. Side effects include dry mouth, epigastric distress, constipation, tachycardia, palpitations, blurred vision, urinary retention, hypotension, and arrhythmias.

Metabolism
  Hepatic, CYP2D6, and CYP2C19 (both major), CYP1A2, CYP3A4, and CYP2B6 (all minor)
Disease
  Hyperlipoproteinemia: $PB\uparrow$
  MI: $PB\uparrow$
Age
  Elderly: $Cl_T\downarrow$
Dialysis
  Hemodialysis $(-)$
  Peritoneal $(-)$

Drug interactions: Imipramine is a moderate inhibitor of CYP2D6 and a weak inhibitor of the following enzyme systems: CYP1A2, CYP2C19, and CYP2E1, and may increase the levels/effects of substrates of these systems. Inhibitors of CYP2C19 and CYP2D6 may increase the levels/effects of imipramine.

Therapeutic and toxic concentrations include the concentration of imipramine's active metabolite, desipramine. There is wide intersubject variation in bioavailability, owing to extensive first-pass metabolism. Side effects include dry mouth, epigastric distress, constipation, tachycardia, palpitations, blurred vision, urinary retention, hypertension, and arrhythmias.

See *Desipramine.*

TEST NAME AND METHOD	SPECIMEN	REFERENCE (THERAPEUTIC) INTERVAL, CONVENTIONAL [INTERNATIONAL RECOMMENDED UNITS]			KINETIC VALUES	

Antidepressants, Tricyclic—CONT

TEST NAME AND METHOD	SPECIMEN				KINETIC VALUES	
Nortriptyline (*Aventyl, Pamelor*) HPLC, GC, GC-MS, IA MW: 263.4	Serum, plasma Therapeutic concentration: Toxic concentration:	*ng/mL* 50-150 >500	× 3.80	*nmol/L* [190-570] [>1900]	$t_{1/2}$: V_d: Cl_T: PB: F:	18-56 hr 15-23 L/kg 7.2 ± 1.8 mL/min/kg 93-95% [× 0.01 = 0.93-0.95, protein-bound mole fraction] 46-70% [× 0.01 = 0.46-0.70, bioavailable mole fraction]
Protriptyline (*Vivactil*) HPLC, GC, GC-MS MW: 263.4	Serum, plasma Therapeutic concentration: Toxic concentration:	*ng/mL* 70-250 >500	× 3.80	*nmol/L* [266-950] [>1900]	$t_{1/2}$: V_d: Cl_T: PB: F:	54-92 hr 22 ± 1 L/kg 3.6 ± 0.6 mL/min/kg 92% 77-93%
Trimipramine (*Surmontil*) GC, HPLC, GC-MS MW: 294.4	Serum, plasma Therapeutic concentration: Toxic concentration:	*ng/mL* 10-250 >500	× 3.40	*nmol/L* [34-850] [>1700]	$t_{1/2}$: V_d: Cl_T: PB: F:	16-40 hr 17-48 L/kg 40-105 L/hr 93-97% 18-63%

1.   Baselt RC: *Disposition of toxic drugs and chemicals in man,* ed 7, Foster City, CA, 2004, Biomedical Publications.
2.   Hardman JG, Limbird LE, Gilman AG: *Goodman and Gilman's the pharmacological basis of therapeutics,* ed 10, New York, 2001, McGraw-Hill.
3.   *Physicians desk reference,* ed 58, Montvale, NJ, 2004, Thomson PDR.
4.   Cannon DJ: Doxepin, *AACC Inservice Training Cont Educ* 12:3-4, 1991.

FACTORS INFLUENCING DRUG DISPOSITION	REMARKS AND INTERFERENCES

Metabolism
  Hepatic, CYP2D6 (major), CYP1A2,
  CYP2C19, and CYP3A4 (all minor)
Disease
  Hyperlipoproteinemia: PB↑
Age
  Elderly: $t_{1/2}$↑ (up to 90 hr), Cl_T↓
Dialysis
  Hemodialysis (−)
  Peritoneal (−)

Drug interactions: Nortriptyline is a weak inhibitor of the following enzyme systems: CYP2D6 and CYP2E1 and may increase the levels/effects of substrates of these systems. Inhibitors of CYP2D6 may increase the levels/effects of nortiptyline.

Nortriptyline is metabolized to the active metabolite 10-hydroxynortriptyline. Side effects include dry mouth, epigastric distress, constipation, tachycardia, palpitations, blurred vision, urinary retention, hypotension, eosinophilia, and arrhythmias.

Metabolism
  Hepatic, CYP2D6
Dialysis
  Hemodialysis (−)
  Peritoneal (−)

Drug interactions: Inhibitors of CYP2D6 may increase the levels/effects of protriptyline.

Side effects include dry mouth, epigastric distress, constipation, tachycardia, palpitations, blurred vision, urinary retention, hypotension, and arrhythmias.

Metabolism
  Hepatic, CYP2D6, CYP3A4, and CYP2C19
  (all major)
Dialysis
  Hemodialysis (−)
  Peritoneal (−)

Drug interactions: CYP2D6, CYP3A4, and CYP2C19 inhibitors may increase levels/effects of trimipramine, and CYP2D6, CYP3A4, and CYP2C19 inducers may decrease its levels/effects.

Trimipramine is used primarily in the treatment of endogenous depression. Side effects include agranulocytosis, eosinophilia, purpura, thrombocytopenia, tachycardia, hypotension, drowsiness, somnolence, agitation, headache, dizziness, tremors, epigastric distress, dry mouth, constipation, weight gain, and seizures.

---

5.   Toney G, Ereshefsky L: The pharmacokinetics of cyclic antidepressants and their relationship to therapeutic drug monitoring, *AACC Inservice Training Cont Educ* 12:9-20, 1990.

6.   Evans WE, Schentag JJ, Jusko WJ, editors: *Applied pharmacokinetics—principles of therapeutic drug monitoring,* ed 3, Vancouver, WA, 1992, Applied Therapeutics Inc.

7.   Clarke EGC: *Clarke's isolation and identification of drugs in pharmaceuticals, body fluids, and post-mortem material,* London, 1986, The Pharmaceutical Press.

TEST NAME AND METHOD	SPECIMEN	REFERENCE (THERAPEUTIC) INTERVAL, CONVENTIONAL [INTERNATIONAL RECOMMENDED UNITS]				KINETIC VALUES	

Antidepressants, Tricyclic—CONT

8. Schulz M, Schmoldt A: Therapeutic and toxic blood concentrations of more than 800 drugs and other xenobiotics, *Pharmazie* 58:447-474, 2003.

9. Frahnert C, Rao ML, Grasmader K: Analysis of eighteen antidepressants, four atypical antipsychotics and active metabolites in serum by liquid chromatography: a simple tool for therapeutic drug monitoring, *J Chromatogr B Analyt Technol Biomed Life Sci* 794:35-47, 2003.

10. ACP's PIER: *Physicians' information and education resource (online version)*, Philadelphia, PA, 2004, American College of Physicians.

11. McEvoy GK, editor: *AHFS drug information (online version)*, Bethesda, MD, 2004, American Society of Health-System Pharmacists Inc.

12. *USP DI drug information for the health care professional*, ed 24, (online version), Taunton, MA, 2004, Micromedex Inc.

13. Martinez MA, Sanchez de la Torre C, Almarza E: A comparative solid-phase extraction study for the simultaneous determination of fluoxetine, amitriptyline, nortriptyline, trimipramine, maprotiline, clomipramine, and trazodone in whole blood by capillary gas-liquid chromatography with nitrogen-phosphorus detection, *J Anal Toxicol* 27:353-358, 2003.

TEST NAME AND METHOD	SPECIMEN		ng/mL		nmol/L	KINETIC VALUES	
Antidepressants, Unicyclic[1-12]	Plasma (heparin, EDTA). Bupropion is unstable in human plasma. Freeze soon after collection.	Therapeutic concentration:	25-100	× 4.17	[104-417]	$t_{1/2}$:	10-20 hr
						V_d:	27-63 L/kg
						Cl_T:	126-140 L/hr
Bupropion		Toxic concentration:	>1200		[5004]	PB:	82-88%
(Wellbutrin)						F:	≥ 90%
HPLC, TLC, GC, IA							
MW: 239.74							
Fluvoxamine	Serum, plasma		ng/mL		nmol/L	$t_{1/2}$:	15-22 hr
(Luvox)		Therapeutic concentration:	150-250	× 3.14	[471-785]	V_d:	25 L/kg
						Cl_T:	21.4 L/hr
HPLC, GC, GC-MS, TLC		Toxic concentration:	>600		[1884]	PB:	77%
						F:	≥ 90%
MW: 318.3							

| FACTORS INFLUENCING DRUG DISPOSITION | REMARKS AND INTERFERENCES |

14. Taylor PJ, Charles BG, Norris R, et al: Measurement of dothiepin and its major metabolites in plasma by high performance liquid chromatography, *J Chromatogr Biomed Appl* 119:152-155, 1992.

15. Hackett LP, Dusci LJ, Ilett KF: A comparison of high-performance liquid chromatography and fluorescence polarization immunoassay for therapeutic drug monitoring of tricyclic antidepressants, *Ther Drug Monit* 20:30-34, 1998.

16. Gutteck U, Rentsch KM: Therapeutic drug monitoring of 13 antidepressant and five neuroleptic drugs in serum with liquid chromatography-electrospray ionization mass spectrometry, *Clin Chem Lab Med* 41:1571-1579, 2003.

17. Keller T, Schneider A, Tutsch-Bauer E: Fatal intoxication due to dothiepin, *Forensic Sci Int* 109:159-166, 2000.

18. Matsumoto K, Kanba S, Kubo H, et al: Automated determination of drugs in serum by column-switching high-performance liquid chromatography IV. Separation of tricyclic antidepressants and their metabolites, *Clin Chem* 35:453-456, 1989.

19. Gulaid AA, Jahn GA, Maslen C, et al: Simultaneous determination of trimipramine and its major metabolites by high-performance liquid chromatography, *J Chromatogr* 566:228-233, 1991.

Metabolism
  Hepatic, CYP2B6 (major), CYP1A2,
  CYP2A6, CYP2C8/9, CYP2D6, CYP2E1,
  and CYP3A4 (all minor)
Dialysis
  Hemodialysis (−)
  Peritoneal (−)

Drug interactions: Bupropion is a weak inhibitor of CYP2D6 enzyme system and may ↑ levels and risk of toxicity from antidepressants (SSRIs and tricyclic), some β-blockers, antiarrhythmics, and antipsychotics. Medications that affect CYP2B6 may interact with bupropion.

Bupropion is used in the treatment of major depressive disorder and, in the form of extended-release tablets (Zyban), as an adjunct in the cessation of smoking. It is metabolized to three active metabolites: hydroxybupropion, erythrohydrobupropion, and threohydrobupropion. Side effects include nonspecific rashes, nausea, vomiting, headache, sleep disorders, agitation, abnormalities in mental status, and seizures. After an overdose, seizure is the most common neurologic effect, whereas cardiac abnormalities are rarely observed.

Metabolism
  Hepatic, CYP2D6, and CYP1A2
Elimination
  Renal (94% within 71 hr)

Drug interactions: Fluvoxamine is a strong inhibitor of CYP1A2 and CYP2C19 and a weak inhibitor of CYP2B6, CYP2C8/9, CYP2D6, and CYP3A4. CYP1A2 and CYP2D6 inhibitors may increase the levels/effects of fluvoxamine. Fluvoxamine may increase the levels/effects of CYP2C19 and CYP1A2 substrates. Fluvoxamine should not be given in combination with MAO inhibitors because of the possibility of a fatal serotonergic syndrome.

Fluvoxamine, a selective serotonin reuptake inhibitor (SSRI), is used for treatment of obsessive-compulsive disorder (OCD) in children ≥8 yr of age and adults and to relieve symptoms of depression. Fluvoxamine exhibits nonlinear, time-dependent kinetics; Cl decreases and $t_{1/2}$ increases with multiple doses >50 mg/day. Side effects include somnolence, headache, agitation, insomnia, nausea, vomiting, dry mouth, constipation, anorexia, sexual dysfunction, and seizures. Fluvoxamine is metabolized to at least 9 metabolites, none of which are active.

TEST NAME AND METHOD	SPECIMEN	REFERENCE (THERAPEUTIC) INTERVAL, CONVENTIONAL [INTERNATIONAL RECOMMENDED UNITS]	KINETIC VALUES

Antidepressants, Unicyclic—CONT

1. Schulz M, Schmoldt A: Therapeutic and toxic blood concentrations of more than 800 drugs and other xenobiotics, *Pharmazie* 58:447-474, 2003.

2. Goldberger BA: Buproprion, *AACC Inservice Training Cont Educ* 13:3-4, 1992.

3. Schatzburg A, DeBattista C, Overman G, et al: 1998 black book of psychotropic dosing and monitoring, adapted from *Prim Psychiatry* 4:July, 1997.

4. Frahnert C, Rao ML, Grasmader K: Analysis of eighteen antidepressants, four atypical antipsychotics and active metabolites in serum by liquid chromatography: a simple tool for therapeutic drug monitoring, *J Chromatogr B Analyt Technol Biomed Life Sci* 794:35-47, 2003.

5. McEvoy GK, editor: *AHFS drug information (online version)*, Bethesda, MD, 2004, American Society of Health-System Pharmacists Inc.

6. Ohkubo T, Shimoyama R, Otani K, et al: High-performance liquid chromatographic determination of fluvoxamine and fluvoxamino acid in human plasma, *Anal Sci* 19:859-864, 2003.

TEST NAME AND METHOD	SPECIMEN			$t_{1/2}$ (hr)	V_d (L/kg)	PB (%)
Antihistamines (H$_1$-blocking agents)[1-6]	Serum	*ng/mL*	*nmol/L*			
		Therapeutic concentration				
		Brompheniramine: 8-15 × 3.13 [25-47]		12-35	9-15	NA
		Chlorpheniramine: 4-17 × 3.64 [15-62]		12-15	5.9	72
GC, HPLC, GC-MS		Diphenhydramine: 9-112 × 3.92 [35-440]		3-14	3-4	98
		Methapyrilene: 6-50 × 3.83 [23-192]		1.1-2.1	2.1-6.6	NA
		Orphenadrine: 50-200 × 3.71 [186-742]		13-20	4.3-7.8	20
		Tripelennamine: 20-60 × 3.92 [78-235]		2.9-5.3	9-12	NA

Toxic concentration for all above

(variable):	>0.5 mcg/mL
[Brompheniramine:	>1.57 μmol/L]
[Chlorpheniramine:	>1.82 μmol/L]
[Diphenhydramine:	>1.96 μmol/L]
[Methapyrilene:	>1.92 μmol/L]
[Orphenadrine:	>1.86 μmol/L]
[Tripelennamine:	>1.96 μmol/L]

1. Baselt C: *Disposition of toxic drugs and chemicals in man,* ed 7, Foster City, CA, 2004, Biomedical Publications.

2. Howarth PH: Assessment of antihistamine efficacy and potency, *Clin Exp Allergy* 29(suppl 3):87-97, 1999.

3. Boland DM, Rein J, Lew EO, et al: Fatal cold medication intoxication in an infant, *J Anal Toxicol* 27:523-526, 2003.

4. Chen X, Zhang Y, Zhong D: Simultaneous determination of chlorpheniramine and pseudoephedrine in human plasma by liquid chromatography-tandem mass spectrometry, *Biomed Chromatogr* 18:248-253, 2004.

5. Barbas C, Garcia A, Saavedra L, et al: Optimization and validation of a method for the determination of caffeine, 8-chlorotheophylline and diphenhydramine by isocratic high-performance liquid chromatography. Stress test for stability evaluation, *J Chromatogr A* 870:97-103, 2000.

6. Simons FE, Simons KJ: Clinical pharmacology of H1-antihistamines, *Clin Allergy Immunol* 17:141-178, 2002.

7. Jan MW, ZumBrunnen TL, Kazmi YR, et al: Pharmacokinetics of fluvoxamine in relation to CYP2C19 phenotype and genotype, *Drug Metabol Drug Interact* 19:1-11, 2002.

8. Palego L, Marazziti D, Biondi L, et al: Simultaneous plasma level analysis of clomipramine, N-desmethylclomipramine, and fluvoxamine by reversed-phase liquid chromatography, *Ther Drug Monit* 22:190-194, 2000.

9. Eap CB, Gaillard N, Powell K, et al: Simultaneous determination of plasma levels of fluvoxamine and of the enantiomers of fluoxetine and norfluoxetine by gas chromatography mass spectrometry, *J Chromatogr B Biomed Appl* 682:265-272, 1996.

10. Spigset O, Axelsson S, Norstrom A, et al: The major fluvoxamine metabolite in urine is formed by CYP2D6, *Eur J Clin Pharmacol* 57:653-658, 2001.

11. Spigset O, Granberg K, Hagg S, et al: Relationship between fluvoxamine pharmacokinetics and CYP2D6/CYP2C19 phenotype polymorphisms, *Eur J Clin Pharmacol* 52:129-133, 1997.

12. van Harten J: Overview of the pharmacokinetics of fluvoxamine, *Clin Pharmacokin* 29(suppl 1):1-9, 1995.

| *Metabolism* Hepatic *Excretion* Renal | These drugs are widely prescribed and available in OTC preparations. They are weakly basic tertiary amines with low serum concentrations. Metabolites and parent drugs are excreted primarily by the kidney. Side effects include drowsiness, which is intensified by ethanol or other CNS depressants. High doses (pediatric and adults) can cause hallucinations, excitement, ataxia, lack of coordination, athetosis, and convulsions. Fixed, dilated pupils with a flushed face and fever are common (atropine-like reaction). Overdose can produce coma and death. |

TEST NAME AND METHOD	SPECIMEN	REFERENCE (THERAPEUTIC) INTERVAL, CONVENTIONAL [INTERNATIONAL RECOMMENDED UNITS]		KINETIC VALUES
Atenolol **(Tenormin)**[1] *GC, HPLC* *MW: 266.34*	Serum, plasma (EDTA, heparin)	Therapeutic concentration: 200-500 ng/mL [$\times$ 0.00375 = 0.75-1.88 μmol/L] Toxic concentration: Not well defined	PK[2-6]: $t_{1/2}$: V_d: Cl_T: PB: F:	6-9 hr 0.55 $\pm$ 0.29 L/kg Calculation from creatinine clearance (0.77 $\times$ CrCl) + 0.05 mL/min/kg <5% [$\times$ 0.01 = <0.05, protein-bound mole fraction] 46-60% [$\times$ 0.01 = 0.46-0.60, bioavailable mole fraction]

1. Baselt RC: *Disposition of toxic drugs and chemicals in man,* ed 7, Foster City, CA, 2004, Chemical Toxicology Institute.
2. Evans WE, Schentag JJ, Jusko WJ: *Applied pharmacokinetics—principles of therapeutic drug monitoring,* ed 3, Vancouver, WA, 1992, Applied Therapeutics, Inc.
3. Gilman A, Hardman J, Limbird L: *The pharmacological basis of therapeutics,* ed 10, New York, 2001, Pergamon Press, Inc.
4. Kirch W, Kohler H, Axthelm T: Clinical pharmacokinetics of atenolol—a review, *Eur J Drug Metab Pharmacokinet* 7:81-91, 1982.
5. Lexi-Comp, Inc.: *Up-to-date online 12.2, drug information,* Hudson, OH, 2004, Lexi-Comp, Inc.
6. Johnsson G, Regardh CG: Clinical pharmacokinetics of β-adrenoreceptor blocking drugs, *Clin Pharmacokinet* 1:233-263, 1976.

| **Azathioprine** **(Imuran)** *HPLC,*[1] *LC-MS*[2] *MW: 277.27* | RBC | Therapeutic concentration: Not defined Toxic concentration: Not defined There are some HPLC and LC-MS methods for measuring major metabolites of azathioprine (6-thioguanine and 6-methylmercaptopurine) in RBC[1,2] mainly as research assays. Currently there are no routine clinical assays or need for drug monitoring. However, there is a need to genotype thiopurine methyltransferase (TPMT) to identify individuals who are deficient in this enzyme so as to use the right dose of aza-thioprine (6-MP).[3] | PK: $t_{1/2}$: V_d: Cl_T: PB: | 3 hr[4] Not available Not available 30%[5] |

FACTORS INFLUENCING DRUG DISPOSITION	REMARKS AND INTERFERENCES

Metabolism
  Hepatic
Excretion
  Urine (primary)
  Feces (secondary)
Disease
  Renal: $t_{1/2}\uparrow$, $V_d\rightarrow$, $Cl_T\uparrow$
Dialysis
  Hemodialysis (+)

Drug interactions: Hydroxide-containing antacids appear to reduce atenolol bioavailability. Phenothiazines may increase plasma atenolol concentrations. Hypertensive crisis may occur after or during withdrawal of either clonidine or atenolol. Atenolol may blunt the hyperglycemic action of glucagon. Atenolol can mask the tachycardia that usually accompanies hypoglycemia when insulin or hypoglycemic agents are used. NSAIDS and salicylates may reduce the antihypertensive effect of atenolol.[5]

This drug is a β-adrenergic receptor antagonist. Serum concentrations that produce minimal β-blockade vary widely. Therapeutic concentrations are expressed in terms of serum concentrations producing β-blockade. However, there is no good correlation between serum concentrations and therapeutic effects. Thus determination of serum levels is of limited value in routine therapy.

Cl_T correlates well with creatinine clearance (CrCl).

Metabolism
  Hepatic
Excretion
  Urine
Disease
  Renal: $t_{1/2}\uparrow$, $Cl\downarrow$
Age
  Neonate: Not available
Dialysis
  Hemodialysis (+)

Drug interactions: Allopurinol may increase serum levels of azathioprine's active metabolite (mercaptopurine). Decrease azathioprine dose to one third to one fourth of normal dose.

Azathioprine is a prodrug of 6-mercaptopurine. It is an immunosuppressant used for prevention of rejection in kidney transplantation and severe rheumatoid arthritis or inflammatory bowel disease that has not responded to other therapies.[6] It is extensively metabolized in the liver via xanthine oxidase to mercaptopurine (active), and mercaptopurine requires detoxification by thiopurine methyltransferase (TPMT).[1,6] TPMT is highly polymorphic and shows a wide range of activity in the normal population, which results in highly variable responses of the individual to azathioprine.[3,7]

Because this TPMT genetic polymorphism causes marked pharmacokinetic differences, patients inheriting this enzyme deficiency must be put on very different doses of affected medications (e.g., 5-10% of standard thiopurine dose).[3]

Side effects of azathioprine include bone marrow suppression and gastrointestinal disturbances.[6]

TEST NAME AND METHOD	SPECIMEN	REFERENCE (THERAPEUTIC) INTERVAL, CONVENTIONAL [INTERNATIONAL RECOMMENDED UNITS]		KINETIC VALUES	
Azathioprine (Imuran)—CONT					

1. Dervieux T, Boulieu R: Simultaneous determination of 6-thioguanine and methyl 6-mercaptopurine nucleotides of azathioprine in red blood cells by HPLC, *Clin Chem* 44:551-555, 1998.

2. Dervieux T, Boulieu R: Identification of 6-methylmercaptopurine derivative formed during acid hydrolysis of thiopurine nucleotides in erythrocytes, using liquid chromatography–mass spectrometry, infrared spectroscopy, and nuclear magnetic resonance assay, *Clin Chem* 44:2511-2515, 1998.

3. Evans WE: Pharmacogenetics of thiopurine S-methyltransferase and thiopurine therapy, *Ther Drug Monit* 26:186-191, 2004.

4. Gaffney K, Scott DG: Azathioprine and cyclophosphamide in the treatment of rheumatoid arthritis, *Br J Rheumatol* 37:824-836, 1998.

5. Lexi-Comp, Inc.: *Up-to-date online 12.2, drug information,* Hudson, OH, 2004, Lexi-Comp, Inc.

6. Micromedex: *Micromedex Healthcare series 2004,* Greenwood Village, CO, 2004, Thomson Micromedex.

7. Weinshalboum R, Slodek S: Mercaptopurine pharmacogenetics: monogenic inheritance of erythrocyte thiopurine methyltransferase activity, *Am J Human Genet* 32:651-662, 1980.

TEST NAME AND METHOD	SPECIMEN	REFERENCE (THERAPEUTIC) INTERVAL, CONVENTIONAL [INTERNATIONAL RECOMMENDED UNITS]		KINETIC VALUES	
Bretylium **(Bretylol)** *GLC* *MW: 414.37* *(as the tosylate)*	Serum, plasma (EDTA, heparin). Stable for 4 days at room temperature.[1]	Therapeutic concentration: Toxic concentration:	Not defined Not defined	PK[2,3]: $t_{1/2}$: V_d: Cl_T: PB: F:	7-15 hr 5.9 ± 0.8 L/kg 10.2 ± 1.9 mL/min/kg 1-6% ~35%

1. Lai CM, Kamath BL, Carter JE, et al: GLC determination of bretylium in biological fluids, *J Pharm Sci* 69:681-683, 1980.

2. Hardman JG, Limbird LE, Gilman AG: *The pharmacological basis of therapeutics,* ed 10, New York, 2001, Pergamon Press, Inc.

3. Lexi-Comp, Inc.: *Up-to-date online 12.2, drug information,* Hudson, OH, 2004, Lexi-Comp, Inc.

FACTORS INFLUENCING DRUG DISPOSITION	REMARKS AND INTERFERENCES

Aminosalicylates (olsalazine, mesalamine, sulfasalazine) may inhibit TPMT, increasing toxicity/myelosuppression of azathioprine. Azathioprine may decrease the effect of warfarin, and concomitant use of ACE inhibitors may induce leukopenia.[5]

See Table II-5.

Metabolism
   None
Excretion
   Urine
Disease
   Renal: $t_{1/2}\uparrow$, $V_d\downarrow$, $Cl_T\downarrow$
Dialysis
   Hemodialysis (+)

Drug interactions: Amphetamines abolish the hypotensive actions of bretylium. Tricyclic antidepressants may inhibit bretylium uptake by the myocardium. Increased toxicity when used with pressor catecholamines and digitalis. Risk of cardiotoxicity is increased with concurrent use of sparfloxacin, moxifloxacin, or gatifloxacin may increase toxicity because of the potential to prolong QT interval.

Bretylium is a class III antiarrhythmic used to manage serious and refractory ventricular arrhythmias. No correlation exists between plasma concentrations and bretylium's cardiac effects. The side effects are hypotension secondary to bretylium's adrenergic blocking action and gastrointestinal, nausea, and vomiting.

TEST NAME AND METHOD	SPECIMEN	REFERENCE (THERAPEUTIC) INTERVAL, CONVENTIONAL [INTERNATIONAL RECOMMENDED UNITS]		KINETIC VALUES	
Buspirone (Buspar)[1-5] GC/MS, HPLC MW: 386	Serum, plasma (EDTA)	*mcg/mL* Therapeutic concentration: 0.001-0.004 Toxic concentration: Not defined	*μmol/L* × 2.59 [0.003-0.01]	$t_{1/2}$: V_d: Cl_T: PB: F: T_{max}:	1.3-6.6 hr 2.7-7.9 L/kg 18-39 mL/min/kg 86->95% (albumin, α_1-acid glycoprotein) [× 0.01 = >0.95, protein-bound mole fraction] 1.5-13% [× 0.01 = 0.015-0.13, bioavailable mole fraction] 0.6-1.5 hr

1. Baselt C: *Disposition of toxic drugs and chemicals in man,* ed 7, Foster City, CA, 2004, Biomedical Publications.
2. Foroutan SM, Zarghi A, Shafaati AR, et al: Simple high-performance liquid chromatographic determination of buspirone in human plasma, *Farmaco* 59:739-742, 2004.
3. Jajoo HK, Mayol RF, LaBudde JA, et al: Metabolism of the antianxiety drug buspirone in human subjects, *Drug Metab Dispos* 17:634-640, 1989.
4. Schulz M, Schmoldt A: Therapeutic and toxic blood concentrations of more than 800 drugs and other xenobiotics, *Pharmazie* 58:447-474, 2003.
5. Sciacca MA, Duncan GF, Shea JP, et al: Simultaneous quantitation of buspirone and 1-(2-pyrimidinyl)piperazine in human plasma and urine by capillary gas chromatography-mass spectrometry, *J Chromatogr* 428:265-274, 1988.

| **Caffeine**[1-5] HPLC, GC, IA, LCMS MW: 194 | Serum, plasma (heparin, EDTA) | *mcg/mL* Therapeutic concentration: Infant: Toxic concentration: | 5-25 8-20 >50 | *μmol/L* × 5.15 | $t_{1/2}$ Premature infant: 52-96 hr [26-129] Adult: 3-5 hr [41-103] V_d Premature infant: 0.8 L/kg [>258] Adult: 0.6-0.7 L/kg Cl_T: 1.6-2.1 mL/min/kg PB: 29-43% [× 0.01 = 0.29-0.43, protein-bound mole fraction] T_{max}: 0.5-0.6 hr |

1. Cook DG, Peacock JL, Feyerabend C, et al: Relation of caffeine intake and blood caffeine concentrations during pregnancy to fetal growth: prospective population based study, *BMJ* 313:1358-1362, 1996.
2. Haller CA, Jacob P 3rd, Benowitz NL: Pharmacology of ephedra alkaloids and caffeine after single-dose dietary supplement use, *Clin Pharmacol Ther* 71:421-432, 2002.
3. Kaplan GB, Greenblatt DJ, Ehrenberg BL, et al: Dose-dependent pharmacokinetics and psychomotor effects of caffeine in humans, *J Clin Pharmacol* 37:693-703, 1997.

FACTORS INFLUENCING DRUG DISPOSITION	REMARKS AND INTERFERENCES

Metabolism
  Hepatic, CYP3A4
Excretion
  Renal, fecal
Disease
  Cirrhosis, renal: $t_{1/2}\uparrow$, $Cl_T\downarrow$
Dialysis
  Hemodialysis ($-$)

Buspirone is an anxiolytic with little apparent potential for abuse; it does not impair psychomotor function and produces minimal sedation. Age and gender do not appear to alter its kinetics significantly. Bioavailability is linear with respect to administered dose. For a given dose of drug, plasma levels in a group of subjects may vary $\sim$10-fold. May follow nonlinear kinetics.

Metabolism
  Hepatic, CPY1A2 (adult)
Excretion
  Renal
Age
  Neonate: $t_{1/2}\uparrow$, $Cl_T\downarrow$
Smoking: $Cl_T\uparrow$
Pregnancy: $t_{1/2}\uparrow$, $Cl_T\downarrow$

Caffeine, found naturally in or added to many foods and beverages, is used therapeutically for treating infants with apnea. It is often combined with analgesic preparations for the treatment of headaches and is used as a stimulant. Caffeine is metabolized to a series of partially demethylated xanthines and methyluric acids. Caffeine is also a minor metabolite of theophylline.

4. Kress M, Meissner D, Kaiser P, et al: Determination of theophylline by HPLC and GC-IDMS, the effect of chemically similar xanthine derivatives on the specificity of the method and the possibility of paracetamol as interfering substance, *Clin Lab* 48:541-551, 2002.

5. Pesce AJ, Rashkin M, Kotagal U: Standards of laboratory practice: theophylline and caffeine monitoring, *Clin Chem* 44:1124-1128, 1998.

TEST NAME AND METHOD	SPECIMEN	REFERENCE (THERAPEUTIC) INTERVAL, CONVENTIONAL [INTERNATIONAL RECOMMENDED UNITS]	KINETIC VALUES	
Cannabinoids[1-16]	Plasma	Negative	$t_{1/2}$:	14-38 hr
			V_d:	4-14 L/kg
GC, GC-MS, HPLC-MS, IA, LC-MS-MS TLC		Peak THC concentration After smoking	PB:	97-99%

		ng/mL		*nmol/L*	
	1.75% cigarette:	50-129	× 3.18	[159-410]	

TEST NAME AND METHOD	SPECIMEN	REFERENCE		
MW: 314.47 (as THC)	Urine	Negative		
	Alternative matrices: Hair, sweat, and oral fluid	Negative		

1. Huestis MA, Mitchell JM, Cone EJ: Urinary excretion profiles of 11-nor-9-carboxy-delta 9-tetrahydrocannabinoid in humans after single smoked doses of marijuana, *J Anal Toxicol* 20:441-452, 1996.

2. Huestis MA, Henningfield JE, Cone EJ: Blood cannabinoids. I. Absorption of THC and formation of 11-OH-THC and TJCCOOH during and after smoking marijuana, *J Anal Toxicol* 16:276-282, 1992.

3. Huestis MA: Marijuana. In Shaw LS, Kwong T, Rosano T, et al, editors: *The clinical toxicology laboratory: contemporary practice of poisoning evaluation,* Washington DC, 2001, AACC Press.

4. McEvoy GK, editor: *AHFS drug information (online version),* Bethesda, MD, 2004, American Society of Health-System Pharmacists Inc.

5. Gustafson RA, Moolchan ET, Barnes A, et al: Validated method for the simultaneous determination of delta 9-tetrahydrocannabinol (THC), 11-hydroxy-THC and 11-nor-9-carboxy-THC in human plasma using solid phase extraction and gas chromatography-mass spectrometry with positive chemical ionization, *J Chromatogr B Anal Tecnol Biomed Life Sci* 798:145-154, 2003.

6. Weinmann W, Vogt S, Goerke R, et al: Simultaneous determination of THC-COOH and THC-COOH-glucuronide in urine samples by LC/MS/MS, *Forensic Sci Int* 113:381-387, 2000.

7. Baselt RC: *Analytical procedures for therapeutic drug monitoring and emergency toxicology,* ed 2, Davis, CA, 1987, Biomedical Publications.

8. Kerrigan S, Phillips Jr WH Jr: Comparison of ELISAs for opiates, methamphetamine, cocaine metabolite, benzodiazepines, phencyclidine, and cannabinoids in whole blood and urine, *Clin Chem* 47:540-547, 2001.

9. Yonamine M, Tawil N, Moreau RL, et al: Solid-phase micro-extraction-gas chromatography-mass spectrometry and headspace-gas chromatography of tetrahydrocannabinol, amphetamine, methamphetamine, cocaine and ethanol in saliva samples, *J Chromatogr B Analyt Technol Biomed Life Sci* 789:73-78, 2003.

10. Strano-Rossi S, Chiarotti M: Solid-phase microextraction for cannabinoids analysis in hair and its possible application to other drugs, *J Anal Toxicol* 23:7-10, 1999.

11. Musshoff F, Lachenmeier DW, Kroener L, et al: Automated headspace solid-phase dynamic extraction for the determination of cannabinoids in hair samples, *Forensic Sci Int* 133:32-38, 2003.

12. Musshoff F, Junker HP, Lachenmeier DW, et al: Fully automated determination of cannabinoids in hair samples using headspace solid-phase microextraction and gas chromatography-mass spectrometry, *J Anal Toxicol* 26:554-560, 2002.

FACTORS INFLUENCING DRUG DISPOSITION	REMARKS AND INTERFERENCES

Metabolism
  Hepatic, active metabolite
  11-OH-THC
Elimination
  65% in feces, primary metabolite 11-OH-THC
  20% in urine, THCCOOH glucuronide primary metabolite

Peak plasma levels are achieved 10 min after smoking or 3 hr after ingestion. About 80-90% of a dose is excreted within 5 days.

Of the many related substances found in marijuana *(Cannabis sativa),* tetrahydrocannabinol (THC) is the most potent. Unusual doses affect mood, memory, motor coordination, cognitive ability, sensorium, time sense, and self-perception. THC is widely abused but is thought by some to be useful in mitigating the side effects of cancer therapy or the pain of glaucoma.

See also *Dronabinol.*

Most commercial immunoassay kits use antibodies directed toward 11-nor-D9-tetrahydrocannabinol-9-carboxylic acid, the most abundant metabolite. This metabolite may persist in urine for several weeks after last use, depending on the frequency and duration of use because THC is stored in adipose tissue. Commonly used cutoff concentrations are 20, 50, or 100 ng/mL [$\times$ 2.90 = 58, 145, or 290 nmol/L] 11-nor-Δ-9-tetrahydrocannabinol-9-carboxylic acid (THC-COOH). With a lower cutoff concentration (20 ng/mL [58 nmol/L]), individuals may occasionally test positive because of passive inhalation of side-stream marijuana cigarette smoke (generally under rather unrealistic conditions). The cutoff concentrations for SAMHSA-regulated drug testing are 50 ng/mL for screening and 15 ng/mL [44 nmol/L] THC-COOH for GC-MS confirmation.

13. Baptista MJ, Monsanto PV, Pinho Marques EG, et al: Hair analysis for delta(9)-THC, delta(9)-THC-COOH, CBN and CBD, by GC/MS-EI. Comparison with GC/MS-NCI for delta(9)-THC-COOH, *Forensic Sci Int* 128:66-78, 2002.

14. Staub C: Chromatographic procedures for determination of cannabinoids in biological samples, with special attention to blood and alternative matrices like hair, saliva, sweat and meconium, *J Chromatogr B Biomed Sci Appl* 733:119-126, 1999.

15. Hall BJ, Satterfield-Doerr M, Parikh AR, et al: Determination of cannabinoids in water and human saliva by solid-phase microextraction and quadrupole ion trap gas chromatography/mass spectrometry, *Anal Chem* 70:1788-1796, 1998.

16. Mieczkowski T: A research note: the outcome of GC/MS/MS confirmation of hair assays on 93 cannabinoid (+) cases, *Forensic Sci Int* 70:83-91, 1995.

TEST NAME AND METHOD	SPECIMEN	REFERENCE (THERAPEUTIC) INTERVAL, CONVENTIONAL [INTERNATIONAL RECOMMENDED UNITS]				KINETIC VALUES	
Carbamazepine **(Tegretol)**[1,2] *HPLC, GLC, GC-MS, EIA, FPIA, FIA* *MW: 236.27*	Serum, plasma (heparin, EDTA). Collect at trough concentration. Avoid hemolysis, especially with EIA assay. Stable at room temperature for several hours. Stable for 1 yr at −20° C.		*mg/mL* Therapeutic concentration: Toxic concentration:	4-12 >15	× 4.23	*mmol/L* 17-51 [>63]	PK[3-6]: $t_{1/2}$ Single dose: Multiple dose: V_d Child: Adult: Cl_T: PB: F:
							18-55 hr 12-17 hr 1.9 L/kg 0.59-2.00 L/kg 0.39 mL/min/kg 75-90% [× 0.01 = 0.75-0.90, protein-bound mole fraction] >70%

1. Sadée W, Beelen GCM: *Drug level monitoring,* New York, 1980, John Wiley and Sons.
2. Baselt RC: *Disposition of toxic drugs and chemicals in man,* ed 7, Foster City, CA, 2004, Chemical Toxicology Institute.
3. Warner A, Privitera M, Bates D: Standards of laboratory practice: antiepileptic drug monitoring, *Clin Chem* 44:1085-1095, 1998.
4. Bertilsson L: Clinical pharmacokinetics of carbamazepine, *Clin Pharmacokinet* 3:128-143, 1978.
5. Evans WE, Schentag JJ, Jusko WJ: *Applied pharmacokinetics—principles of therapeutic drug monitoring,* ed 3, Vancouver, WA, 1992, Applied Therapeutics, Inc.
6. Lexi-Comp, Inc.: *Up-to-date online 12.2, drug information,* Hudson, OH, 2004, Lexi-Comp, Inc.
7. Micromedex: *Micromedex Healthcare series 2004,* Greenwood Village, CO, 2004, Thomson Micromedex.
8. Endocrine Sciences: *Pediatric laboratory services,* Tarzana, CA, 1993, Endocrine Sciences.
9. Lee CS, Wang LH, Marbury TC, et al: Hemodialysis clearance and total body elimination of carbamazepine during chronic hemodialysis, *Clin Toxicol* 17:429-438, 1980.
10. Hansten PD, Horn JR: *Drug interactions,* ed 6, Philadelphia, 1989, Lea & Febiger.

FACTORS INFLUENCING DRUG DISPOSITION	REMARKS AND INTERFERENCES

Metabolism
  Hepatic
Excretion
  Urine (primary)
  Feces (secondary)[7]
Disease or condition
  Hepatic: $t_{1/2}\uparrow$, $Cl_T\downarrow$
  Pregnancy: $Cl_T\uparrow$
Dialysis[8]
  Hemodialysis $(+)$[9]

Drug interactions: Carbamazepine is a hepatic enzyme inducer and may enhance the elimination of ethosuximide, warfarin, and benzodiazepines that undergo hydroxylation. Cimetidine, diltiazem, erythromycin, isoniazid, propoxyphene, and verapamil may increase carbamazepine levels. Phenobarbital, primidone, and phenytoin have been shown to increase the metabolism of carbamazepine. The phenytoin-carbamazepine interaction is variable (i.e., phenytoin levels may increase, decrease, or stay the same, whereas carbamazepine levels usually decrease). Valproic acid may increase the $t_{1/2}$ and decrease protein binding of carbamazepine.[10] Carbamazepine may decrease the effect of CYP1A2, CYP2BCYP2C8/9, CYP2C19, and CYP3A4 substrates. CYP3A4 inducers may decrease the effects of carbamazepine, whereas CYP3A4 inducers may increase the effects.[6]

Carbamazepine increases its own metabolism by enzyme induction. It is metabolized to an active metabolite (10,11-epoxide), which may accumulate in renal failure and may contribute to the therapeutic and toxic concentrations of carbamazepine. Although the significance of this metabolite is not well established, simultaneous monitoring of the parent drug and metabolite by HPLC methods may be occasionally indicated for a patient who may exhibit toxic symptoms in view of an apparently normal parent drug level[3]. The $t_{1/2}$ of the epoxide is $\sim$17 hr.

Concentration-related toxic effects include blurred vision, nystagmus, ataxia, dizziness, drowsiness, and diplopia. Side effects generally unrelated to concentration include urticarial rash, hepatic dysfunction, eosinophilia, and hematological depression.

Carbamazepine has modest human teratogenic potential. It is not clear whether this is idiosyncratic or related to serum levels. Nonetheless, serum levels should be kept as low as possible, consistent with the desired therapeutic effect, in women at risk for pregnancy and throughout pregnancy.

See Table II-5.

TEST NAME AND METHOD	SPECIMEN	REFERENCE (THERAPEUTIC) INTERVAL, CONVENTIONAL [INTERNATIONAL RECOMMENDED UNITS]		KINETIC VALUES	
Carbenicillin (Geopen)[1] *MB, HPLC* *MW: 378.41*	Serum, plasma (heparin, EDTA). Stable in solution for 15 days at 5° C.[2]	Therapeutic concentration: Toxic concentration (neurotoxicity):	Dependent on minimum inhibitory concentration of specific organism[3] >250 mcg/mL [× 2.64 = >660 µmol/L]	PK[4-6]: $t_{1/2}$: V_d: Cl_T: PB:	1.1 hr 0.18 L/kg Calculation from creatinine clearance (0.68 × CrCl) + 0.15 mL/min/kg 50%

1. Sadée W, Beelen GCM: *Drug level monitoring,* New York, 1980, John Wiley and Sons.

2. Gupta VD, Stewart KR: Quantitation of carbenicillin disodium, cefazolin sodium, cephalothin sodium, nafcillin sodium and ticarcillin disodium by high-pressure liquid chromatography, *J Pharm Sci* 69:1264-1267, 1980.

3. Kucers A, Bennett N: *The dose of antibiotics,* ed 4, Philadelphia, 1987, JB Lippincott.

4. Bennett WM, Aronoff GR, Golper TA: *Drug prescribing in renal failure,* ed 3, Philadelphia, 1994, American College of Physicians.

5. Gilman AG, Rall TW, Nies AS, et al: *The pharmacological basis of therapeutics,* ed 8, New York, 1990, Pergamon Press, Inc.

6. Libke RD, Clarke JT, Ralph ED, et al: Ticarcillin vs. carbenicillin: clinical pharmacokinetics, *Clin Pharmacol Ther* 17:441-446, 1975.

7. Hoffman TA, Cestero R, Bullock WE: Pharmacodynamics of carbenicillin in hepatic and renal failure, *Ann Intern Med* 73:173-178, 1970.

8. Eastwood JB, Curtis JR: Carbenicillin administration in patients with severe renal failure, *BMJ* 1:486, 1968.

9. Lexi-Comp, Inc.: *Up-to-date online 12.2, drug information,* Hudson, OH, 2004, Lexi-Comp, Inc.

Cefamandole (Mandol)[1,2] *HPLC, MB* *MW: 462.51*	Serum. Keep specimen in ice water. Centrifuge at 4° C; remove cells as soon as possible. Freeze at −70° C until assayed.	Therapeutic concentration: Toxic concentration:	Not defined Not defined	PK[3-8]: $t_{1/2}$: V_d: Cl_T: PB:	1 hr 0.16 L/kg 2.8 ± 1.0 mL/min/kg 56-78%

FACTORS INFLUENCING DRUG DISPOSITION	REMARKS AND INTERFERENCES

Metabolism
  None
Excretion
  Urine
Disease
  Renal, Oliguria: $t_{1/2}\uparrow$ (15.7 hr)
  Oliguria and hepatic dysfunction:
    $t_{1/2}\uparrow$ (23.2 hr)
Age
  Premature: $t_{1/2}\uparrow$
  Neonate: $t_{1/2}\uparrow$
Dialysis
  Hemodialysis (+)[7]
  Peritoneal (+)[8]

Drug interactions: Probenecid delays active renal tubular secretion and increases the $t_{1/2}$ of the drug. Tetracyclines may decrease effectiveness of carbenicillin. Carbenicillin may increase the effect of warfarin.[9]

Carbenicillin is a broad-spectrum penicillin antibiotic. Half-life and total body clearance values correlate strongly with creatinine clearance (CrCl). Hepatic dysfunction appears to be significant only in the presence of renal failure. Side effects include diarrhea, nausea, vomiting,[9] hypersensitivity, hepatotoxicity, electrolyte and acid-base disturbances, and hematological disorders, including bleeding diathesis, eosinophilia, and reversible granulocytopenia. Neurotoxicity has been observed at concentrations of 320 mcg/mL [845 μmol/L] plasma and 37 mcg/mL [98 μmol/L] spinal fluid.

Metabolism
  None
Excretion
  Urine
Disease
  Uremia: $t_{1/2}\uparrow$, $V_d\rightarrow$, $Cl_T\downarrow$, PB$\rightarrow$
Age
  Neonates: $t_{1/2}\uparrow$
Dialysis
  Hemodialysis (+)

Cefamandole is a second-generation cephalosporin antibiotic. Side effects include allergic urticarial rash, eosinophilia, positive direct Coombs test, fever, $\uparrow$AST, $\uparrow$CK, diarrhea, thrombophlebitis, thrombocytopenia, and granulocytopenia. Cefamandole has a methylthiotetrazole side chain that has been implicated in causing disulfiram-like reactions and occasional bleeding problems (decreases vitamin K synthesis).

TEST NAME AND METHOD	SPECIMEN	REFERENCE (THERAPEUTIC) INTERVAL, CONVENTIONAL [INTERNATIONAL RECOMMENDED UNITS]		KINETIC VALUES

Cefamandole (Mandol)—CONT

1. Winely C, Spears J, Scott J: Comparison of cefamandole nafate to cefamandole by microbiological assay, *Antimicrob Agents Chemother* 16:424-426, 1979.

2. Bliss M, Mayersohn M: Liquid-chromatographic assay of cefamandole in serum, urine, and dialysis fluid, *Clin Chem* 32:197-200, 1986.

3. Bennett WM, Aronoff GR, Golper TA, et al: *Drug prescribing in renal failure. Dosing guidelines for adults,* ed 2, Philadelphia, 1991, American College of Physicians.

4. Evans WE, Schentag JJ, Jusko WJ: *Applied pharmacokinetics—principles of therapeutic drug monitoring,* ed 3, Vancouver, WA, 1992, Applied Therapeutics, Inc.

5. Hardman JG, Limbird LE, Gilman AG: *Goodman & Gilman's the pharmacological basis of therapeutics,* ed 10, New York, 2001, McGraw-Hill.

6. Mellin HE, Welling PG, Madsen PO: Pharmacokinetics of cefamandole in patients with normal and impaired renal function, *Antimicrob Agents Chemother* 11:262-266, 1977.

7. Nightingale CH, Greene DS, Quintiliani R: Pharmacokinetics and clinical use of cephalosporin antibiotics, *J Pharm Sci* 64:1899-1927, 1975.

8. Micromedex: *Micromedex Healthcare series 2004,* Greenwood Village, CO, 2004, Thomson Micromedex.

9. Lexi-Comp, Inc.: *Up-to-date online 12.2, drug information,* Hudson, OH, 2004, Lexi-Comp, Inc.

TEST NAME AND METHOD	SPECIMEN	REFERENCE (THERAPEUTIC) INTERVAL, CONVENTIONAL		KINETIC VALUES
Cefazolin[1,2] **(Kefzol, Ancef)** *HPLC, MB* *MW: 454.51*	Serum. Keep specimen in ice water. Centrifuge at 4° C; remove cells as soon as possible. Freeze at −70° C until assayed.	Therapeutic concentration: Toxic concentration:	Not defined Not defined	PK[3-6]: $t_{1/2}$: 1.8 hr V_d: 0.13-0.22 L/kg Cl_T: 0.95 ± 0.17 mL/min/kg PB: 80-86%

FACTORS INFLUENCING DRUG DISPOSITION	REMARKS AND INTERFERENCES

Drug interactions: Concomitant administration of aminoglycosides and cefamandole can lead to increased risk of nephrotoxicity. There is an increased risk of bleeding when cefamandole is used in patients taking warfarin or heparin.[8] Probenecid may increase cefamandole plasma levels.[9]

Metabolism
  None
Excretion
  Urine
Disease
  Uremia: $t_{1/2}\uparrow$, $V_d\uparrow$, $Cl_T\downarrow$, $PB\downarrow$
Dialysis
  Hemodialysis (+)
  Peritoneal (+)[7]

Side effects include eosinophilia, allergic rashes, fever, malaise, and joint and muscle pain. Gastrointestinal side effects like nausea, vomiting, diarrhea, or pseudomembranous colitis may occur.[6] AST, alkaline phosphatase, and bilirubin may be increased, and direct Coombs test may be positive.

Drug interactions: Concomitant administration of aminoglycosides and cefazolin can lead to increased risk of nephrotoxicity. Probenecid can reduce the renal clearance of cefazolin, increasing the risk of neuromuscular and CNS toxicity. Cefazolin may produce hypoprothrombinemia and may enhance the anticoagulant effect of warfarin.[6]

TEST NAME AND METHOD	SPECIMEN	REFERENCE (THERAPEUTIC) INTERVAL, CONVENTIONAL [INTERNATIONAL RECOMMENDED UNITS]		KINETIC VALUES

Cefazolin—CONT

1. Pitkin D, Actor P, Holl W, et al: Semiautomated turbidimetric microbiological assay for determination of cefazolin, *Antimicrob Agents Chemother* 5:223-227, 1974.

2. Wold JS: Rapid analysis of cefazolin in serum by high-pressure liquid chromatography, *Antimicrob Agents Chemother* 11:105-109, 1997.

3. Hardman JG, Limbird LE, Gilman AG: *Goodman & Gilman's the pharmacological basis of therapeutics,* ed 10, New York, 2001, McGraw-Hill.

4. Nightingale CH, Greene DS, Quintiliani R: Pharmacokinetics and clinical use of cephalosporin antibiotics, *J Pharm Sci* 64:1899-1927, 1975.

TEST NAME AND METHOD	SPECIMEN	REFERENCE (THERAPEUTIC) INTERVAL		KINETIC VALUES	
Cefepime (**Maxipime**)[1]	Serum	Therapeutic concentration:	Not defined	PK[2-4]:	
		Toxic concentration:	Not defined	$t_{1/2}$:	2 hr
		Peak serum concentration:	(2 g IV every 12 hr):	V_d:	14-20 L
HPLC			126-193 mcg/mL[2]	Cl_T:	120-140 mL/min
				PB:	16-19%
MW: 480.57					

1. Bugnon D, Giannoni E, Majcherczyk P, et al: Pitfalls in cefepime titration from human plasma: plasma- and temperature-related drug degradation in vitro, *Antimicrob Agents Chemother* 46:3654-3656, 2002.

2. Hardman JG, Limbird LE, Gilman AG: *Goodman & Gilman's the pharmacological basis of therapeutics,* ed 10, New York, 2001, McGraw-Hill.

3. Barbhaiya RH, Knupp CA, Forgue ST, et al: Pharmacokinetics of cefepime in subjects with renal insufficiency, *Clin Pharmacol Ther* 48:268-276, 1990.

4. Lexi-Comp, Inc.: *Up-to-date online 12.2, drug information,* Hudson, OH, 2004, Lexi-Comp, Inc.

5. Tam VH, McKinnon PS, Akins RL, et al: Pharmacodynamics of cefepime in patients with gram-negative infections, *J Antimicrob Chemother* 50:425-428, 2002.

6. Micromedex: *Micromedex Healthcare series 2004,* Greenwood Village, CO, 2004, Thomson Micromedex.

TEST NAME AND METHOD	SPECIMEN	REFERENCE (THERAPEUTIC) INTERVAL		KINETIC VALUES	
Cefoperazone (**Cefobid**)[1]	Serum. Keep specimen in ice water. Centrifuge at 4° C;	Therapeutic concentration:	Not defined	PK[2-5]:	
		Toxic concentration:	Not defined	$t_{1/2}$:	2.1 ± 0.3 hr
				V_d:	0.14-0.2 L/kg
MB, HPLC	remove cells as soon as possible.			Cl_T:	1.2 ± 0.1 mL/min/kg
				PB:	93% at 25 mcg/mL
MW: 645.68	Freeze at −70° C until assayed.				90% at 250 mcg/mL

FACTORS INFLUENCING DRUG DISPOSITION	REMARKS AND INTERFERENCES

5. Low CL, Gopalakrishna K, Lye WC: Pharmacokinetics of once daily intraperitoneal cefazolin in continuous ambulatory peritoneal dialysis patients, *J Am Soc Nephrol* 11:1117-1121, 2000.

6. Micromedex: *Micromedex Healthcare series 2004,* Greenwood Village, CO, 2004, Thomson Micromedex.

7. Manley HJ, Bailie GR, Asher RD, et al: Pharmacokinetics of intermittent intraperitoneal cefazolin in continuous ambulatory peritoneal dialysis patients, *Perit Dial Int* 19:65-70, 1999.

Metabolism
Hepatic (small amount)
Excretion
Urine
Disease
Renal: $Cl_T \downarrow$, $t_{1/2} \uparrow$[5]
Dialysis
Hemodialysis (+)

Drug interactions: High-dose probenecid may decrease clearance of cefepime, causing an increased drug effect. Concomitant use of aminoglycosides may increase nephrotoxicity.[4]

This drug is a fourth-generation cephalosporin antibiotic.

Side effects of cefepime include headache, blurred vision, lightheadedness, rash, urticaria, fever, dyspepsia, nausea, and antibiotic-associated diarrhea. Phlebitis may occur with intravenous cefepime, and transient elevations in serum transaminases may occur.[6]

Metabolism
Hepatic
Excretion
Bile (primary)
Urine (secondary)
Disease
Hepatitis: $t_{1/2}\uparrow$, $V_d\rightarrow$, $Cl_T\downarrow$
Cirrhosis: $t_{1/2}\uparrow$, $V_d\uparrow$, $Cl_T\rightarrow$
Dialysis
Hemodialysis (+)

Cefoperazone, a third-generation cephalosporin, has a methylthiotetrazole side-chain at the 3-position of the molecule that has been implicated in disulfiram-like reactions and occasional bleeding problems. Nonrenal clearance of cefoperazone may be increased in renal failure patients.

An increase in ALT, AST, and eosinophilia has been reported with cefoperazone, and a positive Coombs test may occur.

TEST NAME AND METHOD	SPECIMEN	REFERENCE (THERAPEUTIC) INTERVAL, CONVENTIONAL [INTERNATIONAL RECOMMENDED UNITS]		KINETIC VALUES

Cefoperazone (Cefobid)—CONT

1. Cowlishaw M, Sharman J: Liquid-chromatographic assay of cefoperazone from plasma and bile, *Clin Chem* 32:894, 1986.
2. Balant L, Dayer P, Auckenthaler R: Clinical pharmacokinetics of the third generation cephalosporins, *Clin Pharmacokinet* 10:101-143, 1985.
3. Bennett WM, Aronoff GR, Golper TA, et al: *Drug prescribing in renal failure. Dosing guidelines for adults,* ed 2, Philadelphia, 1991, American College of Physicians.
4. Bennett WM, Aronoff GR, Golper TA: *Drug prescribing in renal failure,* ed 3, Philadelphia, 1994, American College of Physicians.
5. Hardman JG, Limbird LE, Gilman AG: *Goodman & Gilman's the pharmacological basis of therapeutics,* ed 10, New York, 2001, McGraw-Hill.
6. Micromedex: *Micromedex Healthcare series 2004,* Greenwood Village, 2004, Thomson Micromedex.

TEST NAME AND METHOD	SPECIMEN	REFERENCE (THERAPEUTIC) INTERVAL, CONVENTIONAL		KINETIC VALUES
Cefotaxime[1] **(Claforan)**	Serum. Keep specimen in ice water. Centrifuge at 4° C; remove cells as soon as possible. Freeze at −70° C until assayed.	Therapeutic concentration: Toxic concentration:	Not defined Not defined	PK[2-5]: $t_{1/2}$: 1.1 ± 0.2 hr V_d: 0.24 ± 0.03 L/kg Cl_T: Calculation from creatinine clearance (1.34 × CrCl) + 1.81 mL/min/kg PB: 27-38%
MB, HPLC				
MW: 455.47				

1. Bergan T, Solberg R: Assay of cefotaxime by high-pressure-liquid chromatography, *Chemotherapy* 27:155-165, 1981.
2. Balant L, Dayer P, Auckenthaler R: Clinical pharmacokinetics of the third generation cephalosporins, *Clin Pharmacokinet* 10:101-143, 1985.

| FACTORS INFLUENCING DRUG DISPOSITION | REMARKS AND INTERFERENCES |

Drug interactions: Concomitant administration of aminoglycosides and cefoperazone can increase the risk of nephrotoxicity. Cefoperazone can cause hypoprothrombinemia and reduce vitamin K production, leading to increased risk of bleeding when used together with heparin or warfarin.[6]

Metabolism
  Hepatic
Excretion
  Urine
Disease
  Renal: $t_{1/2}\uparrow$, $V_d\rightarrow$
  Cirrhosis: $t_{1/2}\uparrow$
Age
  Neonate: $V_d\uparrow$
  Elderly: $t_{1/2}\uparrow$
Dialysis
  Hemodialysis (+)

This is a third-generation cephalosporin that undergoes significant renal tubular secretion. Side effects include eosinophilia, granulocytopenia, and thrombocytopenia. Coombs test may be positive.

Interferences: The presence of the microbiologically active desacetyl metabolite may interfere with interpretation of microbiologic assays. (Overestimation of cefotaxime's $t_{1/2}$ can result with organisms partially susceptible to desacetylcefotaxime.)

Drug interactions: Probenecid decreases the renal clearance of cefotaxime by almost 50%. Concomitant administration of furosemide or aminoglycosides can lead to increased risk of nephrotoxicity.[6]

3. Bennett WM, Aronoff GR, Golper TA, et al: *Drug prescribing in renal failure. Dosing guidelines for adults,* ed 2, Philadelphia, 1991, American College of Physicians.

4. Hardman JG, Limbird LE, Gilman AG: *Goodman & Gilman's the pharmacological basis of therapeutics,* ed 10, New York, 2001, McGraw-Hill.

TEST NAME AND METHOD	SPECIMEN	REFERENCE (THERAPEUTIC) INTERVAL, CONVENTIONAL [INTERNATIONAL RECOMMENDED UNITS]		KINETIC VALUES	

Cefotaxime—CONT

5. Patel KB, Nicolau DP, Nightingale CH, et al: Pharmacokinetics of cefotaxime in healthy volunteers and patients, *Diagn Microbiol Infect Dis* 22:49-55, 1995.

Cefoxitin[1]	Serum. Keep specimen in ice water.	Therapeutic concentration:	Not defined	PK^{2-6}:	
(Mefoxin)		Toxic concentration:	Not defined	$t_{1/2}$:	45-60 min
	Centrifuge at 4° C;			V_d:	0.2 L/kg
HPLC, MB	remove cells as			Cl_T:	5.6 mL/min/kg
	soon as possible.			PB:	65-80%
MW: 427.46	Freeze at −70° C until assayed.				

1. Charles B, Ravenscroft P: Rapid HPLC analysis of cefoxitin in plasma and urine, *J Antimicrob Chemother* 13:291-294, 1984.
2. Brogden RN, Heel RC, Speight TM, et al: Cefoxitin: a review of its antibacterial activity, pharmacological properties and therapeutic use, *Drugs* 17:1-37, 1979.
3. Evans WE, Schentag JJ, Jusko WJ: *Applied pharmacokinetics—principles of therapeutic drug monitoring,* ed 3, Vancouver, WA, 1992, Applied Therapeutics, Inc.
4. Garcia MJ, Dominguez-Gil A, Tabernero JM, et al: Pharmacokinetics of cefoxitin in patients with normal or impaired renal function, *Eur J Clin Pharmacol* 116:119-124, 1979.
5. Bennett WM, Aronoff GR, Golper TA: *Drug prescribing in renal failure,* ed 3, Philadelphia, 1994, American College of Physicians.
6. Lexi-Comp, Inc.: *Up-to-date online 12.2, drug information,* Hudson, OH, 2004, Lexi-Comp, Inc.
7. Micromedex: *Micromedex Healthcare series 2004,* Greenwood Village, CO, 2004, Thomson Micromedex.

Ceftazidime[1]	Serum. Keep specimen in ice water.	Therapeutic concentration:	Not defined	PK^{2-4}:	
(Fortaz)		Toxic concentration:	Not defined	$t_{1/2}$:	1.6 ± 0.1 hr
	Centrifuge at 4° C;			V_d:	0.28-0.40 L/kg
MB, HPLC	remove cells as			Cl_T:	Calculation from creatinine clearance
	soon as possible.				(1.05 × CrCl) +
MW: 546.58	Freeze at −70° C until assayed.				0.12 mL/min/kg
				PB:	17%

FACTORS INFLUENCING DRUG DISPOSITION	REMARKS AND INTERFERENCES

6. Lexi-Comp, Inc.: *Up-to-date online 12.2, drug information,* Hudson, OH, 2004, Lexi-Comp, Inc.

Metabolism
    None
Excretion
    Urine
Disease
    Uremia: $t_{1/2}\uparrow$, $V_d\uparrow$, $Cl_T\downarrow$, $PB\downarrow$
Age
    Newborn: $t_{1/2}\uparrow$, $V_d\uparrow$
    Child: $t_{1/2}\downarrow$, $V_d\rightarrow$
Dialysis
    Hemodialysis (+)
    Peritoneal (−)

Drug interactions: Probenecid may decrease clearance of cefoxitin. Anticoagulant effect of warfarin may be enhanced by cefoxitin.[6]

Concomitant administration of furosemide or aminoglycosides may lead to increased risk of nephrotoxicity.[7]

Cefoxitin is a second-generation cephalosporin antibiotic. Side effects include skin rash, eosinophilia, thrombocytopenia, neutropenia, leukopenia, GI upset, pseudomembranous colitis,[7] and thrombophlebitis. Positive direct Coombs test and increases in AST, ALT, alkaline phosphatase, urea nitrogen, and creatinine are also observed.

Interferences: Cefoxitin reacts with picrate in Jaffé reactions for creatinine determination.

Metabolism
    None
Excretion
    Urine
Disease
    Renal: $t_{1/2}\uparrow$, $V_d\rightarrow$, $Cl_T\downarrow$
Age
    Neonate: $t_{1/2}\uparrow$

Ceftazidime is a third-generation cephalosporin that does not undergo significant renal tubular secretion. Side effects include diarrhea, pseudomembranous colitis,[6] eosinophilia, and thrombocytopenia. Increased serum creatinine concentration and lowered glomerular filtration rate have been reported. Coombs test may be positive.

TEST NAME AND METHOD	SPECIMEN	REFERENCE (THERAPEUTIC) INTERVAL, CONVENTIONAL [INTERNATIONAL RECOMMENDED UNITS]		KINETIC VALUES	

Ceftazidime—CONT

1. Ayrton J: Assay of ceftazidime in biological fluids using high pressure liquid chromatography, *J Antimicrob Chemother* 8(suppl B):227-231, 1981.

2. Balant L, Dayer P, Auckenthaler R: Clinical pharmacokinetics of the third generation cephalosporins, *Clin Pharmacokinet* 10:101-143, 1985.

3. Grabe D, Bailie GR, Eisele G, et al: Pharmacokinetics of intermittent intraperitoneal ceftazidime, *Am J Kidney Dis* 33:111-117, 1999.

4. Hardman JG, Limbird LE, Gilman AG: *Goodman & Gilman's the pharmacological basis of therapeutics,* ed 10, New York, 2001, McGraw-Hill.

5. Lexi-Comp, Inc.: *Up-to-date online 12.2, drug information,* Hudson, OH, 2004, Lexi-Comp, Inc.

6. Micromedex: *Micromedex Healthcare series 2004,* Greenwood Village, CO, 2004, Thomson Micromedex.

TEST NAME AND METHOD	SPECIMEN	REFERENCE (THERAPEUTIC)		KINETIC VALUES	
Ceftizoxime[1] **(Cefizox)**	Serum. Keep specimen in ice water. Centrifuge at 4° C; remove cells as soon as possible. Freeze at −70° C until assayed.	Therapeutic concentration: Toxic concentration:	Not defined Not defined	PK[2-4]: $t_{1/2}$: V_d: Cl_T:	1.8 ± 0.7 hr 0.36 ± 0.19 L/kg Calculation from creatinine clearance (1.1 × CrCl) + 0.07 mL/min/kg
MB, HPLC *MW: 383.41*				PB:	28-50%

1. Fasching C, Peterson LR, Bettin KM, et al: High-pressure liquid chromatographic assay of ceftizoxime with an anion-exchange extraction technique, *Antimicrob Agents Chemother* 22:336-337, 1982.

FACTORS INFLUENCING DRUG DISPOSITION	REMARKS AND INTERFERENCES

Dialysis
  Hemodialysis (+)
  Peritoneal (+)

Drug interactions: Probenecid may decrease
clearance of ceftazidime. Concomitant administration of furosemide or aminoglycosides
with ceftazidime may lead to increased risk of
nephrotoxicity.[5]

Metabolism
  Liver (negligible amount)
Excretion
  Urine (primary)
  Bile (secondary)
Disease
  Renal: $t_{1/2}\uparrow$, $V_d\rightarrow$, $Cl_T\downarrow$
Age
  Elderly: $t_{1/2}\uparrow$
Dialysis
  Hemodialysis (+)
  Peritoneal (+)[5]

Drug interactions: Probenecid may decrease
clearance of ceftizoxime. Concomitant administration of furosemide or aminoglycosides
with ceftizoxime may lead to increased risk of
nephrotoxicity.[6]

Ceftizoxime is a third-generation cephalosporin that does not undergo significant renal tubular secretion. Side effects include eosinophilia and thrombocytopenia. Coombs test may be positive. Ceftizoxime is associated with transient
elevation of ALT, AST, and CK in the pediatric population.

---

2. Balant L, Dayer P, Auckenthaler R: Clinical pharmacokinetics of the third generation cephalosporins, *Clin Pharmacokinet* 10:101-143, 1985.

TEST NAME AND METHOD	SPECIMEN	REFERENCE (THERAPEUTIC) INTERVAL, CONVENTIONAL [INTERNATIONAL RECOMMENDED UNITS]		KINETIC VALUES	

Ceftizoxime—CONT

3. Hardman JG, Limbird LE, Gilman AG: *Goodman & Gilman's the pharmacological basis of therapeutics,* ed 10, New York, 2001, McGraw-Hill.

4. Bennett WM, Aronoff GR, Golper TA: *Drug prescribing in renal failure,* ed 3, Philadelphia, 1994, American College of Physicians.

| **Ceftriaxone**[1] **(Rocephin)** *MB, HPLC* *MW: 554.59* | Serum. Keep specimen in ice water. Centrifuge at 4° C; remove cells as soon as possible. Freeze at −70° C until assayed. | Therapeutic concentration: Toxic concentration: | Not defined Not defined | PK[2,3]: $t_{1/2}$: V_d: Cl_T: PB: | 6-9 hr 0.10-0.18 L/kg 0.14-0.29 mL/min/kg 95% at <70 mcg/mL 84% at 300 mcg/mL 58% at 600 mcg/mL |

1. Granich G, Krogstad D: Ion pair high-performance liquid chromatographic assay for ceftriaxone, *Antimicrob Agents Chemother* 31:385-388, 1987.

2. Balant L, Dayer P, Auckenthaler R, et al: Clinical pharmacokinetics of the third generation cephalosporins, *Clin Pharmacokinet* 10:101-143, 1985.

3. Patel IH, Chen S, Parsonnet M, et al: Pharmacokinetics of ceftriaxone in humans, *Antimicrob Agents Chemother* 20:634-641, 1981.

4. Matzke GR, Frye RF, Joy MS, et al: Determinants of ceftriaxone clearance by continuous venovenous hemofiltration and hemodialysis, *Pharmacotherapy* 20:635-643, 2000.

5. Lexi-Comp, Inc.: *Up-to-date online 12.2, drug information,* Hudson, OH, 2004, Lexi-Comp, Inc.

| **Cephalexin**[1] **(Keflex)** *HPLC, MB* *MW: 347.39* | Serum. Keep specimen in ice water. Centrifuge at 4° C; remove cells as soon as possible. Freeze at −70° C until assayed. | Therapeutic concentration: Toxic concentration: | Not defined Not defined | PK[2-6]: $t_{1/2}$: V_d: Cl_T: PB: | 0.5-1.2 hr 0.26 L/kg 4.3 ± 1.1 mL/min/kg 15-20% |

FACTORS INFLUENCING DRUG DISPOSITION	REMARKS AND INTERFERENCES

5. Gross ML, Somani P, Ribner BS, et al: Ceftizoxime elimination kinetics in continuous ambulatory peritoneal dialysis, *Clin Pharmacol Ther* 34:673-680, 1983.

6. Lexi-Comp, Inc.: *Up-to-date online 12.2, drug information,* Hudson, OH, 2004, Lexi-Comp, Inc.

Metabolism
  Intestinal wall (negligible amount)
Excretion
  Urine (primary)
  Bile (secondary)
Disease
  Renal: $t_{1/2}\uparrow$
  Hepatic: $t_{1/2}\uparrow$
Age
  Child: $t_{1/2}\downarrow$, $V_d\uparrow$, $Cl_T\uparrow$
  Elderly: $Cl_T\downarrow$, $PB\downarrow$
Dialysis
  Hemodialysis $(+)$[4]
  Peritoneal $(-)$

Drug interactions: Probenecid may decrease clearance of ceftriaxone. Concomitant administration of furosemide or aminoglycosides with ceftriaxone may lead to increased risk of nephrotoxicity.[5]

Ceftriaxone, a third-generation cephalosporin, does not undergo significant renal tubular secretion. Plasma protein binding is saturable; the peak plasma and tissue concentrations of free (unbound) drug increase disproportionately with increasing doses. Coombs test may be positive. Ceftriaxone is highly protein-bound and should be used with caution in hyperbilirubinemic neonates because of the displacement of bilirubin from serum albumin. Ceftriaxone is also associated with "biliary sludge" or pseudolithiasis.

Metabolism
  None
Excretion
  Urine
Disease
  Uremia: $t_{1/2}\uparrow$, $V_d\rightarrow$, $Cl_T\downarrow$
Age
  Neonates: $t_{1/2}\uparrow$[6]

Side effects include diarrhea, vomiting, abdominal cramps, pruritus, hypersensitivity reactions (skin rashes, eosinophilia, myalgia), hepatic disturbances, diplopia, headache, tinnitus, and at very high serum levels, seizures. Direct Coombs test may be positive. Anemia, granulocytopenia, and thrombocytopenia have also been reported.

TEST NAME AND METHOD	SPECIMEN	REFERENCE (THERAPEUTIC) INTERVAL, CONVENTIONAL [INTERNATIONAL RECOMMENDED UNITS]		KINETIC VALUES

Cephalexin—CONT

1. Lecaillon JB, Rouan MC, Souppart C, et al: Determination of cefsulodin, cefotiam, cephalexin, cefotaxime, desacetyl-cefotaxime and cefroxadin in plasma and in urine by high-performance liquid chromatography, *J Chromatogr* 228:257-267, 1982.

2. Spyker DA, Thomas BL, Sande BA, et al: Pharmacokinetics of cefaclor and cephalexin: dosage nomograms for impaired renal function, *Antimicrob Agents Chemother* 14:172-177, 1978.

3. Hardman JG, Limbird LE, Gilman AG: *Goodman & Gilman's the pharmacological basis of therapeutics,* ed 10, New York, 2001, McGraw-Hill.

4. Evans WE, Schentag JJ, Jusko WJ: *Applied pharmacokinetics—principles of therapeutic drug monitoring,* ed 3, Vancouver, WA, 1992, Applied Therapeutics, Inc.

5. Bennett WM, Aronoff GR, Golper TA: *Drug prescribing in renal failure,* ed 3, Philadelphia, 1994, American College of Physicians.

6. Lexi-Comp, Inc.: *Up-to-date online 12.2, drug information,* Hudson, OH, 2004, Lexi-Comp, Inc.

7. Speight TM, Brogden RN, Avery GS: Cephalexin: a review of its antibacterial, pharmacological and therapeutic properties, *Drugs* 3:9-78, 1972.

| **Cephalothin**[1] **(Keflin)** *HPLC, MB* *MW: 396.44* | Serum. Keep specimen in ice water. Centrifuge at 4° C; remove cells as soon as possible. Freeze at −70° C until assayed. | Therapeutic concentration: Toxic concentration: | Not defined Not defined | PK^{2-4}: $t_{1/2}$: 0.5-1 hr V_d: 0.26 L/kg Cl_T: 6.7 ± 1.7 mL/min/kg PB: 65-80% |

FACTORS INFLUENCING DRUG DISPOSITION	REMARKS AND INTERFERENCES

Dialysis
 Hemodialysis (+)
 Peritoneal (+)[7]

Drug interactions: Probenecid may decrease clearance of cephalexin. Concomitant administration of aminoglycosides with cephalexin may lead to increased risk of nephrotoxicity.[6]

Metabolism
 Liver (negligible amount)
Excretion
 Urine
Disease
 Renal: $t_{1/2}\uparrow$ (3-15 hr); $Cl_T\downarrow$
 Cardiopulmonary bypass surgery: $t_{1/2}\uparrow$, $Cl_T\downarrow$
Age
 Neonate: $t_{1/2}\uparrow$
 Child: $V_d\uparrow$
Dialysis
 Hemodialysis (+)
 Peritoneal (+)

Drug interactions: Probenecid may decrease clearance of cephalothin. Concomitant administration of aminoglycosides with cephalothin may lead to increased risk of nephrotoxicity.[5]

Cephalothin is a first-generation cephalosporin antibiotic. About 22-32% of cephalothin is metabolized to a desacetyl derivative that is 20% as active as cephalothin. In renal failure, the metabolite accumulates along with the parent compound. Toxicity of the metabolite is not fully understood. Side effects include hypersensitive reactions (fever, malaise, weakness, skin rash, and eosinophilia) and hypersensitive interstitial nephritis. Positive direct Coombs test, $\uparrow$AST, platelet aggregation, thrombocytopenia, granulocytopenia, hemolytic anemia, and diarrhea may accompany cephalothin administration.

Interferences: There are reports concerning cephalothin interference in creatinine determination with the Jaffé reaction.

TEST NAME AND METHOD	SPECIMEN	REFERENCE (THERAPEUTIC) INTERVAL, CONVENTIONAL [INTERNATIONAL RECOMMENDED UNITS]		KINETIC VALUES	

Cephalothin—CONT

1. Nilsson-Ehle I, Yoshikawa TT, Schotz MC, et al: Quantitation of antibiotics by high-pressure liquid chromatography: cephalothin, *Antimicrob Agents Chemother* 13:221-227, 1978.

2. Evans WE, Schentag JJ, Jusko WJ: *Applied pharmacokinetics—principles of therapeutic drug monitoring,* ed 3, Vancouver, WA, 1992, Applied Therapeutics, Inc.

3. Hardman JG, Limbird LE, Gilman AG: *Goodman & Gilman's the pharmacological basis of therapeutics,* ed 10, New York, 2001, McGraw-Hill.

TEST NAME AND METHOD	SPECIMEN	REFERENCE		KINETIC VALUES	
Cephapirin[1] **(Cefadyl)** *HPLC, MB* *MW: 445.45*	Serum. Keep specimen in ice water. Centrifuge at 4° C; remove cells as soon as possible. Freeze at −70° C until assayed.	Therapeutic concentration: Toxic concentration:	Not defined Not defined	PK[2-4]: $t_{1/2}$: V_d: Cl_T: PB:	36-48 min 0.22 L/kg 4.3 mL/min/kg 58%

1. Fasching C, Peterson L: Anion-exchange extraction of cephapirin, cefotaxime, and cefoxitin from serum for liquid chromatography, *Antimicrob Agents Chemother* 21:628-633, 1982.

2. Hardman JG, Limbird LE, Gilman AG: *Goodman & Gilman's the pharmacological basis of therapeutics,* ed 10, New York, 2001, McGraw-Hill.

3. Bennett WM, Aronoff GR, Golper TA, et al: *Drug prescribing in renal failure. Dosing guidelines for adults,* ed 2, Philadelphia, 1991, American College of Physicians.

4. Gilbert DN, Bennett WM: Use of antimicrobial agents in renal failure, *Infect Dis Clin North Am* 3:517-531, 1989.

5. Lexi-Comp, Inc.: *Up-to-date online 12.2, drug information,* Hudson, OH, 2004, Lexi-Comp, Inc.

TEST NAME AND METHOD	SPECIMEN	REFERENCE		KINETIC VALUES	
Cephradine[1] **(Anspor, Velosef)** *HPLC, MB* *MW: 349.41*	Serum. Keep specimen in ice water. Centrifuge at 4° C; remove cells as soon as possible. Freeze at −70° C until assayed.	Therapeutic concentration: Toxic concentration:	Not defined Not defined	PK[2-5]: $t_{1/2}$: V_d: Cl_T: PB:	1-2 hr 0.25 L/kg 5.1 mL/min/kg 8-20%

| FACTORS INFLUENCING DRUG DISPOSITION | REMARKS AND INTERFERENCES |

4. Nightingale CH, Greene DS, Quintiliani R: Pharmacokinetics and clinical use of cephalosporin antibiotics, *J Pharm Sci* 64:1899-1927, 1975.
5. Lexi-Comp, Inc.: *Up-to-date online 12.2, drug information,* Hudson, OH, 2004, Lexi-Comp, Inc.

Metabolism
  Hepatic
Excretion
  Urine
Disease
  Uremia: $t_{1/2}\uparrow$, $Cl_T\downarrow$
Dialysis
  Hemodialysis (+)
  Peritoneal (−)

Drug interactions: Probenecid may decrease clearance of cephapirin. Concomitant administration of aminoglycosides with cephapirin may lead to increased risk of nephrotoxicity.[5]

Cephapirin is metabolized to an active metabolite that possesses 54% of the microbiological activity of the parent drug. In renal failure, the metabolite may accumulate along with the parent compound. Toxicity of the metabolite is not fully understood. Side effects include eosinophilia, allergic rashes, fever, malaise, headache, joint and muscle pain, drug fever, neutropenia, and positive direct Coombs test. Increases in AST, ALT, and alkaline phosphatase are transient.

Metabolism
  None
Excretion
  Urine
Disease
  Uremia: $t_{1/2}\uparrow$, $Cl_T\downarrow$[6]
Dialysis
  Hemodialysis (+)
  Peritoneal (+)

Cephradine is a first-generation cephalosporin antibiotic. Side effects include nausea, vomiting, diarrhea, abdominal cramps, skin rashes, joint pains, headache, dizziness, and slight increase in serum urea nitrogen. Eosinophilia and granulocytopenia have been reported. With large doses, a positive Coombs test may occur.

TEST NAME AND METHOD	SPECIMEN	REFERENCE (THERAPEUTIC) INTERVAL, CONVENTIONAL [INTERNATIONAL RECOMMENDED UNITS]		KINETIC VALUES	

Cephradine—CONT

1. McAteer J, Hiltke MF, Silber BM, et al: Liquid-chromatographic determination of five orally active cephalosporins— cefixime, cefaclor, cefadroxil, cephalexin, and cephradine—in human serum, *Clin Chem* 33:1788-1790, 1987.
2. Evans WE, Schentag JJ, Jusko WJ: *Applied pharmacokinetics—principles of therapeutic drug monitoring,* ed 3, Vancouver, WA, 1992, Applied Therapeutics, Inc.
3. Hardman JG, Limbird LE, Gilman AG: *Goodman & Gilman's the pharmacological basis of therapeutics,* ed 10, New York, 2001, McGraw-Hill.
4. Nightingale CH, Greene DS, Quintiliani R: Pharmacokinetics and clinical use of cephalosporin antibiotics, *J Pharm Sci* 64:1899-1927, 1975.
5. Lexi-Comp, Inc.: *Up-to-date online 12.2, drug information,* Hudson, OH, 2004, Lexi-Comp, Inc.
6. Solomon AE, Briggs JD: The administration of cephradine to patients in renal failure, *Br J Clin Pharmacol* 2:443-448, 1975.

TEST NAME AND METHOD	SPECIMEN	REFERENCE (THERAPEUTIC) INTERVAL, CONVENTIONAL	[INTERNATIONAL RECOMMENDED UNITS]	KINETIC VALUES	
Chloral Hydrate[1-4] **(Somnote)**	Serum	Trichloroethanol (active metabolite) Therapeutic	*mcg/mL*	$\mu mol/L$	$t_{1/2}$ Chloral hydrate: 4 min Trichloroethanol: 4-13.6 hr Acute overdose: ~35 hr
GC, GCMS		concentration:	1.5-15 × 6.06	[9.1-91]	V_d Trichloroethanol,
MW: 165		Toxic concentration:	>30	[>181]	Acute overdose: ~1.6 L/kg PB Trichloroethanol: 35% [× 0.01 = 0.35, protein-bound mole fraction] Trichloroacetic acid: 94% [× 0.01 = 0.94, protein-bound mole fraction]

1. Baselt C: *Disposition of toxic drugs and chemicals in man,* ed 7, Foster City, CA, 2004, Biomedical Publications.
2. Gaulier JM, Merle G, Lacassie E, et al: Fatal intoxications with chloral hydrate, *J Forensic Sci* 46:1507-1509, 2001.
3. Jacqz-Aigrain E, Burtin P: Clinical pharmacokinetics of sedatives in neonates, *Clin Pharmacokinet* 31:423-443, 1996.
4. Schulz M, Schmoldt A: Therapeutic and toxic blood concentrations of more than 800 drugs and other xenobiotics, *Pharmazie* 58:447-474, 2003.

FACTORS INFLUENCING DRUG DISPOSITION	REMARKS AND INTERFERENCES

Drug interactions: Probenecid may decrease clearance of cephradine. Concomitant administration of aminoglycosides with cephradine may lead to increased risk of nephrotoxicity.[5]

Metabolism
  Hepatic (primary), alcohol dehydrogenase
Age:
  Neonates: $t_{1/2}\uparrow$ (TCE)

Chloral hydrate was formerly widely prescribed as a sedative-hypnotic. It is a CNS depressant, and any effect is intensified with ethanol or other CNS-depressant drugs. Chloral hydrate is rapidly reduced to trichloroethanol (TCE) by alcohol dehydrogenase in the liver. TCE is then conjugated with glucuronic acid, and the product is excreted in the urine and bile. Variable amounts of chloral hydrate and TCE are oxidized to trichloroacetic acid. TCE is principally responsible for the CNS depressant effects. Adverse effects include drowsiness, gastrointestinal disturbances, hypotension, miosis, jaundice (overdose), coma, and death (principally because of respiratory depression). Metabolites of chloral hydrate may alter the protein binding of acidic drugs.

TEST NAME AND METHOD	SPECIMEN	REFERENCE (THERAPEUTIC) INTERVAL, CONVENTIONAL [INTERNATIONAL RECOMMENDED UNITS]			KINETIC VALUES	
Chloramphenicol[1,2] **(Chloromycetin)**	Serum, plasma (heparin, EDTA). Collect at trough concentration.		*mcg/mL*	$\mu mol/L$	PK^{3-5}: $t_{1/2}$	
HPLC, GLC, MB, colorimetric, EIA	Sample should be centrifuged, sepa-	Therapeutic concentration: Toxic concentration:	10-25	$\times$ 3.09	[31-77]	<2 wk: 24 hr
			>25		[>77]	2-4 wk: 12 hr
MW: 323.13	rated, and frozen if not analyzed immediately.	Gray baby syndrome:	40-100		[124-309]	Adult: 1.6-3.3 hr V_d: 0.50-1.0 L/kg Cl_T: 4.7 ± 1.1 mL/min/kg PB: 50-60% F: 75-90%

1. Sample RH, Glick MR, Kleiman MB, et al: High-pressure liquid chromatographic assay of chloramphenicol in biological fluids, *Antimicrob Agents Chemother* 15:491-493, 1979.
2. Baselt RC: *Disposition of toxic drugs and chemicals in man,* ed 7, Foster City, CA, 2004, Chemical Toxicology Institute.
3. Ambrose PJ: Clinical pharmacokinetics of chloramphenicol and chloramphenicol succinate, *Clin Pharmacokinet* 9:222-238, 1984.
4. Bennett WM, Aronoff GR, Golper TA: *Drug prescribing in renal failure,* ed 3, Philadelphia, 1994, American College of Physicians.
5. Koup JR, Lau AH, Brodsky B, et al: Chloramphenicol pharmacokinetics in hospitalized patients, *Antimicrob Agents Chemother* 15:651-657, 1979.
6. Blouin RA, Erwin WG, Dutro MP, et al: Chloramphenicol hemodialysis clearance, *Ther Drug Monit* 2:351-354, 1980.
7. Lexi-Comp, Inc.: *Up-to-date online 12.2, drug information,* Hudson, OH, 2004, Lexi-Comp, Inc.
8. Micromedex: *Micromedex Healthcare series 2004,* Greenwood Village, CO, 2004, Thomson Micromedex.

FACTORS INFLUENCING DRUG DISPOSITION	REMARKS AND INTERFERENCES

Metabolism
  Hepatic
Excretion
  Bile and feces
  (primary)
  Urine (secondary)
Disease
  Cirrhosis: $t_{1/2}\uparrow$, 4.05 ± 1.39 hr $Cl_T\downarrow$, 2.78 ± 1.02 mL/min/kg[5] 1.99 ± 1.49 mL/min/kg[5]
  PB$\downarrow$, 42.2 ± 6.8%
  [× 0.01 = 0.42 ± 0.07, protein-bound mole fraction]
Age
  Premature: $t_{1/2}\uparrow$, $Cl_T\downarrow$, PB$\downarrow$
  Neonate: $t_{1/2}\uparrow$, $Cl_T\downarrow$, PB$\downarrow$, 32.4 ± 8.2%
  [× 0.01 = 0.32 ± 0.08, protein-bound mole fraction]
Dialysis
  Hemodialysis (↓)[6]
  Peritoneal (−)

Drug interactions: Chloramphenicol weakly inhibits CYP2C8/9 and CYP3A4. It may decrease the metabolism of anticonvulsants, barbiturates, and sulfonylureas. Rifampin may increase the metabolism of chloramphenicol.[7] There is an increased risk of bleeding when chloramphenicol is used concomitantly with warfarin because of inhibition of hepatic metabolism of warfarin and reduction of vitamin K production.[8]

Chloramphenicol palmitate and succinate require in vivo hydrolysis to chloramphenicol (the microbiologically active form). Side effects include bone marrow suppression (leukopenia, thrombocytopenia, and aplasia of marrow with fatal pancytopenia). These represent a hypersensitivity or idiosyncratic reaction. Dose-dependent leukopenia and thrombocytopenia may also occur. Nausea, vomiting, unpleasant taste, diarrhea, and perineal irritation may accompany chloramphenicol administration. Hepatic disturbances are rare.

Interferences: Colorimetric assay may not distinguish between biologically active and inactive forms of chloramphenicol.

See Table II-5.

TEST NAME AND METHOD	SPECIMEN	REFERENCE (THERAPEUTIC) INTERVAL, CONVENTIONAL [INTERNATIONAL RECOMMENDED UNITS]			KINETIC VALUES	
Chlordiazepoxide **(Librium)**[1-6] *HPLC, GC-MS, GC* *MW: 299.8*	Serum, urine Unstable	Therapeutic concentration: Toxic concentration:	*mcg/mL* 0.4-3 >3.5	× 3.34	*μmol/L* [1.3-10] [>11.7]	$t_{1/2}$: 6-48 hr V_d: 0.3-0.5 L/kg Cl_T: 150 mL/min PB: 90-98% F: >95% T_{max}: 0.5-2 hr

1. Baselt C: *Disposition of toxic drugs and chemicals in man,* ed 7, Foster City, CA, 2004, Biomedical Publications.
2. Fraser AD: Use and abuse of the benzodiazepines, *Ther Drug Monit* 20:481-489, 1998.
3. Haver VM, Porter WH, Dorie LD, et al: Simplified high performance liquid chromatographic method for the determination of clonazepam and other benzodiazepines in serum, *Ther Drug Monit* 8:352-357, 1986.
4. Needleman SB, Porvaznik M: Identification of parent benzodiazepines by gas chromotography/mass spectroscopy (GC/MS) from urinary extracts treated with B-glucuronidase, *Forensic Sci Int* 73:49-60, 1995.

TEST NAME AND METHOD	SPECIMEN	REFERENCE (THERAPEUTIC) INTERVAL, CONVENTIONAL [INTERNATIONAL RECOMMENDED UNITS]			KINETIC VALUES	
Chlorpromazine **(Thorazine)**[1-12] *GC, GC-MS,* *HPLC, IA* *MW: 318.9*	Serum, plasma	Therapeutic concentration Child: Adult: Toxic concentration:	*ng/mL* 40-80 50-300 >1000	× 3.14	*nmol/L* [126-251] [157-942] [>3140]	$t_{1/2}$: 10-30 hr V_d: 20 L/kg Cl_T: 8.6 ± 2.9 mL/min/kg PB: 92-97% [× 0.01 = 0.92-0.97, protein-bound mole fraction] F: 30% (highly variable) [× 0.01 = 0.30, bioavail-able mole fraction]

FACTORS INFLUENCING DRUG DISPOSITION	REMARKS AND INTERFERENCES

Metabolism
  Hepatic, CYP3A4
Excretion
  Renal (minimal)
  Active metabolites: desmethylchlordiazepoxide, demoxepam
Disease
  Hepatic: $t_{1/2}\uparrow$
Age
  Elderly: $t_{1/2}\uparrow$
  Smoking: $t_{1/2}\downarrow$
Dialysis
  Hemodialysis (−)

Drug Interactions: Numerous drug interactions are reported and are related to inhibition or induction of CYP3A4.

Chlordiazepoxide is a long-acting benzodiazepine used primarily for the treatment of anxiety and alcohol withdrawal. Its mechanism of action is not well defined. The drug is addictive, and symptoms if abruptly discontinued include sweating, abdominal pain, tremors, and seizures. Symptoms of overdose include somnolence, hyperreflexia, confusion, and coma.

Using immunoassay techniques, urine may be used to screen for benzodiazepine use. Confirmation of the presence of chlordiazepoxide and its metabolites can be performed using GC/MS.

5. Peppers MP: Benzodiazepines for alcohol withdrawal in the elderly and in patients with liver disease, *Pharmacotherapy* 16:49-57, 1996.
6. Schulz M, Schmoldt A: Therapeutic and toxic blood concentrations of more than 800 drugs and other xenobiotics, *Pharmazie* 58:447-474, 2003.

Metabolism
  Hepatic, CYP2D6 (major), and CYP1A2, CYP3A4 (minor)
Age
  Child: $Cl_T\downarrow$
  Elderly: $Cl_T\downarrow$
Dialysis
  Hemodialysis (−)
  Peritoneal (−)

Drug interactions: CYP2D6 inhibitors may increase the levels/effects of clorpromazine. Clorpromazine may increase the levels/effects of CYP2D6 substrates and decrease the levels/effects of CYP2D6 prodrug substrates. Chlorpromazine is a strong inhibitor of CYP2D6 and a weak inhibitor of CYP2E1.

Chlorpromazine is a phenothiazine commonly used for the symptomatic management of psychotic disorders. It is also used for prevention and treatment of nausea and vomiting, relief of restlessness and apprehension before surgery, and for relief of intractable hiccups. Several metabolites are formed and significantly complicate the interpretation of serum concentrations. Side effects include faintness, palpitations, nasal stuffiness, dry mouth, constipation, orthostatic hypotension, hyperthermia and hypothermia, extrapyramidal effects (parkinsonian syndrome), acute dystonic reactions, tardive dyskinesia, jaundice, leukocytosis, thrombocytopenia, leukopenia, and eosinophilia,. Chlorpromazine is extensively metabolized, and 10-12 metabolites have been identified.

TEST NAME AND METHOD	SPECIMEN	REFERENCE (THERAPEUTIC) INTERVAL, CONVENTIONAL [INTERNATIONAL RECOMMENDED UNITS]		KINETIC VALUES

Chlorpromazine (Thorazine)—CONT

1. Baselt R: *Disposition of toxic drugs and chemicals in man,* ed 7, Foster City, CA, 2004, Biomedical Publications.
2. Schulz M, Schmoldt A: Therapeutic and toxic blood concentrations of more than 800 drugs and other xenobiotics, *Pharmazie* 58:447-474, 2003.
3. Hardman JG, Limbird LE, Gilman AG: *Goodman and Gilman's the pharmacological basis of therapeutics,* ed 10, New York, 2001, McGraw-Hill.
4. *Physicians desk reference,* ed 58, Montvale, NJ, 2004, Thomson PDR.
5. Clarke EGC: *Clarke's isolation and identification of drugs in pharmaceuticals, body fluids, and post-mortem material,* London, 1986, The Pharmaceutical Press.
6. ACP's PIER: *Physicians' information and education resource* (online version), Philadelphia, 2004, American College of Physicians.
7. McEvoy GK, editor: *AHFS drug information* (online version), Bethesda, MD, 2004, American Society of Health-System Pharmacists Inc.

Chlorpropamide	Serum		*mcg/mL*	*µmol/L*	$t_{1/2}$: 25-60 hr
(Diabinese)[1-4]		Therapeutic			V_d: 0.1-0.3 L/kg
		concentration:	30-150 × 3.62	[109-543]	Cl_T: 0.025-0.035 mL/min/kg
CZE, LC MS,		Toxic			PB: 60-95%
HPLC, GC		concentration:	200-750	[724-2715]	[× 0.01 = 0.60-0.95, protein-bound mole
MW: 276					fraction]
					F: NA
					T_{max}: 2-5 hr

1. Hardman JG, Limbird LE, Molinoff PB, et al: *Goodman and Gilman's the pharmacological basis of therapeutics,* ed 9, New York, 1996, McGraw-Hill.
2. Magni F, Marazzini L, Pereira S, et al: Identification of sulfonylureas in serum by electrospray mass spectrometry, *Anal Biochem* 282:136-141, 2000.
3. Paroni R, Comuzzi B, Arcelloni C, et al: Comparison of capillary electrophoresis with HPLC for diagnosis of factitious hypoglycemia, *Clin Chem* 46:1773-1780, 2000.
4. Schulz M, Schmoldt A: Therapeutic and toxic blood concentrations of more than 800 drugs and other xenobiotics, *Pharmazie* 58:447-474, 2003.

Chlorprothixene	Serum		*mcg/mL*	*µmol/L*	$t_{1/2}$: 8-12 hr (chlorprothixene)
(Taractan)[1-5]		Therapeutic			20-40 hr (chlorprothix-
		concentration:	0.02-0.2 × 3.16	[0.063-0.634]	ene sulfoxide)
HPLC, CZE		Toxic			V_d: 10-25 L/kg
		concentration:	>0.4	[>1.26]	Cl_T: 14-20 mL/min/kg
MW: 316					PB: >99%

8. *USP DI drug information for the health care professional,* ed 24, (online version), Taunton, MA, 2004, Micromedex Inc.
9. Baselt RC: *Analytical procedures for therapeutic drug monitoring and emergency toxicology,* ed 2, Davis, CA, 1987, Biomedical Publications.
10. Ohkubo T, Shimoyama R, Sugawara K: Determination of chlorpromazine in human breast milk and serum by high-performance liquid chromatography, *J Chromatogr A* 614:328-332, 1993.
11. Valoti M, Palmi M, Della Corte L, et al: Dehalogenation and N-dealkylation of chlorpromazine as revealed by plasma concentrations of metabolites in a population of chronically medicated schizophrenics, *Methods Findings Exp Clin Pharma* 14:445-450, 1992.
12. Smith CS, Morgan SL, Greene SV, et al: Solid-phase extraction and high-performance liquid chromatographic method for chlorpromazine and thirteen metabolites, *J Chromatogr A* 423:207-216, 1987.

FACTORS INFLUENCING DRUG DISPOSITION	REMARKS AND INTERFERENCES

Metabolism
  Hepatic
Excretion
  Renal
Disease
  Renal: $t_{1/2}\uparrow$
Age
  Elderly: $t_{1/2}\downarrow$, $Cl_T\uparrow$
Dialysis
  Peritoneal $(-)$

Chlorpropamide is an oral hypoglycemic agent. Like other sulfonylureas, the mechanism of action involves stimulation of the pancreatic islets to secrete insulin through the binding of the drug to the ATP-sensitive potassium channel receptors. Chloropromide has the longest $t_{1/2}$ and duration of activity of this group of drugs. Adverse effects include transient leukopenia, thrombocytopenia, hemolytic anemia, pancytopenia, eosinophilia, gastrointestinal disturbances, headache, tinnitus, photosensitivity, allergic skin reactions, and intolerance to alcohol. The most serious side effects include hypoglycemia (which may progress to coma and death) and hepatic dysfunction.

Metabolism
  Hepatic
Excretion
  Fecal, renal

Chlorprothixene, an antipsychotic drug related to chlorpromazine, continues to be used in Europe to treat schizophrenia. The pharmacology of the drug is not well described despite its long use. Adverse effects include sedation, extrapyramidal effects, and hypotension. Hepatic dysfunction and eosinophilia, leukopenia, and thrombocytopenia have been reported.

TEST NAME AND METHOD	SPECIMEN	REFERENCE (THERAPEUTIC) INTERVAL, CONVENTIONAL [INTERNATIONAL RECOMMENDED UNITS]	KINETIC VALUES

Chlorprothixene (Taractan)—CONT

F: 10-17%
[× 0.01 = 0.10-0.17, bioavailable mole fraction]

T_{max}: 2.5-3 hr

1. Bagli M, Rao ML, Hoflich G, et al: Pharmacokinetics of chlorprothixene after single intravenous and oral administration of three galenic preparations, *Arzneimittelforschung* 46:247-250, 1996.
2. Bagli M, Suverkrup R, Quadflieg R, et al: Pharmacokinetic-pharmacodynamic modeling of tolerance to the prolactin-secreting effect of chlorprothixene after different modes of drug administration, *J Pharmacol Exp Ther* 29:547-554, 1999.
3. Baselt C: *Disposition of toxic drugs and chemicals in man,* ed 7, Foster City, CA, 2004, Biomedical Publications.
4. Karpinska J, Starczewska B: Simultaneous LC determination of some antidepressants combined with neuroleptics, *J Pharm Biomed Anal* 29:519-525, 2002.
5. Sokoliess T, Gronau M, Menyes U, et al: Separation of (Z)- and (E)-isomers of thioxanthene and dibenz[b,e]oxepin derivatives with calixarenes and resorcinarenes as additives in nonaqueous capillary electrophoresis, *Electrophoresis* 24:1648-1657, 2003.

TEST NAME AND METHOD	SPECIMEN					KINETIC VALUES
Cimetidine[1-5]	Serum, plasma		*mcg/mL*		μ*mol/L*	$t_{1/2}$: 1.7-2.1 hr (adults)
(Tagamet)	(heparin, EDTA).	Therapeutic				2.1-3.6 hr (pediatrics)
	Collect as trough.	concentration:	0.78-3.9	× 3.97	[3.1-15.5]	V_d: 0.8-1.2 L/kg (adults)
HPLC, LCMS		Toxic				2.13 L/kg (pediatrics)
		concentration:	>30		[>119]	Cl_T: 30-48 L/hr
MW: 252						PB: 15-26%
						[× 0.01 = 0.15-0.26, protein-bound mole fraction]
						F: 60-76% (oral)
						[× 0.01 = 0.60-0.76, bioavailable mole fraction]
						T_{max}: 0.75-1.5 hr

1. Gladziwa U, Klotz U: Pharmacokinetics and pharmacodynamics of H(2)-receptor antagonists in patients with renal insufficiency, *Clin Pharmacokinet* 24:319-332, 1993.

FACTORS INFLUENCING DRUG DISPOSITION	REMARKS AND INTERFERENCES

Metabolism
  Hepatic
Excretion
  Renal
Disease
  Renal: $t_{1/2}\uparrow$, $V_d\rightarrow$, $Cl_T\downarrow$
  Hepatic: $t_{1/2}\uparrow$
  Burns: $t_{1/2}\downarrow$
Age
  Elderly: $t_{1/2}\uparrow$, $V_d\downarrow$, $Cl_T\downarrow$
  Children: $V_d\uparrow$
Dialysis
  Hemodialysis ($\pm$)
  Peritoneal ($-$)
  Hemoperfusion ($+$)

Cimetidine is a histamine H_2-receptor antagonist. Side effects include headache, dizziness, fatigue, muscle pains, constipation, diarrhea, skin rashes, confusion, slurred speech, delirium, hallucinations, gynecomastia, and coma. Most of these effects have been observed in renal failure and/or elderly patients. Rare cases of pancytopenia, granulocytopenia, and thrombocytopenia have been reported.

See Table II-5.

Drug interactions: Cimetidine has been implicated in numerous drug interactions occurring through three different mechanisms: (1) metabolic inhibition of compounds metabolized via CYP1A2, CYP2C19, CYP2D6, and CYP3A4, (2) alteration of gastric pH, and (3) inhibition of renal tubular transport of other basic compounds.

2. Gugler R, Fuchs G, Dieckmann M, et al: Cimetidine plasma concentration-response relationships, *Clin Pharmacol Ther* 29:744-774, 1981.

TEST NAME AND METHOD	SPECIMEN	REFERENCE (THERAPEUTIC) INTERVAL, CONVENTIONAL [INTERNATIONAL RECOMMENDED UNITS]	KINETIC VALUES

Cimetidine—CONT

3. Lambert J, Mobassaleh M, Grand RJ: Efficacy of cimetidine for gastric acid suppression in pediatric patients, *J Pediatr* 120:474-478, 1992.
4. Schulz M, Schmoldt A: Therapeutic and toxic blood concentrations of more than 800 drugs and other xenobiotics, *Pharmazie* 58:447-474, 2003.

TEST NAME AND METHOD	SPECIMEN	REFERENCE	KINETIC VALUES
Ciprofloxacin[1-3] **(Cipro)** *HPLC, Bioassay* *MW: 331.35*	Serum, urine. Stable for 20 wk at $-20°$ C.[4]	See Remarks.	PK[5-7]: $t_{1/2}$: 3-5 hr V_d: 2.1-2.7 L/kg Cl_T: 24-72 L/hr Fb: 20-40% F: 70%

1. Jehl F, Gallion C, Debs J, et al: High-performance liquid chromatographic method for determination of ciprofloxacin in biological fluids, *J Chromatogr* 339:347-357, 1985.
2. Joos B, Ledergerber B, Flepp M, et al: Comparison of high pressure liquid chromatography and bioassay for determination of ciprofloxacin in serum and urine, *Antimicrob Agents Chemother* 27:353-356, 1985.
3. Vallee F, LeBel M, Bergeron MG: Determination of ciprofloxacin in biologic samples by reverse phase high performance liquid chromatography, *Ther Drug Monit* 8:340-345, 1986.
4. Pou-Clave L, Campos-Barreda F, Pascual-Mostaza C: Determination of ciprofloxacin in human serum by liquid chromatography, *J Chromatogr* 563:211-215, 1991.
5. Lexi-Comp, Inc.: *Up-to-date online 12.2, drug information,* Hudson, OH, 2004, Lexi-Comp, Inc.
6. Bennett WM, Aronoff GR, Golper TA: *Drug prescribing in renal failure,* ed 3, Philadelphia, 1994, American College of Physicians.
7. Vance-Bryan K, Guay D, Rotschafer JC: Clinical pharmacokinetics of ciprofloxacin, *Clin Pharmacokinet* 19:434-461, 1990.
8. Barrie JR, Mousdale S: Ciprofloxacin levels in a patient undergoing veno-venous haemodiafiltration, *Intensive Care Med* 18:437-438, 1992.

5. Xu K, Arora VK, Chaudhary AK, et al: Quantitative analysis of cimetidine in human plasma using LC/APCI/SRM/MS, *Biomed Chromatogr* 13:455-461, 1999.

Metabolism
  Hepatic
Excretion
  Urine (primary)
  Feces (secondary)
Disease or condition
  Cystic fibrosis: $t_{1/2}\downarrow\rightarrow$, $V_d\downarrow\rightarrow$
  Renal failure: $t_{1/2}\uparrow$, $Cl_T\downarrow$
Age
  Elderly: $t_{1/2}\uparrow$, $V_d\downarrow$, $Cl_T\downarrow$
Dialysis
  Hemodialysis (+)[8]
  Peritoneal (+)[8]

Drug interactions: Sucralfate, aluminum- and magnesium-containing antacids, and products containing iron or zinc decrease bioavailability. Probenecid decreases renal clearance of ciprofloxacin. Ciprofloxacin reduces the metabolism of xanthines (theophylline, caffeine) and may increase prothrombin time in patients receiving concurrent warfarin therapy. Ciprofloxacin is a strong inhibitor of CYP1A2 and a weak inhibitor of CYP3A4. It may increase the effects of CYP1A2 substrates like fluvoxamine.[5]

Ciprofloxacin is a fluoroquinolone antibiotic. Therapeutic concentrations of ciprofloxacin are dependent on the MIC of the organism being treated. In vitro MIC susceptibility breakpoints are recommended as $\leq$1 mg/L [$\times$ 3.02 = $\leq$3 μmol/L] (susceptible), $\leq$2 mg/L [$\leq$6 μmol/L] (moderately susceptible), and $\geq$4 mg/L [$\geq$12 μmol/L] (resistant organisms). Metabolites of ciprofloxacin may have biological activity. A dose of 250 mg given orally leads to peak plasma concentrations of 0.94-1.53 mcg/mL [$\times$ 3.02 = 2.8-4.6 μmol/L], whereas a 500-mg dose given orally leads to peak plasma concentrations of 2.0-2.9 mcg/mL [6.0-8.8 μmol/L].

Interferences: The presence of other antimicrobials may interfere with bioassays.

TEST NAME AND METHOD	SPECIMEN	REFERENCE (THERAPEUTIC) INTERVAL, CONVENTIONAL [INTERNATIONAL RECOMMENDED UNITS]			KINETIC VALUES	
Citalopram	Serum, plasma		*mcg/mL*	µ*mol/L*	$t_{1/2}$:	25-40 hr
(Celexa,		Therapeutic			V_d:	12-16 L/kg
Lexapro)[1-7]		concentration:	0.01-0.2 ×3.08	[0.03-0.62]	Cl_T:	0.33-0.4 L/min
		Toxic			PB:	50-80%
HPLC, GC-MS, GC		concentration:	>5	[>15.4]	F:	80%
					T_{max}:	2-4 hr
MW: 324.4						

1. Baselt C: *Disposition of toxic drugs and chemicals in man*, ed 7, Foster City, CA, 2004, Biomedical Publications.
2. Frahnert C, Rao ML, Grasmader K: Analysis of eighteen antidepressants, four atypical antipsychotics and active metabolites in serum by liquid chromatography: a simple tool for therapeutic drug monitoring, *J Chromatogr B Analyt Technol Biomed Life Sci* 794:35-47, 2003.
3. Hemeryck A, Belpaire FM: Selective serotonin reuptake inhibitors and cytochrome P-450 mediated drug-drug interactions: an update, *Curr Drug Metab* 3:13-37, 2002.
4. Isbister GK, Bowe SJ, Dawson A, et al: Relative toxicity of selective serotonin reuptake inhibitors (SSRIs) in overdose, *J Toxicol Clin Toxicol* 42:277-285, 2004.
5. Milne RJ, Goa KL: Citalopram: a review of its pharmacodynamic and pharmacokinetic properties, and therapeutic potential in depressive illness, *Drugs* 41:450-477, 1991.
6. Schulz M, Schmoldt A: Therapeutic and toxic blood concentrations of more than 800 drugs and other xenobiotics, *Pharmazie* 58:447-474, 2003.
7. Tournel G, Houdret N, Hedouin V, et al: High-performance liquid chromatographic method to screen and quantitate seven selective serotonin reuptake inhibitors in human serum, *J Chromatogr B Biomed Sci Appl* 761:147-158, 2001.

TEST NAME AND METHOD	SPECIMEN	REFERENCE (THERAPEUTIC) INTERVAL, CONVENTIONAL [INTERNATIONAL RECOMMENDED UNITS]			KINETIC VALUES	
Clonazepam	Serum, plasma		*ng/mL*	*nmol/L*	$t_{1/2}$:	20-60 hr
(Klonopin)[1-14]		Therapeutic			V_d:	1.5-4.4 L/kg
		concentration:	20-80 ×3.17	[63-254]	Cl_T:	0.92 ± 0.25 mL/min/kg
HPLC, GC, IA		Toxic			PB:	86%
		concentration:	>80	[>254]		[× 0.01 = 0.86, protein-
MW: 315.7						bound mole fraction]
					F:	70-98%
						[× 0.01 = 0.70-0.98,
						bioavailable mole
						fraction]
					T_{max}:	2-4 hr

1. Schulz M, Schmoldt A: Therapeutic and toxic blood concentrations of more than 800 drugs and other xenobiotics, *Pharmazie* 58:447-474, 2003.
2. Hardman JG, Limbird LE, Gilman AG: *Goodman and Gilman's the pharmacological basis of therapeutics*, ed 10, New York, 2001, McGraw-Hill.

FACTORS INFLUENCING DRUG DISPOSITION	REMARKS AND INTERFERENCES

Metabolism
Hepatic, CYP2C19, CYP3A4, and CYP2D6
Active (weak) metabolite: *N*-desmethylcitalopram

Excretion
Renal (minimal)
Hemodialysis (−)
Hemoperfusion (−)

Drug interactions: Numerous drug interactions are reported related to citalopram's mechanism of action or metabolism by CYP450.

Citalopram is an antidepressant that acts by selectively inhibiting serotonin reuptake. Of this group of drugs, it is the most selective in terms of this action. Although it is sold as a racemic mixture, the S-enantiomer has greater activity and is also sold as escitalopram (Lexapro). Common adverse effects reported include nausea, diarrhea, tremor, sweating, and sexual dysfunction. More serious adverse effects reported include suicidal ideologies, seizures, and hyponatremia. Serotonin syndrome may be life-threatening if unrecognized. SSRIs should not be abruptly stopped but tapered.

Metabolism
Hepatic, CYP3A4

Disease
Hepatic: $Cl_T\downarrow$

Age
Child: $Cl_T\downarrow$

Drug interactions: CYP3A4 inducers may decrease levels/effects of clonazepam, and CYP3A4 inhibitors may increase its levels/effects.

Clonazepam, a benzodiazepine, is used alone or as an adjunct in the treatment of seizures (petit mal and myoclonic) and panic disorder. Clonazepam owes its long $t_{1/2}$ and large V_d to its high lipid solubility. Side effects include drowsiness, fatigue, lethargy, lack of muscular coordination, ataxia, behavioral disturbances, anorexia, and hyperphagia. Clonazepam is metabolized to 7-aminoclonazepam, 7-acetaminoclonazepam, and 3-hydroxy derivatives of these metabolites.

3. McEvoy GK, editor: *AHFS drug information (online version)*, Bethesda, MD, 2004, American Society of Health-System Pharmacists Inc.

4. Tanaka E, Terada M, Misawa S, et al: Simultaneous determination of twelve benzodiazepines in human serum using a new reversed-phase chromatographic column on a 2-microns porous microspherical silica gel, *J Chromatogr B Biomed Appl* 682:173-178, 1996.

TEST NAME AND METHOD	SPECIMEN	REFERENCE (THERAPEUTIC) INTERVAL, CONVENTIONAL [INTERNATIONAL RECOMMENDED UNITS]		KINETIC VALUES

Clonazepam (Klonopin)—CONT

5. El Mahjoub A, Staub C: Semiautomated high-performance liquid chromatographic method for the determination of benzodiazepines in whole blood, *J Anal Toxicol* 25:209-214, 2001.

6. Goldfrank LR, editor: *Goldfrank's toxicological emergencies,* ed 7, (online version), New York, 2002, The McGraw-Hill Companies Inc.

7. Valentine JL, Middleton R, Sparks C: Identification of urinary benzodiazepines and their metabolites: comparison of automated HPLC and GC-MS after immunoassay screening of clinical specimens, *J Anal Toxicol* 20:416-424, 1996.

8. de Carvalho D, Lanchote VL: Measurement of plasma clonazepam for therapeutic control: a comparison of chromatographic methods, *Ther Drug Monit* 13:55-63, 1991.

9. Song D, Zhang S, Kohlhof K: Quantitative determination of clonazepam in plasma by gas chromatography-negative ion chemical ionization mass spectrometry, *J Chromatogr B Biomed Sci Appl* 686:199-204, 1996.

TEST NAME AND METHOD	SPECIMEN	REFERENCE INTERVAL		KINETIC VALUES	
Clonidine[1,2]	Serum, plasma	Therapeutic		PK^{3-6}:	
(Catapres)	(heparin, EDTA)	concentration:	1.0-2.0 ng/mL	$t_{1/2}$:	6-20 hr
			[$\times$ 4.35 = 4.4-8.7 nmol/L]	V_d:	2.1 $\pm$ 0.4 L/kg
GC-MS, GLC		Toxic		Cl_T:	9.94 mL/min/kg
		concentration:	Not well defined	PB:	20-40%
MW: 230.10				F:	~75%

1. Clarke EGC: *Clarke's isolation and identification of drugs in pharmaceuticals, body fluids, and post-mortem material,* London, 1986, The Pharmaceutical Press.

2. Baselt RC: *Disposition of toxic drugs and chemicals in man,* ed 7, Foster City, CA, 2004, Chemical Toxicology Institute.

3. Arndts D: New aspects of the pharmacokinetics and pharmacodynamics of clonidine in man, *Eur J Clin Pharmacokinet* 24:21-30, 1983.

4. Frisk-Holmberg M, Edlund PO, Paalzow L: Pharmacokinetics of clonidine and its relationship to the hypotensive effect in patients, *Br J Clin Pharmacol* 6:227-232, 1978.

5. Frisk-Holmberg M, Paalzow L, Edlund PO: Clonidine kinetics in man—evidence for dose dependency and changed pharmacokinetics during chronic therapy, *Br J Clin Pharmacol* 12:653-658, 1981.

6. Lexi-Comp, Inc.: *Up-to-date online 12.2, drug information,* Hudson, OH, 2004, Lexi-Comp, Inc.

7. Bennett WM, Aronoff GR, Golper TA, et al: *Drug prescribing in renal failure. Dosing guidelines for adults,* ed 2, Philadelphia, 1991, American College of Physicians.

FACTORS INFLUENCING DRUG DISPOSITION	REMARKS AND INTERFERENCES

10. LeGuellec C, Gaudet ML, Breteau M: Improved selectivity for high-performance liquid chromatographic determination of clonazepam in plasma of epileptic patients, *J Chromatogr B Biomed Sci Appl* 719:227-233, 1998.

11. Elian AA: ELISA detection of clonazepam and 7-aminoclonazepam in whole blood and urine, *Forensic Sci Int* 134:54-56, 2003.

12. Salem AA, Barsoum BN, Izake EL: Spectrophotometric and fluorimetric determination of diazepam, bromazepam and clonazepam in pharmaceutical and urine samples, *Spectrochim Acta A* 60:771-780, 2004.

13. Rasanen I, Ojanpera I, Vuori E: Quantitative screening for benzodiazepines in blood by dual-column gas chromatography and comparison of the results with urine immunoassay, *J Anal Toxicol* 24:46-51, 2000.

Metabolism
  Hepatic
Excretion
  Urine (primary)
  Feces (secondary)
Dialysis[7]
  Hemodialysis (−)

Drug interactions:
Antihypertensive effects of clonidine may be antagonized by mirtazapine. Tricyclic antidepressants may diminish the hypotensive effect of clonidine. β-Blockers may enhance the rebound hypertensive effect of clonidine if it is withdrawn abruptly.[6]

Clonidine is a potent antihypertensive agent, with α-adrenergic agonist activity. Dry mouth is associated with serum concentrations >1.0 ng/mL [4.4 nmol/L], and sedation with levels >1.5 ng/mL [6.6 nmol/L]. A linear relationship exists between serum concentration and change in mean arterial pressure. Side effects include dry mouth, sedation, impotence, orthostatic hypotension, bradycardia, convulsions, and coma. Hypertensive crisis has been seen with sudden withdrawal.

TEST NAME AND METHOD	SPECIMEN	REFERENCE (THERAPEUTIC) INTERVAL, CONVENTIONAL [INTERNATIONAL RECOMMENDED UNITS]			KINETIC VALUES	
Clorazepate	Serum, plasma		*mcg/mL*	*μmol/L*	$t_{1/2}$:	40-100 hr
(Tranxene)[1-9]		Therapeutic			V_d:	0.93-1.27 L/kg
		concentration:	0.12-1.00 × 3.01	0.36-3.01	Cl_T:	0.28 mL/min/kg
HPLC, GC		Toxic			PB:	97%
		concentration: Not defined			[× 0.01 = 0.97, protein-	
MW: 332		Desmethyldiazepam (active metabolite)			bound mole fraction]	

1. Baselt R: *Disposition of toxic drugs and chemicals in man,* ed 7, Foster City, CA, 2004, Biomedical Publications.
2. Schulz M, Schmoldt A: Therapeutic and toxic blood concentrations of more than 800 drugs and other xenobiotics, *Pharmazie* 58:447-474, 2003.
3. Hardman JG, Limbird LE, Gilman AG: *Goodman and Gilman's the pharmacological basis of therapeutics,* ed 10, New York, 2001, McGraw-Hill.
4. *Physicians desk reference,* ed 58, Montvale, NJ, 2004, Thomson PDR.
5. Clarke EGC: *Clarke's isolation and identification of drugs in pharmaceuticals, body fluids, and post-mortem material,* London, 1986, The Pharmaceutical Press.
6. ACP's PIER: *Physicians' information and education resource (online version),* Philadelphia, PA, 2004, American College of Physicians.
7. McEvoy GK, editor: *AHFS drug information (online version),* Bethesda, MD, 2004, American Society of Health-System Pharmacists Inc.
8. *USP DI drug information for the health care professional,* ed 24, (online version), Taunton, MA, 2004, Micromedex Inc.
9. Colin P, Sirois G, Lelorier J: High-performance liquid chromatography determination of dipotassium clorazepate and its major metabolite nordiazepam in plasma, *J Chromatogr A* 273:367-377, 1983.

Cocaine[1-30]	Whole blood		*ng/mL*	*nmol/L*	$t_{1/2}$:	0.5-1.5 hr
	(oxalate fluoride),	Therapeutic			V_d:	3-5 L/kg
IA, GC, HPLC,	refrigerate	concentration:	100-500 × 3.3	[330-1650]	Cl_T:	10-30 mL/min/kg
GC-MS,		Toxic				
LC-MS-MS		concentration:	>1000	[>3300]		
MW: 303.3	Urine	Negative				
	Alternative matrices: Oral fluid, sweat, and hair	Negative				

1. Cailleux A, Le Bouil A, Auger B, et al: Determination of opiates and cocaine and its metabolites in biological fluids by high-performance liquid chromatography with electrospray tandem mass spectrometry, *J Anal Toxicol* 23:620-624, 1999.

FACTORS INFLUENCING DRUG DISPOSITION	REMARKS AND INTERFERENCES

Metabolism
  Hepatic, CYP3A4
Disease or condition
  Liver: $t_{1/2}\uparrow$, $V_d\rightarrow$, $Cl_T\downarrow$
  Pregnancy: $t_{1/2}\downarrow$, $V_d\rightarrow$, $Cl_T\uparrow$

Drug interactions: CYP3A4 inducers may decrease levels/effects of clorazepate, and CYP3A4 inhibitors may increase its levels/effects.

Clorazepate, a benzodiazepine, is a prodrug for desmethyldiazepam (nordiazepam), an active metabolite that is rapidly formed in the acidic stomach before absorption. It is used for the treatment of generalized anxiety disorder, management of ethanol withdrawal, and as an adjunct anticonvulsant in management of partial seizures. Side effects include confusion, ataxia, excitement, agitation, transient hypotension, vertigo, fever, GI upset, leukopenia, and liver disease.

Metabolism
  Hepatic, CYP3A4 (major)
Excretion
  Renal

Drug interactions: CYP3A4 inhibitors may increase the levels/effects of cocaine. Cocaine may increase the levels/effects of CYP2D6 substrates and decrease the levels/effects of CYP2D6 prodrug substrates.

Cocaine, a naturally occurring alkaloid, is used as a topical anesthetic for mucous membranes and is a frequently abused drug. The principal cocaine metabolites in urine are benzoylecgonine and ecgonine methyl ester. Coabuse of ethanol and cocaine leads to formation of cocaethylene (ethylcocaine), detectable in urine; cocaethylene inhibits neuronal dopamine reuptake and may contribute to enhanced euphoria of concurrent ethanol and cocaine use.

Immunoassays used for drug screens detect the metabolites rather than the parent drug. For workplace drug testing, the widely accepted immunoassay cutoff concentration to separate positive and negative specimens is 300 ng/mL benzoylecgonine; for GC-MS confirmation, 150 ng/mL benzoylecgonine (mandated by SAMHSA, formerly NIDA).

Alternative matrices used for nonfederally regulated workplace drug testing and being considered for regulated testing include hair, oral fluid, and sweat.

2. Smith FP, Lora-Tamayo C, Carvajal R, et al: Assessment of an automated immunoassay based on kinetic interaction of microparticles in solution for determination of opiates and cocaine metabolite in urine, *Ann Clin Biochem* 34:81-84, 1997.

TEST NAME AND METHOD	SPECIMEN	REFERENCE (THERAPEUTIC) INTERVAL, CONVENTIONAL [INTERNATIONAL RECOMMENDED UNITS]	KINETIC VALUES

Cocaine—CONT

3. Kerrigan S, Phillips Jr WH Jr: Comparison of ELISAs for opiates, methamphetamine, cocaine metabolite, benzodiazepines, phencyclidine, and cannabinoids in whole blood and urine, *Clin Chem* 47:540-547, 2001.

4. Spiehler V, Isenschmid DS, Matthews P, et al: Performance of a microtiter plate ELISA for screening of postmortem blood for cocaine and metabolites, *J Anal Toxicol* 27:587-591, 2003.

5. Kolbrich EA, Kim L, Barnes AJ, et al: Cozart RapiScan Oral Fluid Drug Testing System: an evaluation of sensitivity, specificity, and efficiency for cocaine detection compared with ELISA and GC-MS following controlled cocaine administration, *J Anal Toxicol* 27:407-411, 2003.

6. de Toledo FC, Yonamine M, de Moraes Moreau RL, et al: Determination of cocaine, benzoylecgonine and cocaethylene in human hair by solid-phase microextraction and gas chromatography-mass spectrometry, *J Chromatogr B* 798:361-365, 2003.

7. Romolo FS, Rotolo MC, Palmi I, et al: Optimized conditions for simultaneous determination of opiates, cocaine and benzoylecgonine in hair samples by GC-MS, *Forensic Sci Int* 138:17-26, 2003.

8. Kim I, Barnes AJ, Schepers R, et al: Sensitivity and specificity of the Cozart microplate EIA cocaine oral fluid at proposed screening and confirmation cutoffs, *Clin Chem* 49:1498-1503, 2003.

9. Brunetto R, Gutierrez L, Delgado Y, et al: High-performance liquid chromatographic determination of cocaine and benzolyecgonine by direct injection of human blood plasma sample into an alkyl-diol-silica (ADS) precolumn, *Anal Bioanal Chem* 375:534-538, 2003.

10. Stout PR, Gehlhausen JM, Horn CK, et al: Evaluation of a solid-phase extraction method for benzoylecgonine urine analysis in a high-throughput forensic urine drug-testing laboratory, *J Anal Toxicol* 26:401-405, 2002.

11. Mortier KA, Maudens KE, Lambert WE, et al: Simultaneous, quantitative determination of opiates, amphetamines, cocaine and benzoylecgonine in oral fluid by liquid chromatography quadrupole-time-of-flight mass spectrometry, *J Chromatogr B Analyt Technol Biomed Life Sci* 779:321-330, 2002.

12. Farina M, Yonamine M, Silva OA: One-step liquid-liquid extraction of cocaine from urine samples for gas chromatographic analysis, *Forensic Sci Int* 127:203-207, 2002.

13. Lin SN, Moody DE, Bigelow GE, et al: A validated liquid chromatography-atmospheric pressure chemical ionization-tandem mass spectrometry method for quantitation of cocaine and benzoylecgonine in human plasma, *J Anal Toxicol* 25:497-503, 2001.

14. Klingmann A, Skopp G, Aderjan R: Analysis of cocaine, benzoylecgonine, ecogonine methyl ester, and ecgonine by high-pressure liquid chromatography-API mass spectrometry and application to a short-term degradation study of cocaine in plasma, *J Anal Toxicol* 25:425-430, 2001.

15. deJager LS, Andrews AR: Development of a screening method for cocaine and cocaine metabolites in urine using solvent microextraction in conjunction with gas chromatography, *J Chromatogr A* 911:97-105, 2001.

16. Jeanville PM, Estape ES, Torres-Negron I, et al: Rapid confirmation/quantitation of ecgonine methyl ester, benzoylecgonine, and cocaine in urine using on-line extraction coupled with fast HPLC and tandem mass spectrometry, *J Anal Toxicol* 25:69-75, 2001.

TEST NAME AND METHOD	SPECIMEN	REFERENCE (THERAPEUTIC) INTERVAL, CONVENTIONAL [INTERNATIONAL RECOMMENDED UNITS]			KINETIC VALUES
Codeine[1-23]	Serum, plasma, and blood		*ng/mL*	*nmol/L*	$t_{1/2}$: 2.5-3 hr
		Therapeutic			V_d: ~3.5 L/kg
GC, GC-MS, IA,		concentration:	10-100 $\times$ 3.34	[33-334]	Cl_T: 10-15 mL/min/kg
HPLC, CE,	Urine	Toxic			PB: 7-25%
LC-MS-MS, LC-MS		concentration:	>200	[>668]	[$\times$ 0.01 = 0.07-0.25,
	Alternative				protein-bound mole
MW: 317.4	matrices:	Negative			fraction]
	Hair, oral fluid, and sweat	Negative			

FACTORS INFLUENCING DRUG DISPOSITION	REMARKS AND INTERFERENCES

17. Bourland JA, Hayes EF, Kelly RC, et al: Quantitation of cocaine, benzoylecgonine, cocaethylene, methylecgonine, and norcocaine in human hair by positive ion chemical ionization (PICI) gas chromatography-tandem mass spectrometry, *J Anal Toxicol* 24:489-495, 2000.

18. Pichini S, Pacifici R, Altieri I, et al: Determination of opiates and cocaine in hair as trimethylsilyl derivatives using gas chromatography-tandem mass spectrometry, *J Anal Toxicol* 23:343-348, 1999.

19. Uemura N, Nath RP, Harkey MR, et al: Cocaine levels in sweat collection patches vary by location of patch placement and decline over time, *J Anal Toxicol* 28:253-259, 2004.

20. Campora P, Bermejo AM, Tabernero MJ, et al: Quantitation of cocaine and its major metabolites in human saliva using gas chromatography-positive chemical ionization-mass spectrometry (GC-PCI-MS), *J Anal Toxicol* 27:270-274, 2003.

21. Yonamine M, Tawil N, Moreau RL, et al: Solid-phase micro-extraction-gas chromatography-mass spectrometry and headspace-gas chromatography of tetrahydrocannabinol, amphetamine, methamphetamine, cocaine and ethanol in saliva samples, *J Chromatogr B Analyt Technol Biomed Life Sci* 789:73-78, 2003.

22. Moody DE, Cheever ML: Evaluation of immunoassays for semiquantitative detection of cocaine and metabolites or heroin and metabolites in extracts of sweat patches, *J Anal Toxicol* 25:190-197, 2001.

23. Clauwaert KM, Van Bocxlaer JF, Lambert WE, et al: Segmental analysis for cocaine and metabolites by HPLC in hair of suspected drug overdose cases, *Forensic Sci Int* 110:157-166, 2000.

24. Joseph RE Jr, Hold KM, Wilkins DG, et al: Drug testing with alternative matrices II. Mechanisms of cocaine and codeine deposition in hair, *J Anal Toxicol* 23:396-408, 1999.

25. Moore C, Deitermann D, Lewis D, et al: The detection of cocaine in hair specimens using micro-plate enzyme immunoassay, *J Forensic Sci* 44:609-612, 1999.

26. Huestis MA, Oyler JM, Cone EJ, et al: Sweat testing for cocaine, codeine and metabolites by gas chromatography-mass spectrometry, *J Chromatogr B Biomed Sci Appl* 733:247-264, 1999.

27. Skender L, Karacic V, Brcic I, et al: Quantitative determination of amphetamines, cocaine, and opiates in human hair by gas chromatography/mass spectrometry, *Forensic Sci Int* 125:120-126, 2002.

28. Kidwell DA: Analysis of phencyclidine and cocaine in human hair by tandem mass spectrometry, *J Forensic Sci* 38:272-284, 1993.

29. Brewer WE, Galipo RC, Sellers KW, et al: Analysis of cocaine, benzoylecgonine, codeine, and morphine in hair by supercritical fluid extraction with carbon dioxide modified with methanol, *Anal Chem* 73:2371-2376, 2001.

30. *Fed Register,* 53:11963, April 11, 1988; *Fed Register,* 62:51118, September 30, 1997; *Fed Register,* 69:19673, April 13, 2004.

Metabolism
  Hepatic, CYP2D6 (major), and CYP3A4 (minor)
Excretion
  Renal

Codeine is a morphine derivative with potent analgesic properties. CNS depression and adverse reactions to the drug are similar to those of morphine. Codeine is partially metabolized to morphine and norcodeine. Concentrations of hydrocodone as high as 11% of parent drug have been detected, although hydrocodone is typically considered a minor metabolite.

Drug interactions: CYP2D6 inducers may decrease levels/effects of codeine, and CYP2D6 inhibitors may increase its levels/effects. Codeine is a weak inhibitor of CYP2D6.

For federally regulated workplace drug testing (SAMHSA), the immunoassay cutoff concentration to separate positive and negative specimens for opiates is 2000 ng/mL [7000 nmol/L] morphine equivalents; for GC-MS confirmation, 2000 ng/mL [7000 nmol/L] codeine.

TEST NAME AND METHOD	SPECIMEN	REFERENCE (THERAPEUTIC) INTERVAL, CONVENTIONAL [INTERNATIONAL RECOMMENDED UNITS]	KINETIC VALUES

Codeine—CONT

1. Cailleux A, Le Bouil A, Auger B, et al: Determination of opiates and cocaine and its metabolites in biological fluids by high-performance liquid chromatography with electrospray tandem mass spectrometry, *J Anal Toxicol* 23:620-624, 1999.

2. Ropero-Miller JD, Lambing MK, Winecker RE: Simultaneous quantitation of opioids in blood by GC-EI-MS analysis following deproteination, detautomerization of keto analytes, solid-phase extraction, and trimethylsilyl derivatization, *J Anal Toxicol* 26:524-528, 2002.

3. Levine B, editor: *Principles of forensic toxicology,* Washington, DC, 1999, AACC Press.

4. Haffen E, Paintaud G, Berard M, et al: On the assessment of drug metabolism by assays of codeine and its main metabolites, *Ther Drug Monit* 22:258-265, 2000.

5. Broussard LA, Presley LC, Pittman T, et al: Simultaneous identification and quantitation of codeine, morphine, hydrocodone and hydromorphone in urine as trimethylsilyl and oxime derivatives by gas chromatography-mass spectrometry, *Clin Chem* 43:1029-1032, 1997.

6. Baselt RC: *Analytical procedures for therapeutic drug monitoring and emergency toxicology,* ed 2, Davis, CA, 1987, Biomedical Publications.

7. Zhou T, Yu H, Hu Q, et al: Determination of codeine and its metabolite in human urine by CE with amperometric detection, *J Pharmaceut Biomed Anal* 30:13-19, 2002.

8. Svensson JO, Yue QY, Sawe J: Determination of codeine and metabolites in plasma and urine using ion-pair high-performance liquid chromatography, *J Chromatogr B Biomed Appl* 674:49-55, 1995.

9. Dienes-Nagy A, Rivier L, Giroud C, et al: Method for quantification of morphine and its 3- and 6-glucuronides, codeine, codeine glucuronide and 6-monoacetylmorphine in human blood by liquid chromatography-electrospray mass spectrometry for routine analysis in forensic toxicology, *J Chromatogr A* 854:109-118, 1999.

10. Oyler JM, Cone EJ, Joseph RE Jr, et al: Identification of hydrocodone in human urine following controlled codeine administration, *J Anal Toxicol* 24:530-535, 2000.

11. Mykkanen S, Seppala J, Ariniemi K, et al: GCD quantitation of opiates as propionyl derivatives in blood, *J Anal Toxicol* 24:122-126, 2000.

12. Fraser AD, Worth D: Experience with a urine opiate screening and confirmation cutoff of 2000 ng/mL, *J Anal Toxicol* 23:549-551, 1999.

13. He H, Shay SD, Caraco Y, et al: Simultaneous determination of codeine and its seven metabolites in plasma and urine by high-performance liquid chromatography with ultraviolet and electrochemical detection, *J Chromatogr B Biomed Sci Appl* 708:185-193, 1998.

14. Bogusz MJ, Maier RD, Erkens M, et al: Determination of morphine and its 3- and 6-glucuronides, codeine, codeine-glucuronide and 6-monoacetylmorphine in body fluids by liquid chromatography atmospheric pressure chemical ionization mass spectrometry, *J Chromatogr B Biomed Sci Appl* 703:115-127, 1997.

15. Smith FP, Lora-Tamayo C, Carvajal R, et al: Assessment of an automated immunoassay based on kinetic interaction of microparticles in solution for determination of opiates and cocaine metabolite in urine, *Ann Clin Biochem* 34:81-84, 1997.

16. Seno H, Hattori H, Kurono S, et al: Gas chromatography with surface ionization detection: a highly sensitive method for determining underivatized codeine and dihydrocodeine in body fluids, *J Chromatogr B Biomed Appl* 673:189-195, 1995.

17. Joseph RE Jr, Hold KM, Wilkins DG, et al: Drug testing with alternative matrices II. Mechanisms of cocaine and codeine deposition in hair, *J Anal Toxicol* 23:396-408, 1999.

18. Pichini S, Pacifici R, Altieri I, et al: Determination of opiates and cocaine in hair as trimethylsilyl derivatives using gas chromatography-tandem mass spectrometry, *J Anal Toxicol* 23:343-348, 1999.

FACTORS INFLUENCING DRUG DISPOSITION	REMARKS AND INTERFERENCES
	Alternative matrices used for nonfederally regulated workplace drug testing and being considered for regulated testing include hair, oral fluid, and sweat.
	See *Morphine.*

19. Huestis MA, Oyler JM, Cone EJ, et al: Sweat testing for cocaine, codeine and metabolites by gas chromatography-mass spectrometry, *J Chromatogr B Biomed Sci Appl* 733:247-264, 1999.

20. Skender L, Karacic V, Brcic I, et al: Quantitative determination of amphetamines, cocaine, and opiates in human hair by gas chromatography/mass spectrometry, *Forensic Sci Int* 125:120-126, 2002.

21. Brewer WE, Galipo RC, Sellers KW, et al: Analysis of cocaine, benzoylecgonine, codeine, and morphine in hair by super-critical fluid extraction with carbon dioxide modified with methanol, *Anal Chem* 73:2371-2376, 2001.

22. Romolo FS, Rotolo MC, Palmi I, et al: Optimized conditions for simultaneous determination of opiates, cocaine and benzoylecgonine in hair samples by GC—MS, *Forensic Sci Int* 138:17-26, 2003.

23. *Fed Register,* 53:11963, April 11, 1988; *Fed Register,* 62:51118, September 30, 1997; *Fed Register,* 69:19673, April 13, 2004.

TEST NAME AND METHOD	SPECIMEN	REFERENCE (THERAPEUTIC) INTERVAL, CONVENTIONAL [INTERNATIONAL RECOMMENDED UNITS]		KINETIC VALUES
Cotinine[1-4]	Plasma	*ng/mL*	*nmol/L*	None found.
		Cotinine		
GC, GCMS, HPLC,		Smokers: 16-145 × 5.68	[91-823]	
LCMS, IA		Nonsmokers: 1-8	[6-45]	
MW: 176.22		Nicotine		
		Smokers: 2-10 × 6.16	[12-62]	
		Nonsmokers: 1-4	[6-25]	
	Urine	Cotinine		
		Smokers: 300-1300 × 5.68	[1703-7378]	
		Nonsmokers: 1-20	[6-114]	
		Nicotine		
		Smokers: 200-700 × 6.16	[1233-4315]	
		Nonsmokers: 2-17	[12-105]	

1. Bernert JT Jr, McGuffey JE, Morrison MA, et al: Comparison of serum and salivary cotinine measurements by a sensitive high-performance liquid chromatography-tandem mass spectrometry method as an indicator of exposure to tobacco smoke among smokers and nonsmokers, *J Anal Toxicol* 24:333-339, 2000.

2. Bramer SL, Kallungal BA: Clinical considerations in study designs that use cotinine as a biomarker, *Biomarkers* 8:187-203. 2003.

3. Hansen AM, Garde AH, Christensen JM, et al: Reference interval and subject variation in excretion of urinary metabolites of nicotine from non-smoking healthy subjects in Denmark, *Clin Chim Acta* 304:125-132, 2001.

4. Yildiz D: Nicotine, its metabolism and an overview of its biological effects, *Toxicon* 43:619-632, 2004.

Cyclosporine	Serum (This speci-		*ng/mL*	*nmol/L*	PK[5-7]:	
(Sandimmune)	men is no longer	Renal transplant			$t_{1/2}$ (blood):	16 ± 8 hr
	recommended.)	Therapeutic			V_d (blood):	3.5 ± 2.7 L/kg
FPIA, EIA		concentration			Cl_T (blood):	9.3 ± 1.0
		12 hr after dose: 100-400 × 0.832	[83-333]			mL/min/kg
MW: 1201		24 hr after dose: 100-200		[83-166]	PB:	96%
		Cardiac transplant			F:	23-45%
		Therapeutic				
		concentration				
		12 hr after dose: 100-300		[83-250]		
		24 hr after dose: 100-200		[83-166]		
		Bone marrow				
		transplant				
		Therapeutic				
		concentration				
		12 hr after dose: 100-250		[83-208]		
		Toxic				
		concentration: >400		[>333]		

FACTORS INFLUENCING DRUG DISPOSITION	REMARKS AND INTERFERENCES

See *Nicotine*.

Cotinine, a metabolite of nicotine, is used as a specific indicator of nicotine exposure. Unlike carboxyhemoglobin and thiocyanate, cotinine is derived *only* from the metabolism of nicotine. Its concentration is not influenced by diet or environment, and it is stable in body fluids. Cotinine has an added advantage of a longer $t_{1/2}$ (7-40 hr) compared with the parent drug.

Metabolism
  Hepatic
  Kidney (small amount)
  Intestinal wall (small amount)
Excretion
  Bile (primary)
  Urine (secondary)
Disease
  Hepatic: $Cl_T\downarrow$
Age
  Child: $Cl_T\uparrow$
Dialysis
  Hemodialysis ($-$)
  Peritoneal ($-$)

Drug interactions: Cyclosporine is a major substrate of CYP3A4. It moderately inhibits CYP3A4 and weakly inhibits CYP2C8/9.[8]

Cyclosporine is an immunosuppressant. It is highly bound to erythrocytes and plasma lipoproteins; the binding is temperature dependent in vitro and concentration dependent in vivo. Its main adverse reaction is dose-related nephrotoxicity. Other adverse effects include hirsutism, gingival hyperplasia, hepatotoxicity, hypertension, anaphylaxis, neurotoxicity, and lymphoproliferative disorders. Enterohepatic recycling has been reported for cyclosporine.

Interferences: HPLC is highly specific for parent drug and considered as the gold standard assay. Immunoassays are less specific, with metabolites cross-reacting to varying degrees with antisera. (Cross-reactivity with the major active metabolite, M17, is ~45% but may vary.) The polyclonal FPIA assay is relatively nonspecific and measures both parent drug and metabolites. The new monoclonal FPIA is more specific than the polyclonal assay. In terms of specificity, EMIT<CEDIA<AxSYM[9]. Because CsA metabolite formation can be highly variable in individual patient samples, immunoassays can potentially show small to very large bias, when compared with HPLC, and may have an impact on CsA monitoring[1]. More recently, simpler and rapid LC-MS-MS methods are available for specific monitoring of CsA parent drug.[2,10]

TEST NAME AND METHOD	SPECIMEN	REFERENCE (THERAPEUTIC) INTERVAL, CONVENTIONAL [INTERNATIONAL RECOMMENDED UNITS]	KINETIC VALUES

Cyclosporine (Sandimmune)—CONT

HPLC, RIA, FPIA, EMIT, CEDIA, LC-MS-MS[1-4]	Whole blood (EDTA)	*ng/mL*	*nmol/L*
		Renal transplant Therapeutic concentration	
		12 hr after dose: 100-200 × 0.832 [83-166]	
		Cardiac transplant Therapeutic concentration,	
		12 hr after dose: 150-250	[125-208]
		Hepatic transplant Therapeutic concentration,	
		12 hr after dose: 100-400	[83-333]
		Bone marrow transplant Therapeutic concentration,	
		12 hr after dose: 100-300	[83-250]
		Toxic concentration: >400	[>333]

1. Steimer W: Performance and specificity of monoclonal immunoassays for cyclosporine monitoring: how specific is specific? *Clin Chem* 45:371-381, 1999.

2. Keevil BG, Tierney DP, Cooper DP, et al: Rapid liquid chromatography-tandem mass spectrometry method for routine analysis of cyclosporin A over an extended concentration range, *Clin Chem* 44:69-76, 2002.

3. Lensmeyer G, Wiebe DA, Carlson IH, et al: Three commercial polyclonal immunoassays for cyclosporine in whole blood compared: 2. Cross-reactivity of the antisera with cyclosporine metabolites, *Clin Chem* 36:119-123, 1990.

4. Terrell AR, Daly TM, Hock KG, et al: Evaluation of a no-pretreatment cyclosporin A assay on the Dade Behring Dimension RxL Clinical Chemistry Analyzer, *Clin Chem* 48:1059-1065, 2002.

5. Evans WE, Schentag JJ, Jusko WJ: Applied pharmacokinetics-principles of therapeutic drug monitoring, ed 3, Vancouver, WA, 1992, Applied Therapeutics, Inc.

6. Ptachcinski RJ, Venkataramanan R, Burckart GJ, et al: Clinical pharmacokinetics of cyclosporin, *Clin Pharmacokinet* 11:107-132, 1986.

7. Hardman JG, Limbird LE, Gilman AG: *Goodman & Gilman's the pharmacological basis of therapeutics*, ed 10, New York, 2001, McGraw-Hill.

8. Lexi-Comp, Inc.: *Up-to-date online 12.2, drug information*, Hudson, OH, 2004, Lexi-Comp, Inc.

9. Schutz E, Svinarov D, Shipkova M, et al: Cyclosporin whole blood immunoassays (AxSYM, CEDIA, and EMIT): a critical overview of performance characteristics and comparison with HPLC, *Clin Chem* 44:2158-2164, 1998.

10. Baselt RC: *Disposition of toxic drugs and chemicals in man*, ed 7, Foster City, CA, 2004, Chemical Toxicology Institute.

FACTORS INFLUENCING DRUG DISPOSITION	REMARKS AND INTERFERENCES

Androgens, cimetidine, danazol, diltiazem, erythromycin, estrogens, ketoconazole, and miconazole have been reported to increase cyclosporine plasma concentrations. Phenytoin, the rifampin-isoniazid combination, cotrimoxazole, and phenobarbital increase Cl_T. Long-term steroid therapy may increase Cl_T of cyclosporine. Aminoglycosides, amphotericin B, cotrimoxazole, melphalan, furosemide, and nonsteroidal antiinflammatory drugs may potentiate cyclosporine nephrotoxicity. Oral absorption of cyclosporine may be affected by elapsed time after surgery, dose administered, gastrointestinal dysfunction, external bile drainage, liver disease, and food.

See Tables II-5 and II-6.

TEST NAME AND METHOD	SPECIMEN	REFERENCE (THERAPEUTIC) INTERVAL, CONVENTIONAL [INTERNATIONAL RECOMMENDED UNITS]			KINETIC VALUES	
Dantrolene[1-3] **(Dantrium)**	Serum		*mcg/mL*		$\mu mol/L$	$t_{1/2}$:	4-22 hr
		Therapeutic				V_d:	NA
		concentration:	0.1-3.0	× 3.18	[3.2-9.5]	Cl_T:	NA
HPLC		Toxic				Pb:	>95% (albumin)
		concentration:	Not established			F:	70%
MW: 314.26						T_{max}:	4-8 hr

1. Baselt C: *Disposition of toxic drugs and chemicals in man,* ed 7, Foster City, CA, 2004, Biomedical Publications.
2. Krause T, Gerbershagen MU, Fiege M, et al: Dantrolene—a review of its pharmacology, therapeutic use and new developments, *Anaesthesia* 59:364-373, 2004.
3. Wuis EW, Janssen MG, Vree TB, et al: Determination of a dantrolene metabolite, 5-(p-nitrophenyl)-2-furoic acid, in plasma and urine by high-performance liquid chromatography, *J Chromatogr* 526:575-580, 1999.

TEST NAME AND METHOD	SPECIMEN	REFERENCE (THERAPEUTIC) INTERVAL			KINETIC VALUES	
Diazepam (Valium)[1-11]	Serum, plasma		*ng/mL*		*mmol/L*	$t_{1/2}$:	24-48 hr
		Therapeutic				V_d:	1.2 L/kg
		concentration:	200-1500	× 0.00351	[0.70-5.27]	Cl_T:	0.32 ± 0.06 mL/min/kg
HPLC, GC, IA,		Toxic				PB:	96-99%
LC-MS		concentration:	>3000		[>10.53]		[× 0.01 = 0.96-0.99,
							protein-bound mole
MW: 284.7							fraction]

1. McEvoy GK, editor: *AHFS drug information (online version),* Bethesda, MD, 2004, American Society of Health-System Pharmacists Inc.

FACTORS INFLUENCING DRUG DISPOSITION	REMARKS AND INTERFERENCES

Metabolism
  Hepatic
Excretion
  Renal, biliary

Dantrolene is a peripherally acting skeletal muscle relaxant used to treat malignant hyperthermia, spasticity, and heat stroke. The drug is alkaline and chemically unstable (light-sensitive). Adverse effects include weakness, phlebitis, respiratory failure, drowsiness, and fatigue. Reports of hepatotoxicity after oral administration. Coma can be produced by overdose. Its metabolite, 5-hydroxydantrolene, is also active.

See Table II-5.

Metabolism
  Hepatic, CYP3A4, CYP2C19 (major), CYP1A2, CYP2B6, CYP2C8/9 (minor)
  Active metabolites: desmethyldiazepam, oxazepam.
Disease or condition
  Hepatic: $t_{1/2}\uparrow$, 59.7-112 hr
  $V_d\uparrow$, 1.74 ± 0.21 L/kg
  $Cl_1\downarrow$, 0.20 mL/min/kg
  $PB\downarrow$
  Hypoalbuminemia: $PB\downarrow$, $Cl_T\uparrow$, $V_d\uparrow$
  Pregnancy: $PB\downarrow$
Age
  Premature newborn: $t_{1/2}\uparrow$, 75 hr; $PB\downarrow$
  Child: $t_{1/2}\downarrow$, 18 hr
  $V_d\uparrow$, 2.6 L/kg
  $Cl_T\uparrow$, 1.67 mL/min/kg
  Elderly: $t_{1/2}\uparrow$, $V_d\uparrow$, $Cl_T\rightarrow\downarrow$, $PB\rightarrow$
Dialysis
  Hemodialysis (−)

Drug interactions: CYP3A4 and CYP2C19 inducers may decrease diazepam levels/effects, and CYP3A4 and CYP2C19 inhibitors may increase diazepam levels/effects. Diazepam is a weak inhibitor of CYP2C19 and CYP3A4.

Diazepam is a benzodiazepine used in the treatment of anxiety, status epilepticus, and acute alcohol withdrawal. The drug has a high lipid solubility and is extensively distributed to adipose tissue. Side effects include drowsiness, fatigue, lethargy, muscular incoordination and ataxia, behavioral disturbances, anorexia, and hyperphagia.

Acute CNS toxicity may be treated by administering the benzodiazepine antagonist flumazenil. Half-life of desmethyldiazepam (major metabolite): 50-100 hr.

See also *Oxazepam*.

---

2.   *USP DI drug information for the health care professional,* ed 24, (online version), Taunton, MA, 2004, Micromedex Inc.

TEST NAME AND METHOD	SPECIMEN	REFERENCE (THERAPEUTIC) INTERVAL, CONVENTIONAL [INTERNATIONAL RECOMMENDED UNITS]				KINETIC VALUES	

Diazepam (Valium)—CONT

3. Kratzsch C, Tenberken O, Peters FT, et al: Screening, library-assisted identification and validated quantification of 23 benzodiazepines, flumazenil, zaleplone, zolpidem and zopiclone in plasma by liquid chromatography/mass spectrometry with atmospheric pressure chemical ionization, *J Mass Spectrom* 39:856-872, 2004.

4. Reubsaet KJ, Ragnar Norli H, Hemmersbach P, et al: Determination of benzodiazepines in human urine and plasma with solvent modified solid phase micro extraction and gas chromatography; rationalization of method development using experimental design strategies, *J Pharma Biomed Anal* 18:667-680, 1998.

5. Tanaka E, Terada M, Misawa S, et al: Simultaneous determination of twelve benzodiazepines in human serum using a new reversed-phase chromatographic column on a 2-microns porous microspherical silica gel, *J Chromatogr B Biomed Appl* 682:173-178, 1996.

6. Salem AA, Barsoum BN, Izake EL: Spectrophotometric and fluorimetric determination of diazepam, bromazepam and clonazepam in pharmaceutical and urine samples, *Spectrochim Acta A* 60:771-780, 2004.

7. Capella-Peiro ME, Bose D, Martinavarro-Dominguez A, et al: Direct injection micellar liquid chromatographic determination of benzodiazepines in serum, *J Chromatogr B Analyt Technol Biomed Life Sci* 780:241-249, 2002.

TEST NAME AND METHOD	SPECIMEN	REFERENCE				KINETIC VALUES	
Digitoxin **(Crystodigin)**[1-5] *RIA, FPIA, EIA, HPLC, LC-MS* *MW: 764.95*	Serum (no SST tubes), plasma (heparin, fluoride, oxalate), affected by EDTA or citrate plasma. Sample should ideally be collected at trough level, but at least 8 hr after a dose.	Therapeutic concentration: Toxic concentration:	*ng/mL* 10-30 >45	× 1.31	*nmol/L* [13-39] [>59]	PK[5,6]: $t_{1/2}$: V_d: Cl_T: PB: F:	4-10 days 0.6 L/kg ~0.04 mL/min/kg ~90% 90%

1. Guan F, Ishii A, Seno H, et al: Identification and quantification of cardiac glycosides in blood and urine samples by HPLC/MS/MS, *Anal Chem* 71:4034-4043, 1999.

FACTORS INFLUENCING

DRUG DISPOSITION   **REMARKS AND INTERFERENCES**

8. Kerrigan S, Phillips WH Jr: Comparison of ELISAs for opiates, methamphetamine, cocaine metabolite, benzodiazepines, phencyclidine, and cannabinoids in whole blood and urine, *Clin Chem* 47:540-547, 2001.

9. Needleman SB, Provaznik M: Identification of parent benzodiazepines by gas chromatography/mass spectroscopy (GC/MS) from urinary extracts treated with B-glucuronidase, *Forensic Sci Int* 73:49-60, 1995.

10. Ugland HG, Krogh M, Rasmussen KE: Liquid-phase microextraction as a sample preparation technique prior to capillary gas chromatographic-determination of benzodiazepines in biological matrices, *J Chromatogr B Biomed Sci Appl* 749:85-92, 2000.

11. Rasanen I, Ojanpera I, Vuori E: Quantitative screening for benzodiazepines in blood by dual-column gas chromatography and comparison of the results with urine immunoassay, *J Anal Toxicol* 24:46-51, 2000.

Metabolism
  Hepatic
Excretion
  Urine
  Feces
Disease
  Nephrotic syndrome: $t_{1/2}\downarrow$, $Cl_T\uparrow$, $PB\downarrow$
  Uremia: $t_{1/2}\rightarrow$, $V_d\rightarrow$, $Cl_T\rightarrow$, $PB\downarrow$
Age
  Child: $t_{1/2}\rightarrow$, $V_d\uparrow$, $Cl_T\uparrow$, $PB\rightarrow$
Dialysis
  Hemodialysis $(-)$
  Peritoneal dialysis $(-)$

Drug interactions: Digitoxin is a major substrate of CYP3A4.[7] Metabolism of digitoxin may be enhanced by phenylbutazone, phenobarbital, phenytoin, and rifampin (induction of hepatic microsomal enzymes). Plasma digitoxin is increased during coadministration with amiodarone, quinidine, verapamil, and diltiazem. Cholestyramine and colestipol (binding resins) have been shown to reduce the enterohepatic circulation of digitoxin (may decrease the drug's half-life). Antacids, cholestyramine, colestipol, kaolin-pectin, metoclopramide, neomycin, and sulfasalazine may decrease digitoxin absorption.

Digitoxin is a cardiac glycoside used in the treatment of congestive heart failure and to control ventricular rate in patients with atrial fibrillation or flutter. The drug undergoes significant enterohepatic circulation. The effect of disease states on the kinetics of digitoxin is not well described. Side effects include anorexia, nausea, vomiting, abdominal discomfort and pain, blurred vision, cardiac anomalies (arrhythmias, A-V conduction defects, and, occasionally, impaired conduction in the atria), multifocal PVCs, ventricular tachycardia, A-V block, sinus bradycardia, SA block, atrial fibrillation, and accelerated A-V junctional rhythms. Eosinophilia and thrombocytopenia have been reported.

Interferences: Metabolites may interfere with some RIA procedures. Digitoxin cannot be measured accurately by immunoassay in patients being switched from digoxin. Digitalis-like immunoreactive substances may interfere with FPIA but not chemiluminescent IA assays.[8]

2. Jortani SA, Trepanier D, Yatscoff RW, et al: Convergence of three methods to resolve discrepant immunoassay digitoxin results, *Clin Chem* 43:1805-1808, 1997.

TEST NAME AND METHOD	SPECIMEN	REFERENCE (THERAPEUTIC) INTERVAL, CONVENTIONAL [INTERNATIONAL RECOMMENDED UNITS]			KINETIC VALUES	

Digitoxin (Crystodigin)—CONT

3. Valdes R Jr, Jortani SA, Gheorghiade M: Standards of laboratory practice: cardiac drug monitoring, *Clin Chem* 44:1096-1109, 1998.

4. Jurgens G, Graudal NA, Kampmann JP: Therapeutic drug monitoring of antiarrhythmic drugs, *Clin Pharmacokinet* 42:647-663, 2003.

5. Baselt RC: *Disposition of toxic drugs and chemicals in man,* ed 7, Foster City, CA, 2004, Chemical Toxicology Institute.

6. Hardman JG, Limbird LE, Gilman AG: *Goodman & Gilman's the pharmacological basis of therapeutics,* ed 10, New York, 2001, McGraw-Hill.

TEST NAME AND METHOD	SPECIMEN	REFERENCE INTERVAL	ng/mL	×1.28	nmol/L	KINETIC VALUES	
Digoxin **(Lanoxin)**[1-4] *HPLC, RIA, FPIA, EMIT, CEDIA, ITA* *MW: 780.95*	Serum, plasma (heparin, EDTA); SST should not be used. Collect specimen ≥8-12 hr after dose.	Therapeutic concentration CHF: Arrhythmias: Toxic concentration Adult: Child:	0.8-1.5 1.5-2.0 >2.5 >3.0	×1.28	[1.0-1.9] [1.9-2.6] [>3.2] [>3.8]	PK^{2-5}: $t_{1/2}$: V_d: Cl_T: PB: F:	26-52 hr 5.1-7.4L/kg (IBW) 2.29 mL/min/kg (IBW) 23% 75% (tablets), 85% (elixir)

1. Azzazy HME, Duh SH, Maturen A, et al: Multicenter study of Abbott AxSYM® Digoxin II assay and comparison with 6 methods for susceptibility to digoxin-like immunoreactive factors, *Clin Chem* 43:635-1640, 1997.

2. Baselt RC: *Disposition of toxic drugs and chemicals in man,* ed 7, Foster City, CA, 2004, Chemical Toxicology Institute.

3. Valdes R Jr, Jortani SA, Gheorghiade M: Standards of laboratory practice: cardiac drug monitoring, *Clin Chem* 44:1096-1109, 1998.

4. Jurgens G, Graudal NA, Kampmann JP: Therapeutic drug monitoring of antiarrhythmic drugs, *Clin Pharmacokinet* 42:647-663, 2003.

5. Hardman JG, Limbird LE, Gilman AG: *Goodman & Gilman's the pharmacological basis of therapeutics,* ed 10, New York, 2001, McGraw-Hill.

6. Lexi-Comp, Inc.: *Up-to-date online 12.2, drug information,* Hudson, OH, 2004, Lexi-Comp, Inc.

7. Steimer W, Muller C, Eber B: Digoxin assays: frequent, substantial, and potentially dangerous interference by spironolactone, canrenone, and other steroids, *Clin Chem* 48:507-516, 2002.

8. Soldin S: Digoxin-issues and controversies, *Clin Chem* 32:5-12, 1986.

FACTORS INFLUENCING DRUG DISPOSITION	REMARKS AND INTERFERENCES

7. Lexi-Comp, Inc.: *Up-to-date online 12.2, Drug information,* Hudson, OH, 2004, Lexi-Comp, Inc.
8. Biddle DA, Datta P, Wells A, et al: Falsely elevated serum digitoxin concentrations due to cross-reactivity of water-extractable digitoxin-like immunoreactivity of Chinese medicine Chan SU: elimination of interference by use of a chemiluminescent assay, *Clin Chim Acta* 300:151-158, 2000.

Drug interactions: Digoxin is a minor substrate of CYP3A4.[6] Drugs associated with decreased digoxin absorption include antacids, cholestyramine, colestipol, kaolin-pectin, metoclopramide, neomycin, and sulfasalazine. Quinidine decreases digoxin clearance and has been reported to double steady-state digoxin concentration. Other drugs reported to decrease digoxin clearance include verapamil, spironolactone, nifedipine, and amiodarone. Mexiletine, procainamide, disopyramide, ibuprofen, and quinine may increase plasma digoxin concentrations. Rifampin, phenytoin, and phenylbutazone may decrease plasma digoxin concentrations.

Digoxin is commonly used in the treatment of congestive heart failure and to decrease ventricular response in atrial flutter and fibrillation. A strong correlation exists between creatinine clearance and Cl_T. Side effects include anorexia, nausea, vomiting, abdominal discomfort and pain, blurred vision, and cardiac anomalies (arrhythmias, impaired A-V conduction, and, occasionally, impaired conduction in the atria). Severe toxicity may be treated by digoxin Fab antibody (Digibind) administration.

Biological activity of digoxin is linked to serum K^+ concentration. Digoxin overdose may cause hyperkalemia. In cases of suspected digoxin overdose, it is important to measure potassium in whole blood or serum.

Interferences: Spironolactone, canrenone, and other steroids may cause falsely low digoxin results by MEIA.[7] Patients not on digoxin therapy, but with renal failure or combined renal and hepatic failure, as well as pregnant women, neonates, and infants, exhibit assayable levels of DLIS (digoxin-like immunoreactive substance). The degree of DLIS interference varies widely from patient to patient and from one immunoassay method to another.[1,8,9] Fosinopril may cause a falsely low level with the Digi-Tab RIA kit. Digibind may falsely increase digoxin values by immunoassay, and monitoring by free digoxin assays may be useful post-Digibind administration.[10]

9. Valdes R, Jr: Endogenous digoxin-like immunoreactive factors: impact on digoxin measurements and potential physiological implications, *Clin Chem* 31:1525-1532, 1985.
10. McMillin GA, Owen WE, Lambert TL, et al: Comparable effects of DIGIBIND and DigiFab in thirteen digoxin immunoassays, *Clin Chem* 48:1580-1584, 2002.

TEST NAME AND METHOD	SPECIMEN	REFERENCE (THERAPEUTIC) INTERVAL, CONVENTIONAL [INTERNATIONAL RECOMMENDED UNITS]				KINETIC VALUES	
Diltiazem **(Cardizem)**[1-12] *TLC, GC, HPLC, LC-MS, CE* *MW: 414.53*	Serum, plasma	Therapeutic concentration: Toxic concentration:	*ng/mL* 40-200 >800	× 2.41	*nmol/L* [96-482] [1928]	$t_{1/2}$: V_d: Cl_T Single dose: Multiple dose: PB: F:	3-4.5 hr 5.3 ± 1.7 L/kg 11.5 ± 1.8 mL/min/kg >Twofold ↓ 77-85% [× 0.01 = 0.77-0.85, protein-bound mole fraction] 44 ± 10% [× 0.01 = 0.44 ± 0.10, bioavailable mole fraction]

1. Baselt R: *Disposition of toxic drugs and chemicals in man,* ed 7, Foster City, CA, 2004, Biomedical Publications.
2. Schulz M, Schmoldt A: Therapeutic and toxic blood concentrations of more than 800 drugs and other xenobiotics, *Pharmazie* 58:447-474, 2003.
3. Hardman JG, Limbird LE, Gilman AG: *Goodman and Gilman's the pharmacological basis of therapeutics,* ed 10, New York, 2001, McGraw-Hill.
4. *Physicians desk reference,* ed 58, Montvale, NJ, 2004, Thomson PDR.
5. ACP's PIER: *Physicians' information and education resource (online version),* Philadelphia, 2004, American College of Physicians.
6. McEvoy GK, editor: *AHFS drug information (online version),* Bethesda, MD, 2004, American Society of Health-System Pharmacists Inc.
7. *USP DI drug information for the health care professional,* ed 24, Taunton, MA, 2004, Micromedex Inc.
8. Alebic-Kolbah T, Plavsic F: Determination of serum diltiazem concentrations in a pharmacokinetic study using gas chromatography with electron capture detection, *J Pharm Biomed Analy* 8:915-918, 1990.
9. Li K, Zhang X, Zhao F: HPLC determination of diltiazem in human plasma and its application to pharmacokinetics in humans, *Biomed Chromatogr* 17:522-525, 2003.
10. Coors C, Schulz HG, Stache F: Development and validation of a bioanalytical method for the quantification of diltiazem and desacetyldiltiazem in plasma by capillary zone electrophoresis, *J Chromatogr A* 717:235-243, 1995.
11. Zendelovska D, Stafilov T, Stefova M: High-performance liquid chromatographic determination of diltiazem in human plasma after solid-phase and liquid-liquid extraction, *Anal Bioanal Chem* 376:848-853, 2003.
12. Molden E, Helen Boe G, Christensen H: High-performance liquid chromatography-mass spectrometry analysis of diltiazem and 11 of its phase I metabolites in human plasma, *J Pharm Biomed Anal* 33:275-285, 2003.

Disopyramide **(Norpace)**[1-5] *GC-MS, GLC, HPLC, FPIA, EIA* *MW: 339.48*	Serum, plasma (heparin, EDTA). SST tubes should not be used. Collect at trough concentration.	Therapeutic concentration Arrhythmias, Arterial: Ventricular: Toxic concentration:	*mcg/mL* 2.8-3.2 3.3-7.5 >7	× 2.95	*µmol/L* [8.2-9.4] [9.7-22.1] [>20.6]	PK[3,5,7]: $t_{1/2}$: V_d: Cl_T: PB: F	3-11 hr (dose-dependent) 0.6-1.3 L/kg 1.3 mL/min/kg 28-68% 80%

FACTORS INFLUENCING DRUG DISPOSITION	REMARKS AND INTERFERENCES

Metabolism
  Hepatic, CYP3A4 (major); CYP2C8/9 and CYP2D6 (both minor)

Drug interactions: CYP3A4 inducers may decrease diltiazem levels/effects, and CYP3A4 inhibitors may increase diltiazem levels/effects. Diltiazem is a moderate inhibitor of CYP3A4 and a weak inhibitor of CYP2C8/9 and CYP2D6.

Diltiazem, a calcium channel blocker, is a class IV antiarrhythmic. Hepatic first-pass metabolism appears to be saturable with long-term administration. Desacetyldiltiazem accumulates with multiple oral dosing and appears to contribute to the therapeutic effect.

Metabolism
  Hepatic
Excretion
  Urine (primary)
  Feces (secondary)
Disease
  Uremia: $t_{1/2}\uparrow$, $V_d\downarrow$, $Cl_T\downarrow$
  CHF: $t_{1/2}\uparrow$, $V_d\rightarrow$, $Cl_T\downarrow$
  MI: $t_{1/2}\uparrow$, $V_d\rightarrow$, $Cl_T\downarrow$, $PB\uparrow$
  Tachyarrhythmias: $Cl_T\downarrow$

Protein binding of disopyramide is concentration dependent. Renal clearance of disopyramide has been shown to vary with time, which is partly the result of the concentration-dependent change in protein binding. Side effects include nausea, vomiting, urinary retention, and impotence. Cardiac toxicity (atrioventricular node block, bradycardia, asystole) is associated with concentrations >10 mcg/mL [>29.5 μmol/L]. Rare cases of cholestatic jaundice and leukopenia (reversible) have been reported. Metabolized largely by *N*-dealkylation to nordisopyramide, which has ~50% activity of parent drug. For renal failure patients, unbound drug should be monitored.

TEST NAME AND METHOD	SPECIMEN	REFERENCE (THERAPEUTIC) INTERVAL, CONVENTIONAL [INTERNATIONAL RECOMMENDED UNITS]	KINETIC VALUES

Disopyramide (Norpace)—CONT

1. Flood J, Bowers G, McComb R: Simultaneous liquid-chromatographic determination of three antiarrhythmic drugs: disopyramide, lidocaine, and quinidine, *Clin Chem* 26:197-200, 1980.

2. Pape B: Enzyme immunoassay of disopyramide in serum, *Clin Chem* 27:2038-2040, 1981.

3. Baselt RC: *Disposition of toxic drugs and chemicals in man,* ed 7, Foster City, CA, 2004, Chemical Toxicology Institute.

4. Jurgens G, Graudal NA, Kampmann JP: Therapeutic drug monitoring of antiarrhythmic drugs, *Clin Pharmacokinet* 42:647-663, 2003.

5. Valdes R Jr, Jortani SA, Gheorghiade M: Standards of laboratory practice: cardiac drug monitoring, *Clin Chem* 44:1096-1109, 1998.

6. Hardman JG, Limbird LE, Gilman AG: *Goodman & Gilman's the pharmacological basis of therapeutics,* ed 10, New York, 2003, McGraw-Hill.

7. Lexi-Comp, Inc: *Up-to-date online 12.2, Drug information,* Hudson, OH, 2004, Lexi-Comp, Inc.

Disulfiram[1-5]

GC, HPLC

MW: 296

Plasma. Analyze promptly.

Therapeutic concentration of metabolites

Diethyldithio-carbamate: 0.3-1.4 $\times$ 6.70 [2.0-9.4]

Carbon disulfide: 0.02-0.60 $\times$ 13.13 [0.26-7.88]

mcg/mL   *µmol/L*

$t_{1/2}$

Disulfiram:	7-12 hr
Diethyldithiocarbamate:	15 hr
Diethylamine:	14 hr
Carbon disulfide:	9 hr
Cl_T:	NA
F:	80-90%
PB:	96%
T_{max}:	1-2 hr

1. Chick J: Safety issues concerning the use of disulfiram in treating alcohol dependence, *Drug Saf* 20:427-435, 1999.

2. Brewer C: Recent developments in disulfiram treatment, *Alcohol Alcohol* 28:383-395, 1993.

3. Johansson B: A review of the pharmacokinetics and pharmacodynamics of disulfiram and its metabolites, *Acta Psychiatr Scand* 86:15-26, 1992.

4. Johnson DJ, Amarnath V, Amarnath K, et al: Characterizing the influence of structure and route of exposure on the disposition of dithiocarbamates using toluene-3,4-dithiol analysis of blood and urinary carbon disulfide metabolites, *Toxicol Sci* 76:65-74, 2003.

FACTORS INFLUENCING DRUG DISPOSITION	REMARKS AND INTERFERENCES

Age
  Neonate: PB↓
  Elderly: PB↑
Dialysis[6]
  Hemodialysis (+)

Drug interactions: Disopyramide is a major substrate of CYP3A4.[7] Hepatic enzyme inducers (such as barbiturates) may reduce plasma concentrations.

Metabolism
   Hepatic
 Excretion
   Renal (70-76%), fecal (20%), and
   pulmonary (20-30%)
 	
 Drug interactions: Multiple drug interactions reported because of inhibition of CYP2E1.
	For many years disulfiram was the primary treatment of alcoholism. Because of its adverse risks, other treatment options have been developed. The drug is rapidly metabolized and stored as the diethyldithiocarbamate in fat. Adverse effects include allergic dermatitis, urticaria, drowsiness, fatigue, restlessness, and hepatotoxicity. In combination with alcohol, mild reactions have been reported with blood alcohol concentrations as low as 5 mg/dL. Symptoms are typical when alcohol concentrations are >50 mg/dL, and the patient may become unconscious when alcohol concentrations are >125 mg/dL.
	
	 See Table II-5.

---

5. Zhang Y, Wade KL, Prestera T, et al: Quantitative determination of isothiocyanates, dithiocarbamates, carbon disulfide, and related thiocarbonyl compounds by cyclocondensation with 1,2-benzenedithiol, *Anal Biochem* 239:160-167, 1996.

TEST NAME AND METHOD	SPECIMEN	REFERENCE (THERAPEUTIC) INTERVAL, CONVENTIONAL [INTERNATIONAL RECOMMENDED UNITS]		KINETIC VALUES	
Dronabinol (**Δ-9-Tetra-hydrocannabinol, Marinol**)[1-13] *GC, GC-MS, LC-MS, TLC, IA, LC-MS-MS* *MW: 314.5*	Plasma	*mcg/mL* Therapeutic concentration: 0.005-0.01 Toxic concentration: Not determined	*µmol/L* × 3.18 0.016-0.032	$t_{1/2}$: V_d: PB: F, PO: F, Smoking:	25-36 hr 2.5-6.4 L/kg 97-99% [× 0.01 = 0.97-0.99, protein-bound mole fraction] 6-20% [× 0.01 = 0.06-0.20, bioavailable mole fraction] 18% [× 0.01 = 0.18, bioavailable mole fraction]

1. Baselt R: *Disposition of toxic drugs and chemicals in man,* ed 7, Foster City, CA, 2004, Biomedical Publications.
2. Schulz M, Schmoldt A: Therapeutic and toxic blood concentrations of more than 800 drugs and other xenobiotics, *Pharmazie* 58:447-474, 2003.
3. Hardman JG, Limbird LE, Gilman AG: *Goodman and Gilman's the pharmacological basis of therapeutics,* ed 10, New York, 2001, McGraw-Hill.
4. *Physicians desk reference,* ed 58, Montvale, NJ, 2004, Thomson PDR.
5. Clarke EGC: *Clarke's isolation and identification of drugs in pharmaceuticals, body fluids, and post-mortem material,* London, 1986, The Pharmaceutical Press.
6. ACP's PIER: *Physicians' information and education resource (online version),* Philadelphia, 2004, American College of Physicians.
7. McEvoy GK, editor: *AHFS drug information (online version),* Bethesda, MD, 2004, American Society of Health-System Pharmacists Inc.
8. *USP DI drug information for the health care professional,* ed 24, (online version), Taunton, MA, 2004, Micromedex Inc.
9. Gustafson RA, Moolchan ET, Barnes A, et al: Validated method for the simultaneous determination of delta 9-tetrahydrocannabinol (THC), 11-hydroxy-THC and 11-nor-9-carboxy-THC in human plasma using solid phase extraction and gas chromatography-mass spectrometry with positive chemical ionization, *J Chromatogr B Anal Tech Biomed Life Sci* 798:145-154, 2003.
10. Weinmann W, Vogt S, Goerke R, et al: Simultaneous determination of THC-COOH and THC-COOH-glucuronide in urine samples by LC/MS/MS, *Forensic Sci Int* 113:381-387, 2000.
11. Baselt RC: *Analytical procedures for therapeutic drug monitoring and emergency toxicology,* ed 2, Davis, CA, 1987, Biomedical Publications.
12. Kerrigan S, Phillips Jr W Jr: Comparison of ELISAs for opiates, methamphetamine, cocaine metabolite, benzodiazepines, phencyclidine, and cannabinoids in whole blood and urine, *Clin Chem* 47:540-547, 2001.
13. Staub C: Chromatographic procedures for determination of cannabinoids in biological samples, with special attention to blood and alternative matrices like hair, saliva, sweat and meconium, *J Chromatogr B Biomed Sci Appl* 733:119-126, 1999.

| FACTORS INFLUENCING | |
| DRUG DISPOSITION | REMARKS AND INTERFERENCES |

FACTORS INFLUENCING DRUG DISPOSITION	REMARKS AND INTERFERENCES
Metabolism Hepatic, at least 50 metabolites, major metabolite is 11-OH-THC (psychoactive); extensive first-pass effect; primary urinary metabolite is 11-nor-Δ-9-THC-9-carboxylic acid. *Excretion* Fecal, renal	Δ-9-Tetrahydrocannabinol (THC), the principal psychoactive constituent of marijuana, is highly lipophilic and is widely distributed in the body. Dronabinol (Marinol) is used for treatment of nausea and vomiting associated with cancer chemotherapy in patients who have failed to respond adequately to conventional antiemetic treatments and as an appetite stimulant for AIDS- and cancer-related anorexia. Adverse reactions include drowsiness, sedation, confusion, mood change, and xerostomia.

See *Cannabinoids.*

TEST NAME AND METHOD	SPECIMEN	REFERENCE (THERAPEUTIC) INTERVAL, CONVENTIONAL [INTERNATIONAL RECOMMENDED UNITS]		KINETIC VALUES
Drug Abuse Screen[1] *IA, TLC, GC, HPLC, GC-MS*	Random urine	None detected.		See Table IV-1 for panels recommended in National Academy of Clinical Biochemistry (NACB) Laboratory Medicine Practice Guidelines.

1. Wu AHB, McKay C, Broussard LA, et al: National Academy of Clinical Biochemistry Laboratory Medicine Practice Guidelines: Recommendations for the use of laboratory tests to support poisoned patients who present to the emergency department, *Clin Chem* 49:357-379, 2003.

TEST NAME AND METHOD	SPECIMEN	REFERENCE (THERAPEUTIC) INTERVAL, CONVENTIONAL [INTERNATIONAL RECOMMENDED UNITS]		KINETIC VALUES	
Encainide (Enkaid) *HPLC*[1-3] *MW: 352.48*	Serum, plasma (EDTA, heparin)	Therapeutic concentration:	1-400 ng/mL [$\times 2.84 = 3\text{-}1136$ nmol/L]	PK[4,5]: $t_{1/2}$:	1.5-11.3 hr[6]
		Toxic concentration:	Not defined	V_d: Cl_T: PB: F:	2.7 L/kg 13.2 ± 5.6 mL/min/kg 70.5-78.1% 7-82%
		O-Demethylencainide (active metabolite) Therapeutic concentration:	100-300 ng/mL [$\times 2.95 = 295\text{-}885$ nmol/L]		
		3-Methoxy-*O*-demethylencainide (active metabolite) Therapeutic concentration:	60-280 ng/mL [$\times 2.71 = 163\text{-}759$ nmol/L]		

1. Follath F, Ganzinger U, Schuetz E: Reliability of antiarrhythmic drug plasma concentration monitoring, *Clin Pharmacokinet* 8:63-82, 1983.

2. Turgeon J, Funck-Brentano C, Gray H, et al: Improved high-performance liquid chromatographic assay for encainide and its metabolites in human body fluids, *J Chromatogr* 490:165-174, 1989.

3. Dasgupta A, Rosenzweig IB, Turgeon J, et al: Encainide and metabolites analysis in serum or plasma using a reversed-phase high-performance liquid chromatographic technique, *J Chromatogr* 526:260-265, 1990.

4. Bergstrand RH, Wang T, Roden DM, et al: Encainide disposition in patients with renal failure, *Clin Pharmacol Ther* 40:64-70, 1986.

5. Gillis AM, Kates RE: Clinical pharmacokinetics of the newer antiarrhythmic agents, *Clin Pharmacokinet* 9:375-403, 1984.

6. Wehmeyer AE, Thomas RL: Encainide: a new antiarrhythmic agent, *Drug Intell Clin Pharm* 20:9-13, 1986.

7. Micromedex: *Micromedex healthcare series 2004,* Greenwood Village, CO, 2004, Thomson Micromedex.

8. Woosley RL, Roden DM, Dai GH, et al: Co-inheritance of the polymorphic metabolism of encainide and debrisoquin, *Clin Pharmacol Ther* 39:282-287, 1986.

FACTORS INFLUENCING DRUG DISPOSITION	REMARKS AND INTERFERENCES

Tests to support poisoned patients who present to the emergency department include a combination of qualitative screens in urine and quantitative measurements of selected drugs in serum.

Metabolism
  Hepatic
Excretion
  Urine
Disease
  Cirrhosis: $Cl_T\downarrow$, $F\uparrow$
  Renal: $t_{1/2}\downarrow$, $V_d\downarrow$, $Cl_T\downarrow$, $PB\uparrow$

Drug interactions: Cimetidine may increase plasma concentrations of encainide and its active metabolites. Concurrent use of other antiarrhythmic drugs, adenosine, antipsychotics, foscarnet, and antibiotics like clindamycin and erythromycin can lead to an increased risk in cardiotoxicity.[7]

Encainide is a class IC antiarrhythmic. Its two major metabolites, *O*-demethylencainide (ODE) and 3-methoxy-*O*-demethylencainide (MODE), possess antiarrhythmic activity and are largely excreted by the kidney. Seven to 9% of people are poor metabolizers incapable of rapidly forming ODE. These subjects accumulate very high concentrations of encainide in plasma and have prolonged $t_{1/2}$ (8.7 hr). Antiarrhythmic efficacy appears to be predicted well by plasma ODE concentrations in most patients. Adverse effects include hypotension, bradycardia, seizures, chest pain, ventricular arrhythmias, and death.[8]

Interferences: Maximum cross-reactivity with NDE (the *N*-demethyl metabolite) is reported to be 18% with RIA.

TEST NAME AND METHOD	SPECIMEN	REFERENCE (THERAPEUTIC) INTERVAL, CONVENTIONAL [INTERNATIONAL RECOMMENDED UNITS]		KINETIC VALUES	
Erythropoietin,	Serum, urine		*U/L*	$t_{1/2}$:	4-13 hr (SC),
(Epoetin alfa,		Endogenous concentration:	3-30		27 hr (IV)
Epogen,		Therapeutic concentration:	Not defined	V_d:	0.021-0.063 L/kg
Procrit)[1-11]		Toxic concentration:	Not defined	Cl_T:	0.25-0.4 mL/min/kg
				PB:	NA
HPLC, GC-MS,				F:	22-31% (SC)
GC, CZE, isoelec-				T_{max}:	5-24 hr (SC)
tric focusing elec-					
trophoresis					

1. Abellan R, Ventura R, Pichini S, et al: Evaluation of immunoassays for the measurement of erythropoietin (EPO) as an indirect biomarker of recombinant human EPO misuse in sport, *J Pharm Biomed Anal* 35:1169-1177, 2004.

2. Baselt C: *Disposition of toxic drugs and chemicals in man,* ed 7, Foster City, CA, 2004, Biomedical Publications.

3. Biedback A, Catlin DH, Green GA, et al: Detection of recombinant human erythropoietin in urine by isoelectric focusing, *Clin Chem* 49:901-907, 2003.

4. Bietlot HP, Girard M: Analysis of recombinant human erythropoietin in drug formulations by high-performance capillary electrophoresis, *J Chromatogr A* 759:177-184, 1997.

5. Breymann C: Erythropoietin test methods, *Baillieres Best Pract Res Clin Endocrinol Metab* 14:135-145, 2000.

6. Cascio S, Solari V, Reen DJ, et al: The significance of serum erythropoietin levels in assessing the severity of renal damage in children with reflux nephropathy, *J Urol* 172:1607-1609, 2004.

7. Congote LF: High-performance liquid chromatographic separation of serum erythrotropin and erythropoietin, *J Chromatogr* 310:396-400, 1984.

8. Grimm A, Kendall JD, Mauro LS, et al: *Drugdex drug evaluations: erythropoietins,* Greenwood Village, CO, 2004, Thomson Micromedex.

9. Macdougall IC, Roberts DE, Coles GA, et al: Clinical pharmacokinetics of epoetin (recombinant human erythropoietin), *Clin Pharmacokinet* 20:99-113, 1991.

10. Markham A, Bryson HM: Epoetin alfa: a review of its pharmacodynamic and pharmacokinetic properties and therapeutic use in nonrenal applications, *Drugs* 49:232-254, 1995.

11. Mossuz P, Girodon F, Donnard M, et al: Diagnostic value of serum erythropoietin level in patients with absolute erythrocytosis, *Haematologica* 89:1194-1198, 2004.

Ethanol[1-5]	Serum, whole			*mg/dL*		*mmol/L*	$t_{1/2}$: 25 min (variable)
	blood (oxalate, flu-	Relaxed state		<50	× 0.217	[<10.9]	V_d: 0.6 L/kg
GC, enzymatic	oride). See also	Legally					Cl_T: 6.54 ± 0.05 mL/min/kg
(ADH)	*Remarks.*	intoxicated		> 80		[17.4]	
MW: 46.07	Alcohol swabs	Flushing,					
	should not be used	sensory-motor					
	in collecting the	impairment:		80-100		[17.4-21.7]	
	blood sample; use	Cognitive					
	Betadyne or other	impairment					
	alcohol-free swabs.	Depression of					
		CNS:		>100		[>21.7]	
	Urine	Fatalities					
		reported:		>400		[>86.8]	
	Breath						

FACTORS INFLUENCING DRUG DISPOSITION	REMARKS AND INTERFERENCES
	Epoetin alfa is a recombinant form of human erythropoietin. This protein, normally produced primarily by the kidneys and to a lesser extent by the liver, serves to stimulate erythrocyte production. The drug is used to treat anemia resulting from cancer and HIV chemotherapy and chronic renal failure. Erythropoiesis occurs as rapidly as 7-10 days after initiation of therapy. The increase in hemoglobin and reticulocyte count is proportional to the dose and the duration of therapy. Common side effects include headache and arthralgias, whereas more serious events include hypertension, hyperfibrinogenemia, hyperkalemia, and hyperphosphatemia. The drug is also abused to enhance athletic performance.

Metabolism:
  Hepatic, alcohol dehydrogenase, microsomal ethanol oxidizing system, and peroxides-catalase
Excretion:
  Renal, pulmonary
 	
$\uparrow V_d$ after ingestion of alcohol, aspirin (1 g), and cimetidine.
	Ethanol is a CNS depressant. Acute toxicity ranges from inebriation to seizures, coma, and death. Toxicity from chronic ingestion/exposure includes addiction, malnutrition, dementia, hepatic dysfunction, and pancreatitis. Ethanol consumption during pregnancy is associated with fetal alcohol syndrome.
	
	Medical-legal cases: Proper collection, handling, and storage of the blood alcohol specimen are essential. Blood is the specimen of choice. Concentration determined in a specimen other than whole blood cannot always be converted to blood alcohol concentration. Specimen storage: Blood specimen without sodium fluoride is stable (not opened) at 25° C up to 2 days, at 5° C up to 2 wk, and at −15° C up to 4 wk. With 1% sodium fluoride preservative, specimen is reliable at 25° C up to 2 wk, at 5° C up to 3 mo, and at −15° C up to 6 mo.

TEST NAME AND METHOD	SPECIMEN	REFERENCE (THERAPEUTIC) INTERVAL, CONVENTIONAL [INTERNATIONAL RECOMMENDED UNITS]	KINETIC VALUES

Ethanol—CONT

Serum concentration is 1.2-1.3 times higher than blood.

Values in postabsorptive state are similar to those of serum.

Most states have designated 80 mg/dL as the legal limit for intoxication.

1. Jones AW: Reference limits for urine/blood ratios of ethanol in two successive voids from drinking drivers, *J Anal Toxicol* 26:333-339, 2002.

2. Otsuka M: Determination of ethanol in biological samples by gas chromatography with an electron-capture detection, *Biol Pharm Bull* 25:1639-1641, 2002.

3. Ropero-Miller JD, Winecker RE: Alcoholism. In Kaplan LA, Pesce AJ, Kazmierczak SC, editors: *Clinical chemistry theory, analysis, correlation,* ed 4, St. Louis, 2003, Mosby.

4. Winek CL, Wahba WW, Windisch RM, et al: Serum alcohol concentrations in trauma patients determined by immunoassay versus gas chromatography, *Forensic Sci Int* 139:1-3, 2004.

5. Zuba D, Parczewski A, Reichenbacher M: Optimization of solid-phase microextraction conditions for gas chromatographic determination of ethanol and other volatile compounds in blood, *J Chromatogr B Analyt Technol Biomed Life Sci* 773:75-82, 2002.

TEST NAME AND METHOD	SPECIMEN				KINETIC VALUES	
Ethchlorvynol (Placidyl)[1,2]	Serum, plasma (heparin, EDTA).	Therapeutic	*mcg/mL*	*μmol/L*	$t_{1/2}$:	10-25 hr
	Collect during post-	concentration:	0.5-8	[3.5-55]	V_d:	3-4 L/kg
GLC	distribution phase	Toxic			Cl_T:	NA
	to correlate with	concentration:	>20	$\times$ 6.92	PB:	35-50%
MW: 144.6	toxicity. Stable sev-			[>138]		[$\times$ 0.01 = 0.35-0.5, protein-bound mole fraction]
	eral days at 2-6° C. Freeze for longer storage.				T_{max}:	1.5 hr

1. Bailey DN, Shaw RFL: Ethchlorvynol ingestion in San Diego County: a 14-year review of cases with blood concentrations and findings, *J Anal Toxicol* 14:348-352, 1990.

2. Yell RP: Ethchlorvynol overdose, *Am J Emerg Med* 8:246-250, 1990.

FACTORS INFLUENCING DRUG DISPOSITION	REMARKS AND INTERFERENCES

When using a less-specific method, i.e., enzymatic, other alcohols (e.g., isopropyl and long-chain alcohols) may serve as a substrate in the ADH method and interfere. Environmental contamination of a high-glucose specimen (urine) by yeast may cause a falsely increased ethanol level.

Drug interactions: Coingestion of ethanol and acetaminophen leads to increased risk of hepatotoxicity. Coingestion of ethanol and cocaine leads to production of cocathylene, an active metabolite. Coingestion with sedative, opioids, hypnotics, antidepressants, and antiepileptics may lead to increased CNS depression.

See Table II-5.

Metabolism
  Hepatic
Excretion
  Renal
Dialysis
  Hemodialysis (+)
  Peritoneal (+)

Food slightly delays absorption.

Ethchlorvynol is a hypnotic agent used for short-term relief of insomnia. Because of its potential for abuse, the drug has generally been replaced with safer, more efficacious drugs. Side effects include dizziness, nausea, vomiting, and hypotension. Deep coma, respiratory depression, hypotension, bradycardia, and hypothermia are observed with toxic concentrations.

The $t_{1/2}$ may be prolonged in overdose, ~35 hr.

TEST NAME AND METHOD	SPECIMEN	REFERENCE (THERAPEUTIC) INTERVAL, CONVENTIONAL [INTERNATIONAL RECOMMENDED UNITS]				KINETIC VALUES	
Ethosuximide **(Zarontin)**[1] *HPLC,*[2] *GLC,*[3] *EIA,*[4] *FPIA*[5] *MW: 141.17*	Serum, plasma (heparin, EDTA). Collect at trough concentration. Stable for several hours at room temperature, for 1 yr at −20° C.	Therapeutic concentration: Toxic concentration:	*mcg/mL* 40-100 >150	× 7.08	μ*mol/L* [283-708] [>1062]	PK[6,7]: $t_{1/2}$ Child: Adult: V_d: Cl_T: PB:	30 hr 50-60 hr 0.7 L/kg 0.26 ± 0.05 mL/min/kg Negligible

1. Sadée W: *Drug level monitoring,* New York, 1980, John Wiley and Sons.

2. Galan-Valiente J, Soto-Otero R, Sierra-Marcuno G: Simultaneous measurement of ethosuximide and phenobarbital in brain tissue, serum and urine by HPLC, *Biomed Chromatogr* 3:49-52, 1989.

3. Beam R: Broad-spectrum simultaneous GLC assay of nonderivatized antiepileptic drugs, *Am J Med Technol* 40:211-218, 1974.

4. Dietzler DN, Hoelting CR, Leckie MP, et al: Emit assays for five major anticonvulsant drugs. An evaluation of adaptations to two discrete kinetic analyzers, *Am J Clin Pathol* 74:41-50, 1980.

5. Stewart C, Bottorff M: Fluorescence polarization immunoassay for ethosuximide evaluated and compared with two other immunoassay techniques, *Clin Chem* 32:1781-1783, 1986.

6. Gilman A, Hardman J, Limbird L: *The pharmacological basis of therapeutics,* ed 10, New York, 2001, Pergamon Press, Inc.

7. Lexi-Comp, Inc: *Up-to-date online 12.2. Drug information,* Hudson, OH, 2004, Lexi-Comp, Inc.

8. Bennett WM, Aronoff GR, Golper TA, et al: *Drug prescribing in renal failure. Dosing guidelines for adults,* ed 2, Philadelphia, 1991, American College of Physicians.

9. Browne TR, Dreifuss FE, Dyken PR, et al: Ethosuximide in the treatment of absence (petit mal) seizures, *Neurology* 25:515-524, 1975.

| FACTORS INFLUENCING DRUG DISPOSITION | REMARKS AND INTERFERENCES |

Metabolism
  Hepatic
Excretion
  Feces (primary)
  Urine (secondary)
Age
  Child: $t_{1/2}\downarrow$, $V_d\rightarrow$, $Cl_T\uparrow$
Dialysis[8]
  Hemodialysis (+)

Drug interactions: Ethosuximide is a major substrate of CYP3A4. CYP3A4 inducers like carbamazepine, phenobarbital, phenytoin, and rifamycins may decrease the levels/effects of ethosuximide by increasing its metabolism. CYP3A4 inhibitors like azole antifungals, ciprofloxacin, clarithromycin, diclofenac, doxycycline, erythromycin, imatinib, isoniazid, nefazodone, nicardipine, propofol, protease inhibitors, quinidine, and verapamil may increase the levels/effects of ethosuximide.[7] Valproic acid may increase or decrease plasma ethosuximide concentrations.

Ethosuximide is an antiepileptic agent.[9] Toxic effects are not highly correlated with serum concentration. Concentration-related side effects include nausea, vomiting, anorexia, headache, fatigue, lethargy, and dizziness. The drug may also cause aplastic anemia, leukopenia, and thrombocytopenia. Ethosuximide has been reported to cause a positive Coombs test and an increased antinuclear antibody titer. Serum AST can be elevated.

TEST NAME AND METHOD	SPECIMEN	REFERENCE (THERAPEUTIC) INTERVAL, CONVENTIONAL [INTERNATIONAL RECOMMENDED UNITS]		KINETIC VALUES	
Ethylene Glycol	Serum, plasma (EDTA)	Negative Level for hemodialysis:		$t_{1/2}$:	3-8.6 hr 17-18 hr (with ethanol infusion)
GC, HPLC,					
Fluorimetric,		*mg/dL*	*mmol/L*		2.3-3.5 hr (ethanol and
Enzymatic, GC-MS		>25* × 1.61	4.03		dialysis)
		*With acidosis or renal insufficiency.		V_d:	0.5-0.8 L/kg
MW: 62.07					
	Urine	Negative			

1. Wu AHB, McKay C, Broussard LA, et al: National Academy of Clinical Biochemistry Laboratory Medicine Practice Guidelines: Recommendations for the use of laboratory tests to support poisoned patients who present to the emergency department, *Clin Chem* 49:357-379, 2003.

2. Goldfrank LR, editor: *Goldfrank's toxicological emergencies,* ed 7, (online version), New York, 2002, The McGraw-Hill Companies Inc.

3. Baselt R: *Disposition of toxic drugs and chemicals in man,* ed 7, Foster City, CA, 2004, Biomedical Publications.

4. Schulz M, Schmoldt A: Therapeutic and toxic blood concentrations of more than 800 drugs and other xenobiotics, *Pharmazie* 58:447-474, 2003.

5. Hardman JG, Limbird LE, Gilman AG: *Goodman and Gilman's the pharmacological basis of therapeutics,* ed 10, New York, 2001, McGraw-Hill.

6. *Physicians desk reference,* ed 58, Montvale, NJ, 2004, Thomson PDR.

7. Clarke EGC: *Clarke's isolation and identification of drugs in pharmaceuticals, body fluids, and post-mortem material,* London, 1986, The Pharmaceutical Press.

8. ACP's PIER: *Physicians' information and education resource (online version),* Philadelphia, 2004, American College of Physicians.

9. McEvoy GK, editor: *AHFS drug information (online version),* Bethesda, MD, 2004, American Society of Health-System Pharmacists Inc.

10. *USP DI drug information for the health care professional,* ed 24 (online version), Taunton, MA, 2004, Micromedex Inc.

11. Livesey JF, Perkins SL, Tokessy NE, et al: Simultaneous determination of alcohols and ethylene glycol in serum by packed- or capillary-column gas chromatography, *Clin Chem* 41:300-305, 1995.

12. Williams RH, Shah SM, Maggiore JA, et al: Simultaneous detection and quantitation of diethylene glycol, ethylene glycol, and the toxic alcohols in serum using capillary column gas chromatography, *J Anal Toxicol* 24:621-626, 2000.

13. Eder AF, McGrath CM, Dowdy YG, et al: Ethylene glycol poisoning: toxicokinetic and analytical factors affecting laboratory diagnosis, *Clin Chem* 44:168-177, 1998.

14. Porter WH, Rutter PW, Bush BA, et al: Ethylene glycol toxicity: the role of serum glycolic acid in hemodialysis, *J Toxicol Clin Toxicol* 39:607-615, 2001.

15. Fraser AD: Importance of glycolic acid analysis in ethylene glycol poisoning, *Clin Chem* 44:1769-1770, 1998.

16. Yao HH, Porter WH: Simultaneous determination of ethylene glycol and its major toxic metabolite, glycolic acid, in serum by gas chromatography, *Clin Chem* 42:292-297, 1998.

17. Porter WH, Rutter PW, Yao HH: Simultaneous determination of ethylene glycol and glycolic acid in serum by gas chromatography-mass spectrometry, *J Anal Toxicol* 23:591-597, 1999.

18. Ochs ML, Glick MR, Ryder KW, et al: Improved method for emergency screening for ethylene glycol in serum, *Clin Chem* 34:1507-1508, 1988.

Metabolism
  Hepatic

Alcohol Dehydrogenase (ADH) to the principal toxic metabolite, glycolic acid, and other
acidic compounds, resulting in a metabolic
acidosis.

Ethylene glycol, a component of antifreeze and other products, may be ingested
accidentally or intentionally (by alcoholics). Adverse effects include signs of
intoxication, abdominal pain, metabolic acidosis, CNS depression, tetany, and
renal failure. Oxalate crystals are found in only 33-65% of known ethylene glycol cases. Any amount of ethylene glycol in plasma may be associated with toxicity. Monitoring of ethylene glycol-poisoned patients should include determination of ethylene glycol and glycolic acid levels. One treatment is the
administration of ethanol to saturate the enzyme with a preferred substrate. In
such cases, ethanol levels and glycol levels must be monitored.

See also *Glycolic Acid* and Table II-6.

19. Gupta RN, Smith PT, Eng F: Liquid-chromatographic determination of ethylene glycol in plasma, *Clin Chem* 28:32-33,
    1982.
20. Meola JM, Rosano TG, Swift TA: Fluorometry of ethylene glycol in serum, *Clin Chem* 26:1709, 1980.

TEST NAME AND METHOD	SPECIMEN	REFERENCE (THERAPEUTIC) INTERVAL, CONVENTIONAL [INTERNATIONAL RECOMMENDED UNITS]				KINETIC VALUES	
Fentanyl	Serum, plasma		*ng/mL*		*nmol/L*	$t_{1/2}$:	1-3.5 hr
(Duragesic,		Therapeutic				V_d:	3-8 L/kg
Sublimaze)[1-11]		concentration:	1-3	× 3.08	[3-9.2]	Cl_T:	1.83 ± 0.49 L/kg/hr
		Toxic				(elderly)	2.95 ± 0.92 L/kg/hr
GC, HPLC,		concentration:	>3		[>9]	PB:	80-85%
GC-MS,						T_{max}:	40 min
LC-MS-MS							
MW: 324.8							

1. Ariano RE, Duke PC, Sitar DS: Population pharmacokinetics of fentanyl in healthy volunteers, *J Clin Pharmacol* 41:757-763, 2001.

2. Streisand JB, Busch MA, Egan TD, et al: Dose proportionality and pharmacokinetics of oral transmucosal fentanyl citrate, *Anesthesiology* 88:305-309, 1998.

3. Ohta H, Suzuki S, Ogasawara K: Studies on fentanyl and related compounds IV. Chromatographic and spectrometric discrimination of fentanyl and its derivatives, *J Anal Toxicol* 23:280-285, 1999.

4. Scholz J, Steinfath M, Schulz M: Clinical pharmacokinetics of alfentanil, fentanyl and sufentanil. An update, *Clin Pharmacokinet* 31:275-292, 1996.

5. Palleschi L, Lucentini L, Ferretti E, et al: Quantitative determination of sufentanil in human plasma by liquid chromatography-tandem mass spectrometry, *J Pharmaceut Biomed Anal* 32:329-336, 2003.

6. Levine B, editor: *Principles of forensic toxicology,* Washington DC, 1999, AACC Press.

7. Day J, Slawson M, Lugo RA, et al: Analysis of fentanyl and norfentanyl in human plasma by liquid chromatography-tandem mass spectrometry using electrospray ionization, *J Anal Toxicol* 27:513-516, 2003.

8. Shou WZ, Jiang X, Beato BD, et al: A highly automated 96-well solid phase extraction and liquid chromatography/tandem mass spectrometry method for the determination of fentanyl in human plasma, *Rapid Commun Mass Spectrom* 15:466-476, 2001.

9. Portier EJ, de Blok K, Butter JJ, et al: Simultaneous determination of fentanyl and midazolam using high-performance liquid chromatography with ultraviolet detection, *J Chromatogr B* 723:313-318, 1999.

10. Valaer AK, Huber T, Andurkar SV, et al: Development of a gas chromatographic-mass spectrometric drug screening method for the N-dealkylated metabolites of fentanyl, sufentanil, and alfentanil, *J Chromatogr Sci* 35:461-466, 1997.

11. Kumar K, Ballantyne JA, Baker AB: A sensitive assay for the simultaneous measurement of alfentanil and fentanyl in plasma, *J Pharmaceut Biomed Anal* 14:667-673, 1996.

Flecainide[1-6]	Serum, plasma		*mcg/mL*		*μmol/L*	PK:	
(Tambocor)	(heparin, EDTA).	Therapeutic				$t_{1/2}$:	12-27 hr
	Collect at trough	concentration:	0.2-1.0	× 2.41	[0.5-2.4]	V_d:	9-10 L/kg
GLC, HPLC,	concentration. SST	Toxic				Cl_T:	4.6-12.1 mL/min/kg
GC/MS, IA	tubes should not be	concentration:	>1.0		[>2.4]	PB:	48-68% (α-1 glycoprotein)
	used.					F:	90-95%
MW: 414.35							

FACTORS INFLUENCING DRUG DISPOSITION	REMARKS AND INTERFERENCES

Metabolism
  Hepatic, CYP3A4
Excretion
  Renal (minimal)
  Hemodialysis (−)
  Hemoperfusion (−)

Drug interactions: CYP3A4 inhibitors may increase the levels/effects of fentanyl. Fentanyl is a weak inhibitor of CYP3A4. Not recommended to use fentanyl within 14 days of use of MAO inhibitors.

Fentanyl is a strong analgesic used preoperatively, during surgery, and postoperatively. It is also used intrabuccally in the management of breakthrough cancer pain in patients who are tolerant to opioid therapy. It is 50-100 times as potent as morphine and has a time to peak analgesia of 5 min compared with 15 min for morphine and meperidine. Side effects include hypotension, CNS depression, nausea, respiratory depression, bradycardia, and vomiting. Congeners of fentanyl used as analgesics are sufentanil (Sufenta), alfentanil (Alfenta), and remifentanil (Ultiva). Sufentanil's properties are similar to those of fentanyl. Alfentanil and remifentanil have a more rapid onset of action than fentanyl and sufentanil and are used for short, painful procedures that require intense analgesia and blunting of stress responses. α-Methylfentanyl (China White) is one of several illicit fentanyl derivatives.

Metabolism
  Hepatic[7]
Excretion
  Urine
Disease
  Renal: $t_{1/2}\uparrow$, $Cl_T\downarrow$
  CHF: $t_{1/2}\uparrow$, $Cl_T\downarrow$
Age
  Elderly: $t_{1/2}\uparrow$
Dialysis
  Hemodialysis (−)

Flecainide is a class IC antiarrhythmic used in the treatment of ventricular tachycardia and premature ventricular contractions when other treatment is ineffective. The antiarrhythmic effect appears to be linearly related to plasma flecainide concentrations. The rate of drug excretion is dependent on urinary pH. Flecainide can cause new or worsened arrhythmias. Toxic effects include nausea, vomiting, hypotension, syncope, bradycardia, sinus pause, and heart failure.

Interferences: Propranolol and quinidine cause interference with the spectrofluorometric method.

TEST NAME AND METHOD	SPECIMEN	REFERENCE (THERAPEUTIC) INTERVAL, CONVENTIONAL [INTERNATIONAL RECOMMENDED UNITS]				KINETIC VALUES

Flecainide—CONT

1. Baselt RC: *Disposition of toxic drugs and chemicals in man,* ed 7, Foster City, CA, 2004, Chemical Toxicology Institute.

2. Hardman JG, Limbird LE, Gilman AG: *Goodman & Gilman's the pharmacological basis of therapeutics,* ed 10, New York, 2001, McGraw-Hill.

3. Valdes R Jr, Jortani SA, Gheorghiade M: Standards of laboratory practice: cardiac drug monitoring, *Clin Chem* 44:1096-1109, 1998.

4. Warner A, Annesley T, editors: *Guidelines for therapeutic drug monitoring services,* Washington, DC, 1999, National Academy of Clinical Biochemistry.

5. Lexi-Comp, Inc.: *Up-to-date online 12.2, drug information,* Hudson, OH, 2004, Lexi-Comp, Inc.

6. Lewis GP, Holtzman JL: Interaction of flecainide with digoxin and propranolol, *Am J Cardiol* 53:52B-57B, 1984.

7. Conard GJ, Ober RE: Metabolism of flecainide, *Am J Cardiol* 53:41B, 1984.

TEST NAME AND METHOD	SPECIMEN	REFERENCE (THERAPEUTIC) INTERVAL, CONVENTIONAL		[INTERNATIONAL RECOMMENDED UNITS]	KINETIC VALUES	
Fluconazole	Serum, plasma		*mcg/mL*	μ*mol/L*	$t_{1/2}$:	22-31 hr
(Diflucan)[1-8]		Therapeutic			V_d:	0.58-0.82 L/kg
		concentration			Cl_T:	0.25-0.4 mL/min/kg
HPLC, GC-MS, GC		Meningitis:	2.5-15.1 × 3.26	[8.2-49]	PB:	~12%
		Fungal			F:	>90%
MW: 306.27		infections:	1.9-8	[6.2-26]	T_{max}:	0.5-6 hr (oral)
		Toxic				(dependent on route: oral, topical,
		concentration:	>25	[>82]		intrapericardial, and intravenous)

1. Baselt C: *Disposition of toxic drugs and chemicals in man,* ed 7, Foster City, CA, 2004, Biomedical Publications.

2. Colaluca DM, Hermes AE: *Drugdex drug evaluations: fluconazole,* Greenwood Village, CO, 2004, Thomson Micromedex.

3. Feldmesser M: New and emerging antifungal agents: impact on respiratory infections, *Am J Respir Med* 2:371-383, 2003.

FACTORS INFLUENCING DRUG DISPOSITION	REMARKS AND INTERFERENCES

Drug interactions: Flecainide is a major substrate of CYP2D6 and minor substrate of CYP1A2. It inhibits CYP2D6 weakly.[5] Cimetidine may decrease flecainide clearance, thereby increasing flecainide plasma concentrations. Amiodarone may also increase flecainide concentrations. Coadministration with digoxin may cause a 24% increase in digoxin levels. Coadministration with propranolol may result in slightly elevated plasma levels of both drugs. Acidification of the urine may increase flecainide elimination, whereas alkalinization may decrease it.

Metabolism
  Hepatic, poor
Excretion
  Renal
Age
  Premature infants and neonates: $t_{1/2}\uparrow$
  Hemodialysis (+)
  Peritoneal dialysis (+)
  Hemofiltration (+)

Drug interactions: Fluconazole is known to inhibit CYP2C9 and CYP3A4, leading to numerous potential drug interactions.

Fluconazole is an antifungal drug used to treat candidiasis and cryptococcal meningitis. Resistance by some *Candida* species has developed with long-term use. The most common adverse effects involve the gastrointestinal tract (diarrhea, nausea, and pain). Thrombocytopenia, hyperlipidemia, and increased liver function tests are also reported.

Fluconazole is considered teratogenic.

See Table II-5.

4. Harris SC, Wallace JE, Foulds G, et al: Assay of fluconazole by megabore capillary gas-liquid chromatography with nitrogen-selective detection, *Antimicrob Agents Chemother* 33:714-716, 1989.

TEST NAME AND METHOD	SPECIMEN	REFERENCE (THERAPEUTIC) INTERVAL, CONVENTIONAL [INTERNATIONAL RECOMMENDED UNITS]			KINETIC VALUES	

Fluconazole (Diflucan)—CONT

5. Moraes LA, Lerner FE, Moraes ME, et al: Fluconazole bioequivalence study: quantification by tandem mass spectrometry, *Ther Drug Monit* 21:200-207, 1999.
6. Ng TK, Chan RC, Adeyemi-Doro FA, et al: Rapid high performance liquid chromatographic assay for antifungal agents in human sera, *J Antimicrob Chemother* 37:465-472, 1996.

Flumazenil	Serum, plasma		*mcg/mL*	μ*mol/L*	$t_{1/2}$:	41-79 min
(Romazicon)[1-13]		Therapeutic			V_d:	0.8-1.6 L/kg
		concentration:	0.02-0.1 × 3.08	[0.06-0.31]	PB:	40-50%
HPLC, GC-MS,		Toxic			T_{max}:	3 min (IV)
GC, LC-MS		concentration:	>0.5	[>1.5]		20-90 min (oral)

MW: 303.3

1. Fisher LE, Perch S, Bonfiglio MF, et al: Simultaneous determination of midazolam and flumazenil concentrations in human plasma by gas chromatography, *J Chromatogr B Biomed Appl* 665:217-221, 1995.
2. Song D, Khaykis V, Kohlhof K: Determination of flumazenil in plasma by gas chromatography-negative ion chemical ionization mass spectrometry, *J Chromatogr B Biomed Appl* 663:263-273, 1995.
3. Baselt R: *Disposition of toxic drugs and chemicals in man,* ed 7, Foster City, CA, 2004, Biomedical Publications.
4. Schulz M, Schmoldt A: Therapeutic and toxic blood concentrations of more than 800 drugs and other xenobiotics, *Pharmazie* 58:447-474, 2003.
5. Hardman JG, Limbird LE, Gilman AG: *Goodman and Gilman's the pharmacological basis of therapeutics,* ed 10, New York, 2001, McGraw-Hill.
6. *Physicians desk reference,* ed 58, Montvale, NJ, 2004, Thomson PDR.
7. *Poisindex Management (Internet version), Thomson Micromedex Healthcare series, vol 122,* Greenwood Village, CO, Thomson Micromedex.
8. Zedkova L, Rauw GA, Baker GB, et al: A rapid high-pressure liquid-chromatographic procedure for determination of flumazenil in plasma, *J Pharmacol Toxicol Methods* 46:57-60, 2001.
9. ACP's PIER: *Physicians' information and education resource (online version),* Philadelphia, 2004, American College of Physicians.
10. McEvoy GK, editor: *AHFS drug information (online version),* Bethesda, MD, 2004, American Society of Health-System Pharmacists Inc.
11. *USP DI drug information for the health care professional,* ed 24, (online version), Taunton, MA, 2004, Micromedex Inc.
12. Kratzsch C, Tenberken O, Peters FT, et al: Screening, library-assisted identification and validated quantification of 23 benzodiazepines, flumazenil, zaleplone, zolpidem and zopiclone in plasma by liquid chromatography/mass spectrometry with atmospheric pressure chemical ionization, *J Mass Spectrom* 39:856-872, 2004.
13. Fukuda EK, Choma N, Davis PP: Quantitation of the benzodiazepine antagonist flumazenil in human plasma by gas chromatography-mass spectrometry, *J Chromatogr* 491:97-106, 1989.

FACTORS INFLUENCING DRUG DISPOSITION	REMARKS AND INTERFERENCES

7. Pfaller MA, Diekema DJ: Twelve years of fluconazole in clinical practice: global trends in species distribution and fluconazole susceptibility of bloodstream isolates of Candida, *Clin Microbiol Infect* 10(suppl 1):11-23, 2004.
8. Schulz M, Schmoldt A: Therapeutic and toxic blood concentrations of more than 800 drugs and other xenobiotics, *Pharmazie* 58:447-474, 2003.

Metabolism
  Hepatic
Excretion
  Renal (minimal)
  Hemodialysis (−)
  Hemoperfusion (−)

Flumazenil, an imidazobenzodiazepine derivative, is an antagonist used to reverse benzodiazepine-induced sedation. It is administered IV as a 0.1 mg/mL solution (initial dose 0.2 mg/30 sec) with a maximum recommended cumulative dose of 5 mg total. It should not be used in patients with serious cyclic antidepressant poisoning. Flumazenil is rapidly metabolized to inactive metabolites, including *N*-desmethylflumazenil.

TEST NAME AND METHOD	SPECIMEN	REFERENCE (THERAPEUTIC) INTERVAL, CONVENTIONAL [INTERNATIONAL RECOMMENDED UNITS]			KINETIC VALUES	
Flunitrazepam	Serum, plasma	*mcg/mL*	*μmol/L*		$t_{1/2}$:	16-35 hr
(Rohypnol)[1-14]		Therapeutic			V_d:	3.4-5.5 L/kg
		concentration: 0.005-0.015 × 3.19 [0.016-0.048]			PB:	80%
GC, HPLC, LC-		Toxic				
MS, GC-MS		concentration: >0.05	[>0.16]			
MW: 313.3	Urine					

1. Capella-Peiro ME, Bose D, Martinavarro-Dominguez A, et al: Direct injection micellar liquid chromatographic determination of benzodiazepines in serum, *J Chromatogr B Analyt Technol Biomed Life Sci* 780:241-249, 2002.

2. Terada M, Masui S, Hayashi T, et al: Simultaneous determination of flunitrazepam and 7-aminoflunitrazepam in human serum by ion trap gas chromatography-tandem mass spectrometry, *Legal Med (Tokyo)* 5:S96-S100, 2003.

3. Wang PH, Liu C, Tsay WI, et al: Improved screen and confirmation test of 7-aminoflunitrazepam in urine specimens for monitoring flunitrazepam (Rohypnol) exposure, *J Anal Toxicol* 26:411-418, 2002.

4. Kollroser M, Schober C: Simultaneous analysis of flunitrazepam and its major metabolites in human plasma by high performance liquid chromatography tandem mass spectrometry, *J Pharmaceut Biomed Anal* 28:1173-1182, 2002.

5. Walshe K, Barrett AM, Kavanagh PV, et al: A sensitive immunoassay for flunitrazepam and metabolites, *J Anal Toxicol* 24:296-299, 2000.

6. Rasanen I, Ojanpera I, Vuori E: Quantitative screening for benzodiazepines in blood by dual-column gas chromatography and comparison of the results with urine immunoassay, *J Anal Toxicol* 24:46-51, 2000.

7. Kilicarslan T, Haining RL, Rettie AE, et al: Flunitrazepam metabolism by cytochrome P450S 2C19 and 3A4, *Drug Metab Dispos* 29:460-465, 2001.

8. Drouet-Coassolo C, Iliadis A, Coassolo P, et al: Pharmacokinetics of flunitrazepam following single dose oral administration in liver disease patients compared with healthy volunteers, *Fundam Clin Pharmacol* 4:643-651, 1990.

9. Gafni I, Busto UE, Tyndale RF, et al: The role of cytochrome P450 2C19 activity in flunitrazepam metabolism in vivo, *J Clin Psychopharmacol* 23:169-175, 2003.

10. Kratzsch C, Tenberken O, Peters FT, et al: Screening, library-assisted identification and validated quantification of 23 benzodiazepines, flumazenil, zaleplon, zolpidem and zopiclone in plasma by liquid chromatography/mass spectrometry with atmospheric pressure chemical ionization, *J Mass Spectrom* 39:856-872, 2004.

11. Borrey D, Meyer E, Lambert W, et al: Simultaneous determination of fifteen low-dosed benzodiazepines in human urine by solid-phase extraction and gas chromatography-mass spectrometry, *J Chromatogr B Biomed Sci Appl* 765:187-197, 2001.

12. Reubsaet KJ, Ragnar Norli H, Hemmersbach P, et al: Determination of benzodiazepines in human urine and plasma with solvent modified solid phase micro extraction and gas chromatography; rationalization of method development using experimental design strategies, *J Pharma Biomed Anal* 18:667-680, 1998.

13. El Mahjoub A, Staub C: Semiautomated high-performance liquid chromatographic method for the determination of benzodiazepines in whole blood, *J Anal Toxicol* 25:209-214, 2001.

14. Maurer HH, Kraemer T, Kratzsch C, et al: Negative ion chemical ionization gas chromatography-mass spectrometry and atmospheric pressure chemical ionization liquid-chromatography-mass spectrometry of low-dosed and/or polar drugs in plasma, *Ther Drug Monit* 24:117-124, 2002.

FACTORS INFLUENCING DRUG DISPOSITION	REMARKS AND INTERFERENCES

Metabolism
  Hepatic, CYP3A4 (major), and
  CYP2C19 (minor)
  Principal metabolite:
  7-aminoflunitrazepam (active)
Excretion
  Renal

Flunitrazepam, an intermediate-acting benzodiazepine sedative-hypnotic, is used for the treatment of insomnia and as a preanesthetic. It is illicit in Canada and the U.S. and has been used with alcohol as a "date rape" drug because of its ability to cause disinhibition and amnesia. Adverse effects include hypotension, drowsiness, visual disturbances, dizziness, confusion, gastrointestinal disturbances, and urinary retention.

TEST NAME AND METHOD	SPECIMEN	REFERENCE (THERAPEUTIC) INTERVAL, CONVENTIONAL [INTERNATIONAL RECOMMENDED UNITS]			KINETIC VALUES	
Fluorouracil	Serum		*mcg/mL*	$\mu mol/L$	$t_{1/2}$:	6-22 min
(5-FU, Efudex,		Therapeutic			V_d:	0.1-0.4 L/kg
Adrucil)[1-13]		concentration:			Cl_T:	170-180 mL/min
		Variable depending			PB:	90-98%
HPLC, LCMS,		on protocol			F:	Variable
GC-MS, CZE		and cancer			T_{max}:	0.5-1 hr (dependent on
		Colorectal				route: topical, intraperi-
MW: 246.2		cancer:	2-3	$\times$ 4.06 [8.1-12.2]		cardial, and intravenous)
		Toxic				
		concentration:	>3	[>12.2]		

1. Abel R, Bjornson DC, Corrigan B, et al: *Drugdex drug evaluations: fluorouracil,* Greenwood Village, 2004, Thomson Micromedex.

2. Baselt C: *Disposition of toxic drugs and chemicals in man,* ed 7, Foster City, CA, 2004, Biomedical Publications.

3. Ciccolini J, Mercier C, Blachon MF, et al: A simple and rapid high-performance liquid chromatographic (HPLC) method for 5-fluorouracil (5-FU) assay in plasma and possible detection of patients with impaired dihydropyrimidine dehydrogenase (DPD) activity, *J Clin Pharm Ther* 29:307-315, 2004.

4. Di Paolo A, Ibrahim T, Danesi R, et al: Relationship between plasma concentrations of 5-fluorouracil and 5-fluoro-5,6-dihydrouracil and toxicity of 5-fluorouracil infusions in cancer patients, *Ther Drug Monit* 24:588-593, 2002.

5. Eliason JF, Megyeri A: Potential for predicting toxicity and response of fluoropyrimidines in patients, *Curr Drug Targets* 5:383-388, 2004.

6. Gamelin E, Boisdron-Celle M, Delva R, et al: Long-term weekly treatment of colorectal metastatic cancer with fluorouracil and leucovorin: results of a multicentric prospective trial of fluorouracil dosage optimization by pharmacokinetic monitoring in 152 patients, *J Clin Oncol* 16:1470-1478, 1998.

7. Gamelin E, Boisdron-Celle M, Guerin-Meyer V, et al: Correlation between uracil and dihydrouracil plasma ratio, fluorouracil (5-FU) pharmacokinetic parameters, and tolerance in patients with advanced colorectal cancer: a potential interest for predicting 5-FU toxicity and determining optimal 5-FU dosage, *J Clin Oncol* 17:1105, 1999.

8. Iyer L, Ratain MJ: 5-fluorouracil pharmacokinetics: causes for variability and strategies for modulation in cancer chemotherapy, *Cancer Invest* 17:494-506, 1999.

9. Jiang H, Jiang J, Hu P, et al: Measurement of endogenous uracil and dihydrouracil in plasma and urine of normal subjects by liquid chromatography-tandem mass spectrometry, *J Chromatogr B Analyt Technol Biomed Life Sci* 769:169-176, 2002.

10. Lu HJ, Guo YL, Zhang H, et al: Rapid determination of 5-fluorouracil in plasma using capillary electrophoresis, *J Chromatogr B Analyt Technol Biomed Life Sci* 788:291-296, 2003.

11. Milano G, Ferrero JM, Francois E: Comparative pharmacology of oral fluoropyrimidines: a focus on pharmacokinetics, pharmacodynamics and pharmacomodulation, *Br J Cancer* 91:613-617, 2004.

12. Schulz M, Schmoldt A: Therapeutic and toxic blood concentrations of more than 800 drugs and other xenobiotics, *Pharmazie* 58:447-474, 2003.

13. Siethoff C, Orth M, Ortling A, et al: Simultaneous determination of capecitabine and its metabolite 5-fluorouracil by column switching and liquid chromatographic/tandem mass spectrometry, *J Mass Spectrom* 39:884-889, 2004.

FACTORS INFLUENCING DRUG DISPOSITION	REMARKS AND INTERFERENCES

Metabolism
    Hepatic
Excretion
    Renal
	5-Fluorouracil is a fluorinated pyrimidine antimetabolite used as an antineoplastic agent. The drug is used in the palliative management of breast, colon, stomach, and pancreatic cancers. It is also used to treat dermatological cancers, such as actinic keratoses and basal cell carcinomas.

Drug interactions: Prolonged prothrombin time and INR with coadministration of 5-FU and warfarin. Increased risk of hepatotoxicity with coadministration of 5-FU and levamisole.	The conversion of 5-FU to 5,6-dihydrofluorouracil, a possibly active metabolite, is governed by dihydropyrimidine dehydrogenase (DPD). Patients with a genetic deficiency of DPD may experience severe toxicity. Adverse and toxic effects include alopecia, photosensitivity, anorexia, diarrhea, bleeding, myelosuppression, thrombophlebitis, and myocardial ischemia.

TEST NAME AND METHOD	SPECIMEN	REFERENCE (THERAPEUTIC) INTERVAL, CONVENTIONAL [INTERNATIONAL RECOMMENDED UNITS]			KINETIC VALUES	
Fluoxetine (Prozac)[1-7]	Serum		*mcg/mL*	*µmol/L*	$t_{1/2}$:	4-6 days
		Therapeutic			V_d:	12-42 L/kg
		concentration			Cl_T:	2.7-16.5 mL/min/kg
HPLC, GC-MS, GC		Fluoxetine:	0.03-0.5 ×3.23	[0.1-1.62]	PB:	95% (albumin, α_1 acid
		Norfluoxetine:	0.02-0.47			glycoprotein)
MW: 309.8		Toxic			F:	100%
		concentration:	>1	[>3.23]	T_{max}:	6-8 hr

1. Baselt C: *Disposition of toxic drugs and chemicals in man,* ed 7, Foster City, CA, 2004, Biomedical Publications.
2. Frahnert C, Rao ML, Grasmader K: Analysis of eighteen antidepressants, four atypical antipsychotics and active metabolites in serum by liquid chromatography: a simple tool for therapeutic drug monitoring, *J Chromatogr B Analyt Technol Biomed Life Sci* 794:35-47, 2003.
3. Hemeryck A, Belpaire FM: Selective serotonin reuptake inhibitors and cytochrome P-450 mediated drug-drug interactions: an update, *Curr Drug Metab* 3:13-37, 2002.
4. Isbister GK, Bowe SJ, Dawson A, et al: Relative toxicity of selective serotonin reuptake inhibitors (SSRIs) in overdose, *J Toxicol Clin Toxicol* 42:277-285, 2004.
5. Lacassie E, Gaulier JM, Marquet P, et al: Methods for the determination of seven selective serotonin reuptake inhibitors and three active metabolites in human serum using high-performance liquid chromatography and gas chromatography, *J Chromatogr B Biomed Sci Appl* 742:229-238, 2000.
6. Schulz M, Schmoldt A: Therapeutic and toxic blood concentrations of more than 800 drugs and other xenobiotics, *Pharmazie* 58:447-474, 2003.
7. Tournel G, Houdret N, Hedouin V, et al: High-performance liquid chromatographic method to screen and quantitate seven selective serotonin reuptake inhibitors in human serum, *J Chromatogr B Biomed Sci Appl* 761:147-158, 2001.

TEST NAME AND METHOD	SPECIMEN	REFERENCE (THERAPEUTIC) INTERVAL, CONVENTIONAL [INTERNATIONAL RECOMMENDED UNITS]			KINETIC VALUES	
Fluphenazine (Prolixin, Permitil)[1-4]	Plasma (heparin). Stable for at least 3 wk at −20° C.	Therapeutic concentration:	*ng/mL* 0.2-4.0 ×2.28	*nmol/L* [0.46-9.12]	$t_{1/2}$: Cl_T: V_d: F:	13-58 hr NA 220 L/kg NA
GC, GC-MS, HPLC, LCMS	Fluphenazine may be displaced from protein binding				PB:	91-99% (α_1-acid glycoprotein)
MW: 438	sites by plasticizers in collecting devices.				T_{max}:	1.5-2 hr

| FACTORS INFLUENCING DRUG DISPOSITION | REMARKS AND INTERFERENCES |

Metabolism
  Hepatic, CYP2D6, CYP3A4, CYP2C9, and CYP2C19
  Active metabolite: norfluoxetine
Excretion
  Renal
Dialysis
  Hemodialysis (−)

Drug interactions: Fluoxetine is an inhibitor of CYP2D6, CYP3A4, CYP2C9, and CYP2C19. Numerous interactions are reported, including with desipramine, methadone, alprazolam, triazolam, carbamazepine, throphylline, clozapine, and warfarin. The metabolites contribute to the reported interactions.

Fluoxetine belongs to the group of antidepressants that act by selectively inhibiting neuronal reuptake of serotonin. It is used to treat other psychiatric disorders, including obsessive-compulsive disorder, posttraumatic stress disorder, premenstrual dysphoric disorder, and anxiety disorders. The S- and R-enantiomers exhibit equivalent pharmacological activity. The enantiomers are metabolized to active S- and R-norfluoxetine, which have half-lives of 4-16 days.

Elimination
  Hepatic, active metabolites
Disease or condition
  Smoking: $Cl_T\uparrow$

Drug interactions: Fluphenazine may inhibit the metabolism of some β-blockers. Cyclic antidepressants may inhibit the metabolism of fluphenazine.

Fluphenazine is a neuroleptic agent used to treat schizophrenia and psychotic disorders. The drug has a high frequency of extrapyramidal side effects. The time to peak plasma concentrations and the duration of action vary with drug formulation. Adverse effects include faintness, palpitations, nasal stuffiness, dry mouth, constipation, orthostatic hypotension, hyperthermia and hypothermia, extrapyramidal effects (parkinsonian syndrome), acute dystonic reactions, tardive dyskinesia, jaundice, leukocytosis, thrombocytopenia, leukopenia, eosinophilia, skin reactions, a positive Coombs test, and an increase in serum aminotransferases.

TEST NAME AND METHOD	SPECIMEN	REFERENCE (THERAPEUTIC) INTERVAL, CONVENTIONAL [INTERNATIONAL RECOMMENDED UNITS]			KINETIC VALUES

Fluphenazine (Prolixin, Permitil)—CONT

1. Gutteck U, Rentsch KM: Therapeutic drug monitoring of 13 antidepressant and five neuroleptic drugs in serum with liquid chromatography-electrospray ionization mass spectrometry, *Clin Chem Lab Med* 41:1571-1579, 2003.
2. Desai HD, Seabolt J, Jann MW: Smoking in patients receiving psychotropic medications: a pharmacokinetic perspective, *CNS Drugs* 15:469-494, 2001.

TEST NAME AND METHOD	SPECIMEN	REFERENCE INTERVAL *mcg/mL*		µ*mol/L*	KINETIC VALUES
Flurazepam	Serum, plasma				$t_{1/2}$: 74 ± 24 hr
(Dalmane)		Therapeutic			V_d/F: 22 ± 7 L/kg
		concentration: 0.02-0.1	× 2.58	[0.05-0.26]	Cl_T/F: 4.5 ± 2.3 mL/min/kg
Fluorimetric, GC,		Toxic			PB: 96-98%
HPLC, IA, LC-MS		concentration: >0.2		[>0.5]	[× 0.01 = 0.96-0.98,
					protein-bound mole
MW: 387.9					fraction]
GC-MS	Urine				*Kinetic values represent those of the active metabolite, desalkylflu-razepam, for which flurazepam acts as a prodrug.

1. Rasanen I, Ojanpera I, Vuori E, et al: Quantitative screening for benzodiazepines in blood by dual-column gas chromatography and comparison of the results with urine immunoassay, *J Anal Toxicol* 24:46-51, 2000.
2. Baselt R: *Disposition of toxic drugs and chemicals in man,* ed 7, Foster City, CA, 2004, Biomedical Publications.
3. Schulz M, Schmoldt A: Therapeutic and toxic blood concentrations of more than 800 drugs and other xenobiotics, *Pharmazie* 58:447-474, 2003.
4. Hardman JG, Limbird LE, Gilman AG: *Goodman and Gilman's the pharmacological basis of therapeutics,* ed 10, New York, 2001, McGraw-Hill.
5. *Physicians desk reference,* ed 58, Montvale, NJ, 2004, Thomson PDR.
6. Clarke EGC: *Clarke's isolation and identification of drugs in pharmaceuticals, body fluids, and post-mortem material,* London, 1986, The Pharmaceutical Press.
7. ACP's PIER: *Physicians' information and education resource (online version),* Philadelphia, 2004, American College of Physicians.
8. McEvoy GK, editor: *AHFS drug information (online version),* Bethesda, MD, 2004, American Society of Health-System Pharmacists Inc.
9. *USP DI drug information for the health care professional,* ed 24, (online version), Taunton, MA, 2004, Micromedex Inc.
10. Kratzsch C, Tenberken O, Peters FT, et al: Screening, library-assisted identification and validated quantification of 23 benzodiazepines, flumazenil, zaleplone, zolpidem and zopiclone in plasma by liquid chromatography/mass spectrometry with atmospheric pressure chemical ionization, *J Mass Spectrom* 39:856-872, 2004.
11. Borrey D, Meyer E, Lambert W, et al: Simultaneous determination of fifteen low-dosed benzodiazepines in human urine by solid-phase extraction and gas chromatography-mass spectrometry, *J Chromatogr B Biomed Sci Appl* 765:187-197, 2001.

3. Midha KK, McKay G, Edom R, et al: Kinetics of oral fluphenazine disposition in humans by GC-MS, *Eur J Clin Pharmacol* 25:709-711, 1983.

4. Marder SR, Van Putten T, Aravagiri M, et al: Plasma levels of parent drug and metabolites in patients receiving oral and depot fluphenazine, *Psychopharmacol Bull* 25:479-482, 1989.

Metabolism
  Hepatic, CYP3A4, weak inhibitor of
  CYP2E1
Age
  Elderly: $t_{1/2}\uparrow$
Dialysis
  Hemodialysis ($-$)

Drug interactions: Carbamazepine and other CYP3A4 inducers may increase hepatic metabolism. CYP3A4 inhibitors such as azole antifungals, antibiotics such as erythromycin, and so on, may inhibit hepatic metabolism of flurazepam.

Flurazepam, a benzodiazepine, is used as a hypnotic agent in the short-term treatment of insomnia. Overdose symptoms include respiratory depression, unsteady gait, hypotension, and hypoactive reflexes. Steady-state plasma concentrations are usually attained in 7-10 days.

TEST NAME AND METHOD	SPECIMEN	REFERENCE (THERAPEUTIC) INTERVAL, CONVENTIONAL [INTERNATIONAL RECOMMENDED UNITS]			KINETIC VALUES	
Formaldehyde[1-4]	Blood (fluoride/ oxalate), serum,		*mg/L*	*mol/L*	$t_{1/2}$	
GC, HPLC, LCMS	and urine	Occupational exposure:	0.6-4.0 × 33.3	[20-133]	Formaldehyde: Formic acid:	1.5 min 1.3-1.5 hr
MW: 30.03		Formic acid:	<17 × 21.7	[<369]		
		Exposure:	3-4 times normal formic acid excretion			

1. Burkhart KK, Kulig KW, McMartin KE: Formate levels following a formalin ingestion, *Vet Hum Toxicol* 32:135-137, 1990.
2. Lee XP, Kumazawa T, Kondo K, et al: Analysis of methanol or formic acid in body fluids by headspace solid-phase microextraction and capillary gas chromatography, *J Chromatogr B Biomed Sci Appl* 734:155-162, 1999.
3. Luo W, Li H, Zhang Y, et al: Determination of formaldehyde in blood plasma by high-performance liquid chromatography with fluorescence detection, *J Chromatogr B Biomed Sci Appl* 753:253-257, 2001.
4. Klasco RK, editor: *POISINDEX System,* Greenwood Village, CO, 2004, Thomson Micromedex.

Gabapentin (Neurontin)[1-10]	Serum	Not well established.			$t_{1/2}$: V_d:	5-7 hr 58-61 L
HPLC, LC-MS, LC		Therapeutic	*mcg/mL*	*μmol/L*	Cl_T: PB:	150 mL/min <3%
MW: 171.2		concentration: Toxic	5.9-21 × 5.84	[34.5-123]	F: T_{max}:	50-60% 1.5-4 hr
		concentration:	>85	[>327]		

1. Btaiche IF, Woster PS: Gabapentin and lamotrigine: novel antiepileptic drugs, *Am J Health Syst Pharm* 52:61-69, 1995.
2. Elwes RDC, Binnie CD: Clinical pharmacokinetics of newer antiepileptic drugs: lamotrigine, vigabatrin, gabapentin and oxcarbazepine, *Clin Pharmacokinet* 30:403-415, 1996.
3. Haig GM, Bockbrader HN, Wesche DL, et al: Single-dose gabapentin pharmacokinetics and safety in healthy infants and children, *J Clin Pharmacol* 41:507-514, 2001.
4. Johannessen SI, Battino D, Berry DJ, et al: Therapeutic drug monitoring of the newer antiepileptic drugs, *Ther Drug Monit* 25:347-363, 2003.
5. Kushnir MM, Crossett J, Brown PI, et al: Analysis of gabapentin in serum and plasma by solid-phase extraction and gas chromatography-mass spectrometry for therapeutic drug monitoring, *J Anal Toxicol* 23:1-6, 1999.
6. Lindberger M, Luhr O, Johannessen SI, et al: Serum concentrations and effects of gabapentin and vigabatrin: observations from a dose titration study, *Ther Drug Monit* 25:457-462, 2003.
7. Pappagallo M: Newer antiepileptic drugs: possible uses in the treatment of neuropathic pain and migraine, *Clin Ther* 25:2506-2538, 2003.
8. Schulz M, Schmoldt A: Therapeutic and toxic blood concentrations of more than 800 drugs and other xenobiotics, *Pharmazie* 58:447-474, 2003.

FACTORS INFLUENCING DRUG DISPOSITION	REMARKS AND INTERFERENCES

Metabolism
  Hepatic
Excretion
  Renal, pulmonary (CO_2)
	Formaldehyde is a gas at room temperature but is commonly used as a 37% (v/v) aqueous solution known as formalin, which may be used either as a preservative in embalming or as a fixative in histology. It is widely used in industry and as a constituent of foamed insulation in homes. Formaldehyde is an irritant for eyes and mucous membranes, and adverse effects include lacrimation, cough, pulmonary edema, and contact dermatitis with sensitization occurring in some individuals.
	
	Formaldehyde is rapidly oxidized to formic acid in the erythrocytes and liver. It is further degraded to carbon dioxide and water. Formic acid is the major toxic product from formaldehyde; it is particularly damaging to the retina.

Metabolism
  Not metabolized
Excretion
  Renal, fecal
Disease
  Renal: $t_{1/2}$, Cl_T directly proportional to creatine clearance.
Dialysis
  Hemodialysis (+)
	Gabapentin is an antiepileptic whose use extends beyond the treatment of seizures. It is also used to treat bipolar disorder, migraine headaches, neuropathic pain, and several other neuromuscular disorders. Common adverse effects include fatigue, somnolence, and ataxia.

9.   Tang PH, Miles MV, Glauser TA, et al: Automated microanalysis of gabapentin in human serum by high-performance liquid chromatography with fluorometric detection, *J Chromatogr B Biomed Sci Appl* 727:125-129, 1999.

10.   Wolf CE, Saady JJ, Poklis A: Determination of gabapentin in serum using solid-phase extraction and gas-liquid chromatography, *J Anal Toxicol* 20:498-501, 1996.

TEST NAME AND METHOD	SPECIMEN	REFERENCE (THERAPEUTIC) INTERVAL, CONVENTIONAL [INTERNATIONAL RECOMMENDED UNITS]			KINETIC VALUES	
Gamma Hydroxybutyrate (GHB) (Xyrem)[1-7]	Serum, plasma	*mcg/mL*		$\mu mol/L$	$t_{1/2}$:	0.3-1.0 hr
	Endogenous				V_d:	0.4 L/kg
	concentration:	<10	× 9.62	[<96]	PB:	<1%
	Toxic				T_{max}:	0.5-1.25 hr
GLC, IA,	concentration:	>80		[>770]		
colorimetric,						
GC-MS, CE-MS						
MW: 104.11	Urine					

1. Baldacci A, Theurillat R, Caslavska J, et al: Determination of gamma-hydroxybutyric acid in human urine by capillary electrophoresis with indirect UV detection and confirmation with electrospray ionization ion-trap mass spectrometry, *J Chromatogr A* 990:99-110, 2003.

2. Alston WC 2nd, Ng K: Rapid colorimetric screening test for gamma-hydroxybutyric acid (liquid X) in human urine, *Forensic Sci Int* 126:114-117, 2002.

3. Villain M, Cirimele V, Ludes B, et al: Ultra-rapid procedure to test for gamma-hydroxybutyric acid in blood and urine by gas chromatography-mass spectrometry, *J Chromatogr B Analyt Technol Biomed Life Sci* 792:83-87, 2003.

4. Elian AA: GC-MS determination of gamma-hydroxybutyric acid (GHB) in blood, *Forensic Sci Int* 122:43-47, 2001.

5. Bravo DT, Harris DO, Parsons SM: Reliable, sensitive, rapid and quantitative enzyme-based assay for gamma-hydroxybutyric acid (GHB), *J Forensic Sci* 49:379-387, 2004.

6. Badcock NR, Zotti R: Rapid screening test for gamma-hydroxybutyric acid (GHB, Fantasy) in urine, *Ther Drug Monit* 21:376-377, 1999.

7. Cobaugh DJ, Kerrigan S: Gamma-hydroxybutyrate. In Shaw L, editor: *The clinical toxicology laboratory: contemporary practice of poisoning evaluation,* Washington DC, 2001, AACC Press, pp. 127-144.

Gentamicin[1-6] **(Garamycin)**	Serum, plasma (EDTA). For patients on penicillin		*mcg/mL*	$\mu mol/L$	PK[7-9]:	
	or its derivatives,	Therapeutic concentration			$t_{1/2}$:	1.5-4 hr[10]
MB, HPLC, GLC,	freeze sample if not	Peak			V_d:	0.26 L/kg
RIA, EIA, FPIA	analyzed within 4-6	Less severe			Cl_T:	1.3 mL/min/kg
	hr. Routine collec-	infections:	5-8	× 2.09 [10.5-16.7]	PB:	Negligible
MB assays have	tion of specimen	Severe			F, IM:	100%
been largely re-	should be at trough	infections:	8-10	[16.7-20.9]	F, PO:	Negligible
placed by more	and peak concen-	Trough				
sensitive and spe-	trations (end of a	Less severe				
cific immunoas-	1-hr constant infu-	infections:	<1	[<2.1]		
says.	sion, 30 min after	Moderate				
	the end of a 30-min	infections:	<2	[<4.2]		
	constant infusion,	Severe				
	or 1 hr after an IM	infections:	<2-4	[<4.2-8.4]		
	dose).	Toxic				
		concentration				
		Peak:	>10-12	[>20.9-25.1]		
		Trough:	>2-4	[>4.2-8.4]		

FACTORS INFLUENCING DRUG DISPOSITION	REMARKS AND INTERFERENCES

Metabolism

  Hepatic, metabolized to succinic acid, which enters the TCA (Krebs) cycle

Excretion

  Expired as carbon dioxide.

Drug interactions: GHB should not be used with alcohol or other CNS depressants.

Gamma hydroxybutyrate (GHB), a naturally occurring metabolite of GABA, is thought to function as a neurotransmitter. Xyrem (sodium oxybate) is the first and only FDA-approved medication for cataplexy associated with narcolepsy. Its use is very restricted and regulated. Even at recommended doses, the use of Xyrem has been associated with confusion, depression, neuropsychiatric events, and respiratory depression. The most commonly observed adverse events associated with the use of sodium oxybate were headache, nausea, dizziness, pain, somnolence, pharyngitis, and infection.

GHB and its precursors gamma butyrolactone (GBL) and 1,4-butanediol have emerged as recreational euphoriants. GHB has been used as a "date rape" drug and has been designated as an illicit intoxicant in many states.

Metabolism

  None

Excretion

  Urine

Disease

  Renal: $t_{1/2}\uparrow$, $V_d\rightarrow$, $Cl_T\downarrow$

  Burns: $Cl_T\uparrow$

  Cystic fibrosis: $V_d\rightarrow$, $Cl_T\uparrow$

  Obesity: $V_d\uparrow$ (based on IBW)

  $Cl_T\uparrow$ (based on IBW)

Age

  Newborn: $t_{1/2}\uparrow$, $V_d\uparrow$, $Cl_T\downarrow$

  Child: $t_{1/2}\downarrow$, $V_d\uparrow$, $Cl_T\downarrow$

  Elderly: $t_{1/2}\rightarrow$, $V_d\rightarrow$, $Cl_T\rightarrow$

Dialysis

  Hemodialysis (+)

  Peritoneal (+)[11]

Gentamicin is an aminoglycoside antibiotic. Therapeutic and toxic concentrations should be considered highly variable and individualized for the patient's condition. Penicillin and its derivatives inactivate gentamicin in vivo and in vitro. A definitive cause-and-effect relationship between trough concentration and the incidence of nephrotoxicity has not been established. Cl_T and $t_{1/2}$ are strongly correlated with glomerular filtration rate. Side effects include vestibular and auditory dysfunction (principally vestibular), nephrotoxicity, cholestasis, leukopenia, eosinophilia, and neuromuscular blockade. Gentamicin may cause decreased serum calcium, potassium, and magnesium concentrations.

Interferences: When patient is also taking other antibiotics (penicillins, cephalosporins, tetracyclines, clindamycin, and chloramphenicol), the MB method may lack specificity. Penicillins and cephalosporins can be inactivated with a commercially available β-lactamase to minimize this interference. Heparin has been implicated in the formation of an inactive complex with gentamicin, thereby deactivating the antibiotic.

TEST NAME AND METHOD	SPECIMEN	REFERENCE (THERAPEUTIC) INTERVAL, CONVENTIONAL [INTERNATIONAL RECOMMENDED UNITS]	KINETIC VALUES
Gentamicin—CONT			

1. Maitra S, Yoshikawa T, Hansen J, et al: Serum gentamicin assay by high-performance liquid chromatography, *Clin Chem* 23:2275-2278, 1977.

2. Maitra S, Yoshikawa T, Guze L, et al: Determination of aminoglycoside antibiotics in biological fluids: a review, *Clin Chem* 25:1361-1367, 1979.

3. Mayhew JW, Gorbach SL: Gas-liquid chromatographic method for the assay of aminoglycoside antibiotics in serum, *J Chromatogr* 151:133-146, 1978.

4. O'Leary TD, Ratcliff RM, Geary TD: Evaluation of an enzyme immunoassay for serum gentamicin, *Antimicrob Agents Chemother* 17:776-778, 1980.

5. Oeltgen PR, Shank WA Jr, Blouin RA, et al: Clinical evaluation of the Abbott TDx fluorescence polarization immunoassay analyzer, *Ther Drug Monit* 6:360-367, 1984.

6. Baselt RC: *Disposition of toxic drugs and chemicals in man,* ed 7, Foster City, CA, 2004, Chemical Toxicology Institute.

7. Bauer LA, Blouin RA: Gentamicin pharmacokinetics: effect of aging in patients with normal renal function, *J Am Geriatr Soc* 30:309-311, 1982.

8. Evans WE, Schentag JJ, Jusko WJ: *Applied pharmacokinetics—principles of therapeutic drug monitoring,* ed 3, Vancouver, WA, 1992, Applied Therapeutics, Inc.

9. Pechere JC, Dugal R: Clinical pharmacokinetics of aminoglycoside antibiotics, *Clin Pharmacokinet* 4:170-199, 1979.

10. Postovsky S, Ben Arush MW, Kassis E, et al: Pharmacokinetic analysis of gentamicin thrice and single daily dosage in pediatric cancer patients, *Pediatr Hematol Oncol* 14:547-554, 1997.

11. Jusko WJ, Baliah T, Kim KH, et al: Pharmacokinetics of gentamicin during peritoneal dialysis in children, *Kidney Int* 9:430, 1976.

12. Micromedex: *Micromedex Healthcare series 2004,* Greenwood Village, CO, 2004, Thomson Micromedex.

TEST NAME AND METHOD	SPECIMEN	REFERENCE (THERAPEUTIC) INTERVAL, CONVENTIONAL [INTERNATIONAL RECOMMENDED UNITS]		KINETIC VALUES	
Glutethimide (Doriden)[1-3]	Serum	*mcg/mL*	$\mu mol/L$	$t_{1/2}$:	Biphasic, initial ~4 hr, terminal ~12 hr acute overdose: >40 hr
		Therapeutic concentration: 0.2-5 × 4.60	[0.92-23]		
GC, HPLC, GC-MS		Toxic		V_d:	~3 L/kg
		concentration: >10	[>46]	Cl_T:	NA
MW: 217.3				F:	NA
				PB:	45-60% [× 0.01 = 0.45-0.6, protein-bound mole fraction]
				T_{max}:	1-6 hr

FACTORS INFLUENCING DRUG DISPOSITION	REMARKS AND INTERFERENCES

Drug interactions: Concomitant use of gentamicin with neuromuscular blockers may lead to aminoglycoside-induced respiratory paralysis. Coadministration of cyclosporine or tacrolimus with gentamicin may lead to increased risk of nephrotoxicity. Concomitant usage of furosemide with gentamicin is associated with a risk of ototoxicity and nephrotoxicity.[12]

See Table II-6.

Metabolism
  Hepatic, active metabolites
  (4-hydroxyglutethimide and
  2-phenylglutarimide)
Dialysis
  Hemodialysis (−)
  Peritoneal (−)
  Hemoperfusion (+)

This drug is a highly lipid-soluble sedative, a hypnotic agent producing CNS depression. Because of its high abuse potential, the drug has been replaced by less addictive and more efficacious drugs. Absorption from the intestinal tract is erratic. Approximately 2% of a dose is excreted unchanged into the urine. This drug undergoes extensive enterohepatic recirculation. Additionally, glutethimide is a potent stimulator of the hepatic microsomal enzyme system. Side effects include excitement, blurring of vision, gastric irritation, headache, and skin rashes. Respiratory depression, circulatory collapse, and coma accompany acute overdosage. Osteomalacia has been reported after chronic use.

In some patients, toxicity may occur within the therapeutic range.

TEST NAME AND METHOD	SPECIMEN	REFERENCE (THERAPEUTIC) INTERVAL, CONVENTIONAL [INTERNATIONAL RECOMMENDED UNITS]			KINETIC VALUES	

Glutethimide (Doriden)—CONT

1. Bailey DN, Shaw RF: Interpretation of blood glutethimide, meprobamate, and methyprylon concentrations in nonfatal and fatal intoxications involving a single drug, *J Toxicol Clin Toxicol* 20:133-145, 1983.
2. Baselt C: *Disposition of toxic drugs and chemicals in man,* ed 7, Foster City, CA, 2004, Biomedical Publications.

Test name and method	Specimen	Reference interval	ng/mL		nmol/L	Kinetic values	
Haloperidol (Haldol)[1-5]	Serum, plasma (heparin, EDTA)		*ng/mL*		*nmol/L*	$t_{1/2}$:	14-41 hr (lactate) 14-28 days (decanoate)
		Therapeutic concentration:	5-15	× 2.66	[13.3-39.9]	V_d:	10-22 L/kg
GLC, IA, HPLC, LCMS		Toxic concentration:	> 50		[>133]	Cl_T: PB:	8-17 mL/min/kg 92%
MW: 375.9							[× 0.01 = 0.92, protein-bound mole fraction], (α_1-acid glycoprotein)
						F:	60-70% [× 0.01 = 0.60-0.70, bioavailable mole fraction]
						T_{max}:	2-6 hr

1. Angelo HR, Petersen A: Therapeutic drug monitoring of haloperidol, perphenazine, and zuclopenthixol in serum by a fully automated sequential solid phase extraction followed by high-performance liquid chromatography, *Ther Drug Monit* 23:157-162, 2001.
2. Arinobu T, Hattori H, Iwai M, et al: Liquid chromatographic-mass spectrometric determination of haloperidol and its metabolites in human plasma and urine, *J Chromatogr B Analyt Technol Biomed Life Sci* 776:107-113, 2002.
3. Kratzsch C, Peters FT, Kraemer T, et al: Screening, library-assisted identification and validated quantification of fifteen neuroleptics and three of their metabolites in plasma by liquid chromatography/mass spectrometry with atmospheric pressure chemical ionization, *J Mass Spectrom* 38:283-295, 2003.
4. Kudo S, Ishizaki T: Pharmacokinetics of haloperidol: an update, *Clin Pharmacokinet* 37:435-456, 1999.
5. Ulrich S, Wurthmann C, Brosz M, et al: The relationship between serum concentration and therapeutic effect of haloperidol in patients with acute schizophrenia, *Clin Pharmacokinet* 34:227-263, 1998.

Test name and method	Specimen	Reference interval		Kinetic values	
Heroin (Diamorphine, Diacetylmorphine)	Serum, plasma, and blood	Therapeutic concentration: Toxic concentration:	Not determined Not determined	$t_{1/2}$:	2-6 min (heroin) 6-25 min (6-AM) 2-3 hr
GLC, HPLC, IA,	Urine	Negative		V_d: PB:	25 L/kg 25-35%
GC-MS, fluorimetric, LC-MS-MS, CE, LC-MS	Alternative matrices: Hair, oral fluid, and sweat	Negative			
MW: 303.4					

| FACTORS INFLUENCING DRUG DISPOSITION | REMARKS AND INTERFERENCES |

3. Svinarov DA, Dotchev DC: Simultaneous liquid-chromatographic determination of some bronchodilators, anticonvulsants, chloramphenicol, and hypnotic agents, with Chromosorb P columns used for sample preparation, *Clin Chem* 35:1615-1618, 1989.

Metabolism
  Hepatic, CYP2D6, CYP1A2, and CYP3A4
Excretion
  Renal, fecal
Dialysis
  Hemodialysis ($-$)
  Peritoneal ($-$)

Haloperidol is an antipsychotic drug used in the treatment of schizophrenia and also in reducing tics and vocal utterances of Tourette's syndrome. It is also used to control the choreiform movements of Huntington's disease. Adverse effects frequently seen include blurred vision, tardive dyskinesia, muscular rigidity, tachycardia, hypotension, and arrhythmias, sedation. Rare cases of hepatic dysfunction and leukopenia have been reported.

Metabolism
  Rapid deacetylation by blood and tissue esterases to 6-acetylmorphine (6-AM) and then morphine
Elimination
  Renal as morphine glucuronides

Diacetylmorphine or heroin, the most widely abused opioid, is synthesized by the acetylation of morphine. It has two to three times the potency of morphine and has better penetration across the blood-brain barrier because of the 2-acetyl groups. In some countries, medical prescription of diacetylmorphine is being used or considered as a treatment option for heavily dependent addicts and for the management of chronic pain during terminal illness. It can be administered orally, by intramuscular, intravenous, or subcutaneous injection, intranasal insufflation, or smoking. The analgesic effects of heroin are principally caused by the effect of 6-AM and morphine.

For federally regulated workplace drug testing (SAMHSA), the presence of morphine at immunoassay and GC-MS cutoff concentrations of 2000 ng/mL [7000 nmol/L] morphine equivalents plus 6-AM at a cutoff concentration >10 ng/mL are considered unequivocal evidence of heroin use.

TEST NAME AND METHOD	SPECIMEN	REFERENCE (THERAPEUTIC) INTERVAL, CONVENTIONAL [INTERNATIONAL RECOMMENDED UNITS]	KINETIC VALUES

Heroin (Diamorphine, Diacetylmorphine)—CONT

1. *Fed Register,* 53:11963, April 11, 1988; *Fed Register,* 62:51118, September 30, 1997; *Fed Register,* 69:19673, April 13, 2004.

2. Baselt RC: *Analytical procedures for therapeutic drug monitoring and emergency toxicology,* ed 2, Davis, CA, 1987, Biomedical Publications.

3. Pacifici R, Pichini S, Altieri I, et al: High-performance liquid chromatographic-electrospray mass spectrometric determination of morphine and its 3- and 6-glucuronides: application to pharmacokinetic studies, *J Chromatogr B Biomed Appl* 664:329-334, 1995.

4. Jenkins AJ, Keenan RM, Henningfield JE, et al: Pharmacokinetics and pharmacodynamics of smoked heroin, *J Anal Toxicol* 18:317-330, 1994.

5. Cone EJ, Holicky BA, Grant TM, et al: Pharmacokinetics and pharmacodynamics of intranasal "snorted" heroin, *J Anal Toxicol* 17:327-337, 1993.

6. Cone EJ, Welch P, Mitchell JM, et al: Forensic drug testing of opiates: I. Detection of 6-acetylmorphine in urine as an indicator of recent heroin exposure; drug and assay considerations and detection times, *J Anal Toxicol* 15:1-7, 1991.

7. Zuccaro P, Ricciarello R, Pichini S, et al: Simultaneous determination of heroin 6-monoacetylmorphine, morphine, and its glucuronides by liquid chromatography—atmospheric pressure ionspray-mass spectrometry, *J Anal Toxicol* 21:268-277, 1997.

8. Gyr E, Brenneisen R, Bourquin D, et al: Pharmacodynamics and pharmacokinetics of intravenously, orally and rectally administered diacetylmorphine in opioid dependents, a two-patient pilot study within a heroin-assisted treatment program, *Int J Clin Pharmacol Ther* 38:486-491, 2000.

9. Beike J, Kohler H, Brinkmann B, et al: Immunoaffinity extraction of morphine, morphine-3-glucuronide and morphine-6-glucuronide from blood of heroin victims for simultaneous high-performance liquid chromatographic determination, *J Chromatogr B Biomed Sci Appl* 726:111-119, 1999.

10. Narongchai P, Sribanditmonkol P, Thampithug S, et al: The duration time of urine morphine detection in heroin addicts by radioimmunoassay, *J Med Assoc Thailand* 85:82-86, 2002.

11. Bogusz MJ, Maier RD, Erkens M, et al: Detection of non-prescription heroin markers in urine with liquid chromatography-atmospheric pressure chemical ionization mass spectrometry, *J Anal Toxicol* 25:431-438, 2001.

12. Girardin F, Rentsch KM, Schwab MA, et al: Pharmacokinetics of high doses of intramuscular and oral heroin in narcotic addicts, *Clin Pharmacol Ther* 74:341-352, 2003.

13. Ropero-Miller JD, Goldberger BA: Opioids. In Shaw L, editor: *The clinical toxicology laboratory: contemporary practice of poisoning evaluation,* Washington DC, 2001, AACC Press.

14. Kendall JM, Latter VS: Intranasal diamorphine as an alternative to intramuscular morphine: pharmacokinetic and pharmacodynamic aspects, *Clin Pharmacokinet* 42:501-513, 2003.

15. Smith ML, Shimomura ET, Summers J, et al: Urinary excretion profiles for total morphine, free morphine, and 6-acetylmorphine following smoked and intravenous heroin, *J Anal Toxicol* 25:504-514, 2001.

16. Nakahara Y, Kikura R, Takahashi K: Hair analysis for drugs of abuse. VIII. Effective extraction and determination of 6-acetylmorphine and morphine in hair with trifluoroacetic acid-methanol for the confirmation of retrospective heroin use by gas chromatography-mass spectrometry, *J Chromatogr B Biomed Appl* 657:93-101, 1994.

FACTORS INFLUENCING DRUG DISPOSITION	REMARKS AND INTERFERENCES

Alternative matrices used for nonfederally regulated workplace drug testing and being considered for regulated testing include hair, oral fluid, and sweat.

See *Morphine*.

TEST NAME AND METHOD	SPECIMEN	REFERENCE (THERAPEUTIC) INTERVAL, CONVENTIONAL [INTERNATIONAL RECOMMENDED UNITS]					KINETIC VALUES	
Hydromorphone (Dilaudid)[1-6]	Serum		*ng/mL*			*nmol/L*	$t_{1/2}$:	2.6-4 hr
							V_d:	2.9 L/kg
		Therapeutic concentration:	1-30	× 3.50	[4-105]		PB:	14%
GC, GC-MS,		Toxic						[× 0.01 = 0.14, protein-
HPLC, IA,		concentration:	>100			[>350]		bound mole fraction]
LC-MS-MS								
MW: 285.3								
IA, GC-MS	Urine							

1. Bouquillon AI, Freeman D, Moulin DE, et al: Simultaneous solid-phase extraction and chromatographic analysis of morphine and hydromorphone in plasma by high-performance liquid chromatography with electrochemical detection, *J Chromatogr A* 577:354-357, 1992.

2. Chen YL, Hanson GD, Jiang X: Simultaneous solid-phase extraction and chromatographic analysis of morphine and hydromorphone in human plasma by liquid chromatography with tandem mass spectrometric detection, *J Chromatogr B Analyt Technol Biomed Life Sci* 769:55-64, 2002.

3. Ropero-Miller JD, Lambing MK, Winecker RE: Simultaneous quantitation of opioids in blood by GC-EI-MS analysis following deproteination, detautomerization of keto analytes, solid-phase extraction, and trimethylsilyl derivatization, *J Anal Toxicol* 26:524-528, 2002.

4. Broussard LA, Presley LC, Pittman T, et al: Simultaneous identification and quantitation of codeine, morphine, hydrocodone and hydromorphone in urine as trimethylsilyl and oxime derivatives by gas chromatography-mass spectrometry, *Clin Chem* 43:1029-1032, 1997.

5. Naidong W, Jiang X, Newland K, et al: Development and validation of a sensitive method for hydromorphone in human plasma by normal phase liquid chromatography-tandem mass spectrometry, *J Pharmaceut Biomed Anal* 23:697-704, 2000.

6. Smith ML, Hughes RO, Levine B, et al: Forensic drug testing for opiates. VI. Urine testing for hydromorphone, hydrocodone, oxymorphone, and oxycodone with commercial opiate immunoassays and gas chromatography-mass spectrometry, *J Anal Toxicol* 19:18-26, 1995.

Isoniazid (Hyzyd, Nydrazid)[1-5]	Serum, plasma (heparin, EDTA).		*mcg/mL*			$\mu mol/L$	$t_{1/2}$
		Therapeutic concentration					Fast acetylators: 0.5-1.6 hr
							Slow acetylators: 2-5 hr
GC, HPLC	Collected as peak, 2 hr postdose.	2 hr, 300 mg dose:	3-6	× 7.29	[22-44]		V_d: 0.57-0.75 L/kg Cl_T
MW: 137.1	Process immediately and store at	2 hr, 900 mg dose:	9-18		[66-131]		Fast acetylators: 7.0 mL/min/kg
	−70° C; *N*-acetyl-	Toxic					Slow acetylators: 2.5 mL/min/kg
	isoniazid is extremely unstable,	concentration:	>20		[>146]		F: 90%
	even when frozen.						PB: 4-30%
							T_{max}: 1-2 hr

FACTORS INFLUENCING DRUG DISPOSITION	REMARKS AND INTERFERENCES
Metabolism Hepatic	Hydromorphone is a strong analgesic used to treat moderate to severe pain. It also has antitussive activity. It is subject to abuse. CNS depression and adverse reactions are similar to those of morphine.

Metabolism
  Hepatic (N-acetyltransferase)
Excretion
  Renal
Disease
  Hepatic: $t_{1/2}\uparrow$
  Hepatitis (acute viral): $t_{1/2}\uparrow$
  Renal: $Cl_T\downarrow t_{1/2}\uparrow$ (significant in slow acety-
  lators)
Dialysis
  Hemodialysis (+)
  Peritoneal (+)
 	
Drug/food interactions: Food, particularly a fatty meal, can decrease C_{max} ~50%.
	Isoniazid, used to treat tuberculosis primarily, is metabolized by N-acetyltransferase in the liver. Genetic polymorphism is the cause of the high interindividual variation observed in the rate of metabolism of the drug. Rapid acetylators are not as responsive to the drug. Side effects in slow acetylators include SLE, drowsiness, nausea, polyneuropathy, and CNS toxicity caused by the intact drug. Severe hepatic toxicity is well described and may be more prominent in fast acetylators. The mechanism of toxicity may be related to metabolites. Serum ALT and AST are often increased. Cases of eosinophilia, anemia, and leukopenia have been reported.

TEST NAME AND METHOD	SPECIMEN	REFERENCE (THERAPEUTIC) INTERVAL, CONVENTIONAL [INTERNATIONAL RECOMMENDED UNITS]			KINETIC VALUES	

Isoniazid (Hyzyd, Nydrazid)—CONT

1. American Thoracic Society, Centers for Disease Control, and the Infectious Diseases Society of America: Treatment of tuberculosis, *MMWR* 52:1-77, 2003.

2. Bennett WM, Aronoff GR, Golper TA, et al: *Drug prescribing in renal failure,* ed 3, Philadelphia, 1994, American College of Physicians.

3. Peloquin CA, Namdar R, Dodge AA, et al: Pharmacokinetics of isoniazid under fasting conditions, with food, and with antacids, *Int J Tuberc Lung Dis* 3:703-710, 1999.

4. Peloquin CA: Therapeutic drug monitoring in the treatment of tuberculosis, *Drugs* 62:2169-2183, 2002.

5. Ray J, Gardiner I, Marriott D: Managing antituberculosis drug therapy by therapeutic drug monitoring of rifampicin and isoniazid, *Intern Med J* 33:229-234, 2003.

TEST NAME AND METHOD	SPECIMEN	REFERENCE INTERVAL				KINETIC VALUES	
Isopropanol (2-Propanol)[1-5]	Plasma (fluoride/oxalate), serum, blood, and urine	None detected.	*mg/dL*		*mmol/L*	$t_{1/2}$: Isoprop:	2-8 hr
						Acetone:	10-22 hr
GC		Toxic concentration:	>200	× 0.0166	[>3.32]	V_d:	0.6-0.7 L/kg
MW: 60.09						Cl_T:	NA
						T_{max}:	1-3 hr
						F:	Readily absorbed

1. Abramson S, Singh AK: Treatment of the alcohol intoxications: ethylene glycol, methanol and isopropanol, *Curr Opin Nephrol Hypertens* 9:695-701, 2000.

2. Church AS, Witting MD: Laboratory testing in ethanol, methanol, ethylene glycol, and isopropanol toxicities, *J Emerg Med* 15:687-692, 1997.

3. Ernstgard L, Sjogren B, Warholm M, et al: Sex differences in the toxicokinetics of inhaled solvent vapors in humans 2. 2-propanol, *Toxicol Appl Pharmacol* 193:158-167, 2003.

4. Livesey JF, Perkins SL, Tokessy NE, et al: Simultaneous determination of alcohols and ethylene glycol in serum by packed- or capillary-column gas chromatography, *Clin Chem* 41:300-305, 1995.

5. Williams RH, Shah SM, Maggiore JA, et al: Simultaneous detection and quantitation of diethylene glycol, ethylene glycol, and the toxic alcohols in serum using capillary column gas chromatography, *J Anal Toxicol* 24:621-626, 2000.

FACTORS INFLUENCING DRUG DISPOSITION	REMARKS AND INTERFERENCES

Phenobarbital, ethanol, and corticosteroids may increase the metabolism of isoniazid. p-Aminosalicylic acid, procainamide, and chlorpromazine have been reported to increase isoniazid's $t_{1/2}$. Multiple interactions are related to the inhibition of CYP2C9 by isoniazid.

See Table II-5.

Metabolism
  Hepatic, alcohol dehydrogenase
Excretion
  Renal, pulmonary
Dialysis
  Hemodialysis (+)
  Peritoneal (~)

Isopropanol is a common solvent readily available in 70% solution as rubbing alcohol. The compound is a CNS depressant about twice as potent as ethanol and producing similar effects. Routes of ingestion include oral, dermal, and inhalation. An acute lethal dose in an adult is ~240 mL. Isopropanol is slowly metabolized by alcohol dehydrogenase to acetone. Both are excreted to a small degree in breath and urine. Acetone may be detected in serum ~0.5 hr and in urine ~3 hr after ingestion. Acetone may remain elevated after isopropanol is undetectable. Hypoglycemia and increased osmolar gap are commonly found.

TEST NAME AND METHOD	SPECIMEN	REFERENCE (THERAPEUTIC) INTERVAL, CONVENTIONAL [INTERNATIONAL RECOMMENDED UNITS]			KINETIC VALUES	
Kanamycin[1-5] **(Kantrex)** *RIA, MB, HPLC, GLC, EIA, FPIA* MB assays have been largely replaced by more sensitive and specific immunoassays.	Serum, plasma (EDTA). For patients on penicillin or its derivatives, freeze sample if not analyzed within 4-6 hr. Collect specimen at trough and peak concentration (end of a 1-hr constant infusion, 30 min after the end of a 30-min constant infusion, or 1 hr after an IM dose).		*mg/mL*	*mmol/L*	$PK^{6,7}$: $t_{1/2}$: V_d: Cl_T: Fb: F, IM: F, PO:	2-3 hr 0.26 L/kg 1.3 mL/min/kg Negligible 100% Negligible
		Therapeutic concentration Peak: Trough Less severe infection: Life-threatening infection: Toxic concentration Peak: Trough:	25-35 1-4 4-8 >35-40 >10-15	× 2.06 [52-72] [2-8] [8-17] [>72-82] [>21-31]		

1. Mayhew JW, Gorbach SL: Gas-liquid chromatographic method for the assay of aminoglycoside antibiotics in serum, *J Chromatogr* 151:133-146, 1978.

2. Maitra S, Yoshikawa T, Guze L, et al: Determination of aminoglycoside antibiotics in biological fluids: a review, *Clin Chem* 25:1361-1367, 1979.

3. Kubo H, Kobayashi Y, Nishikawa T: Rapid method for determination of kanamycin and dibekacin in serum by use of high-pressure liquid chromatography, *Antimicrob Agents Chemother* 28:521-523, 1985.

4. Kim BH, Lee SC, Lee HJ, et al: Reversed-phase liquid chromatographic method for the analysis of aminoglycoside antibiotics using pre-column derivatization with phenylisocyanate, *Biomed Chromatogr* 17:396-403, 2003.

5. Baselt RC: *Disposition of toxic drugs and chemicals in man,* ed 7, Foster City, CA, 2004, Chemical Toxicology Institute.

6. Evans WE, Schentag JJ, Jusko WJ: *Applied pharmacokinetics—principles of therapeutic drug monitoring,* ed 3, Vancouver, WA, 1992, Applied Therapeutics, Inc.

7. Pechere JC, Dugal R: Clinical pharmacokinetics of aminoglycoside antibiotics, *Clin Pharmacokinet* 4:170-199, 1979.

8. Danish M, Schultz R, Jusko W: Pharmacokinetics of gentamicin and kanamycin during hemodialysis, *Antimicrob Agents Chemother* 6:841-847, 1974.

9. Micromedex: *Micromedex Healthcare series 2004,* Greenwood Village, CO, 2004, Thomson Micromedex.

Ketamine **(Ketalar)**[1-5] *GC, HPLC, GC-MS* *MW: 238.2*	Serum, urine		*mcg/mL*	*μmol/L*	$t_{1/2}$: V_d: Cl_T: PB: F: T_{max}:	2-3 hr 2-3 L/kg 12-17 mL/min/kg ~45% 16% (oral) 0.25-0.5 hr (IM) ~0.5 hr (oral)
		Therapeutic concentration: Analgesia Anesthesia Toxic concentration:	0.040-0.200 1.1-6 >7	× 4.2 [0.17-0.84] [5.1-25] [>29]		

FACTORS INFLUENCING DRUG DISPOSITION	REMARKS AND INTERFERENCES

Metabolism
  None
Excretion
  Urine
Disease
  Renal: $t_{1/2}\uparrow$, $Cl_T\downarrow$
Age
  Newborn: $t_{1/2}\uparrow$, $V_d\uparrow$, $Cl_T\downarrow$
  Child: $t_{1/2}\downarrow$, $V_d\uparrow$, $Cl_T\uparrow$
Dialysis
  Hemodialysis (+)
  Peritoneal (+)[8]

Drug interactions: Concomitant use of kanamycin with neuromuscular blockers may lead to aminoglycoside-induced respiratory paralysis. Coadministration of cyclosporine or tacrolimus with kanamycin may lead to increased risk of nephrotoxicity. Concomitant usage of loop diuretics with kanamycin is associated with a risk of ototoxicity.[9]

Kanamycin is an aminoglycoside antibiotic. Therapeutic and toxic concentrations should be considered highly variable and individualized for the patient's condition. Penicillin and its derivatives inactivate kanamycin in vivo and in vitro. A definitive cause-and-effect relationship between the trough concentration and the incidence of nephrotoxicity has not as yet been established. Cl_T and $t_{1/2}$ are strongly correlated with the glomerular filtration rate. Side effects include vestibular and auditory dysfunction (principally auditory), nephrotoxicity, eosinophilia, leukopenia, cholestasis, and neuromuscular blockade.

Interferences: When the patient is also taking another antibiotic (penicillin, cephalosporin, tetracycline, clindamycin, or chloramphenicol), the MB method may lack specificity. Penicillins and cephalosporins can be inactivated with a commercially available β-lactamase to minimize this interference.

See Table II-6.

Metabolism
  Hepatic
  Active metabolite: norketamine
Excretion
  Renal
Age
  Children: $t_{1/2}\downarrow$, $Cl_T\uparrow$

Ketamine is an anesthetic agent, administered as a racemic mixture, that has minimal respiratory effects. However, the drug induces a state referred to as "dissociative anesthesia," in which the patient may appear awake or cataleptic. During emergence, they may also experience a series of symptoms that include hallucinations that may be visual, auditory, or proprioceptive. Ketamine is abused for these hallucinative effects (as a "club-drug"). Additional adverse effects include tachycardia, arrhythmias, and hypertension. The drug undergoes

TEST NAME AND METHOD	SPECIMEN	REFERENCE (THERAPEUTIC) INTERVAL, CONVENTIONAL [INTERNATIONAL RECOMMENDED UNITS]		KINETIC VALUES

Ketamine (Ketalar)—CONT

1. Calvey TN: Isomerism and anaesthetic drugs, *Acta Anaesthesiol Scand Suppl* 106:83-90, 1995.

2. Cheng JY, Mok VK: Rapid determination of ketamine in urine by liquid chromatography-tandem mass spectrometry for a high throughput laboratory, *Forensic Sci Int* 142:9-15, 2004.

3. Chou SL, Yang MH, Ling YC, et al: Gas chromatography-isotope dilution mass spectrometry preceded by liquid-liquid extraction and chemical derivatization for the determination of ketamine and norketamine in urine, *J Chromatogr B Analyt Technol Biomed Life Sci* 799:37-50, 2004.

4. Lin HR, Lua AC: Detection of acid-labile conjugates of ketamine and its metabolites in urine samples collected from pub participants, *J Anal Toxicol* 28:181-186, 2004.

5. Rodriguez Rosas ME, Patel S, Wainer IW: Determination of the enantiomers of ketamine and norketamine in human plasma by enantioselective liquid chromatography-mass spectrometry, *J Chromatogr B Analyt Technol Biomed Life Sci* 794:99-108, 2003.

Labetalol[1,2]	Serum, plasma	Therapeutic concentration:	Not well defined	PK[3-6]:
(Normodyne,	(EDTA, heparin)	Toxic concentration:	Not well defined	$t_{1/2}$: 5-8 hr
Trandate)				V_d: 5.1-9.4 L/kg
				Cl_T: 22 ± 9 mL/min/kg
HPLC				PB: 50%
				F: 10-80%
MW: 328.41				

1. Dusci L, Hackett L: Determination of labetalol in human plasma by high-performance liquid chromatography, *J Chromatogr* 175:208-210, 1979.

2. Baselt RC: *Disposition of toxic drugs and chemicals in man,* ed 7, Foster City, CA, 2004, Chemical Toxicology Institute.

3. Hardman JG, Limbird LE, Gilman AG: *Goodman & Gilman's the pharmacological basis of therapeutics,* ed 10, New York, 2001, McGraw-Hill.

FACTORS INFLUENCING DRUG DISPOSITION	REMARKS AND INTERFERENCES

Dialysis
  Hemodialysis (+)
  Peritoneal (−)

considerable first-pass effect. When given orally, the concentration of norketamine is reported to be twice as high as with IM administration.

Metabolism
  Hepatic
Excretion
  Urine (primary)[7]
  Feces (secondary)[7]
Disease
  Cirrhosis: $t_{1/2}{\rightarrow}$, $Cl_T{\rightarrow}$, F↑
Age
  Elderly: F↑

Drug interactions: Major substrate of CYP2D6 and weakly inhibits CYP2D6. CYP2D6 inhibitors like chlorpromazine, fluoxetine, miconazole, paroxetine, pergolide, quinidine, quinine, and ritonavir may increase the effect of labetalol. Phenothiazines and cimetidine may increase labetalol plasma concentrations, probably through their effect on hepatic metabolism. NSAIDs, salicylates, and sulphonylureas may decrease the antihypertensive effect of labetalol.[8]

Labetalol is an antihypertensive with α- and β-adrenoreceptor-blocking properties. The clinical formulation contains equal proportions of four optical isomers; the RR* and SR* isomers produce most of the β- and α-blockade, respectively. Bioavailability exhibits wide interpatient variability. Rare cases of increased serum aminotransferases have been reported.

*Designations for diastereoisomeric configuration: R = right (Latin "rectus"), S = left (Latin "sinister").

---

4. McNeil JJ, Louis WJ: Clinical pharmacokinetics of labetalol, *Clin Pharmacokinet* 9:157-167, 1984.

5. Micromedex: *Micromedex Healthcare series 2004*, Greenwood Village, CO, 2004, Thomson Micromedex.

6. Kanto J, Allonen H, Kleimola T, et al: Pharmacokinetics of labetalol in healthy volunteers, *Int J Clin Pharmacol Ther Toxicol* 19:41-44, 1981.

TEST NAME AND METHOD	SPECIMEN	REFERENCE (THERAPEUTIC) INTERVAL, CONVENTIONAL [INTERNATIONAL RECOMMENDED UNITS]	KINETIC VALUES

Labetalol—CONT

7. Martin LE, Hopkins R, Bland R: Metabolism of labetalol by animals and man, *Br J Clin Pharmacol* 3(suppl 3):695-710, 1976.

Levorphanol (**Levo-Dromoran**)[1-12]	Serum, plasma	*ng/mL* *nmol/L* Therapeutic concentration: 7-20 × 3.89 [27-78] Toxic concentration: >100 [389]	$t_{1/2}$: 11-16 hr V_d: 10-13 L/kg PB: 50% [× 0.01 = 0.50, protein-bound mole fraction]
GC, GC-MS, IA, HPLC			
MW: 257.4			

1. Baselt R: *Disposition of toxic drugs and chemicals in man,* ed 7, Foster City, CA, 2004, Biomedical Publications.

2. Schulz M, Schmoldt A: Therapeutic and toxic blood concentrations of more than 800 drugs and other xenobiotics, *Pharmazie* 58:447-474, 2003.

3. Hardman JG, Limbird LE, Gilman AG: *Goodman and Gilman's the pharmacological basis of therapeutics,* ed 10, New York, 2001, McGraw-Hill.

4. *Physicians desk reference,* ed 58, Montvale, NJ, 2004, Thomson PDR.

5. Clarke EGC: *Clarke's isolation and identification of drugs in pharmaceuticals, body fluids, and post-mortem material,* London, 1986, The Pharmaceutical Press.

6. ACP's PIER: *Physicians' information and education resource (online version),* Philadelphia, 2004, American College of Physicians.

7. McEvoy GK, editor: *AHFS drug information (online version),* Bethesda, MD, 2004, American Society of Health-System Pharmacists Inc.

8. *USP DI drug information for the health care professional,* ed 24, (online version), Taunton, MA, 2004, Micromedex Inc.

9. Everhart ET, Shwonek P, Jacob P 3rd, et al: Quantitation of levorphanol in human plasma at subnanogram per milliliter levels using capillary gas chromatography with electron-capture detection, *J Chromatogr B Biomed Sci Appl* 729:173-181, 1999.

10. Lucek R, Dixon R: Quantitation of levorphanol in plasma using high-performance liquid chromatography with electrochemical detection, *J Chromatogr A* 341:239-243, 1985.

11. Min BH, Garland WA, Pao J: Determination of levorphanol (Levo-Dromoran) in human plasma by combined gas chromatography—negative ion chemical ionization mass spectrometry, *J Chromatogr A* 231:194-199, 1982.

12. Dixon R, Crews T, Mohacsi E, et al: Levorphanol: a simplified radioimmunoassay for clinical use, *Res Commun Chem Pathol Pharmacol* 32:545-548, 1981.

8.   Lexi-Comp, Inc.: *Up-to-date online 12.2, drug information,* Hudson, OH, 2004, Lexi-Comp, Inc.

Metabolism
  Hepatic, conjugation with glucuronic acid

Levorphanol is used for relief of moderate to severe pain, parenterally for pre-operative sedation, and as an adjunct to nitrous oxide/oxygen anesthesia. It is excreted primarily as the glucuronide conjugate. CNS depression and adverse reactions are similar to those of morphine.

TEST NAME AND METHOD	SPECIMEN	REFERENCE (THERAPEUTIC) INTERVAL, CONVENTIONAL [INTERNATIONAL RECOMMENDED UNITS]			KINETIC VALUES	
Lidocaine[1-8] **(Xylocaine)** LC-MS-MS, GLC, GC-MS, EIA, FPIA MW: 234.34	Serum, plasma (heparin, EDTA). No SST tubes. Collect >30 min after a bolus intravenous dose; up to 5-10 hr after start of drug administration. Stable at neutral pH for 24 hr at 2-8° C and 1-2 yr at −20° C. Samples should not be collected in serum separator tubes because lidocaine may be extracted by the separator gel.[9]	Therapeutic concentration: Toxic concentration CNS, cardiovascular depression: Seizures, obtundation, decreased cardiac output:	*mg/mL* 2.0-6.0 6-8 >8	× 4.27	*mmol/L* [6.4-25.6] [25.6-34.2] [>34.2]	PK[1,10]: $t_{1/2}$: 1.5-2.0 hr V_d: 1.3 L/kg Cl_T: 9.2 ± 2.5 mL/min/kg PB: 30-80% (to α_1-acid glycoprotein)

1. Baselt RC: *Disposition of toxic drugs and chemicals in man,* ed 7, Foster City, CA, 2004, Chemical Toxicology Institute.

2. Jurgens G, Graudal N, Kampmann J: Therapeutic drug monitoring of antiarrhythmic drugs, *Clin Pharmacokinet* 42:647-663, 2003.

3. Valdes Jr R, Jortani S, Gheorghiade M: Standards of laboratory practice: cardiac drug monitoring, *Clin Chem* 44:1096-1109, 1988.

4. Warner A, Annesley T: *Guidelines for therapeutic drug monitoring services,* Washington, DC, 1999, National Academy of Clinical Biochemistry.

5. Karch F, Chmielewski K: GLC assay for lidocaine in human plasma, *J Pharm Sci* 70:229-230, 1982.

6. Liu-Allison L, Hui R, Schwenzer K: Analysis of lidocaine on the COBAS INTEGRA, *Ann Clin Lab Sci* 27:105-115, 1997.

7. Watanabe T, Namera A, Yashiki M, et al: Simple analysis of local anaesthetics in human blood using headspace solid-phase microextraction and gas chromatography-mass spectrometry-electron impact ionization selected ion monitoring, *J Chromatogr B* 709:225-232, 1998.

8. Abdel-Rehim M, Bielenstein M, Askemark Y, et al: High-performance liquid chromatography-tandem electrospray mass spectrometry for the determination of lidocaine and its metabolites in human plasma and urine, *J Chromatogr B* 741:175-188, 2000.

9. Koch T, Platoff G: Suitability of collection tubes with separator gels for therapeutic drug monitoring, *Ther Drug Monit* 12:277-280, 1990.

FACTORS INFLUENCING DRUG DISPOSITION	REMARKS AND INTERFERENCES

Metabolism
  Hepatic, active metabolite: mono-
  ethylglycinexylidide (MEGX) and
  glycinexylidide (GX).
Excretion
  Feces (primary)
  Urine (secondary)
Disease
  Hepatic: $t_{1/2}\uparrow$, $V_d\uparrow$, $Cl_T\downarrow$
  CHF: $V_d\downarrow$, $Cl_T\downarrow$
  MI: $t_{1/2}\uparrow$, $Cl_T\downarrow$, $PB\uparrow$
  Shock: $Cl_T\downarrow$
  Uremia: $PB\uparrow$
  Cardiopulmonary bypass surgery: $t_{1/2}\rightarrow$,
  $V_d\downarrow$, $Cl_T\downarrow$, $PB\uparrow$
Age
  Neonate: $t_{1/2}\uparrow$, $V_d\uparrow$, $Cl_T\downarrow$, $PB\downarrow$
  Elderly: $t_{1/2}\rightarrow$, $V_d\rightarrow$, $Cl_T\rightarrow$
Dialysis
  Hemodialysis $(-)$

Drug interactions: Enzyme inducers phenobarbital and phenytoin may increase the metabolism of lidocaine, whereas drugs that decrease cardiac output or hepatic blood flow
(e.g., propranolol, anesthetics, and norepinephrine) probably decrease the drug's clearance. Cimetidine may decrease the hepatic
clearance of lidocaine.

Lidocaine has both antiarrhythmic (class Ib) and local anesthetic activity. When used as an antiarrhythmic agent, the drug is administered intravenously. Lidocaine undergoes first-pass metabolism and is dependent on hepatic blood flow for its elimination. An increase in the $t_{1/2}$ with prolonged administration has been observed. Protein binding is concentration and pH dependent and is strongly correlated to α_1-acid glycoprotein concentration, a protein often elevated in response to inflammation or body stress.[11] Side effects include dissociation, paresthesias, drowsiness, agitation, impaired hearing, disorientation, muscle twitching, convulsions, hypotension, asystole, arrhythmias, and respiratory arrest. Both MEGX and GX are potential contributors to toxicity.

Interferences: Lidocaine may be displaced from protein binding sites by plasticizers in collecting devices. Immunoassays fail to quantitate important metabolites monoethylglycinexylidide (MEGX) and glycinexylidide (GX). Some GLC methods lack specificity and sensitivity.

10. Hardman JG, Limbird LE, Gilman AG: *Goodman & Gilman's the pharmacological basis of therapeutics,* ed 10, New York, 2001, McGraw-Hill.

11. Edwards D, Lalka D, Cerra F, et al: 1-Acid glycoprotein concentration and protein binding in trauma, *Clin Pharmacol Ther* 3:62-67, 1982.

TEST NAME AND METHOD	SPECIMEN	REFERENCE (THERAPEUTIC) INTERVAL, CONVENTIONAL [INTERNATIONAL RECOMMENDED UNITS]				KINETIC VALUES	
Lithium **(Eskalith)**[1-9]	Whole blood, serum, and plasma	Therapeutic concentration:	*mEq/L* 0.4-1.2	× 1.0	*mmol/L* [0.4-1.2]	$t_{1/2}$: V_d: Cl_T:	15-30 hr 0.79 L/kg 0.35 mL/min/kg
FES, AAS, ISE		Toxic concentration:	>1.5		[>1.5]	PB: F:	Negligible 100%
MW: 73.9 *(carbonate)*							[× 0.01 = 1.00, bioavailable mole fraction]
AW: 6.9						T_{max}:	1-3 hr

1. Baselt R: *Disposition of toxic drugs and chemicals in man,* ed 7, Foster City, CA, 2004, Biomedical Publications.
2. Schulz M, Schmoldt A: Therapeutic and toxic blood concentrations of more than 800 drugs and other xenobiotics, *Pharmazie* 58:447-474, 2003.
3. Hardman JG, Limbird LE, Gilman AG: *Goodman and Gilman's the pharmacological basis of therapeutics,* ed 10, New York, 2001, McGraw-Hill.
4. *Physicians desk reference,* ed 58, Montvale, NJ, 2004, Thomson PDR.
5. ACP's PIER: *Physicians' information and education resource (online version),* Philadelphia, 2004, American College of Physicians.
6. McEvoy GK, editor: *AHFS drug information (online version),* Bethesda, MD, 2004, American Society of Health-System Pharmacists Inc.
7. *USP DI drug information for the health care professional,* ed 24, (online version), Taunton, MA, 2004, Micromedex Inc.
8. Clarke EGC: *Clarke's isolation and identification of drugs in pharmaceuticals, body fluids, and post-mortem material,* London, 1986, The Pharmaceutical Press.
9. Dol I, Knochen M, Vieras E: Determination of lithium at ultratrace levels in biological fluids by flame atomic emission spectrometry. Use of first-derivative spectrometry, *Analyst* 117:1373-1376, 1992.

Lorazepam **(Ativan)**[1-7]	Serum, plasma	Therapeutic concentration:	*ng/mL* 50-240	× 3.11	*nmol/L* [156-746]	$t_{1/2}$: V_d: Cl_T:	10-20 hr 1.0-1.3 L/kg 0.7-1.2 mL/min/kg
GC, GC-MS, *HPLC, LC-MS*		Toxic concentration:	>300		[>933]	PB:	85-90% [× 0.01 = 0.85-0.90, protein-bound mole fraction]
MW: 321.2						F:	90%
GC-MS	Urine						[× 0.01 = 0.90, bioavailable mole fraction]

FACTORS INFLUENCING DRUG DISPOSITION	REMARKS AND INTERFERENCES

Metabolism
  Renal, excreted unchanged
Disease or condition
  Renal: $t_{1/2}\uparrow$, $Cl_T\downarrow$
  Hyponatremia: $t_{1/2}\uparrow$, $Cl_T\downarrow$
  Hypernatremia: $t_{1/2}\downarrow$, $Cl_T\uparrow$
  Dehydration: $t_{1/2}\uparrow$, $Cl_T\downarrow$
  Pregnancy: $Cl_T\uparrow$
Age
  Elderly: $t_{1/2}\uparrow$, $Cl_T\downarrow$

Drug interactions: Natriuretic diuretics and nonsteroidal antiinflammatory drugs will significantly reduce the renal clearance of lithium, whereas acetazolamide may increase urinary excretion.

Lithium is commonly used in the treatment of bipolar disorders. The elimination kinetics of lithium can be described by a biphasic decline in the serum concentration/time curve. Sampling before 12 hr after the dose results in poor correlation of serum concentration. Levels obtained at 24 hr have been shown to be a good indicator of maintenance doses. Side effects include weakness, fatigue, tremor, anorexia, ataxia, confusion, coma, weight loss, nausea, and unsteady gait. Thyroid function should be evaluated before lithium therapy is initiated and at 6-mo intervals during therapy.

See Table II-6.

Metabolism
  Hepatic
Disease
  Hepatic: $t_{1/2}\uparrow$, $V_d\uparrow$, $PB\downarrow$
Age
  Neonate: $t_{1/2}\uparrow$
  Elderly: $t_{1/2}\rightarrow$, $V_d\rightarrow$, $Cl_T\rightarrow$, $PB\rightarrow$

Drug interactions: Probenecid may impair glucuronide conjugation. Drugs that affect the CNS may have additive effects when used concomitantly with lorazepam.

Lorazepam, an intermediate-acting benzodiazepine, is used for the management of anxiety disorders. It is metabolized to an inactive glucuronide conjugate. Side effects include ataxia, confusion, excitement, agitation, transient hypotension, vertigo, fever, GI upset, leukopenia, and liver disease.

TEST NAME AND METHOD	SPECIMEN	REFERENCE (THERAPEUTIC) INTERVAL, CONVENTIONAL [INTERNATIONAL RECOMMENDED UNITS]			KINETIC VALUES

Lorazepam (Ativan)—CONT

1. Egan JM, Abernethy DR: Lorazepam analysis using liquid chromatography: improved sensitivity for single-dose pharmacokinetic studies, *J Chromatogr* 380:196-201, 1986.

2. Goldfrank LR, editor: *Goldfrank's toxicological emergencies,* ed 7, (online version), New York, 2002, The McGraw-Hill Companies Inc.

3. Kratzsch C: Screening, library-assisted identification and validated quantification of 23 benzodiazepines, flumazenil, zaleplone, zolpidem and zopiclone in plasma by liquid chromatography/mass spectrometry with atmospheric pressure chemical ionization, *J Mass Spectrom* 39:856-872, 2004.

4. Borrey D, Meyer E, Lambert W, et al: Simultaneous determination of fifteen low-dosed benzodiazepines in human urine by solid-phase extraction and gas chromatography-mass spectrometry, *J Chromatogr B Biomed Sci Appl* 765:187-197, 2001.

Lysergic Acid Di-ethylamide (LSD)[1-12]	Plasma	*ng/mL*		*nmol/L*	$t_{1/2}$:	3.5-4 hr
		Therapeutic			V_d:	0.3 L/kg
		concentration: 0.5-5.0	$\times 3.09$	[1.54-15.4]	PB:	90%
IA, LC-MS, GC-MS		Toxic concentration: >1.0		[>3.09]		[$\times 0.01 = 0.90$, protein-bound mole fraction]

MW: 323.4

GC-MS	Urine	*ng/mL*		*nmol/L*
		After hallucinogenic dose: 1-50	$\times 3.09$	[3-155]

1. Baselt R: *Disposition of toxic drugs and chemicals in man,* ed 7, Foster City, CA, 2004, Biomedical Publications.

2. Schulz M, Schmoldt A: Therapeutic and toxic blood concentrations of more than 800 drugs and other xenobiotics, *Pharmazie* 58:447-474, 2003.

3. Hardman JG, Limbird LE, Gilman AG: *Goodman and Gilman's the pharmacological basis of therapeutics,* ed 10, New York, 2001, McGraw-Hill.

4. *Physicians desk reference,* ed 58, Montvale, NJ, 2004, Thomson PDR.

5. ACP's PIER: *Physicians' information and education resource (online version),* Philadelphia, 2004, American College of Physicians.

6. *USP DI drug information for the health care professional,* ed 24, (online version), Taunton, MA, 2004, Micromedex Inc.

7. Clarke EGC: *Clarke's isolation and identification of drugs in pharmaceuticals, body fluids, and post-mortem material,* London, 1986, The Pharmaceutical Press.

8. McEvoy GK, editor: *AHFS drug information (online version),* Bethesda, 2004, American Society of Health-System Pharmacists Inc.

9. Canezin J, Cailleux A, Turcant A, et al: Determination of LSD and its metabolites in human biological fluids by high-performance liquid chromatography with electrospray tandem mass spectrometry, *J Chromatogr B Biomed Appl* 765:15-27, 2001.

10. Burnley BT, George S: The development and application of a gas chromatography-mass spectrometric (GC-MS) assay to determine the presence of 2-oxo-3-hydroxy-LSD in urine, *J Anal Toxicol* 27:249-252, 2003.

11. Papac DI, Foltz RL: Measurement of lysergic acid diethylamide (LSD) in human plasma by gas chromatography/negative ion chemical ionization mass spectrometry, *J Anal Toxicol* 14:189-190, 1990.

12. Sklerov JH, Kalasinsky KS, Ehorn CA: Detection of lysergic acid diethylamide (LSD) in urine by gas chromatography-ion trap tandem mass spectrometry, *J Anal Toxicol* 23:474-478, 1999.

FACTORS INFLUENCING DRUG DISPOSITION	REMARKS AND INTERFERENCES

5. Tanaka E, Terada M, Misawa S, et al: Simultaneous determination of twelve benzodiazepines in human serum using a new reversed-phase chromatographic column on a 2-microns porous microspherical silica gel, *J Chromatogr B Biomed Appl* 682:173-178, 1996.

6. Pistos C, Stewart JT: Direct injection HPLC method for the determination of selected benzodiazepines in plasma using a Hisep column, *J Pharma Biomed Anal* 33:1135-1142, 2003.

7. Rasanen I, Ojanpera I, Vuori E: Quantitative screening for benzodiazepines in blood by dual-column gas chromatography and comparison of the results with urine immunoassay, *J Anal Toxicol* 24:46-51, 2000.

LSD is classified as a schedule I agent with high abuse potential, no known use in medical treatment, and lack of established safety even under medical supervision. LSD and other indoleamines act at multiple sites in the CNS. Mydriasis, tachycardia, tremor, weakness, paresthesias, and labile mood are produced. Euphoria may result with bizarre effects characterized by synesthesias. Adverse effects are primarily psychological in nature. There may be unpredictable recurrence of hallucination for weeks or months after the last dose. Hysterical behavior, hyperactivity, hyperthermia, and psychotic reactions may be delayed. Protein binding decreases to ~65% in overdose subjects.

TEST NAME AND METHOD	SPECIMEN	REFERENCE (THERAPEUTIC) INTERVAL, CONVENTIONAL [INTERNATIONAL RECOMMENDED UNITS]			KINETIC VALUES	
Maprotiline	Serum, plasma		*mcg/mL*	*µmol/L*	$t_{1/2}$:	20-60 hr
		Therapeutic			V_d:	22.6 L/kg
(Ludiomil)[1-5]		concentration:	0.1-0.25 ×3.60	[0.36-0.9]	Cl_T:	NA
		Toxic			PB:	88%
HPLC, GC-MS, GC		concentration:	>0.3	[>1.08]	F:	100%
					T_{max}:	12 hr
MW: 277.4						

1. Baselt C: *Disposition of toxic drugs and chemicals in man,* ed 7, Foster City, CA, 2004, Biomedical Publications.
2. Crome P, Ali C: Clinical features and management of self-poisoning with newer antidepressants, *Med Toxicol* 1:411-420, 1986.
3. Martinez MA, Sanchez de la Torre C, Almarza E: A comparative solid-phase extraction study for the simultaneous determination of fluoxetine, amitriptyline, nortriptyline, trimipramine, maprotiline, clomipramine, and trazodone in whole blood by capillary gas-liquid chromatography with nitrogen-phosphorus detection, *J Anal Toxicol* 27:353-358, 2003.
4. Namera A, Watanabe T, Yashiki M, et al: Simple analysis of tetracyclic antidepressants in blood using headspace-solid-phase microextraction and GC-MS, *J Anal Toxicol* 22:396-400, 1998.
5. Schulz M, Schmoldt A: Therapeutic and toxic blood concentrations of more than 800 drugs and other xenobiotics, *Pharmazie* 58:447-474, 2003.

TEST NAME AND METHOD	SPECIMEN	REFERENCE (THERAPEUTIC) INTERVAL, CONVENTIONAL [INTERNATIONAL RECOMMENDED UNITS]			KINETIC VALUES	
Meperidine	Serum, plasma		*ng/mL*	*nmol/L*	$t_{1/2}$:	3-6 hr
(pethidine)		Therapeutic			V_d:	3.8 L/kg
(Demerol)[1-11]		concentration:	70-500 ×4.04	[283-2020]	Cl_T:	17 ± 5 mL/min/kg
		Toxic			PB:	60-80%
GLC, colorimetric,		concentration:	>1000	[>4040]		[× 0.01 = 0.60-0.80,
fluorimetric,						protein-bound mole
HPLC, GC-MS,						fraction]
GC-MS-MS					F:	52%
						[× 0.01 = 0.52,
MW: 247.4						bioavailable mole
						fraction]
					T_{max}:	1-2 hr

1. Baselt R: *Disposition of toxic drugs and chemicals in man,* ed 7, Foster City, CA, 2004, Biomedical Publications.
2. Schulz M, Schmoldt A: Therapeutic and toxic blood concentrations of more than 800 drugs and other xenobiotics, *Pharmazie* 58:447-474, 2003.
3. Hardman JG, Limbird LE, Gilman AG: *Goodman and Gilman's the pharmacological basis of therapeutics,* ed 10, New York, 2001, McGraw-Hill.
4. *Physicians desk reference,* ed 58, Montvale, NJ, 2004, Thomson PDR.
5. ACP's PIER: *Physicians' information and education resource (online version),* Philadelphia, 2004, American College of Physicians.
6. McEvoy GK, editor: *AHFS drug information (online version),* Bethesda, MD, 2004, American Society of Health-System Pharmacists Inc.

FACTORS INFLUENCING DRUG DISPOSITION	REMARKS AND INTERFERENCES

Metabolism
  Hepatic, CYP2D6
  Active metabolites: desmethylmaprotiline,
  maprotiline-*N*-oxide
Excretion
  Renal (minimal)
Age
  Elderly: $t_{1/2} \downarrow$

Drug interactions: Cisapride, monoamine oxidase inhibitors, in addition to those related to inhibition or induction of CYP2D6.

Maprotiline is a tetracyclic antidepressant. Adverse effects include hypotension, tachycardia, gastrointestinal distress, and tremor. In overdose, more serious effects encountered include seizures, respiratory arrest, and severe tachycardia, arrhythmias, and hypotension.

Metabolism
  Hepatic
Disease
  Hepatic: $t_{1/2} \uparrow$, 6 hr; $V_d \rightarrow$, $Cl_T \downarrow$, $F \uparrow$
Age
  Elderly: $t_{1/2} \uparrow$, $V_d \uparrow$, $Cl_T \rightarrow$, $PB \downarrow$

Drug interactions: Meperidine is contraindicated in patients who have received MAO inhibitors during the previous 14 days. Serotonin agonists may enhance adverse effects of meperidine leading to serotonin syndrome.

Meperidine is a strong analgesic used for relief of moderate to severe pain. It is metabolized to an active metabolite (normeperidine), which may accumulate in renal failure. Normeperidine has been shown to possess half the analgesic potency of meperidine but twice the seizure-inducing properties of its parent compound. Side effects include nausea, vomiting, tremors, muscular twitches, dilated pupils, hyperactive reflexes, and convulsions. Naloxone is a specific antagonist of meperidine.

7. *USP DI drug information for the health care professional,* ed 24, (online version), Taunton, MA, 2004, Micromedex Inc.
8. Meatherall RC, Guay DR, Chalmers JL: Analysis of meperidine and normeperidine in serum and urine by high-performance liquid chromatography, *J Chromatogr* 338:141-149, 1985.
9. Ishii A, Kurihara R, Watanabe-Suzuki K, et al: Sensitive determination of pethidine in body fluids by surface ionization organic mass spectrometry, *J Chromatogr B Biomed Sci Appl* 758:117-121, 2001.
10. Kintz P, Godelar B, Mangin P, et al: Simultaneous determination of pethidine (meperidine), phenoperidine, and norpethidine (normeperidine), their common metabolite, by gas chromatography with selective nitrogen detection, *Forensic Sci Int* 43:267-273, 1989.
11. Ishii A, Tanaka M, Kurihara R, et al: Sensitive determination of pethidine in body fluids by gas chromatography-tandem mass spectrometry, *J Chromatogr B Analyt Technol Biomed Life Sci* 792:117-121, 2003.

TEST NAME AND METHOD	SPECIMEN	REFERENCE (THERAPEUTIC) INTERVAL, CONVENTIONAL [INTERNATIONAL RECOMMENDED UNITS]			KINETIC VALUES	
Meprobamate (Miltown)[1-11]	Serum, plasma		*mcg/mL*	*μmol/L*	$t_{1/2}$:	6-17 hr
		Therapeutic			V_d:	0.7 L/kg
		concentration:	5-10 × 4.58	[23-46]	PB:	20%
GLC, HPLC,		Toxic				
GCMS,		concentration:	>10-25	[>46-115]		
colorimetric						
MW: 218.3						

1. Baselt R: *Disposition of toxic drugs and chemicals in man,* ed 7, Foster City, CA, 2004, Biomedical Publications.
2. Schulz M, Schmoldt A: Therapeutic and toxic blood concentrations of more than 800 drugs and other xenobiotics, *Pharmazie* 58:447-474, 2003.
3. Hardman JG, Limbird LE, Gilman AG: *Goodman and Gilman's the pharmacological basis of therapeutics,* ed 10, New York, 2001, McGraw-Hill.
4. *Physicians desk reference,* ed 58, Montvale, NJ, 2004, Thomson PDR.
5. Clarke EGC: *Clarke's isolation and identification of drugs in pharmaceuticals, body fluids, and post-mortem material,* London, 1986, The Pharmaceutical Press.
6. ACP's PIER: *Physicians' information and education resource (online version),* Philadelphia, 2004, American College of Physicians.
7. McEvoy GK, editor: *AHFS drug information (online version),* Bethesda, MD, 2004, American Society of Health-System Pharmacists Inc.
8. *USP DI drug information for the health care professional,* ed 24, (online version), Taunton, MA, 2004, Micromedex Inc.
9. Kintz P, Mangin P: Determination of meprobamate in human plasma, urine and hair by gas chromatography and electron impact mass spectrometry, *J Anal Toxicol* 71:408-410, 1993.
10. Gaillard Y, Pepin G, Cabrera B: Rapid, simple and sensitive identification of meprobamate in plasma or urine using Toxi-Tube-B zero from Toxi-Lab and colored reaction on filter paper, *Ann Biol Clin (Paris)* 53:361-362, 1995.
11. Gaillard Y, Gay-Montchamp JP, Ollagnier M: Gas chromatographic determination of meprobamate in serum or plasma after solid-phase extraction, *J Chromatogr A* 577:171-173, 1992.

TEST NAME AND METHOD	SPECIMEN	REFERENCE (THERAPEUTIC) INTERVAL, CONVENTIONAL [INTERNATIONAL RECOMMENDED UNITS]			KINETIC VALUES	
Methadone (Dolophine)[1-10]	Serum, plasma		*ng/mL*	*μmol/L*	$t_{1/2}$:	15-25 hr
		Therapeutic			V_d:	2-9 L/kg
		concentration:	100-400 × 0.00323	[0.32-1.29]	Cl_T:	2 mL/min/kg
GC, IA, HPLC,		Toxic			PB:	60-90%
fluorimetric,		concentration:	>2000	[>6.46]		[× 0.01 = 0.60-0.90,
GC-MS,						protein-bound mole
colorimetric						fraction]
					T_{max}:	1-6 hr
MW: 309.5						
TLC, IA, CE	Urine	Negative				

1. Ferrari A, Coccia CP, Bertolini A, et al: Methadone—metabolism, pharmacokinetics and interactions, *Pharmacol Res* 50:551-559, 2004.

FACTORS INFLUENCING DRUG DISPOSITION	REMARKS AND INTERFERENCES

Metabolism
  Hepatic
Dialysis
  Hemodialysis (+)
  Peritoneal (+)

Meprobamate is a sedative used for management of anxiety disorders. It is rapidly metabolized in the liver to inactive metabolites excreted in urine. Up to 19% is excreted unchanged. The drug induces some hepatic microsomal enzymes. Adverse effects include drowsiness, ataxia, confusion, hypotension, and weakness.

Metabolism
  Hepatic, CYP3A4 (major); CYP2D6 (minor); CYP1A2 (probable)
Dialysis
  Hemodialysis (−)
  Peritoneal (−)

Drug interactions: CYP3A4 inhibitors may increase the effects of methadone. Methadone is a moderate inhibitor of CYP2D6 and may increase the effects of CYP2D6 substrates. It is also a weak inhibitor of CYP3A4.

Methadone is an opiate analgesic, but its primary use is for detoxification and maintenance treatment of narcotic addiction. Adverse reactions include excessive sweating, bradycardia, nausea, vomiting, constipation, thrombocytopenia, and weakness. Toxic effects are similar to those of morphine; diminished pulmonary ventilation predominates. Treatment is similar to that for morphine toxicity, specifically the use of naloxone.

2. Ramseier A, Caslavska J, Thormann W: Stereoselective screening for and confirmation of urinary enantiomers of amphetamine, methamphetamine, designer drugs, methadone and selected metabolites by capillary electrophoresis, *Electrophoresis* 20:2726-2738, 1999.

TEST NAME AND METHOD	SPECIMEN	REFERENCE (THERAPEUTIC) INTERVAL, CONVENTIONAL [INTERNATIONAL RECOMMENDED UNITS]	KINETIC VALUES

Methadone (Dolophine)—CONT

3. Myung SW, Kim S, Park JH, et al: Solid-phase microextraction for the determination of pethidine and methadone in human urine using gas chromatography with nitrogen-phosphorus detection, *Analyst* 124:1283-1286, 1999.

4. Thormann W, Lanz M, Caslavska J, et al: Screening for urinary methadone by capillary electrophoretic immunoassays and confirmation by capillary electrophoresis-mass spectrometry, *Electrophoresis* 19:57-65, 1998.

5. Cheever ML, Armendariz GA, Moody DE: Detection of methadone, LAAM, and their metabolites by methadone immunoassays, *J Anal Toxicol* 23:500-505, 1999.

6. Angelo HR, Beck N, Kristensen K: Enantioselective high-performance liquid chromatographic method for the determination of methadone and its main metabolite in urine using an AGP and a C8 column coupled serially, *J Chromatogr B Biomed Sci Appl* 724:35-40, 1999.

Methamphetamine (Desoxyn)[1-21]

GC, fluorimetric, colorimetric, GC-MS, IA, CE, HPLC, LC-MS-MS
MW: 149.2

	Specimen				
	Serum, plasma		*mcg/mL*	*μmol/L*	$t_{1/2}$: 7-8 hr (acidic urine) 11-12 hr (uncontrolled urine pH)
		Therapeutic concentration:	0.01-0.05 × 6.70	[0.07-0.34]	
		Toxic concentration:	>0.5	[>3.350]	V_d: 3-7 L/kg PB: NA [× 0.01 = protein-bound mole fraction]
	Urine	Negative			
	Alternative matrices: Hair, oral fluid, and sweat	Negative			

1. Jenkins KM, Young MS, Mallet CR, et al: Mixed-mode solid-phase extraction procedures for the determination of MDMA and metabolites in urine using LC-MS, LC-UV, or GC-NPD, *J Anal Toxicol* 28:50-58, 2004.

2. Paul BD, Jemionek J, Lesser D, et al: Enantiomeric separation and quantitation of (+/−)-amphetamine, (+/−)-methamphetamine, (+/−)-MDA, (+/−)-MDMA, and (+/−)-MDEA in urine specimens by GC-EI-MS after derivatization with (R)-(−) or (S)-(+)-alpha-methoxy-alpha-(trifluoromethy)phenylacetyl chloride (MTPA), *J Anal Toxicol* 28:449-455, 2004.

3. Furesz J, Kocsis G, Gachalyi A, et al: Mass selective detection of amphetamine, methamphetamine, and related compounds in urine, *J Chromatogr Sci* 42:259-262, 2004.

4. Baselt RC: *Analytical procedures for therapeutic drug monitoring and emergency toxicology,* ed 2, Davis, CA, 1987, Biomedical Publications.

FACTORS INFLUENCING DRUG DISPOSITION	REMARKS AND INTERFERENCES

7. Moore C, Guzaldo F, Hussain MJ, et al: Determination of methadone in urine using ion trap GC/MS in positive ion chemical ionization mode, *Forensic Sci Int* 119:155-160, 2001.
8. Souverain S, Eap C, Veuthey JL, et al: Automated LC-MS method for the fast stereoselective determination of methadone in plasma, *Clin Chem Lab Med* 41:1615-1621, 2003.
9. Kintz P, Tracqui A, Lugnier AJ, et al: Simultaneous screening and quantification of several nonopiate narcotic analgesics and phencyclidine in human plasma using capillary gas chromatography, *Methods Find Exp Clin Pharmacol* 12:193-196, 1990.
10. Shinderman M, Maxwell S, Brawand-Amey M, et al: Cytochrome P4503A4 metabolic activity, methadone blood concentrations, and methadone doses, *Drug Alcohol Depend* 69:205-211, 2003.

Metabolism
  Hepatic, CYP2D6
Excretion
  Renal, excreted as unchanged parent drug (up to 45%) and metabolites including amphetamine (~7%)

Drug interactions: CYP2D6 inhibitors may increase levels/effects of methamphetamine. Acidification of the urine will enhance the renal excretion of methamphetamine, whereas alkalinization will reduce it.

Amphetamine is a common drug of abuse. Methamphetamine (d isomer) is used for treatment of attention deficit disorder with hyperactivity and as a short-term adjunct for exogenous obesity. Symptoms of acute toxicity with methamphetamine include seizures, hyperactivity, hypertension, and coma.

For federally regulated workplace drug testing (SAMHSA), the widely accepted immunoassay cutoff concentration to separate positive and negative specimens for methamphetamine is 1000 ng/mL [7400 nmol/L] for amphetamine screening and 500 ng/mL [3700 nmol/L] for GC-MS confirmation. In addition, amphetamine (metabolite of methamphetamine) must be detected at a cutoff concentration of 200 ng/mL to report a specimen as positive for methamphetamine. At these cutoff concentrations, methamphetamine may generally be detected in urine for 1-3 days after use.

Alternative matrices used for nonfederally regulated workplace drug testing and being considered for regulated testing include hair, oral fluid, and sweat.

See *Phenethylamines and Amphetamine.*

Interferences: Nonprescription decongestants and diet aids containing ephedrine and phenylpropanolamine and prescription drugs including selegiline, benzphetamine, fenfluramine, mephentermine, phenmetrazine, and phentermine may cause positive IA results.

5. Jacob P 3rd, Tisdale EC, Panganiban K, et al: Gas chromatographic determination of methamphetamine and its metabolite amphetamine in human plasma and urine following conversion to N-propyl derivatives, *J Chromatogr B Biomed Appl* 664:449-457, 1995.
6. Al-Dirbashi OY, Wada M, Kuroda N, et al: Achiral and chiral quantification of methamphetamine and amphetamine in human urine by semi-micro column high-performance liquid chromatography and fluorescence detection, *J Forensic Sci* 45:708-714, 2000.
7. Stout PR, Klette KL, Wiegand R: Comparison and evaluation of DRI methamphetamine, DRI ecstasy, Abuscreen ONLINE amphetamine, and a modified Abuscreen ONLINE amphetamine screening immunoassays for the detection of amphetamine (AMP), methamphetamine (MTH), 3,4-methylenedioxyamphetamine (MDA), and 3,4-methylenedioxymethamphetamine (MDMA) in human urine, *J Anal Toxicol* 27:265-269, 2003.

TEST NAME AND METHOD	SPECIMEN	REFERENCE (THERAPEUTIC) INTERVAL, CONVENTIONAL [INTERNATIONAL RECOMMENDED UNITS]		KINETIC VALUES

Methamphetamine (Desoxyn)—CONT

8. Wood M, De Boeck G, Samyn N, et al: Development of a rapid and sensitive method for the quantitation of amphetamines in human plasma and oral fluid by LC-MS-MS, *J Anal Toxicol* 27:78-87, 2003.

9. Stout PR, Horn CK, Klette KL: Rapid simultaneous determination of amphetamine, methamphetamine, 3,4-methylene-dioxyamphetamine, 3,4-methylenedioxymethamphetamine, and 3,4-methylenedioxyethylamphetamine in urine by solid-phase extraction and GC-MS: a method optimized for high-volume laboratories, *J Anal Toxicol* 26:253-261, 2002.

10. Mortier KA, Dams R, Lambert WE, et al: Determination of paramethoxyamphetamine and other amphetamine-related designer drugs by liquid chromatography/sonic spray ionization mass spectrometry, *Rapid Commun Mass Spectrom* 16:865-870, 2002.

11. Peters FT, Kraemer T, Maurer HH: Drug testing in blood: validated negative-ion chemical ionization gas chromatographic-mass spectrometric assay for determination of amphetamine and methamphetamine enantiomers and its application to toxicology cases, *Clin Chem* 48:1472-1485, 2002.

12. Ramseier A, Caslavska J, Thormann W: Stereoselective screening for and confirmation of urinary enantiomers of amphetamine, methamphetamine, designer drugs, methadone and selected metabolites by capillary electrophoresis, *Electrophoresis* 20:2726-2738, 1999.

13. Nishida M, Namera A, Yashiki M, et al: On-column derivatization for determination of amphetamine and methamphetamine in human blood by gas chromatography-mass spectrometry, *Forensic Sci Int* 125:156-162, 2002.

14. Mortier KA, Maudens KE, Lambert WE, et al: Simultaneous, quantitative determination of opiates, amphetamines, cocaine and benzoylecgonine in oral fluid by liquid chromatography quadrupole-time-of-flight mass spectrometry, *J Chromatogr B Analyt Technol Biomed Life Sci* 779:321-330, 2002.

TEST NAME AND METHOD	SPECIMEN		REFERENCE			KINETIC VALUES	
Methanol[1-9]	Whole blood (fluo-ride/oxalate), serum	Endogenous	*mg/L*		*mmol/L*	$t_{1/2}$:	2-24 hr
						V_d:	0.6 L/kg
GC		production:	<1.5	× 0.0312	[<0.047]	PB:	0%
		Toxic				T_{max}:	0.5-1 hr
MW: 32.04		concentration:	>200		[>6.24]		
		Lethal					
		concentration:	>400		[>12.48]		
	Urine	Occupational					
		exposure:	<50	× 0.0312	[<1.56]		
	Breath		*ppm*		*nmol/L*		
			0.8	× 0.0312	[0.03]		
		Occupational					
		exposure:	2.5		[0.08]		

1. Barceloux DG, Bond GR, Krenzelok EP, et al: American Academy of Clinical Toxicology practice guidelines on the treatment of methanol poisoning, *J Toxicol Clin Toxicol* 40:415-446, 2002.

2. Church AS, Witting MD: Laboratory testing in ethanol, methanol, ethylene glycol, and isopropanol toxicities, *J Emerg Med* 15:687-692, 1997.

| FACTORS INFLUENCING
DRUG DISPOSITION | REMARKS AND INTERFERENCES |

15. Moore KA: Amphetamines. In Shaw L, editor: *The clinical toxicology laboratory: contemporary practice of poisoning evaluation,* Washington, DC, 2001, AACC Press.

16. Stanaszek R, Piekoszewski W: Simultaneous determination of eight underivatized amphetamines in hair by high-performance liquid chromatography-atmospheric pressure chemical ionization mass spectrometry (HPLC-APCI-MS), *J Anal Toxicol* 28:77-85, 2004.

17. Nakashima K, Kaddoumi A, Ishida Y, et al: Determination of methamphetamine and amphetamine in abusers' plasma and hair samples with HPLC-FL, *Biomed Chromatogr* 17:471-476, 2003.

18. Musshoff F, Junker HP, Lachenmeier DW, et al: Fully automated determination of amphetamines and synthetic designer drugs in hair samples using headspace solid-phase microextraction and gas chromatography-mass spectrometry, *J Anal Toxicol* 26:554-560, 2002.

19. Skender L, Karacic V, Brcic I, et al: Quantitative determination of amphetamines, cocaine, and opiates in human hair by gas chromatography/mass spectrometry, *Forensic Sci Int* 125:120-126, 2002.

20. *Fed Register,* 53:11963, April 11, 1988; *Fed Register,* 62:51118, September 30, 1997; *Fed Register,* 69:19673, April 13, 2004.

21. Soares ME, Carvalho M, Carmo H, et al: Simultaneous determination of amphetamine derivatives in human urine after SPE extraction and HPLC-UV analysis, *Biomed Chromatogr* 18:125-131, 2004.

Metabolism
  Hepatic, alcohol dehydrogenase
Excretion
  Renal, pulmonary
Dialysis
  Hemodialysis (+)
  Perotineal (·~)
	Methanol (wood alcohol) is a widely used solvent, a denaturing agent, an antifreeze constituent, and a fuel in internal combustion engines or cooking appliances. Absorption occurs by inhalation, skin contact, and ingestion. Trace amounts are occasionally found and may be the result of bacterial metabolism or food ingestion (fermented fruit). Some alcoholic beverages (e.g., wine, bourbons) may contain methanol. Serum concentrations of up to ~3 mg/dL have been reported after ingestion of these products.

Intoxication effects are milder than those associated with ethanol toxicity, but accumulation of formic acid leads to optic nerve damage, blindness, and severe acidosis. Methanol is metabolized by liver alcohol dehydrogenase to formaldehyde, which does not accumulate but is converted to formic acid. Ten to 20% of methanol is eliminated by lungs, 3% by the kidneys, and up to 60% is oxidized. Urine formic acid (normal, 17 mg/L [0.37 mmol/L]) should not exceed 100 mg/L [2.17 mmol/L] in exposed workers. A high anion gap and osmolar gap are typically found.

Ethanol competitively inhibits the metabolism of methanol and is administered as one form of treatment of methanol toxicity. 4-Methylpyrazole (fomepizole) also inhibits methanol metabolism and is used as an antedote.

3. Ferrari LA, Arado MG, Nardo CA, et al: Post-mortem analysis of formic acid disposition in acute methanol intoxication, *Forensic Sci Int* 133:152-158, 2003.

4. Kerns W 2nd, Tomaszewski C, McMartin K, et al: Formate kinetics in methanol poisoning, *J Toxicol Clin Toxicol* 40:137-143, 2002.

TEST NAME AND METHOD	SPECIMEN	REFERENCE (THERAPEUTIC) INTERVAL, CONVENTIONAL [INTERNATIONAL RECOMMENDED UNITS]		KINETIC VALUES

Methanol—CONT

5. Kostic MA, Dart RC: Rethinking the toxic methanol level, *J Toxicol Clin Toxicol* 41:793-800, 2003.

6. Livesey JF, Perkins SL, Tokessy NE, et al: Simultaneous determination of alcohols and ethylene glycol in serum by packed- or capillary-column gas chromatography, *Clin Chem* 41:300-305, 1995.

7. Roy M, Bailey B, Chalut D, et al: What are the adverse effects of ethanol used as an antidote in the treatment of suspected methanol poisoning in children? *J Toxicol Clin Toxicol* 41:155-161, 2003.

Methaqualone	Serum, plasma		*mcg/mL*	$\mu mol/L$	$t_{1/2}$: 10-42 hr
(Quaalude)[1-6]		Therapeutic			V_d: 6 L/kg
	Urine	concentration:	1-3 ×4.00	[4-12]	PB: 70-90%
GLC, GC-MS, IA		Toxic			[× 0.01 = 0.70-0.90,
HPLC, colorimet-		concentration:	>3-5	[>12-20]	protein-bound mole
ric, CE					fraction]
					F: 100%
MW: 250.3					[× 0.01 = 1.00,
					bioavailable mole
					fraction]
					T_{max}: 2 hr

1. Puopolo PR, Pothier ME, Volpicelli SA, et al: Single procedure for detection, confirmation, and quantification of benzodiazepines in serum by liquid chromatography with photo-array detection, *Clin Chem* 37:701-706, 1991.

2. Prost F, Thormann W: Enantiomeric analysis of the five major monohydroxylated metabolites of methaqualone in human urine by chiral capillary electrophoresis, *Electrophoresis* 22:3270-3280, 2001.

3. Plaut O, Girod C, Staub C: Analysis of methaqualone in biological matrices by micellar electrokinetic capillary chromatography. Comparison with gas chromatography-mass spectrometry, *Forensic Sci Int* 92:219-227, 1998.

4. Liu F, Liu YT, Feng CL, et al: Determination of methaqualone and its metabolites in urine and blood by UV, GC/FID and GC/MS, *Yao Xue Xue Bao* 29:610-616, 1994.

5. Brenner C, Hui R, Passarelli J, et al: Comparison of methaqualone excretion patterns using Abuscreen ONLINE and EMIT II immunoassays and GC/MS, *Forensic Sci Int* 79:31-41, 1996.

6. Singh V, Shukla SK, Mahanwal JS, et al: Methaqualone analysis by derivative UV spectrophotometry, *Pharmazie* 44:229-230, 1989.

Methotrexate[1-4]	Serum, plasma	*Therapeutic concentration*	$\mu mol/L$	$t_{1/2}$: 3-10 hr, low dose
	(heparin, EDTA),	Choriocarcinoma:	1.0	8-15 hr, high dose
HPLC, IA	and cerebrospinal	Head/neck epidermoid carcinoma,		V_d: 0.4-0.8 L/kg
	fluid.	lymphoma:	10.0	Cl_T: 1.5 mL/min/kg
MW: 454		Large cell adenocarcinoma:	100.0	PB: 50-70% (albumin)
	Collect specimen at	Osteosarcoma:	1000.0	[× 0.01 = 0.50-0.70,
	0.5 or 2 hr after			protein-bound mole
	IV or PO low dose,	*Toxic concentration*	$\mu mol/L$	fraction]
	respectively. Col-	1-2 wk after low-dose therapy:	>0.02	F: 20-90%
	lect specimen at 24,	24 hr after high-dose therapy:	≥5	[× 0.01 = 0.2-0.90,
	48, and 72 hr after	48 hr after high-dose therapy:	≥0.5	bioavailable mole
	high-dose infusion.	72 hr after high-dose therapy:	≥0.05	fraction]
				T_{max}: 0.7-4 hr (oral)
				0.5-1 hr (IM)

| FACTORS INFLUENCING DRUG DISPOSITION | REMARKS AND INTERFERENCES |

8. Starr TB, Festa JL: A proposed inhalation reference concentration for methanol, *Regul Toxicol Pharmacol* 38:224-331, 2003.
9. Williams RH, Shah SM, Maggiore JA, et al: Simultaneous detection and quantitation of diethylene glycol, ethylene glycol, and the toxic alcohols in serum using capillary column gas chromatography, *J Anal Toxicol* 24:621-626, 2000.

Metabolism
  Hepatic
Dialysis
  Hemodialysis (−)
  Peritoneal (−)
  Hemoperfusion (+)

This drug is highly lipophilic. Side effects include CNS depression, delirium, pyramidal signs, confusion, coma, and cardiovascular and respiratory depression. The estimated minimum lethal dose for nontolerant subjects is 5 g [20 mmol].

Metabolism
  Intracellular, hepatic
Excretion
  Renal
Disease
  Renal: $Cl_T\downarrow$, $t_{1/2}\uparrow$
  Ascites: $Cl_T\downarrow$
Dialysis
  Hemodialysis (+)
  Peritoneal (−)
  Hemoperfusion (+)

Methotrexate is a folate antimetabolite used to treat numerous malignancies including childhood acute lymphocytic leukemia, osteoscarcoma, and non-Hodgkin's lymphoma, as well as cancers of the head, neck, breast, and lung. It is one of the few chemotherapeutic drugs to be given intrathecally. Methotrexate is also used to treat noncancerous diseases such as rheumatoid arthritis and psoriasis because of its immunosuppressive and antiinflammatory actions. Therapeutic concentrations depend on the treatment protocol. High-dose therapy is usually followed by leucovorin rescue depending on the concentration at 24, 48, and 72 hr.

TEST NAME AND METHOD	SPECIMEN	REFERENCE (THERAPEUTIC) INTERVAL, CONVENTIONAL [INTERNATIONAL RECOMMENDED UNITS]			KINETIC VALUES	
Methotrexate—CONT						
		Stable at 4° C for at least 24 hr and at −20° C for 1 mo. Photodegradation of methotrexate is reported: avoid long exposure to light.				

1. Limelette N, Ferry M, Branger S, et al: In vitro stability study of methotrexate in blood and plasma samples for routine monitoring, *Ther Drug Monit* 25:81-87, 2003.
2. McElnay JC, Elliott DS, Cartwright-Shamoon J, et al: Stability of methotrexate and vinblastine in burette administration sets, *Int J Pharmaceut* 47:239-247, 1988.
3. Rubino FM: Separation methods for methotrexate, its structural analogues and metabolites, *J Chromatogr B Biomed Sci Appl* 764:217-254, 2001.
4. Treon SP, Chabner BA: Concepts in use of high-dose methotrexate therapy, *Clin Chem* 42:1322-1329, 1996.

TEST NAME AND METHOD	SPECIMEN	REFERENCE			KINETIC VALUES	
Methsuximide (Celontin)[1-4]	Serum		*mcg/mL*	*μmol/L*	$t_{1/2}$	
		Therapeutic concentration:	10-40	[53-212]	Methsuximide:	1-3 hr
HPLC, GC, IA	*N*-Desmethyl-methsuximide	Toxic	×5.29		*N*-Desmethylmeth-suximide:	35-45 hr
	(active metabolite)	concentration:	>40	[>212]	Cl_T:	NA
MW: 203.24					F:	NA
					PB:	
					N-Desmethylmeth-suximide:	45-60%
					T_{max}:	1-3 hr

1. Battino D, Estienne M, Avanzini G: Clinical pharmacokinetics of antiepileptic drugs in paediatric patients. Part I: phenobarbital, primidone, valproic acid, ethosuximide and mesuximide, *Clin Pharmacokinet* 29:257-286, 1995.
2. Romanyshyn LA, Wichmann JK, Kucharczyk N, et al: Simultaneous determination of felbamate, primidone, phenobarbital, carbamazepine, two carbamazepine metabolites, phenytoin, and one phenytoin metabolite in human plasma by high-performance liquid chromatography, *Ther Drug Monit* 16:90-99, 1994.
3. Schulz M, Schmoldt A: Therapeutic and toxic blood concentrations of more than 800 drugs and other xenobiotics, *Pharmazie* 58:447-474, 2003.
4. Sigler M, Strassburg HM, Boenigk HE: Effective and safe but forgotten: methsuximide in intractable epilepsies in childhood, *Seizure* 10:120-124, 2001.

FACTORS INFLUENCING DRUG DISPOSITION	REMARKS AND INTERFERENCES

Bioavailability is related to drug dose.

Drug interactions: Methotrexate is weakly acidic. Most reported drug interactions occur when the drug displaces another drug from protein binding (e.g., phenytoin, salicylates, tetracyclins, and chloramphenicol). Weakly acidic drugs such as probenecid and salicylates may reduce renal excretion of methotrexate.

Side effects include bone marrow depression, reversible nephrotoxicity, leukopenia, thrombocytopenia, anemia, stomatitis, mucositis, nausea, vomiting, diarrhea, maculopapular rash, fever, pneumothorax, and cholestasis. AST, ALT, and serum creatinine may be increased. Serum glutamyltransferase may be increased in psoriatic patients.

See Tables II-5 and II-6.

Metabolism
  Hepatic

Drug interactions: Interactions with other AEDs are well documented. Carbamazepine, phenobarbital, phenytoin, and primidone may increase metabolism. Methsuximide decreases topiramate, valproic acid, and lamotrigine. Valproic acid may increase or decrease plasma ethosuximide concentrations.

Methsuximide is used to control petit mal seizures unresponsive to other antiepileptic drugs. It is extensively metabolized to an active metabolite, *N*-desmethylmethsuximide, which contributes to the therapeutic concentration. Side effects include nausea, vomiting, anorexia, drowsiness, lethargy, euphoria, dizziness, and headache. Severe depression, skin rash, fever, periorbital edema, leukopenia, aplastic anemia, nephropathy, and hepatotoxicity have been reported.

TEST NAME AND METHOD	SPECIMEN	REFERENCE (THERAPEUTIC) INTERVAL, CONVENTIONAL [INTERNATIONAL RECOMMENDED UNITS]				KINETIC VALUES	
Methyldopa (Aldomet)[1-6] *HPLC, LC-MS* *MW: 211.22*	Serum, plasma (heparin, EDTA)	Therapeutic concentration: Toxic concentration:	*mcg/mL* 1-5 >7	× 4.73	μ*mol/L* [4.7-24] [>33]	$t_{1/2, alpha}$: V_d: Cl_T: F: PB: T_{max}:	1.3–2.7 hr 0.3-0.6 L/kg 268 mL/min 25-50% [× 0.01 = 0.25-0.5, bioavailable mole fraction] <20% [× 0.01 = ~0.20, protein-bound mole fraction] ~3 hr

1. Campbell NR, Patrick W: Increases in methyldopa absorption and renal excretion after multiple doses, *J Clin Pharmacol* 32:450-454, 1992.
2. Oliveira CH, Barrientos-Astigarraga RE, Sucupira M, et al: Quantification of methyldopa in human plasma by high-performance liquid chromatography-electrospray tandem mass spectrometry application to a bioequivalence study, *J Chromatogr B Analyt Technol Biomed Life Sci* 768:341-348, 2002.
3. Saxer C, Niina M, Nakashima A, et al: Simultaneous determination of levodopa and 3-O-methyldopa in human plasma by liquid chromatography with electrochemical detection, *J Chromatogr B Analyt Technol Biomed Life Sci* 802:299-305, 2004.
4. Schulz M, Schmoldt A: Therapeutic and toxic blood concentrations of more than 800 drugs and other xenobiotics, *Pharmazie* 58:447-474, 2003.
5. Skerjanec A, Campbell NR, Robertson S, et al: Pharmacokinetics and presystemic gut metabolism of methyldopa in healthy human subjects, *J Clin Pharmacol* 35:275-280, 1995.
6. Zarifis J, Lip GY, Ferner RE: Poisoning with anti-hypertensive drugs: methyldopa and clonidine, *J Hum Hypertens* 9:787-790, 1995.

TEST NAME AND METHOD	SPECIMEN					KINETIC VALUES	
Methylene-dioxyamphetamine (MDA, "Love Pills")[1-16] *IA, HPLC, GC, GC-MS, CE, LC-MS, LC-MS-MS* *MW: 179.2*	Serum, plasma	Toxic concentration:	*mcg/mL* > 1.5	× 5.58	μ*mol/L* [>8.37]	$t_{1/2}$: PB: T_{max}:	6-28 hr 40% (in dogs) 3-10 hr
	Urine	Negative					

1. de la Torre R, Farre M, Roset PN, et al: Human pharmacology of MDMA: pharmacokinetics, metabolism, and disposition, *Ther Drug Monit* 26:137-144, 2004.

FACTORS INFLUENCING DRUG DISPOSITION	REMARKS AND INTERFERENCES

Metabolism
  Hepatic
Excretion
  Renal,
  intraneuronal, and fecal
Disease
  Renal: $t_{1/2}\uparrow$, $Cl_T\downarrow$
Age
  Neonate: $t_{1/2}\uparrow$
Dialysis
  Hemodialysis (+)
  Peritoneal (+)

Methyldopa is an antihypertensive that undergoes metabolism intraneurally through successive decarboxylation and *p*-hydroxylation reactions to form the pharmacologically active α-methyldopamine and α-methylnorepinephrine. First-pass metabolism and enterohepatic recirculation have been suggested. Increased sensitivity to methyldopa in renal failure may be attributable to the accumulation of α-methyldopamine, the sulfate conjugate, as well as to methyldopa itself. Side effects include systemic lupus-like syndrome and hepatic disturbances (increased ALT and AST, jaundice). Direct Coombs test can be positive. Cases of hemolytic anemia, eosinophilia, and leukopenia have been reported. CNS side effects include sedation, vertigo, nightmares, and depression.

See Table II-5.

Metabolism
  CYP2D6, CYP3A4
Excretion
  Renal

Drug interactions: Antiretroviral drugs and MAO inhibitors reported to cause life-threatening interactions.

MDA, an illicit psychostimulant drug, is a potent releaser and/or reuptake inhibitor of serotonin, dopamine, and norepinephrine. It is structurally similar to methamphetamine, mescaline, and other designer ring-substituted amphetamines (RSA), such as 3,4-methylenedioxymethamphetamine (MDMA, ecstasy) and 3,4-methylenedioxyethylamphetamine (MDEA, eve). The name ecstasy primarily denotes MDMA but is sometimes used for all of the RSAs, and some ecstasy pills contain mixtures of several RSAs. MDA is also a metabolite of both MDMA and MDEA. Effects of overdose are similar to those of amphetamine overdose and include agitation, tachycardia, hyperthermia, delirium, seizures, muscle rigidity, rapid breathing, and coma.

Most immunoassays for amphetamines do not detect MDA.

See *MDMA.*

---

2. Pizarro N, Ortuno J, Farre M, et al: Determination of MDMA and its metabolites in blood and urine by gas chromatography-mass spectrometry and analysis of enantiomers by capillary electrophoresis, *J Anal Toxicol* 26:157-165, 2002.

TEST NAME AND METHOD	SPECIMEN	REFERENCE (THERAPEUTIC) INTERVAL, CONVENTIONAL [INTERNATIONAL RECOMMENDED UNITS]	KINETIC VALUES

Methylenedioxyamphetamine—CONT

3. Nordgren HK, Beck O: Direct screening of urine for MDMA and MDA by liquid chromatography-tandem mass spectrometry, *J Anal Toxicol* 27:15-19, 2003.

4. Raikos N, Christopoulou K, Theodoridis G, et al: Determination of amphetamines in human urine by headspace solid-phase microextraction and gas chromatography, *J Chromatogr B Analyt Technol Biomed Life Sci* 789:59-63, 2003.

5. Jenkins KM, Young MS, Mallet CR, et al: Mixed-mode solid-phase extraction procedures for the determination of MDMA and metabolites in urine using LC-MS, LC-UV, or GC-NPD, *J Anal Toxicol* 28:50-58, 2004.

6. Paul BD, Jemionek J, Lesser D, et al: Enantiomeric separation and quantitation of (+/−)-amphetamine, (+/−)-methamphetamine, (+/−)-MDA, (+/−)-MDMA, and (+/−)-MDEA in urine specimens by GC-EI-MS after derivatization with (R)-(−) or (S)-(+)-alpha-methoxy-alpha-(trifluoromethy)phenylacetyl chloride (MTPA), *J Anal Toxicol* 28:449-455, 2004.

7. Peters FT, Samyn N, Wahl M, et al: Concentrations and ratios of amphetamine, methamphetamine, MDA, MDMA, and MDEA enantiomers determined in plasma samples from clinical toxicology and driving under the influence of drugs cases by GC-NICI-MS, *J Anal Toxicol* 27:552-559, 2003.

8. Stout PR, Klette KL, Wiegand R: Comparison and evaluation of DRI methamphetamine, DRI ecstasy, Abuscreen ONLINE amphetamine, and a modified Abuscreen ONLINE amphetamine screening immunoassays for the detection of amphetamine (AMP), methamphetamine (MTH), 3,4-methylenedioxyamphetamine (MDA), and 3,4-methylenedioxymethamphetamine (MDMA) in human urine, *J Anal Toxicol* 27:265-269, 2003.

9. Wood M, De Boeck G, Samyn N, et al: Development of a rapid and sensitive method for the quantitation of amphetamines in human plasma and oral fluid by LC-MS-MS, *J Anal Toxicol* 27:78-87, 2003.

TEST NAME AND METHOD	SPECIMEN	REFERENCE INTERVAL	KINETIC VALUES
Methylene-dioxymethamphetamine (MDMA, Ecstasy)[1-17]	Serum, plasma	*mcg/mL* μ*mol/L*	$t_{1/2}$: 9-10 hr
		C_{max}	V_d: 5-8 L/kg
		After 75 mg dose: 0.13 × 5.18 [0.67]	PB: 34% (in dogs)
		After 125 mg dose: 0.23 [1.19]	T_{max}: 2 hr
		Toxic concentration: > 0.35-0.50 [>1.81-2.59]	
IA, HPLC, GC, GC-MS, CE,LC-MS, LC-MS-MS	Urine	Negative	
MW: 193.23			

1. de la Torre R, Farre M, Roset PN, et al: Human pharmacology of MDMA: pharmacokinetics, metabolism, and disposition, *Ther Drug Monit* 26:137-144, 2004.

2. Pizarro N, Ortuno J, Farre M, et al: Determination of MDMA and its metabolites in blood and urine by gas chromatography-mass spectrometry and analysis of enantiomers by capillary electrophoresis, *J Anal Toxicol* 26:157-165, 2002.

3. Nordgren HK, Beck O: Direct screening of urine for MDMA and MDA by liquid chromatography-tandem mass spectrometry, *J Anal Toxicol* 27:15-19, 2003.

4. Raikos N, Christopoulou K, Theodoridis G, et al: Determination of amphetamines in human urine by headspace solid-phase microextraction and gas chromatography, *J Chromatogr B Analyt Technol Biomed Life Sci* 789:59-63, 2003.

5. Kaddoumi A, Kikura-Hanajiri R, Nakashima K: High-performance liquid chromatography with fluorescence detection for the simultaneous determination of 3,4-methylenedioxymethamphetamine, methamphetamine and their metabolites in human hair using DIB-CI as a label, *Biomed Chromatogr* 18:202-204, 2004.

6. Jenkins KM, Young MS, Mallet CR, et al: Mixed-mode solid-phase extraction procedures for the determination of MDMA and metabolites in urine using LC-MS, LC-UV, or GC-NPD, *J Anal Toxicol* 28:50-58, 2004.

FACTORS INFLUENCING DRUG DISPOSITION	REMARKS AND INTERFERENCES

10. Stout PR, Horn CK, Klette KL: Rapid simultaneous determination of amphetamine, methamphetamine, 3,4-methylene-dioxyamphetamine, 3,4-methylenedioxymethamphetamine, and 3,4-methylenedioxyethylamphetamine in urine by solid-phase extraction and GC-MS: a method optimized for high-volume laboratories, *J Anal Toxicol* 26:253-261, 2002.

11. Mortier KA, Dams R, Lambert WE, et al: Determination of paramethoxyamphetamine and other amphetamine-related designer drugs by liquid chromatography/sonic spray ionization mass spectrometry, *Rapid Commun Mass Spectrom* 16:865-870, 2002.

12. Ramseier A, Caslavska J, Thormann W: Stereoselective screening for and confirmation of urinary enantiomers of amphetamine, methamphetamine, designer drugs, methadone and selected metabolites by capillary electrophoresis, *Electrophresis* 20:2726-2738, 1999.

13. Soares ME, Carvalho M, Carmo H, et al: Simultaneous determination of amphetamine derivatives in human urine after SPE extraction and HPLC-UV analysis, *Biomed Chromatogr* 18:125-131, 2004.

14. Maurer HH: On the metabolism and the toxicological analysis of methylenedioxyphenylalkylamine designer drugs by gas chromatography-mass spectrometry, *Ther Drug Monit* 18:465-470, 1996.

15. Clauwaert KM, Van Bocxlaer JF, De Letter EA, et al: Determination of the designer drugs 3,4-methylenedioxymethamphetamine, 3-4-methylenedioxyethylamphetamine, and 3-4-methylenedioxyamphetamine with HPLC and fluorescence detection in whole blood, serum, vitreous humor, and urine, *Clin Chem* 46.1968-1977, 2000.

16. Buechler J, Schwab M, Mikus G, et al: Enantioselective quantitation of the ecstasy compound (R)- and (S)-N-ethyl-3,4-methylenedioxyamphetamine and its major metabolites in human plasma and urine, *J Chromatogr B Analyt Technol Biomed Life Sci* 793:207-222, 2003.

Metabolism

CYP2B6, CYP1A2, CYP2D6, and CYP3A4 Metabolites include MDA (8-9%). Nonlinear pharmacokinetics apparently are caused by autoinhibition of CYP2D6.

Excretion

Renal

Drug interactions: Antiretroviral drugs and MAO inhibitors are reported to cause life-threatening interactions.

MDMA, an illicit psychostimulant drug, is a potent releaser and/or reuptake inhibitor of serotonin, dopamine, and norepinephrine. It is structurally similar to methamphetamine and mescaline. The racemic mixture is consumed. Psychostimulant and empathic effects result from S(+) isomer, and hallucinogenic effects result from R(−) isomer. Common side effects include jaw clenching, dry mouth, palpitations, cold sensitivity, drowsiness, and tremor. Effects of severe overdose include hyperthermia, delirium, seizures, hypotension, tachydysrhythmias, coma, and renal failure.

Most immunoassays for amphetamines do not detect MDMA.

See *MDA* and *Methamphetamine*.

7. Paul BD, Jemionek J, Lesser D, et al: Enantiomeric separation and quantitation of (+/−)-amphetamine, (+/−)-methamphetamine, (+/−)-MDA, (+/−)-MDMA, and (+/−)-MDEA in urine specimens by GC-EI-MS after derivatization with (R)-(−) or (S)-(+)-alpha-methoxy-alpha-(trifluoromethyl)phenylacetyl chloride (MTPA), *J Anal Toxicol* 28:449-455, 2004.

8. Furesz J, Kocsis G, Gachalgi A, et al: Mass selective detection of amphetamine, methamphetamine, and related compounds in urine, *J Chromatogr Sci* 42:259-262, 2003.

9. Peters FT, Samyn N, Wahl M, et al: Concentrations and ratios of amphetamine, methamphetamine, MDA, MDMA, and MDEA enantiomers determined in plasma samples from clinical toxicology and driving under the influence of drugs cases by GC-NICI-MS, *J Anal Toxicol* 27:552-559, 2003.

10. Stout PR, Klette KL, Wiegand R: Comparison and evaluation of DRI methamphetamine, DRI ecstasy, Abuscreen ONLINE amphetamine, and a modified Abuscreen ONLINE amphetamine screening immunoassays for the detection of amphetamine (AMP), methamphetamine (MTH), 3,4-methylenedioxyamphetamine (MDA), and 3,4-methylenedioxymethamphetamine (MDMA) in human urine, *J Anal Toxicol* 27:265-269, 2003.

TEST NAME AND METHOD	SPECIMEN	REFERENCE (THERAPEUTIC) INTERVAL, CONVENTIONAL [INTERNATIONAL RECOMMENDED UNITS]			KINETIC VALUES	

Methylenedioxymethamphetamine—CONT

11. Wood M, De Boeck G, Samyn N, et al: Development of a rapid and sensitive method for the quantitation of amphetamines in human plasma and oral fluid by LC-MS-MS, *J Anal Toxicol* 27:78-87, 2003.

12. Stout PR, Horn CK, Klette KL, et al: Rapid simultaneous determination of amphetamine, methamphetamine, 3,4-methylenedioxyamphetamine, 3,4-methylenedioxymethamphetamine, and 3,4-methylenedioxyethylamphetamine in urine by solid-phase extraction and GC-MS: a method optimized for high-volume laboratories, *J Anal Toxicol* 26:253-261, 2002.

13. Mortier KA, Dams R, Lambert WE, et al: Determination of paramethoxyamphetamine and other amphetamine-related designer drugs by liquid chromatography/sonic spray ionization mass spectrometry, *Rapid Commun Mass Spectrom* 16:865-870, 2002.

14. Ramseier A, Caslavska J, Thormann W: Stereoselective screening for and confirmation of urinary enantiomers of amphetamine, methamphetamine, designer drugs, methadone and selected metabolites by capillary electrophoresis, *Electrophoresis* 20:2726-2738, 1999.

Methyprylon **(Noludar)**[1,2]	Serum		*mcg/mL*		*μmol/L*	$t_{1/2}$: 7-11 hr
		Therapeutic				V_d: 0.97 L/kg
		concenetration:	8-10	× 5.46	[44-55]	Cl_T: NA
GC, HPLC		Toxic				C_{max}: 2 hr
		concentration:	>50		[>273]	PB: 38%
MW: 183.25						F: NA
						T_{max}: 2 hr

1. Contos DA, Dixon KF, Guthrie RM, et al: Nonlinear elimination of methyprylon (noludar) in an overdosed patient: correlation of clinical effects with plasma concentration, *J Pharm Sci* 80:768-771, 1991.

2. Gwilt PR, Pankaskie MC, Thornburg JE, et al: Pharmacokinetics of methyprylon following a single oral dose, *J Pharm Sci* 74:1001-1003, 1985.

Metoprolol **(Lopressor)**[1-3]	Serum, plasma (EDTA, heparin). Stable for 4 mo at	Therapeutic concentration:	75-200 ng/mL [× 3.74 = 281-748 nmol/L]	PK[4-8]: $t_{1/2}$:	3-7 hr
GLC, GC-MS,	−20° C.			V_d:	4.2 ± 0.7 L/kg
HPLC		Toxic		Cl_T:	15 ± 3 mL/min/kg
		concentration:	Not well defined	PB:	13%
				F:	38 ± 14%
MW: 267.37					
HPLC[2]	Urine. Stable for up to 4 mo at −20° C.				

FACTORS INFLUENCING DRUG DISPOSITION	REMARKS AND INTERFERENCES

15. Soares ME, Carvalho M, Carmo H, et al: Simultaneous determination of amphetamine derivatives in human urine after SPE extraction and HPLC-UV analysis, *Biomed Chromatogr* 18:125-131, 2004.

16. Maurer HH: On the metabolism and the toxicological analysis of methylenedioxyphenylalkylamine designer drugs by gas chromatography-mass spectrometry, *Ther Drug Monit* 18:465-470, 1996.

17. Clauwaert KM, Van Boxclaer JF, De Letter EA, et al: Determination of the designer drugs 3,4-methylenedioxymethamphetamine, 3-4-methylenedioxyethylamphetamine, and 3-4-methylenedioxyamphetamine with HPLC and fluorescence detection in whole blood, serum, vitreous humor, and urine, *Clin Chem* 46:1968-1977, 2000.

Metabolism

  Hepatic

Dialysis

  Hemodialysis (+)

  Hemoperfusion (+)

  Peritoneal (±)

Methyprylon is metabolized to a series of products, some of which are active. Only ~3% of unchanged drug is excreted in the urine. This sedative-hypnotic is a CNS depressant and produces drowsiness and ataxia. Acute overdose is generally characterized by coma, apnea, hypotension, shock, and pulmonary edema. The plasma $t_{1/2}$ is prolonged to ~50 hr in acute overdosage. The product is no longer used in the U.S.

Metabolism

  Hepatic

Excretion

  Urine

Disease

  Cirrhosis: $t_{1/2}\uparrow$, $F\uparrow$, $V_d\rightarrow$

  Hyperthyroidism: $t_{1/2}\rightarrow$, $Cl_T\uparrow$

Dialysis[9]

  Hemodialysis (+)

Drug interactions: Metoprolol is a major substrate of CYP2D6 and minor substrate of CYP2C19. Metoprolol weakly inhibits CYP2D6. CYP2D6 inhibitors like chlorpromazine, fluoxetine, miconazole, paroxetine, pergolide, quinidine, quinine, and ritonavir may increase the effects of metoprolol. Barbiturates and other enzyme inducers may enhance metoprolol metabolism. Phenothiazines and cimetidine may increase plasma concen-

Metoprolol exhibits dose-dependent bioavailability secondary to saturable first-pass metabolism. Alterations of dose in renal dysfunction are not warranted. Plasma concentrations that produce minimal β-blockade vary widely. There is no good correlation between serum concentrations and therapeutic effects. Thus determination of serum levels is of limited value in routine therapy.

TEST NAME AND METHOD	SPECIMEN	REFERENCE (THERAPEUTIC) INTERVAL, CONVENTIONAL [INTERNATIONAL RECOMMENDED UNITS]	KINETIC VALUES

Metoprolol (Lopressor)—CONT

1. Ervik M, Kylberg-Hanssen K, Johansson L: Determination of metoprolol in plasma and urine using high-resolution gas chromatography and electron-capture detection, *J Chromatogr* 381:168-174, 1986.

2. Balmer K, Zhong Y, Lagerstrom PO, et al: Determination of metoprolol and two major metabolites in plasma and urine by column liquid chromatography and fluorometric detection, *J Chromatogr* 417:357-365, 1987.

3. Baselt RC: *Disposition of toxic drugs and chemicals in man,* ed 7, Foster City, CA, 2004, Chemical Toxicology Institute.

4. Evans WE, Schentag JJ, Jusko WJ: *Applied pharmacokinetics—principles of therapeutic drug monitoring,* ed 3, Vancouver, WA, 1992, Applied Therapeutics, Inc.

5. Hardman JG, Limbird LE, Gilman AG: *Goodman & Gilman's the pharmacological basis of therapeutics,* ed 10, New York, 2001, McGraw-Hill.

6. Johnsson G, Regårdh C: Clinical pharmacokinetics of β-adrenoreceptor blocking drugs, *Clin Pharmacokinet* 1:233-263, 1976.

7. Regårdh C, Johnsson G: Clinical pharmacokinetics of metoprolol, *Clin Pharmacokinet* 5:557-569, 1980.

8. Micromedex: *Micromedex healthcare series 2004,* Greenwood Village, CO, 2004, Thomson Micromedex.

9. Bennett W, Aronof G, Golper T, et al: *Drug prescribing in renal failure. Dosing guidelines for adults,* ed 2, Philadelphia, 1994, American College of Physicians.

10. Lexi-Comp, Inc: *Up-to-date online 12.2. Drug information,* Hudson, OH, 2004, Lexi-Comp, Inc.

Mexiletine	Serum, plasma		*mg/mL*		*mmol/L*	PK[3,4]:	
(Mexitil)[1-3]	(EDTA heparin).	Therapeutic				$t_{1/2}$:	8-17 hr (urine
	Stable for 10 mo at	concentration:	0.5-2.0	× 5.58	[2.79-11.2]		pH-dependent)
GC-MS, HPLC	−25° C.[2]	Toxic				V_d:	6-12 L/kg
		concentration:	>2.0		[>11.2]	Cl_T:	7.2-12.1 mL/min/kg
MW: 179.26						PB:	50-70%
						F	74-100%

| FACTORS INFLUENCING DRUG DISPOSITION | REMARKS AND INTERFERENCES |

trations, probably through an effect on hepatic metabolism. NSAIDs and salicylates may reduce the antihypertensive effects of metoprolol.[10]

Metabolism
  Hepatic
Excretion
  Feces (primary)
  Urine (secondary)
Disease
  Renal (CrCl <10 mL/min): $t_{1/2}\uparrow$, $Cl_T\downarrow$
  CHF: $t_{1/2}\uparrow$, $Cl_T\rightarrow$
  MI: $t_{1/2}\uparrow$, $V_d\rightarrow$, $Cl_T\downarrow$
  Hepatic: $t_{1/2}\uparrow$

Drug interactions[4]: Mexiletine is a major substrate of CYP1A2 and CYP2D6. It inhibits CYP1A2 strongly. Phenytoin and rifampin or cigarette smoking can induce mexiletine metabolism, thereby decreasing its plasma concentrations and $t_{1/2}$. Cimetidine appears to slow absorbtion of mexiletine slightly. Metoclopramide may increase the rate of mexiletine absorption. Mexiletine may increase plasma digoxin concentration.

Mexiletine is a class Ib antiarrhythmic. Metabolites are not pharmacologically active. Adverse effects include hypotension, vomiting, tremor, toxic confusional states, and atrioventricular dissociation. Can be proarrhythmic. May cause acute hepatic injury. Use cautiously in patients with first-degree block, preexisting sinus node dysfunction, intraventricular conduction delays, significant hepatic dysfunction, hypotension, or severe CHF.

TEST NAME AND METHOD	SPECIMEN	REFERENCE (THERAPEUTIC) INTERVAL, CONVENTIONAL [INTERNATIONAL RECOMMENDED UNITS]			KINETIC VALUES	

Mexiletine—CONT

1. Dasgupta A, Yousef O: Gas chromatographic-mass spectrometric determination of serum mexiletine concentration after derivatization with perfluorooctanoyl chloride, a new derivative, *J Chromatogr B Biomed Sci Appl* 705:283-288, 1998.
2. Paczkowski D, Filipek M, Mielniczuk Z, et al: Simultaneous determination of mexiletine and four hydroxylated metabolites in human serum by high-performance liquid chromatography and its application to pharmacokinetic studies, *J Chromatogr* 573:235-246, 1992.

TEST NAME AND METHOD	SPECIMEN	REFERENCE (THERAPEUTIC) INTERVAL		KINETIC VALUES	
Midazolam **(Versed)**[1-7]	Serum, plasma	*mcg/mL*	*μmol/L*	$t_{1/2}$:	1-4 hr
		Therapeutic		V_d:	0.8-2.5 L/kg
		concentration: 0.04-0.15 × 3.07	[0.12-0.46]	Cl_T:	4.0-8.1 mL/min/kg
GC, HPLC,		Toxic		PB:	97%
GC-MS, LC-MS		concentration: >1.0	[>3.07]		[× 0.01 = 0.97, protein-bound mole fraction]
MW: 325.8				F:	30-50%
					[× 0.01 = 0.30-0.50, bioavailable mole fraction]

1. McEvoy GK, editor: *AHFS drug information (online version),* Bethesda, MD, 2004, American Society of Health-System Pharmacists Inc.
2. *USP DI drug information for the health care professional,* ed 24, (online version), Taunton, MA, 2004, Micromedex Inc.
3. Frison G, Tedeschi L, Maietti S, et al: Determination of midazolam in human plasma by solid-phase microextraction and gas chromatography/mass spectrometry, *Rapid Commun Mass Spectrom* 15:2497-2501, 2001.
4. Kratzsch C, Tenberken O, Peters FT, et al: Screening, library-assisted identification and validated quantification of 23 benzodiazepines, flumazenil, zaleplone, zolpidem and zopiclone in plasma by liquid chromatography/mass spectrometry with atmospheric pressure chemical ionization, *J Mass Spectrom* 39:856-872, 2004.
5. El Mahjoub A, Staub C: Semiautomated high-performance liquid chromatographic method for the determination of benzodiazepines in whole blood, *J Anal Toxicol* 25:209-214, 2001.
6. Portier EJ, de Blok K, Butter JJ, et al: Simultaneous determination of fentanyl and midazolam using high-performance liquid chromatography with ultraviolet detection, *J Chromatogr B Biomed Sci Appl* 723:313-318, 1999.
7. Rasanen I, Ojanpera I, Vuori E: Quantitative screening for benzodiazepines in blood by dual-column gas chromatography and comparison of the results with urine immunoassay, *J Anal Toxicol* 24:46-51, 2000.

3. Baselt RC: *Disposition of toxic drugs and chemicals in man,* ed 7, Foster City, CA, 2004, Chemical Toxicology Institute.
4. Hardman JG, Limbird LE, Gilman AG: *Goodman & Gilman's the pharmacological basis of therapeutics,* ed 10, New York, 2001, McGraw-Hill.
5. Lexi-Comp, Inc: *Up-to-date online 12.2. Drug information,* Hudson, OH, 2004, Lexi-Comp, Inc.

Metabolism
  Hepatic, CYP3A4, CYP2B6 (minor)
  Weak inhibitor of CYP2c8/9 and CYP3A4
Disease
  Obesity: $t_{1/2}\uparrow$, $V_d\uparrow$, $Cl_T\rightarrow$
Age
  Elderly: $t_{1/2}\uparrow$, $V_d\rightarrow$, $Cl_T\downarrow$, $PB\rightarrow$, $F\uparrow$

Drug interactions: CYP3A4 inducers (e.g., carbamazepine, rifampin, and phenytoin) may increase hepatic metabolism. CYP3A4 inhibitors (e.g., diltiazem, azole antifungals, and erythromycin) may inhibit hepatic metabolism.

Midazolam is an ultra-short-acting imidazole used for preoperative sedation, anxiolysis, and anterograde amnesia. It is extensively metabolized in the liver and intestine with the principal metabolite being 1-hydroxymidazolam. Adverse reactions of midazolam include decreased respiration, hypotension, drowsiness, headache, nausea, and vomiting.

TEST NAME AND METHOD	SPECIMEN	REFERENCE (THERAPEUTIC) INTERVAL, CONVENTIONAL [INTERNATIONAL RECOMMENDED UNITS]				KINETIC VALUES	
Morphine[1-30]	Serum, plasma, and blood		*ng/mL*		*nmol/L*	$t_{1/2}$:	2-4 hr
		Therapeutic				V_d:	3.2 ± 0.7 L/kg
GC, HPLC, IA,		concentration:	10-80	$\times 3.50$	[35-280]	Cl_T:	15 ± 2 mL/min/kg
GC-MS, fluorimet-		Toxic				PB:	35%
ric, LC-MS-MS,		concentration:	>200		[>700]		[$\times 0.01 = 0.35$, protein-
CE, LC-MS							bound mole fraction]
	Urine	Negative				F:	20-33%
MW: 303.4							[$\times 0.01 = 0.20$-0.33,
	Alternative matrices: Hair, oral fluid, and sweat	Negative					bioavailable mole fraction]

1. Schanzle G, Li S, Mikus G, et al: Rapid, highly sensitive method for the determination of morphine and its metabolites in body fluids by liquid chromatography-mass spectrometry, *J Chromatogr B Biomed Sci Appl* 721:55-65, 1999.

2. Pacifici R, Pichini S, Altieri I, et al: High-performance liquid chromatographic-electrospray mass spectrometric determination of morphine and its 3- and 6-glucuronides: application to pharmacokinetic studies, *J Chromatogr B Biomed Appl* 664:329-334, 1995.

3. Cailleux A, Le Bouil A, Auger B, et al: Determination of opiates and cocaine and its metabolites in biological fluids by high-performance liquid chromatography with electrospray tandem mass spectrometry, *J Anal Toxicol* 23:620-624, 1999.

4. Ropero-Miller JD, Lambing MK, Winecker RE: Simultaneous quantitation of opioids in blood by GC-EI-MS analysis following deproteination, detautomerization of keto analytes, solid-phase extraction, and trimethylsilyl derivatization, *J Anal Toxicol* 26:524-528, 2002.

5. Emara S, Darwish I, Youssef D, et al: On the perspectives of capillary electrophoresis modes for the determination of morphine in human plasma without sample pretreatment, *Biomed Chromatogr* 18:21-27, 2004.

6. Whittington D, Kharasch ED: Determination of morphine and morphine glucuronides in human plasma by 96-well plate solid-phase extraction and liquid chromatography-electrospray ionization mass spectrometry, *J Chromatogr B Analyt Technol Biomed Life Sci* 796:95-103, 2003.

7. Thevis M, Opfermann G, Schanzer W: Urinary concentrations of morphine and codeine after consumption of poppy seeds, *J Anal Toxicol* 27:53-56, 2003.

8. Chen YL, Hanson GD, Jiang X, et al: Simultaneous solid-phase extraction and chromatographic analysis of morphine and hydromorphone in human plasma by liquid chromatography with tandem mass spectrometric detection, *J Chromatogr B Analyt Technol Biomed Life Sci* 769:55-64, 2002.

9. Ary K, Rona K: LC determination of morphine and morphine glucuronides in human plasma by coulometric and UV detection, *J Pharmaceut Biomed Anal* 26:179-187, 2001.

10. Broussard LA, Presley LC, Pittman T, et al: Simultaneous identification and quantitation of codeine, morphine, hydrocodone and hydromorphone in urine as trimethylsilyl and oxime derivatives by gas chromatography-mass spectrometry, *Clin Chem* 43:1029-1032, 1997.

11. Haffen E, Paintaud G, Berard M, et al: On the assessment of drug metabolism by assays of codeine and its main metabolites, *Ther Drug Monit* 22:258-265, 2000.

12. Zhou T, Yu H, Hu Q, et al: Determination of codeine and its metabolite in human urine by CE with amperometric detection, *J Pharmaceut Biomed Anal* 30:13-19, 2002.

13. Svensson JO, Yue QY, Sawe J: Determination of codeine and metabolites in plasma and urine using ion-pair high-performance liquid chromatography, *J Chromatogr B Biomed Appl* 674:49-55, 1995.

FACTORS INFLUENCING DRUG DISPOSITION	REMARKS AND INTERFERENCES

Metabolism
  Hepatic, CYP2D6 (minor)
Elimination
  Renal, fecal (7-10%)
Disease
  Hepatic: $t_{1/2}\rightarrow$, $V_d\rightarrow$, $Cl_T\rightarrow$, PB$\downarrow$
  Hypoalbuminemia: PB$\downarrow$
  Hyperbilirubinemia: PB$\downarrow$
Dialysis
  Hemodialysis ($-$)

Drug interactions: CNS depressants, tricyclic antidepressants, and dextroamphetamine potentiate effect. Avoid concurrent use of MAO inhibitors.

Morphine, the principal alkaloid of opium, is a narcotic analgesic used to relieve severe, acute, and chronic pain. Side effects include drowsiness, mood changes, mental clouding, nausea, vomiting, miosis, and respiratory depression. Two major metabolites are morphine-6-glucuronide (active) and morphine-3-glucuronide. For federally regulated workplace drug testing (SAMHSA), the immunoassay cutoff concentration to separate positive and negative specimens for opiates is 2000 ng/mL [7000 nmol/L] morphine equivalents; for GC-MS confirmation, 2000 ng/mL [7000 nmol/L] morphine with analysis of 6-acetyl morphine (10 ng/mL cutoff) is also mandated.

Alternative matrices used for nonfederally regulated workplace drug testing and being considered for regulated testing include hair, oral fluid, and sweat.

Interferences: Ingestion of a large amount of poppy seeds may produce a positive result for up to 60 hr with immunoassay procedures using a 300 ng/mL cutoff.

14. Dienes-Nagy A, Rivier L, Giroud C, et al. Method for quantification of morphine and its 3- and 6-glucuronides, codeine, codeine glucuronide and 6-monoacetylmorphine in human blood by liquid chromatography-electrospray mass spectrometry for routine analysis in forensic toxicology, *J Chromatogr A* 854:109-118, 1999.

15. Mykkanen S, Seppala J, Ariniemi K, et al: GCD quantitation of opiates as propionyl derivatives in blood, *J Anal Toxicol* 24:122-126, 2000.

16. Fraser AD, Worth D: Experience with a urine opiate screening and confirmation cutoff of 2000 ng/Ml, *J Anal Toxicol* 23:549-551, 1999.

17. He H, Shay SD, Caraco Y, et al: Simultaneous determination of codeine and its seven metabolites in plasma and urine by high-performance liquid chromatography with ultraviolet and electrochemical detection, *J Chromatogr B Biomed Sci Appl* 708:185-193, 1998.

18. Bogusz MJ, Maier RD, Erkens M, et al: Determination of morphine and its 3- and 6-glucuronides, codeine, codeine-glucuronide and 6-monoacetylmorphine in body fluids by liquid chromatography atmospheric pressure chemical ionization mass spectrometry, *J Chromatogr B Biomed Sci Appl* 703:115-127, 1997.

19. Smith FP, Lora-Tamayo C, Carvajal R, et al: Assessment of an automated immunoassay based on kinetic interaction of microparticles in solution for determination of opiates and cocaine metabolite in urine, *Ann Clin Biochem* 34:81-84, 1997.

20. Kemp P, Sneed G, Kupiec T, et al: Validation of a microtiter plate ELISA for screening of postmortem blood for opiates and benzodiazepines, *J Anal Toxicol* 26:504-512, 2002.

21. Kerrigan S, Phillips Jr W Jr: Comparison of ELISAs for opiates, methamphetamine, cocaine metabolite, benzodiazepines, phencyclidine, and cannabinoids in whole blood and urine, *Clin Chem* 47:540-547, 2001.

22. Pichini S, Pacifici R, Altieri I, et al: Determination of opiates and cocaine in hair as trimethylsilyl derivatives using gas chromatography-tandem mass spectrometry, *J Anal Toxicol* 23:343-348, 1999.

23. Mortier KA, Maudens KE, Lambert WE, et al: Simultaneous, quantitative determination of opiates, amphetamines, cocaine and benzoylecgonine in oral fluid by liquid chromatography quadrupole-time-of-flight mass spectrometry, *J Chromatogr B Analyt Technol Biomed Life Sci* 779:321-330, 2002.

24. Skender L, Karacic V, Brcic I, et al: Quantitative determination of amphetamines, cocaine, and opiates in human hair by gas chromatography/mass spectrometry, *Forensic Sci Int* 125:120-126, 2002.

25. Presley L, Lehrer M, Seiter W, et al: High prevalence of 6-acetylmorphine in morphine-positive oral fluid specimens, *Forensic Sci Int* 133:22-25, 2003.

26. Brewer WE, Galipo RC, Sellers KW, et al: Analysis of cocaine, benzoylecgonine, codeine, and morphine in hair by supercritical fluid extraction with carbon dioxide modified with methanol, *Anal Chem* 73:2371-2376, 2001.

TEST NAME AND METHOD	SPECIMEN	REFERENCE (THERAPEUTIC) INTERVAL, CONVENTIONAL [INTERNATIONAL RECOMMENDED UNITS]		KINETIC VALUES	

Morphine—CONT

27. Sabzevari O, Abdi K, Amini M, et al: Application of a simple and sensitive GC-MS method for determination of morphine in the hair of opium abusers, *Anal Bioanal Chem* 379:120-124, 2004.

28. Nakahara Y, Kikura R, Takahashi K: Hair analysis for drugs of abuse. VIII. Effective extraction and determination of 6-acetylmorphine and morphine in hair with trifluoroacetic acid-methanol for the confirmation of retrospective heroin use by gas chromatography-mass spectrometry, *J Chromatogr B Biomed Appl* 657:93-101, 1994.

TEST NAME AND METHOD	SPECIMEN	REFERENCE (THERAPEUTIC) INTERVAL		KINETIC VALUES	
Muromonab-CD3 (OKT3)[1]	Serum	Therapeutic concentration:	Not available	PK[3]:	
		Toxic concentration:	Not available	$t_{1/2}$:	18 hr[4,5]
				V_d:	6.5 L[5]
ELISA		In most centers using OKT3, therapeutic monitoring of OKT3 is not in widespread use.[2]		Cl_T:	Not available
				PB:	Not available

1. Schroeder T, Michael AT, First MR, et al: Variations in serum OKT3 concentration based upon age, sex, transplanted organ, treatment regimen, and anti-OKT3 antibody status, *Ther Drug Monit* 16:361-367, 1994.

2. Johnston A, Holt DW: Therapeutic drug monitoring of immunosuppressant drugs, *Br J Clin Pharmacol* 47:339-350, 1999.

3. Meijer RT, Koopmans RP, ten Berge IJ, et al: Pharmacokinetics of murine anti-human CD3 antibodies in man are determined by the disappearance of target antigen, *J Pharmacol Exp Ther* 300:346-353, 2002.

4. Hooks MA, Wade CS, Millikan WJ Jr: Muromonab CD-3: a review of its pharmacology, pharmacokinetics, and clinical use in transplantation, *Pharmacotherapy* 11:26-37, 1991.

5. Roitt IM: OKT3: immunology, production, purification, and pharmacokinetics, *Clin Transplant* 7:367-373, 1993.

6. Lexi-Comp, Inc: *Up-to-date online 12.2. Drug information,* Hudson, OH, 2004, Lexi-Comp, Inc.

7. Micromedex: *Micromedex healthcare series 2004,* Greenwood Village, CO, 2004, Thomson Micromedex.

TEST NAME AND METHOD	SPECIMEN	REFERENCE (THERAPEUTIC) INTERVAL		KINETIC VALUES	
Mycophenolic Acid (CellCept)[1-5]	Plasma,[7] serum (red top, no SST)	Therapeutic concentration[2,6,8-10]:	*Trough: 1.0-3.5 mcg/mL	PK[3,8,12,13]: $t_{1/2}$: V_d:	16-18 hr 3.6-4.0 L/kg
HPLC, EMIT, LC-MS-MS	Stable at −20° C for 3 wk; 4° C for 96 hr	Toxic concentration:	Not available	Cl_T:	140-193 mL/min
EMIT shows a positive bias compared with HPLC because the antibody detects acyl glucuronide, an active metabolite of MPA.[6]		Although therapeutic trough levels remain to be conclusively defined, MPA AUC data are more significantly correlated with toxicity/efficacy; a study showed 12-hr AUCs >40 mcg/mL/hr were correlated with efficacy and decreased episodes of rejection, whereas another study showed 12-hr AUC of 32.2-60.6 mcg/mL/hr was correlated to a rejection rate of <10%.[11]		PB: F:	97% 94%

29.   Romolo FS, Rotolo MC, Palmi I, et al: Optimized conditions for simultaneous determination of opiates, cocaine and ben-zoylecgonine in hair samples by GC—MS, *Forensic Sci Int* 138:17-26, 2003.

30.   Moody DE, Cheever ML: Evaluation of immunoassays for semiquantitative detection of cocaine and metabolites or heroin and metabolites in extracts of sweat patches, *J Anal Toxicol* 25:190-197, 2001.

FACTORS INFLUENCING DRUG DISPOSITION	REMARKS AND INTERFERENCES

Metabolism
   Unknown
Excretion
   Binding to T lymphocytes
Dialysis
   Hemodialysis (+)
   Plasmapheresis (+)
 	
Drug interactions: Muromonab-CD3 may en-hance the adverse/toxic effect of vaccines (live organisms). Echinacea may antagonize the im-munosuppressive effect of muromonab CD3 and decrease its effectiveness.[6]
	OKT3 is a murine monoclonal antibody directed against the CD3 receptor on human T lymphocytes and is given in the treatment of allograft rejection in re-nal and other solid organ transplant patients. It is also used for the treatment of acute hepatic and pancreatic rejection episodes, as well as acute graft-versus-host disease after bone marrow transplantation resistant to conventional treat-ment.[1,7]
	
	Side effects of parenteral muromonab-CD3 include headaches, diarrhea, nau-sea, and vomiting.[7] First-dose effect (cytokine release syndrome) may occur 1-3 hr after the first dose and may last for 12-16 hr. Symptoms include mild flulike symptoms to life-threatening anaphylactic shock. Reactions tend to decrease with repeated doses.[6]

Metabolism
   Hepatic
   GI tract
Excretion
   Urine (primary)
   Feces (secondary)
Dialysis
   Hemodialysis (−)
   Peritoneal dialysis (−)
 	
Drug interactions[8]**:** When acyclovir, ganci-clovir, or probenecid is coadministered with mycophenolic acid, levels of both drugs may
	Mycophenolic acid is an immunosuppressive agent used for prophylaxis of or-gan rejection in patients undergoing heart, kidney, and liver transplantation.[12] Its use in combination with cyclosporine and steroids has decreased incidences of acute rejection in renal transplant patients.[2]
	
	The prodrug mycophenolate mofetil is completely hydrolyzed in the liver to the active metabolite, MPA; it is converted to its primary inactive glucuronide metabolite, MPAG, which is predominantly excreted renally.[2,3]
	
	Side effects include nausea, diarrhea, constipation, anemia, leukopenia, headache, weakness, urinary tract infection, liver function test abnormalities, infection related to immunosuppression, and skin rash. Hemorrhagic gastritis and pancreatitis have been reported in a few cases.[12]

TEST NAME AND METHOD	SPECIMEN	REFERENCE (THERAPEUTIC) INTERVAL, CONVENTIONAL [INTERNATIONAL RECOMMENDED UNITS]	KINETIC VALUES

Mycophenolic Acid—CONT

MW: 320.34

*Trough MPA concentration encountered in normal therapy is typically between 1.0-3.5 mcg/mL but remains to be conclusively established.

1. Beal J, Jones C, Taylor P, et al: Evaluation of an immunoassay (EMIT) for mycophenolic acid in plasma from renal transplant recipients compared with a high-performance liquid chromatography assay, *Ther Drug Monit* 20:685-690, 1998.

2. Shaw LM, Holt DW, Keown P, et al: Current opinions on therapeutic drug monitoring of immunosuppressive drugs, *Clin Ther* 21:1632-1652, 1999.

3. Shaw LM, Kaplan B, Brayman KL: Prospective investigations of concentration-clinical response for immunosuppressive drugs provide the scientific basis for therapeutic drug monitoring, *Clin Chem* 44:381-387, 1998.

4. Premaud A, Rousseau A, Le Meur Y, et al: Comparison of liquid chromatography-tandem mass spectrometry with a commercial enzyme-multiplied immunoassay for the determination of plasma MPA in renal transplant recipients and consequences for therapeutic drug monitoring, *Ther Drug Monit* 26:609-619, 2004.

5. Patel CG, Mendonza AE, Akhlaghi F, et al: Determination of total mycophenolic acid and its glucuronide metabolite using liquid chromatography with ultraviolet detection and unbound mycophenolic acid using tandem mass spectrometry, *J Chromatogr* B 813:287-294, 2004.

6. Holt D, Armstrong V, Griesmacher A, et al: International Federation of Clinical Chemistry/International Association of Therapeutic Drug Monitoring and Clinical Toxicology working group on immunosuppressive drug monitoring, *Ther Drug Monit* 24:59-67, 2002.

7. Pawinski T, Shaw L: Stability of mycophenolic acid in plasma samples from patients during mycophenolate mofetil therapy, *Acta Pol Pharm* 60:121-124, 2003.

8. Lexi-Comp, Inc: *Up-to-date online 12.2. Drug information,* Hudson, OH, 2004, Lexi-Comp, Inc.

9. Smak Gregoor PJH, Hesse CJ, van Gelder T, et al: Relation of mycophenolic acid trough levels and adverse events in kidney allograft recipients, *Transplant Proc* 30:1192-1193, 1998.

10. Tredger J, Brown N, Adams J, et al: Monitoring mycophenolate in liver transplant recipients: toward a therapeutic range, *Liver Transpl* 10:503-505, 2004.

11. Wong SHY: Therapeutic drug monitoring for immunosuppressants, *Clin Chim Acta* 313:241-253, 2001.

12. Micromedex: *Micromedex healthcare series 2004,* Greenwood Village, CO, 2004, Thomson Micromedex.

13. Pisupati J, Jain A, Burckart G, et al: Intraindividual and interindividual variations in the pharmacokinetics of mycophenolic acid in liver transplant patients, *J Clin Pharmacol* 455:34-41, 2005.

FACTORS INFLUENCING DRUG DISPOSITION	REMARKS AND INTERFERENCES

increase because of competition for tubular secretion. Cholestyramine and antacids should not be administered together with mycophenolic acid because its absorption can be reduced.

Food can cause C_{max} decreases by ~40%; should avoid Cat's Claw and Echinacea herbal supplementation, which have immunosuppressant activities.[8]

Most PK data on MPA relate to use of MMF after renal transplantation in combination with CsA. Concomitant therapy with tacrolimus or sirolimus can affect MPA AUCs and trough levels differently; it remains to be established whether different drug therapies affect interpretations of trough or target AUC values.[6]

TEST NAME AND METHOD	SPECIMEN	REFERENCE (THERAPEUTIC) INTERVAL, CONVENTIONAL [INTERNATIONAL RECOMMENDED UNITS]		KINETIC VALUES	
Nadolol **(Corgard)**[1-4] *Fluorimetric,* *GC-MS, HPLC* *MW: 309.41*	Serum, plasma (EDTA, heparin)	Therapeutic concentration: Toxic concentration:	Not defined Not defined	PK^{5-9}: $t_{1/2}$: V_d: Cl_T: PB: F:	20-24 hr 2.1 ± 1.0 L/kg 2.9 ± 0.6 mL/min/kg 28-30% [× 0.01 = 0.28-0.30, protein-bound mole fraction] 34 ± 5%

1. Ivashkiv I: Fluorometric determination of nadolol in human serum and urine, *J Pharm Sci* 66:1168-1171, 1977.
2. Ribick M, Ivashkiv E, Jemal M, et al: Use of an inexpensive mass-selective detector for the high-sensitivity gas chromatographic determination of nadolol in plasma, *J Chromatogr* 381:419-423, 1986.
3. Noguchi H, Yoshida K, Murano M, et al: Determination of nadolol in serum by high-performance liquid chromatography with fluorimetric detection, *J Chromatogr* 573:336-338, 1992.
4. Baselt RC: *Disposition of toxic drugs and chemicals in man,* ed 7, Foster City, CA, 2004, Chemical Toxicology Institute.
5. Evans WE, Schentag JJ, Jusko WJ: *Applied pharmacokinetics—principles of therapeutic drug monitoring,* ed 3, Vancouver, WA, 1992, Applied Therapeutics, Inc.
6. Hardman JG, Limbird LE, Gilman AG: *Goodman & Gilman's the pharmacological basis of therapeutics,* ed 10, New York 2001, McGraw-Hill.
7. Johnsson G, Regårdh C: Clinical pharmacokinetics of β-adrenoreceptor blocking drugs, *Clin Pharmacokinet* 1:233-263, 1976.
8. Dreyfuss J, Brannick LJ, Vukovich RA, et al: Metabolic studies in patients with nadolol: oral and intravenous administration, *J Clin Pharmacol* 17:300-307, 1977.
9. Micromedex: *Micromedex healthcare series 2004,* Greenwood Village, CO, 2004, Thomson Micromedex.
10. Lexi-Comp, Inc: *Up-to-date online 12.2. Drug information,* Hudson, OH, 2004, Lexi-Comp, Inc.

TEST NAME AND METHOD	SPECIMEN	REFERENCE (THERAPEUTIC) INTERVAL, CONVENTIONAL *mcg/mL*		*μmol/L*	KINETIC VALUES	
Netilmicin **(Netromycin)**[1-6] *MB, EIA, FPIA,* *HPLC, GLC* *MW: 475.59*	Serum, plasma (EDTA). For patients taking penicillin or its derivatives, freeze samples if not analyzed within 4-6 hr. Collect at trough and peak concentration (end of a 1-hr constant infusion, 30 min after the end of a 30-min constant infusion, or 1 hr after an IM dose).	Therapeutic concentration Peak, Less severe infections: Severe infections: Trough, Less severe infections: Moderate infections: Severe infections:	5-8 8-10 <1 <2 <2-4	× 2.10	[10-17] [17-21] [<2] [<4] [<4-8]	PK^{7-10}: $t_{1/2}$: V_d: Cl_T: PB:	2.3 ± 0.7 hr 37 ± 6 hr (terminal) 0.20 ± 0.02 L/kg 1.3 ± 0.2 mL/min/kg <30%

FACTORS INFLUENCING DRUG DISPOSITION	REMARKS AND INTERFERENCES

Metabolism
  Hepatic
Excretion
  Urine (primary)
  Hepatic (secondary)[8]
Disease
  Renal: $t_{1/2}\uparrow$
Dialysis
  Hemodialysis (+)

Drug interactions: Phenothiazines may increase plasma concentrations, probably through their effect on hepatic metabolism. NSAIDs and salicylates may reduce the antihypertensive effects of nadolol.[10]

Biliary secretion may account for up to 41% of elimination. Nadolol appears to be eliminated via the biliary system in anephric patients. Plasma concentrations that produce minimal β-blockade vary widely. There is no good correlation between serum concentrations and therapeutic effects. Thus determination of serum levels is of limited value in routine therapy.

Metabolism
  None
Excretion
  Urine
Diseases
  Renal: $t_{1/2}\uparrow$, $V_d\rightarrow$, $Cl_T\downarrow$
  Cystic fibrosis: $t_{1/2}\downarrow$, $Cl_T\rightarrow$
Age
  Neonate: $t_{1/2}\uparrow$
Dialysis
  Hemodialysis (+)
  Peritoneal (+)

Netilmicin is an aminoglycoside antibiotic. Therapeutic and toxic concentrations are highly variable and therefore should be individualized for the patient's condition. Penicillin and its derivatives inactivate netilmicin in vivo and in vitro. Cl_T and $t_{1/2}$ are strongly correlated with glomerular filtration rate. Netilmicin appears to have less incidence of ototoxicity than other aminoglycosides.

Interferences: When patient is also taking other antibiotics (penicillins, cephalosporins, tetracyclines, clindamycin, chloramphenicol), the MB method may lack specificity. Penicillins and cephalosporins can be inactivated with a commercially available β-lactamase to minimize this interference.

TEST NAME AND METHOD	SPECIMEN	REFERENCE (THERAPEUTIC) INTERVAL, CONVENTIONAL [INTERNATIONAL RECOMMENDED UNITS]		KINETIC VALUES

Netilmicin (Netromycin)—CONT

		Toxic concentration		
		Peak:	>10-12	[>21-25]
		Trough:	>2-4	[>4-8]

1. Stead D, Richards R: Sensitive high-performance liquid chromatographic assay for aminoglycosides in biological matrices enables the direct estimation of bacterial drug uptake, *J Chromatogr B* 693:415-421, 1997.

2. Marples J, Oates M: Serum gentamicin, netilmicin and tobramycin assays by high performance liquid chromatography, *J Antimicrob Chemother* 10:311-318, 1982.

3. Wenk M, Hemmann R, Follath F: Homogeneous enzyme immunoassay for netilmicin, *Antimicrob Agents Chemother* 22:954-957, 1982.

4. White LO: UK NEQAS in antibiotic assays, *J Clin Pathol* 53:829-834, 2000.

5. Fujimoto T, Tsuda Y, Tawa R, et al: Fluorescence polarization immunoassay of gentamicin or netilmicin in blood spotted on filter paper, *Clin Chem* 35:867-869, 1989.

6. Forest J, Mailhot C, Cartier P, et al: Comparison of a fluorescence polarization immunoassay of netilmicin in plasma, peritoneal dialysate, and urine with a high-performance liquid chromatographic method, *Ther Drug Monit* 19:74-78, 1997.

7. Hardman JG, Limbird LE, Gilman AG: *Goodman & Gilman's the pharmacological basis of therapeutics,* ed 10, New York, 2001, McGraw-Hill.

8. Bennett W, Aronof G, Golper T, et al: *Drug prescribing in renal failure. Dosing guidelines for adults,* ed 2, Philadelphia, 1994, American College of Physicians.

9. Evans WE, Schentag JJ, Jusko WJ: *Applied pharmacokinetics—principles of therapeutic drug monitoring,* ed 3, Vancouver, WA, 1992, Applied Therapeutics, Inc.

10. Micromedex: *Micromedex healthcare series 2004,* Greenwood Village, CO, 2004, Thomson Micromedex.

Nicotine (Nicotrol)[1-9]	Plasma	Nonsmokers (transdermal patch)		$t_{1/2}$:	1-4 hr nonsmokers ~2 hr smokers
Colorimetric, IA	Urine	*mcg/mL*	*μmol/L*	V_d:	1 L/kg
GLC, CE-MS		Therapeutic		PB:	5-20%
HPLC, LC-MS		concentration: 0.005-0.020 × 6.16 [0.031-0.123]			
		Toxic			
MW: 162.2		concentration: >0.4	[>2.46]		

1. Shin HS, Kim JG, Shin YJ, et al: Sensitive and simple method for the determination of nicotine and cotinine in human urine, plasma and saliva by gas chromatography-mass spectrometry, *J Chromatogr B Analyt Technol Biomed Life Sci* 769:177-183, 2002.

FACTORS INFLUENCING DRUG DISPOSITION	REMARKS AND INTERFERENCES

Drug interactions: Concomitant use of netilmicin with neuromuscular blockers may lead to aminoglycoside-induced respiratory paralysis. Coadministration of cyclosporine or tacrolimus with netilmicin may lead to increased risk of nephrotoxicity.[11]

Metabolism
  Hepatic, minor substrate of CYP1A2, CYP2A6, CYP2B6, CYP2C8/9, CYP2C19, CYP2D6, CYP2E1, and CYP3A4
Excretion
  Renal

Nicotine is used as an aid in smoking cessation. It may be delivered by over-the-counter and prescription means, including chewing gum, lozenge, patch, intranasal spray, and oral inhaler. Early effects of nicotine overdose include nausea, vomiting, abdominal pain, cold sweat, confusion, and weakness. Late effects of toxicity include hypotension, breathing difficulty, seizures, and possible death.

Nicotine is metabolized to >20 metabolites, the principal ones being cotinine and nicotine-1'-*N*-oxide. The nicotine metabolite, cotinine, is a sensitive and specific biochemical marker of exposure (direct and passive) to cigarette smoke.

See also *Cotinine.*

2.   Goldfrank LR, editor: *Goldfrank's toxicological emergencies,* ed 7, (online version), New York, 2002, The McGraw-Hill Companies Inc.

TEST NAME AND METHOD	SPECIMEN	REFERENCE (THERAPEUTIC) INTERVAL, CONVENTIONAL [INTERNATIONAL RECOMMENDED UNITS]	KINETIC VALUES

Nicotine (Nicotrol)—CONT

3. Dhar P: Measuring tobacco smoke exposure: quantifying nicotine/cotinine concentration in biological samples by colorimetry, chromatography and immunoassay methods, *J Pharm Biomed Anal* 35:155-168, 2004.

4. Baidoo EE, Clench MR, Smith RF, et al: Determination of nicotine and its metabolites in urine by solid-phase extraction and sample stacking capillary electrophoresis-mass spectrometry, *J Chromatogr B Analyt Technol Biomed Life Sci* 796:303-313, 2003.

5. Cognard E, Staub C: Determination of nicotine and its major metabolite cotinine in plasma or serum by gas chromatography-mass spectrometry using ion-trap detection, *Clin Chem Lab Med* 41:1599-1607, 2003.

6. Meger M, Meger-Kossien I, Schuler-Metz A, et al: Simultaneous determination of nicotine and eight nicotine metabolites in urine of smokers using liquid-tandem mass spectrometry, *J Chromatogr B Analyt Technol Biomed Life Sci* 778:251-261, 2002.

Nifedipine	Serum, plasma	Therapeutic concentration: Not well defined	PK^{4-8}:	
(Procardia)[1-3]	(EDTA)	Toxic concentration: Not well defined	$t_{1/2}$:	2-2.5 hr
			V_d:	1.42-2.21 L/kg
GC-MS, HPLC		Steady-state concentrations on a small number of	Cl_T:	4.3 mL/min/kg
		patients on daily dosage of 30-120 mg showed a	PB:	96-98%
MW: 346.34		mean serum concentration of 115 ng/mL.[3]	F:	17-73%

1. Martens J, Banditt P, Meyer F: Determination of nifedipine in human serum by gas chromatography-mass spectrometry: validation of the method and its use in bioavailability studies, *J Chromatogr B* 660:297-302, 1994.

2. Abou-Auda HS, Najjar TA, Al-Khamis KI, et al: Liquid chromatographic assay of nifedipine in human plasma and its application to pharmacokinetic studies, *J Pharm Biomed Anal* 22:241-249, 2000.

3. Baselt RC: *Disposition of toxic drugs and chemicals in man,* ed 7, Foster City, CA, 2004, Chemical Toxicology Institute.

4. Echizen H, Eichelbaum M: Clinical pharmacokinetics of verapamil, nifedipine, and diltiazem, *Clin Pharmacokinet* 11:425-449, 1986.

| FACTORS INFLUENCING DRUG DISPOSITION | REMARKS AND INTERFERENCES |

7. Moyer TP, Charlson JR, Enger RJ, et al: Simultaneous analysis of nicotine, nicotine metabolites, and tobacco alkaloids in serum or urine by tandem mass spectrometry, with clinically relevant metabolic profiles, *Clin Chem* 48:1460-1471, 2002.

8. Nakajima M, Yamamoto T, Kuroiwa Y, et al: Improved highly sensitive method for determination of nicotine and cotinine in human plasma by high-performance liquid chromatography, *J Chromatogr B Biomed Sci Appl* 742:211-215, 2000.

9. Leischow SJ, Merikle EP, Cook G, et al: An evaluation of NicCheck I: a dipstick method for analyzing nicotine and its metabolites, *Addict Behav* 24:145-148, 1999.

Metabolism
  Hepatic
Excretion
  Urine (primary)
  Bile/feces (secondary)
Disease[9]
  Cirrhosis: $t_{1/2}\uparrow$, $V_d\uparrow$, $Cl_T\downarrow$, $PB\downarrow$, $F\uparrow$
  Renal: $t_{1/2}\uparrow$, $V_d\uparrow$, $Cl_T\rightarrow$, $PB\downarrow$, $F\rightarrow$
Dialysis
  Hemodialysis $(-)$

Drug interactions: Nifedipine is a major substrate of CYP3A4 and minor substrate of CYP2D6. Nifedipine moderately inhibits CYP1A2. CYP3A4 inducers like carbamazepine, phenobarbital, phenytoin, and rifamycins may decrease the effects of nifedipine. CYP3A4 inhibitors like azole antifungals, ciprofloxacin, clarithromycin, and erythromycin may increase the effects of nifedipine.[10] Cimetidine may increase nifedipine serum concentrations by inhibiting hepatic metabolism. Concomitant administration of nifedipine and digoxin occasionally results in up to 50% increase in serum digoxin concentrations.[11]

Nifedipine is a calcium channel blocker with potent vasodilator activity. Its metabolism appears to exhibit oxidative polymorphism; thus there are two phenotypes (rapid and slow metabolizers) in the general population.

Nifedipine may be displaced from protein binding sites by plasticizers in collection devices. Rare cases of hepatic dysfunction have been reported.

5. Hardman JG, Limbird LE, Gilman AG: *Goodman & Gilman's the pharmacological basis of therapeutics,* ed 10, New York, 2001, McGraw-Hill.

6. Palma-Aguirre JA, Montoya-Cabrera MA, du Souich P, et al: Discrepancy between bioavailability and hypotensive effect of oral and sublingual nifedipine, *Am J Ther* 2:3-9, 1995.

7. Grundy JS, Foster RT: The nifedipine gastrointestinal therapeutic system (GITS): evaluation of pharmaceutical, pharmacokinetic and pharmacological properties, *Clin Pharmacokinet* 30:28-51, 1996.

TEST NAME AND METHOD	SPECIMEN	REFERENCE (THERAPEUTIC) INTERVAL, CONVENTIONAL [INTERNATIONAL RECOMMENDED UNITS]				KINETIC VALUES	

Nifedipine—CONT

8. Castaneda-Hernandez G, Palma-Aguirre JA, Montoya-Cabrera MA, et al: Interethnic variability in nifedipine disposition: reduced systemic plasma clearance in Mexican subjects (letter), *Br J Clin Pharmacol* 41:433-434, 1996.

9. Kleinbloesem CH, Van Brummelen P, van Harten J, et al: Nifedipine: influence of renal function on pharmacokinetic/hemodynamic relationship, *Clin Pharmacol Ther* 37:563-574, 1985.

Nitrous Oxide	Whole blood	Anesthetic concentration:	17-22 mL/dL [$\times$ 10 = 170-220 mL/L] or 17-22 volume %		$t_{1/2}$: 5 min
GC-MS,[1] *GLC*[2]					
MW: 44.01		Toxic concentration:	Sedation and confusion occur with 40% N_2O inhalation; 80% results in unconciousness.		

1. Baselt RC: *Disposition of toxic drugs and chemicals in man,* ed 7, Foster City, CA, 2004, Chemical Toxicology Institute.

2. Baselt RC: *Analytic procedures for therapeutic drug monitoring and emergency toxicology,* ed 2, Davis, CA, 1987, Biomedical Publications.

3. Micromedex: *Micromedex healthcare series 2004,* Greenwood Village, CO, 2004, Thomson Micromedex.

Nonsteroidal Antiinflammatory Drugs (NSAIDs)[1-17]

Diclofenac	Serum, plasma		*mcg/mL*		*µmol/L*	$t_{1/2}$:	2 hr
(Voltaren)	(EDTA)	Therapeutic concentration:	0.5-3	$\times$ 3.34	[1.67-10]	V_d:	0.12-0.55 L/kg
HPLC, GC,		Toxic				Cl_T:	266 mL/min
LC-MS, GC, MS		concentration:	>60		[>200]	PB:	>99%
						F:	50%
MW: 318.13						T_{max}:	1-2 hr
GC, LC-MS, GC-MS	Urine						

FACTORS INFLUENCING DRUG DISPOSITION	REMARKS AND INTERFERENCES

10. Lexi-Comp, Inc: *Up-to-date online 12.2. Drug information,* Hudson, OH, 2004, Lexi-Comp, Inc.
11. Micromedex: *Micromedex healthcare series 2004,* Greenwood Village, CO, 2004, Thomson Micromedex.

The gas is eliminated very rapidly by pulmonary diffusion. There is no evidence of biotransformation.[1]

Drug interactions: Nitrous oxide can increase the neuromuscular blocking effect of nondepolarizing muscle relaxants (e.g., pancuronium, gallamine, tubocurarine, vecuronium), leading to respiratory depression.[3]

This is a nonflammable, nearly odorless gas that is a good analgesic at safe concentrations. It is sometimes abused, and fatalities have occurred as a result of simple asphyxia.[1]

Metabolism
   Hepatic
Excretion
   Renal, biliary
Disease
   Rheumatic disease: $C_{max}\downarrow$
Dialysis
   Hemodialysis $(-)$
   Peritoneal $(-)$

Drug interactions: Aluminum or magnesium hydroxide containing antacids may decrease the rate of absorption of diclofenac. Diclofenac may decrease the renal elimination of lithium, digoxin, and methotrexate, causing increases in serum concentrations. The drug may decrease the antihypertensive and diuretic effects of hydrochlorothiazide and furosemide and may increase renal toxicity of cyclosporine.

Food decreases the rate but not the extent of absorption of diclofenac. Age does not appear to affect diclofenac disposition. Side effects include nausea, vomiting, dizziness, drowsiness, edema, rash, peptic ulceration, and gastrointestinal bleeding. The mean peak plasma concentrations of diclofenac after oral doses of 50 mg and 75 mg are 1.5 and 1.9 mg/L [$\times$ 3.14 = 4.7 and 6.0 μmol/L], respectively.

TEST NAME AND METHOD	SPECIMEN	REFERENCE (THERAPEUTIC) INTERVAL, CONVENTIONAL [INTERNATIONAL RECOMMENDED UNITS]				KINETIC VALUES	

Nonsteroidal Antiinflammatory Drugs—CONT

Diflunisal (*Dolobid*) HPLC, GC, LC-MS MW: 250.20	Serum, plasma (EDTA). Stable for at least 14 days at −20° C.		*mcg/mL*		µ*mol/L*	$t_{1/2}$: V_d: Cl_T:	5-20 hr 0.1 L/kg dose-dependent (8 mL/min for 500-mg dose)
		Therapeutic concentration:	40-200	× 4.00	[160-800]		
		Toxic concentration:	>300		[1200]		
						PB:	99%
						T_{max}:	1-2 hr
GC, HPLC, LC-MS	Urine						

Fenoprofen (*Nalfon*) GLC, HPLC, CZE MW: 242.27	Serum, plasma (heparin, EDTA)		*mcg/mL*		µ*mol/L*	$t_{1/2}$: V_d: Cl_T: PB:	1.5-3 hr 0.18-0.1 L/kg 0.69 mL/min/kg 99% [× 0.01 = 0.99, protein-bound mole fraction]
		Therapeutic concentration:	25-60	× 4.13	[103-248]		
						F:	80-85% [× 0.01 = 0.80-0.85, bioavailable mole fraction]
						T_{max}:	0.5-2 hr

Ibuprofen (*Motrin, Rufen, Advil, Nuprin, others*) HPLC, GC, GC-MS, CZE MW: 206.28	Serum, plasma (EDTA)		*mcg/mL*		µ*mol/L*	$t_{1/2}$: V_d: Cl_T/F: PB:	1.8-2 hr 0.11-0.18 L/kg 0.55-0.95 mL/min/kg ≥99% [× 0.01 = 0.99, protein-bound mole fraction]
		Therapeutic concentration:	15-30	× 4.85	[73-146]		
		Toxic concentration:	>200		[970]		
						F:	58-70% racemic mixture [× 0.01 = >0.80, bioavailable mole fraction] 92%, S-ibuprofen [× 0.01 = 0.92, bio-available mole fraction]
						T_{max}:	1.4-1.9 hr

FACTORS INFLUENCING DRUG DISPOSITION	REMARKS AND INTERFERENCES

Metabolism
  Hepatic
Excretion
  Renal
Disease
  Renal failure: $Cl_T\downarrow$, $PB\downarrow$
Dialysis
  Hemodialysis ($-$)
  Peritoneal ($-$)

Drug interactions: Aluminum hydroxide containing antacids decrease the extent of absorption of this drug, and the bioavailability of diflunisal is decreased with the concomitant administration of aspirin. Diflunisal decreases steady-state warfarin concentrations, but it does not appear to affect anticoagulant response. Diflunisal may decrease the renal elimination of digoxin, lithium, and methotrexate.

Food decreases the rate but not the extent of diflunisal absorption. Diflunisal elimination is dose-dependent, and the time to reach steady-state increases with dose. Side effects include nausea, vomiting, peptic ulceration, gastrointestinal bleeding, dizziness, drowsiness, and edema.

Interferences: Diflunisal interferes with the FPIA assay for salicylic acid.

Metabolism
  Hepatic
Excretion
  Renal
Dialysis
  Hemodialysis ($-$)
  Peritoneal ($-$)

Drug interactions: Aspirin decreases plasma fenoprofen concentrations. Probenecid may increase plasma fenoprofen concentrations. Fenoprofen may increase plasma concentrations of digoxin, lithium, and methotrexate.

Fenoprofen is metabolized in the liver to form 4-hydroxyfenoprofen glucuronide and fenoprofen glucuronide. Food decreases both the rate and extent of absorption. Adverse effects include gastrointestinal disturbance, skin eruptions, tinnitus, confusion, and anorexia. Rare cases of leukopenia and thrombocytopenia and cases of nephrotoxicity and hepatotoxicity have occurred.

Metabolism
  Hepatic
Excretion
  Renal
Disease
  Cirrhosis: $t_{1/2}\uparrow$
Dialysis
  Hemodialysis ($-$)
  Peritoneal ($-$)

Drug interactions: Ibuprofen may cause an increase in plasma concentrations of digoxin, lithium, and methotrexate.

Ibuprofen is administered as both a racemic mixture and as the active S-enantiomer, dexibuprofen. Some inactive R-ibuprofen is metabolized to the active isomer. Disposition is stereoselective, and the drug follows nonlinear kinetics, which is probably because of saturable protein binding. Concentrations may remain elevated in synovial fluid long after plasma levels have declined. Adverse effects include gastrointestinal disturbances, thrombocytopenia, leukopenia, skin eruptions, and blurred vision. Hepatic dysfunction and nephrotoxicity have been reported. Rarely, cases of aseptic meningitis have occurred. High-dose ibuprofen therapy is used in treating children with cystic fibrosis.

TEST NAME AND METHOD	SPECIMEN	REFERENCE (THERAPEUTIC) INTERVAL, CONVENTIONAL [INTERNATIONAL RECOMMENDED UNITS]				KINETIC VALUES	

Nonsteroidal Antiinflammatory Drugs—CONT

Indomethacin	Serum, plasma		*mcg/mL*		μ*mol/L*	$t_{1/2}$:	5-10 hr, adults
(Indocin)	(EDTA). Stable for	Therapeutic					10-33 hr, neonates
	at least 14 days at	concentration:	0.3-3.0	× 2.79	[0.84-8.4]	V_d:	0.34-1.57 L/kg
HPLC, GC,	−20° C.	Toxic				Cl_T:	70-140 mL/min
GC-MS, CZE		concentration:	>4		[11]	PB:	99%
						F:	100%
GC, HPLC	Urine					T_{max}:	2 hr

MW: 357.79

Ketoprofen	Serum, plasma		*mcg/mL*		μ*mol/L*	$t_{1/2}$:	2-4 hr
(Orudis)	(EDTA)	Therapeutic				V_d:	0.1-0.5 L/kg
		concentration:	1-20	× 3.93	[3.9-79]	Cl_T:	87 mL/min
MW: 254.29		Toxic				PB:	98.7%
		concentration:	>1100		[4323]	F:	90%
						T_{max}:	0.5-2 hr

FACTORS INFLUENCING DRUG DISPOSITION	REMARKS AND INTERFERENCES

Metabolism
  Hepatic
Excretion
  Renal, biliary, and fecal
Age
  Premature newborns: $t_{1/2}\uparrow$
Elderly: $t_{1/2}\uparrow$
Dialysis
  Hemodialysis ($-$)
  Peritoneal ($-$)

Drug interactions: Magnesium- and aluminum-containing antacids may decrease the rate of absorption but not extent. Sodium bicarbonate increases the absorption rate of indomethacin. Probenecid increases plasma indomethacin concentrations. Indomethacin may increase plasma concentrations of digoxin, lithium, and methotrexate by decreasing renal excretion. Indomethacin may inhibit the diuretic effect of furosemide.

A dose-response relationship has been demonstrated for the inhibition of prostaglandin synthesis, but in rheumatoid arthritis patients, no significant differences in mean steady-state plasma indomethacin concentrations were seen between responders and nonresponders. Indomethacin is almost completely absorbed after oral administration. It undergoes extensive enterohepatic recirculation, which may account for its variable elimination $t_{1/2}$. Adverse effects include peptic ulceration, leukopenia, agranulocytosis, thrombocytopenia, nausea, vomiting, dizziness, and tinnitus. Adverse effects increase with increasing plasma indomethacin concentrations.

Metabolism
  Hepatic
Excretion
  Renal
Dialysis
  Hemodialysis ($-$)
  Peritoneal ($-$)

Drug interactions: Salicylates may reduce ketoprofen's conjugative metabolism while increasing the drug's conversion to nonconjugated metabolites. Salicylates also displace ketoprofen from plasma protein binding sites. Probenecid may inhibit the conjugation of ketoprofen. In addition, probenecid inhibits the renal excretion of ketoprofen conjugates. Ketoprofen may increase plasma concentrations of digoxin, lithium, and methotrexate by decreasing their renal elimination.

Administering probenecid along with ketoprofen may decrease the peak to trough variation seen with ketoprofen. Mean steady-state C_{max} of ketoprofen after a 50-mg dose given four times a day are ~5.6 mcg/mL [$\times$ 3.93 = 22 μmol/L]. Side effects include dyspepsia, peptic ulceration, gastrointestinal bleeding, headache, insomnia, anxiety, thrombocytopenia, anemia, agranulocytosis, rash, and edema. Rare cases of nephrotoxicity and hepatotoxicity have been reported.

TEST NAME AND METHOD	SPECIMEN	REFERENCE (THERAPEUTIC) INTERVAL, CONVENTIONAL [INTERNATIONAL RECOMMENDED UNITS]			KINETIC VALUES	

Nonsteroidal Antiinflammatory Drugs—CONT

Ketorolac	Serum, plasma		*mcg/mL*		μ*mol/L*	$t_{1/2}$:	4-10 hr
(Toradol)		Therapeutic				V_d:	0.17-0.5 L/kg
		concentration:	0.5-3	× 2.66	[1.33-8]	Cl_T:	0.35-0.55 mL/min/kg
HPLC, LC-MS		Toxic				PB:	>99%
		concentration:	>5		[13.3]	F:	100%
MW: 255.27						T_{max}:	0.3-1.0 hr

Mefenamic acid	Plasma	No generally recognized therapeutic range.	$t_{1/2}$:	2-4 hr
(Ponstel)			V_d:	1.3 L/kg
			T_{max}:	1-3 hr
HPLC, GC				
MW: 241.29				

Naproxen	Serum, plasma		*mcg/mL*		μ*mol/L*	$t_{1/2}$:	12-15 hr
(Naprosyn,	(heparin). Stable	Therapeutic				V_d:	0.1-0.3 L/kg
Anaprox)	for at least 14 days	concentration,				Cl_T:	5 mL/min
	at −20° C.	trough:	20-100	× 4.34	[87-434]	PB:	99%
HPLC, GC, LC-		Toxic				F:	100%
MS, CZE, GC-MS		concentration:	>200		[868]	T_{max}:	2-4 hr
MW: 230.26							
HPLC, GC-MS,	Urine						
LC-MS							

FACTORS INFLUENCING DRUG DISPOSITION	REMARKS AND INTERFERENCES

Metabolism
  Hepatic
Excretion
  Renal
Disease
  Renal dysfunction: $t_{1/2}\uparrow$, $Cl_T\downarrow$
Age
  Elderly: $t_{1/2}\uparrow$, $Cl_T\downarrow$
Dialysis
  Hemodialysis $(-)$
  Peritoneal $(-)$

Drug interactions: Ketorolac may enhance the activity of nondepolarizing muscle relaxants. Additionally, the drug may increase plasma concentrations of lithium and methotrexate.

Maximum concentrations after a 10-mg oral and 30-mg IM dose of ketorolac are 0.86 and 3.0 mg/L [$\times 2.66 = 2.3$-8.0 μmol/L], respectively. Up to 60% of ketorolac may be excreted unchanged in the urine. Adverse effects include dyspepsia, nausea, gastrointestinal pain, diarrhea, flatulence, vomiting, peptic ulcer, and gastrointestinal bleeding. Thrombocytopenia, nephrotoxicity, and hepatotoxicity have been reported.

Metabolism
  Hepatic
Excretion
  Renal
Dialysis
  Hemodialysis $(-)$
  Peritoneal $(-)$

Drug interactions: As with other NSAIDs, mefenamic acid may increase plasma concentrations of digoxin, lithium, and methotrexate. Mefenamic acid may increase the anticoagulant effect of warfarin.

Most mefenamic acid is metabolized to 3′-hydroxymethyl and 3′-carboxyl metabolites. A 1-g dose of mefenamic acid given orally yields a mean C_{max} of 10 mcg/mL [$\times 4.14 = 41$ μmol/L]. Plasma concentrations of mefenamic acid >10 mcg/mL [>41 μmol/L] may be associated with toxicity. Side effects are similar to other NSAIDs, with diarrhea being the most common. Occasional incidences of leukopenia, eosinophilia, agranulocytosis, nephrotoxicity, and hepatotoxicity are reported. The drug may cause a false-positive result for urinary bile with the diazo tablet test.

Metabolism
  Hepatic
Excretion
  Renal
Disease
  Renal insufficiency: $V_d\uparrow$, $Cl_T\uparrow$
Dialysis
  Hemodialysis $(-)$
  Peritoneal $(-)$

Drug interactions: Sodium bicarbonate increases the rate of absorption of this drug, whereas antacids containing magnesium and aluminum hydroxide decrease its absorption rate. Probenecid increases plasma naproxen concentrations. Like other NSAIDs, naproxen increases plasma concentrations of digoxin, lithium, and methotrexate.

The conjugated metabolite of naproxen may undergo hydrolysis in the urine. Freezing and thawing of the urine sample may promote more rapid hydrolysis than occurs at room temperature. The concentration of naproxen in the synovial fluid is $\sim 50\%$ that of plasma concentrations. Naproxen exhibits saturable plasma protein binding and therefore exhibits a nonlinear plasma concentration response at high doses and increased renal clearance at high plasma concentrations. Side effects include heartburn, abdominal pain, nausea, constipation, diarrhea, flatulence, peptic ulceration, gastrointestinal bleeding, thrombocytopenia, leukopenia, granulocytopenia, and eosinophilia. Nephrotoxicity and hepatotoxicity have been reported.

TEST NAME AND METHOD	SPECIMEN	REFERENCE (THERAPEUTIC) INTERVAL, CONVENTIONAL [INTERNATIONAL RECOMMENDED UNITS]			KINETIC VALUES	

Nonsteroidal Antiinflammatory Drugs—CONT

Phenylbutazone	Serum, plasma		*mcg/mL*	µ*mol/L*	$t_{1/2}$:	50-72 hr
(Butazolidin)	(EDTA). Unstable	Therapeutic			V_d:	0.097-0.17 L/kg
	in solution.	concentration: 50-100	× 3.24	[162-324]	Cl_T:	0.03 mL/min/kg
GC, HPLC, LC-MS		Toxic			PB:	87-99%
		concentration: >100		[>324]		[× 0.01 = 0.87-0.99,
MW: 308.38						protein-bound mole
		Oxyphenbutazone (active metabolite)				fraction]
		Therapeutic concentration: 25-50 mcg/mL			T_{max}:	2-3 hr
		[× 3.08 = 77-154 µmol/L]				

Piroxicam	Serum, plasma.		*mcg/mL*	µ*mol/L*	$t_{1/2}$:	31-57 hr
(Feldene)	Plasma samples	Therapeutic			V_d:	0.12-0.14 L/kg
	stable for at least	concentration: 2-6	× 3.02	[6-18]	Cl_T:	2-3 mL/min
HPLC	14 days at −20° C.	Toxic concentration: >14		[42]	PB:	≥99%
					T_{max}:	2-3 hr
MW: 331.35						

HPLC	Urine

FACTORS INFLUENCING DRUG DISPOSITION	REMARKS AND INTERFERENCES

Metabolism
  Hepatic
Excretion
  Renal
Disease
  Cirrhosis: $t_{1/2}\uparrow\rightarrow$, $Cl_T/F\downarrow$, $PB\downarrow$
  Renal: $V_d/F\uparrow$, $PB\downarrow$
Age
  Child: $t_{1/2}\downarrow$
  Elderly: $t_{1/2}\rightarrow$, $Cl_T\downarrow$
Malnutrition
  $t_{1/2}\downarrow$, 35.9 ± 3.3 hr
  $V_d/F\uparrow$, 0.145 ± 0.010 L/kg
  $Cl_T/F\uparrow$, 0.055 ± 0.0073 mL/min/kg
  $PB\downarrow$, 85 ± 2.51%

Drug interactions: Phenylbutazone enhances the anticoagulant effects of warfarin. The drug may also enhance the hypoglycemic effect of some sulfonylureas. In addition, the drug may decrease the concentrations of digoxin and digitoxin.

Phenylbutazone is metabolized to the pharmacologically active metabolites oxyphenbutazone ($t_{1/2}$ = 72 hr) and 3-hydroxyphenylbutazone (possesses primarily uricosuric properties). Because of extensive metabolism, protein binding, and passive reabsorption in the distal renal tubule, only traces are excreted in urine.

After a single dose, glucuronidation seems to be the dominant reaction, whereas oxidation reactions increase with multiple dosing (i.e., clearance increases with multiple dosing to 0.03 mL/min/kg). Adverse effects include peptic ulcer, hypersensitivity reactions, ulcerative stomatitis, hepatitis, nephritis, aplastic anemia, leukopenia, agranulocytosis, and thrombocytopenia. The $t_{1/2}$ is dose dependent. Spectrophotometry measures the drug and its metabolites; GLC measures the drug only. HPLC measures the drug but has poor response to the metabolite.

Metabolism
  Hepatic
Excretion
  Renal
Dialysis
  Hemodialysis (−)
  Peritoneal (−)

Drug interactions: Concomitant aspirin administration may decrease piroxicam concentrations. Piroxicam may increase plasma digoxin, lithium, and methotrexate concentrations.

With a dose of 20 mg/day, the peak concentration at steady state is in the range of 4.5-8.0 mcg/mL [14-24 μmol/L]. There is no correlation between toxic effects and plasma piroxicam concentrations. Food decreases the rate of absorption and may decrease the extent. Piroxicam undergoes enterhepatic recirculation. The therapeutic threshold (6.7 mcg/mL [20 μmol/L]) is not well defined. Side effects include epigastric distress, nausea, constipation, stomatitis, diarrhea, flatulence, peptic ulceration, and gastrointestinal bleeding. Less frequent adverse effects include anemia, leukopenia, eosinophilia, thrombocytopenia, nephrotoxicity, and hepatotoxicity.

TEST NAME AND METHOD	SPECIMEN	REFERENCE (THERAPEUTIC) INTERVAL, CONVENTIONAL [INTERNATIONAL RECOMMENDED UNITS]		KINETIC VALUES	

Nonsteroidal Antiinflammatory Drugs—CONT

Salicylic acid	Serum, plasma (EDTA). Collect at trough concentration.		*mcg/mL* *mmol/L*	$t_{1/2}$:	2.4-3.0 hr
HPLC, GC, IA, CZE		Therapeutic concentration		V_d:	0.15-0.20 L/kg
				PB:	90-95% at <100 mcg/mL
MW: 138.12		Analgesia, antipyresis:	<100 × 0.00724 [<0.72]		[× 0.01 = 0.90-0.95, protein-bound mole fraction at <0.72 mmol/L]
HPLC, CZE	Urine	Antiinflammatory:	150-300 [1.09-2.17]		50% at >400 mcg/mL [× 0.01 = 0.50, protein-bound mole fraction at >2.90 mmol/L]
		Toxic concentration		F:	100%
		Gastric intolerance, impaired hemostasis:	>100 [>0.72]		[× 0.01 = 1.00, bioavailable mole fraction]
		Deafness, headache, vertigo, tinnitus:	150-300 × 0.00724 [1.09-2.17]		
		Nausea, vomiting, hyperventilation:	250-400 [1.81-2.90]		
		Intoxication:	>500 [>3.62]		

Sulindac (Clinoril)	Serum, plasma (EDTA). Stable for at least 14 days at −20° C.	No generally recognized therapeutic range.	$t_{1/2}$:	7 hr (active sulfide, 16 hr)
HPLC, EIA			V_d:	0.12-0.17 L/kg
			PB:	≥93%
MW: 356.42			F:	≥88%
			T_{max}:	1-2 hr

| FACTORS INFLUENCING DRUG DISPOSITION | REMARKS AND INTERFERENCES |

Metabolism
  Hepatic
Excretion
  Renal (secondary)
Disease or condition
  Hepatic: $Cl_T\downarrow\rightarrow$, PB$\downarrow$
  Renal: $Cl_T\uparrow$, PB$\downarrow$
  Pregnancy: PB$\uparrow$
  Hypoalbuminemia: PB$\downarrow$
Age
  Newborn: $t_{1/2}\uparrow$, $Cl_T\downarrow$, PB$\downarrow$

Drug interactions: Alkalinization of the urine (pH 8) will increase the renal clearance, whereas acidification will decrease it. Plasma concentrations of salicylic acid may be decreased by aluminum or magnesium hydroxides.

Salicylic acid is the major hydrolysis product of acetylsalicylic acid (ASA, aspirin) metabolism. Its kinetic parameters ($t_{1/2}$, V_d, Cl_T, PB) are dose or concentration dependent. As the concentration increases, the apparent $t_{1/2}\uparrow$, $V_d\uparrow$, $Cl_T\downarrow\rightarrow$, and PB$\downarrow$.

See Tables II-5 and II-6.

Salicyluric acid and salicylphenolic glucuronide undergo dose/concentration-dependent metabolism and follow Michaelis-Menten kinetics. The renal excretion of salicylic acid is dependent on urinary pH. Severe toxicity is characterized by CNS disturbances (EEG abnormalities), skin eruptions, and marked alterations in acid-base balance. A respiratory alkalosis is produced that may revert to metabolic acidosis, particularly in young children. High doses of the drug may increase liver enzymes and may cause acidosis. The estimated minimum lethal adult dose is 15 g. Cases of leukopenia and thrombocytopenia have been reported.

Interferences: Colorimetric and fluorometric methods are subject to a number of interferences but are useful as emergency procedures. Diflunisal interferes with the FPIA and colorimetric methods. Other drugs and metabolites may interfere. Lipemic, icteric, or hemolyzed specimens may yield false-positive results with colorimetric methods.[21]

Metabolismn
  Hepatic
Dialysis
  Hemodialysis ($-$)
  Peritoneal ($-$)

Drug interactions: Sulindac may increase plasma concentrations of digoxin, lithium, and methotrexate. Aspirin may decrease plasma concentrations of sulindac's active sulfide metabolite. Probenecid increases plasma concentrations of sulindac and its sulfone metabolite.

Sulindac is metabolized to its active metabolite sulindac sulfide, which has a longer $t_{1/2}$ than the parent drug. The active metabolite reaches its maximum plasma concentration in ~2 hr. A 200-mg dose of sulindac leads to a mean C_{max} of 4 mcg/mL [11 μmol/L], 3 mcg/mL [8 μmol/L], and 2 mcg/mL [6 μmol/L] for sulindac and its sulfide and sulfone metabolites, respectively. Oxidation to the sulfone metabolite is irreversible, whereas reduction to sulindac sulfide is reversible. Adverse effects include dyspepsia, gastrointestinal distress, flatulence, diarrhea, constipation, vomiting, gastritis, peptic ulceration, and gastrointestinal bleeding. Cases of leukopenia, thrombocytopenia, hemolytic anemia, nephrotoxicity, and hepatotoxicity have been reported.

TEST NAME AND METHOD	SPECIMEN	REFERENCE (THERAPEUTIC) INTERVAL, CONVENTIONAL [INTERNATIONAL RECOMMENDED UNITS]			KINETIC VALUES	

Nonsteroidal Antiinflammatory Drugs—CONT

Tolmetin (*Tolectin*)	Serum, plasma		*mcg/mL*	*mmol/L*	$t_{1/2}$:	4-6 hr
		Therapeutic			V_d:	0.1-0.14 L/kg
HPLC, GC		concentration:	10-80 × 3.90	[39-312]	Cl_T:	125 mL/min
					PB:	99%
MW: 257.29					T_{max}:	0.5-1.0 hr

TLC	Urine

1. Arranz I, Martin-Suarez A, Lanao JM, et al: Population pharmacokinetics of high dose ibuprofen in cystic fibrosis, *Arch Dis Child* 88:1128-1130, 2003.

2. Baselt C: *Disposition of toxic drugs and chemicals in man,* ed 7, Foster City, CA, 2004, Biomedical Publications.

3. Bonato PS, Del Lama MP, de Carvalho R: Enantioselective determination of ibuprofen in plasma by high-performance liquid chromatography-electrospray mass spectrometry, *J Chromatogr B Analyt Technol Biomed Life Sci* 796:413-420, 2003.

4. Kokki H, Tuomilehto H, Karvinen M: Pharmacokinetics of ketoprofen following oral and intramuscular administration in young children, *Eur J Clin Pharmacol* 57:643-647, 2001.

5. Borenstein MR, Xue Y, Cooper S, et al: Sensitive capillary gas chromatographic-mass spectrometric-selected-ion monitoring method for the determination of diclofenac concentrations in human plasma, *J Chromatogr B Biomed Appl* 685:59-66, 1996.

6. Davies NM, Anderson KE: Clinical pharmacokinetics of diclofenac. Therapeutic insights and pitfalls, *Clin Pharmacokinet* 33:184-213, 1997.

7. Davies NM: Clinical pharmacokinetics of ibuprofen: the first 30 years, *Clin Pharmacokinet* 34:101-154, 1998.

8. Dionne RA, Gordon SM, Tahara M, et al: Analgesic efficacy and pharmacokinetics of ketoprofen administered into a surgical site, *J Clin Pharmacol* 39:131-138, 1999.

9. Kincaid RL, McMullin MM, Sanders D, et al: Sensitive, selective detection and differentiation of salicylates and metabolites in urine by a simple HPTLC method, *J Anal Toxicol* 15:270-271, 1991.

10. Makino K, Itoh Y, Teshima D, et al: Determination of nonsteroidal anti-inflammatory drugs in human specimens by capillary zone electrophoresis and micellar electrokinetic chromatography, *Electrophoresis* 25:1488-1495, 2004.

11. Makino K, Yano T, Maiguma T, et al: A rapid and simultaneous determination of several analgesic antiinflammatory agents by capillary zone electrophoresis, *Ther Drug Monit* 25:574-580, 2003.

12. Maurer HH, Tauvel FX, Kraemer T: Screening procedure for detection of non-steroidal anti-inflammatory drugs and their metabolites in urine as part of a systematic toxicological analysis procedure for acidic drugs and poisons by gas chromatography-mass spectrometry after extractive methylation, *J Anal Toxicol* 25:237-244, 2001.

13. Pai YF, Liu CY: Capillary electrochromatographic separation of non-steroidal anti-inflammatory drugs with a histidine bonded phase, *J Chromatogr A* 982:293-301, 2001.

14. Sadecka J, Hercegova A, Polonsky J: Determination of fenoprofen in serum by capillary isotachophoresis, *J Chromatogr B Biomed Sci Appl* 729:11-17, 1999.

15. Schulz M, Schmoldt A: Therapeutic and toxic blood concentrations of more than 800 drugs and other xenobiotics, *Pharmazie* 58:447-474, 2003.

16. Vane JR, Botting RM: The mechanism of action of aspirin, *Thromb Res* 110:255-258, 2003.

| FACTORS INFLUENCING DRUG DISPOSITION | REMARKS AND INTERFERENCES |

Metabolism
  Hepatic
Excretion
  Renal
Dialysis
  Hemodialysis (−)
  Peritoneal (−)

Drug interactions: Aspirin may reduce plasma tolmetin concentrations. Tolmetin may increase plasma digoxin, lithium, and methotrexate concentrations.

Tolmetin is primarily metabolized by oxidation. A 300-mg dose of tolmetin led to a C_{max} of 29 mcg/mL [113 μmol/L]. Plasma tolmetin concentrations >60 mcg/mL [>233 μmol/L] are associated with toxic effects. Adverse effects include dyspepsia, abdominal pain, gastrointestinal distress, flatulence, diarrhea, constipation, vomiting, gastritis, anorexia, peptic ulcer, and gastrointestinal bleeding. Cases of leukopenia, thrombocytopenia, and hemolytic anemia have been reported rarely. Severe hepatic reactions and nephrotoxicity have been reported.

17. Hirai T, Matsumoto S, Kishi I: Simultaneous analysis of several non-steroidal anti-inflammatory drugs in human urine by high-performance liquid chromatography with normal solid-phase extraction, *J Chromatogr B Biomed Sci Appl* 692:375-388, 1997.

18. White S, Wong SH: Standards of laboratory practice: analgesic drug monitoring. National Academy of Clinical Biochemistry, *Clin Chem* 44:1110-1123, 1998.

19. Wu KK: Aspirin and other cyclooxygenase inhibitors: new therapeutic insights, *Semin Vasc Med* 3:107-112, 2003.

TEST NAME AND METHOD	SPECIMEN	REFERENCE (THERAPEUTIC) INTERVAL, CONVENTIONAL [INTERNATIONAL RECOMMENDED UNITS]	KINETIC VALUES
Ofloxacin **(Floxin)**[1-3] *HPLC, MB* *MW: 361.37*	Serum, plasma (heparin)	See *Remarks*.	PK^{4-6}: $t_{1/2}$: 5-8 hr V_d: 2.4-3.5 L/kg Cl_T: 230-280 mL/min PB: 25% F: 95-100%

1. Ohkubo T, Kudo M, Sugawara K: Determination of ofloxacin in human serum by high-performance liquid chromatography with column switching, *J Chromatogr* 573:289-293, 1992.
2. Immanuel C, Hemanth Kumar AK: Simple and rapid high-performance liquid chromatography method for the determination of ofloxacin concentrations in plasma and urine, *J Chromatogr B Biomed Sci Appl* 760:91-95, 2001.
3. Kalager T, Diagranes A, Bergan T, et al: Ofloxacin serum and skin blister fluid pharmacokinetics in the fasting and non-fasting states, *J Antimicrob Chemother* 17:795-800, 1986.
4. Guay DR, Opsahl JA, McMahon FG, et al: Safety and pharmacokinetics of multiple doses of intravenous ofloxacin in healthy volunteers, *Antimicrob Agents Chemother* 36:308-312, 1992.
5. Lamp KC, Bailey EM, Rybak MJ: Ofloxacin clinical pharmacokinetics, *Clin Pharmacokinet* 22:32-46, 1992.
6. Micromedex: *Micromedex healthcare series 2004,* Greenwood Village, CO, 2004, Thomson Micromedex.
7. Lexi-Comp, Inc: *Up-to-date online 12.2. Drug information,* Hudson, OH, 2004, Lexi-Comp, Inc.

TEST NAME AND METHOD	SPECIMEN					KINETIC VALUES
Oxazepam **(Serax)**[1-8] *GC, HPLC, GC-MS, LC-MS* *MW: 286.7*	Serum, plasma (EDTA)	Therapeutic concentration: Toxic concentration:	*mcg/mL* 0.2-1.4 >2.0	× 3.49	*μmol/L* [0.7-4.9] [6.98]	$t_{1/2}$: 5-15 hr V_d: 0.6-2.0 L/kg Cl_T: 0.9-2.0 mL/min/kg PB: 86-99% [× 0.01 = 0.86-0.99, protein-bound mole fraction] T_{max}: 4 hr
IA, GC-MS	Urine					

FACTORS INFLUENCING DRUG DISPOSITION	REMARKS AND INTERFERENCES

Metabolism
  Hepatic (small amount)
Excretion
  Urine (primary)
  Feces (secondary)
Disease or condition
  Renal dysfunction: $t_{1/2}\uparrow$, $Cl_T\downarrow$
Age
  Elderly: $t_{1/2}\uparrow$
Dialysis
  Hemodialysis (+)

Drug interactions: Ofloxacin is a strong inhibitor of CYP1A2. Ofloxacin may increase the effects of CYP1A2 substrates like theophylline and fluvoxamine.[7] Sucralfate, aluminum- and magnesium-containing antacids, and products containing calcium, iron, or zinc may decrease the bioavailability of ofloxacin. Probenecid may decrease renal clearance of ofloxacin. Ofloxacin may increase the degree of warfarin-induced anticoagulation.

Ofloxacin is a fluoroquinolone antibiotic. Therapeutic concentrations of ofloxacin are dependent on the MIC of the organism being treated. MIC values ≤4 mg/L [× 2.77 = ≤11 μmol/L] are considered susceptible to moderately susceptible. Doses of 200 mg, 400 mg, and 600 mg lead to plasma C_{max} of 1.6-2.2 mg/L [4.4-6.1 μmol/L], 3.2-4.3 mg/L [8.9-11.9 μmol/L], and 6.7-8.1 mg/L [18.5-22.4 μmol/L], respectively.

Interferences: The presence of other antimicrobials may interfere with bioassays.

Metabolism
  Hepatic
Excretion
  Renal, glucuronide
Disease
  Renal: $t_{1/2}\uparrow$, $V_d\uparrow$, $Cl_T\uparrow$, $PB\uparrow$
  Liver: $t_{1/2}\rightarrow$, $V_d\rightarrow$, $Cl_T\rightarrow$, $PB\rightarrow$
  Hyperthyroidism: $t_{1/2}\downarrow$, $Cl_T\uparrow$
Age
  Neonate: $t_{1/2}\uparrow$
  Elderly: $t_{1/2}\rightarrow$, $V_d\rightarrow$, $Cl_T\rightarrow$, $PB\rightarrow$
Dialysis[9]
  Hemodialysis (−)

Oxazepam is a short-acting benzodiazepine used for the management of anxiety disorders, alcohol withdrawal agitation, or for short-term relief of anxiety symptoms. It is conjugated directly and not metabolized like many other benzodiazepines (CYP3A4, CYP2c19). Side effects include confusion, ataxia, excitement, agitation, transient hypotension, vertigo, fever, and GI upset. Other side effects include leukopenia and liver damage. Oxazepam is a common metabolite of diazepam, chlordiazepoxide, clorazepate, halazepam, prazepam, medazepam, and temazepam.

See also *Diazepam*.

TEST NAME AND METHOD	SPECIMEN	REFERENCE (THERAPEUTIC) INTERVAL, CONVENTIONAL [INTERNATIONAL RECOMMENDED UNITS]		KINETIC VALUES

Oxazepam—CONT

1. Kratzsch C, Tenberken O, Peters FT, et al: Screening, library-assisted identification and validated quantification of 23 benzodiazepines, flumazenil, zaleplone, zolpidem and zopiclone in plasma by liquid chromatography/mass spectrometry with atmospheric pressure chemical ionization, *J Mass Spectrom* 39:856-872, 2004.

2. Borrey D, Meyer E, Lambert W, et al: Simultaneous determination of fifteen low-dosed benzodiazepines in human urine by solid-phase extraction and gas chromatography-mass spectrometry, *J Chromatogr B Biomed Sci Appl* 765:187-197, 2001.

3. Reubsaet KJ, Ragnar Norli H, Hemmersbach P, et al: Determination of benzodiazepines in human urine and plasma with solvent modified solid phase micro extraction and gas chromatography; rationalization of method development using experimental design strategies, *J Pharm Biomed Anal* 18:667-680, 1998.

4. El Mahjoub A, Staub C: Semiautomated high-performance liquid chromatographic method for the determination of benzodiazepines in whole blood, *J Anal Toxicol* 25:209-214, 2001.

5. Pistos C, Stewart JT: Direct injection HPLC method for the determination of selected benzodiazepines in plasma using a Hisep column, *J Pharm Biomed Anal* 33:1135-1142, 2003.

6. Capella-Peiro ME, Bose D, Martinavarro-Dominguez A, et al: Direct injection micellar liquid chromatographic determination of benzodiazepines in serum, *J Chromatogr B Analyt Technol Biomed Life Sci* 780:241-249, 2002.

7. Needleman SB, Porvaznik M: Identification of parent benzodiazepines by gas chromatography/mass spectroscopy (GC/MS) from urinary extracts treated with B-glucuronidase, *Forensic Sci Int* 73:49-60, 1995.

8. Rasanen I, Ojanpera I, Vuori E: Quantitative screening for benzodiazepines in blood by dual-column gas chromatography and comparison of the results with urine immunoassay, *J Anal Toxicol* 24:46-51, 2000.

TEST NAME AND METHOD	SPECIMEN	REFERENCE (THERAPEUTIC) INTERVAL, CONVENTIONAL			[INTERNATIONAL RECOMMENDED UNITS]	KINETIC VALUES	
Oxycodone (Percodan)[1-8]	Serum, plasma, and blood		*ng/mL*		*nmol/L*	$t_{1/2}$:	4-5 hr
		Therapeutic concentration:	10-100	× 3.17	[32-317]	V_d:	3.2 ± 0.7 L/kg
GC, GC-MS, IA,		Toxic				Cl_T:	15 ± 2 mL/min/kg
HPLC		concentration:	>200		[>634]	PB:	35%
							[× 0.01 = 0.35, protein-bound mole fraction]
MW: 315.4						F:	20-33%
							[× 0.01 = 0.20-0.33, bioavailable mole fraction]
IA, GC-MS, CE, CE-MS	Urine						

1. Ropero-Miller JD, Lambing MK, Winecker RE: Simultaneous quantitation of opioids in blood by GC-EI-MS analysis following deproteination, detautomerization of keto analytes, solid-phase extraction, and trimethylsilyl derivatization, *J Anal Toxicol* 26:524-528, 2002.

2. Smith ML, Hughes RO, Levine B, et al: Forensic drug testing for opiates. VI. Urine testing for hydromorphone, hydrocodone, oxymorphone, and oxycodone with commercial opiate immunoassays and gas chromatography-mass spectrometry, *J Anal Toxicol* 19:18-26, 1995.

3. Spiehler VR, DeCicco L, McCutcheon JR, et al: Screening postmortem whole blood for oxycodone by ELISA response ratios, *J Forensic Sci* 49:621-626, 2004.

4. Von Seggern RL, Fitzgerald CP, Adelman LC, et al: Laboratory monitoring of OxyContin (oxycodone): clinical pitfalls, *Headache* 44:44-47, 2004.

FACTORS INFLUENCING DRUG DISPOSITION	REMARKS AND INTERFERENCES

Drug interactions: Probenecid may impair glucuronide conjugation.

9. Bennett WM, Aronoff GR, Golper TA, et al: *Drug prescribing in renal failure: dosing guidelines for adults,* ed 2, Philadelphia, 1991, American College of Physicians.

Metabolism
  Hepatic, CYP2D6 (major)

Drug interactions: CNS depressants, MAO inhibitors, general anesthetics, and tricyclic antidepressants may potentiate the effect.

Oxycodone, a synthetic phenanthrene-derivative opiate agonist, is used orally for the management of moderate to moderately severe pain. Sustained-release oxycodone (Oxycontin) is often abused by crushing the tablet to release the oxycodone and negate the sustained-release properties. CNS depressant and adverse reactions are similar to those of morphine. Naloxone is a specific antidote. Most immunoassays for opiates do not detect oxycodone.

5. Moore KA, Ramcharitar V, Levine B, et al: Tentative identification of novel oxycodone metabolites in human urine, *J Anal Toxicol* 27:346-352, 2003.

6. Wey AB, Thormann W: Capillary electrophoresis and capillary electrophoresis-ion trap multiple-stage mass spectrometry for the differentiation and identification of oxycodone and its major metabolites in human urine, *J Chromatogr B Analyt Technol Biomed Life Sci* 770:191-205, 2002.

7. Wright AW, Lawrence JA, Iu M, et al: Solid-phase extraction method with high-performance liquid chromatography and electrochemical detection for the quantitative analysis of oxycodone in human plasma, *J Chromatogr B Biomed Appl* 712:169-175, 1998.

8. Kapil RP, Padovani PK, King SY, et al: Nanogram level quantitation of oxycodone in human plasma by capillary gas chromatography using nitrogen-phosphorus selective detection, *J Chromatogr A* 577:283-287, 1992.

TEST NAME AND METHOD	SPECIMEN	REFERENCE (THERAPEUTIC) INTERVAL, CONVENTIONAL [INTERNATIONAL RECOMMENDED UNITS]				KINETIC VALUES	
Pancuronium **(Pavulon)**[1-5]	Plasma.		*mcg/mL*		*μmol/L*	$t_{1/2}$:	1.9-2.2 hr
		50% paralysis:	0.09	× 1.36	[0.12]	V_d:	0.18-0.32 L/kg
	Unstable at room	80% paralysis:	0.17		[0.23]	Cl_T:	0.8-1.9 mL/min/kg
GC, LC-MS	temperature and	99% paralysis:	0.22		[0.30]	PB:	7-29% (albumin, globu-
	pH 7.4. Stable for	Toxic					lin)
MW: 732.68 (as the	20 hr at 23° C and	concentration:	>0.4		[0.54]		[× 0.01 = 0.07-0.29,
dibromide)	pH 5.4.						protein-bound mole
							fraction]
						T_{max}:	2-3 min

1. Atherton DP, Hunter JM: Clinical pharmacokinetics of the newer neuromuscular blocking drugs, *Clin Pharmacokinet* 36:169-189, 1999.
2. Fisher DM: Clinical pharmacology of neuromuscular blocking agents, *Am J Health Syst Pharm* 56(suppl 1):S4-9, 1999.
3. Klys M, Bialka J, Bujak-Gizycka B: A case of suicide by intravenous injection of pancuronium, *Leg Med (Tokyo)* 2:93-100, 2000.
4. Ramzan MI, Somogyi AA, Walker JS, et al: Clinical pharmacokinetics of the non-depolarising muscle relaxants, *Clin Pharmacokinet* 6:25-60, 1981.
5. Sayer H, Quintela O, Marquet P, et al: Identification and quantitation of six non-depolarizing neuromuscular blocking agents by LC-MS in biological fluids, *J Anal Toxicol* 28:105-110, 2004.

TEST NAME AND METHOD	SPECIMEN					KINETIC VALUES	
Paraldehyde[1-4]	Serum, plasma		*mcg/mL*		*μmol/L*	$t_{1/2}$:	4-10 hr
	(heparin, EDTA)	Therapeutic				V_d:	0.9 L/kg
GC		concentration				Cl_T:	~2 mL/min/kg
		Seizure control:	30-150	× 7.57	[227-1136]	PB:	NA
MW: 132		Sedation:	10-100		[76-757]	T_{max}:	0.5-1 hr (IM)
		Anesthesia:	>200		[>1514]		
		Toxic					
		concentration:	>200		[>1514]		
		Lethal					
		concentration:	>400		[>3785]		

1. Githiga IM, Muchohi SN, Ogutu BR, et al: Determination of paraldehyde by gas chromatography in whole blood from children, *J Chromatogr B Analyt Technol Biomed Life Sci* 805:365-369, 2004.
2. Ramsay RE: Pharmacokinetics and clinical use of parenteral phenytoin, phenobarbital, and paraldehyde, *Epilepsia* 30(suppl 2):S1-3, 1989.
3. Streete PJ, Ruprah M, Ramsey JD, et al: Detection and identification of volatile substances by headspace capillary gas chromatography to aid the diagnosis of acute poisoning, *Analyst* 117:1111-1127, 1992.
4. Von Burg R, Stout T: Paraldehyde, *J Appl Toxicol* 11:379-381, 1991.

FACTORS INFLUENCING DRUG DISPOSITION	REMARKS AND INTERFERENCES
Metabolism Hepatic *Excretion* Renal, biliary *Disease* Uremia: $t_{1/2}\uparrow$, $Cl_T\downarrow$ Cirrhosis: $V_d\uparrow$, $t_{1/2}\uparrow$, $Cl_T\downarrow$ *Age* Elderly: $t_{1/2}\uparrow$, $Cl_T\downarrow$	Pancuronium is used as a nondepolarizing neuromuscular blocking agent as an alternative to d-tubocurarine. The drug is metabolized to less active products, which are typically measured along with the parent drug.
Metabolism Hepatic *Excretion* Pulmonary	Paraldehyde may be occasionally used to treat delirium tremens and seizures. Adverse effects include disagreeable taste, irritation to the throat and stomach, cyanosis, cough, hypotension, respiratory depression, acidosis, hepatitis, nephrosis, pulmonary hemorrhage and edema, and dilation of the right ventricle. About 25% is excreted via the pulmonary route, leading to a characteristic smell to the breath. Some GC methods measure the paraldehyde metabolite, acetaldehyde.

TEST NAME AND METHOD	SPECIMEN	REFERENCE (THERAPEUTIC) INTERVAL, CONVENTIONAL [INTERNATIONAL RECOMMENDED UNITS]			KINETIC VALUES	
Paroxetine **(Paxil)**[1-6] *HPLC, GC-MS, GC* *MW: 329.4*	Serum, plasma	Therapeutic concentration: Toxic concentration:	*mcg/mL* <0.01-0.05 × 3.04 >0.35	μ*mol/L* [0.03-0.15] [>1.06]	$t_{1/2}$: V_d: Cl_T: PB: F: T_{max}:	15-22 hr 8.7 L/kg 0.5-1 L/kg 95% NA 1-2 hr

1. Isbister GK, Bowe SJ, Dawson A, et al: Relative toxicity of selective serotonin reuptake inhibitors (SSRIs) in overdose, *J Toxicol Clin Toxicol* 42:277-285, 2004.
2. Lacassie E, Gaulier JM, Marquet P, et al: Methods for the determination of seven selective serotonin reuptake inhibitors and three active metabolites in human serum using high-performance liquid chromatography and gas chromatography, *J Chromatogr B Biomed Sci Appl* 742:229-238, 2000.
3. Richelson E: Pharmacokinetic drug interactions of new antidepressants: a review of the effects on the metabolism of other drugs, *Mayo Clin Proc* 72:835-847, 1997.
4. Schulz M, Schmoldt A: Therapeutic and toxic blood concentrations of more than 800 drugs and other xenobiotics, *Pharmazie* 58:447-474, 2003.
5. Vitiello B, Swedo S: Antidepressant medications in children, *N Engl J Med* 350:1489-1491, 2004.
6. Tournel G, Houdret N, Hedouin V, et al: High-performance liquid chromatographic method to screen and quantitate seven selective serotonin reuptake inhibitors in human serum, *J Chromatogr B Biomed Sci Appl* 761:147-158, 2001.

TEST NAME AND METHOD	SPECIMEN	REFERENCE INTERVAL	KINETIC VALUES	
Pentamidine **(Pentam,** **Nebupent)** *HPLC,*[1] *bioassay,*[2] *LSIMS*[3] *MW: 340.43*	Plasma, serum. Stable at −70° C (or −20° C) for 6 days.	See *Remarks*.	PK: $t_{1/2}$: V_d: Cl_T: See *Remarks*.	6.4-9.0 hr[4] 38.2 ± 27.3 L 268 ± 70 L/hr
HPLC[1]	Whole blood			
HPLC,[1-9] *bioassay*[2]	Urine			

| FACTORS INFLUENCING DRUG DISPOSITION | REMARKS AND INTERFERENCES |

Metabolism
  Hepatic, CYP2D6
  Saturatable kinetics
Excretion
  Renal, fecal

Drug interactions: Paroxetine is a potent inhibitor of CYP2D6 (the same CYP responsible for its metabolism) and possibly CYP3A4. Multiple drug interactions are possible.

Paroxetine belongs to the group of antidepressants that act by selectively inhibiting the reuptake of serotonin. Of this group, it is the most potent but least selective in its interaction with serotonin inhibition. It also exhibits an affinity for the muscarinic acetylcholine receptors similar to that of the tricyclic antidepressants. Paroxetine is also used to treat other psychiatric diorders such as obsessive compulsive disorders, panic disorders, posttraumatic stress disorders, anxiety, and premenstrual dysphoric disorder. Common side effects include anorexia, gastrointestinal disturbances, insomnia, sweating, blurred vision, drowsiness, tachycardia, and weight gain. More serious adverse effects reported include suicide, hyponatremia, and seizures. Potentially lethal events include the development of serotonin syndrome and the syndrome of inappropriate antidiuretic hormone secretion.

Metabolism[5]
  Hepatic
Excretion
  Urine
Disease or condition
  Renal dysfunction: $t_{1/2}\uparrow$

Drug interactions: Pentamidine is a major substrate of CYP2C19 and weakly inhibits CYP2C8/9, CYP2C19, CYP2D6, and CYP3A4. CYP2C19 inducers like carbamazepine, phenytoin, and rifampin may decrease the effects of pentamidine. CYP2C19 inhibitors like fluconazole, fluvoxamine, gemfibrozil, isoniazid, and omeprazole may increase the effects of pentamidine.[6] Concomitant usage of cisapride or droperidol with pentamidine may lead to an increased risk in cardiotoxicity.[7]

Pentamidine is primarily used in the treatment of infections caused by *Pneumocystis carinii*. A 3-mg/kg dose led to a mean C_{max} of 249 ± 80 ng/mL [$\times 2.94 = 732 \pm 235$ nmol/L].[8] Although <5% of pentamidine is renally excreted, the $t_{1/2}$ is prolonged in dialysis patients (i.e., terminal half-life measured after the last dose of a multiple dosing regimen: 12.5 ± 2.4 days).[8] Heating pentamidine samples to 56° C for 1 hr (for HIV deactivation) does not appear to affect pentamidine concentrations. Adverse effects are rare with inhaled pentamidine therapy; chest pain, congestion, cough, dyspnea, wheezing, pharyngitis, skin rash, and extrapulmonary pneumocytosis have been reported. Adverse effects reported with parenteral administration include hyperglycemia, hypoglycemia, leukopenia or neutropenia, elevated liver function tests, nephrotoxicity, thrombocytopenia, anemia, pancreatitis, and hypotension. Rapid intravenous infusion may lead to a precipitous decrease in blood pressure.

TEST NAME AND METHOD	SPECIMEN	REFERENCE (THERAPEUTIC) INTERVAL, CONVENTIONAL [INTERNATIONAL RECOMMENDED UNITS]			KINETIC VALUES

Pentamidine—CONT

1. Ericsson O, Rais M: Determination of pentamidine in whole blood, plasma, and urine by high-performance liquid chromatography, *Ther Drug Monit* 12:362-365, 1990.
2. Bernard EM, Donnelly HJ, Maher MP, et al: Use of a new bioassay to study pentamidine pharmacokinetics, *J Infect Dis* 152:750-754, 1985.
3. Berger BJ, Henry L, Hall JE, et al: Problems and pitfalls in the assay of pentamidine: implications for clinical use, *Clin Pharmacokinet* 22:163-168, 1992.
4. Conte JE, Upton RA, Phelps RT, et al: Use of a specific and sensitive assay to determine pentamidine pharmacokinetics in patients with AIDS, *J Infect Dis* 154:923-929, 1986.

TEST NAME AND METHOD	SPECIMEN	REFERENCE (THERAPEUTIC) INTERVAL, CONVENTIONAL		[INTERNATIONAL RECOMMENDED UNITS]	KINETIC VALUES	
Pentazocine (Talwin)[1-8]	Serum, plasma		*mcg/mL*	*μmol/L*	$t_{1/2}$:	2.0 hr[1]
		Therapeutic concentration:	0.05-0.2 × 3.50	[0.2-0.7]	IV:	5.7 ± 1.4 hr
GC, GC-MS,		Toxic			PO:	3.4 ± 1.2 hr
fluorimetric, IA		concentration:	>1.0	[>3.5]	V_d:	2.9 ± 0.6 hr
					Cl_T:	5.56 ± 1.63 L/kg
MW: 285.4					PB:	10.9 ± 1.86 mL/min/kg
						60-70%
						[× 0.01 = 0.60-0.70, protein-bound mole fraction]
					F:	21 ± 0.7%
						[× 0.01 = 0.21 ± 0.007, bioavailable mole fraction]

1. Baselt R: *Disposition of toxic drugs and chemicals in man,* ed 7, Foster City, CA, 2004, Biomedical Publications.
2. Schulz M, Schmoldt A: Therapeutic and toxic blood concentrations of more than 800 drugs and other xenobiotics, *Pharmazie* 58:447-474, 2003.
3. Hardman JG, Limbird LE, Gilman AG: *Goodman and Gilman's the pharmacological basis of therapeutics,* ed 10, New York, 2001, McGraw-Hill.
4. *Physicians desk reference,* ed 58, Montvale, NJ, 2004, Thomson PDR.
5. Clarke EGC: *Clarke's isolation and identification of drugs in pharmaceuticals, body fluids, and post-mortem material,* London, 1986, The Pharmaceutical Press.
6. McEvoy GK, editor: *AHFS drug information (online version),* Bethesda, MD, 2004, American Society of Health-System Pharmacists Inc.
7. Seno H, Kumazawa T, Ishii A, et al: Determination of pentazocine in human whole blood and urine by gas chromatography/surface ionization organic mass spectrometry, *J Mass Spectrom* 35:33-38, 2000.
8. Ameyibor E, Stewart JT: Resolution and quantitation of pentazocine enantiomers in human serum by reversed-phase high-performance liquid chromatography using sulfated beta-cyclodextrin as chiral mobile phase additive and solid-phase extraction, *J Chromatogr B Biomed Sci Appl* 703:273-278, 1997.

FACTORS INFLUENCING DRUG DISPOSITION	REMARKS AND INTERFERENCES

5. Berger BJ, Lombardy RJ, Marbury GD, et al: Metabolic N-hydroxylation of pentamidine in vitro, *Antimicrob Agents Chemother* 34:1678-1684, 1990.
6. Lexi-Comp, Inc: *Up-to-date online 12.2. Drug information,* Hudson, OH, 2004, Lexi-Comp, Inc.
7. Micromedex: *Micromedex healthcare series 2004,* Greenwood Village, CO, 2004, Thomson Micromedex.
8. Conte JE Jr: Pharmacokinetics of intravenous pentamidine in patients with normal renal function or receiving hemodialysis, *J Infect Dis* 163:169-175, 1991.
9. Berger BJ, Hall JE, Tidwell RR: A high performance liquid chromatographic method for the quantification of several diamidine compounds with potential chemotherapeutic value, *J Chromatogr* 494:191-200, 1989.

Metabolism
Hepatic (primary)
Disease
Cirrhosis: $t_{1/2}\uparrow$, 12.0 ± 3.0 hr
$Cl_T\downarrow$, 5.69 ± 1.23 mL/min/kg
F↑, 70.0 ± 19.0%
Dialysis
Hemodialysis (+)

Drug interactions: Concurrent use with fluoxetine may cause serotonin syndrome.

Pentazocine is a synthetic opiate (1/2 to 1/6 as potent as morphine) used as an analgesic for relief of moderate to severe pain. Pentazocine is extensively metabolized; 3-15% of the unchanged drug is excreted in the urine. First-pass metabolism in the liver is extensive and influences bioavailability. Adverse effects include sedation, sweating, dizziness, nausea, and psychotomimetic effects. Respiratory depression with tachycardia and hypertensive effects is seen at high dosage. Treatment of severe toxicity with naloxone is specific.

Interferences: Metabolites interfere in the fluorometric assay. Acid hydrolysis modifies the structure; therefore deconjugation must be performed enzymatically.

TEST NAME AND METHOD	SPECIMEN	REFERENCE (THERAPEUTIC) INTERVAL, CONVENTIONAL [INTERNATIONAL RECOMMENDED UNITS]				KINETIC VALUES	
Pentobarbital (Nembutal)[1-11]	Serum, plasma		*mcg/mL*		μ*mol/L*	$t_{1/2}$:	20-40 hr
		Therapeutic concentration,				V_d:	1.0 L/kg
						Cl_T:	0.53 mL/min/kg
GC, GC-MS,		hypnotic:	1-5	× 4.42	[4-22]	PB:	35-55%
HPLC, IA		Therapeutic					[× 0.01 = 0.35-0.55,
		coma:	20-50		[88-221]		protein-bound mole
MW: 226.3		Toxic					fraction]
		concentration:	>10		[>44]	F:	99%
							[× 0.01 = 0.99, bioavail-able mole fraction]

1. Baselt R: *Disposition of toxic drugs and chemicals in man,* ed 7, Foster City, CA, 2004, Biomedical Publications.

2. Schulz M, Schmoldt A: Therapeutic and toxic blood concentrations of more than 800 drugs and other xenobiotics, *Pharmazie* 58:447-474, 2003.

3. Hardman JG, Limbird LE, Gilman AG: *Goodman and Gilman's the pharmacological basis of therapeutics,* ed 10, New York, 2001, McGraw-Hill.

4. *Physicians desk reference,* ed 58, Montvale, NJ, 2004, Thomson PDR.

5. Clarke EGC: *Clarke's isolation and identification of drugs in pharmaceuticals, body fluids, and post-mortem material,* London, 1986, The Pharmaceutical Press.

6. Tanaka E, Terada M, Tanno K, et al: Forensic analysis of 10 barbiturates in human biological samples using a new reversed-phase chromatographic column packed with 2-micrometre porous microspherical silica-gel, *Forensic Sci Int* 85:73-82, 1997.

7. Meatherall R: GC/MS confirmation of barbiturates in blood and urine, *J Forensic Sci* 42:1160-1170, 1997.

8. ACP's PIER: *Physicians' information and education resource (online version),* Philadelphia, 2004, American College of Physicians.

9. McEvoy GK, editor: *AHFS drug information (online version),* Bethesda, MD, 2004, American Society of Health-System Pharmacists Inc.

10. *USP DI drug information for the health care professional,* ed 24, (online version), Taunton, MA, 2004, Micromedex Inc.

11. Ferslew KE, Hagardorn AN, McCormick WF: Application of micellar electrokinetic capillary chromatography to forensic analysis of barbiturates in biological fluids, *J Forensic Sci* 40:245-249, 1995.

Phenacetin[1-4]	Plasma (EDTA), urine		*mcg/mL*		μ*mol/L*	$t_{1/2}$:	0.6-3 hr
		Therapeutic				Cl_T:	NA
GC, HPLC, GC-MS		concentration:	5-20	× 5.58	[6-167]	V_d:	1-2 L/kg
		Toxic				PB:	33%
MW: 179.22		concentration:	>50		[>279]		[× 0.01 = 0.33, protein-bound mole fraction]

1. Abbott FV, Fraser MI: Use and abuse of over-the-counter analgesic agents, *J Psychiatry Neurosci* 23:13-34, 1998.

2. Fucci N: Phenacetin and cocaine in a body packer, *Forensic Sci Int* 141:59-61, 2004.

3. McLaughlin JK, Lipworth L, Chow WH, et al: Analgesic use and chronic renal failure: a critical review of the epidemiologic literature, *Kidney Int* 54:679-686, 1998.

FACTORS INFLUENCING DRUG DISPOSITION	REMARKS AND INTERFERENCES

Metabolism
  Hepatic
Disease
  Hepatic: $t_{1/2}\uparrow\rightarrow$
  Renal: PB$\downarrow$
Dialysis
  Hemodialysis $(-)$
  Hemoperfusion $(+)$
 	
Drug interactions: Pentobarbital is a strong CYP2A6 and CYP3A4 inducer and may decrease the levels of CYP2A6 and CYP3A4 substrates.
	Pentobarbital is used primarily as a hypnotic in the short-term (up to 2 wk) treatment of insomnia. High doses are used parenterally to induce coma in the management of cerebral ischemia and increased intracranial pressure associated with head trauma, stroke, and other situations in which reduction of cerebral edema and/or intracranial pressure is desired. Side effects include CNS depression, confusion, drowsiness, ataxia, coma, respiratory depression, shock, and urticaria.

Metabolism
  Hepatic
Excretion
  Renal
	Phenacetin is an analgesic that has been removed from over-the-counter and prescriptive preparations in many countries because of its adverse effects. For many years it was found in combination with analgesics such as acetaminophen, aspirin, and caffeine. It is metabolized to acetaminophen. (See *Acetaminophen.*) Adverse effects include nephrotoxicity (including capillary necrosis), hemolytic effects, thrombocytopenia, and methemoglobin formation. Additionally there is some evidence of addictive properties.

4. Murray S, Boobis AR: Combined assay for phenacetin and paracetamol in plasma using capillary column gas chromatography-negative-ion mass spectrometry, *J Chromatogr* 568:341-350, 1991.

TEST NAME AND METHOD	SPECIMEN	REFERENCE (THERAPEUTIC) INTERVAL, CONVENTIONAL [INTERNATIONAL RECOMMENDED UNITS]			KINETIC VALUES	
Phencyclidine **(Sernylan)**[1-11]	Serum, plasma	*mcg/mL*		*μmol/L*	$t_{1/2}$:	1-12 hr
		Toxic			V_d:	6.2 L/kg
		concentration			PB:	65-80%
GC, MS, GC-MS,		Nonfatal:	0.02-0.100 × 4.11	[0.08-0.41]		[× 0.01 = 0.65-0.80,
IA, TLC		Fatal:	0.5-4.0	[2.06-16.44]		protein-bound mole
						fraction]
MW: 243.4	Urine	Negative				
	Alternative matrices: Hair, oral fluid, and sweat	Negative				

1. Baselt R: *Disposition of toxic drugs and chemicals in man,* ed 7, Foster City, CA, 2004, Biomedical Publications.

2. Schulz M, Schmoldt A: Therapeutic and toxic blood concentrations of more than 800 drugs and other xenobiotics, *Pharmazie* 58:447-474, 2003.

3. Hardman JG, Limbird LE, Gilman AG: *Goodman and Gilman's the pharmacological basis of therapeutics,* ed 10, New York, 2001, McGraw-Hill.

4. *Physicians desk reference,* ed 58, Montvale, NJ, 2004, Thomson PDR.

5. Clarke EGC: *Clarke's isolation and identification of drugs in pharmaceuticals, body fluids, and post-mortem material,* London, 1986, The Pharmaceutical Press.

6. ACP's PIER: *Physicians' information and education resource (online version),* Philadelphia, 2004, American College of Physicians.

7. Goldfrank LR, editor: *Goldfrank's toxicological emergencies,* ed 7, (online version), New York, 2002, The McGraw-Hill Companies Inc.

8. Kerrigan S, Phillips Jr WH: Comparison of ELISAs for opiates, methamphetamine, cocaine metabolite, benzodiazepines, phencyclidine, and cannabinoids in whole blood and urine, *Clin Chem* 47:540-547, 2001.

9. Ishii A, Seno H, Kumazawa T, et al: Simple and sensitive detection of phencyclidine in body fluids by gas chromatography with surface ionization detection, *Int J Legal Med* 108:244-247, 1996.

10. Kidwell DA: Analysis of phencyclidine and cocaine in human hair by tandem mass spectrometry, *J Forensic Sci* 38:272-284, 1993.

11. Nakahara Y, Takahashi K, Sakamoto T, et al: Hair analysis for drugs of abuse. XVII. Simultaneous detection of PCP, PCHP, and PCPdiol in human hair for confirmation of PCP use, *J Anal Toxicol* 21:356-362, 1997.

FACTORS INFLUENCING DRUG DISPOSITION	REMARKS AND INTERFERENCES

Metabolism
  Hepatic, CYP3A4

Drug interactions: CYP3A4 inhibitors may increase the levels/effects of PCP. PCP is a weak inhibitor of CYP3A4. Acidification of the urine (pH <5) significantly accelerates renal excretion.

Phencyclidine (PCP) is a highly lipophilic basic amine and appears to affect all neurotransmitter systems. Side and toxic effects include staggering gait, slurred speech, nystagmus, increased sensitivity to stimuli, mood elevation, agitation, increased blood pressure, hallucinations, paranoia, violent behavior, status asthmaticus, and coma. For workplace and drug abuse testing, the widely accepted immunoassay and GC-MS confirmation cutoff concentration to separate positive and negative specimens for phencyclidine (PCP) is 25 ng/mL [103 nmol/L]. At these cutoff concentrations, PCP may generally be detected in urine for 1-2 wk after use.

Alternative matrices used for nonfederally regulated workplace drug testing and being considered for regulated testing include hair, oral fluid, and sweat.

TEST NAME AND METHOD	SPECIMEN	REFERENCE (THERAPEUTIC) INTERVAL, CONVENTIONAL [INTERNATIONAL RECOMMENDED UNITS]		KINETIC VALUES	
Phenethylamines[1-8]	Serum			$t_{1/2}$	
				Chlorphentermine:	35-44 hr
GC, GC-MS, IA,		*mcg/mL*	*μmol/L*	Diethylpropion:	NA
LC-MS	*Chlorphentermine*			Ephedrine:	4-10 hr
	Therapeutic concentration:	0.1-0.4 × 5.44	[0.54-2.2]	Fenfluramine:	13-30 hr
	Toxic concentration:	>5	[>27.2]	d-Methamphetamine:	6-15 hr
	Diethylpropion			p-Methoxyam-	
	Therapeutic concentration:	0.001-0.01 × 4.87	[0.005-0.049]	phetamine:	NA
	Toxic concentration:	>1	[>5]	Methylemedi-	
	Ephedrine			oxyamphetamine:	NA
	Therapeutic concentration:	0.05-0.10 × 6.05	[0.30-0.61]	Methylphenidate:	1.4-4.2 hr
	Toxic concentration:	>2	[>12.1]	Phendimetrazine:	NA
	Fenfluramine			Phenmetrazine:	8 hr
	Therapeutic concentration:	0.03-0.30 × 4.32	[0.13-1.30]	Phentermine:	19-24 hr
	Toxic concentration:	>1	[>4.32]	Phenylpropanola-	
	Methamphetamine			mine:	3-4.4 hr
	Therapeutic concentration:	0.01-0.05 × 6.70	[0.07-0.34]	Tranylcypromine:	1.5-3.5 hr
	Toxic concentration:	>0.5	[>3.350]		
	p-Methoxyamphetamine				
	Therapeutic concentration:	<0.2 × 6.05	[<1.2]		
	Toxic concentration:	>5	[>30.3]		
	Methylenedioxyamphetamine				
	Therapeutic concentration:	<0.4 × 5.52	[<2.2]		
	Toxic concentration:	>10	[>55.2]		
	Methylphenidate				
	Therapeutic concentration:	0.01-0.04 × 4.29	[0.04-0.17]		
	Phendimetrazine				
	Therapeutic concentration:	0.03-0.25 × 5.23	[0.16-1.31]		
	Toxic concentration:	>1	[>5.23]		
	Phenmetrazine				
	Therapeutic concentration:	0.06-0.25 × 5.64	[0.34-1.41]		
	Toxic concentration:	>5	[>28.20]		
	Phentermine				
	Therapeutic concentration:	0.03-0.09 × 6.70	[0.20-0.60]		
	Toxic concentration:	>5	[>33.50]		
	Phenylpropanolamine				
	Therapeutic concentration:	0.05-0.10 × 6.61	[0.33-0.66]		
	Toxic concentration:	>5	[>33.07]		
	Tranylcypromine				
	Therapeutic concentration:	0.01-0.10 × 7.51	[0.075-0.75]		
	Toxic concentration:	>0.2	[>1.50]		

1. Baselt R: *Disposition of toxic drugs and chemicals in man,* ed 7, Foster City, CA, 2004, Biomedical Publications.
2. Bohn AM, Khodaee M, Schwenk TL: Ephedrine and other stimulants as ergogenic aids, *Curr Sports Med Rep* 2:220-225, 2003.
3. Furesz J, Kocsis G, Gachalyi A, et al: Mass selective detection of amphetamine, methamphetamine, and related compounds in urine, *J Chromatogr Sci* 42:259-262, 2003.
4. Halpern A, Mancini MC: Treatment of obesity: an update on anti-obesity medications, *Obes Rev* 4:25-42, 2003.
5. Kollins SH: Comparing the abuse potential of methylphenidate versus other stimulants: a review of available evidence and relevance to the ADHD patient, *J Clin Psychiatry* 64(suppl 11):14-18, 2003.

FACTORS INFLUENCING DRUG DISPOSITION	REMARKS AND INTERFERENCES
Acidic urine increases the rate of urinary excretion of phenethylamines.	These drugs are CNS stimulants, anorexigenic agents (fenfluramine, phenmetrazine), antidepressants (methylphenidate, tranylcypromine), decongestants (ephedrine, phenylpropanolamine), and hallucinogenics (*p*-methoxyamphetamine, methylenedioxyamphetamine). Many are widely abused. They are metabolized to a variety of derivatives that are largely inactive and primarily excreted by the kidney. Adverse effects include insomnia, agitation, nervousness, hyperthermia, hyperventilation, hypertension, and convulsions. The cross-reactivity of amphetamine immunoassays varies. A positive result may be obtained with those of broader cross-reactivity when some phenethylamines such as ephedrine, pseudoephedrine, phenylpropanolamine, or phentermine are present in sufficient concentration. See also *Amphetamine*.

6. Shekelle PG, Hardy ML, Morton SC, et al: Efficacy and safety of ephedra and ephedrine for weight loss and athletic performance: a meta-analysis, *JAMA* 289:1537-1545, 2003.

7. Soares ME, Carvalho M, Carmo H, et al: Simultaneous determination of amphetamine derivatives in human urine after SPE extraction and HPLC-UV analysis, *Biomed Chromatogr* 18:125-131, 2004.

8. Stout PR, Klette KL, Horn CK: Evaluation of ephedrine, pseudoephedrine and phenylpropanolamine concentrations in human urine samples and a comparison of the specificity of DRI amphetamines and Abuscreen online (KIMS) amphetamines screening immunoassays, *J Forensic Sci* 49:160-164, 2004.

TEST NAME AND METHOD	SPECIMEN	REFERENCE (THERAPEUTIC) INTERVAL, CONVENTIONAL [INTERNATIONAL RECOMMENDED UNITS]		KINETIC VALUES	
Phenobarbital **(Luminal)**[1-8]	Serum, plasma		*mcg/mL*	*μmol/L*	$t_{1/2}$
		Therapeutic			0-4 wk: 118 ± 16 hr
		concentration:	15-40 × 4.31	[65-172]	4-12 mo: 63 ± 4.2 hr
GC, HPLC, IA, CE		Toxic			Child: 40-70 hr
		concentration			Adult: 50-140 hr
MW: 232.2		Slowness,			V_d: 0.7 L/kg
		ataxia,			Cl_T: 0.093 ± 0.044
		nystagmus:	35-80	[151-345]	mL/min/kg
		Coma with			PB: 40-60%
		reflexes:	65-117	[280-504]	[× 0.01 =
		Coma without			0.40-0.60, protein-
		reflexes:	>100	[>431]	bound mole
					fraction]
					F, PO/IM: 80-100%
					[× 0.01 =
					0.80-1.00,
					bioavailable mole
					fraction]
					T_{max}
					PO: 6-18 hr
					IM: 1-2 hr

1. Baselt R: *Disposition of toxic drugs and chemicals in man,* ed 7, Foster City, CA, 2004, Biomedical Publications.

2. Schulz M, Schmoldt A: Therapeutic and toxic blood concentrations of more than 800 drugs and other xenobiotics, *Pharmazie* 58:447-474, 2003.

3. Hardman JG, Limbird LE, Gilman AG: *Goodman and Gilman's the pharmacological basis of therapeutics,* ed 10, New York, 2001, McGraw-Hill.

4. *Physicians desk reference,* ed 58, Montvale, NJ, 2004, Thomson PDR.

5. Clarke EGC: *Clarke's isolation and identification of drugs in pharmaceuticals, body fluids, and post-mortem material,* London, 1986, The Pharmaceutical Press.

6. Tanaka E, Terada M, Tanno K, et al: Forensic analysis of 10 barbiturates in human biological samples using a new reversed-phase chromatographic column packed with 2-micrometre porous microspherical silica-gel, *Forensic Sci Int* 85:73-82, 1997.

7. Meatherall R: GC/MS confirmation of barbiturates in blood and urine, *J Forensic Sci* 42:1160-1170, 1997.

8. McEvoy GK, editor: *AHFS drug information (online version),* Bethesda, MD, 2004, American Society of Health-System Pharmacists Inc.

9. Ohyama K, Wada M, Lord GA, et al: Capillary electrochromatographic analysis of barbiturates in serum, *Electrophoresis* 25:594-599, 2004.

FACTORS INFLUENCING DRUG DISPOSITION	REMARKS AND INTERFERENCES

Metabolism
  Hepatic, CYP2C9; minor: CYP2C19, CYP3E1
Excretion
  Renal, 75% as glucuronide and sulfate conjugates of p-hydroxyphenobarbital
Disease or condition
  Hepatic: $t_{1/2}\uparrow$, $Cl_T\downarrow$
  Pregnancy: $Cl_T\uparrow$
Age
  Neonate: $t_{1/2}\rightarrow$, $V_d\uparrow$, $Cl_T\uparrow$, $PB\downarrow$
  Child: $t_{1/2}\downarrow$, $Cl_T\uparrow$
  Elderly: $t_{1/2}\uparrow$, $PB\rightarrow$
Dialysis
  Hemodialysis (+)
  Hemoperfusion (+)
  Peritoneal (±)

Drug Interactions: Valproic acid and salicylates may increase phenobarbital levels by as much as 40%. Alkalinization of the urine will result in an increased Cl_T of phenobarbital. Alkalinization increases the ionization of the drug and thus reduces its renal tubular reabsorption. Phenobarbital induces uridine diphosphate glucuronosyl transferase (UGT) enzymes and CYP2C and CYP3A subfamilies of cytochrome P450. Drugs metabolized by these enzymes would be metabolized more rapidly when coadministered with phenobarbital.

Phenobarbital is commonly used in the treatment of generalized tonic-clonic and partial seizures. Sedation is the most frequent side effect on initiation of therapy; however, tolerance usually develops with time. Toxic symptoms include CNS depression, coma, and respiratory depression. It is hydroxylated to form p-hydroxyphenobarbital, an inactive metabolite. Because the drug has a long half-life, it may take several weeks to achieve a new steady-state level.

See also *Primidone.*

See Table II-5.

TEST NAME AND METHOD	SPECIMEN	REFERENCE (THERAPEUTIC) INTERVAL, CONVENTIONAL [INTERNATIONAL RECOMMENDED UNITS]		KINETIC VALUES
Phensuximide (Milontin)[1,2] *GC, GC-MS* *MW: 189.21*	Serum, plasma (heparin, EDTA)	Parent drug and metabolite, *N*-desmethylphensuximide, Therapeutic concentration: 40-60 mcg/mL [× 5.71* = 228-343 mmol/L] *Conversion factor based on MW of *N*-desmethylphensuximide of 175.2.		PK[3,4]: $t_{1/2}$: 5-12 hr PB: Negligible

1. Bonitati J: Gas-chromatographic analysis for succinimide anticonvulsants in serum: macro- and micro-scale methods, *Clin Chem* 22:341-345, 1976.
2. Baselt RC: *Disposition of toxic drugs and chemicals in man,* ed 7, Foster City, CA, 2004, Chemical Toxicology Institute.
3. Hardman JG, Limbird LE, Gilman AG: *Goodman & Gilman's the pharmacological basis of therapeutics,* ed 10, New York, 2001, McGraw-Hill.
4. Porter RJ, Penry JK, Lacy JR, et al: Plasma concentrations of phensuximide, methsuximide, and their metabolites in relation to clinical efficacy, *Neurology* 29:1509-1513, 1979.

			mcg/mL		µ*mol/L*		
Phenytoin (Dilantin)[1-5] *HPLC, EIA, FPIA, CEDIA* *MW: 252.27*	Serum, plasma (EDTA). SST tubes should not be used. Collect at steady-state trough concentration. Stable at room temperature for several hours, for 1 yr at −20° C.	Therapeutic concentration: Free phenytoin: Toxic concentration Far lateral nystagmus: Nystagmus at 45° lateral gaze; ataxia: Depressed mental capacity: Death:	10-20 1-2.5 >20 >30 >40 >100	× 3.96	[40-79] [4-10] [>79] [>119] [>158] [>396]	PK[5]: $t_{1/2}$: V_d: PB: F:	8-60 hr 0.5-0.8 L/kg 87-93% 70-90%

FACTORS INFLUENCING DRUG DISPOSITION	REMARKS AND INTERFERENCES

Metabolism
  Hepatic
Excretion
  Bile/feces

Drug interactions: Carbamazepine, phenobarbital, phenytoin, and primidone may increase phensuximide metabolism. Valproic acid may increase or decrease plasma concentrations.

Phensuximide is used in the treatment of seizure disorders. Limited pharmacokinetic and pharmacologic data are available. Side effects include nausea, vomiting, anorexia, headache, fatigue, lethargy, and dizziness. The drug is rapidly absorbed and converted to the *N*-desmethyl metabolite, an active species.

Metabolism:
  Hepatic
Excretion:
  Urine
Disease or condition
  Hepatic: $t_{1/2}\uparrow$, $Cl_T\downarrow$, $PB\downarrow$
  Renal: $t_{1/2}\downarrow$; $V_d\uparrow$, 1.0 L/kg; $PB\downarrow$, 70%
  Pregnancy: $Cl_T\uparrow$, $PB\downarrow$
  Burn: $PB\downarrow$
Age
  Premature: $t_{1/2}\uparrow$, $Cl_T\downarrow$
  Newborn: $t_{1/2}\uparrow$, $V_d\uparrow$, $Cl_T\downarrow$, $PB\downarrow$
  Child: $t_{1/2}\downarrow$, $V_d\uparrow$, $Cl_T\uparrow$
  Elderly: $Cl_T\downarrow$
Dialysis
  Hemodialysis ($-$)
  Peritoneal ($-$)

Drug interactions: Phenytoin is a major substrate of CYP2C8/9 and CYP2C19 and a minor substrate of CYP3A4. It induces CYP2B6, CYP2C8/9, CYP2C19, and CYP3A4 strongly.[6] Metabolism is inhibited by isoniazid, chloramphenicol, dicumarol, warfarin, disulfiram, and amiodarone.

Thioridazine and imipramine may increase plasma phenytoin concentrations. More rapid metabolism is induced by carbamazepine, clon-

Phenytoin is commonly used in the treatment of seizure disorders. It is also used unlabeled/investigational as an antiarrhythmic agent (class Ib) for ventricular arrhythmias. The metabolism and, consequently, $t_{1/2}$ of phenytoin are dose/concentration dependent, making it difficult to titrate dosages based on serum or plasma concentration. Dosage increases should therefore be made gradually. Wide interproduct variability in the bioavailability of the drug has been demonstrated.[7] Side effects include behavioral changes, GI symptoms, gingival hyperplasia, osteomalacia, megaloblastic anemia, hepatic disturbances, and hirsutism. Rare cases of thrombocytopenia, leukopenia, and eosinophilia have been reported. Additionally, when IV is given at an excessive rate (>50 mg/min; >198 μmol/min), cardiovascular collapse or CNS depression has been reported. Total phenytoin plasma concentrations >35 mcg/mL [>139 μmol/L] have been shown to precipitate seizure activity. Free drug may be monitored using ultracentrifugation to separate free drug from bound drug. Phenytoin binding is temperature dependent, and the therapeutic range for free drug is 1-2 mg/L at 37° C at a total level of 10-20 mg/L. The free drug level is the pharmacologically active fraction, and various factors like hypoalbuminemia, uremia, illness, pregnancy, and coadministration of other drugs can unpredictably affect the free fraction in these states. Thus free drug level may be indicated in these complex clinical cases.[8]

Phenytoin is a known human teratogen. Serum levels should be kept as low as possible, consistent with the desired therapeutic effect, in women at risk for pregnancy and throughout pregnancy.

TEST NAME AND METHOD	SPECIMEN	REFERENCE (THERAPEUTIC) INTERVAL, CONVENTIONAL [INTERNATIONAL RECOMMENDED UNITS]	KINETIC VALUES

Phenytoin—CONT

1. Lu-Steffes M, Pittluck G, Jolley M, et al: Fluorescence polarization immunoassay IV. Determination of phenytoin and phenobarbital in human serum and plasma, *Clin Chem* 28:2278-2282, 1982.

2. Haver V, Audino N, Burris S, et al: Four fluorescence polarization immunoassays for therapeutic drug monitoring evaluated, *Clin Chem* 35:138-140, 1989.

3. Hamlin C, Sullivan P: Adaptation of EMIT reagents to the Cobas Bio centrifugal analyzer, *Clin Chem* 30:314-315, 1984.

4. Martinavarro-Dominguez A, Capella-Peiro ME, Gil-Agusti M, et al: Therapeutic drug monitoring of anticonvulsant drugs by micellar HPLC with direct injection of serum samples, *Clin Chem* 48:1696-1702, 2002.

5. Baselt RC: *Disposition of toxic drugs and chemicals in man,* ed 7, Foster City, CA, 2004, Chemical Toxicology Institute.

6. Lexi-Comp, Inc: *Up-to-date online 12.2. Drug information,* Hudson, OH, 2004, Lexi-Comp, Inc.

7. Neuvonen PJ: Bioavailability of phenytoin: clinical pharmacokinetic and therapeutic implications, *Clin Pharmacokinet* 4:91-103, 1979.

8. Burt M, Anderson DC, Kloss J, et al: Evidence-based implementation of free phenytoin therapeutic drug monitoring, *Clin Chem* 46:1132-1135, 2000.

TEST NAME AND METHOD	SPECIMEN	REFERENCE (THERAPEUTIC) INTERVAL, CONVENTIONAL [INTERNATIONAL RECOMMENDED UNITS]		KINETIC VALUES	
Pindolol (Visken)[1]	Serum, plasma (EDTA, heparin)	Therapeutic concentration:	0.5-6.2 ng/mL [× 4.03 = 2.0-25.0 nmol/L]	PK^{2-5}: $t_{1/2}$: V_d:	3.6 ± 0.6 hr 1.2-2.0 L/kg
Fluorimetric, GLC, HPLC		Toxic concentration:	Not well defined	Cl_T: PB:	8.3 ± 1.8 mL/min/kg 51 ± 3%
MW: 248.33				F:	75 ± 9%

FACTORS INFLUENCING DRUG DISPOSITION	REMARKS AND INTERFERENCES

azepam, phenobarbital, rifampin, and alcohol. Salicylates, phenylbutazone, and sulfonylureas compete with phenytoin for serum protein binding sites. The end result is decreased total serum concentration of phenytoin with no change in free phenytoin concentration or pharmacologic effect. Sodium valproate displaces phenytoin from protein binding sites and inhibits its metabolism. Antacids and sucralfate may decrease phenytoin bioavailability.

Interferences: The principal metabolite of phenytoin, 5-(p-hydroxyphenyl)-5-phenylhydantoin, may cross-react with phenytoin in the RIA and EIA methods. Cross-reactivity may be of significance only in the presence of renal failure.

Specimens should not be collected in serum separator tubes because phenytoin may be extracted by the separator gel.

Metabolism
　Hepatic
Excretion
　Urine, bile/feces
Diseases
　Renal: $t_{1/2}\uparrow$, $V_d\rightarrow$, $Cl_T\downarrow$, $F\downarrow$
　Hepatic[6]
　Acute hepatitis: $Cl_T\uparrow$
　Cirrhosis: $Cl_T\downarrow\rightarrow$

Drug interactions: Pindolol is a major substrate of CYP2D6. CYP2D6 inhibitors like chlorpromazine, fluoxetine, miconazole, quinidine, quinine, and ritonavir may increase the effects of pindolol.[7] Phenothiazines and cimetidine may increase plasma concentrations, probably through an effect on hepatic metabolism.

This β-blocker possesses intrinsic sympathomimetic activity (ISA). Plasma concentrations that produce minimal β-blockade vary widely. Therapeutic concentrations are expressed in terms of plasma concentrations that produce β-blockade. However, there is no good correlation between plasma concentrations and therapeutic effects. Thus determination of serum levels is of limited value in routine therapy. Slight but persistent increases in liver enzymes, without injury, have been reported.

TEST NAME AND METHOD	SPECIMEN	REFERENCE (THERAPEUTIC) INTERVAL, CONVENTIONAL [INTERNATIONAL RECOMMENDED UNITS]	KINETIC VALUES

Pindolol—CONT

1. Baselt RC: *Disposition of toxic drugs and chemicals in man,* ed 7, Foster City, CA, 2004, Chemical Toxicology Institute.
2. Johnsson G, Regårdh C: Clinical pharmacokinetics of β-adrenoreceptor blocking drugs, *Clin Pharmacokinet* 1:233-263,1976.
3. Evans WE, Schentag JJ, Jusko WJ: *Applied pharmacokinetics—principles of therapeutic drug monitoring,* ed 3, Vancouver, WA, 1992, Applied Therapeutics, Inc.
4. Hardman JG, Limbird LE, Gilman AG: *Goodman & Gilman's the pharmacological basis of therapeutic,* ed 10, New York, 2001, McGraw-Hill.

Prazepam (Centrax)[1-9]

HPLC, GC, LC-MS

MW: 324.8

Serum, plasma

Desmethyldiazepam (active metabolite)

	mcg/mL		μmol/L
Therapeutic concentration:	0.12-1.0	× 3.08	[0.4-3.1]
Toxic concentration:	>1.0		[1.0]

$t_{1/2}$: 40-120 hr
V_d: 9.3-19.5 L/kg
Cl_T: 0.1-0.3 mL/min/kg
PB: 95-98%
[× 0.01 = 0.95-0.98, protein-bound mole fraction]

1. Baselt R: *Disposition of toxic drugs and chemicals in man,* ed 7, Foster City, CA, 2004, Biomedical Publications.
2. Schulz M, Schmoldt A: Therapeutic and toxic blood concentrations of more than 800 drugs and other xenobiotics, *Pharmazie* 58:447-474, 2003.
3. Hardman JG, Limbird LE, Gilman AG: *Goodman and Gilman's the pharmacological basis of therapeutics,* ed 10, New York, 2001, McGraw-Hill.
4. *Physicians desk reference,* ed 58, Montvale, NJ, 2004, Thomson PDR.
5. Clarke EGC: *Clarke's isolation and identification of drugs in pharmaceuticals, body fluids, and post-mortem material,* London, 1986, The Pharmaceutical Press.
6. ACP's PIER: *Physicians' information and education resource (online version),* Philadelphia, 2004, American College of Physicians.
7. *USP DI drug information for the health care professional,* ed 24, (online version), Taunton, MA, 2004, Micromedex Inc.
8. Kratzsch C, Tenberken O, Peters FT, et al: Screening, library-assisted identification and validated quantification of 23 benzodiazepines, flumazenil, zaleplone, zolpidem and zopiclone in plasma by liquid chromatography/mass spectrometry with atmospheric pressure chemical ionization, *J Mass Spectrom* 39:856-872, 2004.
9. Rasanen I, Ojanpera I, Vuori E: Quantitative screening for benzodiazepines in blood by dual-column gas chromatography and comparison of the results with urine immunoassay, *J Anal Toxicol* 24:46-51, 2000.

Primidone (Mysoline)[1-6]

HPLC, GLC, EIA, FPIA

MW: 218.26

Serum, plasma (heparin, EDTA). Collect at trough concentration. Stable at room temperature for several hours, for 1 yr at −20° C.

	mcg/mL		μmol/L
Therapeutic concentration:	5-12	× 4.58	[23-55]
Toxic concentration:	>15		[>69]

PK[7,8]:
$t_{1/2}$: 3.3-7 hr[9]
V_d: 2-3 L/kg[10]
Cl_T: 0.78 ± 0.62 mL/min/kg
PB: 20-30%[11]
F: 92 ± 18%

FACTORS INFLUENCING DRUG DISPOSITION	REMARKS AND INTERFERENCES

5. Meier J: Pharmacokinetic comparison of pindolol with other beta-adrenoceptor-blocking agents, *Am Heart J* 104:364-373, 1982.
6. Ohnhaus EE, Münch U, Meier J: Elimination of pindolol in liver disease, *Eur J Clin Pharmacol* 22:247-251, 1982.
7. Lexi-Comp, Inc: *Up-to-date online 12.2. Drug information,* Hudson, OH, 2004, Lexi-Comp, Inc.

Metabolism
  Hepatic, CYP3A4 (minor)
Disease
  Liver: $t_{1/2}\uparrow$, $Cl_T\downarrow$, $V_d\rightarrow$
  Renal: $Cl_T\rightarrow$

Drug interactions: Sedative effects and/or respiratory depression may be additive with CNS depressants

Prazepam is a prodrug for desmethyldiazepam and undergoes almost complete first-pass dealkylation by the liver to form desmethyldiazepam. Side effects include confusion, ataxia, excitement, agitation, transient hypotension, vertigo, drug fever, GI upset, leukopenia, and liver disease. Abuse of prazepam may be monitored by urine drug testing with a benzodiazepine-class assay; confirmation of positive specimens is performed by GC-MS determination of the metabolite oxazepam. See *Oxazepam.*

Metabolism
  Hepatic
Excretion
  Bile/feces (primary)
  Urine (secondary)
Disease or condition
  Uremia: $t_{1/2}\uparrow$, $Cl_T\downarrow$
  Pregnancy: $Cl_T\uparrow$

Primidone is used in the treatment of seizure disorders. The drug is metabolized to the active metabolites phenobarbital ($t_{1/2}$: 50-140 hr) and phenylethylmalonamide ($t_{1/2}$: 25-30 hr). Concurrent monitoring of phenobarbital concentrations is required. Side effects include sedation, nystagmus, dizziness, ataxia, and leukopenia.

See also *Phenobarbital.*

TEST NAME AND METHOD	SPECIMEN	REFERENCE (THERAPEUTIC) INTERVAL, CONVENTIONAL [INTERNATIONAL RECOMMENDED UNITS]	KINETIC VALUES

Primidone—CONT

1. Nishina T, Okoshi K, Kitamura M: Improved method for measurement of serum levels of phenobarbital, carbamazepine, primidone and diphenylhydantoin by gas-liquid chromatography, *Clin Chim Acta* 73:463-468, 1976.

2. Dietzler DN, Hoelting CR, Leckie MP, et al: Emit assays for five major anticonvulsant drugs. An evaluation of adaptations to two discrete kinetic analyzers, *Am J Clin Pathol* 74:41-50, 1980.

3. Smith DB, Carl GF: Fluorescent immunoassay for determining antiepileptic drug concentrations: clinical usefulness, *Arch Neurol* 39:363-366, 1982.

4. Sadée W, Beelen GCM: *Drug level monitoring,* New York, 1980, John Wiley and Sons.

5. Chan K, Lok S, Teoh R: The simultaneous determination of five anti-epileptic drugs in plasma by high performance liquid chromatography, *Methods Find Exp Clin Pharmacol* 6:701-704, 1984.

6. Baselt RC: *Disposition of toxic drugs and chemicals in man,* ed 7, Foster City, CA, 2004, Chemical Toxicology Institute.

7. Evans WE, Schentag JJ, Jusko WJ: *Applied pharmacokinetics—principles of therapeutic drug monitoring,* ed 3, Vancouver, WA, 1992, Applied Therapeutics, Inc.

8. Hardman JG, Limbird LE, Gilman AG: *Goodman & Gilman's the pharmacological basis of therapeutics,* ed 10, New York, 2001, McGraw-Hill.

9. Micromedex: *Micromedex healthcare series 2004,* Greenwood Village, CO, 2004, Thomson Micromedex.

10. Lexi-Comp, Inc: *Up-to-date online 12.2. Drug information,* Hudson, OH, 2004, Lexi-Comp, Inc.

11. Hvidberg EF, Dam M: Clinical pharmacokinetics of anticonvulsants, *Clin Pharmacokinet* 1:161-188, 1976.

TEST NAME AND METHOD	SPECIMEN	REFERENCE (THERAPEUTIC) INTERVAL, CONVENTIONAL [INTERNATIONAL RECOMMENDED UNITS]			KINETIC VALUES	
Procainamide (Pronestyl)[1-7]	Serum, plasma (heparin, EDTA, and oxalate). Stable for 2 wk at 2-8° C, 6 mo at −20° C. Collect a trough concentration for assay of procainamide and N-acetylprocainamide.		*mcg/mL*		*μmol/L*	PK[7-10]:
		Therapeutic concentration*:	4-8	× 4.23	[17-33]	$t_{1/2}$: 2.5-5.0 hr
GC, HPLC, EIA, FPIA		Toxic concentration:	>10		[>42]	V_d: 1.5-4.3 L/kg
						Cl_T
MW: 235.33		*Should be analyzed in conjunction with N-acetylprocainamide.				Fast acetylators: 9.8 ± 2.3 mL/min/kg
						Slow acetylators: 8.6 ± 3.1 mL/min/kg
						PB: 15%
						F: 80-90%

| FACTORS INFLUENCING
DRUG DISPOSITION | REMARKS AND INTERFERENCES |

Age
   Neonate: $t_{1/2}\uparrow$
   Child: $t_{1/2}\rightarrow$, $Cl_T\rightarrow$
Dialysis[12]
   Hemodialysis (+)

Drug interactions: Primidone is a strong inducer of CYP1A2, CYP2B6, CYP2C8/9, and CYP3A4.[10]

---

12.   Bennett WM, Aronoff GR, Golper TA, et al: *Drug prescribing in renal failure: dosing guidelines for adults,* ed 2, Philadelphia, 1991, American College of Physicians.

Metabolism:
   Hepatic
   (Active metabolite: *N*-acetylprocainamide
   [NAPA])
Excretion
   Urine
Disease
   Renal: $t_{1/2}\uparrow$, 11.3 hr
   $Cl_T\downarrow$, 5.2 ± 1.7 mL/min/kg[11]
   CHF: $V_d\downarrow$, $Cl_T\downarrow$
   MI: $t_{1/2}\uparrow$, $Cl_T\downarrow$
   Obesity: $t_{1/2}\rightarrow$, $V_d\downarrow$
Age
   Child: $t_{1/2}\downarrow$, $V_d\rightarrow$, $Cl_T\uparrow$
Dialysis
   Hemodialysis (+)

Procainamide is a class IA antiarrhythmic agent. The drug undergoes metabolism by hepatic *N*-acetyltransferase. This metabolic reaction is distributed bimodally (i.e., as rapid and slow metabolizers). *N*-acetylprocainamide (NAPA), procainamide's major metabolite, possesses significant pharmacologic activity and should also be monitored. Side effects include anorexia, nausea, vomiting, diarrhea, giddiness, psychosis, hallucinations, mental depression, and cardiac anomalies. Hypersensitivity reactions include fever, hepatic disturbances, agranulocytosis, and SLE-like syndrome. Slow acetylators are at a greater risk of developing procainamide-induced SLE.

Procainamide concentrations should be evaluated in conjunction with NAPA concentrations. When the sum of procainamide and NAPA concentrations is >25-30 mcg/mL, the risk of toxicity is increased.

See also *N-Acetylprocainamide* (active metabolite).

TEST NAME AND METHOD	SPECIMEN	REFERENCE (THERAPEUTIC) INTERVAL, CONVENTIONAL [INTERNATIONAL RECOMMENDED UNITS]	KINETIC VALUES

Procainamide—CONT

1. Walberg C, Wan S: Clinical evaluation of the EMIT procainamide and N-acetylprocainamide assay, *Ther Drug Monit* 1:47-56, 1979.
2. Bridges R, Jennison T: An HPLC method for the simultaneous quantitation of quinidine, procainamide, *N*-acetylprocainamide, and disopyramide, *J Anal Toxicol* 7:65-68, 1983.
3. Follath F, Ganzinger U, Schuetz E: Reliability of antiarrhythmic drug plasma concentration monitoring, *Clin Pharmacokinet* 8:63-82, 1983.
4. Haver V, Audino N, Burris S, et al: Four fluorescence polarization immunoassays for therapeutic drug monitoring evaluated, *Clin Chem* 35:138-140, 1989.
5. Azzazy HME, Chou PP, Poklis A, et al: Multicenter evaluation of the Abbott AxSYM procainamide and *N*-acetylprocainamide assays: comparison with Abbott TDx/TDxFLx, Syva EMIT 2000, DuPont ACA, and HPLC methods, *Clin Biochem* 31:55-58, 1998.
6. Warner A, Annesley T: Guidelines for therapeutic drug monitoring services: National Academy of Clinical Biochemistry, *Am Assoc Clin Chem,* Washington, DC, 1999.
7. Baselt RC: *Disposition of toxic drugs and chemicals in man,* ed 7, Foster City, CA, 2004, Chemical Toxicology Institute.
8. Hardman JG, Limbird LE, Gilman AG: *Goodman & Gilman's the pharmacological basis of therapeutics,* ed 10, New York, 2001, McGraw-Hill.
9. Lima JJ, Goldfarb AL, Conti DR, et al: Safety and efficacy of procainamide infusions, *Am J Cardiol* 43:98-105, 1979.

TEST NAME AND METHOD	SPECIMEN	REFERENCE INTERVAL		KINETIC VALUES
Procaine **(Novocain)**[1,2] *GC-MS, HPLC* MW: 236.31	Plasma (heparin). Add 2 drops 50% sodium arsenite (or 1 mg echothiopate)[3] per mL blood.	Therapeutic concentration: Toxic concentration:	*mcg/mL* <11 >21	×4.23	*μmol/L* [<47] [>89]	PK[4]: $t_{1/2}$: 7.69 ± 0.99 min V_d: 0.79 ± 0.14 L/kg (1.0 mg/kg/min infusion) V_d: 0.34 ± 0.70 L/kg (1.5 mg/kg/min infusion) Cl_T: 80.0 mL/min/kg (1.0 mg/kg/min infusion) Cl_T: 40.0 mL/min/kg (1.5 mg/kg/min infusion)

1. Storms ML, Stewart JT: Stability-indicating HPLC assays for the determination of prilocaine and procaine drug combinations, *J Pharm Biomed Anal* 30:49-58, 2002.
2. Baselt RC: *Disposition of toxic drugs and chemicals in man,* ed 7, Foster City, CA, 2004, Chemical Toxicology Institute.
3. Smith RH, Brewster MA, MacDonald JA, et al: Measurement of chloroprocaine and procaine in plasma by flame ionization gas-liquid chromatography, *Clin Chem* 24:1599-1602, 1978.

FACTORS INFLUENCING DRUG DISPOSITION	REMARKS AND INTERFERENCES

Drug interactions: Procainamide levels may be increased during coadministration with amiodarone, cimetidine, and ranitidine.

Interferences: Fluorometry and spectrophotometry generally lack specificity and should be avoided. Hemolysis, icterus, and lipemia interfere with assays other than GLC and HPLC.

See Table II-5.

10. Karlsson E: Clinical pharmacokinetics of procainamide, *Clin Pharmacokinet* 3:97-107, 1978.
11. Gibson TP, Atkinson AJ Jr, Matusik E, et al: Kinetics of procainamide and N-acetylprocainamide in renal failure, *Kidney Int* 12:422-429, 1977.

Metabolism
  Plasma hydrolysis
Excretion
  Urine

Drug interactions: Concurrent use of succinylcholine with procaine can lead to prolonged neuromuscular blockade. Procaine is a PABA derivative, and it can antagonize sulfonamide's antibacterial effects.[5]

Procaine is rapidly hydrolyzed in plasma by cholinesterase. Sodium arsenite or echothiopate added to drawn blood minimizes in vitro hydrolysis. Although procaine is rarely administered except as a spinal, topical, or nerve-blocking agent, monitoring the drug or metabolite assesses the degree of peripheral absorption. Adverse effects include hypertension, tachycardia, mydriasis, and convulsions. Colorimetric methods are nonspecific.

4. Seifen AB, Ferrari AA, Seifen EE, et al: Pharmacokinetics of intravenous procaine infusions in humans, *Anesth Analg* 58:382-386, 1979.
5. Micromedex: *Micromedex healthcare series 2004,* Greenwood Village, CO, 2004, Thomson Micromedex.

TEST NAME AND METHOD	SPECIMEN	REFERENCE (THERAPEUTIC) INTERVAL, CONVENTIONAL [INTERNATIONAL RECOMMENDED UNITS]	KINETIC VALUES	
Propafenone (Rythmol)[1] *GC-MS, HPLC* *MW: 341.45*	Serum	Therapeutic concentration: 176-1648 ng/mL[2] Toxic concentration: Not well defined Well absorbed orally with plasma C_{max} occurring 2-3 hr. Although reported effective plasma concentration range from 40-3000 ng/mL, plasma concentration appears to correlate poorly with antiarrhythmic effects. Thus efficacy and toxicity should be monitored more by echocardiographic parameters (QRS prolongation) and suppression of dysrhythmias.[3]	PK[1,3-6]: $t_{1/2}$: V_d: PB: F:	2-10 hr (normal metabolizers) 10-32 hr (slow metabolizers) 1.9-3.0 L/kg 85-97% 10-20%

1. Baselt RC: *Disposition of toxic drugs and chemicals in man,* ed 7, Foster City, CA, 2004, Chemical Toxicology Institute.
2. Hammill S, Sorenson PB, Wood DL, et al: Propafenone for the treatment of refractory complex ventricular ectopic activity, *Mayo Clin Proc* 61:98-103, 1986.
3. Campbell TJ, Williams KM: Therapeutic drug monitoring: antiarrhythmic drugs, *Br J Clin Pharmacol* 46:307-319, 1998.
4. Mason WD, Lanman RC, Kirsten EB: Plasma and saliva propafenone concentrations at steady state, *J Pharm Sci* 76:437-440, 1987.
5. Siddoway LA, Roden DM, Woosley RL: Clinical pharmacology of propafenone: pharmacokinetics, metabolism and concentration-response relations, *Am J Cardiol* 54:9D-12D, 1984.
6. Gillis AM, Yee YG, Kates RE: Binding of antiarrhythmic drug to purified human alpha 1-acid glycoprotein, *Biochem Pharmacol* 34:4279-4282, 1985.
7. Lexi-Comp, Inc: *Up-to-date online 12.2. Drug information,* Hudson, OH, 2004, Lexi-Comp, Inc.
8. Micromedex: *Micromedex healthcare series 2004,* Greenwood Village, CO, 2004, Thomson Micromedex.

TEST NAME AND METHOD	SPECIMEN		*mcg/mL*		*μmol/L*	KINETIC VALUES	
Propoxyphene (Darvon)[1-3] *GC, IA, HPLC, GC-MS* *MW: 339.5*	Serum	Therapeutic concentration: Toxic concentration:	0.05-0.4 >0.5	× 2.95	[0.3-1.2] [>1.5]	$t_{1/2}$: V_d: Cl_T Systemic: Oral: PB: F: C_{max}:	6-12 hr 10-25.7 L/kg 8.57-17.14 mL/min/kg 18.57-51.4 mL/min/kg 76-80% [× 0.01 = 0.76-0.8, protein-bound mole fraction] 30-70% 2-4 hr

FACTORS INFLUENCING DRUG DISPOSITION	REMARKS AND INTERFERENCES

Metabolism
  Hepatic
Excretion
  Feces (primary)
  Urine (secondary)
Dialysis
  Hemodialysis (−)
  Peritoneal dialysis (−)

Drug interactions: Propafenone is a major substrate of CYP2D6 and a minor substrate of CYP1A2 and CYP3A4. It inhibits CYP1A2, CYP2C8/9, and CYP2D6 weakly. CYP2D6 inhibitors like chlorpromazine, fluoxetine, and miconazole may increase the effects of propafenone.[7]

Propafenone is a class 1C antiarrhythmic agent with structural similarities to propranolol. Propafenone has demonstrated efficacy in both ventricular and supraventricular arrhythmias but should be reserved for use in ventricular arrhythmias deemed to be life threatening.[8]

Side effects include dizziness, unusual taste, first-degree atrioventricular block, intraventricular conduction delay, nausea and/or vomiting, and constipation. Dyspnea, congestive heart failure, proarrhythmia hepatotoxicity, agranulocytosis, leukopenia, positive antinuclear antibody, and sexual dysfunction have been reported.[8]

Interpretation of serum propafenone is complex because it is a racemic drug, with the enantiomers having differing activities, and the metabolite 5-hydroxypropafenone has antiarrhythmic activity.[3]

Metabolism
  Hepatic
Excretion
  Renal
Disease
  Cirrhosis, Propoxyphene, Norpropoxyphene:
  PB↓
  Renal, Propoxyphene, Norpropoxyphene:
  Cl_T↓
Age
  $t_{1/2}$↑

Drug interactions: Smoking may increase the hepatic metabolism of propoxyphene.

Propoxyphene is a synthetic opiate agonist. The dextrorotary isomer is a synthetic narcotic analgesic; the levorotary isomer is antitussive. The drug undergoes extensive first-pass metabolism (*N*-demethylation) to an active metabolite, norpropoxyphene. The metabolite is thought to contribute significantly to the toxic effects reported. Propoxyphene is a CNS depressant and has a potential for abuse. Acute overdose is characterized by a rapid onset of coma, severe respiratory depression, convulsions, pulmonary edema, and death. Nephrogenic diabetes insipidus and various ECG abnormalities may be seen. Naloxone and nalorphine are specific antidotes.

Abuse of propoxyphene may be monitored using urine. Samples can be screened using immunoassays. The presence of propoxyphene and norpropoxyphene can be confirmed using GC-MS.

TEST NAME AND METHOD	SPECIMEN	REFERENCE (THERAPEUTIC) INTERVAL, CONVENTIONAL [INTERNATIONAL RECOMMENDED UNITS]			KINETIC VALUES	

Propoxyphene—CONT

	Urine (monitoring)	Norpropoxyphene (metabolite)			$t_{1/2}$:	30-36 hr
					PB:	74%
			mcg/mL	*μmol/L*		[× 0.01 = 0.74,
		Therapeutic				protein-bound
		concentration:	0.1-1.5 × 3.07	[0.3-4.6]		mole fraction]
		Toxic				
		concentration:	>1.5	[>6.1]		

1. Amalfitano G, Bessard J, Vincent F, et al: Gas chromatographic quantitation of dextropropoxyphene and norpropoxyphene in urine after solid-phase extraction, *J Anal Toxicol* 20:547-554, 1996.

2. Pettersson KJ, Nilsson LB: Determination of dextropropoxyphene and norpropoxyphene in plasma by high-performance liquid chromatography, *J Chromatogr* 581:161-164, 1992.

3. Schulz M, Schmoldt A: Therapeutic and toxic blood concentrations of more than 800 drugs and other xenobiotics, *Pharmazie* 58:447-474, 2003.

Propranolol (Inderal)[1-3] *HPLC, GC-MS* *MW: 259.35*	Serum, plasma (heparin, EDTA). Stable at room temperature for ~1 wk. Stabilization of the labile metabolite 4-hydroxypropranolol can be accomplished with the addition of sodium metabisulfite. Collect the specimen at trough concentration.	Therapeutic concentration: Toxic concentration:	50-100 ng/mL [× 3.86 = 193-386 nmol/L] Not defined	PK[3-6]: $t_{1/2}$ Adult: Child: V_d: Cl_T: PB: F:	4-6 hr 2-4 hr 3.6 L/kg 11.4 mL/min/kg 90-95% 30%

FACTORS INFLUENCING DRUG DISPOSITION	REMARKS AND INTERFERENCES

Metabolism
  Hepatic
Excretion
  Urine
Disease or condition
  Hepatic: $t_{1/2}\uparrow$, $V_d\uparrow$, $Cl_T\downarrow$
  Renal failure: $Cl_T\downarrow$
  Hyperthyroidism: $V_d\uparrow$, $Cl_T\uparrow$
  Smoking: $Cl_T\uparrow$
  Malnutrition: $Cl_T\downarrow$
  Hypothermia: $Cl_T\downarrow$
  Inflammation: $PB\uparrow$
  Obesity: $PB\uparrow$
  Pregnancy: $PB\uparrow$
Age
  Elderly: $t_{1/2}\rightarrow$, $V_d\rightarrow$, $Cl_T\rightarrow$
Dialysis[10]
  Hemodialysis ($-$)

Drug interactions: Propranolol is a major substrate of CYP1A2 and CYP2D6 and a minor substrate of CYP2C19 and CYP3A4. It inhibits CYP1A2 and CYP2D6 weakly.[7] Aluminum hydroxide gel appears to decrease GI absorption. Barbiturates and other enzyme inducers may enhance propranolol metabolism. Phenothiazines and cimetidine may increase plasma concentrations, probably through an effect on hepatic metabolism.[8]

Propranolol may be displaced from protein binding sites by plasticizers in collection devices. Propranolol undergoes significant first-pass metabolism. 4-Hydroxypropranolol, its principal metabolite, is reported to have equal β-blocking activity. It is found in animals only after oral administration. Chronic oral dosing results in a saturation of this pathway, causing decreased Cl_T and increased F. Protein binding is strongly correlated to α_1-acid glycoprotein (protein often elevated in response to inflammation or body stress).[9] Side effects include nausea, vomiting, mild diarrhea, constipation, hallucinations, nightmares, insomnia, lassitude, dizziness, depression, heart failure, increased airway resistance, and, rarely, hepatic disturbances with liver enzyme increases. There is no good correlation between plasma concentrations and therapeutic effects.

The fluorometric method is associated with high and variable backgrounds.

TEST NAME AND METHOD	SPECIMEN	REFERENCE (THERAPEUTIC) INTERVAL, CONVENTIONAL [INTERNATIONAL RECOMMENDED UNITS]				KINETIC VALUES

Propranolol—CONT

1. Fu C, Mason W: Determination of propranolol and 4-hydroxypropranolol in human plasma by high-performance liquid chromatography, *Analyst* 114:1219-1223, 1989.

2. Quaglio M, Bellini A, Minozzi L, et al: Simultaneous determination of propranolol or metoprolol in the presence of butyrophenones in human plasma by gas chromatography with mass spectrometry, *J Pharm Sci* 82:87-90, 1993.

3. Baselt RC: *Disposition of toxic drugs and chemicals in man,* ed 7, Foster City, CA, 2004, Chemical Toxicology Institute.

4. Johnsson G, Regårdh C: Clinical pharmacokinetics of β-adrenoreceptor blocking drugs, *Clin Pharmacokinet* 1:233-263, 1976.

5. Hardman JG, Limbird LE, Gilman AG: *Goodman & Gilman's the pharmacological basis of therapeutics,* ed 10, New York, 2001, McGraw-Hill.

Quinidine[1-4]	Serum, plasma (EDTA). Collect at	*mcg/mL*		*μmol/L*	PK[4,6-8]:	
	Therapeutic				$t_{1/2}$:	4-7 hr
GC, HPLC,	trough concentration. Freeze if not	concentration:	2-5	× 3.08	[6.2-15.4]	V_d:	2.4 L/kg
fluorimetric, EIA,	Toxic				Cl_T:	4.7 mL/min/kg
FPIA, FIA	assayed within 24 hr. Stable for	concentration:	>6		[>18.5]	PB:	80-90%
					F:	Gluconate: 71%
MW: 324.42	~1 mo at −5° C.[5]					Sulfate: 80%

1. Lehmann C, Boran K, Pierson W, et al: Quinidine assays: enzyme immunoassay versus high performance liquid chromatography, *Ther Drug Monit* 8:336-339, 1986.

2. Zaninotto M, Secchiero S, Paleari C, et al: Performance of a fluorescence polarization immunoassay system evaluated by therapeutic monitoring of four drugs, *Ther Drug Monit* 14:301-305, 1992.

6. Evans WE, Schentag JJ, Jusko WJ: *Applied pharmacokinetics—principles of therapeutic drug monitoring,* ed 3, Vancouver, WA, 1992, Applied Therapeutics, Inc.

7. Lexi-Comp, Inc: *Up-to-date online 12.2. Drug information,* Hudson, OH, 2004, Lexi-Comp, Inc.

8. Hansten PD, Horu SR, et al: *Drug interactions,* ed 6, Philadelphia, 1989, Lea & Febiger.

9. Edwards D, Lalka D, Cerra F, et al: 1-Acid glycoprotein concentration and protein binding in trauma, *Clin Pharmacol Ther* 3:62-67, 1982.

10. Bennett WM, Aronoff GR, Golper TA, et al: *Drug prescribing in renal failure: dosing guidelines for adults,* ed 2, Philadelphia, 1991, American College of Physicians.

FACTORS INFLUENCING DRUG DISPOSITION	REMARKS AND INTERFERENCES

Metabolism
  Hepatic
Excretion
  Bile/feces (primary)
  Urine (secondary)
Disease
  Hepatic: $t_{1/2}\uparrow$, $V_d\uparrow$, $Cl_T\downarrow$, $PB\downarrow$
  CHF: $t_{1/2}\rightarrow$, $V_d\downarrow$, $Cl_T\downarrow$
  Renal: $Cl_T\downarrow$
  Hyperlipoproteinemia: $PB\rightarrow$
Age[9]
  Elderly: $t_{1/2}\uparrow$, $V_d\rightarrow$, $Cl_T\downarrow$, $PB\rightarrow$
Dialysis[10]
  Hemodialysis $(+)$
  Peritoneal $(+)$

Drug interactions: Quinidine is a major substrate of CYP3A4 and a minor substrate of CYP2C8/9 and CYP2E1. It strongly inhibits CYP2D6 and CYP3A4 and weakly inhibits CYP2C8/9.[11] Enzyme inducers (rifampin, phenobarbital, and phenytoin) may enhance the metabolism of quinidine. Quinidine levels may also be decreased by disopyramide and nifedipine. Plasma quinidine levels may be increased during coadministration with amiodarone, cimetidine, verapamil, and thiazides. Renal quinidine clearance can be enhanced by acidifying the urine. Antacids (sodium bicarbonate, acetazolamide) tend to increase renal reabsorption and elevate plasma or serum concentration.

Quinidine is a class IA antiarrhythmic agent. The drug is metabolized to 3-hydroxyquinidine, 2'-oxoquinidinone, and *O*-desmethylquinidine. These metabolites may contribute to quinidine's antiarrhythmic and toxic effects. Earlier studies should be interpreted with caution because of lack of assay specificity. The optimal therapeutic concentration of quinidine is method dependent because of interference by metabolites and by dihydroquinidine. The optimal therapeutic concentration by double-extraction fluorometric procedures and by EIA is 2-5 mcg/mL [6.2-15.4 μmol/L]; by liquid chromatography it is 1.5-4.5 mcg/mL [4.6-13.9 μmol/L]. Side effects include nausea, vomiting, diarrhea, tinnitus, loss of hearing, blurring of vision, headache, diplopia, photophobia, hypotension, tachycardia, ventricular fibrillation, hemolytic anemia, leukopenia, thrombocytopenia, hepatic dysfunction, and cardiac anomalies.

Quinidine may be displaced from protein binding sites by plasticizers in collecting devices. Increased protein binding of quinidine to α_1-acid glycoprotein after myocardial infarction or other stressful events may increase total quinidine concentrations.[12] However, free quinidine concentrations may remain unaltered, and dosage adjustment may not be warranted.

Interferences: EIA and FPIA assays do not differentiate quinidine from dihydroquinidine (a naturally occurring analog of quinidine found in all drug products). Metabolites of quinidine may cross-react and cause false increases in quinidine concentration. (This may be important in renal failure patients, who have lower clearance of quinidine and metabolites.) The fluorometric technique without extraction and separation is nonspecific and should not be used. Quinine and other drugs that fluoresce may interfere.[13]

Specimens should not be collected in serum separator tubes because quinidine may be extracted by the separator gel.

See Table II-5.

3. Haver V, Audino N, Burris S, et al: Four fluorescence polarization immunoassays for therapeutic drug monitoring evaluated, *Clin Chem* 35:138-140, 1989.

4. Baselt RC: *Disposition of toxic drugs and chemicals in man,* ed 7, Foster City, CA, 2004, Chemical Toxicology Institute.

TEST NAME AND METHOD	SPECIMEN	REFERENCE (THERAPEUTIC) INTERVAL, CONVENTIONAL [INTERNATIONAL RECOMMENDED UNITS]		KINETIC VALUES

Quinidine—CONT

5. Koch T, Platoff G: Suitability of collection tubes with separator gels for therapeutic drug monitoring, *Ther Drug Monit* 12:277-280, 1990.

6. Ueda CT, Hirschfeld DS, Scheinman MM, et al: Disposition kinetics of quinidine, *Clin Pharmacol Ther* 19:30-36, 1976.

7. Ochs HR, Greenblatt DJ, Woo E: Clinical pharmacokinetics of quinidine, *Clin Pharmacokinet* 5:150-168, 1980.

8. Evans WE, Schentag JJ, Jusko WJ: *Applied pharmacokinetics—principles of therapeutic drug monitoring,* ed 3, Vancouver, WA, 1992, Applied Therapeutics, Inc.

9. Ochs HR, Greenblatt DJ, Woo E, et al: Reduced quinidine clearance in elderly persons, *Am J Cardiol* 42:481-485, 1978.

Quinine[1-3]	Plasma (EDTA)	*mcg/mL*	*μmol/L*	PK[3,4]:
		Tonic water		$t_{1/2}$: 3-15 hr
LC, GC-MS,		ingestion: <0.3 × 3.08 [<0.9]		V_d: 1.8 ± 0.4 L/kg
Fluorimetric UV		Therapeutic		Cl_T: 1.9 ± 0.5 mL/min/kg
spectrophotometry		concentration: 5-10	[15.4-30.8]	PB: 93-95%[5]
		Toxic		
MW: 324.42		concentration: >10	[>30.8]	

1. Bannon P, Yu P, Cook JM, et al: Identification of quinine metabolites in urine after oral dosing in humans, *J Chromatogr B Biomed Sci Appl* 715:387-393, 1998.

2. Mirghani RA, Ericsson O, Cook J, et al: Simultaneous determination of quinine and four metabolites in plasma and urine by high-performance liquid chromatography, *J Chromatogr B Biomed Sci Appl* 754:57-64, 2001.

3. Baselt RC: *Disposition of toxic drugs and chemicals in man,* ed 7, Foster City, CA, 2004, Chemical Toxicology Institute.

4. Hardman JG, Limbird LE, Gilman AG: *Goodman & Gilman's the pharmacological basis of therapeutics,* ed 10, New York, 2001, McGraw-Hill.

5. Wanwimolruk S, Denton JR: Plasma protein binding of quinine: binding to human serum albumin, alpha-1-acid glycoprotein and plasma from patients with malaria, *J Pharm Pharmacol* 44:806-811, 1992.

6. Lexi-Comp, Inc: *Up-to-date online 12.2. Drug information,* Hudson, OH, 2004, Lexi-Comp, Inc.

7. Gilman AG, Rall TW, Nies AS, et al: *The pharmacological basis of therapeutics,* ed 8, New York, 1990, Pergamon Press, Inc.

8. Baselt RC: *Disposition of toxic drugs and chemicals in man,* ed 2, Davis, CA, 1982, Biomedical Publications.

| FACTORS INFLUENCING DRUG DISPOSITION | REMARKS AND INTERFERENCES |

10. Bennett W, Aronof G, Golper T, et al; *Drug prescribing in renal failure. Dosing guidelines for adults,* ed 2, Philadelphia, 1994, American College of Physicians.

11. Lexi-Comp, Inc: *Up-to-date online 12.2. Drug information,* Hudson, OH, 2004, Lexi-Comp, Inc.

12. Edwards D, Lalka D, Cerra F, et al: 1-Acid glycoprotein concentration and protein binding in trauma, *Clin Pharmacol Ther* 3:62-67, 1982.

13. Baselt RC: *Analytic procedures for therapeutic drug monitoring and emergency toxicology,* ed 2, Davis, CA, 1987, Biomedical Publications.

Metabolism
  Hepatic
Excretion
  Feces (primary)
  Saliva (secondary)
  Urine (secondary)

Quinine is metabolized by oxidation to more polar metabolites. Blood concentrations up to 11 mcg/mL [33.9 μmol/L] are found in heroin fatalities. An old treatment for malaria, this drug is encountered now as a diluent in heroin and as a flavoring agent in beverages. Adverse effects include tinnitus, headache, nausea, visual disturbances, decreased body temperature, coma, and death as a result of respiratory arrest.[7] Cases of hemolysis and thrombocytopenia may occur.

Drug interactions: Quinine is a minor substrate of CYP1A2, CYP2C19, and CYP3A4. It strongly inhibits CYP2D6, moderately inhibits CYP2C8/9, and weakly inhibits CYP3A4.[6] Plasma quinine concentrations may be decreased by rifampin. Aluminum-containing antacids may decrease or delay absorption of quinine.

Interferences: TLC can separate quinine and quinidine.[8] In most other assays, quinidine is not differentiated.

See Table II-6.

TEST NAME AND METHOD	SPECIMEN	REFERENCE (THERAPEUTIC) INTERVAL, CONVENTIONAL [INTERNATIONAL RECOMMENDED UNITS]			KINETIC VALUES	
Ranitidine (Zantac)[1-5] *HPLC* *MW: 314.4*	Serum, plasma (heparin, EDTA)	Therapeutic concentration: Peptic ulcer disease Hypersecretory disease Toxic concentration:	*ng/mL* 36-94 71-376 Not well defined	$\times 3.18$	*nmol/L* [114-299] [226-1196]	$t_{1/2}$: V_d: Cl_T: PB: F: T_{max}:	2-3 hr 1.4-4.09 L/kg 1.29-1.44 L/hr/kg 12-18% [$\times 0.01 = 0.12$-0.18, protein-bound mole fraction] 50-60% [$\times 0.01 = 0.50$-0.60, bioavailable mole fraction] 0.5-2 hr

1. Castro A, Arancibia A, Romero P, et al: Validated HPLC method for the determination of ranitidine in plasma, *Pharmazie* 58:696-698, 2003.
2. Fontana M, Massironi E, Rossi A, et al: Ranitidine pharmacokinetics in newborn infants, *Arch Dis Child* 68:602-603, 1993.
3. Kataoka H, Lord HL, Pawliszyn J: Automated in-tube solid-phase microextraction-liquid chromatography-electrospray ionization mass spectrometry for the determination of ranitidine, *J Chromatogr B Biomed Sci Appl* 731:353-359, 1999.
4. Wormsley KG: Safety profile of ranitidine: a review, *Drugs* 46:976-985, 1993.
5. Zendelovska D, Stafilov T: Development of an HPLC method for the determination of ranitidine and cimetidine in human plasma following SPE, *J Pharm Biomed Anal* 33:165-173, 2003.

TEST NAME AND METHOD	SPECIMEN	REFERENCE (THERAPEUTIC) INTERVAL			KINETIC VALUES	
Rifampin, rafampicin (Rifadin)[1-6] *HPLC, LC-MS* *MW: 822.9*	Serum, plasma (heparin, EDTA). Collected as peak, 2 hr after dose. Process immediately and store at −70° C.	Therapeutic concentration: Toxic concentration:	*mcg/mL* 2.6-41 >55	$\times 1.22$	*μmol/L* [3.17-50] [67]	$t_{1/2}$: V_d: Cl_T: PB: F: T_{max}:	1.5-5.1 hr 0.9-1.6 L/kg 7.9-9.7 mL/min/kg 60-90% [$\times 0.01 = 0.75$-0.90, protein-bound mole fraction] 90-95% 1-4 hr

| FACTORS INFLUENCING DRUG DISPOSITION | REMARKS AND INTERFERENCES |

Metabolism
  Hepatic
Excretion
  Renal, fecal
Disease
  Renal: $t_{1/2}\uparrow$, $Cl_T\downarrow$
  Cirrhosis: $t_{1/2}\uparrow$, $F\uparrow$
Age
  Elderly: $t_{1/2}\uparrow$, $Cl_T\downarrow$
Dialysis
  Hemodialysis (+)
  Peritoneal (+)

Drug interactions: Inhibitor of CYP2D6. Ranitidine increases the bioavailability of midazolam. Ranitidine appears to compete with the renal tubular secretion of procainamide (decreasing the renal clearance of procainamide).

Ranitidine is a histamine H_2-receptor antagonist that is adminstered orally or parenterally. Reported adverse effects include severe headaches, mental confusion, visual disturbances, hepatotoxicity, and hepatitis. Rare cases of leukopenia and aplastic anemia have been reported. A slight increase in liver enzymes and serum creatinine may be found. Wide interpatient variability exists in the relationship between plasma concentration and degree of acid suppression.

Metabolism
  Hepatic
Excretion
  Renal, biliary, and fecal
Disease
  Cirrhosis: $t_{1/2}\uparrow$, $Cl_T\downarrow$
  Renal: $t_{1/2}\uparrow$, $Cl_T\downarrow$
Age
  Neonate: $V_d\uparrow$, $Cl_T\uparrow$
Dialysis
  Hemodialysis (−)
  Peritoneal (−)

Drug interactions: Rifampin induces CYP2B6, CYP2C9, CYP2D6, and CYP3A4.

Rifampin is used to treat tuberculosis, as well as Hanson's disease and other infections. The metabolite, desacctylrifampicin, possesses less microbiological activity than the parent compound. Side effects include rash, fever, nausea, vomiting, thrombocytopenia, jaundice, hepatorenal syndrome, eosinophilia, anemia, leukopenia, uremia, immunosuppression, and discoloration of body fluids (e.g., urine, sweat, and tears).

See Tables II-5 and II-6.

TEST NAME AND METHOD	SPECIMEN	REFERENCE (THERAPEUTIC) INTERVAL, CONVENTIONAL [INTERNATIONAL RECOMMENDED UNITS]			KINETIC VALUES	

Rifampin, rafampicin—CONT

1. Boffito M, Tija J, Reynolds HE, et al: Simultaneous determination of rifampicin and efavirenz in plasma, *Ther Drug Monit* 24:670-674, 2002.
2. Calleja I, Blanco-Prieto MJ, Ruz N, et al: High-performance liquid-chromatographic determination of rifampicin in plasma and tissues, *J Chromatogr A* 1031:289-294, 2004.
3. Naidon W, Shou WZ, Addison T, et al: Liquid chromatography/tandem mass spectrometric bioanalysis using normal-phase columns with aqueous/organic mobile phases—a novel approach of eliminating evaporation and reconstitution steps in 96-well SPE, *Rapid Commun Mass Spectrom* 16:1965-1975, 2002.

TEST NAME AND METHOD	SPECIMEN	REFERENCE (THERAPEUTIC)			KINETIC VALUES	
Risperidone (Resperdal)[1-6]	Serum	Therapeutic concentration	*mcg/mL*	*μmol/L*	$t_{1/2}$ Extensive metabolizers:	3 hr
HPLC		Not well established	0.02-0.06 × 2.43	[0.05-0.15]	Poor metabolizers:	20 hr
MW: 410.5		Toxic concentration:			V_d:	1-2 L/kg
		Variable	> 0.06	[>0.15]	Cl_T:	3.2-114 L/hg
					PB:	~90%
					F:	70-90%
					T_{max}:	1 hr

1. Acri AA, Henretig FM: Effects of risperidone in overdose, *Am J Emerg Med* 16:498-501, 1998.
2. Androniki EBG, Gex-Fabry M, Genet C, et al: Therapeutic drug monitoring or risperidone using a new, rapid HPLC method: reappraisal of interindividual variability factors, *Ther Drug Monit* 21:105-115, 1999.
3. Baselt R: *Disposition of toxic drugs and chemicals in man,* ed 7, Foster City, CA, 2004, Biomedical Publications.
4. Frahnert C, Rao ML, Grasmader K: Analysis of eighteen antidepressants, four atypical antipsychotics and active metabolites in serum by liquid chromatography: a simple tool for therapeutic drug monitoring, *J Chromatogr B Analyt Technol Biomed Life Sci* 794:35-47, 2003.
5. Tune LE: Risperidone for the treatment of behavioral and psychological symptoms of dementia, *J Clin Psychiatry* 62(suppl 21):29-32, 2001.
6. Zhou Z, Li X, Li K, et al: Simultaneous determination of clozapine, olanzapine, risperidone and quetiapine in plasma by high-performance liquid chromatography-electrospray ionization mass spectrometry, *J Chromatogr B Analyt Technol Biomed Life Sci* 802:257-262, 2004.

TEST NAME AND METHOD	SPECIMEN	REFERENCE (THERAPEUTIC)	KINETIC VALUES	
Salicylamide[1,2]	Plasma, serum	See *Nonsteroidal Antiinflammatory Drugs, Salicylic Acid.*	$t_{1/2}$:	0.5-1.2 hr
GC, HPLC, fluorescence				
MW: 137.1				

1. Pulgarin JA, Bermejo LF: Simultaneous determination of salicylamide and salsalate in serum and urine by first derivative variable-angle synchronous fluorescence spectrometry, *Anal Biochem* 265:331-339, 1998.
2. Xu X, Pang KS: High-performance liquid chromatographic method for the quantitation of salicylamide and its metabolites in biological fluids, *J Chromatogr* 420:313-327, 1987.

FACTORS INFLUENCING DRUG DISPOSITION	REMARKS AND INTERFERENCES

4. Peloquin CA, Namdar R, Dodge AA, et al: Pharmacokinetics of isoniazid under fasting conditions, with food, and with antacids, *Int J Tuberc Lung Dis* 3:703-710, 1999.
5. Peloquin CA: Therapeutic drug monitoring in the treatment of tuberculosis, *Drugs* 62:2169-2183, 2002.
6. Ray J, Gardiner I, Marriott D: Managing antituberculosis drug therapy by therapeutic drug monitoring of rifampicin and isoniazid, *Intern Med J* 33:229-234, 2003.

Metabolism
  Hepatic, CYP2D6, and *N*-dealkylation
  Active metabolite: 9-hydroxyrisperidone

Drug interactions: Numerous drug interactions are reported.

Resperidone, a benzisoxazole derivative, is an antipsychotic used to treat bipolar disorders and schizophrenia. The drug has high affinity for serotonin and dopamine D2 receptors, as well as α_1- and α_2-adrenoreceptors. Common adverse effects include agitation, extrapyramidal symptoms, somnolence, rhinitis, dizziness, anxiety, and constipation. More serious adverse effects reported include neuroleptic malignant syndrome, seizures, stroke, syncope, and transient ischemic attacks.

Salicylamide is an analgesic-antipyretic compound; however, because of its questionable effectiveness the drug is seldom used (even in over-the-counter preparations). It is not metabolized to salicylate but to inactive metabolites that are rapidly excreted. See *Nonsteroidal Antiinflammatory Drugs, Salicylic Acid*.

TEST NAME AND METHOD	SPECIMEN	REFERENCE (THERAPEUTIC) INTERVAL, CONVENTIONAL [INTERNATIONAL RECOMMENDED UNITS]			KINETIC VALUES	
Salicylic Acid See *Nonsteroidal Antiinflammatory Drugs.*						
Secobarbital **(Seconal)** *Colorimetric, GC, HPLC, IA, CE* *MW: 238.3*	Serum, plasma	*mcg/mL* Therapeutic concentration: 1.5-5.0 Toxic concentration: >7.0	× 4.20	μ*mol/L* [6.3-21.0] [>29.4]	$t_{1/2}$: V_d: PB:	19-34 hr 1.6-1.9 L/kg 30-45% [× 0.01 =0.30-0.45, protein-bound mole fraction]

1. Baselt R: *Disposition of toxic drugs and chemicals in man,* ed 7, Foster City, CA, 2004, Biomedical Publications.

2. Schulz M, Schmoldt A: Therapeutic and toxic blood concentrations of more than 800 drugs and other xenobiotics, *Pharmazie* 58:447-474, 2003.

3. Hardman JG, Limbird, LE, Gilman AG: *Goodman and Gilman's the pharmacological basis of therapeutics,* ed 10, New York, 2001, McGraw-Hill.

4. *Physicians desk reference,* ed 58, Montvale, NJ, 2004, Thomson PDR.

5. Meatherall R: GC/MS confirmation of barbiturates in blood and urine, *J Forensic Sci* 42:1160-1170, 1997.

6. ACP's PIER: *Physicians' information and education resource (online version),* Philadelphia, 2004, American College of Physicians.

7. McEvoy GK, editor: *AHFS drug information (online version),* Bethesda, MD, 2004, American Society of Health-System Pharmacists Inc.

8. Tanaka E, Terada M, Tanno K, et al: Forensic analysis of 10 barbiturates in human biological samples using a new reversed-phase chromatographic column packed with 2-micrometre porous microspherical silica-gel, *Forensic Sci Int* 85:73-82, 1997.

9. Ohyama K, Wada M, Lord GA, et al: Capillary electrochromatographic analysis of barbiturates in serum, *Electrophoresis* 25:594-599, 2004.

10. Quinones-Torrelo C, Martin-Biosca Y, Sagrado S, et al: Determination of amobarbital and secobarbital in plasma samples using micellar liquid chromatography, *Biomed Chromatog* 14:287-292, 2000.

11. Ferslew KE, Hagardorn AN, McCormick WF: Application of micellar electrokinetic capillary chromatography to forensic analysis of barbiturates in biological fluids, *J Forensic Sci* 40:245-249, 1995.

FACTORS INFLUENCING DRUG DISPOSITION	REMARKS AND INTERFERENCES

Metabolism
  Hepatic

Drug interactions: Secobarbital is a strong CYP2A6 and CYP2C8/9 inducer and may decrease the levels of CYP2A6 and CYP2C8/9 substrates. MAO inhibitors and valproic acid may inhibit metabolism of barbiturates, increasing the clinical effect or toxicity.

Secobarbital is a short-acting barbiturate used primarily as a hypnotic in the short-term (up to 2 wk) treatment of insomnia. Adverse effects include hypnosis, sedation, coma, respiratory arrest, and death. Toxicity is intensified when the drug is combined with alcohol or other CNS depressants. Secobarbital is metabolized to several inactive metabolites.

TEST NAME AND METHOD	SPECIMEN	REFERENCE (THERAPEUTIC) INTERVAL, CONVENTIONAL [INTERNATIONAL RECOMMENDED UNITS]			KINETIC VALUES	
Sertraline	Serum, plasma		*mcg/mL*	$\mu mol/L$	$t_{1/2}$:	24-26 hr
(Zoloft)[1-7]		Therapeutic			V_d:	20 L/kg
		concentration:	0.05-0.25 $\times$ 3.26	[0.163-0.82]	Cl_T:	96 mL/min
HPLC, GC-MS,GC		Toxic			PB:	99%
		concentration:	>0.3	[>0.98]	F:	100%
MW: 306.7					T_{max}:	4-8 hr

1. Baselt R: *Disposition of toxic drugs and chemicals in man,* ed 7, Foster City, CA, 2004, Biomedical Publications.

2. Frahnert C, Rao ML, Grasmader K: Analysis of eighteen antidepressants, four atypical antipsychotics and active metabolites in serum by liquid chromatography: a simple tool for therapeutic drug monitoring, *J Chromatogr B Analyt Technol Biomed Life Sci* 794:35-47, 2003.

3. Hemeryck A, Belpaire FM: Selective serotonin reuptake inhibitors and cytochrome P-450 mediated drug-drug interactions: an update, *Curr Drug Metab* 3:13-37, 2002.

4. Isbister GK, Bowe SJ, Dawson A, et al: Relative toxicity of selective serotonin reuptake inhibitors (SSRIs) in overdose, *J Toxicol Clin Toxicol* 42:277-285, 2004.

5. Rogowsky D, Marr M, Long G, et al: Determination of sertraline and desmethylsertraline in human serum using copolymeric bonded-phase extraction, liquid chromatography and gas chromatography-mass spectrometry, *J Chromatogr B Biomed Appl* 655:138-141, 1994.

6. Schulz M, Schmoldt A: Therapeutic and toxic blood concentrations of more than 800 drugs and other xenobiotics, *Pharmazie* 58:447-474, 2003.

7. Tournel G, Houdret N, Hedouin V, et al: High-performance liquid chromatographic method to screen and quantitate seven selective serotonin reuptake inhibitors in human serum, *J Chromatogr B Biomed Sci Appl* 761:147-158, 2001.

Sirolimus	Whole blood	Therapeutic		PK^6:		
(Rapamune,	(EDTA).	trough		$t_{1/2}$:	62 hr[7]	
Rapamycin)		concentration:	5-15 ng/mL if cyclosporine A	V_d:	12.0 L/kg[7]	
	Stable up to 24 hr		is used at a target trough con-	Cl_T:	127-240 mL/kg/hr[7]	
HPLC,[1]	at room tempera-		centration of 75-150 ng/mL.[4,5]	PB:	92%	
LC-MS-MS,[2]	ture, 7 days at	Toxic		F:	15%[8]	
MEIA (premarket	2-8° C, and 3 mo at	concentration:	>15 ng/mL predicts the			
version, no longer	−20° C.[4]		occurrence of adverse drug			
available)[3]			reactions.[5]			
MW: 914.2						

FACTORS INFLUENCING DRUG DISPOSITION	REMARKS AND INTERFERENCES

Metabolism
  Hepatic, Active (weakly) metabolite:
  desmethylsertraline
Excretion
  Renal, fecal
  Hemodialysis (−)

Drug interactions: Sertraline is known to inhibit CYP2D6 and CYP2C9, giving rise to possible drug interactions.

Sertraline is an antidepressant also used to treat other psychiatric disorders such as obsessive-compulsive disorder. The drug acts by selectively inhibiting the reuptake of serotonin. Common adverse effects reported include nausea, diarrhea, tremor, sweating, and sexual dysfunction. More serious adverse effects reported include suicidal ideologies, seizures, and hyponatremia. SSRIs should not be abruptly stopped, but tapered. Increased transaminases have been observed during the first 9 wk of treatment.

Metabolism
  Hepatic
Excretion
  Feces (primary)
  Urine (secondary)
Disease
  Hepatic dysfunction increases concentration of sirolimus and metabolites.
Dialysis
  Hemodialysis (−)
  Peritoneal dialysis (−)

Drug interactions[4]: Sirolimus is a major substrate and weak inhibitor of CYP3A4. Drugs affecting CYP3A4 and P-glycoprotein activities are expected to modulate sirolimus levels.

Sirolimus, a macrocyclic lactone, is an immunosuppressant used in combination with cyclosporine and corticosteroids for prophylaxis of organ rejection after kidney transplantation.[10]

Side effects include anemia, thrombocytopenia, hyperlipidemia, and hypertension. When used in combination with cyclosporine, careful monitoring of renal function is required because this combination has been associated with increases in serum creatinine.[10]

Parent drug appears to contribute to clinical effects because there is no current evidence that metabolites are active; thus most current clinical assays are LC-MS-MS techniques that can specifically measure the parent compound. The MEIA automated immunoassay used in Phase III clinical trials can overestimate sirolimus concentrations by ~43% because of cross-reactivity with the metabolites.[4] Future immunoassays require that the antibodies be relatively specific for the parent drug and have minimal cross-reactivity to its metabolites.

TEST NAME AND METHOD	SPECIMEN	REFERENCE (THERAPEUTIC) INTERVAL, CONVENTIONAL [INTERNATIONAL RECOMMENDED UNITS]	KINETIC VALUES

Sirolimus—CONT

1. Holt D, Lee T, Johnston A: Measurement of sirolimus in whole blood using high-performance liquid chromatography with ultraviolet detection, *Clin Ther* 22(suppl B):B38-48, 2000.

2. Holt DW, Lee T, Jones K, et al: Validation of an assay for routine monitoring of sirolimus using HPLC with mass spectrometric detection, *Clin Chem* 46:1179-1183, 2000.

3. Salm P, Taylor PJ, Pillans PI: Analytical performance of microparticle enzyme immunoassay and HPLC-tandem mass spectrometry in the determination of sirolimus in whole blood, *Clin Chem* 45:2278-2280, 1999.

4. Mahalati K, Kahan B: Clinical pharmacokinetics of sirolimus, *Clin Pharmacokinet* 40:573-585, 2001.

5. Kahan B, Napoli K, Kelly P, et al: Therapeutic drug monitoring of sirolimus: correlations with efficacy and toxicity, *Clin Transplant* 14:97-109, 2000.

6. Lexi-Comp, Inc: *Up-to-date online 12.2. Drug information,* Hudson, OH, 2004, Lexi-Comp, Inc.

7. Zimmerman JJ, Kahan BD: Pharmacokinetics of sirolimus in stable renal transplant patients after multiple oral dose administration, *J Clin Pharmacol* 37:405-415, 1997.

8. Yatscoff RW: Pharmacokinetics of rapamycin, *Transplant Proc* 28:970-973, 1996.

9. Cattaneo D, Merlini S, Pellegrino M, et al: Therapeutic drug monitoring of sirolimus: effect of concomitant immunosuppressive therapy and optimization of drug dosing, *Am J Transplant* 4:1345-1351, 2004.

10. Micromedex: *Micromedex healthcare series 2004,* Greenwood Village, CO, 2004, Thomson Micromedex.

TEST NAME AND METHOD	SPECIMEN	REFERENCE (THERAPEUTIC) INTERVAL, CONVENTIONAL [INTERNATIONAL RECOMMENDED UNITS]	KINETIC VALUES
Strychnine[1-6] *GC, HPLC,* *LC-MS, GC-MS* *MW: 334.4*	Whole blood (fluoride/oxalate), serum, and urine.	None detected. Toxic concentration: >0.75 mcg/mL × 2.99 [>2.24 μmol/L]	$t_{1/2}$: 10-16 hr V_d: 13 L/kg

1. Baselt R: *Disposition of toxic drugs and chemicals in man,* ed 7, Foster City, CA, 2004, Biomedical Publications.

2. Duverneuil C, de la Grandmaison GL, de Mazancourt P, et al: Liquid chromatography/photodiode array detection for determination of strychnine in blood: a fatal case report, *Forensic Sci Int* 141:17-21, 2004.

3. Rosano TG, Hubbard JD, Meola JM, et al: Fatal strychnine poisoning: application of gas chromatography and tandem mass spectrometry, *J Anal Toxicol* 24:642-647, 2000.

FACTORS INFLUENCING DRUG DISPOSITION	**REMARKS AND INTERFERENCES**

Cyclosporine clearance may be reduced if taken concurrently with sirolimus.[6] Concomitant therapy with other immunosuppressives, especially CsA, will lead to higher sirolimus trough levels.[9]

Strychnine is an alkaloid found in the seeds of *Strychnos nuxvomica*. By blocking the inhibition of postsynaptic neuronal impulses, it stimulates the CNS. For this reason, it was historically used as a tonic and, more recently, to treat impotence, nonketotic hyperglycemia, and sleep apnea. It is no longer used in medicine. Currently, its primary use is as a pesticide. Additionally, it has been found as an adulterant of street drugs such as cocaine, heroin, and amphetamines, and of alternative (herbal) medications. Ingestion of 60-100 mg may result in death (adult). Tachycardia, hypertension, tachypnea, convulsions, and hyperthermia may be seen. The patient usually remains alert during the convulsions. Twenty percent of strychnine is excreted in urine unchanged. Little metabolic information is available. Strychnine may be found in urine, blood, gastric fluid, and organs, but the levels do not correlate well with clinical toxicity.

4. Schulz M, Schmoldt A: Therapeutic and toxic blood concentrations of more than 800 drugs and other xenobiotics, *Pharmazie* 58:447-474, 2003.

5. Smith BA: Strychnine poisoning, *J Emerg Med* 8:321-325, 1990.

6. Wang Z, Zhao J, Xing J, et al: Analysis of strychnine and brucine in postmortem specimens by RP-HPLC: a case report of fatal intoxication, *J Anal Toxicol* 28:141-144, 2004.

TEST NAME AND METHOD	SPECIMEN	REFERENCE (THERAPEUTIC) INTERVAL, CONVENTIONAL [INTERNATIONAL RECOMMENDED UNITS]		KINETIC VALUES	
Tacrolimus **(Prograf, FK506)**	Whole blood (EDTA).	Therapeutic concentration: Toxic	5-20 ng/mL (trough)[7,8]	PK[9,10]: $t_{1/2}$: V_d:	8.7-11.3 hr[11] 0.6-1.6 L/kg[2]
LC-MS-MS,[1,2] *FPIA,*[3,4] *ELISA*[5]	Stable for 1 wk at room temperature.[6]	concentration:	Not well defined; acute oral overdose is associated with	Cl_T: PB:	60 mL/kg/hr[7] 75-99%[8]
MW: 804.03			blood tacrolimus concentrations of 19-197 ng/mL.[2]	F:	5-67%[8]

1. Taylor P, Jones A, Balderson G, et al: Sensitive, specific quantitative analysis of tacrolimus (FK506) in blood by liquid chromatography-electrospray tandem mass spectrometry, *Clin Chem* 42:279-285, 1996.

2. Baselt RC: *Disposition of toxic drugs and chemicals in man,* ed 7, Foster City, CA, 2004, Chemical Toxicology Institute.

3. Wallemacq PE, Leal T, Besse T, et al: IMx tacrolimus II vs IMx tacrolimus microparticle enzyme immunoassay evaluated in renal and hepatic transplant patients, *Clin Chem* 43:1989-1991, 1997.

4. Tredger JM, Gilkes CD, Gonde CE: Performance of the IMx tacrolimus II assay and practical limits of detection, *Clin Chem* 45:1881-1882, 1999.

5. Cao ZT, Linder MW, Jevans AW, et al: Comparison of tacrolimus concentrations measured by the IMx tacrolimus II vs the PRO-TRAC II FK506 ELISA assays, *Clin Chem* 45:1868-1870, 1999.

6. Ingels S, Koenig J, Scott M: Stability of FK506 (tacrolimus) in whole-blood specimens, *Clin Chem* 41:1320-1321, 1995.

7. Venkataramanan R, Swaminathan A, Prasad T, et al: Clinical pharmacokinetics of tacrolimus, *Clin Pharmacokinet* 29:404-430, 1995.

8. Wong SHY: Therapeutic drug monitoring for immunosuppressants, *Clin Chim Acta* 313:241-253, 2001.

9. Lexi-Comp, Inc: *Up-to-date online 12.2. Drug information,* Hudson, OH, 2004, Lexi-Comp, Inc.

10. Micromedex: *Micromedex healthcare series 2004,* Greenwood, CO, 2004, Thomson Micromedex.

11. Venkataramanan R, Jain A, Warty VW, et al: Pharmacokinetics of FK 506 following oral administration: a comparison of FK 506 and cyclosporine, *Transplant Proc* 23:931-933, 1991.

12. Holt D, Armstrong V, Griesmacher A, et al: International Federation of Clinical Chemistry/International Association of Therapeutic Drug Monitoring and Clinical Toxicology working group on immunosuppressive drug monitoring, *Ther Drug Monit* 24:59-67, 2002.

Teicoplanin **(Targocid)**	Serum. Stable for 1 yr at $-20°$ C.[3]	Therapeutic concentration, trough:	5-10 mg/L	PK: $t_{1/2}$: V_d:	32-130 hr 0.5-1.0 L/kg
Bioassay,[1] *SPERA,*[1] *RASA,*[2] *FPIA,*[3] *HPLC*[4,5]		See *Remarks.*		Cl_T: PB:	0.006-0.016 L/hr/kg 88-91%
Bioassay,[1] *SPERA*[1] *HPLC*[4]	Urine				

| FACTORS INFLUENCING DRUG DISPOSITION | REMARKS AND INTERFERENCES |

Metabolism
  Hepatic
Excretion
  Feces (primary)
  Urine (secondary)
Dialysis
  Hemodialysis (−)
  Peritoneal dialysis (−)

Tacrolimus is a macrolide compound with potent immunosuppressant properties. It is used for prophylaxis of organ rejection in adult patients undergoing liver or kidney transplantion and in pediatric patients undergoing liver transplantion. It has also been used to prevent rejection in heart, small bowel, and allogeneic bone marrow transplant patients and to treat autoimmune diseases. Tacrolimus is extensively metabolized in the liver to 10 possible metabolites, and some of the major metabolites are active.[10]

Drug interactions: Tacrolimus is a major substrate and weak inhibitor of CYP3A4. Concomitant use with cyclosporine or ganciclovir can lead to increased risk of nephrotoxicity. Antacid or sucralfate administration should be separated by at least 2 hr.[9]

Side effects include tremor, headache, diarrhea, hypertension, nausea, and renal dysfunction.[10]

Immunoassays typically cross-react with tacrolimus metabolites as compared with LC-MS-MS method that can identify the parent compound. Thus patients with hepatic impairment may show unacceptable bias when drug is determined by immunoassay.[12]

Metabolism
  None
Excretion
  Urine
Disease or condition
  Renal disease: $t_{1/2}\uparrow$, $V_d\rightarrow$, $Cl_T\downarrow$
Age
  Children: $t_{1/2}\downarrow$, $Cl_T\uparrow$
Dialysis
  Hemodialysis (−)

Teicoplanin is an investigational glycopeptide antibiotic. An initial 6 mg/kg dose generally led to a C_{max} of 60 mg/L and a C_{min} of 4 mg/L.[6] Mean steady-state concentrations for C_{max} and C_{min} after 6 mg/kg/day are 75 mg/L and 14 mg/L, respectively.[6] Trough concentrations should be kept >5 mg/L for most gram-positive infections and not <10 mg/L for severe infections. Teicoplanin is a mixture of six components designated A2-1, A2-2, A2-3, A2-4, A2-5, and A3-1. It is highly soluble in water at pH >7, but it is poorly soluble in organic solvents. Only the HPLC method is able to discern the components of teicoplanin.

TEST NAME AND METHOD	SPECIMEN	REFERENCE (THERAPEUTIC) INTERVAL, CONVENTIONAL [INTERNATIONAL RECOMMENDED UNITS]	KINETIC VALUES

Teicoplanin—CONT

1. Cavenaghi L, Corti A, Cassani G: Comparison of the solid phase enzyme receptor (SPERA) and the microbiological assay for teicoplanin, *J Hosp Infect* 7:85-89, 1986.
2. Corti A, Cavenaghi L, Giani E, et al: A receptor-antibody sandwich assay for teicoplanin, *Clin Chem* 33:1615-1618, 1987.
3. Rybak MJ, Bailey EM, Reddy VN: Clinical evaluation of teicoplanin fluorescence polarization immunoassay, *Antimicrob Agents Chemother* 35:1586-1590, 1991.
4. Jehl F, Monteil H, Tarral A: HPLC quantitation of the six main components of teicoplanin in biological fluids, *J Antimicrob Chemother* 21:53-59, 1988.
5. Joos B, Luthy R: Determination of teicoplanin concentrations in serum by high pressure liquid chromatography, *Antimicrob Agents Chemother* 31:1222-1224, 1987.
6. Rowland M: Pharmacokinetics of teicoplanin, *Clin Pharmacokinet* 18:184-209, 1990.

			mcg/mL		μ*mol/L*		
Temazepam **(Restoril)**[1-14]	Serum, plasma					$t_{1/2}$:	6-25 hr
		Therapeutic concentration:	0.02-0.15	× 3.33	[0.07-0.50]	V_d/F:	1.4 L/kg
GC, HPLC, LC-MS		Toxic concentration:	>1.0		[3.33]	Cl_T/F:	0.87 ± 0.18 mL/min/kg
						PB:	96%
MW: 300.7							[× 0.01 = 0.96, protein-bound mole fraction]
						F:	>80% [× 0.01 = >0.80, bioavailable mole fraction]

1. Baselt R: *Disposition of toxic drugs and chemicals in man,* ed 7, Foster City, 2004, Biomedical Publications.
2. Schulz M, Schmoldt A: Therapeutic and toxic blood concentrations of more than 800 drugs and other xenobiotics, *Pharmazie* 58:447-474, 2003.
3. Hardman JG, Limbird LE, Gilman AG: *Goodman and Gilman's the pharmacological basis of therapeutics,* ed 10, New York, 2001, McGraw-Hill.
4. *Physicians desk reference,* ed 58, Montvale, NJ, 2004, Thomson PDR.
5. Clarke EGC: *Clarke's isolation and identification of drugs in pharmaceuticals, body fluids, and post-mortem material,* London, 1986, The Pharmaceutical Press.
6. ACP's PIER: *Physicians' information and education resource (online version),* Philadelphia, 2004, American College of Physicians.
7. McEvoy GK, editor: *AHFS drug information (online version),* Bethesda, MD, 2004, American Society of Health-System Pharmacists Inc.
8. *USP DI drug information for the health care professional,* ed 24, (online version), Taunton, MA, 2004, Micromedex Inc.
9. Kratzsch C, Tenberken O, Peters FT, et al: Screening, library-assisted identification and validated quantification of 23 benzodiazepines, flumazenil, zaleplone, zolpidem and zopiclone in plasma by liquid chromatography/mass spectrometry with atmospheric pressure chemical ionization, *J Mass Spectrom* 39:856-872, 2004.

FACTORS INFLUENCING DRUG DISPOSITION	REMARKS AND INTERFERENCES

Drug interactions: Teicoplanin and amino-glycosides are incompatible in solution.

Interferences: Lysed erythrocytes and the presence of other antibiotics interfere with the bioassay.

Metabolism
  Hepatic, CYP2B6, CYP2C8/9, CYP2C19, and CYP3A4 (all minor)
Disease
  Cirrhosis: $t_{1/2}\rightarrow$, $V_d\rightarrow$, $Cl_T\rightarrow$, PB$\downarrow$
Age
  Elderly: $t_{1/2}\rightarrow$, $V_d\rightarrow$, $Cl_T\rightarrow$, PB$\downarrow$

Temazepam, a 3-hydroxy benzodiazepine derivative, is a hypnotic agent used in short-term treatment of insomnia for up to 5 wk. The primary metabolic pathway is conjugation. Adverse reactions include confusion, dizziness, drowsiness, anxiety, rash, blurred vision, diarrhea, weakness, and diaphoresis.

---

10. Puopolo PR, Pothier ME, Volpicelli SA, et al: Single procedure for detection, confirmation, and quantification of benzodiazepines in serum by liquid chromatography with photo-array detection, *Clin Chem* 37:701-706, 1991.

11. Kemp P, Sneed G, Kupiec T, et al: Validation of a microtiter plate ELISA for screening of postmortem blood for opiates and benzodiazepines, *J Anal Toxicol* 26:504-512, 2002.

12. Chiba K, Horii H, Chiba T, et al: Development and preliminary application of high-performance liquid chromatographic assay of urinary metabolites of diazepam in humans, *J Chromatogr B Analyt Technol Biomed Life Sci* 668:77-84, 1995.

13. Scott KS, Oliver JS: Development of a supercritical fluid extraction method for the determination of temazepam in whole blood, *J Anal Toxicol* 2:297-300, 1997.

14. Rasanen I, Ojanpera I, Vuori E: Quantitative screening for benzodiazepines in blood by dual-column gas chromatography and comparison of the results with urine immunoassay, *J Anal Toxicol* 24:46-51, 2000.

TEST NAME AND METHOD	SPECIMEN	REFERENCE (THERAPEUTIC) INTERVAL, CONVENTIONAL [INTERNATIONAL RECOMMENDED UNITS]			KINETIC VALUES	
Theophylline[1-6]	Serum, plasma (heparin, EDTA).		*mcg/mL*	*μmol/L*	$t_{1/2}$	
GC, HPLC, IA,		Therapeutic concentration			Premature neonate:	54-76 hr
LC-MS, CZE	Trough collection.	Bronchodilator:	10-20 $\times$ 5.55	[56-111]	Child:	1-7 hr
		Premature			Adult:	6-12 hr
MW: 180.17		apnea:	6-13	[33-72]	V_d:	0.3-0.7 L/kg
		Toxic			Cl_T:	0.3-1.45
		concentration:	>20	[>111]		mL/min/kg
					PB:	40-56%
						[$\times$ 0.01 = 0.4-0.56, protein-bound mole fraction]
					F:	Variable, dependent on formula
					T_{max}:	Variable

1. Barnes PJ: Therapy for chronic obstructive pulmonary disease in the 21st century, *Drugs* 63:1973-1998, 2003.

2. Emara S: Simultaneous determination of caffeine, theophylline and theobromine in human plasma by on-line solid-phase extraction coupled to reversed-phase chromatography, *Biomed Chromatogr* 18:479-485, 2004.

3. Hansel TT, Tennant RC, Tan AJ, et al: Theophylline: mechanism of action and use in asthma and chronic obstructive pulmonary disease, *Drugs Today (Barc)* 40:55-69, 2004.

4. Millar D, Schmidt B: Controversies surrounding xanthine therapy, *Semin Neonatol* 9:239-244, 2004.

5. Pesce AJ, Rashkin M, Kotagal U: Standards of laboratory practice: theophylline and caffeine monitoring, *Clin Chem* 44:1124-1128, 1998.

6. Watson DG, Oliveira EJ, Boyter AC, et al: A rapid and sensitive method for the determination of the amount of theophylline in blood spots, *J Pharm Pharmacol* 53:413-416, 2001.

FACTORS INFLUENCING DRUG DISPOSITION	REMARKS AND INTERFERENCES

Metabolism
Hepatic, CYP1A2, and CYP2E1
Disease
Cirrhosis: $t_{1/2}\uparrow$, $Cl_T\downarrow$, $PB\downarrow$
CHF: $Cl_T\downarrow$
Pulmonary edema: $t_{1/2}\uparrow$, $Cl_T\downarrow$
Cor pulmonale: $t_{1/2}\uparrow$, $Cl_T\downarrow$
Obesity: $t_{1/2}\uparrow$, $Cl_T\downarrow$ (based on IBW)
Smoking: $Cl_1\uparrow$
Age
Premature: $t_{1/2}\uparrow$, $V_d\uparrow$, $Cl_T\downarrow$
Neonate: $t_{1/2}\uparrow$, $Cl_T\downarrow$, $PB\downarrow$
Elderly: $PB\downarrow$
Dialysis
Hemodialysis (+)
Hemoperfusion (+)
Peritoneal (−)

Drug interactions: Numerous drug interactions are reported because of induction or inhibition of metabolic pathways. There is evidence that theophylline blocks adenosine receptors, thereby decreasing the sedative effects of the benzodiazepines. Theophylline decreases the clearance of cetirizine.

Theophylline is a methylxanthine that acts to relax bronchial smooth muscles. It is used in the treatment of chronic asthma and bronchospasm associated with chronic obstructive pulmonary disease. The metabolism of theophylline to 3-methylxanthine (its primary metabolite) follows Michaelis-Menton kinetics.

Adverse and toxic effects are usually concentration related and include nausea, vomiting, tachycardia, arrhythmias, and seizures. In the premature neonate, ~50% of theophylline is excreted unchanged in the urine, and the remaining 50% undergoes metabolism to caffeine and 1,3-dimethyluric acid. In older children and adults, caffeine is a minor metabolite.

See also *Caffeine* (related compound).

TEST NAME AND METHOD	SPECIMEN	REFERENCE (THERAPEUTIC) INTERVAL, CONVENTIONAL [INTERNATIONAL RECOMMENDED UNITS]				KINETIC VALUES	
Thiopental **(Pentothal)**[1-7] *GC, GC-MS, HPLC* *MW: 242*	Serum, plasma (heparin, EDTA). Collect at trough concentration. Stable for at least 24 hr at room temperature and 8 wk at −20° C.	Therapeutic concentration Hypnotic: Therapeutic coma: Anesthesia: Toxic concentration: (See *Remarks*.)	*mcg/mL* 1-5 30-100 7-130 >10	× 4.13	µ*mol/L* [4-21] [124-413] [29-537] [>41]	$t_{1/2}$: V_d: Cl_T: PB:	3-18 hr 2.2-3.2 L/kg 1-4 mL/min/kg 60-96% [× 0.01 = 0.60-0.96, protein-bound mole fraction]

1. Hart AP, Mazarr-Proo S, Blackwell W, et al: A rapid cost-effective high-performance liquid chromatographic (HPLC) assay of serum lamotrigine after liquid-liquid extraction and using HPLC conditions routinely used for analysis of barbiturates, *Ther Drug Monit* 19:431-435, 1997.

2. Kingston HGG, Kendrick A, Sommer KM, et al: Binding of thiopental in neonatal serum, *Anesthesiology* 72:428-431, 1990.

3. Meier P, Thormann W: Determination of thiopental in human serum and plasma by high-performance capillary electrophoresis-micellar electrokinetic chromatography, *J Chromatogr* 59:505-513, 1991.

4. Ohyama K, Wada M, Lord GA, et al: Capillary electrochromatographic analysis of barbiturates in serum, *Electrophoresis* 25:594-599, 2004.

5. Russo H, Bressolle F: Pharmacodynamics and pharmacokinetics of thiopental, *Clin Pharmacokinet* 35:95-134, 1998.

6. Spell JC, Srinivasan K, Stewart JT, et al: Supercritical fluid extraction and negative ion electrospray liquid chromatography tandem mass spectrometry analysis of phenobarbital, butalbital, pentobarbital and thiopental in human serum, *Rapid Commun Mass Spectrom* 12:890-894, 1998.

7. Woster PS, LeBlanc KL: Management of elevated intracranial pressure, *Clin Pharm* 9:762-772, 1990.

TEST NAME AND METHOD	SPECIMEN	REFERENCE (THERAPEUTIC) INTERVAL, CONVENTIONAL [INTERNATIONAL RECOMMENDED UNITS]				KINETIC VALUES	
Thioridazine **(Mellaril)**[1-5] *GC, HPLC* *MW: 370.58*	Serum, plasma (EDTA)	Therapeutic concentration: Toxic concentration: *Mesoridazine*	*mcg/mL* 0.1-2 >2.5 0.2-1.6	× 2.70	µ*mol/L* [0.27-5.4] [>6.75]	$t_{1/2}$: Cl_T: V_d: F: PB:	7-13 hr NA 18 L/kg NA 90-99% (α_1-acid glycoprotein) [× 0.01 = 0.9-0.99, protein-bound mole fraction]

1. Gutteck U, Rentsch KM: Therapeutic drug monitoring of 13 antidepressant and five neuroleptic drugs in serum with liquid chromatography-electrospray ionization mass spectrometry, *Clin Chem Lab Med* 41:1571-1579, 2003.

2. Kilts CD, Patrick KS, Breese GR, et al: Simultaneous determination of thioridazine and its S-oxidized and N-demethylated metabolites using high-performance liquid-chromatography on radially compressed silica, *J Chromatogr* 231:377-391, 1982.

3. Kirchner V, Kelly CA, Harvey RJ: Thioridazine for dementia, *Cochrane Database Syst Rev* 3:CD000464, 2001.

4. Menkes DB, Knight JC: Cardiotoxicity and prescription of thioridazine in N. Zealand, *Aust NZ J Psychiatry* 36:492-498, 2002.

5. Schulz M, Schmoldt A: Therapeutic and toxic blood concentrations of more than 800 drugs and other xenobiotics, *Pharmazie* 58:447-474, 2003.

FACTORS INFLUENCING DRUG DISPOSITION	REMARKS AND INTERFERENCES

Metabolism
  Hepatic
Excretion
  Renal
Disease
  Hepatic: $t_{1/2}\uparrow\rightarrow$, PB$\downarrow$
  Obesity: $t_{1/2}\uparrow$, $V_d\uparrow$
Age
  Elderly: $t_{1/2}\uparrow$, $V_d\uparrow$, $Cl_T\uparrow$, PB$\downarrow$
  Neonates: $t_{1/2}\uparrow$
  Children: PB$\downarrow$

Thiopental is administered as an intravenous, ultrashort-acting anesthetic agent. When used to induce coma, cardiac and pulmonary support are required. Thiopental is highly lipid soluble and distributes extensively to adipose tissue. Pentobarbital is a metabolite and may be detected at low concentrations. The principal toxic effect involves CNS depression. At high concentrations, e.g., 60 mcg/mL [248 μmol/L], the elimination kinetics become nonlinear, and a $t_{1/2}$ of 60 hr may be seen. Rare cases of hepatic dysfunction have been reported.

Metabolism
  Hepatic, CYP2D6
Excretion
  Minimal in urine

Thioridazine is a neuroleptic agent used to treat psychosis, schizophrenia, and some anxiety disorders. The drug is extensively metabolized in the liver and gastric mucosa. At least two pharmacologically active metabolites are known, with mesoridazine having greater activity than the parent compound. Kinetic values are not well defined. Side effects may include orthostatic hypotension, CNS effects (particularly extrapyramidal effects), pigmentation, and cardiac effects. Cases of anemia, leukopenia, and thrombocytopenia, as well as rare cases of hepatic dysfunction, have been reported.

TEST NAME AND METHOD	SPECIMEN	REFERENCE (THERAPEUTIC) INTERVAL, CONVENTIONAL [INTERNATIONAL RECOMMENDED UNITS]			KINETIC VALUES	
Thiothixene	Serum	*mcg/mL*	µ*mol/L*	$t_{1/2}$:	α, ~3.4 hr	
(Navane)[1-4]		Therapeutic			β, ~34 hr	
		concentration: 0.001-0.03 × 2.25 [0.0025-0.07]	T_{max}:	1-3 hr		
GC-MS, HPLC		Toxic				
		concentration: >0.1	[>0.225]			
MW: 443.63						

1. Bergling R, Mjorndal T, Oreland L, et al: Plasma levels and clinical effects of thioridazine and thiothixene, *J Clin Pharmacol* 15:178-186, 1975.
2. Hariharan M, VanNoord T, Kindt EK, et al: A simple, sensitive liquid chromatographic assay of cis-thiothixene in plasma with coulometric detection, *Ther Drug Monit* 13:79-85, 1991.
3. Hobbs DC, Welch WM, Short MJ, et al: Pharmacokinetics of thiothixene in man, *Clin Pharmacol Ther* 16:473-478, 1974.
4. Milton GV, Jann MW: Emergency treatment of psychotic symptoms. Pharmacokinetic considerations for antipsychotic drugs, *Clin Pharmacokinet* 28:494-504, 1995.

TEST NAME AND METHOD	SPECIMEN	REFERENCE	KINETIC VALUES	
Ticarcillin	Serum, plasma	See *Carbenicillin* (related compound).	PK^{3-5}:	
(Ticar)[1,2]	(heparin, EDTA)		$t_{1/2}$:	1.2 hr
			V_d:	0.20 L/kg
MB, HPLC			Cl_T:	1.9 mL/min/kg
			PB:	45-65%
MW: 384.43				

1. Bannatyne R, Cheung R: Ticarcillin bioassay, *Antimicrob Agents Chemother* 20:493-495, 1981.
2. Kwan R, MacLeod S, Spino M, et al: High-pressure liquid chromatographic assays for ticarcillin in serum and urine, *J Pharm Sci* 71:1118-1121, 1982.
3. Libke RD, Clarke JT, Ralph ED, et al: Ticarcillin vs. carbenicillin: clinical pharmacokinetics, *Clin Pharmacol Ther* 17:441-446, 1975.
4. Hardman JG, Limbird LE, Gilman AG: *Goodman & Gilman's the pharmacological basis of therapeutics,* ed 10, New York, 2001, McGraw-Hill.
5. Bennett W, Aronof G, Golper T, et al: *Drug prescribing in renal failure. Dosing guidelines for adults,* ed 2, Philadelphia, 1994, American College of Physicians.
6. Micromedex: *Micromedex healthcare series 2004,* Greenwood Village, CO, 2004, Thomson Micromedex.
7. Parry MF, Neu HC: Pharmacokinetics of ticarcillin patients with abnormal renal function, *J Infect Dis* 133:46, 1976.

FACTORS INFLUENCING DRUG DISPOSITION	REMARKS AND INTERFERENCES

Metabolism
  Hepatic
Excretion
  Biliary

Thiothixene is a potent antipsychotic drug used to treat schizophrenia and other psychotic disorders. Adverse effects include sedation, extrapyramidal effects, tachycardia, and hypotension. The exact mechanism of action of thiothixene is unknown.

Metabolism
  Hepatic (minimal amount)
Excretion
  Urine (primary)
  Bile/feces (secondary)
Disease
  Renal
  Oliguria: $t_{1/2}\uparrow$, 15.7 hr; $Cl_T\downarrow$
  Oliguria and hepatic dysfunction:
  $t_{1/2}\uparrow$, 23.2 hr
Dialysis
  Hemodialysis (+)[6]
  Peritoneal (+)[7]

Drug interactions: Probenecid delays active renal tubular secretion and increases the drug's half-life. Concomitant administration of ticarcillin and an aminoglycoside can lead to loss of aminoglycoside efficacy.[6]

Values for half-life and total body clearance of ticarcillin correlate strongly with creatinine clearance. Hepatic dysfunction appears to be significant only in the presence of renal failure. Side effects include hypersensitivity, hepatotoxicity, electrolyte and acid-base disturbances, hematological disorders (including diathesis and reversible granulocytopenia), and neurotoxicity (observed with plasma concentrations ≥ 320 mcg/mL [$\times 2.60 = \geq 832$ μmol/L] and with CSF concentrations ≥ 37 mcg/mL [≥ 96 μmol/L]). Ticarcillin has a lighter sodium load than carbenicillin. It generally possesses at least 2-4 times more activity against *Pseudomonas* than carbenicillin.

TEST NAME AND METHOD	SPECIMEN	REFERENCE (THERAPEUTIC) INTERVAL, CONVENTIONAL [INTERNATIONAL RECOMMENDED UNITS]		KINETIC VALUES	
Timolol **(Blocadren)**[1,2] *GC-MS, HPLC* *MW: 316.42*	Serum, plasma (EDTA, heparin)	Therapeutic concentration: Toxic concentration:	3-56 ng/mL [× 3.16 = 9-177 nmol/L] Not well defined.	PK[3-6]: $t_{1/2}$: V_d: Cl_T: PB: F:	2-4 hr[7] 2.1 ± 0.8 L/kg 7.3 ± 3.3 mL/min/kg 60% 50-75%

1. Sutton B, Richardson R: Assay of timolol in human plasma using gas chromatography with electron-capture detection, *J Chromatogr* 581:277-280, 1992.
2. He H, Edeki TI, Wood AJJ: Determination of low plasma timolol concentrations following topical application of timolol eye drops in humans by high-performance liquid chromatography with electrochemical detection, *J Chromatogr. B Biomed Sci Appl* 661:351-356, 1994.
3. Johnsson G, Regårdh C: Clinical pharmacokinetics of β-adrenoreceptor blocking drugs, *Clin Pharmacokinet* 1:233-263, 1976.
4. Hardman JG, Limbird LE, Gilman AG: *Goodman & Gilman's the pharmacological basis of therapeutics,* ed 10, New York, 2001, McGraw-Hill.
5. Bennett W, Aronof G, Golper T, et al: *Drug prescribing in renal failure. Dosing guidelines for adults,* ed 2, Philadelphia, 1994, American College of Physicians.
6. Evans WE, Schentag JJ, Jusko WJ: *Applied pharmacokinetics—principles of therapeutic drug monitoring,* ed 3, Vancouver, WA, 1992, Applied Therapeutics, Inc.
7. Kaila T, Karhuvaara S, Huupponen R, et al: The analysis of plasma kinetics and B-receptor binding and -blocking activity of timolol following its small intravenous dose, *Int J Clin Pharmacol Ther Toxicol* 31:351-357, 1993.
8. Lexi-Comp, Inc: *Up-to-date online 12.2. Drug information,* Hudson, OH, 2004, Lexi-Comp, Inc.

| **Tobramycin** **(Nebcin)**[1-6] *HPLC, GC, EIA, FPIA* | Serum, plasma (EDTA). For patients on penicillin or its derivatives, freeze sample if not analyzed within 4-6 hr. Routine collection should be at | *mcg/mL* Therapeutic concentration Peak Less severe infections: Severe infections: | μ*mol/L* 5-8 × 2.14 [10-17] 8-10 [17-21] | PK[6-8]: $t_{1/2}$: V_d: Cl_T: PB: F: | 2-3 hr 0.26 L/kg 1.3 mL/min/kg 0-30%[9] IM: 100% PO: Negligible |

FACTORS INFLUENCING DRUG DISPOSITION	REMARKS AND INTERFERENCES

Metabolism
  Hepatic
Excretion
  Bile/feces (primary)
  Urine (secondary)
Dialysis
  Hemodialysis ($-$)

Drug interactions: Timolol is a major substrate of CYP2D6 and weakly inhibits it. CYP2D6 inhibitors like chlorpromazine, fluoxetine, miconazole, quinidine, quinine, and ritonavir may increase the effects of timolol.[8] Phenothiazines and cimetidine may increase plasma concentrations, probably because of their effect on hepatic metabolism.

Plasma concentrations that produce minimal β-blockade vary widely. Therapeutic concentrations are expressed in terms of plasma concentrations producing β-blockade. However, there is no good correlation between serum concentrations and therapeutic effects. Thus determination of plasma levels is of limited value in routine therapy.

Metabolism
  None
Excretion
  Urine (primary)
  Bile/feces (secondary)
Disease
  Renal: $t_{1/2}\uparrow$, $Cl_T\downarrow$
  Burns: $Cl_T\uparrow$
  Cystic fibrosis: $Cl_T\uparrow$
  Obesity: $V_d\uparrow$ (based on IBW), $Cl_T\uparrow$ (based on IBW)

Tobramycin is an aminoglycoside antibiotic. Therapeutic and toxic concentrations should be considered highly variable, differing with each patient's condition. Penicillin and its derivatives inactivate tobramycin in vivo and in vitro. A definitive cause-and-effect relationship between the trough concentration and the incidence of nephrotoxicity has not been established. Cl_T and $t_{1/2}$ are strongly correlated with the glomerular filtration rate. Side effects include vestibular and auditory dysfunction, nephrotoxicity, and neuromuscular blockade. Very rare cases of anemia, leukopenia, and thrombocytopenia have been reported.

TEST NAME AND METHOD	SPECIMEN	REFERENCE (THERAPEUTIC) INTERVAL, CONVENTIONAL [INTERNATIONAL RECOMMENDED UNITS]		KINETIC VALUES

Tobramycin—CONT

trough and peak concentrations (end of a 1-hr constant infusion, 30 min after the end of a 30-min constant infusion, or 1 hr after an IM dose).		Trough		
		Less severe infections:	<1	[<2]
		Moderate infections:	<2	[<4]
		Severe infections:	2-4	[4-9]
		Toxic concentration		
		Peak:	>10-12	[>21-26]
		Trough:	>2-4	[>4-9]

1. Mayhew JW, Gorlach SL: Gas-liquid chromatographic method for the assay of aminoglycoside antibiotics in serum, *J Chromatogr* 151:133-146, 1978.

2. Maitra S, Yoshikawa T, Guze L, et al: Determination of aminoglycoside antibiotics in biological fluids: a review, *Clin Chem* 25:1361-1367, 1979.

3. Marples J, Oates M: Serum gentamicin, netilmicin and tobramycin assays by high performance liquid chromatography, *J Antimicrob Chemother* 10:311-318, 1982.

4. Redmond L, Chang A, Lynch M: Gentamicin and tobramycin EMIT assays in the CentrifiChem 500, *Clin Chem* 31:1408-1409, 1985.

5. White L, Holt H, Reeves D, et al: Evaluation of Innofluour fluorescence polarization immunoassay kits for the determination of serum concentrations of gentamicin, tobramycin, amikacin and vancomycin, *J Antimicrob Chemother* 39:355-361, 1997.

6. Baselt RC: *Disposition of toxic drugs and chemicals in man*, ed 7, Foster City, CA, 2004, Chemical Toxicology Institute.

7. Pechere J, Dugal R: Clinical pharmacokinetics of aminoglycoside antibiotics, *Clin Pharmacokinet* 4:170-199, 1979.

8. Evans WE, Schentag JJ, Jusko WJ: *Applied pharmacokinetics—principles of therapeutic drug monitoring*, ed 3, Vancouver, WA, 1992, Applied Therapeutics, Inc.

9. Micromedex: *Micromedex healthcare series 2004*, Greenwood Village, CO, 2004, Thomson Micromedex.

TEST NAME AND METHOD	SPECIMEN	REFERENCE (THERAPEUTIC)		KINETIC VALUES
Tocainide **(Tonocard)**[1-3]	Serum, plasma (EDTA, heparin)	Therapeutic concentration:	4-10 mcg/mL [× 5.20 = 21-52 µmol/L]	PK[4-7]: $t_{1/2}$: 13.5 ± 2.3 hr V_d: 3.0 ± 0.2 L/kg
GC, HPLC		Toxic concentration:	Not well defined.	Cl_T: 2.6 ± 0.5 mL/min/kg PB: 4-22%[8]
MW: 192.26				F: 89 ± 5%

FACTORS INFLUENCING DRUG DISPOSITION	REMARKS AND INTERFERENCES

Age
  Newborn: $t_{1/2}\uparrow$, $V_d\uparrow$, $Cl_T\downarrow$
  Child: $t_{1/2}\downarrow$, $V_d\uparrow$, $Cl_T\uparrow$
Dialysis
  Hemodialysis (+)
  Peritoneal (+)[9]

Drug interactions: Coadministration of cyclosporine or tacrolimus with tobramycin may lead to increased risk of nephrotoxicity. Concomitant usage of loop diuretics with tobramycin is associated with a risk of ototoxicity.[9]

Interferences: When a patient is also taking other antibiotics (penicillins, cephalosporins, tetracyclines, clindamycin, chloramphenicol), the MB method may lack specificity. Penicillins and cephalosporins can be inactivated with a commercially available β-lactamase to minimize this interference.

See Table II-6.

Metabolism
  Hepatic
Excretion
  Bile/feces (primary)
  Urine (secondary)
Disease
  Renal: $t_{1/2}\uparrow$, $V_d\rightarrow$, $Cl_T\downarrow$
  CHF: $t_{1/2}\rightarrow$, $V_d\downarrow$, $Cl_T\downarrow$
  Cirrhosis: $t_{1/2}\uparrow$, $V_d\uparrow$, $Cl_T\downarrow$
Dialysis
  Hemodialysis (+)

Tocainide, a class IB antiarrhythmic, is a racemic compound. R(−) tocainide and S(+) tocainide demonstrate significant differences in kinetic parameters. The toxic range is not well defined because central nervous system side effects can occur at tocainide plasma concentrations <10 mcg/mL [<52 μmol/L].

TEST NAME AND METHOD	SPECIMEN	REFERENCE (THERAPEUTIC) INTERVAL, CONVENTIONAL [INTERNATIONAL RECOMMENDED UNITS]				KINETIC VALUES	
Tocainide—CONT							

1. Reece P, Stanley P: High-performance liquid chromatographic assay for tocainide in human plasma: comparison with gas-liquid chromatographic assay, *J Chromatogr* 183:109-114, 1980.

2. Smith P: Measurement of tocainide in serum by capillary gas chromatography, *Ther Drug Monit* 8:361-364, 1986.

3. Baselt RC: *Disposition of toxic drugs and chemicals in man,* ed 7, Foster City, CA, 2004, Chemical Toxicology Institute.

4. Holmes B, Heel RC: Flecainide: a preliminary review of its pharmacodynamic properties and therapeutic efficacy, *Drugs* 29:1-33, 1985.

5. Hardman JG, Limbird LE, Gilman AG: *Goodman & Gilman's the pharmacological basis of therapeutics,* ed 10, New York, 2001, McGraw-Hill.

6. Gillis AM, Yee YG, Kates RE: Binding of antiarrhythmic drug to purified human alpha1-acid glycoprotein, *Biochem Pharmacol* 34:4279-4282, 1985.

7. Alpert JS, Haffajee CI, Young MD: Chemistry, pharmacology, antiarrhythmic efficacy and adverse effects of tocainide hydrochloride, an oral active structural analog of lidocaine, *Pharmacotherapy* 3:316-323, 1983.

8. Elvin AT, Axelson JE, Lalka D: Tocainide protein binding in normal volunteers and trauma patients, *Br J Clin Pharmacol* 13:872, 1982.

9. Micromedex: *Micromedex healthcare series 2004,* Greenwood Village, CO, 2004, Thomson Micromedex.

TEST NAME AND METHOD	SPECIMEN	REFERENCE (THERAPEUTIC) INTERVAL, CONVENTIONAL [INTERNATIONAL RECOMMENDED UNITS]			KINETIC VALUES	
Tolbutamide (Orinase)[1-4]	Serum		*mcg/mL*	*μmol/L*	$t_{1/2}$:	4-12 hr
		Therapeutic			V_d:	6-10 L/kg
		concentration:	50-100 × 3.70	[185-370]	Cl_T:	0.30 mL/min/kg
HPLC, GC, CZE		Toxic			PB:	80-99% (albumin)
		concentration:	>400	[>1480]		[× 0.01 = 0.0.8-99,
MW: 270.3						protein-bound mole fraction]
					F:	93%
						[× 0.01 = 0.93, bioavailable mole fraction]
					T_{max}:	3-5 hr

1. Ferner RE, Chaplin S: The relationship between the pharmacokinetics and pharmacodynamic effects of oral hypoglycemic drugs, *Clin Pharmacokinet* 12:379-401, 1987.

2. Magni F, Marazzini L, Pereira S, et al: Identification of sulfonylureas in serum by electrospray mass spectrometry, *Anal Biochem* 282:136-141, 2000.

3. Paroni R, Comuzzi B, Arcelloni C, et al: Comparison of capillary electrophoresis with HPLC for diagnosis of factitious hypoglycemia, *Clin Chem* 46:1773-1780, 2000.

| **FACTORS INFLUENCING DRUG DISPOSITION** | **REMARKS AND INTERFERENCES** |

Drug interactions: Concurrent use of cimetidine or rifampin can result in a decreased tocainide effectiveness. Administering lidocaine to a patient receiving tocainide can result in serious CNS toxicity.[9]

Metabolism
 Hepatic, CYP2C9
Excretion
 Renal
Disease
 Cirrhosis: $t_{1/2}\downarrow$, $Cl_T\uparrow$, $PB\downarrow$
 Acute viral hepatitis: $t_{1/2}\downarrow$, $Cl_T\uparrow$, $PB\downarrow$
 Hypoalbuminemia: $PB\downarrow$
 Respiratory disease: $t_{1/2}\downarrow$
Age
 Elderly: $PB\downarrow$
Dialysis
 Hemodialysis $(-)$

Tolbutamide is the shortest acting and least potent of the sulfonylureas used to treat type II diabetes. The drug is useful in treating diabetic patients with renal disease because it is extensively metabolized to inactive metabolites. Adverse effects include transient leukopenia, thrombocytopenia, hemolytic anemia, pancytopenia, gastrointestinal disturbances, headache, tinnitus, photosensitivity, allergic skin reactions, and intolerance to alcohol. Most serious effects include hypoglycemia (may progress to coma and death) and hepatic dysfunction.

See Table II-5.

4. Schulz M, Schmoldt A: Therapeutic and toxic blood concentrations of more than 800 drugs and other xenobiotics, *Pharmazie* 58:447-474, 2003.

TEST NAME AND METHOD	SPECIMEN	REFERENCE (THERAPEUTIC) INTERVAL, CONVENTIONAL [INTERNATIONAL RECOMMENDED UNITS]		KINETIC VALUES	
Topiramate **(Topamax)**[1-3]	Serum	Therapeutic concentration:	2.4-8.0 mg/L for daily doses of 125-400 mg.[3]	PK^4: $t_{1/2}$: V_d:	21 hr^5 0.6-0.8 L/kg^5
GC, LC-MS		Toxic concentration:	Not well defined.	Cl_T: PB:	0.30-0.39 mL/min/kg^6 13-17%[4]
MW: 339.37				F:	80%

1. Contin M, Riva R, Albani F, et al: Simple and rapid liquid chromatographic-turbo ion spray mass spectrometric determination of topiramate in human plasma, *J Chromatogr B Biomed Sci Appl* 761:133-137, 2001.

2. Britzi M, Soback S, Isoherranen N, et al: Analysis of topiramate and its metabolites in plasma and urine of healthy subjects and patients with epilepsy by use of a novel liquid chromatography-mass spectrometry assay, *Ther Drug Monit* 25:314-322, 2003.

3. Baselt RC: *Disposition of toxic drugs and chemicals in man*, ed 7, Foster City, CA, 2004, Chemical Toxicology Institute.

4. Lexi-Comp, Inc: *Up-to-date online 12.2. Drug information*, Hudson, OH, 2004, Lexi-Comp, Inc.

5. Bialer M: Comparative pharmacokinetics of the newer antiepileptic drugs, *Clin Pharmacokinet* 24:441-452, 1993.

6. Doose DR, Walker SA, Gisclon LG, et al: Single-dose pharmacokinetics and effect of food on the bioavailability of topiramate, a novel antiepileptic drug, *J Clin Pharmacol* 36:884-891, 1996.

7. Curry W, Kulling D: Newer antiepileptic drugs: gabapentin, lamotrigine, felbamate, topiramate and fosphenytoin, *Am Fam Physician* 57:513-520, 1998.

8. Micromedex: *Micromedex healthcare series 2004*, Greenwood Village, CO, 2004, Thomson Micromedex.

TEST NAME AND METHOD	SPECIMEN			KINETIC VALUES	
Triazolam[1-10] **(Halcion)**	Serum, plasma	*mcg/mL* Therapeutic concentration: 0.002-0.02	$\mu mol/L$ ×2.91 [0.006-0.058]	$t_{1/2}$: V_d/F: Cl_T/F:	2-5 hr 1.1 ± 0.4 L/kg 8.3 ± 1.8 mL/min/kg
GC, HPLC, LC-MS		Toxic concentration: 0.04	[0.12]	PB:	90.1 ± 1.5% [× 0.01 = 0.90 ± 0.02, protein-bound mole fraction]
MW: 343.2					
IA, GC-MS	Urine			F:	55% [× 0.01 = 0.55, bioavailable bound mole fraction]

FACTORS INFLUENCING DRUG DISPOSITION	REMARKS AND INTERFERENCES

Metabolism
  Hepatic (small amount)
Excretion
  Urine
Disease
  Renal: Patients with impaired renal function should use one half of the recommended dosage.[7]
Age
  Neonate: $t_{1/2}\downarrow$, $Cl_T\uparrow$
Dialysis
  Hemodialysis (+)

Drug interactions: Topiramate weakly inhibits CYP2C19 and induces CYP3A4. Concomitant use of CNS depressants may lead to increased sedation. Other anticonvulsants (phenytoin, carbamazepine, valproic acid) may decrease the serum level of topiramate. Effectiveness of oral contraceptives (estrogens) may be reduced by topiramate.[4]

This drug is a sulfamate-substituted monosaccharide used for the treatment of epilepsy.[8] Topiramate may decrease serum bicarbonate concentrations because of inhibition of carbonic anhydrase and increased renal bicarbonate loss, leading to metabolic acidosis.[4]

Side effects of topiramate include cognitive dysfunction, paresthesias, sedation, dizziness, fatigue, weight loss, diarrhea, urolithiasis, oligohidrosis, and hyperthermia.

Metabolism
  Hepatic, CYP3A4
Disease
  Obesity: $t_{1/2}\uparrow$, $V_d\downarrow$, $Cl_T\downarrow$
Age
  Elderly: $t_{1/2}\rightarrow$, $Cl_T\downarrow$

Drug interactions: Triazolam inhibits CYP2C8/9 (weak). Concomitant use with drugs or foods (e.g., grapefruit juice) that inhibit CYP3A isoenzymes may cause increased

Triazolam is an ultrashort-acting oral benzodiazepine hypnotic used for treatment of insomnia. Its primary pathway of metabolism is oxidation (hydroxylation). Adverse reactions include drowsiness, anterograde amnesia, dizziness, ataxia, headache, nausea, and vomiting.

TEST NAME AND METHOD	SPECIMEN	REFERENCE (THERAPEUTIC) INTERVAL, CONVENTIONAL [INTERNATIONAL RECOMMENDED UNITS]				KINETIC VALUES	

Triazolam—CONT

1. Baselt R: *Disposition of toxic drugs and chemicals in man,* ed 7, Foster City, CA, 2004, Biomedical Publications.
2. Schulz M, Schmoldt A: Therapeutic and toxic blood concentrations of more than 800 drugs and other xenobiotics, *Pharmazie* 58:447-474, 2003.
3. Hardman JG, Limbird LE, Gilman AG: *Goodman and Gilman's the pharmacological basis of therapeutics,* ed 10, New York, 2001, McGraw-Hill.
4. *Physicians desk reference,* ed 58, Montvale, NJ, 2004, Thomson PDR.
5. Clarke EGC: *Clarke's isolation and identification of drugs in pharmaceuticals, body fluids, and post-mortem material,* London, 1986, The Pharmaceutical Press.
6. McEvoy GK, editor: *AHFS drug information (online version),* Bethesda, MD, 2004, American Society of Health-System Pharmacists Inc.
7. Kratzsch C, Tenberken O, Peters FT, et al: Screening, library-assisted identification and validated quantification of 23 benzodiazepines, flumazenil, zaleplone, zolpidem and zopiclone in plasma by liquid chromatography/mass spectrometry with atmospheric pressure chemical ionization, *J Mass Spectrom* 39:856-872, 2004.
8. Borrey D, Meyer E, Lambert W, et al: Simultaneous determination of fifteen low-dosed benzodiazepines in human urine by solid-phase extraction and gas chromatography-mass spectrometry, *J Chromatogr B Biomed Sci Appl* 765:187-197, 2001.
9. Tanaka E, Terada M, Misawa S, et al: Simultaneous determination of twelve benzodiazepines in human serum using a new reversed-phase chromatographic column on a 2-microns porous microspherical silica gel, *J Chromatogr B Biomed Appl* 682:173-178, 1996.
10. Rasanen I, Ojanpera I, Vuori E: Quantitative screening for benzodiazepines in blood by dual-column gas chromatography and comparison of the results with urine immunoassay, *J Anal Toxicol* 24:46-51, 2000.

Tubocurarine	Serum, plasma		*mcg/mL*		*μmol/L*	$t_{1/2}$:	1.5-3.8 hr
(Tubarine)[1-6]	(EDTA)	Therapeutic				V_d:	0.3-0.74 L/kg
		concentration:	0.4-6	× 1.47	[0.59-8.8]	Cl_T:	2.5-3.9 mL/min/kg
HPLC, LC-MS						PB:	30-50% (albumin, IgG)
							[× 0.01 = 0.30-0.50,
MW: 681.7							protein-bound mole fraction]
						F:	Poor
						T_{max}:	Minutes

FACTORS INFLUENCING DRUG DISPOSITION	REMARKS AND INTERFERENCES

triazolam concentrations. Cimetidine, erythromycin, or isoniazid coadministration may cause an increase in F but no change in $t_{1/2}$ of triazolam.

Metabolism
  Minimal, hepatic
Excretion
  Renal, biliary
Disease
  Uremia: $t_{1/2}\uparrow$, $Cl_T\downarrow$
  Burn: $PB\uparrow$, $Cl_T\uparrow$
Age
  Neonates, children: $t_{1/2}\uparrow$, $V_d\uparrow$
  Elderly: $t_{1/2}\uparrow$, $V_d\downarrow$, $Cl_T\downarrow$

Drug interactions: Aminoglycoside antibiotics and cimetidine enhance neuromuscular blockade activity. Glucocorticoids are reported to antagonize neuromuscular blockade.

Tubocurarine is a nondepolarizing skeletal muscle relaxant typically. It produces muscular weakness and paralysis, particularly in respiratory muscles. Reported adverse effects include hypotension, tachycardia, bronchospasm, apnea, and hypersensitivity reactions.

TEST NAME AND METHOD	SPECIMEN	REFERENCE (THERAPEUTIC) INTERVAL, CONVENTIONAL [INTERNATIONAL RECOMMENDED UNITS]			KINETIC VALUES	

Tubocurarine—CONT

1. Bjorksten AR, Beemer GH, Crankshaw DP: Simple high-performance liquid chromatographic method for the analysis of the non-depolarizing neuromuscular blocking drugs in clinical anaesthesia, *J Chromatogr* 533:241-247, 1990.

2. Cirimele V, Villain M, Pepin G, et al: Screening procedure for eight quaternary nitrogen muscle relaxants in blood by high-performance liquid chromatography-electrospray ionization mass spectrometry, *J Chromatogr B Analyt Technol Biomed Life Sci* 789:107-113, 2003.

3. McManus MC: Neuromuscular blockers in surgery and intensive care, part 2, *Am J Health Syst Pharm* 58:2381-2395, 2001.

Valproic Acid (Depakene)[1-3] *HPLC, GLC, GC-MS, EIA, FPIA* *MW: 144.21*	Serum, plasma (EDTA). Collect at trough concentration. Stable at room temperature for several hours, for 1 yr at −20° C.	*mcg/mL* Therapeutic concentration: 50-100 Toxic concentration: >100	× 6.93	$\mu mol/L$ [346-693] [>693]	PK[4-7]: $t_{1/2}$ Newborn: Child: Adult: V_d: Cl_T: PB: F:	40 hr 8-11 hr 8-15 hr 0.1-0.4 L/kg 0.12 mL/min/kg 90% 100%

1. Leroux M, Budnik D, Hall K, et al: Comparison of gas-liquid chromatography and EMIT assay for serum valproic acid, *Clin Biochem* 14:87-90, 1981.

2. Chan S: Monitoring serum valproic acid by gas chromatography with electron-capture detection, *Clin Chem* 26:1528-1530, 1980.

3. Baselt RC: *Disposition of toxic drugs and chemicals in man,* ed 7, Foster City, CA, 2004, Chemical Toxicology Institute.

4. Klotz U, Antonin KH: Pharmacokinetics and bioavailability of sodium valproate, *Clin Pharmacol Ther* 21:736-743, 1977.

5. Gugler R, von Unruh GE: Clinical pharmacokinetics of valproic acid, *Clin Pharmacokinet* 5:67-83, 1980.

6. Hardman JG, Limbird LE, Gilman AG: *Goodman & Gilman's the pharmacological basis of therapeutics,* ed 10, New York, 2001, McGraw-Hill.

FACTORS INFLUENCING DRUG DISPOSITION	REMARKS AND INTERFERENCES

4. McManus MC: Neuromuscular blockers in surgery and intensive care, part 1, *Am J Health Syst Pharm* 58:2287-2299, 2001.
5. Tuba Z, Maho S, Vizi ES: Synthesis and structure-activity relationships of neuromuscular blocking agents, *Curr Med Chem* 9:1507-1536, 2002.
6. Utt JK, Ward ME: *Drugdex drug evaluations: tubocurarine,* Greenwood Village, CO, 2003, Thomson Micromedex.

Metabolism
  Hepatic
Excretion
  Bile/feces
Disease or condition
  Cirrhosis: $V_d\uparrow$, $t_{1/2}\uparrow$, $Cl_T\rightarrow$, $PB\downarrow$, 70%[8]
  Renal failure: $PB\downarrow$, 80%
  Burn: $PB\downarrow$
  Hypoalbuminemia: $PB\downarrow$
  Pregnancy: $PB\downarrow$
Age
  Neonate: $t_{1/2}\uparrow$, $V_d\uparrow$, $PB\downarrow$
  Child: $t_{1/2}\downarrow$, $V_d\uparrow$, $Cl_T\uparrow$
  Elderly: $t_{1/2}\rightarrow$, $V_d\rightarrow$, $Cl_T\rightarrow$, $PB\downarrow$
Dialysis[9]
  Hemodialysis $(+)$[10]
  Peritoneal $(+)$[11]

Drug interactions: Valproic acid is a minor substrate of CYP2A6, CYP2B6, CYP2C8/9, CYP2C19, and CYP2E1. It weakly inhibits CYP2C8/9, CYP2C19, CYP2D6, and CYP3A4. It weakly induces CYP2A6.[12] Enzyme inducers (i.e., phenobarbital, phenytoin, and carbamazepine) have been shown to increase the metabolism of valproic acid. Mefloquine may decrease valproic acid plasma concentrations.

Valproic acid is commonly used in the treatment of seizure disorders. Studies in epileptic patients suggest a $t_{1/2}\downarrow$, $V_d\uparrow$, and $Cl_T\uparrow$ compared with healthy control populations. Side effects are of low incidence but may include anorexia, nausea, vomiting, CNS depression, leukopenia, thrombocytopenia, and hepatotoxicity. Protein binding is concentration dependent and will decrease with increasing concentration. Free drug concentrations may be monitored using ultrafiltration to separate free from bound drug. Therapeutic free valproic acid serum concentrations are 2.5-11 mcg/mL [17-76 μmol/L]. Patients on polymedicines or homeopathic medicines and those who are hypoalbuminemic may have elevated free drug level.[13,14]

Valproic acid is a known human teratogen that produces a 10-fold increase in the incidence of neural tube defects. Its use in women at risk for pregnancy must be weighed against its benefits. Fetuses exposed during organogenesis should be studied for evidence of neural tube defects.

See Table II-5.

7. Evans WE, Schentag JJ, Jusko WJ: *Applied pharmacokinetics—principles of therapeutic drug monitoring,* ed 3, Vancouver, WA, 1992, Applied Therapeutics, Inc.
8. Klotz U, Rapp T, Muller WA: Disposition of valproic acid in patients with liver disease, *Eur J Clin Pharmacol* 13:55-60, 1978.
9. Bennett W, Aronoff G, Golper T, et al: *Drug prescribing in renal failure. Dosing guidelines for adults,* ed 2, Philadelphia, 1994, American College of Physicians.
10. Johnson LZ, Martinez I, Fernandez MC, et al: Successful treatment of valproic acid overdose with hemodialysis, *Am J Kidney Dis* 33:786-789, 1999.

TEST NAME AND METHOD	SPECIMEN	REFERENCE (THERAPEUTIC) INTERVAL, CONVENTIONAL [INTERNATIONAL RECOMMENDED UNITS]			KINETIC VALUES	

Valproic Acid—CONT

11. Orr JM, Farrell K, Abbott FS, et al: The effects of peritoneal dialysis on the single dose and steady state pharmacokinetics of valproic acid in a uremic epileptic child, *Eur J Clin Pharmacol* 24:387-390, 1983.

12. Lexi-Comp, Inc: *Up-to-date online 12.2. Drug information,* Hudson, OH, 2004, Lexi-Comp, Inc.

TEST NAME AND METHOD	SPECIMEN	REFERENCE (THERAPEUTIC) INTERVAL, CONVENTIONAL [INTERNATIONAL RECOMMENDED UNITS]			KINETIC VALUES	
Vancomycin (Vancocin)[1-4] *HPLC, FPIA, EIA*	Serum, plasma (heparin, EDTA). Trough concentration should be drawn within 30 min before the dose.	*mcg/mL* Therapeutic concentration Peak: Trough: Toxic concentration: Not well established.	20-40 5-10 >80-100	$\mu mol/L$ × 0.690 [14-28] [3-7] [>55-69]	PK[5-7]: $t_{1/2}$: V_d: Cl_T: PB:	4-6 hr[8] 0.4-1.25 L/kg 1.085 mL/min/kg ~55%

1. Yeo K, Traverse W, Horowitz G: Clinical performance of the EMIT vancomycin assay, *Clin Chem* 35:1504-1507, 1989.

2. Saunders N, Want S, Adams D: Assay of vancomycin by fluorescence polarisation immunoassay and EMIT in patients with renal failure, *J Antimicrob Chemother* 36:2411-2415, 1995.

3. Smith P, Morse G: Accuracy of measured vancomycin serum concentrations in patients with end-stage renal disease, *Ann Pharmacother* 33:1329-1335, 1999.

4. Baselt RC: *Disposition of toxic drugs and chemicals in man,* ed 7, Foster City, CA, 2004, Chemical Toxicology Institute.

5. Matzke GR, McGory RW, Halstenson CE, et al: Pharmacokinetics of vancomycin in patients with varying degrees of renal function, *Antimicrob Agents Chemother* 25:433-437, 1984.

6. Krogstad DJ, Moellering RC Jr, Greenblatt DJ: Single-dose kinetics of intravenous vancomycin, *J Clin Pharmacol* 20:197-201, 1980.

7. Cunha BA, Ristuccia AM: Clinical usefulness of vancomycin, *Clin Pharm* 2:417-424, 1983.

8. Micromedex: *Micromedex healthcare series 2004,* Greenwood Village, CO, 2004, Thomson Micromedex.

| FACTORS INFLUENCING DRUG DISPOSITION | REMARKS AND INTERFERENCES |

13. Dasgupta A, McLemore J: Elevated free phenytoin and free valproic acid concentrations in sera of patients infected with human immunodeficiency virus, *Ther Drug Monit* 20:63-67, 1998.
14. Dasgupta A: Clinical utility of free drug monitoring, *Clin Chem Lab Med* 40:986-993, 2002.

Metabolism
  None
Excretion
  Urine
Disease
  Renal: $t_{1/2}\uparrow$, $V_d\rightarrow$, $Cl_T\downarrow$
  Obesity
  $t_{1/2}\downarrow$ (3.15-4.75 hr)
  $V_d\uparrow$ (based on IBW)
  $Cl_T\uparrow$ (based on IBW)
Age
  Elderly: $Cl_T\downarrow$
Dialysis
  Hemodialysis (−)
  Peritoneal (−)

Drug interactions: Coadministration of vancomycin and an aminoglycoside can lead to increased risk of nephrotoxicity. Concomitant use of vancomycin with metformin can lead to increased plasma concentration of metformin. There may be an increased risk of bleeding when vancomycin is used in patients taking warfarin.[8]

Vancomycin is primarily used in the treatment of infections caused by β-lactam-resistant, aerobic gram-positive bacteria. Therapeutic and toxic concentrations are not well established. Vancomycin declines in a triexponential manner with distribution not completed until ~6 hr. Therefore specimens drawn before 6 hr may not be representative of the drug's concentration in the target organ. Half-life and total body clearance are strongly correlated with creatinine clearance. Primary side effects include ototoxicity, nephrotoxicity, leukopenia, eosinophilia, thrombocytopenia, and hypersensitivity reactions. Liver enzymes may be increased.

Appropriate dosing and monitoring may be challenging in patients with end-stage renal disease (ESRD). Various polyclonal immunoassays may give falsely higher results because of cross reactivity with vancomycin pseudometabolite, termed vancomycin crystalline degradation product (CDP), which accumulates in renal failure patients.[1-3] Immunoassays using monoclonal antibodies (EMIT or FPIA Vancomycin II), are less sensitive to CDP cross-reactivity.[3]

See Table II-6.

TEST NAME AND METHOD	SPECIMEN	REFERENCE (THERAPEUTIC) INTERVAL, CONVENTIONAL [INTERNATIONAL RECOMMENDED UNITS]		KINETIC VALUES	
Verapamil **(Calan, Isoptin)**[1-3] *GC-MS, HPLC* *MW: 454.61*	Serum, plasma (EDTA, heparin)	Therapeutic concentration: Toxic concentration:	100-500 ng/mL [× 2.2 = 220-1100 nmol/L] Not defined.	PK[4-6]: $t_{1/2}$ Single dose: Multiple dose: V_d: Cl_T Single dose: Multiple dose: PB: F:	4.8 ± 2.4 hr >2-fold ↑ 4.0 ± 0.9 L/kg 11.8 ± 5.0 mL/min/kg >2-fold ↓ 90 ± 2% 19 ± 12%

1. Spiegelhalder B, Eichelbaum M: Determination of verapamil in human plasma by mass fragementography using stable isotope-labelled verapamil as internal standard, *Arz Forsch* 27:94-97, 1977.
2. Todd G, Bourne D, McAllister RJ: Measurement of verapamil concentrations in plasma by gas chromatography and high pressure liquid chromatography, *Ther Drug Monit* 2:411-416, 1980.
3. Baselt RC: *Disposition of toxic drugs and chemicals in man,* ed 7, Foster City, CA, 2004, Chemical Toxicology Institute.
4. Hamann SR, Blouin RA, McAllister RG Jr: Clinical pharmacokinetics of verapamil, *Clin Pharmacokinet* 9:26-41, 1984.
5. Hardman JG, Limbird LE, Gilman AG: *Goodman & Gilman's the pharmacological basis of therapeutics,* ed 10, New York, 2001, McGraw-Hill.
6. Echizen H, Eichelbaum M: Clinical pharmacokinetics of verapamil, nifedipine, and diltiazem, *Clin Pharmacokinet* 11:425-449, 1986.
7. Lexi-Comp, Inc: *Up-to-date online 12.2. Drug information,* Hudson, OH, 2004, Lexi-Comp, Inc.

Warfarin **(Coumadin)**[1-8] *HPLC, GC,* *GC-MS, LC-MS,* *CZE, IA* *MW: 308.33*	Serum, plasma (EDTA, citrate)	Therapeutic concentration*: *International normalized ratio (INR) of 1.5-5.0 (2-3 for most indications). Toxic concentration:	*mcg/mL* 1-10 >10	μ*mol/L* × 3.24 [3.2-32.4] [>32.4]	$t_{1/2}$: V_d: Cl_T: PB: F: T_{max}:	S, 21-43 hr R, 37-87 hr 0.11-0.2 L/kg 0.04-0.36 mL/min/kg 99% (albumin, α_1 acid glycoprotein) [× 0.01 = 0.99, protein-bound mole fraction] 77.6-100% [× 0.01 = 0.776-1.00, bioavailable mole fraction] 0.3-4 hr

FACTORS INFLUENCING DRUG DISPOSITION	REMARKS AND INTERFERENCES

Metabolism
  Hepatic
Excretion
  Urine (primary)
  Bile/feces (secondary)
Disease
  Cirrhosis: $t_{1/2}\uparrow$, $V_d\uparrow$, $Cl_T\downarrow$
Age
  Elderly: $Cl_T\downarrow$

Drug interactions: Verapamil is a major substrate of CYP3A4 and a minor substrate of CYP1A2, CYP2B6, CYP2C8/9, CYP2C18, and CYP2E1.[7] Verapamil causes a significant increase in plasma digoxin concentrations and also appears to inhibit the metabolism of quinidine. Concomitant administration of verapamil and β-blockers may result in severe cardiovascular depression. Rifampin may decrease the bioavailability of verapamil.

Verapamil, a calcium channel blocker, is a racemic compound. The dextrorotary and levorotary isomers show pronounced differences in disposition and first-pass metabolism. Two- to three-fold greater plasma verapamil concentrations are required after oral dosing, as compared with IV dosing, to elicit the same increase in A-V conduction time. This is caused by presystemic stereoselective elimination of the pharmacologically more active levorotary isomer.

Nonlinear accumulation is observed after multiple oral dosing. Norverapamil, the *N*-demethylated metabolite, possesses some vasodilatory activity. Verapamil is bound to albumin (60%), but α_1-acid glycoprotein accounts for ~70% of protein-binding variability. Side effects include rare hepatic dysfunction and eosinophilia. Constipation is the common side effect. Toxic effects include nausea, weakness, bradycardia, hypotension, and A-V block.

Interferences: After oral administration, fluorescent methods are unsatisfactory for quantitation of verapamil plasma concentrations because of the appearance of fluorescent metabolites.

Metabolism
  Hepatic, CYP2C9, and isomers are metabolized through different pathways.
Disease
  Renal failure: $V_d\uparrow$, $Cl_T\uparrow$, $PB\downarrow$
  Cancer: $PB\downarrow$

Drug interactions: Multiple drug interactions occur because of competition for albumin binding sites, polymorphisms of CYP2C9, and induction or inhibition of metabolic pathways.

Warfarin, an anticoagulant, is administered as a racemic mixture. The S-enantiomer is two to five times more active than the R-enantiomer. The pharmacologic effect (indicated by the prothrombin time) is more useful for the purpose of drug monitoring than is serum concentration. Plasma protein binding is a major determinant of warfarin elimination and an important cause of interindividual variations in drug clearance. An increase in the free fraction of warfarin in plasma will result in increased drug clearance. Factors that enhance hypoprothrombinemia include inadequate diet, disease of the small bowel, disease associated with vitamin K deficiency, hepatic disease, chronic alcoholism, fever, hyperthyroidism, and aging. Factors decreasing pharmacologic response to warfarin include pregnancy, hypothyroidism, and hereditary resistance. Side effects include hemorrhage, anorexia, nausea, vomiting, and various cutaneous lesions (purpura, urticaria, and alopecia). Reversible increases in liver enzymes

TEST NAME AND METHOD	SPECIMEN	REFERENCE (THERAPEUTIC) INTERVAL, CONVENTIONAL [INTERNATIONAL RECOMMENDED UNITS]	KINETIC VALUES

Warfarin—CONT

1. Daly AK, King BP: Pharmacogenetics of oral anticoagulants, *Pharmacogenetics* 13:247-252, 2003.
2. Fitzpatrick B, O'Kennedy R: The development and application of a surface plasmon resonance-based inhibition immunoassay for the determination of warfarin in plasma ultrafiltrate, *J Immunol Methods* 291:11-25, 2004.
3. Kammerer B, Kahlich R, Ufer M, et al: Determination of (R)- and (S)-phenprocoumon in human plasma by enantioselective liquid chromatography/electrospray ionisation tandem mass spectrometry, *Rapid Commun Mass Spectrom* 18:458-464, 2004.
4. Lombardi R, Chantarangkul V, Cattaneo M, et al: Measurement of warfarin in plasma by high performance liquid chromatography (HPLC) and its correlation with the international normalized ratio, *Thromb Res* 111:281-284, 2003.
5. Maurer HH, Arlt JW: Detection of 4-hydroxycoumarin anticoagulants and their metabolites in urine as part of a systematic toxicological analysis procedure for acidic drugs and poisons by gas chromatography-mass spectrometry after extractive methylation, *J Chromatogr B Biomed Sci Appl* 714:181-195, 1998.
6. Naidong W, Ring PR, Midtlien C, et al: Development and validation of a sensitive and robust LC-tandem MS method for the analysis of warfarin enantiomers in human plasma, *J Pharm Biomed Anal* 25:219-226, 2001.
7. Wittkowsky AK: Warfarin and other coumarin derivatives: pharmacokinetics, pharmacodynamics, and drug interactions, *Semin Vasc Med* 3:221-230, 2003.
8. Zhou Q, Yau WP, Chan E: Enantioseparation of warfarin and its metabolites by capillary zone electrophoresis, *Electrophoresis* 24:2617-2626, 2003.

TEST NAME AND METHOD	SPECIMEN	REFERENCE (THERAPEUTIC) INTERVAL	KINETIC VALUES
Workplace Drug Screen[1-3]	Random urine	None detected.	See Table IV-2 for a listing of drugs commonly included in a workplace drug screen.
IA, GC-MS TLC, GC, HPLC	Alternative matrices: Hair, oral fluid, and sweat	None detected.	See *Amphetamine, Methamphetamine, Codeine, Morphine, Cannabinoids, PCP,* and *Cocaine.*

1. *Fed Register,* 53:11963, April 11, 1988.
2. *Fed Register,* 62:51118, September 30, 1997.
3. *Fed Register,* 69:19673, April 13, 2004.

FACTORS INFLUENCING DRUG DISPOSITION	REMARKS AND INTERFERENCES

have been noticed during warfarin therapy. Treatment of severe toxicity with vitamin K is specific.

Warfarin is a known human teratogen. Its use during pregnancy should be avoided.

See Table II-5.

Workplace drug screens are considered nonspecific, and any positive result must be confirmed with a specific technique. The forensic application GC-MS is used for this purpose. Federally regulated (SAMHSA, formerly NIDA) workplace drug testing mandates screening with immunoassays and confirmation by GC-MS.

Alternative matrices used for nonfederally regulated workplace drug testing and being considered for regulated testing include hair, oral fluid, and sweat.

TEST NAME AND METHOD	SPECIMEN	REFERENCE (THERAPEUTIC) INTERVAL, CONVENTIONAL [INTERNATIONAL RECOMMENDED UNITS]		KINETIC VALUES	
Zidovudine (Retrovir, AZT)[1-2] *HPLC,*[3,4] *RIA, FPIA, DPV,*[5] *LC-MS-MS*[6] MW: 267.24	Serum, plasma (heparin, EDTA). Stable at least 1 hr at both room temperature and 60° C.[7] Stable for 60 days when stored at −20° C.	Therapeutic concentration:	0.15-0.27 mcg/mL[8] [× 3.74 = 0.56-1.01 μmol/L]	PK[9,10]: $t_{1/2}$: V_d: Cl_T: PB: F:	0.5-3 hr 1.4 L/kg 27-30 mL/min/kg[11] 30% 60-65%
HPLC[4]	Urine				
DPV[5]	Whole blood				

1. McLeod GX, Hammer SM: Zidovudine: five years later, *Ann Intern Med* 117:487-501, 1992.
2. Baselt RC: *Disposition of toxic drugs and chemicals in man,* ed 7, Foster City, CA, 2004, Chemical Toxicology Institute.
3. Sadrzadeh SMH, Ainardi V, Gorden C, et al: A simple and rapid HPLC procedure for measuring zidovudine (AZT) in serum, *Clin Chem* 35:1181, 1989.
4. Hedaya MA, Sawchuk RJ: A sensitive liquid chromatographic method for determination of 3′-azido-3′-deoxythymidine (AZT) in plasma and urine, *Clin Chem* 34:1565-1568, 1988.
5. Barone GC III, Pesce AJ, Halsall HB, et al: Electrochemical determination of azidothymidine in human whole blood, *Anal Biochem* 198:6-9, 1991.
6. de Cassia R, Estrela E, Salvadori M, et al: A rapid and sensitive method for simultaneous determination of lamivudine and zidovudine in human serum by on-line solid-phase extraction coupled to liquid chromatography/tandem mass spectrometry detection, *Rapid Commun Mass Spect* 18:1147-1155, 2004.
7. Kamali F, Rawlins MD: Simple and rapid assay for zidovudine and zidovudine glucuronide in plasma using high performance liquid chromatography, *J Chromatogr* 530:474-479, 1990.
8. Paoli I, Dave M, Cohen BD: Pharmacodynamics of zidovudine in patients with end stage renal disease, *N Engl J Med* 326:839-840, 1992.
9. Stagg MP, Cretton EM, Kidd L, et al: Clinical pharmacokinetics of 3′-azido-3′-deoxythymidine (zidovudine) and catabolites with formation of a toxic catabolite, 3′-amino-3′-deoxythymidine, *Clin Pharmacol Ther* 51:668-676, 1992.
10. Blum MR, Liao SHT, Good SS, et al: Pharmacokinetics and bioavailability of zidovudine in humans, *Am J Med* 85(suppl 2A):189-194, 1988.
11. Rodman JH, Flynn PM, Robbins B, et al: Systemic pharmacokinetics and cellular pharmacology of zidovudine in human immunodeficiency virus type I-infected women and newborn infants, *J Infect Dis* 180:1844-1850, 1999.
12. Lexi-Comp, Inc: *Up-to-date online 12.2. Drug information,* Hudson, OH, 2004, Lexi-Comp, Inc.
13. Stretcher B: Monitoring AZT, *AACC Inservice Training Cont Educ* 11:9-16, 1989.

FACTORS INFLUENCING DRUG DISPOSITION	REMARKS AND INTERFERENCES

Metabolism
  Hepatic
Excretion
  Bile/feces (primary)
  Urine (secondary)
Disease or condition
  Cirrhosis: $t_{1/2}\uparrow$, $Cl_T\downarrow$, $C_{max}\uparrow$
  Uremia: $t_{1/2}\uparrow$, $Cl_T\downarrow$, $C_{max}\uparrow$

Drug interactions: Zidovudine is a minor substrate of CYP2A6, CYP2C8/9, CYP2C19, and CYP3A4.[12] Probenecid increases plasma zidovudine (AZT) concentrations. Morphine may inhibit hepatic glucuronidation. Clarithromycin may decrease peak plasma concentrations and area under the curve.

The therapeutic range of zidovudine, a synthetic dideoxynucleoside antiviral agent, is not well established. Serum containing HIV may be treated to kill the virus before AZT concentrations are measured. Heating HIV-infected serum to 58-60° C for 1 hr will reduce virus reverse transcriptase activity below detectable levels with no effect on AZT.[13] Spills on work surfaces may be disinfected with bleach or 70% ethanol.[13] No extraction of samples is required for RIA. Measurement of intracellular forms of AZT may be important in the near future. Only HPLC allows for concurrent measurement of AZT-glucuronide (GAZT).

Patients started on antiretroviral AZT therapy are typically monitored for CD4 counts and HIV viral loads. The HIV viral load should be measured at 4 wk after initial therapy, again at 8-12 wk, and approximately every 6-8 wk until the viral load is undetectable on standard assays (<50 copies/mL). At that point, the viral load can be measured every 3 mo.[12]

Interferences: The antibodies used in RIA and FPIA show limited cross-reactivity with GAZT. DPV requires a fasting specimen because lipemia interferes. Because AZT has activity against Enterobacteriaceae and may interfere with antimicrobial susceptibility testing, metronidazole may interfere with the peak of β-hydroxyethyl-theophylline used as an internal standard in HPLC.

| TABLE IV-1 | DRUG SCREENS RECOMMENDED TO SUPPORT POISONED PATIENTS PRESENTING TO EMERGENCY DEPARTMENT (NACB LABORATORY MEDICINE PRACTICE GUIDELINES)[1] |

STAT (TURNAROUND TIME <1 HR) QUALITATIVE URINE TOXICOLOGY ASSAYS

Cocaine
Opiates
Barbiturates
Amphetamines (based on regional prevalence of abuse)
Propoxyphene (based on regional prevalence of abuse)
PCP (based on regional prevalence of abuse)
Tricyclic antidepressants (TCAs) (in conjunction with ECG)

STAT (TURNAROUND TIME <1 HR) QUANTITATIVE SERUM TOXICOLOGY ASSAYS

Acetaminophen (paracetamol)
Lithium
Salicylate
Cooximetry for oxygen saturation, carboxyhemoglobin, and methemoglobin
Theophylline
Valproic acid
Carbamazepine
Digoxin
Phenobarbital (if urine barbiturates positive)
Iron
Transferrin (or UIBC assay if transferrin not available)
Ethyl alcohol
Methyl alcohol (realistic turnaround time: 2-4 hr; not needed in countries where these agents not available)
Ethylene glycol (realistic turnaround time: 2-4 hr; not needed in countries where these agents not available)

1. Wu AHB, Broussard LA, Hoffman RS, et al: National Academy of Clinical Biochemistry. Laboratory Medicine Practice Guidelines. Recommendations for the Use of Laboratory Tests to Support the Impaired and Overdosed Patients from the Emergency Department, *Clin Chem* 49:357-379, 2003.

TABLE IV-2 WORKPLACE DRUG SCREENS

FEDERALLY REGULATED (SAMHSA, FORMERLY NIDA)

DRUGS (CLASS)	SCREENING CUTOFF, NG/ML	CONFIRMATION CUTOFF, NG/ML
Amphetamines	1000	Amphetamine 500
		Methamphetamine 500
		(plus amp ≥200)
Cannabinoids	50	THC metabolite 15
Cocaine metabolite	300	Benzoylecgonine 150
Opiates	2000	Codeine 2000
		Morphine 2000
		6-acetyl morphine (6-AM) 10
PCP	25	25

SPECIMEN VALIDITY TESTING

Creatinine, specific gravity (when creatinine <20 mg/dL), pH, nitrites, oxidizing agents

NONFEDERALLY REGULATED

Testing typically includes the drugs listed above ("NIDA 5") plus combinations of drugs listed below. Cutoffs may be at lower levels, and samples analyzed may include alternative matrices such as hair, oral fluid, or sweat instead of urine.
Barbiturates
Benzodiazepines
Ethyl alcohol
Methadone
Methaqualone
Propoxyphene

SECTION V
CLINICAL MICROBIOLOGY

A: MICROBIOLOGY TESTS

TEST NAME AND METHOD	SPECIMEN AND SPECIAL REQUIREMENTS	CLINICAL COMMENTS AND REMARKS
Acid-Fast Stain for Mycobacteria (Ziehl-Neelsen, Fluorochrome Stain, AFB Stain, TB Stain)[1-4] (See *Mycobacteria Culture*.)	Specimen used for culture.	Smears should preferably be prepared from concentrated specimens, screened using a fluorochrome stain, and results reported with quantitation within 24 hr of specimen receipt. Organisms appear yellow to orange using a fluorochrome stain. Specimens and colonies may also be stained using either a Cold Kinyoun or Ziehl-Neelsen stain. Acid-fast organisms appear as red-staining bacilli. Observation of only one or two acid-fast bacilli per specimen should warrant specimen recollection. Smears should only be used as an adjunct to culture.

Smears for AFB may not correlate with corresponding cultures and/or molecular tests. For example, some mycobacteria other than tuberculosis do not stain well, if at all, with a fluorochrome stain, yet they will grow in culture. In contrast, some organisms may be detected on the smear that are not recovered in culture, either because of too harsh decontamination procedure, the patient may be receiving antituberculous medications, or the culture conditions may not be appropriate for the species of mycobacterium present. Therefore AFB smears can be used as a quality control measure.

The presence of acid-fast bacilli may be caused by pathogenic or saprophytic acid-fast bacilli. In urine, for example, the saprophyte *Mycobacterium smegmatis* may appear in the acid-fast preparation.

An AFB stain may be used to monitor patients on therapy for purposes of infection control.

1. Forbes BA, Sahm DF, Weissfeld AS: *Bailey & Scott's diagnostic microbiology,* ed 10, St. Louis, 1998, Mosby.
2. Isenberg HD: *Clinical microbiology procedures handbook,* ed 2, Washington, DC, 2004, ASM Press.
3. Murray PR, Baron EJ, Jorgensen JH, et al: *Manual of clinical microbiology,* ed 8, Washington, DC, 2003, ASM Press.
4. Winn W Jr, Allen S, Janda W, et al: *Koneman's color atlas and textbook of diagnostic microbiology,* ed 6, Philadelphia, 2006, Lippincott Williams & Wilkins.

Acid-Fast Stain (Modified) for *Nocardia* spp.[1]	Same specimen used for *Nocardia* culture.	*Nocardia* spp. are partially acid-fast, requiring a shorter or less harsh decolorization process than that of the *Mycobacterium* spp. The acid-fast characteristic is variable; thus a negative result may not rule out *Nocardia*. The stain is most helpful in distinguishing *Nocardia* spp. from *Actinomyces* spp.

1. Isenberg HD: *Clinical microbiology procedures handbook,* ed 2, Washington, DC, 2004, ASM Press.

TEST NAME AND METHOD	SPECIMEN AND SPECIAL REQUIREMENTS	CLINICAL COMMENTS AND REMARKS
***Actinomyces* spp.**[1] *Culture*	Exudate from draining sinuses; pleural fluid; and tissues such as lung. See *Anaerobic Culture* for specific requirements for anaerobic cultures. Notify the laboratory if actinomycosis is suspected.	Actinomycosis is a suppurative disease characterized by the formation of draining sinuses and the presence of granules ("sulfur" granules) composed of aggregates of filamentous, branching, gram-positive bacteria in the exudate. The granules are ~5 mm in diameter, firm in consistency, and usually white or yellow in color. Infections generally involve areas in the respiratory tract because the organisms involved are part of the normal oral flora. An association has also been made between infections and the use of IUDs. Suppurative exudates and pleural fluid should be examined for the presence of granules, as should the gauze dressings applied to draining sinus tracts. Other organisms, however, such as *Staphylococcus aureus* and agents of fungal mycetoma, can also produce granules. Specimens may require up to 14 days of incubation in culture for isolation of *Actinomyces* spp., and thus the laboratory should be made aware of the organisms that are suspected to provide for this extended anaerobic incubation. *Actinomyces* spp. are part of the normal flora of the oral cavity; therefore the isolation of the organism without a corresponding clinical picture of actinomycosis should be evaluated carefully. A Gram stain of the exudate, with or without granules, is helpful in making a presumptive identification of the *Actinomyces* spp. *Nocardia* can also produce granules, but *Nocardia* spp. may be ruled out by performing a partial acid-fast stain. A direct fluorescent antibody stain for *Actinomyces* spp. is available at certain large referral laboratories for use in selected specimens.

1.   Albers AC, Fletcher RD: Accuracy of calibrated-loop transfer, *J Clin Microbiol* 18:40-42, 1983.

TEST NAME AND METHOD	SPECIMEN AND SPECIAL REQUIREMENTS	CLINICAL COMMENTS AND REMARKS
Adenovirus, Direct Test for Antigen[1,2] *EM, IFA , LA, EIA, DNA probe, DNA amplification*	Respiratory secretions, urine, tissue, and stool. Rectal swabs are not acceptable. If not processed immediately, freeze at −70° C.	EM and IEM have been used to detect adenovirus in a variety of specimens, including respiratory secretions, urine, stool and tissue. Adenovirus types 40 and 41 associated with infantile gastroenteritis were first identified by this method. IFA are widely used for direct detection of adenovirus and other pathogens in respiratory specimens. EIA and LA have been shown to be very useful for detection of enteric adenovirus antigens in stool specimens. Similarly, DNA probe assays have been successful for detection of enteric adenoviruses. Several PCR-based assays that amplify hexon gene for detection of all adenoviruses are available in some reference laboratories.

1.   Lennette EH, Smith TF, editors: *Laboratory diagnosis of viral infection,* ed 3, New York, 1999, Marcel Dekker.

2.   Murray PR, Baron EJ, Jorgensen JH, et al, editors: *Manual of clinical microbiology,* ed 8, Washington, DC, 2003, American Society for Microbiology.

TEST NAME AND METHOD	SPECIMEN AND SPECIAL REQUIREMENTS	CLINICAL COMMENTS AND REMARKS
Adenovirus Serological Test[1,2] *CF, EIA, HI, NT*	Serum, acute and convalescent. See *General Information*.	Adenoviruses are endemic throughout the year among all age groups but are most common among children. They are responsible for many clinical syndromes including lower and upper respiratory tract infections (primarily school-aged children but accounting for ~2-5% of all ages); >50% of the cases of acute respiratory disease in military recruits; a pertussis-like syndrome; pharyngoconjunctival fever, epidemic kerato-conjunctivitis, acute hemorrhagic conjunctivitis, cystitis, infantile gastroenteritis, meningitis, and diseases of the immunocompromised patient (diarrhea, pneumonia, and upper respiratory tract infections). There are 51 known serotypes of adenovirus. Serotypes 1-8, 11, 21, 31, 35, 37, 40, and 41 are responsible for the majority of clinical diseases. Serotypes 31, 40, and 41 are specifically associated with infantile gastroenteritis. Serological diagnosis of adenovirus includes the genus-specific CF and EIA assays and the type-specific HI and NT assays. In most cases, the genus-specific assays are sufficient. EIA is more sensitive, standardized, and automated than CF and hence the more widely used assay. HI and NT are usually available only in larger reference laboratories. IgM assays may be more appropriate for the diagnosis of acute disease, but these are not commercially available. Serological procedures alone may not be used to establish the diagnosis without concomitant viral isolation or associated epidemiologic factors. Infants and children may especially present with falsely negative serological tests. Antigen detection, specifically for serotypes 40 and 41, is available for cases of infantile gastroenteritis and may enhance sensitivity and specificity.

1. Murray PR, Baron EJ, Jorgensen JH, et al, editors: *Manual of clinical microbiology,* ed 8, Washington, DC, 2003, American Society for Microbiology.
2. Rose NR, Hamilton RG, Detrick B, editors: *Manual of clinical laboratory immunology,* ed 6, Washington, DC, 2002, American Society for Microbiology.

TEST NAME AND METHOD	SPECIMEN AND SPECIAL REQUIREMENTS	CLINICAL COMMENTS AND REMARKS
Agar Screening Tests[1-4] *High-level aminoglycoside resistance (HLR) Enterococci* (See *Disk Diffusion.*)	*Enterococcus* isolate.	BHI broth containing 500 mg/mL of gentamicin or 1000 µg/mL of streptomycin is inoculated with a 0.5 McFarland suspension of *Enterococcus* spp. that has been prepared by direct colony or broth inoculation according to CLSI (NCCLS) guidelines. As an alternative, BHI agar containing 500 mg/mL of gentamicin or 2000 µg/mL of streptomycin is spot inoculated with 10 µL of a 0.5 McFarland suspension of *Enterococcus* spp. Any growth in the BHI broth or >1 colony or a haze of growth on agar after 24 hr of incubation indicates resistance, i.e., the agent will

TEST NAME AND METHOD	SPECIMEN AND SPECIAL REQUIREMENTS	CLINICAL COMMENTS AND REMARKS

Agar Screening Tests—CONT

| | | not be synergistic with cell-wall active agents. Enterococci that are resistant to gentamicin should be considered resistant to tobramycin and amikacin. Streptomycin must be tested separately because resistance is mediated by a different mechanism.

Aminoglycosides have poor activity against enterococci and cannot be used as monotherapy. However, an aminoglycoside plus a cell wall-active agent such as a penicillin or vancomycin act synergistically to enhance bacterial killing and may be used together in treating systemic enterococcal infections such as endocarditis. Acquired aminoglycoside resistance in enterococci accounts for high-level aminoglycoside resistance (HLR) and generally corresponds to MICs above concentrations normally tested, e.g., ≥ 1000 μg/mL for streptomycin and ≥ 500 μg/mL for gentamicin. |
|---|---|---|
| *Vancomycin-resistant Enterococci (VRE) Screen* (See *Minimum Inhibitory Concentration; Etest.*) | *Enterococcus* isolate. | One to 10 μL of a 0.5 McFarland enterococcal suspension is spot inoculated onto brain heart infusion (BHI) agar containing 6 μg/mL of vancomycin to screen for VRE. Isolates that grow on the screening plate should be confirmed by MIC using CLSI guidelines.

Presence of VRE does not indicate infection because this organism may colonize the intestine. Positive results should be telephoned immediately to infection control to ensure that the patient is placed on appropriate precautions. Patients infected or colonized with high-level (Van A phenotype) and moderate- to high-level vancomycin (Van B phenotype) resistant *Enterococci* spp. should be placed on Contact Precautions in contrast to those with an isolate expressing intrinsic low-level resistance caused by vanC gene.

Three negative specimens collected on separate days are generally required to remove previously positive patients from Contact Precautions. For surveillance purposes, specimens submitted for *Clostridium difficile* testing may be used to screen for VRE. |
| *Oxacillin/ Methicillin-resistant Staphylococcus aureus (ORSA/MRSA) Screen* | *S. aureus* isolate. | Mueller Hinton Agar (MHA) with NaCl and 6 μg/mL of oxacillin is spot inoculated with a 1-μL loop of 0.5 McFarland prepared by direct colony inoculation or from broth. Growth of >1 colony indicates oxacillin/methicillin resistance. The isolate should be considered resistant to all B-lactam agents.

Positive results should be telephoned immediately to infection control. Patients colonized or infected with ORSA should be placed on Contact Precautions. Three negative specimens collected on separate days are generally required to remove a patient from isolation. For surveillance purposes, specimens should be collected from the anterior nares and the site of infection as appropriate. |

TEST NAME AND METHOD	SPECIMEN AND SPECIAL REQUIREMENTS	CLINICAL COMMENTS AND REMARKS

Agar Screening Tests—CONT

Vancomycin-resistant S. aureus Screen

BHI agar containing 6 μg/mL of vancomycin is spot inoculated as above with a 0.5 McFarland suspension prepared by direct colony inoculation or from broth. Growth of >1 colony indicates high-level vancomycin resistance. Results should be telephoned immediately to infection control to ensure appropriate precautions are followed, and to other individuals as appropriate. Identification and at least two other AST methods should be used to confirm the results, and isolates should be sent to a reference laboratory for confirmation. This procedure may not detect VISA using the new CLSI breakpoint of 4-8 mcg/mL.

1. Isenberg HD: *Clinical microbiology procedures handbook,* ed 2, Washington, DC, 2004, ASM Press.
2. Murray PR, Baron EJ, Jorgensen JH, et al: *Manual of clinical microbiology,* ed 8, Washington, DC, 2003, ASM Press.
3. Clinical Laboratory Standards Institute (CLSI): *Performance standards for antimicrobial susceptibility testing; 16th informational supplement, M100-S16,* Wayne, PA, 2006, Clinical Laboratory Standards Institute (CLSI).
4. Winn W Jr, Allen S, Janda W, et al: *Koneman's color atlas and textbook of diagnostic microbiology,* ed 6, Philadelphia, 2006, Lippincott Williams & Wilkins.

Amebiasis Serological Test[1,2]

IHA, EIA, IFA

Serum, acute and convalescent, 1-3 wk apart.

Test is used to support the diagnosis of amebiasis caused by *Entamoeba histolytica.* Eighty-five percent of patients with proven intestinal amebiasis will have a detectable antibody response, whereas 99% of those with extraintestinal disease will demonstrate antibodies. Persons with *E. dispar* (morphologically indistinguishable from *E. histolytica*) do not produce detectable antibodies. Titers may persist for up to 10 years after cure of invasive amebiasis.

A fourfold increase in titer is the most indicative result. False-positive results in amebic liver disease rarely occur when the titers are ≥1:256. With acute presentation of <7 days, however, antibody tests may be negative; repeat examination in 7 days should be positive in amebic liver disease.[3]

EIA for antigen[2]

Stool. See *Cultures, General Instructions,* above.

Test demonstrates antigen of *E. histolytica* in the stool, if present. Sensitivity has been reported between 87-100% and specificity at 97-99%.

1. Garcia LS: *Diagnostic medical parasitology,* ed 4, Washington, DC, 2001, ASM Press.
2. Murray PR, Baron EJ, Jorgensen JH, et al, editors: *Manual of clinical microbiology,* ed 8, Washington, DC, 2003, ASM Press.
3. Katzenstein D, Rickerson V, Braude A: New concepts of amebic liver abscess derived from hepatic imaging, serodiagnosis, and hepatic enzymes in 67 consecutive cases in San Diego, *Medicine (Baltimore)* 61:237-246, 1982.

TEST NAME AND METHOD	SPECIMEN AND SPECIAL REQUIREMENTS	CLINICAL COMMENTS AND REMARKS
Amebic Meningoencephalitis Primary Test (PAM; Naegleria, Acanthamoeba, Free-Living Pathogenic Ameba)[1,2] *Direct examination, culture*	CSF. See *CSF Culture, Routine.* Tissue, e.g., brain, lung, and corneal biopsy. See *Miscellaneous Sites Culture, Routine.* Do not refrigerate or freeze specimens. Notify the laboratory before collection so that specific media can be prepared if culture is requested.	*Naegleria* spp. can cause a fulminant and often fatal meningoencephalitis in children and young adults, called primary amebic meningoencephalitis (PAM). CSF examination may have a normal or slightly decreased glucose and increased protein similar to bacterial meningitis. Gram stains will be negative. The portal of entry is through the nasal passages after exposure to the organisms in fresh water (lakes or swimming pools). *Acanthamoeba* spp. cause subacute or chronic meningoencephalitis with focal granulomatous lesions in the brain referred to as granulomatous amebic encephalitis (GAE). The route of invasion into the CNS is believed to be hematogenous from a primary focus in the respiratory tract or skin. No exposure to water sources is necessary preceding the infection, and most patients have reported previous trauma or underlying diseases, such as alcoholism, diabetes, Hodgkin's disease, pregnancy, or steroid use. In addition, keratitis and corneal ulcerations have been produced by species of *Acanthamoeba* after use of soft or hard contact lenses (primarily daily-wear or extended-wear soft lenses). For either etiology, direct examination of the CSF or involved tissue is part of the diagnostic workup. CSF should be placed on a slide, not in a counting chamber, because amebas resemble leukocytes. Stains such as Giemsa or Trichrome for *Naegleria,* and GMS, calcofluor white, or PAS for acanthamoeba should be utilized because Gram staining is not useful. Cultures for both of these amebas may be done on nonnutrient agar to which a suspension of *Escherichia coli* or *Enterobacter aerogenes* has been overlaid. These cultures are examined daily for 7 days. All personnel working with specimens that might contain these amebas should wear surgical masks and gloves, and processing should be carried out in a biological safety cabinet to ensure safety. Serological tests are not widely available.

1. Ash LR, Orihel TC: *A guide to laboratory procedures and identification,* Chicago, 1987, American Society for Clinical Pathologists.
2. Murray PR, Baron EJ, Jorgensen JH, et al, editors: *Manual of clinical microbiology,* ed 8, Washington, DC, 2003, ASM Press.

TEST NAME AND METHOD	SPECIMEN AND SPECIAL REQUIREMENTS	CLINICAL COMMENTS AND REMARKS
Anaerobic Culture[1-8]	Body fluid aspirate, e.g., pleural, synovial, peritoneal, and pericardial (See *Body Fluid Culture, Routine*); surgical tissue or biopsy sample, sulfur granules (See *Miscellaneous Site Culture, Routine*).	Transport all specimens for anaerobes in an anaerobic transport vial or container as soon as possible for processing, e.g., $\leq$10 min to $\leq$30 min for <1.0 mL to 1.0 mL of aspirated fluid, respectively. Tissue may be placed in a sterile container, which is then placed in a sealable plastic bag with an anaerobic atmosphere. Large specimen volumes and large pieces of tissue may be placed in a sterile container and hand-delivered to the laboratory for immediate processing. Ensure that the sample is collected from the active site of infection. Do not refrigerate specimens.

The microbiology laboratory should provide guidelines for the collection of acceptable specimens for anaerobic culture. Unacceptable specimens from sites that normally contain anaerobic flora should be rejected, e.g., throat, rectal, cervicovaginal swabs, sputum, and feces, because they may give misleading results.

Clinical clues to the presence of an anaerobic infection include putrid-smelling discharge; infections adjacent to a mucosal surface; presence of gas or infection in necrotic avascular tissue; Gram stain revealing mixed, pleomorphic bacterial flora; negative aerobic culture with positive Gram stain; infection following the use of aminoglycosides; septic thrombophlebitis; and a clinical setting suggestive of an anaerobic infection, e.g., septic abortion or after gastrointestinal surgery.

A Gram stain and culture for aerobes should be performed whenever an anaerobic culture is requested. Specimens collected on swabs are inferior and should only be used in rare instances when a very small quantity of specimen is obtained. At least two swabs, one for a Gram stain and the other to inoculate media, should be submitted in an anaerobic transport container. Processing of swab specimens should be limited to a Gram stain and solid media. Abbreviated identification schemes may be used to report results, e.g., "anaerobic gram-negative bacilli." A disclaimer should be recorded on reports generated from swab specimens that state the preferred specimens for optimal recovery of anaerobes are fluid and tissue. |

1. Brook I: *Pediatric anaerobic infections diagnosis and management,* ed 3, New York, 2002, Marcel Dekker, Inc.
2. Forbes BA, Sahm DF, Weissfeld AS: *Bailey & Scott's diagnostic microbiology,* ed 10, St. Louis, 1998, Mosby.
3. Hindlych M, Acevedo V, Carroll KC: Comparison of three transport systems (Starplex StarSwab H, the new Copan Vi-Pak Amies agar gel collection and transport swabs, and BBL Port-A-Cul) for maintenance of anaerobic and fastidious aerobic organisms, *J Clin Microbiol* 39:377-380, 2001.
4. Isenberg HD: *Clinical microbiology procedures handbook,* ed 2, Washington, DC, 2004, ASM Press.
5. Mandell GL, Bennett JE, Dolin R: *Principles and practice of infectious diseases,* ed 6, Philadelphia, 2005, Elsevier Churchill Livingstone.
6. NCCLS: *Methods for antimicrobial susceptibility testing of anaerobic bacteria. Approved standard,* ed 6, M11-A6, Wayne, PA, 2004, NCCLS.
7. Rodloff AC, Appelbaum PC, Zabransky RJ: *Cumitech 5A—practical anaerobic bacteriology,* Washington, DC, 1991, American Society for Microbiology.
8. Winn W Jr, Allen S, Janda W, et al: *Koneman's color atlas and textbook of diagnostic microbiology,* ed 6, Philadelphia, 2006, Lippincott Williams & Wilkins.

TEST NAME AND METHOD	SPECIMEN AND SPECIAL REQUIREMENTS	CLINICAL COMMENTS AND REMARKS
Antideoxyribonuclease B Serological Test (ADN-B Titer, Anti-DNase Titer, Antibody Titer for Group A Beta-Hemolytic Streptococci)[1,2]	Serum	More reliable than the antistreptolysin O (ASO) in identifying patients with pyoderma or post-impetigo nephritis caused by group A streptococcus (GAS). Used to identify GAS infection in patients who lack documentation of recent infection but present with nonsuppurative sequelae of *Streptococcus pyogenes* infection, e.g., acute rheumatic fever, Sydenham's chorea, and acute glomerulonephritis. Serum antibody titers do not peak until 4-6 wk after onset and, in contrast to antistreptolysin O (ASO), remain elevated for several months. Therefore this test may be used to support a diagnosis of Sydenham's chorea because of the associated latency of 3-12 mo between infection and onset of disease. Measurement of ASO and DNAse B antibodies reduces the percentage of false-negative results. Values of 1:60, 1:170, and 1:85 are considered normal for preschool children, school-aged children, and adults, respectively.

1.   Isenberg HD: *Clinical microbiology procedures handbook,* ed 2, Washington, DC, 2004, ASM Press.
2.   Murray PR, Baron EJ, Jorgensen JH, et al: *Manual of clinical microbiology,* ed 8, Washington, DC, 2003, ASM Press.

TEST NAME AND METHOD	SPECIMEN AND SPECIAL REQUIREMENTS	CLINICAL COMMENTS AND REMARKS
Antihyaluronidase Serological Test (AH Titer, Antibody Titer for Group A B-Hemolytic Streptococci)[1,2]	Serum	Test is used to document exposure to group A streptococcal antigens. Titers of AH increase in the second week of infection and decrease after 3-5 wk. The AH titer is elevated in ~60% of the cases of streptococcal pharyngitis, less often in streptococcal pyoderma. When this test is used in conjunction with the antistreptolysin O (ASO) titer, 90-95% of individuals with streptococcal pharyngitis will have an elevated titer against at least one of the group A streptococcal antigens. Values <128 U/mL are considered normal. The AH titer is not influenced by factors that may cause false-positive titers in the ASO test. However, reproducibility of the AH test is not as good as that of the ASO or antideoxyribonuclease B (ADN-B) test.

1.   Albers AC, Fletcher RD: Accuracy of calibrated-loop transfer, *J Clin Microbiol* 18:40-42, 1983.
2.   Meredith FT, Phillips HK, Reller LB: Clinical utility of broth cultures of cerebrospinal fluid from patients at risk for shunt infections, *J Clin Microbiol* 35:3109-3111, 1997.

TEST NAME AND METHOD	SPECIMEN AND SPECIAL REQUIREMENTS	CLINICAL COMMENTS AND REMARKS
Antistreptolysin O Titer (ASO Titer, Antibody Titer for Group A B-Hemolytic Streptococci)[1]	Serum	The most common acute group A *Streptococcus pyogenes* (GAS) suppurative illnesses are pharyngitis and pyoderma, and the most common nonsuppurative complications are acute rheumatic fever, Sydenham's chorea, and acute glomerulonephritis. Rheumatic fever may occur after pharyngitis but not after pyoderma, whereas glomerulonephritis may follow either pharyngitis or pyoderma. Although culture provides a definite laboratory diagnosis during a suppurative GAS illness, serologic tests are useful in providing evidence of antecedent streptococcal infections.
		Increased ASO titers are found in ~85% of patients with rheumatic fever or pharyngitis. The test is less reliable compared with the anti-DNase B test in patients with post-pyoderma nephritis. Titers increase as early as 1 wk after infection, peak in 3-5 wk, and return to baseline in 6-12 mo. A value of ~166 Todd units (TU) is considered normal; however, each laboratory should establish the upper limit of normal applicable to the region. An increase in titer of at least two dilution increments over a 1- to 2-wk period is of greater clinical value than results obtained from one random sample.

1.   Murray PR, Baron EJ, Jorgensen JH, et al: *Manual of clinical microbiology,* ed 8, Washington, DC, 2003, ASM Press.

Aspergillosis Serological Tests[1-3]	Serum	Patients with allergic bronchopulmonary aspergillosis or suspected aspergilloma, immunocompetent patients with unexplained pulmonary or meningeal symptoms, and patients on immunosuppressive therapy with unexplained fever should be tested using a serological test for aspergillosis.
Antibody Test *ID, CIE*		The ID test is sensitive and specific for the diagnosis of aspergillosis in immunocompetent patients. ID precipitins can be found in >90% of patients with aspergillomas and 70% of patients with allergic bronchopulmonary aspergillosis. ID precipitins are less frequent in patients with invasive disease. In the ID test, ≥1 precipitin band is suggestive of infection; ≥3 bands are indicative of an aspergilloma or invasive disease.
		The ID assay is 100% specific when used with reference sera to confirm the identity of bands. Nonspecific bands may be formed as a result of components such as C-reactive protein present in serum. However, these bands can be eliminated during testing. A culture may support the serological results.
		Tests for antibodies in invasive aspergillosis have a poor predictive value in high-risk immunosuppressed patients; instead antigen testing is recommended for these patients.

TEST NAME AND METHOD	SPECIMEN AND SPECIAL REQUIREMENTS	CLINICAL COMMENTS AND REMARKS

Aspergillosis Serological Tests—CONT

Antigen Test *EIA*	Serum	The sensitivity and specificity of the EIA for *Aspergillus* galactomannan are 90% and 84%, respectively. False-positive reactions may be the result of subclinical infection, intestinal colonization, or absorption of galactomannan from a damaged gut. False-negative reactions have been associated with previous amphotericin B therapy, limited blood vessel invasion, and high antibody titers. The disappearance of the antigen appears to correlate with good clinical outcome, whereas the persistence of antigen indicates a poorer prognosis. Urine is an unacceptable specimen because of the presence of an unknown cross-reacting substance.

1. Murray PR, Baron EJ, Jorgensen JH, et al, editors: *Manual of clinical microbiology,* ed 8, Washington, DC, 2003, ASM Press.
2. Yeo SF, Wong B: Current status of nonculture methods for diagnosis of invasive fungal infections, *Clin Microbiol Rev* 15:465-484, 2002.
3. Rose NR, Hamilton RG, Detrick B, et al, editors: *Manual of clinical immunology,* ed 6, Washington, DC, 2002, ASM Press.

Astrovirus, Direct Test for Antigen[1,2] *EM, RT-PCR*	Stool. If not processed immediately, freeze at $-70°$ C. Rectal swabs are not acceptable.	Astrovirus may be responsible for up to 5% of the cases of infantile gastroenteritis. It can also cause gastroenteritis in adults. Whereas EM has traditionally been used to detect this virus, experimental EIA and RT-PCR that amplify conserved 3′ terminus of the Astrovirus genome are now used to detect Astrovirus RNA in clinical specimens.

1. Lennette EH, Smith TF, editors: *Laboratory diagnosis of viral infection,* ed 3, New York, 1999, Marcel Dekker.
2. Murray PR, Baron EJ, Jorgensen JH, et al, editors: *Manual of clinical microbiology,* ed 8, Washington, DC, 2003, American Society for Microbiology.

Bartonella Culture[1-5]	Blood collected in EDTA or Isolator tube (Wampole): lymph node, liver, spleen, and skin tissue.	The most common cause of cat scratch disease (CSD) is *Bartonella henselae.* Humans become infected after the bite or scratch of a cat, a natural reservoir of *B. henselae,* or as a result of autoinoculation when scratch-infected flea blood or feces enters into their skin. Approximately 80% of cases are in individuals aged <21 yr. Patients most commonly present with tender, regional lymphadenopathy. Most immunocompetent patients experience a self-limiting infection. In 14% of patients with CSD, complications will develop, including Parinaud's ocular syndrome, hepatosplenic abscesses, encephalopathy, endocarditis, myocarditis, and occasionally osteomyelitis. In immunodeficient patients, *B. henselae* and *B. quintana* may cause a vascular proliferative disease known as bacillary angiomatosis, peliosis hepatis, or bacteremia.

TEST NAME AND METHOD	SPECIMEN AND SPECIAL REQUIREMENTS	CLINICAL COMMENTS AND REMARKS

Bartonella—CONT

Routine bacterial cultures are not suitable for recovery of *Bartonella* spp. because the majority of isolates require >7 days of incubation. Culture is indicated in the following settings: atypical cat scratch disease; fever of unknown origin with a cat exposure history; fever or lymphadenitis in an immunocompromised patient; and bacillary angiomatosis and peliosis. Culture is not recommended for most cases of cat scratch disease. Specimens should be collected before the initiation of antimicrobial therapy.

Blood cultures from patients with endocarditis are rarely positive; however, *Bartonella* may be recovered from patients with other bacteremic conditions. *B. henselae* is susceptible to concentrations of sodium polyanethol sulfonate (SPS) found in commercial blood culture media. Therefore the use of lytic blood culture systems, such as the Isolator system, is preferred for optimal recovery.

Culture may require up to 30 days.

Histological examination, PCR, and/or serology are generally more productive. A fourfold or greater increase in IgG-specific antibody titer between a serum specimen collected early in the course of infection and a second specimen collected in 7-8 wk is becoming a mainstay of diagnosis for CSD and CNS infection.

See *Bartonella serological test.*

1. Isenberg HD: *Clinical microbiology procedures handbook,* ed 2, Washington, DC, 2004, ASM Press.
2. Centers for Disease Control and Prevention: Cat scratch disease in children—Texas, September 2000-August 2001, *MMWR Morb Mortal Wkly Rep* 51:212-214, 2002.
3. Mandell GL, Bennett JE, Dolin R, editors: *Principles and practice of infectious diseases,* ed 5, New York, 2000, Churchill Livingstone.
4. Murray PR, Baron EJ, Jorgensen JH, et al: *Manual of clinical microbiology,* ed 8, Washington, DC, 2003, ASM Press.
5. Winn W Jr, Allen S, Janda W, et al: *Koneman's color atlas and textbook of diagnostic microbiology,* ed 6, Philadelphia, 2006, Lippincott Williams & Wilkins.

TEST NAME AND METHOD	SPECIMEN AND SPECIAL REQUIREMENTS	CLINICAL COMMENTS AND REMARKS
Bartonella Serological Test (Cat Scratch Disease Titer, *Bartonella henselae* Titer, *Bartonella* Antibody Titer, *Bartonella quintana* Titer)[1-3] *IFA, EIA*	Serum drawn at onset of disease and 2-3 wk later.	Infection with *Bartonella henselae* and *B. quintana* produce a variety of clinical manifestations, including fever and bacteremia, endocarditis, bacillary angiomatosis, and bacillary peliosis. In addition, *B. henselae* is also the causative agent of cat scratch disease. *Bartonella* infection is most frequently seen in immunocompromised patients, especially HIV-infected patients. *Bartonella* species may represent important pathogens in culture-negative endocarditis. Cat scratch disease is the most commonly recognized manifestation of human infection with *Bartonella* species and is most commonly associated with regional lymphadenopathy after a cat scratch or bite. IgG antibody responses among *Bartonella* species are largely cross-reactive; however, differentiation between *B. henselae* and *B. quintana* may be possible based on the magnitude of the antibody response to each organism. Serologic cross-reactions have also been reported with *Coxiella burnetii* and *Chlamydia* spp. IFA IgG titers ≥1:64 and IgM titers ≥1:20 are suggestive of infection. See *Bartonella*.

1. Murray PR, Baron EJ, Jorgensen JH, et al, editors: *Manual of clinical microbiology,* ed 8, Washington, DC, 2003, ASM Press.
2. Rose NR, Hamilton RG, Detrick B, editors: *Manual of clinical immunology,* ed 6, Washington, DC, 2002, ASM Press.
3. Mandell GL, Bennett JE, Dolin R, editors: *Principles and practice of infectious diseases,* ed 5, New York, 2000, Churchill Livingstone.

TEST NAME AND METHOD	SPECIMEN AND SPECIAL REQUIREMENTS	CLINICAL COMMENTS AND REMARKS
***Blastocystis hominis* Examination**[1,2]	Stool See *Ova and Parasite Examination.*	*Blastocystis hominis* inhabits the large intestine and is passed in the feces. Although up to 10-20% of stool specimens examined may be positive for this parasite, only occasionally will patients develop clinical symptoms. The role of *B. hominis* in human disease is still controversial, thus when detected in large numbers in stool samples, and in the absence of other parasites, bacteria, or viral agents, *B. hominis* may be the cause of symptoms and therapy may be required. *B. hominis* can reportedly cause diarrhea, cramps, nausea, vomiting, and abdominal pain with or without fever. Routine stool examinations will adequately detect the central-body forms (or vacuolar forms) of the parasites, which can vary in size from 6-40 μm. Reports should include a quantitation (rare, few, moderate, or many) of the organisms seen in the examination. It is important to remember that other causative pathogens must be ruled out before treatment of this parasite.

1. Murray PR, Baron EJ, Jorgensen JH, et al, editors: *Manual of clinical microbiology,* ed 8, Washington, DC, 2003, ASM Press.
2. Garcia LS: *Diagnostic medical parasitology,* ed 4, Washington, DC, 2001, ASM Press.

TEST NAME AND METHOD	SPECIMEN AND SPECIAL REQUIREMENTS	CLINICAL COMMENTS AND REMARKS
Blastomycosis Serological Test (*Blastomyces dermatitidis* Titer)[1,2] *ID, CF*	Serum collected at onset of disease and 3-4 wk later. In patients with negative results, additional samples may be collected at 3-wk intervals.	This test is used to support the clinical diagnosis of blastomycosis in patients with gradually progressive respiratory disease, fever, weight loss, cough and purulent sputum, and/or suggestive skin lesions. The ID test has been shown to have a sensitivity of ~70-80%; the CF test has a considerably lower sensitivity. In recent studies, the ID test detected 79% of patients with proven disease. A fourfold change in titer indicates probable infection. Decreasing titers indicate a favorable prognosis. Cross-reactions may occur in patients with histoplasmosis, paracoccidioidomycosis, or coccidioidomycosis. Negative test results do not rule out the diagnosis of blastomycosis. Definitive diagnosis is usually made by identification of the organism in tissues or fluids by microscopy and/or culture.

1. Yeo SF, Wong B: Current status of nonculture methods for diagnosis of invasive fungal infections, *Clin Microbiol Rev* 15:465-484, 2002.
2. Rose NR, Hamilton RG, Detrick B, editors: *Manual of clinical immunology,* ed 6, Washington, DC, 2002, ASM Press.

Blood Culture[1-26] (See *Brucella Culture.*) *Routine*	Recommended volume of blood is based on age/body weight. Children aged <1 yr (<9 lb) = 1.0 mL; 1-6 yr 1 mL for each year divided between two blood cultures; children (30-80 lb) = 10-20 mL divided between two blood cultures; adults and older children (>80 lb) = at least 30-40 mL divided between two blood cultures. The minimum collection is two draws totaling 20-30 mL of blood. Bottles should not be overfilled because excess leukocytes may cause automated systems to flag bottles as positive.	Blood volume is the most important factor in optimizing the recovery of pathogens. With the exception of neonates, two or three separate venipunctures are required to document sepsis and to distinguish a significant positive from contamination. If bacterial endocarditis is present, most patients will have a continuous bacteremia and all blood cultures will be positive. For other sources of bacteremia, there may be intermittent shedding of organisms into the blood, requiring three or more blood cultures. There are no standards to support collection of blood at specific intervals, e.g., 30 min apart. Two blood cultures should be collected consecutively from separate venipuncture sites from patients requiring immediate delivery of antimicrobial therapy. Blood cultures should be collected just before the next dose in patients receiving antimicrobial agents. To decrease blood culture contamination, specimens should preferably be drawn from a peripheral site rather than from an indwelling catheter port. Meticulous collection of blood using either tincture of iodine or chlorhexidine skin disinfectant should be used according to manufacturer's directions. The septum of the blood culture bottles should also be disinfected. If poor access requires that blood be drawn through a catheter port, the second blood culture should be collected by venipuncture. The catheter hub connection should be scrubbed with two separate

TEST NAME AND METHOD	SPECIMEN AND SPECIAL REQUIREMENTS	CLINICAL COMMENTS AND REMARKS

Blood Culture—CONT

70% alcohol pledgets and allowed to air dry. Once the tubing or cap of the catheter is disconnected, a syringe is used to collect 3 mL of discard blood in adults and 0.2 mL in children. Blood is then collected for culture through the hub using a new syringe.

Each automated blood culture system uses different media formulations. Media with resins or dematiaceous earth may be used to enhance recovery of organisms, particularly from patients who have already received antimicrobials. Sodium polyanethol sulfonate (0.025-0.05% SPS) is generally incorporated into media as an anticoagulant, antiphagocytic agent, and antimicrobial neutralizing agent. However, SPS may inhibit recovery of *Neisseria* spp., *Peptostreptococcus,* and *Gardnerella vaginalis.* Depending on the patient population, each blood collection is generally inoculated into an aerobic, anaerobic, and/or fungal blood culture bottle. The aerobic bottle should be inoculated first. Anaerobic bottles should be included when collecting blood from febrile neutropenic patients and patients with diabetes or wound infections. Alternatives to automated blood culture systems include manual broth cultures, biphasic media with agar and broth in one bottle, and lysis-centrifugation for colony quantitation. When using the later system, both pediatric and adult collection tubes are available for blood processing before inoculation onto solid media.

Blood cultures should not be refrigerated, even if there is a delay in sending the inoculated bottles to the laboratory. Preferably, incubation and monitoring of blood cultures should begin within 4 hr of specimen collection. Although credentialing agencies may require routine monitoring of blood cultures for 5 days, some laboratories have performed documented verification studies supporting reduction in monitoring to 3 or 4 days. Positive blood cultures are Gram stained and called to the ordering physician or patient-care nurse as soon as possible, and subcultured based on the morphotypes seen on the Gram stain. All blood subcultures should be performed in a biosafety cabinet. Terminal subcultures are not required when using an automated system.

Intense training and annual competency testing of phlebotomy staff are helpful to ensure the appropriate safety precautions are followed, including the use of safety needles, disposal of needles in labeled sharps containers, use of personal protective equipment, handwashing after phlebotomy, reducing blood culture contamination rate to ≤3%, and increasing the true-positive rate to 6-12%. Each laboratory that processes blood cultures should develop a quality assessment program that tracks the contamination rate for the hospital (and possibly for each unit and phlebotomist) and the true-positive rate.

TEST NAME AND METHOD	SPECIMEN AND SPECIAL REQUIREMENTS	CLINICAL COMMENTS AND REMARKS

Blood Culture—CONT

1. Bannatyne RM, Jackson MC, Memish Z: Rapid detection of *Brucella* bacteremia by using the BACTEC 9240 system, *J Clin Microbiol* 35:2673-2674, 1997.

2. Bates DW, Goldmann L, Lee TH: Contaminant blood cultures and resource utilization: the true consequences of false-positive results, *JAMA* 265:365-369, 1991.

3. Blot F, Nitenberg G, Chachaty E, et al: Diagnosis of catheter-related bacteraemia: a prospective comparison of the time to positivity of hub-blood vs peripheral-blood cultures, *Lancet* 354:1071-1077, 1999.

4. Blot F, Schmidt E, Nitenberg G, et al: Earlier positivity of central-venous vs. peripheral-blood cultures is highly predictive of catheter-related sepsis, *J Clin Microbiol* 36:105-109, 1998.

5. Bourbeau PP, Foltzer M: Routine incubation of Bact/ALERT FA and FN blood culture bottles for more than 3 days may not be necessary, *J Clin Microbiol* 43(5):2506-2509, 2005.

6. Bryant JK, Strand CL: Reliability of blood cultures collected from intravascular catheter versus venipuncture, *Am J Clin Pathol* 88:113-116, 1987.

7. Collignon PJ, Neil S, Pearson IY, et al: Is semi-quantitative culture of central vein catheter tips useful in the diagnosis of catheter-associated bacteremia? *J Clin Microbiol* 24:532-535, 1986.

8. Doern G, Brueggemann A, Dunne WM, et al: Four-day incubation period for blood culture bottles processed with the Difco ESP blood culture system, *J Clin Microbiol* 35(5):1290-1292, 1997.

9. Dunne Jr WM, Nolte FS, Wilson ML: In Hindler JA, editor: *Cumitech 1B-blood cultures III,* Washington, DC, 1997, ASM Press.

10. Forbes BA, Sahm DF, Weissfeld AS: *Bailey & Scott's diagnostic microbiology,* ed 10, St. Louis, 1998, Mosby.

11. Gaur AH, Flynn PM, Grannini MA, et al: Difference in time to detection: a simple method to differentiate catheter-related from non-catheter-related bloodstream infection in immunocompromised pediatric patients, *Clin Infect Dis* 37:469-475, 2003.

12. Isaacman DJ, Karasic RR, Reynolds EA, et al: Effect of number of blood cultures and volume of blood on detection of bacteremia in children, *J Pediatr* 128:190-195, 1996.

13. Isenberg HD: *Clinical microbiology procedures handbook,* ed 2, Washington, DC, 2004, ASM Press.

14. Li J, Plorde JJ, Carlson LG: Effects of volume and periodicity on blood cultures, *J Clin Microbiol* 32:2829-2831, 1994.

15. Little JR, Murray PR, Traynor PS, et al: A randomized trial of povidone iodine compared with iodine tincture for venipuncture site disinfection: effects on rates of blood culture contamination, *Am J Med* 107:119-125, 1999.

16. Maki DG, Weise CE, Sarafin HW: A semiquantitative culture method for identifying intravenous catheter-related infection, *N Engl J Med* 296:1305-1309, 1977.

17. Mandell GL, Bennett JE, Dolin R: *Principles and practice of infectious diseases,* ed 6, Philadelphia, 2005, Elsevier Churchill Livingstone.

18. Mensa J, Almela M, Casals C, et al: Yield of blood cultures in relation to the cultured blood volume in BACTEC 6A bottles, *Med Clin (Barc)* 108:512-513, 1997.

19. Miller JM: *A guide to specimen management in clinical microbiology,* ed 2, Washington DC, 1998, ASM Press.

20. Mimoz O, Karim A, Mercat A, et al: Chlorahexidine compared with povidone-iodine as skin preparation before blood culture: a randomized, control study, *Ann Intern Med* 131:834-837, 1999.

21. Murray PR, Baron EJ, Jorgensen JH, et al: *Manual of clinical microbiology,* ed 8, Washington, DC, 2003, ASM Press.

22. NCCLS: *Procedures for the collection of diagnostic blood specimens by venipuncture. Approved guideline, H3-A5,* Wayne, PA, 2003, NCCLS.

23. Schiffmann RB, Strand CL, Meier FA, et al: Blood culture contamination: A College of American Pathologists Q-Probes study involving 640 institutions and 497,134 specimens from adult patients, *Arch Pathol Lab Med* 122:218-220, 1998.

24. Shafazand S, Weinacker AB: Blood cultures in the critical care unit; improving utilization and yield, *Chest* 122:1727-1736, 2002.

25. Smith JA: *Cumitech 23—infections of the skin and subcutaneous tissues,* Washington, DC, 1988, ASM Press.

26. Winn W Jr, Allen S, Janda W, et al: *Koneman's color atlas and textbook of diagnostic microbiology,* ed 6, Philadelphia, 2006, Lippincott Williams & Wilkins.

TEST NAME AND METHOD	SPECIMEN AND SPECIAL REQUIREMENTS	CLINICAL COMMENTS AND REMARKS
Blood Culture for Fungus[1-3]	Blood, 5 mL per 40-mL blood culture bottle (with SPS) or 10 mL per Wampole Isolator tube. See *Blood Culture, Routine.*	The presence of fungi in blood may be an indication of invasive or disseminated fungal disease. An increase in fungemia is found in patients receiving immunosuppressive agents or hyperalimentation and in patients with malignancies or implanted intravascular devices. Continuous monitoring blood culture systems with media to enhance fungal recovery, biphasic blood culture systems and lysis centrifugation systems (Isolator) are available. The ratio of blood to culture medium in bottles should be 1:5-1:10. A higher concentration of blood may reduce the chance of isolating the organism; therefore blood culture bottles should not be overfilled. All of the above methods provide adequate detection of bloodstream infections caused by yeasts. The lysis centrifugation system is the most sensitive for the recovery of filamentous fungi, especially *Histoplasma capsulatum* and other dimorphic fungi. A single negative culture does not rule out the diagnosis of fungemia. Recovery of fungi increases with volume of blood cultured. Because fungal sepsis may be intermittent, at least two samples should be separately collected and cultured. Cultures are usually held up to 4 wk, and isolation may require >2 wk.

1. Murray PR, Baron EJ, Jorgensen JH, et al, editors: *Manual of clinical microbiology,* ed 8, Washington, DC, 2003, ASM Press.
2. Larone DH: *Medically important fungi: a guide to identification,* ed 4, Washington, DC, 2002, ASM Press.
3. Dunne WM Jr, Nolte FS, Wilson ML: In Hindler JA, coordinating editor: *Blood cultures III,* Washington, DC, 1997, American Society for Microbiology.

TEST NAME AND METHOD	SPECIMEN AND SPECIAL REQUIREMENTS	CLINICAL COMMENTS AND REMARKS
Body Fluid Culture, Routine[1-3] **and for Fungus**	Amniotic, cul-de-sac, synovial, pericardial, peritoneal, and pleural.	As much fluid as possible should be collected for culture by percutaneous aspiration using a safety needle and syringe. Culture of more than one large volume specimen processed both aerobically and anaerobically tends to increase the possibility of obtaining a laboratory diagnosis. Synovial and peritoneal fluid should be inoculated directly into aerobic and anaerobic blood culture bottles, as opposed to using the lysis-centrifugation method. Some fluid should be retained for Gram stain preparation. Small volume fluid may be submitted in an anaerobic transport vial, sterile screw-capped container, sterile blood collection tube, preferably without an anticoagulant, or in a Leur Lok-capped syringe that is hand-delivered to the laboratory for immediate processing. Drainage fluids in place >2 days, specimens collected on swabs, and routine cultures for acid-fast bacilli (AFB) and fungi are discouraged. Do not refrigerate specimens.
Fungus[4,5]	Body fluids, e.g., synovial, pleural, pericardial.	Swab specimens are not recommended. Submit as much fluid as possible for culturing fungi. Collection of fluids with heparin may prevent clotting. Alternatively the lysis centrifugation (Isolater) system may be used.

TEST NAME AND METHOD	SPECIMEN AND SPECIAL REQUIREMENTS	CLINICAL COMMENTS AND REMARKS

Body Fluid Culture, Routine—CONT

1. Bourbeau P, Riley J, Heiter BJ, et al: Use of the BacT/Alert blood culture system for culture of sterile body fluids other than blood, *J Clin Microbiol* 36:3273-3277, 1998.

2. Isenberg HD: *Clinical microbiology procedures handbook,* ed 2, Washington, DC, 2004, ASM Press.

3. Miller JM: *A guide to specimen management in clinical microbiology,* ed 2, Washington, DC, 1998, ASM Press.

4. Balous A, Hausler WJ, Hermann KL, et al, eds: *Manual of clinical microbiology,* ed 5, Washington, DC, 1991, American Society for Microbiology.

5. Haley LD, Tandel J, Coyle MB: Cumitech II: *Practical methods for culture and identification of fungi in the clinical microbiology laboratory,* Washington, DC, 1980, American Society for Microbiology.

Bone Marrow Culture for Fungus[1,2]	Bone marrow biopsy or aspirate. A minimum of 0.5 mL should be collected in a heparinized syringe and may be inoculated at bedside onto brain-heart infusion, Sabouraud, or yeast extract phosphate agar. Inoculation into pediatric Isolator tubes is preferable. If specimen is to be sent to laboratory for processing, it must be sent immediately.	This is the specimen of choice for isolation of *Histoplasma capsulatum*. The culture may also be useful in the diagnosis of disseminated candidiasis and cryptococcosis. Routine blood culture bottles are not recommended for bone marrow culturing. See *General Comments* above.

---

1. Murray PR, Baron EJ, Jorgensen JH, et al, editors: *Manual of clinical microbiology,* ed 8, Washington, DC, 2003, ASM Press.

2. Larone DH: *Medically important fungi: a guide to identification,* ed 4, Washington, DC, 2002, ASM Press.

Bordetella pertussis (Whooping Cough)[1-6]	Nasopharyngeal specimens, e.g., nasal aspirates or washings, collected within 4 wk of onset.	Direct examination of nasopharyngeal specimens by DFA can be of value, especially in seriously ill children, because the results are rapidly available. The technique should be used in conjunction with appropriate cultures, owing to frequent false-negative results. Likewise, cross-reactions with other organisms, including *Legionella* spp., may give false-positive results. Serological studies to demonstrate antibodies are generally not helpful in diagnosing pertussis.
Molecular methods, e.g., PCR, are now considered the test of choice because of the higher sensitivity and more rapid turnaround time to results compared with culture. In June 1996, the	Vacuum-assisted nasopharyngeal aspirates, bulb- or syringe-collected nasopharyngeal washings, or transtracheal aspirates provide a higher yield on culture than swabs. If nasopharyngeal swabs are collected for culture, calcium alginate or Dacron tip swabs on a fine flexible wire should be used. Use	The diagnosis of whooping cough is frequently made on clinical grounds alone. Although knowledge of contact is helpful, the appearance of a paroxysmal cough and the typical "whoop" after a brief upper respiratory tract syndrome are strongly suggestive. In infants aged <6 mo, however, the typical whoop may be absent, whereas in adults, they generally only demonstrate catarrhal symptoms, a mild bronchitis, or both. Adults may serve as the reservoir for *B. pertussis*.

TEST NAME AND METHOD	SPECIMEN AND SPECIAL REQUIREMENTS	CLINICAL COMMENTS AND REMARKS

Bordetella pertussis—CONT

Council for State and Territorial Epidemiologists revised laboratory criteria to include positive PCR assays for *B. pertussis* as the official laboratory confirmation of pertussis. If PCR is not available, culture and direct fluorescent antibody (DFA) tests may be used.

flocked pernasal swabs if nasopharyngeal swab specimens are collected for PCR assays. With the patient's head immobilized, gently insert a swab through one nostril to the posterior nasopharynx, rotate, and leave in place 15-30 sec. A second swab should be collected in the same manner for a DFA test for pertussis. Kits including the appropriate swabs, appropriate transport medium, slides for DFA, and instructions for specimen collection have been found to be helpful to ensure that specimens are collected in a manner that will maximize the sensitivity of culture and DFA.

Specimens should be transported to the laboratory without delay. If ≤ 2 hr, use 0.5-1% casein hydrolysate (casamino acid) solution; if <24 hr, use Amies medium with charcoal; and if >24 hr but ≤ 3 days, use Regan-Lowe transport medium. Specimens should be plated as soon as possible on Regan-Lowe charcoal agar and incubated at 35° C without 5% CO_2 for 5-12 days. Colonies consistent with *B. pertussis* are confirmed using DFA.

1. Isenberg HD: *Clinical microbiology procedures handbook,* ed 2, Washington, DC, 2004, ASM Press.

2. Loeffelholz MJ, Thompson CJ, Ong KS, et al: Comparison of PCR, culture, and direct fluorescent-antibody testing for detection of *Bordetella pertussis, J Clin Microbiol* 37:2872-2876, 1999.

3. Meade BD, Bollen A: Recommendations for the use of the polymerase chain reaction in the diagnosis of *Bordetella pertussis* infections, *J Med Microbiol* 41:51-55, 1994.

4. Miller FD, Hoppe JE, Wirsing von Konig CH: Laboratory diagnosis of pertussis: state of the art in 1997, *J Clin Microbiol* 35:2433-2443, 1997.

5. Murray PR, Baron EJ, Jorgensen JH, et al: *Manual of clinical microbiology,* ed 8, Washington, DC, 2003, ASM Press.

6. Winn W Jr, Allen S, Janda W, et al: *Koneman's color atlas and textbook of diagnostic microbiology,* ed 6, Philadelphia, 2006, Lippincott Williams & Wilkins.

TEST NAME AND METHOD	SPECIMEN AND SPECIAL REQUIREMENTS	CLINICAL COMMENTS AND REMARKS
Borrelia burgdorferi **Culture** (Lyme disease agent)[1,2]	Skin biopsy of area of erythema migrans, CSF.	*Borrelia burgdorferi* is the causative agent of Lyme disease. Skin biopsy specimens taken close to the expanding border of the erythema migrans lesion are the best for culture; however, organisms can also be cultured from CSF. Blood and synovial fluid cultures are usually negative. Culture is performed using Barbour-Stoenner-Kelly II medium or modified Kelly medium Preac-Mursic. Because of the complexity and relatively low yield of culture, it is not performed in most clinical laboratories. Most isolates require several weeks of incubation. Negative cultures should be monitored for 6 wk.

1. Murray PR, Baron EJ, Jorgensen JH, et al, editors: *Manual of clinical microbiology,* ed 8, Washington, DC, 2003, ASM Press.
2. Winn W Jr, Allen SD, Janda WM, et al, editors: *Koneman's color atlas and textbook of diagnostic microbiology,* ed 6, Philadelphia, 2006, Lippincott Williams & Wilkins.

Borrelia burgdorferi **Serological Test**[1,2]		*Borrelia burgdorferi* is the etiologic agent of Lyme disease, an inflammatory disorder transmitted to humans by the tick *Ixodes scapularis.* The vector is prevalent in the northeastern and western U.S. IFA or EIA tests can be performed to detect IgM and IgG antibodies. False-negative results may occur early in disease. Serum cross-reactivity occurs with other spirochetal diseases, e.g., syphilis and relapsing fever and in patients with infectious mononucleosis and bacterial endocarditis.
IFA, EIA	Serum, CSF	
Western blot	Serum, CSF, and synovial fluid	A two-step protocol is currently recommended for the testing of patients with suspected Lyme disease. Serum specimens should first be evaluated with a sensitive EIA or IFA. Specimens positive or equivocal by this test should be further evaluated using Western blot.

Western immunoblotting is most frequently used as a supplemental test for equivocal and positive EIA or IFA results. It is not a quantitative test and should only be used to test specimens containing a significant amount of antibody. Ten proteins are currently recognized as useful in Lyme disease serodiagnosis. Positive blots are interpreted as follows:

IgM: 2 of 3 of the following bands—21/25, 39, and 41

IgG: 5 of the following 10 bands—18, 21/25, 28, 30, 39, 41, 45, 58, 66, and 93

1. Murray PR, Baron EJ, Jorgensen JH, et al, editors: *Manual of clinical microbiology,* ed 8, Washington, DC, 2003, ASM Press.
2. Rose NR, Hamilton RG, Detrick B, editors: *Manual of clinical immunology,* ed 6, Washington, DC, 2002, ASM Press.

TEST NAME AND METHOD	SPECIMEN AND SPECIAL REQUIREMENTS	CLINICAL COMMENTS AND REMARKS
Brucella[1-6] (See *Blood Cultures.*)	Blood or bone marrow: acute and convalescent serum specimens.	*Brucella* is a fastidious, slow-growing, gram-negative coccobacillus. Individuals at risk include unvaccinated animal workers who contract the organism directly or by aerosol from infected tissue and those who ingest unpasteurized dairy products contaminated with brucellae. This organism is also categorized as a biothreat level B agent having a moderate chance of transmission and morbidity, but a low rate of mortality. Biphasic broth culture bottles are inoculated, inverted twice daily for the first 2 days and then daily for 21 days. If an automated blood culture system is used, bottles should be monitored for 7-10 days. They may require a terminal subculture with incubation in 5-10% CO_2 for at least 72 hr. Suspected positive cultures should be handled in a biosafety cabinet because of the danger to laboratory workers handling these cultures. Antimicrobial susceptibility tests are unreliable and should not be performed because they erroneously show susceptibility to some agents. As an adjunct to culture, serologic testing such as a Wright's tube agglutination test may be performed. A titer $\geq 1:160$ is considered significant.

1. Bannatyne RM, Jackson MC, Memish Z: Rapid detection of *Brucella* bacteremia by using the BACTEC 9240 system, *J Clin Microbiol* 35:2673-2674, 1997.
2. Gotuzzo E, Carrillo C, Guerra J, et al: An evaluation of diagnostic methods for brucellosis—the value of bone marrow culture, *J Infect Dis* 153:122-125, 1986.
3. Isenberg HD: *Clinical microbiology procedures handbook,* ed 2, Washington, DC, 2004, ASM Press.
4. Murray PR, Baron EJ, Jorgensen JH, et al: *Manual of clinical microbiology,* ed 8, Washington, DC, 2003, ASM Press.
5. Yagupsky P: Detection of *Brucellae* in blood cultures, *J Clin Microbiol* 37:3437-3442, 1999.
6. Winn W Jr, Allen S, Janda W, et al: *Koneman's color atlas and textbook of diagnostic microbiology,* ed 6, Philadelphia, 2006, Lippincott Williams & Wilkins.

TEST NAME AND METHOD	SPECIMEN AND SPECIAL REQUIREMENTS	CLINICAL COMMENTS AND REMARKS
Brucella spp. Serological Test (Agglutinins for Brucellosis)[1]	Serum, drawn the first week of illness and 3-6 wk later.	*Brucella* antibodies are detected during the second week in acute cases and peak in 3-6 wk. An increasing titer is considered positive. A single titer of $\geq 1:160$ is suggestive of infection if there is a compatible history. Rarely are antibodies absent in patients with bacteriologically proven disease. Higher titers of IgG than IgM suggest late disease, localized infection, relapse, or chronic infection. The febrile agglutinin test for *Brucella* is no longer recommended. Detection of *Brucella* antibodies in CSF indicates central nervous system infection, although results must be interpreted carefully to rule out CSF contamination by blood.

Because of cross-reacting antibodies, *B. abortus* antigen will also detect infection with *B. suis* and *B. melitensis* but not with *B. canis*. |

1. Morris AJ, Wilson SJ, Marx CE, et al: Clinical impact of bacteria and fungi recovered only from broth cultures, *J Clin Microbiol* 33:161-165, 1995.

TEST NAME AND METHOD	SPECIMEN AND SPECIAL REQUIREMENTS	CLINICAL COMMENTS AND REMARKS
Calcofluor White Stain for Fungi[1,2]	Appropriate specimen is the same as that for culture of the corresponding site.	Stain is useful for direct microscopic examination of specimens to identify fungal elements. It can be used alone or in conjunction with KOH to clear the specimen for easier observation. Calcofluor white is used to stain fungi in clinical specimens. It is a colorless dye that binds to cellulose and chitin in fungal cell walls and fluoresces when exposed to UV light. *Pneumocystis jiroveci (carinii)* can also be observed in specimens with this stain.

1. Murray PR. Baron EJ, Jorgensen JH, et al, editors: *Manual of clinical microbiology,* ed 8, Washington, DC, 2003, ASM Press.
2. Larone DH: *Medically important fungi: a guide to identification,* ed 4, Washington, DC, 2002, ASM Press.

TEST NAME AND METHOD	SPECIMEN AND SPECIAL REQUIREMENTS	CLINICAL COMMENTS AND REMARKS
Calicivirus, Direct Test for Antigen[1,2] *EM, RT-PCR*	Stool. If not processed immediately, freeze at −70° C. Rectal swabs are not acceptable.	Caliciviruses, which includes Norwalk-like viruses and Sapporo-like viruses, are responsible for gastroenteritis in children and infants. Although present all year, the virus infection peaks in winter months. Symptoms are generally milder in Sapporo-like than in Norwalk-like infections. Sapporo-like outbreaks tend to last 3-5 days longer than those of Norwalk-like virus infections do. RT-PCR is the most sensitive method for the diagnosis of caliciviruses. EM was the most widely used detection method before RT-PCR.

1. Lennette EH, Smith TF, editors: *Laboratory diagnosis of viral infection,* ed 3, New York, 1999, Marcel Dekker.
2. Murray PR, Baron EJ, Jorgensen JH, et al, editors: *Manual of clinical microbiology,* ed 8, Washington, DC, 2003, American Society for Microbiology.

TEST NAME AND METHOD	SPECIMEN AND SPECIAL REQUIREMENTS	CLINICAL COMMENTS AND REMARKS
California Encephalitis Serological Test (LaCrosse Titer)[1,2] *IF*	Serum, acute and convalescent. See *General Information.*	California encephalitis virus is a member of the Group C arboviruses, the bunyavirus. The vector of transmission is the mosquito. Common animal hosts include squirrels, horses, deer, rabbits, and cows. The disease occurs throughout the U.S., but most cases have been found in the north central states during the summer months. Most commonly it occurs in children. The virus has been found to be an important cause of mild meningoencephalitis, with fatalities of <1%. Commercially produced indirect immunofluorescent (IF) antibody tests for both IgG and IgM are now available in the U.S.

TEST NAME AND METHOD	SPECIMEN AND SPECIAL REQUIREMENTS	CLINICAL COMMENTS AND REMARKS

California Encephalitis Serological Test—CONT

Up to 50% of individuals with infection by California serogroups do not develop detectable CF antibodies.

See *Encephalitis Virus Serological Test.*

1. Murray PR, Baron EJ, Jorgensen JH, et al, editors: *Manual of clinical microbiology,* ed 8, Washington, DC, 2003, American Society for Microbiology.
2. Rose NR, Hamilton RG, Detrick B, editors: *Manual of clinical laboratory immunology,* ed 6, Washington, DC, 2002, American Society for Microbiology.

Candidiasis Serological Tests[1-3]

Antibody test

ID, LA, CIE

Serum at onset of disease and 2-3 wk later (if required).

This assay is used to support the diagnosis of systemic (invasive) candidiasis in the immunocompetent host. Immunosuppressed patients may fail to produce antibody; therefore a negative test does not rule out the presence of disease.

The diagnosis of invasive candidiasis is often very difficult to make in the laboratory. LA, ID, and CIE are available to detect antibodies. The production of ≥1 ID precipitin band constitutes a positive test. LA and CIE titers ≥1:8 are presumptive evidence of systemic candidiasis. LA titers of 1:4 and a positive ID test are regarded as evidence of early stages of candidiasis or of colonization with *Candida* spp. A fourfold increase in titer between acute and convalescent sera is presumptive evidence of infection. A fourfold decrease may indicate successful chemotherapy or elimination of the *Candida* colonization. In the immunocompetent host, sensitivity of these antibody tests may reach 80%.

Positive tests may occur as a result of colonization with *Candida* spp. Severe cases of vaginitis or mucocutaneous candidiasis can also produce falsely positive results.

Antigen test

EIA

Serum

The assay is used to detect mannan, a candidal antigen, in the sera of patients with invasive candidiasis. This test should be more specific than determination of the presence of candidal antibodies.

Concentrations of >2 ng of serum mannan by EIA is suggestive of invasive candidiasis. Sensitivity in cancer patients is 65-70%, with a specificity of 100%. Mannanemia appears to be transient and is rapidly cleared from the body; therefore it has been recommended that weekly or twice-weekly assays be performed along with routine blood cultures for *Candida* spp. to best detect the presence of the disease in susceptible patients.

TEST NAME AND METHOD	SPECIMEN AND SPECIAL REQUIREMENTS	CLINICAL COMMENTS AND REMARKS

Candidiasis Serological Tests—CONT

Another antigen assay, Cand-Tec (RAMCO Labs, Houston, TX), measures a heat-labile antigen. Recent studies demonstrated a sensitivity and specificity of 50% and 73%, respectively.

1. Murray PR, Baron EJ, Jorgensen JH, et al, editors: *Manual of clinical microbiology,* ed 8, Washington, DC, 2003, ASM Press.
2. Yeo SF, Wong B: Current status of nonculture methods for diagnosis of invasive fungal infections, *Clin Microbiol Rev* 15:465-484, 2002.
3. Rose NR, Hamilton RG, Detrick B, editors: *Manual of clinical immunology,* ed 6, Washington, DC, 2002, ASM Press.

Catheter Cultures[1-6] — Catheter tip, blood

Several methods are available to provide quantitative or semiquantitative colony counts.

(1) The semiquantitative roll technique is commonly used to distinguish infection ($\geq$15 colonies) from contamination. (2) Quantitative catheter flush and sonication cultures are based on a criterion of $\geq$100 colonies as a reflection of infection. Quantitation with sonication appears to be more sensitive than the semiquantitative method because it detects lumen colonization. A peripheral blood culture should be submitted along with the catheter.

Note: Because catheter tip cultures without a concomitant blood culture have a low specificity, full identification and susceptibility testing is not indicated unless specifically requested.

(3) To avoid removal of the catheter, two blood specimens (one peripheral and one through the catheter) can be submitted together to compare time to positive signal by an automated blood culture instrument. The infection is considered catheter related if the culture through the catheter is positive with the same organism at least 2 hr before the peripherally collected blood culture.

(4) Blood can be collected peripherally and through the catheter and placed in Isolator tubes (Wampole). Catheter sepsis is likely if the blood collected through the catheter has a 5- to 10-fold higher colony count.

1. Blot F, Nitenberg G, Chachaty E, et al: Diagnosis of catheter-related bacteraemia: a prospective comparison of the time to positivity of hub-blood versus peripheral-blood cultures, *Lancet* 354:1071-1077, 1999.
2. Blot F, Schmidt E, Nitenberg G, et al: Earlier positivity of central-venous versus peripheral-blood cultures is highly predictive of catheter-related sepsis, *J Clin Microbiol* 36:105-109, 1998.
3. Collignon PJ, Soni N, Pearson IY, et al: Is semi-quantitative culture of central vein catheter tips useful in the diagnosis of catheter-associated bacteremia? *J Clin Microbiol* 24:532-535, 1986.

TEST NAME AND METHOD	SPECIMEN AND SPECIAL REQUIREMENTS	CLINICAL COMMENTS AND REMARKS

Catheter Cultures—CONT

4. Gaur AH, Flynn PM, Grannini MA, et al: Difference in time to detection: a simple method to differentiate catheter-related from non-catheter-related bloodstream infection in immunocompromised pediatric patients, *Clin Infect Dis* 37:469-475, 2003.

5. Isenberg HD: *Clinical microbiology procedures handbook,* ed 2, Washington, DC, 2004, ASM Press.

6. Maki DG, Weise CE, Sarafin HW: A semiquantitative culture method for identifying intravenous catheter-related infection, *N Engl J Med* 296:1305-1309, 1977.

Chlamydia Group Antibody Serological Test [Genus-Specific Test for Psittacosis or Lymphogranuloma Venereum (LGV)][1-3] *CF*	Acute and convalescent sera drawn 2-4 wk apart.	A fourfold increase in titer between acute and convalescent sera is necessary for confirmation. A single titer ≥1:64 is considered indicative of psittacosis or LGV. Titers in LGV may not increase in paired sera because most patients are tested after the acute phase of illness. For a diagnosis of psittacosis, previous contact with sick birds or employment in a poultry business or pet shop should be documented. The antigen is not species specific; thus a high titer can support the diagnosis of psittacosis or LGV. Titers ≤1:16 may be found in the general population, depending on geographic location. There is no cross-reactivity of CF antibodies with those of syphilis, yaws, gonorrhea, or leprosy. The CF test is not useful in diagnosing trachoma, adult inclusion conjunctivitis, genital tract infections, or neonatal infections.

1. Murray PR, Baron EJ, Jorgensen JH, et al, editors: *Manual of clinical microbiology,* ed 8, Washington, DC, 2003, ASM Press.

2. Black CM: Current methods of laboratory diagnosis of *Chlamydia trachomatis* infections, *Clin Microbiol Rev* 10:160-184, 1997.

3. Rose NR, Hamilton RG, Detrick B, editors: *Manual of clinical immunology,* ed 6, Washington, DC, 2002, ASM Press.

Chlamydophila (Chlamydia) pneumoniae **Culture**[1,2]	Oropharyngeal or nasopharyngeal swabs/aspirates, bronchoalveolar lavage fluid, ear aspirates, and lung tissue Transport to the laboratory immediately in special transport medium such as 2SP or multi-	*C. pneumoniae* is a common cause of community-acquired acute respiratory infection. It is spread person to person via respiratory secretions. Clinically inapparent infection is common, and carriers likely serve as reservoirs for organism dissemination. Because *C. pneumoniae* is fastidious and slow growing, serologic diagnosis or detection via nucleic acid amplification testing is preferred.

TEST NAME AND METHOD	SPECIMEN AND SPECIAL REQUIREMENTS	CLINICAL COMMENTS AND REMARKS

Chlamydophila (Chlamydia) pneumoniae **Culture**—CONT

| | purpose transport medium specific for *Chlamydia,* virus, and mycoplasma. Antibiotics should be included in transport medium to reduce bacterial contamination. | |

1. Murray PR, Baron EJ, Jorgensen JH, et al, editors: *Manual of clinical microbiology,* ed 8, Washington, DC, 2003, ASM Press.
2. Mandell GL, Bennett JE, Dolin R, editors: *Principles and practice of infectious diseases,* ed 5, New York, 2000, Churchill Livingstone.

| *Chlamydophila (Chlamydia) pneumoniae* **Serological Test**[1,2]

MIF, CF | Acute and convalescent sera drawn 2-4 wk apart. | MIF is more sensitive than CF and has the added advantage of being able to discriminate between chlamydial species.

C. pneumoniae differs morphologically and genetically from both *C. trachomatis* and *C. psittaci.* It has been associated with pneumonia in young adults, older adults, and individuals with chronic diseases that require hospitalization. The prevalence of antibodies in the adult population is >50%, but antibodies are uncommon in young children. It may be difficult to demonstrate increasing MIF titers because seroconversion may take >4 wk. In primary infection, an IgM titer >1:32 supports the diagnosis. |

1. Murray PR, Baron EJ, Jorgensen JH, et al, editors: *Manual of clinical microbiology,* ed 8, Washington, DC, 2003, ASM Press.
2. Rose NR, Hamilton RG, Detrick B, editors: *Manual of clinical immunology,* ed 6, Washington, DC, 2002, ASM Press.

| *Chlamydophila (Chlamydia) psittaci* **Culture**[1,2] | Respiratory secretions: Lung tissue; transtracheal aspirates, bronchial washings/brushings, and sputum. See *Sputum Culture, Routine.* Blood.

Transport to laboratory immediately in special transport medium such as 2SP or multipurpose transport medium specific for *Chlamydia,* virus, and mycoplasma. Antibiotics | *Chlamydophila (Chlamydia) psittaci* pneumonia is associated with exposure to infected birds. It may be an occupational hazard of pet shop workers, pigeon handlers, or poultry workers. Organism recovery is optimal when specimens are collected during the first 2 wk of illness; however, isolation should only be attempted by laboratories experienced with this organism and with adequate containment facilities.

Because isolation of *C. psittaci* is particularly hazardous to laboratory workers operating under standard conditions, serologic diagnosis is preferred. |

TEST NAME* AND METHOD	SPECIMEN AND SPECIAL REQUIREMENTS	CLINICAL COMMENTS AND REMARKS

Chlamydophila (Chlamydia) psittaci Culture—CONT

| | should be included in transport
medium to reduce bacterial
contamination. | |

1. Murray PR, Baron EJ, Jorgensen JH, et al, editors: *Manual of clinical microbiology,* ed 8, Washington, DC, 2003, ASM Press.
2. Mandell GL, Bennett JE, Dolin R, editors: *Principles and practice of infectious diseases,* ed 5, New York, 2000, Churchill Livingstone.

| **Chlamydia
trachomatis
Serological Test**[1-4]

MIF | Acute and convalescent sera
drawn 2-4 wk apart; single
acute serum from infant with
pneumonia. | A fourfold increase in titer between acute and convalescent sera is necessary for diagnosis, although very high ($\geq$1:2000) titers occur in patients with LGV. High IgM titers ($\geq$1:256) occur in *C. trachomatis* pneumonia in infants.

MIF is more sensitive than the genus-specific CF test and is specific for *C. trachomatis;* however, a fourfold increase in antibodies is difficult to demonstrate because of the chronic and persistent nature of some infections. Antibodies also may persist from previous infection, and the background prevalence of antibodies will vary among geographic areas. |

1. Murray PR, Baron EJ, Jorgensen JH, et al, editors: *Manual of clinical microbiology,* ed 8, Washington, DC, 2003, ASM Press.
2. Warford A, Chernesky M, Peterson EM: In Gleaves CA, coordinating editor: *Cumitech 19A laboratory diagnosis of Chlamydia trachomatis infections,* Washington, DC, 1999, American Society for Microbiology.
3. Black CM: Current methods of laboratory diagnosis of *Chlamydia trachomatis* infections, *Clin Microbiol Rev* 10:160-184, 1997.
4. Rose NR, Hamilton RG, Detrick B, editors: *Manual of clinical immunology,* ed 6, Washington, DC, 2002, ASM Press.

| **Chromoblastomy-
cosis Examination
and Culture**[1-3] | Aspirates, biopsy material,
scrapings, and tissue. Tissue
should be placed between sterile gauze, and sterile nonbacteriostatic saline should be added
to retain moisture. Send to laboratory immediately. Swab
specimens are not effective for
specimen collection and should
be avoided. | Chromoblastomycosis, or chromomycosis, is a localized chronic mycosis of the skin and subcutaneous tissue leading to the development of warty nodules, tumor-like masses and raised, rough cauliflower-like lesions, primarily on the lower extremities. It is widespread in tropical and subtropical areas among barefooted agricultural workers, although occasionally it is found in temperate climates. The most common agents of chromoblastomycosis include *Exophiala jeanselmei, Fonsecaea pedrosoi, Fonsecaea compacta, Rhinocladiella aquaspersa, Phialophora verrucosa,* and *Cladosporium carrionii.* |

Chlamydia trachomatis Identification can be found in the Appendix on p. 1761.

TEST NAME AND METHOD	SPECIMEN AND SPECIAL REQUIREMENTS	CLINICAL COMMENTS AND REMARKS

Chromoblastomycosis Examination and Culture—CONT

| | | Diagnosis can be made by direct microscopic examination of the specimen and visualization of brown "sclerotic bodies." The presence of sclerotic bodies is diagnostic of chromoblastomycosis. Darkly pigmented hyphae may also be seen near the surface of the lesions. Definitive identification of the organism causing disease requires culture. If cultures are performed, the organisms may require up to 4 wk for growth. Culture is not, however, required for diagnosis. |

1. Murray PR, Baron EJ, Jorgensen JH, et al, editors: *Manual of clinical microbiology,* ed 8, Washington, DC, 2003, ASM Press.
2. Larone DH: *Medically important fungi: a guide to identification,* ed 4, Washington, DC, 2002, ASM Press.
3. Mandell GL, Bennett JE, Dolin R, editors: *Principles and practice of infectious diseases,* ed 5, New York, 2000, Churchill Livingstone.

| *Clostridium botulinum*[1,2] | 25-50 g stool, 15-20 mL serum and suspected food(s). If wound botulism is suspected, collect serum, feces, tissue, exudate, or swab of wound. If infant botulism is suspected, collect stool. | Botulism has been classified into four categories:

(1) Classic food-borne botulism caused by ingestion of toxin in contaminated food.

(2) Wound botulism caused by elaboration of toxin in vivo after growth of *C. botulinum* in an infected wound. Toxigenic strains of *C. botulinum* have been isolated from wounds in the absence of clinical evidence of wound botulism.

(3) Infant botulism in which the toxin is elaborated in vivo in the GI tract of an infant (22 days to 8 mo of age) colonized with *C. botulinum.* In these cases, mild illness to sudden death may occur. Honey has been found to be a source of *C. botulinum.*

(4) Unclassified botulism in individuals ~12 mo old in which no food or wound source is implicated.

In all cases of suspected botulism, the state laboratory or Centers for Disease Control and Prevention should be contacted for specific directions with regard to specimen handling. |

1. Isenberg HD: *Clinical microbiology procedures handbook,* ed 2, Washington, DC, 2004, ASM Press.
2. Murray PR, Baron EJ, Jorgensen JH, et al: *Manual of clinical microbiology,* ed 8, Washington, DC, 2003, ASM Press.

TEST NAME AND METHOD	SPECIMEN AND SPECIAL REQUIREMENTS	CLINICAL COMMENTS AND REMARKS
Clostridium difficile[1] *Toxin assay*	Stool, fresh	Transport immediately to laboratory in leak-proof container without preservative. Refrigerate if delay in transport is anticipated. If referred to another laboratory, send on dry ice because the toxins are unstable. *Clostridium difficile*-associated diarrhea (CDAD) occurs after antimicrobial therapy. The organism produces two toxins, toxin A (enterotoxin, causing extensive tissue damage) and toxin B (cytotoxin, causing cytopathic effect in cell culture). A more virulent strain of C. *difficile* has been identified that is associated with increased toxin production and may not respond to antimicrobial therapy. *C. difficile* can be isolated in culture but does not necessarily reflect a toxigenic strain. For that reason and the fact that there is a delay in turnaround time to results, cultures are generally reserved for research-orientated laboratories. The reference method for the laboratory diagnosis of CDAD has been a cytotoxin cell culture assay for toxin B. Because cell culture results are generally not available for 24-48 hr, several rapid methods have been developed. These tests are available to detect toxin A only, toxin A and B, and toxin A plus a nontoxin protein called glutamate dehydrogenase associated with the organism. Individuals with three unformed stools per day or abdominal pain and a history of antimicrobial therapy within the previous 30-day period should be tested to confirm the diagnosis of CDAD or pseudomembranous colitis caused by *C. difficile*. CDAD rather than a parasitic or enteric pathogen should be considered in patients with diarrhea ≥3 days of hospitalization.

1. Isenberg HD: *Clinical microbiology procedures handbook,* ed 2, Washington, DC, 2004, ASM Press.

TEST NAME AND METHOD	SPECIMEN AND SPECIAL REQUIREMENTS	CLINICAL COMMENTS AND REMARKS
Coccidioidomyco-sis Serological Test (Serological Test for *Coccidioides immitis*)[1-3] *CF, ID, tube precipitin (TP), LA*	Serum or CSF	Serologic tests for coccidioidomysosis should be considered in patients with symptoms of pulmonary or meningeal involvement who have lived or traveled in an endemic area. The TP test provides early evidence of acute coccidioidomysosis. TP antibodies appear early, within 1-3 wk after a primary infection, but disappear by 6 mo. The CF test is diagnostic and prognostic; antibody titers increase in proportion to disease severity and decrease in response to therapy. CF antibodies appear later than TP but remain throughout the course of the disease. Any CF titer should be considered presumptive evidence of infection. Titers ≤1:4 usually indicate early, residual, or meningeal disease. CF titers >1:16 should raise concern about disseminated infection. LA and ID tests yield results similar to the TP and CF test, respectively. The TP test is best for diagnosis of early, primary disease and for diagnosis in endemic areas. CF is best for diagnosis of disseminated disease or to follow treatment effectiveness. The combination of CF and TP has a sensitivity of >90% for primary symptomatic disease.

TEST NAME AND METHOD	SPECIMEN AND SPECIAL REQUIREMENTS	CLINICAL COMMENTS AND REMARKS

Coccidioidomycosis Serological Test—CONT

1. Murray PR, Baron EJ, Jorgensen JH, et al, editors: *Manual of clinical microbiology,* ed 8, Washington, DC, 2003, ASM Press.
2. Yeo SF, Wong B: Current status of nonculture methods for diagnosis of invasive fungal infections, *Clin Microbiol Rev* 15:465-484, 2002.
3. Rose NR, Hamilton RG, Detrick B, editors: *Manual of clinical immunology,* ed 6, Washington, DC, 2002, ASM Press.

Cold Agglutinins (CA) Serological Test[1-3]   Serum

Detection of cold agglutinins was one of the first serologic assays for detection of *Mycoplasma pneumoniae* infection. Only 30-50% of patients with *M. pneumoniae* infection will develop cold agglutinins. Therefore a negative test does not rule out infection. In addition a positive result may be associated with other infectious or collagen vascular diseases. Cold agglutinin testing is no longer recommended for the diagnosis of *M. pneumoniae* infections because of the availability of more sensitive and specific mycoplasma-specific antibody tests.

---

1. Murray PR, Baron EJ, Jorgensen JH, et al, editors: *Manual of clinical microbiology,* ed 8, Washington, DC, 2003, ASM Press.
2. Sharp SE, Robinson A, Saubolle M, et al, editors: In Sharp SE, coordinating editor: *Cumitech 7B, lower respiratory infections,* Washington, DC, 2004, ASM Press.
3. Waites KB, Bebear CM, Robertson JA, et al: In Nolte FS, coordinating editor: *Cumitech 34, laboratory diagnosis of mycoplasmal infections,* Washington, DC, 2001, American Society for Microbiology.

Cryptococcus neoformans **Serological Tests**[1-4]   Serum

Antibody Test

TA, IFA

Serologic tests for *C. neoformans* should be considered in patients with symptoms of pulmonary or meningeal infection. TA and IFA antibody tests are reactive in ~50% of patients with active cases of extrameningeal cryptococcosis. The IFA test has a specificity of 77% and the TA ~89%, both lower than the cryptococcal antigen test. Although the IFA has a lower specificity, it is useful for detection of cryptococcosis when the cryptococcal antigen test is negative. The TA test is useful in the early stages of CNS disease. TA titers of ≥1:2 are suggestive of infection. Titers may decrease as the antigen concentration increases. With effective chemotherapy, antibodies should reappear and may persist for long periods after therapy has ended. Negative serological assays do not rule out the diagnosis of cryptococcosis.

Antigen Test   Serum, CSF

LA, EIA

Serologic tests for *C. neoformans* should be considered in patients with symptoms of pulmonary or meningeal infection. Detection of cryptococcal polysaccharide capsular antigen is the only serologic procedure that is clinically useful on a routine basis and detects both active meningeal and nonmeningeal infection. Detection of cryptococcal antigen is more sensitive than the India ink preparation and more specific than detection of cryptococcal antibodies.

TEST NAME AND METHOD	SPECIMEN AND SPECIAL REQUIREMENTS	CLINICAL COMMENTS AND REMARKS

Cryptococcus neoformans Serological Tests—CONT

The LA test has both diagnostic and prognostic value. A positive reaction in an untreated patient is suggestive of cryptococcal disease. LA titers $\geq$1:8 are suggestive of active disease. The antigen titer is usually proportional to the extent of disease, increasing titers reflecting progressive infection and poorer prognosis. Declining titers generally indicate a favorable prognosis. False-positive reactions are uncommon but may occur in patients with disseminated *Trichosporon beigelii* and *Capnocytophaga canimorsus* infection and rheumatoid arthritis (test includes neutralization of rheumatoid factor). False-negative serum results are rare but may occur in cases of single, usually pulmonary, lesions in which sufficient antigen is not produced for detection.

The EIA test is capable of detecting lower antigen concentrations than the LA test. The reported sensitivity of the EIA is 93% and 100% in serum and CSF, respectively.

1. Murray PR, Baron EJ, Jorgensen JII, et al, editors: *Manual of clinical microbiology,* ed 8, Washington, DC, 2003, ASM Press.
2. Yeo SF, Wong B: Current status of nonculture methods for diagnosis of invasive fungal infections, *Clin Microbiol Rev* 15:465-484, 2002.
3. Rose NR, Hamilton RG, Detrick B, editors: *Manual of clinical immunology,* ed 6, Washington, DC, 2002, ASM Press.
4. Mandell GL, Bennett JE, Dolin R, editors: *Principles and practice of infectious diseases,* ed 5, New York, 2000, Churchill Livingstone.

TEST NAME AND METHOD	SPECIMEN AND SPECIAL REQUIREMENTS	CLINICAL COMMENTS AND REMARKS
Cryptosporidium spp. Stool Examination[1,2] *Acid-fast stain; fluorochrome or Ziehl-Neelsen stain*	Stool See *Ova and Parasite Examination.*	*Cryptosporidium* spp. infect the brush border of intestinal epithelial cells but in immunocompromised patients may also infect cells of other areas, including the respiratory tract, biliary tree, liver, pancreas, or the stomach lining. Immunocompetent individuals develop a profuse, watery diarrhea that is self-limited (10-15 days), whereas immunocompromised hosts develop a more severe, long-lasting diarrhea that can last months to years. Infection with these organisms is associated with travel, exposure to farm animals, attending a day care center, or living in a medical institution.

The organisms are very small (4-5 mm) and are best detected using the routine stool formalin-ethyl acetate concentration technique and acid-fast staining, or by simply centrifuging the specimen and using the newer immunoassay kits. Antigen detection assays are also commercially available. Permanent trichrome stains do not adequately stain *Cryptosporidium* spp. Several specimens may need to be examined to diagnose cryptosporidiosis.

1. Murray PR, Baron EJ, Jorgensen JH, et al, editors: *Manual of clinical microbiology,* ed 8, Washington, DC, 2003, ASM Press.
2. Garcia LS: *Diagnostic medical parasitology,* ed 4, Washington, DC, 2001, ASM Press.

TEST NAME AND METHOD	SPECIMEN AND SPECIAL REQUIREMENTS	CLINICAL COMMENTS AND REMARKS
CSF Culture, Cryptococcus Fungus[1-3]	CSF. As much CSF as possible (preferably >10 mL) should be delivered to the laboratory immediately. See *CSF Culture, Routine.*	This specimen is particularly useful for isolation of bacterial pathogens and *Cryptococcus neoformans.* The number of organisms per milliliter of CSF may be small. Thus a small volume of CSF may be inadequate. A concentration procedure should be performed if the volume of CSF is ≥2 mL. All CSF specimens for fungi should also be tested for the presence of cryptococcal antigen. See *General Comments.*

1. Murray PR, Baron EJ, Jorgensen JH, et al, editors: *Manual of clinical microbiology,* ed 8, Washington, DC, 2003, ASM Press.
2. Larone DH: *Medically important fungi: a guide to identification,* ed 4, Washington, DC, 2002, ASM Press.
3. Winn W Jr, Allen SD, Janda WM, et al, editors: *Koneman's color atlas and textbook of diagnostic microbiology,* ed 6, Philadelphia, 2006, Lippincott Williams & Wilkins.

TEST NAME AND METHOD	SPECIMEN AND SPECIAL REQUIREMENTS	CLINICAL COMMENTS AND REMARKS
CSF Culture, Routine[1-4]	Cerebrospinal fluid (CSF).	Collect in sterile, screw-capped tubes. Tube number 2 or 3 should be hand-delivered to the microbiology laboratory immediately. For optimal recovery, the following volume guidelines should be used: routine culture, ≥1 mL; fungal culture, ≥2 mL; and AFB, ≥2 mL. Do not refrigerate; if there is a delay in processing, incubate at 35-37° C. CSF culture is used to aid in the diagnosis of bacterial meningitis. In infants and neonates, the signs of meningitis may be vague. An unexplained febrile illness in an irritable infant who is doing poorly should lead one to suspect a diagnosis of meningitis. Specimens should be Gram stained preferably by cytocentrifugation and cultured immediately on receipt in the laboratory. Gram stain results should be phoned without delay to guide empiric therapy. The specimen may contain fastidious organisms such as *Haemophilus* spp. or *Neisseria* spp. *All organisms should be identified.* Routine anaerobic cultures of CSF should be ordered only in select cases because the yield of anaerobic isolates from CSF in patients with meningitis is extremely low (<1%).

1. Isenberg HD: *Clinical microbiology procedures handbook,* ed 2, Washington, DC, 2004, ASM Press.
2. Meredith FT, Phillips HK, Reller LB: Clinical utility of broth cultures of cerebrospinal fluid from patients at risk for shunt infections, *J Clin Microbiol* 35:3109-3111, 1997.
3. Miller JM: *A guide to specimen management in clinical microbiology,* ed 2, Washington, DC, 1998, ASM Press.
4. Murray PR, Baron EJ, Jorgensen JH, et al: *Manual of clinical microbiology,* ed 8, Washington, DC, 2003, ASM Press.

TEST NAME AND METHOD	SPECIMEN AND SPECIAL REQUIREMENTS	CLINICAL COMMENTS AND REMARKS
Cysticercosis Serological Test[1,2] *EIA, IB*	Serum, CSF. Collect serum in separation tube and freeze if not assayed immediately.	These tests are used to aid in the diagnosis of cysticercosis. The IB or EITB (enzyme-linked immunoelectrotransfer blot) is the diagnostic test of choice for cystericercosis. It is 100% specific and extremely sensitive. The test may be more sensitive with serum, and CSF may not need to be tested. In patients with multiple cysts, the test has a sensitivity of ≥90%. Sensitivity is lower for patients with calcified cysts or with a single cyst. This test is offered at the CDC and some commercial facilities. The EIA test is 75-100% sensitive in serum and CSF. Cross-reactions with sera from patients infected with other cestodes have been reported. Serological tests do not distinguish active from inactive infections; therefore they have no value in predicting outcome or in following the progress of therapy. See *General Comment*.

1. Ash LR, Orihel TC: *A guide to laboratory procedures and identification,* Chicago, 1987, American Society for Clinical Pathologists.
2. Garcia LS: *Diagnostic medical parasitology,* ed 4, Washington, DC, 2001, ASM Press.

TEST NAME AND METHOD	SPECIMEN AND SPECIAL REQUIREMENTS	CLINICAL COMMENTS AND REMARKS
Cytomegalovirus, Direct Test for Antigen[1,2] *EM, FA, Antigenemia test, PCR, bDNA, Hybrid Capture Assay*	Same as specimens for CMV culture. See *Cytomegalovirus Culture*.	The direct examination of specimen using EM has shown to be laborious and unproductive. Fluorescent conjugated monoclonal antibodies can be used in FA of lung tissue or bronchoalveolar lavage (BAL) fluid for diagnosis of CMV pneumonia. However, in most cases FA is less sensitive than culture or shell vial. CMV antigenemia test is based on the use of monoclonal antibodies to detect CMV antigens directly in leukocytes of the patient's blood. The antibody reacts with CMV structural protein pp65 and product of UL 83. Horseradish peroxidase-labeled antimouse antibodies are added, followed by a substrate solution. The cells are examined under light microscope for dark brown nuclear staining. The test is fairly rapid, quantitative, and can detect CMV infection 5 days before development of the disease. Both quantitative and qualitative PCR assays that are based on traditional PCR or real-time PCR assays are available in most reference laboratories. PCR is shown to detect CMV 17 days in advance of disease development. Quantitative PCR assay provides better interpretation and monitors disease prognosis. bDNA signal amplification test, which is based on hybridization of branched DNA probes to CMV gb gene, also provides a reliable way to monitor disease progression in a CMV-infected individual.

TEST NAME AND METHOD	SPECIMEN AND SPECIAL REQUIREMENTS	CLINICAL COMMENTS AND REMARKS

Cytomegalovirus, Direct Test for Antigen—CONT

| | | Hybrid capture assay is a solution hybridization that is based on hybridizing RNA probes to CMV, followed by detection of RNA:DNA complex with a labeled anti-DNA:RNA antibody.

See also *Cytomegalovirus*. |

1. Lennette EH, Smith TF, editors: *Laboratory diagnosis of viral infection,* ed 3, New York, 1999, Marcel Dekker.
2. Murray PR, Baron EJ, Jorgensen JH, et al, editors: *Manual of clinical microbiology,* ed 8, Washington, DC, 2003, American Society for Microbiology.

| **Cytomegalovirus (CMV) Culture**[1-3] | Urine, saliva, throat swab, BAL, blood (buffy coat), and tissue

Clinical samples for viral isolation should be processed as soon as possible. Specimen may be stored at 4° C for 1-4 days. If prolonged storage is required, freeze at −70° C in the presence of cryopreservative such as sorbitol. Urine and other fluids should be added to equivalent volume of antibiotic-containing solution. | Human CMV is rarely pathogenic in healthy adults but can be associated with severe disease in immunocompromised individuals. CMV is also the most common cause of congenital infection. The disease may be congenital or acquired during the first year of life. Viruria during the first 3 wk of life usually indicates congenital CMV infection; viruria after 4 wk is usually an indication of postpartum or intrapartum infection.

Urine or saliva may be used to diagnose congenital or perinatal infection with CMV. In adults, urine and buffy coat are used to detect CMV in blood as possible predictor of disseminated CMV disease. Detection of CMV in leukocytes is often a better indicator of symptomatic infection than is shedding of virus in urine or throat. Recovery of CMV in urine from adults may reflect asymptomatic viral replication or may indicate an active infection.

In healthy adults, the asymptomatic excretion rate is <1%. During late pregnancy, excretion of virus from urine or uterine or cervical specimens is 2-13%. CMV infection is very common in organ transplant patients. It is recommended that weekly blood and urine be monitored for CMV infection. |

1. Koneman EW, Allan SD, Janda WM, et al, editors: *Color atlas and textbook of diagnostic microbiology,* ed 5, Philadelphia, 1997, JB Lippincott.
2. Lennette EH, Smith TF, editors: *Laboratory diagnosis of viral infection,* ed 3, New York, 1999, Marcel Dekker.
3. Richman DD, Whitely RJ, Hayden FG, editors: *Clinical virology,* ed 2, Washington, DC, 2002, American Society for Microbiology.

TEST NAME AND METHOD	SPECIMEN AND SPECIAL REQUIREMENTS	CLINICAL COMMENTS AND REMARKS

Cytomegalovirus (CMV) Serological Test[1,2]

EIA, IFA, LA, CF, N, IHA

Serum, acute and convalescent. See *General Information.*

CMV is a ubiquitous virus causing primary, acute, and reactivation infections. Active infections include mononucleosis, hepatitis, and pneumonitis in the immunocompetent host and more life-threatening diseases in the immunocompromised individual. Active infections occurring during pregnancy can be transmitted to the fetus or infant, and the result can be asymptomatic infection, mild infection, or severe CNS damage. Isolation of the virus may indicate active infection or chronic viral shedding.

Serological testing can be helpful in conjunction with the culture results and the clinical symptoms. However, serology alone is not conclusive because CMV antibody prevalence in a population aged >30 yr may range between 40% and 100%.

EIA, IFA, or ACIF (anticomplement immunofluorescence) are the most widely used for detecting CMV antibody. ACIF is as sensitive and specific as EIA and IFA, but the methodology is more cumbersome. Passive latex agglutination (LA) is a fairly simple and rapid mean to screen for CMV antibodies.

Determination of IgM levels may be more appropriate for the diagnosis of primary infection and can be performed by EIA, IHA, or IFA. False-positive results may occur in the presence of rheumatoid factor, heterophil antibodies, and varicella. A negative test does not necessarily indicate absence of infection because the assays are not 100% sensitive. Newborn serum with large quantities of maternal IgG antibodies and only small amounts of infant IgM may yield a false-negative result (for IgM anti-CMV) because IgG can compete in the assay. Sera can be adsorbed with protein A to remove IgG, but unless there is sufficient IgM present, it too may be adsorbed. CF, IHA, and NT test are other tests that may be used to measure CMV antibody.

1.   Lennette EH, Smith TF, editors: *Laboratory diagnosis of viral infection,* ed 3, New York, 1999, Marcel Dekker.
2.   Rose NR, Hamilton RG, Detrick B, editors: *Manual of clinical laboratory immunology,* ed 6, Washington, DC, 2002, American Society for Microbiology.

Dengue Virus[1]

ELISA

Serum, acute and convalescent. See *General Information.*

Dengue virus is a mosquito-borne flavivirus and the most prevalent arbovirus in tropical and subtropical regions of the world. It causes dengue fever (DF) and its more serious forms, dengue hemorrhagic fever (DHF) and dengue shock syndrome (DSS). The World Health Organization estimates that there may be 50 million to 100 million cases of dengue virus infections worldwide every year, which result in 250,000-500,000 cases of DHF and 24,000 deaths. There are four distinct serotypes, serotypes 1-4. Infection induces a life-long protective immunity to the homologous serotype but confers only partial and transient protection against subsequent infections by the other three serotypes. In fact, it has generally been accepted that secondary infection with different serotype of dengue virus serotypes is a major risk factor for DHF-DSS because of antibody-dependent enhancement.

TEST NAME AND METHOD	SPECIMEN AND SPECIAL REQUIREMENTS	CLINICAL COMMENTS AND REMARKS

Dengue Virus—CONT

At present, the three basic methods used by most laboratories for the diagnosis of dengue virus infection are viral isolation, detection of the genomic sequence by a nucleic acid amplification assay, or detection of dengue virus-specific antibodies. Two patterns of serological response can be observed: primary and secondary antibody responses, depending on the immunological status of the infected individuals. A primary antibody response is seen in individuals who are not immune to flaviviruses. A secondary antibody response is seen in individuals who have had a previous flavivirus infection. For acute- and convalescent-phase sera, serological detection of antibodies based on capture IgM and IgG ELISA is the standard for the detection and differentiation of primary and secondary dengue virus infections.

1. Shu PY, Huang JH: Current advances in dengue diagnosis, *Clin Diag Lab Immunol* 11(4):642-647, 2004.

Echinococcosis Serological Test[1-3]

IHA, IFA, EIA, IB

Serum. Collect in separation tube and freeze if not assayed immediately.

The immune response often depends on the location and viability of the cysts. IB serology is 80-100% sensitive and 88-96% specific for liver disease but is less sensitive for lung and other organ involvement (25-56%). IHA and EIA assays have a sensitivity of ~60-90%. It is recommended that all positive EIA or IHA assays be confirmed by IB. Because serologic cross-reactions have been noted in low titers in patients with other cestode infections, the IB can by useful to help rule out false-positive results. Imaging remains more sensitive than serology, and a characteristic scan together with negative serology results should still suggest a diagnosis of echinococcus.

See *General Comment.*

1. Ash LR, Orihel TC: *A guide to laboratory procedures and identification,* Chicago, 1987, American Society for Clinical Pathologists.
2. Garcia LS: *Diagnostic medical parasitology,* ed 4, Washington, DC, 2001, ASM Press.
3. Mandell GL, Bennett JE, Dolin R: *Principles and practice of infectious diseases,* ed 5, New York, 2000, Churchill Livingstone.

Encephalitis Virus Serological Test[1,2]

MAC-ELISA, IF, CF, HI

Serum, acute and convalescent. See *General Information.*

Of >525 recognized arboviruses, only a handful are known to cause encephalitis in humans. All but one are mosquito borne. They include Eastern equine encephalitis (EEE), Western equine encephalitis (WEE), Venezuelan equine encephalitis (VEE), St. Louis encephalitis (SLE), Japanese encephalitis (JE), Murray Valley encephalitis (MVE), Rocio (ROC), California encephalitis (LAC), Rift Valley fever (RVF), tick-borne encephalitis (TBE), and West Nile virus encephalitis.

TEST NAME AND METHOD	SPECIMEN AND SPECIAL REQUIREMENTS	CLINICAL COMMENTS AND REMARKS

Encephalitis Virus Serological Test—CONT

Antibodies to one virus may be heterologous to those of other encephalitis viruses. Definitive diagnosis involves isolation or amplification of the viral nucleic acid causing the infection.

Antibody-capture ELISA for IgM (MAC-ELISA) is the test of choice for detecting antibody in cases of acute infection. Double-sandwich ELISA IgG or IF is recommended for serosurvey. HI and CF are used to supplement these tests, and the neutralization test is used for definitive and confirmatory determination of infecting agent.

1. Murray PR, Baron EJ, Jorgensen JH, et al, editors: *Manual of clinical microbiology,* ed 8, Washington, DC, 2003, American Society for Microbiology.
2. Rose NR, Hamilton RG, Detrick B, editors: *Manual of clinical laboratory immunology,* ed 6, Washington, DC, 2002, American Society for Microbiology.

Enterovirus Group Serological Test (Enterovirus Group Titers)[1,2]

CF, NT

Serum, acute and convalescent. See *General Information.*

The enterovirus group includes many serotypes of coxsackie, polio, echovirus, and enterovirus 69-71. They are found in the alimentary tract and produce varied clinical symptomatology.

Group-specific antigens are not available; thus serotype-specific assays are performed when considering the diagnosis. Hence, serological assays are not generally used but may be used in outbreak situations for epidemiological purposes.

A fourfold increase in titer by means of CF or NT usually indicates active infection. The presence of a single high IgM titer may also indicate active infection. NT titers persist for years; CF antibodies are short-lived (3-4 mo).

Isolation or amplification of the viral nucleic acid from blood, CSF, oropharynx, or feces is the usual mode for confirmation of the diagnosis.

1. Murray PR, Baron EJ, Jorgensen JH, et al, editors: *Manual of clinical microbiology,* ed 8, Washington, DC, 2003, American Society for Microbiology.
2. Rose NR, Hamilton RG, Detrick B, editors: *Manual of clinical laboratory immunology,* ed 6, Washington, DC, 2002, American Society for Microbiology.

TEST NAME AND METHOD	SPECIMEN AND SPECIAL REQUIREMENTS	CLINICAL COMMENTS AND REMARKS
Epstein-Barr Virus (Manual, Clin Micro, and Immuno, CDLI 7:451, 2000) Serological Test (EBV Titer)[1-3] *IFA, EIA, CF, IHA*	Serum, acute and convalescent. See *General Information.*	EBV is a ubiquitous virus that infects B lymphocytes and establishes latent infections. EBV syndromes include mononucleosis and tumors such as Burkitt's lymphoma, nasopharyngeal carcinoma, and B-cell lymphoma. EBV may develop into encephalitis in adult AIDS patients and into interstitial pneumonitis in children with AIDS. Ninety to 95% of infectious mononucleosis (IM) is associated with EBV; the remaining cases are associated with CMV, *Toxoplasma gondii* and HIV, adenovirus, or rubella. These latter are generally heterophile antibody negative.

Serological assays are utilized for the following purposes: to determine susceptibility to, immunity to, or primary infection with EBV; to aid in determining the significance of heterophile antibody-negative mononucleosis syndrome; to show the possible association of EBV with other syndromes; and to conduct epidemiological studies.

Heterophile IgM antibodies peak in 2-3 wk and are detectable for several months. Currently, there are several commercially manufactured ELISA, immune adherence hemagglutination, and latex agglutination assays with similar sensitivity and specificity available in the U.S. They are generally more sensitive than traditional Paul-Bunnell for the diagnosis of IM but offer no advantage over the conventional slide test. The slide test is 90% sensitive in adults and <50% in children <4 yr. In individuals who fail to develop heterophile antibodies but who have the clinical and hematological criteria for IM, EBV titers by means of IFA, EIA, or IHA may be of value.

The EBV antibodies that are detected by means of serological assays are:

Antibody to the EBV nuclear antigen (EBNA). EBNA antibody appears weeks to months after onset of illness and lasts for life except in the immunocompromised individual.

Viral capsid antigen (VCA) antibodies. IgM and IgG appear during the acute stage; IgM decreases within 1-3 mo; IgG may persist at low levels for life. High titers of IgG-VCA are noted in Burkitt's lymphoma and nasopharyngeal carcinoma and in immunosuppressed patients. In addition, individuals with nasopharyngeal carcinoma demonstrate high IgA-VCA titers. *Early antigen (EA) antibodies.* Most patients with IM have a transient antibody response to early antigen. IgG-EA lasts several months to several years after infection with EBV.

Positive titers for IgG-VCA, IgM-VCA, and IgG-EA are diagnostic for acute IM. If there has been a past EBV infection, IgM-VCA will be negative, but IgG-VCA and antibody to EBNA will be present. IgG-EA will be negative or in low numbers if there has been a past EBV infection.

1. Bruu A, Hjetland R, Holter E, et al: Evaluation of 12 commercial tests for detection of Epstein-Barr virus specific and heterophile antibodies, *J Clin Microbiol* 7:451-456, 2000.

TEST NAME AND METHOD	SPECIMEN AND SPECIAL REQUIREMENTS	CLINICAL COMMENTS AND REMARKS

Epstein-Barr Virus (Manual, Clin Micro, and Immuno, CDLI 7:451, 2000) Serological Test—CONT

2. Murray PR, Baron EJ, Jorgensen JH, et al, editors: *Manual of clinical microbiology,* ed 8, Washington, DC, 2003, American Society for Microbiology.

3. Rose NR, Hamilton RG, Detrick B, editors: *Manual of clinical laboratory immunology,* ed 6, Washington, DC, 2002, American Society for Microbiology.

Equine Encephalitis Serological Tests

Serum, acute and convalescent. See *General Information.*

EEE virus is a member of the group A arboviruses, the alphaviruses. The vector of transmission is the mosquito. Common animal hosts include birds, ducks, fowl, and horses. This virus has caused epidemics in the eastern U.S. from New Hampshire to Texas. The mortality rate is one of the highest of the viral encephalitides in the U.S. (65-75%). CAUTION: This organism has caused serious infection in laboratory workers involved in its isolation.

Eastern Equine Encephalitis Titer (EEE Titer)[1,2]

IFA, CF

SLE virus is a member of the group B arboviruses, the flaviviruses. The vector of transmission is the mosquito. The common animal host is the bird. Cases of SLE have occurred in the western, central, and southern U.S. Approximately 10-15% of patients with SLE do not develop CF antibodies.

St. Louis Equine Encephalitis Titer (EEE Titer)[1,2]

IFA

VEE virus is a member of the group A arboviruses, the alphaviruses. The vector of transmission is the mosquito. Common animal hosts are the horse and rodent.

Venezuelan Equine Encephalitis Titer (VEE Titer)[2]

VEE has occurred in South and Central America, but the virus has also been isolated in Florida and Texas.

ELISA

WEE virus is a member of the group A arboviruses, the alphaviruses. The vector of transmission is the mosquito. Common animal hosts include birds, snakes, horses, and squirrels. Cases of WEE have been diagnosed all over the U.S. west of the Mississippi. It is endemic in the Central Valley of California.

Western Equine Encephalitis Titer (WEE Titer)[2]

IFA

See *Encephalitis Virus Serological Test.*

---

1. Murray PR, Baron EJ, Jorgensen JH, et al, editors: *Manual of clinical microbiology,* ed 8, Washington, DC, 2003, American Society for Microbiology.

2. Rose NR, Hamilton RG, Detrick B, editors: *Manual of clinical laboratory immunology,* ed 6, Washington, DC, 2002, American Society for Microbiology.

TEST NAME AND METHOD	SPECIMEN AND SPECIAL REQUIREMENTS	CLINICAL COMMENTS AND REMARKS
Exoantigen Assay for Culture Confirmation of *Blastomyces dermatitidis, Histoplasma capsulatum, Coccidioides immitis*, and *Paracoccidioides brasiliensis*[1,2]	Isolates of molds, consistent with a systemic dimorphic fungus.	These assays are used when a white to tan mold is suspected of being one of the systemic dimorphic fungi, especially when direct examination of the specimen is consistent with suspicion. Historically, conversion of the mold form to the yeast phase was required to confirm organism identification. In vitro conversion can be exceedingly difficult and slow; therefore the use of exoantigen tests or DNA probes is preferred for identification confirmation.

The exoantigen technique detects the presence of cell-free antigens in an immunodiffusion test. Lines of precipitin identity indicate the correct identification as indicated below:

Organism	Exoantigens
B. dermatitidis	A
H. capsulatum	h, m
C. immitis	HS, F, HL
P. brasiliensis	1, 2, 3	

1. Murray PR, Baron EJ, Jorgensen JH, et al, editors: *Manual of clinical microbiology,* ed 8, Washington, DC, 2003, ASM Press.
2. Larone DH: *Medically important fungi: a guide to identification,* ed 4, Washington, DC, 2002, ASM Press.

Eye Culture for Fungus[1,2]	Corneal scrapings collected using a platinum spatula inoculated directly onto agar plates (blood or Sabouraud agar).	Septate filamentous fungi, especially *Fusarium solanae,* are the most common cause of fungal keratitis. The most common predisposing factor is corneal trauma in an otherwise healthy patient. *Candida* keratitis usually occurs in patients with preexistent disease.

1. Murray PR, Baron EJ, Jorgensen JH, et al, editors: *Manual of clinical microbiology,* ed 8, Washington, DC, 2003, ASM Press.
2. Larone DH: *Medically important fungi: a guide to identification,* ed 4, Washington, DC, 2002, ASM Press.

FA Direct Stains for Fungi[1,2]	Clinical specimens, biopsy material, and paraffin-fixed tissue sections	Available from the CDC and a few research laboratories. The test is used to stain tissue and clinical material directly for the presence of these fungi: *Blastomyces dermatitidis, Candida* spp., *Coccidioides immitis, Cryptococcus neoformans, Histoplasma capsulatum, Paracoccidioides brasiliensis, Pseudallescheria boydii,* and *Sporothrix schenckii.*

1. Murray PR, Baron EJ, Jorgensen JH, et al, editors: *Manual of clinical microbiology,* ed 8, Washington, DC, 2003, ASM Press.
2. Rose NR, Hamilton RG, Detrick B, editors: *Manual of clinical immunology,* ed 6, Washington, DC, 2002, ASM Press.

TEST NAME AND METHOD	SPECIMEN AND SPECIAL REQUIREMENTS	CLINICAL COMMENTS AND REMARKS
Farmer's Lung Disease, Serological Test/Hypersensitivity Pneumonitis Serological Test (Serological Test for Farmer's Lung Disease, Serological Test for Allergic Bronchopulmonary Aspergillosis)[1,2] *ID, EIA*	Serum	Hypersensitivity pneumonitis, or extrinsic allergic alveolitis, is an allergic lung disease that results from exposure and sensitization to antigens in organic dust. ID precipitins are usually present during the acute stage of the disease, especially when it is caused by inhalation of thermophilic actinomycetes such as *Saccharopolyspora rectivirgula, S. viridis, Thermoactinomyces vulgaris,* or *T. candidus* or spores of various *Aspergillus* spp., including *A. fumigatus.* EIA is more sensitive than ID especially in the serodiagnosis of aspergillosis but has more associated false-positive results. A negative test does not rule out the diagnosis. Clinical presentation, X-rays, and biopsy results should be considered along with the results of serological assays.

1. Murray PR, Baron EJ, Jorgensen JH, et al, editors: *Manual of clinical microbiology,* ed 8, Washington, DC, 2003, ASM Press.
2. Rose NR, Hamilton RG, Detrick B, editors: *Manual of clinical immunology,* ed 6, Washington, DC, 2002, ASM Press.

TEST NAME AND METHOD	SPECIMEN AND SPECIAL REQUIREMENTS	CLINICAL COMMENTS AND REMARKS
Fascioliasis/ Fasciolopsiasis Serological Test[1,2] *EIA, IB*	Serum. Collect in separation tube and freeze if not assayed immediately.	The test is used to support the diagnosis of *Fasciola hepatica* or *Fasciolopsis buski* infection, in conjunction with demonstration of eggs passed in the stool. The sensitivity of the FAST-EIA is reported to be 95%, whereas that of the IB is 100%. The test is best applied in the early stages of the disease or in chronic fascioliasis, when a paucity of eggs may be present. Antibodies usually appear 2-4 wk after infection. Levels decrease shortly after chemotherapy (within 6-12 mo), and their decline can be used to monitor chemotherapy. Titers of 1:128 by EIA are considered significant. Positive EIA assays can be followed up with more specific IB assays to rule out false-positive results, such as may occur in schistosomiasis. See *General Comment.*

1. Rose NR, deMarcario EC, Fahey JL, et al, editors: *Manual of clinical laboratory immunology,* ed 4, Washington, DC, 1992, American Society for Microbiology.
2. Garcia LS: *Diagnostic medical parasitology,* ed 4, Washington, DC, 2001, ASM Press.

TEST NAME AND METHOD	SPECIMEN AND SPECIAL REQUIREMENTS	CLINICAL COMMENTS AND REMARKS
Filariasis Serological Test[1-3] *EIA*	Serum. Collect in separation tube and freeze if not assayed immediately.	Filariasis is rarely seen in the U.S. except in visitors, immigrants, or U.S. citizens who visit endemic areas. It is caused by *Wuchereria* spp. or *Brugia* spp. Serologic tests may be of some use but do not determine between recent and past infections, nor do they discriminate between species of parasites. In addition, antibody tests have little value in endemic areas but may be helpful if a positive result is seen in someone who has traveled to an endemic area. A negative serological test may suggest no infection. See *General Comment.*

1. Rose NR, deMarcario EC, Fahey JL, et al, editors: *Manual of clinical laboratory immunology,* ed 4, Washington, DC, 1992, American Society for Microbiology.
2. Garcia LS: *Diagnostic medical parasitology,* ed 4, Washington, DC, 2001, ASM Press.
3. Mandell GL, Bennett JE, Dolin R: *Principles and practice of infectious diseases,* ed 5, New York, 2000, Churchill Livingstone.

TEST NAME AND METHOD	SPECIMEN AND SPECIAL REQUIREMENTS	CLINICAL COMMENTS AND REMARKS
Genital Culture[1-11]	Amniotic fluid, transvaginal aspirate of endometrium, Bartholin gland, Skene's gland, or lymph node aspirate, endocervical, vaginal, vulval, urethral swab from epididymis, testicles, prostate fluid, and culdocentesis Swab of urethral exudate (males), urethral scrapings with swab or loop, cervical swabs, vaginal/rectal swabs to rule out group B *Streptococcus,* scrapings of skin lesions; ≥1 mL fluid, e.g., amniotic, bartholin, prostate in anaerobic transport system. Transport to the laboratory immediately in transport system or sterile tube. Do not refrigerate.	Indigenous organisms are age related in females. For prepubescent females, diphtheroids and coagulase-negative *Staphylococcus* predominate; in female adults, lactobacilli predominate; and in postmenopausal women, fewer lactobacilli and a greater number of *Enterobacteriaceae* are generally detected. Male urethra contains relatively few skin flora. Specific organism requests rather than a routine genital culture are advised because genital pathogens, e.g., *Neisseria gonorrhoeae,* group B *Streptococcus agalactiae, Haemophilus ducreyi, Staphylococcus aureus,* group A *Streptococcus pyogenes,* yeast, and genital mycoplasma, generally have specific growth requirements. Vulvovaginitis and bacterial vaginosis (BV) can generally be diagnosed by Gram stain or wet mount for clue cells, i.e., epithelial cells coated with bacteria, or a DNA probe assay for the identification of yeast, *Trichomonas,* and *Gardnerella vaginalis* as a marker of BV.
***Neisseria gonorrhoeae* (GC) Culture**[5,6,8,12-14]	Cervical, urethral	There is excellent correlation between presumptive diagnosis of uncomplicated gonorrhea in the male, based on Gram-stained smear of urethral exudate, and confirmation by culture. In the female, the Gram-stained smear may not be as reliable, and culturing is required. Visualize the cervix with a speculum without lubricant. Remove mucus with a large swab and discard. Inoculate transport medium with noncotton swab collected from the endocervical canal, and deliver promptly to

TEST NAME AND METHOD	SPECIMEN AND SPECIAL REQUIREMENTS	CLINICAL COMMENTS AND REMARKS

Genital Culture—CONT

the laboratory. Urethral specimens are collected after removing exudate from the urethral orifice. In males, insert urethrogenital swab ~1 in. into the urethral lumen, rotate swab, leave in place for several seconds, and inoculate transport medium. Specimens should never be refrigerated and should be plated within 2 hr of collection for optimal recovery.

Gram stain of specimens from the urethra is 95% sensitive and 100% specific for the diagnosis of gonococcal urethritis in males when intracellular gram-negative diplococci are detected. In females, endocervical smears are 65% sensitive compared with culture; therefore specimens must also be cultured.

A selective transport medium, e.g., JEMBEC plate, has been shown to increase positivity by as much as 10% over other methods of transport. Three to 10% of the gonococci are susceptible to vancomycin in selective media used for isolation of *N. gonorrhoeae*. Whenever possible, both a nonselective and a selective medium such as modified Thayer-Martin medium incubated in CO_2 should be inoculated.

Although culture traditionally has been the gold standard for identifying gonococcal infection and is still required for presumed rape cases, several molecular-based tests are currently available with excellent sensitivity and specificity. The advantage of these tests is that one specimen can be collected for both *N. gonorrhoeae* and *Chlamydia trachomatis* detection. Verification of polymerase chain reaction for *N. gonorrhoeae* and *C. trachomatis* from transport fluid used to prepare ThinPrep pap smears is also available.

Group B Strep Culture[3,11,14]	Vaginal + rectal swabs	Specimens collected between 35-37 wk gestation to identify infants at risk for infection and guide antimicrobial prophylaxis are placed in Lim broth or other selective media for 18-24 hr amplification and subcultured onto sheep blood agar for identification. Molecular amplification assays are an excellent sensitive alternative to culture.
Haemophilus ducreyi[4]	Vaginal + rectal swabs	Thoroughly cleanse ulcer base with gauze pad saturated with normal saline. Two methods of collection are recommended.

(1) Irrigate and agitate the genital ulcer base with nonbacteriostatic saline and aspirate. Mix well and use as inoculum. (2) Use a cotton swab moistened with saline to obtain material, prepare Gram stain, inoculate chocolate agar enriched with 1% IsoVitaleX and vancomycin, 5 mg/L, and incubate at 33° C. Cultures may require up to 4 days for isolation of *H. ducreyi*.

The specimen should be transported to the laboratory immediately. Do not refrigerate. On Gram stain, organisms appear in a "school of fish" arrangement.

TEST NAME AND METHOD	SPECIMEN AND SPECIAL REQUIREMENTS	CLINICAL COMMENTS AND REMARKS

Genital Culture—CONT

Chancroid is uncommon in the U.S. but endemic in most of the world. Outbreaks have occurred in the U.S. in recent years, in particular in association with HIV infection.

1. Baron E, et al: In Rubin SJ, coordinating editor: *Cumitech 17A—Laboratory diagnosis of female genital tract infections,* Washington, DC, 1993, ASM Press.

2. Brown HL, Fuller DD, Davis TE, et al: Evaluation of the Affirm Ambient Temperature Transport System for the detection and identification of *Trichomonas vaginalis, Gardnerella vaginalis,* and *Candida* species from vaginal fluid specimens, *J Clin Microbiol* 39:3197-3199, 2001.

3. Centers for Disease Control and Prevention: Prevention of perinatal group B streptococcal disease: revised guidelines from CDC. Recommendations and reports, *Morb Mortal Wkly Rep* 51:1-24, 2002.

4. Dangor Y, Radebe F, Ballard RC: Transport media *for Haemophilus ducreyi, Sex Transm Dis* 20:5-9, 1993.

5. Evangelista A, Beilstein H: In Abramson C, coordinating editor: *Cumitech 4A—Laboratory diagnosis of gonorrhea,* Washington, DC, 1993, ASM Press.

6. Farhat SE, Thibault M, Devlin R: Efficacy of a swab transport system in maintaining viability of *Neisseria gonorrhoeae* and *Streptococcus pneumoniae, J Clin Microbiol* 39:2958-2960, 2001.

7. Forbes BA, Sahm DF, Weissfeld AS: *Bailey & Scott's diagnostic microbiology,* ed 10, St. Louis, 1998, Mosby.

8. Miller JM: *A guide to specimen management in clinical microbiology,* ed 2, Washington, DC, 1998, ASM Press.

9. Murray PR, Baron EJ, Jorgensen JH, et al: *Manual of clinical microbiology,* ed 8, Washington, DC, 2003, ASM Press.

10. Schachter J: DFA, EIA, PCR, LCR and other technologies: what tests should be used for diagnosis of chlamydia infections? *Immunol Investig* 26:157-161, 1997.

11. Schrag S, Gorwitz R, Fultz-Butts K, et al: Prevention of perinatal group B streptococcal disease: revised guidelines from CDC, *MMWR Recomm Rep* 51(RR11):1-22, 2002.

12. Arbique JC, Forward KR, LeBlanc J: Evaluation of four commercial transport media for the survival of *Neisseria gonorrheoae, Diagn Microbiol Infect Dis* 36:163-168, 2000.

13. Mandell GL, Bennett JE, Dolin R: *Principles and practice of infectious diseases,* ed 6, Philadelphia, 2005, Elsevier Churchill Livingstone.

14. Winn W Jr, Allen S, Janda W, et al: *Koneman's color atlas and textbook of diagnostic microbiology,* ed 6, Philadelphia, 2006, Lippincott Williams & Wilkins.

Genital Mycoplasma Culture *(Mycoplasma hominis, Ureaplasma urealyticum)*[1,2]

Males: Urethral swabs, prostatic secretions, semen, and urinary calculi.

Females: Urine, cervical or vaginal swabs, endometrial samples, tubal tissue, amniotic fluid, and placenta.

Neonates: Nasopharyngeal secretions, throat swab, and endotracheal secretions.

Transport to the laboratory immediately. Swabs should be

Ureaplasma urealyticum and *Mycoplasma hominis* can be isolated from the genital tract of healthy, sexually active adults. *U. urealyticum* is a cause of nonchlamydial, nongonococcal urethritis in males. The role of genital mycoplasmas in prostatitis remains controversial. *M. hominis* has been associated with salpingitis. Both *U. urealyticum* and *M. hominis* have been recovered from women with postpartum fever.

Neonates may be colonized during the birthing process or in utero. Pneumonia associated with these organisms has been reported in low birth weight infants.

Concurrent tetracycline therapy prevents organism isolation.

TEST NAME AND METHOD	SPECIMEN AND SPECIAL REQUIREMENTS	CLINICAL COMMENTS AND REMARKS

Genital *Mycoplasma* Culture—CONT

| | placed in special transport medium such as 2SP or multi-purpose transport medium specific for *Chlamydia,* virus, and *Mycoplasma.* Antibiotics should be included in the transport medium to reduce bacterial contamination. The swab should be pressed against the side of the tube to release the material into the medium and discarded before transport to the laboratory. If swabs are used, specimens should be obtained by vigorous rubbing to obtain as many cells as possible. Specimens should be refrigerated if not immediately transported to the laboratory. | |

1. Murray PR, Baron EJ, Jorgensen JH, et al, editors: *Manual of clinical microbiology,* ed 8, Washington, DC, 2003, ASM Press.
2. Waites KB, Bebear CM, Robertson JA, et al, editors: In Nolte FS, coordinating editor: *Cumitech 34, Laboratory diagnosis of mycoplasmal infections,* Washington, DC, 2001, American Society for Microbiology.

TEST NAME AND METHOD	SPECIMEN AND SPECIAL REQUIREMENTS	CLINICAL COMMENTS AND REMARKS
Gomori Methenamine Silver (GMS) Stain[1,2]	Appropriate specimen is the same as that for culture of the corresponding site.	Stain is considered by many to be the most useful for direct microscopic examination of clinical specimens to identify fungal elements. GMS stains the fungal cell wall and is commonly used for the histopathological examination of deparaffinized tissue for fungi. Certain bacteria, including *Nocardia* spp., as well as *Pneumocystis jiroveci (carinii)* can also be observed with this stain.

1. Murray PR, Baron EJ, Jorgensen JH, et al, editors: *Manual of clinical microbiology,* ed 8, Washington, DC, 2003, ASM Press.
2. Larone DH: *Medically important fungi: a guide to identification,* ed 4, Washington, DC, 2002, ASM Press.

TEST NAME AND METHOD	SPECIMEN AND SPECIAL REQUIREMENTS	CLINICAL COMMENTS AND REMARKS
Gram Stain[1-5,7]	Clinical specimens (excluding blood, stool, sputum from cystic fibrosis patients, catheter tips, and throat and nasal swabs), colonies on solid media, and growth in broth or blood. Cultures <24 hr from noninhibitory media and fresh specimens yield the best results. Broth for assessment of morphology and organism arrangement, e.g., streptococci. Broth cultures are preferred.	Select purulent or blood-tinged portion of specimens. If fluid or tissue cannot be obtained, collect two swabs, one for culture and one for Gram stain. Gently roll swab across the surface of a clean slide to maintain cell integrity and bacterial arrangement. For broth cultures and colonies on solid media, transfer 1-2 drops to a slide or emulsify a portion of a colony in 1 drop of sterile saline, respectively.

Slides should be prepared so that newspaper print is visible through the smear. For anaerobes, a modified Kopeloff's Gram stain may be used instead of the traditional modified Hucker Gram stain. Carbol fuchsin or basic fuchsin counterstain is used instead of safranin for detecting weakly staining gram-negative organisms such as *Campylobacter* spp., *Legionella* spp., and *Brucella* spp.

Gram stains are used for (1) presumptive identification of microorganisms, (2) cellular response, and (3) as a quality control measure to ensure recovery of all organisms present in a patient specimen. Poor quality smears resulting from use of unclean slides, too thick of a smear preparation, problems related to fixation, overdecolorization, excessive rinsing, or stain precipitate can lead to inaccurate interpretations. Decolorizers include 95% ethanol, acetone-alcohol, acetone alone, and methanol. The latter tends to maintain the integrity of cell morphology, produces a cleaner background, and prevents liquid specimens from washing off of the slides. Smears may be restained by removing immersion oil with xylene substitute and decolorizing.

Cytocentrifuged slide preparations should ideally be used to concentrate organisms in noncloudy or viscous body fluids and to prepare a monolayer of organisms. This procedure increases Gram stain sensitivity and reduces examination time compared with conventional centrifugation of specimens. Smears should be examined for representative areas of inflammatory white blood cells (WBCs) and squamous epithelial cells (SECs). Using an oil immersion lens, examine 20-40 representative fields to identify the shape and Gram reaction of each morphotype present along with their quantitation. When possible, presumptively identify the organism, e.g., gram-negative bacilli consistent with *Haemophilus*. |
| **Sputum Screen**[2,4-6] (See *Sputum Culture, Routine.*) | | Select portions of a specimen that are blood-tinged or purulent. For extremely viscous specimens, dilute with 1 drop of sterile saline before preparing slide. To ensure that the specimen quality is appropriate for culture, examine 20-40 representative areas under low power field (LPF), and apply one of the rejection criteria based on the number of SECs and WBCs. Likewise, endotracheal aspirates may be rejected using the criteria of ≥10 SECs/LPF or no organisms observed. |

TEST NAME AND METHOD	SPECIMEN AND SPECIAL REQUIREMENTS	CLINICAL COMMENTS AND REMARKS
Gram Stain—CONT		
Urine Screen		The presence of a single morphotype of bacteria in unspun urine is consistent with a colony count of ≥105 CFU/mL and is indicative of infection, particularly in the presence of WBCs. Any number of organisms/mL is considered significant in suprapubic-collected urine specimens.
Vaginal Discharge from Posterior Fornix		Use for women of child-bearing age and postmenopausal women on estrogen replacement therapy. Determine the relative number of lactobacilli compared with gram-negative curved rods and gram-variable coccobacilli using the Kopeloff's Gram stain modification and the presence of vaginal SECs coated with bacteria (clue cells) to aid in the diagnosis of bacterial vaginosis.
CSF (See *CSF Culture, Routine.*)		To avoid potential contamination during specimen collection from a lumbar puncture, the second or third tube of CSF should be submitted for Gram stain and culture. Specimens should be processed immediately on receipt and not refrigerated. The number of organisms/mL may be below the detectable level when examining smears prepared from conventionally centrifuged specimens. To increase the sensitivity of the Gram stain ≥100-fold, a cytocentrifuged specimen should be prepared. Results should be immediately called to the ordering physician.
Acridine Orange Stain[2,3,7]	Gram stain-negative blood cultures, broth, and direct smears.	Acridine orange (AO) is a fluorochromatic dye that stains nucleic acid and can be used to differentiate bacteria and fungi that stain bright orange from cellular material that stains yellow green using a fluorescent microscope.
		This stain is useful in discerning the presence of organisms in a Gram-stained specimen with WBCs but no organisms seen, when growth occurs on solid media, e.g., *Mycoplasma*, but does not Gram stain, and in blood cultures that are flagged positive by an automated system, but no organisms are seen. Gram stains can be performed over AO staining and vice versa, after removing the immersion oil.

1. Forbes BA, Sahm DF, Weissfeld AS: *Bailey & Scott's diagnostic microbiology,* ed 10, St. Louis, 1998, Mosby.

2. Isenberg HD: *Clinical microbiology procedures handbook,* ed 2, Washington, DC, 2004, ASM Press.

3. Lauer BA, Reller LB, Mirrett S: Comparison of acridine orange and Gram stains for detection of microorganisms in cerebrospinal fluid and other clinical specimens, *J Clin Microbiol* 14:201-205, 1981.

4. Murray PR, Baron EJ, Jorgensen JH, et al: *Manual of clinical microbiology,* ed 8, Washington, DC, 2003, ASM Press.

5. Shanholtzer CJ, Schaper PJ, Peterson LR: Concentrated Gram stain smears prepared with a cytospin centrifuge, *J Clin Microbiol* 16:1052-1056, 1982.

6. Murray PR, Washington JA: Microscopic and bacteriologic analysis of expectorated sputum, *Mayo Clin Proc* 50:339-344, 1975.

7. Winn W Jr, Allen S, Janda W, et al: *Koneman's color atlas and textbook of diagnostic microbiology,* ed 6, Philadelphia, 2006, Lippincott Williams & Wilkins.

TEST NAME AND METHOD	SPECIMEN AND SPECIAL REQUIREMENTS	CLINICAL COMMENTS AND REMARKS
Hair, Skin, and Nail Culture for Fungus (Dermatophyte Culture)[1-3]	Hair: Collect basal portion of infected hair with forceps. Infected hairs may be visualized by placing the patient under a UV light. Hairs that are fluorescent, distorted, or fractured should be cultured. Skin: Cleanse area with 70% alcohol. Scrape the active, peripheral edge of the lesion with a scalpel. Nail: Cleanse nail with 70% alcohol. Scrape deeply enough to obtain recently invaded nail tissue; discard initial scrapings. The entire nail is preferable. Nail clippings should not be submitted. All specimens should be submitted in a sterile container.	Dermatophytes are a group of fungi that infect keratinized tissue (hair, skin, and nails). They produce a variety of cutaneous infections commonly referred to as "ringworm." The three genera of fungi associated with dermatophyte infections in humans are *Epidermophyton, Trichophyton,* and *Microsporum.* Direct examination of specimens by means of a KOH preparation or other wet-mount preparation should accompany culturing. Recent studies have shown that swabs and toothbrushes may be useful for obtaining hair and skin samples, especially in pediatric patients. Cultures are held for 2-4 wk, but most cultures will become positive earlier. A negative culture does not rule out the possibility of fungal infection.

1. Murray PR, Baron EJ, Jorgensen JH, et al, editors: *Manual of clinical microbiology,* ed 8, Washington DC, 2003, ASM Press.
2. Larone DH: *Medically important fungi: a guide to identification,* ed 4, Washington, DC, 2002, ASM Press.
3. Koneman EW, Allen SD, Janda WM, et al, editors: *Color atlas and textbook of diagnostic microbiology,* ed 4, Philadelphia, 1992, JB Lippincott.

Helicobacter pylori **Antibodies**[1]	Serum for IgA, IgG, or CagA IgG antibodies	Gastric colonization by *Helicobacter pylori* is implicated in the development of gastritis, duodenal and gastric ulcer disease, and possibly gastric cancer. Tests for *H. pylori* IgG should be used to rule out disease in adults because IgG levels may be detected in a significant percentage of adults without clinical disease. Equivocal results may be resolved by performing a CagA IgG antibody test. There appears to be a correlation between the severity of peptic ulcer disease and antibody to the cytotoxin-associated gene A (CagA) protein. In some patients without detectable IgG levels, IgA levels may be helpful in identifying a *H. pylori* infection. *H. pylori* infections may be successfully treated with antimicrobial agents with subsequent decrease in IgG and IgA antibody levels. Testing for IgM is not helpful.

TEST NAME AND METHOD	SPECIMEN AND SPECIAL REQUIREMENTS	CLINICAL COMMENTS AND REMARKS

Helicobacter pylori **Antibodies**—CONT

Note that *H. pylori* antigen detected in stool by EIA is a highly sensitive, specific, and noninvasive test to identify active infection in symptomatic adult patients, not just exposure as determined by serological tests. The antigen test also can be used to monitor response during and after therapy. Eradication is confirmed by a negative antigen test.

1. Murray PR, Baron EJ, Jorgensen JH, et al: *Manual of clinical microbiology,* ed 8, Washington, DC, 2003, ASM Press.

Helicobacter pylori **Culture and Rapid Urease Test (RUT)**[1-4]

Invasive procedures

Gastric biopsy, duodenal biopsy

Transport specimens for culture within 3 hr in nonbacteriostatic saline on ice or in 1 mL of modified Cary-Blair transport medium. For a rapid urease test (RUT), place several biopsy pieces into a tube of urea test medium, incubate at 35° C, and examine at 30 min, 4 hr, and 24 hr. A color change in the medium constitutes a positive test.

Helicobacter pylori is the primary organism causing gastritis. It is associated with an increased risk for development of peptic ulcer disease, gastric adenocarcinoma, and gastric non-Hodgkin's B-cell lymphoma.

To diagnose *H. pylori* infection, both invasive tests using biopsy specimens, i.e., culture, rapid urease test, and histological examination, and noninvasive tests, i.e., serology, urea breath tests, and a stool EIA antigen test, can be used. Although isolation of the organism is possible if it is appropriately cultured, histological demonstration of the organism and/or a RUT is usually sufficient to make a diagnosis.

H. pylori **Antigen Test**[1-3]

Noninvasive procedure (See *Helicobacter pylori* Antibodies.)

Stool

For initial diagnosis and monitoring of patients on therapy, a stool EIA antigen test has proven reliable.

---

1. Isenberg HD: *Clinical microbiology procedures handbook,* ed 2, Washington, DC, 2004, ASM Press.
2. Mandell GL, Bennett JE, Dolin R: *Principles and practice of infectious diseases,* ed 6, Philadelphia, 2005, Elsevier Churchill Livingstone.
3. Murray PR, Baron EJ, Jorgensen JH, et al: *Manual of clinical microbiology,* ed 8, Washington, DC, 2003, ASM Press.
4. Winn W Jr, Allen S, Janda W, et al: *Koneman's color atlas and textbook of diagnostic microbiology,* ed 6, Philadelphia, 2006, Lippincott Williams & Wilkins.

TEST NAME AND METHOD	SPECIMEN AND SPECIAL REQUIREMENTS	CLINICAL COMMENTS AND REMARKS
Herpesviruses 1 and 2 Serological Tests (Herpes Simplex Titers, HSV-1 and -2 Titers, Herpes Simplex Serological Tests)[1,2] *EIA, IIF, ELISA, Immunoblot*	CSF, serum, acute and convalescent. See *General Information.*	HSV is a ubiquitous virus that can present in humans with variable clinical symptoms ranging from mild pharyngitis to severe disease and death. Major syndromes include gingivostomatitis, keratitis, conjunctivitis, vesicular skin eruptions, aseptic meningitis, encephalitis, genital ulcer disease, and neonatal herpes disease. Serological tests are not used to make the diagnosis of herpesvirus disease but may be confirmatory if clinical signs are present and cultures are positive. Serological tests may also be used epidemiologically. Antibodies for HSV-1 and -2 reach peak titers ~4-6 wk after infection and, although they decline with time, usually persist at low levels. Reinfection in a person with preexisting antibodies does not cause a dramatic change in the titer. Serological confirmation of recurrence or infection with a second virus type is not easily performed. There is cross-reactivity between HSV-1 and HSV-2; thus distinguishing between them serologically may be difficult. There may also be cross-reactivity between HSV and VZV antibodies, but the increase in antibody titer to the infecting virus frequently exceeds the increase in heterologous antibody. HerpeSelect ELISA and HerpeImmunoblot test from Focus Technologies (Cypress, CA) are two assays that are FDA approved for detection of HSV-1 or HSV-2. Antibodies may be present in the CSF of patients with CNS infection. Level of CSF antibodies >6% of level of serum antibodies suggests CNS infection. Some level of antibody may be present in the normal population, and thus paired samples should be tested to demonstrate an increase in titer.

1. Murray PR, Baron EJ, Jorgensen JH, et al, editors: *Manual of clinical microbiology,* ed 8, Washington, DC, 2003, American Society for Microbiology.
2. Rose NR, Hamilton RG, Detrick B, editors: *Manual of clinical laboratory immunology,* ed 6, Washington, DC, 2002, American Society for Microbiology.

TEST NAME AND METHOD	SPECIMEN AND SPECIAL REQUIREMENTS	CLINICAL COMMENTS AND REMARKS
Herpes Simplex, Direct Test for Antigen[1] *IFA, Immunoperoxidase (IP), EIA, DNA probe, PCR*	Genital specimens. See *Virus Culture.*	Direct microscopic examination for HSV antigen in specimens is possible by examining for the presence of multinucleated giant cells; however, all herpes viruses, e.g., CMV and VZV, will induce similar morphologies. FA is more specific and has a sensitivity of 10% for a crusted lesion and 87% for specimen from genital ulcers. Immunoperoxidase test allows demonstration of viral antigen within the infected cells and similar to FA requires skilled reading to recognize the staining patterns. Several commercially produced EIA kits with varying degree of sensitivity (35-100%) are available in the market. They are rapid and may be automated.

TEST NAME AND METHOD	SPECIMEN AND SPECIAL REQUIREMENTS	CLINICAL COMMENTS AND REMARKS

Herpes Simplex, Direct Test for Antigen—CONT

Solid-phase in situ hybridization and solution hybridization assay that detect viral DNA are also available commercially. These assays can provide timely identification and detection of HSV in clinical specimens.

Amplification by means of traditional or real-time PCR is a direct and most sensitive way to detect HSV. PCR is now considered the gold standard for detecting HSV in CSF from patients with HSV encephalitis and neonatal herpes. See also *Herpes Simplex Virus.*

1. Lennette EH, Smith TF, editors: *Laboratory diagnosis of viral infection,* ed 3, New York, 1999, Marcel Dekker.

Histoplasmosis Tests[1-3]

Antibody test

CF, ID, LA

Serum, acute and convalescent collected 2-3 wk apart; CSF.

The standard method for the diagnosis of histoplasmosis remains cultural isolation and identification of the organism. However, culture often requires 2-4 wk. Antibody detection offers a more rapid alternative. CF tests are valuable in the diagnosis of acute, chronic, disseminated, and meningeal histoplasmosis. The antibodies appear within 4 wk after exposure. Sensitivity of the CF may be >90%, depending on the antigen used.

CF titers of ≥1:8 are considered presumptive of infection; single titers ≥1:32 or increasing titers are usually indicative of active infection. The higher the titer, the greater the probability of the disease; however, recent skin testing may cause positive titers in up to 20% of persons tested. The CF test is usually positive with CSF from patients with chronic meningitis.

Cross-reactions may be seen in patients with leishmaniasis, blastomycosis, coccidioidomycosis, and other fungal infections, but these titers are usually lower than those caused by histoplasmosis. Failure to demonstrate CF antibodies does not rule out the diagnosis.

ID is useful as a screening procedure or as an adjunct to CF. ID demonstrates 1 or 2 bands. A positive "H" band indicates active infection but is rarely found alone. The presence of an "M" band indicates acute or chronic infection or previous skin testing. The presence of both M and H bands is highly suggestive of active histoplasmosis.

The LA test is useful for early presumptive detection of acute histoplasmosis. Titers ≥1:16 are usually considered strong evidence for active or recent infection. Skin testing before the test may elevate the titer significantly. Positive LA tests should be confirmed with a CF or ID test. False-positive results have occurred, particularly with low LA titers.

Antibodies may be undetectable in patients with HIV infection.

TEST NAME AND METHOD	SPECIMEN AND SPECIAL REQUIREMENTS	CLINICAL COMMENTS AND REMARKS
Histoplasmosis Tests—CONT		
Antigen test *EIA*	Urine, serum	Detection of *Histoplasma* antigenemia or antigenuria is recommended for the detection of disseminated histoplasmosis and may be useful in the early acute stage of pulmonary histoplasmosis before the appearance of CF and ID antibodies. The test can also be used to monitor therapy or to follow relapses in immunocompromised patients. Sensitivity is ~90% in disseminated histoplasmosis. Urine is a superior specimen to serum. Decreases in antigen concentration indicate response to therapy, whereas increases indicate relapse or treatment failure. False-positive results occurred with blastomycosis and coccidioidal meningitis with the previously used RIA. The EIA has increased specificity.

1. Murray PR, Baron EJ, Jorgensen JH, et al, editors: *Manual of clinical microbiology,* ed 8, Washington, DC, 2003, ASM Press.
2. Yeo SF, Wong B: Current status of nonculture methods for diagnosis of invasive fungal infections, *Clin Microbiol Rev* 15:465-484, 2002.
3. Rose NR, Hamilton RG, Detrick B, editors: *Manual of clinical immunology,* ed 6, Washington, DC, 2002, ASM Press.

TEST NAME AND METHOD	SPECIMEN AND SPECIAL REQUIREMENTS	CLINICAL COMMENTS AND REMARKS
HIV Resistance Testing[1] *LiPA, Sequencing, PhenoSense, Antivirogram* *Phenotypic resistance assays*	Whole blood (citrate or EDTA). Spin to separate plasma and refrigerate at 4° C for up to 4 days. For prolonged storage, freeze at –70° C and transport on dry ice.	HIV resistance testing is an important tool in optimizing the efficacy of the combination therapy to treat HIV infection. The identification of resistance mutations allows the care providers to select antiviral agents with maximum therapeutic benefit and minimum toxic side effects. Phenotypic resistance testing is available from at least two commercial laboratories: ViroLogic, Inc. (San Francisco, CA) and Virco (Mechelen, Belgium). These tests rely on PCR amplification of viral protease and RT gene sequences in lieu of viral isolation. The ViroLogic test (PhenoSense) relies on cloning and expression of the amplified viral RNA in an HIV-1 vector that lacks these regions and contains luciferase reporter gene in place of the viral envelope gene. The replication of the recombinant virus in the presence of antiviral agent is monitored by the amount of expressed luciferase. The Virco-developed phenotypic test (Antivirogram) also relies on amplified viral protease and RT genes. However, a mixture of PCR products and protease and RT-deleted HIV-1 proviral clone is transfected into CD^{4+} cell reporter cell lines. The cells produce recombinant virus containing the patient's viral PR-RT sequence. Susceptibility of resulting chimeric virus is tested in the reporter cell using real-time monitoring of HIV replication by high-resolution optics.

TEST NAME AND METHOD	SPECIMEN AND SPECIAL REQUIREMENTS	CLINICAL COMMENTS AND REMARKS

HIV Resistance Testing—CONT

Genotypic resistance assays

The genotypic resistance assay detects specific mutations in the viral genome that are associated with resistance to various antiretroviral agents. There are several manufacturer- and in-house–developed genotypic assays available in the U.S. The initial step in all of these assays is PCR amplification of viral protease and a 250-400 codon segment of HIV RT gene. This is followed by either direct sequencing or by hybridization-based detection of the amplified products (LiPA assay) to assess the presence of mutations associated with antiviral resistance.

1. Aslanzadeh J: HIV resistance testing: an update, *Ann Clin Lab Sci* 32:406-413, 2002.

Human Granulocytotropic Ehrlichiosis Serological Test (Human Granulocytotropic Ehrlichiosis Titer)[1-3]

IFA

Serum drawn at onset of disease and 3-4 wk later.

Ehrlichiosis is a tick-borne disease caused by rickettsia-like organisms. Human granulocytotropic ehrlichiosis is caused by *Anaplasma phagocytophilum*. HGE produces a clinical syndrome similar to HME. An IFA titer of $\geq$1:80 is considered significant; however, only 20-25% of patients will display a significant titer during the first week of illness. A fourfold increase in titer is considered diagnostic. Characteristic intranuclear inclusions within neutrophils, called morulae, are seen in 20-80% of patients with confirmed infection.

There are minimal cross-reactions between *Ehrlichia chaffeensis* and *A. phagocytophilum* antibodies.

1. Murray PR, Baron EJ, Jorgensen JH, et al, editors: *Manual of clinical microbiology,* ed 8, Washington, DC, 2003, ASM Press.
2. Rose NR, Hamilton RG, Detrick B, editors: *Manual of clinical immunology,* ed 6, Washington, DC, 2002, ASM Press.
3. Mandell GL, Bennett JE, Dolin R, editors: *Principles and practice of infectious diseases,* ed 5, New York, 2000, Churchill Livingstone.

Human Herpes 6, 7, and 8[1]

NT, IFA, ELISA, Immunoblot

Serum

Human herpes 6, 7, and 8 are the newest members of the human herpes virus family. Infection with these viruses is generally mild or subclinical in immunocompetent individuals, but clinically important and often severe disease does occur in immunocompromised persons. A variety of serologic assays has been developed to detect antibody to HHV-6, HHV-7, and HHV-8. They include NT, immunoblot, IFA, and ELISA. The overall performances of these assays for detecting antibody to these viruses are fairly similar, with a small sensitivity advantage for the ELISA and a specificity advantage for the immunoblot.

1. Shu PY, Huang JH: Current advances in dengue diagnosis, *Clin Diag Lab Immunol* 11:642-647, 2004.

TEST NAME AND METHOD	SPECIMEN AND SPECIAL REQUIREMENTS	CLINICAL COMMENTS AND REMARKS
Human Immunodeficiency Virus (HIV) Amplification Methods[1,2] *Viral load, HIV proviral* *DNA*	Whole blood (citrate or EDTA). Refrigerate at 4° C for up to 4 days.	Monitoring HIV-1 RNA level (viral load) in sera of infected patients is used to assess HIV disease progression and patient response to antiviral therapy. Currently, there are three FDA-approved commercially developed assays to monitor HIV viral load. Two assays are based on target amplification (Roche Amplicor HIV Monitor v1.5 RT-PCR Assay and bioMerieux NucliSens HIV-1 RNA QT NASBA Assay), and one is based on signal amplification (Bayer Quantiplex HIV RNA v3.0 bDNA Assay). Comparative studies have shown fairly good correlation among the three assays. Amplicor and bDNA are generally more sensitive than NucleSens. Plasma is the specimen of choice. The bDNA is a signal amplification test that relies on a sandwich nucleic acid hybridization procedure. Initially the HIV genomic RNA is released from the virions and captured on a microwell by a set of specific synthetic oligonucleotide target probes. A second set of target probes hybridizes the viral RNA to the preamplifier probes. The preamplifier probes hybridize to the branched DNA (bDNA) amplifiers. Multiple copies of an alkaline phosphatase-labeled probe are then hybridized to the immobilized complex to amplify the signal. Detection is achieved by incubating the complex with a chemiluminescent substrate and measuring the light emission generated by the bound alkaline phosphatase. Light emission is directly proportional to the amount of HIV RNA present in each sample. The apparent dynamic range of this assay is ~75-500,000 viral particles/mL. NASBA is based on coamplification of HIV-1 sample RNA together with internal calibrators. The quantity of amplified RNA is measured by means of electrochemiluminescence (ECL). Three synthetic RNAs of known concentrations (high, medium, and low) are added to the lysis buffer containing the HIV RNA. The extracted nucleic acid that includes the calibrators is then subjected to amplification. The HIV RNA and the calibrators serve as targets for the primer that hybridize to the gag region of HIV and contain the T7-RNA polymerase recognition site. Avian myeloblastosis virus reverse transcriptase (AMV-RT) extends the primer and generates a DNA/RNA complex. After the extension, enzyme RNase H degrades the RNA template and a second primer hybridizes to the cDNA. Synthesis of the second DNA strand is attained through extension of this primer by AMV-RT. Finally, the enzyme T7-RNA polymerase binds to the T7 promoter site and synthesizes multiple copies of the target RNAs. With the RNA synthesis, the system enters the isothermal cyclic phase, resulting in the accumulation of wild-type and calibrator RNA amplification products. To detect the amplification products, aliquots of the amplified sample are added to four hybridization solutions with specific probe for one of the amplification products. The respective amplification products are hybridized with a bead-oligonucleotide and a ruthenium-

TEST NAME AND METHOD	SPECIMEN AND SPECIAL REQUIREMENTS	CLINICAL COMMENTS AND REMARKS

Human Immunodeficiency Virus (HIV) Amplification Methods—CONT

labeled probe. The magnetic beads carrying the hybridized amplification product/probe complex are captured on the surface of an electrode by means of a magnet. Voltage applied to this electrode triggers the ECL reaction. The light emitted by the hybridized ruthenium-labeled probes is proportional to the amount of amplification product. The next generation of this assay will rely on the use of molecular beacons probe technology for real-time detection of the amplification products.

The Amplicor HIV Monitor v1.5 RT-PCR Assay is an automated amplification and detection assay performed on Roche COBAS Amplicor. In this assay the plasma RNA is extracted with a lysis reagent containing guanidine thiocyanate and quantitation standard (QS) RNA. The QS that is introduced into each sample permits quantitation of HIV RNA by comparison of resulting optical densities after amplification and detection. A 142-base pair sequence in the gag gene of HIV and QS (primers SK145 and SKCC1B) is amplified and detected in a single reaction tube by reverse transcription (RT) and polymerase chain reaction (PCR). The reported dynamic range of this assay is 400-750,000 viral particles/mL. HIV monitor Ultrasensitive is a modified version of this assay that requires initial ultracentrification of the sample for 1 hr before RNA extraction and has a dynamic range of 50-50,000 viral particles/mL. The next generation of PCR-based techniques for monitoring HIV viral load will rely on real-time PCR that utilizes Taqman technologies.

HIV infection usually is documented by detection of HIV-specific antibodies in serum. Serologic assays do not readily identify HIV infection in neonates because of the passively acquired maternal antibodies or in individuals with "indeterminate" antibody profiles. The proviral DNA detect kit allows the detection of rare DNA sequences (1-5 copies) of HIV-1 proviral DNA in infected cells. This PCR-based kit can detect proviral DNA by amplification of a specific sequence in the highly conserved gag region of the HIV genome. The DNA PCR may also help to document HIV infection when routine diagnostic assays are not adequate. In recent years several new assays based on real-time PCR have been reported with similar sensitivities.

See also *Human Immunodeficiency Virus I.*

1. Lennette EH, Smith TF, editors: *Laboratory diagnosis of viral infection,* ed 3, New York, 1999, Marcel Dekker.
2. Murray PR, Baron EJ, Jorgensen JH, et al, editors: *Manual of clinical microbiology,* ed 8, Washington, DC, 2003, American Society for Microbiology.

TEST NAME AND METHOD	SPECIMEN AND SPECIAL REQUIREMENTS	CLINICAL COMMENTS AND REMARKS
Human Immunodeficiency Virus (HIV) Culture[1-2] *VCA, RT*	Peripheral blood mononuclear cells (PBMCs), plasma, CSF, tissue, and other body fluids. Collect blood in citrated tubes; process within 24 hr. Tissues: Transport in viral transport media (see *Virus Culture*); process immediately or freeze at −80° C for further processing. Body fluids: Collect and transport as for virus culture and refrigerate, if needed, before processing.	HIV culture isolation relies on cocultivation of PBMC of HIV-infected patient with PBMC from uninfected blood donors that has been stimulated to replicate with mitogen [usually phytohemagglutinin (PHA) and interleukin-2 (IL-2)]. Culture supernatants are assessed for HIV p24 antigen or reverse transcriptase activities at 3- to 4-day intervals for up to 4 wk. Positive culture is usually seen within 1-2 wk. The sensitivity of HIV culture (65-100%) depends on HIV viral load, CD4 count, and presence of inhibitors and susceptibility of donor PBMCs. The rate of virus isolation is higher among untreated patients with advanced disease. Because HIV culture is very laborious, expensive, and requires long incubation time, HIV culture is rarely used for diagnostic purposes. HIV culture, however, is a valuable tool to assess phenotypic resistance to antiretroviral drugs. See also *Human Immunodeficiency Virus Serological Test.*

1. Murray PR, Baron EJ, Jorgensen JH, et al, editors: *Manual of clinical microbiology,* ed 8, Washington, DC, 2003, American Society for Microbiology.
2. Richman DD, Whitely RJ, Hayden FG, editors: *Clinical virology,* ed 2, Washington, DC, 2002, American Society for Microbiology.

Human Immunodeficiency Virus-1 (HIV-1) Serological Test[1,2] *EIA*	Serum, plasma. See *General Information.*	A number of assays are commercially developed to detect antibody to the HIV-1. EIA is the most common assay for detection of the antibody in adults and children aged >15 mo. The assays can be used to screen blood or blood products, to make the clinical diagnosis of HIV infection, and for epidemiologic purposes. The tests measure antibody presence but cannot be used to predict whether an infected individual has AIDS or will go on to develop AIDS. AIDS is a clinical syndrome and can only be diagnosed clinically.
Western blot	Serum, plasma. Store at 2-8° C for up to 2 wk, −20° C if longer.	The Western blot (WB) is used to confirm EIA reactivity of sera to HIV-1 virus. A positive WB is defined as the presence of two of the following bands: p24, gp41, and either gp120 or gp160. Ten to 20% of patients who are reactive by EIA are indeterminate by WB; in a high-risk population, serial tests by WB may be needed to reach a diagnostic conclusion. Twenty to 30% of patients negative by EIA (as well as PCR) may react in the WB and are probably not HIV positive. The positive predictive value of a WB alone, especially in a low seroprevalence population, is only 29%. The predictive value of the combination of EIA plus WB is ~99.5%. There are some EIA- and WB-negative sera that are found to be positive for HIV by PCR, by antigen-detection assays, or by culture, but these are rare. Infants aged <15 mo may carry maternal antibodies and be falsely positive on EIA and WB.

TEST NAME AND METHOD	SPECIMEN AND SPECIAL REQUIREMENTS	CLINICAL COMMENTS AND REMARKS

Human Immunodeficiency Virus-1 (HIV-1) Serological Test—CONT

IFA	Serum, plasma. See *General Information.*	IFA is performed in some laboratories for screening and/or as a substitute for WB. IFA generally turns positive earlier in the course of infection than ELISA. IFA has also been used to discriminate between HIV-1 and HIV-2. A positive result requires >1+ fluorescence at a 1:20 dilution of the specimen compared with an equivalently treated negative control sample. However, the assay is subjective and requires highly skilled and experienced personnel to interpret the results; it is most useful for resolving indeterminate reactions with WB technique.

1. Lennette EH, Smith TF, editors: *Laboratory diagnosis of viral infection,* ed 3, New York, 1999, Marcel Dekker.
2. Murray PR, Baron EJ, Jorgensen JH, et al, editors: *Manual of clinical microbiology,* ed 8, Washington, DC, 2003, American Society for Microbiology.

Human Immunodeficiency Virus-2 Serological Assay[1-3] *EIA, WB, IFA*	Serum; plasma. See *General Information.*	HIV-2 is a retrovirus, closely related to the simian AIDS virus (SIV). The areas of the highest prevalence are the West African nations and Portugal. There have been a small number of reported cases in the U.S. since 1987. Similar modes of transmission are probable; in the U.S., most cases have had heterosexual contact with a West African-infected individual. HIV-2 cross-reacts with HIV-1 in serological tests; the sensitivity of EIA for HIV-2 is ~60-90%. A negative EIA test for HIV-1 does not exclude HIV-2. A positive EIA for HIV-1 with a negative or indeterminate WB suggests possible HIV-2 infection. Specific EIA and WB tests for HIV-2 are available. Similarly, an IFA test is available for screening and confirming HIV-2 infections. It has been shown to be as sensitive as EIA for screening and superior to WB for discriminating between HIV-1 and HIV-2 infections.

1. Lennette EH, Smith TF, editors: *Laboratory diagnosis of viral infection,* ed 3, New York, 1999, Marcel Dekker.
2. Murray PR, Baron EJ, Jorgensen JH, et al, editors: *Manual of clinical microbiology,* ed 8, Washington, DC, 2003, American Society for Microbiology.
3. Rose NR, Hamilton RG, Detrick B, editors: *Manual of clinical laboratory immunology,* ed 6, Washington, DC, 2002, American Society for Microbiology.

TEST NAME AND METHOD	SPECIMEN AND SPECIAL REQUIREMENTS	CLINICAL COMMENTS AND REMARKS
Human Monocytotropic Ehrlichiosis Serological Test (Human Monocytotropic Ehrlichiosis Titer, *Ehrlichia chaffeensis* Titer)[1-3]	Serum drawn at onset of disease and 3-4 wk later.	Human monocytotropic ehrlichiosis (HME) is caused by *E. chaffeensis,* a rickettsia-like organism. HME is often referred to as "spotless" Rocky Mountain spotted fever. An IFA titer of ≥1:80 is considered significant; however, only 20-25% of patients will display a significant titer during the first week of illness. A fourfold increase in titer is considered diagnostic. Characteristic intranuclear inclusions within monocytes, called morulae, are seen in <10% of patients with confirmed infection.
IFA		There are minimal cross-reactions between *Ehrlichia chaffeensis* and *Anaplasma phagocytophilum* antibodies.

1. Murray PR, Baron EJ, Jorgensen JH, et al, editors: *Manual of clinical microbiology,* ed 8, Washington, DC, 2003, ASM Press.
2. Rose NR, Hamilton RG, Detrick B, editors: *Manual of clinical immunology,* ed 6, Washington, DC, 2002, ASM Press.
3. Mandell GL, Bennett JE, Dolin R, editors: *Principles and practice of infectious diseases,* ed 5, New York, 2000, Churchill Livingstone.

TEST NAME AND METHOD	SPECIMEN AND SPECIAL REQUIREMENTS	CLINICAL COMMENTS AND REMARKS
Human Parvovirus B19[1,2]	Serum. See *General Information.*	Human parvovirus B19 is the etiologic agent of erythema infectiosum (also known as fifth disease) and transient aplastic crisis characterized by the abrupt onset of a severe anemia associated with a decrease in reticulocytes in the peripheral blood.
EIA, RIA, IFA		Serological tests have been the cornerstone of B19 diagnostics. The presence of IgM indicates recent infection. However, low-level IgM may persist from months to even years. The presence of IgG alone indicates past infection and probable immunity.
		RIA was used in the past to detect both IgG and IgM. However, in recent years, EIA has replaced RIA. These assays generally detect antibody to structural proteins VP1 and VP2. Indirect immunofluorescence that relies on insect cells infected with recombinant VP1 antigen is also available in some reference laboratories.

1. Coon D: Parvovirus B19: characteristics, disease, and diagnosis, *Clin Microbiol News* 25:161-167, 2003.
2. Rose NR, Hamilton RG. Detrick B, editors: *Manual of clinical laboratory immunology,* ed 6, Washington, DC, 2002, American Society for Microbiology.

TEST NAME AND METHOD	SPECIMEN AND SPECIAL REQUIREMENTS	CLINICAL COMMENTS AND REMARKS
Human T-Cell Lymphotrophic Virus-I/II (HTLV-I/II) Serological Assay[1] *EIA, WB, Line immunoassay, IFA*	Serum, plasma. See *General Information.*	HTLV-I and HTLV-II are Oncovirinae subfamily. HTLV-I has been associated with adult T-cell leukemia (ATL) and myelopathy/tropical spastic paraparesis (HAM/TSP). HTLV-II has been associated with a neurological disease resembling HAM/TSP. The transmission of these viruses appears to be similar to that of HIV-1 (in utero, via breast-feeding, parentally, through intercourse). Two FDA-approved HTLVI/II EIAs with reported sensitivity of 99.76-100% and specificity of 99.63-99.98% are used for blood donor screening and clinical diagnosis of these infections. WB, line immunoassay, and IFA are supplemental serologic tests that can differentiate between antibody to HTLV-I and HTLV-II.

1. Lennette EH, Smith TF, editors: *Laboratory diagnosis of viral infection,* ed 3, New York, 1999, Marcel Dekker.

TEST NAME AND METHOD	SPECIMEN AND SPECIAL REQUIREMENTS	CLINICAL COMMENTS AND REMARKS
India Ink Preparation (Cryptococcus)[1-3]	CSF, pleural fluid, blood, sputum, and pus.	India ink is a negative stain that allows the visualization of capsular material, especially the capsule of *Cryptococcus neoformans.* The appearance of encapsulated yeast, especially in CSF, is suggestive of *C. neoformans,* but identification must be confirmed by culture. Only 50-70% of culture-proven cases may be positive by this preparation. The cryptococcal antigen latex test is significantly more sensitive than the India ink preparation and is recommended for the initial diagnosis of cryptococcal disease. (See *Cryptococcal neoformans Serological Tests.*)

1. Murray PR, Baron EJ, Jorgensen JH, et al, editors: *Manual of clinical microbiology,* ed 8, Washington, DC, 2003, ASM Press.
2. Larone DH: *Medically important fungi: a guide to identification,* ed 4, Washington, DC, 2002, ASM Press.
3. Koneman E, Roberts GD: *Practical laboratory mycology,* ed 3, Baltimore, 1985, Williams and Wilkins.

TEST NAME AND METHOD	SPECIMEN AND SPECIAL REQUIREMENTS	CLINICAL COMMENTS AND REMARKS
Infectious Mononucleosis (IM) Serological Tests[1-3] *Slide test, Latex agglutination, ELISA*	Serum, plasma. See *General Information.*	In patients with primary EBV infection, demonstration of Paul-Bunnell heterophile antibody is diagnostic. The original Paul-Bunnell test has been largely replaced by rapid tests. They utilize either rapid qualitative agglutination or ELISA tests. They detect 80-85% of IM patients. A negative test should imply the absence of significant IM-specific heterophile antibodies. Heterophile antibodies appear in 60% of patients with IM within the first and second weeks and in 80-90% by the first month. In most cases, titers decline in 3-6 mo. The false-positive rate for the Paul-Bunnell antibodies is ~3%, mostly from individuals with a low but persistent level of antibody after their primary illness. In addition, false-positive tests may be associated with hepatitis A or B, leukemia, lymphoma, and pancreatic carcinoma.

TEST NAME AND METHOD	SPECIMEN AND SPECIAL REQUIREMENTS	CLINICAL COMMENTS AND REMARKS

Infectious Mononucleosis (IM) Serological Tests—CONT

The false-negative rate is 10-15% and is more frequently seen in children than adults. It is estimated that 10% of the patients with EBV-related IM never develop PB antibodies. This number increases to 50% in children aged <4 yr.

1. Bruu A, Hjetland R, Holter E, et al: Evaluation of 12 commercial tests for detection of Epstein-Barr virus specific and heterophile antibodies, *J Clin Microbiol* 7:451-456, 2000.
2. Murray PR, Baron EJ, Jorgensen JH, et al, editors: *Manual of clinical microbiology,* ed 8, Washington, DC, 2003, American Society for Microbiology.
3. Rose NR, Hamilton RG, Detrick B, editors: *Manual of clinical laboratory immunology,* ed 6, Washington, DC, 2002, American Society for Microbiology.

TEST NAME AND METHOD	SPECIMEN AND SPECIAL REQUIREMENTS	CLINICAL COMMENTS AND REMARKS
Influenza A and B Serological Tests (Influenza A and B Titer)[1,2] *HI, CF, NT, EIA*	Serum, acute and convalescent. Acute phase: up to 7 days after infection. Convalescent: 14-60 days later.	Most individuals experience their first influenza infection before school age and may have more than one infection during each decade of life. The presence of antibodies may not indicate recent infection. HI titers are most sensitive for influenza A, and CF titers are most sensitive for influenza B. NT and EIA tests are the most widely used assays in serodiagnosis and epidemiologic studies of influenza. A fourfold increase in titer between the acute and convalescent sera collected at least 10 days apart is considered diagnostic. Although serologic methods are accurate, they rarely provide guidance for patient management and/or timely prophylaxis of contacts. Serology, however, remains an important tool for surveillance and epidemiologic studies.

1. Murray PR, Baron EJ, Jorgensen JH, et al, editors: *Manual of clinical microbiology,* ed 8, Washington, DC, 2003, American Society for Microbiology.
2. Rose NR, Hamilton RG, Detrick B, editors: *Manual of clinical laboratory immunology,* ed 6, Washington, DC, 2002, American Society for Microbiology.

TEST NAME AND METHOD	SPECIMEN AND SPECIAL REQUIREMENTS	CLINICAL COMMENTS AND REMARKS
KOH Preparation for Fungi[1-3]	Specimens are the same as for cultures of the corresponding site, e.g., sputum, urine, and tissue.	Wet mounts prepared in KOH are used to distinguish fungi in thick, mucoid specimens or in specimens containing keratin such as hair, skin, and nails. KOH preparations may be negative even with positive cultures. It can be used alone or in conjunction with calcofluor white to facilitate visualization of fungal elements.

TEST NAME AND METHOD	SPECIMEN AND SPECIAL REQUIREMENTS	CLINICAL COMMENTS AND REMARKS

KOH Preparation for Fungi—CONT

1. Murray PR, Baron EJ, Jorgensen JH, et al, editors: *Manual of clinical microbiology,* ed 8, Washington, DC, 2003, ASM Press.
2. Larone DH: *Medically important fungi: a guide to identification,* ed 4, Washington, DC, 2002, ASM Press.
3. Koneman E, Roberts GD: *Practical laboratory mycology,* ed 3, Baltimore, 1985, Williams and Wilkins.

Leishmaniasis Serological Test[1-4]

EIA, CF, IFA, DA

Serum. Collect in separation tube and freeze if not assayed immediately.

Serological testing for visceral leishmaniasis (kala-azar) normally shows high titers and may aid in the clinical diagnosis for immunocompetent people. Patients with mucosal disease will frequently have demonstrable antibodies, whereas only some patients with cutaneous leishmaniasis will only have low titers of antibodies present.

Antibody tests are usually sensitive (>90%), but lack sensitivity because false-positive results can occur with Chagas' *(Trypanosoma cruzi)* and other trypanosomal diseases, malaria, leprosy, schistosomiasis, and toxoplasmosis.

Antigen tests with good sensitivity and excellent specificity have been described in the literature, but they are not readily available.

See *General Comment.*

1. Ash LR, Orihel TC: *A guide to laboratory procedures and identification,* Chicago, 1987, American Society for Clinical Pathologists.
2. Rose NR, deMarcario EC, Fahey JL, et al editors: *Manual of clinical laboratory immunology,* ed 4 Washington, DC, 1992 American Society for Microbiology.
3. Garcia LS: *Diagnostic medical parasitology,* ed 4, Washington, DC, 2001, ASM Press.
4. Mandell GL, Bennett JE, Dolin R: *Principles and practice of infectious diseases,* ed 5, New York, 2000, Churchill Livingstone.

***Leptospira* sp. Identification**[1-4]

Clinical manifestations of leptospirosis range from mild illness to icteric disease with kidney and liver involvement.

Blood Culture[1-3]

1-3 drops of fresh or SPS anticoagulated blood in each of 3-4 tubes of Fletcher's semisolid medium (5 mL) or Ellinghausen, McCullough, Johnson, Harris medium (10 mL). Heparin, sodium oxalate, or citrate is adequate as an anticoagulant if needed.

Blood cultures are the most reliable means for recovering the organism during the first week of illness, but are rarely successful thereafter. Infection should be suspected in patients with a history of contact with leptospires in the previous 3 wk. Common animal hosts include rats, mice, skunks, opossums, foxes, dogs, cattle, and raccoons. The usual mode of infection is via the skin from contact with an infected animal or its waste products or by means of contaminated food or water. Sporadic cases are seen in sewer workers, farmers, fish cleaners, animal handlers, and construction workers.

TEST NAME AND METHOD	SPECIMEN AND SPECIAL REQUIREMENTS	CLINICAL COMMENTS AND REMARKS
Leptospira **sp. Identification**—CONT		
		Culture usually requires several weeks for isolation, but may be held for up to 13 wk before being considered negative for *Leptospira*. Before drawing the specimen, call the laboratory to ensure that the medium is available. Serum should always be collected for antibody studies.
Urine Culture[1-2]	Urine. See *Urine Culture, Routine, Midvoid*.	Leptospires usually occur in the urine after the first week of illness when they are no longer present in the blood. Shedding in the urine may persist for 2-3 mo.
		Leptospira are susceptible to acid urine and should be processed immediately after collection by neutralization of pH. The number of leptospires in the urine is usually low, and therefore repeat urine cultures should be attempted. Serum should always be collected for antibody studies.
Darkfield Examination[1,3]	Blood, CSF, or urine transported to the laboratory immediately	Blood and CSF should be submitted during the first week of illness; after this time, urine is preferable.
		Direct darkfield examination is relatively insensitive and should not be the only diagnostic procedure performed for leptospires. Diagnosis by microscopic exam should be confirmed by culture or serological methods.
		Leptospires are difficult to demonstrate by darkfield examination. A negative darkfield result does not rule out the presence of organisms since at least 10,000 leptospires/mL are required for visualization. In darkfield examinations of blood, caution should be taken not to confuse filamentous structures derived from erythrocytes ("pseudospirochetes") with *Leptospira* spp.
Serological Test[1-4] *MAT, IHA, IgM dipstick*	Serum drawn at onset of disease and at least 1 wk (preferably 2-3 wk) later	Test is used to support the diagnosis of leptospirosis; it is especially helpful when cultures or darkfield examinations are negative. Antibodies can be detected (MAT, IHA) in the first week of illness and reach a maximum within 4 wk of illness. MAT titers up to 1:25,000 have been found.
		A history of contact during the previous 3 wk with an environment in which leptospires have been present may be important. MAT and IHA titers of ≥1:100 are indicative of acute or recent infection; however, a fourfold increase in titer between acute and convalescent sera is diagnostic. The IgM dipstick assay is designed as a screening test; acute and convalescent samples should be tested. Weakly reactive results should be confirmed by MAT.

TEST NAME AND METHOD	SPECIMEN AND SPECIAL REQUIREMENTS	CLINICAL COMMENTS AND REMARKS

Leptospira sp. Identification—CONT

Acute titers may be delayed or decreased in patients receiving early and intensive antibiotic treatment.

1. Murray PR, Baron EJ, Jorgensen JH, et al, editors: *Manual of clinical microbiology,* ed 8, Washington, DC, 2003, ASM Press.
2. Winn W Jr, Allen S, Janda W, et al: *Koneman's color atlas and textbook of diagnostic microbiology,* ed 6, Philadelphia, 2006, Lippincott Williams & Wilkins.
3. Dunne WM Jr, Nolte FS, Wilson ML: *Blood cultures III.* Hindler JA, coordinating editor, Washington DC, 1997, American Society for Microbiology.
4. Rose NR, Hamilton RG, Detrick, B, editors: *Manual of clinical immunology,* ed 6, Washington, DC, 2002, ASM Press.

Lymphocytic Choriomcningitis (LCM) Virus Serological Test[1,2]

IFA, NT, CF

Serum, acute and convalescent; CSF. See *General Information.*

LCM is a member of Arenaviridae, which includes Lassa fever virus. Humans are infected by contact with infected mice or hamsters. The frequency of infection is greatest among young adults; highest incidence occurs in winter and spring. Outbreaks have been reported in families with new pet hamsters and among persons exposed to infected hamsters in animal care units.

The laboratory diagnosis of LCM can be accomplished by viral culture (blood, CSF) or serology. The accepted serological test today is the IFA to determine IgM. Antibodies last <3 mo. Detection of IgM in the CSF is definitive for LCM.

The appearance of antibodies by IFA usually coincides with the disappearance of viremia. IFA positivity appears first; single titers may be presumptive evidence of the disease. Titers may remain high for years. With IFA there is cross-reactivity among other arenaviruses. NT titers are more specific; they appear after 6-8 wk, rise slowly, and remain for years. CF titers peak at 3-5 wk and are gone early after the disease subsides.

1. Lennette EH, Smith TF, editors: *Laboratory diagnosis of viral infection,* ed 3, New York, 1999, Marcel Dekker.
2. Rose NR, Hamilton RG, Detrick B, editors: *Manual of clinical laboratory immunology,* ed 6 Washington, DC, 2002, American Society for Microbiology.

TEST NAME AND METHOD	SPECIMEN AND SPECIAL REQUIREMENTS	CLINICAL COMMENTS AND REMARKS
Malaria Serological Test[1-3] *IIF*	Serum. Collect in separation tube and freeze if not assayed immediately.	Detection of antibody against malaria parasites is not recommended for the diagnosis of malaria. In a patient highly suspected of having malaria, but who has repeatedly negative blood films for the parasites, serological testing may be processed; however, the presence of antibody cannot distinguish between past or present infections. See *General Comment.*

1. Ash LR, Orihel TC: *A guide to laboratory procedures and identification,* Chicago, 1987, American Society for Clinical Pathologists.
2. Rose NR, deMarcario EC, Fahey JL, et al, editors: *Manual of clinical laboratory immunology,* ed 4, Washington, DC, 1992, American Society for Microbiology.
3. Garcia LS: *Diagnostic medical parasitology,* ed 4, Washington, DC, 2001, ASM Press.

TEST NAME AND METHOD	SPECIMEN AND SPECIAL REQUIREMENTS	CLINICAL COMMENTS AND REMARKS
Malaria Smear (Blood Smear for Malaria, Peripheral Blood Smear for Parasites)[1-3]		The diagnosis of malaria is an urgent matter and all requests should be handled as a "stat." Fingerstick prepared slides or whole blood preserved in EDTA are appropriate specimens to collect. Heparin may also be used as an anticoagulant, but EDTA is preferred. Slides or blood should be transported to lab immediately, and smears made and stained within an hour of collection. Pertinent patient travel history should accompany the test request. Thick and thin blood smears should always be prepared for evaluation. Thick films are considered the "gold standard" for detection of parasites because low numbers may be present in the specimen. Thin films are used to determine the morphology and species of the infecting parasite. One negative result does not necessarily rule out the diagnosis of malaria.

1. Ash LR, Orihel TC: *A guide to laboratory procedures and identification,* Chicago, 1987, American Society for Clinical Pathologists.
2. Garcia LS: *Diagnostic medical parasitology,* ed 4, Washington, DC, 2001, ASM Press.
3. Murray PR, Baron EJ, Jorgensen JH, Pfaller MA, Yolken, RH, editors: *Manual of clinical microbiology,* ed 8, Washington, DC, 2003, ASM Press.

TEST NAME AND METHOD	SPECIMEN AND SPECIAL REQUIREMENTS	CLINICAL COMMENTS AND REMARKS
Measles Virus[1,2] *EIA, PRN assay, HI*	Serum, acute and convalescent. See *General Information.*	Measles remains a formidable disease of children in many parts of the world. WHO estimates 30 million cases with 875,000 deaths occurring each year. Virus is transmitted via aerosol or droplet exposure generated from sneeze or a cough or via contaminated fomites.

TEST NAME AND METHOD	SPECIMEN AND SPECIAL REQUIREMENTS	CLINICAL COMMENTS AND REMARKS

Measles Virus—CONT

The recommended laboratory method for the confirmation of clinically diagnosed measles is a serum-based IgM EIA. The assay is fairly rapid and can be used to diagnose acute measles from the time of rash onset to 4 wk after rash onset. Similarly, EIA is also the recommended test for detecting IgG antibody to measles virus. In fact EIA has replaced the traditional PRN and HI tests that are labor intensive, require paired sera, and may take 5-7 days to complete.

1. Lennette EH, Smith TF, editors: *Laboratory diagnosis of viral infection*, ed 3, New York, 1999, Marcel Dekker.
2. Rose NR, Hamilton RG, Detrick B, editors: *Manual of clinical laboratory immunology*, ed 6, Washington, DC, 2002, American Society for Microbiology.

Methylene Blue Stain for Fecal Leukocytes[1]

Fresh Stool

Process within 2 hr.

This stain is used primarily to detect polymorphonuclear leukocytes in stool specimens collected from community-acquired gastroenteritis (i.e., the test is not useful for diagnosis in patients hospitalized >3days). Presence of leukocytes suggests an invasive infection with organisms, such as *Salmonella, Shigella, Campylobacter, Yersinia,* or *C. difficile.* In contrast, polymorphonuclear leukocytes are generally absent in toxigenic *E. coli, Vibrio cholerae, Staphylococcus,* and viruses. This test has a sensitivity of 50%-60% in gastroenteritis and considerably lower in *C. difficile* colitis.

If a delay in transport is anticipated, a LEUKO-TEST latex agglutination test may be performed to detect lactoferrin, a breakdown product of fecal leukocytes. To prevent false-positive results, this test should not be performed on specimens collected from infants who are being breast-fed.

1. Isenberg HD: *Clinical microbiology procedures handbook*, ed 2, Washington, DC, 2004, ASM Press.

Microfilaria Peripheral Blood Preparation (Blood Smear for Parasites, Peripheral Blood Preparation for Filariasis and Trypanosomiasis)[1,2]

Fingerstick prepared slides or collection of whole blood in EDTA is required for diagnosis. Specimens should be transported to lab as soon as possible. Pertinent travel history of the patient should accompany the specimen if possible. *Wuchereria bancrofti* and *Brugia malayi* have nocturnal periodicity; therefore the optimum time for blood collection is be-

Because *Onchocerca volvulus* lie within the dermis and subcutaneous tissues of their hosts, they are identified from skin snips, not from peripheral blood samples.

As with malaria, one negative result does not rule out the possibility of a parasitic infection.

TEST NAME AND METHOD	SPECIMEN AND SPECIAL REQUIREMENTS	CLINICAL COMMENTS AND REMARKS
Microfilaria Peripheral Blood Preparation—CONT	tween 2200 and 0200 hr. *Loa loa* has diurnal periodicity; an optimum time for blood collection is noon. *Mansonella perstans* and *M. ozzardi* have no evident periodicity.	
***Microsporidian* spp. Direct Examination**[2,3] *EM, GMS*	Biopsy of intestine; tissue (e.g., cornea, body fluids, and stool samples.)	Microsporidiosis is a disease of patients with AIDS or other immunocompromised patients. The best test results are from examination of intestinal biopsy or other infected tissue by means of Gomori's methenamine silver (GMS) stain or electron microscopy. In addition the modified trichrome stain for most specimens or the use of chemofluorescent agents, such as calcofluor, Fungi-Fluor or Uvitex 2B, for nonstool specimens are diagnostic options.

1. Murray PR, Baron EJ, Jorgensen JH, et al, editors: *Manual of clinical microbiology,* ed 8, Washington, DC, 2003, ASM Press.
2. Garcia LS: *Diagnostic medical parasitology,* cd 4, Washington, DC, 2001, ASM Press.

Miscellaneous Sites Culture, Routine[1-2] (See *Anaerobe Culture.*)	Surgical and biopsy tissue, bone, ocular, etc.	Transport to lab in sterile container within 30 min if possible. The isolation of an organism from these sites may indicate the etiological agent of infection. Since contamination with normal flora from skin, rectum, vaginal tract, or other body surfaces may occur, care should be exercised in the proper collection of these specimens. All organisms should be identified. Cultures for acid-fast bacilli and fungi should be considered, especially when invasive procedures for specimen collection are involved. Ocular specimens may need to be inoculated onto blood and chocolate agar at the bedside. For suspected bacterial keratitis, 3-5 corneal scrapings are each inoculated on the media, using a C formation for each scraping. Calcium alginate swabs and Dacron swabs with non-wood shafts should be used to collect specimens for chlamydial and viral cultures, respectively. (See *Eye Culture.*)

1. Isenberg HD: *Clinical microbiology procedures handbook,* ed 2, Washington, DC, 2004, ASM Press.
2. Wilhelmus K, Liesagang T, Osato M, et al: *Cumitech 13A, laboratory diagnosis of ocular infections,* Specter SC, coordinating editor, Washington, DC, 1994, American Society for Microbiology.

TEST NAME AND METHOD	SPECIMEN AND SPECIAL REQUIREMENTS	CLINICAL COMMENTS AND REMARKS
Mumps Virus Serological Test (Mumps Virus Titer)[1-3]	Serum, acute and convalescent; CSF. See *General Information.*	Mumps is an acute systemic infection characterized by bilateral or unilateral parotitis accompanied by high fever and fatigue. Despite availability of mumps vaccine, outbreaks continue to occur in vaccinated and unvaccinated populations.
EIA, HAI, NT, CF, IF		A fourfold rise in titer between acute and convalescent titer is usually indicative of infection. CF, HAI, NT, IF, and EIA assays are used to measure antibody titers. NT although sensitive is labor intensive and costly and so is rarely used. EIA is the preferred method in most laboratories and has supplanted most other serological tests because of the ease and commercial availability of EIA kits and automation. Both IF and EIA may be used to measure IgM.

1. Lennette EH, Smith TF, editors: *Laboratory diagnosis of viral infection,* ed 3, New York, 1999, Marcel Dekker.
2. Murray PR, Baron EJ, Jorgensen JH, et al, editors: *Manual of clinical microbiology,* ed 8, Washington, DC, 2003, American Society for Microbiology.
3. Rose NR, Hamilton RG, Detrick B, editors: *Manual of clinical laboratory immunology,* ed 6, Washington, DC, 2002, American Society for Microbiology.

Mycobacteria[1-5] *Culture*	Decontaminated, concentrated specimens.	Note that smears should optimally be prepared from concentrated specimens and read within 24 hr of receipt (see AFB smears). Both liquid and solid selective and nonselective egg-based (supports growth of most mycobacteria) or agar-based (more rapid detection caused by easier visibility of colonies) are recommended.
Blood, bone marrow, CSF	Blood with specific request for AFB. Collect 10 mL (or 1.5 mL for pediatrics) of blood into an Isolator lysis centrifugation tube (Wampole) or broth designed for AFB isolation using an automated or manual monitoring system. CSF ≥ 3.0 mL, tube #2 or #3 Other body fluids (e.g., pleural, synovial, and pericardial)	Mycobacteremia is most commonly caused by *M. avium-intracellulare* (MAC), particularly in HIV-infected individuals. Positive CSF cultures are uncommon because of a low number of bacteria present and a low volume of CSF submitted. Generally active tuberculosis infection often exists elsewhere in patients with tuberculous meningitis. Deliver as much fluid as possible; swabs are not adequate.
Extrapulmonary	Tissue, wounds	Other species of mycobacteria may be responsible for extrapulmonary disease (e.g., *M. fortuitum* and *M. chelonae* have been associated with endocarditis, *M. scrofulaceum* with cervical adenitis, *M. ulcerans* with chronic granulomatous ulcerations of the skin and underlying tissue [Buruli ulcer], and *M. marinum* with skin lesions). Based on specimen source and clinical presentation, cultures should be processed for *Mycobacteria* other than tuberculosis (MOTT) acid-fast bacilli (e.g., *M. marinum* or *M. haemophilum*).

TEST NAME AND METHOD	SPECIMEN AND SPECIAL REQUIREMENTS	CLINICAL COMMENTS AND REMARKS
Mycobacteria—CONT		
		Smears may be most helpful in cases of disease caused by M. *leprae,* since in vitro culturing is not possible. Sputum, induced sputum, gastric lavage.
Pulmonary	Bronchial/tracheal aspirates	Sputum may be induced by inhalation of a hypertonic salt aerosol. Gastric lavage may be the only way of obtaining adequate material from infants and from children and adults unable to cooperate with sputum induction. If gastric lavage processing will be delayed for 2 hr, add sodium carbonate powder or another alkaline buffer salt. Culture reports should include results of concentrated AFB smears.
Urine	First morning, clean-voided urine specimens are preferred. Do not collect 24-hr specimens.	Renal tuberculosis results from hematogenous spread of the tubercle bacilli. Urinary tract tuberculosis should be suspected whenever there is pyuria without bacteriuria or unexplained hematuria or proteinuria. Diagnosis is dependent upon isolation of *M. tuberculosis* from the urine. Maximum yield is obtained by sending three specimens for culture. Smears of the urine for the presence of acid-fast bacilli may not be helpful owing to the paucity of organisms and may be misleading if, for example, saprophytic *M. smegmatis* is present.

1. Forbes BA, Sahm DF, Weissfeld AS: *Bailey & Scott's diagnostic microbiology,* ed 10, St Louis, 1998, Mosby.
2. Isenberg HD: *Clinical microbiology procedures handbook,* ed 2, Washington, DC, 2004, ASM Press.
3. Mandell GL, Bennett JE, Dolin R: *Principles and practice of infectious diseases,* ed 6, Philadelphia, 2005, Elsevier Churchill Livingstone.
4. Murray PR, Baron EJ, Jorgensen JH, et al: *Manual of clinical microbiology,* ed 8, Washington, DC, 2003, ASM Press.
5. Winn W Jr, Allen S, Janda W, et al: *Koneman's color atlas and textbook of diagnostic microbiology,* ed 6, Philadelphia, 2006, Lippincott Williams & Wilkins.

TEST NAME AND METHOD	SPECIMEN AND SPECIAL REQUIREMENTS	CLINICAL COMMENTS AND REMARKS
***Mycoplasma pneumoniae* Culture**[1-3]	Nasopharyngeal swab, throat swab, endotracheal aspirates; sputum, bronchoalveolar lavage and lung tissue; blood; synovial fluid. See *Bronchial/Tracheal Aspirates Culture, Routine; Sputum Culture, Routine;* and *Miscellaneous Sites Culture, Routine.*	Transport to the laboratory immediately. Swabs should be placed in special transport medium, such as 2SP or multipurpose transport medium specific for Chlamydia, virus, and mycoplasma. Antibiotics should be included in transport medium to reduce bacterial contamination. The swab should be pressed against the side of the tube to release the material into the medium and discarded before transport to the laboratory. Specimens should be refrigerated if not immediately transported to the laboratory.
		Mycoplasma pneumoniae is responsible for at least 20% of community-acquired pneumonias. The disease is usually mild and presents as a tracheobronchitis. Pneumonia develops in approximately one third of patients. *M. pneumoniae* has long been associated with pneumonia in children and young adults; however, recently disease incidence is increasing in young children and older adults.

TEST NAME AND METHOD	SPECIMEN AND SPECIAL REQUIREMENTS	CLINICAL COMMENTS AND REMARKS

Mycoplasma pneumoniae **Culture—CONT**

Culture is relatively insensitive for detection of *M. pneumoniae*. Alternative techniques, such as serology and nucleic acid amplification tests, should be used even if culture is performed.

Cultures are held a minimum of 3 wk.

1. Murray PR, Baron EJ, Jorgensen JH, et al, editors: *Manual of clinical microbiology,* ed 8, Washington, DC, 2003, ASM Press.
2. Sharp SE, Robinson A, Saubolle M, et al: *Cumitech 7B, lower respiratory infections,* coordinating editor, Sharp SE, Washington DC, 2004, ASM Press.
3. Waites KB, Bebear CM, Robertson JA, Talkington DF, Kenny GE: *Cumitech 34, Laboratory diagnosis of mycoplasmal infections.* Nolte FS, coordinating editor, Washington DC, 2001, American Society for Microbiology.

TEST NAME AND METHOD	SPECIMEN AND SPECIAL REQUIREMENTS	CLINICAL COMMENTS AND REMARKS

Mycoplasma Serological Test

(Mycoplasma pneumoniae IgG and IgM antibody)[1-3]

CF, EIA, IFA, Particle Agglutination

Serum drawn at onset of disease and 3 wk later.

Serological confirmation of recent infection is based upon the demonstration of a fourfold rise in IgG titer between acute and convalescent sera or the presence of detectable IgM antibody. A single CF titer of $\geq$1:32 serves as presumptive evidence of recent infection. IgM antibody may persist for several months. In addition adults experiencing reinfection may produce a largely IgG response. This confirms the necessity for collection of acute and convalescent phase serum samples.

The CF test may have a false-positive rate $\geq$10% because of cross-reactions with streptococcus antigens and common glycolipid antigens produced in acute inflammatory conditions. For this reason the CF test has been largely replaced with other methodologies.

1. Murray PR, Baron EJ, Jorgensen JH, et al, editors: *Manual of clinical microbiology,* ed 8, Washington, DC, 2003, ASM Press.
2. Rose, NR, Hamilton RG, Detrick B, editors: M*anual of clinical immunology,* ed 6, Washington, DC, 2002, ASM Press.
3. Waites KB, Bebear CM, Robertson JA, et al: *Cumitech 34, laboratory diagnosis of mycoplasmal infections.* Nolte FS, coordinating editor, Washington DC, 2001, American Society for Microbiology.

TEST NAME AND METHOD	SPECIMEN AND SPECIAL REQUIREMENTS	CLINICAL COMMENTS AND REMARKS
Nasal Culture for *Surveillance*[1,2] (See *Agar Screening Tests, ORSA/MRSA Screen.*)	Anterior nares swab specimen.	Used to detect *S. aureus* colonization. Rapid identification of resistant strains of S. *aureus,* particularly oxacillin/methicillin-resistant *S. aureus* (ORSA/MRSA), is important from an infection control perspective. Positive patients should be placed on Contact Precautions. To establish a common source outbreak, a molecular test, such as pulsed-field gel electrophoresis (PFGE), may be used to determine clone (e.g., USA 300) and compare molecular fingerprints of isolates recovered during an outbreak. Likewise, a multiplex polymerase chain reaction (PCR) assay may be used to distinguish community-associated from hospital-associated strains of *S. aureus* (e.g., SCC mec types I-V).
	Nasopharyngeal swab specimen.	Infrequently used to detect *Neisseria meningitidis or Streptococcus pneumoniae* colonization.

1. Isenberg HD: *Clinical microbiology procedures handbook,* ed 2, Washington, DC, 2004, ASM Press.
2. Murray PR, Baron EJ, Jorgensen JH, et al: *Manual of clinical microbiology,* ed 8, Washington, DC, 2003, ASM Press.

***Nocardia* spp.**[1-3] (See *Modified AFB Stain.*) Culture	Sputum, transtracheal aspirates, bronchial washings, surgical specimens (including lung and brain biopsy material), exudate, body fluids (CSF, urine, and blood), scrapings from ulcers, and granules sent on sterile gauze for microscopic examination and culture.	Nocardiosis, most commonly found in immunosuppressed or transplant patients, may present as a suppurative or cavitary pneumonia resembling tuberculosis, lymphocutaneous abscesses, cellulitis, or as a mycetoma with granule formation. The organism has a marked tropism for the CNS with dissemination from a primary pulmonary infection.
		The etiological agents are primarily *N. asteroides, N. brasiliensis,* or *N. caviae,* and all are found as saprophytes in the soil. Humans may contract the organism via inhalation or traumatic implantation. The organisms are probably not part of the normal flora, although they are occasionally isolated from sputum, for example, without clinical evidence of disease. *Nocardia* spp. are aerobic bacteria that require 2-5 days or more for isolation. Direct Gram stains of specimens including granules, demonstrate delicate, beaded, branching, filamentous gram-positive organisms. *Nocardia* spp. are acid-fast using a modified Kinyoun acid-fast stain, a characteristic that helps to differentiate it from *Actinomyces* spp.

1. Isenberg HD: *Clinical microbiology procedures handbook,* ed 2, Washington, DC, 2004, ASM Press.
2. Mandell GL, Bennett JE, Dolin R: *Principles and practice of infectious diseases,* ed 6, Philadelphia, 2005, Elsevier Churchill Livingstone.
3. Murray PR, Baron EJ, Jorgensen JH, et al: *Manual of clinical microbiology,* ed 8, Washington, DC, 2003, ASM Press.

TEST NAME AND METHOD	SPECIMEN AND SPECIAL REQUIREMENTS	CLINICAL COMMENTS AND REMARKS
Norwalk-like Viruses Direct Examination[1-3] *IEM, RIA, EIA, RT-PCR*	See *Rotavirus Direct Examination.*	Outbreaks of gastroenteritis caused by Norwalk-like viruses including the classical Norwalk virus has occurred worldwide. The source of outbreak is often contaminated water or food. The epidemics of gastroenteritis usually occur in closed communities, such as schools, nursing homes, and recreational camps and cruise ships. It is a common pathogen of older children and adults. There is a wide range of symptomatology. Some patients have a mild case of vomiting or diarrhea; others have severe attacks. Cramps, headache, malaise, myalgias, low-grade fever, and nausea are common findings. The disease lasts 24-48 hr. Viral shedding is observed from onset to about 72 hr. Traditionally, direct examination has been the method of choice since the virus has not been directly cultured in cell culture. The direct examination may be performed by means of immune electron microscopy (IEM) or recombinant EIA. Today RT-PCR assays with excellent sensitivity and specificity are available in some reference and research laboratories See also *Norwalk Virus Serological Test.*

1. Lennette EH, Smith TF, editors: *Laboratory diagnosis of viral infection,* ed 3, New York, 1999, Marcel Dekker.
2. Murray PR, Baron EJ, Jorgensen JH, et al, editors: *Manual of clinical microbiology,* ed 8, Washington, DC, 2003, American Society for Microbiology.
3. Richman DD, Whitely RJ, Hayden FG, editors: *Clinical virology,* ed 2, Washington DC, 2002, American Society for Microbiology.

TEST NAME AND METHOD	SPECIMEN AND SPECIAL REQUIREMENTS	CLINICAL COMMENTS AND REMARKS
Norwalk Virus Serological Test[1,2] *ELISA*	Serum, acute and convalescent. See *General Information.*	Norwalk-like viruses, which include classical Norwalk virus, are members of Caliciviridae. They are nonenveloped single-stranded RNA viruses. The prevalence of the antibody among adults may reach as high as 98%. In developed countries the antibody is not commonly acquired until the first or second decade of life. In contrast in developing countries, antibody to NV may be present by the age of 2-5 yr. Norwalk virus has been associated with epidemics of gastrointestinal illness occurring in families, schools, and cruise ships. Because Norwalk virus does not grow in routine cell cultures or animals, all the current ELISA assays used to detect antibody response to NV are based on recombinant viral protein, such as rVLPs. The rELISA is highly sensitive in detecting similar NV, but because of significant variability among the genotypes, the assay may not detect antibody to strains with less than 80% homology.

1. Murray PR, Baron EJ, Jorgensen JH, et al, editors: *Manual of clinical microbiology,* ed 8, Washington, DC, 2003, American Society for Microbiology.
2. Rose NR, Hamilton RG, Detrick B, editors: *Manual of clinical laboratory immunology,* ed 6, Washington, DC, 2002, American Society for Microbiology.

TEST NAME AND METHOD	SPECIMEN AND SPECIAL REQUIREMENTS	CLINICAL COMMENTS AND REMARKS
Ova and Parasite Examination (routine)[1-3]	Fresh sputum (or induced), bronchial alveolar lavage fluid, aspirates, or biopsy material. Keep all specimens at RT.	One negative result does not rule out the possibility of a parasitic infection. See *General Instructions, Parasite Culture.*
	Fresh random stool, preserved stool, sigmoidoscopy material, and duodenal contents. Transport to lab (immediately if unpreserved) in a leak-proof container. Generally, up to three specimens taken on separate days over a 10-day period is recommended. Specimens should be free of urine, water, and soil. Patients should not have taken mineral oil; bismuth; nonabsorbable antidiarrheal medications; antimalarials; some antibiotics, such as the tetracyclines; or have undergone barium studies of the intestinal tract for 1 wk before examination.	Sputum and other respiratory specimens may be used for the detection of *Strongyloides stercoralis, Cryptosporidium* spp., *Echinococcus* spp., and *Paragonimus* spp. Fecal specimens can be used for the detection of many parasites, including protozoans, such as *Entamoeba histolytica* and *Giardia lamblia;* helminths, such as *Strongyloides stercoralis, Ascaris lumbricoides,* and hookworms; tapeworms; and trematodes, such as *Schistosoma* spp. For each stool examination, three components should be considered: A direct wet mount should be performed if the stool specimen is received fresh (within ½ hr of collection), and an examination of the stool concentrate should routinely be performed and an examination of a direct permanent stained preparation. The latter is essential for the recovery and identification of protozoans. If fresh specimens cannot be examined within 1 hr of collection, the stool material should be preserved. More than one stool should be examined before ruling out a parasite infection.
	Urine specimens. Collect a single unpreserved specimen, a 24-hr unpreserved specimen, or an early morning or midday specimen for 2-3 consecutive days.	Urine specimens can be used to detect *Trichomonas vaginalis,* eggs of *Schistosoma haematobium,* microsporidia, and microfilaria.

1. Ash LR, Orihel TC: *A guide to laboratory procedures and identification,* Chicago, 1987, American Society for Clinical Pathologists.
2. Murray PR, Baron EJ, Jorgensen JH, et al, editors: *Manual of clinical microbiology,* ed 8, Washington, DC, 2003, ASM Press.
3. Garcia LS: *Diagnostic medical parasitology,* ed 4, Washington, DC, 2001, ASM Press.

TEST NAME AND METHOD	SPECIMEN AND SPECIAL REQUIREMENTS	CLINICAL COMMENTS AND REMARKS
Paracoccid-ioidomycosis Serological Test (Serological Test for *Paracoccidioides brasiliensis*)[1,2] *ID, CF, EIA*	Serum	Serological tests for *Paracoccidioides brasiliensis* should be considered in patients with chronic disease with lung involvement or ulcerative lesions of the mucosae and skin. A history of living or traveling in Latin America is suggestive. Overall antibodies are difficult to detect in AIDS patients; however, in other patients antibody tests are useful especially in disseminated disease. The CF test will detect antibodies in 80%-96% of infected patients. CF titers ≥1:8 with yeast antigen is considered presumptive evidence of infection. Titers ≥1:32 indicate active disease. High titers are usually

TEST NAME AND METHOD	SPECIMEN AND SPECIAL REQUIREMENTS	CLINICAL COMMENTS AND REMARKS

Paracoccidioidomycosis Serological Test—CONT

found in patients with pulmonary lesions or multifocal disease. CF titers are prognostic and decline in response to therapy. Relapses are accompanied by high titers, and high, fluctuating titers suggest a poor prognosis. Titers may be negative when small, isolated lesions are the only physical findings and in young children. Cross-reactions may occur in patients with histoplasmosis or blastomycosis.

The ID test is excellent for the diagnosis of acute unifocal pulmonary, progressive pulmonary, and multifocal disease. Concurrent use of the CF and ID tests is recommended for establishing the diagnosis and can increase the sensitivity to more than 95%.

1. Yeo SF, Wong B: Current status of nonculture methods for diagnosis of invasive fungal infections, *Clin Microbi Rev* *15*:465-484, 2002.
2. Rose NR, Hamilton RG, Detrick B, editors: *Manual of clinical immunology,* ed 6, Washington, DC, 2002, ASM Press.

Paragonimiasis Serological Test (Lung Fluke Serological Test)[1,2] *EIA, IB, CF*	Serum. Collect in separation tube and freeze if not assayed immediately.	Test is used to support the diagnosis of pulmonary and extrapulmonary infections. Testing is not readily available, and many of these assays are nonstandardized. See *General Comment.*

1. Rose NR, deMarcario EC, Fahey JL, et al, editors: *Manual of clinical laboratory immunology,* ed 4, Washington, DC, 1992, American Society for Microbiology.
2. Garcia LS: *Diagnostic medical parasitology,* ed 4, Washington, DC, 2001, ASM Press.

Parainfluenza Viruses 1, 2, and 3 Serological Tests (Parainfluenza Virus 1, 2, 3 Titer)[1-3] *CF, HI, EIA, NT, IF*	Serum, acute and convalescent. See *General Information.*	Traditional serological diagnosis of parainfluenza virus is based on demonstration of a fourfold increase in titer between the acute and convalescent sera. Demonstration of IgM antibody in acute sera may provide timely diagnosis. However, the serological test is secondary to antigen detection and culture of the virus. Most individuals experience many parainfluenza infections throughout their lives; they will probably have antibodies to at least one serotype. In addition, there may be cross-reactivity among the parainfluenza and mumps viruses. Serological tests are primarily used to make a retrospective diagnosis or to obtain seroepidemiological data. EIA has replaced the traditional HI and CF and IF tests in most laboratories. NT although specific is too cumbersome and not very cost effective.

TEST NAME AND METHOD	SPECIMEN AND SPECIAL REQUIREMENTS	CLINICAL COMMENTS AND REMARKS

Parainfluenza Viruses 1, 2, and 3 Serological Tests—CONT

1. Lennette EH, Smith TF, editors: *Laboratory diagnosis of viral infection,* ed 3, New York, 1999, Marcel Dekker.
2. Murray PR, Baron EJ, Jorgensen JH, et al, editors: *Manual of clinical microbiology,* ed 8, Washington, DC, 2002, American Society for Microbiology.
3. Rose NR, Hamilton RG, Detrick B, editors: *Manual of clinical laboratory immunology,* ed 6, Washington, DC, 2002, American Society for Microbiology.

Parasite Culture[1-3]		Cultures can be performed only for a few parasitic organisms, including *Acanthamoeba* species, *Naegleria fowleri,* some intestinal amebae, *Leishmania* species and *Trypanosoma* species. These tests are not readily available in most clinical laboratories, but may be done at large referral centers or research laboratories. Culture for *Trichomonas vaginalis* is the exception (see below).
Amoeba Culture *(Culture for Parasites, Protozoa)*[1,2]	Stool. See *General Instructions* above. Alternatively, collect liver aspirate, biopsy, or proctoscopic material.	See *General Instructions* above. A direct wet preparation and permanent stain should also be performed.
Nematode Culture *(Agar plate culture; Harada-Mori filter paper strip culture; Baermann culture)*[1,3]	Stool. See *General Instructions* above.	Test is used as a means of detecting light infections with hookworm, *Strongyloides* spp. or *Trichostrongylus* spp. Tests other than the agar plate culture are normally only available in reference or research laboratories.
Toxoplasma gondii Culture[3]	Buffy coat; CSF; placenta	Specimens are inoculated into human embryonic lung fibroblasts (MRC-5) cells and observed for evidence of a cytopathic effect. Test is relatively slow, lacks sensitivity, and not routinely available in clinical laboratories. However, it may be more practical and may be used in place of mouse inoculation.
Trichomonas Culture[1,2]	Urine sediment or a swab of vaginal secretions. See *Trichomonas Preparation.*	Test is used to culture *Trichomonas vaginalis.* Culture is more sensitive than wet mounts for the diagnosis of trichomoniasis. Culture systems are readily available commercially.

1. Ash LR, Orihel TC: *A guide to laboratory procedures and identification,* Chicago, 1987, American Society for Clinical Pathologists.
2. Garcia LS: *Diagnostic medical parasitology,* ed 4, Washington, DC, 2001 ASM Press.
3. Murray PR, Baron EJ, Jorgensen JH, et al, editors: *Manual of clinical microbiology,* ed 8, Washington DC, 2003, ASM Press.

TEST NAME AND METHOD	SPECIMEN AND SPECIAL REQUIREMENTS	CLINICAL COMMENTS AND REMARKS
Periodic Acid Schiff–Stain (PAS Stain)[1]	Appropriate specimen is the same as that for culture of the corresponding site.	The PAS stain is used to detect fungi in clinical specimens especially yeast cells and hyphae in tissue.
		PAS stains polysaccharides in the cell walls of fungi. It is an excellent stain; however, the staining procedure is complex and time consuming. The PAS stain has been replaced in many laboratories by the calcofluor white stain.

1. Murray PR, Baron EJ, Jorgensen JH, et al, editors: *Manual of clinical microbiology,* ed 8, Washington, DC, 2003, ASM Press.

TEST NAME AND METHOD	SPECIMEN AND SPECIAL REQUIREMENTS	CLINICAL COMMENTS AND REMARKS
Pinworm Preparation (Scotch Tape Preparation, *Enterobius vermicularis* Preparation)[1,2]		Late in the evening or early in the morning before bathing or going to the bathroom, a short piece of adhesive tape is applied sticky side down to the perianal folds where the anal canal joins the perianal skin. The tape is then transferred to the laboratory for examination for eggs and/or adult worms. Commercially available paddles with sticky adhesive on one side may also be used for this purpose.
		Approximately 5% of infected patients pass demonstrable eggs into their stool. The Scotch tape preparation yields more accurate results.
		One negative result does not rule out the possibility of a pinworm infection and up to 4-6 pinworm preparations may be necessary to rule out infection. Pinworm eggs are very infectious, and total prevention is not possible. Caution should be used to prevent cross-contaminating individuals involved in handling the pinworm preparation.

1. Rose NR, deMarcario EC, Fahey JL, et al, editors: *Manual of clinical laboratory immunology,* ed 4, Washington, DC, 1992, American Society for Microbiology.
2. Garcia LS: *Diagnostic medical parasitology,* ed 4, Washington, DC, 2001, ASM Press.

TEST NAME AND METHOD	SPECIMEN AND SPECIAL REQUIREMENTS	CLINICAL COMMENTS AND REMARKS
***Pneumocystis jiroveci (carinii)* Examination**[1-3] *GMS, Giemsa, toluidine blue, calcofluor white* *Monoclonal Ab, DFA*	Induced sputum, bronchoalveolar lavage, or bronchial brush. See *Bronchial /Tracheal Aspirates Culture, Routine.* ──────────── Lung tissue. See *Miscellaneous Sites Culture, Routine.* Transport to lab immediately.	*P. jiroveci* is an important cause of pneumonia in patients who are immunocompromised. The gold standard for diagnosis is examination of open lung biopsy material. However, much less invasive procedures, such as induced sputum or bronchoalveolar lavage, may be helpful to demonstrate the organism. Silver, Giemsa, toluidine blue, or calcofluor white stains may be used to visualize the organism. Fluorescent monoclonal antibody stains can also be used to detect *P. jiroveci.*

TEST NAME AND METHOD	SPECIMEN AND SPECIAL REQUIREMENTS	CLINICAL COMMENTS AND REMARKS

Pneumocystis jiroveci (carinii) **Examination**—CONT

Serological diagnosis is of little value since many seemingly noninfected individuals may be positive.

1. Ash LR, Orihel TC: *A guide to laboratory procedures and identification,* Chicago, 1987, American Society for Clinical Pathologists.
2. Garcia LS, Bruckner DA: *Diagnostic medical parasitology,* New York, 1988, Elsevier Science Publishing.
3. Garcia LS: *Diagnostic medical parasitology,* ed 4, Washington, DC, 2001, ASM Press.

Probe Assay for Culture Confirmation of *Blastomyces dermatitidis, Coccidioides immitis,* and *Histoplasma capsulatum*[1]

Isolates of molds or yeasts, consistent with *C. immitis, H. capsulatum,* or *B. dermatitidis.*

These probes, known as Accuprobes (Gen-Probe, San Diego, Calif.), are chemiluminescent-labeled probes that measure the presence of specific ribosomal RNA and can be performed on either the mold or yeast form. They cannot be applied directly to clinical specimens because the sensitivity is no better than the direct stains of these specimens. This has become the method of choice for confirming the identity of molds with typical morphology. Rapid results can be obtained from young cultures using very small amounts of the fungus. Test specificity is nearly 100%.

1. Murray PR, Baron EJ, Jorgensen JH, et al, editors: *Manual of clinical microbiology,* ed 8, Washington, DC, 2003, ASM Press.

Q Fever Serological Test (*Coxiella burnetii* Titer)[1,2]

IFA, MIF

Serum drawn at onset of disease and 2-3 wk later

This test is used to aid in the diagnosis of Q fever pneumonia or its complications (e.g., endocarditis or hepatitis). Humans acquire the organism, *Coxiella burnetii,* a rickettsia, by inhaling aerosolized particles containing the organism, usually from contact with cattle or sheep. Tick bites (ixodid ticks) may also be a mode of transmission.

Phase I and phase II antibodies are produced in response to the organism; phase II antibodies appearing first and phase I antibodies weeks to months later. Antibodies are usually detectable 2-4 wk after the onset of infection. The diagnosis of acute Q fever is confirmed by a fourfold rise in titer between acute and convalescent sera or the presence of an IgM titer to *C. burnetii.* In chronic Q fever, a single sample is diagnostic when high antibody titers are detected against phase I antigens. Recent vaccinations will cause a rise equal to that seen in infection.

Since antibodies for Q fever do not cross-react with other rickettsial antibodies, a rise in titer is considered diagnostic for recent infection in the absence of prior vaccination.

TEST NAME AND METHOD	SPECIMEN AND SPECIAL REQUIREMENTS	CLINICAL COMMENTS AND REMARKS

Q Fever Serological Test—CONT

1. Murray PR, Baron EJ, Jorgensen JH, et al, editors: *Manual of clinical microbiology,* ed 8, Washington, DC, 2003, ASM Press.
2. Rose NR, Hamilton RG, Detrick B, editors: *Manual of clinical immunology,* ed 6, Washington, DC, 2002, ASM Press.

Rabies Virus[1] *NT*	Serum, CSF. See *General Information.*	Rabies is a fatal infection of central nervous system acquired most often through virus-contaminated saliva by the bite of a rabid animal. Fortunately, cases of human rabies infection are rare in part because of vaccination programs and availability of rabies immune globulin and potent vaccine for postexposure treatment. Laboratories in the U.S. are required by the Advisory Committee on Immunization Practices to use NT to determine the antibody titer in an immunized individual. NT measures the antibody response to G protein that neutralizes a challenge inoculum. This is demonstrated by a reduction in the number of fluorescent antibody-stained microscopic foci of infected cells.

1. Murray PR, Baron EJ, Jorgensen JH, et al, editors: *Manual of clinical microbiology,* ed 8, Washington, DC, 2003, American Society for Microbiology.

Rapid HIV Antibody Tests[1,2] *Membrane EIA*	Whole blood, plasma, serum	Rapid HIV antibody test provides timely detection of antibody to HIV in cases of needle stick injury or exposure to potentially HIV-contaminated materials. There are at least three rapid HIV tests approved by the U.S. Food and Drug Administration (FDA) and commercially available for use in the U.S. OraQuick Rapid HIV-1 Antibody Test (OraSure Technologies, Inc.), Reveal Rapid HIV-1 Antibody Test (MedMira, Inc.), and Uni-Gold Recombigen HIV Test (Trinity Biotech, Inc.). OraQuick Rapid HIV-1/2 Antibody Test is approved for use with whole blood specimens obtained by fingerstick or by venipuncture. It is intended for use at point of care in medical and nonmedical settings. OraQuick is a CLIA waived test. Reveal Rapid HIV-1 Antibody Test is also intended for use as a point-of-care test, but it requires some laboratory equipment. The Reveal test does not contain an internal procedural control. External controls (known HIV positive and negative specimens) must be run with each test or batch of tests to monitor test performance. The test is performed on serum or plasma and requires centrifuging the whole blood first to separate cells from the serum or plasma.

TEST NAME AND METHOD	SPECIMEN AND SPECIAL REQUIREMENTS	CLINICAL COMMENTS AND REMARKS

Rapid HIV Antibody Tests—CONT

The Uni-Gold test is a single-use rapid test for the detection of HIV-1 antibodies in plasma, serum, and whole blood (venipuncture). It is intended for use as a point-of-care test as well. CLIA considers both Reveal Rapid HIV-1 Antibody Test and the Uni-Gold Test as moderate complexity tests.

1. Murray PR, Baron EJ, Jorgensen JH, et al, editors: *Manual of clinical microbiology,* ed 8, Washington, DC, 2003, American Society for Microbiology.
2. Truong HM, Klausner JD: Diagnostic assays for HIV-1 infection, *Med Lab Observ* 36:12-20, 2004.

Rapid Influenza Antigen Test[1,2]

EIA antigen detection, RT-PCR

Nasopharyngeal aspirate, NP wash, NP swab, throat swab, BAL

The availability of antiviral drugs to treat influenza is associated with increased demand for rapid detection and diagnosis of influenza virus infections. They are also thought to be useful in hospitals and nursing homes to detect nosocomial outbreaks. The rapid influenza tests currently available in the U.S. detect either viral NP or NA antigens and will generate laboratory results within 30 min. A positive result may be obtained with as few as 20 influenza infected cells. Based on the timing and type of the collected specimen the reported sensitivity of rapid influenza tests range from 40%-100% and specificity from 52%-100%. BAL, NP washes/aspirates and NP swabs are the most productive. Throat swab is least productive and is not recommended.

In recent years, a rapid real time RT-PCR assay that amplifies unique sequences within viral RNA is shown to have sensitivity greater than that of traditional viral culture. With this assay a laboratory diagnosis may be made within 4 hr.

1. Murray PR, Baron EJ, Jorgensen JH, et al, editors: *Manual of clinical microbiology,* ed 8, Washington, DC, 2003, American Society for Microbiology.
2. Richman DD, Whitely RJ, Hayden FG, editors: *Clinical virology,* ed 2, Washington DC, 2002, American Society for Microbiology.

Respiratory Syncytial Virus (RSV) Antigen[1-2]

EIA, DFA, RT-PCR

Nasal wash, nasopharyngeal swab

RSV is an important cause of lower respiratory tract infections during the first 6 mo of life. Reinfection may occur in older children and adults in the form of a mild upper respiratory tract infection. Occasionally, RSV can cause severe respiratory infection in aged adults confined to nursing homes.

DFA is a highly reliable test for detecting RSV in exfoliated nasopharyngeal epithelial cells with sensitivity ranging from 80%-97%. A good specimen should have more than 100 cells on the slide. The titer of the virus is higher in wash than in swab specimens.

TEST NAME AND METHOD	SPECIMEN AND SPECIAL REQUIREMENTS	CLINICAL COMMENTS AND REMARKS

Respiratory Syncytial Virus (RSV) Antigen—CONT

EIA are generally less sensitive than DFA, but technically very simple with an assay time of 15-20 min.

RT-PCR is available in some reference and research laboratories. However, RT-PCR generally does not provide much advantage over DFA.

1. Lennette EH, Smith TF, editors: *Laboratory diagnosis of viral infection,* ed 3, New York, 1999, Marcel Dekker.
2. Murray PR, Baron EJ, Jorgensen JH, et al, editors: *Manual of clinical microbiology,* ed 8, Washington, DC, 2003, American Society for Microbiology.

Respiratory Syncytial Virus (RSV) Serological Test[1,2]

NT, IF, EIA, Immunoblot assay

Serum, acute and convalescent. See *General Information.*

RSV is the most common viral agent causing lower respiratory tract infection in infancy. By the first year of life, 50% of all infants experience a primary RSV infection; by 2 yr, nearly all have contracted RSV disease. Young infants do not always respond serologically; the reaction may be very slow, and significant changes may be missed if convalescent serum is drawn too early. In addition, neonates may possess titers caused by passive transfer of maternal antibody. For older children and adults, the presence of antibodies may indicate previous infection, but antibody titers will also rise with occurrence of recent infections.

Neutralization antibody is the only antibody test that correlates with protection against reinfection with RSV. IF and EIA are much more rapid and are nearly as accurate as NT for detecting increase in antibody titer. Immunoblot assays are used in research laboratories. In any event the absence of a significant rise in antibody titer does not rule out infection. The preferred method of diagnosing RSV is the use of viral culture and/or direct examination of specimen by immunofluorescence procedures.

1. Murray PR, Baron EJ, Jorgensen JH, et al, editors: *Manual of clinical microbiology,* ed 8, Washington, DC, 2003, American Society for Microbiology.
2. Rose NR, Hamilton RG, Detrick B, editors: *Manual of clinical laboratory immunology,* ed 6, Washington, DC, 2002, American Society for Microbiology.

Respiratory Tract, Lower Culture for Fungus[1-3]

Sputum, bronchial/tracheal aspirates. See *Respiratory Tract, Lower Culture, Routine*

Sputum is the most frequently submitted specimen for the diagnosis of systemic mycoses. Since contamination by airborne spores and normal mouth flora is common, the results of this procedure must be interpreted cautiously.

TEST NAME AND METHOD	SPECIMEN AND SPECIAL REQUIREMENTS	CLINICAL COMMENTS AND REMARKS

Respiratory Tract, Lower Culture for Fungus—CONT

The isolation of a fungus, e.g., *Aspergillus fumigatus,* from bronchial or tracheal aspirates may be difficult to interpret, owing to the ubiquitous nature of the spores of these organisms. Isolation may indicate colonization rather than infection. The same may be true for isolation of *Candida* spp., especially in hospitalized patients. The method of choice for diagnosis of *Candida* pneumonia is demonstration of tissue invasion by histopathologic examination.

See *General Comments.*

1. Murray PR, Baron EJ, Jorgensen JH, et al, editors: *Manual of clinical microbiology,* ed 8, Washington, DC, 2003, ASM Press.
2. Larone DH: *Medically important fungi: a guide to identification,* ed 4, Washington, DC, 2002, ASM Press.
3. Winn W Jr, Allen SD, Janda WM, et al, editors: *Koneman's color atlas and textbook of diagnostic microbiology,* ed 6, Philadelphia, 2006, Lippincott Williams & Wilkins.

Respiratory Tract, Lower[1-17]

Culture, Routine

Sputum (expectorated or induced), bronchial washings or bronchoalveolar lavage (BAL), protected bronchial brushing (PBB), pleural fluid, transbronchial biopsy, transtracheal aspirate (TTA).

The following methods of specimen collection are used to obtain specimens for routine, mycobacteria, and fungal cultures as appropriate. Induced sputum and BAL are particularly useful for detecting *Pneumocystis jiroveci.* Anaerobic cultures are generally reserved for TTA, pleural fluid, and biopsy specimens. For optimal results, specimens must be processed within 2 hr of collection (preferred) or refrigerated for <24 hr.

Expectorated sputum: The patient should be instructed to rinse mouth with water, discard, and cough deeply into a sterile container to obtain lower respiratory tract secretions. The

Transport specimen to lab immediately in a sterile container or Leukin's trap and refrigerate until processed. Fastidious organisms may not be recovered if there is a delay of >2 hr in specimen processing. The laboratory should be notified if fastidious organisms are suspected. Select the most purulent or blood-tinged portion of the specimen for culture and Gram stain.

Quantitative cultures of PBB and BAL specimens may be helpful in distinguishing pathogens from contaminants; the isolation of $\geq 10^4$ CFU/mL of BAL likely represents pneumonia, whereas by PBB, $\geq 10^3$ CFU/mL is consistent with bacterial pneumonia. Quantitative cultures can be performed using either a calibrated pipette or loop method, are useful in the diagnosis of ventilator-associated pneumonia, pneumonia in immunocompromised and cystic fibrosis patients, acute episodes in chronic obstructive pulmonary disease, and even in community-acquired pneumonia. Repeat cultures submitted within 48 hr should be rejected.

TEST NAME AND METHOD	SPECIMEN AND SPECIAL REQUIREMENTS	CLINICAL COMMENTS AND REMARKS

Respiratory Tract, Lower—CONT

specimen should be processed for Gram stain and culture.

Induced sputum: The patient should rinse mouth with water and discard. Patients should inhale ~25 mL of 3%-10% hypertonic sterile saline using a nebulizer. The specimen is collected in a sterile container for immediate transport to the laboratory.

BAL: Patients aspirate ~20 mL saline in a suction device, and the lavage fluid is collected into a sterile container. This procedure is repeated five times, and the total collection (40-70 mL) is transported immediately to the laboratory for Gram stain (cytocentrifuged preferred), other special stains, and quantitative aerobic culture.

Single or protected double-lumen brush catheter: Following premedication with atropine and topical anesthesia, a catheter is introduced through a bronchoscope. The brush is advanced to obtain secretions that are used to prepare slides for Gram and other stains and then placed in 1 mL of sterile non-bacteriostatic saline for quantitative aerobic culture.

TTA: Rarely performed. Patients are placed in a supine position with neck hyperextended. A needle with attached catheter is placed through the cricoid membrane to obtain a transtracheal aspirate that bypasses normal respiratory flora.

TEST NAME AND METHOD	SPECIMEN AND SPECIAL REQUIREMENTS	CLINICAL COMMENTS AND REMARKS

Respiratory Tract, Lower—CONT

Legionella Culture[5,14,16]		*Legionella* spp. survive for extended periods of time in the refrigerator. Specimens should not be rejected using Gram stain criteria for routine sputa since most patients with Legionnaires' disease produce sputum that contains few WBCs. Legionellae do not stain with Gram stain reagents. Specimens should be plated on buffered media (e.g., buffered charcoal yeast extract agar [BCYE-a], without increased CO_2 at 35° C for 7 days and adequate humidity). Direct immunofluorescent antibody (IFA) testing of respiratory specimens, although rapid, lacks sensitivity and should always be performed along with a culture. Serology at best will only provide a retrospective lab diagnosis since it generally takes more than 3 wk to mount a detectable antibody response.
Legionella Urine Antigen[16]	Urine	Urine antigen testing is a helpful adjunct to Legionella cultures since it provides a rapid turnaround for results. Although the specificity is excellent, the sensitivity ranges between 70%-90% since it detects primarily *L. pneumophila* serogroup 1 infections.

1. Baron E, et al: *Cumitech 17A-laboratory diagnosis of female genital tract infections.* Rubin SJ, coordinating editor, Washington, DC, 1993, ASM Press.

2. Bryant JK, Strand CL: Reliability of blood cultures collected from intravascular catheter versus venipuncture, *Am J Clin Pathol* 88:113-116, 1987.

3. Farhat SE, Thibault M, Devlin R: Efficacy of a swab transport system in maintaining viability of *Neisseria gonorrhoeae* and *Streptococcus pneumoniae*, *J Clin Microbiol* 39:2958-2960, 2001.

4. Isaacman DJ, Karasic RR, Reynolds EA, et al: Effect of number of blood cultures and volume of blood on detection of bacteremia in children, *J Pediatr* 128(2):190-195, 1996

5. Isenberg HD: *Clinical microbiology procedures handbook,* ed 2, Washington, DC, 2004, ASM Press.

6. Jousimies-Somer HR, Summanen P, Citron DM, et al: *Wadsworth-KTL Anaerobic Bacteriology Manual,* ed 6, Belmont, Calif, 2002, Star Publishing.

7. Little JR, Murray PR, Traynor PS, et al: A randomized trial of povidone iodine compared with iodine tincture for venipuncture site disinfection: effects on rates of blood culture contamination, *Am J Med* 107:119-125, 1999.

8. Maki DG, et al: A semiquantitative culture method for identifying intravenous catheter-related infection, *N Engl J Med* 296:1305-1309, 1977.

9. Mandell GL, Bennett JE, Dolin R: *Principles and practice of infectious diseases,* ed 6, Philadelphia, 2005, Elsevier Churchill Livingstone.

10. Marquette CH, Georges H, Waller F, et al: Diagnostic efficiency of endotracheal aspirates with quantitative bacterial cultures in intubated patients with suspected pneumonia: comparison with the protected specimen brush, *Am Rev Respir Dis* 148:138-144, 1993.

11. Mermel LA, et al: Detection of bacteremia in adults: consequences of culturing an inadequate volume of blood, *Ann Intern Med* 119:270-272, 1993.

12. Miller FD, Hoppe JE, Wirsing von Konig CH: Laboratory diagnosis of pertussis: state of the art in 1997, *J Clin Microbiol* 35:2435-2443, 1997.

13. Morris AJ, Wilson SJ, Marx CE, et al: Clinical impact of bacteria and fungi recovered only from broth cultures, *J Clin Microbiol* 33:161-165, 1995.

14. Murray PR, Baron EJ, Jorgensen JH, et al: *Manual of clinical microbiology,* ed 8, Washington, DC, 2003, ASM Press.

TEST NAME AND METHOD	SPECIMEN AND SPECIAL REQUIREMENTS	CLINICAL COMMENTS AND REMARKS

Respiratory Tract, Lower—CONT

15. Schrag S, et al: Prevention of perinatal group B streptococcal disease: revised guidelines from CDC, *Morb Mortal Wkly Rep* 51(RR11):1-22, 2002.

16. Yzerman EPF, den Boer JW, Lettings KD, et al: Sensitivity of three urinary antigen tests associated with clinical severity in a large outbreak of Legionnaires' disease in The Netherlands, *J Clin Microbiol* 40:3232-3236, 2002.

17. Winn W Jr, Allen S, Janda W, et al: *Koneman's color atlas and textbook of diagnostic microbiology,* ed 6, Philadelphia, 2006, Lippincott Williams & Wilkins.

Rhinosporidiosis Examination[1-3]	Mucocutaneous tissue. Send to the laboratory in a sterile container. Swab specimens are unacceptable.	Rhinosporidiosis is a chronic granulomatous, usually painless, localized infection of the mucous membrane. The lesion increases in size over months to years to form a friable pedunculated mass. Lesions typically appear in the nose, upper airway, or conjunctiva. Children and young adults are most commonly affected, but the disease can occur at any age. Generally the incidence is higher in males than in females. The patient's history will usually indicate exposure to streams or pools. The presence of a pink-to-purple friable lesion in which sporangia may be macroscopically visible in the polyps is indicative of the disease.

Direct examination of the lesion for the presence of sporangia, indicative of the agent *Rhinosporidium seeberi*, is the only means of diagnosis. Cultures have thus far been unsuccessful. If the lesion is processed for histopathology, the diagnosis can be made by hematoxylin-eosin (H&E) staining. |

---

1. Murray PR, Baron EJ, Jorgensen JH, et al, editors: *Manual of clinical microbiology,* ed 8, Washington, DC, 2003, ASM Press.

2. Larone DH: *Medically important fungi: a guide to identification,* ed 4, Washington, DC, 2002, ASM Press.

3. Mandell GL, Bennett JE, Dolin R, editors: *Principles and practice of infectious diseases,* ed 5, New York, 2000, Churchill Livingstone.

Rotavirus Direct Examination[1-3]

EM, LA, EIA, RT-PCR | Stool specimen. Deliver to lab immediately in closed container. If not examined immediately, store specimen at $-70°$ C. If shipped to another laboratory, send on dry ice. | Rotavirus is known to cause sporadic and epidemic cases of gastroenteritis in infants and young children, in particular during the winter months. Approximately one half of the infants and young children hospitalized with diarrhea are found to be infected with a rotavirus. The diarrhea lasts 5-8 days and is frequently accompanied by vomiting and fever. The virus is maximally present in the first 3 days of illness and generally shedding of virus is greatly diminished by the eighth day. Adult contacts may have a mild-to-asymptomatic infection; however, epidemics of gastroenteritis among adults have been described.

For many years the direct examination of stool by EM was the only method to diagnose rotavirus infections and was considered the gold standard. Today several commercial EIA, LA, and dot blot kits are available. The sensitivity and specificity of EIA are about 95% (results may vary according to type of kit used). LA is not considered as sensitive as EIA, but they are rapid and highly specific assays. Unlike EM that detects all groups of rotavirus (A, B, C), EIA and LA only detect group A rotavirus. |

TEST NAME AND METHOD	SPECIMEN AND SPECIAL REQUIREMENTS	CLINICAL COMMENTS AND REMARKS

Rotavirus Direct Examination—CONT

In recent years several PCR-based assays that amplify unique sequences of genes 6, 4, and 9 have proven to be very useful in diagnosing this infection. However, because of cost and turnaround time, the test is limited to reference laboratories.

See also *Rotavirus.*

1. Lennette EH, Smith TF, editors: *Laboratory diagnosis of viral infection,* ed 3, New York, 1999, Marcel Dekker.
2. Murray PR, Baron EJ, Jorgensen JH, et al, editors: *Manual of clinical microbiology,* ed 8, Washington, DC, 2003, American Society for Microbiology.
3. Rose NR, Hamilton RG, Detrick B, editors: *Manual of clinical laboratory immunology,* ed 6, Washington, DC, 2002, American Society for Microbiology.

TEST NAME AND METHOD	SPECIMEN AND SPECIAL REQUIREMENTS	CLINICAL COMMENTS AND REMARKS
Rotavirus Serological Test[1,2] *EIA, RIA*	Serum, acute and convalescent. See *General Information.*	Rotavirus is a major cause of infectious gastroenteritis in infants and young children with a peak incidence during the winter months.

In developing countries rotavirus accounts for 10% to 20% of gastroenteritis-associated death. Virtually all the children in both developed and developing counties are infected with rotavirus by 2 to 3 yr of age. There are three rotavirus groups (A, B, and C) that cause disease in humans. Rotavirus Group A accounts for majority of the outbreaks.

Estimated incubation period is 24-48 hr. Serum antibodies are rapidly acquired between the ages of 6 and 24 mo. Approximately 90% of the population have various levels of preexisting rotavirus-specific serum antibody. A fourfold rise in titer of antibodies is needed for diagnosis.

Direct examination of stool specimens is the primary mode of diagnosis since the isolation of rotavirus in routine cell culture is a relatively slow and laborious process.

RIA and EIA have proved most sensitive for the detection of seroconversion. These tests are not readily available in most clinical laboratories.

1. Murray PR, Baron EJ, Jorgensen JH, et al, editors: *Manual of clinical microbiology,* ed 8, Washington, DC, 2003, American Society for Microbiology.
2. Rose NR, Hamilton RG, Detrick B, editors: *Manual of clinical laboratory immunology,* ed 6, Washington, DC, 2002, American Society for Microbiology.

TEST NAME AND METHOD	SPECIMEN AND SPECIAL REQUIREMENTS	CLINICAL COMMENTS AND REMARKS
Rubella Virus Serological Test (German Measles Titer)[1-3] *HI, EIA, CF, PHA, LA*	Serum, acute and convalescent. See *General Information*.	Rubella is transmitted directly by contact or by droplets from the nasopharynx of infected individuals. The peak incidence is in late winter or early spring. Communicability of the virus is generally felt to have occurred a few days before rash development or 5-7 days after rash has developed. Most cases today occur in the U.S. in young unvaccinated and undervaccinated adults. Infants with congenital rubella may shed virus from nasopharynx or urine for up to 1 yr. Serological tests are used to determine the immune status of the individual, to diagnose postnatal rubella, and occasionally to support the diagnosis of rubella. IgM antibody disappears within 4-5 wk; IgG antibody remains for life. Demonstration of a fourfold rise in titer between acute and convalescent sera may be indicative of a recent infection. Single titers, even >1:256, cannot be interpreted as evidence of recent infection; they are more likely to indicate immune status. For diagnosis EIA is the preferred method, although HAI, CF, or FIAX are also acceptable. LA is useful as a stat assay. PHA is good only for determination of the immune status of a patient, not for diagnosis. In addition, any of the other assays are appropriate for evaluation of immune status. For any reactivity of the assay above a standard cutoff value is considered indicative of immunity. For the diagnosis of congenital rubella in an infant less than 6 mo old, HAI, EIA, or specific IgM assays are necessary. Between 6 and 12 mo old any of the following assays are acceptable: HAI, EIA, LA, or CF.

1. Lennette EH, Smith TF, editors: *Laboratory diagnosis of viral infection,* ed 3, New York, 1999, Marcel Dekker.
2. Murray PR, Baron EJ, Jorgensen JH, et al, editors: *Manual of clinical microbiology,* ed 8, Washington, DC, 2003, American Society for Microbiology.
3. Rose NR, Hamilton RG, Detrick B, editors: *Manual of clinical laboratory immunology,* ed 6, Washington, DC, 2002, American Society for Microbiology.

TEST NAME AND METHOD	SPECIMEN AND SPECIAL REQUIREMENTS	CLINICAL COMMENTS AND REMARKS
Rubeola Virus Serological Test (Measles Encephalitis Serological Test, Subacute Sclerosing Panencephalitis [SSPE] Titer)[1-3] *EIA, IFA, HAI, NT, CF*	Serum, acute and convalescent. See *General Information*. CSF. See *CSF Culture, Routine*.	The readily distinguishable clinical symptoms of measles make laboratory diagnosis unnecessary in most instances. Antibodies as demonstrated by EIA, HAI, CF, or NT appear with development of the rash and peak in about 10 days (about 4 wk postvaccination). EIA and IFA can be used to detect either IgG or IgM; the other methods detect total response and do not distinguish between IgG and IgM. WHO and Pan American Health Organization recommend the use of EIA IgM for laboratory diagnosis of measles. In cases of SSPE, serology reveals increased antibody titers in both CSF and serum. A serum titer >1:1000 or an NT titer >1:4000 in the absence of a recent measles infection is suggestive of SSPE. If the CSF

TEST NAME AND METHOD	SPECIMEN AND SPECIAL REQUIREMENTS	CLINICAL COMMENTS AND REMARKS

Rubeola Virus Serological Test—CONT

titer by HAI is >50 (NT >20), the diagnosis is enhanced. IgM antibody invariably appears and thus cannot be used as a marker for persistent infection.

Cross-reactions, as shown by increasing measles titers, have been demonstrated with other diseases, such as chronic active hepatitis, systemic lupus erythematosus, and infectious mononucleosis.

Patients with multiple sclerosis have had increased CSF titers (not false positives); however, increased titers against other enveloped viruses have also been observed.

1. Lennette EH, Smith TF, editors: *Laboratory diagnosis of viral infection,* ed 3, New York, 1999, Marcel Dekker.
2. Murray PR, Baron EJ, Jorgensen JH, et al, editors: *Manual of clinical microbiology,* ed 8, Washington, DC, 2003, American Society for Microbiology.
3. Rose NR, Hamilton RG, Detrick B, editors: *Manual of clinical laboratory immunology,* ed 6, Washington, DC, 2002, American Society for Microbiology.

TEST NAME AND METHOD	SPECIMEN AND SPECIAL REQUIREMENTS	CLINICAL COMMENTS AND REMARKS
Schistosomiasis Serological Test[1,2] *EIA, IFA, IB, IHA, Circumoval precipitin test, cercaria-Hullen reaction*	Serum. Collect in separation tube and freeze if not assayed immediately.	Test is used to support the diagnosis of infection with *Schistosoma* spp. Presence of antibodies is indicative of schistosomiasis, but cannot be correlated with worm burden, egg production, clinical status, or prognosis; however, it is possible that high titers posttherapy correlate with reinfection or treatment failure. The sensitivity of the assays range from >50%-99% (species dependent), but may be decreased in children or individuals with chronic schistosomiasis. Sensitivity appears to be best for *S. mansoni* and *S. haemotobium* infections, but less for *S. japonicum* infections. Specificity is 99%. See *General Comment.*

1. Garcia LS: *Diagnostic medical parasitology,* ed 4, Washington, DC, 2001, ASM Press.
2. Rose NR, deMarcario EC, Fahey JL, et al, editors: *Manual of clinical laboratory immunology,* ed 4, Washington, DC, 1992, American Society for Microbiology.

TEST NAME AND METHOD	SPECIMEN AND SPECIAL REQUIREMENTS	CLINICAL COMMENTS AND REMARKS
Scrub Typhus Serological Test (*Orientia tsutsugamushi* Titer)[1-3] *IFA*	Serum drawn at onset of disease and 2-3 wk later.	*O. tsutsugamushi* is transmitted by the trombiculid mite. The disease is found in Asia, the Indian subcontinent, Australia, and the Pacific Islands. Indirect fluorescent antibody (IFA) test is the preferred testing method. Antibodies appear in 5-6 days in 50%-60% of the cases; they rise significantly in 18-20 days. Titers peak by the fourth week and then decline over the next few months. A fourfold rise in titer between acute and convalescent sera is diagnostic. Failure to demonstrate antibodies does not rule out the diagnosis of scrub typhus. Antibiotic therapy in the first several days of illness may blunt or delay the serological response.

1. Murray PR, Baron EJ, Jorgensen JH, et al, editors: *Manual of clinical microbiology,* ed 8, Washington, DC, 2003, ASM Press.
2. Rose NR, Hamilton RG, Detrick B, editors: *Manual of clinical immunology,* ed 6, Washington, DC, 2002, ASM Press.
3. Mandell GL, Bennett JE, Dolin R, editors: *Principles and practice of infectious diseases,* ed 5, New York, 2000, Churchill Livingstone.

TEST NAME AND METHOD	SPECIMEN AND SPECIAL REQUIREMENTS	CLINICAL COMMENTS AND REMARKS
Severe Acute Respiratory Syndrome (SARS) Serological diagnosis[1,2] *ELISA*	Serum, acute and convalescent. See *General Information.*	Severe acute respiratory syndrome (SARS) is a viral respiratory illness caused by a coronavirus, called SARS-associated coronavirus (SARS-CoV). SARS was first reported in Asia in February 2003. According to the World Health Organization (WHO), a total of 8098 persons worldwide became sick with SARS during the 2003 outbreak. Of these, 774 died. SARS spreads by close person-to-person contact. SARS virus may be cultivated in vitro or detected using molecular-based assays that detect viral RNA. Commercial kits for detecting antibody response to SARS are in development in many countries. An ELISA test with high sensitivity and specificity is available from CDC for serological diagnosis of SARS in the U.S.

1. Thai HTC, Le MQ, Vung CD, et al: Development and evaluation of a novel loop-mediated isothermal amplification method for rapid detection of SARS coronavirus, *J Clin Microbiol* 42:1956-61, 2004.
2. Woo PCY, Lau SKP, Wong BHL, et al: Detection of specific antibodies to severe acute respiratory syndrome (SARS) coronavirus nucleocapsid protein for serodiagnosis of SARS coronavirus pneumonia, *J Clin Microbiol* 42:2306-2309, 2004.

TEST NAME AND METHOD	SPECIMEN AND SPECIAL REQUIREMENTS	CLINICAL COMMENTS AND REMARKS
Sporotrichosis Serological Test *(Sporothrix schenckii* Titer)[1] *EIA, LA, TA*	Serum, CSF	Serological tests are useful in the diagnosis of extracutaneous or disseminated forms of sporotrichosis especially in patients who have a history of handling thorny plants, moss, or timber. LA titers ≥1:8 are considered presumptive of sporotrichosis. Titers may reach as high as 1:512. Increasing or sustained high titers are helpful in the diagnosis of pulmonary sporotrichosis. CSF LA titers of ≥1:8 are presumptive evidence of meningeal sporotrichosis. LA titers are of limited prognostic value since levels show little change during convalescence. False-positive test results, especially in the range of 1:4 to 1:8, may occur with the LA test in patients with nonfungal diseases. An EIA titer ≥1:16 in serum and ≥1:8 in CSF is considered positive. Unlike LA titers, EIA titers decline with successful treatment. Antibodies frequently appear before cultures are positive for *S. schenckii*. The TA test demonstrates good sensitivity; however, false-positive reactions have been seen in patients with leishmaniasis. A negative test result does not rule out the diagnosis.

1. Rose NR, Hamilton RG, Detrick B, editors: *Manual of clinical immunology,* ed 6, Washington, DC, 2002, ASM Press.

TEST NAME AND METHOD	SPECIMEN AND SPECIAL REQUIREMENTS	CLINICAL COMMENTS AND REMARKS
Spotted Fever Group Serological Test (Rocky Mountain Spotted Fever Titer, Rickettsialpox Titer, *Rickettsia rickettsii* Titer, *Rickettsia akari* Titer)[1-3] IFA, LA, EIA, MIF	Serum drawn at onset of disease and 2-3 wk later. Convalescent specimen should be collected at 6-8 wk if acute specimen is negative.	Spotted fever group rickettsiae include *R. rickettsii* (Rocky Mountain spotted fever), *R. conorii* (boutonneuse fever), *R. africae* (African tick bite fever), *R. sibirica* (North Asian tick typhus), *R. australis* (North Queensland tick typhus), *R. honei* (Flinders Island spotted fever), *R. japonica* (Japanese spotted fever, and *R. akari* (rickettsialpox). Group-specific serology does not allow discrimination of a particular causative organism. A fourfold rise in titer between acute and convalescent sera is diagnostic for one of the spotted fever diseases; however, an IFA or LA titer ≥1:64 is highly suggestive of infection. Antibiotic therapy blunts and delays the antibody response.

1. Murray PR, Baron EJ, Jorgensen JH, et al, editors: *Manual of clinical microbiology,* ed 8, Washington, DC, 2003, ASM Press.
2. Rose NR, Hamilton RG, Detrick B, editors: *Manual of clinical immunology,* ed 6, Washington, DC, 2002, ASM Press.
3. Mandell GL, Bennett JE, Dolin R, editors: *Principles and practice of infectious diseases,* ed 5, New York, 2000, Churchill Livingstone.

TEST NAME AND METHOD	SPECIMEN AND SPECIAL REQUIREMENTS	CLINICAL COMMENTS AND REMARKS
Sputum Culture, Routine[1-6] (See *Respiratory Tract, Lower.*)	Sputum.	Patient should be instructed to remove dentures (if present), rinse mouth, and gargle with sterile saline or water, then cough deeply and expectorate sputum into a sterile container. A first morning specimen is preferred. Transport to lab immediately for processing.
		If the specimen is microscopically consistent with saliva rather than sputum (more than 10 squamous epithelial cells per low power field and few or no leukocytes), the specimen should be rejected for bacterial culture and another obtained. Results of culture should be interpreted in conjunction with Gram stain findings and clinical condition of the patient. Anaerobic cultures should not be performed.

1. Forbes BA, Sahm DF, Weissfeld AS: *Bailey & Scott's diagnostic microbiology,* ed 10, St Louis, 1998, Mosby.
2. Isenberg HD: *Clinical microbiology procedures handbook,* ed 2, Washington, DC, 2004, ASM Press.
3. Miller JM: *A guide to specimen management in clinical microbiology,* ed 2, Washington DC, 1998, ASM Press.
4. Murray PR, Baron EJ, Jorgensen JH, et al: *Manual of clinical microbiology,* ed 8, Washington, DC, 2003, ASM Press.
5. Murray PR, Washington JA: Microscopic and bacteriologic analysis of expectorated sputum, *Mayo Clin. Proc* 50:339-344, 1975.
6. Shanholtzer CJ, et al: Concentrated Gram stain smears prepared with a cytospin centrifuge, *J Clin. Microbiol* 16:1052-1056, 1982.

TEST NAME AND METHOD	SPECIMEN AND SPECIAL REQUIREMENTS	CLINICAL COMMENTS AND REMARKS
Stool Culture for Enteric Pathogens[1-8]	Stool, rectal swabs	**General Comments.** Freshly passed stool delivered to lab immediately in container with tightly fitting lid. Do not refrigerate specimen. If a delay of >30 min in processing is anticipated, transfer stool to transport vial containing Modified Cary-Blair medium with reduced agar content according to manufacturer's direction. Overfilling vial will lead to unsatisfactory preservation of enteric pathogens. Rectal swabs are collected by passing a swab tip approximately 1 inch beyond the anal sphincter, rotating to obtain a good sample, and placing the swab(s) in appropriate transport medium. Duodenal, colostomy, or ileostomy contents may be submitted in either a leakproof container or transport vial.
		Two stools collected from different days may be necessary to diagnose bacterial gastroenteritis. Specimens should be collected during the acute stage of disease. When specimens are submitted in a transport container with preservative or on swabs, the request should include information regarding specimen appearance (e.g., bloody, liquid, formed, solid, or mucoid). Bloody stools are generally associated with illness caused by either *Campylobacter* or strains of enterohemorrhagic *E. coli.*
		As part of the lab's rejection policy, stools should be rejected if: (1) stool is in transport >2 hr, but not in transport medium; (2) in transport medium longer than 24 hr at 25° C or 3 days at 4° C; (3) stool is hard or contains barium; (4) transport medium is yellow, indicating a low pH, which may kill *Shigella* spp.; (5) transport container is overfilled with stool; (6) specimen collected from patient hospitalized >3 days unless

TEST NAME AND METHOD	SPECIMEN AND SPECIAL REQUIREMENTS	CLINICAL COMMENTS AND REMARKS

Stool Culture for Enteric Pathogens—CONT

they are immunocompromised or are part of an institutional cluster epidemic; (7) swabs are dry or (8) more than three stools are submitted within a 3-wk period or more than one specimen is submitted within 1 day.

This procedure is used as a screen for the common enteric pathogens (e.g., *Salmonella* spp., *Shigella* spp., and *Campylobacter* spp.). Specify if other pathogens (e.g., *Vibrio* spp., *Yersinia* spp., enterohemorrhagic strains of *E. coli* [EHEC], including 0157:H7 that produce verotoxin, or *Clostridium difficile*) are suspected. Detection of large quantities of *Pseudomonas aeruginosa, S. aureus, Bacillus cereus,* yeast, or DF-3 should be reported without susceptibility testing. Antimicrobial susceptibility test (AST) should be performed on all enteric pathogens except: (1) EHEC since therapy can induce bacterial lysis, toxin release, and development of hemolytic uremic syndrome (HUS) and (2) *Salmonella* spp. since therapy may prolong the carrier state. The only instances when ASTs of *Salmonella* should be performed are when *Salmonella serovar typhi* is isolated, when the isolate is identified in urine or normally sterile closed body site fluid (i.e., extraintestinal site), in children less than 6 mo of age, or upon request.

Both differential and selective stool culture media should be inoculated to increase the chance of recovering the pathogen causing gastroenteritis. Because of the inhibitory properties of selective media, it should be inoculated heavily with a stool specimen. To increase recovery of small numbers of *Salmonella* or *Shigella,* enrichment broth may be inoculated and incubated for 6-24 hr before subculturing, depending on the broth selected. The method to minimize the number of plates of solid media used per specimen with little compromise in turnaround time to detection is to initially inoculate a MacConkey plate and GN broth. This broth is then subcultured in 6 hr onto selective media (e.g., XLD and Hektoen agar).

To recover campylobacter, avoid phosphate buffered glycerol transport media. Inoculate medium containing cefoperazone incubated at 42° C in a microaerobic environment. A wet mount of a fresh stool received within 30 min of collection may be useful to rapidly identify motile, darting curved rods moving in a zigzag fashion across the microscopic field. The use of a filtration technique that allows passage of motile campylobacters through pores of a filter for selective separation of campylobacters from nonmotile organisms and enrichment broth cultures may be helpful in recovering campylobacter after the acute stage of disease.

For hospitalized patients, positive results for enteric pathogens should be conveyed immediately to the infection control professional to place these patients on Contact Precautions. For cases suspected of life-threatening illness (e.g., *Salmonella serovar typhi* or *paratyphi C, V. cholerae,* or EHEC), the ordering physician should be notified immediately.

TEST NAME AND METHOD	SPECIMEN AND SPECIAL REQUIREMENTS	CLINICAL COMMENTS AND REMARKS

Stool Culture for Enteric Pathogens—CONT

Escherichia coli **0157:H7** *Culture* (*Verotoxin-producing* E. coli or VTEC)[3]		VTEC, also known as Shiga toxin-producing or enterohemorrhagic *E. coli* (EHEC), produces a toxin that is implicated in causing hemorrhagic colitis (HC) and is associated with hemolytic uremic syndrome (HUS), particularly in pediatric patients. Outbreaks have occurred with consumption of improperly cooked meat (e.g., hamburger). The most common toxin-producing strain is *E. coli* 0157:H7, although other *E. coli* serotypes can also produce toxin and have been related to disease. At a minimum, all bloody stools should be screened for *E. coli* 0157 using cefixime tellurite sorbitol MacConkey (MAC) agar (CT-SMAC). Sorbitol-negative colorless colonies are then tested by latex agglutination, and positive results generally can be confirmed with H7 flagellar antiserum and toxin testing at a public health lab. Preferably stool is inoculated into MAC broth for 24 hr at 35° C-37° C and tested using an EHEC EIA to detect verotoxin from *E. coli* 0157 and from other strains.
Vibrio parahaemolyticus[3]		*V. parahaemolyticus* is a marine bacterium that may produce an explosive, watery diarrhea with abdominal cramps and nausea 15-24 hr after ingestion of contaminated seafood. The symptoms may last several hours to 10 days, but usually subside without treatment in 3 days.
Vibrio cholerae[3]		Crab, lobster, shrimp, and seafood cocktail have been implicated in outbreaks in the U.S. The bacterium is transmitted when these foods are improperly refrigerated, insufficiently cooked, or cross-contaminated.
		Specimens should be collected within the first 24 hr of illness before the administration of antimicrobial agents. *V. cholerae* is very sensitive to desiccation, thus specimens must not be allowed to dry out.
		Rectal swabs may be adequate in the acute stage, but are less satisfactory than stool specimens. If there will be a delay in specimen processing, transport specimens in Cary-Blair transport medium or alkaline peptone water. Do not use glycerol-buffered saline for transport; glycerol may be toxic to *Vibrio* spp.
		The most common form of the disease is an acute gastroenteritis with abdominal pain, with or without bloody diarrhea, and fever. Specimens are best taken during the acute stage of the illness.
		A stool positive for *V. cholerae* is typically rice watery in appearance with a fishy odor. The clinical symptom of very severe cases is massive loss of fluid and electrolytes. For every severe case, there are 25-100 mild-to-asymptomatic infections. During the 1980s, both epidemic and environmental strains of *V. cholerae* were isolated in the U.S. In 1991 cases of cholera were identified in the U.S. subsequent to an outbreak in South America.
Yersinia enterocolitica[3]		Selective CIN medium or MacConkey agar incubated at room temperature or a cold enrichment procedure at 4° C with subculturing for 3-4 wk may be needed for isolation of the organism. Most outbreaks have occurred in northern Europe and Canada; however, there have been sporadic cases in the U.S.

TEST NAME AND METHOD	SPECIMEN AND SPECIAL REQUIREMENTS	CLINICAL COMMENTS AND REMARKS

Stool Culture for Enteric Pathogens—CONT

Clostridium difficile **Culture**[1] (See *Toxin Identification for Bacteriological Diseases, Clostridium difficile*)

Nonpreserved stool

Isolation of *C. difficile* from stool in suspected cases of antibiotic-associated diarrhea (AAD) or pseudomembranous colitis (PMC) may support the diagnosis, but demonstration of the specific toxin involved is necessary for confirmation.

C. difficile has been recovered from stool of patients with diarrhea who have received antimicrobial therapy without a clinical diagnosis of PMC. In healthy adults, the rate of isolation of *C. difficile* is 4%; in infants and young children, rates may be significantly higher. Carrier rates may also be high in seriously ill hospitalized patients.

1. Blot F, Nitenberg G, Chachaty E, et al: Diagnosis of catheter-related bacteremia: a prospective comparison of the time to positivity of hub-blood vs peripheral-blood cultures, *Lancet* 354:1071-1077, 1999.
2. Forbes BA, Sahm DF, Weissfeld AS: *Bailey & Scott's diagnostic microbiology,* ed 10, St Louis, 1998, Mosby.
3. Isenberg HD: *Clinical microbiology procedures handbook,* ed 2, Washington, DC, 2004, ASM Press.
4. Miller JM: *A guide to specimen management in clinical microbiology,* ed 2, Washington DC, 1998, ASM Press.
5. Morris AJ, Smith LK, Mirrett S, et al: Cost and time savings following introduction of rejection criteria for clinical specimens, *J Clin Microbiol* 34:355-357, 1996.
6. Murray PR, Baron EJ, Jorgensen JH, et al: *Manual of clinical microbiology,* ed 8, Washington, DC, 2003, ASM Press.
7. Nolte F: *Cumitech 12A-laboratory diagnosis of bacterial diarrhea,* Washington, DC, 1998, ASM Press.
8. Winn W Jr, Allen S, Janda W, et al: *Koneman's color atlas and textbook of diagnostic microbiology,* ed 6, Philadelphia, 2006, Lippincott Williams & Wilkins.

Stool Culture for Fungus[1,2]

Stool. (See *Stool Culture for Enteric Pathogens.*)

Rectal swabs are inadequate specimens.

Stool specimens are not recommended for the isolation of fungi. Colonization by yeasts is very common in both healthy and compromised individuals. If fungal infection of the gastrointestinal tract is suspected, tissue (biopsy) specimens are required for diagnosis.

See *General Comments.*

1. Murray PR, Baron EJ, Jorgensen JH, et al, editors: *Manual of clinical microbiology,* ed 8, Washington, DC, 2003, ASM Press.
2. Larone DH: *Medically important fungi: a guide to identification,* ed 4, Washington, DC, 2002, ASM Press.

Strongyloidiasis Serological Test[1,2]

EIA, IB

Serum. Collect in separation tube and freeze if not assayed immediately.

Test is helpful in supporting the diagnosis of *Strongyloides stercoralis* infection. The test is best applied when the organisms are not seen in the stool or duodenal examination. EIA is recommended with a sensitivity of 84%-92%, although both EIA and IB are reported to be both sensitive and specific. These assays have been shown to be of assistance in the determination of therapeutic response with an accompanying decrease in

TEST NAME AND METHOD	SPECIMEN AND SPECIAL REQUIREMENTS	CLINICAL COMMENTS AND REMARKS

Strongyloidiasis Serological Test—CONT

antibody titers posttherapy. Up to 16% of carriers may be seronegative with these assays. A single antibody titer can not be used to differentiate between current and past infection.

See *General Comment.*

1. Garcia LS: *Diagnostic medical parasitology,* ed 4, Washington, DC, 2001, ASM Press.
2. Rose NR, deMarcario EC, Fahey JL, et al, editors: *Manual of clinical laboratory immunology,* ed 4, Washington, DC, 1992, American Society for Microbiology.

Superficial Wound Culture for Fungus[1-3]

Pus, exudates, and drainage. See *Superficial Wound Culture, Routine.*

The skin over pustular lesions should be disinfected and exudates aspirated using a sterile needle and syringe. Aspirates should be placed in a sterile container for transport to the laboratory. Biopsy of the lesion may be required if the aspirate fails to yield fungi. Swab specimens are not recommended.

If present, granules may signify an actinomycotic infection or may indicate a eumycotic mycetoma associated with *Pseudallescheria boydii, Acremonium* spp., *Madurella* spp., or a variety of other fungi.

See *General Comments.*

1. Murray PR, Baron EJ, Jorgensen JH, et al, editors: *Manual of clinical microbiology,* ed 8, Washington, DC, 2003, ASM Press.
2. Larone DH: *Medically important fungi: a guide to identification,* ed 4, Washington, DC, 2002, ASM Press.
3. Koneman EW, Allen SD, Janda WM, et al, editors: *Color atlas and textbook of diagnostic microbiology,* ed 4, Philadelphia, 1992, JB Lippincott.

Superficial Wound Culture, Routine[1-8]

Aspirate (preferred) of material from wound, abscess, cellulitis

An aspirate ≥ 1 mL from a previously undrained abscess, if properly collected and transported, will be of greatest value. Swabs of deep wounds or abscesses are of limited value. Transport to lab as soon as possible in an anaerobic system or, in a transport system if a swab is used.

Repeated cultures of open, draining wounds or of large areas of devitalized tissue frequently yield many microorganisms of questionable significance. Histopathological examination of biopsy material may be a necessary adjunct to culture, in particular when a chronic, localized infection occurs.

TEST NAME AND METHOD	SPECIMEN AND SPECIAL REQUIREMENTS	CLINICAL COMMENTS AND REMARKS

Superficial Wound Culture, Routine—CONT

1. Isenberg HD: *Clinical microbiology procedures handbook,* ed 2, Washington, DC, 2004, ASM Press.
2. Mandell GL, Bennett JE, Dolin R: *Principles and practice of infectious diseases,* ed 6, Philadelphia, 2005, Elsevier Churchill Livingstone.
3. Miller JM: *A guide to specimen management in clinical microbiology,* ed 2, Washington DC, 1998, ASM Press.
4. Morris AJ, Wilson SJ, Marx CE, et al Clinical impact of bacteria and fungi recovered only from broth cultures, *J Clin Microbiol* 33:161-165, 1995.
5. Murray PR, Baron EJ, Jorgensen JH, et al: *Manual of clinical microbiology,* ed 8, Washington, DC, 2003, ASM Press.
6. Smith, JA: *Cumitech 23-Infections of the skin and subcutaneous tissues,* Washington, DC, 1988, ASM Press.
7. Woolfrey BF, Fox JM, Quall CO: An evaluation of burn wound quantitative microbiology: I. Quantitative eschar cultures, *Am J Clin Pathol* 75:532-537, 1981.
8. Winn W Jr, Allen S, Janda W, et al: *Koneman's color atlas and textbook of diagnostic microbiology,* ed 6, Philadelphia, 2006, Lippincott Williams & Wilkins.

Syphilis
**(*Treponema*
pallidum) Tests**

Direct Examination (Darkfield Examination, DFA-TP)[1,2]	Darkfield examination: genital lesions. DFA-TP: oral, genital, and rectal lesions; amniotic fluid; placenta; umbilicus; skin lesions.	To obtain scrapings superficial debris should be cleaned before collection. Gently abrade the base of the cleansed chancre with saline-moistened gauze to obtain serous fluid. Specimens for darkfield microscopy should be collected on a glass slide, covered with a coverslip, and transported to the laboratory immediately. Specimens for DFA-TP should be collected on a glass slide and allowed to air-dry. Direct examination is useful for the diagnosis of primary, secondary, and early congenital syphilis. Serological tests are often not positive for 14-21 days after infection, and the direct detection of spirochetes may be the only way to establish an early diagnosis. Darkfield examinations should be performed within 30 min of specimen collection to ensure the presence of motile spirochetes. In addition darkfield examination is of no value for oral lesions due to the presence of nonpathogenic spirochetes in the normal oral flora. DFA-TP of tissue and body fluid is especially valuable in the diagnosis of congenital syphilis.
Treponemal Specific Tests	Serum. Reactive specimens must be reported to the state health department.	A negative direct examination of scrapings is not adequate to rule out infection with *Treponema pallidum.* Treponema lesions frequently exude infectious material; therefore care should be taken when handling these specimens.
Fluorescent Treponemal Antibody Absorption (FTA-ABS)[1,2]		The test should be used only to confirm reactive nontreponemal (RPR, VDRL) serological tests for syphilis. Only when late syphilis is suspected should an FTA-ABS be performed when the nontreponemal test is nonreactive.

TEST NAME AND METHOD	SPECIMEN AND SPECIAL REQUIREMENTS	CLINICAL COMMENTS AND REMARKS
Syphilis—CONT		
		The sensitivity of the FTA-ABS is as follows: Primary syphilis 84% (range: 70%-100%) Secondary syphilis 100 Latent syphilis 100 Late syphilis 96
		False-positive results may occur in cases of collagen vascular disease.
		The test is not to be used as a screen for syphilis and is not recommended for CSF specimens.
Treponema pallidum Passive Particle Agglutination (TP-PA)[1,2]	Serum. Reactive specimens must be reported to the state health department.	The test should be used only to confirm reactive nontreponemal (RPR, VDRL) serological tests for syphilis. Only when late syphilis is suspected should a TP-PA be performed when the nontreponemal test is nonreactive.
		The sensitivity of the TP-PA is as follows: Primary syphilis 86% (range: 86%-100%) Secondary syphilis 100 Latent syphilis 100
		False-positive results have occurred in patients with connective tissue disease, leprosy, and infectious mononucleosis.
		The TP-PA, like the FTA-ABS test, is not to be used as a screen for syphilis and is not recommended for CSF specimens.
Nontreponemal Tests *Rapid Plasma Reagin (RPR) Screening Test*[1,2]	Serum.	The RPR test is used as a screening test for primary and secondary syphilis. Sensitivity of the test varies in primary syphilis, but by 2 mo test sensitivity is 100%. Reactive RPR tests should be confirmed with an FTA-ABS or TP-PA. In addition reactive specimens should be titered to monitor therapy or establish reinfection. The titer should decline following successful therapy. A fourfold increase in titer usually indicates treatment failure or reinfection.
		Biological false-positive results may occur in cases of collagen diseases, such as rheumatoid arthritis and lupus erythematosus; in infections, such as infectious mononucleosis, leprosy, and malaria; in pregnancy; and in addiction.

TEST NAME AND METHOD	SPECIMEN AND SPECIAL REQUIREMENTS	CLINICAL COMMENTS AND REMARKS

Syphilis—CONT

TEST NAME AND METHOD	SPECIMEN AND SPECIAL REQUIREMENTS	CLINICAL COMMENTS AND REMARKS
VDRL (Venereal Disease Research Laboratory) Test[1,2]	Serum, CSF (Grossly bloody specimens are unacceptable.)	The serum VDRL test is used as a screening test for primary and secondary syphilis. Sensitivity of the test varies in primary syphilis, but by 2 mo test sensitivity is 100%. Reactive serum VDRL tests should be confirmed with an FTA-ABS or TP-PA. In addition reactive specimens should be titered to monitor therapy or establish reinfection. The titer should decline following successful therapy. A fourfold increase in titer usually indicates treatment failure or reinfection.

Biological false-positive results may occur as with the RPR. (See *Rapid Plasma Reagin Screening Test, serum,* above.)

The CSF VDRL test is used for the diagnosis of neurosyphilis. The test has a specificity of 99.8%, but a sensitivity of 50%. Therefore a negative test result does not rule out the presence of neurosyphilis. Reactive specimens should be titered to monitor therapy or establish reinfection. The titer should decline following successful therapy. Reactive CSF VDRL tests are not confirmed with a treponemal-specific test. |

1.   Murray PR, Baron EJ, Jorgensen JH, et al, editors: *Manual of clinical microbiology,* ed 8, Washington, DC, 2003, ASM Press.
2.   Rose NR, Hamilton RG, Detrick B, editors: *Manual of clinical immunology,* ed 6, Washington, DC, 2002, ASM Press.

TEST NAME AND METHOD	SPECIMEN AND SPECIAL REQUIREMENTS	CLINICAL COMMENTS AND REMARKS
Throat Culture[1] *Routine*	Throat swab	With the exception of deep pharyngeal cultures collected from patients with cystic fibrosis, throat specimens should not be routinely cultured. Only cultures to diagnose specific pathogens (e.g., group A *Streptococcus pyogenes, Corynebacterium diphtheriae, Neisseria gonorrhoeae, Arcanobacterium haemolyticum*) should be processed.
Group A Streptococcus (GAS) Screen[2,3] *Rapid* EIA, Probe, PCR	Swab of oropharynx, tonsillar exudate	Select a rapid group A strep (GAS) antigen test that has high sensitivity since even low numbers of organisms may reflect infection. Because of the difficulty in obtaining good specimens from young children, the American Academy of Pediatrics recommends that negative rapid antigen tests be confirmed by culture for beta-hemolytic GAS. In contrast negative GAS antigen screening tests on specimens collected from adults do not require a reflex culture if the sensitivity of the antigen test exceeds 80%.

Colony quantitation should not be included on the report to distinguish colonization from infection. This distinction should be made on clinical grounds. |

TEST NAME AND METHOD	SPECIMEN AND SPECIAL REQUIREMENTS	CLINICAL COMMENTS AND REMARKS

Throat Culture—CONT

Corynebacterium diphtheriae[1] — Nasopharyngeal swab from inflamed areas and beneath pseudomembrane, if present

It is a requirement of the College of American Pathologists (CAP) that laboratories have a mechanism to culture *C. diphtheriae* in-house or to refer specimens when requested.

The microbiology laboratory should be contacted before specimen collection to ensure appropriate processing of the specimen on special media. Specimens should be collected on cotton-tipped or polyester-tipped swabs. If delay in inoculation of media is anticipated beyond 24 hr, silica gel-containing transport containers should be used to maintain viability. If cutaneous diphtheria is suspected, throat, nasopharyngeal, and skin swabs or aspirates should be collected for culture.

Specimens should be processed in a biosafety cabinet and inoculated media (e.g., blood agar, cystine tellurite blood agar) should be incubated aerobically without CO_2. Direct smears are not reliable for diagnosis since metachromatic granules are seen in other bacteria as well.

If biochemical results are consistent with *C. diphtheriae,* a presumptive report may be issued without quantitation and the isolate forwarded to a public health laboratory for diphtheria confirmation based on a positive toxin test result. A less severe form of diphtheria with pharyngitis, endocarditis, septic arthritis, or other systemic manifestations may occur when the patient is infected with a nontoxigenic strain.

Neisseria gonorrhoeae[1] (See *Genital Culture.*) — Throat swab from tonsillar regions and posterior pharynx

Plate at bedside or transport swabs to lab immediately following specimen collection.

Oropharyngeal infection is generally asymptomatic and occurs preponderantly in homosexual males. A few patients, however, may have acute pharyngitis and tonsillitis.

A Gram stain of the specimen is noncontributory. A culture of anorectal genital sites should also be requested. Inoculate specimens onto modified Thayer-Martin medium. Isolates must be confirmed biochemically since *N. meningitidis* may be present without symptoms.

---

1. Isenberg HD: *Clinical microbiology procedures handbook,* ed 2, Washington, DC, 2004, ASM Press.
2. Forbes BA, Sahm DF, Weissfeld AS: *Bailey & Scott's diagnostic microbiology,* ed 10, St Louis, 1998, Mosby.
3. Gerber MA: Diagnosis of group A beta-hemolytic streptococcal pharyngitis. Use of antigen detection tests, *Diagn Microbiol Infect Dis* 4(3 suppl):5S-15S, 1986.

TEST NAME AND METHOD	SPECIMEN AND SPECIAL REQUIREMENTS	CLINICAL COMMENTS AND REMARKS
Throat, Mouth, Ear, Nose Culture for Fungus[1]	Throat, mouth, ear, nose swabs. Swab the area of exudate or plaque. Deliver to laboratory immediately in a swab transport system. For suspected cases of thrush, scrapings of the lesions are preferred.	Patients with a high incidence of oral candidiasis (thrush) include: newborns, patients on steroids, and cancer and AIDS patients. Plaques or patches consisting of masses of mycelial and yeast forms are found on the buccal mucosa, tongue, palate, and other mucous membranes. The plaques may remain discrete or coalesce to form a continuous white-to-gray pseudomembrane. The diagnosis of thrush is made by the clinical appearance of the lesion and by direct examination of the scraping showing masses of pseudohyphae and yeast cells. Culture alone does not solidify the diagnosis since *Candida* can be isolated from the oral cavity of normal healthy persons. Culture may be particularly helpful in refractory cases.

1. Murray PR, Baron EJ, Jorgensen JH, et al, editors: *Manual of clinical microbiology,* ed 8, Washington, DC, 2003, ASM Press.

TEST NAME AND METHOD	SPECIMEN AND SPECIAL REQUIREMENTS	CLINICAL COMMENTS AND REMARKS
Tissue Culture for Fungus[1-3]	Tissue. If possible portions of the wall, base, and center of the lesion should be collected and placed between gauze moistened with sterile water or 0.85% nonbacteriostatic saline in a sterile container.	If present in subcutaneous tissue, granules may signify an actinomycotic infection or may indicate a eumycotic mycetoma associated with *Pseudallescheria boydii, Acremonium* spp., *Madurella* spp., or a variety of other fungi. See *General Comments.*

1. Murray PR, Baron EJ, Jorgensen JH, et al, editors: *Manual of clinical microbiology,* ed 8, Washington, DC, 2003, ASM Press.
2. Larone DH: *Medically important fungi: a guide to identification,* ed 4, Washington, DC, 2002, ASM Press.
3. Winn W Jr, Allen S, Janda W, et al: *Koneman's color atlas and textbook of diagnostic microbiology,* ed 6, Philadelphia, 2006, Lippincott Williams & Wilkins.

TEST NAME AND METHOD	SPECIMEN AND SPECIAL REQUIREMENTS	CLINICAL COMMENTS AND REMARKS
Toxocariasis Serological Test (Visceral Larva Migrans Serological Test)[1-3] *EIA*	Serum. Collect in separation tube and freeze if not assayed immediately.	The causative organism is *Toxocara canis,* which is transmitted to the human by ingestion of infectious eggs in canine stools. Visceral larva migrans (VLM) and ocular larva migrans (OLM) are seen primarily in young children. A diagnostic EIA titer of 1:32 is considered significant for VLM, and for OLM a titer of 1:8 is considered diagnostic. For VLM and OLM, the sensitivity is 78% and 90%, respectively.

TEST NAME AND METHOD	SPECIMEN AND SPECIAL REQUIREMENTS	CLINICAL COMMENTS AND REMARKS

Toxocariasis Serological Test—CONT

EIA is highly specific and does commonly not give cross-reactions with sera from patients with other helminth infections, but titers may be positive in patients with asymptomatic *Toxocara* infections or ocular infections of other organisms.

See *General Comment.*

1. Garcia LS: *Diagnostic medical parasitology,* ed 4, Washington, DC, 2001, ASM Press.
2. Rose NR, deMarcario EC, Fahey JL, et al, editors: *Manual of clinical laboratory immunology,* ed 4, Washington, DC, 1992, American Society for Microbiology.
3. Ash LR, Orihel TC: *A guide to laboratory procedures and identification,* Chicago, 1987, American Society for Clinical Pathologists.

Toxoplasmosis Serological Test (Toxoplasmosis Titer)[1-4]

EIA, IFA

Serum. Collect in separation tube and freeze if not assayed immediately.

Individuals with detectable antibodies to *Toxoplasma gondii* are in high numbers in most populations around the world making serodiagnosis troublesome. EIA and IFA are the preferred methods of testing in the U.S.

Elevation in IgG specific titers may suggest recent infection, although high titers can be present for a number of years after primary infection. Although this rarely occurs in practice, the demonstration of a conversion from a negative to a positive result or a fourfold rise in IgG titer over a period of several weeks will confirm a diagnosis. When IgG antibodies are present, a positive IgM result is suggestive of acute infection within the last 12 mo. However, one must keep in mind that although IgM titers normally return to undetectable levels within 6-9 mo, it can be detected for as long as 18 mo postinfection.

See *General Comment.*

1. Rose NR, deMarcario EC, Fahey JL, et al, editors: *Manual of clinical laboratory immunology,* ed 4, Washington, DC, 1992, American Society for Microbiology.
2. Murray PR, Baron EJ, Jorgensen JH, et al, editors: *Manual of clinical microbiology,* ed 8, Washington, DC, 2003, ASM Press.
3. Mandell GL, Bennett JE, Dolin R: *Principles and practice of infectious diseases,* ed 5, New York, 2000, Churchill Livingstone.
4. Garcia L.S: *Diagnostic medical parasitology,* ed 4, Washington, DC, 2001, ASM Press.

TEST NAME AND METHOD	SPECIMEN AND SPECIAL REQUIREMENTS	CLINICAL COMMENTS AND REMARKS
Trichinosis Serological Test (Trichinosis Titer)[1-4] *BF, EIA*	Serum. Collect in separation tube and freeze if not assayed immediately.	These tests are used to support the clinical diagnosis of trichinosis caused by *Trichinella spiralis.* A positive EIA test result is confirmed with the BF test. A positive reaction in both tests indicated infection within the past few years. Antibodies are usually not detected for the first 3-5 wk of infection, peak in 2-3 mo, and then decline over a few years. Positive serological reactions are seen in 80%-100% of infected persons at some point during symptomatic disease. See *General Comment.*

1. Rose NR, deMarcario EC, Fahey JL, et al, editors: *Manual of clinical laboratory immunology,* ed 4, Washington, DC, 1992, American Society for Microbiology.
2. Garcia L S: *Diagnostic medical parasitology,* ed 4, Washington, DC, 2001, ASM Press.
3. Mandell GL, Bennett JE, Dolin R: *Principles and practice of infectious diseases,* ed 5, New York, 2000, Churchill Livingstone.
4. Ash LR, Orihel TC: *A guide to laboratory procedures and identification,* Chicago, 1987, American Society for Clinical Pathologists.

Trichomonas Preparation (Trichomonas Smear, Trichomonas Wet Preparation)[1-3]	Adequate volume of freshly voided urine (use sediment for examination). Secretions of vaginal, urethral, or prostatic fluid transported to lab immediately in a transport system or on a moist swab. Do not refrigerate specimen.	The procedure is used to detect infection with *Trichomonas vaginalis.* Specimens should be diluted with a drop of saline and examined immediately to note active motility. One negative examination does not rule out the diagnosis of trichomonad infection. Douching should not be done 3 days before collection of vaginal specimens. Culture of the organism is the definitive method of diagnosis and can be used when infection is suspected and smears are negative. Commercial systems are available for culture of *T. vaginalis.* Other diagnostic tests include permanent stains, such as Giemsa or Papanicolaou's and fluorescent stains. Several diagnostic tests for molecular or immunodetection of *T. vaginalis* are also commercially available. Serological tests are not routinely available.

1. Rose NR, deMarcario EC, Fahey JL, et al, editors: *Manual of clinical laboratory immunology,* ed 4, Washington, DC, 1992, American Society for Microbiology.
2. Garcia L S: *Diagnostic medical parasitology,* ed 4, Washington, DC, 2001, ASM Press.
3. Murray PR, Baron EJ, Jorgensen JH, et al, editors: *Manual of clinical microbiology,* ed 8, Washington, DC, 2003, ASM Press.

TEST NAME AND METHOD	SPECIMEN AND SPECIAL REQUIREMENTS	CLINICAL COMMENTS AND REMARKS
Trypanosomiasis Serological Test (Trypanosomiasis Serum Titer, Chagas' Disease Serological Test, Chagas' Disease Titer)[1-4] *CF, IFA, IHA, EIA*	Serum. Collect in separation tube and freeze if not assayed immediately.	This test is used to support the diagnosis of Chagas' disease caused by *Trypanosoma cruzi*. Endemic areas for Chagas' disease are Central and South America. In the acute stage of the disease, serological testing is unnecessary because of the good sensitivity of the examination of blood films; however, in the chronic forms of the disease and in the immunosuppressed patient, serological tests are of greater assistance. Current serodiagnostic assays for *T. cruzi* are prone to cross-reactions with other infectious diseases, such as malaria, leishmania, syphilis, toxoplasmosis, hepatitis, leprosy, schistosomiasis, infectious mononucleosis, systemic lupus erythematosus, and rheumatoid arthritis. Thus it is recommended that at least two, and perhaps three, different conventional tests be positive before accepting a diagnosis. Screening of donated blood for *T. cruzi* antibodies is performed in areas where Chagas' disease is endemic. See *General Comment*.

1. Rose NR, deMarcario EC, Fahey JL, et al, editors: *Manual of clinical laboratory immunology,* ed 4, Washington, DC, 1992, American Society for Microbiology.
2. Garcia L S: *Diagnostic medical parasitology,* ed 4, Washington, DC, 2001, ASM Press.
3. Mandell GL, Bennett JE, Dolin R: *Principles and practice of infectious diseases,* ed 5, New York, 2000, Churchill Livingstone.
4. Ash LR, Orihel TC: *A guide to laboratory procedures and identification,* Chicago, 1987, American Society for Clinical Pathologists.

TEST NAME AND METHOD	SPECIMEN AND SPECIAL REQUIREMENTS	CLINICAL COMMENTS AND REMARKS
Tularemia Antibody Test *(Francisella tularensis)*[1]	Serum, drawn the first wk of illness and 5 wk later	A positive test result supports a clinical diagnosis of tularemia. A history of contact with rabbits, ticks, dogs, cats, or skunks is suggestive, but a negative history does not rule out the diagnosis. *Francisella tularensis* antibodies appear in 2-3 wk after onset and peak in ~5 wk. A fourfold increase in titer is indicative of active disease.

1. Murray PR, Baron EJ, Jorgensen JH, et al: *Manual of clinical microbiology,* ed 8, Washington, DC, 2003, ASM Press.

TEST NAME AND METHOD	SPECIMEN AND SPECIAL REQUIREMENTS	CLINICAL COMMENTS AND REMARKS
Typhus Group Serological Test (Epidemic Typhus Titer, Murine Typhus Titer, *Rickettsia prowazekii* Titer, *Rickettsia typhi* Titer)[1-3] *IFA, LA, EIA, MIF*	Serum drawn at onset of disease and 2-3 wk later	Typhus group rickettsiae include *R. prowazekii* (epidemic or louse-borne typhus, including the recrudescent form Brill-Zinsser disease) and *R. typhi* (murine typhus). Since typhus rickettsiae share antigens, serological evaluation will not distinguish between epidemic and murine typhus. *R. typhi* antibodies are rarely present during acute illness. Diagnostic titers are present in only 50% of patients with murine typhus at day 7, and 100% of patients are positive at day 15. Cross-reacting antibody reactions may be observed between the typhus groups and spotted fever group rickettsiae. A fourfold rise in titer between acute and convalescent sera is considered diagnostic.

1. Murray PR, Baron EJ, Jorgensen JH, et al, editors: *Manual of clinical microbiology,* ed 8, Washington, DC, 2003, ASM Press.
2. Rose NR, Hamilton RG, Detrick B, editors: *Manual of clinical immunology,* ed 6, Washington, DC, 2002, ASM Press.
3. Mandell GL, Bennett JE, Dolin R, editors: *Principles and practice of infectious diseases,* ed 5, New York, 2000, Churchill Livingstone.

TEST NAME AND METHOD	SPECIMEN AND SPECIAL REQUIREMENTS	CLINICAL COMMENTS AND REMARKS
Urine Culture for Fungus[1-3]	Urine. See *Urine Culture, Routine (Catheterized, Midvoid, Suprapubic).* Collection of a first morning "midstream" specimen is best. 24-hr urines are unacceptable.	The specimen should be collected in a sterile container, and the total volume of the urine sample should be delivered to the laboratory. *Cryptococcus neoformans* may be isolated from the urine of a patient with cryptococcal pyelonephritis or prostatitis. Infections of the upper urinary tract may sometimes require collection of urine from each kidney through a urethral catheter. Quantitation of yeast isolates in urine does not have the same interpretive value as that of bacteria and does not adequately correlate with clinical disease. See *General Comments.*

1. Murray PR, Baron EJ, Jorgensen JH, et al, editors: *Manual of clinical microbiology,* ed 8, Washington, DC, 2003, ASM Press.
2. Larone DH: *Medically important fungi: a guide to identification,* ed 4, Washington, DC, 2002, ASM Press.
3. Koneman EW, Allen SD, Janda WM, et al, editors: *Color atlas and textbook of diagnostic microbiology,* ed 4, Philadelphia, 1992, JB Lippincott.

TEST NAME AND METHOD	SPECIMEN AND SPECIAL REQUIREMENTS	CLINICAL COMMENTS AND REMARKS
Urine Culture, Routine[1-17]	First morning midstream and clean voided	Process specimen aerobically within 2 hr. If a delay in processing is anticipated, refrigerate the specimen or preferably place the urine in a transport device to preserve the colony count. *Anaerobic cultures and culture of urine in broth are inappropriate.*
	Female: Clean meatus with green soap and gauze pads by spreading the labia and washing from front to back. Four pads should be used, one stroke per pad. Rinse the outer genitalia and area around the meatus with sterile water. Patients should urinate into commode and without interrupting the flow of urine collect the middle portion of the void.	One morphotype with a colony count of 10^5/mL from a properly collected urine specimen that has been incubating in the bladder for at least 5 hr is considered significant. Lower colony counts may be significant in young females with urethritis. There are several good references for quantitative interpretation of urine specimens.[13 16]
	Males: Clean the urethral meatus with soap and rinse with sterile water.	
	Catheterized	1. Clamp drainage tubing for 10 min below the level of urine sample port. 2. Cleanse the urine sample port with an alcohol pledget. 3. Insert needle into urine sample port. 4. Withdraw 4 mL of urine. 5. Place specimen in sterile container. 6. Unclamp tubing.
		Deliver urine to lab within 2 hr, refrigerate, or place in transport device for delivery to the laboratory.
Urine Screen		A urine screening procedure may be used to rapidly detect bacteriuria/pyuria with a sensitivity of $\geq 10^5$. Lower counts may be considered significant and require culture confirmation. There are several methods for urine screens including Gram stain, dipsticks to detect leukocyte esterase that reflect white blood cells caused by pyuria, nitrate reduction; blood, and bacteria; and photometric, bioluminescence, and colorimetric filtration procedures. If approved by the medical staff, urine specimens may be screened and reflexed for culture in the event that a positive threshold is met.
Suprapubic	Aspirated urine	Puncture bladder through lower abdominal wall using a sterile needle and syringe. Deliver to lab immediately for processing.
		Suprapubic aspirates are indicated for patients with equivocal colony counts, clinical evidence of urinary tract infection, and for neonates and young children. The presence of all organisms are identified, with the exception of obvious skin contaminants. Urine collected in this manner is the only acceptable urine specimen for anaerobic culture.
		Culture of Foley catheter tips is inappropriate.

TEST NAME AND METHOD	SPECIMEN AND SPECIAL REQUIREMENTS	CLINICAL COMMENTS AND REMARKS

Urine Culture, Routine—CONT

1. Albers AC, Fletcher RD: Accuracy of calibrated-loop transfer, *J Clin Microbiol* 18:40-42, 1983.

2. Clarridge JE, Pezzlo MT, Vosti KL: *Cumitech 2A-laboratory diagnosis of urinary tract infections,* vol. 2A, coordinating editor, Weissfeld AS, Washington, DC, 1987, ASM Press.

3. Forbes BA, Sahm DF, Weissfeld AS: *Bailey & Scott's diagnostic microbiology,* ed 10, St Louis, 1998, Mosby.

4. Hooton TM, Stamm WE: Diagnosis and treatment of uncomplicated urinary tract infection, *Infect Dis Clin N Am* 11:551-581, 1997.

5. Isenberg HD: *Clinical microbiology procedures handbook,* ed 2, Washington, DC, 2004, ASM Press.

6. Kass FH: Asymptomatic infections of the urinary tract, *Trans Assoc Am Phys* 69:56-64, 1956.

7. Lifshitz E, Kramer L: Outpatient urine culture: does collection technique matter? *Arch Intern Med* 160:2537-2540, 2000.

8. Mandell GL, Bennett JE, Dolin R: *Principles and practice of infectious diseases,* ed 6, Philadelphia, 2005, Elsevier Churchill Livingstone.

9. Miller JM: *A guide to specimen management in clinical microbiology,* ed 2, Washington DC, 1998, ASM Press.

10. Murray PR, Baron EJ, Jorgensen JH, et al: *Manual of clinical microbiology,* ed 8, Washington, DC, 2003, ASM Press.

11. Valenstein P, Meier F: Urine culture contamination: a College of American Pathologists Q-Probes study of contaminated urine cultures in 906 institutions, *Arch Pathol Lab Med* 122:123-129, 1998.

12. Weissfeld AC: *Cumitech 2B-laboratory diagnosis of urinary tract infections,* Washington, DC, 1998, ASM Press.

13. Bannatyne RM, et al: Rapid detection of *Brucella* bacteremia by using the BACTEC 9240 system, *J Clin Microbiol* 35:2673-2674, 1997.

14. Blot F, et al: Diagnosis of catheter-related bacteremia: a prospective comparison of the time to positivity of hub-blood vs peripheral-blood cultures, *Lancet* 354:1071-1077, 1999.

15. Cantral, DE, Tape TG, Reed EC, et al: Quantitative culture of bronchoalveolar lavage fluid for the diagnosis of bacterial pneumonia, *Am J Med* 5:601-607, 1993.

16. Gerber MA: Diagnosis of group A beta-hemolytic streptococcal pharyngitis: use of antigen detection tests, *Diagn Microbiol Infect Dis* 4:5S-15S, 1986.

17. Winn W Jr, Allen S, Janda W, et al: *Koneman's color atlas and textbook of diagnostic microbiology,* ed 6, Philadelphia, 2006, Lippincott Williams & Wilkins.

Vaginal Culture for Fungus[1]	Swab of vagina, vulva, or labia placed into a transport system and delivered to the laboratory immediately.	Vaginal candidiasis is usually diagnosed based on clinical symptoms and direct microscopic examination of vaginal secretions. Since *Candida* spp. are part of the normal vaginal flora in up to 20% of healthy females, the recovery of *Candida* spp. is of little value. Cultures are useful in monitoring therapy in refractory disease. See *General Comments*.

1. Murray PR, Baron EJ, Jorgensen JH, et al, editors: *Manual of clinical microbiology,* ed 8, Washington, DC, 2003, ASM Press.

TEST NAME AND METHOD	SPECIMEN AND SPECIAL REQUIREMENTS	CLINICAL COMMENTS AND REMARKS
Varicella-Zoster, Direct Test[6] *Tzanck prep,* *EM, IFA, PCR*	Skin scrapings from base of fresh lesions. Vesicular fluid is collected in capillary pipette or aspirated with tuberculin syringe.	Varicella is a highly communicable disease. Incubation period ranges from 10-23 days (average of 14 days). A history of previous varicella infection indicates immunity. Tzanck preparation is used for the direct examination of herpes virus in skin scrapings but cannot distinguish VZV from HSV. EM can also be used as well but not for distinguishing between VZV and HSV. IFA uses a monoclonal antibody and is specific for VZV. Specimens with too few epithelial cells should be considered unsatisfactory for examination. Real time and traditional PCR tests are highly reliable for detection of VZV from variety of sources, but the main use of PCR is to distinguish between WT and vaccine strains. PCR products from a WT virus contains *Pst*I restriction site. Vaccine strains do not contain PstI restriction site. PCR is often used to investigate cases of possible transmission of vaccine and WT VZV to susceptible contacts.

1. Lennette EH, Smith TF, editors: *Laboratory diagnosis of viral infection,* ed 3, New York, 1999, Marcel Dekker.

TEST NAME AND METHOD	SPECIMEN AND SPECIAL REQUIREMENTS	CLINICAL COMMENTS AND REMARKS
Varicella-Zoster Virus Serological Test (Herpes Zoster Virus, Chickenpox)[1-3] *EIA, NT, FAMA, CF*	Serum, acute and convalescent. See *General Information.*	VZV is a highly contagious virus that causes two distinct clinical illnesses. A generalized vesicular rash characterizes primary infection, chickenpox. VZV may also reactivate decades after primary infection to cause a dermatomally distributed rash also known as shingles. The EIA test is the preferred assay for diagnosis and determination of immune status. The antibody can be detected within 48 hr after onset of rash. Passively acquired antibody can be detected up to 8 wk following VZ immune globulin administration. The CF test cannot be used to determine immune status of exposed patients, especially adults, since titers fall within 12 mo. Neutralization tests are useful, and the antibodies persist for life; however, the tests are not readily available. The fluorescent antibody to membrane antigen (FAMA) is a specific and sensitive test to determine immune status and to measure IgG, IgM, and IgA. The major disadvantage of FEMA is that live virus-infected cells are required

1. Lennette EH, Smith TF, editors: *Laboratory diagnosis of viral infection,* ed 3, New York, 1999, Marcel Dekker.

2. Murray, PR, Baron EJ, Jorgensen JH, et al, editors: *Manual of clinical microbiology,* ed 8, Washington, DC, 2003, American Society for Microbiology.

3. Rose NR, Hamilton RG, Detrick B, editors: *Manual of clinical laboratory immunology,* ed 6, Washington, DC, 2002, American Society for Microbiology.

TEST NAME AND METHOD	SPECIMEN AND SPECIAL REQUIREMENTS	CLINICAL COMMENTS AND REMARKS
Virus Culture[1-2]	Adequate specimen is mandatory. Aspirates, scrapings, and tissue are superior to swab specimens. If swabs are used, they should be cotton or Dacron, not calcium alginate. See Table IV-2 for appropriate specimens for viral isolation in selected clinical syndromes.	The ability to propagate viral particles in cultivated mammalian cells has been the backbone of clinical virology laboratories. Over the years several, primary, diploid, and continuous cell lines have been established to grow most viral agents. Based on suspected pathogen and the source of the specimen, one or more of these cell lines are used to detect the infecting viral agent. Despite these efforts a large number of viral agents either do not grow in vitro or requires several weeks to generate CPE. For many years direct examination of the specimen by electron microscopy (EM) had complemented the traditional viral culture. In recent years, however, highly sensitive and rapid EIA, IFA, and similar assays have virtually replaced EM in the diagnostic laboratories. More recently the introduction of molecular-based techniques, such as direct probe, traditional PCR, real time PCR, bDNA, and NASBA, into the clinical laboratories have transformed and provided a theoretical mean for the laboratories to detect virtually any viral agent. Using these techniques it is now possible to detect, monitor, and predict antiviral resistance and therapeutic outcomes for most viral infections.
Shell vial culture	Specimens should be processed as quickly as possible. For short-term transit or storage (>24 hr) of most viral suspensions, the specimen should be held at 4° C rather than frozen. If longer delays are expected, freeze at −60° C; when ready to process, thaw the sample slowly, raising the temperature about 2-5° C/min.	Shell vial assay is based on inoculating the specimen onto a shell vial, which contains a coverslip that has a monolayer of susceptible cells. Vials are centrifuged, media added, and incubated 16-24 to 48 hr. Following the incubation, the medium is aspirated, and the monolayer is removed and stained to detect viral antigen by FA. Shell vial was originally developed to detect CMV. The new generation of shell vial that is using hybrid cell lines, such as R-Mix (mink lung and A549), which detects all the respiratory viruses; E-Mix (A549 and Buffalo green monkey kidney), which detects enterovirus; H and V-Mix (MRC-5 and African green monkey kidney), which detects CMV, VZV, and HSV. In fact shell vial has begun to replace the traditional viral culture in some laboratories. Shell vial provides the advantage of amplifying low-level virus particles in a specimen by enhanced infection of monolayer and the use of monoclonal antibodies to detect viral antigens instead of viral CPE. Shell vial has greatly reduced the turnaround time for viral detection with sensitivity in most cases equivalent to culture.
The Enzyme-Linked Virus Inducible System (ELVIS®)	Cultures should only be sent during the first week of illness. The yield of a virus rapidly decreases >4 days after onset of illness.	ELVIS is a recently developed shell vial assay that uses genetically engineered cell lines for detecting HSV infection. The assay is based on an HSV-specific gene promoter sequence linked to the reporter gene galactosidase. When the cell monolayers are infected with HSV-1 or HSV-2, proteins produced by HSV-1 and HSV-2 shortly after infection of the cell by the virus turn on the HSV promoter sequence of the cells. The protein product from the transcribed LacZ message is β-galactosidase (β-gal), an enzyme cloned from *E. coli,* which accumulates inside the affected cell and serves as the reporter molecule, which are readily detected by the intense blue color after cells are fixed and stained with the histochemical staining kit.

TEST NAME AND METHOD	SPECIMEN AND SPECIAL REQUIREMENTS	CLINICAL COMMENTS AND REMARKS

Virus Culture—CONT

1. Lennette EH, Smith TF, editors: *Laboratory diagnosis of viral infection,* ed 3, New York, 1999, Marcel Dekker.
2. Murray PR, Baron EJ, Jorgensen JH, et al, editors: *Manual of clinical microbiology,* ed 8, Washington, DC, 2003, American Society for Microbiology.

Virus Direct Detection[1-2] *FA, PCR*	Nasopharyngeal swab, throat swab, nasal aspirate, transtracheal aspirate, bronchoalveolar lavage (BAL), lung tissue, lesions, exanthems, urine, CSF. See *Virus Culture.*	Many monoclonal and polyclonal antibodies are available for direct detection of viral agents in clinical specimens by means of immunofluorescence stain. FA stains are available for direct detection of the following viruses: adenovirus, cytomegalovirus, enterovirus, herpes simplex, influenza, measles, mumps, parainfluenza, rabies, respiratory syncytial virus, and varicella-zoster virus. Similarly, amplification-based assays, such as PCR, with excellent sensitivity and specificity are also available for direct detection of virtually all viral agents in clinical specimens. In fact the availability of real time PCR and other automated "closed" amplification systems that are not prone to amplification carry-over contamination have eliminated most of the initial concerns (except for cost) that had limited the use of these assays in clinical laboratories. Sensitivity of these tests depends on the amount of antigen and/or viral DNA or RNA in the collected sample. Selection of one or more of these assays depends upon the clinical history, patient presentation, history of exposures, and the epidemiology of the area. Knowledge of local outbreaks is necessary as well.

---

1. Forbes BA, Sahm DF, Weissfeld AS, editors: *Bailey and Scott's diagnostic microbiology,* ed 11, St Louis, 2002, Mosby.
2. Lennette EH, and Smith TF, editiors: *Laboratory diagnosis of viral infection,* ed 3, New York, 1999, Marcel Dekker.

Weil-Felix Agglutinins Serological Test (Rickettsial Disease Agglutinins)[1,2]	Serum drawn at onset of disease and 2-3 wk later	The Weil-Felix test is a nonspecific test that uses various *Proteus* species antigens (*OX-19, OX-2,* and *OX-K*) as a surrogate to serodiagnose patients infected with spotted fever group (except rickettsial pox), typhus group, and scrub typhus rickettsiae. The Weil-Felix test has been largely abandoned since currently available methods are more sensitive and specific.

---

1. Murray PR, Baron EJ, Jorgensen JH, et al, editors: *Manual of clinical microbiology,* ed 8, Washington, DC, 2003, ASM Press.
2. Rose NR, Hamilton RG, Detrick B, editors: *Manual of clinical immunology,* ed 6, Washington, DC, 2002, ASM Press.

TEST NAME AND METHOD	SPECIMEN AND SPECIAL REQUIREMENTS	CLINICAL COMMENTS AND REMARKS
West Nile Virus (WNV) Serological Test[1] *ELISA, Plaque reduction neutralization test (PRNT)*	CSF, Serum, acute and convalescent. See *General Information*.	WNV is a member of the family Flaviviridae (genus *Flavivirus*). Serologically, it is a member of the Japanese encephalitis virus antigenic complex, which includes St. Louis, Japanese, Kunjin, and Murray Valley encephalitis viruses. WNV was first isolated in the WN province of Uganda in 1937. In 1999 the first domestically acquired human cases of West Nile encephalitis (WNE) were documented in the U.S. Serological testing IgM and IgG ELISA are available from CDC, public health laboratories, and few commercial reference laboratories. The West Nile virus IgM is usually detected early when symptoms appear. IgG may not be detectable for 4-5 days of the illness. Because ELISA can cross-react between flaviviruses (e.g., SLE, dengue, and yellow fever), it should be viewed as a screening test only. Initial serologically positive samples should be confirmed by neutralization test.

1. Makar RS: West Nile Virus: an emerging infection in transfusion medicine, *Clin Microbiol News* 26:65-70, 2004.

Zygomycosis Serological Test[1] *EIA, ID*	CSF, serum	Patients with diabetic ketoacidosis, evidence of rhinocerebral disease, immunocompromised patients with renal disease, patients with acute leukemia, and debilitated patients with symptoms of pulmonary or systemic infection can be tested. Both EIA and ID tests can be used to detect antibodies in patients with active zygomycosis. The ID and EIA demonstrate a sensitivity of 70% and 80%, respectively. ID and EIA specificity are 90% and 94%, respectively. More sensitive methods would be more useful, but available assays may aid in the diagnosis of zygomycosis in patients with signs of pulmonary or systemic infection.

1. Rose NR, Hamilton RG, Detrick B, editors: *Manual of clinical immunology,* ed 6, Washington, DC, 2002, ASM Press.

PART B: SUSCEPTIBILITY TESTS

Disk Diffusion for Antimicrobial Susceptibility Test (AST) (Bauer-Kirby Test)[1-4]	Isolate of bacteria causing the infection	A qualitative test performed and interpreted according to CLSI guidelines. Zones of growth inhibition for each antimicrobial agent tested are interpreted as susceptible (S), intermediate (I), or resistant (R).

TEST NAME AND METHOD	SPECIMEN AND SPECIAL REQUIREMENTS	CLINICAL COMMENTS AND REMARKS
Cefoxitin Disk Diffusion Test for Prediction of *mec*A-mediated Oxacillin/Methicillin Resistance in Staph[4] **(ORSA/MRSA)**	*Staphylococcus aureus* or coagulase-negative staph isolate	30-μg cefoxitin disk is used with alternate breakpoints to predict *mec*A-mediated resistance to oxacillin/methicillin in *Staph* spp. *S. aureus* and coagulase-negative staph with zone sizes ≤19 mm and ≤24 mm, respectively, should be reported as oxacillin resistant. Note that the same zone interpretation used for *S. aureus* should be applied to *S. lugdenensis*. Other tests, such as a latex agglutination test, to detect protein binding site (PBP) 2′ (product of *mec*A gene); molecular tests including polymerase chain reaction and CHROMagar designed to detect ORSA/MRSA generally provide more rapid results. As a surveillance and infection control tool, the Cepheid Smart Cycler may be used to directly test nasal swabs for ORSA without prior culturing. Patients who are colonized or infected with ORSA should be placed on Contact Precautions. Patients treated with clindamysin may not respond to this therapy.
D-Zone or Blunting Test for Inducible Clindamycin Resistance[4]	*Staphylococcus* spp. isolate	According to CLSI, erythromycin and clindamycin disks are used to identify inducible *erm* gene positive, clindamycin resistant isolates that would otherwise be reported as susceptible. A blunted or D-zone of inhibition around the clindamycin disk is interpreted as resistant. These isolates express the methylase enzyme that blocks the antibiotic binding site on the bacterial ribosome. Patients treated with clindamycin may not respond to this therapy.
Oxacillin Disk Diffusion Test for Penicillin and Cephalosporin Resistant *S. pneumoniae*[4]	*Streptococcus pneumoniae* isolate	According to CLSI guidelines, this test is used to predict penicillin resistance in *S. pneumoniae*. Zone sizes ≤19 mm are interpreted as resistant to B-lactam drugs. Results should be confirmed using an MIC method before reporting isolates as penicillin resistant.
Chromogenic Cefinase Disk Test[1-3]	Aerobic or anaerobic bacterial isolate	A chromogenic cephalosporin substrate is used to identify the production of a B-lactamase enzyme in organisms, such as *Staphylococcus, Haemophilus, Neisseria,* and *Bacteroides*. Organisms that are positive should be considered resistant to all of the B-lactam drugs.
ESBL Confirmatory Synergy Disk Diffusion Test[2,4,5]	*Klebsiella pneumoniae, K. oxytoca, Escherichia coli, Proteus mirabilis* isolate	According to CLSI guidelines, all *Klebsiella* and *E. coli* isolates, as well as *Proteus mirabilis* isolates from closed body sites, should be screened to determine if they are extended-spectrum B-lactamase enzyme (ESBL) producers. Resistance to a third-generation cephalosporin constitutes a positive screening test result for an ESBL and should be confirmed using a synergy test. According to CLSI guidelines, an isolate can be confirmed as a B-lactamase producer by testing ceftazidime and cefotaxime disks with and without the B-lactamase inhibitor clavulanic acid. An increase in zone size of at least ≥5 mm in the presence of clavulanic acid confirms the presence of an ESBL.

TEST NAME AND METHOD	SPECIMEN AND SPECIAL REQUIREMENTS	CLINICAL COMMENTS AND REMARKS
		If a screening result has been confirmed, all cephalosporins, penicillins, and aztreonam should be reported as resistant even if the initial susceptibility test result was susceptible. Since these isolates are multidrug resistant, patients should be placed on Contact Precautions, and an infectious disease specialist may be consulted.

1. Forbes BA, Sahm DF, Weissfeld AS: *Bailey & Scott's diagnostic microbiology,* ed 10, St Louis, 1998, Mosby.
2. Isenberg HD: *Clinical microbiology procedures handbook,* ed 2, Washington, DC, 2004, ASM Press.
3. Murray PR, Baron EJ, Jorgensen JH, et al, editors: *Manual of clinical microbiology,* ed 8, Washington, DC, 2003, ASM Press.
4. CLSI: Performance standards for antimicrobial susceptibility testing: 14th informational supplement, M100-S14, Wayne, PA, 2006.
5. Winn W Jr, Allen S, Janda W, et al: *Koneman's color atlas and textbook of diagnostic microbiology,* ed 6, Philadelphia, 2006, Lippincott Williams & Wilkins.

TEST NAME AND METHOD	SPECIMEN AND SPECIAL REQUIREMENTS	CLINICAL COMMENTS AND REMARKS
Etest[1,5]	An aerobic or anaerobic isolate	A quantitative continuous concentration gradient of an antimicrobial agent applied to one side of a numerically labeled plastic strip. Appropriate Etest strips are placed on a seeded agar plate similar to the Disk Diffusion Test and incubated for 18-24 hr depending on the organism being tested. The minimum inhibitory concentration (MIC) value can be obtained by determining where the elliptical zone of growth inhibition intercepts the Etest strip.
ESBL Confirmatory Synergy Test[1,2] **(see ESBL** *Confirmatory Synergy Disk Diffusion Test.*)	*Klebsiella pneumoniae, K. oxytoca, Escherichia coli,* or *Proteus mirabilis* isolate	A synergy test is performed to confirm a positive ESBL screening test result based on resistance to one or more of the third-generation cephalosporins. At least two Etest strips, each containing a third-generation cephalosporin (e.g., ceftazidime and cefotaxime) with and without a B-lactamase inhibitor (e.g., clavulanic acid) are used. A screening result is confirmed for the presence of an ESBL, if there is at least a 3 twofold decrease in MIC for either agent tested in combination with clavulanic acid versus the MIC when tested alone.
		Additional markers to identify an ESBL-producing organism include susceptibility to one or more cephamycins, such as cefoxitin or cefotetan, and to the carbapenems (i.e., imipenem, merapenem, or ertapenem).
		ESBL-producing organisms are multidrug resistant. Patients with these organisms should be placed on Contact Precautions. An infectious disease consult may be indicated.

1. Isenberg HD: *Clinical microbiology procedures handbook,* ed 2, Washington, DC, 2004, ASM Press.
2. Winn W Jr, Allen S, Janda W, et al: *Koneman's color atlas and textbook of diagnostic microbiology,* ed 6, Philadelphia, 2006, Lippincott Williams & Wilkins.

TEST NAME AND METHOD	SPECIMEN AND SPECIAL REQUIREMENTS	CLINICAL COMMENTS AND REMARKS
Minimum Bactericidal (MBC) Concentration[1-4] (See *Minimum Inhibitory Concentration.*)	Log phase bacterial isolate	The MBC is the minimum concentration of an antimicrobial agent that will kill ≥99.9% of the initial inoculum of the organism being tested. Initially a macrodilution or microdilution minimum inhibitory concentration (MIC) test is performed. After 18-24 hr, the tubes or wells with no visible growth are subcultured onto solid medium and incubated 18-24 hr. The lowest antimicrobial concentration showing bactericidal activity for ≥99.9% of the test inoculum is defined as the MBC and is expressed in μg/mL. Results obtained from MBC tests may be used to predict bacterial eradication in patients with certain conditions, e.g., endocarditis, osteomyelitis, and neutropenia. A significant discrepancy (MBC/MIC ≥32) between the MIC and MBC for typical bactericidal drugs, e.g., the B-lactams and aminoglycosides, has been termed "tolerance." There is no evidence that tolerance in microorganisms other than enterococci has any predictive value for clinical outcome.

1. Forbes BA, Sahm DF, Weissfeld AS: *Bailey & Scott's diagnostic microbiology,* ed 10, St Louis, 1998, Mosby.
2. Isenberg HD: *Clinical microbiology procedures handbook,* ed 2, Washington, DC, 2004, ASM Press.
3. Murray PR, Baron EJ, Jorgensen JH, et al, editors: *Manual of clinical microbiology,* ed 8, Washington, DC, 2003, ASM Press.
4. NCCLS: Performance standards for antimicrobial susceptibility testing: 14th informational supplement, M100-S14, Wayne, PA, 2004.

TEST NAME AND METHOD	SPECIMEN AND SPECIAL REQUIREMENTS	CLINICAL COMMENTS AND REMARKS
Minimum Inhibitory Concentration (MIC)[1-3]	Log phase or stationary phase bacterial isolate	A semiquantitative test using CLSI (NCCLS) guidelines to determine the minimum inhibitory concentration (MIC) of an antimicrobial agent tested against an isolate and expressed as the concentration of an antimicrobial that will inhibit the growth of the test organism. Results can be reported in μg/mL, and using CLSI interpretation, as susceptible, intermediate, or resistant. Tests may be performed using agar dilution, Etest gradient agar diffusion, a manual or automated broth dilution test. Either a full-range MIC test using five to eight antimicrobial dilutions or breakpoint MICs using one to three concentrations of each agent may be used. The test is performed by adding known concentrations of an antimicrobial agent into a series of tubes or microwells when performing a broth microdilution or by employing a series of agar plates, each with a different concentration of the antimicrobial. A standard inoculum is then added to each antimicrobial concentration. In the case of an agar dilution test, up to 36 different isolates may be inoculated onto each plate using a replicator. The agar dilution test is considered the "gold standard," but is quite laborious and generally reserved for research-orientated laboratories.

1. Isenberg HD: *Clinical microbiology procedures handbook,* ed 2, Washington, DC, 2004, ASM Press.
2. Murray PR, Baron EJ, Jorgensen JH, et al, editors: *Manual of clinical microbiology,* ed 8, Washington, DC, 2003, ASM Press.
3. NCCLS: Performance standards for antimicrobial susceptibility testing: 14th informational supplement, M100-S14, Wayne, Pa, 2004.

TEST NAME AND METHOD	SPECIMEN AND SPECIAL REQUIREMENTS	CLINICAL COMMENTS AND REMARKS
Schlichter Test (Serum Inhibitory and Bactericidal Titers, SIT and SBT)[1-3]	2-5 mL of serum or body fluid and an isolate of bacteria causing the infection	Patient's isolate and sera collected no more than 30 min before the next dose (trough), 60 min after a 30-min intravenous infusion, 60 min after an intramuscular dose, or 90 min after an oral dose of the antimicrobial agent. Schlichter tests are used to determine the efficacy of treatment by testing the patient's serum bacteriostatic (SIT) and bactericidal (SBT) activities of an antimicrobial agent(s) when tested against the patient's isolate. The SIT is defined as the highest dilution of serum that inhibits visible growth following incubation for 24 hr. Tubes showing no growth are subcultured and incubated for 24-72 hr. The SBT is the highest dilution of serum or body fluid that kills ≥99.9% of the patient's isolate. An approved CLSI (NCCLS) document is available for performing this test although there is controversy regarding the choice of diluent used in the test (e.g., patient serum versus broth). Clinical indications for performing this test are limited to monitoring effective therapy in patients with osteomyelitis; closed-space infections, such as meningitis; and the use of oral agents after intravenous therapy. The precise value of the SBT is controversial since there has not been a clear-cut correlation between any particular titer and efficacy. Most often this assay is used for the following: to monitor therapy of infections that require bactericidal activity (e.g., endocarditis, osteomyelitis, and meningitis), to evaluate antimicrobial combinations subsequent to their administration, and to monitor the antibacterial activity of serum after changing from parenteral to oral therapy.

1. Isenberg, H.D: *Clinical microbiology procedures handbook,* ed 2, Washington, DC, 2004, ASM Press.
2. Murray PR, Baron EJ, Jorgensen JH, et al, editors: *Manual of clinical microbiology,* ed 8, Washington, DC, 2003, ASM Press.
3. NCCLS. Methodology for the serum bactericidal test: Approved Guideline, M21-A, Wayne, Pa, 1999.

TABLE V-1 NORMAL MICROBIAL FLORA

Microorganisms normally residing on body surfaces or in various cavities of the body without invasion or harm to the host are referred to as "normal flora." The types and numbers vary according to the environment of the surfaces and cavities. These organisms help prevent colonization, invasion, and infection by pathogenic microorganisms. Some of the normal flora in the alimentary tract synthesize vitamin K, aid in nutrient absorption, and help convert bile pigments and acids in the intestine. Although harmless in their usual sites, normal flora may produce disease if introduced into other areas (especially those cavities that are normally sterile) as opportunists.

The following is a compilation of microorganisms that constitute normal flora encountered in various body sites.[1]

MOUTH AND OROPHARYNX

Viridans streptococci
Coagulase-negative
  staphylococci
Veillonella spp.
Fusobacterium spp.
Treponema spp.
Bacteroides spp.
Prevotella spp.
Propionibacterium spp.
Peptostreptococcus spp.
Neisseria spp. and *Moraxella*
  catarrhalis
Streptococcus pneumoniae
β-Hemolytic streptococci (not
  group A)
Candida spp.
Haemophilus spp.
Diphtheroids
Actinomyces spp.
Eikenella corrodens
Staphylococcus aureus
Lactobacillus spp.

NOSE AND NASOPHARYNX

Coagulase-negative
  staphylococci
Viridans streptococci
Staphylococcus aureus
Neisseria spp.
Haemophilus spp.
Streptococcus pneumoniae

OUTER EAR

Coagulase-negative
  staphylococci
Diphtheroids
Bacillus spp. (occasionally)
Micrococcus spp.
Saprophytic *Neisseria* spp.
  (occasionally)
Saprophytic *Mycobacterium*
  spp. (occasionally)
Aspergillus spp.
Alternaria spp.
Penicillium spp.
Candida spp.

CONJUNCTIVAE

Coagulase-negative
  staphylococci
Diphtheroids
Saprophytic *Neisseria* spp.
  (occasionally)
Viridans streptococci

SKIN

Coagulase-negative
  staphylococci
Diphtheroids (including
  Propionibacterium acnes)
Micrococcus spp.
Staphylococcus aureus
Streptococci (various species)
Bacillus spp.
Acinetobacter spp.
Malassezia spp.
Candida spp.
Saprophytic *Mycobacterium*
  spp. (occasionally)

URETHRA

Coagulase-negative
  staphylococci
Diphtheroids
Streptococci (various species)
Enterococcus spp.
Enterobacteriaceae
Lactobacillus spp.
Mycobacterium smegmatis
Bacteroides spp.
Peptostreptococcus spp.
Candida spp.

VAGINA

Lactobacillus spp.
Peptostreptococcus spp.
Diphtheroids
Micrococcus spp.
Coagulase-negative
  staphylococci
Streptococci (various species)
Enterococcus spp.
Clostridium spp.
Bacteroides spp.
Candida spp.
Gardnerella vaginalis

GASTROINTESTINAL TRACT

Small Intestine

Lactobacillus spp.
Bacteroides spp.
Clostridium spp.
Enterococcus spp.
Enterobacteriaceae
Peptostreptococcus spp.
Candida spp.

Large Intestine

Bacteroides spp.
Prevotella spp.
Porphyromonas spp
Fusobacterium spp.
Clostridium spp.
Bifidobacterium spp.
Eubacterium spp.
Peptostreptococcus spp.
Escherichia coli
Klebsiella spp.
Proteus spp.
Lactobacillus spp.
Enterococcus spp.
Streptococci (various species)
Coagulase-negative
  staphylococci
Staphylococcus aureus
Actinomyces spp.
Candida spp.

---

1. Murray PR, Baron EJ, Jorgensen JH, et al, editors: *Manual of clinical microbiology,* ed 8, Washington, DC, 2003 ASM Press.

TABLE V-2 SPECIMENS FOR VIRAL ISOLATION IN SELECTED CLINICAL SYNDROMES

INFECTION	VIRUS	PREFERRED SPECIMEN
Central nervous system (encephalitis, aseptic meningitis)	Enterovirus	Throat or rectal swab, CSF
	HSV	CSF, vesicle fluid, brain biopsy
	Mumps	Throat swab, urine, CSF
	Rabies, arbovirus	Usually not cultured
Congenital/perinatal	CMV	Throat swab, urine, blood (leukocytes)
	Enterovirus	Throat, stool, or rectal swab; CSF
	HSV	Throat swab, CSF, vesicle fluid
Eye (conjunctivitis, keratitis)	Adenovirus, enterovirus, HSV	Throat or conjunctival swab, corneal scrapings
Gastrointestinal tract	Adenovirus	Stool or rectal swab
	Rotavirus, Norwalk agent	Usually not cultured; EIA or EM on stool
Genital tract	HSV	Vesicle fluid, endocervical swab
Heart	Coxsackievirus B	Throat, stool, or rectal swab; pericardial fluid
	CMV	
	Influenza A, B	Throat swab, urine, pericardial fluid throat swab
Hepatitis	EBV; Hepatitis A, B, and C	Not cultured
	CMV	Throat, urine, liver
Mononucleosis	CMV, HIV	Urine, throat wash, blood
	EBV	Not cultured
Rash Maculopapular	Adenovirus, enterovirus	Throat or rectal swab, stool
	Parainfluenza, RSV	Nasopharyngeal aspirate
	Rubella, rubeola	Usually not cultured
	Coxsackievirus A, echovirus	Throat or rectal swab, stool, vesicle fluid
Vesicular	HSV, VZV, vaccinia	Vesicle fluid
Respiratory tract	Adenovirus, coxsackievirus, echovirus	Throat swab or wash
	HSV	Oral swab
	CMV	Throat swab, urine
	Enterovirus	Throat swab
	Influenza	Throat swab and nasal wash
	Parainfluenza, RSV	Nasopharyngeal aspirates
	Rhinovirus	Nasal swab or wash
Urinary tract	Adenovirus, CMV	Urine

HSV, herpes simplex virus; *CMV,* cytomegalovirus; *EBV,* Epstein-Barr virus; *HIV,* human immunodeficiency virus; *VZV,* varicella-zoster virus; *RSV,* respiratory syncytial virus; *CSF,* cerebospinal fluid; *EIA,* enzyme immnoassay; *EM,* electron microscopy.

SECTION VI
IMMUNOPHENOTYPING
MARKERS

INTRODUCTION

The evaluation of hematopoietic and lymphoid neoplasms requires a variety of methods. Although morphological features remain the cornerstone of the evaluation of leukemias and malignant lymphomas, ancillary studies including immunophenotyping, cytogenetics, and/or molecular genetic testing are needed in most, if not all, cases.

Immunophenotyping, by multiparameter flow cytometry and/or immunohistochemistry, now is an integral part of the modern diagnosis and classification systems for leukemias and malignant lymphomas. There is a growing list of immunophenotyping markers, and many of them are currently used in clinical flow cytometry and immunohistology laboratories. Knowledge of these markers, its normal distribution and biological functions in particular, is essential for appropriate interpretation of immunophenotyping test results.

The majority of immunophenotyping markers are the cluster of differentiation antigens, or CD antigens. All cells involved in hematopoietic, immune, and phagocytic functions express a number of surface and cytoplasmic antigens unique to the cell lineage and stage of development. For standardization purposes, international workshops were held to assign a cluster of differentiation numbers, or CD number, to each antigen that is recognized by a cluster of monoclonal antibodies. If only one antibody defines a cluster or if all antibodies defining a cluster originate from the same laboratory, a suffix *w* is added to the CD designation. All CD antigens defined at the first to seventh international workshops on Human Leukocyte Differentiation Antigens (HLDA) are presented in Part I, along with any common names used before a CD number was assigned, molecular size, normal tissue distribution, and known or suspected physiological function. A few key primary papers and review articles for each CD antigen are also included. The eighth HLDA workshop was held in Adelaide, Australia in December 2004, and an additional 95 molecules were assigned CD numbers which are not included in this section.

In addition to the CD antigens, other commonly used immunophenotyping markers are also presented in Part I. It is worth noting that ZAP-70 is a new marker and currently not available in most flow cytometry laboratories, but is on the horizon to become a key prognostic marker for chronic lymphocytic leukemia and/or small lymphocytic lymphoma.

Typical immunophenotypes of hematopoietic and lymphoid neoplasms are summarized and listed in Part II. A brief summary of clinical, morphological, and/or genetic features of each disease is provided. The lists of diseases are based on the currently used World Health Organization (WHO) classification system, which was published in 2001.

PART I: IMMUNOPHENOTYPING MARKERS

1. THE CLUSTER OF DIFFERENTIATION ANTIGENS (THE CD ANTIGENS)

CD MARKERS	OTHER NAMES	MOLECULAR WEIGHT (KDA)	KNOWN NORMAL DISTRIBUTION	REMARKS
CD1a	R4; HTA1; T6; Leu-6	49	Cortical thymocytes (strong), B-cell subset, dendritic cells, Langerhans cells	CD1 is a member of immunoglobulin superfamily on chromosome 1q22-23. There are five different CD1 isoforms (CD1a-e), all noncovalently associated with a 12 kDa β_2 microglobulin. Each isoform is involved
CD1b		45	Cortical thymocytes (moderate), B-cell subset, dendritic cells, Langerhans cells	in presentation of antigens including lipids, restricting T-cell responses to certain antigens. CD1 may also mediate thymic T-cell development.
CD1c		43	Cortical thymocytes (weak), B-cell subset, dendritic cells, Langerhans cells	*Immunol Rev 147:5, 1995* *Curr Opin Immunol 11:100, 1999*
CD2	E-rosette receptor; LFA-2 (leukocyte function antigen-2); T11	50	Thymocytes, T cell, NK cells	CD2 serves as the ligand for CD58, CD48, and CD59. It binds to CD58 on antigen-presenting cells and induces co-stimulatory signals in T cells. CD2 also regulates T- and NK-mediated cytolysis, induces apoptosis in activated peripheral T cells, mediates T-cell cytokine production, and regulates T-cell energy. *Immunol Rev 163:217, 1998* *Immunol Today 17:177, 1996*
CD3	T3; Leu-4	16, 20, 25-28	T cells, NK cells (cytoplasmic only)	CD3 is considered the lineage-specific T-cell marker. CD3 is composed of a family of proteins (γ, δ, ϵ), which form the membrane signal transduction complex linked to T-cell receptor (TCR). CD3 itself does not bind antigen, but is involved in the transduction of signals into the T cell after the TCR has bound the antigen. *Adv Immunol 72:103, 1999* *Mol Immunol 40:1295, 2004*
CD4	T4; Leu-3	55	Helper and/or inducer T cells, monocytes, macrophages, dendritic cells	CD4 serves as co-receptor in MHC class II-restricted antigen-induced T-cell activation. It binds to MHC class II molecules expressed on antigen-presenting cells, facilitating recognition of peptide antigens. In addition, CD4 is also a co-receptor for HIV gp120.

CD MARKERS	OTHER NAMES	MOLECULAR WEIGHT (KDA)	KNOWN NORMAL DISTRIBUTION	REMARKS
CD4—CONT				
				Transplant Proc 31:820, 1999 *Curr Issues Mol Biol 6:1, 2004*
CD5	Leu-1; B4; Ly-1; Tp67	67	T cells, B-cell subset	CD5 belongs to ancient scavenger receptor family and is physically and functionally coupled with the membrane T-cell receptor (TCR)-CD3 complex. CD5 appears to be ligand for CD72 and serves as a dual receptor, giving either stimulatory or inhibitory signals depending both on the cell type and the development stage. CD5 is a phenotypic marker for some B-cell lymphoproliferative disorders (chronic lymphocytic leukemia and/or small lymphocytic lymphoma, mantle cell lymphoma, etc.). *Int J Biochem Cell Biol 36:2105, 2004* *Immunol Res 26:255, 2002* *Cur Opin Hematol 6:30, 1999* *Immunol Today 19:106, 1998*
CD6	T12	105 or 130	T cells, B-cell subset	CD6 is a cell surface receptor belonging to the scavenger receptor cysteine-rich (SRCR) protein superfamily. It binds cell adhesion molecule CD166 and is involved in T-cell development and activation. *Eur J Immunol 34:930, 2004* *Transplant Proc 31:795, 1999* *Proteins 40:420, 2000* *Immunol Today 18:498, 1997*
CD7	Leu-9; 3A1; Gp40	40	T cells, NK cells, some myeloid precursor cells	CD7 is considered the earliest marker for T-cell differentiation. CD7 is a membrane glycoprotein and Fc receptor for IgM. It associates with PI-3 kinase and is involved in T-cell and NK-cell activation. *Immunol Res 24:31, 2001* *Crit Rev Immunol 19:331, 1999* *J Clin Immunol 17:265, 1997*
CD8	Leu-2; T8; Lyt2/3	68 (32-34)	Cytotoxic and/or suppressor T cells, NK cells, most thymocytes	CD8 serves as co-receptor in T-cell activation. It is composed of α and β chains and facilitates the recognition of cell-bound, MHC class I antigens. *Immunol Rev 182:201, 2001* *Sem Immunol 9:87, 1997* *J Immunol 157:4287, 1996*

CD MARKERS	OTHER NAMES	MOLECULAR WEIGHT (KDA)	KNOWN NORMAL DISTRIBUTION	REMARKS
CD9	p24; MRP-1; BA-2; DRAP-27	24, 26	Megakaryocytes, platelets, monocytes, activated T cells, pre-B cells, eosinophils, basophils, vascular endothelial cells and smooth muscle cells, some epithelia, cardiac muscle cells	CD9 plays role in signal transduction leading to cell activation, adhesion, aggregation, and/or cell migration. *Immunol Today 15:588, 1994* *Mol Biol Cell 7:193, 1996* *Leuk Lymphoma 38:147, 2000*
CD10	Common ALL antigen (CALLA); neutral endopeptidase; enkephalinase	100	Lymphoblasts (pre-B cells and pre-T cells), germinal center B cells (centroblasts and centrocytes), some T cells, neutrophils, intestinal epithelial cells, myoepithelial cells, hepatocytes, etc.	CD10 is a cell membrane zinc-binding metallopeptidase that cleaves peptides on the amino side of hydrophobic amino acids, thereby inactivating bioactive peptides. CD10 is considered the earliest marker for lymphoid differentiation and a characteristic marker for acute lymphoblastic leukemia (ALL), follicular lymphoma, Burkitt's lymphoma and/or leukemia, and angioimmunoblastic T cell lymphoma. CD10 is also used as a marker for breast myoepithelial cells. CD10 is positive in a variety of solid tumors. *J Exp Med 181:2271, 1995* *Blood 82:1052, 1993* *Blood 99:627, 2002*
CD11a	αL chain of β_2 integrins; leukocyte function-associated antigen-1α (LFA-1α) (in complex with CD18)	180	Granulocytes, monocytes, macrophages, lymphocytes	CD11a is an alpha integrin chain that binds to CD18 to form receptor for CD54 (intercellular adhesion molecule-1, ICAM-1) and CD102 (ICAM-2). By forming complex with CD18, it mediates leukocyte adhesion and transendothelial migration and lymphocyte recirculation through lymph nodes. Patients with leukocyte adhesion deficiency (mutations in CD18) often have severe immunodeficiency with recurrent bacterial and/or fungal infections early in life. *Curr Opin Cell Biol 9:643, 1997* *Immunol Rev 146:82, 1995*
CD11b	αM chain of β_2 integrins; complement receptor-3 (CR3); iC3b receptor; Mac-1	170	Granulocytes, monocytes, macrophages, dendritic cells, NK cells, some B cells and T cells	CD11b assembles with CD18 to form a receptor for iC3b, fibrinogen, clotting factor X, and CD54. It facilitates adhesion to endothelium and platelets, phagocytosis of particles opsonized with iC3b, and/or chemotaxis. *Cell 80:631, 1995* *Immunol Res 25:219, 2002*

CD MARKERS	OTHER NAMES	MOLECULAR WEIGHT (KDA)	KNOWN NORMAL DISTRIBUTION	REMARKS
CD11c	αX chain of $β_2$ integrins; Leu-M5; gp150/95; complement receptor-4 (CR4)	150	Granulocytes, monocytes, macrophages, NK cells, some B cells and T cells	CD11c assembles with CD18 to form a receptor for iC3b and fibrinogen. It facilitates the clearance of opsonized particles and immune complex. It also binds to fibrinogen and thereby is involved in adhesion of neutrophils and monocytes to endothelium and induces neutrophil respiratory burst. In addition to most acute myeloid leukemias (AML), CD11c is also positive in hairy cell leukemia and a subset of chronic lymphocytic leukemia and/or small lymphocytic lymphoma (CLL/SLL). *Immunol Today 5:209, 1996* *J Immunol 156:3780, 1996*
CD13	Aminopeptidase N (APN); Leu-M7; My7	150	Myeloid cells (granulocytic cells), monocytes, some NK cells	CD13 is a zinc-binding metalloprotease that catalyzes removal of N-terminal amino acids from peptides, thereby inactivating bioactive peptide hormones. CD13 is considered a characteristic marker for myeloid differentiation, although is less specific than CD33. In addition to most myeloid leukemias, CD13 is positive in some pre-B acute lymphoblastic leukemias and rare pre-T acute lymphoblastic leukemias. CD13 is also positive in bile duct canaliculi, central nervous system synapses, endothelial cells, osteoclasts, small intestinal epithelial cells, etc. *J Exp Med 184:183, 1996* *J Exp Med 194:1183, 1996* *Immunol Today 20:83, 1999*
CD14	LPS receptor, endotoxin receptor; GPI-linked glycoprotein	55	Monocytes, macrophages, dendritic cells, Langerhans cells, some myeloid cells	CD14 is the receptor for lipopolysaccharide (LPS) that can transduce signal(s), leading to oxidative burst and/or synthesis of tumor necrosis factor alpha. CD14 is used as a marker for monocytic differentiation. CD14 may be deficient in patients with paroxysmal nocturnal hemoglobinuria. *Trend Immunol 23:301, 2002* *Curr Opin Immunol 11:19, 1999*
CD15	Leu-M1; Lewis^X (Lex)	185-260	Neutrophils, monocytes, eosinophils, activated T-cells and B cells	CD15 is a carbohydrate determinant that is found on many cell surface glycolipids and glycoproteins (e.g., CD11 and/or CD18, CD66) and is dependent on the activity of

CD MARKERS	OTHER NAMES	MOLECULAR WEIGHT (KDA)	KNOWN NORMAL DISTRIBUTION	REMARKS
CD15—CONT				alpha 3-fucosyltransferase. The sialylated form of CD15 (CD15s) is the ligand for CD62E and CD62P. In addition to myeloid and myelomonocytic leukemias, CD15 is characteristically positive in CALLA (CD10)-negative precursor B acute lymphoblastic leukemia with 11q23 (MLL) abnormalities. CD15 is also positive in the majority of classical Hodgkin's lymphomas. *Arch Pathol Lab Med 125:1227, 2001* *Histo Histopathol 11:1007, 1996* *Histochem J 24:811, 1992*
CD16a	FcRIII A	50-65	NK cells, macrophages, mast cells, neutrophils, some T cells	CD16a is a component of low-affinity Fc receptor for aggregated IgG, mediating phagocytosis, cytokine production, and antibody-dependent cell-mediated cytotoxicity (ADCC). Along with CD56, CD16a is widely used to identify NK cells. *Autoimmune Rev 1:13, 2002* *J Leukoc Biol 67:279, 2000* *J Immunol 162:735, 1999* *Proc Natl Acad Sci USA 96:5640, 1999*
CD16b	FcRIII B	48-60	Neutrophils	CD16b is the GPI-linked isoform of CD16 that is present on neutrophil surface. Cross-linking CD16b may transduce a different signal from that of CD16a. CD16b is deficient in patients with paroxysmal nocturnal hemoglobinuria. *Immunol Res 29:219, 2004* *Transfusion 39:593, 1999*
CDw17	Lactosylceramide (LacCer)		Neutrophils, basophils, monocytes, macrophages, platelets, some peripheral B cells	CDw17 is a cell surface glycosphingolipid that may play a role in granule content packaging, exocytosis, and signaling. It may also function in phagocytosis by binding to bacteria. *J Biol Chem 273:34349, 1998* *Circ Res 82:540, 1998*
CD18	Beta chain of the β_2 integrins	95	Same as CD11a-d combined	CD18 assembles into a heterodimer with one of several alpha chains (CD11a-c) and is essential for neutrophil adhesion and sig-

CD MARKERS	OTHER NAMES	MOLECULAR WEIGHT (KDA)	KNOWN NORMAL DISTRIBUTION	REMARKS
CD18—CONT				nal transduction. Mutations in CD18 gene cause leukocyte adhesion deficiency type 1 (LAD-1). Patients typically have recurrent bacterial or fungal infections, pronounced leukocytosis in the absence of infection, reduced expression of all members of the CD18 or β_2 integrin family on circulating leukocytes, and diminished CD18-dependent leukocyte functions, including cell adhesion, chemotaxis, transendothelial migration, and oxidative burst activation in response to iC3b-coated particles. *Blood 103:1105, 2004* *Int J Biochem Cell Biol 30:179, 1998* *Curr Opin Cell Biol 9:643, 1997*
CD19	B4	95	B cells, B-cell precursors, follicular dendritic cells	CD19 forms a noncovalent complex with CD21, CD81, and CD225 that modulates signal transduction by B-cell antigen receptors. It regulates B-cell development, differentiation, and activation. CD19 is considered the earliest marker for B-cell differentiation. Plasma cells lack CD19. *Science 256:105, 1992* *Sem Immunol 10:267, 1998* *Immunol Res 26:45, 2002*
CD20	B1; L26	95 (33, 35, 37)	B cells	The structure of CD20 is similar to that of an ion channel. It may act as a Ca^{2+} channel involved in regulating cell cycle progression and activation. CD20 is one of the pan–B-cell markers. Its expression is behind CD10 and CD19, but earlier than CD21, CD22, and immunoglobulins. Plasma cells lack CD20. The majority of B-cell non-Hodgkin's lymphomas and nodular lymphocyte predominant Hodgkin's lymphomas are positive for CD20. Monoclonal anti-CD20 antibodies (e.g., rituximab, Bexxar, Zevalin) are currently widely used for the treatment of B-cell lymphomas. *Curr Opin Hematol 5:237, 1998* *Semin Oncol 27(S12):17, 2000* *Semin Cancer Biol 13:211, 2003*

CD MARKERS	OTHER NAMES	MOLECULAR WEIGHT (KDA)	KNOWN NORMAL DISTRIBUTION	REMARKS
CD21	CD2; EBV receptor; C3d receptor	145	B cells, follicular dendritic cells, some epithelial cells, astrocytes, some T cells	CD21 is the cell surface receptor for C3d and Epstein-Barr virus (EBV). It forms a signaling complex with CD19, CD81, and CD225. Binding of C3d to CD21 enhances B-cell antigen receptor signal transduction. EBV-infected B cells trigger a reactive process called infectious mononucleosis with increase in circulating reactive T cells. EBV-infected B cells may also transform into malignant lymphomas. Like CD23, CD21 is used as a dendritic cell marker. Nodular lymphocyte predominant Hodgkin's lymphoma and angioimmunoblastic T-cell lymphoma characteristically demonstrate expansion and/or disruption of follicular dendritic meshwork. *Adv Exp Med Biol 452:181, 1998* *Sem Immunol 10:279, 1998* *Int Rev Immunol 20:739, 2001*
CD22	B lymphocyte cell adhesion molecule (BL-CAM); Leu-14	135	B cells (surface expression), B-cell precursors (cytoplasmic expression)	The CD22 antigen is a transmembrane sialoglycoprotein of the immunoglobulin superfamily. It is initially present in the cytoplasm of developing B cells, but is later expressed on the surface during B-cell maturation once IgD expression occurs. Most circulating IgM^+IgD^+ cells express CD22. CD22 is strongly expressed in follicular, mantle, and marginal zone B cells, but is weakly present in differentiating B cells. CD22 plays a role in a number of biological activities, including cellular adhesion and homing and regulation of the B-cell activation. CD22 is considered a target for immunotherapy. *Adv Exp Med Biol 452:181, 1998* *Ann Rev Immunol 15:481, 1997* *Semin Oncol 30:253-257, 2003*
CD23	Fc epsilon R II (IgE receptor); Leu-20; B6	45	Mature B cells expressing surface IgM and IgD, monocytes, macrophages, T-cell subsets, platelets, eosinophils, follicular dendritic cells	CD23 is a Ca^{2+}-dependent lectin with low affinity for IgE, CD11, and CD21-CD19-CD81 complex, which plays a role in the regulation of IgE synthesis and in cell-cell adhesion. Secreted form of CD23 may act as growth factor. CD23 is also used as a dendritic cell marker. CD23 is characteristically positive in chronic lymphocytic leuke-

CD MARKERS	OTHER NAMES	MOLECULAR WEIGHT (KDA)	KNOWN NORMAL DISTRIBUTION	REMARKS
CD23—CONT				mia and/or small lymphocytic lymphoma (CLL/SLL). *Immunol Today 19:313, 1998* *Cell Mol Life Sci 59:648, 2002*
CD24	Heat stable antigen (HSA); BA-1	35-45	B cells, B-cell precursors, neutrophils, epithelial cells, early T cells	CD24 a cell surface GPI-anchored adhesion protein. It may serve as ligand for CD62p and play a role in antigen-dependent B-cell proliferation and/or differentiation. CD24 is positive in a variety of epithelial carcinomas, and its expression is associated with a worse clinical outcome. *Blood 89:3385, 1997* *Int Immunol 7:155, 1995*
CD25	IL-2 receptor alpha chain; TAC antigen	55	Activated T cells and B cells, some thymocytes, early myeloid cells	CD25 is a low-affinity receptor for interleukin-2 (IL-2). It can associate with CD122 and CD132 to form a heterotrimeric receptor with high affinity for IL-2. CD25 is characteristically positive in hairy cell leukemia and HTLV-1-associated adult T-cell leukemia and/or T-cell lymphoma. *Adv Immunol 59:225, 1995* *Cell 75:5, 1995*
CD26	Depeptidyl peptidase IV; ADA binding protein	110	T-cell subset, macrophages, activated B cells, renal proximal tubular epithelial cells, small intestinal epithelial cells, biliary canaliculi	CD26 is a cell surface serine-type exopeptidase that cleaves dipeptides from the N-terminal of proteins. With an intracellular domain that associates with adenosine deaminase (ADA), CD26 also can function as a T-cell costimulatory molecule. It costimulates both the CD3- and the CD2-dependent T-cell activation and tyrosine phosphorylation of TCR-CD3 signal transduction pathway proteins. CD26 in vivo has integral membrane protein and soluble forms. Soluble CD26 is at significant levels in serum with its levels altered in many diseases. CD26 is also a cofactor of CD4 for HIV entry into cells. Normally, more than 90% of peripheral CD4$^+$ cells are positive for CD26. For patients with Sézary syndrome, CD26 is useful for therapy monitoring since Sézary cells are characteristically

CD MARKERS	OTHER NAMES	MOLECULAR WEIGHT (KDA)	KNOWN NORMAL DISTRIBUTION	REMARKS
CD26—CONT				
				positive for CD4 and negative for CD26. *Crit Rev Clin Lab Sci 40:209, 2003* *Scand J Immunol 54:249-264, 2001*
CD27	S152; T14	110(55)	Medullary thymocytes, T cells, NK cells, memory B cells	CD27 is a ligand for CD70 and a member of the nerve-growth-factor superfamily. CD27-CD70 interactions regulate T- and B-cell activation and differentiation. CD27 is T-cell activation marker. *Immunol Res 21:23, 2000* *Sem Immunol 10:491, 1998* *Immunol Today 15:307, 1994*
CD28	Tp44 antigen	90(44)	95% CD4 T cells, 50% CD8 T cells, activated B cells, plasma cells	CD28 interacts with CD80 (B7-1) and CD86 (B7-2) expressed on antigen-presenting cells and activated B cells. The interactions provide co-stimulatory signal in activation of naïve T cells, and interleukin-2 expression. The opponent of CD28 is CD152 (CTLA-4), which mediates the negative signaling in T-cell activation. *Nat Rev Immunol 3:939, 2003* *Immunol Rev 165:287, 1998* *Crit Rev Immunol 18:389, 1998*
CD29	Platelet gpIIa, integrin β_1 subunit; fibronectin receptor, VLA-beta chain	130	Platelets, all leukocytes with higher levels on memory T cells	CD29 assembles into a heterodimer with one of the several alpha chains (CD49a-f) to form the transmembrane β_1 integrins. The extracellular domains of integrin alpha and/or beta heterodimers mediate cell-matrix and cell-cell contacts, and their cytoplasmic tails associate with the cytoskeleton. Integrins are capable of transducing information in a bidirectional manner, and the beta subunit is recognized to play an important role in the process. *Int J Biochem Cell Biol 30:179, 1998* *J cell Biol 132:211, 1996*
CD30	Ki-1 antigen; Ber-H2	105	Activated T cells, B cells, and NK cells; monocytes	CD30 is a member of the TNF receptor family. CD30 binds to CD30 ligand (CD153) and plays a role in cell activation, differentiation, and/or proliferation. Signal-

CD MARKERS	OTHER NAMES	MOLECULAR WEIGHT (KDA)	KNOWN NORMAL DISTRIBUTION	REMARKS
CD30—CONT				ing via CD30 can lead to proliferation or cell death. CD30 is positive in activated lymphocytes following EBV, HIV, HTLV-1, HHV-8, or HBV infection. Reed-Sternberg cells seen in classical Hodgkin's lymphoma are characteristically positive for CD30. In addition, CD30 is usually positive in anaplastic large cell lymphoma (ALCL), lymphomatoid papulosis (LyP), peripheral T-cell lymphomas, primary effusion lymphoma, and embryonal carcinoma of testis. *Sem Immunol 10:457, 1998* *Autoimmunity 33:45, 2000* *Curr Opin Hematol 10:267, 2003*
CD31	Platelet endothelial cell adhesion molecule-1 (PECAM-1)	130	Platelets, monocytes, macrophages, osteoclasts, neutrophils, T-cell subset, endothelial cells	CD31 is a glycoprotein belonging to the immunoglobulin superfamily of cell adhesion molecules. It interacts with itself (CD31 binds CD31 on the apposing cell) and with integrin $\alpha_v\beta_3$ and glycosaminoglycans. Ligand of CD31 activates leukocyte integrins. It plays an important role in diapedesis step of transendothelial migration of neutrophils. CD31 has also been shown to be involved in mediating signal transduction. CD31 is used as a marker for vascular endothelium and malignant vascular tumors. *J Clin Invest 99:3, 1997* *J Exp Med 184:229, 1996* *N Engl J Med 334:286, 1996*
CD32	FcγRII	40	Monocytes, macrophages, platelets, B cells (B isoform only), neutrophils (A and C isoforms), eosinophils, basophils	CD32 is the low-affinity Fc receptor for aggregated IgG and IgG immune complexes. It triggers IgG-mediated phagocytosis and oxidative burst. In B cells, CD32 transduces an inhibitory signal, rendering B cells to undergo apoptosis. Its expression on placental epithelia suggests a role in transport of IgG. *Ann Rev Immunol 19:275, 2001* *Adv Immunol 57:1, 1994*
CD33	Gp67	67	Cells of myelomonocytic lineage but not stem cells	CD33 is a sialoadhesin that may mediate cell-cell adhesion. It is one of the earliest markers for myeloid differentiation and thereby used for the diagnosis of acute

CD MARKERS	OTHER NAMES	MOLECULAR WEIGHT (KDA)	KNOWN NORMAL DISTRIBUTION	REMARKS
CD33—CONT				myeloid leukemia (AML). It acts as a receptor that inhibits the proliferation of normal and leukemic myeloid cells. CD33 is positive in approximately 90% of AML and has become a therapeutic target. Anti-CD33 antibodies (e.g., gemtuzumab ozogamicin or Mylotarg) are currently used as therapeutic agents for AML in a subset of older patients. *Cancer 98:2095, 2003* *Blood 85:2005, 1995*
CD34	My10; HPCA-2	105-120	Hematopoietic progenitor cells (1%-4% of bone marrow cells), endothelial cells	CD34 is a cell surface glycoprotein that may mediate cell-cell adhesion through its ability to interact with CD62L, CD62P, and CD62E. It may actually mediate the attachment of hematopoietic progenitor cells to their particular microenvironment (extracellular matrix and/or stromal cells), or niche, in the bone marrow. Antibodies against CD34 are widely used to purify and quantify hematopoietic stem cells (progenitor cells) for research and for bone marrow transplantation. It is also one of the most commonly used markers for the diagnosis and monitoring of acute lymphoblastic and myeloid leukemias. *Adv Exp Med Biol 534:107, 2003* *Blood 87:1, 1996* *J Hematother 1:115, 1992*
CD35	Complement receptor-1 (CR1); C3b/C4b receptor; immune adherence receptor	Erythrocytes (160, 190, 220, 250) Leukocytes (165, 195, 225, 255)	Monocytes, neutrophils, eosinophils, follicular dendritic cells, red blood cells, B cells, some T cells and NK cells, some astrocytes, glomerular podocytes	CD35 is the receptor for C3b and C4b. It facilitates phagocytosis and/or binding to immune complexes or cells coated with C3b or C4b. CD35 is one of the few CD antigens with allotypic polymorphism resulting in varied molecular sizes. In addition, the Knops, McCoy, Swain-Langley, and York blood group antigens are located on CD35 molecule. *Immunol Rev 180:112, 2001* *J Hematother 4:357, 1995* *J Biol Chem 269:13273, 1994*

CD MARKERS	OTHER NAMES	MOLECULAR WEIGHT (KDA)	KNOWN NORMAL DISTRIBUTION	REMARKS
CD36	Platelet gpIV or gpIIIb.	88	Platelets, megakaryo-cytes, monocytes, macrophages, adipocytes, some epithelial cells, en-dothelial cells, young red blood cells	CD36 is signal transducing receptor for thrombospondin, collagen, oxidized LDL, fatty acids, anionic phospholipids, and *Plasmodium falciparum*-infected red blood cells. It serves as a scavenger receptor for oxidized LDL, involved in platelet adhesion and aggregation and platelet-monocyte and platelet-tumor cell interaction, and plays a role in the cytoadherence of *Plasmodium falciparum*-infected red cells to microvascu-lar endothelial cells. CD36 also binds thrombospondin-1 and mediates its antian-giogenic activity. CD36 is usually positive in acute myeloid leukemia FAB M4-7. *Front Biosci 8:S874, 2003* *J Clin Invest 108:785, 2001* *J Biol Chem 271:22315, 1996* *Blood 80:1105, 1992*
CD37	Gp40-52	40-52	Mature B cells, some T cells and/or monocytes and/or neutrophils (weak)	CD37 belongs to tetraspanin family. It asso-ciates with MHC class II, CD19, CD21, CD53, CD81, and CD82 in B-cell mem-brane, suggesting a role in signal transduc-tion. CD37 also plays a regulatory role in T-cell proliferation. It is positive in hairy cell leukemia. *J Immunol 172:2953, 2004* *Immunol Today 15:588, 1994* *J Immunol 140:905, 1988*
CD38	T10	45	Plasma cells (strong), early or activated B cells and T cells, thymocytes, monocytes, NK cells, myeloid progenitor cells (blasts), brain	CD38 is NAD (nicotinamide adenine dinu-cleotide) glycohydrolase. It can synthesize cyclic ADP-ribose (cADPR) from NAD and hydrolyze cADPR to ADPR. It serves as both positive and negative regulator of cell activation, proliferation, and survival, de-pending on the cellular environment. It is the target of immunotoxin therapy for mul-tiple myeloma. CD38 is characteristically positive in myeloma and primary effusion lymphoma. It is also positive in a subset of chronic lymphocytic leukemia and/or small lymphocytic lymphoma, and its expression appears to associate with worse clinical out-come. *Leuk Lymphoma 45:455, 2004* *J Leukoc Biol 65:151, 1999* *Faseb J 10:1408, 1996*

CD MARKERS	OTHER NAMES	MOLECULAR WEIGHT (KDA)	KNOWN NORMAL DISTRIBUTION	REMARKS
CD39	Vascular nucleoside triphosphate diphosphohydrolase (NTPDase)	78	Endothelial cells, macrophages, dendritic cells, activated cells of the NK-cell, B-cell, or T-cell lineage (not on resting cells or germinal center B cells); placenta	CD39 is a membrane-bound ectoenzyme that hydrolyzes extracellular ATP and ADP to AMP. It inhibits platelet adhesion and aggregation by digesting ADP. It may also facilitate the homotypic adhesion of B cells and play roles in regulating a variety of vascular and inflammatory processes. *J Biol Chem 271:9898, 1996* *J Immunol 153:3574, 1994*
CD40	Bp50	48	Mature B cells, monocytes, dendritic cells, basal epithelial cells, endothelial cells, fibroblasts, keratinocytes	CD40 is a member of the nerve growth factor receptor superfamily. It binds CD154 (CD40L) expressed on activated T-helper cells and serves as receptor for costimulatory signal for B cells; promotes growth, differentiation, and isotype switching of B cells; and regulates cytokine production by macrophages and dendritic cells. It is worth emphasizing that CD40-CD154 interaction is essential for B-cell differentiation, maturation, and secretion of IgG, IgA, and IgE antibodies. Patients with mutations in CD40L have an immunodeficiency called *X-linked hyper-IgM syndrome.* CD40 is positive in most B-cell lymphomas. *Immunol Res 24:311, 2001* *Immunol Today 19:502, 1998*
CD41	GpIIb of the gpIIb-gpIIIa complex; αIIb integrin	120	Platelets and megakaryocytes	CD41 associates with CD61 (gpIIIa) to form receptor for fibrinogen, fibronectin, vitronectin, vWF, and thrombospondin. It facilitates platelet adhesion and aggregation. Deficiency of CD41 and/or CD61 causes thromboasthenia *(Glanzmann disease).* Patients' platelets do not aggregate with ADP, epinephrine, thrombin, collagen, and arachidonic acid in vitro. CD41 and CD61 are used as markers for megakaryocytic differentiation (e.g., AML FAB-M7). *N Engl J Med 332:1553, 1995* *J Biol Chem 271:6017, 1996* *J Biol Chem 271:18610, 1996*

CD MARKERS	OTHER NAMES	MOLECULAR WEIGHT (KDA)	KNOWN NORMAL DISTRIBUTION	REMARKS
CD42a	GpIX	22	Platelets and megakaryocytes	CD42a associates with CD42b; CD42c and CD42d with 2:2:2:1 stoichiometry to form the gpIb-IX complex that serves as the receptor for subendothelial vWF, allowing for platelet adhesion to damaged blood vessels. Deficiency of gpIb-IX complex causes defective binding to vWF and thereby defective adhesion to exposed subendothelial matrix *(Bernard-Soulier syndrome)*. Patients have variable degree of thrombocytopenia, and their platelets do not aggregate with ristocetin in vitro. CD42 is also used as a marker for megakaryocytic differentiation.
CD42b	CD42b-α; GPIb-α	145	Platelets and megakaryocytes	
CD42c	CD42b-β; GPIb-β	24	Platelets and megakaryocytes	
CD42d	GPV	82	Platelets and megakaryocytes	
				Blood 87:1377, 1996 *Blood 81:2339, 1993* *J Biol Chem 269:23716, 1996* *J Biol Chem 271:22076, 1996*
CD43	Leukosialin; sialophorin	95-115	Thymocytes, T cells, neutrophils, macrophages, monocytes, NK cells, platelets, megakaryocytes, activated B cells (weak), plasma cells, hematopoietic stem cells	CD43 is a sialoglycoprotein that may bind to CD54 (ICAM-1) and/or albumin and function as an antiadhesion molecule. It inhibits T-cell interactions, including T-cell killing. Its expression is defective in Wiskott-Aldrich syndrome, secondary to X-linked genetic defect. CD43 is positive in the majority of T-cell lymphomas. CD43 is usually positive in myeloma, lymphoplasmacytic lymphoma, extranodal marginal zone B-cell lymphoma of mucosa-associated lymphoid tissue (MALT lymphoma), mast cell disease, and myeloid and/or granulocytic sarcomas. It is worthy of emphasis that CD43 is a very useful immunohistochemical marker for the diagnosis of MALT lymphoma (CD20$^+$/CD43$^+$/CD3$^-$) and myeloid sarcomas (CD43$^+$/CD3$^-$/CD20$^-$) in biopsy tissues. *J Exp Med 199:1277, 2004* *Immunol Today 19:546, 1998* *Nature 377:535, 1995*
CD44	Phagocytic glycoprotein-1 (Pgp-1); Hermes antigen; extracellular matrix receptor type III (ECMRIII); Hutch-1	85	Most cell types except platelets, hepatocytes, cardiac muscle, renal tubular epithelium, testis	CD44 is a polymorphic receptor for hyaluronate that facilitates lymphocyte binding to high endothelial venules (HEV). Variant isoforms of CD44 have attached chondroitin sulfate and are able to bind fibronectin, laminin, and collagen. CD44 is

CD MARKERS	OTHER NAMES	MOLECULAR WEIGHT (KDA)	KNOWN NORMAL DISTRIBUTION	REMARKS
CD44—CONT				also a receptor for chemotactic cytokine osteopontin. CD44 and its isoforms have been implicated in many biological processes, such as cell adhesion, cell substrate, cell to cell interactions, including lymphocyte homing hemopoiesis, cell migration, and tumor metastasis. It is worth noting that CD44R (exon 9 of CD44) also serves as the protein backbone of red blood cell Lutheran antigen. *Clin Exp Metastasis 20:195, 2003* *Exp Hematol 27:978, 1999* *Science 271:509, 1996* *Adv Immunol 54:271, 1993*
CD45	Leukocyte common antigen (LCA); T200; B220	180, 200, 210, 220	All leukocytes, all hematopoietic cells	CD45 is a tyrosine phosphatase that modulates signal transduction by surface antigen receptor. It is critical for the antigen-receptor mediated activation of T cells and B cells and other leukocytes. There are multiple isoforms of CD45 that result from alternative splicing. Changes in the extracellular domain do not affect the intracellular phosphatase activity of the cytoplasmic domain. It is worth noting that early hematopoietic precursor cells and plasma cells may be negative for CD45. *Leuk Lymphoma 45:229, 2004* *Ann Rev Immunol 21:107, 2003* *Ann Rev Immunol 12:85, 1993* *Adv Immunol 66:1, 1997* *Immunol Res 16:101, 1997*
CD45RA	B220	220	B cells, subset of naïve CD4 T cells, monocytes	CD45RA is formed by joining the 8-amino acid N-terminal sequence to that encoded by exons A, B, and C and is the largest of the CD45 isoforms. *Immunology 2:246, 1999* *Eur J Immunol 29:2098, 1999*
CD45RB	T200	210, 220	Memory T cells, B cells, monocytes, neutrophils (weak)	CD45RB is formed by joining the 8-amino acid N-terminal sequence to that encoded by exons B and C. *Eur J Immunol 28:3435, 1998* *Cell Immunol 167:56, 1996*

CD MARKERS	OTHER NAMES	MOLECULAR WEIGHT (KDA)	KNOWN NORMAL DISTRIBUTION	REMARKS
CD45RC		190, 210, 220	B cells, some T cells	CD45RC is formed by joining the 8-amino acid N-terminal sequence to that encoded by exon C. *Immunol Rev 146:82, 1995*
CD45RO	UCHL-1	180	Memory and activated T cells, some B cells, gran-ulocytes (weak), macrophages (weak), cortical thymocytes	CD45RO is formed by joining the 8-amino acid N-terminal sequence to the CD45 backbone without A, B, or C and thus is the smallest CD45 isoform. CD45RO is usually positive in T-cell lymphomas, but negative in most B-cell lymphomas. *Eur J Immunol 29:2098, 1999*
CD46	Membrane cofactor protein (MCP)	66, 56	Endothelial cells, epithe-lial cells, fibroblasts, pla-centa, sperm, all blood cells except red cells	CD46 acts as a cofactor for Factor I proteo-lytic cleavage of C3b and C4b. It permits factor I, a serine protease, to convert C3b and C4b into inactive complement frag-ments. CD46 also serves as the receptor for measles virus and human herpes virus-6. CD46 has multiple isoforms. *Trends Immunol 25:496, 2004* *Rev Med Virol 14:217, 2004* *Int J Mol Med 1:809, 1998*
CD47	Integrin-associated pro-tein (IAP); ovarian CA antigen (OV-3); Rh-related antigen	50-55	All hematopoietic cells, epithelial cells, endothe-lial cells, fibroblasts, mesenchymal cells	CD47 associates with CD61 integrins to form receptor for thrombospondin, suggest-ing a role in chemotaxis and cell-cell adhe-sion. It forms part of the Rh antigen com-plex on red cells and is not expressed on Rh_{null} red blood cells. It may also play a role in giant cell creation from macrophage fusion. *Trends Cell Biol 11:130, 2001* *Science 274:795, 1996*
CD48	Blast-1; BCM1; MEM-102; HuLy-m3	45	All hematopoietic cells except neutrophils, platelets, red cells	CD48 is a GPI-anchored, low-affinity ligand for CD2. It also binds to CD244. On T cells its cytoplasmic domain associates with the Lck and Fyn tyrosine kinases. Thus CD48 may play a role in signal transduction. *Immunol Rev 181:234, 2001* *Immunol Today 17:177, 1996*

CD MARKERS	OTHER NAMES	MOLECULAR WEIGHT (KDA)	KNOWN NORMAL DISTRIBUTION	REMARKS
CD49a	Very late activation antigen-1 (VLA-1) α subunit; α_1 integrin	210	Monocytes, endothelium, smooth muscle, activated T cells and B cells	Integrins are integral cell surface proteins composed of an α- and a β-chain. A given chain may combine with multiple partners resulting in different integrins. Very late antigens are a family of integrins originally identified on activated T cells, later on fibroblasts, platelets, monocytes, etc. Six VLA isoforms have been identified (VLA1 to VLA-6), each with distinct α chain (α1-α6) associated with a common β-chain. CD49a assembles into a heterodimer with CD29 to form a receptor for collagen and laminin. *J Biol Chem 168:2989, 1993* *Ann Rev Immunol 8:365, 1990*
CD49b	Very late activation antigen-2 (VLA-2) α subunit; α_2 integrin	160	Monocytes, platelets, T cells, B cells, and NK cells, thymocytes, fibroblasts, endothelium, osteoclasts, epithelium	CD49b assembles with CD29 to form a receptor for laminin, fibronectin, e-cadherin, and collagen types I, II, III, and IV. It is responsible for platelet adhesion to collagen during clotting and plays a role in angiogenesis. *Ann Rev Immunol 114:365, 1990* *Eur J Immunol 22:1109, 1992*
CD49c	Very late activation antigen-3 (VLA-3) α subunit; α_3 integrin	125	Monocytes, T cells and B cells, kidney glomeruli, thyroid, some basement membranes	CD49c assembles with CD29 to form a receptor for laminin and epiligrin (kalinin) that also binds weakly to collagen and fibronectin, suggesting a role in cell-cell adhesion. *Mol Cell Biol 7:194, 1996* *J Biol Chem 268:8651, 1993*
CD49d	Very late activation antigen-4 (VLA-4) α subunit; α_4 integrin	150	T cells, B cells, and NK cells, monocytes, erythroblasts, myeloblasts, thymocytes, mast cells, dendritic cells, eosinophils, basophils	CD49d assembles with CD29 or β_7 integrin to form VLA-4 or $\alpha_4\beta_7$, respectively. These integrins bind VCAM-I (CD106) and some forms of fibronectin. $\alpha_4\beta_7$ also binds mucosal addressin MAdCAM-1. These integrins help mediate lymphocyte adhesion to endothelium and migration into tissue, promote differentiation of hematopoietic precursors by adhesion to bone marrow stromal cells. It is also relevant to tumor progression and metastasis. *J Immunol 156:3727, 1996* *Cell 80:413, 1995* *J Clin Invest 94:1722, 1994*

CD MARKERS	OTHER NAMES	MOLECULAR WEIGHT (KDA)	KNOWN NORMAL DISTRIBUTION	REMARKS
CD49e	Very late activation antigen-5 (VLA-5) α subunit; α_5 integrin	155 (135/25)	Thymocytes, T cells, monocytes, platelets, activated or very early B cells, neutrophils	CD49e assembles with CD29 to form a receptor for fibronectin and invasin via binding to RGD. Upon binding it activates the Na^+-H^+ antiporter and may act as accessory molecule for T-cell activation. *Cell 69:11, 1992* *Ann Rev Immunol 114:365, 1990*
CD49f	Very late activation antigen-6 (VLA-6) α subunit; α_6 integrin; platelet gpIc	140 (120/30)	Platelets, macrophages, monocytes, thymocytes, T cells, adherent epithelia	CD49f assembles with CD29 or the β_4 integrin chain (CD104) to form a receptor for laminin on basement membranes of vessels. It is also important for the formation of hemidesmosomes of stratified squamous and transitional epithelia. *Trends Cell Biol 5:419, 1995* *Proc Natl Acad Sci USA 88:10183, 1991*
CD50	Intercellular adhesion molecule-3 (ICAM-3)	120-140	Thymocytes, T cells and B cells, neutrophils, monocytes, endothelial cells	CD50 serves as a ligand for LFA-1 (CD11a-CD18). *Biochem Soc Trans 26:644, 1998* *J Cell Biol 123:1007, 1993*
CD51	Vitronectin receptor α chain; α_v subunit of $\alpha_v\beta_3$ integrin, vitronectin receptor	150 (125/24)	Endothelial cells, monocytes, macrophages, platelets (weak), some B cells (weak)	CD51 assembles with CD61 (β_3) to form a receptor for vitronectin, vWF, thrombospondin, fibrinogen, and collagen. These receptors facilitate platelet aggregation and/or endothelial cell adhesion and play a role in monocyte migration through subendothelium and in angiogenesis. CD51 also can associate with the β_5 integrin to form an alternate vitronectin receptor. *Curr Opin Cell Biol 13:563, 2001* *Curr Opin Cell Biol 5:864, 1993* *Thromb Haemost 70:87, 1993*
CD52	CAMPATH-1	25-29	Thymocytes, lymphocytes, monocytes, macrophages, eosinophils, epithelial cells lining the male reproductive tract, spermatozoa	CD52 is a GPI-anchored surface glycoprotein with a very short mature protein sequence (composed of only 12 amino acids), but with a large carbohydrate domain. The physiological function of CD52 is largely unknown. CD52 is necessary for spermatozoa to preserve normal motility. Anti-CD52 monoclonal antibodies (MoAb) are lytic for target cells, both with complement and via antibody-dependent cytotoxicity. Anti-CD52 (e.g., alemtuzumab, CAMPATH-1H)

CD MARKERS	OTHER NAMES	MOLECULAR WEIGHT (KDA)	KNOWN NORMAL DISTRIBUTION	REMARKS
CD52—CONT				has been used for the treatment of patients with low-grade lymphoproliferative disorders, refractory chronic lymphocytic leukemia (CLL) in particular. Anti-CD52 is also used for depletion of bone marrow T lymphocytes and tolerance induction in transplantation. *Semin Oncol 30:493, 2003* *Mol Hum Reprod 2:177, 1996* *Biochem Soc Trans 23:1057, 1995* *J Hematother 3:15, 1994*
CD53	OX-44	32-42	Leukocytes	CD53 is a member of the tetraspanin-transmembrane-4 superfamily. CD53 is among several tetraspanins to be expressed differentially on cells at different stages of growth and differentiation. CD53 participates in a series of complexes with other leukocyte surface molecules, including CD2, CD19, CD21 and MHC class II, and other tetraspanins, including CD37, CD81, and CD82. Association between tetraspanins and integrins may be linked to the ability of tetraspanins, such as CD81 and CD9, to influence cell migration and adhesion. CD53 also associates with the β_1 integrin, VLA-4, suggesting a role in cell motility. In addition, CD53 is involved in a variety of signaling events in leukocytes. *Immunol Today 15:588, 1994* *J Biol Chem 273:30537, 1998*
CD54	ICAM-1	90	Leukocytes, endothelial cells, various epithelial cells, expression increased with activation	CD54 functions as a ligand for LFA-1 (CD11a-CD18), Mac-1 (CD11b-CD18), and CD11c-CD18, participating in immune response and inflammation. CD54 also acts as the receptor for rhinovirus and *Plasmodium falciparum*-infected red blood cells. *Adv Drug Deliv Rev 56:763, 2004* *J Exp Med 182:1231, 1995* *Eur J Immunol 154:6080, 1995* *Nature 346:425, 1990*

CD MARKERS	OTHER NAMES	MOLECULAR WEIGHT (KDA)	KNOWN NORMAL DISTRIBUTION	REMARKS
CD55	Decay accelerating factor (DAF)	70	All hematopoietic cells, all cells in contact with serum, CNS, epithelial cells lining body fluid cavities	CD55 neutralizes complement activation on autologous tissue by preventing the assembly of C3 convertase (C3bBb and C4b2a) or accelerating disassembly of preformed convertase. It also serves as the receptors for CD97, echovirus, and Coxsackie B virus. CD55 is deficient in blood cells from patients with paroxysmal nocturnal hemoglobinuria (PNH) and thereby is used as a marker for the diagnosis of PNH. *Clin Lab Sci 17:172, 2004* *J Lab Clin Med 123:485, 1994*
CD56	Neural cell adhesion molecule-1 (N-CAM); Leu-19; NKH1	175-220	NK cells, embryonic cells, muscle, neural cells, epithelium, some activated T cells	CD56 is a cell surface adhesion molecule that facilitates homophilic adhesion and plays a role in contact-dependent growth inhibition, NK-cell cytotoxicity, and neural development. CD56 is the prototypic marker for NK cells. It is also present on subsets of CD4 and CD8 T cells. It is positive in a variety of hematological and/or lymphoid malignancies, such as NK-cell and/or T-cell leukemia and /or NK-cell or T-cell lymphoma, anaplastic large cell lymphoma, and plasma cell myeloma. Plasma cell leukemia is characteristically negative for CD56. *Leuk Lymphoma 45:61, 2004* *Ann Hematol 74:51, 1997* *Proc Natl Acad Sci USA 93:6421, 1996* *Neuron 17:413, 1996*
CD57	Human natural killer-1 (HNK-1); Leu 7	110	Subsets of NK cells, T cells, B cells, and monocytes; some Schwann cells; neuroectodermal tissue; brain; prostate; proximal tubules of kidney	CD57 is a cell surface glycoprotein with cell adhesion functions. It is a NK-and/or T-cell marker and neuroendocrine marker. Cells that are positive for CD56 but not CD57 have substantial NK-cell activities. Cells that are positive for CD56 and CD57 have variable (weak) NK-cell activities. CD57 is usually positive in T-cell large granular lymphocyte leukemia, but is negative in aggressive NK-cell leukemia. *Oncologist 9:247, 2004* *Trend Neurosci 18:183, 1995*

CD MARKERS	OTHER NAMES	MOLECULAR WEIGHT (KDA)	KNOWN NORMAL DISTRIBUTION	REMARKS
CD58	LFA-3	55-70	Most hematopoietic cells, fibroblasts, endothelium, epithelial cells	CD58 is a surface adhesion molecule that binds CD2 and thereby enhances T-cell antigen recognition. The CD58 homologue on sheep red cells allows these cells to form rosettes with human T cells. *Cell 97:791, 1999* *Proc Natl Acad Sci USA 96:4289, 1999* *Ann Rev Immunol 5:223, 1987*
CD59	Complement protectin; membrane inhibitor of reactive lysis (MIRL); H19; MACIF; HRF20; P-18; protectin	19-25	Leukocytes, red cells, endothelial and epithelial cells, placenta, spermatozoa, body fluids	CD59 is a GPI-anchored protein that inhibits complement-mediated lysis by preventing full assembly of the membrane attack complex (MAC). It binds to activated C8 in the C5b-8 complex, preventing C9 polymerization during the final step of MAC formation. It also is a minor ligand for CD2 and may be involved in T-cell signal transduction. Like CD55, CD59 is deficient in blood cells from patients with paroxysmal nocturnal hemoglobinuria (PNH). *Clin Lab Sci 17:172, 2004* *Mol Immunol 38:249, 2001* *Exp Clin Immunogenet 9:33, 1992*
CD60	NeuAc-NeuAc-Gal; UM4D4	120	T-cell subset, platelets, some monocytes, melanocytes, thymic epithelium, glomeruli, smooth muscle cells, astrocytes	CD60 has been identified as the terminal 9-O-acetylated form of ganglioside G_{D3}. The natural ligand for CD60 antigen remains unknown. Both anti-CD60 and anti-G_{D3} antibodies can exert co-stimulatory effects on activation of T cells, implying that the CD60 is an important surface component in the T-cell activation signaling pathway. *Immunol Invest 30:67, 2001* *Cell Immunol 187:117, 1998* *J Exp Med 179:1385, 1994*
CD61	GPIIIa; β_3 integrin; vitronectin receptor β chain	110	Platelets, megakaryocytes, monocytes, macrophages, endothelial cells	CD61 associates with CD41 to form the gpIIb-IIIa heterodimer that facilitates platelet aggregation or with CD51 to form a receptor for vitronectin. Deficiency of CD41 and/or CD61 causes thromboasthenia *(Glanzmann disease)*. Patients' platelets do not aggregate with ADP, epinephrine, thrombin, collagen, and arachidonic acid in

CD MARKERS	OTHER NAMES	MOLECULAR WEIGHT (KDA)	KNOWN NORMAL DISTRIBUTION	REMARKS
CD61—CONT				vitro. CD41 and CD61 are used as markers for megakaryocytic differentiation (e.g., AML FAB-M7). *Curr Pharm Des 10:1567, 2004* *Blood 88:1666, 1996* *Thromb Haemost 2:492, 1994*
CD62E	E-selectin; endothelial leukocytes adhesion molecule-1 (ELAM-1); LECAM-2	115, 97	Endothelium	CD62E mediates leukocyte rolling on activated endothelium at inflammatory sites, facilitates tumor cell adhesion during hematogenous metastasis, and plays a role in angiogenesis. Patients with leukocyte adhesion deficiency-2 (LAD-2) who lack sialyl Lewis^X component of E-selectin receptors suffer recurrent pyogenic infections. *Cells Tissues Organs 172:161, 2002* *Cell 84:563, 1996* *Faseb J 9:866, 1995*
CD62L	L-selectin; TQ1; leukocyte adhesion molecule-1 (LAM-1); Leu-8; LECAM-1; MEL-14	65, 95	B cells, T cells, neutrophils, thymocytes, monocytes, eosinophils, basophils, erythroid and myeloid progenitor cells, NK cells	CD62L mediates lymphocyte homing to high endothelial venules of peripheral lymphoid tissue (e.g., lymph nodes) and leukocyte rolling on activated endothelium at inflammatory sites. *Ann Rev Immunol 22:129, 2004* *Science 272:60, 1996* *Nature 380:720, 1996* *J Clin Invest 98:1081, 1996*
CD62P	P-selectin; GMP-140; LECAM-3; PADGEM	120, 140	Platelets, megakaryocytes, endothelial cells	CD62P interacts with CD162, and thereby mediates tethering and rolling of leukocytes on the surface of activated endothelial cells, the first step in leukocyte extravasation and migration. It also mediates rolling of platelets on endothelial cells and platelet-mediated delivery of lymphocytes to high endothelial venules. *Trends Mol Med 10:179, 2004* *Science 273:252, 1996* *Cell 84:563, 1996*

CD MARKERS	OTHER NAMES	MOLECULAR WEIGHT (KDA)	KNOWN NORMAL DISTRIBUTION	REMARKS
CD63	Platelet 53-kDa activation antigen; ME491; MLA1; PTLGP40; granulophysin; LAMP-3	40-60	Activated platelets, monocytes, macrophages, secretory granules of vascular endothelial cells (Weibel-Palade bodies), platelet dense body granules, fibroblasts, osteoclasts, dendritic cells, synovial lining cells, brain white matter and peripheral nerves	CD63 is a member of the tetraspanin family and may facilitate adhesion to activated endothelium. In human dendritic cells, CD63 appears to be involved in antigen capture and its subsequent processing and/or presentation in the context of MHC class II molecules. It is used as a marker for platelet activation in vivo. It can also be used as a marker for primary melanomas. CD63 is deficient in dense granules of platelets with Hermansky-Pudlak syndrome._Immunol Rev 189:136, 2002_ _Biochem Biophys Res Commun 222:13, 1996_ _J Immunol 157:2039, 1996_
CD64	FcγRI	72	Monocytes, macrophages, dendritic cells, activated neutrophils	CD64 is a high-affinity receptor that binds Fc region of IgG (IgG3>IgG1>IgG4>IgG2) and mediates phagocytosis, antigen capture, antibody-dependent cellular cytotoxicity (ADCC), and release of cytokines and reactive oxygen intermediates. There are at least three isoforms (A, B, and C). Like CD14 and CD4, CD64 is used as a marker for monocytic differentiation and is positive in acute myelomonocytic leukemia (FAB M4) and acute monocytic leukemia (FAB M5)._Mol Immunol 35:989, 1998_ _J Immunol 157:541, 1996_ _Immunol Today 14:215, 1994_
CD65	Ceramide-dodecasaccharide 4c; VIM-2		Myeloid cells, some monocytic cells	CD65 serves as a minor E-selectin (CD62E) ligand. It is used as a marker for myeloid and myelomonocytic differentiation (e.g., acute myeloid leukemias). It is an adhesion molecule that appears to be a significant risk factor for extravascular leukemic infiltration._Leuk Res 25:847, 2001_ _J Biochem 119:456, 1996_
CD65s	Sialylated CD65		Granulocytes, monocytes	CD65s appears when the progenitor antigen CD34 disappears, suggesting that this sialylated carbohydrate antigen marks a turning point in normal myeloid differentiation. CD65s is widely used for acute leukemia cell typing. Low expression of CD65s is a

CD MARKERS	OTHER NAMES	MOLECULAR WEIGHT (KDA)	KNOWN NORMAL DISTRIBUTION	REMARKS
CD65s—CONT				characteristic immunophenotypic feature for undifferentiated or minimally differentiated AML (FAB M0/M1), which occur predominantly in older adults. A subset of B-ALL (CD10-negative early pre-B ALL) may express CD65s and/or CD15. *Leukemia 17:1544, 2003*
CD66a	Phosphorylated glycoprotein; biliary glycoprotein-1 (BGP-1); nonspecific cross-reacting antigen-160 (NCA-160); CEA-related cell adhesion molecule-1 (CEA-CAM-1)	160-180 (113, 96, 74)	Neutrophils, histiocytes, some myeloid progenitor cells, brush border of colonic epithelial cells, prostate glands and ducts, bile canaliculi between liver cells.	The granulocyte activation antigens, CD66a, CD66b, CD66c, and CD66d belong to the family of carcinoembryonic antigen (CEA)-related cell adhesion molecules (CEACAM) and are expressed at low levels on resting blood granulocytes, but their surface expression is up regulated following stimulation. CD66a, in contrast to CD66b and CD66c that are anchored to the membrane via a GPI-linkage, is a transmembrane protein with a cytoplasmic domain. CD66a appears to facilitate Ca^{2+}-independent homotypic and heterotypic adhesion and neutrophil activation. Phosphorylation of CD66a on tyrosine by an associated tyrosine kinase may play a role in the function of CD66a. In addition, CD66a possesses Lewis^X and sialyl Lewis^X determinants. *J Immunol 166:6537, 2001* *Cancer Res 60:1236, 2000* *J Immunol 164:4257, 2000* *Eur J Immunol 28:3664, 1998*
CD66b (CD67)	CD67; CGM6; p100; nonspecific cross-reacting antigen-95 (NCA-95); CEACAM-8	95-100	Neutrophils, eosinophils	CD66b is one GPI-anchored isoform of CD66. It is a highly glycosylated protein expressed only in neutrophils and eosinophils. The precise function of CD66b remains unclear. As a member of the family of CEA, it may play a role in the interaction between granulocytes or between granulocytes and endothelial and/or epithelial cells. Serum CD66b may also serve as a biological marker for active granulocyte activities in vivo. *Clin Diagn Lab Immunol 10:485, 2003* *Blood 91:663, 1998*

CD MARKERS	OTHER NAMES	MOLECULAR WEIGHT (KDA)	KNOWN NORMAL DISTRIBUTION	REMARKS
CD66c	Nonspecific cross-reacting antigen-90 (NCA-90), CEACAM-6	90	Granulocytes (myeloid restricted)	CD66c is another GPI-anchored isoform of CD66. It is a cell adhesion protein on neutrophils, which reveals homophilic adhesion and heterophilic adhesion to other CEA family antigens, including CD66a, CD66b, and CEA (CD66b exhibits only heterophilic adhesion to CD66c). Cross-linking of CD66c induces aggregation and activation possibly via binding to CD62E. CD66c is expressed in a subset of pre-B ALL. *J Leukoc Biol 70:543, 2001* *Leukemia 13:779, 1999* *Tissue Antigens 52:1, 1998*
CD66d	CGM-1, CEACAM-3	30	Neutrophils	CD66d is a member of the CEA family of adhesion molecules that facilitates homotypic adhesion and neutrophil activation. It also functions as a receptor for *Neisseria gonorrhoeae* and *Neisseria meningitidis*. CD66d may play a signaling role and regulate adhesion activity of CD11-CD18 in neutrophils. *J Biol Chem 276:17413, 2001* *J Leukoc Biol 60:106, 1996*
CD66e	CEA	180-200	Tissues derived from all three germ layers during embryogenesis, adult colon epithelial cells (very weak), granulocytes	CD66e is a GPI-anchored glycoprotein, and may facilitate Ca^{2+}-independent homotypic and heterotypic adhesion during embryogenesis. CD66e binds weakly to other nonspecific cross-reacting antigens CD66a-c. It is widely used as a tumor marker for monitoring for disease recurrence in patients with a variety of malignancies, particularly gastrointestinal adenocarcinomas. *Semin Cancer Biol 9:67, 1999* *Cancer Res 56:4805, 1996* *Cancer Res 55:3873, 1995*
CD66f	PSG (pregnancy-specific glyco-protein), Sp-1	54-72	Tissues derived from all three germ layers during embryogenesis, adult colon epithelial cells (very weak), myeloid cell lines	CD66f is a GPI-anchored glycoprotein. Its function is unknown, but appears necessary for successful pregnancy and may be involved in protection of the fetus from maternal immune recognition. Low levels of CD66f in maternal blood predict spontaneous abortion. *Semin Cancer Biol 9:67, 1999* *Cancer Res 56:4805, 1996* *Cancer Res 55:3873, 1995*

CD MARKERS	OTHER NAMES	MOLECULAR WEIGHT (KDA)	KNOWN NORMAL DISTRIBUTION	REMARKS
CD68	Gp110; macrosialin (mouse); KP-1	110	Monocytes, macrophages, osteoclasts, mast cells, dendritic cells, neutrophils, activated platelets, B cells and T cells	CD68 is a sialomucin belonging to a family of highly glycosylated, acidic lysosomal glycoproteins (LGPs) that include LAMP-1 (CD107a) and LAMP-2 (CD107b). It may have role in macrophage phagocytic activities. CD68 is specific to lysosomes, not cell lineage, and functions to protect the lysosomal membranes from attack by hydrolases. CD68 is used as a marker for monocytes and/or macrophages and is positive in a variety of malignancies, including AML-M4/M5, histiocytic sarcoma, interdigitating dendritic cell sarcoma, Langerhans cell histiocytosis, mastocytosis, mast cell disease, etc. *Genomics 54:165, 1998* *Proc Natl Acad Sci USA 93:14833, 1996* *Am J Clin Pathol 103:425, 1995*
CD69	Activation inducer molecule (AIM); early activation antigen (EA-1); MLR-3; Leu-23	60 (28/33)	Platelets, activated T cells (Th1 cells), B cells, NK cells, neutrophils, eosinophils, epidermal Langerhans cells	CD69 is a member of the Ca^{2+}-dependent (C-type) lectin superfamily of type II transmembrane proteins. It forms a homodimer that may function as signal transducer, enhancing cell activation and/or platelet aggregation. It is involved in early events of T-cell, NK-cell, monocyte, and platelet activation. CD69 is highly expressed on T cells from inflammatory infiltrates of rheumatoid arthritis, viral hepatitis, and autoimmune thyroid disorders. It is positive in angioimmunoblastic T-cell lymphoma, Lennert's lymphoma, mycosis fungoides and/or Sézary syndrome, etc. *J Exp Med 197:1093, 2003* *J Immunol 162:3978, 1999* *Scand J Immunol 48:196, 1998*
CD70	CD27 ligand; Ki-24 antigen	29	Activated B cells and some activated T cells, antigen-presenting cells	CD70 is a member of the TNF family that binds CD27 and provides co-stimulatory signal for T- and B-cell activation. It is expressed transiently on activated T cells and B cells. It has been shown that CD70 expression on APCs plays a key role in the CD40-CD154-dependent CD8 T-cell responses. CD70 is expressed constitutively on a subset of B-cell chronic lymphocytic leukemia and large B-cell lymphomas. Reed-Sternberg cells are also positive for CD70. *J Immunol 173:6542, 2004* *Semin Immunol 10:491, 1998*

CD MARKERS	OTHER NAMES	MOLECULAR WEIGHT (KDA)	KNOWN NORMAL DISTRIBUTION	REMARKS
CD71	Transferrin receptor; T9	180 (95/95)	All proliferating cells, cells requiring iron (reticulocytes, erythroid precursors, capillary endothelial cell in brain)	CD71 serves as the receptor for iron-bound transferrin (ferrotransferrin). It is a transmembrane protein that mediates cellular uptake of iron, and the expression on cells reflects iron needs and erythropoietic activity. Transferrin receptors are also shed into plasma in an amount proportional to the amount present on cell surfaces and the concentration of transferrin receptor in serum (sTfR) can be measured. The sTfR level remains unchanged in anaemia arising from chronic disease so that it is a reliable marker to distinguish iron deficiency anemia from the anemia of chronic inflammation and liver disease. Increases in sTfR concentration occur earlier in the development of functional iron deficiency than do changes in free erythrocyte protoporphyrin or mean corpuscular volume. *Int J Hematol 76:213, 2002* *Semin Hematol 35:13, 1998* *Proc Natl Acad Sci USA 93:8175, 1996*
CD72	Lyb-2, Ly-32.2	86 (39/43)	All B cells (except plasma cells), macrophages (weak)	CD72 is a B-cell co-receptor that is expressed in all stages of B-cell development except plasma cells. Ligation of CD72 enhances B-cell growth and differentiation. The class IV semaphoring, CD100, has been identified as the natural ligand for CD72. It appears that CD72 plays a dual signaling role in B-cell function. *Trends Immunol 25:543, 2004* *Immunol Res 25:155, 2002* *Eur J Immunol 28:3003, 1998* *J Immunol 160:4662, 1998*
CD73	Ecto-5′-nucleotidase	70	Some B cells, some T cells, thymocytes (weak), some epithelial and endothelial cells, dendritic cells	CD73 is a GPI-anchored enzyme that catalyzes 5′ dephosphorylation of purine and pyrimidine ribonucleoside and deoxyribonucleoside monophosphates to their corresponding nucleosides. It also mediates costimulatory signals in T-cell activation and lymphocyte adhesion to endothelium. High levels of CD73 expression are poor prognostic factors in leukemia and/or lymphomas (e.g., ALL, CLL and/or SLL).

CD MARKERS	OTHER NAMES	MOLECULAR WEIGHT (KDA)	KNOWN NORMAL DISTRIBUTION	REMARKS
CD73—CONT				
				It is worth noting that the type-I isoform of pyrimidine 5'-nucleotidase (P5N-I) is a cytosolic enzyme encoded by a gene located on chromosome 7p15-14. P5N-I is physiologically important for the RNA degradation during reticulocyte maturation. P5N-I deficiency causes mild hemolytic anemia and basophilic stippling in red cells. P5N-I is a lead-sensitive enzyme. *Br J Haematol 120:375, 2003* *Biomed Pharmacother 56:100, 2002* *Immunol Rev 161:95, 1998*
CD74	Class II-associated invariant chain; Ii; Iγ; LN-2	33/35/41	B cells, activated T cells, monocytes (weak), dendritic cells, activated endothelial and epithelial cells	CD74 associates with the α and β chains of MIIC Class II proteins in the endoplasmic reticulum to block the peptide-binding groove and thus prevent binding of endogenous peptides. It is released from the MHC protein in the acidic lysosomal compartment. CD74 plays a key role in presentation of peptide antigens to T-cell antigen receptors. *Hum Immunol 54:159, 1997* *Immunology 79:331, 1993*
CD75	Lactosamines; LN-1	53 and 87	Mature B cells but not plasma cells, some T cells, red blood cells	CD75 serves as the ligand for CD22. The 'Popcorn cells' (L&H cells) seen in nodular lymphocyte predominant Hodgkin's lymphoma (NLPHL) are characteristically positive for CD75. The formerly known CDw75 is an alpha-2.6-sialylated protein (CD75s) of unknown function. The formerly known CDw76 (now CD75s) was deleted at the 7th HLDA Workshop. *Blood 87:5113, 1996* *J Cell Biol 116:423, 1992*
CD77	Globotriaosylceramide (Gβ3); P^k blood group; Burkitt's lymphoma associated antigen (BLA); ceramide trihexoside		Germinal center B cells, follicular dendritic cells, endothelium, some epithelial cells	CD77, a neutral glycosphingolipid, is the B-cell differentiation antigen. Binding of different ligands of CD77 triggers apoptosis, a key feature of germinal center B cells. CD77 acts as the receptor for Shiga toxin (produced by *Shigella dysenteriae*) and verotoxin-1 (produced by *Escherichia coli*).

CD MARKERS	OTHER NAMES	MOLECULAR WEIGHT (KDA)	KNOWN NORMAL DISTRIBUTION	REMARKS
CD77—CONT				
				It also binds CD19. Burkitt's lymphoma cells are characteristically positive for CD77.
				J Biol Chem 278:45200, 2003 *Eur J Immunol 21:1131, 1991* *J Exp Med 180:191, 1994*
CD79a	MB-1 (Igα)	82-95 (32-33)	B cells	CD79a is the Ig-alpha protein of the B-cell antigen receptor, analogous to CD3 for T cells. It is expressed early in B-cell differentiation and remains positive in mature B cells. It serves as an accessory molecule that mediates surface immunoglobulin expression and signal transduction.
				Appl Immunohistochem Mol Morphol 9:97, 2001 *Curr Opin Cell Biol 7:163, 1995*
CD79b	B29 (Igβ)	82-95 (37-39)	B cells	CD79b is the Ig-beta protein of the B-cell antigen receptor (see remarks for CD79a). CD79b is positive in a subset of plasma cells.
				Appl Immunohistochem Mol Morphol 9:97, 2001 *Immunity 4:145, 1996*
CD80	B7; B7-1; BB1	60	Activated B cells, monocytes, dendritic cells	CD80 is the ligand for T-cell marker CD28 or CD152 (CTLA4). It interacts with CD28 or CD152 for co-stimulation or co-inhibition of T cells with CD86, respectively. CD80-CD28 family molecules have critical roles in autoimmune, humoral, and transplant immune responses and have emerged as potential therapeutic targets.
				Nat Rev Immunol 4:336, 2004 *Trends Immunol 24:314, 2003* *Curr Opin Immunol 9:858, 1997*
CD81	Target of an antiproliferative antibody (TAPA-1)	22	Lymphocytes, endothelial cells, epithelial cells	CD81 is a member of CD19-CD21-Leu-13 (CD225) signal transduction complex that functions to regulate cell growth. It is a molecule involved in signal transduction and cell adhesion in the immune system.

CD MARKERS	OTHER NAMES	MOLECULAR WEIGHT (KDA)	KNOWN NORMAL DISTRIBUTION	REMARKS
CD81—CONT				
				CD81 may also be the receptor for hepatitis C virus. *Ann Rev Immunol 16:89, 1998* *Science 282:938, 1998*
CD82	R2; IA4; 4F9; KAI-1	50-53	Epithelia, endothelium, monocytes, neutrophils, platelets, activated lymphocytes	CD82 is a highly glycosylated protein that belongs to the transmembrane 4 (tetraspanin) superfamily. It associates with CD4 or CD8 and delivers co-stimulatory signals for T-cell receptor pathway. It is down-regulated in tumor progression and may function as a suppressor of tumor metastasis. Its expression appears to correlate with p53 expression. *Eur J Immunol 32:1328, 2002* *Curr Biol 24:1009, 2000* *Immunol Today 15:588, 1994*
CD83	HB15	45	Dendritic cells (not FDC), Langerhans cells, B cells (weak), interdigitating reticular cells	CD83 is involved in antigen presentation and the cellular interactions that follow lymphocyte activation. CD83 is strongly up-regulated together with co-stimulatory molecules, such as CD80 and CD86 during dendritic cell (DC) maturation, and is best known as a marker for mature DCs. Studies with herpes simplex virus type 1 (HSV-1)-infected DCs and the inhibition of the CD83 mRNA-specific transport from the nucleus to the cytoplasm have provided evidence that CD83 is important for DC biology. *Trends Immunol 23:273, 2002* *J Immunol 156:541, 1996*
CD84		72-86	Monocytes, platelets, germinal center B cells (strong), mantle zone B cells (weak), T-cell subset	CD84 is a member of the CD2 subgroup of immunoglobulin receptor superfamily (e.g., CD2, CD48, CD58, 2B4, Ly9, etc.). CD84 is involved in the activation of T cells via an SAP (signaling lymphocyte activation molecule-associated protein)-independent mechanism. In addition, the proliferative potential of CD34$^+$ progenitor cells decreases with increasing CD84 expression, suggesting that CD84 may serve as a

CD MARKERS	OTHER NAMES	MOLECULAR WEIGHT (KDA)	KNOWN NORMAL DISTRIBUTION	REMARKS
CD84—CONT				marker for committed hematopoietic progenitor cells.
				Tissue Antigens 64:132, 2004
				Exp Hematol 31:798, 2003
				J Immunol 171:2485, 2003
CD85	ILT/LIR family	110	Plasma cells (strong), mantle zone and germinal center B cells, subsets of T cells and NK cells, monocytes, dendritic cells	CD85 (isoforms a-m) are inhibitory MHC class I receptors, function to prevent killing by NK cells and T cells. It also inhibits B cells activated by antigen receptor and myelomonocytic cells activated by HLA-DR. CD85 is known as a marker for plasma cells and hairy cell leukemia.
				J Immunol 168:207, 2002
				J Immunol 165:3742, 2000
				J Leukoc Biol 65:841, 1999
CD86	B7-2; B70	80	Monocytes, dendritic cells, activated B cells and T cells, endothelial cells	CD86 is the ligand for CD28 and CD152 (CTLA4). It interacts with CD28 to provide a co-stimulatory signal or with CD152 to provide an inhibitory signal for T-cell activation.
				Trends Immunol 24:314, 2003
				Ann Rev Immunol 14:233, 1996
CD87	Urokinase plasminogen activator receptor (uPAR); Mo3	50-65	Monocytes, neutrophils, activated NK cells and LGL cells, T cells, endothelial cells, fibroblasts, smooth muscle cells, keratinocytes, placenta trophoblasts, hepatocytes	CD87 is the receptor for urokinase plasminogen activator (uPA). It functions to retain and concentrate uPA at the plasma membrane, allowing for local conversion of plasminogen to plasmin. Many tumor cells express CD87 and plasmin receptor, which are implicated in tumor invasion and metastasis.
				Leukemia 18:394, 2004
				J Immunol 156:297, 1996
				J Immunol 152:505, 1994
CD88	Receptor for C5a (C5aR)	40	Neutrophils, monocytes, eosinophils, mast cells, hepatocytes, smooth muscle, endothelial cells, dendritic cells, astrocytes, microglia	CD88 is a G-protein coupled receptor that triggers chemotaxis, activation, respiratory burst, and degranulation upon binding to C5a.
				Nat Rev Immunol 4:133, 2004
				Nature 383:86, 1996
				Ann Rev Immunol 12:785, 1994

CD MARKERS	OTHER NAMES	MOLECULAR WEIGHT (KDA)	KNOWN NORMAL DISTRIBUTION	REMARKS
CD89	Fc receptor for IgA; FcαR	55-75	Neutrophils, monocytes, macrophages, mucosa, activated eosinophils, some B cells and T cells	CD89 binds Fc of IgA_1 or IgA_2 with high affinity to trigger granulocyte responses. As such, it amplifies the protective effects of IgA by inducing phagocytosis, degranulation, respiratory burst, and killing of microorganisms. *Immunol Lett 92:23, 2004* *J Immunol 156.4442, 1996*
CD90	Thy-1; theta	18	Hematopoietic stem cells, thymic stromal cells, prothymocytes, neurons, connective tissue	CD90 mediates differentiation of hematopoietic stem cells and synaptogenesis in the central nervous system. $CD34^+CD90^+$ cells (hematopoietic stem cells) are essential for bone marrow engraftment after transplantation. *Leuk Lymphoma 45:661, 2004* *Nature 379:826, 1996*
CD91	Receptor for α_2 macroglobulin; LDL-receptor associated protein-1	600 (515/85)	Monocytes, macrophages, antigen-presenting cells, astrocytes, fibroblasts, epithelial cells	CD91 is a member of the low density lipoprotein receptor family that binds to α_2 macroglobulin (a neutral protease inhibitor) and apo-E-containing lipoproteins. It mediates chylomicron remnant clearance from plasma. It is also the cell surface receptor for heat shock proteins (HSP), mediating a cascade of events including maturation, activation, and representation of chaperoned foreign peptides with class I molecules on the surface of antigen-presenting cells. *J Antimicrob Chemother 53:1, 2004* *Proc Natl Acad Sci USA 101:6128, 2004* *Ann NY Acad Sci 737:1, 1994*
CD92	GR9	70	Neutrophils, monocytes, platelets, endothelial cells	The function of CD92 is unknown, but it may regulate dendritic cell function.
CD93	C1qRp, GR11	110-120	Neutrophils, monocytes, endothelial cells	CD93 is an O-sialoglycoprotein, which was originally identified as a myeloid cell surface marker. It has been shown to be a phagocytic receptor involved in the in vitro C1q- and IgG-dependent enhancement of phagocytosis. *J Immunol 172:3406, 2004* *J Cell Physiol 196:512, 2003*

CD MARKERS	OTHER NAMES	MOLECULAR WEIGHT (KDA)	KNOWN NORMAL DISTRIBUTION	REMARKS
CD94	Kp43	70 (30,43)	NK cells, T-cell subset	CD94 forms a heterodimer with NKG2, both expressed on NK cells and a small subset of T cells. This receptor varies in function as an inhibitor or activator depending on which isoform of NKG2 is expressed. The ligand for CD94-NKG2 is HLA-E, which is nonclassical class I molecule that binds leader peptide from other class I molecules. *Mol Immunol 42:485, 2005* *J Immunol 157:4741, 1996*
CD95	Apo-1; Fas	42	Activated lymphocytes, fibroblasts, monocytes, neutrophils, liver, breast, vaginal and/or endometrial and/or ovarian epithelium	CD95 induces apoptosis when bound by Fas ligand (Fas-L, CD178). When activated Fas-associated death domain (FADD) recruits caspase-8 to the receptor. The resulting "death-inducing signaling complex" performs caspase-8 proteolytic activation and thereby programmed cell death. *Semin Immunol 15:185, 2003* *Curr Opin Immunol 8:355, 1996*
CD96	T-cell activation increased late expression (TACTILE)	160	Activated T cells and NK cells	CD96 is involved in adhesion of activated T cells and NK cells to target cells in immune responses. *J Immunol 172:3994, 2004* *J Immunol 148:2600, 1992*
CD97	CD55 ligand; GR1	74, 80, 89	Neutrophils, monocytes, activated T cells and B cells, dendritic cells	CD97 acts as an adhesion molecule by binding to its cellular ligand, CD55 (DAF). It is involved in cell adhesion and signaling during leukocyte activation. It is also an EGF-TM7 receptor found on various carcinomas where expression levels correlate with dedifferentiation and tumor stage. *Int J Cancer 112:815, 2004* *J Immunol 172:1125, 2004* *Immunogenetics 55:655, 2004*
CD98	4F2; FRP-1; SLC3A2	120 (40/80) —	Strong on monocytes, activated T cells, and cardiomyocytes; weak on T cells, B cells, and NK cells	CD98 is a cell surface glycoprotein, formed by the covalent linkage of CD98 heavy chain with several different light chains and functions to serve as amino acid transporters. There is a growing literature impli-

CD MARKERS	OTHER NAMES	MOLECULAR WEIGHT (KDA)	KNOWN NORMAL DISTRIBUTION	REMARKS
CD98—CONT				cating CD98 in integrin function and its role in cell growth regulation. *J Membr Biol 173:165, 2000* *J Immunol 155:3585, 1995*
CD99	MIC-2; O13; E2; 12E7; HuLy-m6; FMC29	32	All white blood cells, Xg(a⁺) red blood cells (surface), Xg(a⁻) red blood cells (cytoplasm), ovarian granulose cells, pancreatic islets, infant thymus, Sertoli cells	CD99 is encoded by the MIC2 gene and is a surface antigen with broad cellular expression but with no clear, designated biological function. MIC2Y and MIC2X are expressed in males and females, respectively. MIC2X does not undergo X inactivation. CD99 is involved in rosette formation with sheep red blood cells. CD99 also serves as a nonspecific marker for Ewing's sarcoma, T-cell lymphomas, and Reed-Sternberg cells. It appears to associate with EWS-FLI1 fusion transcript, t(11;22)(q24;q12), causing FLI1 protein overexpression. *Hum Pathol 35:773, 2004* *Faseb J 16:1946, 2002* *Immunol Invest 24:173, 1995* *J Immunol 154:26, 1995*
CD100	Sema4D; GR3	300 (150)	B cells, T cells, and NK cells, most myeloid cells; expression increases upon activation	CD100 is a member of Semaphorin (sema) family that plays a role in monocyte migration, T-cell activation, B-cell survival, and T-cell -B-cell and T-dendritic cell cooperation. It functions by modifying the signaling of other receptors, such as CD40 or CD45. *Cell Mol Life Sci 61:292, 2004* *Crit Rev Immunol 23:65, 2003*
CD101	V7; p126	200 (126)	Monocytes, granulocytes, dendritic cells, activated T cells	CD101 is a member of the immunoglobulin (Ig) superfamily of proteins and plays a co-stimulatory role in T-cell activation. Neoplastic Langerhans cells (e.g., Langerhans cell histiocytosis) are usually positive for CD101. *Histopathology 36:229, 2000* *J Immunol 157:3366, 1996*

CD MARKERS	OTHER NAMES	MOLECULAR WEIGHT (KDA)	KNOWN NORMAL DISTRIBUTION	REMARKS
CD102	ICAM-2	54-68	Endothelial cells (strong), platelets (strong), resting lymphocytes, monocytes, dendritic cells	CD102 acts as a ligand for LFA-1 (CD11a-CD18), but unlike CD54, it does not bind to Mac-1 (CD11b-CD18) or undergo up-regulation upon cellular activation. It provides co-stimulatory signal in immune response and is important in lymphocyte recirculation. *J Biol Chem 268:21474, 1993* *Eur J Immunol 28:1970, 1998*
CD103	Integrin αE subunit; human mucosal lymphocyte antigen-1 (HML-1)	175 (150, 25)	1%-3% peripheral lymphocytes, intraepithelial lymphocytes, some lamina propria T cells, intraepithelial dendritic cells, testis, prostate, ovary, pancreas	CD103 associates with the β_7 integrin to form a receptor that binds E-cadherin to facilitate adhesion to epithelia. It serves as a useful marker for intraepithelial lymphocytes (normal or neoplastic). CD103 is characteristically in hairy cell leukemia, enteropathy-associated T-cell lymphoma, and HTLV-1 associated adult T-cell leukemia and/or lymphoma. *Eur J Immunol 34:2720, 2004* *Curr Opin Hematol 10:258, 2003* *Semin Immunol 7:335, 1995*
CD104	Integrin β_4 chain	210 (220)	Epithelia, CD4 and/or CD8 thymocytes, few neuronal cells, basement membranes, Schwann cells	CD104 associates with α_6 (CD49f) to form a receptor for laminin (and possibly epiligrin), facilitating adhesion of cells to the extracellular matrix. *J Cell Biol 134:559, 1996* *Nature Genet 10:229, 1995*
CD105	Endoglin; receptor for TGF-β	170 (95)	Endothelium, activated monocytes, macrophages, proerythroblasts, follicular dendritic cells, syncytiotrophoblasts, cytotrophoblasts	CD105 has binding activity for TGF-β_1 and TGF-β_3 in association with TGF-β receptors I and II. It is involved in regulation of cell differentiation and migration. It is a useful marker for assessing microvascular density in various malignancies. Mutations in CD105 gene cause hereditary hemorrhagic telangiectasia type I. *Anticancer Res 24:1337, 2004* *Mod Pathol 17:1513, 2004* *J Transl Med 2:18, 2004* *J Immunol 154:4456, 1995*
CD106	VCAM-1; INCAM-110	100-110	Activated endothelial cells, macrophages, follicular dendritic cells	CD106 is the ligand for VLA-4 (CD49d-CD29) that is present in stimulated endothelium and plays a role in migration of white blood cells to sites of inflammation. It is

CD MARKERS	OTHER NAMES	MOLECULAR WEIGHT (KDA)	KNOWN NORMAL DISTRIBUTION	REMARKS
CD106—CONT				
				also involved in lymphocyte-dendritic cell interactions and in myogenesis. *Nature 373:539, 1995* *J Immunol 156:2851, 1996*
CD107a	Lysosome-associated membrane protein-I (LAMP-1)	110	Activated platelets, neutrophils, T cells, macrophages, dendritic cells, endothelial cells, tonsillar epithelium	CD107a serves as ligand for galaptin, an S-type lectin (galectin) in the extracellular matrix. It contains sialylated Lewis^x structures that can bind CD62E. It may play a role in tumor metastasis. *Biochem Biophys Res Commun 215:757, 1995* *J Biol Regul Homeost Agents 16:147, 2002*
CD107b	LAMP-2	120	Activated platelets, neutrophils, activated endothelial cells, tonsillar epithelium	Same as CD107a
CDw108	John-Milton-Hagen blood group antigen; GR2; sema7A	75	Erythrocytes, lymphoblasts, lymphocytes (weak)	CD108 is a GPI-anchored antigen (semaphorin) that is a potent stimulator of cytokine production, chemotaxis, and superoxide release in monocytes. Deficiency may be associated with a rare form of congenital dyserythropoietic anemia (CDA). *J Immunol 162:4094, 1999* *Scand J Immunol 56:270, 2002*
CD109	Gov alloantigen; GR56	175	Endothelium, hematopoietic progenitor cells, platelets, activated T cells	CD109 is a GPI-anchored glycoprotein that carries the biallelic platelet-specific Gov antigen system, which is implicated in refractoriness to platelet transfusion, neonatal alloimmune thrombocytopenia, and post-transfusion purpura. *Exp Hematol 27:1282, 1999*
CD110	Thrombopoietin receptor (TPO-R); myeloproliferative leukemia virus oncogene (MPL)		Hematopoietic stem and progenitor cells, megakaryocytes, platelets (weak)	CD110 is the receptor for thrombopoietin (TPO), which induces megakaryocyte differentiation and proliferation. Mutations in CD110 gene are found in some patients with congenital amegakaryocytic thrombocytopenia. *Semin Hematol 40(S1):6, 2003* *Proc Natl Acad Sci USA 96:3132, 1999*

CD MARKERS	OTHER NAMES	MOLECULAR WEIGHT (KDA)	KNOWN NORMAL DISTRIBUTION	REMARKS
CD111	Nectin-1	64-72	Hematopoietic cells, epithelial cells, endothelial cells, neurons	CD111 is a widely expressed adhesion molecule that is a component of the adherens junction, where it bridges cells through homophilic or heterophilic interactions with other nectins. It also serves as the receptor for HSV-1 and HSV-2. *Leukemia 17:1137, 2003* *Cancer Sci 94:655, 2003* *J Virol 77:8985, 2003*
CD112	Nectin-2	64-72	Same as CD111	Same as CD111
CD114	G-CSF receptor	150	Granulocytes, monocytes, platelets, endothelium, placenta, trophoblast cells	CD114 is a class I cytokine receptor for G-CSF that plays a role in the regulation of myeloid differentiation and proliferation. Mutations in CD114 are found in some patients with severe congenital neutropenia. *Blood 88:761, 1996* *Rev Clin Exp Hematol 7:72, 2003*
CD115	M-CSF receptor, c-fms	150	Monocytes and/or macrophages and their precursors, osteoclasts, placental trophoblasts, neurons, microglia, astrocytes	CD115 is a class III cytokine receptor for M-CSF. M-CSF induces tyrosine phosphorylation of CD115, leading to the differentiation and proliferation of monocytes and its precursors. Deficiency of CD115 causes reduced osteoclasts and macrophages, abnormal bone remodeling and osteopetrosis, abnormal breast development, and decreased fertility. *Growth Factors 17:155, 2000* *Cell 61:203, 1990*
CD116	GM-CSF receptor; CSF-1R; HGM-CSFR	70-85	Monocytes, neutrophils, eosinophils, endothelial cells, dendritic cells, fibroblasts	CD116 is the receptor for GM-CSF. The low affinity of the α subunit for GM-CSF is increased when it forms a heterodimer with a 120-140 kDa β subunit common to the IL-3 receptor (CD123-CD131) and the IL-5 receptor (CD125-CD131). Binding of CD116 to GM-CSF stimulates cell proliferation and differentiation. *Cell 67:1, 1991* *Cytokine Growth Factor Rev 12:19, 2001*

CD MARKERS	OTHER NAMES	MOLECULAR WEIGHT (KDA)	KNOWN NORMAL DISTRIBUTION	REMARKS
CD117	C-kit; stem cell factor receptor; steel factor receptor	145	Hematopoietic progenitors, mast cells, melanocytes, spermatogonia, oocytes, some NK cells, breast epithelium	CD117 is the class III cytokine receptor (receptor tyrosine kinase) and functions to induce its tyrosine kinase activity, leading to cellular proliferation and/or differentiation. It is important for the development and survival of hematopoietic stem cells, mast cells, melanocytes, germ cells, and interstitial cells of Cajal. CD117, like PDGF receptors and Bcr/Abl fusion protein, has become a therapeutic target of tyrosine kinase inhibitor (e.g., Gleevec) for the treatment of gastrointestinal stromal tumor (GIST) and systemic mastocytosis, etc. *Cell Mol Life Sci 61:2535, 2004* *J Allergy Clin Immunol 114:13, 2004*
CD118		90	Broadly expressed	CD118 is the receptor for interferon-α and/or interferon-β
CD119		90	Monocytes, macrophages, T cells, B cells, and NK cells, neutrophils, epithelial cells, endothelial cells, fibroblasts	CD119 is the receptor for interferon-γ. *Ann Rev Immunol 11:571, 1993* *Cell 76:793, 1994*
CD120a	TNFR-1	55	Many cell types (hematopoietic and non-hematopoietic); highest levels on epithelial cells, germinal center dendritic reticulum cells	CD120a is a 55-kDa receptor for TNF-α and TNF-β. *J Biol Chem 266:18324, 1991*
CD120b	TNFR-2	75	Many cell types (hematopoietic and non-hematopoietic); highest levels on myeloid cells	CD120a is a 75-kDa receptor for TNF-α and TNF-β. *J Exp Med 176:1015, 1992*
CD121a	IL-1R type I	80	T cells, thymocytes, fibroblasts, endothelial cells, chondrocytes, synovial cells, keratinocytes, hepatocytes	CD121a is the receptor for interleukin-1 alpha (IL-1α) and interleukin-1 beta (IL-1β) that induces cellular proliferation and/or activation upon binding IL-1. *Proc Natl Acad Sci USA 90:6155, 1993*

CD MARKERS	OTHER NAMES	MOLECULAR WEIGHT (KDA)	KNOWN NORMAL DISTRIBUTION	REMARKS
CD121b	IL-1R type II	68	B cells, monocytes, macrophages, neutrophils	CD121b acts as a decoy receptor (target) for IL-1α and IL-1β and functions to inhibit IL-1 effects by competing with CD121a for IL-1 binding. *Science 261:472, 1993*
CD122	IL-2R-beta	75	Activated T cells, B cells, monocytes, NK cells	CD122 associates with CD25 and CD132 to form a heterotrimeric receptor with high affinity for IL-2. CD122 also associates with the IL-15Rα to form the IL-15 receptor. *Ann Rev Immunol 11:245, 1993* *Cell 73:147, 1993*
CD123	IL-3R-alpha	70	Pluripotent stem cells and committed hematopoietic progenitor cells, granulocytes, monocytes, megakaryocytes	CD123 is a low-affinity receptor for IL-3 that associates with CD131 to form a high-affinity receptor for IL-3 that, upon binding to IL-3, stimulates proliferation and/or differentiation. *Cytokine Growth Factor Rev 12:19, 2001* *J Biol Chem 270:22422, 1995*
CD124	IL-4R-alpha	140	Mature B cells, T cells, epithelia, endothelium, hematopoietic precursors, fibroblasts	CD124 is the subunit of receptor for IL-4 (CD124-CD132) and IL-13 (CD124-CD213a1). *Int Immunol 8:1915, 1996* *Ann Rev Biochem 59:783, 1990*
CD125	IL-5R-alpha	55-60	Eosinophils, basophils, activated B cells	CD125 associates with CD131 to form the IL-5 receptor that stimulates proliferation and/or differentiation of eosinophils and/or basophils upon binding to IL-5. CD125 is the therapeutic target of eosinophilic inflammation involved in bronchial asthma. *Cytokine Growth Factor Rev 12:19, 2001* *Immunity 4:483, 1996*
CD126	IL-6R-alpha	80	Plasma cells (strong), activated B cells (strong), T cells, monocytes, epithelial cells, fibroblasts, neural cells, hepatocytes	CD126 associates with CD130 to form IL-6 receptor that stimulates cell growth and/or differentiation upon binding to IL-6. *Ann Rev Immunol 15:797, 1997* *Int Rev Immunol 16:249, 1998*

CD MARKERS	OTHER NAMES	MOLECULAR WEIGHT (KDA)	KNOWN NORMAL DISTRIBUTION	REMARKS
CD127	IL-7R-alpha; HIL-7R	75	B-cell precursors, thymocytes, mature T cells, monocytes	CD127 associates with CD132 to form a functional high-affinity receptor for IL-7. The IL-7-IL-7R system plays a critical role in lymphoid development. *Blood 99:3892, 2002* *J Leuk Biol 58:623, 1995*
CD128a	IL-8R-alpha; CXCR1	58-67	Neutrophils, basophils, T-cell subset, monocytes, keratinocytes	CD128a associates with CD128b to form the IL-8 receptor that is a G-protein coupled receptor involved in chemotaxis and inflammation. *Semin Immunol 11:95, 1999* *Crit Rev Immunol 19:1, 1999*
CD128b	IL-8R-beta; CXCR2	58-67	Neutrophils, projection neurons, neuroendocrine cells (various)	Same as CD128a
CD129	IL-9 receptor	64	Activated T cells, B cells, myeloid and erythroid precursors, mast cells	CD129 associates with CD132 to form the receptor for IL-9. *J Biol Chem 273:9255, 1998* *Adv Immunol 54:79, 1993*
CD130	Gp130; subunit of receptor for IL-6, oncostatin-M, leukemia inhibitory factor, IL-11, ciliary neurotrophic factor, or cardiotrophin-1	130-140	Almost all cell types (weak)	CD130, together with each respective specific alpha chain, forms high-affinity receptor for IL-6, oncostatin-M, leukemia inhibitory factor, IL-11, ciliary neurotrophic factor, or cardiotrophin-1. IL-6 and oncostatin-M-dependent activation of CD130 are involved in the pathogenesis of multiple myeloma. *Ann Rev Immunol 15:797, 1997* *Science 260:1805 & 1808, 1993*
CD131	IL-3 receptor common beta chain	140	Myeloid cells (early and mature), early B cells	Common beta subunit for IL-3, IL-5, and GM-CSF receptors. Defective CD131 is associated with protein alveolar proteinosis. *Leukemia S3:418, 1997* *Blood 82:1960, 1993*
CD132	IL-2 receptor common gamma chain	64	T cell, B cells, NK cells, monocytes, macrophages, neutrophils	CD132 is the common gamma subunit for IL-2, IL-4, IL-7, IL-9, and IL-15 receptors. Mutations in CD132 cause X-linked severe combined immunodeficiency (no T cells, no

CD MARKERS	OTHER NAMES	MOLECULAR WEIGHT (KDA)	KNOWN NORMAL DISTRIBUTION	REMARKS
CD132—CONT				NK cells). CD132 is a target molecule for gene therapy for X-linked SCID. *Immunol Today 20:71, 1999* *Crit Rev Immunol 18:503, 1998*
CD133	Prominin-1; AC-133	120	CD34$^+$ hematopoietic stem cells and progenitor cells, neural and endothelial stem cells, cytotrophoblasts, syncytiotrophoblasts, retina	CD133 is a five-membrane-span glycoprotein that appears to act as an organizer of plasma membrane protrusions. It serves as a neural and hematopoietic stem cell marker and is an alternative to CD34 in selecting hematopoietic stem and progenitor cells for transplantation studies. *Blood 90:5002, 1997* *Blood 90:5013, 1997*
CD134	MRC OX40; receptor for OX-40 ligand; OX-40	50	Medullary thymocytes, activated CD4 T cells (Th1 cells)	CD134 is a member of the TNF receptor family. It is a co-stimulatory molecule for B-cell activation. *Trends Immunol 23:102, 2002* *J Immunol 163:3007, 1999* *Adv Immunol 61:1, 1996*
CD135	Flt-3; STK-1; Flk-2	130-150	Multipotential, myelomonocytic, and primitive B-cell progenitors	CD135 (fms-like tyrosine kinase-3, flt-3) is a receptor tyrosine kinase present on hematopoietic stem and/or progenitor cells. Presence of the activating length mutation in the juxtamembrane domain or point mutation in the kinase domain of flt-3 mediates ligand-independent progrowth and prosurvival signaling in approximately one third of acute myeloid leukemias and thereby leads to relatively poor prognosis. Flt-3 has become a therapeutic target molecule for AML. *Semin Oncol 31 (2 S4):80, 2004* *Proc Natl Acad Sci USA 91:459, 1994*
CD136	Macrophage stimulating protein receptor (MSP-R); RON	180	Monocytes, epithelial cells, central and peripheral nervous system	CD136 is a heterodimeric receptor tyrosine kinase that provides signal transduction, regulating chemotaxis, phagocytosis, cell growth and differentiation. *Scand J Immunol 56:545, 2002* *J Leukoc Biol 65:345, 1999* *Oncogene 13:2167, 1996*

CD MARKERS	OTHER NAMES	MOLECULAR WEIGHT (KDA)	KNOWN NORMAL DISTRIBUTION	REMARKS
CD137	ILA (induced by lymphocyte activation); 4-1BB	30	T lymphocytes and B lymphocytes, monocytes, some epithelial cells	CD137 is a member of the TNF receptor family that serves as co-stimulatory signal for T-cell proliferation. *Nat Rev Immunol 3:609, 2003* *Semin Immunol 10:481, 1998* *Eur J Immunol 24:2219, 1994* *Blood 85:1053, 1995*
CD138	Syndecan-1; heparin sulfate proteoglycan	80-250	Pre-B cells, immature B cells, plasma cells, stratified squamous epithelium, mesenchymal cells	CD138 is an integral membrane protein that serves as the co-receptor for extracellular matrix. It mediates cell adhesion and growth. CD138 is characteristically positive in primary effusion lymphoma. It is also widely used as a marker for plasma cells and myeloma cells. *Ann Hematol 81:125, 2002* *Leuk Lymphoma 34:35, 1999*
CD139		209 (228)	B cells, monocytes, granulocytes, follicular dendritic cells, endothelial cells	Unknown
CD140a	PDGF-R-alpha	160	Mesenchymal cells, platelets, various cancers (undetectable on most normal cells)	CD140a is a split tyrosine that serves as receptor for PDGF that is involved in signal transduction induced by PDGF binding. *Hematol J 5(S3):133, 2004*
CD140b	PDGF-R-beta	180	Mesenchymal cells, monocytes, neutrophils, subset of endothelial cells, various cancers	Same as CD140a. It is up-regulated in a subtype of chronic myelomonocytic leukemia (CMML) with t(5;12)(q33;p13) and is the therapeutic target of tyrosine kinase inhibitor (e.g., Gleevec). *Blood 93:1707, 1999* *J Biol Chem 269:32023, 1994* *Cell 77:307, 1994*
CD141	Thrombomodulin; fetomodulin	75	Endothelial cells, neutrophils, mesothelial cells, keratinocytes, smooth muscle cells, megakaryocytes, monocytes, synovial lining cells, urothelium	CD141 is a transmembrane glycoprotein and cofactor for the activation of protein C. It is of crucial importance in initiating and activating the endogenous protein C-protein S anticoagulation pathway. Mutations in CD141 cause rare hereditary thromboembolic diseases. D141 is also used as a

CD MARKERS	OTHER NAMES	MOLECULAR WEIGHT (KDA)	KNOWN NORMAL DISTRIBUTION	REMARKS
CD141—CONT				marker for mesotheliomas (vs. adenocarcinoma) and endothelial cells. *Hematol Rev 9:251, 1996* *J Biol Chem 271:16603, 1996*
CD142	Tissue factor; thromboplastin; coagulation factor III	45–47	Epidermal keratinocytes, activated monocytes and endothelial cells, some neutrophils, glomerular epithelial cells and various other epithelia, adventitial cells of blood vessels, astrocytes, myocardium, Schwann cells, stromal cells of the liver, pancreas, spleen, and thyroid	CD142 is a serine protease cofactor that functions as the major initiating factor of clotting. It binds factor VIIa to form a complex, which then activates factors X, IX, and VII. *Arterioscler Thromb Vasc Biol 24:1015, 2004* *Faseb J 9:883, 1995* *Blood Coag Fibrinol 4:281, 1993*
CD143	Peptidyl dipeptidase A; angiotensin-converting enzyme (ACE)	170	Endothelial cells of small and/or medium arteries, pulmonary capillary endothelium, proximal renal tubule brush borders, basal ganglia neurophil, granulose cells, Leydig cells, mesenchymal tissues, activated macrophages, some T cells	CD143 acts as a peptidyl dipeptide hydrolase to metabolize angiotensin, bradykinin, substance P, LH-RH, and other dipeptides. Patients with high ACE activity have DD genotype and are at increased risk for myocardial infarction, strokes, and diabetic nephropathy. Soluble form of CD143 is present in plasma, and its level and/or activity is increased in some cases of active sarcoidosis and decreased in patients having chronic obstructive lung disease, lung cancer, emphysema, and cystic fibrosis. *Clin Chem Lab Med 40:256, 2002* *J Biol Chem 269:26806, 1994*
CD144	VE-cadherin, cadherin-5	135	Endothelial cells	CD144 is endothelial-specific cadherin localized at intercellular junction. *Am J Pathol 155:887, 1999* *Int Arch Allergy Immunol 120:237, 1999* *Blood 87:630, 1996*
CD145		25, 90, 110	Endothelial cells, some stromal cells	Unknown

CD MARKERS	OTHER NAMES	MOLECULAR WEIGHT (KDA)	KNOWN NORMAL DISTRIBUTION	REMARKS
CD146	MCAM; MUC18; S-ENDO; Mel-CAM; A32	118	Endothelium, smooth muscle cells, T-cell subset, follicular dendritic cells, Schwann cells, intermediate trophoblasts	CD146 is an adhesion molecule present at the endothelial junction and is involved in cell-cell cohesion. Soluble form of CD146 is present in plasma, and its level is increased in patients with chronic renal insufficiency. The expression of CD146 in malignant melanoma is associated with tumor progression and the development of metastasis. *J Pathol 189:4, 1999* *Curr Top Microbiol Immunol 213:95, 1996*
CD147	M6; EMMPRIN (extracellular matrix metalloproteinase inducer); neurothelin; basigin; OX-47	31-65	All leukocytes, red blood cells, platelets, endothelial cells	CD147 is a transmembrane glycoprotein with remarkable variations in size (31-65 kDa) because of heterogeneous *N*-glycosylation, with the most highly glycosylated forms functioning to induce matrix metalloproteinase (MMP) production. It is widely expressed on many cell types; appears at especially high levels on human tumor cells. *Curr Top Dev Biol 54:371, 2003* *Cancer Res 55:434, 1995* *Biochem Biophys Res Commun 224:33, 1996*
CD148	HPTP-eta; DEP-1; p260	220-250	Neutrophils, monocytes, eosinophils, platelets, fibroblasts, dendritic cells, neurons, B cells, memory T cells	CD148 is a receptor-like protein tyrosine phosphatase expressed on a wide variety of cell types. Its expression increases on contact between cells and may be involved in contact inhibition, lymphocyte signal transduction, and T-cell activation. It may play an important regulatory role to control immune responses. *Leuk Lymphoma 35:237-243, 1999* *J Immunol 161:3249, 1998*
CD150	Signaling lymphocyte activation molecule (SLAM); IPO-3	70	Thymocytes, CD45RO+ T cells, B cells, NK cells, dendritic cells, endothelial cells	CD150 is a T-cell and/or B-cell and/or dendritic cell surface glycoprotein, acting as a co-stimulatory receptor involved in T- and B-cell activation. It is also identified as the cellular receptor for measles virus. *Rev Med Virol 14:217, 2004* *Microbiol Immunol 46:135, 2002*

CD MARKERS	OTHER NAMES	MOLECULAR WEIGHT (KDA)	KNOWN NORMAL DISTRIBUTION	REMARKS
CD151	PETA-3; SFA-1	27	Platelets, megakaryocytes, monocytes, epithelial and endothelial cells	CD151 is a member of the tetraspanin family that forms complexes with integrins and regulates cell adhesion and migration. *Mol Cell Biol 24:5978, 2004* *Cancer Res 59:3812, 1999*
CD152	CTLA-4	44	Activated CD4 and CD8 T cells	CD152 serves as the ligand for CD80 (B7-1) and CD86 (B7-2) that negatively regulates T-cell activation. Its function is in contrast to that of CD28. *Nat Rev Immunol 4:336, 2004* *Science 271:1734, 1996*
CD153	CD30 ligand	40	Activated T cells, activated macrophages, neutrophils, B cells	CD153 is a TNF family member and serves as ligand for CD30. *Eur J Immunol 32:163, 2002* *Blood 85:3378, 1995*
CD154	CD40 ligand; gp39; TRAP (TNF-related activation protein)	39	Activated CD4 T cells, few activated CD8 T cells	CD154 serves as CD40 ligand that induces activation, proliferation, and/or differentiation of CD40-expressing cells. Note that CD40-CD154 interaction is essential for B-cell differentiation, maturation, immunoglobulin class switch, and secretion of IgG, IgA, and IgE antibodies. Patients with mutations in CD154 have an immunodeficiency called *X-linked hyper-IgM syndrome*. *Immunol Res 24:311, 2001* *Adv Immunol 61:1, 1996*
CD155	Poliovirus receptor	80-90	Monocytes, macrophages, thymocytes, spinal cord anterior horn motor neurons	CD155 localizes in cell-matrix adhesions and cell-cell junctions and plays a role in the regulation of cell adhesion and cell motility. It also serves as the receptor for poliovirus. *Mol Immunol 42:463, 2005* *Virology 195:798, 1993*
CD156a	ADAM8	69	Neutrophils, monocytes	CD156a (A Disintegrin And Metalloprotease 8, ADAM 8) is part of the ADAM family of proteins with the catalytic site consensus sequence of metalloprotease and disintegrins. *J Biol Chem 277:48210, 2002* *Immunol Today 20:278, 1999*

CD MARKERS	OTHER NAMES	MOLECULAR WEIGHT (KDA)	KNOWN NORMAL DISTRIBUTION	REMARKS
CD156b	ADAM17; TACE (TNF alpha converting enzyme)	85	Widely expressed	CD156b (ADAM17) mediates the ectodomain shedding of membrane-bound precursors for TNF-alpha, EGF (epidermal growth factor), heparin-binding EGF (HB-EGF), amphiregulin, etc. This proteolytic processing functions to regulate the availability of active and soluble forms of growth factors, switch receptor signaling from autocrine or juxtacrine modes to paracrine or endocrine mechanisms, and/or influence the nature (e.g., duration) of the signaling events. *Ann NY Acad Sci 995:22, 2003* *Int J Biochem Cell Biol 34:1, 2002*
CD157	Mo5; BST-1; BP-3	42-45	Monocytes, neutrophils, marrow stroma, follicular dendritic cells, endothelial cells, synovial cells, some T cells, early B cells	CD157 is a GPI-anchored cell surface protein, encoded by a member of the CD38 NADase-ADP-ribosyl cyclase gene family. It is an important mediator of neutrophil adhesion and migration. It also facilitates early B-cell proliferation and differentiation. Overexpression of CD157 appears to cause polyclonal B-cell abnormalities in rheumatoid arthritis. *Cell Biochem Funct 20:309, 2002* *Int Immunol 8:183, 1996* *Int Immunol 8:1395, 1996*
CD158a	Killer cell inhibitory receptor (KIR)-c1.42; NKAT1; p58.1 and/or p50.1; EB6-reactive	50, 58	NK cells, some T cells	CD158a is the ligand for HLA-Cw2, 4, 5, and 6 that regulates NK-mediated cytotoxicity (p58.1 is inhibitory, and p50.1 is activating). *Ann Rev Immunol 14:619, 1996* *Science 268:405, 1995*
CD158b	Killer cell inhibitory receptor (KIR)-c1.6; NKAT2; p58.2 and/or p50.2; GL183-reactive	50, 58	NK cells, some T cells	CD158b is the ligand for HLA-Cw1, 3, 7, and 8 that regulates NK-mediated cytotoxicity (p58.2 is inhibitory, and p50.2 is activating). *Ann Rev Immunol 14:619, 1996*
CD159a	NKG2A	43	NK cells	CD94-CD159a (NKG2A) is a heterodimer, lectinlike complex receptor expressed on natural killer (NK) and a small subset of T cells. This receptor varies in function as an inhibitor or activator, depending on which

CD MARKERS	OTHER NAMES	MOLECULAR WEIGHT (KDA)	KNOWN NORMAL DISTRIBUTION	REMARKS
CD159a—CONT				isoform of NKG2 is expressed. The ligand for CD94-NKG2 is HLA-E in human, which are nonclassical class I molecules that bind leader peptides from other class I molecules. CD94-NKG2A is able to inhibit NK-cell and T-cell cytolytic activity. This inhibition of lytic activity is mediated by two immunoreceptor tyrosine inhibitory motifs (ITIMs) in the cytoplasmic domain of NKG2A. *Cancer Biol Ther 2:610, 2003* *Immunol Rev 181:52, 2001*
CD160	By55	26	NK-cell subset (CD56$^+$dim, CD16$^+$), T-cell subset (CD8$^+$)	CD160 is Ig-like, GPI-anchored receptor. Signaling through CD160 triggers NK-cell cytotoxicity after its engagement with an HLA-C molecule. *J Immunol 173:5349, 2004* *Proc Natl Acad Sci USA 99:16963, 2002*
CD161	NKR-P1A	60	NK cells, T-cell subset (CD4$^+$ and/or CD8$^+$ T cells, memory T cells), monocytes	CD161 is a surface receptor, functioning to activate NK cells. *Curr Opin Immunol 14:615, 2002* *Ann Rev Immunol 11:613, 1993*
CD162	P-selectin glycoprotein ligand-1 (PSGL-1)	110	Neutrophils, monocytes, most lymphocytes	CD162 binds to CD62P and helps mediate tethering and rolling of leukocytes on the surface of activated endothelial cells, the first step in leukocyte extravasation and migration-mediating cell migration. *Blood 104:2549, 2004* *J Biol Chem 271:6342, 1996*
CD163	M130 antigen; GHI/61; Ber-Mac3; Ki-M8; SM4	130	Monocytes, macrophages	CD163 is a member of the scavenger receptor cysteine-rich family that plays a regulatory role in inflammatory processes. It is used as a specific marker for macrophages in tissue sections. *Am J Clin Pathol 122:794, 2004* *Int J Biochem Cell Biol 34:309, 2002*

CD MARKERS	OTHER NAMES	MOLECULAR WEIGHT (KDA)	KNOWN NORMAL DISTRIBUTION	REMARKS
CD164	MUC-24; multiglycosylated core protein 24 (MGC-24)	80	Intestinal epithelial cells, thyroid epithelial cells, monocytes, marrow stroma	CD164 is a mucinlike cell surface glycoprotein that facilitates adhesion of CD34$^+$ cells to bone marrow stroma and thereby regulates hematopoietic cell proliferation. *Stem Cells 21:162, 2003* *Blood 92:849, 1998*
CD165	AD2; gp37	37	Platelets, thymocytes, T cells, B cells, and NK cells, few monocytes, neurons, islet cells	CD165 plays a role in intercellular adhesion between thymocytes and thymic epithelial cells. *J Immunol 154:2012, 1995*
CD166	ALCAM; CD6L; BEN; SC-1; DM-GRASP; neurolin; Kg-CAM	105	Thymic epithelial cells, activated T cells and monocytes, CD34$^+$ marrow cells, endothelial cells, fibroblasts, neurons	CD166 is an adhesion molecule, which binds to CD6 and plays a role in T-cell development, embryonic hematopoiesis and angiogenesis, and neuronal neurite extension. *Eur J Immunol 34:930, 2004* *Eur J Cell Biol 81:313, 2002*
CD167a	Discoidin domain receptor-1 (DDR1)	120	Epithelial cells, myoblasts	CD167a is tyrosine kinase receptor activated by collagen and involved in cell-matrix communication. *J Biol Chem 279:31462, 2004* *Febs Lett 514:175, 2002*
CD168	RHAMM	84-88	Thymocytes, T-cell subset, monocytes, bronchial epithelium, CNS neurons	CD168 binds to hyaluronic acid and stimulates ciliary besting. It also plays a role in cell signaling, migration, and adhesion. *Dev Immunol 7:209, 2000* *Biochem Soc Trans 27:135, 1999*
CD169	Sialoadhesin	185	Macrophages (all sites but microglia)	CD169 is a macrophage-restricted membrane glycoprotein that is involved in cell-cell and cell-matrix interactions during inflammatory reactions. Like CD68, it can be used as a marker for tissue macrophages. *Blood 97:288, 2001* *J Leukoc Biol 66:705, 1999*

CD MARKERS	OTHER NAMES	MOLECULAR WEIGHT (KDA)	KNOWN NORMAL DISTRIBUTION	REMARKS
CD170	Siglec-5	140	Neutrophils, macrophage subset	Also known as sialic acid binding immunoglobulin-like lectin (Siglec)-5, which mediates cell-cell interaction. *Br J Haematol 123:420, 2003* *Br J Haematol 119:221, 2002* *J Leukoc Biol 66:705, 1999*
CD171	L1	200	Monocytes, lymphocyte subset, epithelial cell subset, neurons, glia	CD171 is an adhesion molecule required for normal neurohistogenesis. Mutations in CD171 cause CRASH (corpus callosum hypoplasia and/or agenesis, retardation, aphasia, spastic paraplegia and/or shuffling gait and hydrocephalus caused by stenosis of aqueduct of Sylvius), an X-linked neurological disorder. *Cancer Lett 189:237, 2003* *Curr Opin Neurobiol 8:87, 1998*
CD172a	SIRP alpha; SHPS-1; MyD-1	110	Monocytes, dendritic cells, T-cell subset, stem cells	CD172a is a member of the signal regulatory phosphatase (SIRP)-binding protein receptor family. It binds to CD47, an integrin-associated protein. *J Immunol 173:2562, 2004* *J Immunol 168:5823, 2002*
CD173	Blood group H type 2		Hematopoietic progenitor cells	CD173 is the fucosylated histo-blood group antigen H type 2 (blood group O) and may play a role in the homing process of hematopoietic stem cells to the bone marrow. It is a marker for early hematopoiesis. *Glycobiology 11:677, 2001*
CD174	Lewis^Y		Hematopoietic progenitor cells	CD174 is the fucosylated histo-blood group antigen Lewis^Y and may play a role in the homing process of hematopoietic stem cells to the bone marrow. It is a marker for early hematopoiesis. *Glycobiology 11:677, 2001*
CD175	Tn		Stem cell subset	Simple mucin-type carbohydrate antigen produced in the initial steps of mucin biosynthetic pathway caused by aberrant or incomplete glycosylation of mucins. *Acta Biochim Pol 42:11, 1995*

CD MARKERS	OTHER NAMES	MOLECULAR WEIGHT (KDA)	KNOWN NORMAL DISTRIBUTION	REMARKS
CD175s	Sialyl-Tn		Erythroblasts	Sialyl-Tn (STn) is a carbohydrate antigen formed by the premature 2-6 sialylation of N-acetylgalactosamine. It belongs to a family of antigens widely expressed in carcinomas, but only to a limited degree in normal tissue. The expression of STn is associated with prognosis in different tumors. *J Histochem Cytochem 49:1581, 2001* *Acta Biochim Pol 42:11, 1995*
CD176	Thomsen-Friedenreich antigen		Stem cell subset	A cryptic glycoprotein, referred to as tumor antigen or cancer-associated antigen because it is absent or masked by some carbohydrates in normal tissues, but present in many human cancers. *Adv Exp Med Biol 535:147, 2003* *Histol Histopathol 12:263, 1997*
CD177	NB1; HNA-2alpha	58-64	Myeloid cells	CD177 is a GPI-anchored glycoprotein. It is a member of the Ly-6 (leukocyte antigen-6) gene superfamily involved with neutrophil proliferation. It is also a potential marker for polycythemia vera vs. secondary erythrocytosis. *Br J Haematol 126:650, 2004* *J Trans Med 2:8, 2004*
CD178	Fas ligand	38-42	Activated T cells, immune privileged sites (testis, anterior chamber of eye, placenta)	CD95 (Fas) ligand, which plays important role in T-cell-mediated cytotoxicity and induces apoptosis in Fas-expressing target cells. Reed-Sternberg cells are typically positive for CD178. *Biochem Pharmacol 66:1417, 2003*
CD179a	Vpre-B	16	Pro-B cells, pre-B cells	CD179a associates noncovalently with CD179b to form surrogate light chain as component of pre–B-cell receptor (pre-BCR: 2 mu HC/Vpre-B/lambda5), which plays a critical role in early B-cell differentiation. *Mod Pathol 17:423, 2004* *Rev Immunogenet 2:185, 2000*
CD179b	Lambda5	22	Pro-B cells, pre-B cells	Same as 179a

CD MARKERS	OTHER NAMES	MOLECULAR WEIGHT (KDA)	KNOWN NORMAL DISTRIBUTION	REMARKS
CD180	RP105	95-105	B-cell subset (strong on mantle and marginal zone B cells), monocytes, dendritic cells	CD180 is a leucine-rich repeat (LRR) molecule that belongs to the toll-like receptor family of pathogen receptors. It is involved in B-cell recognition and lipopolysaccharide (LPS) signaling. *Blood 99:1699, 2002* *Rheumatology 40:1315, 2001*
CD183	CXCR3	40	Activated T cells (Th1 cells) and NK cells, eosinophils, plasmacytoid dendritic cells, hematopoietic progenitors	CD183 is the chemokine receptor for interferon-inducible protein 10, monokine induced by IFN-γ and IFN-inducible T-cell α-chemoattractant. It plays a major role in Th1 cell-induced inflammatory processes. *Curr Opin Immunol 15:479, 2003* *Hum Immunol 63:1164, 2002*
CD184	CXCR4	45	T-cell subset (Th2 cells), B cells, monocytes, dendritic cells, endothelial cells, epithelial cells, neurons, astrocytes	CD184 and its ligand SDF-1 are an important chemokine receptor-ligand pair, which play a crucial role in numerous biological processes, including hematopoiesis, cardiogenesis, vasculogenesis, neuronal development, and immune cell trafficking. CD184 is also the main co-receptor for T-cell-tropic HIV strain. *AIDS Res Hum Retroviruses 20:111, 2004* *Immunol Rev 195:58, 2003*
CD195	CCR5	45	Monocytes, T-cell subset	CD195 is a chemokine receptor for RANTES, MIP-1α, and MIP-1β. It also serves as the co-receptor for macrophage-tropic HIV strain. *AIDS Res Hum Retroviruses 20:111, 2004* *Int J Biochem Cell Biol 36:35, 2004* *Curr Opin Immunol 15:479, 2003*
CDw197	CCR7	45	T-cell subset	CDw197 is a chemokine receptor that plays a critical role in the coordinate migration of T cells and dendritic cells (DC) into and their localization within secondary lymphoid organs. *Immunol Rev 195:117, 2003* *Immunol Rev 195:58, 2003*

CD MARKERS	OTHER NAMES	MOLECULAR WEIGHT (KDA)	KNOWN NORMAL DISTRIBUTION	REMARKS
CD200	OX-2	45-50	Activated T cells, thymocytes, B cells, follicular dendritic cells, endothelial cells, neurons, syncytiotrophoblasts	CD200 is a broadly distributed cell surface glycoprotein that interacts with its receptor (CD200R), which is restricted to myeloid-derived antigen-presenting cells and certain populations of T cells. CD200 imparts an immunoregulatory signal through CD200R, leading to the suppression of T-cell-mediated immune responses. It may play a role in immune tolerance of peripheral self-antigens. *J Immunol 172:7744, 2004* *Eur J Immunol 34:1688, 2004*
CD201	EPCR (endothelial cell protein C receptor)	50	Endothelial cells (not in liver or kidney)	CD201 (EPCR) is part of the thrombomodulin (TM)-protein C (PC)-EPCR system, which plays a critical role in regulating coagulation and inflammation. TM, a cell surface-expressed glycoprotein, preponderantly synthesized by vascular endothelial cells, is a critical cofactor for thrombin-mediated activation of PC, an event further amplified by EPCR. Activated PC (APC) is best known for its natural anticoagulant properties. TM, APC, and EPCR have activities that impact not only on coagulation, but also on inflammation, fibrinolysis, and cell proliferation. *Arterioscler Thromb Vasc Biol 24:1374, 2004* *Crit Care Med 32:S298, 2004*
CD202b	Tie2; Tek	150	Endothelial cells, hematopoietic stem cells	CD202b is a receptor tyrosine kinase, which binds its ligand, angiopoietin-1 (Ang-1). It plays crucial roles in vein morphogenesis, communication between endothelial cells and smooth muscle cells for remodeling and repair of blood vessels, and maintenance of hematopoietic stem cells in a quiescent sate in the bone marrow niche. It may be the earliest endothelial cell marker. *Front Biosci 10:666, 2005* *Cell 118:139, 2004*
CD203c	E-NPP3; PDNP3	130-250	Basophils, megakaryocytes, mast cells, some myeloid cells	CD203c is an ectoenzyme that catalyzes hydrolysis of oligonucleotides, nucleoside phosphates, and NAD. In basophils and mast cells, cross-linking of the Fc epsilon

CD MARKERS	OTHER NAMES	MOLECULAR WEIGHT (KDA)	KNOWN NORMAL DISTRIBUTION	REMARKS
CD203c—CONT				RI by an allergen or anti-IgE antibody results in a rapid up-regulation of intracellular CD203c molecules to the cell surface and is accompanied by mediator release. CD203c is therefore a potential target molecule for a flow cytometry-based test to analyze sensitized individuals and patients with type I allergy. CD203c is also associated with carcinogenesis of certain human cancers, and serum CD203c may be used as a tumor marker. *Int Arch Allergy Immunol 133:317, 2004* *Int J Mol Med 12:763, 2003*
CD204	Macrophage scavenger receptor 1	220	Macrophages	CD204 is a scavenger receptor that is involved in endocytosis of macromolecules. *Dev Dyn 232:67, 2005* *Glia 40:195, 2002*
CD205	DEC-205	210	Dendritic cells, thymic epithelium	CD205 is antigen-uptake receptor that plays a role in initiating immune responses. *Int Immunol 16:877, 2004* *Immunol 111:262, 2004*
CD206	Macrophage mannose receptor	180	Dendritic cell subset	CD206 plays important roles in phagocytosis and pinocytosis of mannosylated protein antigens, such as glycoproteins derived from bacteria and fungi (e.g., *Malassezia furfur*). *J Invest Dermatol 118:327, 2002* *Clin Exp Allergy 30:1759, 2000* *J Exp Med 172:1785, 1990*
CD207	Langerin (Langerhans cell specific c-type lectin)	40	Immature Langerhans cells (dendritic cells of epidermis and mucosa)	CD207 is localized to Birbeck granules (organelles specific to Langerhans cells). It participates in antigen recognition and uptake, functioning as endocytic receptor. *Immunol Res 28:93, 2003* *Immunity 12:71, 2000*
CD208	DC-LAMP	70-90	Dendritic cell (DC) subset	CD208, dendritic cell-lysosomal associated membrane protein (DC-LAMP), is specifically expressed by DCs on activation and

CD MARKERS	OTHER NAMES	MOLECULAR WEIGHT (KDA)	KNOWN NORMAL DISTRIBUTION	REMARKS
CD208—CONT				therefore serves as marker of DC maturation. It is detected first in activated DCs within MHC class II molecule-containing compartments just before the translocation of MHC class II-peptide complexes to the cell surface, suggesting a possible involvement in this process.
				Immunity 9:325, 1998
				Traffic 3:894, 2002
CD209	DC-SIGN	44	Dendritic cell subset	CD209, DC-SIGN (dendritic cell specific intercellular adhesion molecule-3-grabbing nonintegrin), is one of several C-type lectin receptors expressed by dendritic cell subsets. CD209 binds to highly mannosylated glycoproteins, promoting their endocytosis and potential degradation. It also mediates attachment of HIV, leading to endocytosis or enhancement of CD4- and/or CD195-dependent infection. CD209 also appears to function as capture receptors for hepatitis C virus, Ebola virus, cytomegalovirus, and dengue virus.
				Proc Natl Acad Sci USA 101:14067, 2004
				J Exp Med 197:823, 2003
				Immunity 17:653, 2002
CDw210	IL-10R	90-100	T cells, B cells, NK cells, monocytes, macrophages	This is an IL-10 receptor.
				Ann Rev Immunol 19:683, 2001
CD212	IL-12Rβ₁	100	Activated T cells and NK cells	This is an IL-12 receptor.
				Immunol Rev 170:65, 1999
				Ann Rev Immunol 16:495, 1998
CD213a1	IL-13Rα₁	65	B cells, T cells, endothelial cells, monocytes, fibroblasts	CD213a1 is IL-13 receptor alpha₁ that associates with IL-4 receptor alpha (CD124) to form a functional receptor for IL-13. Polymorphisms in components of the IL-4 and IL-13 cytokine-receptor axes are associated with allergy and asthma.
				Immunology 112:597, 2004
				Immunol Cell Biol 79:332, 2001

CD MARKERS	OTHER NAMES	MOLECULAR WEIGHT (KDA)	KNOWN NORMAL DISTRIBUTION	REMARKS
CD213a2	IL-13Rα_2	65	B cells, monocytes	CD213a2, IL-13 receptor alpha$_2$, is a decoy receptor for IL-13, functioning to inhibit binding of IL-13 to functional IL-13 receptor. *J Allergy Clin Immunol 111:677, 2003* *Blood 97:2673, 2001*
CDw217	IL-17	130	Board	This is an IL-17 receptor. *Cytokine Growth Factor Rev 14:155, 2003*
CD220	Insulin receptor	140 + 70	Board	CD220 is receptor tyrosine kinase for insulin. *J Cell Sci 114:1429, 2001*
CD221	IGF-1R	140 + 70	Board	CD 221 is a receptor tyrosine kinase for insulin-like growth factor-1 with a 70% homology to the insulin receptor (CD220) *Int J Cancer 107:873, 2003* *J Cell Physiol 194:108, 2002* *Endocrine Rev 22:818, 2001*
CD222	IGF-2R; M6P	250	Board	CD222 is a receptor protein that interacts with multiple ligands and plays a significant role in regulation of cell growth and apoptosis by participating in internalization and degradation of IGF-2, the activation of TGF-β, and the binding, transport, and activation of newly synthesized lysosomal enzymes, such as cathepsins. *J Biol Chem 277:40575, 2002* *Ann Rev Biochem 61:307, 1992*
CD223	LAG-3	70	Activated T cells and NK cells	CD223 is a CD4-related transmembrane protein that binds to MHC class II molecules. *J Immunol 173:6806, 2004* *Trends Immunol 24:619, 2003*
CD224	GGT (γ-glutamyl transferase)	27, 68	Leukocytes, platelets, stem cells	CD224 is a transmembrane ectoenzyme that cleaves extracellular glutathione (GSH) to facilitate the recapture of cysteine for synthesis of intracellular GSH.

CD MARKERS	OTHER NAMES	MOLECULAR WEIGHT (KDA)	KNOWN NORMAL DISTRIBUTION	REMARKS
CD225	Leu-13	17	Broad	CD225 is an interferon-inducible protein and is a component of a multimeric complex involved in the transduction of antiproliferative and homotypic adhesion signaling. *J Biol Chem 270:23860, 1995* *J Immunol 150:736, 1993*
CD226	DNAM-1; PTA-1; TLiSA-1	65	T cells, NK cells, monocytes, platelets, subset of B cells	CD226 is an adhesion molecule involved in NK-cell and T-cell-mediated cytotoxicity, etc. Its ligands include CD155 (poliovirus receptor) and CD112 (nectin-2/PRR-2). *Mol Immunol 42:463, 2005* *J Biol Chem 272:21735, 1997*
CD227	MUC-1; EMA; episialin	300	Activated T cells, monocytes, some B cells, follicular dendritic cells, all mucosal epithelial cells	CD227 is a large cell surface and secreted mucin glycoprotein. It is best known as a marker for adenocarcinomas. *J Biol Chem 276:18327, 2001* *J Leukoc Biol 72:692, 2002*
CD228	Melanotransferrin (MTf); p. 97	80-95	Stem cells, melanoma cells	CD228 is a membrane-bound glycoprotein with sequence similarity and iron-binding properties of transferrin superfamily. It is an important iron transporter across the blood-brain barrier. *Febs Lett 483:11, 2000* *Biochim Biophys Acta 1331:1, 1997*
CD229	Ly-9	120	T cells, B cells	CD229 is a cell surface receptor selectively expressed on lymphocytes. It belongs to the CD150 family receptors (CD150, CD229, CD84, CD244, NTB-A, CS1) and interacts with SAP/SH2D1α protein. Receptors of the CD150 family function as co-stimulatory molecules, regulating cytokine production and cytotoxicity. Mutation of CD229 is responsible for a fatal X-linked lymphoproliferative disease. *Blood 97:3513, 2001* *Ann Rev Immunol 19:657, 2001*
CD230	Prion protein	35	Neurons (nonpathogenic isoform)	CD230 is known as prion protein. Mutant and/or aberrant forms can act as an infectious agent that causes Creutzfeldt-Jakob

CD MARKERS	OTHER NAMES	MOLECULAR WEIGHT (KDA)	KNOWN NORMAL DISTRIBUTION	REMARKS
CD230—CONT				
				disease, Gerstmann-Sträussler disease, and Kuru.
				Curr Opin Neurol 17:337, 2004
CD231	TALLA-1; TM4SF2; A15; CCG-B7	30-45	Neurons	CD231 is a member of the tetraspanin protein family, which is known to contribute in molecular complexes including β1 integrins. It may play a role in the control of neurite outgrowth. Mutations in CD231 gene cause X-linked mental retardation. CD231 is characteristically positive in T-cell ALL and desmoplastic small round-cell tumor.
				Am J Pathol 163:2165, 2003
				Int J Cancer 61:706, 1995
CD232	VESPR; Plexin C1	200	Broad	CD232 is a receptor for the GPI-anchored semaphorin Sema7A (Sema-K1) and functions as an immune modulator during virus infection.
				Immunity 8:473, 1998
				Blood 79:1574, 1992
CD233	Band 3	90	Red blood cells	CD233 is a red cell membrane protein that functions as an anion (chloride and/or bicarbonate) exchanger and attachment site for cytoskeleton. Truncated form of CD233 is expressed in renal tubules and involved in acid secretion. Mutations cause hereditary spherocytosis or distal renal tubular acidosis.
				Blood 103:3233, 2004
				Semin Hematol 41:118, 2004
CD234	Duffy	35-45	Red blood cells, postcapillary endothelial cells, cerebellum Purkinje cells	CD234 is the Duffy blood group antigen (Fy glycoprotein). It is a chemokine receptor and also serves as the receptor for *Plasmodium vivax*.
				Immunohematol 20:37, 2004
				Immunogenetics 55:682, 2004

CD MARKERS	OTHER NAMES	MOLECULAR WEIGHT (KDA)	KNOWN NORMAL DISTRIBUTION	REMARKS
CD235a	Glycophorin A	36	Red blood cells	CD235a and CD235b are major sialoglyco-proteins of the human erythrocyte membrane. It carries the MN and Ss blood group antigens. *Immunohematol 17:76, 2001* *Adv Exp Med Biol 491:155, 2001*
CD235b	Glycophorin B	20	Red blood cells	Same as CD235a.
CD236	Glycophorin C and/or D	32/23	Stem cell subset, red blood cells, breast, liver, kidney	CD236, unlike CD235, plays a critical role in mature red cells, functioning to regulate cell shape, membrane deformability, and membrane mechanical stability. It carries blood group Gerbich antigens. *Semin Hematol 30:152, 1993* *Transfus Med Rev 6.63, 1992*
CD236R	Glycophorin C	32	Stem cell subset, red blood cells, breast, liver, kidney	Same as CD236. Glycophorins C and D are produced by a single gene called GE (Gerbich). Compared with glycophorin C, the glycophorin D contains a truncated amino terminal domain.
CD238	Kell blood group antigen	93	Stem cell subset, red blood cells	CD238 is a transmembrane glycoprotein that is surface exposed and shares sequence and structural homology with zinc endopeptidases, which are involved in regulating bioactive peptides. *Immunohematol 20:37, 2004* *Transfus Med Rev 14:93, 2000*
CD239	Lutheran blood group antigen; B-CAM	78-85	Stem cell subset, red blood cells	CD239 is a membrane glycoprotein that acts as adhesion molecule and red cell receptor for laminin. It also directly interacts with spectrin, participating in signaling and/or the linkage of the lipid bilayer to the red cell skeleton. *Baillieres Best Pract Res Clin Haematol 12:729, 1999*
CD240CE	Rh30 CE	30-32	Red blood cells	Rh blood group antigens (Cc and Ee). It associates with Rh50, CD47, and glycophorin B to form the Rh antigens. *Immunohematol 20:23, 2004* *Transfusion 44:1663, 2004*

CD MARKERS	OTHER NAMES	MOLECULAR WEIGHT (KDA)	KNOWN NORMAL DISTRIBUTION	REMARKS
CD240D	Rh30 D	30-32	Red blood cells	CD240D is an Rh blood group D antigen.
CD241	Rh50	50	Red blood cells	CD241 (Rh50 glycoprotein) does not carry Rh antigens (Rh30s), but serves as a co-expressor by forming a membrane complex with Rh30s through protein-protein interactions.
CD242	ICAM-4; Landsteiner-Wiener blood group	42	Red blood cells	CD242 (intercellular adhesion molecule-4) is an adhesion molecule and functions as a ligand for binding the integrins $\alpha_L\beta_2$ (CD11a-CD18), $\alpha_M\beta_2$ (CD11b-CD18), $\alpha_4\beta_1$ (CD49d-CD29), α_V (CD51), and $\alpha_{IIb}\beta_3$ (CD41/CD61). It carries the Lw blood group antigen. *Blood 103:1503, 2004* *Proc Natl Acad Sci USA 91:5306, 1994*
CD243	MDR-1; P-glycoprotein	180	Some hematopoietic stem cells, adrenal cortex, biliary canaliculi, intestinal epithelia, blood-brain endothelium, blood-testicle endothelium, placenta, proximal renal tubules	CD243, P-glycoprotein, is a drug transporter, encoded by the MDR1 gene. It is one of the important determinants in absorption, tissue targeting, and elimination of drugs. Apical (or luminal) expression of CD243 in tissue results in reduced drug absorption from the gastrointestinal tract, enhanced drug elimination into bile and urine, and impeded entry of certain drugs into the central nervous system. In addition to physiological and environmental factors, its expression and function are modified by genetic polymorphisms of the MDR1 gene product. CD243 is also an important prognostic factor in malignant diseases, such as tumors of the gastrointestinal tract. *Gastroenterology 127:339, 2004* *Hematology 9:91, 2004*
CD244	2B4	70	NK cells, T-cell subset, monocytes	CD244 is a member of the CD2 subset of the Ig superfamily molecules expressed on NK cells and other leukocytes. It is the high-affinity ligand for CD48. Engagement of CD244 on NK-cell surfaces with specific antibodies or CD48 can trigger cell-mediated cytotoxicity, interferon gamma secretion, phosphoinositol turnover, and NK-cell invasiveness. *Mol Immunol 42:489, 2005* *Immunol Rev 181:234, 2001*

CD MARKERS	OTHER NAMES	MOLECULAR WEIGHT (KDA)	KNOWN NORMAL DISTRIBUTION	REMARKS
CD246	ALK1	80	Weakly positive in brain, colon, and prostate	CD246, anaplastic large cell lymphoma (ALCL) kinase (ALK), is a receptor tyrosine kinase belonging to the insulin receptor superfamily. It appears to function as the receptor for pleiotrophin. CD246 normally is silent and/or negative in lymphoid cells, but is characteristically positive in ALCL because of t(2;5)(p23;q35) or other variant chromosomal translocations involving the ALK gene locus on chromosome 2. Although ALK may play a role in neural development, the normal functions of full-length ALK remain to be elucidated. *Blood 91:2076, 1998*
CD247	TCR zeta chain	16	T cells	CD247 (TCR-CD3 ζ chain) forms the TCR-CD3 complex together with TCRα/β (or γ/δ) heterodimer and CD3 γ, δ, and ε subunits. CD247 has a key role in the receptor assembly, expression, and signaling. Down-regulation of CD247 results in T-cell function impairment. *Cancer Immunol Immunother 53:865, 2004* *Curr Opin Immunol 9:380, 1997*

2. OTHER ANTIGENS USEFUL FOR IMMUNOPHENOTYPING

ANTIGENS	OTHER NAMES	MOLECULAR WEIGHT (KDA)	KNOWN NORMAL DISTRIBUTION	REMARKS
Bcl-1	Cyclin D1; PRAD1; CCND1	36	Some epithelial cells (no expression in normal lymphocytes)	Bcl-1 is one of the cell cycle regulatory proteins involved in restriction point control between G1 and S phase (G1-S transition). It forms complexes with cyclin-dependent kinases (CDK) 4 and 6 and further with retinoblastoma protein (pRB). Phosphorylation of pRB by Bcl-1/CDK4/6 leads to release of the E2F transcription factor, which then leads to progression of the cell cycle into the S phase. The Bcl-1/CDK4/6 activity is inhibited by p15/16, p18/19, p21, and p27. Bcl-1 is characteristically up-regulated in mantle cell lymphoma caused by t(11;14)(q13;q32), where the Bcl-1 gene at 11q13 is brought under the control of IgH gene enhancer. The translocation is also seen in subsets of B-cell prolymphocytic leukemia, plasma cell leukemia, splenic lymphoma with villous lymphocytes, chronic lymphocytic leukemia, and multiple myeloma. *Am J Pathol 154:1449, 1999* *Arch Pathol Lab Med 123:1182, 1999*
Bcl-2	124	26	Resting B cells and T cells, but not normal germinal center B cells, cortical thymocytes, or monocytoid B cells	Bcl-2 is a well-characterized inhibitor of apoptosis. It functions to prevent the release of cytochrome C from mitochondria and sequestrate procaspase-8 and procaspase-9 and thereby to block the signaling pathway leading to activation of the caspase cascades. The Bcl-2 gene is located at chromosome 18q21. Bcl-2 is positive in all cases of follicular lymphoma caused by t(14;18)(q32;q21) or rare t(2;18)(p12;q21). Most other B-cell lymphomas and T-cell lymphomas are also positive for Bcl-2. Clinically, Bcl-2 is a highly sensitive marker for distinguishing follicular hyperplasia from follicular lymphoma and reactive monocytoid B-cell hyperplasia from marginal zone lymphoma, respectively. *Mod Pathol 11:864, 1998* *Am J Clin Pathol 103:472, 1995* *Proc Natl Acad Sci USA 88:6961, 1991*

ANTIGENS	OTHER NAMES	MOLECULAR WEIGHT (KDA)	KNOWN NORMAL DISTRIBUTION	REMARKS
Bcl-6		79	Germinal center B cells and T cells, skeletal muscle cells, keratinocytes	Bcl-6 is a sequence-specific DNA binding transcriptional factor that mediates transcriptional repression by recruiting the SMRT (silencing mediator of retinoid and thyroid receptors), NCoR (nuclear receptor co-repressor), and BCoR (Bcl-6 co-repressor) co-repressors in a mutually exclusive manner. Bcl-6 is required for the formation of germinal centers and the Th2-mediated responses. Its gene is located at chromosome 3q27. Bcl-6 gene is frequently dysregulated in B-cell lymphomas. It is expressed in germinal center cell-derived lymphomas, including follicular lymphoma, diffuse large B-cell lymphoma, nodular lymphocyte predominant Hodgkin's lymphoma, and angioimmunoblastic T-cell lymphoma. *Histol Histopathol 19:637, 2004* *Leuk Lymphoma 44:S5, 2003* *Hum Pathol 30:403, 1999* *N Engl J Med 331:74, 1994*
FMC-7		105	B cells	FMC-7 is a glycoprotein found on circulating B lymphocytes. FMC-7 identifies the same cell type as CD22, but is a superior alternative for characterization of B-cell lymphomas. It is negative to weakly positive in chronic lymphocytic leukemia (CLL), but strongly positive in B-cell prolymphocytic leukemia (PLL), hairy cell leukemia (HCL), and splenic marginal zone lymphoma with villous lymphocytes (SLVL). It is thereby used for the differentiation of PLL from CLL (e.g., progression of CLL to PLL) and for confirmation of the diagnosis of other disorders, such as HCL and SLVL. *Am J Clin Pathol 120:754, 2003* *Am J Clin Pathol 115:285, 2001*
HLA-DR	Ia/7.2	63	B cells and B-cell precursors, activated T cells, monocytes and/or macrophages and their precursors, myeloid precursors, dendritic cells, endothelial cells	HLA-DR is one of the MHC (major histocompatibility complex) class II antigens. It consists of two glycoprotein chains, designated α and β, both of which are attached to the membrane. It is positive in B-cell acute lymphoblastic leukemia (ALL), some T-cell ALL, and acute myeloid leukemias (AML), except acute promyelocytic leukemia.

ANTIGENS	OTHER NAMES	MOLECULAR WEIGHT (KDA)	KNOWN NORMAL DISTRIBUTION	REMARKS
Immuno-globulin (Ig) heavy chains		~50	B cells (surface membrane expression), pre-B cells (cytoplasmic μ chain), plasma cells (cytoplasmic expression)	There are five different heavy (H) chains, μ, δ, γ, α, and ε, which bind to kappa or lambda light (L) chain to form IgM, IgD, IgG, IgA, and IgE, respectively. The five H chains are produced through rearrangement of the Ig H chain gene, located at chromosome 14q32. Each H chain contains about 440 amino acids and is divided into variable (V) and constant (C) regions. Heavy chains are distinguished from each other on the basis of amino acid sequences in their C region (isotypic determinants) and by the number of domains. Molecular testing for Ig H chain gene rearrangement is routinely used for the determination of clonality and diagnosis of B-cell neoplasms. *J Mol Diagn 2:178, 2000* *Leukemia 11:852, 1997*
Immuno-globulin (Ig) light chains		~25	B cells (surface membrane expression), plasma cells (cytoplasmic expression)	There are two different Ig light (L) chains, kappa (κ) and lambda (λ) L chains, encoded by two different genes located on chromosomes 2 and 22, respectively. The L chain contains about 220 amino acids. The κ and λ L chains are distinguished by the amino acid sequences in their C regions (isotypic determinants). The κ L chain has four subgroups, and λ has six subgroups. Each Ig molecule contains either κ or λ L chain, but not both. Neoplastic B cells and plasma cells characteristically express only κ or λ L chain (L chain restriction), an important feature for the confirmation of B-cell neoplasms and plasma cell neoplasms.
Ki-67	MIB-1	320, 359	Proliferating cells	Ki-67 is a nuclear protein involved in cell proliferation regulation. Ki-67 protein is used as a cell proliferation marker in research and diagnostics. It is present in the nuclei of cells in G_1, S, and G_2 phases of cell division and in mitosis. Quiescent or resting cells in the G_0 phase do not express the Ki-67 protein. The fraction of Ki-67-positive tumor cells (the Ki-67 labeling index) is often correlated with the grade and clinical course of the disease. *Histopathology 40:2, 2002* *Cancer 94:2151, 2002* *J Pathol 182:145, 1997*

ANTIGENS	OTHER NAMES	MOLECULAR WEIGHT (KDA)	KNOWN NORMAL DISTRIBUTION	REMARKS
Lysozyme	Muramidase	14	Monocytes, macrophages	Lysozyme is a lysosomal enzyme that hydrolyzes beta-1,4-glucosidic linkages in the mucopolysaccharide cell wall of a variety of microorganisms. It is primarily present in monocytes (macrophages) and is used as a marker for monocytic or myelomonocytic differentiation. *Int J Surg Pathol 11:271, 2003* *Am J Clin Pathol 104:431, 1995*
Myeloperoxidase	MPO	140	Mature and immature myeloid cells, monocytes	Myeloperoxidase (MPO) is an iron-containing, dimeric molecule that is found in the primary (azurophilic) granules of neutrophils (strong) and in the lysosomes of monocytes (weak). The gene for MPO is located on chromosome 17q22-23. The synthesis of MPO primarily occurs during the promyelocytic stage of myeloid differentiation, concurrent with development of primary granules. MPO catalyzes the conversion of hydrogen peroxide and chloride ions into hypochlorous acid, which is much more potent in microbial killing than hydrogen peroxide. Patients with MPO deficiency have impaired microbial killing, but most are asymptomatic, and the condition usually is undiagnosed. MPO is widely used in clinical diagnostics as a marker for myeloid and monocytic differentiation. *Int J Surg Pathol 11:271, 2003* *J Lab Clin Med 134:215, 1999*
Terminal deoxynucleotidyl transferase	TdT	60	Early lymphoid precursor cells	Terminal deoxynucleotidyl transferase (TdT) is a template-independent DNA polymerase, functioning to add 1 to 20 nucleotides to rearranging variable, diversity, and joining gene segments during the immunoglobulin gene rearrangement. The presence of TdT identifies blast cells as probably lymphoid in nature. It is a useful marker for the classification of acute leukemias and for the recognition of lymphoblastic lymphoma. *Semin Hematol 38:124, 2001* *Science 261:1171, 1993* *Nature 311:752, 1984*

ANTIGENS	OTHER NAMES	MOLECULAR WEIGHT (KDA)	KNOWN NORMAL DISTRIBUTION	REMARKS
ZAP-70	Zeta-chain (TCR) associated protein kinase	70	T cells and NK cells (cytoplasmic)	ZAP-70 is a member of the Syk–ZAP-70 protein tyrosine kinase family. It is normally expressed in T cells and natural killer cells and has a critical role in the initiation of T-cell signaling and activation. The expression of ZAP-70 is observed in a subset of chronic lymphocytic leukemia (CLL) and some other B-cell leukemias and/or lymphomas. Of interest, the ZAP-70 expression by CLL cells serves as a surrogate marker for the unmutated status of immunoglobulin heavy-chain variable-region gene (IgV_H). Patients with Binet stage A CLL who had at least 20% ZAP-70–positive leukemic cells had more rapid progression and poorer survival than those with less than 20% ZAP-70–positive cells. Thus, like CD38, ZAP-70 expression appears to be a prognostic marker for CLL. *N Engl J Med 351:893, 2004* *Am J Clin Pathol 122:582, 2004*

PART II: IMMUNOPHENOTYPES OF NEOPLASMS OF HEMATOPOIETIC AND LYMPHOID TISSUES

1. IMMUNOPHENOTYPES OF ACUTE MYELOID LEUKEMIAS

DISEASE	TYPICAL IMMUNOPHENOTYPE	REMARKS
AML with t(8;21)(q22;q22), *(AML1-ETO)*	In addition to CD34 and HLA-DR, the blasts typically express myeloid markers CD13, CD33, CD15, MPO, and CD117. Aberrant expression of CD19 is frequently present. CD56 is often expressed.	The translocation t(8;21)(q22;q22) involves the AML1 gene, which encodes CBFα, and the ETO (8-21) gene. The AML1/ETO fusion transcript is consistently detected in patients with t(8;21) AML. AML with t(8;21) is usually associated with good response to chemotherapy and high complete remission rate with long-term disease-free survival. Some factors appear to adversely affect survival, including CD56 expression and secondary karyotypic abnormalities.
AML with inv(16)(p13;q22) or t(16;16)(p13;q22), *(CBFβ-MYH11)*	In addition to myeloid markers (CD13, CD33, MPO, CD117), the blasts frequently express monocytic markers (CD14, CD4, CD11b, CD11c, CD64, CD36, lysozyme). Co-expression of CD2 is often present.	Inv(16)(p13;q22) and t(16;16)(p13;q22) both result in the fusion of the CBFβ gene at 16q22 to the smooth muscle myosin heavy chain (MYH11) at 16p13. By conventional cytogenetics, the inv(16) is a subtle rearrangement that may be overlooked. Trisomy 22 is a frequent secondary karyotypic abnormality. AML with inv(16) or t(16;16) typically shows myeloid and monocytic differentiation and the presence of eosinophilia, referred to as AMML-Eo. The disease usually responds well to chemotherapy with high complete remission rate.
AML with t(15;17)(q22;q12), *(PML-RARα)* and variants (FAB AML-M3)	The leukemic cells express CD13 (variable), CD33 (bright), MPO, and CD117 (variable). CD34 and HLA-DR are characteristically absent. There is frequent co-expression of CD2 and/or CD9.	AML with t(15;17), acute promyelocytic leukemia (APL), is caused by fusion of the retinoic acid receptor alpha (RARα) gene on 17q12 and the PML gene on 15q22, giving rise to a PML-RARα fusion product. APL has a particular sensitivity to treatment with all-trans retinoic acid (ATRA), which acts as a differentiating agent. APL is frequently associated with DIC. Rare variant translocations seen in APL include t(11;17)(q23;q12) (PLZF-RARα), t(5;17)(q35;q12) (NPM-RARα), and t(11;17)(q13;q12) (NuMA-RARα). APL with PLZF-RARα fusion is resistant to ATRA.
AML with 11q23 (MLL) abnormalities	The leukemic cells variably express CD13, CD33, CD117, and MPO. CD34 is generally absent. Cases with monoblastic morphology usually express monocytic differentiation markers (CD4, CD14, CD11b, CD11, CD64, CD36, lysozyme).	AML with 11q23 (MLL) abnormalities is usually associated with monocytic features. There are two clinical subgroups: one is AML in infants, and the other group is therapy-related AML usually occurring after treatment with DNA topoisomerase II inhibitors. The MLL (mixed lineage leukemia) gene on 11q23 is involved in a number of translocations with different partner chromosomes. AML with 11q23 abnormalities have an intermediate survival.
AML with multilineage dysplasia	Blasts are generally positive for CD34 and HLA-DR and express myeloid markers (CD13, CD33, MPO, CD117). There is frequent aberrant expression of CD56 and/or CD7.	AML with multilineage dysplasia is an acute leukemia with 20% or more blasts in blood or marrow and dysplasia in two or more myeloid cell lines, generally including megakaryocytes. Dysplasia must be present in 50% or more of the cells of at least two lines. These features must be present in a pretreatment specimen. The disease entity may occur de novo or following MDS or MDS/MPD.

DISEASE	TYPICAL IMMUNOPHENOTYPE	REMARKS
AML, therapy related	This AML is alkylating agent and/or radiation related. Blasts are generally positive for CD34 and HLA-DR and express myeloid markers (CD13, CD33, MPO, CD117). There is frequent aberrant expression of CD56 and/or CD7. It is also topoisomerase II inhibitor related. This is same as AML with 11q23 abnormalities.	Alkylating-agent and/or radiation-related AML usually occur 5-6 years following exposure. Cytogenetic abnormalities are primarily unbalanced translocations or deletions involving chromosomes 5 and/or 7. This type of therapy-related AML is generally refractory to chemotherapy and is associated with short survival. Topoisomerase II inhibitor-related AML usually occurs 1-3 years after exposure and characteristically has a significant monocytic component. The primary cytogenetic finding is a balanced translocation involving chromosome 11q23 (the MLL gene). Most cases respond to initial therapy in a manner similar to that of a patient with de novo AML.
AML, minimally differentiated (FAB AML-M0)	Blasts express panmyeloid markers (CD13, CD33, CD117), but not MPO. Most cases express precursor cell-associated antigens (CD34, CD38, HLA-DR). TdT may be positive in some cases.	The differential diagnosis includes ALL, acute megakaryoblastic leukemia, and biphenotypic or mixed lineage acute leukemia. Flow cytometric immunophenotyping is required for the confirmation of the diagnosis.
AML without maturation (FAB AML-M1)	Blasts express myeloid markers (CD13, CD33, CD117) and MPO. CD34 is often positive.	More than 20% blasts in the marrow. At least 3% of the blasts are positive for MPO. Blasts constitute more than 90% of the nonerythroid nucleated marrow cells.
AML with maturation (FAB AML-M2)	Blasts express myeloid markers (CD13, CD33, CD15, CD117) and MPO. CD34 and HLA-DR are often positive.	Blasts constitute more than 20% of all bone marrow cells and 20%-89% of nonerythroid cells. Monocytes constitute less than 20% of bone marrow cells.
Acute myelomonocytic leukemia (FAB AML-M4)	The blasts variably express CD13, CD33, CD117, HLA-DR and show some markers of monocytic differentiation, including CD14, CD4, CD11b, CD11c, CD64, CD36, and lysozyme. A subset of blasts expresses CD34.	Blasts constitute more than 20% of all bone marrow cells and nonerythroid cells. Monocytic component (monoblasts to monocytes) composes 20%-79% of bone marrow cells.
Acute monoblastic leukemia (FAB AML-M5a) and acute monocytic leukemia (FAB AML-M5b)	The leukemic cells variably express CD13, CD33, CD117, HLA-DR and show some markers of monocytic differentiation, including CD4, CD14, CD11b, CD11c, CD64, CD68, CD36, and lysozyme. CD34 is usually negative.	Blasts constitute more than 20% of all bone marrow cells and nonerythroid cells. Monocytic component (monoblasts to monocytes) composes 80% or more of bone marrow cells.

DISEASE	TYPICAL IMMUNOPHENOTYPE	REMARKS
Acute erythroid leukemia (FAB AML-M6) and pure erythroid leukemia	The erythroblasts in acute erythroid leukemia generally lack myeloid markers, but are positive for CD36 and glycophorin A. The myeloblasts express many myeloid antigens, including CD13, CD33, CD117, and MPO, with or without expression of precursor-cell markers, such as CD34 and HLA-DR. The erythroid cells in pure erythroid leukemia express CD36 and glycophorin A, and the more immature forms may also express CD34 and HLA-DR.	The diagnostic criteria for acute erythroid leukemia include: (1) erythroblasts constitute more than 50% of the nucleated marrow cells and (2) myeloblasts compose more than 20% of the nonerythroid cells. Pure erythroid leukemia is defined as a neoplastic proliferation of erythroid precursors (>80% of nucleated marrow cells) without a significant myeloblastic component.
Acute megakaryocytic leukemia (FAB AML-M7)	The blasts express CD36 and one or more of the platelet glycoproteins (CD41, CD61, and CD42). The blasts may or may not express HLA-DR, CD34, CD117, CD13, CD33, CD11c, CD14, and CD15.	Blasts constitute more than 20% of nucleated marrow cells and express one or more of the markers for megakaryocytic differentiation. Flow cytometric immunophenotyping is required for the confirmation of the diagnosis.
Acute leukemia of ambiguous lineage	Undifferentiated acute leukemia: The blasts often express HLA-DR, CD34, CD38 and may express TdT and CD7. The blasts generally lack lineage-specific markers, such as cCD79a, cCD22, cIgM, CD3, and MPO. Bilineal acute leukemia: There is a dual population of blasts with each population expressing markers of a distinct lineage, such as myeloid and lymphoid or B cell and T cell. Biphenotypic acute leukemia: The blasts co-express myeloid and T-cell or B-cell lineage-specific antigens or concurrent B-cell and T-cell antigens.	Cases of bilineal and biphenotypic acute leukemia usually have cytogenetic abnormalities. The common abnormalities include Philadelphia chromosome, t(4;11)(q21;q23) or other 11q23 abnormalities. The prognosis of acute leukemia of ambiguous lineage is unfavorable.

2. IMMUNOPHENOTYPES OF ACUTE LYMPHOBLASTIC LEUKEMIAS AND/OR LYMPHOMAS

DISEASE	TYPICAL IMMUNOPHENOTYPE	REMARKS
Precursor B lymphoblastic leukemia and/or lymphoblastic lymphoma (precursor B-cell acute lymphoblastic leukemia) (B-ALL/LBL)	The lymphoblasts in B-ALL/LBL are generally positive for TdT, HLA-DR, CD19, CD20, cCD79a. CD45 expression is usually dim and may be negative. The blasts in most cases are positive for CD10 and CD34. Cases with t(4;11)(q21;q23) or other 11q23 abnormalities are usually negative for CD10 and CD20, and CD15 is frequently expressed. Aberrant expression of CD13 and/or CD33 may be present. Early precursor B-ALL/LBL: TdT$^+$, HLA-DR$^+$, CD34$^+$ and/or Cd34$^-$, CD10$^-$, CD45$^-$ and/or CD45$^+$, CD19$^+$, cCD22$^+$, CD20$^-$, CD15$^+$, cIg$^-$, sIg$^-$. Common B-ALL/LBL: TdT$^+$, HLA-DR$^+$, CD34$^+$, CD10$^+$, CD45$^+$(dim), CD19$^+$, CD20$^+$, cIg$^-$, sIg$^-$. Pre–B-ALL/LBL: TdT$^-$ and/or TdT$^+$, CD34$^-$ and/or CD34$^+$, HLA-DR$^+$, CD45$^+$(dim), CD19$^+$, CD20$^+$, cIgM$^+$, sIg$^-$.	The cytogenetic abnormalities in B-ALL/LBL include several groups: hypodiploid, hyperdiploid (<50), hyperdiploid (>50), translocations, and pseudodiploid. The commonly seen translocations include t(9;22)(q34;q11) *(BCR-ABL)*, t(12;21)(p13;q22) *(TEL-AML1)*, t(5;14)(q31;q32) *(IL-3-IgH)*, t(1;19)(q23;p13) *(PBX-E2A)*, t(17;19)(q21;p13) *(HLF-E2A)*, t(4;11)(q21;q23) *(AF4-MLL)*, and other translocations involving 11q23. The cytogenetic findings are prognostically important.

DISEASE	TYPICAL IMMUNOPHENOTYPE	REMARKS
Precursor T lymphoblastic leukemia and/or lymphoblastic lymphoma (precursor T-cell acute lymphoblastic leukemia) (T-ALL/LBL)	T-ALL/LBL most often has an immunophenotype that corresponds to the common thymocyte stage of differentiation. The blasts are positive for TdT and often CD10 and variably express CD1a, CD2, CD3, CD4, CD5, CD7, and CD8. CD4 and CD8 are frequently co-expressed on the blasts. Myeloid markers CD13 and CD33 are often present. CD79a and CD117 expression has been observed in some cases. Some T-ALL/LBL has an immunophenotype that corresponds to prothymocyte stage of differentiation. The blasts are positive for TdT and early T-cell antigens (CD7, CD3, CD5 and CD2). Both CD4 and CD8 are characteristically absent. Occasional T-ALL/LBL cases show an immunophenotype that corresponds to that of mature thymocytes. The blasts often expresss TdT, CD2, CD3 (surface expression), CD5 and CD7. However, the blasts express either CD4 or CD8 but not both.	In about one third of T-ALL/LBL, translocations have been detected involving the alpha and delta T-cell receptor loci at 14q11.2, the beta locus at 7q35, and the gamma locus at 7p14-15, with a variety of partner genes. Genes include the transcription factors MYC (8q24), TAL1 (1p32), RBTN1 (11p15), RBTN2 (11p13), and HOX11 (10q24), and the cytoplasmic tyrosine kinase LCK (1p34-35). In most cases these translocations lead to a dysregulation of transcription of the partner gene by juxtaposition with the regulatory region of one of the T-cell receptor loci. It is worth noting that T-ALL/LBL can be part of a unique disease entity known as the 8p11 myeloproliferative syndrome caused by constitutive activation of FGFR1. FGFR1 is a receptor tyrosine kinase for fibroblast growth factors and is encoded by a gene on chromosome 8p11. Disruption of FGFR1 gene is associated with a chronic myeloproliferative disorder that frequently has eosinophilia and associated T-cell lymphoblastic lymphoma. Four gene fusions associated with distinct translocations have been described in this syndrome: the t(8;13)(p11;q12), t(8;9)(p11;q33), t(6;8)(q27;p11), and t(8;22)(p11q22) that fuse ZNF198, CEP110, FOP, and BCR, respectively, to FGFR1. The resulting fusion proteins have constitutive tyrosine kinase activity and activate multiple signal transduction pathways. These pathways and the fusion proteins are attractive targets for targeted signal transduction therapy.

3. IMMUNOPHENOTYPES OF MATURE B-CELL NEOPLASMS

DISEASE	TYPICAL IMMUNOPHENOTYPE	REMARKS
Chronic lymphocytic leukemia and/or small lymphocytic lymphoma (CLL/SLL)	The malignant cells express weak or dim surface IgM or IgM and IgD, but not surface IgG. They express CD5, CD19, CD20 (weak), CD22 (weak), CD79a, CD23, CD43 and are negative for CD10, Bcl-1 (cyclin D1), FMC-7, and CD79b. A subset of cases expresses CD11c (weak). Cases with unmutated Ig variable region genes have been reported to be positive for CD38 and ZAP-70. Some cases may have an atypical immunophenotype (e.g., CD5$^-$ or CD23$^-$, FMC7$^+$ or CD11c$^+$, or strong sIg or CD79b$^+$).	The clinical course is often indolent but incurable. The disease may progress and/or transform to prolymphocytic leukemia (PLL) or large B-cell lymphoma (Richter's syndrome). CD38 and/or ZAP-70 positivity is associated with worse prognosis. About 80% of the CLL/SLL cases have abnormal karyotypes. Trisomy 12 is reported in ~20% of cases and deletions at 13q14 in up to 50% of cases. Trisomy 12 in CLL/SLL correlates with a worse prognosis. In addition to CLL/SLL, aberrant CD5 expression is also characteristic of mantle cell lymphoma and/or leukemia (MCL).
B-cell prolymphocytic leukemia (B-PLL)	The cells of B-PLL strongly express surface IgM and B-cell antigens CD19, CD20, CD22, CD79a, CD79b, and FMC-7. CD5 is present in about one third of cases, and CD23 is typically negative.	B-PLL can be divided into CD5$^+$ B-PLL (arising in CLL/SLL) and CD5$^-$ B-PLL (de novo PLL). CD5$^+$ B-PLL has a longer median survival than CD5$^-$ B-PLL.
Lymphoplasmacytic lymphoma and/or Waldenström's macroglobulinemia (LPL)	The cells express strong surface and cytoplasmic (some cells) immunoglobulin, usually of IgM type (rarely IgG or IgA), are typically IgD$^-$, and express B-cell antigens (CD19, CD20, CD22, CD79a), and are CD5$^-$, CD10$^-$, CD23$^-$, CD43$^+$ and/or CD43$^-$, and CD38$^+$. Lack of CD5 and strong immunoglobulin expression are useful in distinction from CLL/SLL.	Characteristic features include IgM monoclonal gammopathy; spectrum of small lymphocytes, plasmacytoid lymphocytes, and plasma cells, with or without PAS$^+$ intranuclear pseudoinclusions (Dutcher bodies); interstitial, nodular, or diffuse pattern of bone marrow involvement; and typical immunophenotype (sIgM$^+$, CD19$^+$, CD20$^{+,}$ CD5$^-$, CD23$^-$, CD10$^-$).
Splenic marginal zone lymphoma (SMZL)	The tumor cells express surface IgM and are positive for CD19, CD20, CD79a and negative for CD5, CD10, CD23, CD25, CD43, CD103, and Bcl-1 (cyclin D1).	Circulating lymphoma cells are usually, but not always, characterized by the presence of short polar villi (villous lymphocytes). The absence of CD5 and CD43 are useful in excluding CLL/SLL and MCL (mantle cell lymphoma). The absence of CD103 is useful in excluding hairy cell leukemia, and the absence of CD10 is useful in excluding follicular lymphoma. On tissue sections, Bcl-1 (cyclin D1) is also useful in distinguishing between SMZL and MCL. The clinical course is indolent, even with bone marrow involvement. The disease is incurable with available therapy.

DISEASE	TYPICAL IMMUNOPHENOTYPE	REMARKS
Hairy cell leukemia (HCL)	The leukemic cells express surface Ig (IgM, IgD, IgG, or IgA), pan–B-cell markers (CD19, CD20, CD22, CD79a, but usually not CD79b), and are typically negative for CD5, CD10, and CD23. The cells are characteristically positive for CD11c, CD25, FMC-7, and CD103. In tissue sections, the cells are typically positive for DBA-44 and negative for Bcl-1 (cyclin D1).	Patients with HCL usually have splenomegaly, pancytopenia (monocytopenia is characteristic), and may have circulating hairy leukemic cells. The cells in bone marrow biopsy sections may produce a "fried-egg" appearance because of abundant cytoplasm and prominent cell borders. Bone marrow reticulin fibers are characteristically increased, often resulting in "dry tap" during aspirate procedure. Interferon alpha, deoxycoformycin (pentostatin), or 2-chlorodeoxyadenosine (2-CdA, cladribine) can induce long-term remissions.
Plasma cell myeloma and/or plasmacytoma	The malignant cells typically express monotypic cytoplasmic immunoglobulin (Ig) (IgG, IgA, light chain only, rare IgD, IgM, or IgE) and lacks surface Ig. The cells generally lack CD45 and pan–B-cell antigens (CD19, CD20, CD22), but CD79a is positive in the majority of cases. The cells are typically positive for CD38, CD138 and often express CD56, CD43, and rarely CD10. The phenotype of plasma cell leukemia is similar to that of myeloma, but CD56 is characteristically negative.	Plasma cells do not express surface immunoglobulin. For the clonality (or light chain restriction) determination by flow cytometry analysis, cell permeabilization procedure is necessary. The procedure gives antibodies access to intracellular structures and/or molecules and leaves the morphological scatter characteristics of the cells intact.
Extranodal marginal zone B-cell lymphoma of mucosa-associated lymphoid tissue (MALT lymphoma)	The lymphoma cells typically express IgM ± IgD, and less often IgA or IgG and show light chain restriction. The cells are positive for CD19, CD20, CD79a, CD43 and negative for CD5, CD10, CD23, and Bcl-1.	Trisomy 3 is found in ~60%, and t(11;18)(q21;q21) has been detected in 25%-50% of MALT lymphoma cases. Analysis of the t(11;18) breakpoint has shown fusion of the apoptosis-inhibitor gene API2 to a novel gene at 18q21, named MLT. Neither t(14;18) nor t(11;14) is present. Cases with t(11;18) appear to be resistant to *H. pylori* eradication therapy. In small biopsy tissue sections, the co-expression of CD20 and CD43 and lack of CD5, CD10, and Bcl-1 (cyclin D1) are characteristic for MALT lymphoma.
Nodal marginal zone B-cell lymphoma (NMZL)	The immunophenotype of most cases is similar to that of extranodal MALT lymphoma. Some cases are IgD+ and CD43−, similar to SMZL.	NMZL is a primary nodal B-cell neoplasm that morphologically resembles lymph nodes involved by marginal zone lymphomas of extranodal or splenic types, but without evidence of extranodal or splenic disease. Monocytoid B cells may be prominent.

DISEASE	TYPICAL IMMUNOPHENOTYPE	REMARKS
Follicular lymphoma (FL)	The lymphoma cells are usually positive for pan–B-cell antigens (CD19, CD20, CD22, CD79a), sIg (IgM ± IgD, IgG, or rarely IgA), CD10, Bcl-2, Bcl-6 and negative for CD5. Rare cases may express CD5 and/or CD43. Bcl-2 is expressed in the majority of cases, ranging from nearly 100% in grade 1 to 75% in grade 3 FL.	Virtually all cases of FL have cytogenetic abnormalities. The most common translocation, t(14;18)(q32;q21), involving rearrangement of the Bcl-2 gene and IgH gene, is present in 80%-95% of FL. Rare cases have a t(2;18)(p12;q21), which places the Bcl-2 gene with the light chain gene on chromosome 2. Clonal evolution in FL has been reported. FL may transform into precursor B-ALL, and c-myc (8q24) rearrangement is often associated with the transformation. In addition to FL, Bcl-2 is expressed by resting B cells and T cells, but not by normal germinal center cells, cortical thymocytes, or monocytoid B cells. Bcl-2 is particularly useful in distinguishing reactive follicular hyperplasia and FL.
Mantle cell lymphoma (MCL)	The lymphoma cells usually express surface IgM ± IgD, pan–B-cell antigens (CD19, CD20, CD79a), Bcl-2, FMC-7, CD5, CD43 and are typically negative for CD10, CD23, and Bcl-6. Virtually all cases express Bcl-1 (cyclin D1). Rare CD5-negative cases have been reported.	MCL and CLL/SLL are the two common CD5-positive B-cell lymphoproliferative disorders. But unlike CLL/SLL, MCL cells express bright surface immunoglobulin, bright CD20 and FMC-7, and are characteristically CD23 negative. Virtually all MCL cases show rearrangement involving the cyclin D1 (Bcl-1) gene and IgH gene using FISH (fluorescence in situ hybridization). The t(11;14)(q13;q32) translocation is demonstrable in about 75% of MCL cases by conventional cytogenetic study.
Diffuse large B-cell lymphoma (DLBCL)	DLBCL cells typically express various pan–B-cell antigens (CD19, CD20, CD22, CD79a), sIg and/or cIg (IgM>IgG>IgA), Bcl-6, and CD10. Bcl-2 is positive in 30%-50% of cases. CD5 is expressed in about 10% of cases. DLBCL with anaplastic morphology also express CD30.	Morphological variants of DLBCL include centroblastic, immunoblastic, T-cell and/or histiocyte-rich, anaplastic, and plasmablastic DLBCL. Translocation of the Bcl-2 gene (e.g., t[14;18], a hallmark of follicular lymphoma [FL]) occurs in 20%-30% of cases. Up to 30% of cases show abnormalities of 3q27 region involving Bcl-6 gene. Bcl-2 expression has been reported to be associated with an adverse disease-free survival, and expression of Bcl-6 appears to be associated with a better prognosis.
Mediastinal (thymic) large B-cell lymphoma (Med-DLBCL)	The lymphoma cells express CD45 and B-cell antigen (CD19, CD20). Immunoglobulin (Ig) and HLA class I and II molecules (e.g., HLA-DR) are frequently absent. The cells do not express CD5 and CD10 and lack Bcl-2, Bcl-6, and c-myc rearrangements.	Med-DLBCL is a subtype of DLBCL arising in the mediastinum of putative thymic B-cell origin with distinct clinical, immunophenotypic, and genotypic features. Tissue sections usually show diffuse lymphoid proliferation, compartmentalized into groups by fine and/or delicate fibrotic bands.
Intravascular large B-cell lymphoma	The lymphoma cells express pan–B-cell antigens (CD19, CD20, CD22, CD79a). CD5 co-expression is seen in some cases.	Intravascular large B-cell lymphoma is a rare subtype of extranodal DLBCL characterized by the presence of lymphoma cells only in the lumina of small vessels, particularly capillaries. The intravascular growth pattern appears to be due to a defect in homing receptors (e.g., CD29, CD54) on the lymphoma cells.

DISEASE	TYPICAL IMMUNOPHENOTYPE	REMARKS
Primary effusion lymphoma (PEL)	The lymphoma cells usually express CD45, but are usually negative for pan–B-cell markers (CD19, CD20, CD79a). Surface and cytoplasmic immunoglobulin is likewise often absent. Activation and plasma cell-related markers, such as CD30, CD38, and CD138 are usually positive. Aberrant cytoplasmic CD3 expression has been reported.	PEL is a neoplasm of large B cells usually having serous effusions without detectable tumor masses. It is universally associated with human herpes virus 8 (HHV-8), most often occurring in the setting of immunodeficiency. Rare cases of PEL of T-cell origin have been reported.
Lymphomatoid granulomatosis (LYG)	The lymphoma cells usually express CD20 and are variably positive for CD79a and CD30, but negative for CD15. The cells generally lack cytoplasmic and surface immunoglobulin expression. The background small lymphocytes are CD3-positive T cells, with CD4-positive cells more frequent than CD8-positive cells.	LYG is an angiocentric and angiodestructive lymphoproliferative disease involving extranodal sites, comprised of Epstein-Barr virus (EBV)-positive B cells admixed with reactive T cells, which usually are preponderant. LYG may progress to an EBV-positive DLBCL. The common sites of involvement are lung, kidney, brain, liver, and skin.
Burkitt's lymphoma (BL)	The lymphoma cells express surface IgM with light chain restriction, pan–B-cell antigens (CD19, CD20, CD22, CD79a), CD10, CD77, and Bcl-6. The cells are negative for CD5, CD23, CD34, and TdT. Nearly 100% of the cells are positive for Ki-67 (MIB-1). Bcl-2 is not expressed.	All BL cases show a translocation of c-*myc* gene at chromosome 8q24 to the IgH gene at 14q32 or less commonly to light chain loci at 2p12 or 22q11. Genetic abnormalities involving the c-*myc* gene play an essential role in BL pathogenesis. The expression of CD10 and Bcl-6 indicates a germinal center origin of the tumor cells. BL is highly aggressive, but potentially curable.

4. IMMUNOPHENOTYPES OF MATURE T-CELL AND NK-CELL NEOPLASMS

DISEASE	TYPICAL IMMUNOPHENOTYPE	REMARKS
T-cell prolymphocytic leukemia (T-PLL)	The leukemic cells express CD2, CD3, and CD7, but not TdT and CD1a. In about two thirds of patients with T-PLL, the cells are CD4$^+$ and CD8$^-$. In ~25% of cases, the cells co-express CD4 and CD8, a feature almost unique to T-PLL. In ~15% of cases, the cells are CD4$^-$ and CD8$^+$.	T-PLL is an aggressive T-cell leukemia characterized by the proliferation of small to medium sized prolymphocytes with a mature postthymic T-cell phenotype involving the blood, bone marrow, lymph nodes, spleen, and skin. The most frequent chromosome abnormality in T-PLL involves inversion of chromosome 14 with breakpoints in the long arm at q11 and q32, seen in ~80% of patients. In ~10% of cases, there is a reciprocal tandem translocation t(14;14)(q11;q32). These translocations juxtapose the TCR-α/β locus with the oncogenes TCL1 and TCL1b at 14q32, which are activated through the translocation.
T-cell large granular lymphocyte leukemia (T-LGL)	T-LGL cells have a mature T-cell immunophenotype. Based on the predominant cell markers, T-LGL can be subdivided into: 1. Common type (80% of cases): CD3$^+$, TCR$\alpha\beta^+$, CD4$^-$, CD8$^+$ 2. Rare variants: (1) CD3$^+$, TCR$\alpha\beta^+$, CD4$^+$, CD8$^-$ (2) CD3$^+$, TCR$\alpha\beta^+$, CD4$^+$, CD8$^+$ (3) CD3$^+$, TCR$\gamma\delta^+$ CD11b, CD56, and CD57 are variably expressed. CD57 is often expressed in the common type. TIA-1 is usually positive.	T-LGL is a heterogeneous disorder characterized by a persistent (>6 mo) increase in the number of peripheral blood large granular lymphocytes (LGLs), usually between 2-20 $\times$ 10^3/mL, without a clearly identified cause. Severe neutropenia with or without anemia is a characteristic clinical feature. Pure red cell hypoplasia has been reported in association with T-LGL leukemia. Moderate splenomegaly, rheumatoid arthritis, and the presence of autoantibodies are commonly seen in patients with T-LGL.
Aggressive NK-cell leukemia	The leukemic cells are CD2$^+$, surface CD3$^-$, cytoplasmic CD3ϵ^+, CD56$^+$ and positive for cytotoxic molecules (TIA-1, granzyme B, and/or perforin). This immunophenotype is identical to that of extranodal NK- and/or T-cell lymphoma, nasal type. CD11b and CD16 may be expressed, whereas CD57 is usually negative.	Aggressive NK-cell leukemia is characterized by a systemic proliferation of NK cells. The disease has an aggressive clinical course. T-cell receptor (TCR) genes are in germline configuration. Clonality therefore has to be established by other methods, such as cytogenetic studies and pattern of X chromosome inactivation in female patients. A variety of clonal cytogenetic abnormalities have been reported, such as del(6)(q21q25).
Adult T-cell leukemia and/or lymphoma (ATLL)	The tumor cells express T-cell antigens (CD2, CD3, CD5), but usually lack CD7. Most cases are CD4$^+$, CD8$^-$. Rare cases are CD4$^-$, CD8$^+$, or double negative for CD4 and CD8. CD25 is expressed in virtually all cases. TIA-1 and granzyme B are negative.	ATLL is a peripheral T-cell neoplasm most often composed of highly pleomorphic lymphoid cells. The disease is usually widely disseminated and is caused by the human T-cell leukemia virus type 1 (HTLV-1). Clonally integrated HTLV-1 is found in all cases. ATLL is endemic in Japan, the Caribbean basin, and parts of Central Africa. T-cell receptor genes are clonally rearranged.

DISEASE	TYPICAL IMMUNOPHENOTYPE	REMARKS
Extranodal NK/T-cell lymphoma, nasal type	The typical immunophenotype is $CD2^+$, $CD56^+$, surface $CD3^-$, and cytoplasmic $CD3\epsilon^+$. Most cases are positive for cytotoxic molecules (TIA-1, granzyme B, perforin). The tumor cells are usually negative for CD4, CD5, CD8, CD16, and CD57. But CD43, CD45RO, HLA-DR, CD95 are commonly expressed.	The disease entity is designated NK/T-(rather than NK) cell lymphoma because although most cases appear to be NK-cell neoplasms (EBV^+, $CD56^+$), rare cases show an EBV^+, $CD56^-$ cytotoxic T-cell phenotype. T-cell receptor and immunoglobulin genes are in germline configuration in a majority of cases. EBV can be demonstrated in the tumor cells in nearly all cases. The prognosis is variable, with some patients responding well to therapy and others dying of disseminated disease despite aggressive therapy.
Enteropathy-type T-cell lymphoma	Tumor cells are $CD3^+$, $CD5^-$, $CD7^+$, $CD8^-$ and/or $CD8^+$, $CD4^-$, $CD103^+$ and contain cytotoxic molecules (TIA-1, granzyme B). A varying proportion of the tumor cells express CD30. In a subset of cases, the tumor cells are $CD8^+$ and $CD56^+$.	The lymphoma is a tumor of intraepithelial T lymphocytes, showing varying degrees of transformation, but usually having a tumor composed of large lymphoid cells. TCRβ and TCRγ genes are clonally rearranged. The tumor occurs most commonly in the jejunum or ileum, and there is a clear association with celiac disease. The prognosis is usually poor.
Hepatosplenic T-cell lymphoma	The tumor cells are $CD3^+$, $CD4^-$, $CD8^-$, $CD5^-$, $CD56^+$ and/or $CD56^-$. The cells are usually $TCR\delta1^+$, $TCR\alpha\beta^-$ and express TIA-1.	Hepatosplenic T-cell lymphoma is an extranodal and systemic neoplasm derived from cytotoxic T cells usually of γδ T-cell receptor type, medium in size, demonstrating marked sinusoidal infiltration of spleen, liver, and bone marrow. TCRδ genes are clonally rearranged. TCRβ genes are usually in germline configuration. Isochromosome 7q is present in nearly all cases, sometimes in conjunction with other abnormalities, most commonly trisomy 8. The clinical course is aggressive.
Subcutaneous panniculitis-like T-cell lymphoma (SPTCL)	The tumor cells are usually $CD3^+$, $TCR\alpha\beta^+$, $CD5^-$, $CD4^-$, $CD8^-$ and express cytotoxic molecules, including granzyme B, perforin, and TIA-1 (T-cell intracellular antigen). Cases of γδ origin may express CD56 and CD16.	SPTCL is a cytotoxic T-cell lymphoma, which preferentially infiltrates subcutaneous tissue. It is composed of atypical lymphoid cells of varying size, often with marked tumor necrosis and karyorrhexis. Some patients may have a hemophagocytic syndrome with pancytopenia. The clinical course is aggressive.
Blastic NK-cell lymphoma	The neoplastic cells are $CD4^+$, $CD56^+$, and $CD43^+$. The cells lack surface CD3 and are usually negative for CD2, CD7, cytoplasmic CD3ε, and cytotoxic molecules. All cases studied have been EBV negative.	Blastic NK-cell lymphoma is composed of cells with a lymphoblast-like morphology and evidence of commitment to the NK lineage. TCR genes are germline in configuration. The clinical course is usually aggressive.
Mycosis fungoides and Sézary syndrome (MF/SS)	The typical phenotype is $CD2^+$, $CD3^+$, $TCR\beta^+$, $CD5^+$, $CD4^+$ and $CD8^-$ (rarely $CD4^-$ and $CD8^+$). Virtually all cases are negative for CD26. CD7 is usually negative.	MF is a mature T-cell lymphoma with Th2-like immunophenotype, occurring in the skin with patches and/or plaques and characterized by epidermal and dermal infiltration of small to medium sized T cells with cerebriform nuclei. SS is a generalized mature T-cell lymphoma characterized by the presence of erythroderma, lymphadenopathy, and neoplastic T lymphocytes in the blood ($>1 \times 10^3/\mu l$). Similar to MF, the neoplastic T cells in SS also have cerebriform nuclei. TCR genes are clonally rearranged.

DISEASE	TYPICAL IMMUNOPHENOTYPE	REMARKS
Primary cutaneous CD30-positive T-cell lymphoproliferative disorders	Primary cutaneous anaplastic large cell lymphoma (C-ALCL): The tumors cells express T-cell antigens (CD2, CD3, CD5, CD7) and are usually positive for CD4. CD30 is expressed in the majority (>75%) of the cells. Cytotoxic molecules (granzyme B, perforin, TIA-1) are usually positive. Aberrant T-cell phenotype with loss of one or more T-cell antigens (CD2, CD5, or CD7) is common, but null cell phenotype is rare. CD56 is expressed in some cases. Unlike systemic ALCL, the tumor cells are negative for EMA (epithelial membrane antigen, also called CD227) and ALK (anaplastic large cell lymphoma kinase, also called CD246). Lymphomatoid papulosis (LyP): The atypical T cells are CD4$^+$, CD8$^-$. The cells often express aberrant phenotypes with variable loss of pan–T-cell antigens (e.g., CD2, CD5, or CD7). CD30 is positive in a LyP subtype (type A). Cytotoxic molecules are often expressed, but ALK (CD246) is absent.	LyP and C-ALCL constitute a spectrum of related conditions originating from transformed or activated CD30-positive T lymphocytes. They may co-exist in individual patients; they can be clonally related, and they often show overlapping clinical and/or histological features.
Angioimmunoblastic T-cell lymphoma (AITL)	The neoplastic cells express T-cell antigens (CD2, CD3, CD5, CD7), usually without aberrant antigen loss. The tumor cells are CD4$^+$ and CD8$^-$, but admixed reactive CD8$^+$ T cells are usually present. The neoplastic T cells are characteristically positive for CD10 and Bcl-6. CD21 stain highlights the intact or disrupted follicular dendritic meshwork.	AITL is a T-cell lymphoma with Th1-like immunophenotype. It is characterized by systemic disease, a polymorphous infiltrate involving lymph nodes, with a prominent proliferation of high endothelial venules and follicular dendritic cells. TCR genes are rearranged in the majority (>75%) of cases. Secondary EBV-related B-cell lymphoma may occur. Recent studies showed that almost all cases are positive for CD10 and Bcl-6, suggesting a germinal center derivation of the tumor cells. The clinical course is aggressive with a median survival of less than 3 years.

DISEASE	TYPICAL IMMUNOPHENOTYPE	REMARKS
Peripheral T-cell lymphoma, unspecified	The neoplastic cells express T-cell antigens (CD2, CD3, CD5, CD7), but aberrant T-cell phenotypes with antigen loss (e.g., CD7, CD5) are frequent. Most nodal cases are CD4$^+$, CD8$^-$. CD30 is expressed by a majority of tumor cells in large cell variants. CD56 may be positive in some cases. Expression of cytotoxic molecules is rare.	TCR genes are clonally rearranged in most cases. Complex karyotypes, consistent with clonal evolution, are frequent. Trisomy 3 is frequent in the lymphoepithelioid cell (Lennert's) variant. EBV (Epstein-Barr virus) is usually absent in the tumor cells. The diseases are among the most aggressive of the non-Hodgkin's lymphomas.
Anaplastic large cell lymphoma (ALCL)	The tumor cells express one or more T-cell antigens (CD2, CD3, CD5, CD7), but apparent "null cell" phenotype has been reported. The cells usually express CD30 (membrane and in the Golgi region), ALK (CD246, cytoplasmic and/or nuclear), EMA, cytotoxic molecules (TIA-1, granzyme B, and/or perforin), CD43, and CD45. Clusterin is expressed in all cases of systemic ALCL, but not primary cutaneous ALCL (C-ALCL) or classical Hodgkin's lymphoma.	Nearly all ALCL cases show clonal rearrangement of the T-cell receptor genes irrespective of whether they express T-cell antigens or not. Expression of ALK (CD246) in ALCL is due to genetic alteration of the ALK locus on chromosome 2. The most frequent alteration is t(2;5)(p23;q35), resulting in fusion of the ALK gene and nucleophosmin (NPM) gene on 5q35. The classic t(2;5) leads to positive staining for ALK in both the nucleolus, nucleus, and the cytoplasm. In other variant translocations, often only cytoplasmic staining is observed. ALK positivity is an important prognostic indicator, which is associated with a favorable prognosis.

1. Jaffe ES, Harris NL, Stein H, et al, editors: *World Health Organization classification of tumors: pathology and genetics of tumours of haematopoietic and lymphoid tissues,* Lyon, France, 2001, IARC Press.

2. Chan JKC, Banks PM, Cleary ML, et al: A revised European-American classification of lymphoid neoplasms proposed by the International Lymphoma Study Group: a summary version, *Am J Clin Pathol* 103:543-560, 1995.

3. Harris NL, Jaffe ES, Stein H, et al: A revised European-American classification of lymphoid neoplasms proposed by the International Lymphoma Study Group, *Blood* 84:1361-1392, 1994.

4. Dunphy CH: Applications of flow cytometry and immunohistochemistry to diagnostic hematopathology, *Arch Pathol Lab Med* 128:1004-1022, 2004.

5. Attygalle A, Al-Jehani R, Diss TC, et al: Neoplastic T cells in angioimmunoblastic T-cell lymphoma express CD10, *Blood* 99:627-633, 2002.

SECTION VII
PHARMACOGENOMICS

Pharmacogenomics, a clinical and scientific discipline, is based on the phenotype and genotype and/or haplotype correlation. It uses genetic information to predict the drug efficacy and toxicity and to identify responders and nonresponders.[1-9] Pharmacogenomics may be regarded as one of the tangible outcomes of the completion of the human genome project.[10,11] As such, pharmacogenomics constitutes the genomic component for personalized medicine, which also encompasses personalized laboratory medicine. Other personalized laboratory medicine components would include: clinical chemistry, such as creatinine, as a renal biomarker; TDM biomarker; and possibly future proteomics biomarkers. Together this combination of personalized laboratory medicine tests would enable the benefit of drug therapy and/or discovery based on an individual's genetic, proteomic, and metabolic profiles. Even though pharmacogenomics and pharmacogenetics are used interchangeably, the proposed definition of pharmacogenetic testing is concerned with using genotyping for identifying interindividual DNA sequence variation, whereas pharmacogenomic testing is concerned with identifying variation in whole genomes, haplotypes, and gene expression or inactivation.[11,12] Since FDA-approved pharmacogenomic product is limited, the majority of the testing is performed in " home-brew" settings by developing or adopting published procedures. Currently the testing may be more readily characterized as pharmacogenetics in that the majority of the clinical protocols identify mutations and/or single nucleotide polymorphisms (SNPs). The top ten pharmacogenetic tests, according to a recent AACC survey, are: *CYP 2D6, TPMT, CYP 2C9, CYP 2C19, NAT-2, CYP 3A5, UGT1A1, MDR1, CYP 2B6,* and *MTHFR.*[13] These procedures may be performed by a variety of molecular techniques by using genomic DNA. Readers are referred to review papers for technical details.[14-20] Pharmacogenomics testing for the gene expressions of drug-metabolizing enzymes, transporters, and receptors are limited to drug discovery and clinical research laboratories. Currently, they are not yet offered clinically for patient services.

This section attempts to provide a database for pharmacogenomics and/or pharmacogenetics testing and is divided into four sections: Phase I drug-metabolizing enzymes, phase II drug-metabolizing enzymes, drug transporters, and drug receptors and/or targets. Currently the majority of the interest is focused on phase I and II drug-metabolizing enzymes genes, with emerging interest in drug transporters and receptors and/or targets. The tables are organized by each gene with the known mutations, representative and/or selected drug substrates, inhibitors, inducers, nucleotide changes, amino changes, frequencies, and clinical effects. References are provided to guide the readers. Since the practice of personalized medicine—personalized laboratory medicine—and pharmacogenomics are rapidly evolving, representative websites are listed below:

Websites

http://www.genome.gov/glossary.cfm
http://www.geneclinics.org
http://www.cdc.gov/genomics/hugenet/reviews.htm
http://www.cancer.gov/cancer_information/pdq
http://www.ncbi.nlm.nih.gov/omin/
http://www4.od.nih.gov/oba/sacgt.htm
http://www.nhlbi.nih.gov/resources/docs/cht-book.htm

http://www.nhlbi.nih.gov/about/factpdf.htm
http://www.cardiogenomics.med.harvard.edu
http://www.nhgri.nih.gov/Policy_and _public_ affairs/Legislation/insure.htm
http://medicine.iupui.edu/flockhart/table.htm
http://www.imm.ki.se/CYPalleles/
http;//www.aidsinfonyc.org/tag/science/pgp.html

PART I: PHASE I DRUG-METABOLIZING ENZYMES

PHARMACOGENOMICS

CYTOCHROME P-450	SUBSTRATES[21]			INHIBITORS[21]	INDUCERS[21]
CYP1A2	amitriptyline	methadone	ropivacaine	amiodarone	beta-naphthoflavone
	caffeine	mexiletine	tacrine	cimetidine	insulin
	clomipramine	mirtazapine	theophylline	fluoroquinolones	modafinil
	clozapine	naproxen	verapamil	fluvoxamine	nafcillin
	cyclobenzaprine	olanzapine	warfarin-R	furafylline	omeprazole
	desipramine	ondansetron	zileuton	methoxsalen	tobacco
	diazepam	pentazocine	zolmitriptan	mibefradil	
	estradiol	phenacetin		ticlopidine	
	fluvoxamine	propranolol			
	haloperidol	riluzole			
CYP2B6	bupropion			thiotepa	phenobarbital
	cyclophosphamide			ticlopidine	rifampin
	efavirenz				
	ifosfamide				
	methadone				
CYP2C8	amodiaquine			gemfibrozil	rifampin
	cerivastatin			glitazones	
	paclitaxel			quercetin	
	repaglinide			trimethoprim	
	torsemide				
CYP2C9	amitriptyline	meloxicam		amiodarone	rifampin
	celecoxib	naproxen-S		fluconazole	secobarbital
	diclofenac	nateglinide		fluvastatin	
	fluoxetine	phenytoin		fluvoxamine	
	fluvastatin	piroxicam		isoniazid	
	glibenclamide	rosiglitazone		lovastatin	
	glimepiride	suprofen		phenylbutazone	
	glipizide	tamoxifen		probenicid	
	glyburide	tolbutamide		sertraline	
	ibuprofen	torsemide		sulfamethoxazole	
	irbesartan	warfarin-S		trimethoprim	
	losartan			zafirlukast	
CYP2C19	amitriptyline	nilutamide		chloramphenicol	carbamazepine
	carisoprodol	omeprazole		cimetidine	norethindrone
	citalopram	pantoprazole		felbamate	prednisone
	clomipramine	phenobarbitone		fluoxetine	rifampin
	cyclophosphamide	phenytoin		fluvoxamine	
	diazepam	primidone		indomethacin	
	eniposide	progesterone		ketoconazole	

SELECTED MUTATIONS	PREVALENCE OF VARIANT ALLELES (%, RACE)[22 UNLESS SPECIFIED]	NUCLEOTIDE CHANGE[25]	CLINICAL EFFECT (ENZYME ACTIVITY)
CYP1A2*1A		none wild type	normal in vivo and in vitro[27]
CYP1A2*1B		5347T>C	n/a
CYP1A2*1C	2, Caucasian; 25, Asian[23]	3860G>A	decreased in vivo[28]
CYP1A2*1D		2467delT	n/a
CYP1A2*1E		739T>G	n/a
CYP1A2*1F	68, Caucasian[23]	163C>A	higher inducibility in vivo[29]
CYP1A2*2		63C>G	n/a
CYP1A2*4		2499A>T	n/a
CYP1A2*7		3534G>A	decreased in vivo[30]
CYP1A2*11		558C>A	decreased in vitro[31]
CYP2B6*1A		none wild type	normal in vivo and in vitro[32]
CYP2B6*8	2.6, Caucasian[33]	13072A>G	decreased expression in vitro[33]
CYP2B6*11A		136A>G	decreased expression in vitro[33]
CYP2B6*12		12820G>A;18273G>A	decreased expression in vitro[33]
CYP2B6*14		13076G>A,18273G>A	decreased in vitro[33]
CYP2C8*1A		none wild type	normal in vivo and in vitro[34]
CYP2C8*1B		271C>A	n/a
CYP2C8*1C		370T>G	n/a
CYP2C8*2	18, African American[35]	805A>T	increased Km for paclitaxel 6a-OH in vitro[35]
CYP2C8*3	13, Caucasian[35]	416G>A; 1196A>G	decreased paclitaxel turnover in vitro[35]
CYP2C9*1		none wild type	normal in vivo and in vitro[36]
CYP2C9*2	8-20, Caucasian	430C>T	decreased in vitro[37]
CYP2C9*3	6-9, Caucasian	1075A>C	decreased in vivo and in vitro[38]
CYP2C9*4		1076T>C	n/a
CYP2C9*5		1080C>G	decreased in vitro[39]
CYP2C9*6		818delA	n/a
CYP2C9*7		55C>A	n/a
CYP2C9*8		449G>A	increased in vitro[40]
CYP2C9*9		752A>G	n/a
CYP2C9*10		815A>G	n/a
CYP2C9*11		1003C>T	decreased in vitro[40]
CYP2C9*12		1465C>T	decreased in vitro[40]
CYP2C19*1A		none wild type	normal in vivo & in vitro[41]
CYP2C19*2A	13, Caucasian; 29, Chinese; 25, African American	681G>A; 99C>T;	none in vivo[42]
CYP2C19*3	0.3, Caucasian; 12, Japanese and Korean	990C>T; 991A>G	none in vivo[42]
CYP2C19*4	0.6, Caucasian	636G>A; 991A>G;	none in vivo[43]
CYP2C19*5A		1251A>C	none in vivo[44]
CYP2C19*8		1A>g; 99C>T; 991A>G	decreased in vitro[45]
CYP2C19*9		1297C>T	decreased in vitro[46]

CYTOCHROME P-450	SUBSTRATES[21]		INHIBITORS[21]	INDUCERS[21]
CYP2C19—CONT				
	hexobarbital	proguanil	lansoprazole	
	imipramine	propranolol	modafinil	
	indomethacin	warfarin-R	omeprazole	
	moclobemide		probenicid	
	nelfinavir		ticlopidine	
			topiramate	
CYP2D6	alprenolol	phenacetin	amiodarone	dexamethasone
	amitriptyline	phenformin	bupropion	rifampin
	amphetamine	propafenone	celecoxib	
	atomoxetine	propranolol	chlorpheniramine	
	bufuralol	risperidone	chlorpheniramine	
	carvedilol	sparteine	chlorpromazine	
	chlorpheniramine	tamoxifen	cimetidine	
	chlorpromazine	thioridazine	citalopram	
	clomipramine	timolol	clemastine	
	codeine	tramadol	clomipramine	
	debrisoquine	venlafaxine	cocaine	
	desipramine		diphenhydramine	
	dexfenfluramine		doxorubicin	
	dextromethorphan		escitalopram	
	encainide		fluoxetine	
	flecainide		halofantrine	
	fluoxetine		haloperidol-red	
	fluvoxamine		hydroxyzine	
	haloperidol		levomepromazine	
	imipramine		methadone	
	lidocaine		metoclopramide	
	methoxyamphetamine		mibefradil	
	metoclopramide		moclobemide	
	metoprolol-S		paroxetine	
	mexiletine		perphenazine	
	minaprine		quinidine	
	nortriptyline		ranitidine	
	ondansetron		ritonavir	
	paroxetine		sertraline	
	perhexiline		terbinafine	
	perphenazine		tripelennamine	
CYP2E1	acetaminophen	enflurane	isoflurane	disulfiram	ethanol
	aniline	ethanol	methoxyflurane	isoniazid
	benzene	foramide	sevoflurane	
	chlorzoxazone	halothane	theophylline	

SELECTED MUTATIONS	PREVALENCE OF VARIANT ALLELES (%, RACE)[22] UNLESS SPECIFIED	NUCLEOTIDE CHANGE[25]	CLINICAL EFFECT (ENZYME ACTIVITY)
CYP2C19*10		358T>C	decreased in vitro[46]
CYP2C19*12		99C>T; 680C>T;	unstable in vitro[46]
CYP2C19*13		991A>G	n/a
CYP2C19*14		99C>T; 991A>G;1473	n/a
CYP2C19*15		A>C	n/a
CYP2C19*16		991A>G; 1228C>T	n/a
		50T>C; 99C>T; 991A>G	
		55A>C; 991A>G	
		1324 C>T	
CYP2D6*1A		none wild type	normal in vivo and in vitro[47]
CYP2D6*1XN		2549A>del	increased in vivo[48]
CYP2D6*3A	21, Caucasian	1846G>A	none in vivo and in vitro[49]
CYP2D6*4A	20-23, Caucasian; 7-9, African American;	CYP2D6 deleted	none in vivo and in vitro[49]
	9, African	1707T>del	none in vivo[50]
CYP2D6*5	2-5, Caucasian; 10-13, Japanese	2935A>C	none in vivo[51]
CYP2D6*6A	2, Caucasian	1758G>T	none in vivo[52]
CYP2D6*7	<1-2, Caucasian	2613-2615del AGA	none in vivo[53]
CYP2D6*8	<1, Caucasian	100C>T	decreased in vivo and in vitro[54]
CYP2D6*9	2, Caucasian	883G>C	decreased in vivo[55]
CYP2D6*10A	2-5, Caucasian; 43-51, Chinese; 33-60,	124G>A	none in vivo[56]
	Japanese	1758G>A	none in vivo[57]
CYP2D6*11	<1, Caucasian	138insT	none in vivo[58]
CYP2D6*12	<1, Caucasian	1023C>T; 2850C>T	none in vivo[59]
CYP2D6*14A		4125-4133ins	decreased in vivo and in vitro[60]
CYP2D6*15		GTGCCCACT	none in vivo[61]
CYP2D6*17	26, African American; 9-34, African;	1973insG	none in vivo[62]
	19, Korean	100C>T	decreased in vivo & in vitro[63]
CYP2D6*18		2988G>A	decreased in vivo[64]
CYP2D6*20		2950G>C	none in vivo[65]
CYP2D6*36	9, Korean; 31 Chinese and Japanese		
CYP2D6*41	8.4, Caucasian		
CYP2D6*44			
CYP2E1*1A		none wild type	normal in vivo and in vitro[66]
CYP2E1*2		1132G>A	decreased in vitro[67]
CYP2E1*3		10023G>A	normal in vitro[67]
CYP2E1*4		4768G>A	normal in vitro[68]

CYTOCHROME P-450	SUBSTRATES[21]			INHIBITORS[21]	INDUCERS[21]
CYP3A4,5,7	alfentanil	finasteride	saquinavir	amiodarone	barbiturates
	alprazolam	gleevec	sildenafil	aprepitant	carbamazepine
	amlodipine	haloperidol	simvastatin	chloramphenicol	efavirenz
	astemizole	hydrocortisone	sirolimus	cimetidine	glucocorticoids
	atorvastatin	indinavir	tacrolimus	ciprofloxacin	modafinil
	buspirone	irinotecan	tamoxifen	clarithromycin	nevirapine
	Cafergot	LAAM	taxol	delavirdine	phenobarbital
	caffeine	lercanidipine	telithromycin	diltiazem	phenytoin
	cerivastatin	lidocaine	terfenadine	erythromycin	pioglitazone
	chlorpheniramine	lovastatin	terfenadine	fluconazole	rifabutin
	cilostazol	methadone	testosterone	fluvoxamine	rifampin
	cisapride	midazolam	trazodone	gestodene	St. John's wort
	clarithromycin	nateglinide	triazolam	grapefruit juice	troglitazone
	cocaine	nelfinavir	verapamil	indinavir	
	cyclosporine	nifedipine	vincristine	itraconazole	
	dapsone	nisoldipine	zaleplon	ketoconazole	
	dextromethorphan	nitrendipine	zolpidem	mibefradil	
	diazepam	ondansetron		mifepristone	
	diltiazem	pimozide		nefazodone	
	domperidone	progesterone		nelfinavir	
	eplerenone	propranolol		norfloxacin	
	erythromycin (not 3A5)	quinidine (not 3A5)		norfluoxetine	
	estradiol	quinine		ritonavir	
	felodipine	ritonavir		saquinavir	
	fentanyl	salmeterol		verapamil	
Alcohol dehydrogenase[75]	ethanol methanol				
Aldehyde dehydrogenase	acetaldehyde[78]				
Butyryl-cholinesterase	succinylcholine[24]				
Dihydropyrimidine dehydrogenase	fluorouracil[78]				

SELECTED MUTATIONS	PREVALENCE OF VARIANT ALLELES (%, RACE)[22] UNLESS SPECIFIED	NUCLEOTIDE CHANGE[25]	CLINICAL EFFECT (ENZYME ACTIVITY)
CYP3A4*1A		none wild type	normal in vivo and in vitro[69]
CYP3A4*1B		392A>G	n/a
CYP3A4*2		15713T>C	n/a
CYP3A4*3	4, Caucasian	1334T>C	n/a
CYP3A4*4		352A>G	n/a
CYP3A4*5		653C>G	n/a
CYP3A4*6		831insA	n/a
CYP3A4*7		167G>A	n/a
CYP3A4*8		389G>A	n/a
CYP3A4*9		508G>A	n/a
CYP3A4*10		520G>C	n/a
CYP3A4*11		1088C>T	n/a
CYP3A4*12		1117C>T	n/a
CYP3A4*13		1247C>T	n/a
CYP3A4*14		44T>C	n/a
CYP3A4*17	2, Caucasian	566T>C	decreased in vitro[70]
CYP3A5*1A		none wild type	normal in vivo and in vitro[71]
CYP3A5*2		27289C>A	n/a
CYP3A5*3A		6986A>G, 31611C>T	severely decreased in vitro[72]
CYP3A5*4		14665A>G	n/a
CYP3A5*5		12952T>C	n/a
CYP3A5*6		14690G>A	none or severely decreased in vitro[72]
CYP3A5*7		27131-32insT	n/a
CYP3A5*8		3699C>T	decreased in vitro[73]
CYP3A5*9		19386G>A	decreased in vitro[73]
ADH1B*1	95, Caucasian[79]	none wild type[75]	increased (fast) metabolism[79]
ADH1B*2	34-60, Japanese; 44-55, Chinese; 48-65, Korean[79]	AA substitution: Arg47His[79]	increased (fast) metabolism[79]
ADH1B*3		AA substitution: Arg369Cys[79]	
ADH1C*1	92, Japanese; 80-90, Chinese; 19-40, Caucasian[79]	AA substitution: Arg271, Ile349[75]	
ADH1C*2	40-50, Caucasian[79]	AA substitution: Ile349Val[79]	
ALDH2*1	>95, Caucasian[79]	none wild type[79]	no activity[79]
ALDH2*2	45, Japanese[80]	AA substitution: Glu487Lys[79]	
dibucaine		D70G (Asp70->Gly)[77]	enhanced drug effect[24]
K-variant		A539T (Ala539->Thr)[77]	
sil-1	<1, Caucasian[24]	G117FS (Gly GGT to GGAG)[77]	
flu-1		T243M (Thr243->Met)[77]	
flu-2		G390V (Gly390->Val)[77]	
	<1, Caucasian[5]; 1-2, Finnish; <1, Turkish; 2, Taiwanese[78]	IVS14+ 1G>A	enhanced drug effect[74]

PART II: PHASE II DRUG-METABOLIZING ENZYMES*

DRUG-METABOLIZING ENZYMES	GENES	FREQUENCY
Thiopurine S-methyltransferase (TPMT)	TPMT*1 (wt)[82]	
	TPMT*2	Caucasians 0.002-0.005, African American 0.004, Ghanaian 0, Chinese 0, Japanese 0
	TPMT *3A	Caucasians 0.032-0.045, African American 0.008, Ghanaian 0, Chinese 0, Japanese 0
	TPMT*3C	Caucasians 0.002-0.03, African American 0.02,[4] Ghanaian 0.063, Chinese 0.023, Japanese 0.015[101]
	TPMT*3B[101]	
	TPMT*3D	
	TPMT*4	
	TPMT*5	
	TPMT*6	
	TPMT*7	
	TPMT*8	
Uridine diphosphate-glucuronosyl transferase 1A (TATA-box polymorphism) (UGT)	UGT1A1 UGT1A1*6[107,108] UGT1A1*7[110,111] UGT1A1*27[83] UGT1A1*28[113,114]	European 0.075, Chinese 0.04, Japanese 0.01
N-acetyltransferase[118] NAT2	NAT2*4 (wt) NAT2*5(A-I) NAT2*6(A-E) NAT2*7(A-B) NAT2*10 NAT2*11(A-B) NAT2*13(A-D) NAT2*14(A-G) NAT2*17 NAT2*18 NAT2*19	European 0.75, African 0.71, East Asian 0.37, Central Asians and West Asians 0.74[1]
Catechol O-methyltransferase, COM		Caucasian 0.54, Ghanaian 0.26, Chinese 0.18[128]
Glutathione-S-transferase, GST	GSTP1[130] GST theta[136]	Caucasian 0.39-0.54, Black 0.31, Chinese 0.45-0.49, Japanese 0.51[1]
	GSTM1 and GSTT1	

*Adapted from Weinshilbaum R: Inheritance and drug response, *N Engl J Med* 348:529-537, 2003.

DRUGS	MUTATIONS AND PREVALENCE	CLINICAL EFFECTS
Mercaptopurine[10,81] Azathioprine	These three mutations account for 80%-95% of TPMT deficiency[94-99] 460G>A, Ala154Thr, and 719A>G, Tyr240Cys 100	6-Mercaptopurine (6-MP) is used in the treatment of acute lymphoblastic leukemia (ALL). 6-MP, a prodrug, is converted to both active thioguanine triphosphate nucleotides (6-TGN) and inactive metabolites. TPMT is responsible for metabolism of 6-MP and indirectly regulates 6-TGN.[10, 83-91] TPMT-deficient patients might receive half or fifteenfold reduction in dose.[92,93]
Irinotecan[102] Bilirubin[106]	211G>A, G71R 1456T>G, Y486D 686C>A, P229Q (TA)/TAA, TA insertion	Irinotecan is initially metabolized by carboxylesterase-2 to 7-ethyl-10-hydroxycamptothecin (SN-38), a topoisomerase I inhibitor.[103-105] This is glucuronidated to inactive SN-38G by UGT1A1. UGT1A1 deficiency would result in accumulation of SN-38, causing diarrhea.[109] Enhanced drug effect,[112] Gilbert syndrome,[106,115,116] Crigler-Najjar syndrome[117]
Amonafide[119-121] Isoniazid[122] Hydralazine[123] Procainamide[127]	191G>A 282 C>T 341T>C 481C>T 590G>A 803A>G 857G>A	NAT acetylates amonafide, a topoisomerase II inhibitor, to an active metabolite, N-acetyl-amonafide. Rapid acetylator would result in myelosuppression.[119,120] NAT2 mutants account for 55% of slow acetylator.[124,125] WT has much higher acetylation rate.[126] Enhanced drug effects[128]
Levodopa[81,129]		Enhanced drug effect
Alkylating agents and/or cyclophosphamide metabolites [131] Cisplatin[101] Thiotepa[138]	Duplication Deletion[137] SNP Ile114 Val, Ala 114 Val	Cyclophosphamide metabolites[101,119,120,131-135] Null genotypes correlate to poorer survival of ovarian cancer patients.[139] GSTM increases risks of relapse in childhood acute lymphoblastic leukemias (ALL).[140] GSTT1 genotype affects outcome using prednisone I Berlin-Frankfurt-Munster protocols with null GSTT1 for a 7.6 risk reduction. Null GSTM1, null GSTT1, and GSTp1 Val105 /val105 are "low-risk" genotypes. For acute myeloid leukemia (AML) patients, null GSTT1 genotype results in lower survival and toxic drug deaths.[141]

PART III: DRUG TRANSPORTERS*

PROTEIN TRANSPORTER GENES	PROTEIN TRANSPORTERS	SUBSTRATES	INHIBITORS
Albumin	Albumin	Warfarin, salicylate, diazepam	
Multidrug resistance-associated proteins	MRP1	Anticancer drug glucuronide, sulfate and glutathione conjugates	
	MRP2 Canalicular multidrug resistance-associated protein (cMRP, also known as cMOAT)	Bilirubin glucuronide conjugates,[145] glutathione conjugates, vinblastine,[146] and telmisartan[147]	
	MRP3	Glucuronide and glutathione conjugates,[148,149] MTX,[149] bile acid conjugates,[149] etoposide,[148,150] vincristine[150]	
	MRP4	9-(2-phosphonyl methoxyethyl) adenine PMEA (cytotoxic acyclic nucleoside phosphonate), AZT, 3TC, d4T, MTX,[151] CMP, 6-TG[152]	
	MRP5	PMEA, 6MP, and 6 TG	Sildenafil
	MRP6	Anthracycline	
Multidrug resistance family (MDR)			
Multidrug-resistance gene, human MDR1	P-glycoprotein P-gp[154] (ABCB1)	Lipophilic and/or amphipathic, with one or more aromatic rings	

*Adapted from Tirona RG, Kim RB: Pharmacogenomics of drug transporters; and Fromm MF, Eichelbaum M: The pharmacogenomics of human P-gylycoprotein. In Licinio J, Wong ML, editors: *Pharmacogenomics,* Weinheim, Germany, 2002, Wiley-VCH.

MUTATIONS	GENOTYPING FREQUENCIES	CLINICAL EFFECTS
		Reduced warfarin affinity of some albumin variants[142]
1 gene deletion and 17 SNPs[143]		It may change tissue drug level. Effect pending.[144]
11 mutations: Point mutation, base pair deletion, premature stop codons, and aberrant RNA splicing[143]		Effect pending.[143]
10 SNPs		Effect pending.[143]
2 mutations		High expression results in drug resistance to PMEA and nucleoside analogues. Other effects pending[143]
11 SNPs		High expression results in drug resistance to PMEA and nucleoside analogs. Other effects pending[143,153]
25 mutations: missense, splice, deletions, and insertions		Effects pending.[143]
20 SNPs in Caucasian[155-157]		P-gp, an ATP-binding cassette (ABC) superfamily of membrane proteins and ATP-dependent xenobiotics exporter from cells, is expressed in intestine, liver, kidneys, brain, placenta and testis.[154,158-165] and protects against xenobiotics. Intestinal P-gp limits absorption of immunosuppressants, cardiac glycoside and some β-adrenoceptor antagonists. Drug interactions may be caused by P-gp induction and inhibition.

PROTEIN TRANSPORTER GENES	PROTEIN TRANSPORTERS	SUBSTRATES	INHIBITORS
		Chemotherapeutics[154] Actinomycin D[168] Etoposide[169] Daunorubicin[170] Docetaxel[171] Doxorubicin[170] Irinotecan[172] Mitomycin C[173] Mitoxantrone[173] Paclitaxel[174] Teniposide[173] Topotecan[173] Vinblastine[175] Vincristine[176]	
		Immunosuppressants[154] Cyclosporine A[177] FK 506[177] Rapamycin(?) RAD (?)	**Immunosuppressants** Cyclosporine A[19,154]
		Steroids[154] Aldosterone[19] Hydrocortisone[19] Cortisol[19] Corticosterone[19] Dexamethasone[19]	**Antiestrogen** Tamoxifen[19] Mefipristone[19,154]
		HIV protease inhibitors[154] Amprenavir[178] Indinavir[179] Nelfinavir[179] Ritonavir[179] Saquinavir[180]	Nelfinavir[19,154] Ritonavir[19,154] Saquinavir[19,154]
		Digitalis glycoside[154,181] Digoxin[182]	**Antifungal agent** Ketoconazole[19,154]
		Antiarrhythmic agent[154] Quinidine[165]	**Sedative agent** Midazolam[19,154]

MUTATIONS	GENOTYPING FREQUENCIES				CLINICAL EFFECTS
Wobble 3435C>T at exon 26		CC	CT	TT	This silent mutation results in al-
	African American[166,167]	0.61-0.68	0.31-0.34	0.01-0.05	tered P-gp function. TT geno-
	Caucasian, German[156,157]	0.21-0.28	0.48-0.51	0.24-0.29	type results in lower expression
	Chinese[166]	0.32	0.42	0.26	of P-gp in intestine and kidneys,
	Japanese[167]	0.34	0.46	0.2	and higher plasma concentration
	Kenyan[166]	0.7	0.26	0.04	of P-gp substrate such as digoxin[156]

2677G>T at exon 21		Ala893Ser or Ala893Thr, effect not established.
61G>A at exon 2		Asn21Asp, effect not established.
1199G>A at exon 11		Ser400Asn, effect not established.
2995G>A at exon 24		Ala999Thr, effect not established.
3320A>C at exon 26		Gln1107Pro, rare
3421T>A at exon 26		Ser1141Thr, rare

P-gp deficiency does not seem to affect CsA bioavailablity, but CYP 3A4/5 deficicency increases immunosuppressants bioavailbility

PROTEIN TRANSPORTER GENES	PROTEIN TRANSPORTERS	SUBSTRATES	INHIBITORS
		Antibiotic[154,183-185] Erythromycin[183]	Warfarin
		Antituberculous agent Rifampin[187] Rhodamine[19]	
MDR3		Digoxin, paclitaxel, and vinblastine[188]	
Sister of P-glycoprotein	SPGP	Vinblastine[195] and sulindac[196]?	
Novel organic cation transporters	OCTN1	Tetraethylammonium (TEA), quinidine, pyrilamine, and verapamil[199]	
	OCTN2	TEA,[200] quinidine, verapamil,[201] cephalosporins[207]	
Organic anion polypeptide transporters	OATP-A OATP-B OATP-C	Steroid sulfates,[208,209] fexofenadine[210] Unknown Sulfate and glucuronide conjugates,[211] pravastatin,[212] MTX[213,214]	
	OATP-E	Taurocholate[215]	
	OATP8	Similar to OATP-C	
Organic anion transporter	OAT1 OAT2 OAT3 OAT4	Cidofovir, adefovir[216] Unknown Methotrexate, cimetidine, and setrone sulfate[217] Steroid sulfates and ochratoxin A[218]	
Organic cation transporter	OCT1 OCT2 OCT3 OCTN1 OCTN2	TEA, 1-methyl 1,4-phenylpyridinium (MPP^+) N-1-methylnicotinamide MAOI and amantadine Adrenaline, noradrenaline, MPP^+ TEA, quinidine, pyrilamine, and verapamil[199] TEA,[200] quinidine,[201] verapamil[201] cephalosporins[207]	

MUTATIONS	GENOTYPING FREQUENCIES	CLINICAL EFFECTS
		Variable warfarin affinity of some P-gp varaiants[186]
23 mutations include deletions, insertions, and missense mutations		Polymorphisms result in low or nondetectable MDR3 protein expression in liver, and hence change hepatic drug elimination rate.[184] Mutations cause progressive familial intrahepatic cholestasis type 3 (PFIC3), intrahepatic cholestasis of pregnancy, and cholesterol gallstone disease.[143,189-194]
14 mutations: frameshift, missense and premature stop codon[197,198]		Mutations cause PFIC2.[197] Effect pending on further study.[147]
5 mutations[143]		Effect unknown.[143]
15 mutations[202-206]		Mutations may affect drug metabolism.[143]
Unknown		Unknown
4 mutations		Unknown
16 mutations		Unknown
1 mutation		Unknown
1 mutation		Unknown
5 mutations		Unknown
Unknown		Unknown
Unknown		Unknown
Unknown		Unknown
Unknown		
Unknown		
Unknown		
Unknown		
5 mutations		Unknown
15 mutations		Unknown

PROTEIN TRANSPORTER GENES	PROTEIN TRANSPORTERS	SUBSTRATES	INHIBITORS
Peptide transporter family	PepT1	β-Lactam antibiotics,[219,220] valaciclovir[221] valganciclovir,[222] captopril[223]	
	PepT2	Similar to PepT1 with different affinity[224]	
Serotonin transporter (5-hydroxytryptamine)	5-HTTs (short variant)	Antidepressants: clomipramine, fluoxetine, paroxetine	
	5-HTTl (long variant)		
"White" ABC transporter family	BCRP (or MXR or ABCP) (breast cancer resistance protein)	Topotecan, overlaps with MDR1 and MRPs[228]	

MUTATIONS	GENOTYPING FREQUENCIES	CLINICAL EFFECTS
Unknown		Unknown
6 mutations		Unknown
44 bp deletion		5-Hydroxytryptamine neuro-transmission, antidepressant response.[11,225-227] Reduced transcriptional efficiency and subsequent 5-HTT expression and uptake in lymphoblasts, higher risk of a manic phase in bipolar disorder
44 bp insertion		Higher response to fluvoxamine and paroxetine
34 SNPs[229]		May explain interindividual variability.

PART IV: DRUG RECEPTOR/TARGET SYSTEMS*

RECEPTORS/TARGETS	SUBSTRATES	MUTATIONS/AMINO ACID CHANGES/CLINICAL EFFECT
Angiotensinogen-converting enzyme (ACE)	ACE inhibitors—enalapril, lisinopril, captopril	Renoprotective effects, blood pressure reduction, reduction in left ventricular mass, endothelial function[11,228-236]
	Fluvastatin	Lipid changes, progression or regression of coronary atherosclerosis[11,237]
Angiotensin I (angiotensinogen, AGT)	Salt intake and ACE inhibitors	Variation in the efficacy of reduced sodium intake[238] and of ACE inhibitors in hypertension treatment, susceptibility to hypertension[239]
Apolipoprotein E (APOE)	Cholinesterase inhibitor, tacrine	Variation in cognitive function improvements with tacrine in the treatment of Alzheimer's disease,[240] susceptibility to Alzheimer's disease, increased by the epsilon-4 allele and decreased by epsilon-2 allele[241]
Arachidonate 5-lipoxygenase	Leukotriene inhibitors	Improvement in forced expiratory volume in 1 sec[11,242]
β_2-Adrenergic receptor (ADRB2)	β_2 Agonists, albuterol	16 SNPs,[243] Arg-to-Gly at codon 16, Gln-to-Glu at codon 27,[243-244] bronchodilatation, susceptibility to agonist-induced desensitization, cardiovascular effects[243-250]
Bradykinin B_2 receptor	ACE inhibitors	ACE inhibitor-induced cough[11,251]
Cholesteryl ester transfer protein (CETP)	HMG-CoA reductase inhibitor, pravastatin	Efficacy of pravastatin in the treatment of coronary atherosclerosis and susceptibility to coronary atherosclerosis[252]
Dopamine receptors (D2, D3, D4)	Antipsychotics—haloperidol	Antipsychotic response (D2, D3, D4), antipsychotic-induced tardive dyskinesia (D3), antipsychotic-induced acute akathisia (D3)[11,253-257]
Estrogen receptor-α	Conjugated estrogens	Increase in bone mineral density[11,258]
	Hormone-replacement therapy	Increase in high-density lipoprotein cholesterol[11,259]
Glycoprotein IIIa subunit of glycoprotein IIb/IIIa	Aspirin or glycoprotein IIb/IIIa inhibitors	Antiplatelet effect[11,260]
Guanine nucleotide binding protein[261] (G-protein), α, β, γ subunits		Coupling to opiate receptor to distinct cellular effector system
Opiates[261]—μ, δ, κ μ δ κ	Opiates and endogenous enkephalins and endorphins	Naloxone as antagonist; Asp95Asn reduces δ receptor affinity for DPDPE, DSLET, and SIOM; eliminate buprenorphine as agonist
	Morphine, enkephalins, and endorphins	Asp114 to noncharged amino acid decreases binding of DAMGO and morphine
	Morphine, enkephalins, and endorphins	
	Dynorphin A	

RECEPTORS/TARGETS	SUBSTRATES	MUTATIONS/AMINO ACID CHANGES/CLINICAL EFFECT
Peroxisome proliferator activated receptor (PPAR-GAMMA-2)	Insulin	Variation of insulin efficacy in the treatment of diabetes, susceptibility to type II diabetes[262]
5-hydroxytryptamine 2A receptor HTR2A	Neuroleptics[263]	Variation of clozapine[264] and typical neuroleptics[265] efficacy in schizophrenia treatment, increased susceptibility to schizophrenia[266]
Sulfonylurea receptor 1 (SUR1)	Sulfonylurea (tolbutamide)	Decreased tolbutamide-stimulated insulin secretion in healthy subjects with sequence variants in the high-affinity sulfonylurea receptor gene,[267] susceptibility to type II diabetes[268]
Vitamin D (VDR)	1, 25-dihydroxyvitamin D_3	Vitamin D response in patients affected with rickets, susceptibility to osteoporosis[269] and autosomal dominant rickets disease[270]

*Adapted from Evans WE, McLeod HL: Pharmacogenomics-drug disposition, drug targets and side effects, *N Engl J Med* 348:538-549, 2003; and from Essioux L, Destenaves B, Jais P, et al: Association studies in pharmacogenomics. In Licinio J, Wong M-L. *Pharmacogenomics,* Weinheim, Germany, 2002, Wiley-VCH.

REFERENCES

1. Weber WW: *Pharmacogenetics,* Oxford, UK, 1997, Oxford University Press.

2. Linder MW, Prough RA, Valdes R Jr: Pharmacogenetics: a laboratory tool for optimizing therapeutic efficiency (Review), *Clin Chem* 43:254-266, 1997.

3. Guttmacher AE, Collins FS, Drazen JM, editors: *Genomic medicine—articles form the New England Journal of Medicine,* Baltimore, 2004, Johns Hopkins University Press and Boston, New England Journal of Medicine.

4. Wong SHY, Linder MW, Valdes R Jr: *Pharmacogenomics and proteomics,* Washington, DC, 2006, AACC Press. (In press).

5. White R, Wong SHY: Pharmacogenomics and its clinical applications, *MLO* 37(3):20-27, 2005.

6. Licinio J, Wong ML: Pharmacogenomics, Weinheim, Germany, 2002, Wiley-VCH.

7. McLeod HL, Evans WE: Pharmacogenomics: unlocking the human genome for better drug therapy, *Ann Rev Pharm Tox* 41:101-21, 2001.

8. International Human Genome Sequencing Consortium: Initial sequencing and analysis of the human genome, *Nature* 409:860-921, 2001.

9. Venter JC, Adams MD, Myers EW, et al: The sequence of human genome, *Science* 291:1304-51, 2001.

10. Weinshilboum R: Inheritance and drug response, *N Engl J Med* 348:529-37, 2003.

11. Evans WE, McLeod HL: Pharmacogenomics-drug disposition, drug targets and side effects, *N Engl J Med* 348:538-49, 2003.

12. Biomarkers definitions working group, *Clin Pharm Ther* 69:89-95, 2001.

13. Salerno RA, Lesko LJ: Pharmacogenomics in drug development and regulatory decision-making: the genomic data submission (GDS) proposal, *Pharmacogen* 5(1):25-50, 2004.

14. Auxter-Parham S.: Bringing pharmacogenomic assays to market, *Clin Lab News* 30:1-7, 2004.

15. Jannetto PJ, Laleli-Sahin E, Wong SH: Pharmacogenomics: methodologies for genotyping and phenotyping. In Hempel G, editor: *Drug monitoring and clinical chemistry handbook of analytical separation,* vol 5, St Louis, 2004, Elsevier.

16. Jannetto PJ, Laleli-Sahin E, Schur BC, et al: Enabling pharmacogenomics: methodologies for genotyping. In Wong, SHY, Linder, MW, Valdes R Jr, editors: *Pharmacogenomics and proteomics,* Washington, DC, 2005, AACC Press (in press).

17. Weber WW: Techniques for analyzing pharmacogenetic variation. In Wong SHY, Linder MW, Valdes R Jr, editors: *Pharmacogenomics and proteomics,* Washington, DC, 2005, AACC Press (in press).

18. Steimer W, Muller B, Leucht SK, et al: Pharmacogenetics: a new diagnostic tool in the management of antidepressants drug therapy, *Clin Chim Acta* 308:33-41, 2001.

19. Lazar A., Tomalik-Schartee D, Fuhr U: Applications of genotyping and phenotyping for clinically-relevant polymorphisms of drug metabolizing enzymes and drug transporters. In Hemple G, editor: *Drug monitoring and clinical chemistry: handbook of analytical separations,* Vol 5, St Louis, 2004, Elsevier.

20. Schmitz G, Aslanidis C, Lackner KJ: Pharmacogenomics: implications for laboratory medicine, *Clin Chim Acta* 308:43-53, 2001.

21. http://medicine.iupui.edu/flockhart/table.htm

22. Phillips KA, et al: Potential role of pharmacogenomics in reducing adverse drug reactions, *JAMA* 286: 2270-2279, 2001.

23. Todesco L, et al: Determination of -3858G—>A and 164C—>A genetic polymorphism of CYP1A2 in blood and saliva by rapid allelic discrimination: large difference in the prevalence of the -3858G—>A mutation between Caucasians and Asians, *Eur J Clin Pharmol* 59:343-6, 2003.

24. Lockridge O: Genetic variants of human butyrylcholinesterase influence the metabolism of the muscle relaxant succinylcholine. In Kalow W, editor: *Pharmacogenetics of drug metabolism. International encyclopedia of pharmacology and therapeutics,* New York; 1992, Pergamon Press.

25. Raida M, Schwabe W, Hansler P, et al: Prevalence of a common point mutation in the dihydropyrimidine dehydrogenase (DPD) gene within the 5′-splice donor site of intron 14 inpatients with severe 5-fluorouracil (5-FU) related toxicity compared with controls, *Clin Cancer Res* 7:2832-9, 2001.

26. http://www.imm.ki.se/CYPalleles

27. Ikeya K, Jaiswal AK, Owens RA: Human CYP1A2: sequence, gene structure, comparison with the mouse and rat orthologous gene and differences in liver 1A2 MRNA expression, *Mol Endocrinol* 3:1399-408, 1989.

28. Nakajima M, Yokoi T, Mizutani M, et al: Genetic polymorphism in the 5′-flanking region of human CYP1A2 gene: effect on the CYP1A2 inducibility in humans, *J Biochem* (Tokyo) 125:803-8, 1999.

29. Sachse C, Brockmoller J, Bauer S, et al: Functional significance of a C—A polymorphism in intron 1of the cytochrome P450 CYP1A2 gene tested with caffeine, *Br J Clin Pharmacol* 47:445-9, 1999.

30. Allorge D, Chevalier D, Lo-Guidice JM, et al: Identification of a novel splice-site mutation in the CYP1A2 gene, *Br J Clin Pharmacol* 56:341-4, 2003.

31. Murayama N, Soyama A, Saito Y, et al: Six novel nonsynonymous CYP1A2 gene polymorphisms: catalytic activities of the naturally occurring variant enzymes, *J Pharmacol Exp Ther* 308:1219, 2004.

32. Yamano S, Nhamburo PT, Aoyama T, et al: cDNA cloning and sequence and cDNA-directed expression of human P450 IIB1: identification of a normal and two variant cDNAs derived from the CYP2B locus on chromosome 19 and differential expression of the IIB mRNAs in human liver, *Biochemistry* 28 (5):7340-8, 1989.

33. Multiple novel nonsynonimous CYP2B6 gene polymorphisms in Caucasians: demonstration of phenotypic null alleles, *J Pharmacol Exp Ther* 311:34-43, 2004. electronic publication, June 9, 2004.

34. Klose TS, Blaisdell JA, Goldstein JA: Gene structure of CYP2C8 and extrahepatic distribution of the human CYP2Cs, *J Biochem Mol Toxicol* 3:289-95, 1999.

35. Dai D, Zeldin DC, Blaisdell JA, et al: Polymorphisms in human CYP2C8 decrease metabolism of the anticancer drug paclitaxel and arachidonic acid, *Pharmacogenetics* 11:597-607, 2001.

36. Romkes M, Faletto MB, Blaisdell JA, et al: Cloning and expression of complementary DNAs for multiple members of the human cytochrome P450IIC subfamily, *Biochemistry* 30 (2):3247-55, 1991.

37. King BP, Khan TI, Aithal GP, et al: Upstream and coding region CYP2C9 polymorphisms: correlation with warfarin dose and metabolism, *Pharmacogenetics* 14:813-22, 2004.

38. Shintani M, Ieiri I, Inoue K, et al: Genetic polymorphisms and functional characterization of the 5′-flanking region of the human CYP2C9 gene: in vitro and in vivo studies, *Clin Pharmacol Ther* 70:175-82, 2001.

39. Allabi AC, Gala JL, Horsmans Y, et al: Functional impact of CYP2C95, CYP2C96 CYP2C98 and CYP2C911 in vivo among black Africans, *Clin Pharmacol Ther* 76:113-8, 2004.

40. Blaisdell J, Jorge-Nebert LF, Coulter S, et al: Discovery of new potentially defective alleles of human CYP2C9, *Pharmacogenetics* 14:527-37, 2004.

41. Romkes M, Faletto MB, Blaisdell JA, et al: Cloning and expression of complementary DNAs for multiple members of the human cytochrome P450IIC subfamily, *Biochemistry* 30:3247-55, 1991.

42. de Morais SM, Wilkinson GR, Blaisdell J, et al: The major genetic defect responsible for the polymorphism of S-mephenytoin metabolism in humans, *J Biol Chem* 269:15419-22, 1994.

43. Ferguson RJ, DeMorais SM, Benhamou S, et al: A new genetic defect in human CYP2C19: mutation of the initiation codon is responsible for poor metabolism of S-mephenytoin, *J Pharmacol Exp Ther* 284:356-61, 1998.

44. Xiao ZS, Goldstein JA, Xie HG, et al: Differences in the incidence of the CYP2C19 polymorphism affecting the S-mephenytoin phenotype in Chinese Han and Bai populations and identification of a new rare CYP2C19 mutant allele, *J Pharmacol Exper Ther* 281:604-9, 1997.

45. Ibeanu GC, Blaisdell J, Ferguson RJ, et al: A novel transversion in the intron 5 donor splice junction of CYP2C19 and a sequence polymorphism in exon 3 contribute to the poor metabolizer phenotype for the anticonvulsant drug S-mephenytoin, *J Pharmacol Exp Ther* 290:635-40, 1999.

46. Blaisdell J, Mohrenweiser H, Jackson J, et al: Identification and functional characterization of new potentially defective alleles of human CYP2C19, *Pharmacogenetics* 12:703-11, 2002.

47. Kimura S, Umeno M, Skoda RC, et al: The human debrisoquine 4-hydroxylase (CYP2D) locus: sequence and identification of the polymorphic CYP2D6 gene, a related gene, and a pseudogene, *Am J Hum Genet* 45:889-904, 1989.

48. Dahl ML, Johansson I, Bertilsson L, et al: Ultrarapid hydroxylation of debrisoquine in a Swedish population analysis of the molecular genetic basis, *J Pharmacol Exp Ther* 274:516-20, 1995.

49. Kagimoto M, Heim M, Kagimoto K, et al: Multiple mutations of the human cytochrome P450IID6 gene CYP2D6) in metabolizers of debrisoquine: study of the functional significance of individual mutations by expression of chimeric genes, *J Biol Chem* 265:17209-14, 1990.

50. Gaedigk A, Blum M, Gaedigk R, et al: Deletion of the entire cytochrome P450 CYP2D6 gene as a cause of impaired drug metabolism in poor metabolizers of the debrisoquine/sparteine polymorphism, *Am J Hum Genet* 48:943-50, 1991.

51. Saxena R, Shaw GL, Relling MV, et al: Identification of a new variant CYP2D6 allele with a single base deletion in exon 3 and its association with the poor metabolizer phenotype, *Hum Mol Genet* 3:923-6, 1994.

52. Evert B, Griese EU, Eichelbaum M: A missense mutation in exon 6 of the CYP2D6 gene leading to a histidine 324 to proline exchange is associated with the poor metabolizer phenotype of sparteine, *Naunyn Schmiedebergs Arch Pharmacol* 350:434-9, 1994.

53. Broly F, Marez D, Lo Guidice JM, et al: A nonsense mutation in the cytochrome P450 CYP2D6 gene identified in a Caucasian with an enzyme deficiency, *Hum Genet* 96:601-3, 1995.

54. Tyndale R, Aoyama T, Broly F, et al: Identification of a new variant CYP2D6 allele lacking the codon encoding Lys-281: possible association with the poor metabolizer phenotype, *Pharmacogenetics* 1:26-32, 1991.

55. Yokota H, Tamura S, Furuya H, et al: Evidence for a new variant CYP2D6 allele CYP2D6J in a Japanese population associated with lower in vivo rates of sparteine metabolism, *Pharmacogentics* 3:256-63, 1993.

56. Marez D, Sabbagh N, Legrand M, et al: A novel CYP2D6 allele with an abolished splice recognition site associated with the poor metabolizer phenotype, *Pharmacogenetics* 5:305-11, 1995.

57. Marez D, Legrand M, Sabbagh N, et al: An additional allelic variant of the CYP2D6 gene causing impaired metabolism of sparteine, *Hum Genet* 97:668-70, 1996.

58. Wang SL, Lai MD, Huang JD: G169R mutation diminishes the metabolic activity of CYP2D6 in Chinese, *Drug Metab Dispos* 27:385-8, 1999.

59. Sachse C, Brockmoller J, Bauer S, et al: A rare insertion of T226 in exon 1 of CYP2D6 causes a frameshift and is associated with the poor metabolizer phenotype: CYP2D6*15, *Pharmacogenetics* 6:269-72, 1996.

60. Masimirembwa C, Persson I, Bertilsson L, et al: A novel mutant variant of the CYP2D6 gene (CYP2D6*17) common in black African population: associated with diminished debrisoquine hydroxylase activity, *Br J Clin Pharmacol* 42:713-9, 1996.

61. Yokio T, Losaka Y, Chida M, et al: A new CYP2D6 allele with a nine base insertion in exon 9 in Japanese population associated with poor metabolizer phenotype, *Pharmaocgenetics* 6:395-401, 1996.

62. Marez-Allorge D, Ellis SW, Lo Guidice JM, et al: A rare G2061 insertion affecting the open reading frame of CYP2D6 and responsible for the poor metabolizer phenotype, *Pharmacogenetics* 9:393-6, 1999.

63. Marex D, Legrand M, Sabbagh N, et al: Polymorphism of the cytochrome P450 CYP2D6 gene in a European population: characterization of 48 mutations and 53 alleles, their frequencies and evolution, *Pharmacogenetics* 7:193-202, 1997.

64. Raimundo S, Toscano C, Klein K, et al: A novel intronic mutation, 2988G>A, with high predictivity for impaired function of cytochrome P450 2D6 in white subjects, *Clin Pharmacol Ther* 76:128-38, 2004.

65. Ymazaki H, Kiyotani K, Tsubuko S, et al: Two novel haplotypes of CYP2D6 gene in a Japanese population, *Drug Metab Pharmacokinet* 8:269-71, 2003.

66. Umeno M., McBride OW, Yang CS, et al: Human ethanol-inducible P450IIE1: complete gene sequence, promoter characterization, chromosome mapping, and cDNA-directed expression, *Biochem* 27:9006-13, 1988.

67. Hu Y, Oscarson M, Johansson I, et al: Genetic polymorphism of human CYP2E1: characterization of two variant alleles, *Mol Pharmacol* 1:370-6, 1997.

68. Fairbrother KS, Grove J, de Waziers I, et al: Detection and characterization of novel polymorphisms in the CYP2E1 gene, *Pharmacogenetics* 8:543-52, 1998.

69. Gonzalez FJ, Schmid BJ, Umeno M, et al: Human P450PCN1: sequence chromosome localization and direct evidence through cDNA expression that P450PCN1 is nifedipine oxidase, *DNA* 7:79-86, 1988.

70. Dai D, Tang J, Rose R, et al: Identification of variants of CYP3A4 and characterization of their abilities to metabolize testosterone and chlorpyrifos, *J Pharmacol Exp Ther* 299:825-31, 2001.

71. Aoyama T, Yamano S, Waxman DJ, et al: Cytochrome P-450 hPCN3, a novel cytochrome P-450 IIIA gene product that is differently expressed in adult human liver: cDNA and deduced amino acid sequence and distinct specificities of cDNA-expressed hPCN1 and hPCN3 for the metabolism of steroid hormones and cyclosporine, *J Biol Chem* 264:10388-95, 1989.

72. Kuehl P, Zhang J, Lin Y, et al: Sequence diversity in CYP3A promoters and characterization of the genetic basis of polymorphic CYP3A5 expression, *Nat Genet* 27:383-91, 2001.

73. Lee SJ, Usmani KA, Chanas B, et al: Genetic findings and functional studies of human CYP3A5 single nucleotide polymorphisms in different ethnic groups, *Pharmacogenetics* 13:461-72, 2003.

74. Tuchman M, Stoeckeler JS, Kiang DT, et al: Familial pyrimidinemia and pyrimidinurea associated with severe fluorouracil toxicity, *N Engl J Med* 313:245-9, 1985.

75. Hurley TD, Edenberg HJ, Li TK: Pharmacogenomics of alcoholism. In Licinio J, Wong ML, editors: *Pharmacogenomics, the search for individualized therapies,* Weinheim, Germany, 2002, Wiley-VCH.

76. Neumark YD, Friedlander Y, Durst R, et al: Alcohol dehydrogenase polymorphisms influence alcohol-elimination rates in a male Jewish population, *Alcohol Clin Exp Res* 28:10-14, 2004.

77. Yen T, Nightingale BN, Burns JC, et al: Butyrylcholinesterase (BCHE) genotyping for post-succinylcholine apnea in an Australian population, *Clin Chem* 49 (8):1297-1308, 2003.

78. van Kuilenburg ABP: Dihydropyrimidine dehydrogenase and the efficacy and toxicity of 5-fluorouracil, *Eur J Cancer* 40: 939-950, 2004.

79. Brennan P, Lewis S, Hashibe M, et al: Pooled analysis of alcohol dehydrogenase genotypes and head and neck cancer: a HuGE Review, *Am J Epidemiol* 159:1-16, 2004.

80. Higuchi S, Matsushita S, Masaki T, et al: Influence of genetic variations of ethanol-metabolizing enzymes on phenotypes of alcohol-related disorders, *Ann NY Acad Sci* 1025:472-480, 2004.

81. Weinshilboum RM, Otterness DM, Szumlanski CL: Methylation pharmacogenetics: catechol O-methyltransferase, thiopurine methyltransferase, and histamine N-methyltransferase, *Annu Rev Pharmacol Toxicol* 39:19-52, 1999.

82. McLeod HL, Krynetski EY, Rellig MV, et al: Genetic polymorphism of thiopurine methyltransferase and its clinical revelance for childhood acute lymphoblastic leukemia, *Leukaemia* 14:567-572, 2000.

83. Innocenti FI, Iyer L, Ratan MJ: Pharmacogenomics of chemotherapeutic agents in cancer treatment. In Licinio J, Wong ML, editors: *Pharmacogenomics,* Weinheim, Germany, 2002, Wiley-VCH.

84. Lennard L, Rees CA, Lilleyman JS, et al: Childhood leukaemia: a relationship between intracellular 6-mercaptopurine metabolites and neutropenia, *Br J Clin Pharmacol* 16:359-363, 1983.

85. Schmiegelow K, Bruunshuus I: 6-Thioguanine nucleotide accumulation in red blood cells during maintenance chemotherapy for childhood acute lymphoblastic leukemia, and its relation to leukopenia, *Cancer Chemother Pharmacol* 26:288-292, 1990.

86. Tidd DM, Paterson AR: A biochemical mechanism for the delayed cytotoxic reaction of 6-mercaptopurine, *Cancer Res* 34:738-746, 1974.

87. Ling YH, Chan JY, Beattie KL, et al: Consequences of 6-thioguanine incorporation into DNA on polymerase, ligase, and endonuclease reactions, *Mol Pharmacol* 42:802-807, 1992.

88. Deininger M, Szumlanski CL, Otterness DM et al: Purine substrates for human thiopurine methyltransferase, *Biochem Pharmacol* 48:2135-2138, 1994.

89. Woodson LC, Ames MM, Selassie CD, et al: Thiopurine methyltransferase: aromatic thiol substrates and inhibition by benzoic acid derivatives, *Mol Pharmacol* 24:471-478, 1983.

90. Lennard L, Lilleyman JS, Van Loon J, et al: Genetic variation in response to 6-mercaptopurine for childhood acute lymphoblastic leukaemia, *Lancet* 336:225-229, 1990.

91. Lilleyman JS, Lennard L: Mercaptopurine metabolism and risk of relapse in childhood lymphoblastic leukaemia, *Lancet* 343:1188-1190, 1994.

92. McLeod HL, Coulthard S, Thomas AE, et al: Analysis of thiopurine methyltransferase variant alleles in childhood acute lymphoblastic leukaemia, *Br J Haematol* 105:696-700, 1999.

93. Evans WE, Horner M, Chu YQ, et al: Altered mercaptopurine metabolism toxic effects and dosage requirement in a thiopurine methyltransferase-deficient child with acute lymphocytic leukemia, *J Pediatr* 119:985-989, 1991.

94. Otterness D, Szumlanski C, Lennard L, et al: Human thiopurine methyltransferase pharmacogenetics: gene sequence polymorphisms, *Clin Pharmacol Ther* 62:60-73, 1997.

95. Szumlanski C, Otterness D, Her C, et al: Thiopurine methyltransferase pharmacogenetics: human gene cloning and characterization of a common polymorphism, *DNA Cell Biol* 15:17-30, 1996.

96. Yates CR, Krynetski EY, Loennechen T, et al: Molecular diagnosis of thiopurine S-methyltransferase deficiency: genetic basis for azathioprine and mercaptopurine intolerance, *Ann Intern Med* 126:608-614, 1997.

97. Tai HL, Krynetski EY, Yates CR, et al: Thiopurine S-methyltransferase deficiency: two neucleotide transitions define the most prevalent mutant allele associated with loss of catalytic activity in Caucasians, *Am J Hum Genet* 58:694-702, 1996.

98. Otterness DM, Szumlanski CL, Wood TC, et al: Human thiopurine methyltransferase pharmacogenetics: kindred with a terminal exon splice junction mutation that results in loss of activity, *J Clin Invest* 101:1036-1044, 1998.

99. Hon YY, Fessing MY, Pui CH, et al: Polymorphism of the thiopurine S-methyltransferase gene in African-Americans, *Hum Mol Genet* 8:371-376, 1999.

100. Weinshilboum RM, Sladek SL: Mercaptopurine pharmacogenetics: monogenic inheritance of erythrocyte thiopurine methyltransferase activity, *Am J Hum Genet* 32:651-62, 1980.

101. McLeod HL, Ameyaw MM: Ethnicity and pharmacogenomics. In Licinio J, Wong ML, editors: *Pharmacogenomics,* Weinheim, Germany, 2002, Wiley-VCH.

102. Iyer L, Hall D, Das S, et al: Phenotype-genotype correlation of in vitro SN-38 (active metabolite of irinotecan) and bilirubin glucuronidation in human liver tissue with UGT1A1 promoter polymorphism, *Clin Pharmacol Ther* 65:576-82, 1999.

103. Kawato Y, Furuta T, Aonuma M, et al: Antitumor activity of a camptothecin derivative, CPT-11, against human tumor xenografts in nude mice, *Cancer Chemother Pharmacol* 28:192-198, 1991.

104. Humerickhouse R, Lohrbach K, Li L, et al: Characterization of CPT-11 hydrolysis by human liver carboxylesterase isoforms hCE1 and hCE-2, *Cancer Res* 60:1189-1192, 2000.

105. Rivory LP, Bowles MR, Robert J, et al: Conversion of irinotecan (CPT-11) to its active metabolite, 7-ethyl-10-hydroxycamptothecin (SN-38), by human liver carboxylesterase, *Biochem Pharmacol* 52:1103-1111, 1996.

106. Bosma PJ, Chowdhury JR, Bakker C, et al: The genetic basis of the reduced expression of bilirubin UDP-glucuronosyltransferase 1 in Gilbert's syndrome, *N Engl J Med* 333:1171-5, 1995.

107. Akaba K, Kimura T, Sasaki A, et al: Neonatal hyperbilirubinemia and mutation of the bilirubin uridine diphosphate-glucuronosyltransferase gene: a common missense mutation among Japanese, Koreans, and Chinese, *Biochem MolBiol Int* 46:21-26, 1998.

108. Akaba K, Kimura T, Sasaki A, et al: Neonatal hyperbilirubinemia and a common mutation of the bilirubin uridine diphosphate-glucuronosyltransferase gene in Japanese, *J Hum Genet* 44:22-25, 1999.

109. Araki E, Ishikawa M, Iigo M, et al: Relationship between development of diarrhea and the concentration of SN-38, an active metabolite of CPT-11, in the intestine and the blood plasma of athymic mice following intraperitoneal administration of CPT-11, *Jpn J Cancer Res* 84:697-702, 1993.

110. Huang CS, Luo GA, Huang MJ, et al: Variations of the bilirubin uridine-diphosphoglucuronosyl transferase 1A1 gene in healthy Taiwanese, *Pharmacogenetics* 10:539-544, 2000.

111. Maruo Y, Sato H, Yamano T, et al: Gilbert syndrome caused by a homozygous missense mutation (Tyr486Asp) of bilirubin UDP-glucuronosyltransferase gene, *J Pediatr* 132:1045-1047, 1998.

112. Iyer L, Das S, Janisch L, et al: UGT1A1*28 polymorphism as a determinant of irinotecan disposition and toxicity, *Pharmacogenetics J* 2:43-7, 2002.

113. Juliano RL, Ling V: A surface glycoprotein modulating drug permeability in Chinese hamster ovary cell mutants, *Biochem Biophys Acta* 455:152-162, 1976.

114. Monaghan G, Ryan M, Seddon R, et al: Genetic variation in bilirubin UDP-glycuronyltransferase gene promoter and Gilbert's syndrome, *Lancet* 347:578-581, 1996.

115. Bosma PJ, Chowdhury JR, Bakker C, et al: The genetic basis of the reduced expression of bilirubin UDP-glucuronosyltransferase 1 in Gilbert's syndrome, *N Engl J Med* 333:1171-1175, 1995.

116. Monagham G, Ryan M, Seddon R, et al: Genetic variation in bilirubin UDP-glucuronosyltransferase gene promoter and Gilbert's syndrome, *Lancet* 347:578-581, 1996.

117. van Es HHG, Goldhoorn B, Paul-Abrahamse P, et al: Immunochemical characterization of UDP-glucuronosyltransferase in four patients with the Crigler-Najjar type I syndrome, *J Clin Invest* 85:1199-1205, 1990.

118. Grant DM, Blum F, Beer M, et al: Monomorphics and polymorphic human arylamine N-acetyltransferases: a comparison of lier isozymes and expressed products of two cloned genes, *Mol Pharmacol* 39:184-191, 1991.

119. Ratain MJ, Mick R, Berezin F, et al: Phase I study of amonafide dosing based on acetylator phenotype, *Cancer Res* 53:2304-2308, 1993.

120. Ratain MJ, Mick R, Janisch L, et al: Individualized dosing of amonafide based on a pharmacodynamic model incorporating acetylator phenotype and gender, *Pharmacogenetics* 6:93-101, 1996.

121. Weber WW: *The acetylator genes and drug response,* New York, 1987, Oxford University Press.

122. Price Evans DA, Manley KA, McKusick VA: Genetic control of isoniazid metabolism in man, *Brit Med J* 12:485-91, 1960.

123. Timbrell JA, Harland SJ, Facchini V: Polymorphic acetylation of hydralazine, *Clin Pharmacol Ther* 28:350-5, 1980.

124. Meyer UA, Zanger UM: Molecular mechanisms of genetic polymorphisms of drug metabolism, *Ann Rev Pharmacol Toxicol* 37:269-296, 1997.

125. Grant DM, Goodfellow GH, Sugamori K, et al: Pharmacogenetics of the human arylamine N-acetyltransferases, *Pharmacology* 61:204-211, 2000.

126. Cascorbi I., Drakoulis N, Brockmoller J, et al: Arylamine N-acetyltransferase (NAT2) mutations and their allelic linkage in unrelated Caucasian individuals: correlation with phenotypic activity, *Am J Human Genet* 57:581-592, 1995.

127. Reidenberg MM, Drayer DE, Levy M, et al: Polymorphic acetylation of procainamide in man, *Clin Pharmacol Ther* 17:722-30, 1975.

128. Weinshilboum RM, Otterness DM, Szumlanski CL: Methylation pharmacogenetics: catechol O-methyltransferase, thiopurine methyltransferase, and histamine N-methyltransferase, *Annu Rev Pharmacol Toxicol* 39:19-52, 1999.

129. Reilly DK, Rivera-Calimlim L, Van Dyke D: Catechol-O-methyltransferase activity: a determinant of levodopa response, *Clin Pharmacol Ther* 28:278-86, 1980.

130. Hall AG, Matheson E, Kearns PR, et al: Expression of mu class glutathione S-transferase in childhood acute lymphoblastic leukaemia, *Proc Am Soc Cancer Res* 36:315, 1995.

131. Dirven HAA, van Ommen B, van Bladeren PJ: Involvement of human gluthathione-S-transferease isoenzymes in the conjugation of cyclophosphamide metabolites with glutathione, *Cancer Res* 54:6215-6220, 1994.

132. Board PG, Coggan M, Johnston P, et al: Genetic heterogeneity of the human glutathione transferase: a complex of gene families, *Pharmacol Ther* 48:357-369, 1990.

133. Vatsis KP, Weber WW: Structural heterogeneity of caucasian N-acetyltransferase at the NAT1 locus, *Arch Biochem Biophsy* 301:71-76, 1993.

134. Leiby JM, Malpspeis L, Staubuo AE, et al: Amonafide (NSC 308847): a clinical phase I study of two schedules of administration, *Proc Am Assoc Cancer Res* 29:278, 1988.

135. Ratain MJ, Rosner G, Allen SL, et al: Population pharmacodynamic study of amonafide: a cancer and leukemia group B study, *J Clin Oncol* 13:741-747, 1995.

136. Schroder KR, Wiebel FA, Reich S, et al: Glutathione-S-transferase (GST) theta polymorphism influences background SCE rate, *Arch Toxicol* 69:505-507, 1995.

137. Hayes JD, Strange RC: Glutathione S-transferase polymorphisms and their biological consequences, *Pharmacology* 61:154-166, 2000.

138. Srivastava SK, Singhal SS, Hu X, et al: Differential catalytic efficiency of allelic variants of human glutathione S-transferase Pi in catalyzing the glutathione conjugation of thiotepa, *Arch Biochem Biophys* 366:89-94, 1999.

139. Howells RE, Redman CW, Dhar KK, et al: Association of glutathione S-transferase GSTM1 and GSTT1 null genotypes with clinical outcome in epithelial ovarian cancer, *Clin Cancer Res* 4:2439-2445, 1998.

140. Anderer G, Schrappe M, Brechlin AM, et al: Polymorphisms within glutathione S-transferase genes and initial response to glucocorticoids in childhood acute lymphoblastic leukaemia, *Pharmacogenetics* 10:715-726, 2000.

141. Davies SM, Robison LL, Buckley JD, et al: Glutathione S-transferase polymorphisms and outcomes of chemotherapy in childhood acute myeloid leukemia, *J Clin Oncol* 19:1279-1287, 2001.

142. Kragh-Hansen U, Brennan SO, Calliano M, et al: Binding of warfarin, salicylate, and diazepam to genetic variants of human serum albumin, *Mol Pharmacol* 37:238-242, 1990.

143. Tirona RG, Kim RB: Pharmacogenomics of drug transporters. In Licinio J, Wong ML, editors: *Pharmacogenomics*, Weinheim, Germany, 2002, Wiley-VCH.

144. Flens MJ, Zaman GJ: Tissue distribution of the multidrug resistance protein, *Am J Path* 148:1237-1247, 1996.

145. Kamisako T, Leier I., Cui Y, et al: Transport of monoglucuronosyl and bisglucuronosyl bilirubin by recombinant human and rat multidrug resistance protein 2, *Hepatology* 30:485-490, 1999.

146. Evers R, Kool M, van Deemter L, et al: Drug export activity of the human canalicular multispecific organic anion transporter in polarized kidney MDCK cells expressing cMOAT (MRP2) cDNA, *J Clin Invest* 101:1310-1319, 1998.

147. Nishino A, Kato Y, Igarashi T, et al: Both cMOAT/MRP2 and another unknown transporter (s) are responsible for the biliary excretion of glucuronide conjugate of the nonpeptide angiotensin II antagonist, telmisaltan, *Drug Metab Dispos* 28:1146-1148, 2000.

148. Kool M, van der Linden M, de Haas M, et al: MRP3 an organic anion transporter able to transport anti-cancer drugs, *Proc Natl Acad Sci* (US) 96:6914-6919, 1999.

149. Zeng H, Liu G, Rea PA, et al: Transport of amphipathic anions by human multidrug resistance protein 3, *Cancer Res* 60:4779-4784, 2000.

150. Zeng H, Bain LJ, Belinsky MG, et al: Expression of multidrug resistance protein 3 (multispecific organic anion transporter-D) in human embryonic kidney 293 cells confers resistance to anti-cancer agents, *Cancer Res* 59:5964-5967, 1999.

151. Lee K, Klein-Szanto AJ, Kruh GD: Analysis of the MRP4 drug resistance profile in transfected NIH3T3 cells, *J Natl Cancer Inst* 92:1934-1940, 2000.

152. Chen ZS, Lee K, Kruh GD: Transport of cyclic nucleotides and estradiol 17-beta-D-glucuronide by multidrug resistance protein 4: resistance to 6-mercaptopurine and 6-thioguanine, *J Biol Chem* 276:33747-33754, 2001.

153. Wijnholds J, Mol CA, van Deemter L, et al: Multi-drug-resistance protein 5 is a multi-specific organic anion transporter able to transport nucleotide analogs, *Proc Natl Acad Sci* (US) 97:7476-7481, 2000.

154. Fromm MF, Eichelbaum M: The pharmacogenomics of human P-glycoprotein. In Licinio J, Wong ML, editors: *Pharmacogenomics*, Weinheim Germany, 2002, Wiley-VCH.

155. Mickley LA, Lee JS, Weng Z, et al: Genetic polymorphism in MDR-1: a tool for examining allelic expression in normal cells, unselected and drug-selected cell lines, and human tumors, *Blood* 91:1749-1756, 1998.

156. Hoffmeyer S, Burk O, von Richter O, et al: Functional polymorphisms of the human multidrug-resistance gene: multiple sequence variations and correlation of one allele with P-glycoprotein expression and activity in vivo, *Proc Natl Acad Sci* (US) 97:3473-3478, 2000.

157. Cascorbi I, Gerloff T, Johne A, et al: Frequency of single polymorphisms in P-glycoprotein drug transporter MDR1 gene in white subjects, *Clin Pharmacol Ther* 69:169-174, 2001.

158. Juliano RL, Ling V: A surface glycoprotein modulating drug permeability in Chinese hamster ovary cell mutants, *Biochem Biophys Acta* 455:152-162, 1976.

159. Thiebaut F, Tsuruo T, Hamada H, et al: Cellular localization of the multidrug-resistance gene product P-glycoprotein in normal human tissues, *Proc Natl Acad Sci* (US) 84:7735-7738, 1987.

160. Cordon-Cardo C, O'Brien JP, Casals D, et al: Multidrug-resistance gene (P-glycoprotein) is expressed by endothelial cells at blood-brain barrier sites, *Proc Natl Acad Sci* (US) 86:695-698, 1989.

161. Klimecki WT, Futscher BW, Grogan TM, et al: P-glycoprotein expression and function in circulating blood cells from normal volunteers, *Blood* 83:2451-2458, 1994.

162. Lown KS, Mayo RR, Leichtman AB, et al: Role of intestinal P-glycoprotein (mdr1) in interpatient variation in the oral bioavailability of cyclosporine, *Clin Pharmacol Ther* 62:248-260, 1997.

163. Greiner B, Eichelbaum M, Fritz P, et al: The role of intestinal P-glycoprotein in the interaction of digoxin and rifampin, *J Clin Invest* 104:147-153, 1999.

164. Westphal K, Weinbrenner A, Zschiesche M, et al: Induction of P-glycoprotein by rifampin increases intestinal secretion of talinolol in human beings: a new type of drug/drug interaction, *Clin Pharmacol Ther* 68:345-355, 2000.

165. Fromm MF, Kim RB, Stein CM, et al: Inhibition of P-glycoprotein–mediated drug transport: a unifying mechanism to explain the interaction between digoxin and quinidine, *Circulation* 99:552-557, 1999.

166. Ameyaw MM, Regateiro F, Lit T, et al: MDR1 pharmacogenetics: frequency of the C3435T mutation in exon 26 is significantly influenced by ethnicity, *Pharmacogenetics* 11:217-221, 2001.

167. Schafefeler E, Eichelbaum M, Brinkmann U, et al: Frequency of C3435T polymorphism of MDR1 gene in African people, *Lancet* 358:383-384, 2001.

168. Jette L, Murphy GF, Leclerc JM, et al: Interaction of drugs with P-glycoprotein in brain capillaries, *Biochem Pharmacol* 50:1701-1709, 1995.

169. Schinkel AH, Wagenaar E, Mol CA, et al: P-glycoprotein in the blood-brain barrier of mice influences the brain penetration and pharmacological activity of many drugs, *J Clin Invest* 97:2517-2524, 1996.

170. Bart J, Groen HJ, Hendrikse NH, et al: The blood-brain barrier and oncology: new insights into function and modulation, *Cancer Treat Rev* 26:449-462, 2000.

171. Wils P, Phung-Ba V, Warnery A, et al: Polarized transport of docetaxel and vinblastine mediated by P-glycoprotein in human intestinal epithelial cell monolayers, *Biochem Pharmacol* 48:1528-1530, 1994.

172. Sugiyama Y, Kato Y, Chu X: Multiplicity of biliary excretion mechanisms for the camptothecin derivative irinotecan (CPT-11), its metabolite SN-38, and its glucuronide: role of canalicular multispecific organic anion transporter and P-glycoprotein, *Cancer Chemother Pharmacol Suppl* 42:S44-S49, 1998.

173. Relling MV: Are the major effects of P-glycoprotein modulators due to altered pharmacokinetics of anticancer drugs?, *Ther Drug Monit* 8:350-356, 1996.

174. Sparreboom A, van Asperen J, Mayer U, et al: Limited oral bioavailability and active epithelial excretion of paclitaxel (Taxol) caused by P-glycoprotein in the intestine, *Proc Natl Acad Sci* (US) 94:2031-2035, 1997.

175. Hoki Y, Fujimori A, Pommier Y: Differential cytotoxicity of clinically important camptothecin derivatives in P-glycoprotein-overexpressing cell lines, *Cancer Chemother Pharmacol* 40:433-438, 1997.

176. Schinkel AH, Smit JJ, van Tellingen O, et al: Disruption of the mouse mdr1a P-glycoprotein gene leads to a deficiency in the blood-brain barrier and to increased sensitivity to drugs, *Cell* 77:491-502, 1994.

177. Saeki T, Ueda K, Tanigawara Y, et al: Human P-glycoprotein transports cyclosporin A and FK506, *J Biol Chem* 268:6077-6080, 1993.

178. Polli JW, Jarrett JL, Studenberg SD, et al: Role of P-glycoprotein on the CNS disposition of amprenavir (141W94), an HIV protease inhibitor, *Pharm Res* 16:1206-1212, 1999.

179. Kim RB, Fromm MF, Wandel C, et al: The drug transporter P-glycoprotein limits oral absorption and brain entry of HIV-1 protease inhibitors, *J Clin Invest* 101:289-294, 1998.

180. Alsenz J, Steffen H, Alex R: Active apical y76 secretory efflux of the HIV protease inhibitors saquinavir and ritonavir in Caco-2 cell monolayers, *Pharm Res* 15:423-428, 1998.

181. Pauli-Magnus C, Murdter T, Godel A, et al: P-glycoprotein-mediated transport of digitoxin, alpha-methyldigoxin and beta-acetyldigoxin, *Naunyn Schmiedebergs Arch Pharmacol* 363:337-343, 2001.

182. Schinkel AH, Wagenaar E, van Deemter L, et al: Absence of the mdr1a P-Glycoprotein in mice affects tissue distribution and pharmacokinetics of dexamethasone, digoxin, and cyclosporin A, *J Clin Invest* 96:1698-1705, 1995.

183. Schuetz EG, Yasuda K, Arimori K, et al: Human MDR1 and mouse MDR1a P-glycoprotein alter the cellular retention and disposition of erythromycin, but not of retinoic acid or benzo(a)pyrene, *Arch Biochem Biophys* 350:340-347, 1998.

184. Ito T, Yano I, Tanaka K, et al: Transport of quinolone antibacterial drugs by human P-glycoprotein expressed in a kidney epithelial cell line, LLC-PK1, *J Pharmacol Exp Ther* 282:955-960, 1997.

185. De Lange E, Marchand S, van den Berg D, et al: In vitro and in vivo investigations on fluoroquinolones; effects of the P-glycoprotein efflux transporter on brain distribution of sparfloxacin, *Eur J Pharm Sci* 12:85-93, 2000.

186. Herve F, Gomas E, Duche JC, et al: Evidence for differences in the binding of drugs to the two main genetic variants of human 1-acid-glycoprotein, *Br J Clin Pharmacol* 36:241-249, 1993.

187. Schuetz EG, Schinkel AH, Relling MV, et al: P-glycoprotein: a major determinant of rifampicin-inducible expression of cytochrome P4503A in mice and humans, *Proc Natl Acad Sci* (US) 93:4001-4005, 1996.

188. Smith AJ, van Helvoort A, van Meer G, et al: MDR3 P-glycoprotein, a phosphatidylcholine translocase, transports several cytotoxic drugs and directly interacts with drugs as judged by interference with nucleotide trapping, *J Biol Chem* 275:23530-23539, 2000.

189. De Vree JM, Jaquemin E, Sturm E, et al: Mutations in the MDR3 gene cause progressive familial intrahepatic cholestasis, *Proc Natl Acad Sci* (US) 95:282-287, 1998.

190. Jacquemin E, de Vree JM, Cresteil D, et al: The wide spectrum of multidrug resistance 3 deficiency: from neonatal cholestasis to cirrhosis of adulthood, *Gastroenterology* 120:1448-1458, 2001.

191. Chen HL, Chang PS, Hsu HC, et al: Progressive familial intrahepatic cholestasis with high gamma glutamyltranspeptidase levels in Taiwanese infants: role of MDR3 gene defect?, *Pediatr Res* 50:50-55, 2001.

192. Jacquemin E, Cresteil D, Manouvrier S, et al: Heterozygous non-sense mutation of the MDR3 gene in familial intrahepatic cholestasis of pregnancy, *Lancet* 353 (9140):210-211, 1999.

193. Dixon PH, Weerasekera N, Linton KJ, et al: Heterozygous MDR3 missense mutation associated with intrahepatic cholestasis of pregnancy: evidence for a defect in protein trafficking, *Hum Mol Genet* 9:1209-1217, 2000.

194. Rosmorduc O, Hermelin B, Poupon R: MDR3 gene defect in adult with symptomatic intrahepatic and gallbladder cholesterol cholelithiasis, *Gastroenterology* 120:1459-1467, 2001.

195. Lecureur V, Sun D, Hargrove P, et al: Cloning and expression of murine sister of P-glycoprotein reveals a more discriminating transporter than MDR1/P-glycoprotein, *Mol Pharmacol* 57:24-35, 2000.

196. Bolder U, Trang NV, Hagey LR, et al: Sulindac is excreted into bile by a canalicular bile salt pump and undergoes a cholehepatic circulation in rats, *Gastroenterology* 117:962-971, 1999.

197. Strautnieks SS, Bull LN, Knisely AS, et al: A gene encoding a liver specific ABC transporter is mutated in progressive familial intrahepatic cholestasis, *Nature Genet* 20:233-238, 1998.

198. Jansen PL, Strautnieks SS, Jacquemin E, et al: Hepatocanalicular bile salt export pump deficiency in patients with progressive familial intrahepatic cholestasis, *Gastroenterology* 117:1370-1379, 1999.

199. Yabuuchi H, Tamai I, Nezu J, et al: Novel membrane transporter OCTN1 mediates multispecific, bidirectional, and pH-dependent transport of organic cations, *J Pharmacol Exp Ther* 289:768-773, 1999.

200. Wu X, Prasad PD, Leibach FH, et al: cDNA sequence, transport function, and genomic organization of human OCTN2, a new member of the organic cation transporter family, *Biochem Biophys Res Commun* 246:589-595, 1998.

201. Ohashi R, Tamai I, Yabuuchi H, et al: Na$^+$ dependent carnitine transport by organic cation transporter (OCTN2): its pharmacological and toxicological relevance, *J Pharmacol Exp Ther* 291:778-784, 1999.

202. Mayatepek E, Nezu J, Tamai I, et al: Two novel missense mutations of the OCTN2 gene (W283R and V446F) in a patient with primary systemic carnitine deficiency, *Hum Mutat* 15:118, 2000.

203. Wang Y, Taroni F, Garavaglia B, et al: Functional analysis of mutations in the OCTN2 transporter causing primary carnitine deficiency: lack of genotype-phenotype correlation, *Hum Mutat* 16:401-407, 2000.

204. Wang Y, Kelly MA, Cowan TM, et al: A missense mutation in the OCTN2 gene associated with residual carnitine transport activity, *Hum Mutat* 15:238-245, 2000.

205. Vaz FM, Scholte HR, Ruiter J, et al: Identification of two novel mutations in OCTN2 of three patients with systemic carnitine deficiency, *Hum Genet* 105 (1-2):157-161, 1999.

206. Burwinkel B, Kreuder J, Schweitzer S, et al: Carnitine transporter OCTN2 mutations in systemic primary carnitine deficiency: a novel Arg169Gn mutation and a recurrent Arg282ter mutation associated with an unconventional splicing abnormality, *Biochem Biophys Res Commun* 261:484-487, 1999.

207. Ganapathy ME, Huang W, Rajan DP, et al: β-lactam antibiotics as substrates for OCTN2, an organic cation/carnitine transporter, *J Biol Chem* 275:1699-1707, 2000.

208. Miyake K,. Michley L, Litman T, et al: Molecular cloning of cDNAs which are highly overexpressed in mitoxantrone-resistant cells: demonstration of homology to ABC transport genes, *Cancer Res* 59:4559-4563, 1999.

209. Bossuyt X, Muller M, Meier PH: Multi-specific amphipathic substrate transport by an organic anion transporter of human lier, *J Hepatol* 25:733-738, 1996.

210. Cvetkovic M, Leake B, Fromme MF, et al: OATP and P-glycoprotein transporters mediate the cellular uptake and excretion of fexofenadine, *Drug Metab Dispos* 27:866-871, 1999.

211. Konig J, Cui Y, Nies AT, et al: A novel human organic anion transporting polypeptide localized to the basolateral hepatocyte membrane, *Am J Physiol Gastrointest Liver Physiol* 278:G156-G164, 2000.

212. Hsiang B, Zhu Y, Wang Z, et al: A novel human hepatic organic anion transporting polypeptide (OATP2): identification of a liver-specific human oraganic anion transporting polypeptide and identification of rat and human hydroxymethylglutaryl-CoA reductase inhibitor transporters, *J Bio Chem* 274:37161-37168, 1999.

213. Abe T, Unno, M, Onogawa T, et al: Lst-2, a human liver-specific organic anion transporter, determines methotrexate sensitivity in gastrointestinal cancers, *Gastroenterology* 120:1689-1699, 2001.

214. Tirona RG, Leake BF, Merino G, et al: Polymorphism in OAT P-C: identification of multiple allelic variants associated with altered transport activity among European- and African-Americans, *J Biol Chem* 276:35669-35675, 2001.

215. Fujiwara K, Adachi H, Nishio T, et al: Identification of thyroid hormone transporters in humans: different molecules are involved in a tissue-specific manner, *Endocrinology* 142:2005-2012, 2001.

216. Cihlar T, Lin DC, Pritchard JB, et al: The antiviral nucleotide analogs cidofovir and adefovir are novel substrates for human and rat renal organic anion transporter 1, *Mol Pharmacol* 56:570-580, 1999.

217. Cha SH, Sekine T, Fukushima JI, et al: Identification and characterization of human organic anion transporter 3 expressing predominantly in the kidney, *Mol Pharmacol* 59:1277-1286, 2001.

218. Cha SH, Sekine T, Kushuhara H, et al: Molecular cloning and characterization of multispecific organic anion transporter 4 expressed in the placenta, *J Biol Chem* 275:4507-4512, 2000.

219. Fey YJ, Kana Y, Nussberger S, et al: Expression cloning of a mammalian proton-coupled oligopeptide transporter, *Nature* 368(6471):563-566, 1994.

220. Ganapathy ME, Brandsch M, Prasad PD, et al: Differential recognition of beta-lactam antibiotics by intestinal and renal peptide transporters: PEPT1 and PEPT 2, *J Biol Chem* 270:25672-25677, 1995.

221. Ganapathy ME, Huang W, Wang H, et al: Valacyclovir: a substrate for the intestinal and renal peptide transporters PEPT1 and PEPT2, *Biochem Biophys Res Commun* 246:470-475, 1998.

222. Groneberg DA, Nickolaus M, Springer J, et al: Localization of the peptide transporter PEPT2 in the lung: implications for pulmonary oligopeptide uptake, *Am J Pathol* 158:707-714, 2001.

223. Zhu T, Chen XZ, Steel A, et al: Differential recognition of ACE inhibitors in *Xenopus laevis* oocytes expressing rat PEPT1 and PEPT2, *Pharm Res* 17:526-532, 2000.

224. Inui K, Terada T, Masuda S, et al: Physiological and pharmacological implications of peptide transporters, PEPT1 and PEPT2, *Nephrol Dial Transplant* 15 (Suppl 6):11-13, 2000.

225. Kim DK, Lim SW, Lee S, et al: Serotonin transporter gene polymorphism and antidepressant response, *Neuroreport* 11:215-9, 2000.

226. Smeraldi E, Zanardi R, Benedetti F, et al: Polymorphism within the promoter of the serotonin transporter gene and antidepressant efficacy of fluvoxamine, *Mol Psychiatry* 3:508-11, 1998.

227. Whale R, Quested DJ, Laver D, et al: Serotonin transporter (5-HTT) promoter genotype may influence the prolactin response to clomipramine, *Psychopharmacology* (Berl) 150:120-2, 2000.

228. Litman T, Brangi M, Hudson R, et al: The multidrug-resistant phenotype associated with overexpression of the new ABC half-transporter, MXR (ABCG2), *J Cell Sci* 113 (Pt11):2011-2021, 2000.

229. Stephens JC, Schneider JA, Tanguay DA, et al: Haplotype variation and linkage disequilibrium in 313 human genes, *Science* 293 (5529):489-493, 2001.

230. Ohmichi N, Iwai N, Uchida Y, et al: Relationship between the response to the angiotensin converting enzyme inhibitor imidapril and the angiotensin converting enzyme genotype, *Am J Hypertens* 10:951-5, 1997.

231. Okamura A, Ohishi M, Rakugi H, et al: Pharmacogenetic analysis of the effect of angiotensin converting enzyme inhibitor on restenosis after percutaneous transluminal coronary angioplasty, *Angiology* 50:811-22, 1999.

232. Penno G, Chaturvedi N, Talmud PJ, et al: Effect of angiotensin-converting enzyme (ACE) gene polymorphism on progression of renal disease and the influence of ACE inhibition in IDDM patients: findings from the EUCLID Randomized Controlled Trial: EURODIAB Controlled Trial of Lisinopril in IDDM, *Diabetes* 47:1507-11, 1998.

233. Perna A, Ruggenenti P, Testa A, et al: ACE genotype and ACE inhibitors induced renoprotection in chronic proteinuric nephropathies, *Kidney Int* 57:274-81, 2000.

234. Prasad A, Narayanan S, Husain S, et al: Insertion-deletion polymorphism of the ACE gene modulates reversibility of endothelial dysfunction with ACE inhibition, *Circulation* 102:35-41, 2000.

235. Sasaki M, Oki T, Iuchi A, et al: Relationship between the angiotensin converting enzyme gene polymorphism and the effects of enalapril on left ventricular hypertrophy and impaired diastolic filling in essential hypertension: M-mode and pulsed Doppler echocardiographic studies, *J Hypertens* 14:1403-8, 1996.

236. Stavroulakis GA, Makris TK, Krespi PG, et al: Predicting response to chronic antihypertensive treatment with fosinopril: the role of angiotensin-converting enzyme gene polymorphism, *Cardiovasc Drugs Ther* 14:427-32, 2000.

237. Marian AJ, Safaavi F, Ferlic L, et al: Interactions between angiotensin-I converting enzyme insertion/deletion polymorphism and response of plasma lipids and coronary atherosclerosis to treatment with fluvastatin: The Lipoprotein and Coronary Atherosclerosis Study, *J Am Coll Cardiol* 35:89-95, 2000.

238. Hunt SC, Geleijnse JM, Wu LL, et al: Enhanced blood pressure response to mild sodium reduction in subjects with the 235T variant of the angiotensinogen gene, *Am J Hypertens* 12:460-466, 1999.

239. Jeunemaitre X, Inoue I, Williams C, et al: Haplotypes of angiotensinogen in essential hypertension, *Am J HumGenet* 60:1448-1460, 1997.

240. Poirier J, Delisle MC, Quirion R, et al: Apolipoprotein E4 allele as a predictor of cholinergic deficits and treatment outcome in Alzheimer disease, *Proc Natl Acad Sci* (US) 92:12260-12264, 1995.

241. Amouyel P, Vidal O, Launay JM, et al: The apolipoprotein E alleles as major susceptibility factors for Creutzfeldt-Jakob disease: The French Research Group on Epidemiology of Human Spongiform Encephalopathies, *Lancet* 344(8933):1315-1318, 1994.

242. Lander ES, Schork NJ: Genetic dissection of complex traits, *Science* 265(5181):259-265, 1994.

243. Drysdale CM, McGraw DW, Stack CB, et al: Complex promoter and coding region beta 2-adrenergic receptor and haplotypes alter receptor expression and predict in vivo responsiveness, *Proc Natl Acad Sci* (US) 97:10483-8, 2000.

244. Drazen JM, Yandava CN, Dub L, et al: Pharmacogenetics association between ALOX5 promoter genotype and the response to anti-asthma treatment, *Nat Genet* 22:168-70, 1999.

245. Dishy V, Sofowora GG, Xie HG, et al: The effect of common polymorphisms of the β_2-adrenergic receptor on agonist-mediated vascular desensitization, *N Engl J Med* 345:1030-5, 2001.

246. Cockcroft JR, Gazis AG, Cross DJ, et al: Beta (2)-adrenoceptor polymorphism determines vascular reactivity in humans, *Hypertension* 36:371-5, 2000.

247. Israel E, Drazen JM, Liggett SB, et al: Effect of polymorphism of the beta (2)-adrenergic receptor on response to regular use of albuterol in asthma, *Int Arch Allergy Immunol* 124:183-6, 2001.

248. Lima JJ, Thomason DB, Mohamed MH, et al: Impact of genetic polymorphisms of the beta2-adrenergic receptor on albuterol bronchodilator pharmacodynamics, *Clin Pharmacol Ther* 65:519-25, 1999.

249. Martinez FD, Graves PE, Baldini M, et al: Association between genetic polymorphisms of the beta 2-adrenoceptor and response to albuterol in children with and without a history of wheezing, *J Clin Invest* 100:3184-8, 1997.

250. Tan S, Hall IP, Dewar J, et al: Association between beta 2-adrenoceptor polymorphism and susceptibility to bronchodilator desensitization in moderately severe stable asthmatics, *Lancet* 350:995-9, 1997.

251. Mukae S, Aoki S, Itoh S, et al: Bradykinin B_2 receptor gene polymorphism is associated with angiotensin-converting enzyme inhibitor-related cough, *Hypertension* 36:127-31, 2000.

252. Kuivenhoven JA, Jukema JW, Zwinderman AH, et al: The role of common variant of the cholesteryl ester transfer protein gene in the progression of coronary atherosclerosis: The Regression Growth Evaluation Statin Study Group, *N Engl J Med* 338:86-93, 1998.

253. Arranz MJ, Munro J, Birkett J, et al: Pharmacogenetic prediction of clozapine response, *Lancet* 355:1615-6, 2000.

254. Basile VS, Masellis M, Badri F, et al: Association of the MscI polymorphism of the dopamine D3 receptor gene with tardive dyskinesia in schizophrenia, *Neuropsychopharmacol* 21:17-27, 1999.

255. Eichhammer P, Albus M, Borrmann-Hassenbach M, et al: Association of dopamine D3-receptor gene variants with neuroleptic induced akathisia in schizophrenic patients: a generalization of Steen's study on DRD3 and tardive dyskinesia, *Am J Med Genet* 96:187-91, 2000.

256. Hwu HG, Hong CJ, Lee YL, et al: Dopamine D4 receptor gene polymorphisms and neuroleptic response in schizophrenia, *Biol Psychiatry* 44:483-7, 1998.

257. Kaiser R, Konneker M, Henneken M, et al: Dopamine D4 receptor 48-bp repeat polymorphism: no association with response to antipsychotic treatment, but association with catatonic schizophrenia, *Mol Psychiatry* 5:418-24, 2000.

258. Ongphiphadhanakul B, Chanprasertyothin S, Payatikul P, et al: Oestrogen-receptor-alpha gene polymorphism affects response in bone mineral density to oestrogen in post-menopausal women, *Clin Endocrinol* (Oxf) 52:581-5, 2000.

259. Herrington DM, Howard TD, Hawkins GA, et al: Estrogen-receptor polymorphisms and effects of estrogen replacement on high-density lipoprotein cholesterol in women with coronary disease, *N Engl J Med* 346:967-74, 2000.

260. Michelson AD, Furman MI, Goldschmidt-Clermont P, et al: Platelet GP IIIa PI(A) polymorphisms display different sensitivities to agonists, *Circulation* 101:1013-8, 2000.

261. Reisine T: Pharmacogenomics of opioid systems. In Licinio J, Wong ML, editors: *Pharmacogenomics,* Weinheim, Germany, 2002, Wiley-VCH.

262. Deeb SS, Fajas L, Nemoto M, et al: A Pro 12A1a substitution in PPARgamma2 associated with decreased receptor activity, lower body mass index and improved insulin sensitivity, *Nature Genet* 20:284-287, 1998.

263. Essioux L, Destenaves B, Jais P, et al: Association studies in pharmacogenomics. In Licinio J, Wong ML, editors: *Pharmacogenomics,* Weinheim, Germany, 2002, Wiley-VCH.

264. Aranz MJ, Munro J, Birkett J, et al: Pharmacogenetic prediction of clozapine response, *Lancet* 355(9215):1615-1616, 2000.

265. Joober R, Benkelfat C, Brisebois K, et al: T102C polymorphism in the 5HT2A gene and schizophrenia: relation to phenotype and drug response variability, *J Psychiatry Neurosci* 24:141-146, 1999.

266. Inayama Y, Yoneda H, Sakai T, et al: Positive association between a DNA sequence variant in the serotonin 2A receptor gene and schizophrenia, *Am J Med Genet* 67:103-105, 1996.

267. Hansen T, Echwald SM, Hansen L, et al: Decreased tolbutamide-stimulated insulin secretion in healthy subjects with sequence variants in the high-affinity sulfonylurea receptor gene, *Diabetes* 47:598-605, 1998.

268. Reis AF, Ye WZ, DuBoise-Laforgue D, et al: Association of a variant in exon 31 of the sulfonylurea receptor 1 (SUR1) gene with type 2 diabetes mellitus in French Caucasians, *Hum Genet* 107:138-144, 2000.

269. Lucotte G, Mercier G, Burckel A: The vitamin D receptor FokI start codon polymorphism and bone mineral density in osteoporotic postmenopausal French women, *Clin Genet* 56:221-224, 1999.

270. Malloy PJ, Eccleshall T, Gross C, et al: Hereditary vitamin D resistant rickets caused by a novel mutation in the vitamin D receptor that results in decreased affinity for hormone and cellular hyporesponsiveness, *J Clin Invest* 99:297-304, 1997.

SECTION VIII
ALLERGY TESTING

BACKGROUND AND INTRODUCTION

Allergic Disease: Significance and Extent of Disease

The allergic diseases include a spectrum of disorders: asthma, rhinitis, anaphylaxis, atopic dermatitis, and sinusitis. These diseases affect up to 20% of the population. Although there are a number of immunologic mechanisms that may be involved in the various disorders, the primary focus of this chapter is those allergic reactions that are classified as type I (or immediate-type hypersensitivities) according to the classical Gel Coombs scheme. These usually involve a special immunoglobulin, IgE, which circulates in the serum at low concentrations and is present on mast cells and basophils.[1]

Allergy Diagnostics

Diagnostic testing for allergy has evolved over the years. Skin testing has been the primary method to confirm allergic sensitization since the early 1900s. With this method a small quantity of allergen extract is injected into the skin where it reacts with IgE on the surface of the tissue mast cells. The cross-linking of IgE on the surface of mast cells by the multivalent allergen results in rapid cellular changes, including degranulation. This degranulation event leads to a release of chemical mediators such as histamine in the skin. Histamine causes a visible wheal and flare reaction at the site of allergen injection. These reactions in the skin can be graded according to size.[2] The skin test method is a very sensitive bioassay for allergic sensitization and is still widely used, especially by allergy specialists in the United States.

The most common laboratory test methods to assess allergic sensitization are based on the measurement of allergen-specific IgE in serum rather than IgE on the surface of cells. The development of these in vitro methods followed the discovery of IgE in 1967.[3] In these laboratory test methods, the allergenic proteins are usually coupled to a solid-phase (e.g., cellulose) or a soluble matrix polymer.[4,5] Serum from the patient is incubated with the coupled allergen of interest so that the allergen-specific IgE can bind. After this incubation period, a washing step is used to remove any unbound IgE, and the amount of specific IgE is then measured by one of several methods with a labeled antihuman IgE antibody.[6] The most widely used methods are outlined in the following section.

ALLERGENS

A variety of substances, derived from many different sources, can sensitize an individual and cause allergic disease. In the vast majority of cases, allergens are protein molecules, usually in the molecular weight range of 10,000 to 40,000 Da. The various types of allergenic substances are outlined and organized in Tables VIII-1 and VIII-2 by source (e.g., pollen, foods). The selection of the appropriate allergens for testing requires knowledge of the patient's environmental exposure, age, and clinical history. A limited selection or panel of indoor allergens (e.g., mites, animal dander, and fungi) and pollens (weeds, trees, and grasses) can be useful to the primary care physician who is trying to evaluate the possibility of allergy in patients with symptoms suggestive of allergy. Although there are literally hundreds of tests that may be ordered, large screening panels are seldom indicated. In general, because of both specific geographic exposure charts and cross-reaction considerations, the panel of allergens should not need to total >12 to 15 tests. Laboratories should advise physicians to limit the number of allergy tests in screening evaluations. However, if foods are to be investigated, an additional 5 to 10 allergens may be appropriate. Often the clinical laboratory will have designed regional panels that can be used by the primary care physician.

REFERENCES

1. Homburger HA: Diagnostic allergy testing, *Clin Lab News* 30:12-14, 2004.
2. Hamilton RG: Assessment of human allergic disease. In Rich RR, Fleisher TA, Shearer WT, et al, editors: *Clinical immunology, principles and practice,* London, 2003, Mosby. ci. 40:208-211, 1995.
3. Wide L, Bennich H, Johansson SGO: Diagnosis of allergy by an in vitro test for allergen-specific IgE antibodies, *Lancet* 2:1105-1107, 1967.
4. Hamilton RG, Adkinson NF Jr: In vitro assays for the diagnosis of IgE-mediated disorders, *J Allergy Clin Immunol* 114:213-225, 2004.
5. Hamilton RG, Adkinson NF Jr: Immunological tests for diagnosis and management of human allergic disease: total and allergen-specific IgE and allergen-specific IgG. In Rose NR, de Macario EC, Folds JD, et al, editors: *Manual of clinical laboratory immunology,* Washington, DC, 1997, ASM Press.
6. Valcour A: Allergy testing for the 21st century, *Advances for Administrators of the Laboratory* 12:68-73, 2003.

TABLE VIII-1	INDIVIDUAL ALLERGENS AVAILABLE FOR ALLERGEN-SPECIFIC IgE TESTING*

CATEGORY OF ALLERGEN AND ALLERGEN NAME	USUAL EXPOSURE

GRASS POLLENS

Sweet vernal grass *(Anthoxanthum odoratum)*   Inhalation
Bermuda grass *(Cynodon dactylon)*
Orchard grass *(Dactylis glomerata)*
Meadow fescue *(Festuca elatior)*
Rye grass *(Lolium perenne)*
Timothy grass *(Phleum pratense)*
Common reed grass *(Phragmites communis)*
Kentucky blue grass *(Poa pratensis)*
Redtop or Bent grass *(Agrostis stolonifera)*
Johnson grass *(Sorghum halepense)*
Brome grass *(Bromus inermis)*
Cultivated rye grass *(Secale cereale)*
Velvet grass *(Holcus lanatus)*
Cultivated oat *(Avena sativa)*
Cultivated wheat *(Triticum sativum)*
Meadow foxtail grass *(Alopercurus pratensis)*
Bahia grass *(Paspalum notatum)*
Wild rye grass *(Elymus triticoides)*
Canary grass *(Phalaris arundinacea)*
Barley *(Hordeum vulgare)*
Maize or corn *(Zea mays)*

WEED POLLENS

Common ragweed *(Ambrosia elatior)*   Inhalation
Western ragweed *(Ambrosia psilostachya)*
Giant ragweed *(Ambrosia trifida)*
False ragweed *(Franseria acanthicarpa)*
Wormwood *(Artemisia absinthium)*
Mugwort *(Artemisia vulgaris)*
Ox-eye daisy *(chrysanthemum leucanthemum)*
Dandelion *(Taraxacum vulgare)*
English plantain *(Plantago lanceolata)*
Lamb's quarters *(Chenopodium album)*
Russian thistle *(Salsola kali)*
Golden rod *(Solidago virgaurea)*
Cocklebur *(Xanthium commune)*
Wall pellitory *(Parietaria judaica)*

CATEGORY OF ALLERGEN AND ALLERGEN NAME	USUAL EXPOSURE

TREE POLLENS

Box-elder *(Acer negundo)*   Inhalation
Grey alder *(Alnus incana)*
Common silver birch *(Betula verrucosa)*
Hazel *(Corylus avellana)*
American beech *(Fagus grandifolia)*
Mountain juniper *(Juniperus sabinoides)*
Oak *(Quercus alba)*
Elm *(Ulmus americana)*
Olive *(Olea europaea)*
Walnut *(Juglans californica)*
Maple leaf sycamore, London plane *(Platanus acerifolia)*
Willow *(Salix caprea)*
Cottonwood *(Populus deltoides)*
White ash *(Fraxinus Americana)*
White pine *(Pinus strobes)*
Japanese cedar *(Cryptomeria japonica)*
Eucalyptus, Gum tree *(Eucalyptus* spp.)
Acacia *(Acacia longifolia)*
Mesquite *(Prosopis juliflora)*
Melaleuca, Cajeput-tree *(Melaleuca leucadendron)*
Pecan, Hickory *(Carya pecan)*
Italian/Funeral cypress *(Cupressus sempervirens)*
Mulberry *(Morus alba)*
Queen palm *(Arecastrum romanzoffianum)*
Australian pine *(Casaurina equisetifolia)*
Linden *(Tilia cordata)*
Privet *(Ligustrum vulgare)*

MOLDS AND YEASTS

Penicillium notatum   Usually inhalation of spores
Cladosporium herbarum (Hormodendrum)
Aspergillus fumigatus
Mucor racemosus
Candida albicans
Alternaria alternata (A. tenuis)
Botrytis cinerea
Helminthosporium halodes
Fusarium moniliforme
Stemphylium botryosum
Rhizopus nigricans
Aureobasidium pullulans
Phoma betae
Epicoccum purpurascens
Trichoderma viride
Curvularia lunata
Pityrosporum orbiculare
Cephalosporium acremonium
Trichophyton rubrum
Aspergillus niger

CATEGORY OF ALLERGEN AND ALLERGEN NAME	USUAL EXPOSURE

MITES

House dust mite *(Dermatophagoides pteronyssinus)*   Inhalation
House dust mite *(Dermatophagoides farinae)*
House dust mite *(Dermatophagoides microceras)*
Storage mite *(Acarus siro)*
Storage mite *(Lepidoglyphus destructor)*
Storage mite *(Typrophagus putrescentiae)*
Storage mite *(Glycyphagus domesticus)*
House dust mite *(Euroglyphus maynei)*

HOUSE DUST

House dust, Greer Labs, Inc   Inhalation
House dust, Hollister-Stier Labs

ANIMAL EPIDERMALS AND PROTEINS

Cat dander   Inhalation
Dog epithelium
Horse dander
Cow dander
Dog dander
Guinea pig epithelium
Pigeon droppings
Goose feathers
Mouse urine proteins
Rat epithelium
Rat urine proteins
Rat serum proteins
Mouse serum proteins
Budgerigar droppings
Budgerigar feathers
Budgerigar serum proteins
Goat epithelium
Sheep epithelium
Rabbit epithelium
Swine epithelium
Hamster epithelium
Chicken feathers
Duck feathers
Canary bird feathers
Parrot feathers

CATEGORY OF ALLERGEN AND ALLERGEN NAME	USUAL EXPOSURE

FOODS

Egg white   Ingestion
Milk
Fish, cod *(Gadus morhua)*
Wheat *(Triticum aestivum)*
Rye *(Secale cereale)*
Barley *(Hordeum vulgare)*
Oat *(Avena sativa)*
Maize, corn *(Zea mays)*
Rice *(Oryza sativa)*
Sesame seed *(Sesamum indicum)*
Buckwheat *(Fagopyrum esculentum)*
Pea *(Pisum sativum)*
Peanut *(Arachis hypogaea)*
Soybean *(Glycine max)*
White bean *(Phaseolus vulgaris)*
Hazelnut *(Corylus avellana)*
Brazil nut *(Bertholletia excelsa)*
Almond *(Amygdalus communis)*
Crab *(Cancer pagurus)*
Shrimp *(Pandalus borealis)*
Tomato *(Lycopersicon lycopersicum)*
Pork *(Sus* spp.)
Beef *(Bos* spp.)
Carrot *(Daucus carota)*
Orange *(Citrus sinensis)*
Potato *(Solanum tuberosum)*
Coconut *(Cocos nucifera)*
Blue mussel *(Mytilus edulis)*
Tuna *(Thunnus albacares)*
Salmon *(Salmo salar)*
Strawberry *(Fragaria vesca)*
Yeast *(Saccaromyces cerevisiae)*
Garlic *(Allium sativum)*
Onion *(Allium cepa)*
Apple *(Malus sylvestris)*
Chub mackerel *(Scomber japonicus)*
Bamboo shoot *(Phyllostachys pubescens)*
Sweet potato *(Ipomoea batatas)*
Common millet *(Panicum milliaceum)*
Foxtail millet *(Setaria italica)*
Japanese millet *(Echinochloa crusgalli)*
Pacific squid *(Todarodes pacificus)*
Octopus *(Octopus vulgaris)*
Jack mackerel, scad *(Trachurus japonicus)*
Sardine, pilchard *(Sardinops melanosticta)*
Egg yolk
α-Lactalbumin
β-Lactoglobulin
Casein
Gluten

CATEGORY OF ALLERGEN AND ALLERGEN NAME	USUAL EXPOSURE

FOODS—CONT

Lobster *(Homarus gammarus)*
Cheese, cheddar type
Cheese, mold type
Chicken meat *(Gallus* spp.)
Kiwi fruit *(Actinidia chinensis)*
Celery *(Apium graveolens)*
Parsley *(Petrosilenum crispum)*
Melon *(Cucumis melo* spp.)
Mutton *(Ovis* spp.)
Mustard *(Brassica/Sinapis* spp.)
Malt
Mango fruit
Banana *(Musa* spp.)
Cacao *(Theobroma cacao)*
Pear *(Pyrus communis)*
Peach *(Prunus persica)*
Avocado *(Persea americana)*
Pecan nut *(Carya illinoensis)*
Cashew nut *(Anacardium occidentale)*
Pistachio *(Pistacia vera)*
Trout *(Oncorhynchus mykiss) (Salmo gairdnieri)*
Herring *(Clupea harengus)*
Clam *(Ruditapes* spp.)
Lemon *(Citrus limon)*
Grapefruit *(Citrus paradisis)*
Pineapple *(Ananas comosus)*
Rabbit meat *(Oryctolagus* spp.)
Spinach *(Spinacia oleracea)*
Lettuce *(Lactuca sativa)*
Cabbage *(Brassica oleracea var capitata)*
Paprika, sweet pepper *(Capsicum annuum)*
Pumpkin *(Cucurbita pepo)*
Milk, boiled
Ovalbumin
Ovomucoid
Lentil *(Lens esculenta)*
Apricot *(Prunus armeniaca)*
Cherry *(Prunus avium)*
Cucumber *(Cucumis sativus)*
Egg (yolk and white)
Plaice *(Pleuronectes platessa)*
Plum *(Prunus domestica)*
Walnut *(Juglans* spp.)
Grape *(Vitis vinifera)*
Broccoli *(Brassica oleracea var italica)*
Black pepper *(Piper nigrum)*
Turkey meat *(Meleagris gallopavo)*
Oyster *(Ostrea edulis)*
Chestnut, sweet *(Castanea sativa)*

CATEGORY OF ALLERGEN AND ALLERGEN NAME	USUAL EXPOSURE

INSECTS

Cockroach *(Blatella germanica)*   Inhalation or biting
Moth *(Bombyx mori)*
Mosquito *(Aedes communis)*
Green nimitti *(Cladotanytarsus lewisi)*
Blood worm *(Chironomus riparious)*
Berlin beetle *(Trogoderma angustum)*
Horse botfly *(Gasterophilus intestinalis)*

STINGING INSECT VENOMS

Honey bee *(Apis mellifera)*   Venom injection by sting
White-faced hornet *(Dolichovespula maculata)*
Common wasp, Yellow jacket *(Vespula* spp.)
Paper wasp *(Polistes* spp.)
Yellow hornet *(Dolichovespula arenaria)*
European hornet *(Vespa crabro)*
Fire ant *(Solenopsis invicta)*

PARASITES AND MICROBIALS

Ascaris   Ingestion
Echinococcus   Ingestion
Anisakis   Ingestion
Staphylococcal enterotoxin A   Skin
Staphylococcal enterotoxin B   Skin

DRUGS AND BIOLOGICALS

Penicilloyl G   Ingestion or injection
Penicilloyl V
Ampicillin
Amoxicillin
Human insulin
Gelatin

CATEGORY OF ALLERGEN AND ALLERGEN NAME	USUAL EXPOSURE

OCCUPATIONAL AND MISCELLANEOUS

Green coffee beans	Inhalation
Castor bean	Inhalation or ingestion
Ispaghula	Inhalation or ingestion
Silk waste	Inhalation
Silk *(Bombyx mori)*	Inhalation or contact
Isocyanate TDI	Inhalation
Isocyanate MDI	Inhalation
Isocyanate HDI	Inhalation
Ethylene oxide	Inhalation or contact
Phthalic anhydride	Inhalation
Formaldehyde/formalin	Inhalation
Ficus spp.	Contact
Latex *(Hevea braziliensis)*	Inhalation, contact, or injection
Cotton seed	Inhalation
Sunflower seed	Inhalation or ingestion
Chloramin T	Inhalation
Trimellitic anhydride, TMA	Inhalation
α-Amylase	Inhalation or ingestion
Cotton, crude fibers	Inhalation
Seminal fluid	Contact

*The allergens included in the above list are only those that have been cleared by the FDA for in vitro diagnostic use. Laboratories that specialize in allergy testing may offer additional allergen-specific IgE tests.

TEST NAME AND METHOD	SPECIMEN REQUIREMENTS	REFERENCE INTERVAL, CONVENTIONAL [INTERNATIONAL RECOMMENDED UNITS]			CHEMICAL INTERFERENCES AND IN VIVO EFFECTS
Allergen-Specific IgE	Serum/plasma	$k_A U/L$	Class	Interpretation	Seasonal exposures fre-
		<0.35	0	Undetectable	quently result in eleva-
		0.35-0.69	I	Low	tions of allergen-specific
FEIA		0.70-3.49	II	Moderate	IgE in sensitized individu-
		3.50-17.49	III	High	als.[1] Antihistamine drugs
		17.5-49.9	IV	Very high	do not interfere with the
		50.0-99.99	V	Very high	measurement of IgE.
		≥100	VI	Very high	
CEIA	Serum	kU/L	Class	Interpretation	
		<0.35	0	Undetectable	
		0.35-0.69	I	Low	
		0.70-3.49	II	Moderate	
		3.50-17.49	III	High	
		17.5-52.49	IV	Very high	
		52.5-99.99	V	Very high	
		≥100	VI	Very high	
RIA (or RAST)	Serum	IU/mL	Class	Interpretation	
		<0.05	0	Below detection	
		0.05-0.08	0/I	Equivocal	
		0.08-0.15	I		
		0.15-0.50	II	Increasing	
		0.50-2.50	III	levels of	
		2.50-12.5	IV	antigen-specific	
		12.5-62.50	V	IgE antibodies	
		>62.50	VI		

1. Hamilton RG, Adkinson NF Jr: Immunological tests for diagnosis and management of human allergic disease: total and allergen-specific IgE and allergen-specific IgG. In Rose NR, de Macario EC, Folds JD, et al, editors: *Manual of clinical laboratory immunology,* Washington, DC, 1997, ASM Press.

2. Hamilton RG, Adkinson NF Jr: In vitro assays for the diagnosis of IgE-mediated disorders, *J Allergy Clin Immunol* 114:213-225, 2004.

3. Hamilton RG, Adkinson NJ Jr: In vitro assays for the diagnosis of IgE-mediated disorders, *J Allergy Clin Immunol* 114:213-225, 2004.

Eosinophil Cationic Protein (ECP)	Serum	FEIA	Normal <18 ng/mL	[<18 mcg/L]
	Serum	CEIA	Normal <24 ng/mL	[<24 mcg/L]
	Specimen processing is critical. Collect the blood in a 4-mL Vacutainer Hemogard SST tube. The tube should be completely filled			

DIAGNOSTIC INFORMATION	REMARKS
See *Background and Introduction to Allergy Testing.*	There are many different scoring schemes used to report allergen-specific IgE.[3] Most academic investigators now prefer quantitative units (kU/L) rather than the use of class scores in reporting specific IgE results. However, most laboratories still report both class and quantitative units.
See *Background and Introduction to Allergy Testing.*	The reference range for ECP is the 95% confidence interval for a normal healthy population. Serum ECP measurements may be used to monitor asthma therapies and optimize drug dosing.[1]

TEST NAME AND METHOD	SPECIMEN REQUIREMENTS	REFERENCE INTERVAL, CONVENTIONAL [INTERNATIONAL RECOMMENDED UNITS]		CHEMICAL INTERFERENCES AND IN VIVO EFFECTS
Eosinophil Cationic Protein—CONT				
	and then gently inverted five times. Allow the blood to clot at room temperature (20-24° C) for 60 min (±5 min). Centrifuge the serum at 1000-1300*g* for 10 min at room temperature. If not tested immediately, the serum should be stored frozen.			

1. Zimmerman B: Clinical experience with the measurement of ECP: usefulness in the management of children with asthma, *Clin Exp Allergy* 51:245-250, 1993.

TEST NAME AND METHOD	SPECIMEN REQUIREMENTS	REFERENCE INTERVAL, CONVENTIONAL [INTERNATIONAL RECOMMENDED UNITS]		CHEMICAL INTERFERENCES AND IN VIVO EFFECTS
Histamine	Plasma	<1.0 ng/mL	[<1.0 mcg/L]	See *Background and Introduction to Allergy Testing.*
EIA	Collect blood in an EDTA tube (Lavender Top). Cool immediately on ice. Centrifuge at 1500 rpm for 10 min at 4° C. The centrifugation should be performed within 20 min of collection. Carefully remove plasma from tube and transfer to a plastic vial (not glass) and freeze.			
	Blood	20-200 ng/mL	[20-200 mcg/L]	
	Collect blood into a heparin tube (Green Top). Do not use EDTA. Freeze immediately.			
	Random urine	<88 ng/mL	[<88 mcg/L]	
	24-hr urine	<118 mcg/24 hr		

Histamine measurement is often useful in evaluating patients with suspected anaphylaxis, mastocytosis, gastrointestinal disease, reactions to radiocontrast media, and drug-induced anaphylactoid reactions.[1]

TEST NAME AND METHOD	SPECIMEN REQUIREMENTS	REFERENCE INTERVAL, CONVENTIONAL [INTERNATIONAL RECOMMENDED UNITS]		CHEMICAL INTERFERENCES AND IN VIVO EFFECTS

Histamine—CONT

An aliquot (e.g., 5 mL) of urine should be sent to the laboratory. If the specimen is from a 24-hr urine collection, indicate the total 24-hr volume on the tube. Do not use a glass container to ship or collect the specimen. Freeze.

1. McBride P, Bradley D, Kaliner M: Evaluation of a radioimmunoassay for histamine measurement in biologic fluids, *J Allergy Clin Immunol* 82:638-646, 1988.

Immunoglobulin E (IgE)

Serum/plasma

Upper 95% Limit

Avoid repeated freeze-thaw cycles.

FEIA

Age	kU/L		mcg/L
3 mo	4.1	× 2.4	[9.84]
6 mo	7.3		[17.5]
9 mo	10		[24.0]
12 mo	13		[31.2]
2 yr	23		[55.2]
3 yr	32		[76.8]
4 yr	40		[96.0]
5 yr	48		[115]
6 yr	56		[134]
7 yr	63		[151]
8 yr	71		[170]
9 yr	78		[187]
10 yr	85		[204]
Adult	64		[154]

CEIA (Immulite 2000)

Serum/plasma

Upper 95% Limit

Avoid repeated freeze-thaw cycles.

Age	U/mL		mcg/L
0-1 yr	29	× 2.4	[69.6]
1-2 yr	49		[118]
2-3 yr	45		[108]
3-9 yr	52		[125]
Adult	87		[209]

CEIA (Access)

Serum/plasma

Upper 95% Limit

Avoid repeated freeze-thaw cycles. Human anti-mouse antibody may interfere.

Age	U/mL		mcg/L
Adults	<165.3	× 2.4	[<397]

DIAGNOSTIC INFORMATION	REMARKS

See *Background and Introduction to Allergy Testing.*

Reference value reported for this total IgE method is the geometric mean + 1 SD.

There is significant overlap in total IgE between allergic and nonallergic individuals. For this reason, the measurement of a total IgE is not very useful as a stand-alone screen for allergy disease.[1] After increasing up to the early teens (ages 10-15 yr), the total serum IgE declines in the later years.[1,2] Low total IgE can aid the exclusion of allergic bronchopulmonary aspergillosis or ABPA.[1]

TEST NAME AND METHOD	SPECIMEN REQUIREMENTS	REFERENCE INTERVAL, CONVENTIONAL [INTERNATIONAL RECOMMENDED UNITS]			CHEMICAL INTERFERENCES AND IN VIVO EFFECTS

Immunoglobulin E—CONT

CEIA (Advia Centaur)	Serum	95% Range			Avoid hemolysis, lipemic and icteric serum.
		Age	*U/mL*	*mcg/L*	
		<1 yr	1.4-52.3 × 2.4	[3.4-126]	
		1-4 yr	0.4-351.6	[1.0-844]	
		5-10 yr	0.5-393.0	[1.2-943]	
		11-15 yr	1.9-170.0	[4.6-408]	
		Adult	<158	[<379]	
Nephelometry (BN System)	Serum/plasma	*Age*	*U/mL*	*mcg/L*	High turbidity from rheumatoid factor may interfere.
		Neonates	<1.5 × 2.4	[<3.6]	
		<1 yr	<15	[<36]	
		1-5 yr	<60	[<144]	
		6-9 yr	<90	[<216]	
		10-15 yr	<200	[480]	
		Adults	<100	[240]	

1. Hamilton RG: Assessment of human allergic disease. In Rich RR, Fleisher TA, Shearer WT, et al, editors: *Clinical immunology, principles and practice,* London, 2003, Mosby.

2. Hamilton RG, Adkinson NF Jr: In vitro assays for the diagnosis of IgE-mediated disorders, *J Allergy Clin Immunol* 114:213-225, 2004.

Tryptase	Serum/plasma	<11.4 ng/mL	[11.4 mcg/L]	
FEIA	Stable for 3 wk at 4-25° C.[1]			

1. Randall BB, Butts J, Halsey JF: Elevated postmortem tryptase in the absence of anaphylaxis, *J Forensic Sci* 40:208-211, 1995.

2. Hamilton RG: Assessment of human allergic disease. In Rich RR, Fleisher TA, Shearer WT, et al, editors: *Clinical immunology, principles and practice,* London, 2003, Mosby.

3. Schwartz LB, Metcalfe DD, Miller JS, et al: Tryptase levels as an indicator of mast-cell activation in systemic anaphylaxis and mastocytosis, *N Engl J Med* 316:1622-1626, 1987.

4. Horn KD, Halsey JF, Zumwalt RE: Utilization of serum tryptase and immunoglobulin E in the postmortem diagnosis of anaphylaxis, *Am J Forensic Med Pathol* 25:37-43, 2004.

| **DIAGNOSTIC INFORMATION** | **REMARKS** |

See *Background and Introduction to Allergy Testing.*

The commercially available assay for tryptase measures both the α and β forms of this mast cell enzyme. Constitutively elevated tryptase is a useful finding in the diagnosis of mastocytosis, and transiently high levels of tryptase are used to confirm the occurrence of a systemic mast cell event or anaphylaxis.[2,3] The tryptase in the blood peaks within the initial 30-40 min after an anaphylactic event and decays with a half-life of ~2 hr. Elevations in tryptase that are unrelated to an anaphylactic event have been reported in postmortem bloods.[4] Therefore caution is necessary in the interpretation of test results with postmortem bloods.

APPENDIX

TEST NAME AND METHOD	SPECIMEN REQUIREMENTS	REFERENCE INTERVAL, CONVENTIONAL [INTERNATIONAL RECOMMENDED UNITS]		CHEMICAL INTERFERENCES AND IN VIVO EFFECTS
Alanine (Ala)[1-6] *Ion-exchange chromatography*	Plasma (heparin) or serum, fasting. Place blood in ice water immediately; separate and freeze within 1 hr of collection. Stable for 1 wk at −20° C; for longer periods, deproteinize and store at −70° C.[7,8]	*mg/dL* Premature (first 6 wk) 1.89-4.49 0-1 mo: 1.17-6.33 1-24 mo: 1.28-3.92 2-18 yr: 1.35-4.88 Adult 1.58-5.21	× 112	*μmol/L* [212-504] [131-710] [143-439] [152-547] [177-583]	P ↑ V Glucose (load), glutamic acid, histidine (after oral load), and valproic acid P ↓ V Ethanol, oral contraceptives, and progesterone (high doses)
	Urine, 24 hr. Add 20 mL of toluene at start of collection. (Alternatively, refrigerate specimen during collection.) Store frozen at −20° C.	*mg/day* 10 days-7 wk: 4.1-9.3 3-12 yr: 9.1-39.2 Adult: 7.9-48.3 or 14 ± 6 mg/g creatinine (SD) [× 1.27 = 17.8 ± 7.6 mmol/mol creatinine]	× 11.2	*μmol/day*[10] [46-104] [102-439] [88-541]	U ↑ V Ascorbic acid (after large intake)
		μmol/g creatinine[11] 0-1 mo: 554-2957 1-6 mo: 613-2874 6 mo-1 yr: 428-2064 1-2 yr: 389-1497 2-3 yr: 255-1726	× 0.113	*mmol/mol creatinine* [62.6-334.1] [69.3-324.8] [48.4-233.2] [44.0-169.2] [28.8-195.0]	
	CSF. Collect in sterile tubes; store frozen. Stable at −20° C for 1 wk or at −70° C for 2 mo.[9]	*mg/dL* Neonate: 0.537 ± 0.225 (SEM) 3 mo-2 yr: 0.169 ± 0.044 (SD) 2-10 yr: 0.149 ± 0.039 Adult: 0.291 ± 0.019	×112.2	*μmol/L* [60.2 ± 25.2][9] [19.0 ± 4.9][12] [16.7 ± 4.4][12] [32.7 ± 2.1][10]	

1. Friedman RB, Young DS: *Effects of disease on clinical laboratory tests,* ed 4, Washington, DC, 2001, American Association of Clinical Chemistry.

2. Scriver CR, Beaudet AL, Valle D, et al, editors: *The metabolic and molecular bases of inherited disease,* ed 8, New York, 2001, McGraw-Hill.

3. Young DS: *Effects of drugs on clinical laboratory tests,* ed 5, Washington, DC, 2000, American Association of Clinical Chemistry.

4. Bremer HJ, Duran M, Kamerling JP, et al: *Disturbances of amino acid metabolism: clinical chemistry and diagnosis,* Baltimore, 1981, Urban and Schwarzenburg.

5. Nyhan W, Sakait N: *Diagnostic recognition of genetic disease,* Philadelphia, 1987, Lea & Febiger.

6. Slocum RH, Cummings JG: Amino acid analysis of physiological samples. In *Techniques in human biochemical genetics,* New York, 1991, Wiley-Liss, pp. 87-126.

7. Cummings JG: Routine amino acids analysis in the clinical laboratory, *Am Clin Products Rev* Feb: 20-25, 1988.

8. Schaefer A, Piquard F, Haberey P: Plasma amino acids analysis: effects of delayed samples preparation and of storage, *Clin Chim Acta* 164:163-169, 1987.

DIAGNOSTIC INFORMATION	REMARKS

P ↑ In hyperalaninemia, mild increase in citrullinemia, Cushing's disease, gout, hyperornithinemia, kwashiorkor, septicemia, urea cycle enzyme defects, pyruvate carboxylase deficiency, and lysinuric protein intolerance

Glycine and proline, as well as alanine, may be increased in kwashiorkor.

P ↓ Chronic renal disease, wasting syndrome of HIV infection, ketotic hypoglycemia, and Huntington's chorea

---

U ↑ Secondary lactic acidosis, acute leukemia, pyruvate dehydrogenase deficiency, glycogen synthase deficiency, other diseases with elevated plasma pyruvic acid, Hartnup disease, histidinemia, rheumatoid arthritis, and lead intoxication

Increase may be seen as a result of bacterial contamination of specimen.

Values in children (3 mo-10 yr) were measured using reversed-phase liquid chromatography.

---

9.   Heiblim DI, Evans HE, Glass L, et al: Amino acid concentrations in cerebrospinal fluid, *Arch Neurol* 35:765-768, 1978.

10. Shih V: *Laboratory techniques for the detection of hereditary metabolic disorders,* Boca Raton, FL, 1973, CRC Press.

11. Mayo Medical Laboratories: *Test catalog,* Rochester, MN, 1993, Mayo Medical Laboratories.

12. Goldsmith RF, Earl JW, Cunningham AM: Determination of δ-aminobutyric acid and other amino acids in cerebrospinal fluid of pediatric patients by reversed-phase liquid chromatography, *Clin Chem* 33:1736-1740, 1987.

TEST NAME AND METHOD	SPECIMEN REQUIREMENTS	REFERENCE INTERVAL, CONVENTIONAL [INTERNATIONAL RECOMMENDED UNITS]				CHEMICAL INTERFERENCES AND IN VIVO EFFECTS
β-Alanine (β-Ala)[1-4] *Ion-exchange chromatography*	Plasma (heparin) or serum, fasting. Place blood in ice water immediately; separate and freeze within 1 hr of collection. Stable for 1 wk at −20° C; for longer periods, deproteinize and store at −70° C.[5,6]	*mg/dL* 0-18 yr Adult	<0.09 <0.11	× 112.2	$\mu mol/L^4$ [<10] [<12]	None found.
	Urine, 24 hr. Add 10 mL of 6 mol/L HCl as preservative at start of collection. (Alternatively, refrigerate specimen during collection.) Store frozen at −20° C.	*mg/day* 3-16 yr Adult or	<3.8 <8.3 <11 mg/g creatinine[8] [× 1.27 = <14 mmol/mol creatinine]	× 11.2	$\mu mol/day^7$ [<42] [<93]	

1. Scriver CR, Beaudet AL,Valle D, et al, editors: *The metabolic and molecular bases of inherited disease,* ed 8, New York, 2001, McGraw-Hill.
2. Bremer HJ, Duran M, Kamerling JP, et al: *Disturbances of amino acid metabolism: clinical chemistry and diagnosis,* Baltimore, 1981, Urban and Schwarzenburg.
3. Nyhan W, Sakait N: *Diagnostic recognition of genetic disease,* Philadelphia, 1987, Lea & Febiger.
4. Slocum RH, Cummings JG: Amino acid analysis of physiological samples. In *Techniques in human biochemical genetics,* New York, 1991, Wiley-Liss, pp. 87-126.
5. Cummings JG: Routine amino acids analysis in the clinical laboratory, *Am Clin Products Rev* Feb:20-25, 1988.
6. Schaefer A, Piquard F, Haberey P: Plasma amino acids analysis: effects of delayed samples preparation and of storage, *Clin Chim Acta* 164:163-169, 1987.
7. Mayo Medical Laboratories: *Test catalog,* Rochester, MN, 1993, Mayo Medical Laboratories.
8. Meites S, editor: *Pediatric clinical chemistry,* ed 2, Washington, DC, 1981, American Association for Clinical Chemistry.

α-Aminoadipic Acid (Aad)[1-4] *Ion-exchange chromatography*	Urine, 24 hr. Add 10 mL of 6 mol/L HCl at start of collection. (Alternatively, refrigerate specimen during collection.) Store frozen at −20° C.	*nmol/mg creatinine* Premature (first 6 wk) 0-1 mo 1-24 mo 2-18 yr Adult	70-460 0-180 45-268 2-88 40-110	None found.

1. Scriver CR, Beaudet AL,Valle D, et al, editors: *The metabolic and molecular bases of inherited disease,* ed 8, New York, 2001, McGraw-Hill.
2. Bremer HJ, Duran M, Kamerling JP, et al: *Disturbances of amino acid metabolism: clinical chemistry and diagnosis,* Baltimore, 1981, Urban and Schwarzenburg.

DIAGNOSTIC INFORMATION	REMARKS
P ↑ Hyper-β-alaninemia	β-Aminoisobutyric acid and taurine are also excreted in the urine in hyper-β-alaninemia; elevated levels of β-alanine and γ-aminobutyric acid (GABA) occur in plasma and CSF.

U ↑ Rejection of kidney transplant, hyper-β-alaninemia

↑ Saccharopinuria, hyperlysinemia, and Reye's syndrome

↑↑ α-Aminoadipic aciduria, α-ketoadipic aciduria

3. Slocum RH, Cummings JG: Amino acid analysis of physiological samples. In *Techniques in human biochemical genetics,* New York, 1991, Wiley-Liss, pp. 87-126.
4. Shapira E, Blitzer MG, Miller JB, et al, editors: *Biochemical genetics: a laboratory manual,* Oxford, UK, 1989, Oxford University Press, pp. 96-97.

TEST NAME AND METHOD	SPECIMEN REQUIREMENTS	REFERENCE INTERVAL, CONVENTIONAL [INTERNATIONAL RECOMMENDED UNITS]			CHEMICAL INTERFERENCES AND IN VIVO EFFECTS
α-Amino-*n*-butyric Acid (Abu)[1-5] *Ion-exchange chromatography*	Plasma (heparin) or serum, fasting. Place blood in ice water immediately; separate and freeze within 1 hr of collection. Stable for 1 wk at −20° C; for longer periods, deproteinize and store at −70° C.[6,7]		*mg/dL*	μ*mol/L*	None found.
		Premature (first 6 wk)	0.14-0.54 × 97.0	14-52	
		0-1 mo	0.08-0.25	8-24	
		1-24 mo	0.03-0.27	3-26	
		2-18 yr	0.04-0.32	4-31	
		Adult	0.05-0.42	5-41	
	Urine, 24 hr. Add 10 mL of 6 mol/L HCl at start of collection. (Alternatively, refrigerate specimen during collection.) Store frozen at −20° C.		*nmol/mg creatinine*		
		Premature (first 6 wk)	50-710		
		0-1 mo	8-65		
		1-24 mo	30-136		
		2-18 yr	0-77		
		Adult	0-90		
	CSF. Collect in sterile tubes; store frozen. Stable at −20° C for 1 wk or at −70° C for 2 mo.[8]		*mg/dL (SD)*	μ*mol/L (SD)*	
		3 mo-2 yr	0.025 ± 0.009 × 97.0	[2.4 ± 0.9][9]	
		2-10 yr	0.019 ± 0.005	[1.8 ± 0.5][9]	
		Adult	0.039 ± 0.006	[3.8 ± 0.6][8]	

1. Scriver CR, Beaudet AL, Valle D, et al, editors: *The metabolic and molecular bases of inherited disease,* ed 8, New York, 2001, McGraw-Hill.

2. Young DS: *Effects of drugs on clinical laboratory tests,* ed 5, Washington, DC, 2000, American Association of Clinical Chemistry.

3. Bremer HJ, Duran M, Kamerling JP, et al: *Disturbances of amino acid metabolism: clinical chemistry and diagnosis,* Baltimore, 1981, Urban and Schwarzenburg.

4. Slocum RH, Cummings JG: Amino acid analysis of physiological samples. In *Techniques in human biochemical genetics,* New York, 1991, Wiley-Liss, pp. 87-126.

5. Shapira E, Blitzer MG, Miller JB, et al, editors: *Biochemical genetics: a laboratory manual,* Oxford, UK, 1989, Oxford University Press, pp. 96-97.

6. Cummings JG: Routine amino acids analysis in the clinical laboratory, *Am Clin Products Rev* Feb: 20-25, 1988.

7. Schaefer A, Piquard F, Haberey P: Plasma amino acids analysis: effects of delayed samples preparation and of storage, *Clin Chim Acta* 164:163-169, 1987.

8. Heiblim DI, Evans HE, Glass L, et al: Amino acid concentrations in cerebrospinal fluid, *Arch Neurol* 35:765-768, 1978.

9. Goldsmith RF, Earl JW, Cunningham AM: Determination of δ-aminobutyric acid and other amino acids in cerebrospinal fluid of pediatric patients by reversed-phase liquid chromatography, *Clin Chem* 33:1736-1740, 1987.

10. Jain KM, Rush BF Jr, Seelig RF, et al: Changes in plasma amino acid profiles following abdominal operations, *Surg Gynecol Obstet* 152:302-306, 1981.

DIAGNOSTIC INFORMATION	REMARKS

P ↑ Starvation

P ↓ After abdominal surgery (day 8)[10]

U ↑ Nonspecific aminoacidurias

Values in children (3 mo-10 yr) were measured using reversed-phase liquid chromatography.

TEST NAME AND METHOD	SPECIMEN REQUIREMENTS	REFERENCE INTERVAL, CONVENTIONAL [INTERNATIONAL RECOMMENDED UNITS]		CHEMICAL INTERFERENCES AND IN VIVO EFFECTS
β-Aminoisobu-tyric Acid (β-AIB)[1-5] *Ion-exchange chromatography*	Urine, 24 hr. Add 10 mL of 6 mol/L HCl at start of collection. (Alternatively, refriger-ate specimen during collection.) Store frozen at −20° C.	*nmol/mg creatinine* Premature (first 6 wk) 0-1 mo 1-24 mo 2-18 yr Adult	50-470 421-3133 802-4160 291-1482 10-510	None found.

1. Scriver CR, Beaudet AL, Valle D, et al, editors: *The metabolic and molecular bases of inherited disease,* ed 8, New York, 2001, McGraw-Hill.

2. Young DS: *Effects of drugs on clinical laboratory tests,* ed 5, Washington, DC, 2000, American Association of Clinical Chemistry.

3. Bremer HJ, Duran M, Kamerling JP, et al: *Disturbances of amino acid metabolism: clinical chemistry and diagnosis,* Balti-more, 1981, Urban and Schwarzenburg.

4. Slocum RH, Cummings JG: Amino acid analysis of physiological samples. In *Techniques in human biochemical genetics,* New York, 1991, Wiley-Liss, pp. 87-126.

5. Shapira E, Blitzer MG, Miller JB, et al, editors: *Biochemical genetics: a laboratory manual,* Oxford, UK, 1989, Oxford University Press, pp. 96-97.

Arginine (Arg)[1-8] *Ion-exchange chromatography*	Plasma (heparin) or serum, fasting. Place blood in ice water im-mediately; separate and freeze within 1 hr of collection. Stable for 1 wk at −20° C; for longer periods, depro-teinize and store at −70° C.[9,10]	*mg/dL* Premature (first 6 wk) 0-1 mo 1-24 mo 2-18 yr Adult	0.56-1.20 0.10-2.44 0.21-2.32 0.17-2.44 0.26-2.23	× 57.4	*μmol/L*[7] [34-96] [6-140] [12-133] [10-140] [15-128]	P ↑ V Histidine (after oral load) P ↓ V Glucose, proges-terone (high doses)

	Urine, 24 hr. Add 10 mL of 6 mol/L HCl at start of collection. (Alternatively, refriger-ate specimen during collection.) Store frozen at −20° C.	*nmol/mg creatinine* Premature (first 6 wk) 0-1 mo 1-24 mo 2-18 yr Adult	190-820 35-214 38-165 31-109 10-90	U ↑ V Cycloleucine

	CSF. Collect in sterile tubes; store frozen. Sta-ble at −20° C for 1 wk or at −70° C for 2 mo.[11]	Neonate 3 mo-2 yr 2-10 yr Adult	*mg/dL* 0.472 ± 0.263 (SEM) 0.327 ± 0.056 (SD) 0.310 ± 0.068 0.376 ± 0.023	× 57.4	*μmol/L* [27.1 ± 15.1][11] [18.8 ± 3.2][12] [17.8 ± 3.9][13] [21.6 ± 1.3][14]

DIAGNOSTIC INFORMATION	REMARKS

↑ Various types of neoplastic disease, diseases associated with excessive tissue breakdown of nucleic acids, Down syndrome, protein malnutrition, hyper-β-alaninemia, β-aminoisobutyric aciduria, and lead poisoning

Both D- and L-isomers occur in human plasma. In urine, only the D-form is found. The disease is a familial recessive expression of altered thymine metabolism.

P ↑ Hyperargininemia, in some cases of type II hyperlysinemia

See Table II-2.

P ↓ 2-3 days after abdominal surgery,[15] chronic renal failure, rheumatoid arthritis, marasmus, and citrullinemia

P ↓↓ In septic patients

U ↑ Dibasic aminoaciduria, cystinuria, and cystinosis

Newborns and young infants show a moderate excretion of arginine; otherwise, urine levels are very low.

CSF ↑ Bacterial meningitis[16]

CSF ↓ Multiple sclerosis

Values in children (3 mo-10 yr) were measured using reversed-phase liquid chromatography.

TEST NAME AND METHOD	SPECIMEN REQUIREMENTS	REFERENCE INTERVAL, CONVENTIONAL [INTERNATIONAL RECOMMENDED UNITS]		CHEMICAL INTERFERENCES AND IN VIVO EFFECTS

Arginine—CONT

1. Friedman RB, Young DS: *Effects of disease on clinical laboratory tests,* ed 4, Washington, DC, 2001, American Association of Clinical Chemistry.

2. Scriver CR, Beaudet AL, Valle D, et al, editors: *The metabolic and molecular bases of inherited disease,* ed 8, New York, 2001, McGraw-Hill.

3. Young DS: *Effects of drugs on clinical laboratory tests,* ed 5, Washington, DC, 2000, American Association of Clinical Chemistry.

4. Bremer HJ, Duran M, Kamerling JP, et al: *Disturbances of amino acid metabolism: clinical chemistry and diagnosis,* Baltimore, 1981, Urban and Schwarzenburg.

5. Freund H, Atamian S, Holyroyde J, et al: Plasma amino acids as predictors of the severity and outcome of sepsis, *Ann Surg* Nov:571-576, 1979.

6. Nyhan W, Sakait N: *Diagnostic recognition of genetic disease,* Philadelphia, 1987, Lea & Febiger.

7. Hommes FA, editor: *Techniques in diagnostic human biochemical genetics,* New York, 1991, Wiley-Liss.

8. Shapira E, Blitzer MG, Miller JB, et al, editors: *Biochemical genetics: a laboratory manual,* Oxford, UK, 1989, Oxford University Press, pp. 96-97.

Asparagine (Asn)[1-5]

Ion-exchange chromatography

Plasma (heparin) or serum, fasting. Place blood in ice water immediately; separate and freeze within 1 hr of collection. Stable for 1 wk at $-20°$ C; for longer periods, deproteinize and store at $-70°$ C.[6,7]

	mg/dL		$\mu mol/L^4$	P ↓ V Asparaginase
Premature (first 6 wk)	1.19-3.90	× 75.7	[90-295]	
0-1 mo	0.38-1.74		[29-132]	
1-24 mo	0.28-1.25		[21-95]	
2-18 yr	0.30-1.48		[23-112]	
Adult	0.46-0.98		[35-74]	

Urine, 24 hr. Add 10 mL of 6 mol/L HCl at start of collection. (Alternatively, refrigerate specimen during collection.) Store frozen at $-20°$ C.

	nmol/mg creatinine
Premature (first 6 wk)	1350-5250
0-1 mo	185-1550
1-24 mo	252-1280
2-18 yr	72-332
Adult	99-470

CSF. Collect in sterile tubes; store frozen. Stable at $-20°$ C for 1 wk or at $-70°$ C for 2 mo.[8]

	mg/dL		$\mu mol/L$
Neonate	0.217 ± 0.071 (SEM)	× 75.7	[16.4 ± 5.4][8]
3 mo-2 yr	0.087 ± 0.024 (SD)		[6.6 ± 1.8][9]
2-10 yr	0.063 ± 0.009		[4.8 ± 0.7][9]
Adult	0.097 ± 0.004		[7.4 ± 0.3][10]

1. Friedman RB, Young DS: *Effects of disease on clinical laboratory tests,* ed 4, Washington, DC, 2001, American Association of Clinical Chemistry.

2. Scriver CR, Beaudet AL, Valle D, et al, editors: *The metabolic and molecular bases of inherited disease,* ed 8, New York, 2001, McGraw-Hill.

9. Cummings JG: Routine amino acids analysis in the clinical laboratory, *Am Clin Products Rev* Feb:20-25, 1988.

10. Schaefer A, Piquard F, Haberey P: Plasma amino acids analysis: effects of delayed samples preparation and of storage, *Clin Chim Acta* 164:163-169, 1987.

11. Heiblim DI, Evans HE, Glass L, et al: Amino acid concentrations in cerebrospinal fluid, *Arch Neurol* 35:765-768, 1978.

12. Goldsmith RF, Earl JW, Cunningham AM: Determination of δ-aminobutyric acid and other amino acids in cerebrospinal fluid of pediatric patients by reversed-phase liquid chromatography, *Clin Chem* 33:1736-1740, 1987.

13. Saifer A: Rapid screening methods for the detection of inherited and acquired aminoacidopathies, *Adv Clin Chem* 14:145-218, 1971.

14. Stabler SP, Alien RH, Savage DG, et al: Clinical spectrum and diagnosis of cobalamin deficiency, *Blood* 76:871, 1990.

15. Jain KM, Rush BF Jr, Seelig RF, et al: Changes in plasma amino acid profiles following abdominal operations, *Surg Gynecol Obstet* 152:302-306, 1981.

16. Schott KJ, Meier D: Free amino acid pattern of cerebrospinal fluid in meningeal pathology, *Acta Neurol Scand* 75:304-309, 1987.

Asparagine is relatively unstable, and aspartic acid is formed quickly when plasma, urine, or CSF is stored at room temperature. Asparagine is the storage form of ammonia in tissues.

U ↑ Burn patients,[11] Hartnup disease, and cystinosis

Values in children (3 mo-10 yr) were measured using reversed-phase liquid chromatography.

3. Bremer HJ, Duran M, Kamerling JP, et al: *Disturbances of amino acid metabolism: clinical chemistry and diagnosis,* Baltimore, 1981, Urban and Schwarzenburg.

4. Hommes FA, editor: *Techniques in diagnostic human biochemical genetics,* New York, 1991, Wiley-Liss.

TEST NAME AND METHOD	SPECIMEN REQUIREMENTS	REFERENCE INTERVAL, CONVENTIONAL [INTERNATIONAL RECOMMENDED UNITS]		CHEMICAL INTERFERENCES AND IN VIVO EFFECTS

Asparagine—CONT

5. Shapira E, Blitzer MG, Miller JB, et al, editors: *Biochemical genetics: a laboratory manual,* Oxford, UK, 1989, Oxford University Press, pp. 96-97.

6. Cummings JG: Routine amino acids analysis in the clinical laboratory, *Am Clin Products Rev* Feb:20-25, 1988.

7. Schaefer A, Piquard F, Haberey P: Plasma amino acids analysis: effects of delayed samples preparation and of storage, *Clin Chim Acta* 164:163-169, 1987.

8. Heiblim DI, Evans HE, Glass L, et al: Amino acid concentrations in cerebrospinal fluid, *Arch Neurol* 35:765-768, 1978.

Aspartic Acid (Asp)[1-7] *Ion-exchange chromatography*	Plasma (heparin) or serum, fasting. Place blood in ice water immediately; separate and freeze within 1 hr of collection. Stable for 1 wk at −20° C; for longer periods, deproteinize and store at −70° C.[8,9]	*mg/dL* Premature (first 6 wk) 0.32-0.67 0-1 mo 0.23-1.72 1-24 mo 0-0.31 2-18 yr 0.01-0.31 Adult 0.01-0.33	× 75.1	$\mu mol/L^6$ P ↑ V Glutamic acid [24-50] [20-129] [0-23] [1-24] [1-25]
	Urine, 24 hr. Add 10 mL of 6 mol/L HCl at start of collection. (Alternatively, refrigerate specimen during collection.) Store frozen at −20° C.	*nmol/mg creatinine* Premature (first 6 wk) 580-1520 0-1 mo 336-810 1-24 mo 230-685 2-18 yr 0-120 Adult 60-240		U ↑ V Ascorbic acid (after large intake)
	CSF. Collect in sterile tubes; store frozen. Stable at −20° C for 1 wk or at −70° C for 2 mo.[10]	*mg/dL* Neonate 0.081 ± 0.024 (SEM) 3 mo-2 yr 0.008 ± 0.004 (SD) 2-10 yr 0.006 ± 0.003 Adult 0.008 ± 0.004	× 75.1	*μmol/L* [6.1 ± 0.18][10] [0.61 ± 0.32][11] [0.46 ± 0.23][11] [0.6 ± 0.3][4]

1. Friedman RB, Young DS: *Effects of disease on clinical laboratory tests,* ed 4, Washington, DC, 2001, American Association of Clinical Chemistry.

2. Scriver CR, Beaudet AL, Valle D, et al, editors: *The metabolic and molecular bases of inherited disease,* ed 8, New York, 2001, McGraw-Hill.

3. Young DS: *Effects of drugs on clinical laboratory tests,* ed 5, Washington, DC, 2000, American Association of Clinical Chemistry.

4. Bremer HJ, Duran M, Kamerling JP, et al: *Disturbances of amino acid metabolism: clinical chemistry and diagnosis,* Baltimore, 1981, Urban and Schwarzenburg.

5. Nyhan W, Sakait N: *Diagnostic recognition of genetic disease,* Philadelphia, 1987, Lea & Febiger.

6. Hommes FA, editor: *Techniques in diagnostic human biochemical genetics,* New York, 1991, Wiley-Liss.

7. Shapira E, Blitzer MG, Miller JB, et al, editors: *Biochemical genetics: a laboratory manual,* Oxford, UK, 1989, Oxford University Press, pp. 96-97.

9. Goldsmith RF, Earl JW, Cunningham AM: Determination of δ-aminobutyric acid and other amino acids in cerebrospinal fluid of pediatric patients by reversed-phase liquid chromatography, *Clin Chem* 33:1736-1740, 1987.

10. Shih V: *Laboratory techniques for the detection of hereditary metabolic disorders,* Boca Raton, FL, 1973, CRC Press.

11. Cynober L, Dinh FN, Blonde F, et al: Plasma and urinary amino acid pattern in severe burn patients: evolution throughout the healing period, *Am J Clin Nutr* 36:416-425, 1982.

P ↓ 1 day after abdominal surgery,[12] amyotrophic lateral sclerosis, and citrullinemia

Aspartic acid (Asp) easily arises from asparagine; improper preservation of plasma, CSF, or urine may lead to false elevations of Asp. Asp is 100 times higher in erythrocytes, leukocytes, and thrombocytes than in plasma.

See also Table II-2.

U ↑ Dicarboxylic aminoaciduria, acute leukemia

Glutamic acid is also significantly increased in dicarboxylic aminoaciduria. (The dicarboxylic acids are aspartic acid and glutamic acid.)

8. Cummings JG: Routine amino acids analysis in the clinical laboratory, *Am Clin Products Rev* Feb:20-25, 1988.

9. Schaefer A, Piquard F, Haberey P: Plasma amino acids analysis: effects of delayed samples preparation and of storage, *Clin Chim Acta* 164:163-169, 1987.

10. Heiblim DI, Evans HE, Glass L, et al: Amino acid concentrations in cerebrospinal fluid, *Arch Neurol* 35:765-768, 1978.

11. Goldsmith RF, Earl JW, Cunningham AM: Determination of δ-aminobutyric acid and other amino acids in cerebrospinal fluid of pediatric patients by reversed-phase liquid chromatography, *Clin Chem* 33:1736-1740, 1987.

12. Jain KM, Rush BF Jr, Seelig RF, et al: Changes in plasma amino acid profiles following abdominal operations, *Surg Gynecol Obstet* 152:302-306, 1981.

TEST NAME AND METHOD	SPECIMEN REQUIREMENTS	REFERENCE INTERVAL, CONVENTIONAL [INTERNATIONAL RECOMMENDED UNITS]		CHEMICAL INTERFERENCES AND IN VIVO EFFECTS
Biotin[1-3]	Whole blood (sodium citrate) or serum	200-500 pg/mL × 0.0041 x̄: 350	[0.82-2.05 nmol/L] [x̄: 1.43]	↑ V Chronic hemodialy- sis, autoimmune hepatitis
MB *(O. dancia)*[4]	Urine, 24 hr	6-50 mcg/day × 4.1 x̄: 29	[25-205 nmol/day] [x̄: 119]	↓ V Antibiotics, anticon- vulsants (e.g., carba- mazepine, phenobarbital,
Solid-phase (cellulose) binding assay[5]	Plasma	285-940 pg/mL × 0.0041 x̄: 590 ± 171	[1.17-3.85 nmol/L] [x̄: 2.42 ± 0.70]	phenytoin, primidone, val- proic acid), levodopa, and excessive consumption of raw egg whites (avidin
Chemilumines- cence[6]	Serum	292-1049 pg/mL x̄: 588 ± 222	[1.20-4.30 nmol/L] [x̄: 2.41 ± 0.91]	binds biotin and renders it unavailable for absorp- tion)

1. Brown ML, editor: *Present knowledge in nutrition,* ed 6, Washington, DC, 1990, International Life Sciences Institute, Nutri- tion Foundation.
2. Kinney JM, Jeejeebhoy KN, Hil GL, et al: *Nutrition and metabolism in patient care,* Philadelphia, 1988, WB Saunders.
3. Shils ME, Olson JA, Shike M, editor: *Modern nutrition in health and disease,* ed 8, Philadelphia, 1994, Lea & Febiger.
4. Baker H, Frank O: *Clinical vitaminology. Methods and interpretation,* New York, 1968, Interscience.
5. Chang PW, Bartlett K: A new solid-phase assay for biotin and biocytin and its application to the study of patients with bio- tinidase deficiency, *Clin Chim Acta* 159:185-196, 1986.
6. Williams EJ, Campbell AK: A homogeneous assay for biotin based on chemiluminescence energy transfer, *Anal Biochem* 155:249-255, 1986.
7. Mock DM, Johnson BB, Holman RT: Effects of biotin deficiency on serum fatty acid composition: evidence for abnormali- ties in humans, *J Nutr* 188:342-348, 1988.

Biotinidase (Indirect Test for Biotin)	Whole blood (dried spot on paper)	Presence of color indicates normal biotinidase ac- tivity, whereas absence of color indicates bio- tinidase deficiency.	↑ C Sulfonamide
Colorimetric (screening test)[1]			
Enzymatic[2,3]	Serum. Samples that are not immediately processed can be frozen and stored at −70° C.	3.5-12.0 nmol *p*-aminobenzoate/min/mL (x̄: 7.10) [× 1.0 = 3.5-12.0 U/L (x̄: 7.10)]	

1. Heard GS, McVoy JRS, Wolf B: A screening method for biotinidase deficiency in newborns, *Clin Chem* 30:125-127, 1984.
2. Weissbecker KA, Gruemer H-D, Heard GS, et al: An automated procedure for measuring biotinidase activity in serum, *Clin Chem* 35:831-833, 1989.

Plasma lactic acid and 15:0 and 17:0 fatty acids are increased in biotin deficiency.

Biotin deficiency has been noted to occur in patients receiving long-term parenteral nutrition unsupplemented with biotin, and particularly in those with short small intestines (biotin is produced by the gut flora). Biotin deficiency also occurs in association with Leiner's disease and in infants with genetic defects of carboxylases and biotinidase. Carboxylase defects are usually multiple; treatment requires 5-10 mg/day of biotin and can be given prenatally. In biotin-deficient infants, urinary excretion of biotin is decreased to <6 mcg/day [<25 nmol/day], whereas excretion of toxic organic acids (methylcitrate, 3-methylcrotonylglycine, 3-OH-isovalerate) is increased. No toxicity to biotin has been described. See *Biotinidase.*

Clinical symptoms include scaly dermatitis, pallor, irritability, lethargy, anorexia, nausea, and loss of hair. Altered T-cell and B-cell immunity can also occur.[7]

Biotinidase acts to recycle biotin by cleaving the covalently bound vitamin from CoA carboxylase enzymes during their degradation. Biotinidase deficiency can cause Leigh syndrome, which may result in death.[4]

3. Dove Pettit DA, Wolf B: Quantitative colorimetric assay of biotinidase activity. In *Techniques in human biochemical genetics,* New York, 1991, Wilcy-Liss, pp. 561-565.

4. Baumgartner ER, Suormala TM, Wick H, et al: Biotinidase deficiency: a cause of subacute necrotizing encephalomyelopathy (Leigh syndrome). Report of a case with lethal outcome, *Pediatr Res* 26:260-266, 1989.

TEST NAME AND METHOD	SPECIMEN REQUIREMENTS	REFERENCE INTERVAL, CONVENTIONAL [INTERNATIONAL RECOMMENDED UNITS]				CHEMICAL INTERFERENCES AND IN VIVO EFFECTS
Carnitine (L-Carnitine), Total[1-3] *Enzymatic* *Tandem mass spectrometry*[4-6]	Serum. Store at 20° C.	$\mu mol/L^2$ Children 8-15 yr 36-41 Adults M 36-83 F 28-75				↑ C Compounds containing sulfhydryl group ↑ V Ethanol ↓ V Carbamazepine, phenobarbital, pivampicillin, pivmecillinam, and valproic acid

	Serum, heparinized plasma. Avoid gel separator tubes.					
	Age	*Total carnitine (TC), μmol/L*	*Free carnitine (FC), μmol/L*	*Acyl carnitine (AC), μmol/L*	*AC/FC ratio*	
	1 day	23-68	12-36	7-37	0.4-1.7	
	2-7 days	17-41	10-21	3-24	0.2-1.4	
	8-31 days	19-59	12-46	4-15	0.1-0.7	
	32 days-12 mo	38-68	27-49	7-19	0.2-0.5	
	13 mo-6 yr	35-84	24-63	4-28	0.1-0.8	
	7-10 yr	28-83	22-66	3-32	0.1-0.9	
	11-17 yr	34-77	22-65	4-29	0.1-0.9	
	>18 yr	34-78	25-54	5-30	0.1-0.8	

	Urine, 24 hr. Store at 20° C.	$\mu mol/day$	
		Infants	
		3 days	5.7-9.3
		6 days	4.7-9.3
		Adults	
		M	306-534
		F	208-324

1. Bazilinski N, Dunea G: Carnitine: an overview, *Int J Artif Organs* 13:720-721, 1990.

2. Haeckel R, Kaiser M, Oellerich M, et al: Carnitine: metabolism, function and clinical application, *J Clin Chem Clin Biochem* 28:291-295, 1990.

3. Hill RE: Carnitine, *JIFCC* 3:66-71, 1991.

4. Ho CS, Cheng BS, Lam WK: Rapid liquid chromatography-electrospray tandem mass spectrometry method for serum free and total carnitine, *Clin Chem* 49:1189-1191, 2003.

5. Schmidt-Sommerfeld E, Werner E, Penn D: Carnitine plasma concentrations in 353 metabolically healthy children, *Eur J Pediatr* 147:356-360, 1988.

6. Chace DH, Pons R, Chiriboga CA: Neonatal blood carnitine concentrations: normative data by electrospray tandem mass spectrometry, *Pediatr Res* 53:823-829, 2003.

DIAGNOSTIC INFORMATION	REMARKS

↓ Carnitine deficiencies either myopathic or systemic. Systemic deficiency presents acutely in early life; symptoms may mimic Reye's syndrome. The condition is frequently associated with inherited organic acidurias but may also be caused by dietary deficiency in infancy. The myopathic type develops later in life with the carnitine deficiency present only in muscle. Serum carnitine levels may be within the reference range.

↑ Severe renal disease

TEST NAME AND METHOD	SPECIMEN REQUIREMENTS	REFERENCE INTERVAL, CONVENTIONAL [INTERNATIONAL RECOMMENDED UNITS]		CHEMICAL INTERFERENCES AND IN VIVO EFFECTS
Citrulline (Cit)[1-7] *Ion-exchange chromatography*	Plasma (heparin) or serum, fasting. Place blood in ice water immediately; separate and freeze within 1 hr of collection. Stable for 1 wk at $-20°$ C; for longer periods, deproteinize and store at $-70°$ C.[8,9]	*mg/dL* Premature (first 6 wk) 0.35-1.52 0-1 mo 0.18-0.79 1-24 mo 0.05-0.61 2-18 yr 0.02-0.81 Adult 0.21-0.96	$\times$ 57.1	$\mu mol/L$[7] 20-87 10-45 3-35 1-46 12-55	P $\uparrow$ Histidine (after oral load) P $\downarrow$ Tranylcypromine, marasmus
	Urine, 24 hr. Add 10 mL of HCl at start of collection. (Alternatively, refrigerate specimen during collection.) Store frozen at $-20°$ C.	*nmol/mg creatinine* Premature (first 6 wk) 240-1320 0-1 mo 27-181 1-24 mo 22-180 2-18 yr 10-99 Adult 8-50		
	CSF. Collect in sterile tubes; store frozen. Stable at $-20°$ C for 1 wk or at $-70°$ C for 2 mo.[10]	*mg/dL* Neonate 0.070 ± 0.028 (SEM) Adult 0.047 ± 0.004 (SD)	$\times$ 57.1	$\mu mol/L$ 4.0 ± 1.6[10] 2.7 ± 0.2[11]	

1. Scriver CR, Beaudet AL, Valle D, et al, editors: *The metabolic and molecular bases of inherited disease,* ed 8, New York, 2001, McGraw-Hill.

2. Young DS: *Effects of drugs on clinical laboratory tests,* ed 5, Washington, DC, 2000, American Association of Clinical Chemistry.

3. Bremer HJ, Duran M, Kamerling JP, et al: *Disturbances of amino acid metabolism: clinical chemistry and diagnosis,* Baltimore, 1981, Urban and Schwarzenburg.

4. Kamoun P, Droin V, Forestier F, et al: Free amino acids in human fetal plasma, *Clin Chim Acta* 150:227-230, 1985.

5. Nyhan W, Sakait N: *Diagnostic recognition of genetic disease,* Philadelphia, 1987, Lea & Febiger.

6. Slocum RH, Cummings JG: Amino acid analysis of physiological samples. In *Techniques in human biochemical genetics,* New York, 1991, Wiley-Liss, pp. 87-126.

7. Shapira E, Blitzer MG, Miller JB, et al, editors: *Biochemical genetics: à laboratory manual,* Oxford, UK, 1989, Oxford University Press, pp. 96-97.

8. Cummings JG: Routine amino acids analysis in the clinical laboratory, *Am Clin Products Rev* Feb:20-25, 1988.

9. Schaefer A, Piquard F, Haberey P: Plasma amino acids analysis: effects of delayed samples preparation and of storage, *Clin Chim Acta* 164:163-169, 1987.

10. Heiblim DI, Evans HE, Glass L, et al: Amino acid concentrations in cerebrospinal fluid, *Arch Neurol* 35:765-768, 1978.

11. Shih V: *Laboratory techniques for the detection of hereditary metabolic disorders,* Boca Raton, FL, 1973, CRC Press.

DIAGNOSTIC INFORMATION	REMARKS

P ↑ Citrullinemia, liver disease, argininosuccinic aciduria, ammonia intoxication, pyruvate carboxylase deficiency, lysinuric protein intolerance, and chronic renal failure

Premature infants show a steady increase in citrulline concentrations during the first month of life. Citrullinemia is caused by a deficiency of arginosuccinate synthetase; however, arginosuccinate levels are not increased.

U ↑ Citrullinemia, Hartnup disease, argininosuccinic aciduria, and glutaric aciduria type II

In urine the concentration may fluctuate greatly, but the absolute amount remains very small.

CSF ↑↑ Citrullinemia

TEST NAME AND METHOD	SPECIMEN REQUIREMENTS	REFERENCE INTERVAL, CONVENTIONAL [INTERNATIONAL RECOMMENDED UNITS]			CHEMICAL INTERFERENCES AND IN VIVO EFFECTS
Cystathionine [Hcy (Ala)][1-4] *Ion-exchange chromatography*	Plasma (heparin) or serum, fasting. Place blood in ice water immediately; separate and freeze within 1 hr of collection. Stable for 1 wk at $-20°$ C; for longer periods, deproteinize and store at $-70°$ C.[5,6]		*mg/dL*	$\mu mol/L^4$	
		Premature (first 6 wk)	0.11-0.22 $\times$ 45.5	5-10	
		0-1 mo	0-0.07	0-3	
		1-24 mo	0-0.11	0-5	
		2-18 yr	0-0.07	0-3	
		Adult	0-0.07	0-3	
	Urine, 24 hr. Add 10 mL of 6 mol/L HCl at start of collection. (Alternatively, refrigerate specimen during collection.) Store frozen at $-20°$ C.		*nmol/mg creatinine*		U ↑ V Vitamin B6 depletion
		Premature (first 6 wk)	260-1160		
		0-1 mo	16-47		
		1-24 mo	33-470		
		2-18 yr	0-26		
		Adult	20-50		

1. Bremer HJ, Duran M, Kamerling JP, et al: *Disturbances of amino acid metabolism: clinical chemistry and diagnosis,* Baltimore, 1981, Urban and Schwarzenburg.

2. Nyhan W, Sakait N: *Diagnostic recognition of genetic disease,* Philadelphia, 1987, Lea & Febiger.

3. Slocum RH, Cummings JG: Amino acid analysis of physiological samples. In *Techniques in human biochemical genetics,* New York, 1991, Wiley-Liss, pp. 87-126.

4. Shapira E, Blitzer MG, Miller JB, et al, editors: *Biochemical genetics: a laboratory manual,* Oxford, UK, 1989, Oxford University Press, pp. 96-97.

5. Cummings JG: Routine amino acids analysis in the clinical laboratory, *Am Clin Products Rev* Feb:20-25, 1988.

6. Schaefer A, Piquard F, Haberey P: Plasma amino acids analysis: effects of delayed samples preparation and of storage, *Clin Chim Acta* 164:163-169, 1987.

DIAGNOSTIC INFORMATION	REMARKS
P ↑ Methylmalonic acidemia, homocystinuria	
U ↑ Cystathioninuria, cystinosis, secondary to pyridoxine deficiency, neuroblastoma, and hepatoblastoma	Excretion of cystathionine is markedly increased in patients with both homocystinuria and methylmalonic aciduria.

TEST METHOD	SPECIMEN AND SPECIAL REQUIREMENTS	CLINICAL COMMENTS AND REMARKS
***Chlamydia trachomatis* Identification** *Culture for Lymphogranuloma venereum (LGV)*[1,2]	Aspiration of bubo or of pus from urethra, endocervix, or infected tissue. Only cotton, rayon, or Dacron swabs should be used for swab collections. In addition, epithelial cell specimens should be collected by vigorous swabbing or scraping of the infected site. Transport to laboratory immediately in special transport medium such as 2SP or multipurpose transport medium specific for Chlamydia, virus and mycoplasma. Antibiotics should be included in transport medium to reduce bacterial contamination.	Isolation of *C. trachomatis* in tissue culture is the most reliable method of making the diagnosis of LGV. The organism is isolated from pus in ~30% of patients with clinical and/or serological evidence of LGV. The disease is relatively uncommon in the U.S.; most cases occur in travelers returning from Southeast Asia or Central or South America. There are, however, sporadic cases in the U.S. in individuals who have not had exposure abroad. When LGV is suspected in a patient with lymphadenopathy, perform a needle aspiration of the node through healthy adjacent tissue rather than directly into the bubo. Fluctuant nodes should yield frank pus, but if they do not, a small amount of sterile saline should be injected and aspirated back into the syringe.
Culture in Neonatal Chlamydia Infections[1,2]	Conjunctival scrapings; nasopharyngeal aspirates; tracheobronchial aspirates. Transport to laboratory immediately at 4° C in special transport medium such as 2SP or multipurpose transport medium specific for Chlamydia, virus and mycoplasma. Antibiotics should be included in transport medium to reduce bacterial contamination.	Inclusion conjunctivitis and pneumonia are the two principal manifestations of neonatal chlamydia infection. Approximately 30% of children born to women with genital chlamydia infection develop inclusion conjunctivitis. The course of this mucopurulent conjunctivitis is generally benign, and the disease resolves spontaneously within a few weeks to several months. Pneumonia occurs in 10-20% of infants born to infected mothers. *C. trachomatis* is responsible for up to 60% of all pneumonias during the first 6 mo of life, making it a major cause of pneumonia in this age group. Pneumonia is usually of mild to moderate severity. Approximately 50% of infants with pneumonia also have conjunctivitis. Culture for *C. trachomatis* routinely requires at least 2-3 days.
Culture for Adult Eye Infections of Chlamydial Origin[1-3]	Scrapings of the conjunctiva.	Ocular trachoma is the leading cause of preventable blindness in underdeveloped countries. Primary infection usually occurs early in life. In endemic areas, trachoma is transmitted via hand to eye contact. In developed countries, infection usually presents in adulthood as adult inclusion conjunctivitis. Spread of the disease depends on transmission from genital tract to eye and likely results from autoinoculation in patients with concurrent genital tract disease. Spread between individuals from eye to eye may also occur in the absence of sexual contact.

TEST METHOD	SPECIMEN AND SPECIAL REQUIREMENTS	CLINICAL COMMENTS AND REMARKS
Culture for Nongonococcal Urethritis (NGU) and Cervicitis[1-3]	Urethral scrapings collected on a swab inserted 2-4 cm into the urethra; endocervical scrapings collected from the transitional zone of the cervix; fluids/aspirates or tissue collected from the epididymis, endometrium, or fallopian tubes. Transport to laboratory immediately at 4° C in special transport medium such as 2SP or multipurpose transport medium specific for Chlamydia, virus and mycoplasma. Antibiotics should be included in transport medium to reduce bacterial contamination.	A definitive diagnosis can only be made by isolation of the organism in tissue culture. In the U.S., trachoma was once a very serious problem, but today it is usually found only in certain groups, such as the American Indians and immigrants from Mexico and the Far East. *C. trachomatis* is the most common cause of nongonococcal urethritis in men. In addition up to 30% of males with gonorrhea may also have chlamydial infection. Asymptomatic urethral infection is also common in young, sexually active males. *C. trachomatis* causes >20% of the cases of mucopurulent cervicitis in females; asymptomatic cases occur more frequently than symptomatic ones. Approximately 50% of women with gonorrhea have a concomitant chlamydial infection. Culture for *C. trachomatis* routinely requires at least 2-3 days. Discharge (pus/mucus) and urine are inadequate specimens for culture. Specimens containing epithelial cells should be collected directly from the surface of the involved tissue.
Direct Fluorescent Antibody (DFA)[1-3]	Conjunctival scrapings, urethral scrapings, and endocervical scrapings. Transport to laboratory on special slides made available for the test.	
Nucleic Acid Hybridization (PACE 2/PACE 2C, Gen-Probe, San Diego, CA; Hybrid Capture II, Digene, Gaithersburg, MD)[1,4,5]	Conjunctival, urethral, and endocervical swabs collected using manufacturer-specific swab collection devices.	The DFA test utilizes a *C. trachomatis*-specific monoclonal antibody to detect the organism directly in clinical specimens. Published studies have shown a sensitivity of 75-85% and a specificity of 98-99% compared with culture and a lower sensitivity compared with nucleic acid amplification tests. Specimen quality greatly affects test performance. It is extremely important that cellular material be obtained. If cellular material is insufficient, the specimen is unsatisfactory.
EIA[1,6]	Conjunctival, urethral, and endocervical swabs collected using manufacturer-specific swab collection devices; urine. Males should not urinate for at least 1 hr before specimen collection.	The GenProbe assay is a probe test that utilizes DNA-RNA hybridization for detection of *C. trachomatis* directly in specimens from the genital tract or eye. Its reported sensitivity ranges from 77-96% depending on prevalence of the disease in the population being tested. The Hybrid Capture II assay utilizes a signal amplification component to improve test sensitivity, which has been reported as >95%. Both assays have the ability to simultaneously test for the presence of *N. gonorrhoeae*. Collection of specimens using these transport devices renders them unacceptable for culture; therefore specimens for culture must be collected separately.

TEST METHOD	SPECIMEN AND SPECIAL REQUIREMENTS	CLINICAL COMMENTS AND REMARKS
		Recent recommendations indicate that confirmatory testing on positive Chlamydia tests should be performed when the patient is from a low incidence population or if there would be adverse consequences of reporting a false-positive result. The sensitivity and specificity of these assays range from 40-80% and 98-100%, respectively. The predictive value will depend on the prevalence of the disease in the population being tested. EIA tests are significantly less sensitive than nucleic acid hybridization or nucleic acid amplification tests.

1. Murray PR, Baron EJ, Jorgensen JH, et al, editors: *Manual of clinical microbiology,* ed 8, Washington, DC, 2003, ASM Press.

2. Warford A, Chernesky M, Peterson EM: Gleaves CA, coordinating editor: *Cumitech 19A laboratory diagnosis of Chlamydia trachomatis infections,* Washington, DC, 1999, American Society for Microbiology.

3. Mandell GL, Bennett JE, Dolin R, editors: *Principles and practice of infectious diseases,* ed 5,New York, 2000, Churchill Livingstone.

4. Iwen PC, Walker RA, Warren KL, et al: Evaluation of nucleic acid based test (PACE 2C) for simultaneous detection of *Chlamydia trachomatis* and *Neisseria gonorrhoeae* in endocervical specimens, *J Clin Microbiol* 33:2587-2591, 1995.

5. Schachter J, Hook EW III, McCormack WM, et al: Ability of the Digene Hybrid Capture II test to identify *Chlamydia trachomatis* and *Neisseria gonorrhoeae* in cervical specimens, *J Clin Microbiol* 37:3668-3671, 1999.

6. VanDyck E, Ieven M, Pattyn S, et al: Detection of *Chlamydia trachomatis* and *Neisseria gonorrhoeae* by enzyme immunoassay, culture and three nucleic acid amplification tests, *J Clin Microbiol* 39:1751-1756, 2001.

TEST INDEX

Alternate immunophenotyping name index

DISEASE INDEX

Acanthosis nigricans, 447

Achlorhydria, 411, 967

Acquired immune deficiency syndrome/human inmmunodeficiency virus, 603, 605, 611, 757, 1194, 1224, 1556, 1570, 1571-1575, 1616

Acrodermatitis enteropathica, 389

Acromegaly, 35, 85, 283, 317, 445, 503, 505, 507, 511, 595, 623, 627, 1039, 1055, 1073, 1099

Addison's disease, 55, 57, 59, 61, 75, 115, 207, 301, 303, 385, 447, 587, 589, 707, 819, 827, 831, 833, 1019

Adrenal adenoma/carcinoma, 343, 589, 891

Adrenogenital syndrome, 59, 113, 303, 335, 337, 339, 341, 371, 589, 591

Adenovirus, 1209, 1522, 1632

Aldosteronism, hypo, idiopathic, 75, 79, 115, 163, 213, 235, 407, 407, 423, 583, 707, 709, 881, 947, 949, 993, 1103

Alkaptonuria, 579, 1165

Allergic bronchopulmonary aspergillosis, 1527

Alport syndrome, 971

Alzheimer's disease, 93, 121, 1137

Amyloidosis, 67, 81, 111, 275, 411, 441, 675, 783, 925, 951, 969, 1103

Amyotrophic lateral sclerosis, 1773

Anaphylaxis, 1755, 1759

Anemias, 1417

    aplastic anemia, 361, 393, 525, 639, 667, 765, 953, 1195

    congenital dyserythropoietic anemia, 1669

    Cooley's anemia, 1220

    Fanconi's syndrome/anemia, 193, 205, 837, 853, 855, 917, 1099, 1107, 1169, 1218

    hemolytic anemia, autoimmune, congenital, 51, 53, 155, 275, 411, 457, 459, 471, 479, 483, 523, 528, 939, 553, 635, 639, 649, 701, 731, 791, 953, 1067, 1141, 1183, 1190, 1473, 1501, 1608

    iron deficiency anemia, 635, 639, 717, 719, 789, 791, 827, 835, 1063, 1183, 1193

    megaloblastic anemia, 411, 533, 639, 643, 649, 653, 701, 711, 719, 835, 939, 1023, 1125, 1186, 1190

    pernicious anemia, 55, 195, 385, 393, 431, 433, 435, 635, 649, 653, 667, 1009, 819, 827, 831, 1069, 1099, 1183

    sickle cell anemia/nephritis, 37, 69, 113, 333, 363, 413, 475, 513, 519, 533, 649, 653, 711, 917, 1099, 1103, 1105, 1153, 1194, 1220, 1221

    sideroblastic anemia, 393, 639, 765, 939, 953, 1155, 1183, 1186

Anencephaly, 401

Angelman Syndrome, 1209

Anorexia nervosa, 35, 117, 277, 375, 413, 503, 627, 695, 767, 835, 881, 891, 983

Argonz Del Castillo syndromes, 901

Astroma, 1210

Ataxia telangiectasia, 601

Autoimmune adrenal disease, 55

Bacillary angiomatosis, 1531

Bartter's syndrome, 75, 237, 423, 881, 947, 995

Benign prostatic hypertrophy, 907, 911, 913

Berger's disease, 601, 971

Bernard-Soulier syndrome, 181, 865, 1647

Biliary atresia, 171, 643, 1141

Blackwater fever, 971

Blastomycosis, 1532

Bloom syndrome, 1211

Botulism, 1546

Brain infarction, 307

Brain tumor, 125

Branched-chain ketonuria, 35, 391, 447, 645, 647, 663, 665, 1107

Brill-Zinsser disease, 1620

Bronchial asthma, 1672, 1687

Cancers

    bladder cancer, 51, 221, 327, 549, 781, 1061, 1211

    breast cancer, 185, 207, 209, 251, 373, 393, 463, 495, 549, 761, 765, 795, 807, 811, 819, 823, 859, 897, 1023, 1099, 1103, 1155, 1217, 1220, 1230

    cervical cancer, 221, 463, 549, 1213

    colorectal cancer, 207, 209, 221, 463, 471, 549, 1214

    endometrial cancer, 1213, 1220

    esophageal cancer, 1232